Procedures

BASIC NURSING

Theory and Practice

BASIC NURSING

Theory and Practice

PATRICIA A. POTTER, RN, MSN
Director of Nursing Practice, Barnes and Jewish Hospitals,
St. Louis, Missouri

ANNE GRIFFIN PERRY, RN, MSN, EdD
Professor, Saint Louis University School of Nursing;
Co-Coordinator, Critical Care Education,
Saint Louis University Health Sciences Center,
St. Louis, Missouri

THIRD EDITION
with 607 *illustrations*

Mosby

St. Louis Baltimore Berlin Boston Carlsbad Chicago London Madrid
Naples New York Philadelphia Sydney Tokyo Toronto

Mosby
Dedicated to Publishing Excellence

Publisher: Nancy L. Coon
Editor: Susan Epstein
Senior Developmental Editor: Beverly J. Copland
Project Manager: John Rogers
Senior Production Editor: Chris Murphy
Designer: Renée Duenow
Manufacturing Supervisor: John Babrick
Cover Design: Renée Duenow, Jason Sonderman

Printed in the United States of America
Composition by Graphic World, Inc.
Printing/binding by Von Hoffmann Press

Mosby–Year Book, Inc.
11830 Westline Industrial Drive
St. Louis, Missouri 63146

Library of Congress Cataloging in Publication Data

Basic nursing : theory and practice / [edited by] Patricia A. Potter,
Anne Griffin Perry. — 3rd ed.
p. cm.
Rev. ed. of: Basic nursing / Patricia A. Potter, Anne G. Perry.
2nd ed., c1991.
Includes bibliographical references and index.
ISBN 0-8016-7876-5
1. Nursing. I. Potter, Patricia Ann. II. Perry, Anne Griffin.
III. Potter, Patrica Ann. Basic nursing.
[DNLM: 1. Nursing. 2. Nursing Care. 3. Nursing Process. WY100
B3117 1995]
RT41.P84 1995
610.73—dc20
DNLM/DLC
for Library of Congress 94-16728
CIP

95 96 97 98 99 / 9 8 7 6 5 4 3 2 1

Contributors

Cynthia Hoppe Allen, RN, MN, MPH
Assistant Professor,
Charity School of Nursing,
Delgado Community College,
New Orleans, Louisiana

Della Aridge, RN, MSN
Clinical Nurse Specialist,
Abdominal Organ Transplant Service,
Saint Louis University Health Sciences Center,
St. Louis, Missouri

Patricia A. Castaldi, RN, BSN, MSN
Assistant Dean,
Elizabeth General Medical Center School of Nursing,
Elizabeth, New Jersey

Judith A. Chaney, RN, BA, BSN, MS, PhD
Associate Professor, School of Nursing,
Southern Illinois University at Edwardsville,
Edwardsville, Illinois

Dorothy McDonnell Cooke, RN, BSN, MSN, PhD
Associate Professor,
Saint Louis University School of Nursing,
St. Louis, Missouri

Deanna S. Cross, RN, BSN, MSN, PhD
Head, Department of Associate Degree Nursing,
Armstrong State College,
Savannah, Georgia

Martha Keene Elkin, RN, BSN, MS
Clinical Instructor,
Lincoln Land Community College,
Springfield, Illinois

Sally M. Featherstone, RN, MN, CS
Clinical Service Line Director,
Barnes-Jewish Psychiatry Service of the BJC Health System,
St. Louis, Missouri

Susan J. Fetzer-Fowler, RN, BA, BSN, MSN, MBA, CCRN
Assistant Professor,
University of New Hampshire,
Durham, New Hampshire

Cathy Franklin, RN, BSN, MA
Dean of Nursing and Allied Health,
Rockingham Community College,
Wentworth, North Carolina

Lois K. Hess, RN, BA, JD
General Counsel,
Jewish Hospital Healthcare Services, Inc.
Louisville, Kentucky

Donna M. Kauffman, RN, MSN
Assistant Professor,
Purdue University School of Nursing,
West Lafayette, Indiana

Pamela A. Lesser, RNC, MS
Manager, Women's Educational Services,
Newborn Service,
Barnes and Jewish Hospitals,
St. Louis, Missouri

Martha Long, RN, MSN, CIC
Infection Control Practitioner,
University of Alabama Hospital,
Birmingham, Alabama

Ruth Ludwick, RNC, MSN, PhD
Assistant Professor,
Kent State University School of Nursing,
Kent, Ohio

Annette Giesler Lueckenotte, RN, MS, CS
Director of Nursing,
Barnes Extended Care,
St. Louis, Missouri

Jeff McManemy, RN, BSN, MSN
Coordinator of Nursing Education/Adjunct Faculty,
Saint Louis University Health Sciences Center,
St. Louis, Missouri

Mary Dee Miller, RN, BSN, MS, CIC
Clinical Nursing Specialist-Infection Control/Epidemiology,
St. Joseph's Hospital and Medical Center,
Phoenix, Arizona;
Nursing Faculty, University of Phoenix,
Phoenix, Arizona

Faye A. Mitchell, RN, MN
Instructor, School of Nursing,
Louisiana State University Medical Center,
New Orleans, Louisiana

Nellie Nelson, RN, MSN, CARN
Nursing Faculty, Scottsdale Community College,
Scottsdale, Arizona;
Nursing Faculty, University of Phoenix,
Phoenix, Arizona

Karen A. Piotrowski, RNC, MSN
Assistant Professor,
D'Youville College,
Buffalo, New York

Janet T. Robuck, BS, MS, RD, LD
Associate Professor,
University of Alabama,
Birmingham, Alabama

Rachel E. Spector, RN, PhD, CTN
Associate Professor,
Boston College School of Nursing,
Chestnut Hill, Massachusetts

Martha A. Spies, RN, BSN, MSN
Assistant Professor,
Deaconess College of Nursing,
St. Louis, Missouri

Victoria McGreevy Steelman, RN, BSN, MA, CNOR
Clinical Nursing Specialist II,
Perioperative Nursing,
The University of Iowa Hospitals and Clinics,
Iowa City, Iowa

Dorothy Thomas, RN, BSN, MSN
Associate Professor,
St. Louis Community College at Florissant Valley,
St. Louis, Missouri

JoEtta A. Vernon, RN, PhD
Consultant,
Omaha, Nebraska

Laurel A. Wiersema, RN, MSN, CS
Clinical Nurse Specialist,
Barnes Hospital at Washington University Medical Center,
St. Louis, Missouri

Valerie J. Yancey, RN, BA, BSN, MS, CCRN
Assistant Professor,
Barnes College,
St. Louis, Missouri

Reviewers

June Allen, RNC, BSN, MSN
Associate Professor,
Lorain County Community College,
Elyria, Ohio

Elizabeth A. Ayello, RN, BSN, MS, PhD, CS, CETN
Clinical Assistant Professor of Nursing,
New York University,
New York, New York

Billie J. Bodo, RNC, MSN
Assistant Professor of Nursing,
Lakeland Community College,
Mentor, Ohio

Jerri Bryant, RN, BSN, MPH, CIC
Clinical Epidemiologist,
Office of Quality Management,
Cleveland Clinic Foundation,
Cleveland, Ohio

Catherine B. Burke, RN, BSN, MS
Nursing Instructor,
Kankakee Community College,
Kankakee, Illinois

Kathlyn Carlson, RN, BSN, MA, CPAN
Staff Nurse, PACU,
Abbott-Northwestern Hospital,
Minneapolis, Minnesota

Patricia A. Castaldi, RN, BSN, MSN
Assistant Dean,
Elizabeth General Medical Center School of Nursing,
Elizabeth, New Jersey

Petrine Churchill, RN, BN
Nursing Instructor,
Yarmouth Regional Hospital School of Nursing,
Yarmouth, Nova Scotia

Janet L. Dougherty, RN, BSN, MSN
Nursing Instructor,
Baptist School of Nursing,
Little Rock, Arkansas

Martha Keene Elkin, RN, BSN, MS
Clinical Instructor,
Lincoln Land Community College,
Springfield, Illinois

Joan O. Ervin, RN, BSN, MS, CCRN
Nursing Instructor,
Florence Darlington Technical College,
Florence, South Carolina

Linda K. Evans, RN, BSN, MSN
Pulmonary Clinical Nurse Specialist,
University of Missouri Hospital and Clinics,
Columbia, Missouri

Ellen Fish-Kingsbury, RN, MS, CS
Psychiatric Clinical Specialist,
Chestnut Hill Counseling Associates,
Dover, New Hampshire

Susan Fetzer-Fowler, RN, BA, BSN, MSN, MBA, CCRN
Assistant Professor,
University of New Hampshire,
Durham, New Hampshire

Carol Flom, RN, BS, MS, MEd
Instructor,
Minneapolis Community College,
Minneapolis, Minnesota

Joyce J. Hamlin, RN, BSN, MSN
Learning Resources Nurse Educator,
Helene Fuld School of Nursing,
Trenton, New Jersey

Renee Covey Harrison, RN, BSN, MS
Assistant Professor,
Tulsa Junior College,
Tulsa, Oklahoma

Pat Hartley, RN, BSN, MEd
Nursing Department Head,
Vancouver Community College–City Centre,
Vancouver, British Columbia

Susan A. Hauser, RN, BA, BSN, MS
Instructor,
Mansfield General Hospital School of Nursing,
Mansfield, Ohio

Mary Reuther Herring, RN, BSN, MSN
Occupational Health Nurse, Motorola,
Nursing Faculty, University of Phoenix,
Phoenix, Arizona

Karen Hill, RN, BSN, MSN
Assistant Professor,
Southeastern Louisiana University,
Hammond, Louisiana

Mary G. Hirsch, RN, MSN, CETN
Director, Medical Services,
St. Louis Medical Supply,
St. Louis, Missouri

Brenda Hoshaw, RN, BSN, MSN, CS, ARNP
Assistant Professor,
Grand View College,
Des Moines, Iowa

Larita Norris Kaspar, RN, BSN, MSN
Certification in Bioethics,
Associate Professor of Nursing,
Lorain County Community College,
Elyria, Ohio

Patricia T. Ketcham, RN, BSN, MSN
Assistant Professor,
Undergraduate Program Director,
Oakland University School of Nursing,
Rochester, Michigan

Judith Ann Kilpatrick, RNC, BSN, MSN
Senior Lecturer, School of Nursing,
Widener University,
Chester, Pennsylvania

Marjorie Knox, RN, BSN, MA, MPA
Professor of Nursing,
Community College of Rhode Island,
Warwick, Rhode Island

Erma McNeill, RN, BSN, MNSc
Nursing Instructor,
Jefferson School of Nursing,
Pine Bluff, Arkansas

Rose Miller, RN, ADN, BSN, MSN, MPA
ADN Instructor,
Wallace College,
Dothan, Alabama

Janet Morgan, RN, AB, BS, MS
Associate Professor of Nursing,
Tompkins-Cortland Community College,
Dryden, New York

Julia R. Popp, RN, BSN, MSN
Nursing Instructor,
Owens Community College,
Toledo, Ohio

Mary Reuland, RN, BSN, MS
Assistant Professor,
College of St. Catherine,
Minneapolis, Minnesota

Candie Ross, RN, BSN, MSN
Gerontological Clinical Nurse Specialist,
St. Louis University Health Sciences Center,
Adjunct Faculty, School of Nursing,
Saint Louis University
St. Louis, Missouri

Patricia P. Shoemaker, RN, BSN, MSN
Chair, Human Services and Health Division,
Davidson County Community College,
Lexington, North Carolina

April Sieh, RN, BSN, MSN
Associate Professor of Nursing,
Delta College,
University Center, Michigan

Kathleen Rice Simpson, RNC, MSN
Perinatal Clinical Nurse Specialist,
St. John's Mercy Medical Center,
St. Louis, Missouri;
Lecturer, School of Nursing,
University of Missouri at St. Louis,
St. Louis, Missouri

Christine E. Smith, RN, BSN, MSN, CNOR
Perioperative Nursing Faculty,
Delaware County Community College,
Media, Pennsylvania

Patricia Sullivan, RN, BSN, MS
Instructor,
Midland College,
Midland, Texas

Dorothy Thomas, RN, BSN, MSN
Assistant Professor of Nursing,
St. Louis Community College at Florissant Valley,
St. Louis, Missouri

B. Jane Threatt, RN, BSN, MSN, CS, ARNP, CCRN
Assistant Professor of Nursing,
University of Florida,
Gainesville, Florida

To Louise Sponsler,
a grand lady who has nursed family,
neighbors, and friends for many years.
Her spirit is inspiring and her love
for her family undying.

PATRICIA A. POTTER

To my husband and children,
for their strength, guidance, and love.

ANNE GRIFFIN PERRY

Preface

The future of nursing promises dynamic change and continual challenge, with exciting health care reform in progress and technologies as yet undreamed on the horizon. Thus the primary focus of this text is to provide students with a solid foundation of knowledge and an understanding of essential nursing principles. *Basic Nursing* presents the fundamental nursing concepts, skills, and techniques that provide a firm foundation for more advanced areas of study.

But nursing is much more than science and technology. We believe that whatever advances the future holds, the heart of nursing practice will, and must, remain the same—humans caring for other humans with knowledge, sensitivity, and compassion. We, therefore, stress the concept of caring throughout this text. The nurse must never forget that each client is an individual with unique needs. And to truly meet those needs, nurses must always remember that the client is a person, not merely a recipient of health care.

Because nursing education addresses changes in practice, so must nursing textbooks. This third edition has been revised and expanded to reflect both current practice and anticipated developments through the end of the century. We are indebted to the many educators and students who have shared their thoughts and ideas with us, and credit each of them as valuable collaborators for this revision.

FEATURES

We have carefully developed this third edition with the student always in mind. We have designed this text to welcome the new student to nursing, communicate our own love for the profession, and promote learning and understanding. Key features of the text include the following:

- The organizing framework of the text embodies a **building block approach:** first, theoretical concepts are presented, followed by the clinical applications of these concepts. This simple-to-complex organization governs the order of presentation of chapters, ensuring that the student continually builds on and reinforces knowledge already mastered.
- Students will appreciate the **clear, engaging writing style.** Even complex technical and theoretical concepts are presented in language that is readily understandable.
- The book's **visual appeal** has been carefully planned as an integral and functional part of the text. Hundreds of large, clear, full-color drawings and photographs illustrate the text, reinforcing and clarifying key concepts and techniques. The clear, readable type and bold headings make the book easy to read and follow. Far more than merely adding bright and attractive colors to the page, each accented special element is consistently color-keyed so that students can immediately identify important information that supports the narrative.
- The **five-step nursing process** serves as the organizing framework for all discussions of clinical content. The process is introduced and clearly explained in Unit 2. In each clinical chapter nursing process is discussed in narrative and enhanced by boxes highlighting NANDA diagnoses and sample care plans. The student learns how the application of the nursing process requires critical thinking, making judgments as to the appropriateness of therapies and the need to revise the plan of care. Both the narrative and care plans focus on client-centered goals and expected outcomes.
- A new chapter, "Promoting Continuity of Care and Home Health Care," addresses the nurse's role in ensuring continuity of care as clients move through the various health care institutions and back to the community. Shorter hospital stays and rapidly expanding community-based health care resources make the nurse's role as teacher and advocate pivotal. Throughout the text, we have integrated principles for community and home care.
- Effective **collaborative care** is the key to a successful outcome for the client. Therefore we have stressed the importance of the nurse working as a member of the health care team, consulting with other professionals and referring clients as appropriate.
- A **health promotion focus** reflects the emphasis of to-

day's practice on maintaining wellness and preventing illness. Activities and interventions that promote health are provided throughout the text to assist the student to identify appropriate strategies.

- Caring for the **older adult client** presents a unique challenge. Gerontologic Practice boxes alert students to special concerns and provide guidelines to help them meet the needs of these clients.
- **Client teaching** is one of the nurse's most vital responsibilities in today's practice. Special boxes highlight what to teach clients and families to ensure that they become knowledgeable, active participants in care.
- Both nurses and clients may be greatly influenced by their **ethnic or cultural heritage.** A separate chapter on multicultural nursing emphasizes the importance of ascertaining each client's cultural beliefs and practices as they pertain to health care. Nurses must also be aware of their own beliefs and should neither assume they are shared by clients nor attempt to promote them.
- Essential **nursing procedures** are presented in a clear, step-by-step, 2-column format with research-based rationales for each step. Large, full-color photos and drawings clarify important or difficult steps to ensure understanding and mastery.
- Vital to professional success is the development of **critical thinking** and **decision-making** skills. Each chapter in the text concludes with a series of critical thinking activities designed to help students learn to apply what they have learned to clinical situations. The Instructor's Resource Manual includes guidelines for directing class discussion for each of these activities.
- **Learning aids** to help students identify, review, and apply important content in each chapter include Learning Objectives, Key Terms, Summary, Key Concepts, Critical Thinking Activities, References, and Bibliography.
- To assist students to learn important terminology, **key terms** are boldfaced and defined in each chapter. In addition, the Glossary at the end of the book provides a convenient resource for reference and study.

NEW AND EXPANDED CONTENT

As the scope of nursing practice broadens, so must the knowledge base for even beginning students. To truly prepare students for today's practice, this knowledge must reflect the most current guidelines and techniques. We have, therefore, totally updated all content and added and expanded coverage in key areas.

Incorporated throughout are the latest standards and guidelines from the JCAHO, OSHA, AHCPR, and NANDA. Current CDC guidelines are highlighted in the totally revised Infection Control chapter. The practice of both Universal Precautions and Body Substance Isolation precautions are stressed throughout the text to reflect their increasing inclusion in agency protocols.

The oxygenation chapter has been expanded to include both cardiovascular and pulmonary conditions. Wound care is also covered in greater depth to address current therapies. The comfort chapter has been updated to reflect the latest guidelines for acute pain management and cancer pain from the AHCPR. A new chapter on skin integrity provides comprehensive coverage of the prevention and care of pressure ulcers, incorporating the latest AHCPR and NPUAP guidelines for risk identification, prevention, and treatment. Quality Initiatives have been incorporated in the Evaluation chapter to emphasize the integral part nurses must play in the day-to-day improvement of nursing care delivery and nursing practice.

TEACHING AND LEARNING PACKAGE

In recognition of the challenges faced by both faculty and students, we have developed an unsurpassed array of teaching/learning materials. For instructors, we offer a totally revised and expanded **Instructor's Resource Manual with Test Bank, Computerized Test Bank, Transparency Acetates,** and a series of **Skills Videos.**

The Instructor's Resource Manual is keyed throughout to the learning objectives in the text, and includes Student Worksheets for each chapter. Performance Checklists are provided to facilitate evaluation and documentation of students' mastery of the procedures in the text. The test bank includes all new questions that reflect the new NCLEX format. The test bank is also available in a computerized format for IBM or MacIntosh.

More than 100 Overhead Transparency Acetates, most in full color, have been selected for effective use in class discussions and for instructional value. Mosby's Nursing Skills Video Series is an ideal complement to the text, providing visual reinforcement to enhance learning. The Instructor's Resources Manual provides a section that details how to maximize the benefit of the videos and includes questions for each to assist in evaluating student learning.

New for this edition is the Student Learning Guide. This guide includes the worksheets and performance checklists from the Instructor's Resource Manual, and is available individually or packaged with the text.

•••

We are pleased to note the growing number of men currently involved in the practice of nursing, and acknowledge their dedication, skill, and professionalism. We have, therefore, made every effort to eliminate any gender-specific pronouns. In a very few instances, we have used "she" to refer to the nurse and "he" to refer to the client in order to clearly communicate to the reader.

ACKNOWLEDGMENTS

The development of this textbook resulted from the combined efforts of many talented professionals committed to excellence. We appreciate their dedication and enthusiasm. Throughout the text we have attempted to acknowledge the contributions of our professional nurse colleagues who make a difference in the lives of their clients and the communities they serve. We are very proud to be associated with such very fine individuals.

We wish to give special recognition to the editorial and production teams who have helped to make this textbook a reality. We especially wish to thank

- Suzi Epstein, Editor, and Beverly Copland, Developmental Editor, for their guidance and support. This text is truly a team effort. Their leadership has ensured a quality textbook with innovative design and informative content. Both Suzi and Bev have committed long hours to keep us on schedule and on target with regard to the objectives for this project. Bev continues to be a first-class tracker of contributors, manuscript, and authors!
- Chris Murphy, Senior Production Editor, for his methodical review and analysis of the text's design and format. His attention to detail helps to make the text readable, interesting, and of high quality.
- Renée Duenow, Book Designer, whose innovative design gives the book its exciting and attractive visual appeal.
- Vicki M. Friedman and Marci H. Hartstein, surgical illustrators, for their meticulous line drawings. Their attention to detail creates appealing visual images second to none.
- Pat Watson, photographer, whose skillful work brings visual life to each page. A special thanks to Michael Clement, MD, Mesa, Arizona, for his photographic contributions, and to Mary Reuther Herring, RN, MSN, and Sue Dodd, RN, MSN, for their time and assistance to Dr. Clement with photography.
- Our contributors and reviewers, whose painstaking critique of content and design ensures a high quality textbook. Their work often goes unnoticed. However, they have helped to set the standard for a comprehensive and accurate text.
- To Dorothy Thomas, RN, MSN, for her continuous assistance and exceptional dedication in reviewing the entire book.
- To the professional managers and nursing staff at Barnes Hospital and the faculty and nursing staff of Saint Louis University Hospital. We hope to capture and reveal the accomplishments they achieve daily within the case studies and clinical examples within the text. Their example of clinical excellence motivates us to develop an instructive textbook.

The creation of a nursing textbook is no small feat. We continue to be very grateful to the faculty and students who use our text. The partnership that we have forged during the last 14 years has been a very rewarding one. We hope to continue to meet the standard of excellence you, our readers, expect.

Patricia A. Potter
Anne Griffin Perry

Contents

unit three
SKILLS BASIC TO NURSING PRACTICE

unit four
PSYCHOSOCIAL AND DEVELOPMENTAL NEEDS

unit five
PROTECTION, SAFETY, AND COMFORT NEEDS

Detailed Contents

unit three
SKILLS BASIC TO NURSING PRACTICE

unit five
PROTECTION, SAFETY, AND COMFORT NEEDS

BASIC NURSING

Theory and Practice

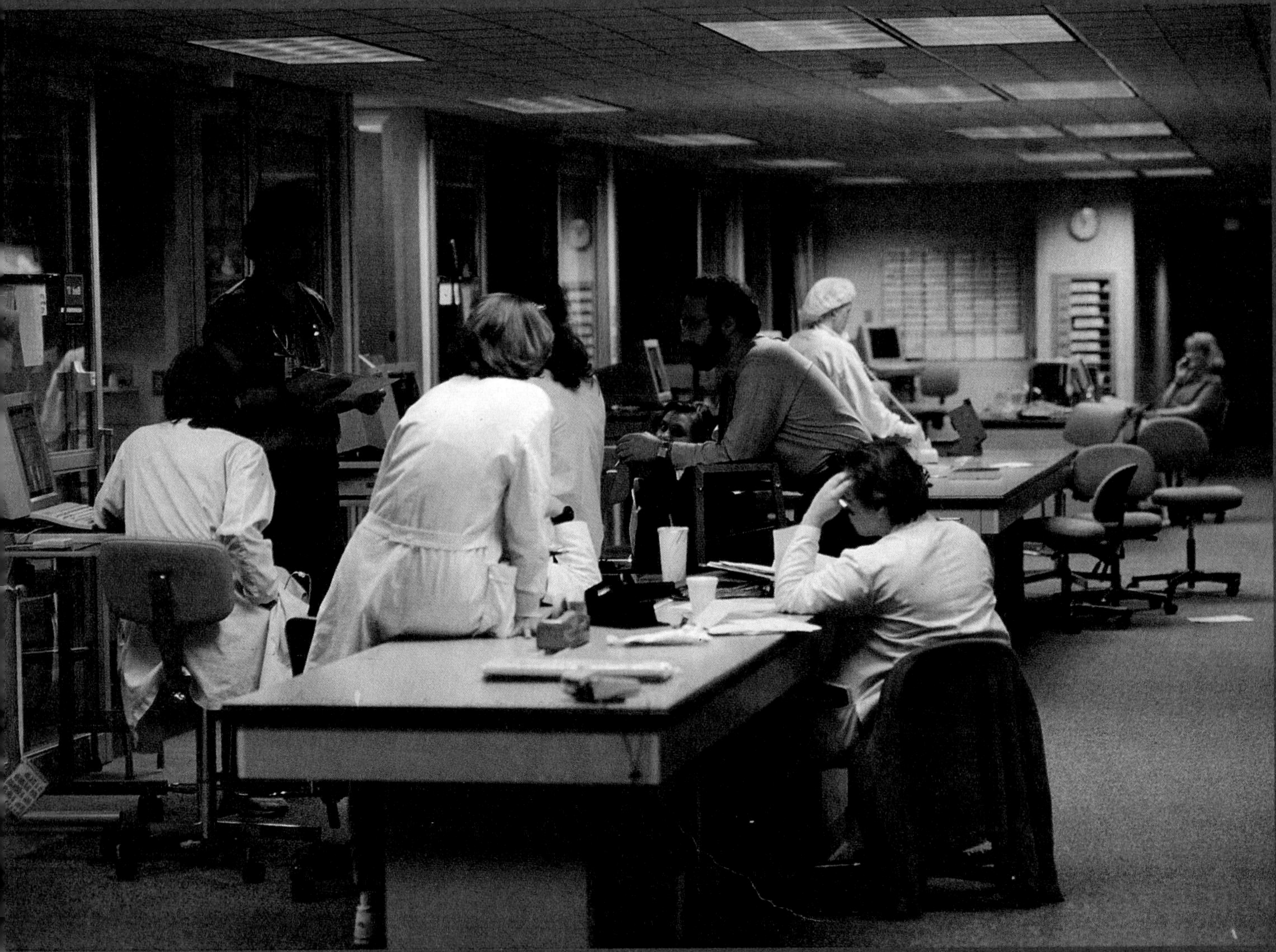

unit one

CONCEPTS BASIC TO NURSING PRACTICE

1

Nursing and the Contemporary Health Care System

OBJECTIVES

Mastery of content in this chapter will enable the student to:

- Define the key terms listed.
- Discuss the modern definitions and philosophies of nursing.
- Describe common practice settings for nurses.
- Discuss the variety of roles available for professional nurses.
- List the five characteristics of a profession.
- Discuss ways in which nursing demonstrates professional characteristics.
- Describe health care trends and their relation to nursing care delivery systems.
- Explain the significance of nursing's agenda for health care reform.

KEY TERMS

autonomy
career roles
case management
certification
code of ethics
community-based nursing
continuing education
credentialing
delivery of care model
differentiated nursing practice
functional nursing
in-service education
licensed practical nurse
nurse practice acts
primary nursing
professional nursing
registered nurse
vocational nurse

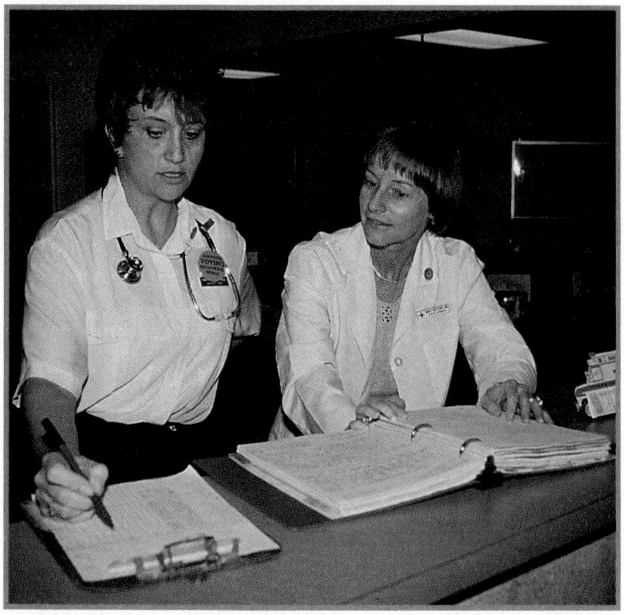

(Courtesy Michael S. Clement, MD, Mesa, Ariz.)

Modern nursing involves many kinds of concepts and skills related to health and social sciences, basic sciences, and contemporary issues. Nursing as a profession is unique because it addresses humanistically and holistically the responses of clients and families to actual and potential health problems.

Nurses have many roles such as care givers, advocates, researchers, and teachers. Because of the diversity of nursing roles, nurses need a philosophy of nursing to guide their practice. Over the years nurses have developed many philosophies, and as a result the profession continues to grow and mature.

There has never been a time in history when nursing has had such an opportunity to make a difference in the quality of life for humanity. The call for health care reform in 1993 by President Clinton has provided a significant opportunity for nurses to change the rules, get more clinical autonomy and power, and take charge of the new health care system (Sharp, 1993). To understand the position nursing is prepared to assume within health care, it is first important to understand its origins, professional standards, and roles within the community.

HISTORICAL PERSPECTIVE

Nursing has always been directed at serving the health care needs of society. Nursing originated with the desire to keep people healthy and provide comfort, care, and assurance to the ill.

Nursing was distinguished in its early history as a form of community service and was originally related to a strong instinct to preserve and protect the family (Donahue, 1985). Although the goals of nursing have remained relatively the same over the centuries, its practice has been influenced by the changing characteristics of society. Thus nursing has gradually evolved into a modern profession.

Nursing is as old as medicine. Throughout history, nursing and medicine have had an interdependent relationship. During the era of Hippocrates, medicine practiced without nursing, and during the Middle Ages, nursing practiced without rational medicine (Donahue, 1985).

In ancient cultures, religious beliefs and myths were the basis for health care and medical practice. Religious leaders were responsible for diagnosis and treatment, and many cultures believed illness was caused by the gods' displeasure. In these cultures, nurses usually had a role subservient to religious leaders.

Many ancient societies did not value human life in the same way Western civilization does today, so the caretakers of life were less respected. Nurses delivered custodial care and depended on physicians or priests for direction (Kelly, 1981). The nurse tended to the hygiene of clients in the home under the direct supervision of a physician. Nurses did not participate in activities to promote health, nor did they teach families how to care for the ill.

One consistent role of the nurse from early civilization is the midwife. Throughout medical and nursing history the midwife has been accepted in a role to assist women during childbirth.

Under the influence of Christianity, nurses gained respect, and the practice of nursing expanded. One of the earliest records of Christian nursing was the formation of the Order of the Deaconesses, a group somewhat like today's public health or visiting nurses.

Although nursing became increasingly humanistic, there was still no formal education or training for nurses. Nurses were often employed as servants, caring for infants and children to free the mistress of the household for social duties. In early institutions for the physically and mentally ill, uneducated nurses administered care as best they could, generally under the orders of a physician.

In the Middle Ages the Crusades were a stimulus for expanded nursing and health care. After the Crusades, with the decline of feudalism, large cities began to develop. Secular groups were formed to meet specific health care needs. The practice of midwifery also flourished in the Middle Ages.

The Sisters of Charity (1633) was founded by St. Vincent de Paul. The sisters cared for people in hospitals, asylums, and poor-houses. The sisters also became widely known as visiting nurses because they cared for sick people in their homes. The first supervisor of the Sisters of Charity was Louise de Gras who established perhaps the first educational program to be associated with a nursing order. The program included experience in the hospital, home visits, and the care of the ill. She recruited intelligent, refined, and compassionate women (Donahue, 1985). The Sisters of Charity were introduced in America by Mother Elizabeth Seton in 1809 and later changed their name to the Daughters of Charity (Donahue, 1985).

In the eighteenth century, the growth of cities brought an increase in the number of hospitals and a greater role for nurses. Smallpox epidemics in the French colonies and the Revolutionary War in the English colonies increased the need for nursing services.

During the nineteenth century, the Deaconess order was revived by Protestant churches. The Deaconess Institute at Kaiserswerth, Germany, was established in 1836 by Pastor Theodor Fliedner (Woodham-Smith, 1983; Donahue, 1985). The regeneration of this nursing order was stimulated by the recognition of the need for the services of women as nurses. In 1853 Florence Nightingale went to Paris to study with the Sisters of Charity and later was appointed superintendent of the English General Hospitals in Turkey. During this period, she brought about major reforms in hygiene, sanitation, and nursing practice and reduced the mortality rate at the Barracks Hospital in Scutari, Turkey, from 42.7% to 2.2% in 6 months (Cohen, 1984; Woodham-Smith, 1983; Donahue, 1985).

In 1860 Nightingale wrote *Notes on Nursing: What It Is and What It Is Not* for the layperson. Her philosophy of nursing practice reflected the changing needs of society. She saw the role of nursing as having "charge of somebody's health" based on the knowledge of "how to put the body in such a state to be free of disease or to recover from disease" (Nightingale, 1860). During the same year she developed the first organized program of training for nurses, the Nightingale Training School for Nurses at St. Thomas' Hospital in London.

The Civil War (1861-1865) stimulated the growth of nursing in the United States. Clara Barton (who founded the American Red Cross in 1882), Harriet Tubman, and others tended soldiers on the battlefields (Figure 1-1). After the Civil War, nursing schools in the United States and Canada began to follow the Nightingale plan. In the 1890s, through the efforts of Mary Agnes Snively and Isabel Hampton Robb, the Nurses' Associated Alumni of the United States and Canada was founded, which later led to the American Nurses Association and the Canadian Nurses Association.

Nursing in hospitals expanded in the late nineteenth century, but nursing in the community did not increase significantly until 1893, when Lillian Wald and Mary Brewster opened the Henry Street Settlement. It was one of the first community health services to focus on the health needs of poor people living in the New York City tenements. Nurses working in this settlement had greater responsibility for their clients than nurses working in hospitals because they frequently encountered situations that required action independent of physicians' orders. The concept of caring was never more important as nurses showed the ability to care for clients with a variety of needs from all walks of society.

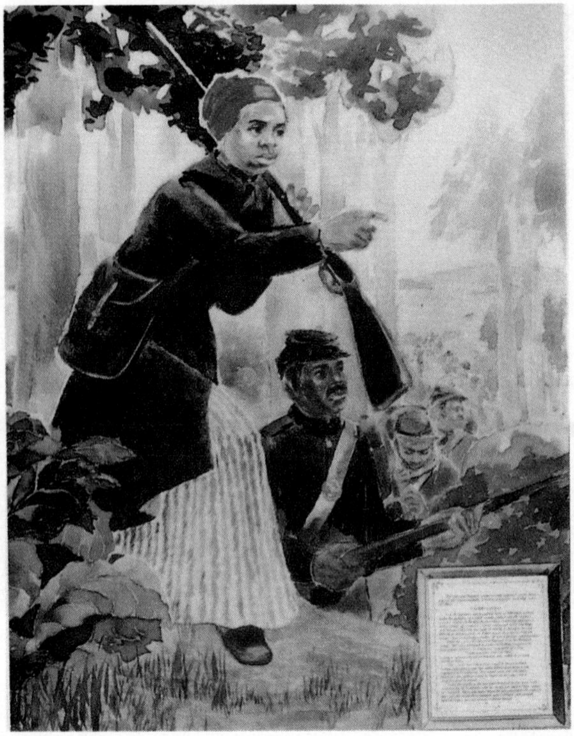

FIGURE 1-1 Harriet Tubman, shown here in a portrait by Joan Maynard, played several important roles in the Civil War, including working in the Underground Railroad movement and attending to the needs of sick and wounded soldiers. (From Defense Audiovisual Agency, Washington, DC.)

Nursing education from 1900 to 1935 was predominately based in hospital diploma programs. Of the more than 1800 diploma programs in existence in the mid-1930s less than 100 baccalaureate nursing programs were available for generic nursing education (NLN, 1990). Early in the twentieth century, Mary Adelaide Nutting was instrumental in the affiliation of nursing education with universities. She became the first professor of nursing in a university in 1907.

In 1923 the Rockefeller Foundation funded a survey of nursing education, the Goldmark Report. The report concluded that nursing education needed increased financial support and suggested that the money be given to university schools of nursing. As a result nursing programs such as those at Yale University and Vanderbilt University received funds for expansion.

As nursing education developed, nursing practice

also expanded. In 1901 the Army Nurse Corps was established, followed in 1908 by the Navy Nurse Corps. Nursing specialization was also developing. In the 1920s graduate nurse-midwifery programs began, and beginning in the 1950s specialty organizations such as the Association of Operating Room Nurses (1949) were formed.

Social events coupled with the impact of world wars from the late 1930s to the late 1940s affected all aspects of nursing education and practice. The classic Brown report of 1948 written by Dr. Esther Lucille Brown, a social scientist, significantly changed the course of nursing education. She examined nursing service and education from a societal perspective. Her report, funded by the Carnegie Foundation, suggested all nursing education programs affiliate with universities and have their own budgets. A broad academic grounding within a university setting and a 2-year nursing program together would help address the nursing shortage. These programs would have a more technical focus.

By 1952 Dr. Mildred Montag expanded current nursing education systems. These systems created the associate degree nursing program, offering a third educational track for the basic nursing student. Nursing students had community college courses linked to a practice setting for strong clinical and technical training. By 1988 only 9% of graduating nurses had a diploma education, 33% had a baccalaureate degree, and the remaining 58% had associate degrees (NLN, 1990).

The 1965 National Commission on Nursing and Nursing Education Report, directed by Jerome Lysaught, further developed the nursing profession. The Lysaught report indicated that nursing roles and responsibilities should be clarified in relation to those of other health care professionals. It also advocated greater financial support for nurses and more career opportunities to attract nurses and retain them in the profession (Lysaught, 1970).

Within 10 years, the American Nurses Association (ANA) and the W.K. Kellogg Foundation jointly produced *From Abstract Into Action.* This was an attempt to implement the recommendations from the Lysaught Report through the creation of the National Joint Practice Commission. Also the early (1953) work of the National League for Nursing (NLN) with universities began to develop graduate nursing education. By 1963 there were 32 Masters of Nursing programs nationwide. Nursing at the doctoral level was initiated by New York University as early as 1934. As of 1988 there were 46 doctoral nursing programs (NLN, 1990).

The 30 years of educational and practice changes from the 1950s to the 1980s expanded specialization for nurses. Margaretta Styles and Inez Hinsvark edited the American Nurses Association Study on Credentialing. It examined these new roles and the credentialing process in the growth of the nursing profession. The latter part of this chapter discusses current and future trends in specialization and certification for professional nursing.

MODERN DEFINITIONS AND PHILOSOPHIES OF NURSING

As nursing has evolved, expanding its roles and concepts, theorists have defined nursing in many ways. Florence Nightingale addressed nursing as a discipline in 1859 and believed that the nature of nursing and the need for nursing knowledge was distinct from medicine (Hayne, 1992). Conceptual and theoretical nursing models provide knowledge to improve practice, guide research and nursing curricula, and identify the goals of nursing practice. Theory provides the nurse with goals for assessment, diagnosis, and intervention. It also provides common ground for communication and for professional autonomy and accountability (Marriner-Tomey, 1994; Chinn, Jacobs, 1991; Meleis, 1991; Hayne, 1992) (see box below). The following sections describe, in chronological order, the general focus of several important theories of the philosophy of nursing. A nursing curriculum will often include one or more of these nursing theories as a part of its conceptual framework. Table 1-1 presents a summary of selected nursing theories for comparison.

Peplau's Theory

Hildegard Peplau's theory (1952) focuses on interpersonal relationships people form as they pass through developmental stages. Nursing's purpose is to educate the client and family and help the client to reach mature personality development (Chinn, Jacobs, 1991). Therefore the nurse develops a nurse-client relationship in which

GOALS OF THEORETICAL NURSING MODELS

- Formulate legislation governing nursing practice and education.
- Formulate regulations interpreting nurse practice acts so that nurses and others better understand the laws.
- Develop curricula for nursing education.
- Establish criteria for measuring the quality of nursing care, education, and research.
- Prepare job descriptions used by employers of nurses.
- Guide the development of nursing care delivery systems.
- Provide knowledge to improve nursing administration, practice, education, and research.
- Guide research to establish an empirical knowledge base for nursing.
- Identify the domain and goals of nursing.

table 1-1

SUMMARY OF NURSING THEORIES

Theorist	Goal of nursing	Framework for practice
Hildegard Peplau (1952)	To develop interpersonal interaction between client and nurse	Interpersonal theoretical model emphasizing relationship between client and nurse
Faye Abdellah (1960)	To deliver nursing care for whole individual	Problem solving based on 21 nursing problems
Ida Orlando (1961)	To respond to client's behavior in terms of immediate needs	Three elements, including client behavior, nurse reaction, and nurse action, composing a nursing situation
Virginia Henderson (1964)	To help client gain independence as rapidly as possible	Henderson's 14 basic needs
Dorothy Johnson (1968)	To reduce stress so that client can recover as quickly as possible	Adaptation model based on seven behavioral subsystems
Martha Rogers (1970)	To help client achieve maximal level of wellness	"Unitary man" evolving along life process
Imogene King (1971)	To use communication to help client to reestablish positive adaptation to environment	Nursing process as dynamic interpersonal state between nurse and client
Dorothea Orem (1971)	To care for and help client to attain self-care	Self-care deficit theory
Betty Neuman (1972)	To assist individuals, families, and groups to attain and maintain maximal level of total wellness by purposeful interventions	Systems model of nursing practice having stress reduction as its goal; nursing actions in one of three levels: primary, secondary, or tertiary
Myra Levine (1973)	To use conservation activities aimed at optimal use of client's resources	Adaptation model of human as integrated whole based on "four conservation principles of nursing"
Sister Callista Roy (1976)	To identify types of demands placed on client and client's adaptation to them	Adaptation model based on four adaptive modes: physiological, psychological, sociological, and independence
Madeleine Leininger (1978)	To care for individuals and groups in a culturally specific method meeting their health conditions	Cultural sensitivity with attention to the social structure through ethnonursing care
Jean Watson (1979)	To promote health, restore clients to health, and prevent illness (Marriner-Tomey, 1989)	Philosophy and science of caring: caring is an interpersonal process comprising interventions that result in meeting human needs (Torres, 1986)

the nurse is a resource person, counselor, and surrogate. When the client seeks help, the nurse discusses the nature of the problem and explains the services available. As the nurse-client relationship develops, the nurse helps the client to identify the problem and potential solutions. The client gains from this relationship by using available services to meet needs. When the original needs have been resolved, new needs may appear.

Abdellah's Theory

The nursing theory developed by Faye Abdellah et al. (1960) emphasizes delivering nursing care for the whole person to meet physical, emotional, intellectual, social, and spiritual needs. The nurse needs knowledge and skills in interpersonal relations, psychology, growth and development, communication, sociology, and the basic sciences, as well as specific nursing skills. The nurse, a problem solver and decision maker, forms an individualized view of the client's needs, which may occur in the following areas:

1. Comfort, hygiene, and safety
2. Physiological balance
3. Psychological and social factors
4. Sociological and community factors

In these areas, Abdellah et al. (1960) identify 21 specific client problems (often referred to as "Abdellah's 21 nursing problems"), which emphasize the physical (e.g., maintenance of elimination or sensory function) and psychological needs (e.g., maintenance of effective verbal and nonverbal communication) of each client. The nurse helps the client meet these needs by facilitating and maintaining a healthy physical condition in the best therapeutic environment possible. The nurse uses interpersonal skills, sound medical knowledge, and community resources to provide individualized holistic care.

Henderson's Theory

Virginia Henderson's nursing theory involves basic needs of the whole person. Henderson (1964a) defines nursing as:

> assisting the individual sick or well in the performance of those activities contributing to health or its recovery (or to a peaceful death) that he would perform unaided if he had the necessary strength, will, or knowledge. And to do this in such a way as to help him gain independence as rapidly as possible.

Henderson (1964) identifies specific needs, often called "Henderson's 14 basic needs," such as breathe normally, sleep, and rest. These emphasize maintaining a safe, healthy way of living, associated with good hygiene, an active social life, and personal development.

Orlando's Theory

To Ida Orlando (1961), the client is an individual with a need that, when met, diminishes distress, increases adequacy, or enhances well-being (Chinn, Jacobs, 1991). Her theory focuses on nurses' reactions to client behavior in terms of the client's immediate need (Torres, 1986). Orlando's theory describes three elements—client behavior, nurse reaction, and nurse actions—that compose the nursing situation (Marriner-Tomey, 1994). After nurses assess the client's needs, they recognize the impact of that need on the client's level of health and then act automatically or deliberately to meet the need. Nursing acts to reduce the client's distress.

Johnson's Theory

Dorothy Johnson's theory of nursing (1968) focuses on how the client adapts to illness and how actual or potential stress can affect the ability to adapt. For Johnson the goal of nursing is to reduce stress so the client can move more easily through the recovery process. Johnson's theory focuses on basic needs in terms of the following categories or subsystems of behavior:

1. Security-seeking behavior
2. Nurturance-seeking behavior
3. Mastery of oneself and one's environment according to internalized standards of excellence
4. Taking nourishment in socially and culturally acceptable ways
5. Ridding the body of waste in socially and culturally acceptable ways
6. Sexual and role identity behavior
7. Self-protective behavior

The nurse assesses the client's needs in these categories. The client is able to function fairly effectively in the environment under normal conditions. When stress disrupts normal adaptation, however, behavior becomes erratic and less purposeful. The nurse identifies the inability to adapt and provides nursing care to resolve problems in meeting the client's needs.

Rogers' Theory

Martha Rogers is known primarily for her contributions to the development of nursing science and the development of nursing as a profession (Gioiella, 1989). In her theory, Rogers (1970) considers man (unitary human being) as an energy field coexisting within the universe. Man is in continuous interaction with his environment. Unitary man is a "four dimensional energy field identified by pattern and manifesting characteristics that are specific to the whole and which cannot be predicted from the knowledge of parts" (Marriner-Tomey, 1994). The four dimensions used in Rogers' theory—energy fields, openness, patterns and organization, and four dimensionality—are used to derive principles about ways in which human beings develop and interact with their environments.

Rogers views nursing as a science and is committed to nursing research. Nursing incorporates knowledge of the basic sciences and physiology, as well as nursing knowledge:

> The science of nursing aims to provide a body of abstract knowledge growing out of scientific research and logical analysis and capable of being translated into nursing practice. Nursing's body of scientific knowledge is a new product specific to nursing. . . . Nursing is a humanistic science.

King's Theory

Imogene King's theory (1971, 1981) also focuses on the interpersonal relationship between the client and nurse. The nurse-client relationship is the vehicle for the nursing process, a dynamic interpersonal process in which the nurse and the client are affected by each other's behavior and the health care system. The nurse communicates to assist the client in reestablishing or maintaining a positive adaptation to the environment.

Orem's Theory

Dorothea Orem's (1971) definition of nursing emphasizes the self-care needs of the client. Orem describes her philosophy of nursing as follows:

> Nursing has as a special concern man's needs for self-care action and the provision and management of it on a continuous basis in order to sustain life and health, recover from disease or injury, and cope with their effects. Self-care is a requirement of every person—man, woman, and child. When self-care is not maintained, illness, disease, or death will occur. Nurses sometimes manage and maintain required self-care continually for persons who are totally incapacitated. In other instances, nurses help persons to maintain required self-care by performing some but not all care measures, by supervising others who assist patients, and by instructing and guiding individuals as they gradually move toward self-care.

The goal of Orem's self-care deficit theory is helping the client achieve self-care. Nursing care is necessary when the client is unable to fulfill biological, psychological, developmental, or social needs. The nurse determines reasons a client is unable to meet self-care needs, actions that will enable the client to meet these needs, and client self-care abilities.

Neuman's Theory

Betty Neuman forms a total-person model by incorporating the holistic concept and the open-system approach (Marriner-Tomey, 1994). Neuman views the person as a dynamic composite of physiological, sociocultural, and developmental variables functioning as an open system (Neuman and Young, 1972). Her goal of nursing is to assist individuals, families, and groups to attain and maintain a maximal level of total wellness.

The nurse assesses, manages, and evaluates client systems and focuses on factors affecting the client's response to stressors. Nursing actions are in one of the following levels of prevention: primary, secondary, and tertiary. Primary prevention strengthens a line of defense through identification of actual or potential risk factors associated with stressors. Secondary prevention strengthens internal defenses and resources by establishing priorities and treatment plans for identified needs. Tertiary prevention focuses on readaptation (Neuman, 1982).

Levine's Theory

Myra Levine's nursing theory (1973) views the client as an integrated being who interacts with and adapts to the environment. Conservation of energy is a primary concern. In this theory, health is viewed in terms of conservation of energy in the following areas, which Levine calls the "four conservation principles of nursing":

1. Conservation of client energy
2. Conservation of structural integrity
3. Conservation of personal integrity
4. Conservation of social integrity

With this approach, nursing care involves conservation activities aimed at optimal use of the client's resources.

Roy's Theory

Sister Callista Roy's adaptation theory (1976) views the client as an adaptive system. Roy believes the need for nursing care arises when the client cannot adapt to internal and external environmental demands. All individuals must adapt to the following demands:

1. Meeting basic physiological needs
2. Developing a positive self-concept
3. Performing social roles
4. Achieving a balance between dependence and independence

The nurse determines what demands are causing problems for a client and assesses adaptation to these demands. Nursing care then helps the client to adapt.

Leininger's Theory

Madeleine Leininger's theory of cultural care diversity and universality is a dramatic change in nursing theory (Belknap, 1993). Her focus is on caring. Care refers to the "assistive, supportive or facilitative acts toward another individual or group with evident or anticipated needs that ameliorate or improve the human condition" (Leininger, 1984). She believes nursing care is learned scientifically, allowing individuals and groups to develop culturally specific care to help meet their health needs.

Watson's Theory

Jean Watson also developed her nursing theory around the principle of caring as a philosophy and science. Caring is an interpersonal process consisting of interventions that result in meeting human needs (Torres, 1986). Nursing goals promote health, restore the client to a state of health, and prevent illness. Watson's model is designed around the caring process, which is defined by 10 "carative" factors. Each factor describes the caring process of how a client attains or maintains health or dies peacefully. Caring is the framework of the process of nursing care.

ANA DEFINITION OF NURSING PRACTICE

The definition of nursing has changed significantly over the last 50 years. In 1955 the ANA published the following official definition of nursing practice:

> The practice of professional nursing means the performance for compensation of any act in the observation, care, and counsel of the ill, injured, or infirm or in the maintenance of health or prevention of illness of others, or in the supervision and teaching of other personnel, or the administration of medications and treatments as prescribed by licensed physician or dentist, requiring substantial specialized judgment and skill

and based on knowledge and application of the principles of biological, physical, and social sciences. The foregoing shall not be deemed to include acts of diagnosis or prescription of therapeutic or corrective measures.

This definition is significant in its attempt to specifically define nursing practice. Nonetheless, it stresses nursing's dependent role, an emphasis no longer accepted. In 1965 the ANA Committee on Education issued a position paper that presents a broader definition of nursing and emphasizes nursing as an independent profession:

Nursing is a helping profession and, as such, provides services which contribute to the health and well-being of people.

Nursing is a vital consequence to the individual receiving services; it fills needs which cannot be met by the person, by the family, or by other persons in the community.

The essential components of professional nursing are care, cure, and coordination. The care aspect is more than "to take care of," it is "caring for" and "caring about" as well. It is dealing with human beings under stress, frequently over long periods of time. It is providing comfort and support in times of anxiety, loneliness, and helplessness. It is listening, evaluating, and intervening appropriately.

The promotion of health and healing is the cure aspect of professional nursing. It is assisting clients to understand their health problems and helping them to cope. It is the administration of treatments and the use of clinical nursing judgment in determining, on the basis of clients' reactions, whether the plan for care needs to be maintained or changed. It is knowing when and how to use existing and potential resources to help clients toward recovery and adjustment by mobilizing their own resources.

Professional nursing practice is this and more. It is sharing responsibility for the health and welfare of all those in the community, and participating in programs designed to prevent illness and maintain health. It is coordinating and synchronizing medical and other professional and technical services since these affect patients. It is supervising, teaching, and directing all those who give nursing care.

In 1980 the ANA Congress for Nursing Practice defined nursing as the diagnosis and treatment of human responses to actual or potential health problems (ANA, 1980). This definition involves the following characteristics of nursing: phenomena, theory application, nursing action, and evaluation of the effects of action. Phenomena are the human responses to actual or potential health problems. The nurse uses nursing theory to understand the client's responses. The nurse takes actions to resolve actual or potential health care problems. The nurse then evaluates the effects of nursing actions on client responses. These characteristics of nursing are related to the nursing process in Figure 1-2.

CNA Definition of Nursing Practice

The Canadian Nurses Association (CNA), founded in 1908, provides leadership to practicing nurses in the Canadian provinces. Its 1980 *Definition of Nursing and Standards of Practice* holds concepts similar to those of the ANA:

The nursing profession exists in response to a need of society and holds ideals related to man's health throughout his life span. Nurses direct their energies toward the promotion, maintenance, and restoration of health; the prevention of illness; the alleviation of suffering, and the ensurance of a peaceful death when life can no longer be sustained. Nurses value a holistic view and regard an individual as a biopsychosocial being who has the capacity to set goals and make decisions and who has the right and responsibility to make informed choices congruent with personal beliefs and values. Nursing, a dynamic and supportive profession guided by its code of ethics, is rooted in caring, a concept evident throughout its four fields of activity: practice, education, administration and research.

EDUCATION AND THE REGULATION OF NURSING PRACTICE

Modern nursing is complex and is expanding its professional roles to meet the needs of the changing health care system. Nurses practice in settings that emphasize educational diversity. The regulation of safe and competent nursing practice is monitored through the licensure process and the specific laws within each state. Various educational programs provide opportunities for nurses to enter many careers within the same profession.

Licensed Practical Nurse Education

A licensed practical or vocational nurse is trained in basic nursing techniques and direct client care. The licensed practical nurse (LPN) practices under the supervision of a registered nurse in a hospital or community health practice. Licensed practical nurses, licensed vocational nurses (LVNs), and, in Canada, registered nurse's assistants (RNAs) generally receive 1 year of education and training in a hospital, community college, or other agency. The licensed practical nurse is licensed by the state board of nursing after completing an educational program and passing the National Council Licensure Examination for Practical Nurses (NCLEX-PN).

Registered Nurse Education

In the United States, an individual can become a **registered nurse** (RN) through the following types of programs: a 2-year associate degree program usually offered by a college or junior college, a 2- or 3-year diploma program usually associated with a hospital, and a 4-year baccalaureate program in a college or university. In Canada, diploma programs are offered in community colleges or hospitals and are usually 2-year pro-

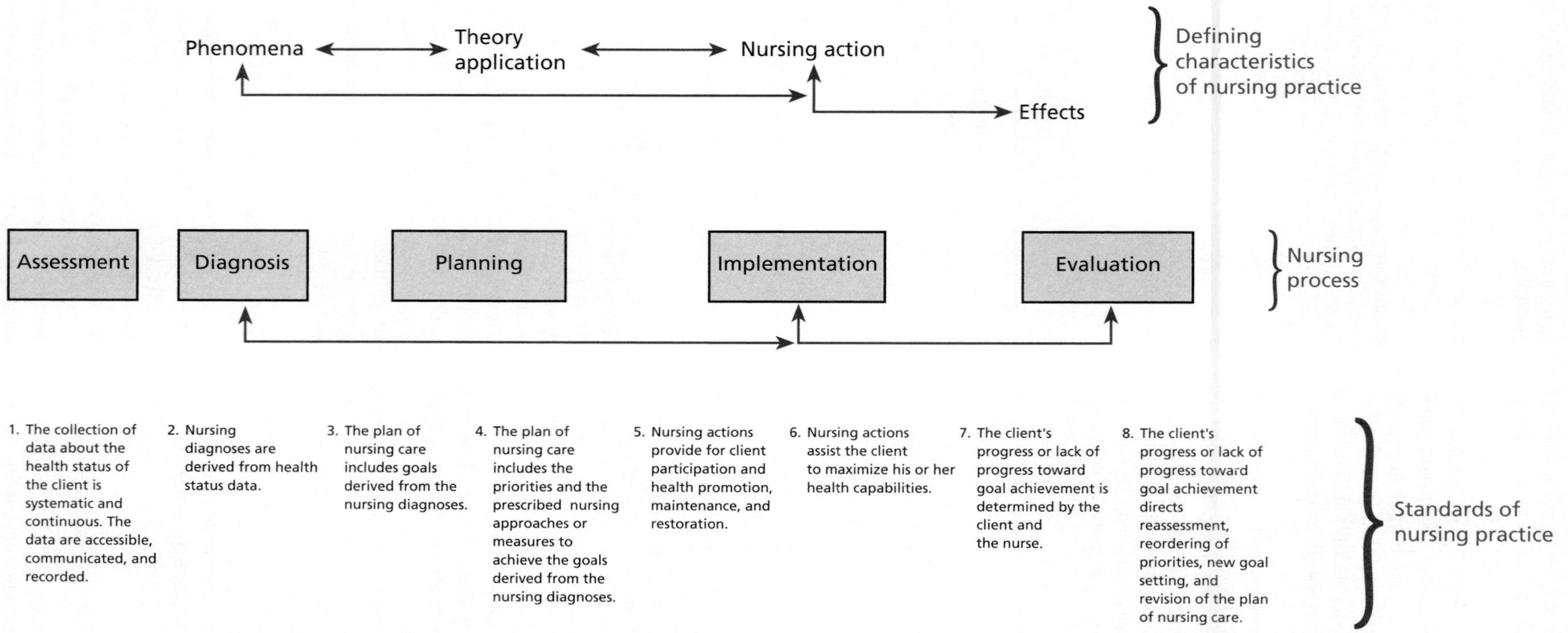

FIGURE 1-2 Summary of defining characteristics of nursing practice: relationship to the nursing process and the standards of nursing practice. (Modified from the American Nurses Association: *Nursing and social policy statement,* Washington, DC, 1980, The Association.)

grams. A Bachelor of Science in Nursing (BScN) in Canada is the equivalent to the Bachelor of Science in Nursing (BSN) in the United States. Within recent years, many universities have developed agreements with community colleges to assist the associate degree student to move into the baccalaureate program following NCLEX-RN licensure.

RN licensure for practice in most states and provinces requires the student to complete a prescribed course of study from an approved program. In the United States the program must be approved by the State Board of Nursing in the state in which the student is seeking licensure. In Canada the program must be approved by the Provincial Board of Nursing in the province in which the student seeks licensure.

RN candidates in the United States must pass the National Council Licensure Examination for Registered Nurses (NCLEX-RN). Graduates of all three types of programs take the same licensing examination. In Canada the CNA Testing Service (CNATS) administers the test to qualified candidates in each province. Whether a nurse in the United States or in Canada can practice in a different state or province depends on the reciprocal agreement in effect between the two states or provinces involved. In some instances, reciprocity in Canada is considered individually.

Graduate Nursing Education

As expressed by the ANA (1969), the purpose of a graduate program in nursing is to prepare nurse clinicians capable of improving nursing care through the advancement of nursing theory and sciences. Those completing a graduate program can receive the degree of Master of Arts in Nursing (MA), Master in Nursing (MN), or Master of Science in Nursing (MSN). A master's degree is valuable for nurses who seek expanded roles such as nurse educator, clinical nurse specialist, or advanced nurse practitioner.

The ANA, in the *Social Policy Statement,* defines as a generalist an RN with a basic education who may practice in a special area of nursing. A specialist is a nurse with a graduate degree who practices in a special area of nursing (ANA, 1980). As nursing theory has developed, many nurses have desired the advanced knowledge and research skills required for a doctoral degree to further develop and test nursing theories. The doctoral degree prepares the nurse for education, administration, research, and clinical practice. A few programs in the United States have optional graduate programs so that the student with a baccalaureate degree can obtain a doctorate in nursing.

Continuing Education

Continuing education programs help nurses remain current in nursing skills, knowledge, and theory. They involve formal, organized, educational programs offered by educational and health care institutions. Nursing journals often provide the option of obtaining continuing education by completing written educational units. As expressed by the ANA (1975), the goals of continuing education in nursing are to improve and maintain nursing practice, to promote and exercise leadership in changing health care delivery systems, and to fulfill professional learning needs. Continuing education programs are short term and are designed for all professional nurses. The ANA or the State Board of Nursing is the accrediting agency for continuing education programs called Continuing Education Approval and Recognition Program (CEARP). In 3% of states, continuing education is mandatory for re-licensure. Because of the variation in the hours needed for licensure renewal, the RN is informed of specific requirements at the time of licensure.

In-Service Education

In-service education programs are instruction or training provided by a health care agency or institution in which nurses are employed. An in-service program is designed to increase the knowledge, skills, and competencies of nurses and other health care professionals. Examples of in-service programs include training on how to perform blood glucose monitoring, how to use the hospital's patient care computer functions, and how to use techniques such as the patient controlled analgesia pump (PCA pump) for pain management.

PROFESSIONAL PRACTICE DIMENSIONS

Nurses practice in many settings, in many roles within those settings, and with other care givers in the allied health professions. State and provincial nurse practice acts establish legal regulations for nursing practice, and professional organizations establish standards of nursing practice as criteria for nursing care. The nurse must have knowledge about both ANA generic standards of practice and specialty practice standards to gain current nursing competency.

Standards of Practice

As nursing has become more independent as a profession and the realm of nursing practice has been more clearly defined, a need for standards of nursing practice has evolved. Standards of practice are important as guidelines for nurses to provide care and as criteria for evaluating care. Standards of practice within the agency should be established by nurses with expertise in administering care to groups of clients. When standards are clearly defined and followed, clients can be assured

table 1-2

ANA STANDARDS OF NURSING PRACTICE

Standard	Element
ASSESSMENT	
The nurse collects client health data.	The priority of data collection is determined by the client's immediate condition of needs. Pertinent data are collected using appropriate assessment techniques. Data collection involves the client, significant others, and health care providers when appropriate. The data collection process is systematic and ongoing. Relevant data are documented in a retrievable form.
DIAGNOSIS	
The nurse analyzes the assessment data in determining diagnoses.	Diagnoses are derived from the assessment data. Diagnoses are validated with the client, significant others, and health care providers, when possible. Diagnoses are documented in a manner that facilitates the determination of expected outcomes and plan of care.
The nurse identifies expected outcomes individualized to the client.	Outcomes are derived from the diagnoses. Outcomes are documented as measurable goals. Outcomes are mutually formulated with the client and health care providers, when possible. Outcomes are realistic in relation to client's present and potential capabilities. Outcomes are attainable in relation to resources available to the client. Outcomes include a time estimate for attainment. Outcomes provide direction for continuity of care.
PLANNING	
The nurse develops a plan of care that prescribes interventions to attain expected outcomes.	The plan is individualized to the client's condition or needs. The plan is developed with the client, significant others, and health care providers, when appropriate. The plan reflects current nursing practice. The plan is documented. The plan provides for continuity of care.
IMPLEMENTATION	
The nurse implements the interventions identified in the plan of care.	Interventions are consistent with the established plan of care. Interventions are implemented in a safe and appropriate manner. Interventions are documented.
EVALUATION	
The nurse evaluates the client's progress toward attainment of outcomes.	Evaluation is systematic and ongoing. The client's responses to interventions are documented. The effectiveness of interventions is evaluated in relation to outcomes. Revisions in diagnoses, outcomes, and the plan of care are documented. The client, significant others, and health care providers are involved in the evaluation process, when appropriate.

From ANA: *Standards of clinical practice,* Washington, DC, 1991. The Association.

table 1-3
SUMMARY OF CNA STANDARDS FOR NURSING PRACTICE

Standard	Elements
Nursing practice requires that conceptual models for nursing be the basis for the independent part of that practice.	Nurses are required to: Have a clear idea or conception of the distinct goal of nursing. Have a clear idea or conception of the client. Have a clear idea or conception of their role in response to the health needs of society. Have a clear idea or conception of the source of client difficulty. Have a clear idea or conception of the focus and modes of nursing intervention. Have a clear idea or conception of the expected consequences of nursing activities.
Nursing practice requires the effective use of the nursing process.	Nurses are required to: Collect data in accordance with their conception of the client. Analyze data collected in accordance with their conception of the goal of nursing, their role, and the source of client difficulty. Plan their nursing actions based on the identified actual and potential client problems, in accordance with their conception of the focus and modes of intervention. Perform nursing actions that implement the plan. Evaluate all steps of the nursing process in accordance with their conceptual model(s) for nursing.
Nursing practice requires that the helping relationship be the nature of the client/nurse interaction.	Nurses are required to: Increase the likelihood that the client will perceive the health service experience as understandable, manageable, and meaningful at the outset. Set mutually agreed upon expectations as a means of increasing the likelihood that the client will perceive the health service experience as understandable, manageable, and meaningful. Ensure a successful termination of the helping relationship.
Nursing practice requires nurses to fulfill professional responsibilities.	Nurses are required to: Respect statutes and policies relevant to the profession and the practice setting. Comply with the code of ethics of their profession. Function as members of a health team.

Modified from Canadian Nurses Association: *A definition of nursing practice standards for nursing practice,* Ottawa, 1980 (revised 1987), The Association.

they are receiving high-quality care, nurses know how to give quality care, and administrators can evaluate whether this care meets acceptable standards and whether clients have achieved expected outcomes. Standards of practice may be internal or external. Internal standards are established by a nursing department. External standards are created by outside regulatory and professional agencies such as the ANA or Joint Commission on Accreditation of Healthcare Organizations (JCAHO). Moreover, standards of practice are important if a legal dispute arises (see Chapter 6). The ANA and the Canadian Nurses Association (CNA) have published standards of nursing practice (Tables 1-2 and 1-3). The 1991 ANA *Standards of Clinical Nursing Practice* consists of the standards of care and the standards of professional performance with each section noting measurement goals.

Nurse Practice Acts

In all states in the United States and all provinces in Canada, nurse practice acts regulate the licensure and practice of nursing. Each state or province defines the scope of legal nursing practice. They are usually quite similar. A nurse licensed in a specific state or province is accountable for nursing practice within that state or province. The classic definition of nursing practice published by the ANA in 1955 represents the scope of nursing practice as defined in most states and provinces. In the last decade, however, many states have revised nurse practice acts to reflect nursing's growing autonomy and the expanded roles of nurses in practice. The ANA 1980 definition of nursing, which describes the profession as the "diagnosis and treatment of human response to actual or potential health problems," reflects that expanded focus. The number of advanced clinical practitioners and specialists continues to grow and responds to the public's health care needs. Currently a variety of states are responding to this need by requiring certification of advanced practitioners to ensure they have achieved excellence in practice.

Currently only 17% of all states specify advanced practitioner roles in their nurse practice acts. Currently many advanced practitioners already seek specialty certification credentials. The mandatory licensure could be seen as an additional unnecessary credential. The ANA in 1981 supported the continued regulation of specialties by the professional organization and not by the state (ANA, 1981). The debate will continue as health care delivery needs change and as nursing continues to respond to these needs.

Practice Settings

As nursing's role in the health care system has expanded, the settings in which nurses practice have also increased. More nurses continue to work in hospitals than in any other type of practice setting, but that number is declining. In a 1990 report from the Department of Health and Human Services, a study that examined the RN work force indicated 67% of RNs worked in hospitals; smaller numbers worked in ambulatory care, community health, and nursing home or extended care facilities. Nurses involved in home health care represent a rapidly expanding nursing specialty. Figure 1-3 represents the percentages in the 1990 report.

The roles and responsibilities of nurses in hospitals vary. For example, a nurse in an acute care setting usually cares for clients with severe illnesses and more complex problems. The rapid increase in the number of older adult clients, clients with chronic illnesses, and clients with functional impairments has resulted in the growth of long-term care facilities. Nurses in these facilities take on an additional role of being a rehabilitator.

Hospitalization trends reflect that inpatient acuity rates have increased (Figure 1-4). However, the length

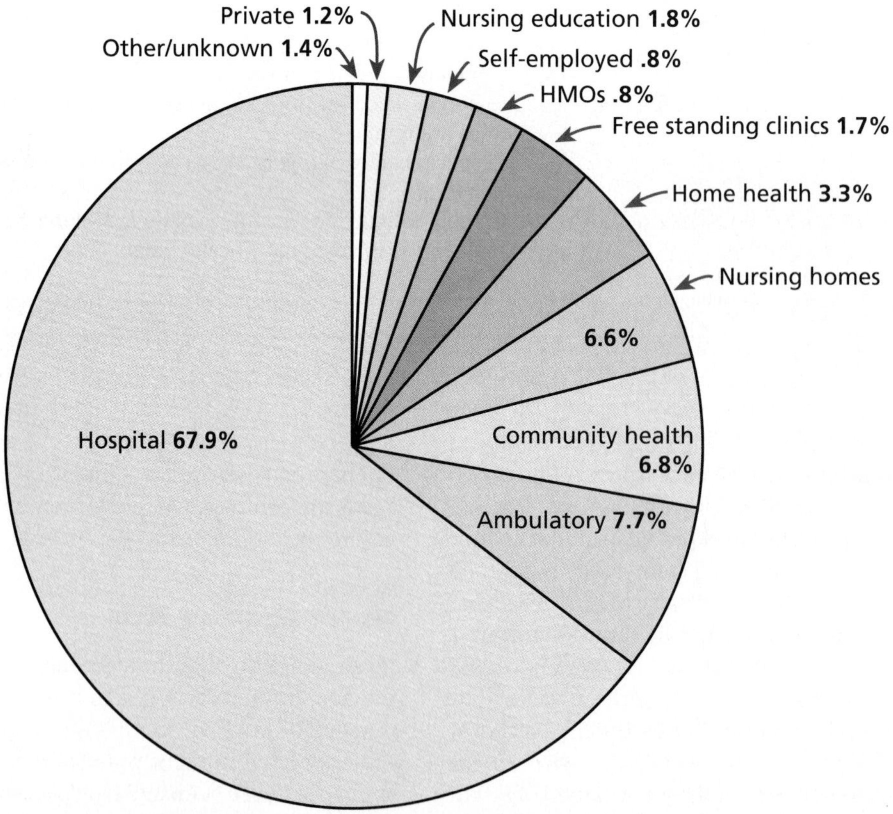

FIGURE 1-3 Percentage of nurses in practice areas. (Modified from U.S. Department of Health and Human Services: *The registered nurse populations: findings from the National sample of RNs,* Washington, DC, 1990, U.S. Government Printing Office.)

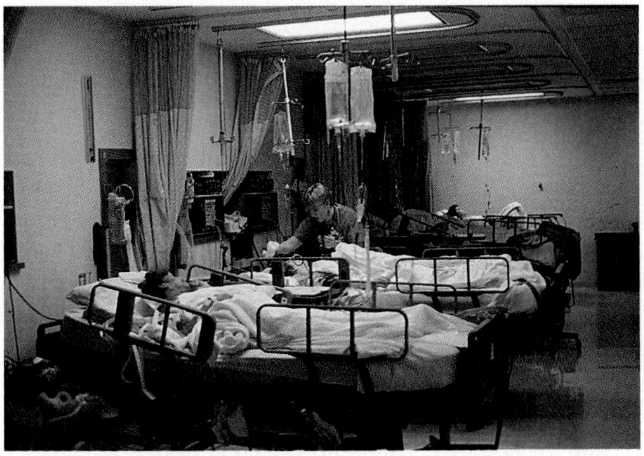

FIGURE 1-4 Nurses in recovery room.

of stay for each client has decreased at the same time. This shift has resulted in part from new disease entities and new forms of supportive therapy, along with changes in insurance payment systems and the movement toward community-based care. Opportunistic infections associated with acquired immunodeficiency syndrome (AIDS), organ transplantation, and technological equipment in the critical care setting are a few factors contributing to a higher percentage of critically ill clients in hospitals. Today's nurses must meet the needs of the client and family within a shorter time during a health crisis as hospitals try to reduce length of stay. Nursing services operate in hospitals 24 hours a day. Hospitals use different staffing patterns such as 8-, 10-, or 12-hour shifts to meet this need.

Since 1974 the number of nurses employed in community-based practice settings has increased. More than 2% of the North American client population is in either acute, long-term, or other institutional settings at any given time. Because of the growing older adult population, 300,000 to 1 million nurses will be needed by the year 2000 to work in nursing home and extended care community-based facilities (Philipose, Tate, and Jacobs, 1992). Nursing in community-based settings has traditionally been focused primarily on health promotion, maintenance, education and management, and coordination and continuity of care. Whereas institutional health care focuses on the individual and the family, community-based nursing is directed toward the health of the community and the interaction of individuals within that community.

Nurses' roles and responsibilities vary widely in other practice settings. A nurse in a physician's office, for example, may have little independent responsibility compared with a nurse practitioner in independent practice or in joint practice with other nurses. Other important opportunities for nurses include careers in college teaching positions, in clinical research, occupational health, nurse paralegal practice, and school nursing.

Delivery of Care Models

Nurses provide care to clients while working under a variety of care-delivery models. A delivery of care model is a philosophy of care delivery and a system for organizing the relationships and roles of all nursing care personnel. A delivery of care model is not a staffing mix, such as number of registered versus licensed practical nurses, nor is it a staffing system that dictates the total number of staff needed for a particular nursing division.

Historically, several delivery of care models have been used in nursing. Each differs in regard to the types of responsibilities assumed by registered nurses and other nursing personnel. The models also differ in the extent to which a registered nurse directly coordinates the care of all clients and the extent to which clients' needs are matched with staff abilities.

Functional Nursing. The functional nursing model indicates that nursing personnel are routinely responsible for selected tasks based on their qualifications and skills. A registered nurse, for example, administers medications and performs complex nursing procedures. A nurse assistant gives a bed bath or assists with feeding. Care is administered in a task-oriented approach and can lead to fragmented nursing care. The registered nurse may not assume responsibility for a client's total plan of care.

Team Nursing. In a team nursing structure, nursing personnel are assigned to groups of clients usually organized by geographical boundaries. For example, one hallway in a nursing division may be assigned to Team I, whereas a second hallway is assigned to Team II. A registered nurse is usually the team leader, coordinating the care delivered by other team members such as registered and licensed practical nurses or nurse assistants. The team leader may administer all medications and select treatments for a team of clients, or an additional nurse may be the medication nurse. In this model, although a registered nurse supervises care on a nursing unit for a particular shift, there is no assurance that he or she personally administers or plans care to selected clients.

Total Client Care or Modified Primary Nursing. In the total client care model, nursing personnel are assigned their own caseload of clients for a single shift or tour of duty. An attempt is made to match the client's needs with the abilities of the available staff. A nurse assumes responsibility for the assigned clients' nursing care, including administration of prescribed therapies for the shift. In many institutions, the registered nurse "covers" the licensed practical nurse for any procedures he or she is not licensed to perform or is restricted from performing because of agency policy, such as intravenous therapy. In total client care, a given client often receives care from many nursing personnel and no single registered nurse is completely responsible for the client's care over time.

Primary Nursing. In a primary nursing model, each client is assigned to a single registered nurse, who is responsible for administering and coordinating the client's nursing care. Primary nursing focuses on the relationship of the nurse and client, who work together to plan care. The client's needs are matched with the nurse's knowledge and skills. By having one nurse direct care there is less fragmentation and improved continuity compared with other traditional delivery of care models. The primary nurse does not work every day or each shift while a client is in the health care setting. However, the primary nurse communicates to all nursing personnel a plan of care so that one consistent plan is followed. An associate nurse (registered or licensed practical) cares for a client and follows the plan communicated by the primary nurse during the primary nurse's absence.

Case Management. Case management is a systematic approach to care that provides a framework that targets the coordination of medical and nursing interventions. Case management is not a true delivery of care model but a system that can be applied to any nursing care delivery system (Zander, 1988). In case management, a nurse functioning as a case manager coordinates care of groups of clients, often of a specific case type. Unlike a primary nurse, the case manager does not typically give direct client care. The case manager will facilitate referrals, discharge planning, and scheduling of testing. In many institutions case managers use critical pathways, developed by nurses, physicians, and other health team members, for selected groups of clients. The critical pathways are guidelines that sequence specific clinical interventions that must be administered to clients. Critical pathways map out client care activities over a projected length of stay. For example, medical paths are activity orders, diagnostic procedures, and medication prescriptions, and nursing paths are teaching protocols, comfort measures, and self-care activities that must be provided by nurses, clients, and other care providers during a specific time frame. This system is useful in many different health care settings.

ROLES AND FUNCTIONS OF THE NURSE

CARE GIVER

The nurse directly helps the client to regain health through the healing process. The nurse addresses the holistic health care of the client, including helping the client and family restore emotional and social well-being.

DECISION MAKER

The nurse, before taking any action, interprets available information and decides the best approach for the individual client. These decisions can be made alone, with the client and family, or with other health care professionals.

PROTECTOR AND CLIENT ADVOCATE

The nurse maintains a safe environment, helps prevent injury, and protects the client from possible adverse effects related to treatment. The nurse also protects the client's human and legal rights and assists him or her in asserting those rights if the need arises.

MANAGER

The nurse delegates responsibility, supervises other health care workers, manages the resources of the practice setting, and coordinates activities.

REHABILITATOR

The nurse assists the client's return to maximal functioning through teaching and helping the client to cope with changes associated with illness or disability.

COMFORTER

The nurse cares for the client as a person through emotional support. The client needs help in reaching therapeutic goals.

COMMUNICATOR

The nurse is continually involved in promoting communication among all people affected by the client's needs. Communication is critical in meeting the needs of clients, families, and communities.

TEACHER

The nurse explains concepts and facts about health care to the client, reinforces learning, and evaluates progress. Teaching is individualized and may be formal or informal.

Roles and Functions of the Nurse

A contemporary nurse possesses knowledge and skills in a variety of areas. In the past, nurses provided care and comfort while they carried out specific nursing functions, but changes in nursing have expanded the roles of nurses to include health promotion, illness prevention, health restoration, and concern for the whole client (see box above).

Career Roles. Career roles are specific employment positions. Most skills required for the expanded roles of the 1980s and 1990s are taught in baccalaureate nursing

CAREER ROLES

NURSE EDUCATOR

Nurse educators work in schools of nursing, staff development departments, and client education departments. They provide educational programs for student nurses and nurses and teach clients about self-care and home care. They usually are required to have graduate nursing education.

CLINICAL NURSE SPECIALIST

Clinical nurse specialists work in critical, acute, long-term, and community health care agencies (Figure 1-5). They often specialize in managing specific diseases, and they function as clinicians, educators, managers, consultants, and researchers. They have master's degrees in nursing.

NURSE PRACTITIONER

Nurse practitioners are certified to provide health care to clients, usually in outpatient or community settings. Adult nurse practitioners provide primary care to adults; family nurse practitioners provide primary care for families; pediatric nurse practitioners provide care for infants and children; gerontologic nurse practitioners provide care to older adults; and obstetrics-gynecology nurse practitioners provide primary care for women. Most have master's degrees in nursing.

CERTIFIED NURSE-MIDWIFE

Certified nurse-midwives are certified by the American College of Nurse-Midwives to provide independent care for women during normal pregnancy, labor, and delivery. They practice in conjunction with a health care agency, which provides assistance.

NURSE ANESTHETIST

Nurse anesthetists are registered nurses who have advanced training in anesthesiology. They provide surgical anesthesia under the supervision of an anesthesiologist and administer anesthetics to clients during minor surgery.

NURSE ADMINISTRATOR

Nurse administrators manage client care within a health care agency. They may hold middle-level (e.g., head nurse) or upper-level (e.g., director) management positions. They usually have baccalaureate degrees in nursing and may have master's degrees.

NURSE RESEARCHER

Nurse researchers investigate nursing problems to improve care and to define and expand the scope of nursing practice. They may be in academic, independent, or community settings. They must have a graduate degree in nursing. In some settings, a doctoral degree is required.

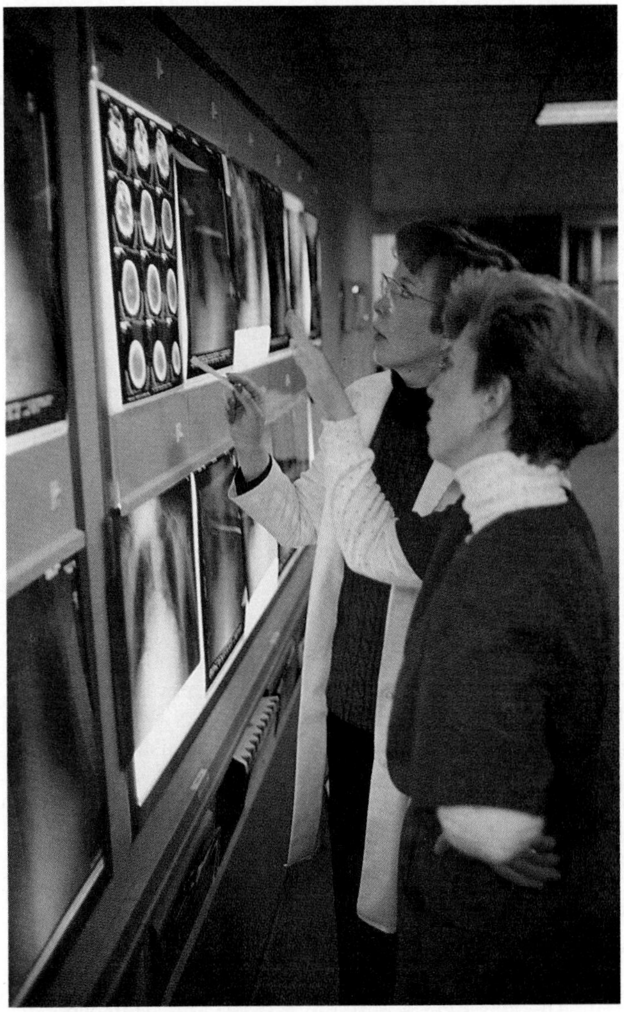

FIGURE 1-5 Nurse specialist consults on difficult client case.

programs. These skills are now directed toward the generalist practitioner. The newer requirements for nursing specialization are redefining the term "expanded role" (Mechanic, 1988). Nursing specialties have input into the educational requirements for these roles and career opportunities (see box at left).

One method of redesigning nursing roles has been the focus of differentiated nursing practice. This practice had early design in the educational setting where graduate-expected competencies were based on different types of educational experiences. Differentiated practice is now expanding into clinical practice as new nursing roles incorporate primary nursing and case management principles (Harkness et al., 1992). Broadly defined, differentiated practice structures roles and functions of nurses according to education, experience, and competence, while recognizing the importance of all roles to create a community of professional nursing practice (Koerner, 1992). For example, in such a system there is a clear difference between the responsibilities of a baccalaureate-prepared nurse versus one with an associate's degree.

Health Care Team

In most practice settings, the nurse works with other health care professionals to provide total care for clients (see box below). The involvement of many persons in the client's health care can pose risks for fragmenting care. Because nurses have the greatest opportunity to interact with all professionals in the health care team, they often coordinate and integrate services within the care plan.

> **OTHER HEALTH CARE TEAM MEMBERS**
>
> **PHYSICIAN**
>
> A physician is a professional who has earned a degree of doctor of medicine or doctor of osteopathy and has passed a licensing examination. Most physicians specialize their practice of medicine. Nurses work closely with physicians under supervision or as collaborators.
>
> **PHYSICIAN ASSISTANT**
>
> Physician assistants have medical training and work under the direction of physicians in hospitals, clinics, and private offices (they do not practice in Canada). Nurses work with them as they do with physicians.
>
> **THERAPIST**
>
> Therapists are licensed to assist in the examination and treatment of clients in special ways (i.e., as physical, occupational, or respiratory therapists). Their education varies but usually involves 4-year programs. Nurses collaborate with them and evaluate their work.
>
> **PHARMACIST**
>
> Pharmacists are licensed to formulate and dispense drugs. They may have bachelor of science degrees or doctorates in pharmacology. Pharmacists provide valuable information to nurses about drugs and their use and effects.
>
> **SOCIAL WORKER**
>
> Social workers are trained to counsel and refer clients to appropriate agencies. They have baccalaureate or master's degrees. Nurses work together with them to identify the best resources for the client, particularly when the client returns home.
>
> **CHAPLAIN**
>
> Chaplains offer spiritual support and guidance to clients and their families. They may be employed by an agency or provided by a church in the community. A client may request a chaplain, or a nurse may refer the client to one.

NURSING AS A PROFESSION

Professionalism

"Professionalism of nursing will be achieved only through the professionalhood of its members" (Margarita Styles, 1982). Nursing is not simply a collection of specific skills, and the nurse is not simply a person trained to perform specific tasks. Nursing continues to evolve into a profession. No one factor absolutely differentiates a job from a profession, but several characteristics are basic to any true profession. Sociologists ranging from Flexner in 1900 to Caplow in 1950, Etzioni in 1960, and Levenstein in 1985 have studied the characteristics of professions. They agree that some core characteristics are true for any profession. These include education, theoretical body of knowledge, the provision of a specific service, the autonomy of members, and a code of ethics. Nursing clearly shares, to some extent, each of these characteristics and faces controversial issues as nurses strive for greater professionalism.

Education. An earlier section describes the three basic types of educational preparation for registered nurses. As a profession, nursing requires that its members possess a significant education, but the issue of educational standardization is a major controversy in nursing today. Most nurses agree that nursing education is of great importance to practice and that nursing education along with continuing education must respond to the changes in health care created by scientific and technological advances.

Theory. Nursing knowledge has been developed through nursing theories. Theoretical models are frameworks for nursing curricula and clinical practice and also lead to research that increases the scientific basis of nursing practice. A theory is a way of understanding a reality, and, in this general sense, all practicing nurses use theories they have learned as a part of their clinical practice. Theoretical frameworks help nurses to understand the scope of their practice and to select interventions most likely to assist clients to an improved state of health.

Service. Nursing, like other professions, provides a specific service. Today, nursing is a vital part of the health care delivery system, providing holistic and comprehensive services to clients with varying needs. Nurses are now the largest group of professionals in this system. Approximately 2 million people are now registered nurses, and one study indicates that approximately 80% of them are employed (Aiken and Millinix, 1987).

Autonomy. Autonomy means that one is reasonably independent and self-governing in decision making and practice. It has been difficult for nurses to attain the degree of autonomy enjoyed by some other professionals. Some data suggest that the history of nursing has been a struggle by nurses for autonomy in the face of different societal expectations (Cohen, 1992). In the past, physicians, hospital administrators, and others in the health care delivery system have found nursing autonomy difficult to understand and support. Through clinical competence and greater educational preparation, however, nurses are increasingly taking on independent roles in nurse-run clinics, collaborative practice, and advanced nursing careers. A 1992 nursing research study indicated a positive relationship between the highest level of nursing education and the autonomy of nursing roles (Schutzenhofer, 1992). Greater responsibility and accountability come with increased autonomy. Accountability means the nurse is answerable, professionally and legally, for the type and quality of nursing care provided to clients. The nursing profession regulates accountability through standards of practice, nurse practice acts, nursing audits, and certification.

Code of Ethics. Nursing has had a code of ethics since 1903. The code of ethics describes the goals and values of the nursing profession and establishes a code of conduct by which nurses function. Ethical principles within the code provide a foundation for nursing practice. In addition, nurses incorporate their own values and ethics into their practice. The American Nurses Association publishes a Code of Ethics and Interpretative Statements (see Chapter 5). Integrated within the code are the five characteristics for a profession. Figure 1-6 summarizes the legal and professional regulations of the nursing profession.

Professional Organizations. A professional organization is created to deal with issues of concern to those practicing in the profession. In North America, major professional nursing organizations are the American Nurses Association (ANA), Canadian Nurses Association (CNA), and the National League for Nursing (NLN). The CNA and the ANA were formed in the late nineteenth century to improve standards of health and the availability of health care, to foster high standards for nursing, and to promote the professional development and general and economic welfare of nurses. The ANA and CNA are part of the International Council of Nurses (ICN). The objectives of the ICN parallel those of the CNA and ANA.

The NLN is concerned with improving nursing education, nursing service, and health care delivery in the United States. It is the credentialing body for accrediting nursing programs. In Canada the Canadian Association of University Schools of Nursing and the Canadian Association of Practical and Nursing Assistants perform similar functions.

Nursing students also take part in organizations such as the National Student Nurses Association (NSNA) in the United States and the Canadian Student Nurses Association (CSNA) in Canada. These organizations consider issues of importance to nursing students and often cooperate in activities and programs with professional organizations.

Specialty Nursing Practice and Organizations. Some professional organizations focus on specific areas of nursing. Their goals are to improve the standards of practice, expand nursing roles, and foster the welfare of nurses within the specialty areas. The greatest expansion for nursing during the past 20 years has been generalist nurses working in clinical specialty areas. More than 40 professional organizations are currently unique to specialty nursing practice. Of these, more than 33 certify the registered nurse in the particular area of nursing specialty.

The American Nurses Association (ANA) is one of those professional organizations. The American Nursing Credentialing Center (ANCC), a part of ANA, has certified more than 70,000 registered nurses as generalists or specialists. Approximately 150,000 nurses now hold certification in specialized areas (ANA, 1993). Certification is a credential reflecting a nationally recognized level of competency. In some special areas of nursing such as a nurse anesthetist or a nurse-midwife, certification is the entry credential into nursing practice. Organizations that support specialty nursing practice in their area of expertise include the Association of Women's Health, Obstetric, and Neonatal Nurses (AWHONN), the Association of Operating Room Nurses (AORN), and the American Association of Critical-Care Nurses (AACN). Nurses obtaining the voluntary credentials of certification in their practice area represent a growing trend. The current movement toward requiring a baccalaureate degree for certification thus could affect many RNs in the future. In 1998 the ANA will require the baccalaureate degree for all certification programs.

HEALTH CARE ISSUES FOR THE 1990S

Throughout its history, nursing has responded to social, economic, and political change. The health care system in the United States today faces many problems: poor access, increased specialization, the demand for cost controls, a rising older adult population, and a public demand for quality. Because nurses make up the largest segment of health care professionals, they have an opportunity to find solutions to these problems through meaningful change.

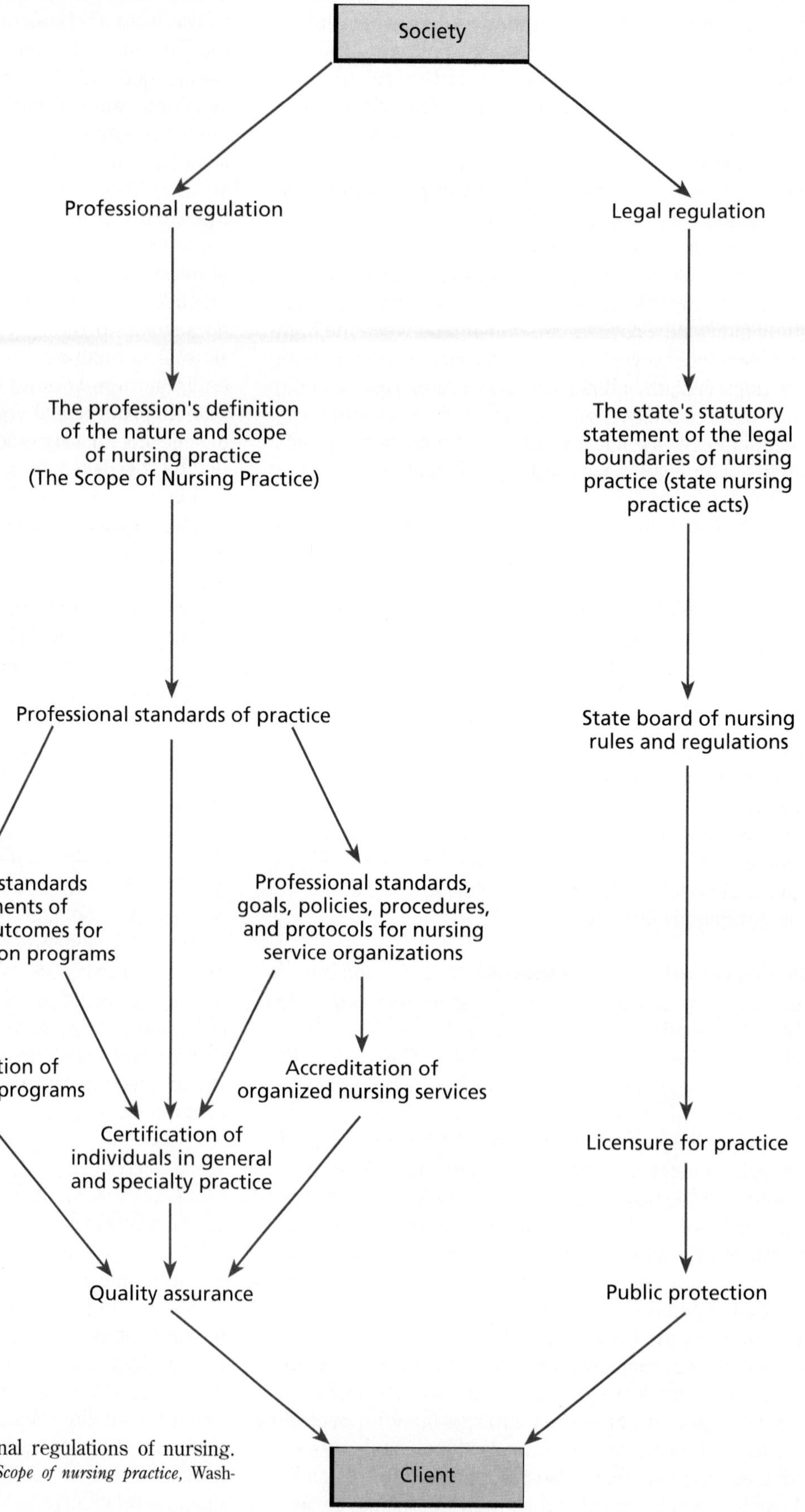

FIGURE 1-6 Legal and professional regulations of nursing. (From American Nursing Association, *Scope of nursing practice,* Washington, DC, 1987, The Association.)

Access

A significant portion of the population has limited access to the health care delivery system. Access is restricted by geographical, financial, and attitudinal barriers. A client may not have a primary care physician in his or her neighborhood. A person's employer may fail to provide health insurance to workers. Failure to value disease prevention often results in clients waiting too late to seek health care.

A true health care delivery system has accessible services that promote health, prevent and treat illness, and rehabilitate the client to a maximal level of functioning (Mitchell et al., 1993). Nursing is in a perfect position to provide such service. The traditional scope of nursing practice embraces a broader perspective of health care. More nurses are going into communities to provide affordable primary care services and to promote the health of the community and society at large.

Specialization

Advanced scientific knowledge and technology have increased specialization of health care in all areas. Although specialization allows each professional to give clients highly advanced care, the delivery of total care is often fragmented. Often, no one is in charge of a client's health. The number of primary physicians has declined. Many families have a different physician for each family member or illness. As a result care is not provided for the family as a unit or for the whole person.

Nursing has always supported a holistic model for health care. This involves providing care to the person, family, community, and society. The present health care system emphasizes curing rather than caring. Nursing can make a difference by becoming more involved in all levels of health care and providing services at a more cost-effective and qualitative level than other providers (Maraldo, 1989).

Cost Control

As health care costs rise because of an increased population, more people with chronic illness, increased cost of technology and specialization, and increased acuity of hospitalized clients, reimbursement for services declines. The challenge is to reduce costs without reducing quality. Physicians and nurses are being asked to use fewer resources such as diagnostic tests, equipment, and even medications. If these resources are reduced without understanding the outcome for clients, serious problems can arise.

Nurses have always been strong collaborators in the health care team. It is becoming increasingly important for nurses to use clinical decision making in the choice of resource use and in coordinating client care. For example, early referral to home health may be the way to reduce costs that would result from an unnecessary extended hospital stay. Selecting the proper support surface early for a client might prevent a pressure ulcer from developing. A pressure ulcer can escalate the costs for a client's care. Looking at the total client and understanding the implications of care are critical in reducing the costs of care.

Older Adult Population

Older adults comprise a significant portion of clients within the health care system. Chronic illnesses affect older adults more often than children or young adults. Because people live longer, the number of clients with chronic disease rises. Quality of life becomes an issue. Should therapies be used that prolong life, when it means prolonged disability as well?

The rapidly growing specialty of gerontologic nursing prepares nurses to design strategies aimed at helping older adults maintain functioning and independence. The collaboration of all health care disciplines is needed for improved care. More long-term care facilities designed to provide safe, functional, and stimulating environments for older adults are needed. This type of health care will support the chronically ill and disabled in an environment that is also less costly.

Quality

As public awareness about health care improves and as statistics for performance of health care systems become available, quality of care becomes a larger issue. Hospital mortality and morbidity rates are now available for public review and raise questions about the efficacy of certain therapies. To determine the quality of health care, a person must ask about the outcomes of care. Outcomes are the result of care delivered (Williams, 1991). The incidence of nosocomial infection is an example of an outcome. More important, outcomes must be looked at in a broader sense. It is not enough to know that a client leaves a hospital without obvious complications. The question must be asked: how quickly does the client return to a functional life-style?

Nursing is again in a good position to influence the quality of health care because of its holistic perspective. With the right health care system in place, clients can be followed from home to clinic to hospital to rehabilitation facility or to any other site, with continuity and an individualized approach to quality. Advanced nurse practitioners have shown the ability to manage clients across various settings and to achieve a higher level of wellness for clients.

NURSING RESPONSES TO SOCIAL CHANGES IN HEALTH CARE

One of the most significant documents to guide nursing responses to health care changes for the 1990s is *Nursing's Agenda for Health Care Reform* (see box below). This document was compiled from more than 50 nursing organizations and promotes primary health care as the focus of a restructured health care system. Successful achievement of this agenda will shift the focus of health care from illness and cure to wellness and care.

Nursing will have a role in the greater emphasis on health promotion and illness prevention. This trend is mirrored in the consumer movement. The agenda proposes that consumers would have access to nurses as cost-effective providers in community-based settings. Nursing's response to this concern ranges from programs in the community to specific health promotion and teaching activities for clients in hospitals and other health care settings.

SUMMARY

The nursing profession is poised to be a significant contributor to a reforming health care system in the United States. Just as the nursing profession has grown and changed to meet the demands of a complex society, it must continue to participate in current changes. The roles of nurses and the functions they perform are essential to providing optimal care for clients. Nursing as a profession has become a critical part of the health care delivery system. As a result of the rapid growth of the health care industry, patterns of use by clients have changed, and new emphases are emerging. The costs of health care are growing as rapidly as the health care system itself. Some projected changes include the following:

- Increased consumerism with emphasis on illness prevention and health promotion
- A shift to a community-based system of care with a variety of health care providers, including more nonphysician providers

NURSING'S AGENDA FOR HEALTH CARE REFORM

The basic components of nursing's "core of care" include:

- A restructured health care system that:
  - Enhances consumer access to services by delivering primary health care in community settings
  - Fosters consumer responsibility for personal health, self-care, and informed decision making in selecting health care services
  - Facilitates the use of the most cost-effective providers and therapeutic options
- A federally-defined standard package of essential health care services available to all citizens and residents of the United States, provided and financed through an integration of public and private plans and sources.
- A phase-in of essential services, so that the health care delivery system can be fiscally responsible in the:
  - Coverage of pregnant women and children, which is critical
  - Design of services that specifically assist vulnerable populations who have had limited access to the health care delivery system. (A "Healthstart Plan" is proposed to improve the health status of these individuals.)
- Planned change to anticipate health care service needs that correlate with changing national demographics
- Steps to reduce health care costs, including:
  - Required use of managed care in a public health plan and encouraged in private plans
  - Incentives for consumers and providers to use managed-care arrangements
  - Controlled growth of the health care delivery system through planning and prudent resource allocation
  - Incentives for consumers and providers to be more cost efficient in exercising health care options
  - Development of health care policies based on effectiveness and outcomes research
  - Ensurance of direct access to a full range of qualified providers
  - Elimination of unnecessary bureaucratic controls and administrative procedures
- Case management required for clients with continuing health care needs
- Provisions for long-term care, including:
  - Public and private funding for services of short duration to prevent personal impoverishment
  - Public funding for extended care
  - Emphasis on the consumers' responsibility to financially plan for long-term care needs
- Insurance reforms to ensure improved access to coverage
- Access to services ensured by no payment at the point of service and elimination of balance billing in public and private plans
- Establishment of public or private-sector review—operating under federal guidelines and including payers, providers, and consumers—to determine resource allocation, cost reduction approaches, allowable insurance premiums, and fair and consistent reimbursement levels (This review would progress in a climate sensitive to ethical issues.)

Modified from ANA: *Nursing's agenda for health care reform,* Washington DC, 1991, The Association.

- Changing technology and demographics will change worker's role and increased cultural diversity
- The connection between costs and outcomes will become a major accountability feature in all health care delivery settings, (AONE, 1993).

Dr. Pam Maraldo summarizes the essence of these trends: "The next century will see the nursing model of care integrated more fruitfully into priorities and policies of the health care . . . just as the last century brought clash between autonomy and obedience, the next century will bring unity of nursing leadership and professionalism into every facet of the health care delivery system" (Maraldo, 1992).

KEY CONCEPTS

Nursing responds to the health needs of society, which are influenced by economic, social, and cultural variables.

Nursing philosophies and theories reflect changes in the practice of nursing and help to bring about changes by identifying the domain of nursing practice and guiding research, practice, and education.

A license for a registered nurse is granted after a candidate has completed an accredited program and passed a national licensing examination (NCLEX-RN).

Graduate nursing programs prepare nurse clinicians, educators, researchers, and administrators to improve nursing care through the advancement of nursing theory and sciences.

Continuing education programs help the nurse to remain current in skills, knowledge, and theory.

Nursing standards provide the guidelines for implementing and evaluating care.

The roles and functions of the nurse include care giver, decision maker, client advocate, manager, rehabilitator, comforter, communicator, and teacher.

Employment positions include staff nurse, educator, clinical nurse specialist, nurse practitioner, certified nurse-midwife, nurse anesthetist, administrator, and researcher.

The health care team is multidisciplinary and may include a physician, physician assistant, physical therapist, occupational therapist, respiratory therapist, pharmacist, social worker, and chaplain, as well as the nurse.

Nursing as a profession has educational preparation, nursing theory, a service provided, autonomy, and a code of ethics.

Consumers are requesting more information, especially on services related to illness prevention, health promotion, and health care costs.

Health care services are provided to all-age groups, and for the chronically and acutely ill people in hospital- and community-based settings.

Specialization of nursing practice is a national trend at both the generalist and specialist levels.

CRITICAL THINKING ACTIVITIES

1. Summarize in your own words the nursing theorist(s) that your nursing program uses in the curriculum. Think of an example of how that theory influences your selection of nursing interventions for a client.
2. Having summarized the nursing theorist, discuss two or three points that help you think about it (the theory) having a nursing focus instead of a medical focus.
3. The year is 2000 and you are helping a friend plan for his/her nursing education because he/she wants to be a nurse practitioner and help people with cancer. What educational path would you suggest for that goal and how is that role different from a generalist RN?
4. Why is it important for a profession such as nursing to be regulated? Discuss at least three methods of professional regulation that you understand from reading this chapter.
5. You are a new nurse working in an acute medical-surgical health care setting. Describe some of the health care colleagues that you would encounter in your daily care management for your clients. How critical is your role as "communicator" when working with so many health care colleagues?
6. With the decreasing length of hospital stays for people needing acute care, what are the kinds of things that you could do as a new RN to keep up with these changes and maintain your quality of care but also stay sensitive to the needs of clients who come through your hospital setting so quickly?

References

Abdellah FG et al.: *Patient-centered approaches to nursing,* New York, 1960, Macmillan.

Aiken L and Millinix C: The nursing shortage: myth or reality, *N Engl J Med* 317:641, 1987.

American Nurses Association Committee on Education: *A position paper,* New York, 1965, The Association.

American Nurses Association: *Statement on graduate education in nursing,* New York, 1969, The Association.

American Nurses Association: *Standards for continuing education in nursing,* Kansas City, 1975, The Association.

American Nurses Association: *Nursing and social policy statement,* Kansas City, 1980, The Association.

American Nursing Credentialing Center Catalog, American Nurses Association, Washington, DC, 1993.

American Organization of Nurse Executives: A call for reform of our nursing educational system, *Nurs Management* 21(1):33, 1993.

Belknap R: Care: a significant paradigm shift and focus in nursing for the future, *NLN* publication 1993(14-2510).

Bernd DL: Patient focused care pays hospital wide dividends, *Health Care Strategic Management* 10(12):9, 1992.

Bullough B: Alternative models for special nursing practice, *Nursing and Health Care* 13(5), 1992.

Canadian Nurses Association: *Definition of nursing standards and practice,* Ottawa, 1980, The Association.

Chinn PL and Jacobs MK: Theory and nursing: a systematic approach, ed 3, St. Louis, 1991, Mosby.

Cohen IB: Florence Nightingale, *Sci Am* 250(128):137, 1984.

Cohen L: Power and change in health care: A challenge for nursing, *J Nurs Ed,* vol 31(3), 1992.

Donahue MP: *Nursing: the finest art, an illustrated history,* St. Louis, 1985, Mosby.

Etzioni A: *The semi-professionals and their organizations,* New York, 1961, Free Press.

Gioiella E: Professionalizing nursing: a Rogers legacy, *Nurs Sci Quarterly* 2(2):61, 1989.

Harkness G, Miller J, and Hill N: Differentiated practice: a three dimensional model, *Nursing Management* 23(12): 1992.

Hayne Y: The current status and future significance of nursing as a discipline, *J Adv Nurs* 17:7, 1992.

Henderson V: The nature of nursing, *Am J Nurs* 64:62, 1964a.

Henderson V: *The nature of nursing,* New York, 1964b, Macmillan.

Johnson D: Theory in nursing: borrowed and unique, *Nurs Res* 11:206, 1968.

Kelly LY: *Dimensions of professional nursing,* New York, 1981, Macmillan.

King IM: *A theory for nursing: systems, concepts, process,* New York, 1981, John Wiley & Sons.

King IM: *Toward a theory for nursing,* New York, 1971, John Wiley & Sons.

Koerner JE: Differentiated practice evolution of professional nursing, *J Prof Nurs* 8(6):335, 1992.

Leininger M: *Transcultural nursing: concepts, theories, and practices,* New York, 1978, Wiley.

Leininger M: *Care the essence of nursing and health,* Throughfare, NJ, 1984. Slack.

Levine MC: *An introduction to clinical nursing,* ed 2, Philadelphia, 1973, FA Davis.

Lysaught J: *An abstract for action,* New York, 1970, McGraw-Hill.

Maraldo PJ: The nursing solution, *Health Manage Q* 11(4):18, 1989.

Maraldo P: NLN's first century, *Nursing and Health Care* 13(5):228, 1992.

Marriner-Tomey A: *Nursing theorists and their work,* ed 3, St. Louis, 1994, Mosby.

Mechanic H: Expanded roles, *Nurs Outlook* 36(6):280, 1988.

Meleis AI: *Theoretical nursing: development and progress,* ed 2, Philadelphia, 1991, JB Lippincott.

Minarik P: Second licensure for advanced nursing practice, *Clin Nurs Specialist* 6(4):221, 1992.

Mitchell P and Grippando G: *Nursing perspectives and issues,* Albany, NY, 1993, Delmar.

National League For Nursing: *Nursing data review 1989,* New York, 1990, National League for Nursing.

Neuman BM: *The Neuman systems model: application to nursing education and practice,* New York, 1982, Appleton-Century-Crofts.

Neuman BM and Young RJ: A model for teaching total person approach to patients' problems, *Nurs Res* 21:264, 1972.

Nightingale F: *Notes on nursing: what it is and what it is not,* London, 1860, Harrison & Sons.

Orem DE: *Nursing: concepts of practice,* New York, 1971, McGraw-Hill.

Orlando IJ: *The dynamic nurse-patient relationship, function, process, and principles,* New York, 1961, Putnam.

Peplau HE: *Interpersonal relations in nursing,* New York, 1952, Putnam.

Philipose V, Tate J, and Jacobs S: Evolution of gerontological education in nursing, *Nursing and Health Care* 12(10):528, 1992.

Rogers ME: *An introduction to the theoretical basis of nursing,* Philadelphia, 1970, FA Davis.

Roy C: *An introduction to nursing: an adaptation model,* Englewood Cliffs, NJ, 1976, Prentice-Hall.

Sharp N: Nurses: call to action, *Nurs Manag* 24(7):25, 1993.

Schutzenhofer K: Nursing education and professional autonomy, *Reflections* 18(4), 1992.

Styles M: *Toward new empowerment,* St. Louis, 1982, Mosby.

Torres G: *Theoretical foundations of nursing,* Norwalk, Conn, 1986, Appleton-Century-Crofts.

U.S. Dept. of Health and Human Services: *The registered nurse populations: findings from a national sample of RNs,* 1988, March 1990, U.S. Government Printing Office.

Watson J: *Nursing: the philosophy and science of caring,* Boston, 1979, Little, Brown, & Co.

Williams AD: Development and application of clinical indicators for nursing, *J Nurs Care Qual,* 6(1):1, 1991.

Woodham-Smith C: *Florence Nightingale,* New York, 1983, McGraw-Hill.

Zander K: Why managed care "works," *Definitions* 3(4):1, 1988.

Bibliography

Brink H: Teaching caring in nursing: a needs assessment, *Curationis* 13(1-2):38-43, 1990.

Bevis E: A symphony of caring: shared visions and eloquent futures for nursing education and practice, *NLN Publication* Jan (14-2510) 81-97, 1993.

Booth, RA: Working for patients with further implications for nursing education, *Nurs Educ Today* 12(4):243-251, 1992.

Bowles K: Health care trends: a call for advanced knowledge in baccalaureate graduates, *Focus on Critical Care* 18(6):465-468, 1991.

Jones DL: Education and training—the case for professional bodies and who should have control? *Nursing Times* 86(4):40, 1990.

Mann RE: Preserving humanity in an age of technology, *Intensive Crit Care Nurs* 8(1)54-59, 1992.

Melies AI: Directions for nursing theory development in the 21st century, *Nurs Sci Quart* 5(3):112-117, 1992.

Orem D: *Nursing: concepts of practice,* ed 4, St. Louis, 1991, Mosby.

Salvage J: The theory and practice of the new nursing, *Nursing Times* 86(4):42-45, 1990.

2 Nursing in Health and Illness

OBJECTIVES

Mastery of concepts in this chapter will enable the student to:

- Define the key terms listed.
- Discuss health definitions, models, and concepts.
- Describe health promotion and illness prevention activities.
- Discuss the three levels of preventive care.
- Describe variables influencing health beliefs and practices.
- Describe variables influencing illness behavior.
- Discuss the stages of illness behavior.
- Describe the impact of illness on the client and family.
- Discuss the nurse's role for the client in health and illness.

KEY TERMS

active strategies of health promotion
acute illness
agent
agent-host-environmental model
chronic illness
health
health behaviors
health belief model
health promotion
health-illness continuum
high-level wellness model
host
illness
illness behavior
illness prevention
passive strategies of health promotion
primary prevention
risk factor
secondary prevention
tertiary prevention
wellness

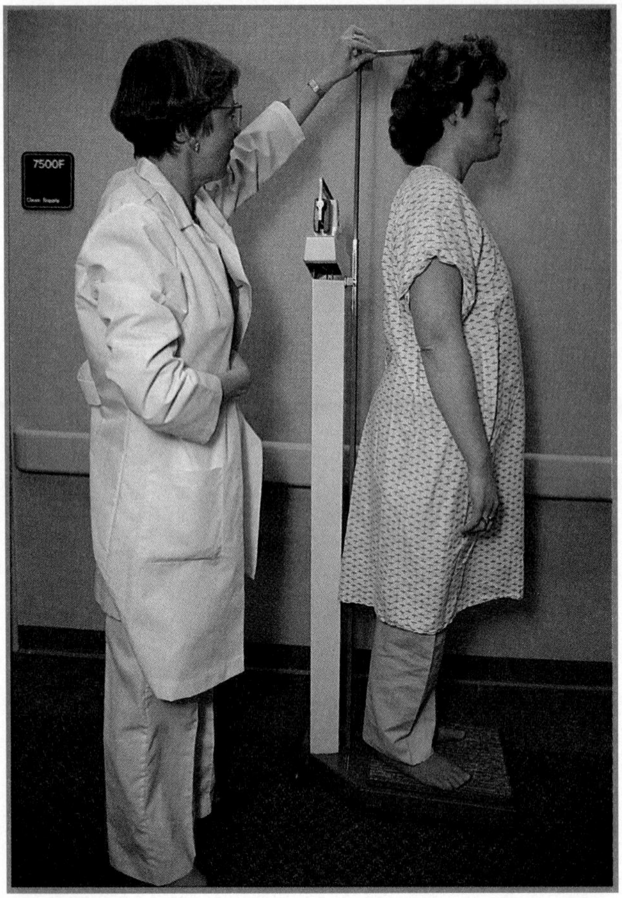

In the past, most people have viewed good health or wellness as the opposite or absence of disease. However, this simple attitude ignores states of health between disease and good health. It also overlooks the complex interrelationships among all human dimensions. Today's health and medical care services are shaped largely by the way health professionals and consumers define *health* and *illness* (Weitzel, 1989; Balog, 1982).

Health care professionals' definitions determine the types and quality of health care services to be provided. Not all health care professionals, however, agree on the definitions. These definitions also may not always correspond with clients' definitions, which are based on life-style, cultural background, spiritual beliefs, and economic and psychosocial status.

People also have different attitudes about illness and react in different ways to illness. Medical sociologists call the reaction to illness, *illness behavior.* The nurse who understands how clients react to illness can minimize the effects of illness and assist the client and family to maintain or return to the highest level of functioning. The nurse also identifies actual and potential risk factors that predispose a person or a group to illness. Nursing actions involving health promotion and illness prevention assist the client to achieve and maintain an optimal level of health. The nurse assesses the whole person in all dimensions and observes all interactions with family and community (Edelman, Mandle, 1990).

DEFINITION OF HEALTH

Health or wellness is not merely the absence of **illness** or disease. Defining health is difficult. Health is a state of being people define in relation to their own values.

No current definition of health is acceptable to all health care workers. The World Health Organization (WHO) defines health as a "state of complete physical, mental and social well-being, not merely the absence of disease or infirmity" (WHO, 1947). Yet this definition of health has not been totally accepted. Those opposed to it believe it is unrealistic because people who are poor or who live in underdeveloped countries would not be considered healthy (Fuchs, 1974). And it is difficult to scientifically determine who is or is not healthy (Breslow, 1972).

The WHO definition, however, has the following characteristics that promote a more holistic concept of health (Edelman, Mandle, 1990):

1. A concern for the individual as a total system
2. A view of health that identifies internal and external environments
3. An acknowledgment of the importance of an individual's role in life

Each client's attitude toward health involves much more than the absence of illness or disability. To help clients identify and reach health goals, the nurse must discover and use information about their concepts of health to set individual health goals.

Health is a dynamic state in which the individual adapts to changes in internal and external environments to maintain a state of well-being. Because both environments continuously change, the person must adapt to maintain this state.

Health and *illness* therefore must be defined in terms of the individual. Health can include conditions previously considered to be illness. For example, a person with epilepsy who has learned to control seizures with medication and who functions at home and at work may now not consider himself ill. Health is also closely related to life-style, and some illnesses can be considered to be the result of that life-style. A health professional's rigid attitude toward health and illness, in which the whole person is not considered, may have little meaning for a client's future health. Therefore, because the client's and nurse's definition of health may not coincide, the nurse works with the client and family to establish individualized nursing care.

MODELS OF HEALTH AND ILLNESS

A *model* is a theoretical way of understanding a concept or idea. Because health and illness are complex concepts, models are used to understand the relationships between these concepts and the client's attitudes toward health and health practices.

Health beliefs are a person's ideas, convictions, and attitudes about health and illness. They may be based on factual information or misinformation, common sense or myths, or reality or false expectations. Because **health behaviors** usually result from health beliefs, they can positively or negatively affect health. Positive health behaviors are activities related to maintaining, attaining, or regaining good health and preventing illness, such as proper sleep patterns, and adequate exercise, diet, and nutrition. Negative health behaviors include practices actually or potentially harmful to health, such as smoking, drug or alcohol abuse, poor diet, and refusal to take necessary medications.

Nurses have developed the following health models to understand clients' health behaviors and beliefs so they can provide effective health care. These models include the health-illness continuum, the high-level wellness, the agent-host-environment, the evolutionary-based, and health-promotion models.

Health-Illness Continuum Model

According to a **health-illness continuum model,** health is a dynamic state that fluctuates as a person adapts to changes in the internal and external environments to maintain a state of total well-being. Because health and illness are relative qualities, existing in varying degrees, it is more accurate to consider health and illness in terms of a scale or continuum rather than as absolute states, as shown in the example in Figure 2-1.

The literature supports the view that health and its attainment is a crucial goal of nursing practice (Meleis, 1990; Pender, 1975, 1986, 1987, 1990; Parse, 1981, 1990; Neuman, 1989, 1990). High-level wellness and severe illness are at opposite ends of the continuum. According to Neuman (1990), "health on a continuum is the degree of client wellness that exists at any point in time, ranging from an optimal wellness condition, with available energy at its maximum, to death, which represents total energy depletion." A nurse can determine a client's level of health at any point on the health-illness continuum. A client's risk factors are important in identifying level of health. Risk factors include genetic and physiological variables such as age, life-style, and environment. As a person progresses through the developmental stages, certain risk factors are more common than others. An adolescent, for example, is more likely than an adult to experience stressors related to body image and self-concept, and an older adult is more likely than a child to develop cardiac illness.

The way clients view their levels of health depends on their attitudes toward health, values, beliefs, and perceptions of their well-being. The nurse helps clients identify their positions on the health-illness continuum to set goals for optimal health (Meleis, 1990).

It is not always easy to describe a client's level of health in terms of one point between two extremes. For example, is a man with a broken leg who has adapted to limited mobility more or less healthy than a physically

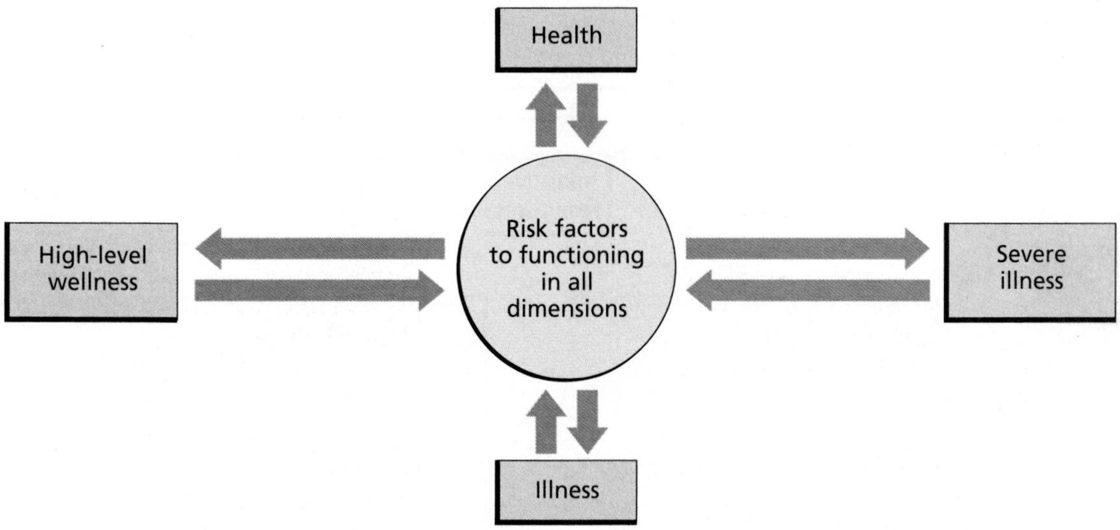

FIGURE 2-1 The health-illness continuum, ranging from high-level wellness to severe illness, provides a method of identifying a client's level of health. Level of health is a reflection of the client's level of functioning in all dimensions.

healthy man experiencing severe depression after the death of his spouse? Health-illness continuums are most effective when used to compare a client's present level of health with previous levels of health.

High-Level Wellness Model

The **high-level wellness model** developed by Dunn (1977) focuses on maximizing the health potential of an individual, family, or community. It requires the individual to maintain a continuum of balance and purposeful direction within the environment. It involves progress toward a higher level of functioning, an open-ended and ever-expanding challenge to live at the fullest potential and an integration of health practices by the individual at increasingly higher levels throughout life (Dunn, 1959, 1977; Pender, 1987).

Nursing models of wellness are directed at behavioral change and have been successful in nurse-managed centers for older adults (Gilpatrick, 1989; Smith, Sorrell, 1989). In the behavioral change approach to wellness, nurses implement nursing interventions that help clients modify selected high-risk behaviors (Gilpatrick, 1989).

Health care directed at helping a client achieve high-level wellness emphasizes health promotion and illness prevention rather than treatment. High-level wellness is a dynamic process, not a passive, static state.

Agent-Host-Environment Model

The **agent-host-environment model** began in the community health work of Leavell et al. (1965) and has been expanded as a model to describe the cause of illness in other health areas. It states that the level of health or illness of an individual or group depends on the dynamic relationship of the agent, any internal or external factor that can lead to illness, the group who may be susceptible to the illness, and the environmental factors that may increase risk of the illness. **Agents** can be

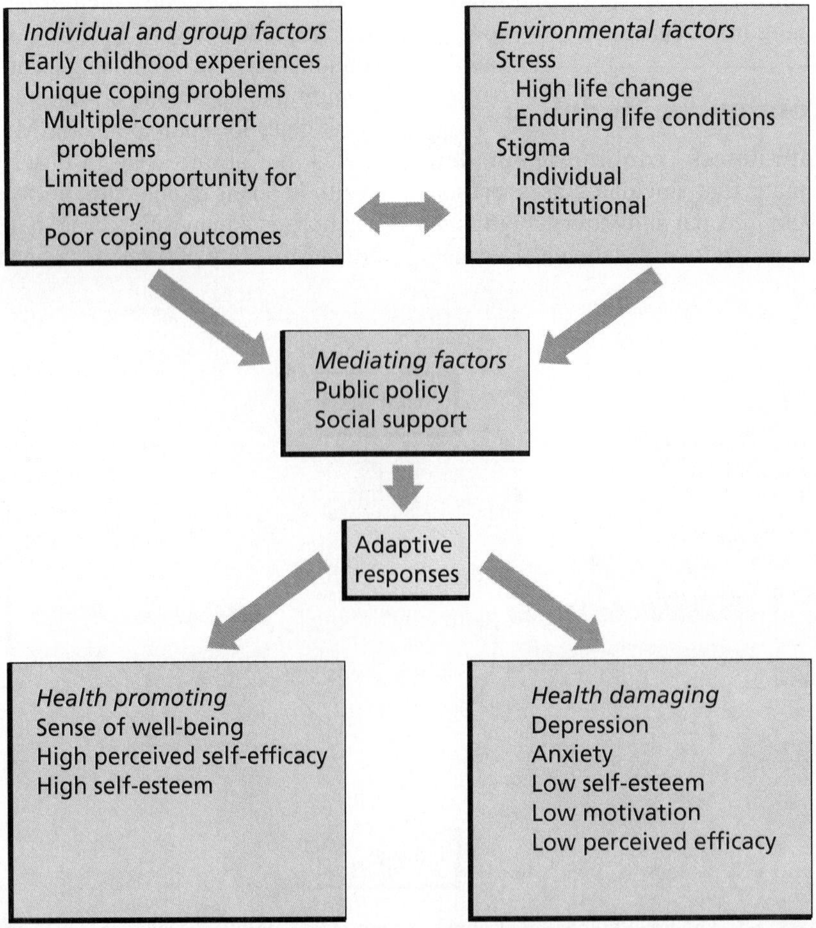

FIGURE 2-2 Adaptational model of poverty. (Modified from Pesznecker BL: *Public Health Nurs* 1[4]:237, 1984.)

biological, chemical, physical, or psychosocial. **Host** factors are physical or psychosocial situations or conditions putting people at risk for illness. **Environment** includes external factors that make illness more or less likely.

Community health nursing has further developed the interactions among agent-host-environment into a model for addressing the health needs for homeless families (Figure 2-2). The agent-host-environment model emphasizes that health and illness depend on the dynamic interaction of all three variables. This model, first developed by Pesznecker (1984) and recently reported by Berne et al. (1990), proposes that health-promoting or health-damaging responses are shaped by interaction between the individual or group and the environment. Public policy also has an effect.

The agent-host-environment model has been expanded into a general theory of the causes of disease. Health care workers now recognize that most diseases have multiple causes, as this model demonstrates. This is important to nurses because nursing emphasizes holistic care of the client, based on knowing about the effects of environmental, psychosocial, and life-style factors.

Health Belief Model

Rosenstoch's (1974) and Becker and Maiman's (1975) **health belief model** (Figure 2-3) addresses the relationship between a person's belief and behaviors. It is a way of understanding and predicting how clients will behave in relation to their health and how they will comply with health care therapies. Use of the model is based on a person's perception of the susceptibility to an illness, the seriousness of the illness, and the benefits of taking action to prevent the illness.

This model helps nurses to understand factors influencing clients' perceptions, beliefs, and behavior and to plan the most effective care. A study by Prewitt (1989) identified relationships between health beliefs and preventive health behaviors and educational materials dealing with acquired immunodeficiency syndrome (AIDS). This study focused on high-risk behaviors and the susceptibility of the illness. Researchers used educational

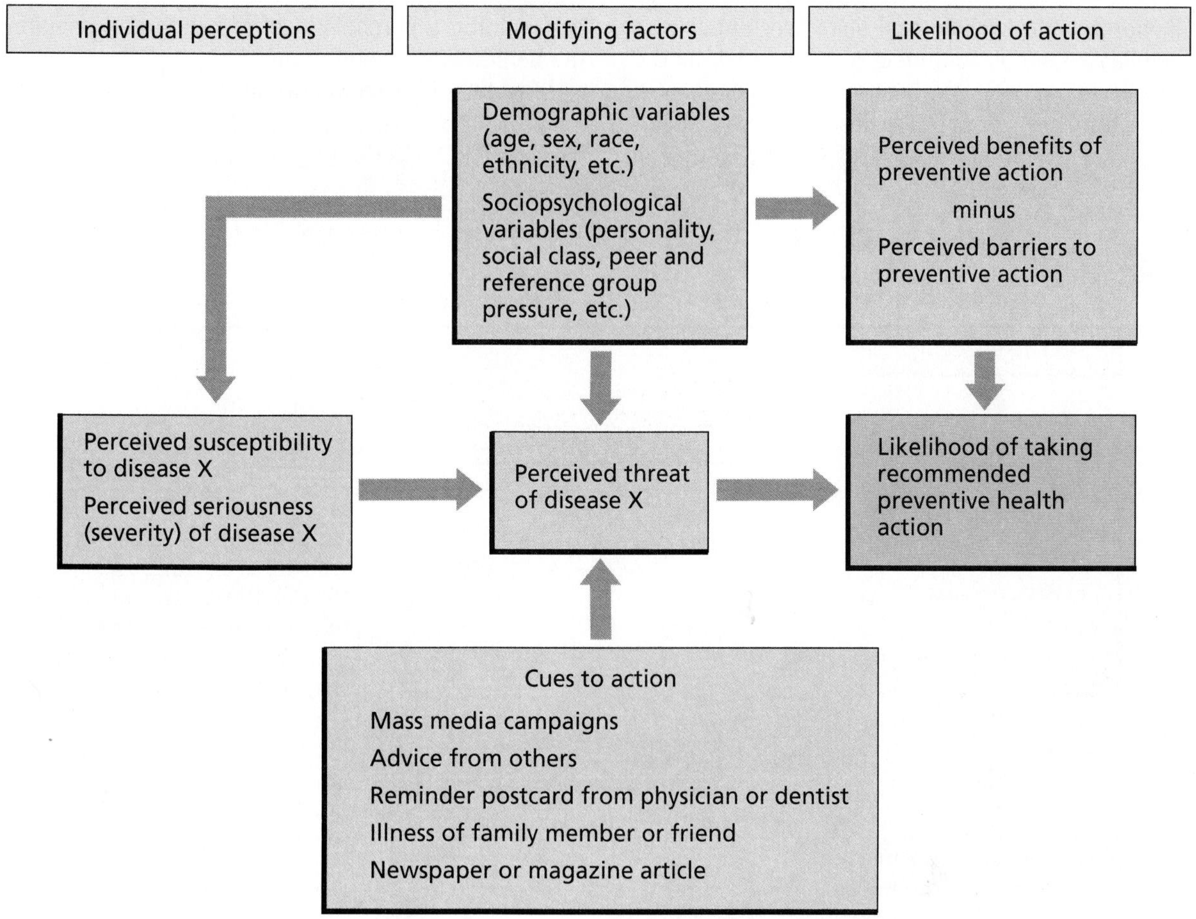

FIGURE 2-3 Health belief model. (Modified from Becker MH, Maiman LA: *Med Care* 13[1]:12, 1975.)

pamphlets to reinforce preventive health behaviors. Results of the study identified that subjects who perceived a threat to their health developed more preventive behaviors.

Evolutionary-Based Model

The **evolutionary-based model** suggests that illness and death sometimes have an evolutionary function (Dixon, Dixon, 1984). The model (Figure 2-4) interrelates the following elements:

1. Life events, which reflect developmental variables and chance variables associated, such as accidents or relocation
2. Life-style determinants, which are personal and learned strategies a person uses to make life-style changes
3. Evolutionary viability, which reflects the extent to which people function to promote survival and well-being (Dixon, Dixon, 1984)
4. Control perceptions, which reflect the extent to which a person can influence life circumstances
5. Viability emotions, which are "affective reactions" developed from life events or life-style determinants
6. Health outcomes, which are the physiological, behavioral, and psychological states resulting from viability emotions and the other factors within the model

With this model, nurses can design holistic health promotion interventions for each of the six elements. This is important because of the potential long-term relationship with the client and family.

Health Promotion Model

Pender's (1982, 1984) **health promotion model** is to be a "complementary counterpart to models of health protection." Health promotion seeks to increase a client's level of well-being (Pender, 1987). The model focuses on the client's cognitive-perceptual factors, modifying factors, and participation in health-promoting behaviors (Figure 2-5). It identifies factors that enhance or decrease health promotion activities. It also organizes cues into a pattern to explain the likelihood of a client's developing health promotion behaviors (Pender, 1990). The model has been tested with many populations and is a reliable indicator of health promotion (Weitzel, 1989; Pender, Walker, et al., 1990).

Basic Human Needs

Basic human needs are elements necessary for human survival and health (e.g., food, water, safety, and love). Although each person has other unique needs, the basic human needs are shared by all people, and the extent to which health needs are met is a major factor in determining a person's level of health and position on the health-illness continuum.

Maslow's **hierarchy of human needs** is a model nurses can use to understand the interrelationships of basic human needs (Figure 2-6). According to this

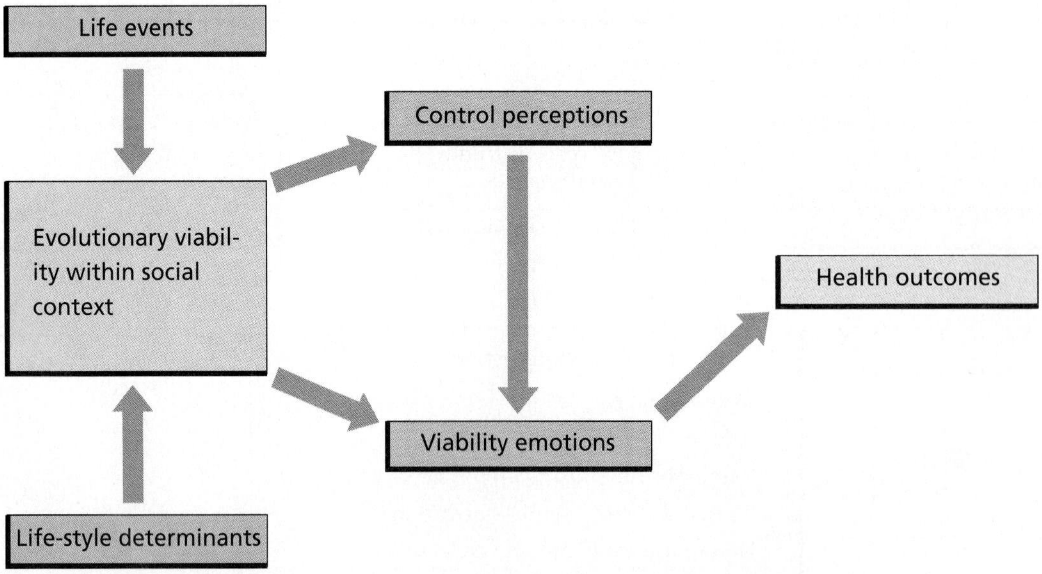

FIGURE 2-4 Evolutionary-based model of viability and health. (Redrawn from Dixon JK, Dixon JP: *ANS* 6[3]:1, 1984.)

model, certain human needs are more basic than others; that is, some needs must be met before other needs (e.g., fulfilling the physiological needs before the needs of love and belonging). The major goal is to restore the client as much as possible to a self-actualized state.

This model can provide a basis for nursing clients of all ages in all health settings. However, when the model is applied, the focus of care is on the client's needs rather than strict adherence to the hierarchy. In all cases, an emergent physiological need takes precedence over a higher-level need. In some situations it is unrealistic to expect a client's basic needs to occur in the fixed hierarchical order. To provide the most effective care, the nurse needs to understand the relationships of different needs and the factors that determine the priorities for the client.

VARIABLES INFLUENCING HEALTH BELIEFS AND PRACTICES

Nurses need to understand the variables influencing clients' health beliefs and practices. Internal and external variables can influence thoughts and actions. Understanding the effects of these variables allows the nurse to plan and deliver individualized care (Pender, 1990; Palank, 1991).

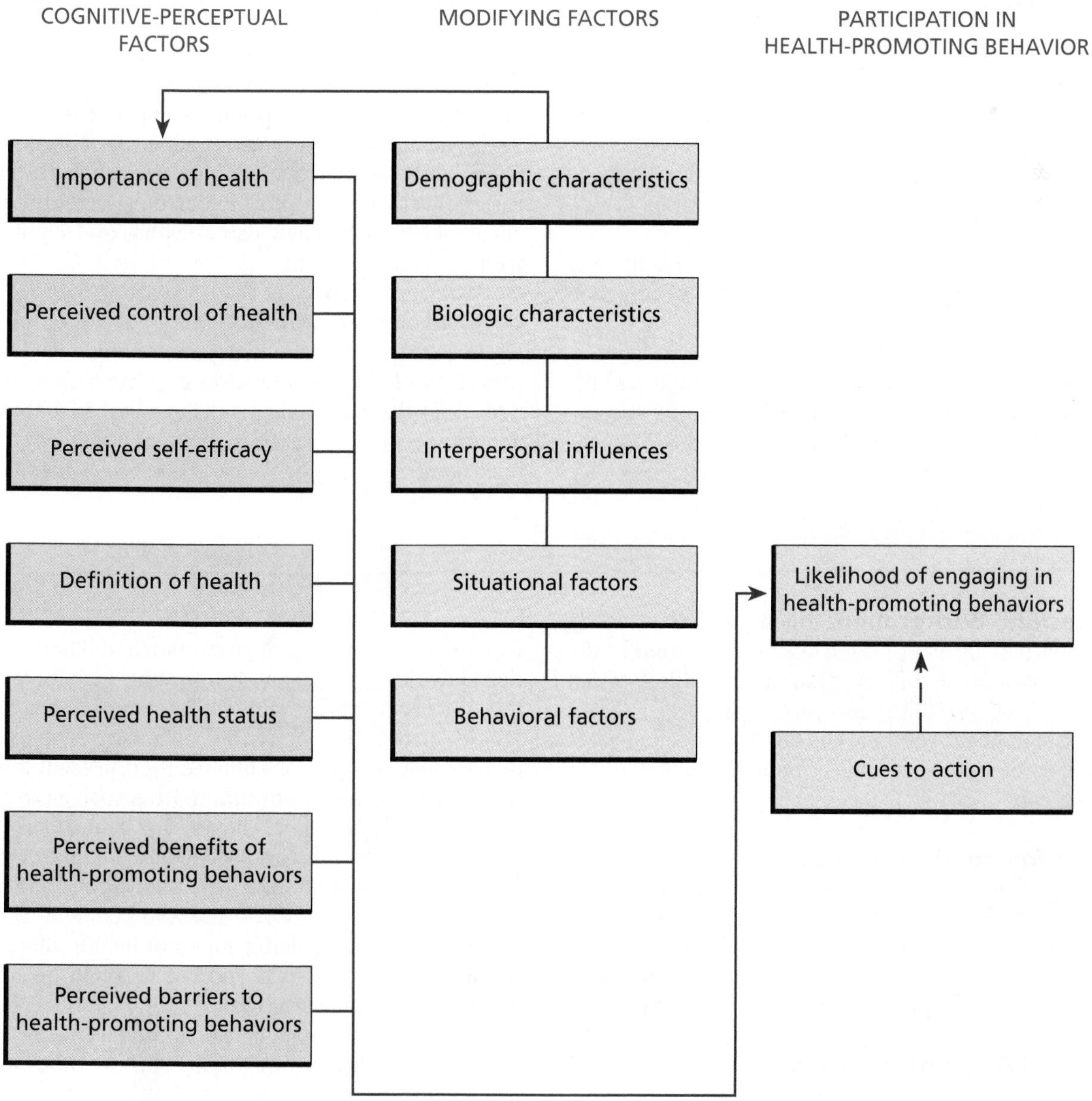

FIGURE 2-5 Health promotion model. (From Pender NJ: *Health promotion in nursing practice,* ed 2, Norwalk, Conn., 1987, Appleton & Lange.)

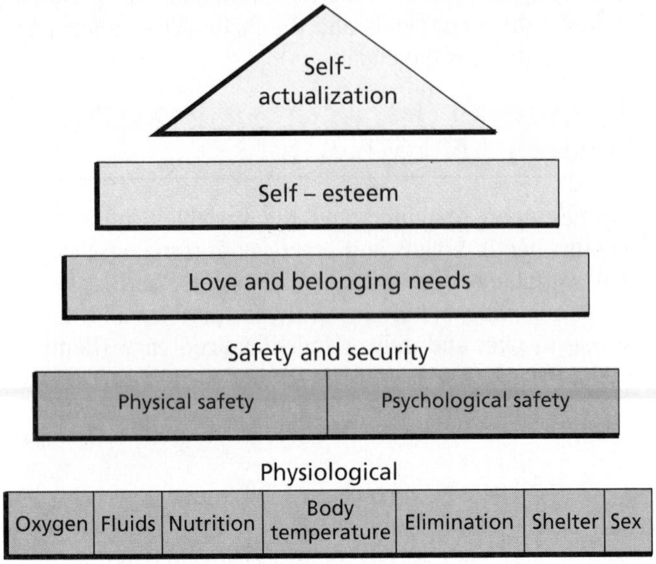

FIGURE 2-6 Maslow's hierarchy of needs.

Internal Variables

Internal variables include a person's developmental stage, intellectual background, perception of functioning, and emotional and spiritual factors.

Developmental Stage. A person's thought and behavior patterns change throughout life. The nurse must consider the client's level of growth and development when using his/her health beliefs and practices as a basis for planning care. The nurse can then predict the client's response to a present illness or the threat of future illness.

Intellectual Background. Knowledge about body functions and illnesses, educational background, and past experiences all influence how a client thinks about health. These variables also shape the *way* a client thinks about health. A nurse considers intellectual background so that these variables can be incorporated into nursing care.

Perception of Functioning. The way people perceive their physical functioning affects health beliefs and practices. When nurses assess a client's level of health, they gather subjective data about the way the client perceives physical functioning (such as level of fatigue) and they obtain objective data about actual functioning (such as blood pressure) to successfully plan and implement individualized care.

Emotional and Spiritual Factors. The client's degree of calm or stress can influence health beliefs and practices. Spiritual beliefs also influence whether and how a client seeks or avoids health behaviors. As with emotional variables, a nurse must understand clients' spiritual values to involve them effectively in nursing care (see Chapter 17).

External Variables

External variables influencing a person's health beliefs and practices include family practices, socioeconomic factors, and cultural background.

Family Practices. The way that clients' families use health care services generally affects their health practices. Their perceptions of the seriousness of diseases and their history of preventive care behaviors (or lack of them) can influence how clients will think about health.

Socioeconomic Factors. Social networks, social relationships, economic level, and psychosocial factors influence the way a client defines and reacts to illness. They can also put the client at risk for specific diseases. Social and economic factors also affect how the health care delivery system provides medical care, the way a client enters the health care system, and compliance with medical treatment.

Cultural Background. Cultural background influences beliefs, values, and customs. It influences the approach to the health care system, personal health practices, and the nurse-client relationship. As with family and socioeconomic variables, cultural variables must be incorporated into a client's care plan (see Chapter 18).

HEALTH PROMOTION AND ILLNESS PREVENTION

Nurses emphasize health promotion and illness prevention activities as important forms of health care because these assist clients in maintaining and improving health. **Health promotion activities** such as routine exercise help clients maintain or enhance their present levels of health. **Illness prevention activities** such as an immunization program protect clients from actual or potential threats to health. Both are focused on the future; the difference between them involves motivations and goals. Health promotion activities motivate people to act positively to reach more stable levels of health. Illness prevention activities motivate people to avoid declines in health or functional levels.

Health-promotion activities can be passive or active. With **passive strategies of health promotion,** individuals gain from the activities of others without acting themselves. The fluoridation of municipal drinking water and the fortification of homogenized milk with vitamin D are examples of passive health promotion strategies.

With **active strategies of health promotion** such as routine exercise and low-fat diets, individuals are motivated to change their risk factors and adopt healthier behaviors (Pender, 1990). Health care has become increasingly focused on health promotion and illness prevention. The rapid rise of health care costs has motivated people to seek ways of decreasing the incidence and minimizing the results of illness or disability.

Pender (1987) has developed the Lifestyle and Health Habits Assessment (LHHA), which may increase clients' awareness of life-style patterns and through nursing interventions assist them in changing behaviors (Pender, 1987; Pender, 1990; Pender, Walker, et al., 1990).

The goal of a total health program is to improve a client's level of well-being in all dimensions. Total health programs are based on the belief that many factors can affect level of health, including individual behaviors, physical and psychological stressors, and environmental factors (Palank, 1991). Total health programs are directed at changing life-style by developing habits that can improve level of health. The following factors affect a client's health status (Edelman, Mandle, 1990):

1. Smoking
2. Nutrition
3. Alcohol use
4. Habituating drug use
5. Driving
6. Exercise
7. Sexuality and contraceptive or barrier use
8. Family relationships
9. Risk-factor modification
10. Coping and adaptation

Some programs such as smoking cessation clinics, exercise programs, and stress-reduction programs seek to help clients make life-style changes to improve their health. Such programs are available to clients in all settings and across all developmental levels. Ruffing-Rahal (1991) identified how changes in exercise and dietary habits improved older adults' level of well-being and their independence in self-care activities. Another author underscores how health/education partnerships in school-based health centers are key in influencing health promoting behaviors (e.g., exercise, good nutrition, and reducing health risk behaviors as opposed to substance abuse or unsafe sexual practices) (Lear, 1992).

Some health promotion and illness prevention programs are operated by health care agencies; others are independently operated. Many corporations, colleges, and community centers offer health promotion and illness prevention programs. Nurses may be actively involved in these programs or may be consultants or give referrals. The goal of these activities is to improve the client's level of health through preventive health services, environmental protection, and health education.

Health promotion and illness prevention activities are important to the consumer and the health care provider. Whether an activity uses the active or passive strategy, the goal is to maintain or improve the level of well-being in all dimensions. Nurses in all areas of practice often have opportunities to assist clients in adopting activities to promote health and decrease risks of illness.

Levels of Preventive Care

Nursing care oriented to health promotion and illness prevention can be understood in terms of health activities on the primary, secondary, and tertiary levels (Table 2-1).

Primary Prevention. **Primary prevention** is true prevention. It is applied to clients who are considered physically and emotionally healthy. It is not therapeutic, does not use therapeutic treatments, and does not involve identifying symptoms (Edelman, Mandle, 1990). Primary prevention includes health education programs, immunization, and physical and nutritional fitness activities. It can be provided to an individual or to a general population.

Secondary Prevention. **Secondary prevention** focuses on individuals with health problems or illnesses and who are at risk for developing complications or worsening conditions. Activities are directed at diagnosis and prompt intervention, to enable the client to return to a maximal level of health as early as possible (Pender, 1987; Edelman, Mandle, 1990). Most secondary level nursing care is delivered in homes, hospitals, or skilled nursing facilities. It includes screening techniques and treating early stages of disease.

Tertiary Prevention. **Tertiary prevention** involves minimizing the effects of long-term disease or disability. Interventions are directed at preventing complications and enhancing rehabilitation (Edelman, Mandle, 1990; Pender, 1987). Care at this level aims to help clients achieve as high a level of functioning as possible. It is called *preventive care* because it involves preventing further disability or reduced functioning.

Acute and Chronic Illness

Acute and chronic illness are two general classifications of illness used in this chapter.

Acute Illness. An **acute illness** is usually short term and severe. The symptoms appear abruptly, are intense, and often subside after a relatively short period. An acute illness may result in a state of recovery compara-

table 2-1
THE THREE LEVELS OF PREVENTION

Primary prevention		Secondary prevention		Tertiary prevention
Health promotion	**Specific protection**	**Early diagnosis and prompt treatment**	**Disability limitations**	**Restoration and rehabilitation**
Health education Good standard of nutrition adjusted to developmental phases of life Attention to personality development Provision of adequate housing and recreation and agreeable working conditions Marriage counseling and sex education Genetic screening Periodic selective examinations	Use of specific immunizations Attention to personal hygiene Use of environmental sanitation Protection against occupational hazards Protection from accidents Use of specific nutrients Protection from carcinogens Avoidance of allergens	Case-finding measures: individual and mass Screening surveys Selective examinations Cure and prevention of disease process to prevent spread of communicable disease, prevent complications, and shorten period of disability	Adequate treatment to arrest disease process and prevent further complications Provision of facilities to limit disability and prevent death	Provision of hospital and community facilities for retraining and education to maximize use of remaining capacities Education of the public and industries to use rehabilitated persons to the fullest possible extent Selective placement Work therapy in hospitals Use of sheltered colony

Modified from Leavell H, Clark AE: *Preventive medicine for doctors in the community,* New York, 1965, McGraw-Hill.

ble to the client's previous level of wellness or it may result in death or develop into a chronic disease process.

Chronic Illness. A **chronic illness** lasts more than 3 months. Presently, 13% of the American population are affected by chronic illness. Also, a significant increase in chronic illness occurs between the ages of 45 and 64 (Edelman, Mandle, 1990). Nurses therefore must provide chronically ill clients with client-centered goals designed to optimize their levels of functioning and their ability to live with the illness (Cooper, 1990).

RISK FACTORS

A **risk factor** is any situation, habit, environmental condition, physiological condition, or other variable that increases the vulnerability of an individual or group to an illness or accident (e.g., a family history of heart disease or exposure to industrial pollution). Risk factors can include variables other than physical conditions (e.g., stress over a long period). The presence of risk factors does not mean that a disease will develop, but risk factors increase a person's susceptibility to a disease. Risk factors can occur in different aspects of a person's internal or external environment. Nurses and other health care professionals are concerned with them for several reasons. Risk factors play a major role in how a nurse identifies a client's health status. They can also influence health beliefs and practices if a person is aware of their presence. Identifying risk factors is also important for health promotion and illness prevention activities because the clients may modify or eliminate the risk factors.

Risk factors can be placed in the following interrelated categories: genetic and physiological factors, age, physical environment, and life-style.

Genetic and Physiological Factors

Physiological risk factors involve the physical functioning of the body. Certain physical conditions, such as being pregnant or overweight, place increased stress on physiological systems (e.g., the circulatory system), increasing susceptibility to illness in these areas. Heredity, or genetic predisposition to specific illness, is a major physical risk factor (e.g., a person with a family history of diabetes mellitus, cancer, or heart disease).

Age

Age increases susceptibility to certain illnesses (e.g., the risk of heart disease increases with age for both sexes). The risks of birth defects and complications of pregnancy increase after age 35. Many kinds of cancer pose a greater risk for persons older than age 45 than for younger persons. Age risk factors are often closely linked to other risk factors such as family history and personal habits.

Environment

The environment in which a person works or lives can increase the likelihood of certain illnesses. For example, some kinds of cancer and other diseases are more likely to develop in industrial workers exposed to certain chemicals or in people who live near toxic waste disposal sites. Screenings for these environmentally based risk factors are directed at the short-term effects of the exposure and the potential for long-term effects (Edelman, Mandle, 1990).

Air, water, and noise pollution, high crime rates, or overcrowding also can increase the risk of illness. In the home, the environment may include conditions that pose risks to an individual or family. Unclean, poorly heated or cooled, or overcrowded dwellings increase the likelihood that infections and other diseases will be contracted and spread. Within the family, conflicts or other problems may create stressors that put individual members or the family as a whole at increased risk of illness.

Life-Style

Many activities, habits, and practices involve risk factors, as do the stresses of life crises and frequent life-style changes. Health practices with potential negative consequences (e.g., poor nutrition, insufficient rest and sleep, poor personal hygiene, smoking, alcohol or drug abuse, and activities that involve a threat of injury) are risk factors.

Any emotional stress can be a risk factor if it is severe or prolonged or the person is unable to cope adequately with it. In such a case, emotional stress may increase the chance of illness. Emotional stress may occur with events such as divorce, pregnancy, and arguments. Any area of life that leads to long-term emotional stress can be a risk factor.

Holmes and Rahe (1967) developed a classic social readjustment rating scale that correlates life changes with the risk of illness. Their research has shown there is a greater risk for illness when a person has encountered a major life event change or multiple changes during a 12-month period. Adjustments that clients must make in health care settings also involve a risk for further illness. Volicer (1974) developed a hospital stress rating scale that closely parallels the Holmes and Rahe scale. This scale seeks to predict the risk of a long hospital stay, complications, and pain. All of these factors may be linked to further disability or prolonged illness. The hospital stress rating scale assigns a numerical value to actual or potential stressors experienced during hospitalization. The higher the total score, the greater the risk. This scale helps a nurse identify risks so that nursing interventions can be developed to reduce hospital stress.

ILLNESS AND ILLNESS BEHAVIOR

Illness is not merely the presence of a disease process. Illness is a state in which a person's physical, emotional, intellectual, social, developmental, or spiritual functioning is diminished or impaired compared with previous experience. Illness is not synonymous with disease; although nurses must be familiar with different kinds of diseases and their treatments, they are concerned more with illness, which may include disease but also the effects on functioning and well-being in all dimensions.

Ill people generally act in a way medical sociologists call **illness behavior.** It involves how people monitor their bodies, define and interpret their symptoms, take remedial actions, and use the health care system (Mechanic, 1982). If people perceive themselves to be ill, illness behaviors can be coping mechanisms. For example, illness behavior may be a means of obtaining reassurance (Lambert, Lambert, 1987). The health team can also support and reassure clients. This support is particularly important for clients with chronic diseases. In addition, illness behavior can result in clients being released from roles, social expectations, or responsibilities.

Variables Influencing Illness Behavior

Just as health behavior is affected by internal and external variables, so is illness behavior. To understand the client's behavior and to plan individualized care, the nurse needs to understand the influences of these variables. They are complex in their origins and effects.

Internal Variables. Internal variables influencing the way clients behave when they are ill include their perceptions of illness, the nature of the illness, and the extent of the symptoms. Clients are more likely to seek out health care if they perceive their symptoms or illnesses to be disruptive or potentially serious. Some clients may also avoid health care assistance because they fear serious illness. Cox (1985) investigated the reliability of the Health Self-Determination Index (HSDI) and noted that the tool could assist nurses in determining and predicting client responses to health problems and needs.

A client's illness behavior can also be affected by the nature of the illness. Acute illnesses may affect functioning in any dimension but are usually short term. Chronic illnesses persist over a long period and can also affect functioning in any dimension. Several variables influence the illness behavior of a client with a chronic illness. If a chronic illness cannot be cured and the symptoms are only partially relieved by therapy, the client may not comply with the therapy plan. In addition, the present health care system is geared to short, intensive client interactions. This reduces continuity of care and may affect how the illness is managed.

Clients with acute illnesses are more likely to seek health care and comply with therapy. Chronically ill clients may become less actively involved and may comply less readily with care. Nurses are often in the unique position of being able to assist chronically ill clients in overcoming problems related to illness behavior.

External Variables. External variables influencing a client's illness behavior include the visibility of symptoms, social group, cultural background, economic variables, accessibility of the health care system, and social support.

The visibility of the symptoms of an illness can affect body image and illness behavior. A client with a visible symptom may be more likely to seek assistance than a client without such a visible symptom.

Clients' social groups may assist them in recognizing the threat of illness or support the denial of potential illness. Families, friends, and co-workers all may influence clients' illness behavior. Cultural and ethnic background teaches a person how to be healthy, recognize illness, and be ill. Meanings attached to health and illness are related to the basic culture-bound values by which a person defines a given experience and perception (Spector, 1991). The effects of disease and its interpretation vary according to cultural circumstances.

Economic variables influence the way a client reacts to illness. Because of economic constraints, a client may delay treatment and in many cases may continue to carry out daily activities. Also, a client with inadequate health insurance may not gain access to the health care system (Larkin, 1987).

Clients' access to the health care system is closely related to economic factors. The health care system is a socioeconomic system that clients must enter, interact within, and exit. For many clients, entry into the system is complex or confusing. The physical proximity of clients to a health care agency often influences how soon they enter the system.

Social support has been linked to health practices such as seat belt use, exercise, nutrition, smoking cessation, and health screening practices (Muhlenkamp, Sayles, 1986). Clients often react positively to social support while practicing positive health behaviors.

These internal and external factors can interact in various ways to influence how clients behave when ill. Mechanic (1982) summarized the influences on illness behavior in a list of 10 primary determinants (see box above). Knowing these determinants can assist the nurse in providing care that uses the clients' resources to restore maximal health.

DETERMINANTS OF ILLNESS BEHAVIOR

The visibility and recognizability of the illness's symptoms

The extent to which the person perceives the symptoms as serious (the person's estimate of the present and future risks)

The person's information, knowledge, and cultural assumptions and understanding related to the perceived symptoms

The extent to which symptoms disrupt family, work, and social activities

The frequency of the appearance of the symptoms and their persistence

The extent to which others exposed to the person tolerate the symptoms

The extent to which basic needs are denied because of the illness

The extent to which meeting other needs competes with illness responses

The extent to which the person gives other possible interpretations to the symptoms

The availability and physical proximity of treatment resources and the psychological and monetary costs of taking action (including costs in time and effort, as well as costs such as stigma, social distance, and feelings of humiliation)

Modified from Mechanic D: The epidemiology of illness behavior and its relationship to physical and psychological distress. In Mechanic D: *Symptoms, illness behavior, and help seeking,* New York, 1982, Prodist.

Stages of Illness Behavior

Clients generally pass through five stages of illness behavior (Figure 2-7). This pattern involves how a client seeks, finds, and uses health care resources.

A nurse encounters clients in various stages of illness behavior. Knowledge of these stages enables the nurse to assess client behavior, determine the stage of illness behavior, and develop interventions to promote optimal functioning in all dimensions throughout the illness.

Stage 1: Symptom Experience. During the initial stage, a client is aware that "something is wrong," recognizing a physical sensation or a limitation in functioning but does not suspect a specific diagnosis.

The client's perception of a symptom includes awareness of a physical change, evaluation of this change, and a decision that it is a symptom of an illness. There is also an emotional response. After noting the presence of

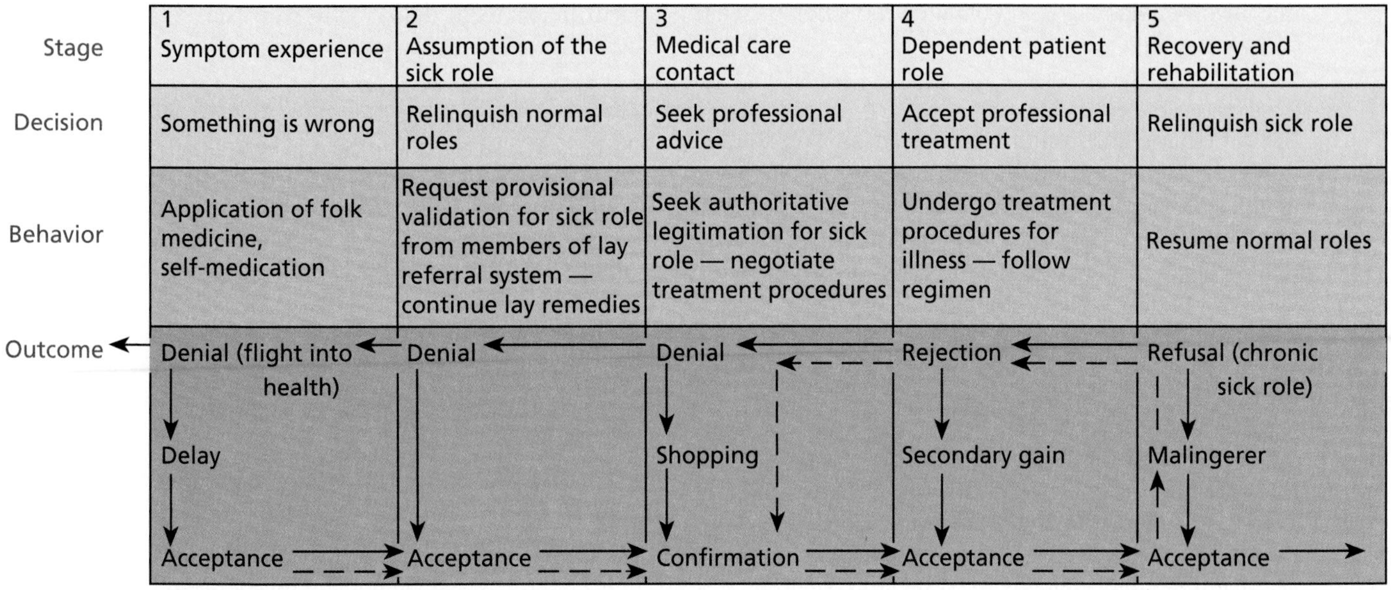
Stage
Decision
Behavior
Outcome
1 Symptom experience
2 Assumption of the sick role
3 Medical care contact
4 Dependent patient role
5 Recovery and rehabilitation
Something is wrong
Relinquish normal roles
Seek professional advice
Accept professional treatment
Relinquish sick role
Application of folk medicine, self-medication
Request provisional validation for sick role from members of lay referral system — continue lay remedies
Seek authoritative legitimation for sick role — negotiate treatment procedures
Undergo treatment procedures for illness — follow regimen
Resume normal roles
Denial (flight into health)
Denial
Denial
Rejection
Refusal (chronic sick role)
Delay
Shopping
Secondary gain
Malingerer
Acceptance
Acceptance
Confirmation
Acceptance
Acceptance

FIGURE 2-7 Stages of illness behavior. (From Suchman EA: *J Health Hum Behav* 6:114, 1965.)

symptoms, a client may behave in many ways. If the symptoms seem mild or not life threatening, self-medication may be the response. If the symptoms seem severe or life threatening, the client may seek care or deny the symptoms exist. The client must first acknowledge the presence of a health problem before moving to the next stage.

Stage 2: Assumption of the Sick Role. If symptoms persist and become severe, clients assume the sick role. At this point the illness becomes a social phenomenon, and clients seek confirmation from their families and social groups that they are ill and should be excused from normal duties and role expectations (Coe, 1978). The social group supports the presence of the illness.

The assumption of the sick role results in emotional changes. They may be simple or complex, depending on the severity of the illness, degree of disability, and anticipated length of the illness.

After accepting the persistent nature of the symptoms or the potential threat to present and future levels of wellness, the client seeks contact with the health care system.

Stage 3: Medical Care Contact. If symptoms persist despite the home remedies, become severe, or require emergency care, the client is motivated to seek professional health services. In this stage the client seeks expert acknowledgment of the illness, its treatment, an explanation of the symptoms, the cause, the course, and the implications of the illness for future health.

The severity of the illness influences how long the client waits before contacting health care professionals. Life-threatening illness or trauma may result in immediate contact. The psychosocial and cultural variables affecting illness behavior may delay contact if the illness does not seem severe.

Clients' illnesses can be validated at any point on the health-illness continuum. A health professional may determine they do not have an illness or that illnesses are present and may be life threatening. Clients then accept or deny this diagnosis, depending on the variables that affect illness behavior. If clients accept the diagnoses, they usually follow the prescribed treatment plan. If they deny the diagnoses, they may consult several health care providers until they find one who makes the desired diagnosis or until they accept the initial diagnoses.

Stage 4: Dependent Client Role. In this stage the client depends on health care professionals to relieve symptoms. The client accepts care, sympathy, and protection from the demands and stresses of life. A client can adopt the dependent role in any setting. It is socially permissible for clients in the dependent role to be relieved of normal obligations and tasks. The client must also adjust to a disrupted daily schedule, which affects most of the client's social roles.

Stage 5: Recovery and Rehabilitation. The final stage of illness behavior—recovery and rehabilitation—can arrive suddenly, such as when a fever subsides. If recovery is not prompt, long-term care may be required before the client is able to resume an optimal level of functioning. With chronic illness, the final stage may involve adjusting to a prolonged reduction in health and functioning.

• • •

Not all clients go through each stage, nor do they all move through them at the same rate or in the same manner. Nonetheless, this pattern of illness behavior occurs in many cases. The nurse who understands all of these stages can identify clients' changing illness behaviors and plan effective nursing care.

IMPACT OF ILLNESS ON CLIENT AND FAMILY

Illness is never an isolated life event. The client and family must deal with changes resulting from illness and treatment. Because each client responds uniquely to illness, nursing interventions must be individualized. The client and family commonly experience changes in behavior and emotions, family roles and dynamics, body image, and self-concept. Environment, personal behaviors, and psychosocial factors all interact in illness and health. Assessments based on these interactions result in more specific nursing diagnoses and interventions (Shaver, 1985).

Behavioral and Emotional Changes

People react differently to illness or the threat of illness, depending on the nature of the illness, the client's attitude toward it, the reaction of others to it, and the variables of illness behavior.

Short-term, relatively minor illnesses evoke few behavioral changes in the functioning of the client or family. Severe illness can lead to more extensive emotional and behavioral changes, such as anxiety, shock, denial, anger, and withdrawal. These are common responses to the stress of illness, and the client and the family may need help in coping with and adapting to these stressors (see Chapter 4).

Anxiety. Anxiety is a feeling of apprehension, uneasiness, agitation, uncertainty, and fear that occurs in anticipation of a threat, such as an illness. Anxiety responses vary from client to client, family to family, and stage to stage in illness behavior.

Shock. The shock response is a powerful emotional state usually arising when a client receives the diagnosis of a severe illness. For some, the state may be an adaptive mechanism. However, for others the shock response triggers inappropriate behavior.

Denial. Denial is a refusal to acknowledge difficult facts. Short-term denial, however, can be an effective way of coping with an illness.

Anger. Anger may be directed toward others, the illness, or health care professionals. Family members may express anger toward the client. This anger might also be directed toward themselves. Anger, like other emotions, may be irrational. It also may have effects on a client's social or spiritual dimensions (see Chapter 17).

Withdrawal. Withdrawal is a refusal to interact with others. It is a symptom of depression and may be an effect of an illness or diagnosis. Family members may also withdraw from the client.

Impact on Family Roles

When an illness occurs, the roles of client and family may change. This change may be subtle and short term or drastic and long term. People generally adjust more easily to subtle, short-term changes. Long-term changes, however, require an adjustment process similar to the grief process (see Chapter 21). The client and family often require specific counseling and guidance to assist them in coping with the role changes. Because changes in a client's role affect the family, nurses must incorporate the family into the care plan (deChesnay, Magnuson, 1988).

Impact on Body Image

Body image is the subjective concept of physical appearance (see Chapter 17). Some illnesses result in changes in physical appearance, and clients and families react differently to these changes. These reactions depend on the type of change, the ability of family members to adapt, the rate of the changes, and support services available. When a change in body image occurs, the client generally adjusts in the following phases: shock, withdrawal, acknowledgment, acceptance, and rehabilitation. Initially the client may be shocked by the change or impending change and may depersonalize it and talk about it as though it were happening to someone else. As the client and family recognize the reality of the change, they become anxious and may withdraw, refusing to discuss it. Withdrawal is an adaptive coping mechanism that can assist the client in making the adjustment. As the client and family acknowledge the change, they move through a period of grieving. At the end of the acknowledgment phase, they accept the loss. During rehabilitation, the client is ready to learn how to adapt to the change in body image through using a prosthesis or changing life-styles and goals.

Impact on Self-Concept

Self-concept is a mental self-image of strengths and weaknesses in all aspects of personality. Self-concept depends in part on body image and roles but also includes other aspects of psychology and spirituality (see Chapter 17). The impact of illness on the self-concepts of clients and family members may be more complex and less readily observed than role changes.

Self-concept is important in relationships with family members. A client whose self-concept changes because of illness may no longer meet family expectations, leading to tension or conflict. In the course of providing care, a nurse is able to observe changes in the client's self-concept—or in the self-concepts of family members—and develop a care plan to help them adjust to the changes resulting from the illness.

Impact on Family Dynamics

Family dynamics is the process by which the family functions, makes decisions, supports family members, and copes with changes. Because of the effects of illness, family dynamics often change. Nursing interventions need to be directed toward the family and client (Reeder, 1991). Family members may delay regular functioning or fail to assume the client's usual roles. In cases of prolonged illness, the family often has to shift to a new pattern of functioning, which can cause emotional stress. Role reversal is common, as parents and children try to adapt to major changes resulting from a family member's illness. Such a reversal also causes stress. The nurse must view the whole family as a client under stress, planning care to help the family regain the maximal level of functioning and well-being (see Chapter 19).

SUMMARY

The concepts of health and illness continuously change. Health is not merely the absence of illness or disability. It is a dynamic state in which people adapt to internal and external environments to maintain well-being. To provide effective nursing care and assist clients in regaining and maintaining high levels of wellness, nurses must understand clients' concepts of health and their health beliefs and practices.

Health care professionals and consumers today emphasize health promotion and illness prevention activi-

KEY CONCEPTS

- A healthy individual adapts to changes in the internal and external environment and thus maintains a state of well-being in all dimensions.
- An illness may be a disease, but it also includes reduced functioning in any human dimension.
- A person's state of health or illness depends on individual values, personality, and life-style.
- According to the health-illness continuum model, health and illness are in a dynamic, relative relationship.
- The high-level wellness model describes health as an integrated method of functioning to maximize well-being.
- The agent-host-environment model describes disease or illness as the result of the dynamic interaction of these three factors.
- The health-belief model considers factors influencing health beliefs.
- The evolutionary-based model suggests that illness and death sometimes have evolutionary functions.
- The health promotion model increases individual well-being and self-actualization.
- Health beliefs and practices are influenced by internal and external variables.
- To individualize care and ensure client's maximal participation, the nurse considers health beliefs and practices when planning care.
- Health promotion activities help maintain or enhance health.
- Illness prevention activities protect against risk factors and thus maintain an optimal level of health.
- Nursing incorporates health promotion and illness prevention activities rather than simply treating illness.
- Risk factors threaten health, influence health practices, and are important considerations in illness prevention activities.
- Risk factors involve genetic or physiological variables, age, environment, and life-style.
- Illness behavior, like health practices, is influenced by many variables and must be considered by the nurse when planning care.
- Although no two clients behave in exactly the same way when ill, most pass through five stages of illness behavior: symptom experience, assumption of the sick role, medical care contact, the dependent role, and recovery and rehabilitation.
- Illness can have many effects on the client and family, including changes in behavior and emotions, family roles and dynamics, body image, and self-concept.
- To plan and implement holistic nursing care that assists in attaining states of maximal functioning and well-being, the nurse must consider all the effects of an illness on clients and their families.

ties designed to help clients reduce the risks of illness and maintain maximal health.

Ill people progress through stages of illness behavior. If the illnesses are serious enough for people to enter the hospital or extended facility, the nurse must identify factors that influence clients' behavior and the impact of illnesses on clients and families. Nursing care is thus directed at preventing illness and promoting health, helping clients adjust to illnesses and their impact, and helping them regain maximal functioning.

CRITICAL THINKING ACTIVITIES

1. In a day-care setting you are asked to design an early education health promotion program for the 4-year-old group. You initially focus on diet and exercise. How do you begin to design the program? What resources do you need?
2. One of the students in your school asks for help in finding a smoking cessation program. How do you identify the best resources? Which program would be suitable? What information does the client need?
3. Assess your own life-style. Identify three areas for change. Select one area, determine what needs to change, how to identify resources to promote change, how to select and implement the resources, and how to evaluate the effectiveness of the change.
4. Think of someone you know who had difficulty adjusting to an illness. Discuss the variables that influenced this person's adjustment.

References

Balog JE: The concepts of health and disease: a relativistic perspective, *Health Values* 6:7, 1982.

Becker MH, Maiman LA: Sociobehavioral determinants of compliance with health and medical care recommendations, *Med Care* 33(1):1021, 1975.

Berne AS et al.: A nursing model for addressing the health needs of homeless families, *Image J Nurs Sch* 22:8, 1990.

Breslow L: A quantitative approach to the World Health Organization definition of health: physical, mental and social well-being, *Int J Epidemiol* 1:347, 1972.

Coe R: *Sociology of medicine,* ed 2, New York, 1978, McGraw-Hill.

Cooper MC: Chronic illness and nursing's ethical challenge, *Holistic Nurs Pract* 5(1):19, 1990.

Cox CL: The health self-determination index, *Nurs Res* 34:177, 1985.

deChesnay M, Magnuson N: How healthy families cope with stress, *AAOHN J* 36:361, 1988.

Dixon JK, Dixon P: An evolutionary based model of health and viability, *ANS* 6(3):1, 1984.

Dunn H: What high level wellness means, *Health Values* 1:9, 1977.

Dunn HL: High-level wellness for man and society, *Am J Public Health* 49:789, 1959.

Edelman CL, Mandle CL: *Health promotion throughout the life span,* ed 2, St Louis, 1990, Mosby.

Fuchs VR: *Who shall live? Health, economics, and social choice,* New York, 1974, Basic Books.

Gilpatrick DM: Moving clients toward wellness: behavioral change, *Clin Nurse Spec* 3(1):25, 1989.

Holmes TH, Rahe RH: Social readjustment rating scale, *J Psychosom Res* 11:213, 1967.

Lambert CE, Lambert VA: Psychosocial impacts created by chronic illness, *Nurs Clin North Am* 22:527, 1987.

Larkin J: Factors influencing one's ability to adapt to chronic illness, *Nurs Clin North Am* 22:535, 1987.

Lear JG: Building a health/education partnership: the role of school-based health centers, *Pediatr Nurs* 18(2):172, 1992.

Leavell HR et al.: *Preventive medicine for the doctor in his community,* ed 3, New York, 1965, McGraw-Hill.

Mechanic D: The epidemiology of illness behavior and its relationship to physical and psychological distress. In Mechanic D: *Symptoms, illness behavior, and help seeking,* New York, 1982, Prodist.

Meleis AI: Being and becoming healthy: the core of nursing knowledge, *Nurs Sci Q* 3:107, 1990.

Muhlenkamp AF, Sayles JA: Self-esteem, social support and positive health practices, *Nurs Res* 35:334, 1986.

Neuman B: Health as a continuum based on the Neuman Systems Model, *Nurs Sci Q* 3:129, 1990.

Neuman B: *The Neuman systems model,* ed 2, Norwalk, Conn, 1989, Appleton & Lange.

Palank CL: Determinants of health-promotive behavior: a review of current research, *Nurs Clin North Am* 26(4):815, 1991.

Parse RR: *Man-living-health: a theory of nursing,* New York, 1981, Wiley.

Pender NJ: A conceptual model for preventive health behavior, *Nurs Outlook* 23:385, 1975.

Pender NJ: *Health promotion and nursing practice,* Norwalk, Conn, 1982, Appleton-Century-Crofts.

Pender NJ: *Health promotion in nursing practice,* ed 2, Norwalk, Conn, 1987, Appleton & Lange.

Pender NJ, Pender AR: Attitudes, subjective norms, and intentions to engage in health behaviors, *Nurs Res* 35(1):15, 1986.

Pender NJ, Walker SN, et al.: Predicting health-promoting lifestyles in the workplace, *Nurs Res* 39:326, 1990.

Pender NJ: Expressing health through lifestyle patterns, *Nurs Sci Q* 3(3):115, 1990.

Prewitt VR: Health beliefs and AIDS educational materials, *Fam Community Health* 12:65, 1989.

Reeder JM: Family perception: a key to intervention. In American Association of Critical-Care Nurses: *AACN clinical issues in critical care nurse,* 1991, The Association.

Ruffing-Rahal MA: Rationale and design for health promotion with older adults, *Pub Health Nurs* 8(4):258, 1991.

Shaver JF: A biopsychosocial view of human health, *Nurs Outlook* 33:186, 1985.

Smith JM, Sorrell V: Developing wellness programs: a nurse-managed stay-well center for senior citizens, *Clin Nurse Spec* 3(1):198, 1989.

Spector RE: *Cultural diversity in health and illness,* ed 3, Norwalk, Conn, 1991, Appleton & Lange.

Suchman EA: Stages of illness and medical care, *J Health Human Behav* 6:114, 1965.

World Health Organization Interim Commission: *Chronicle of WHO,* Geneva, 1947, The Organization.

Bibliography

Aiken LH: Chronic illness and responsive ambulatory care. In Mechanic D: *The growth of bureaucratic medicine,* New York, 1976, Wiley.

Airhihenbuwa CO: Health education for African Americans: a neglected task, *Health Educ* 20:9, 1989.

Allinger RL: Study of illness referral in a Spanish speaking community, *Nurs Res* 26:53, 1977.

Anderson JM: The cultural context of caring, *Can Crit Care Nurs J* 4(4):7, 1987.

Dixon JK, Dixon JP: An evolutionary-based model of health and viability, *ANS* 6(3):1, 1984.

Parse RR: Health: a personal commitment, *Nurs Sci Q* 3:136, 1990.

Parsons T: Definitions of health and illness in light of American values and social structures. In Joco EG, editor: *Patients, physicians, and illness,* New York, 1958, Free Press.

Pender NJ: Expressing health through lifestyle patterns, *Nurs Sci Q* 3:115, 1990.

Pender NJ: Health promotion and illness prevention. In Werley HH and Fitzpatrick JJ, editors: *Annual review of nursing research,* New York, 1984, Springer.

Pesznecker E: The poor: a population at risk, *Public Health Nurs* 1:237, 1984.

Pollock SE: Human responses to chronic illness: physiologic and psychosocial adaptation, *Nurs Res* 35:90, 1986.

Steinfels P: The concept of health: an introduction, *Hastings Cent Rep* 1(3):3, 1973.

Tilden VP, Weinert, C: Social support and the chronically ill individual, *Nurs Clin North Am* 22:613, 1987.

Tripp-Reimer T: Reconceptualizing the construct of health: integrating emic and itic perspectives, *Res Nurs Health* 7:101, 1984.

Volicer BJ: Patient's perceptions of stressful events associated with hospitalization, *Nurs Res* 2(3):235, 1974.

Volicer BJ: Perceived stress levels of events associated with the experience of hospitalization: development and testing of a measurement tool, *Nurs Res* 22:491, 1973.

Volicer BJ, Bahannon MW: A hospital stress rating scale, *Nurs Res* 24:354, 1975.

Walker SN, Sechrist KR, Pender NJ: The health-promoting life-style profile: development and psychometric characteristics, *Nurs Res* 36:76, 1987.

Weitzel MH: A test of the health promotion model with blue-collar workers, *Nurs Res* 38:99, 1989.

Yarcheski A, Mahon N: A causal model of positive health practices: the relationship between approach and replication, *Nurs Res* 38:88, 1989.

Zborowski M: Cultural components in response to pain, *J Soc Issues* 8:16, 1952.

3

Promoting Continuity of Care and Home Health Care

OBJECTIVES

Mastery of content in this chapter will enable the student to:

- Define the key terms listed.
- Describe the nurse's role in maintaining continuity of care throughout hospitalization, including admission, transfer, and discharge.
- Identify components of effective discharge planning involving a multidisciplinary discharge team.
- Identify services provided by home health care agencies.
- Describe roles of nurses in home health care.
- Describe how regulatory standards and quality improvement guidelines affect the clinical practice of home health nursing.
- Identify recent social, economic, technological, and government forces that have influenced the growth of home health nursing.

KEY TERMS

discharge planning
durable medical equipment (DME)
home health care
home health care agencies
home IV therapies
hospice care
private duty agencies

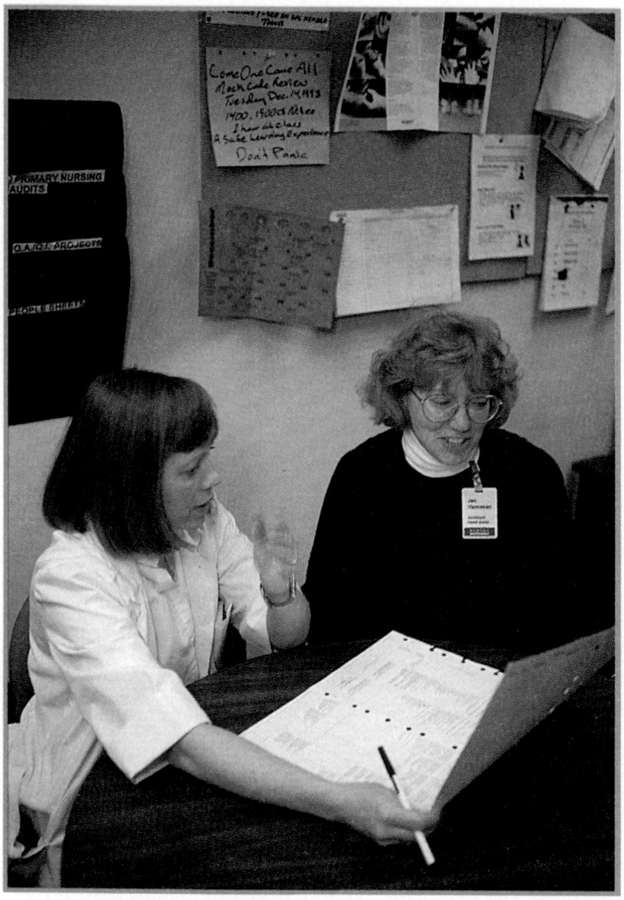

EXAMPLES OF JCAHO STANDARDS FOR ADMISSION AND DISCHARGE

NURSING AND HEALTH TEAM RESPONSIBILITIES

Each client's need for nursing care related to admission is assessed by a registered nurse.

Each client's assessment includes consideration of biophysical, psychosocial, environmental, self-care, educational, and discharge planning factors.

The client and family are involved in care as appropriate.

Nursing staff members collaborate, as appropriate, with physicians and members of other clinical disciplines to make decisions regarding the client's need for nursing care.

In preparation for discharge, continuing care needs are assessed and referrals for such care are documented in the client's medical record.

ADMINISTRATION RESPONSIBILITIES

Each hospital provides policies and procedures on discharge planning. These will include mechanisms to identify a client who requires discharge planning to foster continuity of medical or other care to meet the identified needs.

There are mechanisms to initiate discharge planning on a timely basis.

From Joint Commission on Accreditation of Healthcare Organizations: *Manual of hospital accreditation: 1992 standards,* Chicago 1994, The Commission.

For clients to have their health care needs met holistically and comprehensively and move through the health care system, nurses must provide continuity of care. This means that regardless of where a client is in the health care system, there is a sense that nurses and other health care providers are collaborating on a common plan of care. Whether a client utilizes a hospital outpatient clinic system, community based clinic, rehabilitation center, or hospital, nurses and other care providers must know the client's health care needs and provide effective, appropriate care. Admission into and movement through the health care system involves many complex factors. Hospitals are faced with the challenge of providing clients with the appropriate services to meet their needs, as well as the challenge of doing this as quickly as possible. Reimbursement guidelines require that clients leave hospitals earlier. As a result, clients require continued care within the home or extended health care facilities.

REGULATORY AGENCIES

The purpose of regulatory standards regarding the admission-discharge process is to provide a clear direction for all health care providers. It is believed that a client will receive the best quality of care within shorter time frames if health care is well coordinated from the moment the client enters a hospital. Success in meeting these standards requires collaboration from all professional care givers.

The U.S. government through Medicare and the health departments of all 50 states have created specific standards addressing the importance of **discharge planning** leading to continuity of care from hospital to the home. The Joint Commission on Accreditation of Healthcare Organizations (JCAHO) seeks to improve the quality of health care provided to the public and stimulate health care organizations to meet or exceed standards of practice (JCAHO, 1994). Specific standards pertaining to making a client's admission and discharge a well-coordinated process can be found in the box above.

ADMISSION PROCESS

Whether a client is entering a hospital, a nursing home, or a rehabilitation center, the purposes of the admission process are similar. They include data collection for nursing care and discharge planning, minimizing client and family anxiety, teaching the client and family, providing comfort and safety, and maintaining the client's legal rights as a health care recipient.

The admission process is likely to be an extremely stressful event. Various procedures feel depersonalizing, uncomfortable, and frightening. A client can feel powerless, not knowing what to expect. The nurse's role is to lead the client through the admission process so that the client can become informed and prepared to cope with all care activities. Friends or family members may be included in this process to facilitate the gathering of information. Presence of these persons also provides support and reassurance for the client.

Initial Admitting Procedures

At the time of admission it is necessary to collect information about the client. In many institutions an admissions clerk goes to the client, either in the emergency room or even on a patient care unit. Some hospitals have established admitting stations on their patient care units. In the traditional hospital setting an admitting office is close to the hospital's main entrance. An admitting clerk acquires identifying information, including full legal name, age, birth date, address, next of kin, admitting physician, religion, occupation, and type of insurance. This information ensures correct legal identification of the client. Data are entered into a computer that provides a printout of an admission sheet that is placed within the client's permanent medical record. Each client receives a permanent identification number for the hospital record.

After this identifying information is gathered, the client receives an identification bracelet for use when therapies or procedures such as medication administration or x-ray examinations are performed. The bracelet should be secure so that it remains in place throughout hospitalization. This is especially important for confused or comatose clients and children.

Clients' Legal Rights

The hospital is responsible for informing clients of their legal rights at admission. The admitting clerk will instruct clients or legal guardians about the general consent form for treatment. The signature on the consent form gives the hospital permission to perform routine procedures and selected therapies such as medication administration, blood testing, and noninvasive radiological procedures.

In addition, the hospital must give clients written information about state laws regarding medical care, including the right to accept or refuse medical or surgical treatment. Clients must receive information about their rights to formulate advance directives such as living wills. The Patient Self-Determination Act became effective in December 1991. Each state determines how the law concerning advance directives is to be stated. Also it is important for the client to receive information regarding the *Patient's Bill of Rights* from the American Hospital Association (AHA, 1992). This document must be posted in the admitting office for all clients to see. In addition, most institutions give clients copies of the *Patient's Bill of Rights* in their admission booklets. The bill describes clients' rights to be well informed and receive respectful, competent, continuous, and confidential health care (see Chapter 6).

Institutional Policies and Procedures

Each agency has policies and procedures that the client should know. Usually the client or family is given a brochure explaining available services (e.g., pastoral care and social work), visiting hours, meal time schedules, smoking policies, and any other policies or rules that affect the person's conduct as a client. At admission, a client may be quite anxious and unable to take in a great deal of information. A booklet gives the client a resource that can be used at any time.

In some cases, clients undergo laboratory and x-ray testing at the time of admission. However, the majority of testing is now done on an outpatient basis to control the costs of inpatient care. Pre-admission tests can be performed safely and more cheaply before the client is hospitalized.

Admission to a Nursing Division

The admitting office notifies the nursing division of the client's admission, current status, and room assignment. This allows nursing staff to prepare a room and obtain necessary equipment before the arrival of the client. In some hospitals the nursing department determines room assignments. In addition to routine admission information, the nurse must determine the client's level of consciousness and whether or not the client has an active infection. This ensures that the client who requires frequent observation or special therapy is placed in a room accessible to the nursing staff. In the case of certain infections, such as active tuberculosis, a private room will be necessary.

Members of the admitting office or emergency room transport the client to the nursing division. The client's condition determines whether ambulation or use of a wheelchair or stretcher is most appropriate. On arrival on the division, the client and family are introduced to

> **NURSING DIAGNOSES FOR DISCHARGE PLANNING**
>
> - Altered health maintenance
> - Altered protection
> - Ineffective management of therapeutic regimen
> - Knowledge deficit
> - Noncompliance
> - High risk for infection
> - High risk for injury
> - Health seeking behaviors
> - Self-care deficit

the nurse assuming the client's care. The initial moments spent with a client begin the orientation phase of the nurse-client relationship.

Nursing's Role During Admission

The admission process includes orientation of the client to the room and unit procedures, a nursing history and physical assessment, collection of specimens, and a clarification of client questions and expectations. The nurse must respond appropriately to the client's level of comfort and fatigue. The admission process can be exhausting, especially if there is a delay in the admitting office for a room assignment. When the client is experiencing physical or psychological symptoms, the nurse determines priorities for assessment and if any portion of the admission process can be completed later after therapy has been administered.

An older adult who is to be admitted into a health care facility needs special consideration during the admission procedure. More time is needed to explain and perform procedures. Similarly older adults cannot assume positions necessary during a physical examination as quickly as younger adults. Gradual loss of sensory perception places the older client at risk for sensory alterations that may result in confusion, feelings of isolation, and high risk for injury. Clear explanations must be communicated to older clients with time for feedback and questions.

Clients who live alone, are elderly, and have had repeated hospitalization need additional assessment of the home situation to determine if returning to the home environment is appropriate. Level of functioning needs to be assessed including activities of daily living (ADL) (e.g., bathing, dressing, toileting, transfer, continence, and feeding). In addition, activities such as shopping, housekeeping, taking medication, handling finances, and using the telephone and transportation should be considered (Cookfair, 1991).

As soon as possible after the initial assessment the nurse is responsible for analyzing available data and identifying appropriate individualized nursing diagnoses. Consideration must be given to anxiety related to hospitalization, impending diagnostic or treatment procedures planned, and separation from home and family.

A client may have any of a number of nursing diagnoses. However, when the nurse begins to anticipate discharge planning needs, it is important to consider the client's potential ability to manage personal health care. Specifically the nurse assesses the client's perceived health status and its relevance to current activities and future planning. Nursing diagnoses within this category should be considered at the time of admission as they have definite implications for discharge planning (see box at left).

Individually established specific and measurable goals and outcomes set cooperatively with the client and family often provide motivation and encouragement to clients during hospitalization. Evaluation of outcomes that establishes achievement of goals will signal readiness for discharge.

DISCHARGE PLANNING

Successful discharge planning is a centralized, coordinated, multidisciplinary process that ensures that the client has a plan for continuing care after leaving the hospital (AHA, 1983). Planning for discharge should begin on admission to the agency and continue throughout the experience. The discharge should come as a surprise to no one. The following outcomes must be evaluated for a client's discharge plan:

1. Are the client and family able to explain the diagnosis, anticipated level of functioning, safe and effective use of discharge medications, and anticipated medical follow-up?
2. What specialized instruction or training is needed for the client and family to be able to provide proper care after discharge?
3. What community support systems need to be coordinated to enable the client to return home?
4. Are the client and family able to cope with the client's health status?
5. Is relocation of the client, coordination of support systems, or transfer to another health care facility needed?

Nurses play a key role in coordinating care from admission through discharge and in some cases after discharge into the home or an extended care facility. Nurses often have the opportunity to spend enough time to have a clear perspective of the holistic approach needed in a client's care. Nurses coordinate the many resources required to ensure a well-coordinated transition throughout hospitalization and following discharge.

In some agencies a home health coordinator initiates assessment of clients during hospitalization that facilitates continuity of care and, in many cases, speeds the discharge process (see box on p. 46). A complete dis-

ASSESSMENT FOR DISCHARGE PLANNING

1. Do you want to go home?
2. Do you think you will be able to manage your health care needs in your home?
3. Will you be willing to work with a home health nurse on how to manage your health care needs at home?
4. What new skills will you need to learn for home care?
5. Who is willing to help you with your care after you go home?
6. What special supplies, equipment, or resources will you need when you go home?

Modified from Rice R, *Home health nursing practice: concepts and application*, St. Louis, 1992, Mosby.

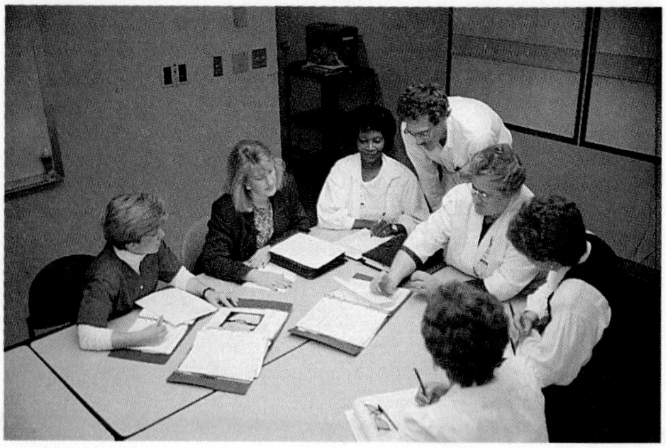

FIGURE 3-1 Staff participating in discharge planning conference.

charge assessment allows home health care nurses to better understand the client's needs and plan accordingly for the very first visit.

Many hospitals also have discharge planning teams. During routine conferences (e.g., daily or weekly), various members of the health care team discuss the status of each client with respect to plans for discharge (Figure 3-1). Multidisciplinary conferences allow all team members to interact and discuss the best options for each client. If special problems are faced by a client, the team may ask members of the family or friends to participate in the conference. Members of discharge planning teams may include nurses, physicians, dietitians, social workers, home health nurses, clinical nurse specialists, and others.

The delivery of care model within a hospital influences how discharge planning is conducted. When the delivery of care model is primary nursing, a single nurse is responsible for coordinating care from admission to discharge. Even though the primary nurse is unable to be with the client daily, it is that nurse's responsibility to identify the client's discharge planning needs and to be sure that all members of the health care team are aware of those needs.

When hospitals use a case management approach, an RN in the role of case manager is responsible for specific client outcomes. Often the case manager does not provide direct nursing care, but instead coordinates discharge planning activities for a case load of clients. Care expected to be delivered by various disciplines throughout a hospital is planned and managed through formal case management plans, sometimes called *critical pathways* (Zander, 1988). The critical pathways are multidisciplinary treatment plans that predict certain interventions over a projected length of stay. Case managers use the paths as tools to improve the delivery of care. The discharge plan is the critical pathway, because it provides clear direction for the care to be delivered to a client.

Staff nurses are the members of the discharge planning team who have contact with clients 24 hours a day and who can best assess mental and emotional status, functional abilities and disabilities (self-care deficits with transfers, ambulation, eating, and toileting). Nurses should assess the client's social support system and their abilities to assist in care. For example, a client may have a very supportive spouse, but if that spouse is elderly and also ill or disabled, the amount of assistance that can be given will be limited (Corkery, 1989).

The nurse and health care team determine whether resources are available to assist clients at home or whether home health care services are required. Clients who require more extensive care may enter skilled nursing facilities or rehabilitation programs or become residents of nursing homes. When health care continues after discharge, health care providers must receive a thorough review of client needs. The hospital nurse may talk directly with care givers in other agencies or provide a detailed summary of the care plan on a discharge document.

Clients at Risk

Every client in a hospital requires discharge planning. There are conditions, however, that place a client at risk for being unable to meet continuing health care needs after discharge such as the terminally ill or clients with permanent disabilities. When clients have one of these conditions, it is especially important to assess their desire and ability to manage health care needs at home (Rice, 1992).

Clients that should be considered for home care include those needing assistance while recovering from acute illness, or to prevent or manage exacerbations of

REFERRALS FOR HEALTH CARE SERVICES

Dietary: Registered dietitian can determine nutrients clients require based on clients' physical condition. Also teaches about prescribed diet plans.

Social worker: Qualified to conduct counseling and assist coping with life crises. Also assists in available community resources and support systems.

Physical therapy: Licensed to assist in examination and treatment of physically disabled or handicapped person. Therapist assists in rehabilitation.

Occupational therapy: Assist in adaptation to physical handicaps by learning new vocational skills or activities of daily living (ADLs).

Speech therapy: Assists with disorders affecting oral communication.

chronic illness, and families needing assistance in the care of the terminally ill (Cookfair, 1991).

Referrals for Health Care Services

Often a client will require the services of various disciplines within a hospital, such as dietary, social work, and/or physical therapy. The nurse often has the best opportunity to identify client's needs. For example, a client may not eat well for several days and reveals to the nurse a dislike for many of the food choices on the menu. A referral to a dietitian could result in identifying food preferences appropriate to the client's diet. It is important to collaborate with other health professionals with specialized skills and knowledge. Referrals should be made as soon as possible after the client's need is identified.

It is ideal to have clients participate in referral processes so that they are involved in decision making. The box above summarizes the role that various disciplines can play in a treatment plan. A physician's order may be needed for a referral, especially when specific therapies are planned (e.g., physical therapy).

When multiple referrals are made for a client's plan of care, the nurse coordinates referral activities. Often it is necessary to have different therapists collaborate so that a client's care is uninterrupted. For example, there may be certain times in the day when a client can better tolerate physical therapy or is most receptive to instruction. The nurse attempts to plan referral activities at these times.

Transfers Within an Agency

Transfer of a client from one nursing division to another creates another challenge for providing continuity of care. Transfers may occur when the client requires a different type of nursing service. For example, a client may be admitted to a medical nursing division for diagnosis of chest pain but is eventually transferred to a surgical nursing division for an open-heart procedure. Transfers to different divisions require considerable preparation. Nurses on the sending division coordinate activities with nurses on the receiving division; these activities include preparing the client's medical record, transporting medications and personal supplies, orienting the client and family to the transfer procedure, and transporting the client to the new division. Before a transfer is initiated, it is critical to determine a client's physical condition. A client who is not stable may require special equipment such as oxygen, a cardiac monitor, or intravenous fluids during transfer to a new division. Receiving nurses must have a clear understanding of the client's status and the plan of care. They receive this information from the transferring nurses in the form of a verbal report and in some institutions a written report as well.

After a client arrives on a new division, the nursing staff is responsible for assessing the client's condition and determining whether revisions to the plan of care are needed. Throughout the transfer process, the client and family need to be kept informed to minimize anxiety and fear.

Teaching as Part of the Discharge Plan

Education of the client, family, and other care givers is the primary responsibility of the nurse in the discharge planning process (Hogstel, 1992). Ultimately the goal is to provide clients and families with the knowledge and skills required to meet ongoing health care needs (JCAHO, 1994). When preparing clients for discharge it is extremely important to identify the support person who will be helping at home. With the advancing age of the general population it is not unusual for clients over the age of 80 to be cared for by persons above 60 years of age who are themselves debilitated. In some situations older adults are left dependent on the teenagers who fill in for parents who are at work. Although this may be manageable, teaching must be at an appropriate level for the capacities and limitations of these care givers.

Nurses today are challenged with providing effective education while often having limited contact with clients. Clients admitted to hospitals for short, 24-hour stays, for example, should receive education before coming to the hospital or be instructed on priority issues just before discharge. It is difficult to provide clients with the information they need the evening before or morning of discharge. Client education ideally is broken into easily digested segments that are taught and reinforced over a period of time. Clients are then provided the opportunity to think about and practice

BARRIERS TO LEARNING COMMON IN OLDER ADULTS

Sensory changes (e.g., decreased vision and hearing)
Pain
Bladder frequency or urgency
Limited endurance
Decreased attention span
Physical inability to perform motor tasks
Environmental noise, which is distracting and disruptive
Environmental temperature, especially drafts or chilling
Depression with low energy levels

Modified from Hogstel M: *Clinical manual of gerontological nursing,* St. Louis, 1992, Mosby.

JCAHO CLIENT AND FAMILY EDUCATION STANDARDS

Information is to be presented in ways understandable to clients and family and is to include:

- The safe and effective use of medication
- The safe and effective use of medical equipment, when applicable
- Instruction on potential drug-food interactions and counseling on nutrition intervention
- Instruction in rehabilitation techniques to facilitate adaptation
- Access to available community resources
- When and how to obtain further treatment
- The client's and family's responsibilities in the client's care

From Joint Commission on Accreditation of Healthcare Organizations: *Manual of hospital accreditation: 1994 standards,* Chicago, 1994, The Association.

self-care skills and ask questions (Chapter 14). A fear of making mistakes or not being capable may block learning and lead to noncompliance.

Before beginning to teach, nurses must determine what information has already been given by the physician or other care givers. By having clients describe what they believe they are to do when they go home, the nurse can identify inconsistencies and concerns that can result from conflicting information from a variety of care givers and provide clarification and consistency in teaching. Nurses need to be alert for possible learning barriers that affect all clients, and especially older adults (see box above). Learning is enhanced if spoken instructions are reinforced with written materials, and a variety of modes of presentation are used, including videotapes, booklets, discussion, and others.

The JCAHO (1994) has set minimum standards for information to be provided to clients and families (see box above, right). Nurses and other members of the team, as appropriate, must document any instruction provided to clients as well as an evaluation of the client's understanding. Many institutions have special teaching checklists to facilitate the documentation process.

Discharge from the Hospital

If discharge planning is successful, the discharge of a client from a hospital should be uneventful. As a client successfully meets expected outcomes of care, goals of care are met and the client is ready for discharge. At discharge, clients must have the knowledge, skill, and resources to meet self-care needs.

On the day of discharge the nurse must complete a number of routine activities. Clients and families anticipate a smooth and quick discharge process. If appropriate discharge planning began early, the day of discharge should be relatively routine. Before clients leave the hospital, the nurse:

- Provides a final chance for client and family or friends to ask questions and discuss concerns. Teaching may be summarized and reinforced
- Checks the physician's final discharge orders
- Assists client with dressing and packing of personal belongings
- Accounts for all client valuables
- Provides client with prescriptions or medications
- Arranges for client to check with billing office (refer to agency policy)
- Assists client in transport to vehicle that will be used for transportation home
- Documents client's status at discharge

Discharge Against Medical Advice. Occasionally a client chooses to leave a hospital against medical advice (AMA). In this situation, there is a risk that the client will suffer complications from leaving the hospital prematurely. The client must sign a form that releases the physicians and hospital from any legal responsibility for the client's health. Before an AMA form is completed, the nurse and/or physician discusses with the client the possible outcomes of the decision. The client must clearly understand possible risks. The AMA form is signed by the client and is witnessed by the physician or nurse (depending on agency policy). Usually staff inform the risk-management department of any AMAs.

Health Promotion

In some cases a brief illness or minor event brings relatively healthy clients into the health care system. Each contact with clients gives nurses the opportunity to promote health and wellness in a holistic sense. Motivation to take action to promote health or to prevent disease is based on how strongly the individual believes that he or she is susceptible to illness, that the illness would have a significant effect on quality of life, and that there are ways to take action that can help prevent the illness or reduce its severity. Clients may seek assistance in areas such as exercise, stress reduction, weight control, and illness and accident prevention (Tripp, 1992).

Health Seeking Behaviors is one nursing diagnosis that is useful when a client is seeking ways to pursue a healthier life-style. When using this diagnosis, the nurse specifies the area of concern the client is motivated to manage (e.g., stress or diet management). Client education (Chapter 14), therapeutic communication (Chapter 13), sleep hygiene (Chapter 27), and relaxation therapies (Chapter 28) are just some interventions the nurse may rely on to assist clients in achieving healthier life-styles.

HOME HEALTH CARE

Home health care is the provision of medically related services and equipment to clients and families in their places of residence for health maintenance, education, illness prevention, diagnosis and treatment of disease, palliation, and rehabilitation. Older adults are eligible for home care services under Medicare provided they meet the eligibility requirements (see box below). The most common services include nursing; medical and social work; physical, occupational, speech, and respiratory therapy; nutrition therapy; and physician care. Of these services nursing is used most often.

Other services include home health aides, housekeepers, and companions. Many of these care givers provide personal care and household support services that prevent the need for costly hospitalization or care in a skilled nursing facility.

Home health care equipment is any medically related product adapted for home use, including highly technical items such as mechanical ventilators and intravenous (IV) infusion pumps and nontechnical items such as hospital beds and walkers.

Home health has extended almost every type of health care service into the client's residence. Health promotion and education are traditionally the primary objectives. The focus is encouragement of client and family independence through teaching of self-care. Recovery and stabilization of illness are addressed in the home, where situations related to life-style, safety, environment, family dynamics, and health care practices can be accurately assessed.

The delivery of home health care requires involvement of the client and family. The client and family are accustomed to having control in their own homes. Client involvement in planning and teaching leads to better goal achievement. The client is urged to take an active role. The following factors must be considered when planning home care:

1. Socioeconomic, cultural, and environmental factors
2. Family and community resources
3. Client teaching
4. Interdisciplinary collaboration between home health care and hospital professionals
5. The client's physician and other health care providers who must be consulted and informed on a regular basis

Outcomes of care must be documented for continuity of care, reimbursement, accreditation, and research. Evaluation of client response to teaching, treatments, and medications results in identification of changes needed in therapy. It also helps identify obstacles that interfere with the effectiveness of the care plan. Effective, ongoing evaluation of outcomes and thorough follow-up for necessary changes are the most important functions of home health care personnel.

ELIGIBILITY FOR HOME CARE SERVICES UNDER MEDICARE

The client is confined to home. Leaving the home would require a considerable and taxing effort. Acceptable absences from home include those that are infrequent, are of short duration, or are for the purpose of receiving medical treatment.

Services are provided under a plan of care established and approved by a physician who is qualified to sign the physician certification and plan of care.

The client needs skilled nursing care on an intermittent basis, needs physical therapy or speech therapy, or has continued need for occupational therapy.

From Department of Health and Human Services: Health Care Financing Administration (1989) *Medicare: Home health agency manual (HCFA Publication 11),* Washington, DC, 1989, U.S. Government Printing Office.

Types of Home Health Care Agencies

Home health agencies provide skilled, intermittent professional and home health aide services, usually once or twice a day up to 7 days a week. Visits usually last 1 hour. Agencies may be hospital based, private or public, and each provides care in the home following a physician-approved plan of treatment. Home health care services are reimbursed by government funds, private insurance, or private pay. Medicare and Medicaid programs have strict and elaborate regulations governing reimbursement for home health care services. Most professional services provided through a Medicare-licensed agency are reimbursed at the costs for providing the service by government programs.

Private-duty agencies provide home health care services on a more continuous basis up to 24 hours a day, usually by registered nurses, licensed practical nurses, housekeepers, companions, or home health aides. The cost for these services is quite high. Government funds will not pay for private-duty nursing care; therefore these services are generally affordable only to people for whom commercial insurance provides reimbursement or to those who can afford to pay privately.

Durable medical equipment (DME) companies provide medical equipment such as hospital beds, home oxygen, ventilators, and disposable supplies. Reimbursement is through government and private insurance. The DME industry is one of the most rapidly growing areas in health care. Nurses and therapists are frequently employed by the agencies. Referrals can be made by any health care professional.

Hospices are programs frequently existing within health care agencies that provide care for the terminally ill. Hospice-related programs have a philosophy of care that exists to provide support and care for persons in the last months of an incurable illness so that life can be lived as fully and comfortably as possible. Nurses working in this specialty require skills related to pain control (Chapter 28) and the psychology of dealing with dying clients and their families. In the United States, approximately 80% of certified hospice care is provided in the homes. Home hospice care is usually preferred over inpatient hospice care for clients whose family members are able to provide home care.

INCREASED DEMAND FOR HOME HEALTH CARE

Home health care has evolved into a challenging and rapidly growing field. Because of recent economic, social, governmental, and technological developments, home health professionals are caring for clients who are more ill, who go home from the hospital sooner, and who have more needs for highly technical care and complex equipment than ever before.

Other forces causing more demand for home health care services include increases in the number of older adults and chronically ill persons, advances in home care technology, and the breakdown of the extended family. Many households require two incomes, which leaves fewer family members at home to care for the older adults and disabled persons. Clients are more acutely ill when discharged from the hospital and require more intensive services.

The U.S. government's health care payment system has resulted in major cutbacks that have made an impact on the home health care industry. Funding for hospital care, especially for older adults, has been drastically cut, resulting in a tremendous increase in the need for home health care services by clients who would have previously been hospitalized. As a result, many of these clients require more highly skilled and technical home-centered services.

RESPONSIBILITIES OF THE HOME HEALTH NURSE

The home health care nurse must apply the nursing process in the community setting and practice with a minimum of supervision. More independent judgment and decision making are needed more than in most other types of nursing practice. It requires skills relating to many age-groups and cultures. The baccalaureate degree in nursing is often required for an RN to assume a position in a home health care agency.

Home health nurses provide creative and adaptive care to clients in the home. A holistic, nonjudgmental, and family-centered philosophy is essential for the nurse in the home. The nurse must understand a client's value systems and beliefs. A sincere commitment to health promotion and maintenance helps clients develop independence. Effective use of the nursing process makes it possible for home health nurses to take the initiative to assess and diagnose client problems, implement appropriate therapies, and evaluate outcomes. Some agencies use the nurse as a case manager, who is the person responsible for initiating the plan of care and ensuring continuous follow-up with progress toward discharge.

Home health care nurses provide individualized care and have one-on-one contact with clients and families. They have greater autonomy in managing their own caseloads, and they help clients adapt to the plan of care and disease processes. Visits may be scheduled as frequently as twice a day, daily, twice a week, weekly, or less frequently. Nurses also help clients adjust to the influences of cultural and environmental factors and have the opportunity to develop the nurse-client relationship more fully than nurses in hospitals.

Home health nursing involves many skilled nursing services (see box on p. 51) including clinical assessment and judgment, clinical procedures, teaching skills, and the ability to coordinate and document care provided (Figure 3-2). A home health care nurse needs a broad knowledge of community resources, cultural and socioeconomic factors, family dynamics, and psychology. Writing skills that include demonstrated knowledge and application of regulatory and reimbursement guidelines are essential abilities. In most settings the home health care nurse is a generalist, one who applies nursing care skills and knowledge for clients of all ages and a wide range of health problems. However, as more technology moves into the home setting and as clients require more complicated levels of care, a need grows for specialists in home care. Agencies are beginning to

HOME HEALTH NURSING SKILLS

Wound care: Sterile dressings, debridement and irrigation of wounds, packing, assessment of drainage, assessment and culture of wounds, and instructing clients and families in wound care.
Respiratory care: Management of oxygen therapy, mechanical ventilation, and suctioning and care of tracheostomies.
Vital signs: Monitoring blood pressure, cardiopulmonary status, and instructing clients and families in pulse taking (when appropriate).
Elimination: Clients with new ostomy appliances often need assistance with irrigation and skin care procedures as well as learning to use specialized equipment. Assessment and teaching, insertion of urinary catheters, irrigation, observation for infection, and instruction of family in intermittent catheterization are also provided.
Nutrition: Assessment of nutrition and hydration status, instruction on prescribed diet, administration of tube feedings, and instructing families in tube feedings.
Rehabilitation: Instructing clients and families in the use of assistive devices, range of motion exercises, ambulation, and transfer techniques.
Medications: Instructing clients and families on medication actions, administration, and side effects. Monitoring compliance and effectiveness of prescribed medications.
Intravenous therapy: Assessment and management of dehydration, giving antibiotic medications, parenteral nutrition, blood products, and analgesic and chemotherapeutic agents.*

Modified from Corkery E: Discharge planning and home health care: what every staff nurse should know, *Orthop Nurs* 8:6, 1989.
*In the United States, many agencies require national certification offered through the Intravenous Nurses Society (INS) for nurses administering home IV therapy. These nurses are usually certified in chemotherapy.

develop specialty nursing teams in areas such as IV and pulmonary therapy, obstetrics, psychiatry, pediatrics, oncology, and diabetes care. Many larger agencies employ clinical nurse specialists to develop and manage specialty nursing programs.

Most nurses in home health care agencies are involved in many educational activities. Nurses determine client and family learning abilities and needs, develop and implement individualized teaching plans, and evaluate the success of the client in meeting learning objectives. It is always important to continue and reinforce teaching that began in the acute care setting. Often the home health nurse must adapt previously established teaching plans to the client's home environment and lifestyle. Government and private insurers pay for visits only until the client and family have had time to learn procedures. Home visits facilitate evaluation of whether clients are successfully applying new knowledge to health care practices.

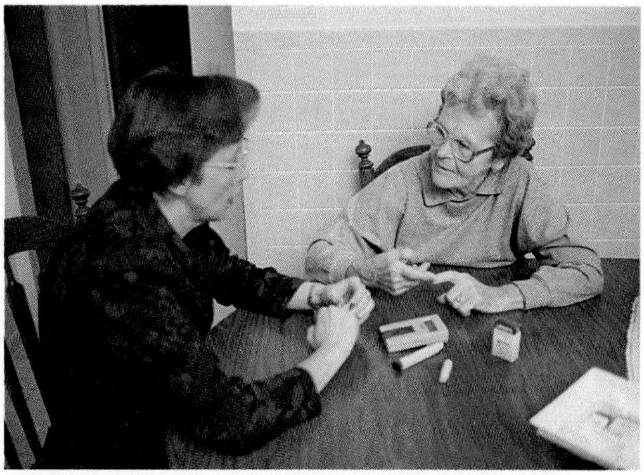

FIGURE 3-2 Nurses teach skilled procedures in the home setting.

Infection control policies and procedures are of considerable importance in home health care. Clients in need of home health care often suffer communicable diseases, require invasive medical devices, or are immunocompromised. While clients are less likely to become infected by microorganisms in their own environment, the threat arises as the nurse moves from home to home. Regulations and recommendations for accreditation and licensure specified by the Occupational Safety and Health Administration (OSHA) and the Centers for Disease Control and Prevention (CDC) are increasingly strict regarding infection control policies (Rice, 1992). This includes use of barrier protection and disposal of infectious materials.

Most home health care agencies coordinate staff educational activities, including orientation, case conferences, monthly in-service workshops, and physical assessment courses. Workshops about specialty services are also important as home care becomes more technical and intensive.

Many agencies are engaged in formalized studies to document cost effectiveness of clinical problems, staffing needs, consumer satisfaction, and quality improvement activities. These research activities will become important as competition and regulations increase and funding sources decrease.

Legal and Ethical Responsibilities

Nurses are legally able to perform independent nursing activities based on educational preparation and experience. Nurses can evaluate clients for home health care services and must provide care under the direction of a written plan of treatment signed by a physician. Home health care nurses often establish the plan of care and then collaborate with the physician. The most controversial legal issues in home health clinical practice include the following:

1. Risks associated with providing highly technical procedures such as administration of IV medication and blood products in the home
2. Legal aspects of client teaching such as liability for errors made by family care givers based on misuse of information provided by the nurse
3. Compliance with Medicare or other government home health care regulations

Because of limited and highly fragmented funding for home care, home health care nurses may need to determine whether to continue providing services when there is risk of inadequate reimbursement for services. When Medicare coverage expires, clients may need ongoing care and be unwilling or unable to pay for it. Many nurses face ethical dilemmas when torn between complying with regulations and caring for the needs of older adults, indigent, and/or chronically ill clients. The nurse must be very knowledgeable about home health care policies to provide clinical documentation that will result in optimal reimbursement for the client. Nursing managers must also be very knowledgeable about regulations and follow the legal steps necessary to overturn coverage denials when appropriate.

QUALITY IMPROVEMENT IN HOME HEALTH CARE

Many government and private regulatory agencies have established standards and guidelines for the operation and reimbursement of home health care agencies. The United States and Canadian governments have established specific reimbursement guidelines for coverage of home health services. Government agencies, specifically the Health Care Financing Administration (HCFA), distribute funds for all claims and monitor for compliance with guidelines.

Two independent organizations, the JCAHO and the Community Health Accreditation Program (CHAP), have established comprehensive standards for home health care. To receive accreditation, all hospital-based home health care agencies must meet JCAHO standards. Other organizations elect to achieve JCAHO or CHAP accreditation for quality improvement and reimbursement purposes. Most states also require licensure of home health care agencies. State guidelines follow those of Medicare but may also include additional regulations. Accreditation standards focus on documentation and case management because they affect the day-to-day practice of home health nurses.

The client's clinical record must contain comprehensive, updated care plans and detailed nursing notes from each visit. Visit reports must contain evidence that a visit was necessary and that skilled care was given (e.g., assessments that reflect medical instability, and client teaching and consultation with physicians). Homebound status, safety measures, progress toward discharge, client comprehension of instruction, and functional limitations must also be well documented.

Each client must be assigned a case manager who coordinates all aspects of care, including planning and collaboration with all home health care disciplines, community resources, and physicians. The case manager plans the client's discharge from a home health care program and implements follow-up as needed. A monthly case conference must be held on each client and followed by written documentation.

The goal of case management is to ensure the quality of interdisciplinary planning and coordination of care. The purpose of quality improvement is to ensure delivery and documentation of quality care and compliance with standards.

FUTURE TRENDS IN HOME HEALTH CARE

Experts anticipate continued growth in home health care. In the competitive managed care environment, hospitals will begin to downsize and more health care will be performed in the home. Trends in the field of home care include a change in the focus of home care to preventive care and the individual's responsibility for health (Griffith, 1987). In addition, government pressure to respond to the needs of the poor and catastrophically ill will affect reimbursement and the development of future home health care programs. Successful health restoration, rehabilitative, and palliative interventions by nurses will increasingly be used by home health nurses. Nurses need to work together to ensure that the needs of the aging population can be met effectively in caring ways.

SUMMARY

The challenge in health care today is to provide clients with appropriate services as quickly as possible. A hospital can be a foreign and threatening place. The nurse plays a key role in helping a client adjust and knowing what to expect from various health care providers. From admission through discharge, the nurse coordinates client care so that there is a smooth transition from hospital to the home or alternative health care facility. A multidisciplinary approach is needed to ensure that clients receive all available resources. Discharge planning ensures a continuum of care after the client leaves the hospital.

As more clients leave hospitals with continuing health care needs, increasing numbers receive health care in the home. Nurses assume many roles in home health care through different types of agencies. Although some aspects of nursing care in the home are the same as practiced in other health care settings, home health care nurses pay particular attention to collaboration among family members, the client, and other members of the health care team. Client independence is a primary goal. Quality improvement activities are conducted to ensure safe and effective care in the home.

KEY CONCEPTS

Admission into a hospital begins with ensuring that a client knows what to expect during the hospital stay.

Prospective reimbursement has created pressure to discharge clients as soon as possible.

Discharge planning begins when a client is admitted to a hospital.

Regulatory agencies have created standards for discharge planning.

During admission, clients are given information about their rights in making decisions about medical care, including the right to refuse treatment.

A variety of factors may indicate the need for thorough discharge planning.

A nurse should refer clients to other health care providers when it becomes apparent that the expertise of other disciplines is needed.

The ultimate outcome of discharge planning is to give clients the knowledge, skills, and resources needed to assume self-care after discharge.

Home health care is a rapidly changing field affected by many forces and trends in society.

Nursing is the essential and predominant component of home health care. Nurses hold many roles from top management to bedside clinician.

Home health care is closely regulated by government and accreditation agencies, which have a tremendous impact on the clinical practice of home health nurses.

The future of home health care nursing will be marked by rapid growth, specialization, high technology, reimbursement reform, and a change in focus to preventive care.

Discharge planning is an integral part of home health nursing.

CRITICAL THINKING ACTIVITIES

1. Mr. Garcia is a 70-year-old man with a neurogenic bladder requiring self-catheterization. His vision is poor. He lives alone and is accustomed to being very independent. He has been shown the technique of self-catheterization. Identify a nursing diagnosis and one goal, and describe your approach to teaching this client.
2. Mrs. Phillips is a 55-year-old woman newly diagnosed with diabetes. You visit her twice a week to evaluate blood glucose measurement and insulin administration. Today, her blood glucose is high, and she tells you she cannot afford her medicine. She has barely enough income to cover living expenses. Identify a nursing diagnosis and one goal and describe interventions for Mrs. Phillips.
3. Mr. Douglas is 66 years old, recovering from a stroke that has left his right side partially paralyzed. His doctor has prescribed four medications to be taken after discharge from the hospital. As the nurse, what would you want to know about Mr. Douglas in order to plan his discharge from the hospital?

References

American Hospital Association: *Patients' bill of rights,* Catalog No. 157759, 1992.

American Hospital Association: *Introduction to discharge planning for hospitals,* Chicago, 1983, American Hospital Publishing.

American Nurses Association: *Standards of nursing care for home health care practice,* Kansas City, Mo, 1986, The Association.

Cookfair JM: *Nursing process and practice in the community,* St. Louis, 1991, Mosby.

Corkery E: Discharge planning and home health care: what every staff nurse should know, *Orthop Nurs,* 8:6, 1989.

Griffith E: Homecare prophecies and predictions. I. *Home Healthcare Nurse* 5(6):10, 1987.

Hogstel MO: *Clinical manual of gerontological nursing,* St. Louis, 1992, Mosby.

Joint Commission on Accreditation of Healthcare Organizations: *Manual of hospital accreditation: 1994 standards,* Chicago, 1994, The Commission.

Rice R: *Home health nursing practice concepts and application,* St. Louis, 1992, Mosby.

Zander K: Managed care within acute care settings, design and implementation via nursing case management, *Health Care Superv* 6(2):27, 1988.

Bibliography

Bullough B, Bullough V: *Nursing in the community,* St. Louis, 1990, Mosby.

Farren E: Discharge planning: quality care: financial savings, *Nursing Health Care: The Supplement,* New York, 1990, National League for Nursing Pub No. 41-2365.

Fredriks CMA: The functional status and utilization of care of elderly people living at home, *J Community Health* 15:5, 1990.

Gordon M: *Manual of nursing diagnosis,* St. Louis, 1993, Mosby.

Handy CM: Home care of patients with technically complex nursing needs, *Nurs Clin North Am* 23(2):315, 1988.

Jacobson JM: Nursing's response to the aging population, *Home Healthcare Nurse* 8:3, 1990.

Kim MJ, McFarland GK, McLane AM: *Pocket guide to nursing diagnoses,* ed 5, St. Louis, 1993, Mosby.

Mitchell MK, Storfield JL, editors: *Standards of excellence for home care organizations: Community Health Accreditation Program (CHAP),* New York, 1989, National League for Nursing.

Ruffing-Rahal MA: Rationale and design for health promotion with older adults, *Pub Health Nurs* 8:4, 1991.

Tripp SL: Health maintenance, health promotion: is there a difference, *Pub Health Nurs* 9:3, 1992.

4

Stress, Adaptation, and Coping

OBJECTIVES

Mastery of content in this chapter will enable the student to:

- Define the key terms listed.
- Describe the five components of adaptation.
- Describe the three phases of the general adaptation syndrome.
- Discuss task-oriented behaviors that are responses to stress.
- Discuss the most common ego-defense mechanisms that are responses to stress.
- Discuss the effects of prolonged stress.
- Discuss the methods of data collection as they pertain to assessing a client under stress.
- Describe stress management techniques beneficial for coping with stress.
- Discuss the process of crisis intervention.
- List three appropriate NANDA-approved nursing diagnoses related to stress.
- Develop a nursing care plan for clients experiencing stress.
- Discuss how stress in the workplace can affect the nurse.

KEY TERMS

adaptation
alarm reaction
burnout
crisis intervention
developmental crises
ego-defense mechanisms
exhaustion stage
"flight-or-fight" response
general adaptation syndrome (GAS)
homeostasis
inflammatory response
local adaptation syndrome (LAS)
mind-body interaction
reflex pain response
resistance stage
situational crisis
stress
stressors
task-oriented behaviors

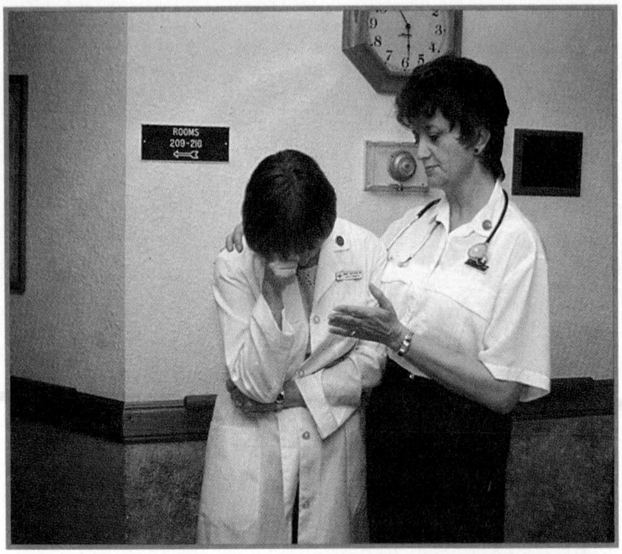

Every person experiences various kinds of stress throughout life. Stress can provide the stimulus for change and growth. In this respect, some stress can be positive. However, too much stress can result in poor judgment, physical and mental illness, and inability to cope with the stressor.

The term **stress** is derived from the Latin word *stringere,* which means "to draw tight" (Skeat, 1958). Claude Bernard, in 1867, was one of the first physiologists to recognize the potential consequences of stress for an organism. He proposed that changes in the internal and external environments disrupted the functioning of an organism. Thus it is essential for an organism to adapt to a stressor to survive. In 1920 Walter Cannon introduced the term *homeostasis* to describe how an organism successfully responds to stress. Cannon studied mechanisms that organisms use to adapt to stress and to maintain a balance, homeostasis, within the internal environment.

Hans Selye developed a biochemical model of stress, the general adaptation syndrome (GAS). The GAS model clearly describes the reactions of the human body during a stress response. Selye also introduced the concept of stressors, internal or external stimuli that cause stress (Selye, 1976). Selye's research into stress and stressors is the primary focus of this chapter. His model applies to all areas of nursing practice. For instance, when planning care for an individual with a fractured arm, the nurse must address the physical and emotional needs of the client. In addition to the obvious physical care required, consideration must also be given to the stress associated with the client's alteration in life-style. Life-style changes may include inability to work and caring for needs of self and family.

(Courtesy Michael S. Clement, MD, Mesa, Ariz.)

CONCEPTS OF STRESS AND ADAPTATION

Stress and Stressors

Unless a person is able to adapt to or cope with the effects of stress, illness can result. Stress threatens a person's physiological and psychological equilibrium. This equilibrium is called homeostasis.

A stressor can be classified as any event, individually interpreted, as either negative or positive. Being diagnosed with a chronic illness is a stressor that can threaten a client's well-being. Stressors can be classified as internal or external. Internal stressors (e.g., a fever, a condition such as pregnancy or menopause, or an emotion such as guilt) originate inside a person. External stressors (e.g., a marked change in environmental temperature, a change in family or social role, or peer rejection) originate outside a person.

Homeostasis

Homeostasis is the body's tendency to maintain a relative state of equilibrium in the body's internal environment. Homeostasis is not the same as *stasis,* a state of absolute nonchange. Our bodily systems continually need to adapt to changes. Throughout life, a person encounters many stressors that challenge the internal homeostatic environment. To adapt to these changes, adequate physiological and psychological ways of coping are essential.

Physiologically, homeostasis is maintained by controlling body mechanisms. The body makes adjustments in heart rate, respiratory rate, blood pressure, temperature, fluid and electrolyte balances, hormone secretions, and level of consciousness. These adjustments are directed at maintaining physiological homeostasis. Psychologically, homeostasis is maintained by cognitive, emotional, and behavioral means such as problem solving, general outlook on life, and a person's hardiness to face stressors.

When a person consciously acknowledges an unmet physiological need, deliberate actions can be taken to meet the need. When a nurse realizes fatigue is due to the demands of the job, the nurse can then offset this by planning time for rest and relaxation. However, homeostasis mostly involves automatic adjustments by the body. Homeostatic mechanisms also function through a process of negative feedback. This is a process by which the controlling mechanism senses an abnormal state and makes an adaptive response to return the state to normal. In this way, homeostatic mechanisms compensate for abnormal conditions.

Major homeostatic mechanisms are controlled by the medulla oblongata, the reticular formation, and the pituitary gland.

The medulla oblongata controls vital functions such as heart rate, blood pressure, and respiration that are necessary for survival. Impulses traveling to and from the medulla oblongata can increase or decrease these vital functions.

The reticular formation, a small cluster of neurons in the brain stem and spinal cord, also controls vital functions but continuously monitors the physiological status of the body through connections with sensory and motor tracts.

The pituitary gland, a small gland attached to the hypothalamus, supplies hormones that control vital functions. The pituitary gland produces hormones necessary for adaptation to stresses (e.g., adrenocorticotrophic hormone [ACTH]), as well as growth hormone. In addition, the pituitary gland regulates the secretion of thyroid, gonadal, and parathyroid hormones. Hormone secretion is normally regulated by a feedback mechanism that continuously monitors hormone levels in the blood. When hormone levels drop, the pituitary gland receives a message to increase hormone secretion.

When hormone levels rise, the pituitary gland decreases hormone production. In a person with an illness or injury, however, the mechanisms may be unable to maintain homeostasis.

Limitations of Homeostatic Control

Homeostatic body mechanisms work through complex relationships among the nervous system, hormone levels, and other body systems to maintain equilibrium. However, homeostatic mechanisms provide only short-term control over the body's equilibrium. Thus illness, injury, or prolonged stress can decrease the adaptive capacity of homeostatic functions. Decreased functioning can result in continued but inadequate homeostatic control or breakdown of the feedback mechanism that allows control. In either situation, the result is illness or death.

In severe stress situations (e.g., traumatic blood loss), the pulse increases to continue vascular perfusion. As this situation continues, however, the adaptive response deteriorates and functioning declines.

Adaptation

Adaptation is the process of change that occurs as a person responds to stress. Because stress is inevitable, the need for adequate adaptation is imperative.

An adaptive response occurs when a stimulus from the internal or external environment threatens a person's well-being. Thus adaptation is an attempt to maintain optimal functioning through physiological and coping mechanisms. A stressor that stimulates adaptation may be short term such as a fever or long term such as paralysis of a limb. To function optimally, a person must be able to adapt to these demands or changes effectively.

Like an individual, families or groups may need to adapt to a stressor. Family adaptation is the process by which a family maintains a balance so it can fulfill its purposes and tasks, deal with stress, and promote the growth of individual members. Successful family adaptation depends on effective communication skills, mutual respect for all members, adequate resources for adaptation, and previous experience with stressors.

The adaptive response of a group is similar to that of a family. Groups vary according to purpose, size, and complexity. When a group encounters a stressor, it must adapt, usually by some type of change in tasks or purpose. Such change maintains an equilibrium within the group.

Components of Human Adaptation

In understanding how a person adapts, the following components of adaptation need to be evaluated.

Physiological Adaptation. Physiological adaptation is the process by which the body responds to a stressor to maintain functioning compatible with survival. A physiological response to stress may be limited to a particular body area or may involve the entire body.

Psychosocial Adaptation. Emotional adaptation involves using psychological coping mechanisms that defend the client in the presence of stress. Although every client has a different personality, basic forms of psychological adaptation are common (McNett, 1989). Within a client's personality is a level of hardiness. The research findings of Maddi and Kobasa (1991) indicate that a sense of commitment, control, and challenge found in early life are the marks of hardiness.

Developmental Adaptation. The developmental component includes not only cognitive development and education but also perceptions of other people and the world in general, problem-solving ability, and communication patterns. Developmental adaptive responses to stress include activities that involve gathering information, solving problems, and communicating. Developmental adaptation can be strongly influenced by emotions. Helping a client to adapt emotionally can lead to more effective developmental adaptation.

Nurses are often in a unique position to assist clients in this way. As seen in Erikson's stage of trust versus mistrust, if this stage is not adequately accomplished the person will have difficulty formulating relationships in later life.

Sociocultural Adaptation. Everyone has social relationships with others. The social network may consist of family members, co-workers, and peers. This group may provide formal or informal psychological support to assist a person adapting to stress. The social component is often closely interrelated with the other components of adaptation.

A client unable to cope emotionally with stress, for example, may withdraw from contact with people who could assist in adaptation. On the other hand, when faced with emotional overload, a person experiencing excessive stress may erect a psychological barrier that enables continued functioning with minimal external distractions (Mitchell and Bray, 1990). Often times nurses need to put up psychological barriers while working. Regardless of the stressors experienced at home, the nurse needs to put these issues aside in order to stay focused on clients' needs.

Spiritual Adaptation. The spiritual component can include beliefs about a supreme being, a feeling of oneness with nature and the world, and a positive sense of life's meaning and purpose. The nurse needs to respect the spiritual beliefs of others and address this during the nursing assessment. These beliefs or attitudes can be powerful resources for adapting to stress as it relates to an illness (see Chapter 17).

OVERVIEW OF THE STRESS RESPONSE

Historically, research was focused on the physiological responses to stress. However, recently more emphasis has been placed on psychological and behavioral responses that are also important to understanding the stress response. When stress occurs, a person uses emotional and physical energy to respond and adapt. The amount of energy required and the effectiveness of the attempt to adapt depends on the intensity, scope, and duration of the stressor and on the number of other stressors present.

Factors Influencing the Response to Stressors

The response to a stressor depends on the individual person and on the nature of the stressor. The nature of the stressor involves the following factors, each influencing how a person responds:

1. **Intensity.** A person may perceive the intensity or magnitude of a stressor as minimal, severe, or somewhere in between. The greater the magnitude of the stressor, the greater the stress response.
2. **Scope.** The range in which stress encompasses a person's total being. The greater the scope of a stressor, the greater the stress response.
3. **Duration.** The duration of stressors varies. The greater the duration, the greater the stress response.
4. **Number and nature of other stressors present.** The presence of and the types of stressors present affect the client's response. An increase in presence of multiple stressors, the greater the stress response.

Physiological Component

The two forms of physiological response to stress are the local adaptation syndrome (LAS) and the general adaptation syndrome (GAS) (Figure 4-1). Through effective assessment skills, the nurse can document to what extent the syndromes are taking place.

Local Adaptation Syndrome. The **local adaptation syndrome (LAS)** is a response of body tissue, an organ, or a part of the body to the stress of trauma, illness, or other physiological change. All forms of the LAS share similar characteristics. The response is localized (not involving entire body systems), and it is a short-term adaptive response. The **reflex pain response,** for example, is a localized response of the central nervous system to the stimulus of pain (see Chapter 26). The reflex pain response is an adaptive response and protects the tissue from further damage. The response involves a sensory receptor, sensory nerve to the spinal cord, connector neuron within the spinal cord, motor nerve from the spinal cord, and effector muscle. An example would be a person's unconscious reflex of removing a hand from a hot surface.

Another LAS, the **inflammatory response,** is stimulated by trauma or infection. The inflammatory response localizes the inflammation. This prevents the spread of the infection and promotes wound healing. It may produce localized pain, swelling, heat, redness, and changes in functioning. It occurs in three phases. The first involves changes in cells and the circulatory system. When trauma occurs, there is an initial narrowing of blood vessels at the site of injury to control bleeding. This narrowing occurs only when trauma causes a break in the skin and underlying blood vessels. Then histamine is released at the site, increasing blood flow to the area and the number of white blood cells to combat infection. The release of kinins, which increase capillary permeability to permit the flow of proteins, fluid, and leukocytes to the site, occurs almost simultaneously with the release of histamine. At this point, the localized blood flow decreases, keeping leukocytes in the area of injury to fight infection.

The second phase of the inflammatory response involves the release of exudate from the wound. Exudate is a combination of fluid, cells, and other substances produced in the area of injury. The type and amount vary from injury to injury and person to person. Exudate is usually released at the site of injury, which may be a cut, laceration, or surgical incision.

The last phase is the repair of tissue by regeneration or scar formation. Regeneration replaces damaged cells by identical or similar cells. Scar formation replaces original tissue but is not functional. The inflammatory response indicates the body is adapting to a local injury. Nursing's responsibility is to note signs of the inflammatory response such as increased white blood cell count, increased temperature, increased pulse and respirations, and swelling, redness, pain, and warmth to

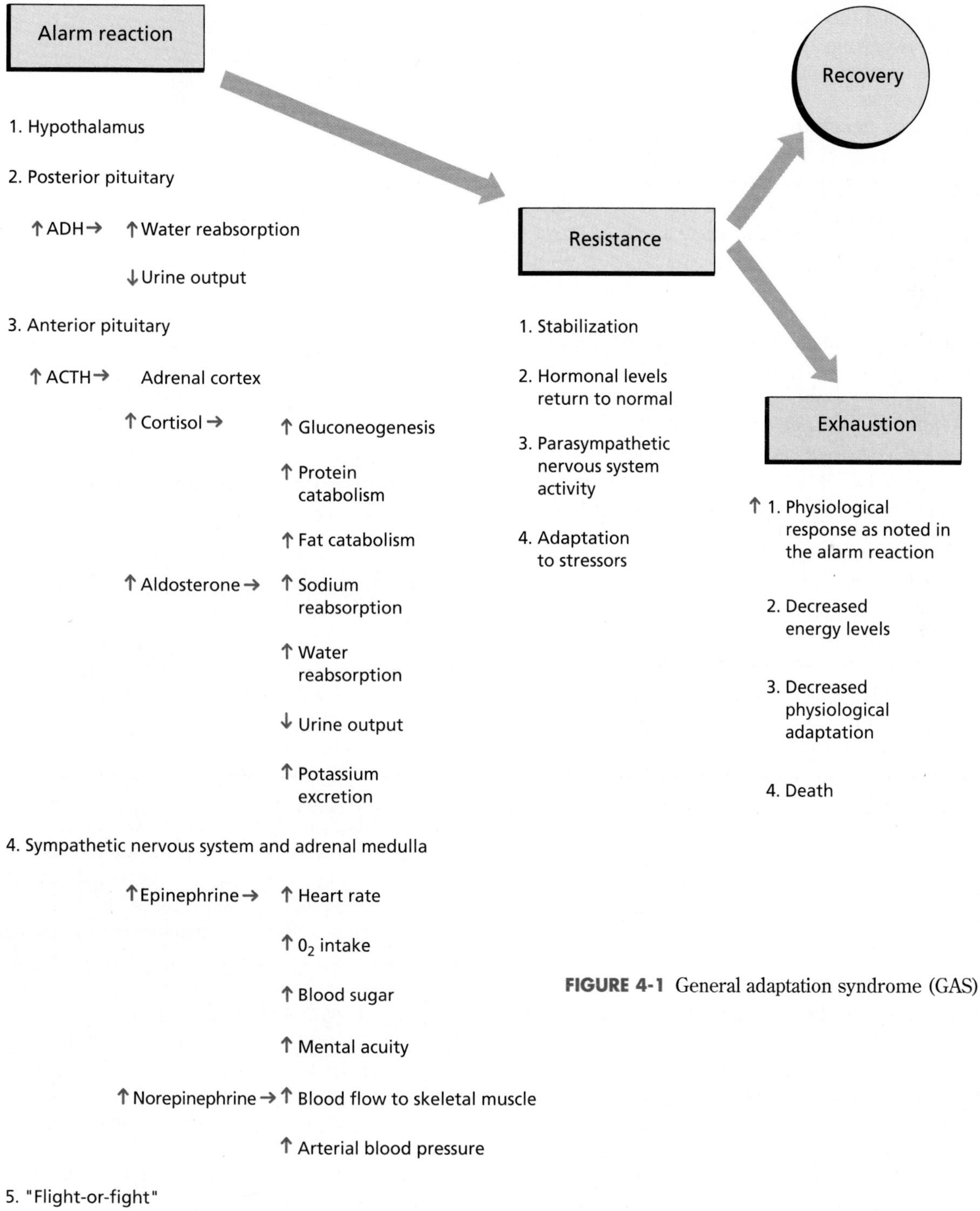

FIGURE 4-1 General adaptation syndrome (GAS).

touch in involved area. During adaptation the inflammatory response protects the body from infection and promotes wound healing.

General Adaptation Syndrome. The **general adaptation syndrome (GAS)** is a physiological response of the whole body to stress and involves several body systems, primarily the autonomic nervous system and the endocrine system. Internal bleeding from an automobile accident can trigger the GAS.

The GAS consists of the alarm reaction, the resistance stage, and the exhaustion stage (see Figure 4-1). Although everyone generally goes through these stages, the duration and effectiveness of each vary from person to person.

The **alarm reaction** is the mobilization of the defense mechanisms of the body or mind to cope with the stressor. Hormone levels rise to increase blood volume and thereby prepare the person to act. Other hormones are released to increase blood sugar levels to make energy available for adaptation. Increased levels of other hormones (epinephrine and norepinephrine) result in increased heart rate, increased blood flow to muscles, increased oxygen intake, and greater mental alertness.

This extensive hormonal activity prepares the person for the **"flight-or-fight" response,** in which cardiac output, oxygen intake, and respiratory rate increase, the pupils of the eyes dilate to produce a greater visual field, the heart rate increases for more muscular and other energy, and other changes occur to prepare the person to act (Figure 4-2). With the increased mental energy and alertness that result, the person is prepared to choose to flee or to fight the stressor.

During the alarm reaction the person is faced with a specific stressor. The physiological response is extensive, involving major systems of the body, and may last from 1 minute to many hours. If the stressor is extreme or remains for a long time, there may be a threat to the person's life. If the stressor is still present after the initial alarm reaction, the person progresses to the second stage, resistance.

During the **resistance stage** the body stabilizes, and hormone levels, heart rate, blood pressure, and cardiac output return to normal. During this stage the person attempts to adapt to the stressor. If the stress can be resolved, the body repairs any damage that may have occurred. However, if the stressor remains, as in continued blood loss, debilitating disease, or long-term severe mental illness, and the person is unable to adapt, he or she enters the third stage, exhaustion.

The **exhaustion stage** occurs when the body can no longer resist the stress and when the energy necessary to maintain adaptation is depleted. The physiological response is intensified, but the person's energy level is compromised, and adaptation to the stressor diminishes. The body is unable to defend itself against the impact of the stressor, physiological regulation diminishes, and, if the stress continues, death may result.

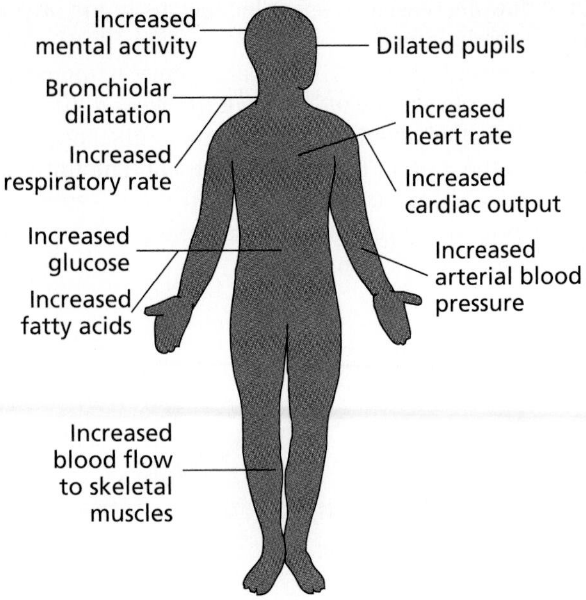

FIGURE 4-2 Physical assessment findings of flight-or-fight response.

Psychological Component

Healthy individuals develop psychological adaptive behaviors to cope with stressors. These behaviors are acquired through learning and experience. Psychological adaptive behaviors, also referred to as "coping mechanisms," are efforts directed at stress management. Such mechanisms can be **task-oriented behaviors,** involving the use of direct problem-solving techniques to cope with the threats, or they can be **ego-defense mechanisms,** which regulate emotional distress and thus protect a person from anxiety and stress (see box on p. 61).

Psychological adaptive behaviors can be constructive or destructive. These behaviors affect reality orientation, problem-solving abilities, personality, and, in severe circumstances, ability to function and level of health (Egger, 1987). Constructive behaviors help an individual to accept the challenge to resolve the conflict causing stress. Destructive behaviors do not help a person to cope with a stressor. For example, a woman experiencing stress related to her new parenting role who actively seeks out resources to help her adapt to this new role would be using constructive behavior. However, if she did not address the reasons for experiencing the stress and the stress continued, she could eventually neglect her needs in addition to the infant's needs. This would be an example of destructive behavior.

PSYCHOLOGICAL ADAPTIVE BEHAVIORS

TASK-ORIENTED BEHAVIORS

Attack behavior.

Acting to remove or overcome a stressor or to satisfy a need.

Withdrawal behavior.

Removing oneself physically or emotionally from the stressor.

Compromise behavior.

Changing the usual method of operating, substituting goals, or omitting the satisfaction of needs to meet other needs or to avoid stress.

EGO-DEFENSE MECHANISMS

Compensation.

Making up for a deficiency in one aspect of self-image by strongly emphasizing a feature considered an asset.

Conversion.

Unconsciously repressing an anxiety-producing emotional conflict and transforming it into nonorganic symptoms.

Denial.

Avoiding emotional conflicts by refusing to acknowledge consciously anything that might cause intolerable emotional pain.

Displacement.

Transferring emotions, ideas, or wishes from a stressful situation to a less anxiety-producing substitute.

Identification.

Patterning behavior after another person and assuming that person's qualities, characteristics, and actions.

Regression.

Coping with a stressor through actions and behaviors associated with an earlier developmental period.

Rationalization.

Contrived excuse for behavior.

Projection.

Noting in others one's own unacceptable behaviors.

When dealing with the hospitalized client, the nurse must remember the client will use defense mechanisms. These should not be viewed as negative because defense mechanisms can occur naturally as a part of illness and can be useful in the healing process. For example, a certain amount of regressive behavior such as staying in bed and assuming a dependency role during hospitalization may relieve some unnecessary stress (Grainger, 1989).

Mind-body Interaction. Health care professionals are becoming aware of the relationship between psychological stress and medical illness, frequently called the **mind-body interaction.** Studies have shown the relationship between stress and disease (Newberry, Jaikins-Madden and Gerstenberger, 1991). Also the leading causes of death have shifted from infectious diseases to diseases related to life-style stressors.

The more intense and the longer the stress situation, the higher the risk for a negative health outcome. Mild stress situations such as minor daily irritations do not usually produce long-lasting physiological damage. Such situations are usually short term and isolated and are unlikely to increase the risk of illness unless a person experiences them continuously.

Moderate stress situations such as conflict with a family member last longer, from several hours to a number of days. These situations can be significant because they increase the risk of physical illness in a person with a predisposition to that illness.

Severe stress situations such as continual marital disagreements or long-term physical illness may last several weeks to several years.

CONSEQUENCES OF PROLONGED STRESS

The consequences of prolonged stress can be physical, developmental, or psychosocial.

Physical. Almost every body system can be damaged by prolonged stress. Several illnesses are closely associated with high levels of stress, including cardiovascular illness, gastrointestinal illness, and cancer. In most cases, stress causes physical changes that could lead to the development of a disease (Newberry, Jaikins-Madden and Gerstenberger, 1991). The box on p. 62 illustrates the diseases that can occur as stress becomes more intense.

Susceptibility to a disease, presence of the disease-producing agent, and the environment determine whether illness is likely to develop in a given person.

Susceptibility is linked to factors such as heredity, personality, life-style, health status, health beliefs, and health practices. Susceptibility is a more important factor in cases of diseases related to chronic stress than in cases of infectious disease.

Developmental. During any specific developmental stage a person normally faces certain characteristic tasks and engages in certain characteristic behaviors.

SYSTEMS AFFECTED BY PROLONGED STRESS

Musculoskeletal	Muscle myopathy Osteoporosis Susceptibility to fractures Slow tissue repair
Cardiovascular	Hypertension, heart damage
Gastrointestinal	Peptic ulcers, colitis, chronic diarrhea
Respiratory	Asthma, bronchitis, other respiratory conditions
Endocrine	Contributes to onset of diabetes
Immune	More susceptible to disease

Prolonged stress can interrupt or impede passage through any of the developmental stages. In extreme forms, prolonged stress can lead to a developmental crisis.

Developmental crises occur when a person is unable to complete the developmental tasks of a psychosocial stage. A developmental crisis can occur at any point in life if circumstances prevent a person from meeting the challenge of a particular stage. This type of crisis is different from situational crisis.

An infant or young child generally encounters stressors within the home. For example, an infant must learn trust through interactions with parents. However, if parental figures are absent or fail to provide the infant with the security needed to develop a sense of trust, this void can become a stressor. In later life the child may experience chronic distrust, resulting in withdrawal and limited interpersonal relationships.

The infant progressing into childhood normally develops a sense of autonomy. If parents or environmental factors prevent the child from developing autonomy, he or she may experience stress and may become overly dependent on others to meet needs. A preschool child normally develops a conscience, begins to explore his surroundings, and determines differences between males and females. The child is ashamed when caught being "bad" and wants to be reinforced when being "good."

A school-age child normally develops a sense of adequacy. Children begin to realize they can accumulate knowledge and master skills to accomplish goals, and self-esteem develops through friendships and sharing with peers.

An adolescent normally develops a strong sense of identity and at the same time has a need to be accepted by a peer group. Some of the many stressors common to this age-group include conflicts involving sexual drive and expected standards of behavior. Prolonged conflict may result in indecision and confusion, rebelliousness, depression, or anxiety. If the conflict is not resolved, it can create problems in later years.

A young adult is in transition from youthful experiences to adult responsibilities. This person must prepare for a career, for living independently, and perhaps for forming a family. Young adults may experience conflict between responsibilities to work and family and the desire to maintain an active social life. Stressors in this developmental stage include conflicts between expectations and desires.

A middle-age adult is usually involved in family building, creating a stable career, and perhaps caring for aging parents. Middle-age adults are generally able to control desires, and in some cases substitute the needs of a spouse, children, or parents for their own needs. Stress can result, however, if they feel too many responsibilities have been placed on them.

An older adult is commonly faced with adapting to family changes and perhaps to the death of a spouse. The older adult must also adjust to changes in physical appearance and physiological functioning. In addition, older adults experience the stress of decreasing social interactions as friends die or become unable to maintain contact. Retirement can often create even more stress. Prolonged fear and stress can make an older adult overly dependent, which may cause further stress on family or social relationships.

Situational crises differ from developmental crises. A **situational crisis** arises suddenly in response to an external event or conflict involving a specific circumstance. Symptoms associated with situational crises are short term and the episodes are brief but can occur suddenly at any time. Any changes such as major life events, acute physical illness, physical assault, and family crises are examples of situational crises.

Psychosocial. Psychosocial changes are a direct and sometimes obvious result of prolonged stress. A nurse can frequently observe the emotional impact of stress through changes in a client's behavior.

Stress affects emotional well-being in many ways. Everyone's personality involves a complex relationship among several factors. These include support systems, prior experience with stressors, coping mechanisms, and overall stress response. Nurses, family members, and friends should be attentive to any changes in behavior. It may often be difficult to anticipate someone's reaction to stress. However, if reactions are anticipated early, preventive measures can be taken.

Prolonged stress can reduce the ability to acquire new knowledge and skills leading to ineffective communication, problem solving, changes in "normal" roles, expectations, and practices. Severe stress may also cause an individual to reevaluate spirituality. For instance, the stress associated with an acute illness or the death of a loved one may threaten one's meaning of life and can lead to spiritual distress.

The nurse needs to be aware that many clients are being diagnosed with posttraumatic stress disorder (PTSD), which is a psychological reaction to an overwhelming traumatic event considered outside the range of normal human experiences (Blair and Hildreth, 1991). PTSD can be considered an example of the effects of prolonged stress when further intervention is necessary.

When caring for clients, nurses must be aware of the ill effects of prolonged stress. Stress not only contributes to physical illness, but it can also lead to developmental and psychosocial changes. Nurses are often able to spend time with clients and their families and friends in a variety of settings. Thus nurses can assist clients in adapting to stressors by using stress management techniques.

NURSING PROCESS

Assessment

Data Collection

When obtaining assessment data, nurses have many resources. Data collection consists of subjective and objective findings. Subjective data include the interview

INDICATORS OF STRESS

PHYSICAL	
Cardiovascular findings	Tightness of chest Increased heart rate Elevated blood pressure
Respiratory findings	Breathing difficulty Tachypnea
Neuro/endocrine findings	Headaches, migraines Fatigue, exhaustion Insomnia, sleep disturbances Feeling uncoordinated Restlessness, hyperactivity Tremors (lips, hands) Profuse sweating (palms) Dry mouth Cold hands and feet
GI/GU findings	Urinary frequency Nausea, diarrhea, vomiting Weight gain or loss more than 10 pounds Change in appetite GI bleeding Diagnostic findings Blood in stools/vomitus Elevated blood sugar
Musculoskeletal findings	Backaches, muscle aches Bruxism (clenched jaw) Slumped posture
Reproductive findings	Amenorrhea Failure to ovulate Impotency in men Loss of libido
Immunological findings	Frequent or prolonged colds/flu
PSYCHOLOGICAL	
Cognitive findings	Forgetfulness/preoccupation Denial Increased fantasy life Poor concentration Inattention to detail Orientation to past instead of present Decreased creativity Slower thinking, reactions Learning difficulties Apathy Uses path of least resistance Confusion Lower attention span Calculation difficulties Memory problems Ruminating Distressing dreams Disruption of logical thinking Blaming others
Emotional findings	Lack of motivation to get up in the morning Crying tendencies Lack of interest Irritability Isolative Diminished initiative Negative thinking Worrying Decreased involvement with others Feeling cynical
Behavioral/lifestyle findings	Change in activity level Withdrawal Suspiciousness Change in communication Change in interactions with others Increased or decreased food intake Increased smoking or alcohol intake Overly vigilant to environment Excessive humor or silence No exercise Type A personality

and health history. Objective data include physical examination, observation of behavior, and data from the medical record, as well as data from the health care team members, family members, and significant others.

With some data it is difficult to distinguish between subjective and objective data (see Chapter 7). The box on p. 63 lists important objective indicators of stress.

Subjective Findings

INTERVIEW. Throughout the interview, the nurse and client can establish a therapeutic relationship. The nurse can also gain insight into what is troubling the client. However, discussing information related to stress and its influence on the client can itself be stressful. Therefore it is wise to address this information after developing a therapeutic relationship (see Chapter 13). When a client is unable to handle a problem or situation by using prior coping strategies, a crisis can occur. Behavior tends to be disorganized, and the client may make only abortive attempts at resolving the problem (Aguilera and Messick, 1989).

To accomplish a successful interview, the nurse needs to respect the confidentiality and sensitivity of the information shared by the client. The nurse should choose an environment conducive to sharing information. The box at left lists suggestions for collecting subjective assessment data. A nurse should be cautioned to use sensitivity and judgment when phrasing the questions.

HEALTH HISTORY. The interview questions in the box at left identify stressors and how the stress manifests within a client. The health history will also evolve from these questions (see Chapter 7).

SAMPLE INTERVIEW QUESTIONS FOR GATHERING SUBJECTIVE DATA

1. In your own words, what has been the most stressful thing for you during this hospitalization?
2. When you have experienced stress in the past, how did you solve the stress?
   - Sought out reasons for those feelings
   - Blamed others
   - Withdrew from family, friends, or co-workers
   - Used distraction
     - Examples of positive distractors (music, exercise, relaxation techniques)
     - Examples of negative distractors (alcohol and drug usage, smoking, changes in eating habits)
   - Talked with others (spouse, clergy, friends, support groups)
3. Describe any stress-related problems for which you have been treated in the past.
4. Describe any recent major life changes (within the last year) related to any of the following.
   - Health (physical and mental)
   - Family
   - Life-style habits
   - Changes in daily activities (eating, sleeping, getting up to go to work)
   - Supportive network
   - Work (Do you enjoy your work?)
   - Financial/legal problems
   - Recent losses or trauma
5. Can you rate how stressful these major life changes have been on a scale of 1 to 10 (from least stressful to most stressful)?
6. How many people are you responsible for (elderly parents, children, other dependents)?
7. Tell me how you spend your leisure time. Are these activities done alone or with a group of friends?
8. How often do you take vacations or mental health days off?

Objective Findings

OBSERVATIONS

PHYSICAL EXAMINATION (see Chapter 16).

MENTAL STATUS EXAMINATION. While conducting the interview and health history, the nurse should observe client behaviors. The nurse must decide whether this behavior is appropriate or inappropriate to the existing situation. A review of the client's mental status may also reveal the effects of stress. The box below lists suggested observations for collecting data on mental status.

SAMPLE OBSERVATIONS FOR COLLECTING MENTAL STATUS DATA

1. Have there been changes in appearance (dress, grooming, posture)?
2. Have there been changes in behavior (eye contact, degree of physical activity)?
3. Have there been changes in speech (rate, tone, degree of spontaneity)?
4. Have there been changes in perception (awareness and interpretation of environment)?
5. Have there been changes in thought patterns (bizarre content, suicidal or homicidal obsessions, illogical thought processes)?
6. Have there been changes in affect (flat, labile, inappropriate)?
7. Have there been changes in mood (sad, happy, angry, calm, depressed, frightened)?
8. Have there been changes in intellectual functioning (orientation, recall, concentration, language, memory, insight, judgment)?

Modified from Lewis, S, et al.: Manual of psychosocial nursing interventions: Promoting mental health in medical surgical settings, Philadelphia, 1989, WB Saunders.

The nurse should also note if the client is using any defense mechanisms as a shield from the stressors (e.g., a client diagnosed with bone cancer insisting that he is experiencing arthritic pain). This client is using the defense mechanisms of denial and rationalization to minimize the severity of the problem as a way of coping in a maladaptive way.

Medical Record. The client's medical record or chart has valuable information that can assist the nurse in completing a nursing assessment (e.g., diagnostic tests can validate whether a client is experiencing a stress-related illness).

Other Resources. Additional assessment data can be obtained from other health care team members, family members, friends, and significant others. They may supplement information or verify information provided by the client. For the very young or for unconscious or confused clients, significant others can provide important data. This information helps to address the client's needs comprehensively in addition to monitoring the effectiveness of the care plan.

Nursing Diagnosis

After reviewing the subjective data, such as reports of increased fatigue, and objective findings, such as elevated pulse rate, the nurse must cluster the data through critical thinking. Wilkinson (1992) states that critical thinking skills are used throughout the nursing process. For example, when clustering data the nurse utilizes critical thinking to distinguish relevant data from irrelevant data and to determine patterns and relationships formulating accurate nursing diagnoses.

Nursing diagnoses as they relate to the client experiencing stress need to be recognized early so that prolonged stress does not result. However, it is sometimes difficult to differentiate among some of the nursing diagnoses. For example, Bruss (1988) illustrates the difficulty of distinguishing between hopelessness and powerlessness, because they share many of the same defining characteristics such as pessimism, decreased social interaction, or decreased problem solving.

Actual nursing diagnoses must be supported by appropriate defining characteristics from the assessment data. When existing data are not apparent, relevant risk factors and client circumstances, along with anticipated changes or needs, should prompt the nurse to consider potential nursing diagnoses.

For any given nursing diagnosis, there can be several "related to" factors. For example, NANDA's nursing diagnosis of "powerlessness" may have several factors related to relinquishing control to others or to the failure to be consulted on health care decisions. Recognizing the appropriate "related to" factor will indicate what type of nursing interventions are appropriate (e.g., providing the client with increased opportunity to be involved in health care decisions or providing the client with choices). After formulating the nursing diagnosis, the nurse is then prepared to develop a care plan (see box above).

NURSING DIAGNOSES FOR STRESS

Activity intolerance
Altered growth and development
Fatigue
Hopelessness
Ineffective family coping: compromised or disabled
Ineffective individual coping
Potential for injury
Sleep pattern disturbance
Anxiety
Fear

Planning

Following nursing diagnoses, the nurse initiates a care plan individualized for the client. Specific developmental considerations need to be addressed with some clients (such as the very young or the older adult). Together, the client and nurse develop realistic, measurable outcomes designed to assist the client in coping with the stressor.

Overall general goals for clients experiencing stress include the following:

Goal: Client verbalizes feelings associated with the stress-producing situation.

Outcomes

- Client able to state feelings of frustration, anger, sadness, etc.
- Client able to identify changes in behavior (e.g., decreased socialization, poor hygiene practices)

Goal: Client is able to identify potential stressors.

Outcomes

- Client able to list prior stressful situations
- Client able to list possible stressors in present situations

Goal: Client develops problem-solving techniques to address and minimize the effects of stress.

Outcomes

- Client able to list at least two methods for reducing each identified stressor

SAMPLE NURSING CARE PLAN
Ineffective Individual Coping

ASSESSMENT

Clinical scenario: Mrs. Kline is a 52-year-old woman who was *widowed 2 months ago.* She has three children, all of whom live out of town. Her contact with her children is consistent; they talk on the phone weekly. She visits each family for 2 weeks during the year. Mrs. Kline *describes herself as lonely.* She has *not made any attempt to meet new friends and has avoided social contact with old friends.* She has *withdrawn from all church and volunteer activities.* When asked how she spends her days, she describes herself as *continually crying, looking outside, and wishing that her husband was there* to take care of her. Throughout the interview, Mrs. Kline *did not smile or cry;* she *continually looked down in her lap.* Although attractive, she wore no makeup, her hair was styled nicely, and she was dressed in black.

NURSING DIAGNOSIS

Ineffective individual coping related to adjustment to widowhood

PLANNING

Goal	Expected Outcomes
Client reports improving adjustment to widowhood.	Client verbalizes feelings of loss, fear, and helplessness. Client acknowledges the relationship between her behavior and stress. Client reports fewer crying spells. Client selects effective relaxation techniques. Client demonstrates an increase in social interactions. Client returns to church or volunteer activities.

IMPLEMENTATION

Steps	Rationale
1. Provide client with information on support groups for newly widowed persons.	Support groups provide common bond with client because stressors are similar and potential solutions are more realistic. In addition, support groups can provide social outlets (Stewart, 1989).
2. Teach client progressive relaxation exercises.	Performing relaxation exercises has a recuperative effect that normalizes physical, mental, and emotional processes (Davis, Eshelman, and McKay, 1988).
3. Assist client in resuming social contact with friends. Begin with friends with whom client is more comfortable.	Strong social supports can provide a realistic cure for loneliness and social isolation (Newberry, Jaikins-Madden, and Gertstenberger, 1991).
4. Encourage verbalization of feelings.	The more specific and concrete the client can be about the stress, the better she will be able to deal with reducing the stress response (Schultz and Dark, 1990).
5. Within calm environment, explore with client ways to deal with stress.	Stressful behavior can be escalated by external stimuli (Schultz and Dark, 1990).
6. Teach client how to recognize early signs of stress.	Early detection of signs and symptoms enables client to resolve stress in a shorter period of time (Schultz and Dark, 1990).
7. Share observations of stressful behaviors with client (may include facial expressions, appearance, and eye contact).	Client may be unaware of relationship between stress and behavior (Schultz and Dark, 1990).

EVALUATIVE MEASURES

Ask client if relaxation exercises reduce crying episodes.
Observe client for positive changes in affect: increased eye contact, smiling, wearing make-up.
Ask client about number and type of social activities.
Ask client to discuss feelings associated with widowhood.

Client evaluates each method of stress reduction

Goal: Client returns to prior level of functioning.

Outcomes

Client maintains an adequate balance of rest and sleep

Client achieves appropriate level of social interaction and daily activities

The nurse must set priorities in the presence of several nursing diagnoses. Stress can magnify the outcome of a physical problem. Therefore the nurse must pay equal attention to both psychosocial and physiological findings. For example, a client's fears and anxieties resulting from a new diagnosis need to be addressed before the nurse can expect the client to assume primary responsibility for daily health care. The client's involvement enhances the probability of a successful outcome.

Other health care team members and family members can help in developing a care plan. Consulting with other health care team members or family members can result in a more concise and comprehensive approach to the care plan. This comprehensive approach is used throughout the client's hospitalization and is incorporated into the discharge plan (see box on p. 66 for a sample nursing care plan regarding stress).

Implementation

Stress is inevitable and must be integrated into the type of care planned for clients of all ages. To implement nursing care, the nurse must respect the individualized nature of the stress and the client's response to it. Therefore intervention strategies must be selected based on the client's unique characteristics as they pertain to level of health, motivation, sources of support, and prior coping experiences.

Because of the increase of the hospitalized older adult population, more emphasis needs to be placed on the older adult client (see box at right). Because older adults increasingly suffer more losses, they often see situations negatively when more positive interpretations are valid (Zerhusen, Boyle, and Wilson, 1991). The nurse should help these clients replace the negative perceptions with more valid positive ones.

GERONTOLOGIC NURSING PRACTICE

Gerontological nursing practices for the client experiencing stress might include:

- Older adults commonly suffer from depression. Suicide rates increase with age, especially among the ill and older, single white males (Mellick, Buckwalter, and Stolley, 1992). Impaired adjustment may occur because of an increase in the number of losses older adults experience.
- Older adults are often taking many prescribed medications. Many commonly prescribed medications for stress and anxiety should be used with caution. Obtaining a careful drug history is necessary because many drugs can mimic depression. Impaired kidney and liver function can lead to medication toxicity.
- Older adults often have alterations in mental alertness. Reasons for decreased mental alertness should be investigated to determine whether they are physiological or symptomatic of prolonged stress.
- Older adults are at increased risk for suicide. Starvation, accidental overdose, and noncompliance with treatment regimens can be subtle signs of suicide.
- Older adults react individually to aging. Do not assume a client over a certain age will become senile, dependent, or no longer sexually active.
- Older adults can benefit from comprehensive discharge planning. For a successful transition from hospital to home, the nurse can minimize the client's stress by gathering a good information base to use for a successful discharge outcome (Naylor and Shaid, 1991).
- Older adults have specific information needs. The nurse should focus on the following client information needs (Naylor and Shaid, 1991): managing present health problem, providing access to community resources, teaching about specific surgical and diagnostic procedures, promoting health, and preventing future health problems.

From Kaufmann N. In Rogers-Seidl F: *Geriatric nursing care plan*, St. Louis, 1991, Mosby.

Health Promotion for Clients and Nurses

To help promote health, individuals should anticipate stressors. Nurses can provide anticipatory guidance before the stress leads to a crisis. Nurses also need to nurture themselves while attending to the needs of the client. However, according to the ANA statistics, a frightening number of practicing nurses are chemically impaired. This is a problem that all nurses need to address for client safety.

Health-enhancing habits can reduce the impact of stress on physical and mental health. These common sense approaches often provide a sound basis for effective, low-stress living. They include regular exercise, good nutrition and diet, adequate rest, a successful support system, and effective time management.

Regular Exercise. A regular exercise program improves muscle tone and posture, controls weight, reduces tension, and promotes relaxation. In addition, exercise reduces the risk of cardiovascular disease and improves cardiopulmonary functioning.

Clients who have a history of a chronic illness, who are at risk for developing an illness, or who are older than 35 years of age should begin a physical exercise program only after discussing the plan with a physician. In general, for a fitness program to have positive physical effects, a person should exercise at least three times a week for 30 to 40 minutes.

Anyone who follows an exercise program should use warm-up exercises before vigorous exercise to stimulate blood flow to the muscles and increase flexibility. Warm-up exercises reduce the risk of damage to the musculoskeletal system. Similarly, after vigorous exercise a person should do cool-down exercises rather than stop abruptly. These allow the cardiovascular, pulmonary, musculoskeletal, and metabolic systems to gradually return to their resting functional states.

Nutrition and Diet. Nutrition and exercise are closely related because diet provides the body with fuel for activity and because increased exercise improves circulation and the delivery of nutrients to body tissues. Everyone is encouraged to maintain a normal weight according to standard ranges for sex, age, and body build. In addition to avoiding overeating or undereating, a person should be aware of the nutritional quality of the food eaten. Too much caffeine, salt, fat, sugar, or deficiencies in vitamins, minerals, and nutrients can upset the body's metabolic functioning. This almost always intensifies stress.

Poor dietary habits can exacerbate a stress response and make a person irritable, hyperactive, and anxious, thus impairing the ability to meet personal, family, and job responsibilities. In general, dietary goals should be based on the following objectives:

1. Reduce the consumption of salt, refined sugar, fat, caffeine, cholesterol, and triglycerides. Read food labels closely to note high levels of salt or sugar that may be hidden.
2. Increase the consumption of fruit, vegetables, and whole grains.
3. Increase intake of poultry and fish while reducing red meat intake and overall consumption of meat.
4. Substitute low-fat or non-fat products for whole milk products.
5. Try to maintain appropriate calorie intake based on energy demands.

Rest. An established, habitual pattern of sufficient rest and sleep is also important to stress management. A client experiencing stress should be encouraged to allow enough time for rest and sleep. Rest and sleep refresh the body and help the client to relax mentally and to be able to use problem-solving methods to deal with stressors and resolve conflicts. A client may need specific help in learning to relax to fall asleep.

Support Systems. A support system of family, friends, and colleagues who will listen and offer advice and emotional support benefits a client experiencing stress. There are many support groups available to individuals such as those sponsored by the American Heart Association or the American Cancer Society. Support systems can reduce stress reactions and promote physical and mental well-being. Thus a client experiencing stress should be encouraged to expand social and personal contacts. Nurses can use many methods, such as therapeutic communication skills, teaching techniques, and supportive behavior, to help clients to build support systems.

Time Management. A person who uses time efficiently generally experiences less stress related to social, family, and job activities. For some clients, time management techniques may include developing a list of tasks to be performed in order of priority (Jones and Kovalcik, 1988). Another time management measure is learning to say "no" to potential disruptions and some requested tasks. Time management may also include realistic scheduled appointments to avoid undue haste.

Health Restoration

When clients are handling stress ineffectively, the nurse is often the first to identify or to address this behavior. The nurse can also help the client adopt restorative activities through stress management techniques (see client teaching box below). These techniques can also be useful to the client as future coping strategies. However, if there is an immediate need for stress re-

CLIENT TEACHING FOR STRESS

General practices for teaching a client experiencing stress might include:

Realize mild stress can be useful and productive.

Mild anxiety can enhance motivation on a daily basis.

Be aware of your own feelings and responses as they relate to stress.

Respect client's perception of stressors by being nonjudgmental.

Remain calm in approach to client to enhance client's sense of security.

Select stress reduction strategies appropriate to individual client and client's needs.

duction, crisis intervention techniques may be required. Before using any method of stress management, however, a nurse assesses the client to understand the amount of stress and the coping mechanisms present.

Other more sophisticated techniques for stress reduction require advanced education and training and should be implemented by experienced nurses or other providers. These techniques include imagery and visualization, biofeedback and autogenic training, muscular relaxation techniques, music therapy, use of humor, and assertiveness training. The nurse may need to consult other health care providers if any of these approaches are outside the nurse's expertise (Davis, Eshelman, and McKay, 1988).

Imagery and Visualization. Emile Cové popularized the belief that a person can significantly reduce stress with imagination. Willing yourself into a relaxed state allows one to visualize a relaxing, peaceful setting.

Biofeedback and Autogenic Training. Autogenic training is a systematic program that teaches individuals how to use their own body and mind in responding quickly and effectively to verbal commands, which will eventually return the body to a balanced state. Autogenic training is used in conjunction with biofeedback. Biofeedback monitors muscle and skin responses as indicators of a person's state of relaxation.

Progressive Muscle Relaxation. In the presence of anxiety-provoking thoughts and events, a common physiological symptom is muscle tension. Physiological tension will be diminished through progressive muscle relaxation.

Music Therapy. For some individuals, music can be beneficial in relaxation. It can be used as an intervention in lessening the stress response, therefore decreasing the anxiety level. Music can be a distraction from the stressor or may act directly on the limbic system through the increased production of endorphins (White, 1992). Music should be carefully selected because it can trigger many different emotions and memories. It is imperative for the nurse to keep the client safe and comfortable.

Use of Humor. The ability to laugh at oneself when faced with situations that are unpleasant and out of one's control reduces stress. Examples of using humor include sharing embarrassing situations, telling jokes, playing noncompetitive games, or using amusing video and audiotapes. The energizing effects of humor can also be stabilizing for the nurse (Buxman, 1991).

Assertiveness Training. Unresolved conflicts cause stress. The ability to resolve conflict with others through assertiveness training is important to reducing stress. When used effectively, these skills can also empower the nurse.

CRISIS INTERVENTION

Crisis intervention is a therapeutic technique for helping a client to resolve an overwhelming stressful event. Crisis intervention does not involve an in-depth analysis of a situation but addresses the immediate urgent need for stress reduction. The goal is to restore the client as quickly as possible to the pre-crisis level of functioning.

After determining that a crisis exists, the nurse plans and implements measures to help resolve it. Resolution depends on the client's realistic perception of the stressful event, having adequate support, and using appropriate coping mechanisms. If the client lacks any of these, the nurse and client set goals to address the crisis. This approach to crisis intervention is based on effective communication between the nurse and the client. The nurse listens to the client's concerns and helps the client to develop new methods of coping with stressors. They choose specific methods (such as priority setting) to restore the client to a pre-crisis level of functioning. After intervention, the nurse uses evaluative measures to determine to what extent the client was able to resolve the crisis.

Evaluation

Evaluation of the expected outcomes will let the nurse know if the nursing interventions were effective. If the nursing interventions have not been effective, the nurse needs to reassess the care plan to determine what needs to be revised.

Based on the general goals for clients experiencing stress, a nurse needs to validate whether the goals have been met.

Goal: Client verbalized feelings associated with stress-producing situation.

Outcome

Client able to state feelings of frustration, anger, sadness, etc.

Evaluative measure

Ask client about feelings of frustration, anger, sadness, etc.

Outcome

Client able to identify changes in behavior, (e.g., decreased socialization, poor hygiene practices).

Evaluative measures

Ask client or family about changes from usual behavior.

Observe client's appearance and affect.

Goal: Client is able to identify potential stressors.

Outcome

Client able to list past stressful situations.

Evaluative measure

Ask client to state past stressful situations.

Outcome

Client able to list possible stressors in present situations.

Evaluative measures

Ask client to identify possible stressors in present situations.

Ask client to identify perceptions of response to stressors.

Goal: Client develops problem-solving techniques to address and minimize the effects of stress.

Outcome

Client able to list at least two methods for reducing each identified stressor.

Evaluative measure

Ask client to list at least two methods for reducing each identified stressor.

Outcome

Client evaluates each method of stress reduction.

Evaluative measures

Ask client to determine the effectiveness of each method of stress reduction.

Obtain client's vital signs.

Observe client's behaviors and interactions.

Goal: Client returns to prior level of functioning.

Outcome

Client maintains an adequate balance of rest and sleep.

Evaluative measures

Client reports adequate balance of rest and sleep.

Observe client for decreased anger, fatigue, crying, etc.

Outcome

Client achieves appropriate level of social interaction and daily activities.

Evaluative measure

Clients and family demonstrate increased social interactions.

If the client had difficulty with a particular step, the nurse can give specific attention to this step through revising the care plan.

STRESS MANAGEMENT FOR NURSES

Rapid changes in society, health care technology, health care knowledge, and the nursing profession can place stress on nurses. Job stress is individually perceived. Most nurses experience stress within the work environment. The reaction to a job-related stressor depends on individual personality and hardiness, health status, previous experience with stress, and coping mechanisms. Perceived job stress and lower levels of personality hardiness are contributing factors to *burnout* (McCranie, Lambert, and Lambert, 1987). Burnout is characterized by emotional, physical, and spiritual exhaustion (Selye, 1979). Another term for burnout is *cumulative stress* (Mitchell and Bray, 1990). This implies that a person is suffering through the buildup of a variety of stressors over time. For example, many nurses work in institutions in which team building is not emphasized. This can build up stress to high levels. Burnout contributes to negative feelings among nurses, increased absenteeism, and nonproductivity.

Nurses sometimes encounter traumatic and unpredicted critical incidents that can be overwhelming and can exhaust the usual coping strategies (Clark and Friedman, 1992). Critical incident stress debriefings are structured group meetings that emphasize ventilating emotions and other reactions to a critical event (Mitchell and Bray, 1990). Some employers offer short, on-site debriefings, initial defusing, and formal, structured critical incident stress debriefings for their employees. The purpose is to reduce the impact of the stress and accelerate the recovery process within the work environment. A nursing supervisor who intervenes with the nursing staff after an incident of verbal abuse is providing an example of informal defusing. The death of a child, serious injuries, or another unusually powerful event, are examples of situations when debriefing would be appropriate.

Employees can also sometimes use free, short-term counseling services available through employee assistance programs (EAP). Individually, nurses can reduce both personal and work-related stresses by using the stress management techniques they teach to clients. Nurses can use the following problem-solving process toward stress reduction and conflict resolution:

1. Define the stress-related problem.
2. Generate a list of alternative solutions that can be used to resolve the problem.
3. Analyze the positive and negative consequences associated with implementing each alternative solution.
4. Select the best alternative solution that has a higher probability of a successful outcome (resolving the problem).
5. Implement the alternative solution.
6. Evaluate the effectiveness of the solution.
7. If the alternative solution did not achieve a successful outcome, select another alternative and begin this process over again.

SUMMARY

Stress exists to some degree in everyone's life. According to the perception of the stressor, personality, prior experience with stress, and use of coping mechanisms, each person reacts differently to stress. Stress can be positive if it results in necessary changes in life-style and work environment. However, prolonged stress can affect a person's level of health, resulting in physical or mental illness. Stress management techniques are directed toward changing the way in which a person reacts to a stressor. Through early detection, health promotion, and health maintenance strategies, nurses can help clients to manage stress successfully.

A nurse, like anyone else, is exposed to stressors. Management of job stress requires an ability to solve problems and to use effective stress management techniques, thus avoiding cumulative stress and job burnout.

KEY CONCEPTS

- Homeostasis is a state of relative constancy in the internal environment.
- Stress is a physiological or psychological tension that can affect a person.
- Stressors are events, situations, or other stimuli an individual may encounter in the internal or external environment.
- Stressors necessitate change or adaptation so a state of equilibrium can be maintained.
- Adaptation is the process through which a person changes in response to stress.
- Physiological adaptation is the body's attempt to maintain optimal functioning.
- The physiological responses to stress are the local and the general adaptation syndromes.
- Psychological responses to stress include task-oriented behaviors and ego-defense mechanisms.
- Stress has an impact on the onset, course, and outcome of illness.
- Prolonged stress decreases the ability to adapt to the stress.
- Stress management techniques include health-enhancing habits, crisis intervention, and methods of reducing job stress.

CRITICAL THINKING ACTIVITIES

1. You are caring for a 30-year-old single mother who has recently been diagnosed as having the HIV virus. She is the sole provider for three young children (all under 7 years of age). Discuss the various stressors that will need to be considered when writing an appropriate discharge plan.
2. A client comes to the emergency room with a hand laceration resulting from an accidental injury. During the health history the client says she is in situational crisis. She is presently experiencing anorexia, poor concentration, neck and back pain, and is having difficulty sleeping. She also says she is working 32 hours per week and attending college. Her husband recently lost his job, which is causing financial and marital strain. Plus, she is having trouble finding reliable child care for her two young children. Develop nursing diagnoses related to this situation.
3. A widowed older adult who lives alone is admitted to the hospital with a fractured hip. She has been independent since her husband died. She has no children who can help her when she returns home. She is concerned not only about who will care for her after she is discharged but also about who will pay the hospital bill. By using the nursing process, determine what nursing care is appropriate for her.
4. Student nurses have many stressors specific to their academic situations. Keep a log of your own nutrition and rest patterns for 7 days. Compare your life-style to the recommendations for a healthy life-style given in the text. Can you recognize modifications necessary to reduce stress?

References

Aguilera DC and Messick JM: *Crisis intervention: theory and methodology,* ed 6, St Louis, 1989, Mosby.

Blair D and Hildreth N: PTSD and the Vietnam veteran: the battle for treatment, *J Psychosoc Nurs* 29(10):15-20, 1991.

Bruss C: Nursing diagnosis of hopelessness, *J Psychosoc Nurs* 26(3):28-31, 1988.

Buxman K: Humor in therapy for the mentally ill, *J Psychosoc Nurs* 29:15-18, 1991.

Clark M and Friedman D: Pulling together: building a community debriefing team, *J Psychosoc Nurs* 30(7):27-32, 1992.

Davis M, Eshelman E, McKay M: *The relaxation and stress reduction workbook,* Oakland, Calif., 1988, New Harbinger Publications.

Egger J: Psychosocial risk factors in cardiovascular diseases, *Theor Med* 7(3):319, 1987.

Grainger R: The patient with anxiety. In Lewis S, Grainger R, Dailey R, McDowell W, Gregory R and Messner R: *Manual of psychosocial nursing interventions: promoting mental health in medical-surgical settings,* Philadelphia, 1989, WB Saunders.

Jones JG and Kovalcik EM: Goal setting: a method to help patients escape the negative effects of stress, *Postgrad Med* 83(1):257, 1988.

Lee EJ, Jacobson JM, and Levanas V: Stressful life events and accidents at school, *Pediatr Nurs* 15:140, 1989.

Lewis S et al.: Manual of psychosocial nursing interventions: promoting mental health in medical-surgical settings, Philadelphia, 1989, WB Saunders.

Maddi SR and Kobasa SC: The development of hardiness. In Monat A and Lazarus R, editors: *Stress and coping,* New York, 1991, Columbia University Press.

McCranie E, Lambert V, and Lambert C Jr: Work stress, hardiness and burnout among hospital staff nurses, *Nurs Res* 36(6):374-377, 1987.

McNett S: Lazarus' theory of stress and coping. In Riegel B and Ehrenreich D: *Psychological aspects of critical care nursing,* Rockville, Md, 1989, Aspen Publishers.

Mellick E, Buckwalter K, and Stolley, J: Suicide among elderly white men: development of a profile, *J Psychosoc Nurs,* 30(2):29-34, 1992.

Mitchell J and Bray G: *Emergency services stress: guidelines for preserving the health and careers of emergency services personnel,* Englewood Cliffs, NJ, 1990, Prentice-Hall.

Naylor M and Shaid E: Content analysis of pre- and post-discharge topics taught to hospitalized elderly by gerontological clinical nurse specialist, *Clin Nurs Special,* 5(2):111-116, 1991.

Newberry B, Jaikins-Madden J, and Gerstenberger, T: *A holistic conceptualization of stress and disease,* New York, 1991, AMS Press.

Schultz JM and Dark SL: *Manual of psychiatric nursing care plans,* ed 3, Glenview, Ill., 1990, Scott, Foresman & Co.

Selye H: *The stress of life,* ed 2, New York, 1976, McGraw-Hill.

Selye H: For emotional well-being, work hard at reducing stress, *Parameters* 4(2):5, 1979.

Skeat WW: *A concise etymological dictionary of the English language,* Oxford, 1958, Oxford University Press.

Stewart MJ: Social support instruments created by nurse investigators, *Nurs Res* 38:268, 1989.

Stuart GW and Sundeen SJ: *Principles and practice of psychiatric nursing,* ed 4, St Louis, 1991, Mosby.

White J: Music therapy: An intervention to reduce anxiety in the myocardial infarction patient, *J Adv Nurs Pract* 6(2):58-63, 1992.

Wilkinson JM: *Nursing process in action: a critical thinking approach,* Redwood City, Calif., 1992, Addison-Wesley Nursing.

Zerhusen J, Boyle K and Wilson W: Out of the darkness: group cognitive therapy for depressed elderly, *J Psychosoc Nurs* 29(9): 16-21, 1991.

Bibliography

Alberti RE and Emmons ML: *Your perfect right: a guide to assertive living,* San Luis Obispo, Calif., 1990, Impact Publishers.

Bargagliottli CA and Trygstad LN: Differences in stress and coping findings: a reflection of social realities or methodologies, *Nurs Res* 36:170, 1987.

Carpenito LJ: *Nursing diagnosis: application to clinical practice,* Philadelphia, 1993, JB Lippincott.

Chenevert M: *Special techniques in assertiveness training STAT,* ed 3, St. Louis, 1988, Mosby.

Davidhizar R: When the nursing student faces discouragement, *Imprint* 40(2):67-69, 1993.

Heuer L: Parental stressors in a pediatric intensive care unit, *Pediatr Nurs* 19(2):128-133, 1993.

Kirkpatrick H, and Forchuk C: Assertiveness training: does it make a difference, *J Nurs Staff Develop* 8(2):60-65, 1992.

Lowery BJ and Jacobsen BS: Attributional analysis of chronic illness outcomes, *Nurs Res* 35:82, 1985.

Martin K: Critical incidents: pulling together to cope with the stress, *Nurs* 23(5):38-41, 1993.

McFarland G, and TM: *Psychiatric mental health nursing: application of the nursing process,* Philadelphia, 1991, JB Lippincott.

Pender NJ: *Health promotion in nursing practice,* ed 2, Norwalk, Conn, 1987, Appleton & Lange.

Roberts JG et al.: Analysis of coping responses and adjustment: stability of conclusions, *Nurs Res* 36:94, 1987.

Walter HJ and Hofman A: Socioeconomic status, ethnic origin, and risk factors for coronary heart disease in children, *Am Heart J* 113(3):812, 1987.

White N, Richter J, and Fry C: Coping, social support and adaptation to chronic illness, *West J Nurs Res* 14(2):211-224, 1992.

5 Values and Ethics

OBJECTIVES

Mastery of content in this chapter will enable the student to:

- Define the key terms listed.
- Describe and differentiate values, ethics, and morals.
- Describe how values influence behavior and attitudes.
- Discuss how values are learned.
- Contrast and compare modes of value transmission.
- Describe how values contribute to different stages of moral development.
- Explain how personal and professional values interrelate.
- Describe the process of values clarification.
- Explain how values clarification strategies can be used to clarify nurses' professional values.
- Discuss the techniques used in client values clarification.
- Describe the role of ethics in nursing practice.
- Describe an ethic of care as nursing's moral foundation.
- Explain how accountability and responsibility are evident in nursing practice.
- Discuss advocacy as a nursing value.
- Discuss the process used to analyze an ethical dilemma.
- Relate the principles of health care ethics to the role they play in ethical decision making.
- Describe the ethical conflicts experienced by nurses in different settings.

KEY TERMS

accountability
advocacy
codes of ethics
ethical principles
ethic of care
ethics
legalism
moral development
moral reasoning
morals
professionalism
responsibility
socialization
value
values clarification

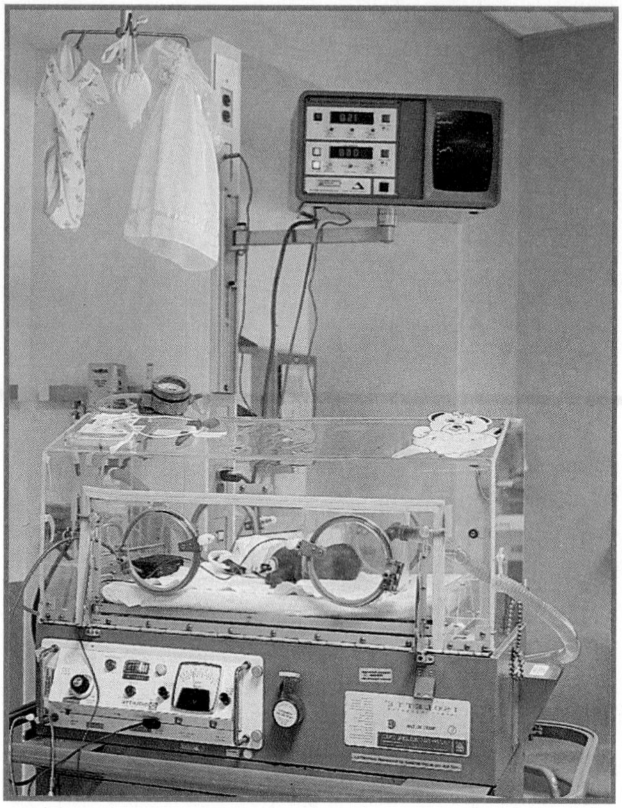

Nursing is a moral enterprise. This means that the nature of nursing concerns itself, in the broadest sense, with what "ought" to be for human beings. In partnership with the client, nurses seek goals that are of value—good health practices, healing after an illness or injury, or a peaceful death. The nurses' professional role relates to clients and their families in the most intimate and vulnerable moments of life and in that role always has the capacity to affect the relationship for good or for ill. Consequently, nothing about nursing is morally neutral. It is impossible to be a nurse without considering what is of value. In birth and death, joy and suffering, healing and illness, the nurse and the client establish a relationship that has meaning for both people.

Good, bad, values, meaning, "ought to," and relationship are words used to describe nursing's moral knowledge. Much of nursing is involved with technical knowledge (i.e., learning the reasons and methods for performing necessary skills). It is important that a nurse, for example, learn the proper theory and techniques for cardiopulmonary resuscitation (CPR). Equally important in using CPR is the nurse's moral knowledge that will help him or her know when and on whom CPR ought to be performed. Inevitably, the nurse may also experience a challenge to his or her personal values in some instances of CPR.

The nurse practices under both personal and professional values when entering relationships with clients. Each client also possesses a unique value system. At times a nurse's values may conflict with those of the client. In these instances, the nurse should understand how his or her values may influence decisions about a client's care. The nurse strives for self-awareness to better understand attitudes, feelings, and behavior in professional relationships. After a nurse becomes aware of the values motivating personal and professional behavior, it becomes easier to assist clients in identifying the values that influence their attitudes and behaviors.

Understanding one's own personal and professional values and the ethical foundation upon which nursing is built helps the nurse confront moral distress and uncertainty, challenges to personal values, and the ethical dilemmas that increasingly influence nursing practice.

DEFINITIONS OF VALUES AND ETHICS

A concept as complicated as value cannot be simply defined. Agreement among the classic writers on values (Kluckhohn, 1951; Maslow, 1959; Rokeach, 1973) is enough to state that a **value** is a personal belief about the worth of a given idea, attitude, custom, or object that sets standards that influence behavior. If a person holds a particular value, he or she has personally chosen, interpreted, justified, and preferred that value over others. The values an individual holds reflect personal needs, cultural and societal influences, and relationships with significant others. Values vary among people, developing and changing over time. A well-developed value system may help reduce conflict during decision making.

Uustal (1992) summarizes the common elements in values definitions. Valuing has cognitive, selective, affective, and action components. A person thinks about, chooses, feels for, and acts on important personal values. Some values are less important than others, depending on the choices a person makes or the way he or she prioritizes.

Like value, ethics is a term with many meanings. Simply stated, **ethics** indicates what a person ought to do and how one ought to be in relation to others. It is concerned with questions of good and bad, right and wrong conduct, character or motives. Defined broadly, **morals** and ethics are often used as interchangeable terms, although some subtle differences in meaning exist in ethics literature. Health care ethics, of which nursing ethics is a part, concerns itself with what is good or right for human health and life.

Ethics can also mean a pattern or way of life. For example, a person can be said to have a good "work ethic." A Western culture work ethic includes the "oughts" of work—punctuality, industriousness, creativity, and compliance with job standards. Nursing's moral way of life has been described by many as an "ethic of care" (Watson, 1988; Bevis, 1988; Leininger, 1991). Care is a moral word, then, that guides the way a nurse should act and be with others.

At times a nurse must engage in a disciplined, critical thought process about an ethical question. Most commonly, ethics refers to thoughtful, studied investigation of moral concerns. Inquiry of this nature helps a person decide what to do in situations in which the right action is not clear. Authors who define ethics as a term different from morals view ethics as the philosophical investigation or study of a particular issue, whereas morals describe the actual behaviors, customs, and beliefs of people groups. Morals have a social character (Davis and Aroskar, 1991).

Like ethics, the law is also concerned with right and wrong and how people ought to behave. A culture's legal system is based on what people value and what they believe to be right. Therefore taking another's property without permission is both illegal and unethical in most cultures. A person's legal rights are guaranteed to them, imposing on others the ethical obligation to uphold those rights.

The law does not always define what is ethical, however. Persons who oppose abortion, for example, do so claiming that what is legal is not necessarily moral. The practice of substituting legal sanction for ethics is called **legalism.** A nurse, of course, must always consider what the law says in a situation but should also remember that what is ethical may require more of the nurse or may even be contrary to a rule or law (see Chapter 6). Rules, codes, and laws give nurses good guidance but instances occur when a nurse should question whether or not simple adherence to a rule or law fulfills his or her moral obligation. For example, according to hospital and professional "rules," a physician is responsible for explaining and obtaining informed consent from the client before surgery. A nurse, aware that obtaining surgical consent is primarily the physician's role, should not knowingly fail to give further information to a client who is confused about the surgery. Many times a nurse must go beyond the guidelines of the professional "rules" to act ethically. Although the nurse may be functioning within the rules or the law, ethical considerations may reach beyond the law.

FORMATION OF VALUES

Values are learned both consciously and unconsciously through observation, reasoning, and experience (Hamilton, 1992). An individual observes behaviors in certain settings and notes the response it evokes. Successful or productive behaviors then become guides to conduct. Nursing students, for example, can learn caring values by observing the clinical instructor at a bedside.

Values are also acquired through experience. After experiencing similar situations, a person reflects upon and evaluates the successes and failures of certain behaviors. The social feedback a person receives upon performing a behavior helps determine whether or not it is acquired permanently. The nursing student who receives an instructor's praise after performing a task will probably continue to perform that task well. Repeated positive reinforcement of values results in the student becoming a skilled clinician.

Modes of Value Transmission

Values are not all consciously chosen by the individual. They are learned in childhood and become a part of the individual through **socialization** in the family, school, church, and other groups. Children observe parents, family, and friends and internalize behaviors that then become part of their value system.

People who influence a child are often unaware of the way they transmit their values. For example, if parents consistently demonstrate honesty in dealings with others, the child will likely value truth telling. The child becomes honest without insistence or threat. However, the process of imposing values can be deliberate, as when a parent says to a child who has lied, "You should be ashamed of yourself. Good children don't lie." Four modes of value transmission, with examples of their effectiveness in different developmental stages, are displayed in Table 5-1. Nurses, as health care professionals, use these same modes of value transmission when working with clients, families, and communities.

Moral Development

Just as a person matures physically, intellectually, spiritually, and emotionally, he or she also grows and changes morally. The formation, modification, and reinforcement of values and moral convictions throughout life is called **moral development.** The classic works of Piaget (1932), Kohlberg (1981), and Gilligan (1982) provide descriptions of this intricate process. Familiarity with developmental levels and corresponding needs better equips the nurse to help clients identify values, understand the effect illness has on values, and modify values as needs arise. Values and morals are often related in actions, as people act out what they value, giving expression to their moral life. Brief descriptions of age-related concerns for moral development, particularly for persons in Western cultures, follow (see also Chapter 20).

table 5-1

MODES OF VALUE TRANSMISSION

Description	Implications
MODELING	
Persons act in a way to show others the preferred way to behave. People acquire values from a variety of role models.	Children initially wish to be like their parents, and thus parents can model values they perceive as significant. Modeling may not lead to socially acceptable behavior (e.g., viewing another person's aggressive behavior). Unless parents point out values that are most desirable, children can follow any role model.
MORALIZING	
Parents and teachers hold standards for right and wrong and rigidly force children to conform to their set of values.	Approach can be very authoritarian. Moralizing parent may be unwilling to consider alternative values for child. Parents' way is often only way. Young persons reared by moralizing adults often have difficulty making independent choices.
LAISSEZ-FAIRE	
People acquire values by behaving informally without restrictions or limitations. No one value system is right for everyone, and child forms values without parent's rigid guidelines.	Parents want children to be free to explore variety of life experiences. Children are encouraged to be inquisitive and learn from experiences. Parents may refrain from discipline. A limitation is that no one assumes responsibility for child's behavior. Conflict and confusion may arise if child has no direction.
RESPONSIBLE CHOICE	
Balance of freedom and restriction allows children to select values that lead to personal satisfaction and parental support. Child's choices are more limited as compared with laissez-faire approach.	Values are not strictly imposed by parents. As child chooses values, parents, other family members, and teachers allow him or her to explore within boundaries new behaviors and their consequences. Child who can freely discuss his or her behavior and its effects will learn to understand personal values.

Infant. The newborn seeks emotional and physical security from parents. Although he or she has no ability to reason, an infant senses the emotions and behaviors of others. The manner in which parents react to and discipline the child expresses their values. For example, a parent who values being in control or having a "perfect" child may reward a baby who does not cry with a smile or a hug. If the child becomes irritable, such a parent may become angry and shout at the child. When the parents' values regarding methods of discipline conflict with the child's needs for security, the child may ultimately express fear, anger, or mistrust. The infant gains emotional security through prompt, predictable, and consistent responses to needs.

Toddler. The toddler learns values by imitating and gaining the approval of others when engaging in acceptable behavior. The child's experimentation and exploration of the environment lead to an understanding of the world. While striving for a sense of self-direction, the toddler begins to form an identity shaped by the values of the people with whom he or she associates. Parents who do not overly criticize or restrict the child's behavior help the child attain a healthy independence. A toddler's need for independence is balanced against the need for parental protection since the child is too young to judge safe behaviors. When parents fail to provide sufficient supervision, the child can get hurt. Restrictions imposed by parents who value a highly protective environment, however, can inhibit the child's testing of normal behaviors and block valuable learning experiences.

Preschool Child. The preschool child begins to form concepts. To this child, concepts are objects, events, and experiences that have acquired meaningful labels (e.g., dogs bark and a mother holds and comforts). The preschooler thinks concretely, not abstractly; that is, the child can name what he or she sees or hears, but hearing the name does not conjure up a mental picture of the object.

The words "right" and "wrong" do not elicit thoughts of acceptable or unacceptable behaviors. Right and wrong are associated only with single acts. Through play, the preschool child strives for a sense of initiative or the ability to set goals independently and act on them. Parents who value a child's need for creative and imaginative play are less likely to instill guilt in the child. Consistent, fair, and kind limits for behavior let the child experience parental care. This developmental stage is a suitable time to direct the child toward behaviors that the parents value.

School-Age Child. The school-age child is influenced by people holding diverse values, such as school personnel, neighborhood peers, school, and church. The school-ager socializes with other children and becomes less self-centered and more aware of the group (Figure 5-1). The child is motivated by peer approval and a desire to satisfy adults. It is important for the school-age child to acquire a sense of industry and contribute to a group effort. The mature school-ager generally comes to value self-motivation and productiveness rather than being manipulated by a peer group. Parents and teachers promote a sense of industry by providing the child with constructive guidance. In teaching values, parents who offer alternative behaviors help the child learn to solve problems and make responsible decisions. As the child seeks opportunities to perform chores around the home, he or she gains the experience of working toward a meaningful goal.

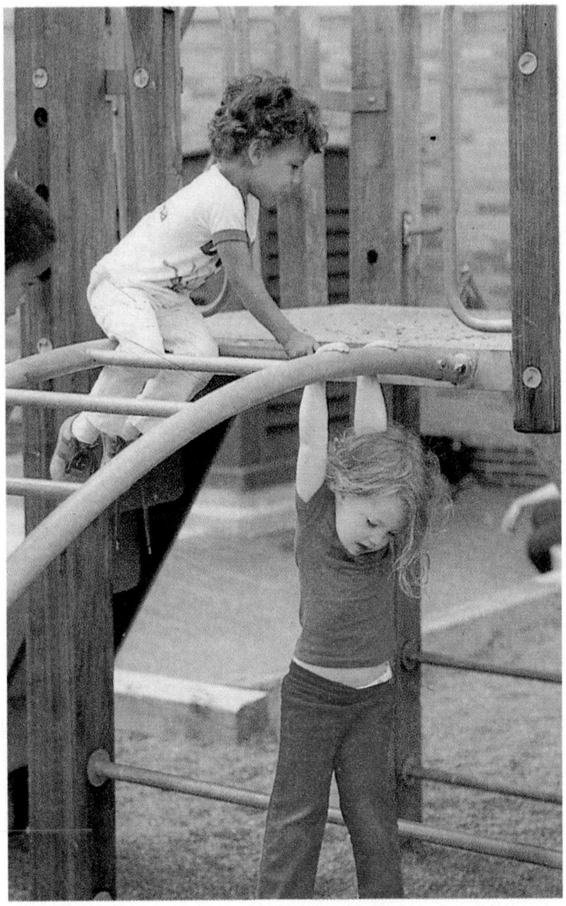

FIGURE 5-1 School-age child learns values through socialized play.

Adolescent. During adolescence, the youth gains greater freedom and responsibility. It is a time of rapid learning; the adolescent is exposed to many ideas and values. The adolescent undergoes dramatic physical changes that may affect the ability to develop a stable self-concept. Parental patience, support, and understanding can help an adolescent meet the need for independence. An adolescent's primary concerns are conformity with peers and the development of an identity that conveys his or her uniqueness. The teenager experiments with a number of roles, often aimlessly, until he or she begins to acquire distinctly personal behaviors. Most adolescents are unable to identify the values or attitudes that compose their identity. However, with maturity, they develop a workable philosophy of life, a personally meaningful set of values, and worthy ideals. Adolescents often adopt the values of their parents, although parents are no longer the only source of direction and support.

Adult. Ideally, the mature adult is able to test values and freely determine acceptable ones. At each level of adulthood (young, middle-age, and elderly) the adult has experiences that lead to confrontations over the most desired values. Marriage, child rearing, and career selection often require the young adult to redefine values. Middle-age adults begin to redefine their self-concepts to suit the needs of later life. As old age approaches, the individual who is satisfied with his or her life and values may experience little turmoil with the aging process. The onset of aging may pose a threat, however, to older adults who value youth and vitality. During late adulthood, an individual faces significant changes in life, including retirement from work, physical alterations of aging, and loss of close friends. Maintaining independent activities and social relationships beyond the immediate family may help the older adult fulfill many significant values. The adult who remains open to new ideas and values continues to have the opportunity to grow.

Sociocultural Influences

The values that contribute to a person's moral development are formed in social settings in which the educational, socioeconomic, spiritual, and cultural backgrounds of people vary (see Chapters 17 and 18). Leininger (1978) describes culture as "a way of life belonging to a designated group of people." Although cultural influences on an individual's value system are extensive, it remains difficult to establish moral norms for any culture because absolute agreement among people about acceptable values does not exist.

A culture's value orientation influences the way its members pursue health care. Persons in certain cultural groups may seek health care for the slightest problems, whereas those in other groups seek care only when their condition is serious. A client's socioeconomic status may determine how he or she values health promotion behaviors. Financial resources, availability of care, and learned behaviors all influence health promotion and are often directly linked to a client's socioeconomic status.

Health care within American society is changing rapidly. As a result, nurses and clients face situations requiring a careful analysis of cultural value systems. For example, along with an aging American population have come rapid advances in technologies for extending life. This raises important cultural questions about quality of life and the use of expensive technologies to prolong an older person's life. Although society may value technological advances and new approaches to client care, nurses also strive to maintain compassionate personal care.

The nurse can deliver more effective care by understanding the influence of cultural values on health behaviors, client stress, use of health care services, and adjustment to illness. At times the nurse's value system may differ from the client's. However, the nurse should work to respect the cultural values of others, realizing that no single culture agrees on what is "right" or "wrong."

VALUES CLARIFICATION

As individuals mature and experience new situations, their values change. It would be unusual if any one value remained the primary motivating factor throughout a person's life. Value changes may involve a reordering of values or the replacement of old values with new ones. As a result of changing values, the person modifies his or her attitudes and behavior. The willingness to change shows a healthy attitude toward life and the ability to adapt to new experiences.

To change values to suit needs and preferences, a person must first be aware of his or her own values. In addition, the individual must realize the ways in which values affect behavior. Yet individuals do not suddenly become aware of their values, and many are unable to define their values clearly and meaningfully. To achieve awareness of personal values, a cognitive process of values clarification can be used.

Values clarification, or valuing, is a process of self-discovery that helps a person gain insight into values. It is not a set of rules designed to interfere with conscientious decision making, and it does not suggest that a specific set of values should be accepted by all persons; it is not a method of indoctrination to religious, moral, or cultural standards. A person clarifying values learns to make choices when alternatives are presented and determines whether choices are carefully made. The result of valuing is greater self-awareness and personal insight.

Louis Raths (Raths, Harmin, and Simon, 1979) pioneered values clarification as an approach to an individual's appraisal of values. Valuing involves the following actions: choosing, prizing, and acting (see box below). In values clarification, the person uses ranked values as a guide for personal conduct, life choices, and interpersonal interactions.

As values are not predetermined, a person should be able to choose them freely. The freedom to select among alternative values allows a person to cherish the final choice. However, the individual must also understand alternatives. For example, an older adult knows that surgery is an option for the treatment of a hip problem. Although the client values independence and mo-

THE THREE ACTIONS OF VALUES CLARIFICATION

Choosing one's beliefs and behaviors
- Choosing from alternatives
- Choosing freely
- Considering all consequences

Prizing one's beliefs and behaviors
- Prizing and cherishing the choice
- Publicly affirming the choice

Acting on one's beliefs
- Making the choice part of one's behavior
- Acting with a pattern of consistency and repetition

Modified from Raths LE, Harmin M, and Simon SB: *Values and teaching,* ed 2, Columbus, Ohio, 1979, Merrill Publishing.

bility, the risks and discomforts of surgery and hospitalization must be considered. The client should ideally examine treatment choices, considering how they will affect the most prized values, and then choose freely without judgment from others.

Prizing is showing private and public satisfaction with the chosen value. This happens when a person reaches a point when he or she is able to affirm values in the presence of significant others. When a terminally ill client chooses to die without emergency resuscitation and shares that decision with family members, he or she is prizing that value. By declaring values, a person reaffirms the importance or relevance of these values.

Acting on a chosen value solidifies its acceptance. The value on which a person acts should be consistently followed in similar experiences or circumstances. For example, a young man permanently disabled by an injury to his leg chooses to retain his independence by living alone. He enters a rehabilitation program and continues to function independently in his work and social life.

Strategies for Values Clarification in Nursing

Certain strategies can be used to make valuing more insightful, practical, and meaningful for any person with unclear values. These exercises help an individual clarify values using the three steps of valuing. The nurse can use the strategies to help clients or to clarify personal values.

A nurse who uses values clarification undergoes personal growth and gains professional satisfaction. During encounters with clients, peers, and health care professionals, the nurse's values are challenged and tested. How does the nurse demonstrate a willingness to be accountable as a professional? How do the nurse's attitudes about a client influence the care provided? The nurse has difficulty assuming the role of a professional if personal values are poorly conceived and unclear. Values clarification helps the nurse explore these values and decide whether to act on beliefs. A clear perspective of personal values permits the nurse to give greater attention to client needs. Values clarification also facilitates decision making and problem solving. The strategies in the box on p. 80 can help the nurse explore attitudes, beliefs, interests and goals, order values, or set value priorities.

Values clarification can be used with an entire health care team. In working relationships, nurses should have confidence in colleagues since they rely on their responses and decisions. The values-aware nurse can assist colleagues to clarify values in dealing with clients and performing health care. Sharing values about clients, families, and colleagues helps professionals recognize commonalities. This sharing also helps team members understand the behavior of colleagues. Open communication facilitates resolution of controversial ethical matters. The quality of working relationships is enhanced as nurses gain insight into themselves and coworkers.

Values Clarification as a Tool in Client Care

Valuing also helps clients and their families adapt to the stress of illness and other health-related problems. Merely encouraging a client to express feelings may provide inadequate information if the real problem is a conflict in values. Values clarification is a consciousness-raising activity through which clients gain an awareness of personal priorities, identify ambiguities in values, and resolve major conflicts between values and behavior. With it, the nurse helps the client clarify the meaning and significance of values and emotions. The end goal of values clarification with a client is effective nurse-client communication leading to health-protecting or health-promoting behaviors. As the client becomes more willing to express problems and true feelings, the nurse can better establish an individualized plan of care. The nurse who learns about client values and needs can devise a successful teaching program to promote well-being.

To assist in client values clarification, the nurse shapes responses to the client's questions or statements in a manner that stimulates introspection. The nurse's clarifying verbal response arises from an awareness that the valuing process will motivate the client to examine his or her own thoughts and actions. When the nurse makes a clarifying response, it should be brief, selective, nonjudgmental, thought provoking, and spontaneous. A good clarifying response is designed to encourage the client to think about personal values after the exchange is over. This way, client self-direction is respected and the nurse's own values are not inappropriately introduced into the conversation. Although values clarification can occur in any setting, it is often most successful when the nurse has repeated contact with the client. As shown in the case study on p. 81, it takes time for the nurse to develop values clarification as a tool for client care.

Ultimately the client gains a perception of how valuing provides personal satisfaction. Values clarification promotes effective reasoning and decision making. The client becomes aware of how values influence actions, an essential component of problem solving.

Behaviors Reflecting the Need for Values Clarification

It may be difficult to determine when a nurse, health care team, or client might benefit from values clarifica-

STRATEGIES FOR VALUES CLARIFICATION

SENTENCE COMPLETION

Complete the following sentences. Use them to examine your feelings and values.

I feel I succeed in caring for a client when . . .
A client has a right to . . .
I wish my clinical supervisor would . . .
Physicians and nurses work together best when . . .
I fail in caring for a client if I cannot . . .
The most difficult client is one who . . .

RANK ORDERING

The following questions require you to make value judgments. Rank the choices to the questions according to your value preferences. Write the number "1" to the left for the most important value. Continue in the same manner until all four values are ranked. Discuss your preferences with a colleague and examine the alternatives.

If I had the time, money, and skill to solve problems for nurses, I would
____ Increase nurses' salaries
____ Enhance staff education
____ Increase the number of nurses to staff the division
____ Give staff more positive feedback

In developing a professional relationship with a physician, I believe a student or nurse should
____ Respond promptly to all requests
____ Demonstrate knowledge of the clients assigned to the physician
____ Look attractive and be neatly dressed
____ Share ideas about the clients' needs

When assigned to a client's care, it is most important to
____ Make him or her as physically comfortable as possible
____ Let him or her know you are interested in his or her ideas and feelings
____ Be competent and skilled in the performance of all procedures
____ Allow the client to make decisions about his or her care

If I had a serious health problem, I would prefer to
____ Not be told
____ Be told immediately by the physician
____ Learn by accident
____ Keep it secret from my family

HEALTH VALUE SCALE

Below you will find 10 values listed in alphabetical order. Arrange the values in order of their importance as guiding principles in your life. Study the list carefully and choose the value that is most important to you. Write the number "1" in the space to the left of that value. Write the number "2" for the value that ranks second in importance. Continue in the same manner for the remaining values until you have included all ranks. Each value will have a different rank.

____ A comfortable life (a prosperous life)
____ An exciting life (a stimulating, active life)
____ A sense of accomplishment (lasting contribution)
____ Freedom (independence, free choice)
____ Happiness (contentedness)
____ Health (physical and mental well-being)
____ Inner harmony (freedom from inner conflict)
____ Pleasure (an enjoyable, leisurely life)
____ Self-respect (self-esteem)
____ Social recognition (respect, admiration)

Modified from Uustal DB: *Am J Nurs* 78:2058, 1978.

tion. Since people do not always share the same values, the nurse should resist the idea that the goal of values clarification is to direct another person's values closer to one's own. In some cases, however, a person's behaviors suggest that his or her values are unclear. Some behaviors in clients (see box on p. 82) could interfere with efforts to promote good health care, signaling the need for values clarification. When client behaviors reflect the need for values clarification, the nurse's role should be to determine whether the client is unhappy with or unsure of his or her value system or is experiencing a conflict of values that could be detrimental to health. When either the nurse or health care team experiences values distress or ethical tension in the work environment, it may be useful to consider a clarification of values.

The Relationship Between Values and Ethics

Values and values clarification are both very personal. Values are freely chosen, prized, and acted on by the person holding them. Values clarification helps persons come to grips with their own competing or unsettled values and feelings. It can also help people understand one another.

Ethics also concerns itself with what people see as good and, in that sense, flows from values. Values clarification is not a substitute for ethics, however (Deloughery, 1991). Ethics should not be reduced to a discussion about what individuals want, feel, or value. Since all people want, feel, and value different things, ethics would then be no more than each person assert-

CASE STUDY

Mrs. James is a 73-year-old woman who fractured her ankle in a fall at home. Her daughter is concerned about her mother's welfare and wants Mrs. James to live with her family. The daughter has voiced concern to the nurse that Mrs. James is incapable of caring for herself. Mrs. James' rehabilitation has progressed well, and one day she asks the nurse, Ms. Fryer, "What should I do? I know my daughter worries about me, but I don't want to be cared for like a child."

Ms. Fryer realizes that Mrs. James is experiencing a conflict in her values for independence, love for her daughter, and health. The nurse thinks the values clarification process would help Mrs. James to make her choice. Ms. Fryer begins by helping Mrs. James to choose from available alternatives.

Choosing from alternatives. The nurse's response depends partly on Mrs. James' age, education, and level of maturity. Mrs. James is an alert woman, knowledgeable about her needs, and capable of making decisions for herself. She has demonstrated motivation in her rehabilitation.

Examining all consequences. Mrs. James loves her daughter and knows that the offer to join the daughter's family is genuine. Mrs. James says that she has many friends in her apartment building and that moving to her daughter's home would make it difficult for her to socialize with her friends. Mrs. James' apartment is on the third floor, which requires her to climb two flights of stairs. A downstairs apartment will soon be vacant.

The nurse says, "Perhaps it would help to weigh the advantages and disadvantages of joining your daughter against moving into the downstairs apartment." In making this suggestion the nurse carefully avoids letting her own values influence Mrs. James' thinking, even though she has a close relationship with her own daughter and has been very happy when they shared her house on extended visits.

Choosing freely. The next day, Ms. Fryer enters Mrs. James' room during breakfast. The nurse's goal is to determine if Mrs. James was able to make a decision of her own. Mrs. James says, "I've decided to move into the downstairs apartment." Ms. Fryer asks, "Was this a difficult choice to make?"

Prizing the choice. Mrs. James acknowledges that she does not want to hurt her daughter's feelings; however, she knows her decision was the best one. "I still have many friends, and they have encouraged me to stay in the apartment. I still feel spry and able to take care of myself." The nurse recognizes that it is important for Mrs. James to be satisfied with her choice.

Affirming the choice. Mrs. James must be able to speak out in support of her decision. She may need assistance from the nurse in thinking of ways to affirm the choice. An appropriate response by Ms. Fryer is, "What will be the best way to share your decision with your daughter?" Mrs. James replies, "My daughter and son-in-law are coming to visit this evening. I've decided to let them know tonight."

Acting on the choice. Mrs. James has made the decision to retain her independence. She is able to share her choice and the rationale for it with her daughter. The nurse, using values clarification, recognizes Mrs. James' need to act on her decision. She asks, "What can you do to begin planning for your move?"

Mrs. James calls the apartment manager to arrange for her new home. She is going to stay with her daughter for a week after discharge from the hospital. Meanwhile, she will have the opportunity to select new paint and wallpaper for the apartment. Mrs. James' value of independence remains alive in the measures she has taken to accomplish her move.

Acting with a pattern. A month after discharge, Mrs. James returns to her physician's office for a checkup. She stops by the nursing division to say hello to Ms. Fryer. Ms. Fryer is interested in learning whether Mrs. James retained her independence. A value must be kept alive. For independence to be meaningful to Mrs. James, it must become integrated into her life-style. Ms. Fryer asks, "Was your choice to remain in the apartment the right one?" Mrs. James responds, "For now, yes. I am feeling much better and there are many friends to help me. My daughter visits every week. You know, though, I do have to be cautious in the way I walk around. I know someday I may have to live with my daughter."

As Mrs. James becomes more physically dependent, a conflict will arise between the independence she prizes and her ability to act on that value. The value of the genuine love and concern expressed by Mrs. James' daughter may become a higher priority than the value of independence. Mrs. James' maturity will be reflected in her eventual ability to modify her values. As she becomes more physically dependent, her values may have to adapt accordingly. The daughter's ability to provide a safe environment for her mother without compromising Mrs. James' ability to make her own decisions should prove to be mutually satisfying.

CLINICAL EXAMPLES: CLIENTS WHO MAY BENEFIT FROM VALUES CLARIFICATION

APATHY

Mr. Smith has reentered the hospital several times for the same health problem. His wife reports that he will not consistently follow his diet restrictions. During a discussion with the nurse, Mr. Smith cannot remember when he should take his medications. He does not seem to care about health promotion activities. When asked if he understands his physician's orders, Mr. Smith replies, "Oh, I suppose so. I just have trouble remembering sometimes. It's hard to always do the right thing."

FLIGHTINESS

Mrs. Jones is visited at home by a public health nurse, who is giving advice on the care of Mrs. Jones' newborn infant. Mrs. Jones tells the nurse, "I'm so glad you are here; I have questions about the baby." Before the nurse is able to answer questions about breastfeeding, Mrs. Jones changes the subject and discusses her new kitchen curtains. Even Mrs. Jones' actions seem poorly directed. She places the infant in bed but returns in a moment and picks the child up again.

UNCERTAINTY

Ms. Nelson has been suffering a gradual loss of vision. Her physician has proposed a new type of experimental surgery. Ms. Nelson has not been able to decide whether to follow the physician's recommendations. She has asked her family and friends for their opinions. She asks each nurse who cares for her whether surgery is the right choice.

INCONSISTENCY

Mr. Wall has had serious heart disease for 3 years. He rarely follows the exercise plan prescribed by his physician. In a conversation with a nurse, Mr. Wall remarks that people should become more concerned about maintaining their health.

DRIFTING

Mr. Rush has had back pain for 3 years. His first physician recommended surgery to correct his problem. Since then, Mr. Rush has also visited a chiropractor and an osteopath. He believes in physical fitness and wants to find a cure for his pain. However, he tries each remedy for only a short time.

OVERCONFORMING

Mrs. Wade has gone to a physician for advice on weight reduction. The physician has ordered a diet of 1500 calories per day and a program of regular exercise. Mrs. Wade has bought four diet books to help her to count calories and a scale to weigh foods. She keeps a chart on the refrigerator door to record each day's meals. After Mrs. Wade eats the limit of 1500 calories, she refuses to eat for the remainder of the day, even if it means missing dinner. Each day she runs a mile at 7:15 AM and 5:45 PM.

ROLE PLAYING

Mrs. Elson might be called the "perfect" client. She always has a smile for the nurses, never talks about her predicament, and rarely complains about pain. This is despite the fact that Mrs. Elson, age 24 and mother of three children, is dying of cancer.

ing his or her own beliefs. Just because a person values something, however sincerely, it does not necessarily make it ethical. Consider, for example, a client with a young family who decides not to have a potentially curative surgery for cancer because he or she values being pain free and independent. The nurse may believe in a client's autonomy but may be unsure if the client has weighed all the relevant ethical considerations.

Ethics, as disciplined reflection on good conduct, character, and motives, also seeks to settle claims of what constitutes the "good" or valuable among people with differences. It strives to go beyond personal preferences to establish norms and standards upon which individuals, professions, and societies agree. Within nursing, specific values and moral imperatives are necessary for the integrity of the profession. An ethical nurse will act and be with others in specific ways, consistent with nursing norms, not just according to an individual nurse's preferences or values.

PROFESSIONAL NURSING ETHICS

To better understand nursing ethics, a discussion of professionalism is first necessary since it has important ethical implications. A profession is made of a group of people with specialized education, knowledge, and skills who serve specific social needs. **Professionalism** is above all a way of life that demands commitment from practitioners (Kelly, 1992). To be a professional means that a person makes a promise to do and be what the profession lays claim to. Nurses, then, promise to care for the chronically and acutely ill and injured, promote wellness, and help people die peacefully. Society, trusting that promise, relies on a nurse to be committed to its ideals. In the end, this comes down to the commitment of the individual practitioner.

Whether or not nursing is a profession has been long debated, although most agree that nursing has made great strides in that direction. Establishing professional autonomy has been difficult for nurses. With professional maturity and expanded practice roles for nurses, the independent realm of nursing care has been more carefully described. It should also be remembered that interdependence is necessary for all professions, particularly in health care (Kelly, 1992).

Nursing has characteristics similar to other health professions. Chitty (1993) summarizes how nursing meets established criteria for a profession. Those social criteria are as follows:

1. A vital human service is provided to the society by the profession.
2. Professions possess a special body of knowledge that is continuously enlarged through research.
3. Practitioners are expected to be accountable and responsible.
4. The education of professionals takes place in institutions for higher education.
5. Practitioners have an independent function and control their own practice.
6. Professionals are committed to their work and are motivated by doing good.
7. A code of ethics guides professional decisions and conduct.
8. A professional organization oversees and supports standards of practice.

This list of criteria points to both values and ethics as necessary for professionalization. Through codes of ethics and the instillation of particular values, a profession fulfills its promises to society. The values of care, accountability, responsibility, and advocacy provide the moral foundation for nursing practice. The codes of ethics give ethical guidance and establish norms of behavior.

Codes of Ethics

The nursing profession has **codes of ethics** that set forth ideals of conduct. A code is a set of ethical principles that are generally accepted by all members of a profession. These principles indicate factors that nurses must consider when deciding on proper conduct. Ethical codes also provide a common foundation for professional nursing curricula. A profession's ethical code is a collective statement about the group's expectations and standards of behavior.

It is difficult to codify all morally relevant principles in a field as ethically complex as nursing. Nurses face ethical situations not always clearly governed by ethical codes. In these instances, nurses have to deliberate, using the code as a guideline. A useful code of ethics must be brief, yet detailed enough to offer clear guidance and attain widespread acceptance. The American Nurses Association (ANA), International Council of Nurses (ICN), and Canadian Nurses Association (CNA) have established widely accepted codes that the professional nurse should attempt to follow (see boxes on pp. 84 and 85). Although these codes differ somewhat in specific emphasis, they reflect the same underlying principles.

Core Values in Nursing

A person entering nursing has a set of personal values that guide actions. These values are the result of personal choice and are learned over time. Persons entering nursing may at first be unable to reconcile themselves with all attributes of a professional nurse. After some time, they find that personal and professional values interact.

The American Association of Colleges of Nursing (1986) identified seven values essential to the practice of professional nursing. These values are aesthetics (qualities of objects, events, and persons that provide satisfaction), altruism (regard for the welfare of others), equality (having the same rights and privileges), freedom (the ability to exercise choice or action), human dignity (inherent worth of an individual), justice (fair treatment through the upholding of moral and legal principles), and truth (faithfulness to fact or reality).

Care is valued in nursing because it encompasses in some way all of the aforementioned values. Advocacy, too, has long been advanced as a fundamental moral stance for nurses because it protects other values. Responsibility and accountability are necessary for the fulfillment of any moral commitment. A brief discussion of these core values follows.

Care as a Central Nursing Value. Care has been called the "central and unifying domain for the body of knowledge and practices in nursing" (Leininger, 1988). Care can be described as an action, a virtue, an ethical principle, or a way of being in the world (Gilligan, 1982; Noddings, 1984; Watson, 1988; Leininger, 1988; Salsberry, 1992). Care as an ethic for nursing is concerned not only with the resolution of ethical dilemmas, sometimes called quandary ethics, but also with the way people behave toward one another. An **ethic of care** is therefore relational and concerned with a practitioner's character and attitude toward others.

To be able to care is part of one's human nature. Caring exchanges early in life give a child a moral knowledge about what it is to care and be cared for. People who do not experience care in their lives often find it difficult to creatively act in caring ways. The care that a person already has for the world can be professionalized. Nurses become experts in caring by learning how to attend to the specific needs of the persons with whom they are in relationship. A professional caring nurse is able to have empathy for another person. The nurse must also understand the client's situation, trying to take into account as much of the person's life as possible. The care giver is able to go from a self-centered to

AMERICAN NURSES ASSOCIATION CODE OF ETHICS

The nurse provides services with respect for human dignity and the uniqueness of the client unrestricted by considerations of social or economic status, personal attributes, or the nature of health problems.

The nurse safeguards the client's right to privacy by judiciously protecting information of a confidential nature.

The nurse acts to safeguard the client and the public when health care and safety are affected by the incompetent, unethical, or illegal practice of any person.

The nurse assumes responsibility and accountability for individual nursing judgments and actions.

The nurse maintains competence in nursing.

The nurse exercises informed judgment and uses individual competence and qualifications as criteria in seeking consultation, accepting responsibilities, and delegating nursing activities to others.

The nurse participates in activities that contribute to the ongoing development of the profession's body of knowledge.

The nurse participates in the profession's efforts to implement and improve standards of nursing.

The nurse participates in the profession's efforts to establish and maintain conditions of employment conducive to high-quality nursing care.

The nurse participates in the profession's effort to protect the public from misinformation and misrepresentation and to maintain the integrity of nursing.

The nurse collaborates with members of the health professions and other citizens in promoting community and national efforts to meet the health needs of the public.

From American Nurses Association: *Code for nurses with interpretive statements,* Kansas City, Mo, 1985, The Association.

CANADIAN NURSES ASSOCIATION CODE OF ETHICS

The body of the code is divided into the following sources of nursing obligations:

CLIENTS

A nurse is obliged to treat clients with respect for their individual needs and values.

Based on respect for clients and regard for their rights to control their own care, nursing care should reflect respect for clients' right of choice.

The nurse is obliged to hold confidential all information about a client learned in the health care setting.

The nurse has an obligation to be guided by consideration for the dignity of clients.

The nurse is obligated to provide competent care to clients.

The nurse is obliged to represent the ethics of nursing before colleagues and others.

The nurse is obligated to advocate clients' interests.

In all professional settings, including education, research, and administration, the nurse retains a commitment to the welfare of clients. The nurse has an obligation to act in a fashion that will maintain trust in nurses and nursing.

HEALTH TEAM

Client care should represent a cooperative effort, drawing on the expertise of nursing and other health professions. By acknowledging personal or professional limitations, the nurse recognizes the perspective and expertise of colleagues from other disciplines.

The nurse, as a member of the health care team, is obliged to take steps to ensure that the client receives competent and ethical care.

SOCIAL CONTEXT OF NURSING

Conditions of employment should contribute to client care and to the professional satisfaction of nurses. Nurses are obliged to work toward securing and maintaining conditions of employment that satisfy these goals.

RESPONSIBILITIES OF THE PROFESSION

Professional nurses' organizations recognize a responsibility to clarify, secure, and sustain ethical nursing conduct. The fulfillment of these tasks requires professional organizations to remain responsive to the rights, needs, and interests of clients and nurses.

From Canadian Nurses Association: *Code of ethics for nursing,* 1985.

INTERNATIONAL COUNCIL OF NURSES CODE FOR NURSES

The fundamental responsibility of the nurse is fourfold: to promote health, to prevent illness, to restore health, and to alleviate suffering.

The need for nursing is universal. Inherent in nursing is respect for life, dignity, and rights of man. It is unrestricted by considerations of nationality, race, creed, color, age, sex, politics, or social status.

Nurses render health services to the individual, the family, and the community and coordinate their services with those of related groups.

NURSES AND PEOPLE

The nurse's primary responsibility is to those people who require nursing care.

The nurse, in providing care, promotes an environment in which the values, customs, and spiritual beliefs of the individual are respected.

The nurse holds in confidence personal information and uses judgment in sharing this information.

NURSES AND PRACTICE

The nurse carries personal responsibility for nursing practice and for maintaining competence by continual learning. The nurse maintains the highest standards of nursing care possible within the reality of a specific situation.

The nurse uses judgment in relation to individual competence when accepting and delegating responsibilities.

The nurse when acting in a professional capacity should at all times maintain standards of personal conduct that reflect credit upon the profession.

NURSES AND SOCIETY

The nurse shares with other citizens the responsibility for initiating and supporting action to meet the health and social needs of the public.

NURSES AND CO-WORKERS

The nurse sustains a cooperative relationship with coworkers in nursing and other fields. The nurse takes appropriate action to safeguard the individual when his care is endangered by a co-worker or any other person.

NURSES AND THE PROFESSION

The nurse plays the major role in determining and implementing desirable standards of nursing practice and nursing education.

The nurse is active in developing a core of professional knowledge.

The nurse, acting through the professional organization, participates in establishing and maintaining equitable social and economic working conditions in nursing.

From International Council of Nurses: *ICN code for nurses: ethical concepts applied to nursing,* Geneva, 1973, Imprimeries Populaires.

an other-centered position, and finally, is willing to take action on behalf of the other person (Brown, Kitson, and McKnight, 1992).

Caring activities cannot be prescribed since they depend on the situation. Care is contextual. A client who has attempted suicide will need different caring behaviors than those appropriate for the care of an older adult with cognitive impairment. Research studies also demonstrate that clients and nurses prioritize caring behaviors differently, underscoring the importance of client participation in nursing plans of care (Cochran and Ganong, 1989; Holmes and Edburn, 1989; Von Essen and Sjoden, 1991). An ethic of care leads a nurse to respond to each situation with technical and moral knowledge, compassion, competence, and personal integrity.

Responsibility and Accountability. A nurse assumes responsibility and accountability for all nursing care delivered. **Responsibility** refers to the execution of duties associated with a nurse's particular role (ANA, 1985). When administering a medication, a nurse is responsible for assessing the client's need for the drug, giving it safely and correctly, and evaluating the response to it. By being responsible the nurse is reliable and worthy of trust from colleagues and clients. A responsible nurse is competent in knowledge and skills and ethically executes duties within the guidelines of the profession.

When nurses perform care, they must be accountable. **Accountability** refers to being answerable for one's own actions. A nurse is accountable to self, the client, the profession, the employing institution, and society. If a nurse knows that a client ready to be discharged is confused about how to self-administer insulin, the nurse is accountable to the client, the physician, the employing institution that sets the standards of expected performance, and society, which demands professional excellence. Being accountable, the nurse will take steps to initiate more teaching or arrange home care to prevent injury to the client. Accountability calls for an evaluation of a nurse's effectiveness in practice.

Professional accountability serves the following basic purposes:

1. To evaluate new professional practices and reassess existing ones
2. To maintain standards of health care
3. To facilitate personal reflection, ethical thought, and personal growth on the part of health professionals
4. To provide a basis for ethical decision making

Nurse as Advocate. Nurses deal with people who, because of illness or injury, are often vulnerable and dependent on professional knowledge and skill. Clients may lose the ability to move freely, communicate, or make clear decisions. Illness may interfere with clients' independence, forcing them to go to nurses for assistance. For clients' rights to be preserved, their decisions cannot be made for them by health care professionals. The nursing profession has set forth and adheres to high ideals of conduct, assuring the public that nurses will enhance client autonomy and promising that nurses will not use their power to exploit persons in need of assistance.

The relationship between nurse and client allows the nurse to be the client's advocate. **Advocacy** involves giving clients the information they need to make decisions and then supporting those decisions. To inform a client properly, a nurse must have accurate information or know where to get it and be able to convey it meaningfully to the client. Nurses may rely on other health professionals as sources of information (Figure 5-2). A nurse advocate also wants the client to have the information. He or she recognizes that many persons—family members, other nurses, physicians, or health care administrators—may not want clients to have information. This situation makes advocacy very difficult. The role of advocate becomes a careful balancing act between telling a client what he or she needs to know and not threatening the client's relationship with the physician or family. It should also be remembered that clients have the right *not* to know something if too much information overwhelms them.

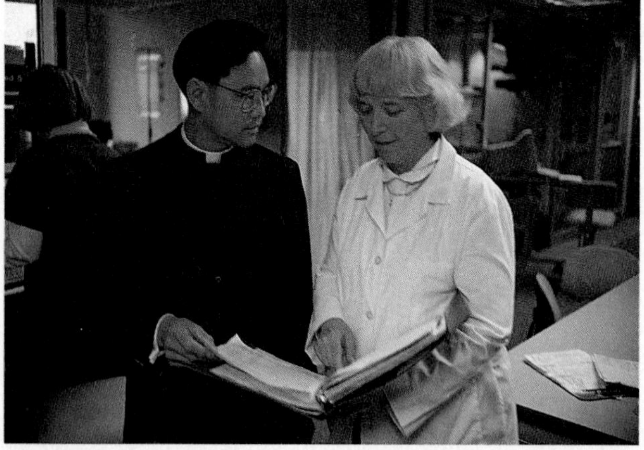

FIGURE 5-2 Nurse and chaplain collaborate on ethical consultation.

The nurse advocates for clients without falling into a defensive or rescuing position. Rescuing or defending a client without the client's request or participation may not really be advocacy but rather a method for the nurse to advance his or her own standing or opinions. This is one of the dangers in advancing unbridled advocacy values in nursing (Bernal, 1992). The responsibility for decision making rests with the client and his or her family. The nurse advocate refrains from assuming that he or she is the only person who can defend clients or help them make decisions. Not all clients require an advocate if they are capable of making their own decisions without support. It is, however, always appropriate for a nurse to share pertinent and meaningful information.

PROCESS FOR RESOLVING ETHICAL PROBLEMS

Ethical problems can cause distress and perplexity for both clients and care givers. Controversy is the very nature of ethical deliberations, and few people like conflict. Ethical decisions are usually very important and are made under stressful circumstances. Ethical issues should be processed carefully so that decisions are not made solely on an emotional level. As discussed previously, an ethical outcome is not obtained by considering only what people want and feel. Therefore having a pattern or a guide for thinking through ethical conflicts or dilemmas is very helpful. Several such guides are in the nursing literature (Uustal, 1990; Husted and Husted, 1992; Potter and Perry, 1993).

Although each pattern or decision-making matrix looks a bit different, they all advocate a similar approach and include the same relevant points. **Moral reasoning** is the thinking that happens after a person recognizes he or she is in an ethical conflict and before he or she takes action on it. It is a form of analysis that encourages thorough consideration of an ethical conflict in light of agreed upon moral norms. It should also be remembered that moral reasoning is not a process that moves in a straight line, even though it is pictured that way. Instead, the steps in the process may be considered simultaneously or in a different order, depending on the situation.

Decision making based on ethical reasoning is similar to the nursing process because it requires deliberate systematic thinking (Figure 5-3). The nurse first determines that an ethical problem exists, in a sense making a diagnosis. There is a data gathering stage, usually followed by a consideration of options based on ethical rationale and principles. After alternatives are considered, persons in an ethical conflict come to a point of action that can be evaluated in an ongoing manner.

Recognition of the Ethical Dilemma

The nurse first distinguishes ethical problems from questions of procedure, legality, or medical diagnosis. To distinguish an ethical problem from other problems, Curtin and Flaherty (1982) recommend that the nurse decide whether the problem has one or more of the following characteristics:

1. It cannot be resolved solely through a review of scientific data.
2. It is perplexing. One cannot easily think logically or make a decision about the problem.
3. The answer to the problem will have a profound relevance for several areas of human concern.

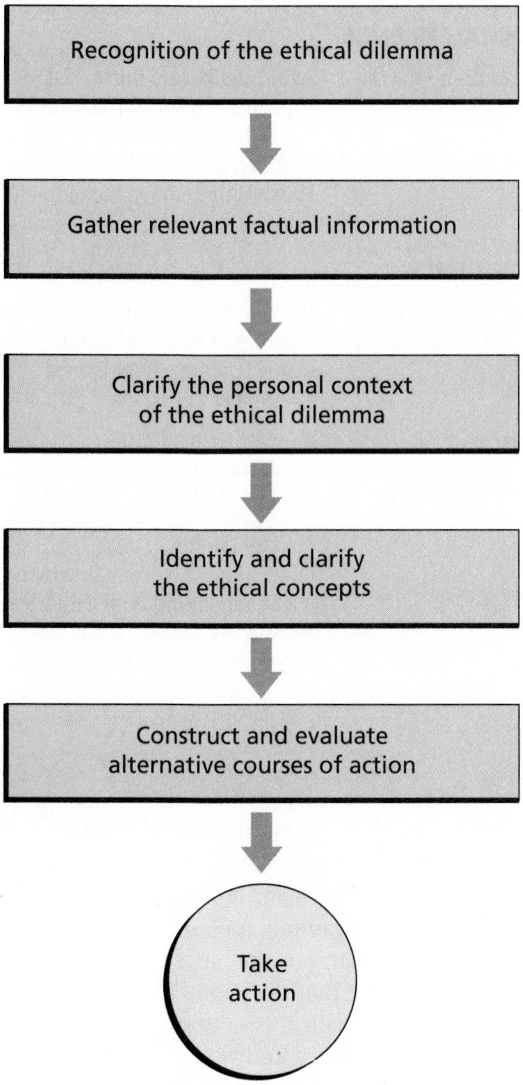

FIGURE 5-3 Process for resolution of ethical dilemmas.

In the following case study, a nurse learns that a young male client diagnosed with AIDS is being discharged after a bout with pneumonia. The client has requested that his family not be informed of his disease, but family members will be involved in the client's care. What health problems are created by the client's decision? Should the client be forced to inform his family? Is it right for the family not to be informed about the client's health care needs? Will the family be exposed to any risks? A conflict in values and ethical principles exists. Either way, the relationship of the client with his family and theirrelationship to others in society could be significantly altered. The dilemma involving this client is an ethical one, and its resolution may be difficult. While there may be some legal issues regarding client confidentiality with HIV infection, the ethical issues are also present.

Gathering Relevant Factual Information

After the nurse recognizes that an ethical dilemma exists, all available information about the situation is collected. Who are all the stakeholders? What are each person's perceptions? It is unwise to make ethical decisions on the basis of another person's opinions or emotions. The nurse gathers information pertinent to the issue and the individuals involved. If clients are involved, this includes medical facts about the situation, knowledge about the client's ability to make decisions, and the meaning of the situation to all affected persons. A client's religious, cultural, and family orientation are part of the nurse's assessment.

In the case study the nurse learns that the client has a history of homosexual contacts about which he states his family is unaware. The nurse suspects that one sister knows about his sexual orientation by the questions she asks. The client and family have always been very close, and he will need extensive care at home. AIDS can be transmitted through contact with blood or body fluids, with the risk of transmission quite low unless a person has direct exposure by a needle stick or a break in the skin. At this time the client does not have any open wounds or bloody secretions, but he does have diarrhea. During the illness, family members have visited often and have shown emotional support. The family believes the client suffers from cancer. The client, capable of making decisions, has expressed a concern that he does not wish to hurt his family especially since he may not live long anyway. His prognosis is uncertain.

Clarifying the Personal Context of the Ethical Dilemma

The next step in ethical problem solving requires the nurse to clarify personal and professional values. Quite likely this step has been addressed all along, but it is important to pause and give it serious consideration. What emotions, attitudes, or values influence the nurse's perception of the dilemma? To clarify the true ethical issues in any situation, a nurse needs to be aware of personal responses.

Because nurses' values can influence clinical decision making, they should understand their own values, how they interact with the values of clients, and the influence nurses' values have on clinical decision making. Sometimes people engaged in ethical conflicts develop distrust for those who see the situation differently from them. It is best to try to enter all conversations with good will toward others in the situation. People come to different conclusions about the same situation with no malice intended toward other people. Remembering this will help the nurse be an effective arbitrator in conversation because when he or she is not defensive, better listening is possible. Using standards clarified within a code of ethics helps the nurse to view dilemmas in a more unbiased manner.

In this situation the nurse recognizes her own bias toward protecting confidentiality. She had a friend with AIDS who lost his job because of careless sharing of information. The nurse also has a personal belief that the family has a right to know about the client's diagnosis and to be protected against any possible risks, even if the risks are few. Furthermore the nurse has had a good relationship with the family and believes they will understand. Despite her feelings the nurse clearly recognizes that the client has the right to keep or share information as he sees appropriate.

Identify and Clarify the Ethical Concepts

When the nurse has as much relevant data as possible, he or she can more clearly define the ethical problem. The nurse frames the problem in ethical language. Here the **ethical principles** of health care are rigorously considered. Principles express what people can agree upon as norms for health care ethics. Like codes of ethics, they are quite general in nature but can provide important guidelines for moral reasoning. Most ethicists agree that principles are binding, meaning that they cannot be just thrown out or not considered. At times principles conflict with one another, making it necessary to give one greater or lesser consideration in a situation.

Five principles are listed most often in health care ethics literature (Beauchamp and Childress, 1989). They include respect for persons, autonomy, nonmaleficence, beneficence, and justice. Definitions of these principles and nursing implications are given in Table 5-2. Many issues arise within health care to challenge a nurse's adherence to each principle. For example, a nurse advocate supports clients' rights to exercise self-determination by allowing them to refuse or accept treatment (respect for autonomy). There are times when the nurse compromises a client's autonomy, however, to prevent harm from coming to the client (nonmaleficence). For example, a client may initially refuse to take a medication; yet the nurse may persuade the client to reconsider that decision. The client's ability to make decisions is critical to a nurse's plan of care, yet the nurse also possesses knowledge and skills that must often be exercised without the client's choice if client welfare is at risk.

table 5-2

PRINCIPLES OF HEALTH CARE ETHICS

Definitions	Nursing implications
RESPECT FOR PERSONS	
Sanctity of life Quality of life Acceptance of death	Display respect for all persons. Support client goals for meaningful life. Care for dying with respect.
AUTONOMY	
Personal liberty of action Independence Self-reliance	Promote client decision making. Support client's right to informed consent. Make decisions when client's choice poses harm. Autonomy is truly exercised when members of the health care team agree to importance of autonomy.
NONMALEFICENCE	
Duty to do no harm	Avoid deliberate harm, risk of harm, and harm that occurs during performance of nursing actions. Prevent or remove harm to client when possible.
BENEFICENCE	
Doing or active promotion of good	Provide health benefits to clients. Balance benefit and harm. Consider how client is best helped.
JUSTICE	
Fairness or equity	Ensure fair allocation of resources such as nursing care to all clients. Determine the order in which clients should be treated; for example, clients at greatest risk are treated first.

In applying principles to the AIDS case study, the issue centers on the client's right to be self-determining in making decisions. Autonomy supports this client's right to choose his course of therapy and to refrain from informing the family about his disease.

The family members have the right to be informed of any potential risks to minimize risks to themselves. The client's freedom should not endanger someone else's life. The nurse must consider the extent to which the family may be at risk. Guided by the principle of nonmaleficence and beneficence, the nurse wants to make sure the family has the information needed to care for the client safely and properly. Furthermore, the nurse may believe that a greater good (beneficence) may be accomplished by having the client tell his family. Perhaps talking would bring them closer because of the trust displayed.

Construct and Evaluate Alternative Courses of Action

With the ethical problem more clearly defined, the nurse can list all options to determine the action that will maintain the client's rights and the nurse's professional integrity. The nurse constructs and reviews alternatives based on ethical principles. In listing alternatives, all options should be considered. Sometimes courses of action that seem unlikely take on new possibilities as they are put to reasoned analysis.

The nurse in the case study is faced with several alternatives. If the family is to be told, the question of who should tell remains. The family could be told by the client, a health care professional, or another support person. They can be told with the client's consent or without it, depending on the risk to the family involved. Another alternative is to remain silent and not inform the family.

The nurse knows that the client loves and respects his family and is trying to protect them from further emotional harm. If the client informs the family about his disease, the family can learn to safely care for the client. A well-educated family can also anticipate the client's needs more effectively. There is a risk, however, that the client's acknowledgment of his condition may cause the family to reject him. The client has already expressed the desire to be cared for in the home. As the client becomes more critically ill, the family might become exposed to body fluids. The nurse considers whether there are ways to protect the family from harm if they remain uninformed.

Take Action

The nurse decides on a course of action after evaluating all alternatives. Regardless of how careful a person is in resolving ethical dilemmas, others may reject the solution or opinion. Involvement of all informed health team members can prove a useful resource.

In this case, the nurse decides to talk with the client about his reasons for not telling his family. She does not believe the risk to the family is great enough at this time to betray client confidentiality. The nurse explains to the client how his disease may progress, the extent to which the family may become involved, and the risks to them. In the end, the client must decide whether to inform his family. The nurse explains the value of having the family informed so that safe supportive care can be given. If the client still chooses not to inform his family, the nurse assures him that his right will be respected and works with the family and a home health nurse to be sure the family learns safe techniques. Procedures can be explained without revealing the client's diagnosis. If the risk to the family should change, the decision can be reevaluated and a new course of action taken.

No two ethical dilemmas are the same. Without a systematic approach to ethical decision making, a nurse cannot resolve ethical issues in a consistent, objective, and professional manner. Ethical decisions are always made, either deliberately or by default. Whether or not nurses contribute to successful outcomes in ethical situations will be determined by their willingness to engage in a disciplined and compassionate dialogue with others.

ETHICAL PROBLEMS IN NURSING

Nursing ethics must keep pace with the diversity in nursing practice. Nursing involves caring for all aspects of a person's health care needs, not just care during a hospitalized illness. More independent roles for nurses are emerging, such as in home health care or clinical nurse specialties. As the professional roles expand, nurses confront a variety of ethical dilemmas. Issues may arise in any of the following areas for which the nurse is accountable: self, profession, client and family, employing institution, and society. In addition, in any practice specialty, a nurse will be confronted with ethical issues unique to that practice (see box on p. 90). The following sections describe some pertinent ethical dilemmas and give one specific situation for several areas of nursing practice.

Community Health Nursing. As providers of primary care, community health nurses work with clients in situations that are often very different from those faced by other health care workers. Clients and their families face difficult decisions regarding diagnosis and treatment and the social implications of disease. The community health nurse is especially concerned with the social and environmental factors in health and wellness.

For example, a concerned mother may seek medical

ETHICAL ISSUES IN NURSING PRACTICE

COMMUNITY HEALTH NURSING

Abortion
Artificial insemination by donor
Contraception
Genetic counseling
Rights to health care

HOME HEALTH NURSING

Reimbursement restrictions for home health care
Undertreatment of terminally ill with analgesic medications
Client's refusal to be hospitalized
Treatments administered by family members

NURSING OF CHILDREN

Allowing severely ill neonates to die
Child abuse
Surrogate decision making for children

MEDICAL-SURGICAL NURSING

Organ and tissue transplantation
Brain death protocols
Disclosure of diagnosis to terminally ill clients
Inadequate staffing
Living wills
Termination of life support
Futile treatment

NURSING HOMES

Elderly abuse
Research involving residents
Use of restraints

MENTAL HEALTH NURSING

Behavior control
Involuntary hospitalization
Informed consent

NURSING RESEARCH

Confidentiality
Informed consent
Rights of human subjects
Identification of risks

NURSE-PHYSICIAN-CLIENT RELATIONSHIPS

Confidentiality
Power relationships
Role conflicts
Verbal or telephone orders
Impaired nurses and physicians

NURSE-NURSE RELATIONSHIPS

Reporting nurses who are impaired or observing incorrect nursing practice
Interdependent roles
Staffing

care for her 15-year-old daughter whom she suspects is sexually active. The daughter's unwillingness to talk with the mother suggests a problem. The mother insists that the daughter be placed on birth control. The nurse is obligated to assess the daughter's needs to determine whether a health problem exists. The risks of pregnancy or exposure to sexually transmitted disease should be shared with the teenager. She has a right to be informed and referred to a physician if she uses birth control. As an advocate, the community health nurse must ensure that the client has sufficient information to make a decision.

Home Health Nursing. Changes in reimbursement have created the incentive for hospitals to discharge clients in a timely and efficient manner. As a result, nurses in hospitals often have less time to educate or prepare clients and families for care needed in the home. More clients return home with pain, chronic illness, ambulation restrictions, new medications, and incompletely healed surgical incisions. Home health nurses may work in settings with clients who have limited financial resources and who need care that is not reimbursable.

Frequently, while caring for a client in the home, the nurse may learn of health problems unrelated to the client's primary diagnosis. For example, a client with limited knowledge of self-care may require several instruction sessions. The nurse has an ethical responsibility to give clients the information they need. Regulations prohibit reimbursement for client education if it is the only service offered by the nurse; the client also must require specific skilled nursing care. The principle of beneficence implies that the client should be given the best help for his or her particular health problem. Failure to give instruction could leave this client uninformed and at risk for medical complications.

Nursing of Children. The ethical question of whether a person should be allowed to die is one of the most difficult faced by health care professionals and society. The issue is of even more value when it involves children; people often find it difficult to understand why a child dies without having had the opportunity to experience a full life. If a child suffers from a terminal illness or a serious brain injury, parents and family members may have to decide between pursuing life at great cost and allowing the child to die. Some people believe that a person should not be forced to endure pain, suffering, or humiliation and that he or she has the right to choose relief in dying. Others, however, believe that hope should never be discarded; they argue that no individual has the right to determine when life is over. The ethical principle of autonomy gives the parents the right to decide their child's fate. Sometimes the parents seek the nurse's advice. The nurse helps the parents clarify their own values and then supports the decision.

Medical-Surgical Nursing. Of all the treatment situations experienced by medical-surgical nurses, few raise as many ethical questions as organ transplantation. Transplantation is now a realistic option for persons suffering chronic and disabling diseases. Organ and tissue recipients are able to resume productive lives after surgery, and their life expectancy may be extended several years.

With the success of organ transplants, ethical concerns have increased. The availability of donor organs is limited, making transplants a scarce resource. What criteria should be used to determine who should be a recipient? Should a transplant be withheld if a client cannot afford it? Nurses care for donors and recipients, and the issues of organ transplantation can become very emotional.

Most states now have "required request" laws making it mandatory for trained staff to inform families of the option for organ donation when a deceased person is a potential organ or tissue donor. The option of organ donation raises many questions. Will the body be disfigured because of organ or tissue removal? Are there donor costs related to organ recovery? Will burial be delayed? (The answer to all these questions is "No.") The nurse learns to be an advocate, giving families the information needed to decide if organ donation is desirable. If families decide against donation, their right to make that decision should be respected and supported.

Nursing Homes. The number of older adults in the United States and Canada is increasing every year—a result, in part, of disease cures, better treatment for chronic illness, and more interest in health promotion. A relatively small percentage of this population lives in nursing homes. Questions of client competence, the use of restraints, advance directives, and issues of quality of life are relevant for nursing home practitioners.

Also, an alarming number of older adults entering nursing homes are victims of abuse from family members. The older adult experiences physical and psychological abuse, financial and personal exploitation, and neglect. A nurse may see symptoms of physical abuse when a client is first admitted to a nursing home or after the client returns from a short visit with family.

Today a majority of states require nurses and other health care professionals to report abuse of older adults regardless of whether that person wishes a report to be made. Many abused older adults are able to make their own decisions, but state laws support the false idea that most older adults are incompetent. The nurse should make a careful assessment of the client's decision making abilities. Complying with the law leaves many nurses believing they have violated the client's autonomy, especially if the nurse's assessment of abuse is wrong. Making the wrong conclusions can seriously threaten the relationship with the client and family, but to allow abuse to continue is a problem of grave concern.

Mental Health Nursing. Controlling a person's behavior can be considered an infringement of liberty. Confinement in a mental institution is an example of depriving persons of freedom. However, mental health care professionals have a variety of less extreme methods to control behavior in the interest of the person's health and welfare and the welfare of society. Tranquilizers, electric shock, psychosurgery (removal or destruction of a portion of brain tissue that controls behavior), and psychotherapy are examples. Many ethical dilemmas arise. Who decides whether behavior is normal or desirable? Who is expert enough to identify normal behavior? If persons have difficulty adjusting to their role in society, whose goals should influence behavior therapy—the client's, family's, therapist's, or society's? Should a person's behavior be changed if he or she does not wish it to be? Should the nurse participate?

Nursing Research. Many opportunities exist for researching the effectiveness of nursing interventions. For example, staff nurses may wish to compare two methods for decubitus ulcer care or two different teaching methods on a group of clients. The studies may prove that one form of care is measurably better than the other. Nursing research can contribute to the body of knowledge influencing nursing practice.

Research involving human subjects can be useful and beneficial. The nurse is ethically responsible for obtaining free and informed (voluntary) consent from persons participating in a study. Informed consent means that all study subjects understand the purpose of the study, research methods (e.g., application of a new type of ulcer dressing), and possible risks or benefits. The nurse who plans the study is responsible for acquiring informed consent.

There is often pressure to complete a study in a timely manner. Clients approached as potential study subjects may not always be totally alert or responsive because of pain, the effects of medication, or the systemic effects of illness. A client who hurriedly signs a consent form without asking questions may not understand the study's purpose and implications. The nurse must be sure that all clients involved are fully informed.

Nurse-Physician-Client Relationships. In addition to clients, nurses are also accountable to families, health care administrators, and physicians. Ethical duties to all of these participants pose unique problems for nurses. These duties may conflict simultaneously. For example, assume that a nurse is caring for a client whose wife has died during his hospitalization. The client asks frequent questions about why his wife has not visited. The client's physician has left orders not to tell the client of his wife's death for fear that an emotional setback would worsen his condition. The nurse's duty to the client's needs conflicts with the duty to follow the physician's orders. The nurse's responsibility to provide psychological support has been made more difficult because the truth cannot be shared with the client. Recent nursing studies reveal that nurses and physicians process ethical questions in different ways, contributing to disagreements in what action to take in a situation of conflict (Grundstein-Amado, 1992; Uden, Norberg, Lindseth and Marhaug, 1992).

The question of a nurse's autonomy is raised here. Although all practitioners depend on one another in the accomplishment of client goals, nurses often find themselves caught in power relationships over which they have no control (Yarling and McElmurry, 1986). They must weigh their obligations to the client, family, physician, and employing institution. Although nurses have tremendous responsibility and accountability to others, they often do not have the authority to carry out their judgments.

The nurse can face a conflict of duty between her loyalty to the client and his or her place of employment. The nurse wants to give compassionate and skilled care. Health care administrators need good consumer relations and a realistic budget. Physicians expect nurses to follow the proposed plans of treatment. If a tight budget results in understaffing, the number of nurses may be inadequate to provide compassionate care. A physician may write an order that a nurse knows to be inappropriate for the staffing situation; yet the nurse faces great pressure to carry out the order. To whom is the nurse most accountable? How can the nurse resolve an ethical dilemma and still retain her professionalism in delivering quality care?

Nurse-Nurse Relationships. In most areas of nursing practice, nurses work together. Because of these interdependent relationships, one nurse's practice affects and is affected by the practice of others. When one nurse acts unethically, questions may be raised about the entire nursing team.

Several factors add to the complexity of ethical issues between nurses. Levels of experience among nurses vary widely. A nurse experienced in one area of practice and informed about current developments in nursing is likely to be more clinically qualified than a recent graduate. Nurses place differing degrees of importance on theoretical models of nursing, as well as on activities involved in the nursing process. It is common to find two nurses correctly performing the same procedure in two entirely different ways.

Regardless of educational preparation and experience, nurses are expected to perform competently. Ethical conflicts between nurses may arise when a nurse's competence is questioned. For example, a hospitalized client complains to the nurse working the evening shift about a nurse on the day shift who was rude and slow to respond to calls. The client does not want the evening nurse to tell anyone about the incident for fear that the day shift nurse will become angry. If the client's report is true, the offending nurse has failed to meet the obligation of an ethic of care. Unless something is done, additional problems may develop between the day nurse and the client. Should the evening nurse report the incident?

If a nurse has been observed by peers to make mistakes and become rude with clients, something must be done about that nurse's behavior. A nurse is not demonstrating responsiblity, accountability, or care if the unethical conduct of a colleague is ignored. Careful judgment is needed to resolve the dilemma of unethical professional relationships.

SUMMARY

A person's unique set of values about ideas and behaviors influences decisions and actions and in part determines identity. A person's conscious awareness of values helps in reaching decisions and avoiding and resolving conflicts. A client conscious of values related to health and health behaviors is able to participate more fully in health care, and a nurse who is conscious of values is better able to help clients clarify values and make decisions.

Ethics consist of the principles that govern proper conduct, character, and motives. Ethical issues are frequently confused with legal issues. Although the law and ethics often overlap, ethics is concerned with what is right or good regardless of its legality. To substitute legal truth for ethical truth is legalism. The terms *ethics* and *morals* are usually used interchangeably. Ethics, however, may mean the study of ethical situations, and morals refers to the behaviors and attitudes people put into practice.

People form values consciously and unconsciously through reasoning, observation, experience, and socialization. Values are acquired in a continuous process that begins in infancy and continues through life. People undergo moral development at different stages in their lives. Nurses have personal and professional values. With socialization into the nursing profession, these values may converge into one.

The process of values clarification can be useful for increasing awareness of the impact personal values have on professional behavior and for resolving conflicts when values are being tested. Values clarification is the use of strategies to explore the meaning of values and behaviors. When values are known, stated, and positively affirmed, the client, nurse, or health care team is more capable of making objective decisions about health care.

A professional commits himself or herself to the profession, taking on its moral obligations. A profession's ethical posture is communicated through the instillation of values and in its codes of ethics. Responsible practitioners of nursing exhibit competence and skill when performing required nursing actions.

Care, advocacy, responsibility, and accountability are primary nursing values. Care is a core value that requires the nurse to be empathic, understanding, and other-directed. Advocacy requires the nurse to uphold the client's autonomy through education and support. Responsibility and accountability are necessary for the moral performance of all nursing functions.

The professional nurse assumes roles in which complex ethical situations develop. To resolve an ethical problem, a nurse uses a systematic process to understand the nature of the problem and to plan a responsible course of action. The ethical principles of respect for person, autonomy, nonmaleficence, beneficence, and justice assist the nurse in clinical decision making. Although ethical dilemmas are not easily resolved, a nurse applying good reasoning skills will be better able to help self and others arrive at meaningful, fair, and humane ethical decisions.

The scope of nursing practice involves caring for all aspects of a person's health care needs. As nursing's professional role expands, a greater variety of ethical dilemmas arise. The nurse's professional activities with clients, families, and other health care professionals will lead to ethical situations that challenge the nurse's moral reasoning skills.

KEY CONCEPTS

- A nurse's values can influence decisions about a client's care.
- People develop morally just as they do physically, emotionally, and spiritually.
- A child is helped to acquire values by observing behaviors that prove successful or productive for others.
- A child acquires values from parents, other family members, school, church, and other social institutions.
- Restrictions that parents set for a child should be balanced with opportunities for the child to explore behaviors and their consequences.
- Values clarification is not an indoctrination method but a process that promotes an individual's understanding of personal values.
- A person should be able to choose values freely from available alternatives and understand the consequences of that choice.
- Values clarification helps a nurse to explore personal values and feelings and decide whether to act on personal beliefs.
- The nurse who learns about client values is better prepared to help the client assume health-protecting or health-promoting behaviors.
- A nurse's values influence decisions made about a client's care.
- Values clarification promotes effective reasoning and decision making.
- A professional nursing code of ethics protects both the public and the professional practitioners by setting standards of conduct.
- Professional nurses have a commitment to clients, the profession, and society to provide high-quality health care.
- An ethical nurse maintains competence in practice and assumes responsibility for nursing judgments.
- The primary functions of advocacy are to inform and to support.
- Advocacy requires a nurse to give a client accurate meaningful information without jeopardizing the client's relationship with physician or family.
- Care is the moral foundation of nursing.
- A nurse guided by an ethic of care will be empathic, understanding, other-centered, and able to take action on behalf of another.
- Ethical problems arise from conflicts in values, changing professional roles, technological advances, and uncertainty in decision making.
- The ethical principles of respect for persons, autonomy, nonmaleficence, beneficence, and justice guide moral reasoning.
- A method for resolving ethical dilemmas helps nurses think through morally perplexing situations.
- Experiences in nursing practice help nurses incorporate professional values into their personal value system.
- Responsibility and accountability demand that when nurses witness acts that may endanger clients, they are obligated to take the action necessary to eliminate the danger.

CRITICAL THINKING ACTIVITIES

1. Write a paragraph or short story that describes a personal caring experience or expresses how you learned to value caring.
2. Complete the values clarification exercise "Health Values Scale" with a group of classmates. Share your rankings and select a person from the group whose health values are different from your own. Determine what that person may need if he or she were a client in your care.
3. You are teaching a recently diagnosed 15-year-old diabetic about his diet when he says: "I'm going to eat whatever I want. It doesn't matter anyway since I have to take this insulin stuff." Regarding this situation, determine what value conflicts may be present, discuss this client's moral/value development needs, and suggest how this nurse may demonstrate accountability and responsibility?
4. A client in a cardiac rehabilitation center has been encouraged to quit smoking and reduce stress in his life. Using the four modes of value transmission, give examples of how a nurse may communicate values to this client regarding smoking and stress reduction. Describe how nurses give messages of which they are unaware.
5. Determine your position on a common ethical issue (e.g., abortion, assisted suicide, euthanasia). Then pose as many arguments as you can **against** your own position.

References

American Association of Colleges of Nursing: *Essentials of college and university education for professional nursing,* Washington, DC, 1986, The Association.

American Nurses Association: *Code for nurses with interpretative statements,* Kansas City, Mo, 1985, The Association.

Beauchamp T and Childress J: *Principles of biomedical ethics,* ed 3, New York, 1989, Oxford University Press.

Bernal E: The nurse as patient advocate, *Hast Cen Rep* 22(4):18-23, 1992.

Bevis E: Caring: a life force. In Leininger M, editor: *Caring: an essential human need,* Detroit, 1988, Wayne State University Press.

Brown J, Kitson A, and McKnight T: *Challenges in caring: explorations in nursing and ethics,* London, 1992, Chapman & Hall.

Canadian Nurses Association: *Code of ethics for nursing,* 1985, The Association.

Chitty K: *Professional nursing: concepts & challenges,* Philadelphia, 1993, WB Saunders.

Cochran J and Ganong L: A comparison of nurses' and patients' perceptions in intensive care unit stressors, *J Adv Nurs* 14(12):1038-1043, 1989.

Curtin L and Flaherty MJ: *Nursing ethics: theories and pragmatics,* Bowie, Md, 1982, Brady.

Davis A and Aroskar M: *Ethical dilemmas and nursing practice,* Norwalk, Conn, 1991, Appleton & Lange.

Deloughery G: *Issues and trends in nursing,* St. Louis, 1991, Mosby.

Gilligan C: *In a different voice,* Cambridge, Mass, 1982, Harvard University Press.

Grundstein-Amado R: Differences in ethical decision-making processes among nurses and doctors, *J Adv Nurs* 17(2):129-137, 1992.

Hamilton P: *Realities of contemporary nursing,* Reading, Mass., 1992, Addison-Wesley Nursing.

Holmes S and Eburn E: Patients' and nurses' perceptions of symptom distress in cancer, *J Adv Nurs* 14(10):840-846, 1989.

Husted G and Husted J: *Ethical decision making in nursing,* St. Louis, 1991, Mosby.

International Council of Nurses: *Ethical concepts applied to nursing,* Geneva, 1973, Imprimeries Popularies.

Kelly L: *The nursing experience: trends, challenges, and transitions,* ed 2, New York, 1992, McGraw-Hill.

Kohlberg L: *Essays on moral development: vol I-III,* San Francisco, 1981, Harper & Row.

Kluckhohn C: Values and value-orientation in the theory of action: an exploration in definition and classification. In Parsons T and Shils E, editors: *Toward a general theory of action,* New York, 1951, Harper & Row.

Leininger M: *Transcultural nursing: concepts, theories, and practices,* New York, 1978, John Wiley & Sons.

Leininger M: *Caring: an essential human need,* Detroit, 1988, Wayne State University Press.

Leininger M: *Culture care diversity and universality: a theory of nursing,* New York, 1991, National League of Nursing Press.

Maslow A: *New knowledge in human values,* New York, 1959, Harper & Row.

Noddings N: *Caring: a feminist approach to ethics and moral education,* Berkeley, Calif., 1984, University of California Press.

Piaget J: *The moral development of the child,* New York, 1932, The Free Press.

Potter P and Perry A: *Fundamentals of nursing: concepts, process, and practice,* ed 3, St. Louis, 1993, Mosby.

Raths LE, Harmin M, and Simon SB: *Values and teaching,* ed 2, Columbus, Ohio, 1979, Merrill Publishing.

Rokeach M: *The nature of human values,* New York, 1973, The Free Press.

Salsberry P: Caring, virtue theory, and a foundation for nursing ethics, *Sch Inq Nurs Prac: Int J* 6(2):155-167, 1992.

Uden G, Norberg A et al. Ethical reasoning in nurses' and physicians' stories about care episodes, *J Adv Nurs* 17(9):1028-1034, 1992.

Uustal D: Enhancing your ethical reasoning, *Crit Care Nurs Clin North Am* 2(3):437-442, 1990.

Uustal D: *Values and ethics in nursing: from theory to practice,* ed 4, East Greenwich, RI, 1992, Educational Resources in Nursing & Holistic Health.

Von Essen L and Sjoden PO: Patient and staff perceptions of caring: review and replication, *J Adv Nurs* 16(1):1363-1374, 1991.

Watson J: *Nursing: human science and human care—a theory of nursing,* New York, 1988, National League of Nursing Press.

Yarling R and McElmurry B: The moral foundation of nursing, *ANS* 8(2):63-73, 1986.

Bibliography

Allmark P: The ethical enterprise of nursing, *J Adv Nurs* 17(1):16-20, 1992.

Anderson SL: Patient advocacy and whistle-blowing in nursing: help for the helpers, *Nurs Forum* 25(3):5-15, 1990.

Bishop A and Scudder J: *Nursing: the practice of caring,* New York, 1990, National League of Nursing Press.

Bishop A and Scudder J: *The practical, moral and personal sense of nursing,* Albany, NY, 1990, State University of New York Press.

Cameron M: Justice, care and virtue, *J Prof Nurs* 7(4):206, 1991.

Chinn P: *Anthology on caring,* New York, 1991, National League of Nursing Press.

Chipman Y: Caring: its meaning and place in the practice of nursing, *J Nurs Ed* 30(4):171-175, 1991.

Cooper MC: Principle-oriented ethics and the ethic of care: a creative tension, *ANS* 14(2):22-31, 1991.

Davis A: Dilemmas in alternative care settings, *West J Nurs Res* 13(5):650-652, 1991.

Diekelmann N: Nursing education: caring, dialogue, and practice, *J Nurs Ed* 29(7):300-305, 1990.

Elliot C: Where ethics comes from and what to do about it, *Hast Cen Rep* 22(2):28-35, 1992.

Erlen JA: Demystifying ethical decision making, *Orthop Nurs* 11(1):49-53, 1992.

Evers S: Nursing ethics: the central concept of nursing education, *Nurs Educ* 9(4):14-18, 1984.

Freitas L: Historical roots and future perspectives related to nursing ethics, *J Prof Nurs* 6(4):197-205, 1990.

Gingerich BS: Values incorporation throughout the organization, *Caring* 12(1):18-23, 1993.

Hunt G: What is nursing ethics? *Nurs Educ Today* 12(5):323-328, 1992.

Jarczewski PH: What is an ethical decision? Ethics for contemporary nursing practice, *Adv Clin Care* 5(3):28, 1990.

Kjervik DK: The connection between law and ethics, *J Prof Nurs* 6(3):138, 1990.

Kurtz R and Wang J: The caring ethic: more than kindness, the core of nursing science, *Nurs For* 26(1):4-8, 1991.

Lund M: Nursing home dilemmas . . . tell us how you manage the day-to-day ethical issues, *Geriatr Nurs* 10(6):298-300, 1989.

May W: *The physician's ordeal,* Bloomington, Ind, 1992, Indiana University Press.

Mayeroff M: *On caring,* New York, 1971, Harper Perennial.

Moccia P: Re-claiming our communities, *Nurs Outlook* 38(2):73-76, 1990.

Pratt RJ: Moral decision making in the age of AIDS, *Nursing (Lond)* 4(34):17-18, 1991.

Reilly D: Ethics and values in nursing: are we opening Pandora's box? *Nurs Health Care* 12:91-95, 1991.

Rogers B: Ethics and research, *AAOHN J* 38(12):588-590, 1990.

Roberts J: Uncovering hidden caring, *Nurs Outlook* 38(2):67-69, 1990.

Thompson JE: Moral development, *Neonat Netw* 9(1):77-78, 1990.

Watson J: The moral failure of the patriarchy, *Nurs Outlook* 38(2):62-66, 1990.

Wuthnow R: *Acts of compassion: caring for others and helping ourselves,* Princeton, NJ, 1991, Princeton University Press.

6

Legal Considerations

OBJECTIVES

Mastery of content in this chapter will enable the student to:

- Define the key terms listed.
- Explain legal concepts that apply to nurses.
- Give examples of legal issues that arise in nursing practice.
- Describe legal responsibilities and obligations of nurses.
- Understand the concept of negligence.
- List sources for standards of care for nurses.
- Define legal aspects of nurse-client, nurse-physician, and nurse-employer relationships.

KEY TERMS

assault
battery
civil law
common law
crime
criminal law
defamation of character
euthanasia
felony
Good Samaritan laws
incident report
informed consent
invasion of privacy
libel
living wills
malpractice
malpractice insurance
misdemeanor
negligence
nursing practice acts
regulatory agencies
slander
standards of care
statutory law
tort

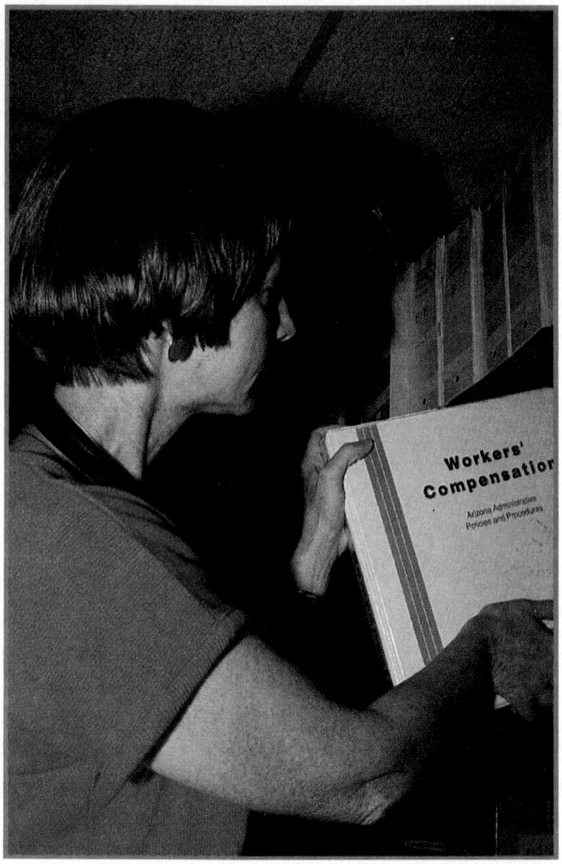

(Courtesy Philip James Acker, Motorola, Inc.)

Contemporary law is a composite of the rules, regulations, mores, and norms by which society governs itself. Without law, society could not deal with disputes and problems in an orderly fashion. The laws of Western society are flexible and ever changing through the legislative process or judicial decisions, in keeping with societal changes.

The law serves many valuable functions when applied to nursing practice. It differentiates nursing practice from the practice of other health care professions, and it describes and protects the rights of clients and nurses. For these reasons, nurses should understand basic legal concepts as they relate to nursing practice (Brown, 1989).

Many nurses view the law with apprehension because they fear being named in a malpractice lawsuit. With increased emphasis on clients' rights, nurses today must understand their legal obligations and responsibilities to clients. Nurses who give competent care based on their education will seldom need to worry about a malpractice lawsuit.

The public is better informed today than in the past about health and illness. Through reports in newspapers, magazines, and on television, more information is available to consumers of health services. Many clients know their rights, and nurses are challenged to become advocates for clients. In 1972 the American Hospital Association (AHA) developed and adopted A Patient's Bill of Rights. It has undergone several revisions, the most recent in 1992 (AHA, 1992). In 1974 the Dying Person's Bill of Rights was completed, and in 1975 the Pregnant Patient's Bill of Rights was written. In addition, the Joint Commission on Accreditation of Health Care Organizations, the organization that surveys and accredits health care facilities such as hospitals and nursing homes, has developed a list of patients' rights and requires the organizations to support those rights (JCAHO, 1993). Although these documents are not considered legally binding, many hospitals use them to provide guidelines for care.

LEGAL LIMITS OF NURSING

Standards of Care

One of the functions of law, as applied to nursing practice, is to define the standards of care the nurse must provide. All U.S. state legislatures and Canadian provincial parliaments have passed **nursing practice acts** that define the scope of nursing practice. These acts define nursing practice and expanded nursing roles, set educational requirements for nurses, and distinguish between nursing practice and medical practice. Each act also defines "registered nursing" or "professional nursing" and "practical or vocational nursing." All nurses are responsible for knowing the provisions of the act for the state or province in which they work.

Professional organizations are another source for defining the standards of care. The American Nurses Association (ANA) and Canadian Nurses Association (CNA) have developed standards for nursing practice, policy statements, and similar resolutions. These standards are very general and include such recommendations as the obligation to provide continuing education programs.

The written policies and procedures of the employing institution detail ways in which the nurse is to perform duties. Such policies are usually quite specific and are set forth in procedure manuals found in most nursing units. For example, a procedure and policy outlining the steps that should be taken when changing a dressing or administering medication gives specific information for nurses to perform these tasks. These policies provide another definition of standards of care. Policies and procedures of institutions may be more restrictive than nurse practice acts, but they can never request a nurse to act beyond the standards of practice allowed by law.

Standards of care are guidelines by which nurses should practice. If nurses do not perform duties within accepted standards of care, they may place themselves in jeopardy of legal action. In a malpractice lawsuit, these standards are used to determine whether the nurse has acted as would any reasonably prudent nurse with the same level of education and experience, and in the same or similar circumstances. Standards of care are thus guidelines for determining whether the nurse performed duties in an appropriate manner. If nurses are named in malpractice lawsuits, and it is shown that neither the accepted standards of care outlined by the state or province nursing practice act nor the policies of the employing institution were followed, the nurses' legal liability is clear.

Standards of care concern nurses' accountability or willingness to answer for their actions. Standards clarify the scope of functions a nurse is responsible to perform (Horting, 1989). General duty nurses are legally responsible for meeting the same standards as other general duty nurses in similar settings. However, specialized nurses such as nurse anesthetists, intensive care nurses, certified nurse midwives, or operating room nurses are held to standards of care and skill exercised by those in the same specialty as defined by applicable standards. Every nurse must know the appropriate standards of care (Hemelt and Mackert, 1981).

One of the first and most important cases to discuss a nurse's liability was *Darling v. Charleston Community Memorial Hospital.* The verdict in the case, decided by the Illinois Supreme Court in 1966, has been adopted by almost every state. It involved an 18-year-old man with a fractured leg. When the cast was applied to the leg, the physician placed insufficient padding under the plaster. The man's toes became swollen and discolored, and he had decreased sensation in them. He complained to the nursing staff many times. Although the nurses recognized the symptoms as signs of impaired circulation, they failed to notify their supervisor that the physician did not respond to their calls or the client's needs. During the next 4 days, gangrene developed, and the man's leg had to be amputated. The physician in the emergency room was liable for applying the cast incorrectly. The nursing staff was also liable because it had not adhered to the standards of care appropriate for the client's symptoms.

Licensure

All registered nurses and licensed practical nurses are licensed by the board of nursing of the state or province in which they practice. The requirements for licensure vary, but requirements for education are in most licensing acts, and the nurse must pass an examination. Licensure permits persons to offer special skills and knowledge to the public, but it also provides legal guidelines for protection of the public. All states use the National Council Licensure Examinations (NCLEX) for registered and licensed practical nurse examinations.

A nurse's license can be suspended or revoked by the board of nursing if conduct violates provisions of the licensing statute. For example, nurses who perform illegal acts such as selling or taking controlled substances jeopardize their license status. Before licenses are revoked, nurses must be notified of the charges and permitted to attend a hearing to present evidence on their own behalf. These hearings are not court proceedings but are usually conducted by the state or provincial board of nursing. Some states and provinces provide for judicial review of such cases if the nurse has exhausted all other forms of appeal.

Student Nurses

If clients suffer harm as a direct result of nursing students' actions, the liability for the incorrect action is generally shared by the student, instructor, and hospital or health care facility. Student nurses should never be assigned to tasks for which they are unprepared and should be carefully supervised by instructors as they learn new procedures. Although student nurses are not considered employees of the hospital, the institution has a responsibility to monitor the acts of nursing students. Student nurses are expected to perform as a professional nurse would; the law does not provide for a difference in quality of care rendered to clients (Ulys, 1988). Faculty members are usually responsible for instructing and observing students, but in some situations staff nurses may share these responsibilities. Every nursing school should provide clear definitions of responsibility.

Sometimes, student nurses are employed as nursing assistants or nurse's aides when they are not attending classes. If student nurses are so employed, they should not perform tasks that do not appear in a job description for a nurse's aide or assistant. For example, even if a student has learned to administer intramuscular medications in class, this task may not be performed by a nurse's aide.

LEGAL LIABILITY IN NURSING

Two basic sources exist for contemporary law. **Statutory law** is created by elected legislative bodies such as state or provincial legislatures, the U.S. Congress, administrative bodies such as state boards of nursing, or the Canadian Parliament. **Common law** is created by judicial decisions made in courts when cases are decided.

Criminal law is concerned with relationships be-

Administrative law made by boards and government boards

tween individuals and governments and with acts that threaten society and its order. Misuse of controlled substances is an example of criminal conduct for nurses.

A **crime** is an offense against society that violates a law. Criminal acts are prosecuted in the criminal justice system (Black, 1979). A **felony** is a crime of a serious nature that usually carries a penalty of imprisonment or death (Black, 1979). A **misdemeanor** is a crime of a less serious nature than a felony, and the penalty is usually a fine or imprisonment for less than a year (Black, 1979). In nursing, there are few crimes a nurse would commit if practicing within accepted standards of care. For purposes of this chapter, flagrant criminal activity such as murder or illegally dispensing controlled substances will not be discussed. Laws pertaining to such offenses apply to nurses as well as all other individuals.

Civil law is concerned with the relationships among people and the protection of a person's rights (Black, 1979). Although violations of civil law might cause harm to an individual or property, society as a whole is usually not affected. For example, defamatory statements made about an individual might lead to interpersonal problems, but they do not threaten society as a whole.

A **tort** is a civil wrong committed against a person or property (Black, 1979). Torts may be subtle and difficult to define; they may be classified as intentional or unintentional. Unintentional torts include negligence. Malpractice is one example of an unintentional tort, or negligence. Intentional torts are willful acts that violate another's rights. Examples are assault, battery, defamation, invasion of privacy, false imprisonment, and fraud.

Negligence

Negligence is conduct that falls below the standard of care. It is established by law for the protection of others against unreasonable risk of harm, and it is characterized chiefly by inadvertence, thoughtlessness, or inattention (Black, 1979).

If nurses give care that does not meet appropriate standards, they may be held liable for negligence. Negligence may involve carelessness, such as failing to check a client's arm band and then administering the wrong drug. Another example of negligence may be administering a medication even when it has been documented that the client has an allergy to that medication. However, carelessness is not always the cause. If nurses attempt a procedure for which they have not been trained and do it carefully but still harm the client, a claim of negligence could be made.

Nurses have been involved in several common negligent acts including the following:

1. Intravenous therapy errors resulting in infiltrations or phlebitis
2. Burns to clients
3. Falls resulting in injury to clients
4. Failure to use aseptic technique where required
5. Errors in sponge, instrument, or needle counts in surgical cases
6. Failure to give a report, or to give an incomplete report, to an oncoming shift

Nurses are responsible for performing all procedures correctly and for exercising professional judgment as they carry out the orders of physicians and duties not ordered but for which they have authority. Any nurse who does not meet accepted standards of care while discharging duties or who performs duties carelessly runs a risk of being found negligent.

Malpractice

Malpractice is one type of negligence. It is defined as professional misconduct, unreasonable lack of skill or fidelity in professional duties, evil practice, or illegal or immoral conduct (Black, 1979). In a malpractice lawsuit against a nurse, the following criteria must be established:

1. The nurse (defendant) owed a *duty* to the client (plaintiff)
2. The nurse *did not carry out that duty*
3. The client was *injured*
4. The client's *injury was a result of* the nurse's *failure to carry out his or her duty*

These are the criteria for every type of tort, not only malpractice (Prosser and Keeton, 1988).

The best way for nurses to avoid being named in lawsuits is to follow standards of care, give competent health care, document assessments, interventions, and evaluations fully, and develop empathetic rapport with the client. Poor client relations are leading causes of lawsuits. A client who believes that the nurse performed duties correctly and was concerned with his or her welfare is unlikely to initiate a lawsuit. In addition, careful, complete, and objective documentation are keys to avoiding malpractice (Neubauer, 1990). Nurses should also know and keep current with the practice of nursing. They should know and follow the policies and procedures of the institution in which they work. Finally, nurses should be sensitive to the common sources of client injury, such as falls and medication errors.

Malpractice Insurance. All nurses should consider purchasing malpractice insurance, even if the employing institution has coverage (Feutz, 1987; Arbeiter, 1986). Such insurance guarantees that nurses are adequately protected in all aspects of professional practice. The nurse employed by an institution may also practice in a noninstitutional setting (e.g., assisting a neighbor or doing volunteer work). Because nurses are professionals, it is difficult, if not impossible, to separate the private person from the professional for purposes of limiting exposure to suits for malpractice.

In nursing practice the nurse deals with many people including the client and family, physicians, other nurses,

A PATIENT'S BILL OF RIGHTS

INTRODUCTION

Effective health care requires collaboration between patients and physicians and other health care professionals. Open and honest communication, respect for personal and professional values, and sensitivity to differences are integral to optimal patient care. As the setting for the provision of health services, hospitals must provide a foundation for understanding and respecting the rights and responsibilities of patients, their families, physicians, and other caregivers. Hospitals must ensure a health care ethic that respects the role of patients in decision making about treatment choices and other aspects of their care. Hospitals must be sensitive to cultural, racial, linguistic, religious, age, gender, and other differences, as well as the needs of persons with disabilities.

The American Hospital Association presents *A Patient's Bill of Rights* with the expectation that it will contribute to more effective patient care and be supported by the hospital on behalf of the institution, its medical staff, employees, and patients. The American Hospital Association encourages health care institutions to tailor this bill of rights to their patient community by translating and/or simplifying the language of this bill of rights as may be necessary to ensure that patients and their families understand their rights and responsibilities.

BILL OF RIGHTS*

1. The patient has the right to considerate and respectful care.
2. The patient has the right to and is encouraged to obtain from physicians and other direct caregivers relevant, current, and understandable information concerning diagnosis, treatment and prognosis.

   Except in emergencies when the patient lacks decision-making capacity and the need for treatment is urgent, the patient is entitled to the opportunity to discuss and request information related to the specific procedures and/or treatments, the risks involved, the possible length of recuperation, and the medically reasonable alternatives and their accompanying risks and benefits.

   Patients have the right to know the identity of physicians, nurses, and others involved in their care, as well as when those involved are students, residents, or other trainees. The patient also has the right to know the immediate and long-term financial implications of treatment choices, insofar as they are known.
3. The patient has the right to make decisions about the plan of care prior to and during the course of treatment and to refuse a recommended treatment or plan of care to the extent permitted by law and hospital policy and to be informed of the medical consequences of this action. In case of such refusal, the patient is entitled to other appropriate care and services that the hospital provides or transfer to another hospital. The hospital should notify patients of any policy that might affect patient choice within the institution.
4. The patient has the right to have an advance directive (such as living will, health care proxy, or durable power of attorney for health care) concerning treatment or designating a surrogate decision maker with the expectation that the hospital will honor the intent of that directive to the extent permitted by law and hospital policy.

   Health care institutions must advise patients of their rights under state law and hospital policy to make informed medical choices, ask if the patient has an advance directive, and include that information in patient records. The patient has the right to timely information about hospital policy that may limit its ability to implement fully a legally valid advance directive.
5. The patient has the right to every consideration of privacy. Case discussion, consultation, examination, and treatment should be conducted so as to protect each patient's privacy.
6. The patient has the right to expect that all communications and records pertaining to his/her care will be treated as confidential by the hospital, except in cases such as suspected abuse and public health hazards when reporting is permitted or required by law. The patient has the right to expect that the hospital will emphasize the confidentiality of this information when it releases it to any other parties entitled to review information in these records.
7. The patient has the right to review the records pertaining to his/her medical care and to have the information explained or interpreted as necessary, except when restricted by law.
8. The patient has the right to expect that, within its capacity and policies, a hospital will make reasonable response to the request of a patient for appropriate and medically indicated care and services. The hospital must provide evaluation, services, and/or referral as indicated by the urgency of the case. When medically appropriate and legally permissible, or when a patient has so requested, a patient may be transferred to another facility. The institution to which the patient is to be transferred must first have accepted the patient for transfer. The patient must also have the benefit of complete information and explanation concerning the need for, risks, benefits, and alternatives to such a transfer.
9. The patient has the right to ask and be informed of the existence of business relationships among the hospital, educational institutions, other health care providers, or payers that may influence the patient's treatment and care.
10. The patient has the right to consent to or decline to participate in proposed research studies or human experimentation affecting care and treatment or requiring direct patient involvement, and to have those studies fully explained prior to consent. A patient who declines to participate in research or experimentation is entitled to the most effective care that the hospital can otherwise provide.

*These rights can be exercised on the patient's behalf by a designated surrogate or proxy decision maker if the patient lacks decision-making capacity, is legally incompetent, or is a minor.

"Floating"

Nurses are sometimes required to "float" from the area in which they normally practice to other nursing units. In one case, a nurse in obstetrics was assigned to an emergency room. A client entered the emergency room and complained of chest pain. He was given a markedly increased dosage of lidocaine by the obstetrical nurse and died after suffering cardiac arrest and subsequent irreversible brain damage. The nurse lost the malpractice lawsuit brought against her (*Goff,* 1989).

Nurses who float should inform the supervisor of any lack of experience in caring for the types of clients on the new nursing unit. They should also request and be given orientation to the unit. Nurses floated to a unit are held to the same standards of care as nurses who regularly work in that area (Murphy, 1988).

Incident Reports

An **incident report** is filed when something arises that could or did cause injury and that was not consistent with good care. For example, if a nurse administers an incorrect dose of medication, a client falls out of bed, or an intravenous solution infiltrates the skin causing sloughing and scar formation, the nurse should complete an incident report (Orlikoff and Vanagunas, 1988). Most institutions provide specific forms for this purpose. The nurse objectively records the details of the incident, and the physician examines the client and reports any untoward effects caused by the error (Figure 6-2). Subjective assumptions should not be included on the incident report nor should statements assigning blame be included.

Many nurses are reluctant to file incident reports because they believe they are detrimental to their employment records. Actually, incident reports are used by the institution's administration for quality assurance and risk management. By reviewing incident reports, administrators can determine areas of client risk (Orlikoff and Vanagunas, 1988). For example, if a certain kind of problem has occurred repeatedly, such as pressure ulcers, educational methods can be used to prevent the problem in the future. In addition, the insurance carrier for a hospital or other institution relies on incident reports to assess liability and possible future claims. Incident reports supplement quality improvement programs to ensure provision of high-quality care. Incident reports are not a part of the client's medical record and should not be mentioned in the nursing documentation because they generally are not admissible in a court of law. However, the nurse is advised to check the appropriate state law.

Risk management is a system of ensuring appropriate nursing care. Steps involved in risk management include identifying possible risks, analyzing them, acting to reduce the risks, and evaluating the steps taken. One tool used in risk management is the incident report.

For nurses in practice, the underlying rationale for quality assurance and risk management programs is the highest possible quality of care. Some insurance companies, medical and nursing organizations, and the JCAHO require the use of quality improvement and risk management procedures (JCAHO, 1993).

Reporting Obligations

Nurses are required to make a report in such situations as child abuse, rape, gunshot wounds, attempted suicide, or certain communicable diseases to the appropriate authorities (Kreitzer, 1981). The nurse may also be required to report unsafe or impaired professionals. Because information that must be reported varies among states and provinces, the nurse should become familiar with the appropriate statutes.

Good Samaritan Laws

Good Samaritan laws have been enacted in almost every state and province to encourage health care professionals to assist in emergency situations. These laws limit liability and offer legal immunity for people who help in an emergency, providing they give the best possible care under the conditions (Northrop, 1990). If a nurse stops at the scene of an automobile accident and gives appropriate emergency care such as using caution when moving the injured person in case of a spinal injury or applying pressure to stop hemorrhage, the nurse is acting within accepted standards, even though proper equipment was not available.

Contracts

A contract is a written or oral agreement between two people in which goods or services are exchanged (Black, 1979). An oral contract is as legally binding as a written one, but it may be more difficult to prove. A breach of contract occurs if either party fails to carry out agreed obligations.

By accepting a job, a nurse enters into an agreement with an employer. The nurse will perform professional duties competently, adhering to the policies and procedures of the institution. In return the employer not only pays for services but also furnishes the facilities and equipment in proper working order to enable the nurse to provide efficient and competent care.

Nurses also enter into contractual agreements with clients (Cushing, 1988). Nurses agree to give competent care, and clients agree to pay for the services. When clients sign admission forms upon entering the hospital or agree to nursing care in any health care agency, they initiated the contract. Private duty nurses have specific written contracts with their clients. It is from such contracts that the duty to perform competently arises and the failure to follow through leads to the concept of negligence.

Controlled Substances

Another legal issue that might arise for nurses involves the use of controlled substances. In 1970 the Comprehensive Drug Abuse Prevention and Control Act was passed in the United States. It controls substances such as narcotics, depressants, stimulants, and hallucinogens. The act regulates hospital distribution systems, rehabilitation programs for drug abuse, and research into the medical treatment of addiction. Canadian law similarly regulates controlled substances. Nurses may administer controlled substances only under the direction of a licensed physician.

Controlled substances should be kept securely locked, and only authorized personnel should have access to them. Criminal penalties for misuse of controlled substances exist. There have been cases in which physicians have illegally prescribed and dispensed controlled substances, and if nurses employed by such physicians fail to report these activities, they may be legally accountable for aiding and abetting the physicians.

LEGAL ISSUES IN PRACTICE

Many legal liabilities exist in all areas of nursing practice (Northrop and Kelly, 1987; Killian, 1990b). A nurse who works in a specialized field should study the legal issues pertaining to it. Space does not permit a complete description of all legal liabilities, but a few issues involved in some practice areas are discussed in the following sections.

Perinatal Nursing

The specialty of perinatal nursing involves care of women before, during, and immediately after pregnancy, as well as care of newborn infants. Many legal issues are involved in the care of a mother and her neonate. These include contraceptive or infertility counseling, fetal monitoring during labor, standards of care for the newborn, documentation of stillbirth, provision of intensive care for ill newborns, and prevention of iatrogenic disease in a neonatal intensive care unit.

Pediatric Nursing

Every state and province with child abuse legislation requires that suspected child abuse or neglect be reported (Kreitzer, 1981). Health care professionals such as nurses are mandated to report suspected cases. To encourage reports of suspected cases, states and provinces provide legal immunity for the reporter if the report is made in good faith and without malice. Health care professionals who do *not* report suspected child abuse or neglect may be held liable for civil or criminal legal action.

As in all areas of nursing practice, negligence involving pediatric clients is possible, as in failing to follow physician's orders and causing harm to the client. A nurse is responsible for preventing a child in his or her care from accidentally coming to harm. Cribs, which sometimes have a restraining device over the top, are designed to keep infants and toddlers from climbing out of bed and injuring themselves. All poisonous substances and sharp objects should be kept out of the reach of small children. When possible, small children should be kept under constant watch to minimize opportunities for accidental harm.

Medical-Surgical Nursing

As in the case of children, adults who are disoriented may require some form of restraint to prevent accidental self-injury. Standards of care, laws, and regulations concerning the use of restraints and supervision apply to nursing practice with medical-surgical and other patients. The federal Food and Drug Administration has recently set forth guidelines in this area (FDA Safety Alert, 1992). Side rails and bed alarms are available on most hospital beds to use with adult clients. Some disoriented clients may also require belt restraints to prevent them from falling out of bed. The nurse must know when and how to use restraints correctly. A physician's order is required to physically restrain a client. After a client is restrained, the nurse is required to make frequent client assessments and to periodically release restraints. For example, the skin under the restraint should be assessed for circulation, signs of abrasions, or irritation. A client who falls out of bed and becomes injured or who suffers injury from improper restraint application may bring a lawsuit against the nurses and institution.

Critical Care Units

Critical care nurses require additional training and ongoing in-service education to provide them with information about advances in care methods.

The staffing ratio in an intensive care setting should be one nurse for each client, or at most, 1:2½, depending on the severity of the clients' conditions. The JCAHO recommended these ratios because of the intensity of care required by such clients. These clients usually require careful observation and assessment of their conditions, and treatments, procedures, and medications. If a nurse is assigned to three or four intensive care clients and is unable to give appropriate care and a client suffers harm, the nurse is liable for accepting the client assignment.

Possible legal problems for critical care nurses are associated with the use of electronic monitoring devices. No monitor is totally reliable, and the nurse must not completely depend on it. Therefore the nurses' continual assessment of a client is necessary to help document accurary of electronic monitoring. There may also be electrical hazards to the nurse and the patient. The equipment should be checked routinely by engineers to ensure that a client will not receive an electrical shock (Killian, 1990a).

Psychiatric Nursing

The primary purpose for hospitalizing a client with mental illness is rehabilitation so he or she may return to society as a useful and healthy citizen. Current principles of treatment suggest that mentally ill clients be given as much freedom as possible. One problem arising from this freedom is the possibility that clients will slip away, or elope. If the nurse fails to prevent the client elopement, the nurse and employer would be liable for any injuries the clients sustain or inflict as a result.

Another concern is the possibility of client injury or suicide. If history and medical records indicate suicidal tendencies, the client must be kept under supervision.

Acquired Immunodeficiency Syndrome

The mention of acquired immunodeficiency syndrome (AIDS) causes fear and panic in many members of society. This lethal disease is found in clients in virtually every segment of nursing practice, from AIDS victims on medical-surgical units, to mothers and infants in perinatal units, to pediatric clients with hemophilia.

Legal questions surround this disease in relation to the civil liberties of the victim (Levine, 1986). An example is whether clients with AIDS have the right to withhold information about the diagnosis from the family members who will care for them (*Beringer,* 1991). Rights of the individual versus protection of public health are debated. In the future, new laws enacted by the legislatures and many court cases addressing this problem will arise. The nurse should treat all clients as if they could be infected. This is referred to as Universal Precautions. Universal Precautions indicate that gloves must be worn when handling blood and other bodily fluids. Gowns, masks, and protective eye wear should also be worn when appropriate. The nurse has the responsibility to safeguard himself or herself and others. Therefore items or areas contaminated with bodily fluids must be appropriately handled, discarded, and/or decontaminated (29 CFR 1910, 1991).

Currently the federal government is considering whether health care workers should disclose to clients that they are HIV positive. At least two court cases have found a compelling need for physicians to disclose their HIV status to the hospitals in which they work and to their clients (*Beringer,* 1991; *Hershey Medical Center,* 1991).

SUMMARY

Many legal issues are confronting a practicing nurse today, but nurses should view the law not with apprehension but as a helpful adjunct to defining nursing practice. Nurses aware of legal rights and obligations are better prepared to care for clients. Nursing standards of care delineate and define appropriate nursing care.

Nursing standards of care set forth to validate that clients receive appropriate care. Some standards are stated in general terms, such as those enacted in nursing practice statutes. More specific standards are defined by a nurse's employing institution. If nurses act within the accepted standards of care, the chances of being involved in lawsuits are reduced. When the nurse does not provide care according to the current standards, the potential for harm and liability increase. All nurses giving care to clients must understand the legal significance of their acts.

CRITICAL THINKING ACTIVITIES

1. Mrs. Kline is a 42-year-old woman admitted with pneumonia. She is placed on IV antibiotics, every 6 hours at 0600, 1200, 1800, and 2400 hours. At 0900 on the second day of treatment, you note a skin rash and notify the physician, who changes her antibiotic. The medication nurse gives the 1200 dose of the original antibiotic, and the client has a severe allergic reaction. Identify the elements of neglect. Establish how such negligence can be avoided.
2. You are arriving at work and are in a crowded elevator. The conversation in the elevator revolves around a college student who was admitted during the night with a drug overdose. You realize that you know the client. How has the client's right to confidentiality been breached. What are your actions?
3. Mr. James is admitted to your division following surgery for an abdominal injury. He received a narcotic analgesic 45 minutes ago. The physician had decided that a CAT scan with contrast is needed, and you need to obtain the client's consent to the procedure. What factors must be considered before obtaining consent?

KEY CONCEPTS

- With the increased emphasis on client rights, a nurse in practice today must understand legal obligations and responsibilities to clients.
- Under the law, the practicing nurse must follow standards of care, which originate in nurse practice acts, the guidelines of professional organizations, and written policies and procedures of employing institutions.
- Nurses are responsible for performing procedures correctly and exercising professional judgment when they carry out physician orders; otherwise they may be guilty of negligence.
- All clients are entitled to confidential health care and freedom from unauthorized release of information; otherwise the nurse may be guilty of invasion of privacy, slander, or libel.
- A nurse can be found guilty of malpractice if the following criteria are established: (1) the nurse (defendant) owed a duty to the client (plaintiff), (2) the nurse did not carry out that duty, (3) the client was injured, and (4) the client's injury resulted from the nurse's failure to carry out that duty.
- Informed consent must meet the following criteria: (1) the person giving consent must be competent and of legal age, (2) the consent must be given voluntarily, (3) the person giving consent must thoroughly understand the procedure and its risks and benefits, as well as alternative procedures, and (4) the person giving consent has a right to have all questions answered satisfactorily.
- The nurse is obligated to follow the physician's order unless he or she believes the order is in error or could be detrimental to the client, in which case the nurse must make a formal report explaining the refusal.
- The nurse must file an incident report in any unusual situation when there is a possibility of a lawsuit; such reports are also used for quality assurance and risk management.
- A legal definition of death aids in determining when it is appropriate to pursue organ donation.

References

AIDS Symposium, *J Hosp Law* 21(10):249, 1988.

Accreditation Manual for Hospitals, 1993 ed., Joint Commission on the Accreditation of Health Care Organizations.

American Hospital Association: *A patient's bill of rights,* Catalog No. 157759, Chicago, 1992, The Association.

American Hospital Association: *Required request legislation: a guide for hospitals in organ and tissue donation,* Chicago, 1988, The Association.

Arbeiter J: A buyer's guide to malpractice insurance, *RN* 49:22, 1986.

The basis for the right of committed patients to refuse psychotropic medication, *J Health Hosp Law* 22(6):176, 1989.

Black HC: *Black's law dictionary,* ed 5, St Paul, Minn., 1979, West Publishing.

Brown CE: The law and your profession, *J Pract Nursing* 39(2):28-31, 1989.

Calloway SD: *Nursing and the law,* Eau Claire, Wis., 1986, Professional Educational Systems.

Cournoyer PR: *The nurse manager and the law,* Aspen Publications, 1989.

Cushing M: Law and orders . . . how you carry out medical orders, *Am J Nurs* 90(5):29-30,32, 1990.

Cushing M: *Nursing jurisprudence,* Norwalk, Conn., 1988, Appleton & Lange.

FDA Safety Alert, United States Food and Drug Administration, Department of Health and Human Services, July 15, 1992.

Feutz SA: Professional liability insurance. In Northrup CE, Kelly ME: *Legal issues in nursing,* St. Louis, 1987, Mosby.

Fiesta J: *The law and liability for nurses,* ed 2, New York, 1988, John Wiley & Sons.

Hemelt MD and Mackert ME: *Dynamics of law in nursing and health care,* ed 2, Reston, Va., 1981, Reston Publishing.

Horsley JE: Short-staffing means increased liability for you, *RN* 44:73, 1981.

Horting M: Understanding professional liability, *Clin Manage Phys Ther,* 9(6):40-41, 43, 45-46, 1989.

Horty, J: Informed consent: nurse as trouble shooter, *OR Manager* 6(2): 10-11, 1990.

Killian W: Equipment mishaps may result in lawsuits, *Am Nurse* 22(6):34, 1990a.

Killian, W: Nurses face increasing liability, *Am Nurse* 22(1):43, 1990b.

Kreitzer M: Legal aspects of child abuse: guidelines for the nurse, *Nurs Clin North Am* 16(1):149, 1981.

Levine C, et al.: AIDS: public health and civil liberties, *Hastings Cent Rep* 16(6):9, 1986.

Murphy EK: Liability exposure when a nurse 'floats' to an unfamiliar area, *AORN J* 48(2):376, 378, 380, 1988.

Neubauer, MP: Careful charting—your best defense, *RN* 53(11):77-78, 81-82, 1990.

Ney CA: Living wills: the ethical dilemmas, *Crit Care Nurse* 9(8):20, 1989.

Northrop CE: How Good Samaritan laws do and don't protect you, *Nursing* 20(9): 50-51, 1990.

Northrop CE and Kelly ME: *Legal issues in nursing,* St Louis, 1987, Mosby.

Orlikoff J and Vanagunas AM: *Malpractice prevention and liability control for hospitals,* ed 2, Chicago, 1988, American Hospital Publishing.

Prosser W and Keeton W: *Prosser and Keeton on the law of torts,* ed 5, St Paul, Minn., 1988, West Publishing.

Rosen LF: Liability for understaffing: who is responsible? *Today's OR Nurse* 12(1): 36, 1990.

Scott DJ: Withholding consent for medical care of a child: the ultimate parental decision, *J Health Hosp Law* 23:3, 1990.

Stark JL et al.: Attitudes affecting organ donation in the intensive care unit, *Heart Lung* 13:400, 1984.

Ulys L: But she's just a student nurse, *Nurs RSA Verpleging* 3(11/12):50, 1988.

Withdrawal of nutrition and hydration symposium I, *J Health and Hosp Law* 23(8):225, 1990.

Younger SJ: Do not resuscitate orders: no longer secret, but still a problem, *Hastings Cent Rep* 17(1):17, 1987.

STATUTES AND CASES

Kentucky Revised Statutes, KRS 446.400 (definition of death).

Kentucky Revised Statutes, KRS 311.225, et seq. (Anatomical Gift Act).

Kentucky Revised Statutes, KRS 311.622, et seq. (Living Will Act).

National Organ Transplant Act, Public Law 98-507, (October 19, 1984).

29 CFR Parts 1910, et al., "Occupational Exposure to Bloodborne Pathogens", Dec. 6, 1991.

42 CFR Parts 417, et al., "Medicare and Medicaid: Advance Directives" March 6, 1992.

"Rights of the Terminally Ill Act," Uniform Laws Annotated (1989).

Cruzan, et al. v. Director, Missouri Department of Health, 58 U.S.L.W. 4916 (1990).

DeGrella v. Elson, et al., 92-CI-825-DG (Ky S. Ct., July 15, 1993).

Darling v. Charleston Community Memorial Hospital, 33 Ill 2d 326 (1966).

Estate of William Beringer, MD v. Medical Center of Princeton, docket no. L88-2550 (Sup. Ct. NJ 1991)

Goff v. St. Luke's Hospital in Kansas City, Mo, 748 SW 2d 557 (1989).

In Re: Application of the Milton S. Hershey Medical Center, Sup Ct No. 361 (Harrisburg, Pa. 1991).

In Re: Schiller, 148 NJ Super 168 (1977).

Mohr v. Williams, 95 Minn 261 (1905).

Schloendorff v. Society of New York Hospital, 211 NY 125 (1914).

Bibliography

Anderson GC et al.: Living wills: do nurses and physicians have them? *Am J Nurs* 86:271, 1986.

Annas GJ: The baby broker boom, *Hastings Cent Rep* 16(3):30, 1986.

Callahan D: How technology is reframing the abortion debate, *Hastings Cent Rep* 16(1):33, 1986.

Creighton H: *Law every nurse should know,* ed 5, Philadelphia, 1986, WB Saunders.

Fenner K: *Ethics and law in nursing: professional perspectives,* New York, 1980, Van Nostrand Reinhold.

Fost N: Putting hospitals on notice, *Hastings Cent Rep* 12(4):5, 1982.

Harris CH: Legal and ethical issues. In Bobak IM, Jensen MD, and Zalar MK, editors: *Maternity and gynecologic care: the nurse and the family,* ed 4, St Louis, 1989, Mosby.

Moskop JC, Saldanha RL: The Baby Doe rule: still a threat, *Hastings Cent Rep* 16(2):8, 1986.

Rhodes A: Issue Update: Baby Doe regulations, *MCN* 15(6):379, 1990.

Whalen ER: Informed consent: the opinions of critical care nurses, *Heart Lung* 13:662, 1984.

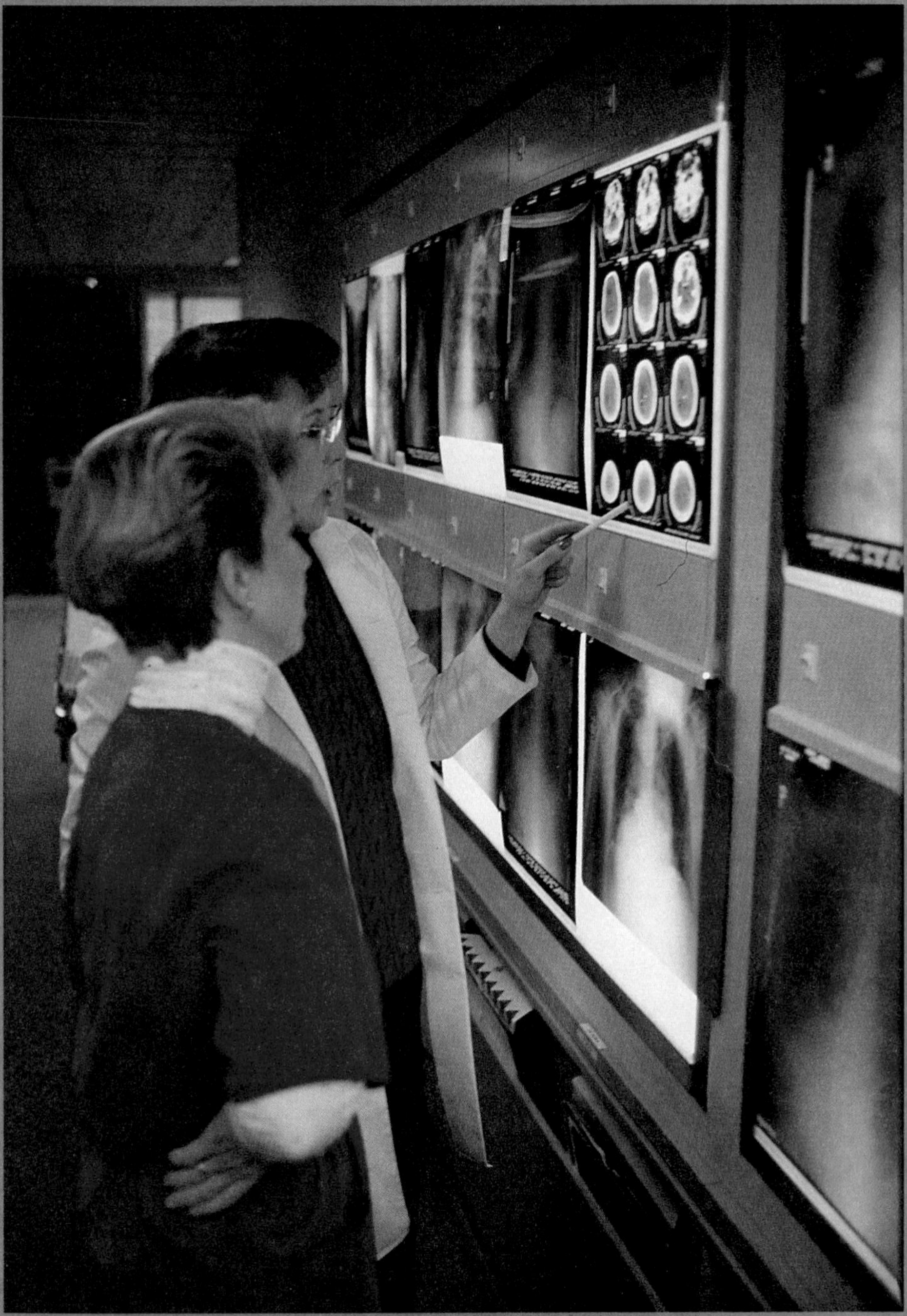

unit two

IMPLEMENTING THE NURSING PROCESS

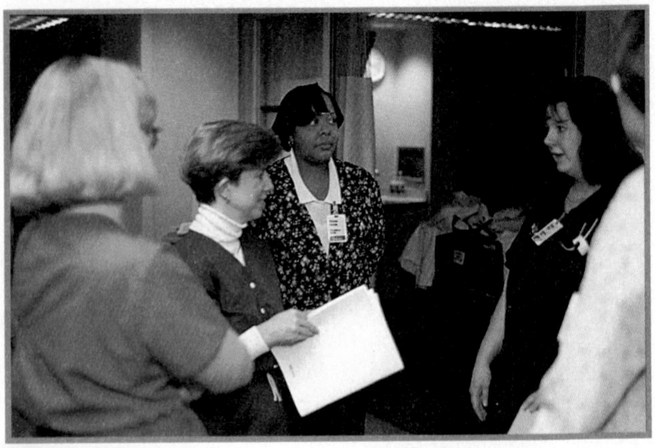

Unit II discusses the nursing process, a systematic problem-solving method for providing individualized care for clients in all states of health. The client is viewed as an individual and a member of a social unit that includes the family and significant others. The nurse includes the client and family and significant others in each step of nursing care. The flexible structure of the nursing process provides a framework enabling nurses in all health care settings to identify and meet client needs (Figure 1).

The nursing process has five interrelated steps: assessment, nursing diagnosis, planning, implementation, and evaluation. During the assessment phase, information about the client is gathered to identify client problems. The collected information is analyzed, and specific client health care problems are stated during the nursing diagnosis step. During the planning step, goals, expected outcomes, and nursing care are planned with the client. Actual nursing care is delivered during the im-

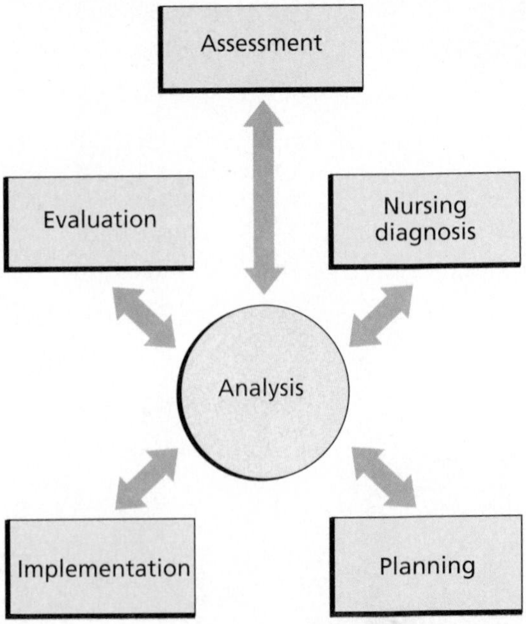

FIGURE 1 Five-step nursing process model that allows nurses in all settings to identify and meet changing client needs. The process is sequential and interrelated, each step depending on the previous.

plementation phase. The evaluation step allows the nurse and client to evaluate the success of nursing care through achievement of client goals and expected outcomes. These sequential steps provide a systematic format that ensures continuity of client care and maintenance of professional standards while assisting clients to regain, maintain, or promote health.

The nursing process is the unifying concept of nursing; it is the method by which nursing is practiced systematically and provides the means by which nurses demonstrate accountability and responsibility to clients and families.

OVERVIEW OF NURSING PROCESS

The purposes of the five-step nursing process are to establish a client data base; identify the client's health care needs; determine priorities of care, goals, and expected outcomes; establish a nursing care plan and provide nursing interventions to meet client needs; and determine the effectiveness of nursing care in achieving client goals (Table 1).

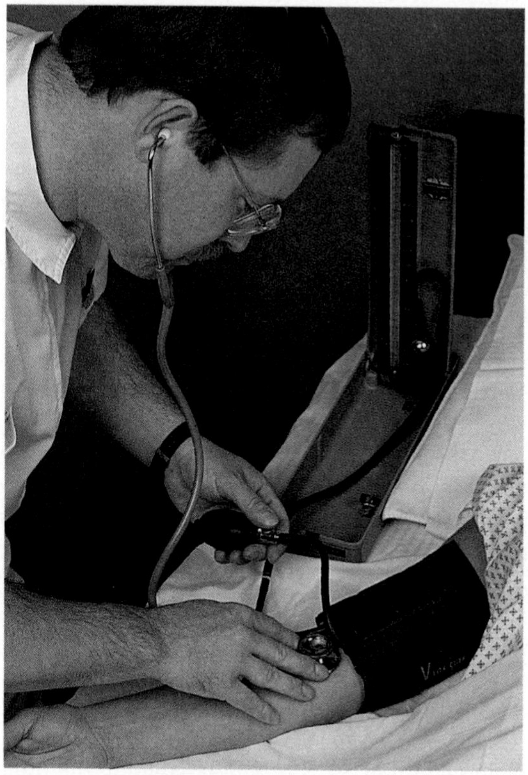

FIGURE 2 Nurse collects blood pressure as part of data collection.

table 1

SUMMARY OF NURSING PROCESS

Component	Purpose	Steps
Assessment	To gather, verify, and communicate data about client so data base is established	1. Collecting nursing health history 2. Performing physical examination 3. Collecting laboratory data 4. Validating data 5. Clustering data 6. Documenting data
Nursing diagnosis	To identify client health care needs and responses to health problems so as to direct nursing care	2. Identifying client problems 3. Formulating nursing diagnoses 4. Documenting nursing diagnoses
Planning	To identify client's goals; to determine priorities of care, to determine expected outcomes, to design nursing strategies to achieve goals of care	1. Identifying client goals 2. Establishing expected outcomes 3. Selecting nursing actions 4. Consulting 5. Delegating actions 6. Writing nursing care plan
Implementation	To complete nursing actions necessary for accomplishing plan	1. Performing nursing actions 2. Reassessing client 3. Reviewing and modifying existing care plan
Evaluation	To determine extent to which goals of care have been achieved	1. Comparing client response to expected outcomes 2. Analyzing reasons for results and conclusions 3. Modifying care plan

Relationship of Steps of Nursing Process

Each step of the nursing process is essential to the problem-solving technique and is closely interrelated with the other four steps. During assessment, the nurse collects data about the client from a variety of sources (Figure 2). This information is used for problem identification so that planning and implementation are appropriate to the client's needs; it is also the basis for accurate evaluation.

Nursing diagnosis involves formulating diagnostic statements that identify the client's health-related problems. The accuracy of these statements depends on the thoroughness of the assessment, including data collection, sorting and clustering, and validation. The identified nursing diagnoses form the framework for the nursing care plan. Nursing diagnoses thus provide the nurse with an individualized client-centered focus.

During the planning step of the process, a care plan is formulated. It is individualized based on the assessment and nursing diagnoses. The care plan contains client goals with expected client outcomes and appropriate nursing interventions. Expected outcomes are the criteria used to evaluate the effectiveness of care.

Implementation is the action step of the nursing process. During this step, individualized client care is delivered according to the care plan. Interventions are continually modified as deemed necessary by an ongoing nursing assessment of the client's responses.

The last step of the process is evaluation. The nurse determines the client's progress toward meeting expected outcomes and achieving goals and the success of the nursing interventions. This step provides for revision of the nursing care plan as necessary to resolve the client's health problems.

The entire process is sequential and interrelated; each step depends on the previous one. The sequence is logical in that client information is gathered before determining the client's health care needs. The plan is established based on client needs. Nursing care is provided according to the plan, and nursing care is evaluated in terms of achievement of expected outcomes. It is dynamic in that any step may be reviewed and revised during evaluation. It is this dynamic flexibility that allows the nurse to respond to changing client needs.

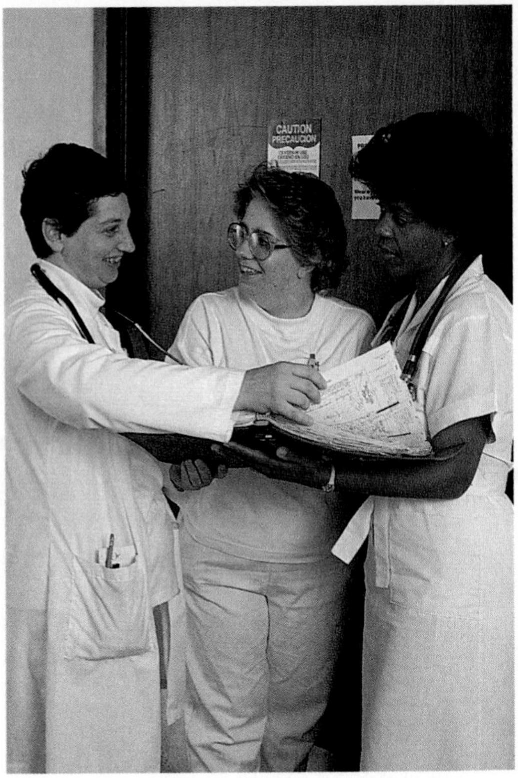

FIGURE 3 One means of problem solving is through collaboration.

table 2

COMPARISON OF STEPS IN PROBLEM SOLVING AND THE SCIENTIFIC METHOD WITH THE NURSING PROCESS

Problem solving	Scientific method	Nursing process
Encountering problem	Recognizing problem	Assessment
Collecting data	Collecting data	
Identifying exact nature of problem	Forming hypothesis	Nursing diagnosis
Determining plan of action	Selecting plan for testing hypothesis	Planning
Carrying out plan	Testing of hypothesis	Implementation
Evaluating plan in new situation	Interpreting results Evaluating hypothesis	Evaluation

Theoretical Comparison

The focus of the nursing process is problem identification and resolution (McHugh, 1986). Problem solving and the scientific method are theoretical approaches used to identify and resolve problems in nursing and other professions (Table 2). The nursing process shares several characteristics with the problem-solving and scientific methods. The components of both can be correlated with each step of the nursing process.

Problem-Solving Method. Problem solving is the foundation for the nursing process. In nursing, a problem arises when a client is unable to meet health care needs. Problem solving is a specific method for obtaining a solution, and it is used by nurses to assist clients in meeting their health needs. The problem-solving method used in clinical nursing practice is a six-step model that enables the nurse to make judgments and be accountable for them (Figure 3).

Scientific Method. The scientific method is a testable, systematic process for solving problems. There are seven steps to this method, which is used in clinical practice when the nurse wants to investigate or research a specific nursing problem.

Benefits

When the nursing process is used to organize and deliver nursing care, the client becomes an active participant in an individualized health care process. Through the planning phase, the care plan communicates to the health care team the client's specific problems, the prescribed interventions, and the expected outcomes of care (Carpenito, 1993). The client receives comprehensive and consistent care. The evaluation of successful achievement of expected outcomes and quality improvement studies document the quality of care promoted by the use of the nursing process. The nursing process also assists in cost containment because nursing care is based on client needs.

The nurse benefits from the structured approach, with economy of time and energies, enhanced professional growth, a sense of profession, and increased job satisfaction. The profession of nursing is advanced through nursing's unique role in overall client care. The nursing process provides the means by which nurses increase their autonomy and fulfill their professional and legal responsibilities (McGillan, 1990). Complete and accurate documentation of each step demonstrates professional competence, responsibility, and accountability in meeting client health care needs.

Historical Perspective

The term *nursing process* was first introduced by Lydia Hall in 1955. During the late 1950s and early 1960s, Dorothy Johnson (1959), Ida Orlando (1961), and Ernestine Wiedenbach (1963) introduced a three-step nursing process model. In 1966 Virginia Henderson identified basic nursing actions as independent functions and stated that the nursing process uses the same steps as the scientific method. In 1967 Lois Knowles presented a process model that she called the "five D's": discover, delve, decide, do, and discriminate (Perry, 1982). In 1967 the Western Interstate Commission of Higher Education (WICHE) and the Catholic University of America studied the nursing process. WICHE listed the steps in the process as perception and communication, interpretation, intervention, and evaluation. The faculty at the Catholic University of America divided the nursing process into four phases: assessment, planning, intervention, and evaluation (Yura and Walsh, 1983).

In 1969 Dolores Little and Doris Carnevali used a four-step process that combined health assessment and designation of the problem into the first step. In 1973 Kristine Gebbie and Mary Ann Lavin at the St. Louis University School of Nursing initiated national conferences on the classification of nursing diagnoses (Gebbie, Lavin, 1975). In addition, nursing educators and clinicians began to use the five-step process model on a regular basis. Since 1973, conferences on the classification of nursing diagnoses have been held every 2 years.

Also in 1973 the American Nurses Association (ANA) published the *Standards of Nursing Practice,* which describes the five-step nursing process model (ANA, 1973). Further commitment by the ANA to the five-step model was documented in the 1980 *A Social Policy Statement* (ANA, 1980), which made this model the standard for professional nursing practice. The 1991 revision of the ANA's *Standards of Clinical Nursing Practice* continues to use the five-step model (ANA, 1991).

In 1982 the professional state board examinations (NCLEX) were revised to include the nursing process as one of the organizational concepts necessary for competent nursing practice.

The Joint Commission on Accreditation of Health Care Organizations (JCAHO) continues to require the nursing process as a means for documenting all phases of client care (JCAHO, 1994). Nursing process continues to be incorporated into the policies and practices of accredited hospitals.

7 Nursing Assessment

OBJECTIVES

Mastery of content in this chapter will enable the student to:

- Define the key terms listed.
- Identify the five steps of the nursing process.
- Discuss the purposes of the nursing process.
- Describe the components of assessment.
- Describe the interrelationship of the steps of the process.
- Differentiate between subjective and objective data.
- State the sources of data for assessment.
- Describe how to assess functional health patterns.
- Discuss the necessity for validating assessment data.
- State the essential characteristics of accurate documentation of assessment.

KEY TERMS

assessment
auscultation
data clustering
data collection
data documentation
functional health patterns
health care team
health history
inspection
interview
medical record
nursing health history
nursing process
objective data
palpation
percussion
physical examination
subjective data
validation

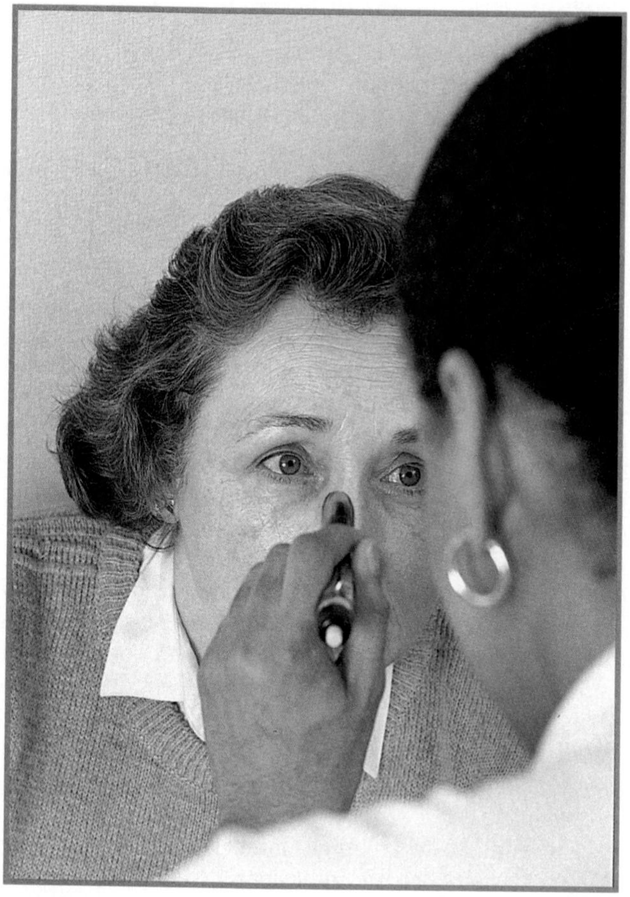

TYPOLOGY OF ELEVEN FUNCTIONAL HEALTH PATTERNS*

Health-perception—health management pattern Describes client's perceived pattern of health and well-being and how health is managed

Nutritional-metabolic pattern Describes pattern of food and fluid consumption relative to metabolic need and pattern indicators of local nutrient supply

Elimination pattern Describes patterns of excretory function (bowel, bladder, and skin)

Activity-exercise pattern Describes pattern of exercise, activity, leisure, and recreation

Cognitive-perceptual pattern Describes sensory-perceptual and cognitive pattern

Sleep-rest pattern Describes patterns of sleep, rest, and relaxation

Self-perception—self-concept pattern Describes self-concept pattern and perceptions of self (e.g., body comfort, body image, feeling state)

Role-relationship pattern Describes pattern of role-engagements and relationships

Sexuality-reproductive pattern Describes client's patterns of satisfaction and dissatisfaction with sexuality pattern; describes reproductive patterns

Coping—stress tolerance pattern Describes general coping pattern and effectiveness of the pattern in terms of stress tolerance

Value-belief pattern Describes patterns of values, beliefs (including spiritual), or goals that guide choices or decisions

From Gordon M: *Nursing diagnosis: process & application,* New York, 1987, McGraw-Hill.

*The pattern areas were identified by the author about 1974 for purposes of teaching assessment and diagnosis at Boston College School of Nursing.

Nursing **assessment** is the first step of the **nursing process.** During assessment, the nurse systematically gathers, verifies, and communicates data about a client to establish a data base about the client's level of wellness, health practices, past illnesses and related experiences, and expectations. The assessment phase includes collecting the data in a systematic manner; validating, sorting, and organizing the data; and documenting the data in an organized format.

Nurses gather client data in a variety of settings using multiple approaches. For example, a community health nurse uses observation of the client's environment to assess for safety and functional limits, while a hospital-based nurse approaches a client in the acute care setting and may eventually focus only on the physiological status.

The format for data collection can be a review of systems format, which is used as an example in Chapter 12, Figures 12-4 and 12-5. In addition a Functional Health Pattern assessment model has been developed. This model provides a guide for an admission assessment and a data base for deriving nursing diagnoses (Gordon, 1993, 1987). For each of the 11 patterns the nurse assesses clients by organizing patterns of behavior and physiological responses that pertain to a functional health category (see box above). Thus this model directs the nurse's assessment to determine the client's level of function within each of the 11 patterns.

DATA COLLECTION

Data collection includes the nursing health history, physical examination, results of laboratory and diagnostic tests, and information from health care team members and the client's family and significant others. Data collected during assessment should be descriptive, concise, and complete, and should not include interpretative statements.

The **nursing health history** is obtained when the nurse interviews the client. To collect data from an interview, the nurse uses communication skills (see Chapter 13) to initiate the nurse-client relationship and progress through the three phases of an interview: orientation, working, and termination. The skills of inspection, palpation, percussion, and auscultation permit the nurse to collect data from the physical examination (see Chapter 16). Laboratory and diagnostic tests further validate the findings of the history and physical examination.

Client information is organized into subjective and objective data. **Subjective data** are clients' perceptions about their health problems. Only clients can provide this kind of information. For example, the presence of pain is a subjective finding. Only the client can provide information about its frequency, duration, location, and intensity. Subjective data usually include feelings of anxiety, physical discomfort, or mental stress. Subjective data are difficult to measure (McNaull et al., 1992). However, while only clients can provide subjective data relevant to these feelings, the nurse must be aware that these problems can result in physiological changes, which are identified through objective data collection.

Objective data are observations or measurements made by the data collector. Identifying the presence of a body rash is an example of observed objective data. The measurement of objective data is based on an accepted standard, such as a thermometer, on which the Fahrenheit or centigrade scale is the standard or unit of measure. Measurements of client's body temperature and blood pressure are examples of objective data.

For efficiency, the nurse should use a systematic "branching" technique during each phase of data collection (Milner, 1992). In branching, the nurse further assesses areas in which a dysfunction or abnormality appears to exist and abbreviates the assessment in areas in which no problem is apparent. For example, if the client indicates problems with indigestion, the nurse should conduct an in-depth nutritional and bowel history and physical examination. Likewise, if the client expressed no problems with headaches, the nurse would not further investigate the neurological portion of the history and examination.

Subjective Data

Interview and Health History. The first step in establishing a data base is to collect subjective information by interviewing the client. An **interview** is an organized conversation with the client to obtain the client's **health history.** The interview includes orientation, working, and termination phases. By doing the interview first, the nurse has an opportunity to do the following:

1. Introduce the client to the nurse as a staff member of an agency or hospital.
2. Establish a therapeutic relationship with the client.
3. Gain insight about the client's concerns and worries.
4. Determine the client's expectations of the health care delivery system.
5. Obtain cues about which parts of the data collection phase require in-depth investigation (branching).

During the orientation phase of the interview, the nurse introduces herself or himself by name and position and states the purpose of the interview. The nurse then assures the client that any information obtained will be used only by health care professionals who participate in the client's care. These courtesies lessen client anxieties about giving personal information to a stranger and enlist the client as a partner in health care management. Demographic data, as specified by the facility, are collected first. Because this information is the least personal, it helps to initiate development of the therapeutic relationship and to ease transition into the working portion of the interview.

The working part of the interview is designed to gather information pertinent to the client's health status. It should be focused and orderly and conducted in an unhurried manner. In the working part of the interview, the current illness and health history are investigated systematically. The general format for a nursing health history contains eight basic components (see box on p. 121).

The admission, or initial, interview is normally the most extensive of all interviews. Major topics that should be covered include biographical data, current illness, and health history. Ongoing interviews do not need to be as extensive; they update the client's status and are more focused toward changes in previously identified and new problems. Many aspects of the admission interview, such as demographic data, are omitted because they are already documented in the client's medical record.

If the client is hospitalized, the nurse caring for the client should conduct a brief ongoing interview at the beginning of each shift to validate any changes in status. In outpatient situations, the nurse should ask the client for health status updates at every visit.

As in the other phases of the interview, termination requires skill on the part of the interviewer. Ideally the client should be given a clue that the interview is coming to an end. For example, the nurse may say, "There are just two more questions," or "We'll be finished in 5 to 6 minutes." With this method, the client can maintain direct attention without being distracted by wondering about when the interview will end. This approach also gives the client an opportunity to ask any questions. When concluding the interview, the nurse summarizes the important points and asks the client whether the summary was accurate. Validation of the interview is essential because it allows the client to clarify or add information.

The nurse should be as organized during this phase

BASIC COMPONENTS FOR A NURSING HEALTH HISTORY

Biographical information: date of birth, sex, address, family members' names and addresses, marital status, religious preference and practices, occupation, source of health care, and insurance

Reasons for seeking health care: goals of care, expectation of the services and care delivered, and expectations of the health care system

Present illness or health concern: onset, symptoms, nature of symptoms (e.g., sudden or gradual), duration, precipitating factors, relief measures, and weight loss or gain

Past health history: prior illnesses throughout development, injuries and hospitalizations, surgeries, blood transfusions, allergies, immunizations, habits (e.g., smoking, caffeine intake, alcohol or drug abuse), prescribed and self-prescribed medications, work habits, relaxation activities, and sleep, exercise, and eating or nutritional patterns

Family history: health status of the immediate family and living relatives, cause of death of relatives, and risk factor analyses for cancer, heart disease, diabetes mellitus, kidney disease, hypertension, or mental disorders

Environmental history: hazards, pollutants, and physical safety

Psychosocial and cultural history: primary language, cultural group, community resources, mood, attention span, and developmental stage

Review of systems (ROS): head-to-toe review of all major body systems, as well as the client's knowledge of and compliance with health care (e.g., frequency of breast or testicular self-examination or last visual acuity examination)

or

Functional health patterns: method for organizing assessment data based on function

COMMUNICATION STRATEGIES

Silence promotes observations about the client and allows time for the client to organize thoughts.

Attentive listening facilitates eye contact with the client and communicates interest in the client's needs, concerns, and problems.

Conveying acceptance promotes a nonjudgmental attitude about the client's life-style, values, and ethics.

Planning related questions provides an organized approach related to a specific topic or system that uses a language understood by the nurse and the client.

Paraphrasing provides an opportunity for the interviewer to validate information from the client in more specific words.

Clarifying facilitates correct communication of information by asking the client to restate information or provide an example.

Focusing eliminates vagueness in communication, limits the area of discussion for the client, and helps the nurse to direct attention to the pertinent aspects of a client's message.

Stating observations provides the client with feedback as to how the message is received.

Offering information and educating the client during the interview.

Summarizing condenses data to further validate information and to end a component of the interview or the interview itself.

as in opening the interview. The interview is terminated in a friendly manner, with the nurse indicating when there will be additional contact.

Interviewing Techniques. The manner in which the interview is conducted is just as important as the questions asked. Attention to environmental aspects and client comfort, as well as communication techniques (see Chapter 13), ensures a successful interview.

Environmental aspects include providing for privacy and eliminating distractions, unnecessary noise, and interruptions. The client is more likely to be candid if the interview is conducted privately, out of earshot of other clients, visitors, and staff. Privacy and quiet may be provided by going to an unoccupied room or drawing the curtains around the bed. Noise and distractions can be reduced by requesting that the television and radio remain off during the interview. Timing is important in avoiding interruptions. If possible, a 15- to 30-minute period should be set aside when no other activities are planned. The client should be made to feel relaxed and unhurried.

Before beginning, the client should be comfortable. This includes adequate light, warmth, and positioning. If possible, the nurse should sit to facilitate eye contact. During the interview, the nurse observes client for signs of discomfort or fatigue.

Good communication starts with a nonjudgmental, interested, and caring attitude. This is conveyed nonverbally if the nurse and client are at approximately the same eye level. The nurse should sit facing the client when possible. Throughout the interview many communication techniques should be used (see the box above). Initially, open questions such as "Tell me about your pain" or "Describe the symptoms you've noticed" prevent stalls and provide the opportunity for the client to indicate major concerns. When more specific information about a topic is needed, closed questions serve best. "Why" questions must be avoided because they are often unanswerable and sometimes make the client defensive. Conducting the interview by only asking questions may make the client feel like a subject of interrogation. Other communication techniques such as making observations and clarifying should be interspersed throughout the interview to encourage the exchange of information. If the client is talkative, the nurse may need to refocus the interview when the client strays from the topic. Summarization and validation are always used when concluding an interview. Active listening is important during the entire interview; it makes the nurse alert to unspoken clues and reinforces the therapeutic relationship.

Objective Data

The remainder of the data collection process involves gathering observable information undistorted by client perceptions.

Physical Examination. During **physical examination,** vital signs and other measurements are taken and all body parts are examined. The examiner looks for abnormalities that may yield information about past, present, and future health problems. Physical assessment is best begun in a nonthreatening manner. This is best accomplished by starting with the familiar procedure of taking vital signs (see Chapter 15).

Actual hands-on physical assessment should be conducted so that the client's anxiety is not aroused. The nurse should explain each step and continue talking throughout, explaining and asking about specific functions and discomforts. The nurse protects the client's privacy, dignity, and warmth; each body part is uncovered and recovered in turn (see Chapter 16).

Physical assessment proceeds in an orderly sequence, using the four techniques of inspection, auscultation, palpation, and percussion (see Chapter 16). **Inspection** begins with the nurse's first contact with the client and continues throughout data collection. During physical examination, the nurse visually examines the client's entire body for structure and function, paying particular attention to deviations or abnormalities. **Auscultation** is the process of listening to sounds produced by the body. A stethoscope is used to auscultate the cardiovascular, respiratory, and gastrointestinal systems. **Palpation** involves using the hands and sense of touch to detect tenderness, temperature, texture, vibration, pulsations, masses, and other changes in body integrity. The client should be instructed to let the nurse know when tenderness, pressure, or pain is experienced during palpation. The nurse should also closely observe the response to palpation for validation of the client's report. **Percussion** is the tapping of the body's surface to produce vibration and sound. The sounds indicate the density of the underlying tissue and thus detect the size and position of the organs. Percussion is most frequently used on the thorax for examining the heart and lungs.

The initial physical assessment is the longest and most extensive part of assessment because it establishes a baseline of normal and abnormal findings. The ongoing physical assessment is briefer, focusing on those areas in which a dysfunction or abnormality was initially found and on those areas in which there was an initial assessment of potential dysfunction. As with the interview, familiarity with the client and previously documented information shortens and improves the process.

Observation of Behavior. During the interview and physical examination, the nurse observes client behavior for level of function, consistency, and congruency. This information adds greater depth to the objective data base.

The level of function includes physical, developmental, psychological, and social aspects. Observation of the level of function differs from the interview in that it is what the nurse sees the client doing rather than what the client says he or she can do. Level of function differs from the physical assessment in that this is the degree of function at which the client is operating, rather than the greatest extent of function present determined by the hands-on physical examination.

Consistency refers to the degree to which the client operates at the same level of functioning (physical, developmental, psychological, and social) throughout the assessment and day by day. Any inconsistency is worthy of further data collection.

Congruency is the matching or agreement between two or more things. The client's statements should match mood and behavior. Subjective and objective data should generally agree. Incongruencies indicate the need for further data collection.

Diagnostic and Laboratory Data. Another source of assessment data are the results of diagnostic and laboratory tests (Figure 7-1). These data can identify or verify alterations questioned or identified during the nursing health history and physical examination. These results include information about the response to illness and information about the effects of later treatment measures.

Laboratory data are compared with the established norms for a particular test, age-group, and sex. These data can also be used to evaluate the success or failure of nursing and medical interventions. Diagnostic and laboratory data are one more source of information the nurse uses in completing the assessment data base.

Medical Record. The **medical record** provides pertinent data about the client's medical history, laboratory tests, diagnostic studies (see the box on p. 123), and the

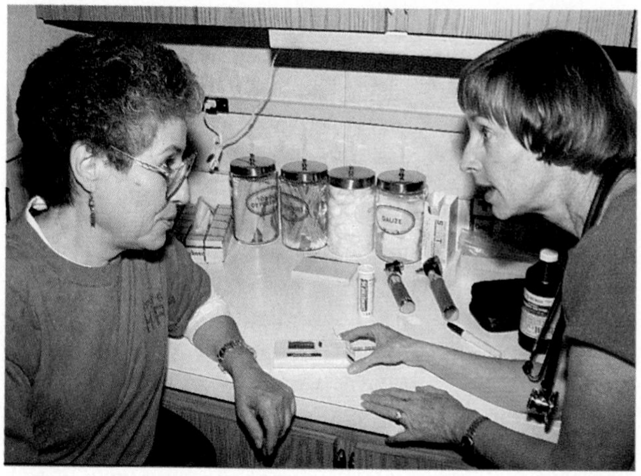

FIGURE 7-1 Nurse teaching client to do blood glucose monitoring. (Courtesy Phillip James Acker, Motorola, Inc.)

physician's proposed treatment plan. The data contained in the medical record are baseline information about the client's response to illness and information about the effects of later treatment measures. The nurse uses the chart as a resource for additional information and as a tool for checking the consistency and congruency of personal observations. Nursing notes, frequently overlooked, are an excellent means for validating assessment.

Other Sources of Data. Health care team members, family and significant others, and nursing and medical literature are important resources for completing the data base.

Health care team members include physicians, nurses, and ancillary staff (see Chapter 1). Team members can provide data about the way the client interacts within the health care environment, reacts to information about diagnostic tests, and responds to visitors. Every member of the team interacting with a client is a source of information and may provide invaluable insights into client behavior and needs.

The client's family and significant others know the client from a point of view unavailable to the health care team. They frequently provide background information essential to understanding the client's situation and responses. In cases of severe illness or emergency situations, or in cases in which the client is an infant, a child, or mentally handicapped, the family or significant others may be the only available source of data about health-illness patterns, current medications, allergies, and onset of illness.

A literature review about the client's illness helps to complete the data base. The review increases the nurse's knowledge about the symptoms, treatment, and prognosis of a specific illness. The knowledgeable nurse researches information pertinent to assessment and planning.

COMMON LABORATORY AND DIAGNOSTIC TESTS

BLOOD

Complete blood count (CBC)
Electrolyte tests: Sequential multiple analyses—SMA_6, SMA_{12}
Arterial blood gas (ABG) analysis
Fasting blood sugar (FBS) test
Glucose tolerance test (GTT)

URINE

Urinalysis (UA)
Urine culture and sensitivity test

RADIOLOGICAL EXAMINATIONS

Chest roentgenogram (CXR)
Upper gastrointestinal (UGI)
Lower gastrointestinal (LGI)
Scans: body, head, chest, and bone

STOOL

Guaiac tests
Ova and parasites tests

SPUTUM

Culture and sensitivity test
Acid-fast bacilli (AFB) test
Cytology tests

OTHER

Electrocardiogram (ECG or EKG)
Stress test
Tuberculosis (TB) skin test

DATA VALIDATION

After gathering the subjective and objective data, the collected information must be validated to ensure its accuracy. **Validation** of each source of assessment data is obtained by comparing the data with another source. The client should be asked to validate the information obtained during the interview and health history. Any additions or corrections should be noted and added to the data base. Findings concerning physical examination and observation of client behavior can be validated by comparing data in the medical record with consultation from another health team member, family member, or significant other. A literature review will confirm that the collected data are consistent with the medical diagnosis.

DATA CLUSTERING

After collecting and validating the subjective and objective data, the nurse needs to organize the information into meaningful and usable clusters, keeping in mind the client's response to illness. The nurse bases this sorting of data on professional knowledge. **Data clustering** organizes the collected data for meaningful documentation and focuses the nurse's attention on functions needing support and assistance for recovery.

DATA DOCUMENTATION

Data documentation is the last part of a complete assessment. Thoroughness and accuracy of facts are necessary when recording client data. If an item is not recorded, it is lost and unavailable to anyone researching the chart. If specific information is not given, the reader is left with only general impressions.

The nurse is thorough for the client's benefit; thoroughness ensures that all information is available to those caring for the client's needs. Even information that does not seem to indicate an abnormality should be recorded. It may become important later, serving as baseline data for a change in status. A general rule of thumb is that if it was assessed, it should be recorded.

The nurse's professional proficiency and nursing license are protected by thoroughness. The nurse practice acts in all states and the ANA Social Policy Statement (1980) mandate accurate data collection and recording as independent functions essential to the role of the professional nurse. Thorough documentation visibly demonstrates professional competence and provides protection of the license by demonstrating that professional responsibilities were met (see Chapter 6).

Being factual is easy after it becomes a habit. The basic rule is to record all observations. When the nurse records data, attention should be paid to facts, and efforts should be made to be as descriptive as possible. Anything heard, seen, touched, and smelled should be reported exactly. The nurse should not generalize or form judgments too early. Conclusions about such observations become nursing diagnoses. Because of a familiarity with the signs and symptoms of a problem, the nurse often immediately assumes the existence of that problem. If the assumption is charted as data, the actual facts are lost. Because assessment includes the collection and documentation of subjective and objective client data, the nurse should make certain that the data base is complete and factual before **data clustering.** Premature clustering can lead to inaccurate nursing diagnoses. In situations in which the client has just been admitted or when the client's status is changing rapidly, it is often better to collect and document the new data continually and delay clustering.

SUMMARY

Nursing assessment is the gathering and verifying of data about a client to establish a data base. Data collec-

KEY CONCEPTS

- The nursing process is a method for organizing and delivering nursing care.
- The purposes of the nursing process are to identify the client's health care needs, establish a nursing care plan, and complete nursing interventions designed to meet the needs.
- The nursing process has five component steps: assessment, nursing diagnosis, planning, implementation, and evaluation.
- Assessment is the collection, validation, sorting, and documentation of data about a client.
- Sources of client data are the client interview and health history, physical examination, observation of client behavior, medical records, consultation with health team members and family or significant others, and medical literature.
- The functional health pattern assessment model enables the nurse to collect data about the clients' level of function in one or all eleven patterns.
- Subjective data are the client's perceptions.
- Objective data are observations or measurements by the data collector.
- The interview comprises three phases: orientation, working, and termination.
- Effective communication skills are essential to the client interview.
- Physical examination requires the skills of inspection, auscultation, palpation, and percussion.
- Data validation ensures accuracy of the assessment.
- Data clustering organizes the assessed information into meaningful clusters for efficient documentation.
- Thoroughness and factualness are essential to accurate data documentation.

tion and documentation are the foundations for the care plan. Therefore the care plan can be only as good as the data on which it is based. Data should be gathered from a variety of sources, including the client interview and health history, physical examination, observation of client behavior, medical record, family or significant others, health team members, and medical literature. The data must be validated by comparing information from all data sources. A complete assessment ensures an accurate view of the client.

After collecting and validating data, the nurse sorts and organizes the information into related groups. Analysis and synthesis are the preparatory steps toward making a nursing diagnosis.

The assessed data should be documented thoroughly and factually, with observations described in measurable terms. Major normal and abnormal findings should be included in each category assessed.

If some pertinent data were not collected, the care plan will be insufficient to meet the client's needs. If all pertinent data were collected but not well documented, the care plan will contain elements not justified in the medical record. Accuracy and thoroughness during assessment are essential to good care planning.

CRITICAL THINKING ACTIVITIES

1. Develop examples of closed and open questions on a similar subject. Practice using them on a classmate and compare the information you gather.
2. You greet Mrs. Jaynes on her first visit to the Family Planning Clinic. You introduce yourself, describe the facility and its purposes, and ask her why she came to the clinic. What aspect of the interview has taken place? What will you do next?
3. Take the following narrative and identify subjective and objective data. Mr. Kantor is lying on his side, grimacing and rubbing his abdomen, and complaining of pain. His vital signs are as follows: BP 140/100, P 120, R 22. He is pale, diaphoretic, and his skin is warm to touch. Oral temperature is 102° F.

References

American Nurses Association: *Nursing: a social policy statement,* Washington, DC, 1980, The Association.

American Nurses Association: *Standards of clinical nursing practice,* Washington, DC, 1991, The Association.

American Nurses Association: *Standards of nursing practice,* Washington DC, 1973, The Association.

Carpenito LJ: *Nuursing diagnosis: application to clinical practice,* ed 5, Philadelphia, 1993, JB Lippincott.

Gebbie K, Lavin MA: *Classification of nursing diagnoses,* St. Louis, 1978, Mosby.

Gordon M: *Manual of nursing diagnosis,* St. Louis, 1993, Mosby.

Gordon M: *Nursing diagnosis: process and application,* New York, 1987, McGraw-Hill.

Joint Commission on Accredidatation of Healthcare Organizations: *Manual of hospital accredidatation: 1993 standards,* Chicago, 1993, The Association.

McGillan PM: Assessment and care planning increase autonomy of practice, *Provider* 16(6):37, 1990.

McHugh M: Nursing process: musings on the method, *Holistic Nurs Pract* 1(1):21, 1986.

McNaull FW, McLees JP, et al.: A comparison of education methods to enhance nursing performance in pain assessment, *J Contin Educ Nurs* 23(6):267, 1992.

Milner EM, Collins MB: Tools to improve systematic client assessment in undergraduate nursing education, *J Nurs Educ* 31(4):186, 1992.

Perry AG: Analysis of the components of the nursing process. In Carlson JH, Craft CA, and McGuire AD, editors: *Nursing diagnosis,* Philadelphia, 1982, WB Saunders.

Yura H and Walsh M: *The nursing process: assessing, planning, implementing, and evaluation,* ed 4, New York, 1983, Appleton-Century-Crofts.

Bibliography

Bellack JP, Bamford DA: *Nursing assessment: a multidimensional approach,* 1984, Belmont, Calif., Wadsworth.

Bermost LS: Interviewing: a key to therapeutic communication in nursing practice, *Nurs Clin North Am* 1:205, 1966.

Bowers AC, Thompson JM: *Clinical manual of health assessment,* ed 3, St. Louis, 1988, Mosby.

Brown MD: Functional assessment of the elderly, *J Gerontol Nurs* 14:13, 1988.

Carpenito LJ: *Handbook of nursing diagnosis,* ed 2, Philadelphia, 1987, JB Lippincott.

Edelman C, Mandle CC: *Health promotion throughout the lifespan,* ed 2, St. Louis, 1990, Mosby.

Fraser C, Filler MJ: The assessment factor most nurses forget, *RN* March 1989, p 32.

Gordon M: *Manual of nursing diagnosis: 1991-1992,* St. Louis, 1991, Mosby.

Haberman MR, Woods NF, Packard NJ: Demands of chronic illness: reliability and validity assessment of a demands-of-illness inventory, *Holistic Nurs Pract* 5(1):25, 1990.

Hickey PW: *Nursing process handbook,* St. Louis, 1990, Mosby.

Ivey AE: *Intentional interviewing and counseling: facilitating client development,* ed 2, Pacific Grove, Calif., 1988, Brooks/Cole Publishing.

Jones DA, Lepley MK, Baker BA: *Health assessment across the life span,* New York, 1984, McGraw-Hill.

Levin RF, Crosley JM: Focused data collection for the generation of nursing diagnoses, *J Staff Development* 2 (2):56, 1986.

Loveridge CE, Heinkeken J: Confirming interactions, *J Gerontol Nurs* 14:27, 1988.

Luekenotte AG: *Pocket guide to gerontologic assessment,* St. Louis, 1990, Mosby.

Malasanos L et al.: *Health assessment,* ed 4, St. Louis, 1989, Mosby.

Marriner A: *The nursing process: a scientific approach to nursing care,* ed 4, St. Louis, 1987, Mosby.

McCain RF: Nursing by assessment, not intuition, *Am J Nurs* 65:82, 1965.

Mengel A: Getting the most from patient interviews, *Nurs 82,* 12(11):46, 1982.

Moss AR: Determinants of patient care: Nursing process or nursing attitudes? *J Adv Nurs* 13:615, 1988.

Norris L: Coaching the question, *Nurs 86* 16(5):100, 1986.

Reed J, Bond S: Nurses' assessment of elderly patients in hospital, *Int J Nurs Studies* 28 (1):55, 1991.

Savage P: Patient assessment in psychiatric nursing, *J Adv Nurs* 16(3): 311, 1991.

Whittenberg RW: Playing by OBRA's new documentation rules, *Geriatric Nursing-American Journal of Care for the Aging* 11(5):251, 1990.

8 Nursing Diagnosis

OBJECTIVES

Mastery of content in this chapter will enable the student to:

- Define the key terms listed.
- Explain the relationship between the nursing diagnosis and the other components of the nursing process.
- Differentiate between medical and nursing diagnoses.
- List the steps of the nursing diagnostic process.
- Discuss the criteria for a nursing diagnosis.
- Identify the format for a nursing diagnosis.
- Discuss the advantages of nursing diagnoses for the client and nursing profession.
- State the importance of prioritizing nursing diagnoses.
- Demonstrate the ability to put a list of nursing diagnoses in order of priority.
- Identify common errors in the formulation of the nursing diagnostic statement.
- Explain how to correct an error in the nursing diagnostic statement.
- Formulate nursing diagnoses from a nursing assessment.

KEY TERMS

actual problems
criteria
data analysis
defining characteristics
diagnostic process
documentation
error of commission
error of omission
health care problems
medical diagnosis
NANDA
nursing diagnosis
potential problems
prioritization
problem
problem identification
related factor
taxonomy

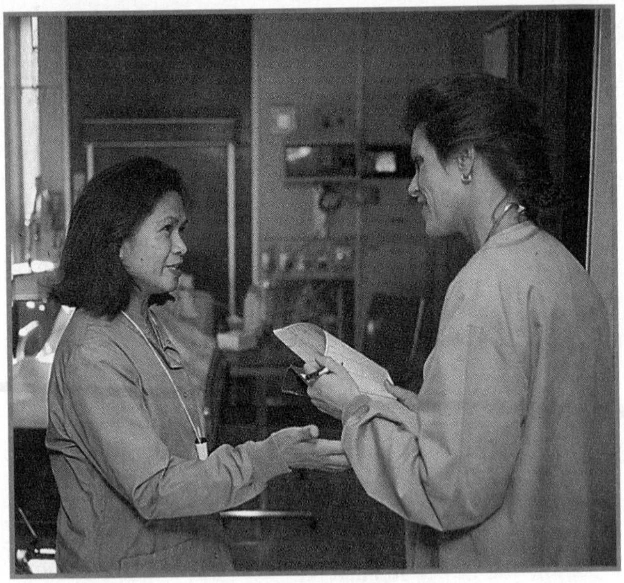

Nursing diagnosis, the second step of the nursing process, begins after assessment is complete. Data collected and sorted into clusters are analyzed to identify the client's **health care problems.** *Diagnosis* means to distinguish or to know. A **nursing diagnosis** is a clinical judgment about individual, family, or community responses to actual and potential health problems or life processes. Nursing diagnoses provide the basis for selection of interventions to achieve outcomes for which the nurse is accountable (NANDA, 1990; Carpenito, 1993). A *nursing diagnosis* is then defined as a statement that describes the client's actual or potential response to a health problem that the nurse is licensed and competent to treat. The client's actual and potential responses are obtained from the assessment data base and a review of literature, client's past medical records, and consultation with other professionals, all of which were collected during assessment. Last, the client's actual or potential responses require interventions from the domain of nursing (Carlson et al., 1991).

DIAGNOSTIC ANALYSIS

Nursing diagnosis is the step of the process that enables the nurse to individualize care for the client. During the diagnostic phase, the nurse analyzes and interprets data collected about the client using scientific and professional knowledge. The nurse then identifies the client's health care problems and writes nursing diagnoses, which form the basis for the care plan.

Historically, the nursing diagnosis step was the last to be clearly identified and defined in the literature. However, the North American Nursing Diagnosis Association (NANDA) has formulated and validated a taxonomy of nursing diagnoses that nurses are educationally and legally competent to treat (Aden, Warren, 1991). NANDA is a body of professional nurses who identify and research nursing diagnostic labels. NANDA meets every 2 years to add new nursing diagnoses and refine the taxonomy.

Use of standard formal nursing diagnostic statements endorsed by NANDA serves several purposes. Each diagnosis has a precise definition that gives all members of the health care team a clear understanding of the client's problem. Also, because the nursing diagnosis deals with the client's response to the illness or condition rather than the **medical diagnosis,** it distinguishes the nurse's role from the physician's role and helps the nurse to focus on the role of nursing.

Diagnostic Process

The **diagnostic process** is the decision making steps the nurse uses to develop a diagnostic statement (Carnevali et al., 1984, Liukkonen, 1992). This process includes analysis and interpretation of data, identification of problems, and formulation of nursing diagnoses (Figure 8-1). Data validation and clustering follow assessment (see Chapter 7) and lead to analysis and interpretation of data.

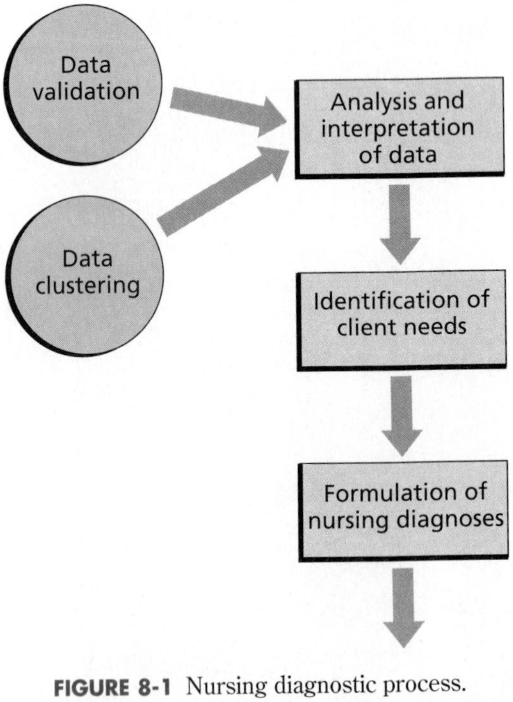

FIGURE 8-1 Nursing diagnostic process.

Analysis and Interpretation of Data

In the assessment phase, data were collected from a variety of sources, validated, and then sorted into clusters or categories. The data base is continually revised to include changes in the client's physical and emotional status and the results of laboratory and diagnostic tests. During this step, the nurse, using knowledge and experience, analyzes and interprets or draws inferences from clusters of data (Figure 8-2).

The analysis involves recognizing patterns or trends, comparing them with normal healthful standards, and coming to a reasoned conclusion about the client's response (see the box below). When looking for patterns or trends, the nurse examines the clusters in the data base. When a relationship among these patterns is identified, a list of client-centered needs begins to emerge. The nurse groups together these clusters and patterns; this grouping consists of defining characteristics. **Defining characteristics** are the clinical criteria that support (validate) the presence of the diagnostic category. Clinical criteria are objective or subjective signs and symptoms, clusters of signs and symptoms, or risk factors (Carpenito, 1989). Multiple defining characteristics resulting from assessment data support the nursing diagnosis (Carpenito, 1987, 1993). The presence of one sign or symptom does not support the nursing diagnostic label. Instead, the clustering of multiple defining characteristics supports the diagnosis. Absence of these characteristics suggests that the diagnosis should be rejected. Defining characteristics support the identification of client needs and actual formulation of the nursing diagnoses (Hurley, 1986).

Identification of patterns is perhaps best demonstrated through the following example. Gray hair does not necessarily indicate that a person is an older adult. However, if gray hair is clustered with wrinkled skin, age spots, and slowed gait, these characteristics indicate that the person is an older adult.

The identified pattern is then compared with normal, healthful standards. The nurse uses widely accepted norms, such as normal laboratory and diagnostic test values, and professional knowledge as the basis for comparison and judgment. When comparing patterns, the nurse judges whether the grouped signs and symptoms are normal for the client and whether they are within the range of healthful responses. Defining characteristics deemed outside healthy norms are isolated and form the basis for problem identification.

Problem Identification

Before formulating the nursing diagnosis, the nurse identifies the client's problems. When identifying these problems, the nurse considers all assessment data and focuses on pertinent and abnormal data. It may help the inexperienced nurse to think of this identification phase as the general health care problem and the formulation of the nursing diagnosis as the specific health care problem. Thus in describing health care problems, the nurse moves from general to specific.

To identify the client's need, the nurse first determines what the client's health problems are and whether they are actual or potential problems. An **actual health problem** is one that is perceived or experienced by the client, such as difficulty in sleeping. A **potential health problem** is one for which the nurse determines that the client is more vulnerable to develop a problem (Carpenito, 1993). For example, an obese client who smokes is at risk for respiratory problems.

The problem-identification step brings the nurse closer to forming a nursing diagnosis and making general analyses of the clustered data; thus this step assists the nurse in making a nursing diagnosis.

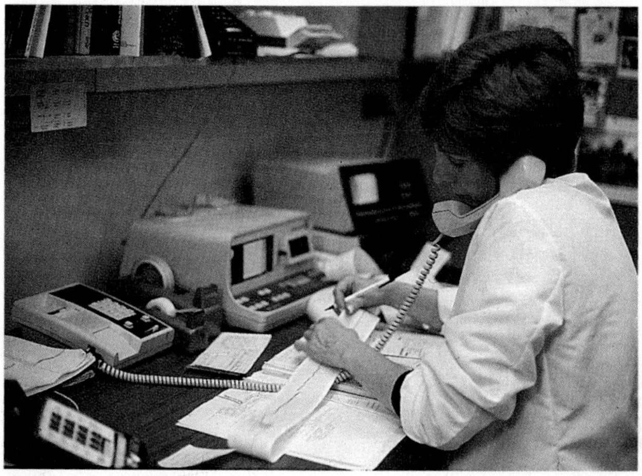

FIGURE 8-2 Nurse analyzes EKG strip with other assessment data.

EXAMPLE OF DATA ANALYSIS

RECOGNIZE PATTERN (POSSIBLE DEFINING CHARACTERISTICS)

No bowel movement for 4 days
Painful defecation with straining
Last stool small and hard
Abdomen firm and distended

COMPARE WITH NORMAL STANDARDS

Soft, formed stool daily
Defecation not painful
Abdomen soft, nondistended

MAKE A REASONED CONCLUSION

Bowel elimination problem

NURSING DIAGNOSIS STATEMENT

Formulation of the nursing diagnosis is based on identification of client problems. Once patterns of assessment begin to reveal problems, the nurse is directed toward selection of appropriate nursing diagnoses. The diagnostic label is supported by defining characteristics, which are present in the client's assessment data. The label should include the problem (e.g., *high risk for injury*) and its related factor (e.g., *related to confusion*). Related factors are etiological or other contributing factors that have influenced the change in the client's health status (Carpenito, 1993).

The connecting phrase "related to" between the diagnostic label and the related factor establishes a relationship between the two parts of the statement. This indicates that the etiology can contribute to or be associated with the problem (Figure 8-3).

The **related factor,** or the second part of the statement, identifies the probable sources of the problem. It may be a direct or contributing factor in the development of the client need and subsequent nursing diagnosis. Related factors are grouped into one of four categories: pathophysiological (physiological or psychological), treatment related, situational, and maturational (Carpenito, 1993). The etiology is represented in the nursing diagnostic statement after the phrase *related to.* Inclusion of the etiology individualizes the nursing diagnosis and subsequent interventions (Table 8-1).

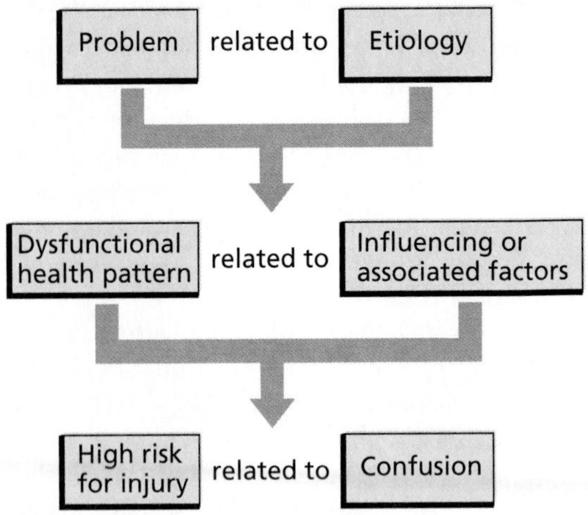

FIGURE 8-3 Relationship between diagnostic statement and format. (Redrawn from Hickey P: *Nursing process handbook,* St. Louis, 1990, Mosby.)

Etiological or related factors are difficult to validate. In some settings, medical diagnoses are recorded as the etiology of the nursing diagnosis, which is incorrect. Nursing interventions cannot change the medical diagnosis. However, nursing interventions can be directed at etiological factors and the diagnostic label. For example, the nursing diagnosis, *pain related to breast cancer,* is incorrect. Nursing actions cannot affect the medical diag-

table 8-1

COMPARISON OF INTERVENTIONS FOR NURSING DIAGNOSES WITH DIFFERENT ETIOLOGIES

Nursing diagnoses	Interventions
CLIENT A	
Ineffective airway clearance related to obesity	Place client in high Fowler's position. Have client cough and deep breathe every 2 hours while awake. Start weight-reduction diet (1200 calories) to decrease obesity.
Feeding self-care deficit related to decreased physical mobility secondary to bilateral arm casts	Encourage family to visit during meals. Be certain staff or family members are available to feed client. Provide high-calorie milk shakes with straw at 3 and 8 PM.
Social isolation related to protective isolation	Plan staffing patterns to include visits to client's room 4 times a day. Offer diversional activities (e.g., cards, music, reading).
CLIENT B	
Ineffective airway clearance related to poor coughing	Teach client deep breathing and coughing. Splint client's abdominal incision during coughing.
Feeding self-care deficit related to inability to grasp feeding utensils	Provide large-handled eating utensils. Offer finger foods cut in large pieces for between-meal snacks: 10-2-8.
Social isolation related to recent move into neighborhood.	Provide client with phone numbers and location of local senior citizen's center. Draw client a map of neighborhood stores, restaurants, and libraries.

nosis of breast cancer. Rewording the diagnosis to read, *pain related to break in skin integrity secondary to mastectomy,* results in nursing interventions directed at improving comfort, controlling pain, and preventing infection. By focusing the intervention on the etiology rather than the diagnostic label, the interventions are even more focused and individualized for the client. Once the etiology is resolved, the problem should disappear.

As the client's needs change, nursing diagnoses are modified. For example, a client's pertinent assessment data includes decreased dietary fiber and limited fluid intake, no bowel movement for 3 days, decreased bowel sounds, distention of the lower abdomen, hard fecal material extracted during digital rectal examination, and a guaiac-negative stool specimen. The nursing diagnosis was *constipation related to limited fiber and fluid intake.* After appropriate nursing intervention, the constipation was resolved, and the nursing diagnosis was modified to read *high risk for constipation related to limited fiber and fluid intake.* The risk exists based on the client's past history of constipation and decreased fiber and fluid intake.

If there is no risk of a resolved health problem reoccurring, the nursing diagnosis for that problem is no longer relevant and must be modified or eliminated. A client's physiological and emotional status may change, resulting in a need to change the etiology even though the problem statement of the nursing diagnosis remains relevant.

The modification of nursing diagnoses is ongoing. As the level of nursing care and level of wellness change, these changes are reflected in the statement of nursing diagnoses. Outdated nursing diagnoses do not accurately reflect the client's current needs and result in a lower quality of nursing care.

Assessment Data and the Diagnostic Statement

As nurses develop nursing diagnoses, they must be sure that the client's assessment data support the diagnostic label and etiology. It may help to identify assessment activities that produce specific kinds of data. For example, asking the client about the quality and perception of pain results in subjective data. However, palpating an area and eliciting a painful grimace provides objective information. Likewise, asking a client to describe the perception of an irregular heartbeat elicits subjective information, and using auscultation to obtain a pulse produces an objective measurement for heart rate and rhythm.

The box below contains a summary of the pertinent assessment data that may lead to the identification of an actual or potential health care problem. Table 8-2 demonstrates data clustering, identification of client need, and formulation of nursing diagnoses from the pertinent assessment data that are presented in the box.

Table 8-3 uses the three nursing diagnoses, *high risk for ineffective airway clearance, high risk for self-esteem disturbance,* and *high risk for ineffective individual coping,* to demonstrate the way that the defining characteristics and probable etiologies assist in the development

SUMMARY OF RELEVANT ASSESSMENT DATA

PHYSICAL AND DEVELOPMENTAL

Diarrhea for 3 weeks
Productive cough on rising each morning
Fifteen-pound weight loss 2 weeks before hospitalization
Hemoglobin 10 g
Slight change in emphysema shown on chest roentgenogram
Crackles in bilateral lung bases
Distended abdomen
Squamous cell cancer of the lung
Smoked for 20 years, 2 packs a day (40 pack-years)
Family history of stomach cancer
Family history of heart attack
Married for 40 years
Self-employed for 20 years
One adult son, 35 years old
Two sisters, 50 and 48, with no major health problems
Temporary sigmoid colostomy
Abdominal incision

INTELLECTUAL

Talkative
Frequently asks nurses if he has cancer
Good attention span

EMOTIONAL

Anxious
Withdrawn after biopsy report of squamous cell cancer
Avoids viewing abdomen
States fear of stomach cancer

SOCIAL

Plays tennis 3 times a week
Active in his neighborhood

SPIRITUAL

Methodist
Attends church weekly
Reads Bible daily

table 8-2

FORMULATION OF NURSING DIAGNOSES

Clustering data	Identification of client need	Nursing diagnoses formulation
Colostomy Distended abdomen Family history of stomach cancer	Alteration in elimination patterns	*Diarrhea related to unknown cause*
Weight loss: 15 pounds Diarrhea Anemia, hemoglobin level of 10 g	Excessive weight loss	*Altered nutrition: high risk for less than body requirements related to chronic diarrhea for 3 weeks*
40 pack-year history of smoking Slight change of emphysema shown on chest x-ray film Crackles auscultated in lung fields	Risk for postoperative respiratory complications	*High risk for ineffective airway clearance after surgery related to incisional pain*
Temporary colostomy Abdominal incision Client resistance to viewing of abdomen	Change in body image	*High risk for self-esteem disturbance related to change in body image*
Client verbalization of fear of stomach cancer Client withdrawal after biopsy report	Changes in interpersonal interactions	*High risk for ineffective individual coping related to fear and anxiety about unknown prognosis*

table 8-3

DEFINING CHARACTERISTICS AND ETIOLOGIES TO SUPPORT NURSING DIAGNOSES

Defining characteristics	Nursing diagnoses	Etiologies ("related to")
Abnormal breath sounds Changes in rate or depth of respiration Cough Cyanosis Dyspnea Smoking history	Actual (or high risk) ineffective airway clearance	Decreased energy/fatigue Tracheobronchial infection, obstruction, secretion Pain
Verbal or nonverbal response to actual or perceived change in structure or function Missing or impaired body part, not looking at or touching body or body part Trauma to body Refusal to acknowledge change	Actual (or high risk) self-esteem disturbance	Biophysical (e.g., amputation or loss of function of extremity) Cognitive/perceptual (e.g., expressions of worthlessness and sorrow) Psychosocial (e.g., withdrawal behavior and excessive crying)
Verbalization of inability to cope Inability to meet role expectations Inability to problem solve Inability to meet basic needs Alteration in societal participation Destructive behavior Inappropriate use of defense mechanisms Verbal manipulation Change in usual communication patterns High rate of illness High rate of accidents	Actual (or high risk) ineffective individual coping	Situational crises (e.g., unexpected illness and financial difficulties) Maturational crises (e.g., marriage and parenthood)

of the total diagnostic label. The defining characteristics and relevant etiologies are from the text *Pocket Guide to Nursing Diagnosis* by Kim, McFarland, and McLane (1993) and are derived from the NANDA classification. A complete list of the current NANDA classification of nursing diagnostic labels is in the box on pp. 134-135).

Diagnostic Errors

Errors can occur in the diagnostic process. Such an error is the failure to identify a client need or the incorrect identification of a need. Errors in the diagnostic process result in the development of an incomplete or inappropriate nursing care plan and adversely affect the quality of care.

Errors can occur during any step of the process and can be errors of omission or commission (Gordon, 1987). An **error of omission** occurs when the nurse fails to identify a health care problem. An incomplete nursing assessment may result in omission of crucial data and failure to identify client problems. Errors in data clustering usually occur when the nurse prematurely groups data before completing assessment; this error results in an inaccurate diagnosis. Incorrect analysis often forces the nurse to make the defining characteristics fit an inappropriate nursing diagnosis (Gordon, 1987; Hickey, 1990).

Errors of commission occur from overdiagnosis or diagnosing nonexistent health care problems. For example, a nurse may prematurely make the diagnosis, *knowledge deficit regarding postoperative regimen,* for a client who enters a hospital for surgery. However, on further assessment the nurse may learn that the client has undergone this type of surgery before and knows postoperative self-care. Another source of error is the manner in which the nursing diagnosis is stated. Incorrect wording results in a vague diagnostic statement or a statement that shifts the focus from the client problem to other areas such as the medical diagnosis or the nurse's needs (Gordon, 1987; Hickey, 1990).

Avoiding and Correcting Errors

Nursing diagnoses are easy to write if the nurse remembers that the problem portion of the statement is concerned with the client's response to the illness or condition and that the problem and etiology portions must be within the scope of nursing to diagnose and treat (see box at right). The following suggestions should help the nurse to avoid the most common errors in formulating nursing diagnoses accurately:

1. Identify the client's response, not the medical diagnosis (Carpenito, 1993). Because the medical diagnosis requires medical interventions, it is legally inadvisable to include it in the nursing diagnosis. The diagnosis, *pain related to myocardial infarction,* may be changed to *pain related to physical exertion.*
2. Identify a NANDA diagnostic statement rather than the symptom. Nursing diagnoses are derived from a cluster of defining characteristics; one symptom is insufficient for problem identification. For example, *cough related to excessive mucus production* should be written as *ineffective breathing pattern related to increased airway secretions.*
3. Identify a treatable etiology rather than a clinical sign or chronic problem. Nursing interventions are directed toward correcting the etiology of the problem. A diagnostic test or a chronic dysfunction is not an etiology or nursing intervention. *Altered respiratory function related to abnormal arterial blood gases* can be correctly stated as *altered peripheral tissue perfusion related to inadequate oxygen intake.*
4. Identify the problem caused by the treatment or diagnostic study rather than the treatment or study itself. Clients experience many responses to diagnostic tests and medical treatment. These responses are the area of nursing concern. The diagnosis, *cardiac catheterization related to angina,* should be restated to read *anxiety related to lack of knowledge about cardiac catheterization.*
5. Identify the client response to the equipment rather than the equipment itself. Clients are often unfamiliar with medical technology. The diagnosis, *anxiety related to cardiac monitor,* can be changed to *knowledge deficit regarding the need for cardiac monitoring.*
6. Identify the client's problems rather than the nurse's problems. Nursing diagnoses are always

AVOIDING DIAGNOSTIC ERRORS

Identify client's response to illness.
State a NANDA diagnostic statement.
Identify an etiology treatable by nursing.
Identify a client need associated with a treatment or test.
Identify client's response to equipment.
Identify client's, not nurse's, problem.
Identify client's problem, not interventions.
Identify client's problem, not goals.
Avoid prejudicial statements.
State the etiology legally.
Identify a problem and an etiology.
Identify only one client problem in a diagnostic statement.

NANDA-APPROVED NURSING DIAGNOSES

Activity intolerance
Altered family processes
Altered growth and development
Altered health maintenance
Altered nutrition: less than body requirements
Altered nutrition: more than body requirements
Altered nutrition: high risk for more than body requirements*
Altered oral mucous membrane
Altered parenting
Altered patterns of urinary elimination
Altered protection
Altered role performance
Altered sexuality patterns
Altered thought processes
Altered (specify type) tissue perfusion (cerebral, cardiopulmonary, renal, gastrointestinal, peripheral)
Anticipatory grieving
Anxiety
Bathing/hygiene self-care deficit
Body-image disturbance
Bowel incontinence
Care giver role strain*
Chronic low self-esteem
Chronic pain
Colonic constipation
Constipation
Decisional conflict (specify)
Decreased cardiac output
Defensive coping
Diarrhea
Diversional activity deficit
Dressing/grooming self-care deficit
Dysfunctional grieving
Dysfunctional ventilatory weaning response (DVWR)*
Dysreflexia
Effective breastfeeding
Family coping: potential for growth
Fatigue
Fear
Feeding self-care deficit
Fluid volume deficit (1)
Fluid volume deficit (2)
Fluid volume excess
Functional incontinence
Health-seeking behaviors (specify) or desire for high-level wellness (specify)
High risk for activity intolerance*
High risk for altered body temperature*
High risk for altered parenting
High risk for care giver role strain*
High risk for fluid volume deficit*
High risk for aspiration*
High risk for disuse syndrome*
High risk for impaired skin integrity*
High risk for infection*
High risk for injury*
High risk for peripheral neurovascular dysfunction*
High risk for poisoning*
High risk for self-mutilation*
High risk for suffocating*
High risk for trauma*
High risk for violence: self-directed or directed at others*
Hopelessness
Hyperthermia
Hypothermia
Impaired adjustment
Impaired gas exchange
Impaired home maintenance management
Impaired physical mobility
Impaired skin integrity
Impaired social interaction
Impaired swallowing
Impaired tissue integrity
Impaired verbal communication
Inability to sustain spontaneous ventilation*
Ineffective airway clearance
Ineffective breastfeeding
Ineffective breathing pattern
Ineffective denial
Ineffective family coping: compromised
Ineffective family coping: disabled
Ineffective individual coping
Ineffective infant feeding pattern*
Ineffective management of therapeutic regimen (individual)*
Ineffective thermoregulation
Interrupted breastfeeding*
Knowledge deficit (specify)
Noncompliance (specify)
Pain
Parental role conflict
Perceived constipation
Personal identity disturbance
Post-trauma response
Powerlessness
Rape-trauma syndrome
Rape-trauma syndrome: compound reaction
Rape-trauma syndrome: silent reaction
Reflex incontinence
Relocation stress syndrome*
Self-esteem disturbance
Sensory/perceptual alterations (specify) (auditory, gustatory, kinesthetic, olfactory, tactile, visual)

*Diagnosis accepted in 1992.

NANDA-APPROVED NURSING DIAGNOSES—cont'd

Sexual dysfunction	Toileting self-care deficit
Situational low self-esteem	Total incontinence
Sleep pattern disturbance	Unilateral neglect
Social isolation	Urge incontinence
Spiritual distress (distress of the human spirit)	Urinary retention
Stress incontinence	

client centered and form the basis for goal-directed care. *Potential IV complications related to poor vascular access* indicates a nursing problem in initiating and maintaining intravenous therapy. The diagnosis, *potential for infection related to presence of invasive lines,* properly centers attention on client needs.

7. Identify the client problem rather than the nursing intervention. Nursing interventions are planned to alleviate client problems. Failure to state a diagnostic label results in an inability to evaluate problem resolution. The statement, *offer bedpan frequently because of altered elimination patterns,* should be changed to identify the problem and etiology. *Diarrhea related to food intolerance* corrects the misstatement and allows proper implementation of the nursing process.
8. Identify the client problem rather than the goal. Goals are established in terms of client problems. If the problem is not identified, evaluation of problem resolution is difficult. *Client needs high-protein diet related to potential alteration in nutrition* should be changed to *potential altered nutrition: less than body requirements related to inadequate nutritional intake* to allow for planning to correct the etiology.
9. Make professional rather than prejudicial judgments. Nursing diagnoses are based on subjective and objective client data and should not include the nurse's personal beliefs and values. The nurse's judgment can be removed from *potential impairment of skin integrity related to poor hygiene habits* by changing the etiology to *lack of knowledge about perineal care.*
10. Avoid legally inadvisable statements (Carpenito, 1993). Statements that imply blame, negligence, or malpractice can result in litigation. The diagnosis, *recurrent angina related to insufficient medication,* implies inadequate prescription by the physician. Correct problem identification might read *pain related to improper use of medications.*
11. Identify the problem and etiology. Be careful to avoid a circular statement. Such statements are vague and give no direction to nursing care. *Alteration in comfort related to pain* can be changed to identify the client problem and the cause: *ineffective breathing pattern related to incisional pain.*
12. Identify only one client problem in the diagnostic statement. Every problem has different specific expected outcomes. Confusion during the planning step occurs when multiple problems are included in a nursing diagnosis. It is, however, permissible to include multiple etiologies contributing to one client problem. *Pain and anxiety related to difficulty in ambulating* should be restated as two nursing diagnoses, such as *impaired mobility related to pain in right knee* and *anxiety related to difficulty in ambulating.*

Nursing Diagnoses: Application to Care Planning. The use of nursing diagnoses is a mechanism for identifying the domain of nursing. The formulated nursing diagnoses provide direction for the planning process and the selection of nursing interventions to achieve the desired outcomes. Thus the expected outcomes are developed for each nursing diagnosis (McFarland, McFarlane, 1989). The care plan (see Chapter 9) is a mechanism for demonstrating accountability (Carlson et al., 1991; Carpenito, 1987, 1989). In addition, the nursing diagnoses and subsequent care plan assist in communicating to other professionals the client-centered problems through the nursing care plan, consultations, discharge planning, and client care conferences (Zink, 1991).

NURSING DIAGNOSES VERSUS MEDICAL DIAGNOSES

A *medical diagnosis* is the identification of a disease condition based on a specific evaluation of physical signs, symptoms, history, diagnostic tests, and procedures. Physicians are licensed to treat these diseases or pathological processes by performing surgery, prescribing medication, and ordering specific invasive and noninva-

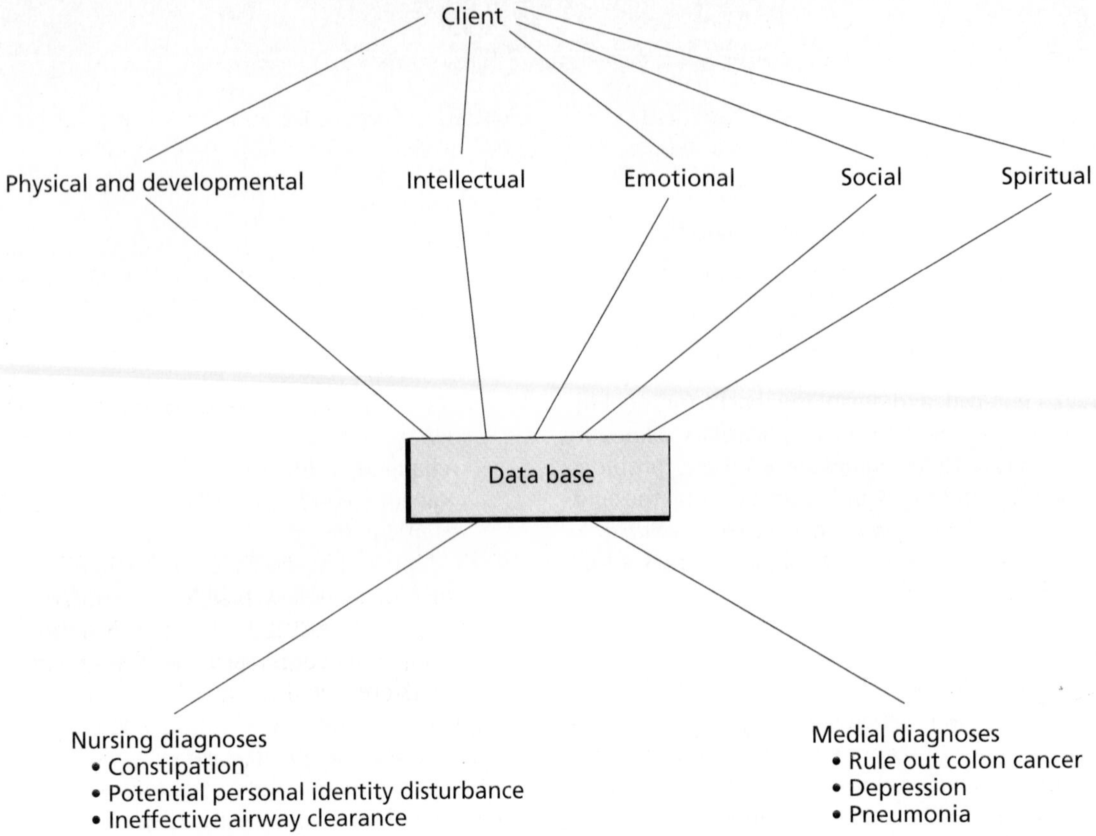

FIGURE 8-4 Comparison of nursing and medical diagnoses using same data base.

sive therapies. Thus the focus of the medical diagnosis is the identification, treatment, and cure of the disease or pathological process.

A *nursing diagnosis* is a statement of a client's actual or potential response to a health problem that the nurse is licensed and competent to treat. It reflects the client's level of health or response to a disease or pathological process. Medical and nursing diagnoses are derived from the physiological, psychological, sociocultural, developmental, and spiritual dimensions of the client (Figure 8-4).

The goals and objectives of a nursing diagnosis differ from those of a medical diagnosis. The goal of a nursing diagnosis is to identify actual and potential client responses, whereas the goals of a medical diagnosis are to identify and design a treatment plan for curing the disease or the pathological process.

The objective of a nursing diagnosis is development of an individualized plan of care so that the client and family can adapt to changes resulting from health problems. The objective of the medical diagnosis is to prescribe treatment. A medical diagnosis of appendicitis, for example, requires the physician to remove the infected appendix. After the appendectomy the client may have a nursing diagnosis of *impaired physical mobility related to painful incision*. The nursing care would be directed at gradually increasing the client's mobility to preoperative levels by decreasing incisional pain.

Advantages

Nursing diagnoses are advantageous for the health care team, nurse, and client. Communication among nurses and other health care providers about a client's level of wellness, current needs, and discharge planning is facilitated by use of standardized NANDA-approved statements. As the list of client problems is modified, client progress becomes readily apparent and the health care team is able to effectively coordinate care.

The nurse benefits from the use of nursing diagnoses in two ways. Efficiency in client care is increased because the client's problems have been identified and the nurse can begin care to solve them. The nurse can then devote energies to ongoing assessment and organized problem resolution.

In addition, well-stated nursing diagnoses help to keep the nurse from straying into the realm of medical practice. Because nursing diagnoses identify responses to the medical illness or treatment, nursing care is directed specifically to actions within the standards of nursing practice. Nursing diagnoses individualized to specific health care needs result in consistent care. Nursing care is client centered, goal directed, and coordinated. The result is personalized care and effective problem resolution that promotes client and family function after discharge and return to the community.

Limitations of Nursing Diagnoses

Nursing diagnoses have limitations. Because of the continuous evolution of the term and use of nursing diagnoses, the language can occasionally be wordy and contain jargon. This may limit the use of nursing diagnoses only to nursing professionals and result in confusion among other members of the health care team (Shamansky, Yanni, 1985).

Imprecise language of the diagnostic label may incorrectly "label" a client. One such diagnostic label is *noncompliance.* The term is value laden and incomplete (Edel, 1985; Stantis, Ryan, 1982).

Priority Setting

Many methods can be used for **priority setting** of nursing diagnoses. One method for setting priorities reflects the biopsychosocial approach and involves looking for the most life-threatening problems, followed by problems that interfere with normal life functioning, and then those concerned with quality of life. A second example for priority setting is according to resource availability. By identifying priority nursing diagnoses, the nurse can best direct health care resources toward attaining client-centered goals (Carpenito, 1993). A final example for priority setting is client preference. For example, a newly diagnosed diabetic may wish the nursing diagnosis ***knowledge deficit regarding insulin self-administration*** have a higher priority than ***knowledge deficit regarding use of a diabetic diet.*** The nurse consults with the client, and, when possible, a collaborative agreement on the priority nursing diagnosis related to the client's desires for return to health and health maintenance and the anticipation of potential problems is reached (Loomis, Conco, 1991).

Documentation

After analyzing assessment data, the nurse identifies client problems and decides how they should be listed on the care plan. In the clinical facility, nursing diagnoses are usually listed chronologically. When initiating the original care plan, the nurse should place the highest priority nursing diagnoses first. Thereafter, additional nursing diagnoses are added to the list. Each nursing diagnosis is dated at the time of entry. This **documentation** system, in addition to changes in the client's status, eventually results in a list of nursing diagnoses that may not be in order of priority. When reviewing the list, the nurse must identify those nursing diagnoses with the greatest priority despite the chronological order.

When completing a care plan class assignment, the student should list the identified nursing diagnoses in descending order of priority. Because school care plans are usually required only once for each client, the problems of ongoing identification and chronological listing of nursing diagnoses are bypassed.

SUMMARY

A nursing diagnosis is a statement of the client's response to an unhealthful condition. Nursing diagnoses are developed through a process in which data are validated, clustered, and analyzed, the client's needs are identified, and specific nursing diagnoses are formulated. Nursing diagnoses are made to identify client problems and to provide a basis for formulating a treatment plan. The diagnosis and treatment plan must be educationally and legally within the domain of nursing practice.

The diagnostic statement has two parts: problem and the related factor. The problem portion is the client's dysfunctional health pattern. The related factor states the etiology or condition associated with or contributing to the problem. These parts are connected by the phrase *related to.*

Writing nursing diagnoses takes practice. In the beginning, the nurse should follow the rules, use the standardized statements formulated by NANDA, and remember that the client's response to the illness or condition should constitute a problem treatable with nursing care. The etiology must be precise and descriptive and cannot contain legal or professional misstatements.

Properly written nursing diagnoses benefit the client, family, and nurse. They focus attention and care on the client's problems in an organized manner, thereby meeting the client's and family's needs more effectively. Nurses benefit by using standardized nursing diagnoses because everyone on the health care team can understand the identified problems in the same way; this understanding facilitates communication and organization of care delivery.

KEY CONCEPTS

The statement of nursing diagnoses is the result of the diagnostic process.

The diagnostic process includes analysis and interpretation of data, identification of client and family needs, and formulation of the nursing diagnostic statement.

Nursing diagnoses state actual or potential problems in the client's health status.

Nursing diagnoses are written for the physical, developmental, intellectual, emotional, social, and spiritual dimensions of the client.

The problem and related factor portions of the nursing diagnostic statement must be within the domain of nursing to identify and treat.

Nursing diagnoses improve communication between nurses and other health professionals.

Nursing diagnoses result in efficient high-quality care for the client.

Nursing diagnostic errors may lead to inadequate nursing care.

Nursing diagnostic errors can occur by omission or commission.

Nursing diagnostic errors can occur during assessment, data clustering, data analysis, or formulation of the diagnostic statement.

A correctly written nursing diagnosis contains a NANDA-approved diagnostic problem statement and a precise statement of the influencing factors contributing to the problem, connected by the phrase *related to.*

CRITICAL THINKING ACTIVITIES

1. Describe the relationship of the nursing diagnosis step to the other steps of the nursing process.
2. During an assessment the nurse notes that a client notes an increase in number of colds, sputum is thick and yellow, and an increase in shortness of breath. Which step of the diagnostic process is taking place?
3. From the three characteristics in the previous question, list the potential client problems.
4. These two nursing diagnoses are worded incorrectly. What is wrong? 1. High risk of ineffective airway clearance due to pneumonia. 2. Body disturbance due to anorexia nervosa.

References

Aden C, Warren J: A validation study of NANDA's Taxonomy I. In Carroll-Johnson RM, editor: *Classification of nursing diagnoses: proceedings of the ninth conference held in Orlando, Fla.,* 1990. Philadelphia, 1991, JB Lippincott.

American Nurses Association: *Nursing: a social policy statement,* Kansas City, Mo., 1980, The Association.

American Nursing Association: *Standards of clinical nursing practice,* Kansas City, Mo., 1991, The Association.

American Nurses Association: *Standards of nursing practice,* Kansas City, Mo., 1973, The Association.

American Nurses Association: *Model nurse practice act,* Kansas City, Mo., 1955, The Association.

Carlson JH et al.: *Nursing diagnosis: a case-study approach,* Philadelphia, 1991, WB Saunders.

Carnevali DL et al.: *Diagnostic reasoning in nursing,* Philadelphia, 1984, JB Lippincott.

Carpenito LJ: *Nursing diagnoses: application to clinical practice,* ed 2, Philadelphia, 1987, JB Lippincott.

Carpenito LJ: *Nursing diagnoses: application to clinical practice,* ed 5, Philadelphia, 1993, JB Lippincott.

Carpenito LJ: *Nursing diagnoses: application to clinical practice,* ed 3, Philadelphia, 1989, JB Lippincott.

Edel MK: Noncompliance: an appropriate nursing diagnosis? *Nurs Outlook* 33:183, 1985.

Gordon M: *Nursing diagnosis: process and application,* ed 2, St. Louis, 1993, Mosby.

Gordon M: Towards theory-based diagnostic categories, *Nursing Diagnoses* 1(1):5, 1990.

Hickey PW: *Nursing process handbook,* St. Louis, 1990, Mosby.

Hurley ME: *Classification of nursing diagnoses,* St. Louis, 1986, Mosby.

Kim MJ, McFarland GK, McLane AM: *Pocket guide to nursing diagnoses,* ed 5, St. Louis, 1993, Mosby.

Liukkonen A: The nurse's decision-making process and the implementation of psychogeriatric nursing in a mental hospital, *J Adv Nurs* 17(3): 356, 1992.

Loomis ME, Conco D: Patients' perceptions of health chronic illness, and nursing diagnoses, *Nurs Diagnosis* 2(4):162, 1991.

North American Nursing Diagnosis Association: *Proceedings of the ninth national conference,* Orlando, Fla., March 17-21, 1990.

Porter EJ: Critical analysis of NANDA nursing diagnoses taxonomy. I. *Image J Nurs Sch* 18:137, 1986.

Shamansky SL, Yanni CR: In opposition to nursing diagnosis: a minority opinion, *Image J Nurs Sch* 17:47, 1985.

Stantis MA, Ryan J: Noncompliance, an unacceptable diagnosis, *Am J Nurs* 82:941, 1982.

Zink MR: Home care nurses' perception of standardized nursing diagnosis, *Home Healthcare Nurse* 9(6):27, 1991.

Bibliography

Anderson JE and Briggs LL: Nursing diagnosis: a study of quality and supportive evidence, *Image* 20:141, 1988.

Aspinall MJ: Nursing diagnosis: the weak link, *Nurs Outlook* 24:433, 1976.

Aspinall MJ: Use of a decision tree to improve diagnostic accuracy, *Nurs Res* 28:182, 1979.

Atkinson LD and Murray ME: *Understanding the nursing process,* ed 3, New York, 1986, Macmillan.

Benner P and Tanner C: How expert nurses use intuition, *Am J Nurs* 87:23, 1987.

Bulechek GM, Kraus VL, et al.: An evaluation guide to assist with implementation of nursing diagnosis, *Nurs Diagnosis* 1(1):18, 1990.

Christensen PJ and Kenney JW: *Nursing process: application of theories, frameworks, and models,* ed 3, St. Louis, 1990, Mosby.

Dalton J: A descriptive study: defining characteristics of the nursing diagnosis: cardiac output, alterations in, decreased, *Image J Nurs Sch* 17:113, 1985.

Fehring RJ: Validating diagnostic labels: standardized methodology. In Hurley M, editor: *Classification of nursing diagnoses: proceedings of the sixth conference (NANDA),* St. Louis, 1986, Mosby.

Gebbie KM, Lavin MA: Classifying nursing diagnoses, *Am J Nurs* 74:250, 1974.

Gleit CJ, Tatro S: Nursing diagnoses for healthy individuals, *Nurs Health Care* 8:456, 1981.

Gordon M: Classification of nursing diagnoses, *J NY State Nurses Assoc* 9:5, 1978.

Gordon M: Nursing diagnoses and the diagnostic process, *Am J Nurs* 76:1298, 1976.

Gordon M: *Nursing diagnoses: process and practice,* New York, 1982, McGraw-Hill.

Gordon M: The concept of nursing diagnoses, *Nurs Clin North Am* 14:487, 1979.

Greenlee KK: The effects of implementation of an operational definition and guidelines for the formulation of nursing diagnoses in a critical care setting. In Carroll-Johnson RM, editor: *Classification of nursing diagnoses: proceedings of the ninth conference held in Orlando, Fla., 1990,* Philadelphia, 1991, JB Lippincott.

Holzmer WL, Henry SB: Nursing care plans for people with HIV/AIDS: confusion or consensus? *J Adv Nurs* 16(3):257, 1991.

Iyer PW, Taptich BJ, and Bernocchi-Losey D: *Nursing process and nursing diagnosis,* Philadelphia, 1986, WB Saunders.

Kim MJ: Nursing diagnoses in critical care, *Dimens Crit Care Nurs* 2:5, 1983.

Kim MJ: Without collaboration, what's left? *Am J Nurs* 85:281, 1985.

King LS: What is a diagnosis? *JAMA* 202:154, 1967.

Levin RF, Crosley JM: Focused data collection for the generation of nursing diagnoses, *Nurs Staff Dev* 2(2):56, 1986.

Lunney M: Nursing diagnoses: refining the system, *Am J Nurs* 82:456, 1986.

Maas M, Hardy M: A challenge for the furtue: expanding knowledge and use of nursing diagnoses, *J Geron Nurs* 14(3):8, 1988.

Martens K: Let's diagnose strengths, not just problems, *Am J Nurs* 86:192, 1986.

McFarland GK, McFarlane EA: *Nursing diagnosis and intervention: planning for patient care,* St. Louis, 1989, Mosby.

McKeehan KM: Nursing diagnosis in a discharge planning program, *Nurs Clin North Am* 14:517, 1979.

Nettle C et al.: Community nursing diagnosis, *J Community Health* 6(3):135, 1989.

Popkess SA: Diagnosing your patient's strengths, *Nurs 81* 11:34, 1981.

Soares O'Hearn CA: Nursing diagnosis: a phenomenological structural description and multidimensional taxonomy or typological redefinition. In Chaska N: *The nursing profession: turning points,* St. Louis, 1990, Mosby.

Thomas NM, Newsome GG: Factors affecting the use of nursing diagnosis, *Nurs Outlook* 40(4):182, 1992.

Walker L: Nursing diagnoses and interventions: new tools to define nursing's unique role, *Nurs Health Care* 7(6):323, 1986.

9

Planning for Nursing Care

OBJECTIVES

Mastery of content in this chapter will enable the student to:

- Define the key terms listed.
- Discuss the process of priority setting.
- Describe goal setting.
- List the seven guidelines of a written outcome statement.
- Discuss the difference between a goal and an expected outcome.
- Discuss the process of selecting nursing interventions.
- Define the three types of interventions.
- Discuss the differences between dependent, independent, and interdependent interventions.
- List the purposes of the nursing care plans used in hospitals and community health settings.
- Describe the differences between care plans used in hospitals and community health settings.
- Develop a care plan from a nursing assessment.
- List the six steps involved in consultation.
- Discuss the consultation process.

KEY TERMS

client-centered goal
collaboration
consultation
dependent interventions
expected outcome
goals
independent interventions
interdependent interventions
Kardex
nursing care plan
planning
scientific rationale

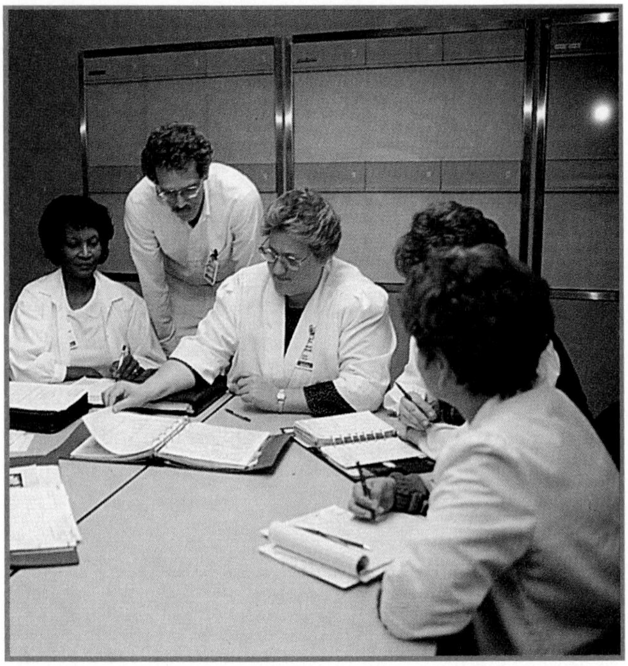

Nursing assessment and the formulation of nursing diagnoses initiate the planning step of the nursing process. **Planning** is a category of nursing behaviors in which client-centered goals are established and strategies are designed to achieve the goals. Planning requires the nurse to use deliberate decision making and problem solving skills to design nursing care for each client (Liukkonen, 1992 and Christensen, Kenney, 1990). During planning, priorities are set, goals are determined, expected outcomes are developed, and a nursing care plan is formulated. In addition to collaborating with the client and family, the nurse consults with other members of the health care team, reviews pertinent literature, modifies care, and records relevant information about the client's health care needs and clinical management.

ESTABLISHING PRIORITIES

After formulating specific nursing diagnoses, the nurse establishes the priorities of the diagnoses by ranking them in order of importance (Christensen, Kinney, 1990). Priorities of care are established so that the nurse can best direct health care resources when a client has multiple problems or alterations (Carpenito, 1989, 1993) (see Chapter 8).

Establishing priorities is not merely a matter of numbering the nursing diagnosis on the basis of severity or physiological importance. Rather, it is a method by which the nurse and the client mutually rank the diagnoses in order of importance based on the client's desires, needs, and safety.

Because clients have multiple diagnoses, the nurse is not able to treat all of them when they are identified. The nurse selects mutually agreed on priorities based on the urgency of the problem, the nature of the treatment indicated, and the interaction among the diagnoses (Gordon, 1987).

Priorities are classified as *high, intermediate,* or *low* (Table 9-1). Nursing diagnoses that, if untreated, could result in harm to the client or others have the highest priorities (Gordon, 1987). High priorities occur in the psychological and physiological dimensions, and the nurse should avoid classifying only physiological nursing diagnoses as high priority.

Intermediate-priority nursing diagnoses involve the nonemergency, non–life-threatening needs of the client. Low-priority nursing diagnoses are client needs that may not be directly related to a specific illness or prognosis but may affect their future well-being.

Whenever possible, the client should be involved in priority setting and subsequent goal setting. In some situations the client and nurse assign different priority

table 9-1

PRIORITY SETTING

Nursing diagnoses	Rationale
HIGH PRIORITY	
High risk for ineffective individual coping related to anxiety about unknown medical diagnosis	Prompt intervention for anxiety will help client prepare for and cope with a diagnostic test, treatment, or diagnosis.
High risk for ineffective airway clearance after surgery related to abdominal incisional pain	Because of the risk of postoperative pulmonary complications, nurse will institute preventive client education early in nursing care.
INTERMEDIATE PRIORITY	
High risk for altered nutrition: less than body requirements related to chronic diarrhea for 3 weeks	This nursing diagnosis does not affect client's immediate physiological or emotional status. Possible surgery will also assist nurse in resolving diagnosis.
LOW PRIORITY	
Knowledge deficit regarding smoking cessation programs	This nursing diagnosis reflects client's long-term needs.

rankings to the nursing diagnoses. If both place a different value on health care needs and treatments, these differences can be resolved through open communication. However, when the client's physiological and emotional needs are at stake, the nurse needs to assume primary responsibility for setting priorities.

ESTABLISHING GOALS AND EXPECTED OUTCOMES

Goals and expected outcomes are specific statements of client behaviors or responses that the nurse anticipates from nursing care. After assessing, diagnosing, and establishing priorities about the client's health care needs, the nurse formulates goals and expected outcomes with the client for each diagnosis (Hickey, 1990 and Christensen, Kinney, 1990).

The purposes for writing goals and expected outcomes are twofold. First, goals and expected outcomes provide direction for the individualized nursing interventions. Second, the goals and outcomes are the focus of the nurses' evaluation to determine the effectiveness of the interventions.

In this text, the terms *goals* and *expected outcomes* are used to indicate anticipated client responses. Figure 9-1 illustrates the relationships between nursing diagnoses, goals, and expected outcomes. Each goal and expected outcome statement must have a time frame for evaluation. The time element depends on the nature of the problem, etiology, overall condition of the client, and treatment setting.

Goals of Care

Individual nursing diagnoses and priority setting help determine the goals of care. Bulechek and McCloskey (1985) define goals as "guideposts to the selection of nursing interventions and criteria in the evaluation of nursing interventions." Setting goals is an activity that includes the client and family or significant others.

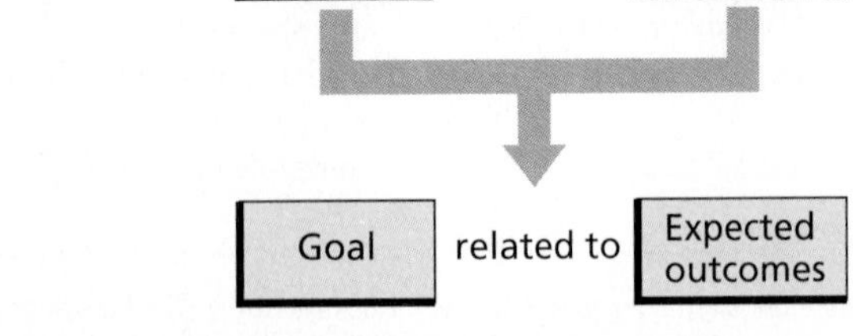

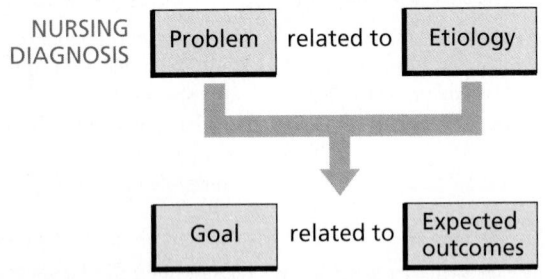

FIGURE 9-1 Relationship of parts of the nursing diagnosis to the goals and expected outcomes. (Redrawn from Hickey P: *Nursing process handbook,* St. Louis, 1991, Mosby.)

Nursing goals are established according to nursing diagnoses and priority setting established by the client and nurse. The nursing diagnoses formulated are based on the client's response and perception of changes in level of wellness, activities of daily living, life-style patterns, and role performance. Because each person responds uniquely to a situation, the nursing diagnoses and client goals of health care are also unique.

Role of the Client in Goal Setting. A **client-centered goal** is a specific and measurable objective designed to reflect the client's highest level of wellness and independence in function. Client-centered goals are mutually set between nurse and client. Mutual goal setting involves the collaboration with the client to identify and prioritize care goals, then develop a plan to attain the goals (McCloskey, Bulechek, 1992).

When developing goals, the nurse can act as an advocate for the client to ensure that the goals are realistic and to prevent further deterioration in the level of wellness or of cognitive and physical functioning (Carpenito, 1993). When clients' cognitive and physical impairments are so severe that they cannot actively participate in goal setting, the nursing team acts in their behalf to develop client-centered goals.

Goals should not only meet the immediate needs of the client but should also include prevention and rehabilitation. Two types of goals—short-term goals and long-term goals—are developed for the client.

Short-Term Goals. A short-term goal is an objective that is expected to be achieved in a short period of time, usually less than a week (Alfaro, 1990; Carpenito, 1993). With the present health care system and shorter hospital stays, short-term goals are the direction for the immediate care plan. A short-term goal for a client with ineffective airway clearance, for example, may be "return of normal lung sounds within 2 days."

Long-Term Goals. A long-term goal is an objective that is expected to be achieved over a longer period of time, usually over weeks or months (Carpenito, 1993). Long-term goals are appropriate for clients in long-term care facilities and for some clients in rehabilitation, mental health, ambulatory care, and community nursing settings (Carpenito, 1993). For example, a long-term goal for a client with an ineffective airway clearance may be to "remain free of upper respiratory infection for 6 months."

Goal setting establishes the framework for the nursing care plan. Table 9-2 shows the progression from nursing diagnoses to goals and expected outcomes, which are individualized to meet client needs. These goals often focus on prevention, rehabilitation, discharge, and health education. Through goals, the nurse is able to provide continuity of care and promote optimal use of time and resources.

Expected Outcomes

Expected outcomes should be specified before an intervention is selected (McCloskey and Bulechek, 1992). An **expected outcome** is the specific, step-by-step objective that leads to attainment of the goal and the resolution of the etiology for the nursing diagnosis (see Table 9-2). An outcome is the measurable criterion against which to judge the success of a nursing intervention (McCloskey, Bulechek, 1992). The outcome represents the observable or measurable client response to nursing care (Alfaro, 1990). Outcomes are the desired response of client condition in the physiological, social, emotional, developmental, or spiritual dimensions.

In addition, expected outcomes have other functions. Projected before nursing actions are formulated, expected outcomes provide a direction for nursing activities (Gordon, 1987). Second, they also provide a projected time span for goal attainment. Finally, the nurse uses expected outcomes as criteria to evaluate the effectiveness of nursing activities.

Multiple expected outcomes are developed for each goal and nursing diagnosis (see Table 9-2). The rationale for the multiple expected outcomes is that few client problems can be resolved by one nursing action. In addition, the listing of the step-by-step expected outcomes gives the nurse practical guidance in planning interventions.

Guidelines for Writing Goals and Expected Outcomes

The goal should be written as a positive measure that indicates the absence of the problem (see Table 9-2). There are seven guidelines for writing goals and expected outcomes. These seven guidelines involve client-centered, singular, observable, measurable, time-limited, mutual, and realistic factors.

Client-Centered Factors. Because nursing care is directed from nursing diagnoses, the goals and expected outcomes focus on the client. These statements

table 9-2

EXAMPLES OF GOAL SETTING

Nursing diagnoses	Goals	Expected outcomes
Ineffective individual coping related to fear of negative prognosis	Client will attend "I Can Cope" classes biweekly.	Client will ask pertinent questions about diagnosis by 6/1. Client will express fears of unfavorable outcome by 6/2. Client will identify at least two strategies for dealing with fear by 6/4.
Potential ineffective airway clearance related to incisional pain	Client's lungs will remain clear throughout postoperative period.	Client's lung will be clear to auscultation 6/2. Client's use of incentive spirometer will remain at baseline or greater 6/2. Client will request pain medication as needed before breathing exercises.
Knowledge deficit regarding postoperative care at home	Client will state four postoperative risks before discharge.	Client will identify need to drink 2 to 3 liters of fluid every day by 6/2. Client will name three signs of infection by 6/3. Client will demonstrate aseptic wound care by 6/4. Client will state home activity restrictions by 6/5.
Potential altered peripheral tissue perfusion related to potential thrombophlebitis secondary to postoperative venous stasis	Client will maintain adequate tissue perfusion by discharge.	Client's skin remains warm and dry 6/1. Client will progressively increase ambulation by 50 feet every day. Client's dorsalis pedis pulse will remain palpable 6/1.

reflect expected client behaviors and responses as a result of nursing interventions.

A common error in writing expected outcomes is to write the statement as an intervention. The correct statement is, "client will ambulate in the hall 3 times a day." A common error is to write, "nursing assistant will ambulate client in the hall 3 times a day."

Singular Factors. Each expected outcome statement should address only *one* behavioral response. This singularity provides a more precise method to evaluate client response to the nursing action. If the statement reads, "client's lungs will be clear to auscultation and respiratory rate will be 22/min by 8/22" and the lungs are clear but the respiratory rate is 28/min after nursing actions, it is difficult to determine whether the expected outcome has been achieved. By splitting the statement into two parts, "lungs will be clear to auscultation by 8/22" and "respiratory rate will be 22/min by 8/22," the nurse can determine specifically the outcome that has been achieved.

Observable Factors. The desired outcome of nursing care must be observable. Through observation, the nurse notes that the change has taken place. Observable changes can occur with changes in physiological findings or in the client's level of knowledge, comfort, or anxiety. The measurable results can be obtained by asking the client directly about the condition or by using assessment skills. Examples of outcomes involving assessment skills are, "lungs will be clear on auscultation by 8/22" and "nonpurulent wound drainage will occur by 9/12."

Measurable Factors. Goals and expected outcomes are written to give the nurse a standard against which to measure the client's response to nursing care. Examples of outcomes are "body temperature will remain 98.6" and "apical pulse will remain between 60 and 100 beats per min." A goal or an outcome that is stated in measurable terms allows the nurse to objectively quantify changes in the client's status.

Common mistakes are made when the nurse uses vague qualifiers such as *"normal, acceptable, stable,* or *sufficient"* in the expected outcome statement. Vague qualifiers have different meanings to different people. Using such terms results in guesswork in determining the client's response to care. Terms specifically describing quality, quantity, frequency, and weight allow the nurse to evaluate that the expected outcome was or was not achieved.

Time-Limited Factors. The time frame for each goal and expected outcome indicates when the expected response should occur. Time frames assist the nurse and client in determining that progress is being made at a reasonable rate.

Time limits assist the nurse in keeping expected outcomes in order. When the date of evaluation arrives, the nurse assesses the client to determine whether that particular expected outcome has been reached. If the expected outcome is still appropriate for the client's care and has not yet been reached, another future evaluation date is set.

Mutual Factors. Mutual setting of goals and expected outcomes ensures that the client and nurse agree on the direction and time limits of care. Mutual goal setting can increase the client's motivation and cooperation.

During this mutual setting of goals and outcomes, the nurse does not impose personal values on the client. However, the nurse must also be aware of client safety and basic human needs. Using experience and acquired knowledge, the nurse may need to direct some of the goals and expected outcomes to keep the client physically and emotionally stable and safe in the environment.

Realistic Factors. Short realistic goals and expected outcomes can quickly provide the client and nurse with a sense of accomplishment. In turn, this sense of accomplishment can increase the client's motivation and cooperation. When establishing realistic goals, the nurse, through assessment, must know the resources of the health care facility, family, and client; the client's physiological, emotional, cognitive, and sociocultural potential; and the economical cost and resources available to reach expected outcomes in a timely manner. Establishing goals and expected outcomes without assessment of client, environment, or resources can be frustrating to the client and nurse because the plan then contains unrealistic goals.

DESIGNING NURSING INTERVENTIONS

Nursing interventions, strategies, or actions are selected after goals and expected outcomes are established. However, implementation of these strategies occurs during the implementation phase of the nursing process (see Chapter 10).

Choosing suitable nursing strategies is a decision making process. The nurse uses assessment data, priority setting, knowledge, and experience to select actions that will successfully meet the established goals and expected outcomes (Prescott, Dennis, Jacox, 1987). In addition, in order to initiate the intervention, the nurse must be competent in three areas: (1) have knowledge

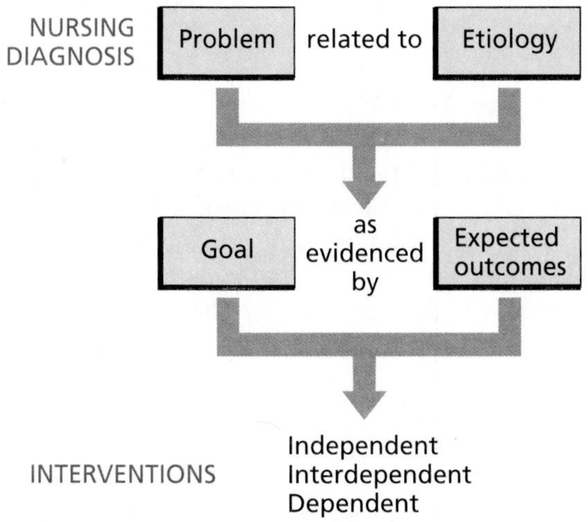

FIGURE 9-2 Relationship of interventions to goals and expected outcomes. (Redrawn from Hickey P: *Nursing process handbook,* St. Louis, 1991, Mosby.)

of the scientific rationale for the intervention; (2) possess the necessary psychomotor and interpersonal skills; and (3) be able to function within a particular setting to use the health care resources effectively (Bulechek and McCloskey, 1992).

The method of intervention selection is always the same, but the types of interventions are individualized to the client's needs. Figure 9-2 illustrates the relationship of interventions to goals and expected outcomes.

Types of Interventions

There are three categories of nursing interventions: independent, interdependent, and dependent. The category selection is based on client needs. One client may have all three categories on the care plan, whereas another client may have only independent and interdependent categories on the care plan.

Independent Factors. Independent interventions involve aspects of professional nursing practice encompassed by applicable licensure and law. These interventions require no supervision or direction from others. For example, designing interventions for increasing a client's knowledge about adequate nutrition or activities of daily living related to hygiene is an independent nursing action.

Independent interventions can solve the client's problems without consultation or collaboration with physicians or other health care professionals (Kim, 1986). Additional examples of independent nursing interventions include progressive relaxation and guided imagery techniques and therapeutic touch and massage (Snyder, 1985).

DELINEATION OF NURSING PRACTICE

Self-care limitations
Impaired functioning in areas such as rest, sleep, ventilation, circulation, activity, nutrition, elimination, skin, or sexuality
Pain and discomfort
Emotional problems related to illness and treatment, life-threatening events, or daily experiences such as anxiety, loss, loneliness, or grief
Distortion of symbolic function, reflected in interpersonal and intellectual processes such as hallucinations
Deficiencies in decision making and the ability to make personal choices
Self-image changes required by health status
Dysfunctional perceptual orientations to health
Strains related to life processes such as birth, growth and development, and death
Problematic affiliative relationships

From American Nurses Association: *Nursing: a social policy statement,* Washington, DC, 1980, The Association.

In delineating the scope of nursing practice, the ANA (1980) listed 10 areas in nursing's domain (see box above). This list, with the continuing work of NANDA and nurse researchers, clarifies and elaborates the realm of independent nursing practice.

Independent nursing interventions do not require a physician's order or an order from another professional. Physicians frequently include in their written orders the specifics of independent nursing interventions. However, according to the nurse practice acts in a majority of states, nursing actions pertaining to activities of daily living, health education, health promotion, and counseling are in the domain of nursing practice. These acts delineate the legal scope of the practice of nursing within the geographical boundaries of the jurisdiction (see Chapter 6).

Interdependent Factors. Interdependent interventions are carried out by the nurse with another health care professional. An example of an interdependent action is implementation of a hypertension protocol, in which the nurse has criteria to change drug and diet therapies when a client's blood pressure rises.

Interdependent interventions also provide a solution to a client's problem in a collaborative manner through judgment and recommendations of the interdisciplinary health care team. The ANA (1980) defines **collaboration** as a partnership in which the power on both sides is valued by both, with recognition and acceptance of separate and combined spheres of activity and responsibility, mutual safeguarding of legitimate interests of each party, and a commonality of goals that is recognized by both parties.

Dependent Factors. **Dependent interventions** are based on the instruction or written orders or another professional. Administering a medication, implementing an invasive procedure, and preparing a client for diagnostic tests are dependent nursing interventions. It is not within the legal practice of nursing for the nurse to prescribe and order these treatments, but it is within the practice of nursing for the nurse to complete such orders.

Each dependent nursing intervention requires specific nursing responsibilities and technical nursing knowledge. When administering medications, the nurse is responsible for knowing the classification of the drug, its physiological action, normal dosage, side effects, and nursing interventions related to its action or side effects (see Chapter 26). Nursing interventions associated with administering medication depend on the physician's written order.

All nursing interventions require nursing judgment and decision making. When encountering an order for a dependent intervention, the nurse does not automatically implement the order but stops to determine whether the requested order is appropriate for the client. Every nurse encounters an inappropriate or incorrect order at some time. The nurse with a strong knowledge base will recognize the error and seek clarification of it. The ability to recognize incorrect orders is particularly important when administering medications or implementing procedures. Clarifying an order is competent nursing practice, and it protects the client and members of the health care delivery system.

Selection of Interventions

When selecting interventions, the nurse deliberates about all possible interventions to achieve the expected outcomes; researches standardized care plans, textbooks, and nursing and related health care literature; and collaborates with other health care professionals. During deliberation, the nurse reviews client needs, priorities, and previous experiences to select nursing interventions that have the best potential for achieving the expected outcomes. As the nurse gains experience, this deliberation process becomes more efficient and experienced based (Benner, 1984).

Research of standardized care plans, textbooks, and nursing and related literature addresses usual problems and nursing actions for given conditions. Although they are written in general terms, the nurse uses these resources to acquire new client care knowledge. This knowledge then assists in the individualization of the intervention.

Usually the nurse will have more interventions than are necessary to meet the desired outcome. Some are discarded as inappropriate, and some are adapted to the client's needs and abilities. As a result, the list of possible interventions is narrowed down to those most suitable to the client and relevant nursing diagnoses (McCloskey and Bulechek, 1992). These interventions are then written on the nursing care plan.

CONSULTING OTHER HEALTH CARE PROFESSIONALS

Consultation may occur at any step in the nursing process but is needed most often in the planning and intervention steps because the nurse is more likely to identify a problem requiring additional knowledge or skills or a need to obtain community or agency resources. **Consultation** is a process in which a specialist's (such as a dietitian or clinical nurse specialist's) help is sought to identify ways to handle problems in client management or the planning and implementation of programs. Consultation is based on the problem-solving approach, and the consultant is the stimulus for change.

Consultation completes the selection of interventions. Through consultation and collaboration the nurse is able to tap the best resources to individualize the nursing actions to meet the expected outcomes (Carpenito, 1993).

When to Consult

The need for consultation in nursing occurs when the nurse has identified a problem that cannot be solved using personal knowledge, skills, and resources. Consultation increases the nurse's knowledge about the problem and helps in learning skills and obtaining the resources needed to solve the problem. After the consultation, the nurse may be able to resolve similar problems in the future.

Consultation is also used when the exact problem remains unclear. A consultant who is objectively entering a situation can more clearly assess and identify the exact nature of the problem, whether it is client oriented, personnel oriented, or equipment oriented. An unbiased consultant can often objectively identify the problem and outline a method for resolving it.

How to Consult

The first step in the consultation process is identification of the general problem area, which will give the consultant a starting point for identifying the problem. Second,

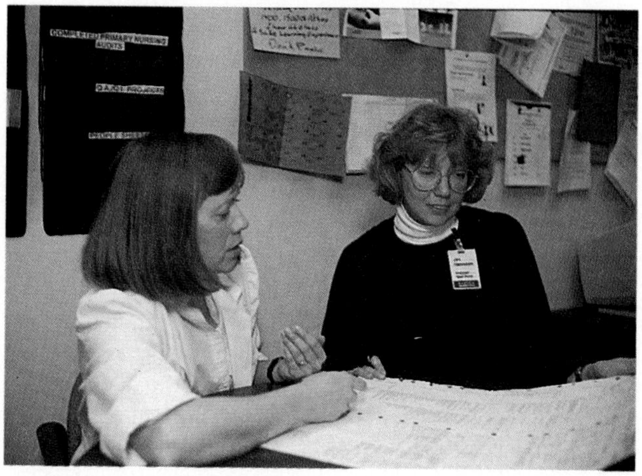

FIGURE 9-3 Consultation with another health care professional.

the consultation should be directed to the appropriate professional, who may be another nurse or another member of the health care team (Figure 9-3). A consultation requested of the wrong individual delays problem solving and diminishes the quality of care delivered to the client.

Third, the nurse provides the consultant with pertinent information and resources about the problem area. Pertinent information includes a brief summary of the problem, methods used to resolve the problem, and outcome of those methods. Other resources can include the client's medical record, nurses and other members of the health team, and the client's family.

Fourth, the nurse should not bias consultants. Consultants are in the clinical setting to identify and resolve a nursing problem, and biasing them can hinder problem resolution. Bias can be avoided by not overloading consultants with subjective and emotional conclusions about the client and problem.

Fifth, the nurse requesting consultation should be available to discuss the findings and recommendations. When a consultation is requested, the nurse provides a private, comfortable atmosphere in which the consultant and client can meet. However, this does not mean that the nurse leaves the environment. A common mistake is turning the whole problem over to the consultant. The consultant is not there to take over the problem but to assist the nurse in resolving it. When possible, the nurse requesting assistance should request the consultation for a day when both are scheduled to work and a time when distractions are minimal. Thus the consultant is available to the nurse, and the nurse is also available to the consultant.

Finally, the nurse incorporates the consultant's recommendations into the care plan. The success of the advice depends on the implementation of the problem-solving techniques suggested.

NURSING CARE PLAN

One product of the planning component is the nursing care plan, which is based on assessment data and the nursing diagnoses, priorities, and goals and expected outcomes. Generally, nursing care plans involve the following areas: nursing diagnoses, goals, expected outcomes, and specific nursing activities and strategies.

Purpose of Care Plans

The **nursing care plan** is a written guideline for client care. Written care plans document the client's health care needs and nursing diagnoses, priorities, and goals and expected outcomes formulated during planning.

The care plan also coordinates nursing care, promotes continuity of care, and lists outcome criteria to be used in the evaluation of nursing care (Christensen, Kenney, 1990). In addition, the written care plan communicates to other nurses and health care professionals pertinent assessment data, a list of problems, and therapies. A written care plan decreases the risk of incomplete, incorrect, or inaccurate care.

The care plan is organized so that any nurse can quickly identify the nursing actions to be delivered. In hospitals and outpatient and community-based settings, the client often receives care from more than one nurse, physician, allied health professional, and health technician. The written nursing care plan makes possible the coordination of nursing care, subspecialty consultations, and scheduling of diagnostic tests.

The care plan can also identify and coordinate resources used to deliver nursing care. The listing of specific equipment and supplies necessary for nursing actions is an economically efficient mechanism for selecting equipment. If all equipment and supplies are included in the care plan, the nurse's time is used more effectively in providing care as opposed to locating supplies.

The nursing care plan enhances the continuity of nursing care by listing specific nursing actions necessary to achieve the goals of care. These nursing activities can be carried out throughout the day and from day to day. A correctly formulated nursing care plan facilitates the continuity of care from one nurse to another. As a result, all nurses have the opportunity to deliver the same quality of care.

Written nursing care plans organize information exchanged by nurses in change-of-shift reports. Nurses focus these reports on nursing care and treatments delineated in care plans. At the end of shifts, nurses discuss care plans with the next care givers. Thus all nurses are able to discuss current and pertinent information about the client's care plan.

The written care plan can also be adapted to the discharge needs of the client. Incorporating the goals of the care plan into discharge planning is particularly important for a client who will be undergoing long-term rehabilitation in the community. The adaptation of the care plan enhances the continuity of nursing care between nurses in the hospital and community.

Same-day surgeries and earlier discharges from hospitals require the nurse to plan discharge needs on the care plan the moment the client enters a health care agency. Mortensen and McMullin (1986) note that incomplete assessments and the absence of measurable outcome criteria extend client stays in short-term, one-day surgical centers. Client stays were lengthened because there were no documented, measurable criteria for discharge readiness on the postoperative nursing care plan, resulting in confusion among all the health care professionals as to when the client could safely be discharged from the setting.

When developing an individualized care plan, the nurse involves the family and client. The family is a resource that can be used to help the client meet health goals. In addition, meeting some of the family's needs can improve the client's level of wellness.

The final component on the nursing care plan is the expected outcome criteria used in evaluation of care. Proper listing of the criteria provides the nurse with objective statements that help determine whether the goals of care have been achieved.

The complete care plan is the blueprint for nursing action. It provides direction for implementation of the plan and a framework for evaluation of the client's response to nursing actions.

Care Plans in Various Settings

The structure of the nursing care plan varies from one health care setting to another. For example, the care plan used in a hospital is different from one used in a community health setting. The nursing care plan developed for the client returning home is usually based solely on long-term health needs. In addition, the client and family are more involved and assume more responsibility for care because the client is receiving nursing care in the home. Although the structure of the care plan varies depending on the setting, its overall purpose is to provide a written guideline for care so that the health care needs of the client and subsequent therapies are communicated among the health care team.

Institutional Care Plans. Institutional (staff) care plans are concise documents that become part of the client's medical record. Many hospitals use the Kardex nursing care plan. **Kardex** is a trade name for a card-filing system that allows quick reference to the particular needs of the client for certain aspects of nursing care. Each card is folded once. Information about medications, activity levels, level of self-care, diet, treatments, and procedures is usually included on the outside of the card. The nursing care plan is commonly placed on the inside (Figure 9-4). Each institution has its own format for the Kardex, but the basic information contained on it is universal. The care plan section of the Kardex also has institutional variations. One institution might use a three-column nursing care plan, which includes the problem, goal, and nursing action. Another institution may incorporate a four-column nursing care plan, which includes the nursing diagnosis, goal, nursing action, and evaluation. As the five-step nursing process has gained popularity, the nursing care plan on the Kardex in many hospitals has been revised to include the following components of the nursing process: assessment, nursing diagnosis, implementation, and evaluation (Figure 9-5).

STANDARDIZED CARE PLANS. The use of computers and the need to efficiently organize the nurse's time have resulted in standardized care plans, which are forms created for a specific clinical problem (e.g., pain, immobility) that is commonly found in a clinical area (e.g., coronary care, abdominal surgery, postpartum, and same-day surgery units). Each care plan lists generalized nursing diagnoses, goals, outcome criteria, and interventions that can apply to specific clients.

After completing a nursing assessment, the nurse, using a standardized format, determines whether it should be used for that particular client. Even if the care plan is generally appropriate for a client, the nurse must add or delete information on the standardized form to individualize it for the client's needs. Failure to do so can result in incomplete and inaccurate care.

Standardized nursing care plans are a method to streamline and augment care planning. They are not intended to replace the nursing care plan process but to avoid a situation in which the nurse must write the same generalized plan repeatedly.

Student Care Plans. Nursing students learn to write and use a nursing care plan as part of their education. The student care plan is essential for learning the problem-solving technique, the nursing process, skills of written and verbal communication, and organizational skills needed for nursing care. Most important, by using the nursing care plan, students can apply the knowledge gained from nursing and medical literature and the classroom to a practice situation.

The student care plan is more elaborate than a care plan in a hospital or community health care agency because its purpose is to teach the process of planning care. To learn the care-planning process, the student must progress in a step-by-step manner, beginning with assessment and ending with evaluation. Student care plans vary from one educational program to another and between beginning and more advanced students. Some educational institutions model the student care plan on the care plan used in the affiliated health care agency.

Medical Diagnosis and other pertinent medical information:
10/25 LBP c̄ RLE SCIATICA
10/26 LAMINECTOMY L4-L5 c̄ BONE GRAFT

1083 13160 23-4
SMITH, PHIL

Condition SATIS — PMH:
Allergies (Drugs, food, other) PCN, ASA, CODEINE — DM

Adm. Date 10/23	Age 64	Religion CATH	Mode of Travel
Service ORTHO	Doctor FORD	Resident KOWALSKI	Intern

Stamp Addressograph Plate Here

FREQUENTLY ORDERED ITEMS		Date	Specimens/Daily Lab	Date	Treatments
Temp. / Pulse & Resp. / BP	q4°	10/25	ADM. BLOOD WORK	10/24	BR AND LOGROLL q 2°
		10/25	UA c̄ MICRO		
I & O	q8°	10/25	BS		
Weights					
Spot Checks					
Chest P.T.					
Incentive Spirometer					
P.T.					

ACTIVITIES		NUTRITION	Date	Diagnostic Procedures
Ad lib		Diet REGULAR		
Ambulate	x 2			
Chair				
BRP				
Bedrest			10/25	MYELOGRAM
Bath		Feedings		CT SCAN
Self			10/25	CXR
Tub		Assist c̄ meals	10/25	EKG
Shower		FLUID BALANCE		
Bed	✓	Force		
Assist.		D E N		
		Restrict		
		D E N		
Orderlies Needed				
Family:				

NURSING CARE PLAN

Date	Nursing Diagnosis	Expected Outcomes	Nursing Plan/Orders
10/26	ALTERED COM-	1. PT. REQUESTS	1. ENCOURAGE PATIENT TO SPLINT INCISION
	FORT, PAIN	FOR PAIN MED.	WHEN TURNING
		DECREASES BY 10/30	2. INSTRUCT PATIENT IN RELAXATION
		2. PT. RESPIRATORY	EXERCISES
		EXPANSION ↑ BY 10/28	
10/27	IMPAIRED	1. PT. INCREASES	1. AMBULATE IN HALL c̄ PT 20 MINUTES
	PHYSICAL MOBILITY	AMBULATION	AFTER ADMINISTRATION OF ANALGESIC
	RELATED TO PAIN	FROM BID TO	2. ENCOURAGE FAMILY TO WALK PATIENT
		QID OR GREATER	
		2. PT. ASSUMES	1. ALLOW PT. EXTRA TIME TO DO SELF CARE
		ADL BY 10/31	FOR HYGIENE NEEDS

Discharge Planning: Destination: Transportation: Probable Date: Referral Agencies: Appointment:
Supplies:

Patient Name

FIGURE 9-4 Nursing care plan on a nursing Kardex.

Assessment	Nursing Diagnosis	Goals	Implementation	Evaluation
Weight loss: 15 lb in 10 days.	Altered nutrition: less than body requirements related to sensation of fullness with meals.	Client will maintain weight during hospitalization.	Weigh daily at 7 AM on scale #3.	Weight remains at 185 lb.
Eats only 10% of meal due to feeling of fullness immediately after beginning meal.		Client will eat 100% of meal by 2/4.	Small, frequent, high-calorie feedings at 08-10-12-14-16-18.	Client consumes all food on meal tray.
			Assist client to high Fowler's position for each meal.	

FIGURE 9-5 Five-column nursing care plan.

table 9-3

SCIENTIFIC RATIONALE FOR THE STUDENT CARE PLAN

Assessment	Goals	Implementation	Rationale	Expected outcomes
Nursing diagnosis: *High risk for impaired skin integrity* related to immobility resulting from coma **Definition:** High risk for impaired skin integrity is the state in which an individual's skin is at risk of being adversely altered.*				
Fever: higher than 102° F for 72 hours Diaphoresis Incontinence of urine	Skin remains intact Skin is free of pressure	Turn client every 2 hours in following sequence: 8 AM—supine 10 AM—left side Noon—prone Repeat, beginning with supine position.	Critical time for skin tissue breakdown is between 1 and 2 hours of constant pressure.†	No skin breakdown is noted. Skin color, temperature, and capillary return are normal.
Decreased skin turgor No skin breakdown noted		Keep client's skin dry at all times.	Moisture increases maceration of skin and promotes bacterial growth‡	Skin remains dry and intact. Skin turgor is improved.

*Data from Kim MJ, McFarland GK, McLane AM: *Pocket guide to nursing diagnoses,* ed 5, St. Louis, 1993, Mosby.
†Data from Bereck KH: *Nurs Clin North Am* 10(1):160, 1975; Braden: 1988.
‡Data from Kavchack-Keys MA: *Nurs* 77(7):60, 1977; Braden: 1988; Bergstrom: 1987; Greenleaf: 1984.

The only modification may be that the instructor requires the beginning student to include the scientific rationale for the nursing actions selected (Table 9-3). A **scientific rationale** is the reason that, based on supporting literature, a specific nursing action was chosen.

WRITING THE NURSING CARE PLAN

As an initial step in planning, the nurse assigns a priority to each nursing diagnosis; priority can be based on Maslow's hierarchy of needs, urgent client physiological and safety needs, and important needs perceived by the client. The nursing diagnosis with the highest priority is the beginning point for the nursing care plan and is followed by other nursing diagnoses in order of assigned priority.

When using the five-column plan (see Figure 9-5), in the assessment column (column 1), the nurse includes all data relevant to the corresponding nursing diagnosis (column 2). The nurse includes the previously developed goals in the next column (column 3). At this point,

table 9-4

FREQUENT ERRORS IN WRITING NURSING INTERVENTIONS

Type of error	Incorrectly stated nursing intervention	Correctly stated nursing intervention
Failure to precisely or completely indicate nursing actions	Primary nurse will turn client every 2 hours.	Primary nurse will turn client every 2 hours, using the following schedule: 2 PM—right side 8 AM—supine 10 AM—left side Noon—prone Repeat at 4 PM and 2 AM
Failure to indicate frequency	Primary nurse will observe client cough and deep breathe.	Primary nurse will observe client cough and deep breath at 10 AM—2 PM—6 PM—10 PM.
Failure to indicate quantity	Primary nurse will provide hydrogen peroxide (H_2O_2) mouthwash to client every 2 hours while awake: 8-10-12-2-4-6-8-10.	Primary nurse will provide 50 ml of H_2O_2 mouthwash to client every 2 hours while awake: 8-10-12-2-4-6-8-10.
Failure to indicate method	Primary nurse will change client's dressing once a shift: 6 AM—2 PM—10 PM.	Primary nurse will replace client's dressing, with Neosporin ointment to wound and two dry 4 × 4 dressings secured with hypoallergenic tape, once a shift: 2 PM—10 PM—6 AM.
Failure to indicate person to perform the action	Irrigate nasogastric (NG) tube every 2 hours (even) around the clock with 30 ml of normal saline (NS).	Primary nurse will irrigate NG tube every 2 hours (even) around the clock with 30 ml NS.

the nurse begins to translate the short- and long-term goals into action plans that anticipate the needs of the client, coordinate nursing care, and select appropriate nursing measures.

The nurse writes the action plan in the implementation column (column 4) of the care plan. Each nursing action is written to include information necessary to implement nursing care. It may help the beginning nurse to ask whether the stated interventions answer the following questions:

1. *What* is the intervention?
2. *When* should each intervention be implemented? For how long?
3. *How* should the intervention be performed?
4. *Who* should be involved in each aspect of intervention?

In addition, the nurse should understand the reason for a specific intervention. Nonspecific nursing interventions result in incomplete or inaccurate nursing care, lack of continuity among care givers, and poor use of resources.

Common omissions in writing nursing interventions include action, frequency, quantity, method, or person to perform them. These errors can occur if the nurse is unfamiliar with the planning process. Table 9-4 illustrates these types of errors by showing incorrect and correct statements of nursing interventions.

Column 5 of the nursing care plan contains the projected outcome criteria previously identified. Listing the criteria on the care plan gives a written estimation of when the goal of care has been achieved, thus indicating when a particular nursing diagnosis is no longer relevant to the client's plan of care.

SUMMARY

The planning component of the nursing process results in the development of the nursing care plan, which details the selected nursing interventions and the appropriate evaluation criteria for each client. The nursing student learns the process of planning care in the educational and the clinical settings. Although the format of the care plan varies from one educational institution to another and from one health care setting to another, the student nurse will encounter the student care plan and the institutional care plan throughout the educational process.

Planning nursing care involves a cognitive and written process. The student learns to solve a client's health care problems by selecting appropriate nursing interventions. In addition, the student learns to communicate the client's health care needs through the written care plan. Individual care plans are the result of the nurse's knowledge and expertise, as well as the knowledge and expertise gained through the use of consultants.

Complete and accurate planning of nursing care results in individualization, coordination, and continuity of nursing care. Planning establishes the framework of nursing care to be delivered during implementation.

KEY CONCEPTS

During the planning component, client goals are determined, priorities are established, expected outcomes of nursing care are developed, and a nursing care plan is written.
Nursing care is planned and organized around specific nursing diagnoses, resulting in an individualized care plan.
When establishing priorities, the nurse ranks nursing diagnoses and goals in order of importance.
The nurse begins the nursing care plan with the nursing diagnoses that have the highest priority.
Goals include prevention, the crisis or urgent, and rehabilitation needs of the client.
Goals can include preventive, rehabilitative, or urgent needs of the client.
Goal setting establishes a framework for the care plan.
Using expected outcomes, the nurse evaluates the effectiveness of the care plan.
In general, care plans include the nursing diagnosis, goals, specific actions by the nurse, and expected outcomes.
The care plan is a written guideline for client care so that the care given can be quickly understood by all members of the health care team.
The care plan increases communication among nurses and facilitates the continuity of care from one nurse to another and from one health care setting to another.
The development of an individualized care plan requires involvement of the client and family during the planning phase.
Care plans become part of a client's medical record.
The care plan is a method for teaching students to transfer knowledge gained from nursing and medical literature and the classroom into practical experience.
Poorly written nursing care plans result in incomplete or inaccurate nursing care, lack of continuity among care givers, and poor use of resources.
Correctly written nursing interventions include actions, frequency, quantity, method, and the person to perform them.
Independent nursing interventions are completed without consultation or collaboration with physicians or other health care professionals.
Interdependent nursing interventions are completed with or without a physician's order or are written at a nurse's suggestion and can provide the solution to the client's problem in a collaborative manner with judgment and recommendations of the interdisciplinary health team.
Dependent nursing interventions are completed with a physician's order but require nursing judgment or decision making.
Planning nursing care often involves consultation with other members of the health care team.
The need for consultation in nursing occurs when a problem that cannot be solved using the nurse's knowledge, skills, and resources is identified.

CRITICAL THINKING ACTIVITIES

1. List the components of the planning phase of the nursing process.
2. Discuss the relationship of the planning phase to the other steps of the nursing process.
3. Correctly write the following incorrect nursing interventions.
   a. Irrigate nasogastric tube with normal saline.
   b. Suction client every 2 hours.
   c. Change client's dressing at 0600, 1400, and 2200 hours.
4. From the following list of goals, select the short-term goals.
   a. Client stops smoking within 2 months.
   b. Client's lungs are free of adventitious sounds in 48 hours.
   c. Client is able to independently care for ostomy by discharge.
   d. Client observes incision on second postoperative day.
   e. Client is able to perform all activities of daily living.

References

Alfaro R: *Application of nursing process: a step by step guide,* ed 2, Philadelphia, 1990, JB Lippincott.
American Nurses Association: *Nursing: a social policy statement,* Kansas City, Mo., 1980, The Association.
Benner P: *From novice to expert: excellence and power in clinical nursing practice,* Menlo Park, Calif., 1984, Addison-Wesley.
Bulechek G, McCloskey J: *Nursing interventions: treatments for nursing diagnoses,* ed 2, Philadelphia, 1992, WB Saunders.
Carpenito LJ: *Nursing diagnosis application to clinical practice,* ed 5, Philadelphia, 1993, JB Lippincott.
Carpenito LJ: *Nursing diagnosis application to clinical practice,* ed 3, Philadelphia, 1989, JB Lippincott.
Christensen PJ, Kenney JW: *Nursing process application of conceptual models,* ed 3, St. Louis, 1990, Mosby.
Gordon M: *Nursing diagnosis: process and application,* ed 3, St. Louis, 1994, Mosby.
Hickey PW: *Nursing process handbook,* St. Louis, 1990, Mosby.
Kim MJ: In Hurley MA, editor: *Classification of nursing diagnoses: proceedings of the sixth conference (NANDA),* St. Louis, 1986, Mosby.
Liukkonen A: The nurse's decision-making process and the implementation of psychogeriatric nursing in a mental hospital, *J Adv Nurs* 17(3):356, 1992.
McCloskey JC, Bulechek GM: *Nursing interventions classification,* St. Louis, 1992, Mosby.
Mortensen M, McMullin C: Discharge score for surgical outpatients, *Am J Nurs* 86:1347, 1986.
Prescott PA, Dennis KE, Jacox AK: Clinical decision-making of staff nurses, *Image* 19:56, 1987.
Snyder M: *Independent nursing interventions,* New York, 1985, Wiley.

Bibliography

Aucamp V: *Nursing care plans for the child bearing family,* Norwalk, Conn., 1984, Appleton-Century-Crofts.
Berkey KM, Hanson SMH: *Pocket guide to family assessment and intervention,* St. Louis, 1991, Mosby.
Carnevali DL: *Nursing care planning: diagnosis and management,* ed 3, Philadelphia, 1983, JB Lippincott.
Carpenito LJ: *Nursing care plans and documentation: nursing diagnoses and collaborative problems,* Philadelphia, 1991, JB Lippincott.
Cookfair JM: *Nursing process and practice in the community,* St. Louis, 1991, Mosby.
Doenges M, Morehouse M, and Geissler A: *Nursing care plans,* Philadelphia, 1989, FA Davis.
Higgins M, McCaughan D, et al.: Assessing the outcomes of nursing care, *J Adv Nurs* 17(5):561, 1992.
Hixon AK, Padios E, et al.: Improving continuity of care by evaluation of post-discharge outcomes, *Sci Nursing* 9(2):42, 1992
Holzmer WL, Henry SB: Computer-supported versus manually-generated nursing care plans: a comparison of patient problems, nursing interventions, and AIDS patient outcomes, *Computers in Nursing* 10(1): 19, 1992.
Kim MJ, McFarland GK, McLane AM: *Pocket guide to nursing diagnoses,* ed 5, St. Louis, 1993, Mosby.
McCormick K: Areas of outcome research for nursing, *J Prof Nurs* 8(2):71, 1992.
Megivern K, Halm MA, Jones G: Measuring patient satisfaction as an outcome of nursing care, *J Nurs Care Quality* 6(4):9, 1992.
Pinkley CL: Exploring NANDA's definition of nursing diagnosis: linking diagnostic judgements with the selection of outcomes and interventions, *Nurs Diagn* 2(1):26, 1991.
Prescott PA, et al.: Changing how nurses spend their time, *Image* 23(1):23, 1991.
Thomas LH, Bond S: Outcomes of nursing care: the case of primary nursing, *Int J Nurs Studies* 28(4):291, 1991.

10

Implementing Nursing Care

OBJECTIVES

Mastery of content in this chapter will enable the student to:

- Define the key terms listed.
- Discuss differences between protocols and standing orders.
- Describe the information-processing model for selecting nursing interventions.
- List and discuss the five steps of the implementation process.
- Select appropriate implementation methods for a client.

KEY TERMS

activities of daily living (ADLs)
adverse reaction
assistive care
counseling
delegation
functional nursing system
implementation
life-saving measure
nursing intervention
preventive nursing actions
primary nursing system
protocol
standing order
supportive care
teaching
team nursing system
total client care

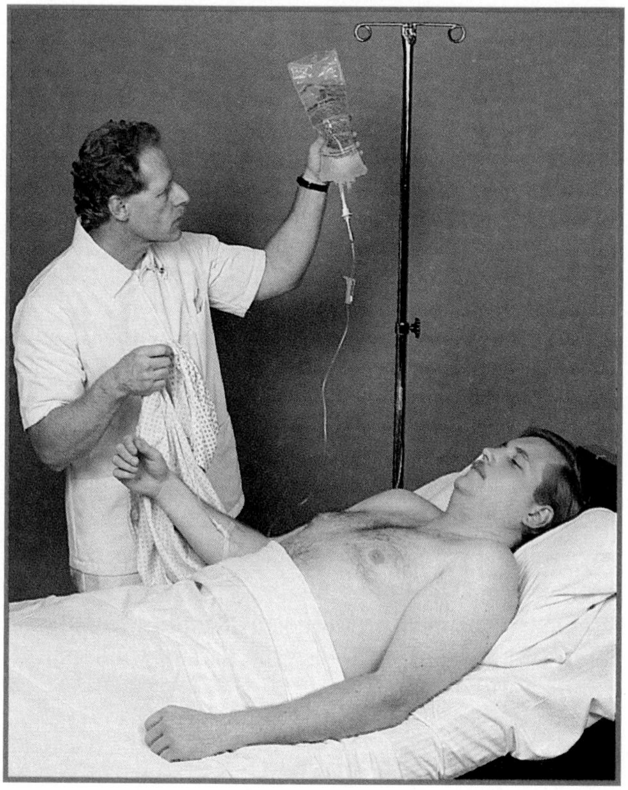

Nursing care is the focus of the implementation step of the nursing process. The purpose of **implementation** is to carry out the nursing care plan developed in the previous component of the nursing process. Implementation is a category of nursing behavior in which the actions necessary for achieving the expected outcomes of nursing care are initiated and completed. Implementation includes performing, assisting, or directing the performance of activities of daily living, counseling and teaching the client or family, giving direct care to achieve client-centered goals, supervising and evaluating the work of staff members, and recording and exchanging information relevant to the client's continued health care.

Implementation begins after the care plan has been developed and focuses on nursing interventions to achieve goals of the care plan. A **nursing intervention** is any act by a nurse that implements the nursing care plan or any specific objective of the plan. The client may require intervention in the form of emotional and physical support, medication, treatment for his or her condition, client-family education, or treatment to prevent future health problems.

Implementation is continuous and interacts with the other components of the nursing process. To complete implementation effectively, the nurse must be knowledgeable about types of interventions, the implementation process, and specific implementation methods.

TYPES OF NURSING INTERVENTIONS

Implementation puts the care plan into action. After the plan has been developed according to client needs and priorities, the nurse performs specific nursing interventions, which can be dependent, independent, or interdependent (see Chapter 9). In addition, nursing interventions may be entirely based on protocols or standing orders. Although these types of interventions may be viewed by some as a form of a dependent or interdependent order, a clear description of each is necessary.

Protocols and Standing Orders

A **protocol** is a written plan specifying the procedures to be followed during an assessment or when providing treatment for a specific condition or nursing care problem. For example, nurses providing primary care for clients in an outpatient setting follow a protocol. In such a setting, nurses assess the client and identify abnormalities. The established protocol delineates the conditions that nurses are permitted to treat and the types of treatment that they are permitted to administer.

A protocol can also be strictly within the framework of nursing such as a protocol for admission and discharge, relaxation training, or pain management. Protocols are also used in interdisciplinary settings for diagnostic testing and physical, occupational, and speech therapies.

A **standing order** dictates a clinical situation and prescribes a standardized intervention. Standing orders are approved and signed by the physician in charge of care before their implementation. They are commonly found in critical care settings, in which clients' needs can change rapidly and require immediate attention. Standing orders are also common in the community health setting, in which the nurse encounters situations that do not permit immediate contact with a physician. Thus standing orders and protocols give the nurse the legal protection to intervene appropriately in the client's best interest.

Before implementing any therapy, including those included in protocols and standing orders, the nurse must use sound judgment in determining whether the intervention is correct and appropriate. Second, the nurse implementing any intervention has the responsibility to obtain correct theoretical knowledge and develop the clinical competency necessary to perform the intervention. Nursing responsibility is equally great for all types of interventions.

DECISION-MAKING STRATEGIES FOR CHOOSING NURSING INTERVENTIONS

Nurses using the nursing process make two major types of decisions. The diagnostic process defines the client's strengths and problems at the conclusion of the assessment and throughout the diagnostic stage (Hickey, 1991; McFarland, McFarlane, 1989). Specific nursing interventions are also selected during the planning stage (Grier, 1981; Gordon, 1987).

The student must carefully select the interventions designed to achieve expected outcomes and know the way that dependent, independent, and interdependent interventions differ. Several factors make decision making more difficult when choosing among independent nursing interventions (Snyder, 1985). One factor is the absence of objective data concerning the probable consequences of the interventions. Another factor is that independent nursing interventions are often not mutually exclusive from medical therapies. For example, the nurse may need to augment relaxation, massage, and guided imagery techniques with prescribed analgesics for pain management (see Chapter 28).

Snyder (1985) proposes an information-processing model of decision making (Table 10-1). The objective of this model is to characterize the sequence of the thought process used by problem solvers. This model focuses on decisions that will be made rather than the ways that they are made. Therefore the information-processing model identifies how decisions are made, and the behavioral decision model denotes the decisions made. Because of the information-processing model, a student uses the following components of decision making when determining nursing interventions (Snyder, 1985):

1. The set of all possible nursing actions
2. A listing of all possible consequences associated with each possible nursing action
3. The determination of the probability that each of the consequences will occur
4. A judgment based on the value of that consequence to the client

IMPLEMENTATION PROCESS

Adequate and thorough preparation before implementing the care plan ensures efficient and effective nursing care. The box on p. 157 lists preparatory nursing activities.

Reassessing the Client

Assessment is a continuous process that occurs each time a nurse interacts with a client. When new data are gathered and a new client need is identified, the nurse modifies the care plan. During the initial phase of im-

table 10-1

INFORMATION-PROCESSING MODEL FOR PAIN RELATED TO ABDOMINAL INCISION HEALING

Possible actions	Possible consequences associated with action	Probability of consequence	Value of consequence to client
Teach relaxation exercises.	Client is able to control perception of pain.	Moderate	Ability to control perception and response to pain
	Pain is unrelieved.	Moderate	
	Pain increases.	Low	
Teach client use of controlled analgesia.	Client is able to control administration of analgesia within preset limits.	High	Ability of client to use analgesia to continuously relieve pain
	Pain is relieved.	High	
	Pain is unrelieved.	Moderate	
	Pain increases.	Low	
Administer narcotic analgesia every 4 hours.	Client is unable to control administration of analgesia.	High	Inability to control administration of analgesia
	Pain increases in intensity before nurse administers narcotic analgesia.	Moderate to high	Increase or decrease of pain perception based on blood levels of narcotic analgesia
	Pain is relieved.	Moderate to high	
	Client is confused after administration of narcotic analgesia.	Low to moderate	

PREPARATION ACTIVITIES

Reassess client
Review and revise care plan
Organize
  Equipment
  Personnel
Prepare
  Environment
  Client and family
Anticipate and prevent complications

plementation, the nurse reassesses the client. This is a partial assessment and may focus on one dimension of the client or on one system. The reassessment will provide a mechanism to determine whether the proposed nursing action is appropriate for the client's level of wellness.

Reviewing and Revising the Care Plan

Although the nursing care plan is developed according to the nursing diagnoses, changes in the client's status can require modification of planned nursing care. Before beginning care, the nurse reviews the plan of care and compares the established plan with assessment to validate stated nursing diagnoses and to determine whether the nursing interventions are the most appropriate for the clinical situation. If the nurse determines that the client's status has changed and the nursing diagnoses and related nursing interventions are no longer appropriate, the nursing care plan needs to be modified (see Chapter 11).

Modification of the existing plan includes several steps (Table 10-2). First, data in the assessment column are revised to reflect the client's status. New data entered in the care plan should be dated to inform the health care team when the change occurred.

Then, nursing diagnoses are revised. Nursing diagnoses that are no longer relevant or that have been resolved by previous interventions are deleted, and new

table 10-2
MODIFIED NURSING CARE PLAN FOR MR. BROWN

Assessment	Goals	Implementation	Evaluation
Nursing diagnosis: *High risk for ineffective airway clearance after surgery* related to abdominal incision			
Definition: High risk for ineffective airway clearance after surgery is the state in which an individual is unable to clear secretions or obstructions from the respiratory tract to maintain airway patency.*			
Smoked two packs/day 20 years; chest x-ray film showing slight change of emphysema; crackles auscultated in lung field; scheduled for abdominal surgery	Client's airway remains patent by 7/1	Demonstrate turn, cough, and deep breathing to client. Have client demonstrate turning, coughing, and deep breathing exercises.	Productive cough produced. Airway clear to auscultation.
MODIFIED 24 HOURS AFTER SURGERY			
Nursing diagnosis: *Ineffective airway clearance* related to decreased inspiratory effort secondary to abdominal incision.			
Decreased chest wall movements; crackles in base that do not clear with coughing fever tachypnea	Client coughs productively by 7/2	Administer chest physiotherapy to all lobes of the lung: 8-12-4-8-12-4.	Lung fields are clear on auscultation. Client becomes afebrile. Sputum: clear
		Ensure that Mr. Brown coughs and deep breathes every 2 hours around the clock.	Chest x-ray film demonstrates atelectasis resolving.
	Client's lungs free of abnormal lung sounds 7/2	Suction nasotracheal area every 2 hours if client is unable to cough productively.	
		Teach client to splint incision with pillow before and during coughing.	Client does not report increased pain during coughing.

*Data from Kim MJ, McFarland GK, McLane AM: *Pocket guide to nursing diagnoses,* ed 5, St. Louis, 1993, Mosby.

nursing diagnoses are added.

Third, specific interventions are revised to correspond to the new nursing diagnoses and goals. The new implementation methods indicate the client's greater independence from or dependence on nursing. In addition, the revised implementation can include the client's specific needs for health care resources.

Finally, the nurse evaluates the client response to the nursing actions. If client response is not consistent with the established expected outcomes, further revisions for the plan of care are needed. For example, a preoperative care plan was developed for Mr. Brown. As he progressed through the postoperative period, his nursing needs changed. New data were noted and dated. The nurse made modifications in the care plan for one nursing diagnosis: *high risk for ineffective airway clearance after surgery related to pain of abdominal incision* (Table 10-2). On the second postoperative day, the nurse assessed Mr. Brown and noted decreased chest wall movements, crackles that were auscultated in the right lower lobes, and an elevated temperature (39° C). Mr. Brown had a standing order for a chest x-ray examination, which was taken immediately and revealed the collapse of alveoli in the right lower lobe. The nursing diagnosis was revised to read *ineffective airway clearance related to pain of abdominal incision.* The goal of "maintaining a patent airway" was still appropriate. Specific nursing interventions were developed to assist in achieving a patent airway. Finally, the projected evaluation criteria were rewritten to reflect the desired level of wellness and indicate when the need had been resolved.

Organizing Resources and Care Delivery

A facility's resources include equipment and skilled personnel. Organization of equipment and personnel makes efficient, skilled client care possible. After a plan of care is determined, the nurse prepares the necessary supplies and decides on the time and provider of care. The last phase of preparing for care delivery involves preparing the environment and client for nursing intervention.

Equipment. Most nursing procedures, from bed making to client teaching, require some equipment or supplies. The nurse must analyze each planned intervention for needed items. Realistic interventions call for only those things available in the facility.

All necessary supplies should be gathered and put in a convenient location, usually where they will be used, before implementation. Extra supplies should be available in case of mishaps. Extra sterile gloves, for example, anticipate the possibility of a break in sterile technique. The nurse also arranges the supplies in the order in which they will be used. Following the procedure the nurse appropriately returns any unused supplies.

Personnel. Nursing care delivery systems vary among facilities and must be considered when allocating resources. The system by which nursing is organized determines the way in which personnel are designated for client care delivery. The most common types of nursing delivery systems are functional, team, primary nursing, and case management.

Three categories of functions are inherent to professional nursing practice: actual client care, **delegation,** and coordination. These functions assume varying levels of importance, depending on the nursing system.

A **functional nursing system** divides client care into a series of tasks, each of which is delegated to the lowest level of personnel having the requisite skill and competence to complete the task. Each staff member then performs this same task for all clients on the unit. Thus the client is cared for by a number of people who concentrate on their own particular assignments.

A **team nursing system** is a method of care delivery in which a small group of personnel, supervised by a professional nurse, delivers care to a number of clients. The team leader is responsible for the client and the care plan, delegates client care to team members, and coordinates the team's efforts. Cooperation and collaboration are hallmarks of good team nursing.

Total client care has a registered nurse who is responsible for the complete care of a number of clients throughout a shift. Client care is totally individualized; the nurse assigned to the client is responsible for direct client care, coordination with other departments for services, and contribution to the care plan.

Direct client care is emphasized. A single nurse provides all aspects of care during the shift. When assigning clients, the unit manager should assign nurses to the same clients to ensure continuity of care. There is no delegation under this system; the nurse on each shift independently gives care and is responsible for the care plan during that time.

A **primary nursing system** has a primary nurse who is responsible for all aspects of a client's nursing care from admission to discharge. When the primary nurse is off duty, an associate nurse assumes care of the client. If a problem arises, the associate nurse confers directly or indirectly with the primary nurse, who retains full authority and responsibility for the client's nursing care plan.

Case management is an organized system for delivering health care to an individual client or a group of clients through an episode of illness. This system includes assessment and development of a plan of care, coordination of all services, referral, and follow-up, usually assigned to one individual.

No matter what the nursing care delivery system, continuity of individualized care is a primary consideration when assigning and organizing personnel.

Environment. Environmental factors influence delivery and reception of care. The surroundings in which nursing activities occur should be safe and conducive to achievement of the goal of the intervention strategy. Safety is always the first concern. If the client has sensory deficits or an alteration in level of consciousness, the environment must be arranged to prevent injury. Special rooms, rearrangement of furniture and equipment, and provision for additional personnel are examples of creating safe surroundings.

The client benefits most from nursing interventions when surroundings are compatible with activities. Privacy promotes relaxation when body parts are exposed. Reducing distractions enhances learning opportunities. Provision of adequate warmth and lighting prevents intrusion of environmental factors.

Client. Before beginning to perform interventions, the nurse should make the client as physically and psychologically comfortable as possible. Pain, for example, frequently interferes with a client's full concentration and cooperation. Comfort measures or medication for pain before initiating interventions enable the client to participate more fully. If client alertness is needed, the dose of pain medication should be sufficient to relieve discomfort but not impair mental faculties.

Even if pain is not a factor, the client should be made physically comfortable during interventions. Controlling environmental factors, positioning, and taking care of other physical needs should precede initiation of the intervention session. The nurse should also consider the client's level of endurance and plan only the amount of activity the client can comfortably tolerate.

Awareness of the client's psychosocial needs helps the nurse to create a favorable emotional climate. Some clients feel reassured by having a significant other present to lend encouragement and moral support. Other strategies include planning sufficient time or multiple opportunities for the client to work through and ventilate feelings and anxieties. Adequate preparations allow the client to benefit from intervention sessions and alleviate the need for many sessions.

Anticipating Complications. Risks to the client arise from the illness and treatment. The nurse must identify these risks, evaluate the relative benefit of the treatment versus the risk, and initiate preventive measures.

Many client conditions place the client at risk for additional complications. The nurse's knowledge of pathophysiology helps in the identification of problems. Scientific rationales help the nurse to evaluate the usefulness of preventive strategies. A confused client, for example, is at risk for pulmonary complications because of extended periods of immobility. The nurse knows that getting the client out of bed will expand the bases of the lungs but also realizes this activity poses a risk to the client's safety. Preventive safety measures may require remaining with the client while out of bed or having the family stay with a client and encouraging deep breathing.

Some nursing procedures also pose risks for the client. The nurse needs to be aware of potential complications and institute precautionary measures. For instance, the client receiving feedings through a nasogastric tube is at risk for aspiration. The nurse should elevate the head of the bed and have pharyngeal suction equipment at the bedside before initiating the feedings.

IDENTIFYING AREAS OF ASSISTANCE. Some nursing situations require the nurse to seek assistance, which can be additional personnel, additional knowledge, and additional nursing skills. Before implementing care, the nurse evaluates the plan to determine the need for assistance and the type required.

Situations requiring additional personnel vary. For example, a nurse assigned to care for an overweight, immobilized client may need additional personnel to help to turn, transfer, and position the client. The nurse also needs to determine when the personnel are needed. He or she must then determine the number of persons needed and must discuss the need for assistance with potential resources.

Some nursing situations require additional knowledge and skills, as well as additional personnel. A nurse needs additional knowledge when administering a new medication or implementing a new procedure. Such information can be obtained from a hospital's formulary or procedure book. If the nurse still is uncertain about the new medication or procedure, other members of the health care team can be consulted.

Because of the continual growth of health care professions and related technology, a nurse may lack the skills to perform a new procedure. When this occurs, information about the procedure is obtained from the literature and the agency's procedure book. Next, all equipment necessary for the procedure is collected. Finally, another nurse who has completed the procedure correctly and safely provides assistance and guidance. The assistance can come from another staff nurse, a supervisor, an educator, or a nurse specialist. Requesting assistance occurs frequently in all types of nursing practice and is a learning process that continues throughout educational experiences and into professional development.

INTERVENTIONS

The primary focus of the implementation step of the nursing process is intervention on the client's behalf. When the preparatory steps have been completed, the nurse can select the appropriate implementation method and intervene as planned.

Implementation Methods

The nurse carries out the nursing care plan by using several implementation methods to achieve the goals of nursing care. The nurse is able to identify the implementation methods needed for each nursing diagnosis. Each method includes specific theoretical knowledge and clinical skills. The nurse is responsible for knowing when one of these methods is preferred over another and for having the necessary theoretical knowledge and skills to implement each.

Assisting With Activities of Daily Living. **Activities of daily living (ADLs)** are usually performed in the course of a normal day, such as eating, dressing, bathing, brushing the teeth, or grooming. Conditions resulting in the need for assistance with ADLs can be acute, chronic, temporary, permanent, or rehabilitative. An acute disease is characterized by symptoms that are usually severe and present for a relatively short period. An episode of acute disease results in recovery to a state of health and activity comparable to that before the disease, passage into a chronic phase of the disease, or death. For example, the postoperative client is unable to complete ADLs independently because of surgery. As the client progresses through the postoperative period, he or she depends less on nurses for completing ADLs.

A chronic disease persists longer. Although the symptoms of chronic disease are usually less severe than those of the acute phase of the same disease, chronic disease may result in complete or partial disability. A client with partial paralysis after a cerebrovascular accident has a chronic impairment requiring long-term assistance with ADLs.

In the case of temporary assistance with ADLs, the client needs assistance during a specific time period, such as after surgery. A client gradually assumes responsibility for ADLs during recovery. A client with a total self-care deficit related to a high spinal cord injury has a permanent need for assistance. It is unrealistic for the nurse to plan a rehabilitation program with the goal of independent client performance of ADLs. Through rehabilitation, the client will learn new ways to perform certain ADLs, thus becoming more independent in performing some aspects of self-care.

Counseling. **Counseling** is an implementation method that helps the client to use a problem-solving process to recognize and manage stress and that facilitates interpersonal relationships between the client and family, significant others, or health care team members. Nurses provide counseling to help the client to accept actual or impending changes resulting from stress. Counseling is emotional, intellectual, spiritual, and psychological support (Dalton, Swenson, 1991). Clients and families in need of nursing counseling have "normal" adjustment difficulties and are upset or frustrated but are not psychologically disabled.

Clients, families, or significant others in need of counseling include persons who must adjust their life-style, cope with chronic or disabling disease, or accept the possibility of death. Counseling encourages individuals to examine available alternatives and to choose useful and appropriate choices. When clients examine alternatives, they develop a sense of control and are able to better manage stress.

Teaching. **Teaching** is an activity closely aligned to counseling. Both involve using communication skills to effect a change in the client (see Chapter 14, Teaching and Learning). Teaching is an implementation method used to present correct principles, procedures, and techniques of health care to clients, to inform clients about their health status, and to refer the client and family to appropriate health or social resources in the community. Health teaching can help the client to promote, maintain, modify, or increase health-related behaviors (Figure 10-1). During the teaching-learning process, specific learning objectives are presented and achieved (Redman, 1988).

Preventing Adverse Reactions. To achieve the therapeutic goals of the client, the nurse initiates interventions to prevent adverse reactions by using precau-

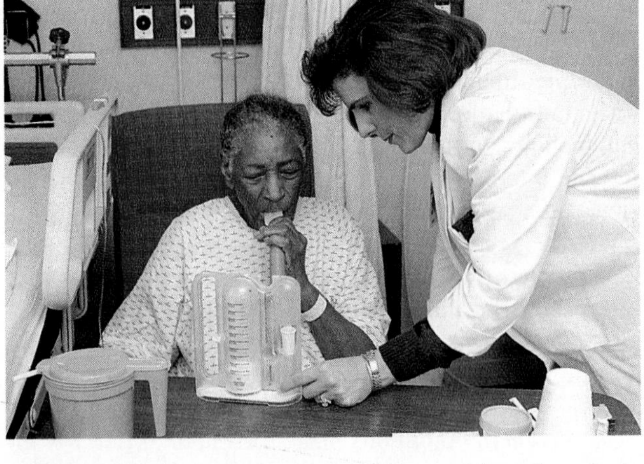

FIGURE 10-1 Explanations assist client to safely and correctly use equipment.

tionary and preventive measures when providing care and applying correct techniques in administering care and preparing the client for special procedures. An **adverse reaction** is a harmful or unintended effect of a medication, diagnostic test, or therapeutic treatment. The nurse is responsible for knowing potential adverse reactions to therapeutic interventions and for instituting appropriate preventive actions. Prevention includes assessment and promotion of the client's health potential; application of prescribed measures such as immunizations, health teaching, early diagnosis and treatment; and development of rehabilitation potential.

In the case of a client with a hypersensitivity to penicillin, the nurse can implement several preventive measures. The nurse indicates the penicillin allergy in the client's medical record, informs the client and family of the need for a Medic-Alert bracelet, and teaches them actions to take if the client is given penicillin again. The nurse also teaches the client and family about the allergy and specific drugs to avoid.

Preventive nursing actions are used to meet the therapeutic goals of the client. Through preventive actions the nurse can help the client to attain the highest level of wellness.

Compensating for Adverse Reactions. Adverse reactions can follow independent, dependent, or interdependent nursing interventions. Nursing actions that compensate for adverse reactions reduce or counteract the reaction. To intervene, the nurse must know about potential undesired effects and the correct course of action to take if an adverse reaction occurs.

When administering a medication, for example, the nurse understands the known potential side effects of the drug. After administration, the nurse assesses the client for side effects. The client with an unknown sensitivity to penicillin, for example, may develop hives after several doses. The nurse records the reaction, stops administration of the drug, consults with the physician for orders, and administers an antipruritic medication to relieve the itching and an antihistamine to reduce the allergic response.

The initiation of life-saving measures is an essential component of nursing practice. A **life-saving measure** is an independent, dependent, or interdependent nursing intervention implemented when a client's physiological or psychological state is threatened. The purpose of such a measure is to restore physiological or psychological equilibrium. These measures include administering emergency medications, instituting cardiopulmonary resuscitation (CPR), and controlling a bleeding wound. As with any procedure, the nurse must know about the life-saving procedure itself, the times to use it, the way in which to do it, and the expected outcome.

Although adverse effects are uncommon, they do occur. The nurse learns potential side effects, is able to recognize the presence of an adverse reaction, and is able to intervene accordingly.

Nursing Implementation Skills

Nursing practice is composed of cognitive, interpersonal, and technical skills. Each skill is needed to implement the four types of implementation methods.

Cognitive Skills. Cognitive skills involve nursing knowledge. The nurse must know the rationale for therapeutic interventions, understand normal and abnormal physiological and psychological responses, be able to identify client learning needs and teach appropriate health care information, and recognize the need for preventive and compensatory nursing actions. The range of nursing knowledge includes the social and biological sciences.

Interpersonal Skills. Interpersonal skills are essential to effective nursing intervention. The nurse needs to communicate clearly with the client, family, significant others, and health care team (Figure 10-2). Client teaching and counseling must be done at the client's level of understanding. The nurse must also be sensitive to the client's emotional responses to the disease process and treatment. The perceptive nurse maintains an awareness of the client's psychological status and promotes client motivation to achieve wellness.

Technical Skills. Technical skills are involved in all client care. In a hospital, the nurse is required to complete many procedures each day. He or she is responsible for correctly performing each procedure. Some of these procedures might be new, so before entering into a new procedure the nurse assesses personal compe-

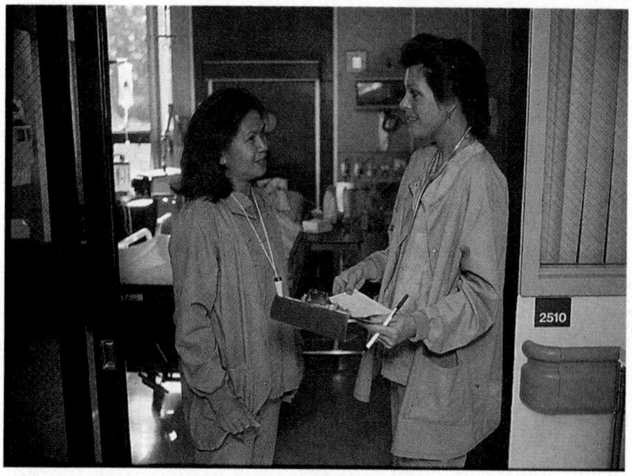

FIGURE 10-2 Collaboration with other health care providers results in efficient interventions.

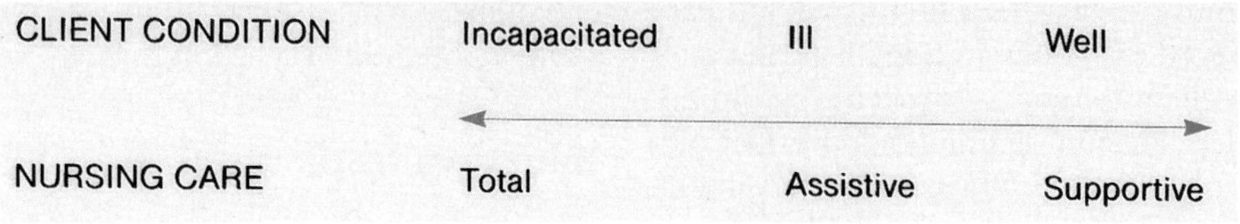

FIGURE 10-3 Continuum of client condition and level of nursing care. (Redrawn from Hickey P: *Nursing process handbook,* St. Louis, 1990, Mosby.)

tencies and determines the need for assistance, new knowledge, or new skills.

Level of Assistance

Even when they have the same medical diagnoses, no two clients are in exactly the same condition or have precisely the same needs, strengths, or weaknesses. Every client must be given care at a level that reflects the individual's precise physical and emotional status and that best promotes attainment of expected outcomes. The level of care the nurse provides a client can be thought of as on a continuum with three basic divisions: total care, assistive care, and supportive care. The continuum of client condition and nursing level of care is illustrated in Figure 10-3.

Total Care. The client who is incapacitated, unconscious, or completely unable to provide self-care requires total care, meaning that the nurse maintains bodily functions and provides all nurturing activities until the client improves enough to participate. Total nursing care may extend to all areas of function (e.g., when the client is unconscious). The nurse, in such cases, does everything for the client, including maintaining autonomic functions (e.g., respiration or blood pressure) as needed. All four types of nursing interventions are used in a manner that differs from other levels of care.

Nursing strategies focus on maintaining life and improving its quality. Client education is limited to explaining procedures as they are performed, even though the client is unconscious. Educational and counseling interventions are also implemented for significant others.

Sometimes a client is conscious but is still unable to participate in one or more areas of care; that is, the client is able to provide some self-care but cannot do some things adequately. Clients with high spinal cord injuries are good examples of this category of infirmity. The client is conscious and retains full intellectual powers but is unable to care for bodily needs. Nursing care is total in respect to this client's physical needs. On the other hand, the client may require only assistive or supportive levels of care for emotional, intellectual, and social needs.

Assistive Care. Most hospitalized clients require **assistive care** during most of their stay. They are able to provide some of their own care but need help in some aspects. At the assistive level, the nurse and client work together; the nurse supplements the client's capabilities when necessary.

This area of the continuum has a wide span, from clients requiring assistance with almost all activity to those needing it in only one or two situations. The nurse must determine the client's capabilities and the amount and kind of assistance required. The focus of care at this level is to decrease or eliminate unhealthy responses and to foster healthy ones.

During the immediate postoperative period, for example, the client requires assistance with almost everything. Generally, recovery is rapid and the client needs less and less assistance for normal activities as time passes. However, the nurse may still do all dressing changes or other technical procedures. In the meantime, the nurse also uses psychosocial and educative measures to assist the client in adapting to a new body image and learning new health care information. The nurse may also confer with the family or make a referral to a home health care agency for care after discharge. The assistive level of care changes frequently for almost all clients. Ongoing assessment is necessary to ensure that the level of care is compatible with client capabilities. As care is given, the client's condition should improve, and the amount of assistance needed should lessen. The client should progress to the supportive level of care.

Supportive Care. Some clients are physically capable of providing their own care but have difficulty doing so because of lack of knowledge or motivation. At this level of care, the client performs all health care measures while the nurse supports, teaches, and guides.

Counseling and teaching are the primary intervention modes. The client may need information and support for decision making or may need anticipatory guidance and emotional support while grieving. Motivational reinforcement may be required; for example, the nurse in a clinic or doctor's office is often a consultative resource. The client needing **supportive care** should soon be self-sufficient. Termination of the helping relationship should be planned and gradual, but it should occur before the client becomes dependent.

Modifications

As interventions are implemented, the client's condition and responses should improve and expected outcomes are achieved. Thus client needs and the level of nursing care should also change, necessitating adjustments in the level, kind, and amount of nursing interventions.

The client's condition must be frequently assessed and the level of care adjusted accordingly. The amount of nursing assistance provided for each concern should be evaluated on a daily basis.

Client responses during implementation may also indicate the need for an adjustment. A negative response is cause for evaluation of the appropriateness of the intervention. If an intervention is not going smoothly, the nurse needs to pause, reassess the situation, and consider changes. The care plan is flexible; it is meant to be altered when the client's status changes.

Supervising and Evaluating the Work of Other Staff Members

The nurse who develops the nursing care plan frequently does not initiate all nursing interventions. This is particularly true in functional and team nursing situations in which some interventions may be delegated to another member of the health care team. The nurse assigning tasks is responsible for ensuring that each task is assigned to an individual skilled to perform it. The nurse is also responsible for ensuring that the delegated task was completed according to the standard of care and for determining the client's status after care delivery. With a busy workload of clients, the nurse must learn to delegate tasks without feeling compelled to perform all tasks alone.

SUMMARY

The implementation step is the action-oriented phase of the nursing process in which the nurse initiates and carries out the objectives of the nursing care plan. The nurse prepares to intervene by reassessing the client; reviewing priorities and modifying the existing care plan; identifying areas of assistance; organizing supplies and personnel; preparing the environment and client; and anticipating and preventing potential complications.

Interventions require cognitive, interpersonal, and technical skills. When implementing care, the nurse must choose the level of care that will result in optimal client and family benefit. The selection of total, assistive, or supportive care is based on the client's condition and capabilities.

The implementation step is the focal point of the nursing process. It is what nursing is about: nursing care delivery for client and family. When properly planned and implemented, the implementation step resolves client problems and assists the client back to wellness.

KEY CONCEPTS

During implementation, the nurse carries out the nursing care plan developed in the planning component of the nursing process.

Preparation for implementation includes reassessing the client; reviewing, setting in order of priority, and modifying the care plan; identifying areas in which assistance is needed; organizing supplies and personnel; and preparing the client, family, and environment.

Implementation methods consist of assisting with ADLs, counseling and teaching, preventing adverse reactions, and compensating for adverse reactions.

Implementation methods require the nurse to use cognitive, interpersonal, and technical skills.

Assisting with ADLs is a nursing strategy that compensates for the client's self-care deficits until he or she can resume normal activity.

Counseling helps the client to use problem solving to recognize and manage stress and facilitates interpersonal relationships between the client, family, significant others, or health care team.

Teaching is used to present correct principles, procedures, and techniques of health care to the client; to inform clients about their health status; and to refer the client and family to appropriate resources.

Nursing actions to achieve therapeutic goals include preventing adverse reactions, using correct techniques for administering care, preparing the client for procedures, and implementing lifesaving measures.

Delegating care to other personnel involves ensuring that the individuals are skilled in the tasks and evaluating that each task was completed according to the standard of care.

To complete any nursing procedure, the nurse must be knowledgeable about the procedure, times it is needed, its steps, and its expected outcome.

CRITICAL THINKING ACTIVITIES

1. Mr. Clark is a 45-year-old man admitted with congestive heart failure. His lung sounds are clear; his vital signs are 130/88, 112, 24. Your interventions include assisting Mr. Clark to ambulate. While walking, the client tells you that he feels that his heart is racing. His vital signs are now 90/60, 136, 28, and he is diaphoretic and pale. What are your interventions?
2. You are assigned to administer all medications. What measures will you take to reduce the incidence of an adverse reaction to clients receiving intravenous piggyback medications?
3. Mrs. Jones is a 240-pound comatose client. You assign your nursing assistant to provide skin and hygiene care. What type of help do you anticipate that the nurse assistant will need in order to provide safe care and reduce the risk of pressure ulcers to this client?

References

Dalton JA, Swenson I, et al.: Brief: counseling hospitalized patients to quit smoking—study of an educational intervention, *J Continuing Education in Nursing* 22(5):209, 1991.

Gordon M: *Nursing diagnosis: process and application,* ed 2, New York, 1987, McGraw-Hill.

Grier M: The need for data in making nursing decisions. In Werley H, Grier M, editors: *Nursing information systems,* New York, 1981, Springer.

Hickey P: *Nursing process handbook,* St. Louis, 1991, Mosby.

Kim MJ, McFarland GK, McLane AM: *Pocket guide to nursing diagnoses,* ed 5, St. Louis, 1993, Mosby.

McFarland GK, McFarlane EA: *Nursing diagnosis and intervention: planning for patient care,* St. Louis, 1989, Mosby.

Redman BK: *The process of patient education,* ed 7, St. Louis, 1992, Mosby.

Stewart BJ, Archbold PG: Nursing intervention studies require outcome measures that are sensitive to change: Part Two. *Res Nurs Health* 16:77, 1993

Bibliography

American Nurses Association: *Nursing: a social policy statement,* Kansas City, Mo., 1980, The Association.

Bulechek GM, McCloskey JM: Defining and validating nursing interventions, *Nurs Clin North Am* 27(2):289, 1992.

Carpenito LJ: *Nursing diagnosis application to clinical practice,* ed 5, Philadelphia, 1993, JB Lippincott.

Carpenito LJ: *Nursing diagnosis: application to clinical practice,* ed 3, Philadelphia, 1989, JB Lippincott.

Kim MJ: Nursing diagnoses: a Janus view. In Hurley ME, editor: *Classification of nursing diagnoses: proceedings of the sixth conference (NANDA),* St. Louis, 1986, Mosby.

Kim MJ: Degree of independence of nursing interventions for nursing diagnoses. In Hurley MA, editor: *Classification of nursing diagnoses: proceedings of the sixth conference (NANDA),* St. Louis, 1986, Mosby.

Marriner A: *The nursing process: a scientific approach to nursing care,* ed 4, St. Louis, 1987, Mosby.

Prescott PA, Dennis KE, and Jacox AK: Clinical decision making of staff nurses, *Image* 19:56, 1987.

11

Evaluation

OBJECTIVES

Mastery of content in this chapter will enable the student to:

- Define the key terms listed.
- Explain the relationship between expected outcomes and goals of care.
- Describe how evaluative measures are used to determine a client's progress.
- Explain the function evaluation plays in improving the quality of client care.
- Give examples of evaluation measures used to determine progress toward expected outcomes.
- Evaluate nursing actions performed for a select client.
- Discuss the differences between structure, process, and outcome quality indicators.
- Explain how quality improvement activities influence the work of a staff nurse.

KEY TERMS

benchmarking
CQI
evaluation
outcome indicators
process indicators
quality assurance
quality improvement
standard of care
structure indicators
threshold

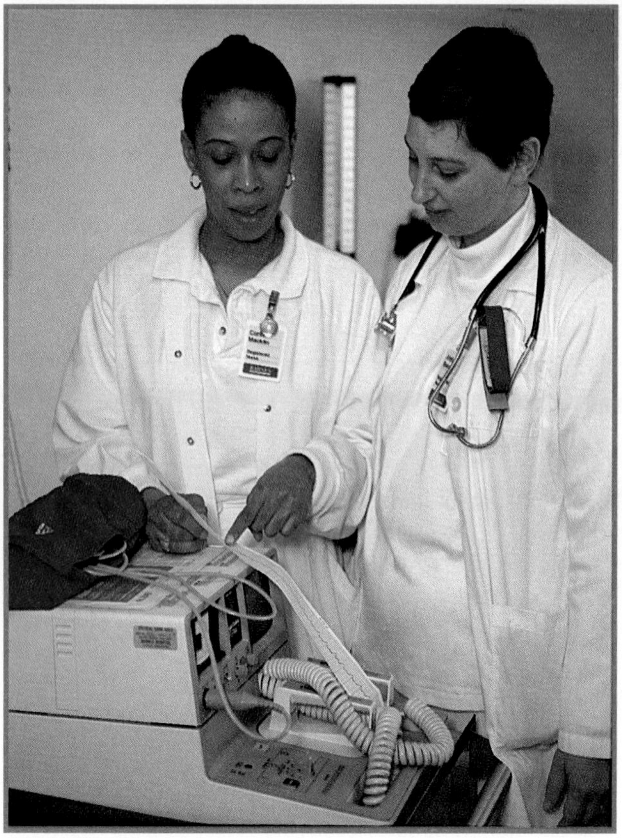

GOAL: CLIENT REMOVES SECRETIONS FROM TRACHEOBRONCHIAL TREE

INTERVENTION	EVALUATION	OUTCOMES
Turn, cough, deep breathe every 2 hours while awake	Observe cough Auscultate lungs bilaterally	Coughs productively after exercises Lung sounds clear in all lung fields

Nurses must be critical thinkers. The nursing process is a series of nursing actions based on and supported by clinical judgments that nurses make to help clients (Bleich, 1990). The previous chapters describing the nursing process have explained how nurses gather essential information, form a diagnostic conclusion about the information, form a plan, and take action. The evaluation component of the nursing process measures the client's response to nursing interventions and the client's progress toward achieving goals (see box above). Put more simply, evaluation determines if a client improves, remains stable, or deteriorates. The nurse evaluates whether the client's behaviors or responses reflect a reversal or improvement in a nursing diagnosis or maintenance of a healthy state. By examining a client's response and comparing it with a behavior stated in an expected outcome, the nurse determines if the client has progressed and if nursing care is effective. It is the one step of the nursing process made to adjust nursing care to a client's changing needs.

Another aspect of evaluation involves measurement of the quality of nursing care provided in health care settings. Institutions are required by external regulating agencies such as the Joint Commission on Accreditation of Health Care Organizations (JCAHO) and Professional Standards Review Organizations (PSROs) to demonstrate the quality, appropriateness, and effectiveness of care delivered to clients. Quality improvement has become the philosophy of many health care organizations. Through the systematic collection of data, institutions monitor the level of performance of processes within the organization, identify areas for improvement, evaluate results, and design new processes. Collectively, the quality improvement effort is designed to improve client care and the functions of health care organizations (JCAHO, 1993). Nurses play an active role in helping organizations prioritize quality improvement efforts.

DYNAMICS OF EVALUATION

While caring for clients, the nurse is more than a casual observer. Constantly the question is asked, "What is happening to my client?" Unless evaluation is applied, the question cannot be answered. The nurse compares observed results (e.g., improved depth of respiration, proper use of a cane) with expected outcomes developed in the plan of care. The nurse uses critical thinking to analyze the findings of evaluative measures. For example, when evaluating a client for a change in vital signs, the nurse applies knowledge of disease processes and physiology to interpret whether a change has occurred. Positive evaluations occur when desired outcomes are met, leading the nurse to conclude that the care plan met client goals. Negative evaluations or undesired outcomes indicate that the problem was not resolved or that potential problems were not avoided. As a result, the nurse changes the care plan and the nursing process sequence is repeated. The sequence continues until problems are resolved.

Evaluation is not always simple, particularly for clients with multiple problems, presenting almost constant changes in status. As nurses mature in their practice, intuition becomes an important characteristic. Benner (1984) has noted that an experienced nurse be-

table 11-1
EXAMPLES OF OBJECTIVE EVALUATION OF GOAL ACHIEVEMENT

Goals	Outcome criteria	Client responses	Evaluation
Client will self-administer insulin by 12/18.	Client prepares insulin dosage in syringe by 12/17. Client demonstrates self-injection by 12/18.	Client prepared accurate dosage in syringe on 12/17. Client administered morning insulin dosage; self-injection was correctly performed on 12/18.	Outcome criteria and client response agree; goal was met.
Client's lungs will be free of secretions by 11/30.	Lungs will be clear to auscultation by 11/30. Coughing will be nonproductive by 11/29. Respirations will be 16-20 per minute by 11/30.	Lungs were clear to auscultation on 11/30. Client coughed frequently but nonproductively on 11/29. Respirations were 18 per minute on 11/29.	Outcome criteria and client response agree; goal was met.
Client will be able to perform self-care measures without discomfort in 3 days.	Client will be able to bathe while reporting pain at 3 on a scale of 10 within 3 days.	Client reports severe right sided abdominal pain at 5 on a scale of 10 while attempting bathing on day 3.	Outcome criteria and client response disagree; goal was not met.

comes keenly aware of nuances or subtle changes in a client's condition, similar to an almost automatic evaluative response. The nurse can see quickly the combination of subtle changes a client experiences and makes the clinical decisions necessary to deliver the right interventions at the right time.

The new nurse must first understand the systematic nursing process and recognize the value of evaluation. Accurate clinical decisions are based on knowing what to look for and evaluating what actually occurs. Over time the nurse acquires more experience and knowledge, so that rapid decisions can benefit a client. Effective evaluation means advancing the client's care and noting outcomes.

GOALS AS THE BASIS FOR EVALUATION

The purpose of nursing care is to assist the client in resolving actual health problems, preventing the occurrence of potential problems, and maintaining a healthy state. Evaluation of goals determines whether these purposes are accomplished. When a plan of care is established, the nurse identifies the goals, specific client behaviors or responses, that will reveal resolution of a nursing diagnosis or maintenance of a healthy state. Over time the nurse matches the client's actual behavior or response (e.g., self-administers insulin or relief of pain) to the behavior or response specified in the goal. Each nursing diagnosis in the plan of care has a goal, and every goal has a time frame for evaluation.

To objectively evaluate the degree of success in achieving a goal, the nurse should use the following steps:

1. Examine the goal statement to identify the exact desired client behavior or response.
2. Assess the client for the presence of that behavior or response.
3. Compare the established outcome criteria with the behavior or response.
4. Judge the degree of agreement between outcome criteria and the behavior or response.

There are different degrees of goal attainment. If the client's response matches or exceeds the outcome criteria, the goal is met. If the client's behavior begins to show changes but does not yet meet specified criteria, the goal is partially met. If there is no progress, the goal is not met (Table 11-1). A clearly defined goal with specific outcomes is easily measured.

Expected Outcomes

The initial assessment of a client provides baseline data to later determine if a client's condition changes. For example, during assessment, a postoperative surgical client may report acute abdominal pain, rate the pain an 8 on a scale from 1 to 10 (see Chapter 28), grimace or hold the abdomen during attempts to move in bed, and refuse to try to sit in a chair. This baseline of data establishes the nursing diagnosis of *activity intolerance related to pain at the surgical site* and establishes the goal, "client will be able to perform self-care measures without discomfort in 4 days." To evaluate whether nursing interventions begin to relieve the client's pain effectively, the nurse measures success at meeting the expected outcomes established during planning.

Expected outcomes are statements of progressive, step-by-step responses or behaviors that measure movement toward goal achievement. A client must meet outcomes in order to remove or modify the etiology of a nursing diagnosis. For example, for the diagnosis *activity intolerance related to pain at surgical site,* the client must be able to continue to be mobile and gradually be able to return to self-care activities while the surgical wound heals. To determine if the client achieves self-care, the nurse establishes outcomes measuring the client's improved mobility. Expected outcomes have short time frames (depending on the health care setting) and include as few as one or two intervention sessions (Hickey, 1991). To provide objective measurements, the outcomes are stated behaviorally and have time frames for evaluation. For example, "client will turn independently by 2nd post op day," and "client will verbalize pain at a 3 on a scale of 1 to 10 by 3rd post op day." After nursing interventions are performed, the nurse evaluates the client by measuring the subjective report of pain and observing body movement. The new data are compared with outcome criteria to determine if predicted changes occurred.

Evaluation of each expected outcome and its place in the sequence of a client's care is essential. Failure to do so results in an inability to determine the place in which the sequence faltered. If the client achieves an expected outcome, the nurse continues with the care plan. If evaluation shows the expected outcome was not met or only partially met, the nurse begins reassessment and revision of the plan of care.

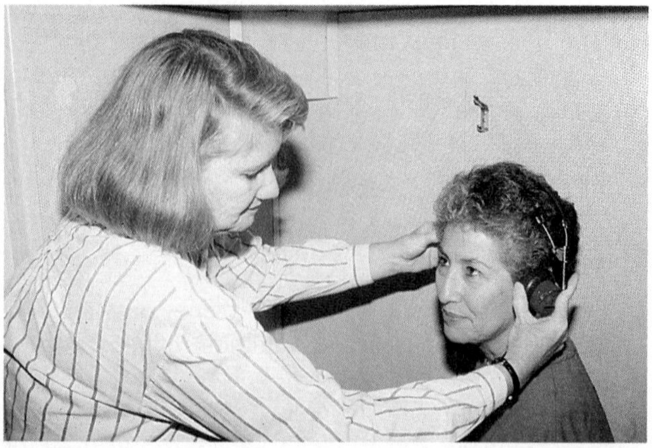

FIGURE 11-1 Nurse evaluates client's hearing acuity. (Courtesy Philip James Acker, Motorola, Inc.)

Evaluative Measures and Sources

Evaluative measures are the assessment skills and techniques used to collect data for evaluation. For example, questioning a client about pain, measuring hearing acuity (Figure 11-1), observing a client's skill performance, and inspecting the skin are all evaluative measures. The new data collected from evaluative measures are compared with expected outcomes to determine if change has occurred and whether the client is moving toward goal achievement (Table 11-2).

The client is a primary source of data; however the nurse also uses the family and other care givers for information. The nurse is better at evaluation after having cared for a client over time. Accuracy of an evaluation improves when the nurse is familiar with the client's behavior and physiological status. Similarly the nurse can respond to problems more quickly and revise the plan of care without undue delay.

Health Team Communication

All members of the health care team must know whether a client is progressing. Accurate and timely documentation and reporting are critical (Figure 11-2).

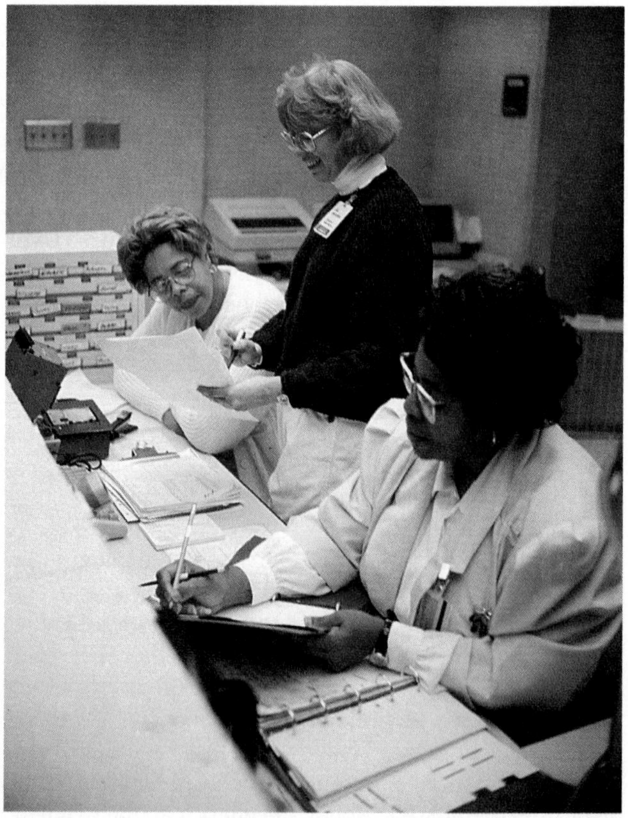

FIGURE 11-2 Staff nurse communicates change in client progress.

Written nursing progress notes are traditionally used to convey evaluative information. Notes organized by the PIE or APIE format lend themselves particularly to evaluation (Chapter 12). The nurse documents progress in meeting expected outcomes set forth in the plan of care. If notes are clear, the nurse's colleagues can determine their role in continuing the plan.

Innovative documentation forms lend themselves to documenting a client's progress. Critical pathways are multidisciplinary treatment plans that predict the interventions and outcomes to be met for select clients over a projected length of stay. Many institutions have made the pathways documentation tools. Each day of the pathway includes the interventions to be performed and outcomes to be achieved. The nurse uses charting by exception (Chapter 12), noting only those interventions or outcomes that are not achieved as predicted. A brief summary note explains why there are variances from the pathway. This approach emphasizes evaluation of the client's progress and keeps all members of the health care team informed and focused.

Information shared between nurses during the change-of-shift report should include the client's progress toward meeting outcomes and goals. The report is a time when nurses can inform colleagues about what interventions are effective or ineffective, how the client responds, and whether goals are achieved. This approach can eventually conserve time for the client and nurse, preventing duplication of interventions that are unnecessary. A report should summarize data about clients so that all team members can contribute to their ongoing progress.

CARE PLAN REVISION

After the nurse evaluates goals, adjustments are made to the care plan. If a goal was successfully met, that portion of the care plan is discontinued. Unmet and partially met goals require the nurse to reactivate the nursing process sequence. After reassessment, modification or addition of nursing diagnoses, goals, expected outcomes, and interventions is made as needed. With revisions to the care plan, priorities are also reestablished. At this point, evaluation begins again to review client progress.

Discontinuing a Care Plan

Once expected outcomes and goals have been met, the nurse confirms this evaluation with the client or family. If both agree that the expected outcomes have been

table 11-2

EVALUATION MEASURES TO DETERMINE THE SUCCESS OF GOALS AND EXPECTED OUTCOMES

Goals	Evaluative measures	Expected outcomes
Client's pressure ulcer will heal within 7 days.	Inspect color, condition, and location of pressure ulcer. Measure diameter of ulcer daily. Note odor and color of drainage from ulcer.	Erythema will be reduced in 2 days. Diameter of ulcer will decrease from 2 cm in 5 days. Ulcer will have no drainage in 2 days. Skin overlying ulcer will be closed in 7 days.
Client will tolerate ambulation to end of hall by 11/20.	Palpate client's radial pulse before exercise. Palpate client's radial pulse 10 minutes after exercise. Observe client for dyspnea or breathlessness during exercise. Assess respiratory rate during exercise.	Pulse will remain below 110 beats per minute during exercise. Pulse rate will return to resting baseline within 10 minutes after exercise. Respiratory rate will remain within 2 breaths of client's baseline rate. Client will deny feeling of breathlessness by 11/20.
Client will self-administer prescribed insulin dosage correctly by 12/18.	Observe client preparing insulin dosage. Have client explain how to prevent infection while preparing a syringe. Observe client administering self-injection.	Client will correctly prepare prescribed dosage of insulin on 12/17. Client will describe 3 ways to prevent infection while preparing syringe and administering injection. Client will perform return demonstration of self-injection correctly on 12/18.

met, the nurse discontinues that portion of the care plan. For example, consider the nursing diagnosis of a client newly diagnosed with diabetes: *high risk for non-compliance with medical regimen related to knowledge deficit.* To achieve the goal of the client accurately administering insulin, the nurse establishes outcomes such as, "client will describe the purpose of insulin and the side effects of hypoglycemia, and client will prepare an insulin dosage correctly by day 3." The nurse discusses the information with the client and determines whether the client understands by asking the client to explain insulin therapy. If the client demonstrates an understanding, it is unnecessary to teach additional information about insulin side effects or the purpose of insulin.

The client's progress will be communicated to other members of the health care team. Staff who assume care for the client will know to focus attention on having the client learn to prepare an insulin dosage. This ensures that other nurses will not unnecessarily continue educating the client about insulin. Continuity of care assumes that care provided is relevant to client needs.

Modifying a Care Plan

When goals are not met, evaluation involves identifying variables or factors that block goal achievement. Usually a change in the client's condition, needs, or abilities makes alteration of the care plan necessary. For example, when teaching self-administration of insulin, the nurse finds that the client has a visual impairment that prevents reading insulin dosages on the syringe. As a result, original outcomes cannot be met. The nurse uses new interventions and revises outcomes to meet the goal of care.

Lack of goal achievement may also result from an error in nursing judgment or a misstep at some point in the nursing process. Clients frequently present very complex situations and problems. The nurse should always remember the possibility of overlooking or misjudging something. When there is failure to achieve a goal, no matter what the reason, the entire nursing process sequence is repeated to discover changes that need to be made to promote, maintain, or restore the client's health.

Reassessment. A complete reassessment of all client factors relating to the nursing diagnosis and etiology is the first step in reactivating the nursing process. Reassessment requires critical thinking when the nurse compares new data about the client's condition with previously assessed information. The nurse may apply intuition and knowledge from previous experience to direct the reassessment process. As in the original assessment, data are collected from all available sources. Depending on the nurse's findings, it may be necessary to assess variables that were not covered previously.

Reassessment ensures that the data base is accurate and current. It may also reveal the missing link; that is, a critical piece of new information may have been previously overlooked and thus interfere with goal achievement. All new data are sorted, validated, and clustered to analyze and interpret differences from the original data base. The nurse documents reassessment to alert other nurses to the client's status.

Nursing Diagnoses. After reassessment, the nurse reviews the appropriateness of all nursing diagnoses. Is the diagnostic statement correct? Are the same etiological factors still present? Are there new nursing diagnoses? The problem list should then be revised to reflect the client's status. If a previous diagnosis no longer accurately reflects the problem, it should be discontinued and a new or modified statement entered. For example, if the nurse finds that the client with diabetes has a serious visual impairment, it may be unlikely that the client will be able to self-administer insulin. High risk for noncompliance remains appropriate, but resolution of it through client education will not guarantee the client receives regular insulin therapy. The nurse's assessment reveals a family member is an available resource. The nurse decides to establish a new diagnosis, *altered health maintenance related to visual impairment,* and develops a plan designed to include the family member during education sessions. The family member's involvement will increase the likelihood of the client receiving regular insulin dosages.

A nurse's care is based on accurate nursing diagnoses. As the client's condition changes, the diagnoses change also.

Goals and Expected Outcomes. Every goal and expected outcome should be evaluated for needed changes. Even the goals for unchanged nursing diagnoses should be examined for appropriateness. Determining that each goal and expected outcome is realistic for the nursing diagnosis, etiology, and time frame is particularly important. Unrealistic outcome criteria and time frames make goal achievement difficult.

Goals and expected outcomes for new or revised nursing diagnoses should be written. When the goal is still appropriate but has not yet been met, the evaluation date may need to be changed to allow for more time. All goals and expected outcomes should be client centered, with realistic expectations for client achievement.

Implementation. The evaluation of interventions must examine two factors: the appropriateness of the interventions selected and the correct application of the implementation process. The appropriateness of care may be based on the **standard of care** for a client's health problem. A standard of care is the minimum required level of care accepted to ensure quality of care to a client. If the client has a nursing diagnosis such as *in-*

effective airway clearance, the standard of care established by a nursing department may include pain control measures with coughing or deep breathing exercises to help a client clear the airway and breathe more comfortably. The nurse reviews the standard of care to determine if the right interventions were chosen or if additional ones are needed.

It may only be necessary to increase or decrease the frequency of interventions. The nurse uses judgment based on past experience, as well as the client's actual response to therapy. For example, if a client continues to have congested lung sounds, the frequency of coughing exercises is increased.

During evaluation, the nurse may determine that some planned interventions are designed for an inappropriate level of nursing care. If the level of care needs to be changed, a different action verb, such as *assist* in place of *provide,* or *demonstrate* instead of *explain,* may be substituted. Sometimes the level of care is appropriate, but the interventions are unsuitable because of a change in the expected outcome. In this case, the interventions should be discontinued and new ones planned.

During implementation, the nurse evaluates the client's response during and immediately after intervention. This is the beginning of the evaluation process. Evaluation is integrated with ongoing nursing care activity. While administering a bath, giving a medication, repositioning a client, or changing a dressing, the nurse is always evaluating. If the response is favorable, implementation continues. Reassessment of implementation occurs when the intervention is evaluated as unsuccessful. The nurse then examines other components of implementation, such as client and environment preparation, anticipated complications, or use of the nurse's personal or technical skills during care delivery (Hickey, 1991).

Changes in implementation should be guided by the nature of the client's response. Consulting with other nurses may yield suggestions for improving the approach to care delivery. Senior nurses are excellent resources because of their experience. Simply changing the care plan is not enough. The nurse must implement the new plan and reevaluate the client's response to the nursing actions. Evaluation of care is a continuous process.

Occasionally an error during care planning and delivery is discovered during evaluation. This should be anticipated. The nursing process is designed to be a systematic, problem-solving approach to individualized client care, but there is a wide variety of variables for each client with health problems. Clients with the same health care problem are not treated the same. As a result, sometimes the nurse makes errors in judgment. Systematic evaluation helps a nurse to catch errors in judgment. The nurse consistently incorporates evaluation into practice to reduce error and ensure that the most appropriate interventions are used.

QUALITY IMPROVEMENT

The evaluation of health care is a process used to improve the quality of care and service to clients. The process seems natural to those professionals who have been involved in the clinical care of clients. However, the process has assumed more importance as health care institutions are challenged to lower their costs for delivering care while ensuring optimal quality.

In the competitive health care environment, the institutions that can successfully demonstrate excellent client outcomes at lower, affordable costs will survive. It has become important for nurses and other health care professionals to understand the nature of their work and how it influences the costs of delivering care and the ability to ensure quality. A health care organization faced with economic pressures must identify the factors that differentiate it from other organizations, with outcomes such as fewer client complications, lower death rate, or more rapid return of clients to their functional status.

Continuous quality improvement (CQI) is a term introduced into health care as a result of the work by Edward Deming, who conducted studies of Japanese management practices following World War II. CQI is defined as meeting or exceeding customer's needs, with the "customer" being the client, family, physician, and anyone else associated with health care delivery (Fanucci et al., 1993). The JCAHO (1994) sets guidelines for health care organizations to assess and improve organizational performance, based on three dimensions:

Performance is *what* is done and *how* well it is done to provide health care.

The level of performance in health care is the degree to which *what* is done is efficacious and appropriate for individual clients.

The degree to which *how* it is done makes it available in a timely manner to clients who need it, is effective, is coordinated with other care and care providers, is safe, is efficient, and is caring and respectful of the client.

How well an institution performs will affect client health outcomes and costs to reach those outcomes. Through the CQI process there is ongoing monitoring of performance and identification of opportunities to improve health care delivery.

Unit-Based QI Programs

The staff nurse plays an important role in quality improvement, simply because the nurse is involved in a majority of client care activities. A unit-based QI program places the responsibility and authority for monitoring and evaluating quality of nursing practice on professional staff nurses. In a unit-based program, each unit has a QI committee whose members identify clinical priorities for their unit, monitor quality indicators, evaluate monitoring results, and recommend changes in nursing practice. The committees are participative, involving all staff in the decision for improving practice, thus increasing autonomy of nursing practice. Quality is a daily expectation of all staff nurses.

With a QI approach, prevention becomes the focus. For example, the nurses on a cardiology unit become concerned over a recent client complaint about not receiving enough information about discharge medications. Using a QI approach, the staff identify the process used to deliver client education on their unit. They discover that a number of elements are involved in successful client education: accurate assessment of educational needs and clients' readiness to learn, availability of teaching resources, appropriate use of resources, teaching skills of staff, documentation of education, and evaluation of client learning. The staff may choose to address one or all factors influencing education in hopes of improving the outcome that clients will be able to explain the purpose of discharge medications and the correct regimen for self-administration.

Monitoring and evaluation activities objectively and systematically define opportunities for continuous improvement in client care. Perhaps the staff learn that they are not proficient in applying adult learning principles or that the documentation forms are not designed for accurate summary of client learning. The QI process is ongoing. Once staff institute change, such as a class on client education or a new documentation form, they will monitor the effects of change and determine if additional changes are necessary.

Components of a QI Program

A well-organized QI program has in place a systematic process for measuring, assessing, and improving organizational performance. Institutions may vary in their approach to how QI programs are structured or organized. However, it is becoming more important for QI programs to have a multidisciplinary focus. There are few instances, except in the case of independent nursing practice, in which disciplines do not interact in the care of clients. Even when nurses use independent interventions, a nurse specialist or educator may be called in to provide expertise. The CQI approach involves all caregivers so that all variables are understood when quality improvements are made.

The JCAHO (1991) offered a 10-step approach for structuring the QI process within an organization (see box above). Although organizations are no longer required to use this specific approach (there are other alternatives), it is very practical. The 10 steps ensure a systematic approach for identifying opportunites to improve quality of health care services and to take action to resolve problems.

JCAHO'S TEN STEPS FOR QI

Establish responsibility and accountability for a QI program.
Define the scope of service for a clinical area.
Define the key aspects of service for the clinical area.
Develop quality indicators to monitor the outcomes and appropriateness of care delivered.
Establish thresholds for evaluation of indicators.
Collect and analyze data from monitoring activities.
Evaluate results of monitoring activities to determine the need for change in practice.
Resolve problems through development of action plans.
Reevaluate to determine if the action plan was successful.
Communicate results of QI to members of the organization.

Responsibility for Program. The chief nurse executive is responsible and accountable for ensuring that nursing service participates in and has a QI program in place. In many institutions this may mean that nursing participates in the overall hospital program. However, nursing must be able to demonstrate ongoing improvement activities within the defined scope of nursing care. A nurse manager such as a head nurse will be responsible for supporting any unit-based program. Individual staff nurses on unit-based committees are responsible for monitoring quality, making decisions about practice, and ensuring quality care.

Scope of Service. Each nursing unit or practice area provides a well-defined set of services to select groups of clients. An analysis of a unit's scope of service reveals the types of clients who receive nursing care. An example might be an orthopedic unit that cares for young, middle-age, and older adults undergoing major joint replacements, back surgery, and repair of traumatic injuries. Understanding the scope of service allows nurses to focus on quality issues related to typical client groups. This begins the prioritization needed in effective CQI.

Key Aspects of Service. The unit-based committee reviews activities or services considered most important in providing quality service to clients. Examples of key aspects of service on the orthopedic unit might include client education, rehabilitation, postoperative monitoring, and pain management. To identify the greatest opportunity for measuring quality, nurses categorize the key aspects of service by **high-volume, high-risk,** and **problem** areas. This creates a second level of prioritizing so that staff may focus on the most important care activities.

Developing Quality Indicators. Schroeder (1991) defines an indicator as that which is measured to demonstrate and improve quality. Staff nurses and their health care colleagues collaborate to select indicators that quantitatively measure an important aspect of care that determines whether quality of service conforms to requirements. There are three types of indicators: structure, process and outcome.

Structure indicators evaluate the structure or systems for delivering care. They include evaluation of the physical setting and equipment, administrative procedure, and the nursing system in use. The rationale is that a good environment promotes quality care. Examples of structure indicators include an emergency cart containing all necessary resuscitative equipment or a staff nurse who attends a critical care course.

Process indicators evaluate the manner in which care is delivered (Williams, 1991). For example, the nurse completes an admission assessment accurately or staff followed the correct procedure for intravenous dressing changes. **Outcome indicators** evaluate the result of nursing interventions and the effectiveness of care in terms of client recovery and survival. They represent measurable changes in a client's status related to receiving nursing care (Marek, 1989). For example, the client's skin remains intact following bed rest or the client is able to demonstrate an insulin injection.

Indicators can be written in a variety of ways. An example of an indicator written as a standard is "all clients will have an admission assessment within 8 hours of admission." Another approach is to write indicators as occurrence screens (e.g. "clients who develop a pressure ulcer while hospitalized"). Finally, indicators are often written as ratios (e.g. "number of clients who have a significant injury over the total number of clients who fall") (Schroeder, 1991).

Most organizations stress the use of outcome indicators for quality monitoring because they focus on the client. However, it may be necessary to combine outcome and process measures to understand the results of monitoring. For example, if staff nurses were only to monitor whether clients can explain the dosage of medications, they would have no data to explain why clients failed to explain dosages. A monitor of the indicator "clients will explain dosages at discharge" might also include a review of documented teaching sessions or distribution of teaching booklets.

Quality is best evaluated when nurses test the standards of care established by their organization. Quality improvement helps to answer whether standards of care help achieve desired client outcomes.

Establishing Thresholds or Benchmarks for Evaluation. After selecting a quality indicator, nurses and colleagues must determine methods for quantitative measurement. Ratios, percentage of times the indicator is observed or frequency of occurrence, are common measures. After the measurement is determined, nurses then establish a threshold, or minimum acceptable level of performance that they choose to reach. The threshold is a standard for determining whether a problem with quality exists. A measurement that falls below a threshold indicates a problem. For example, nurses may set the threshold of 90% of clients explaining self-care instructions. If the threshold is not met, nurses will review factors interfering with successful client education. If indicators are critical to safe client care (e.g., blood administration), a threshold might be set of 100%. Thus in any case when an indicator is not met it would be investigated. When QI is an ongoing process, nurses will continuously work to improve outcomes or performances by raising thresholds.

There are measures available to allow hospitals to compare themselves with other institutions in determining quality. Benchmarks are measures used to establish evaluative standards for excellence. An example might be the national mortality rate for clients who undergo coronary bypass surgery. Another example is the comparisons institutions make for client satisfaction, as measured by standardized surveys. As institutions become better able to define quality outcome measures, more benchmarks will be established.

Data Collection and Analysis. On unit-based committees, nurses monitor criteria for each quality indicator for a predetermined number of clients or cases. It is important to measure a representative sample of clients. Generally a minimum of 25 to 30 is necessary; however this number can vary depending on the indicator being reviewed. The data that are collected must yield an accurate analysis of the appropriateness of care. To make QI easy and less time consuming, staff develop simple checklists for data gathering. Examples of data to gather for the indicator "incidence of skin breakdown in clients with total hip replacement" include number of clients with breakdown, number of clients without breakdown, site of breakdown, client age, mobility status, and degree of breakdown. Collection of relevant data allows accurate analysis of potential problems with quality and their possible causes.

Evaluation of Care. Using monitoring data, nurses evaluate their nursing care. If results exceed or meet the threshold, no problem has been identified. When thresholds for satisfactory performance have not been met, nurses must attempt to determine the cause of problems. For example, staff may set a threshold of 100% of clients having intact skin after total hip procedures. When only 90% of clients meet that goal, nurses must determine the reasons. Collaboration with other care givers is important. Perhaps, in this example, the problem of skin breakdown begins in the operating room because of improper client positioning. Another variable might be the physician's preference of tape used in applying the dressing. Removal of an adherent tape might cause skin blistering. It is critical for all care givers involved in a particular practice problem to meet together to discuss the results of QI findings. Evaluation requires an honest review of practice activities and a pursuit of opportunities to improve.

Resolution of Problems. After evaluating the success in meeting established quality indicators, nurses and their colleagues develop action plans to resolve any problems. It is important to establish actions that will result in success. For example, the action of merely notifying staff about the results of monitoring will unlikely change practice or improve outcomes over time. An action plan should be more direct and have a time frame for implementation.

In the example of the indicator for skin breakdown, staff may decide to use a new support surface on the operating table or try a new type of tape. In addition, formal inservices may be given to improve staff recognition of pressure ulcers.

Evaluation of Improvement. After implementing an action plan to improve quality of care, staff must reevaluate the plan's success. Remonitoring of quality indicators will reveal whether change has occurred. The change may be positive or negative. For example, if the incidence of skin breakdown for clients who have had total hip replacements decreases from previous measures, staff have successfully improved outcomes. Similarly, if the incidence worsens, a new action plan is needed. As is the case with the nursing process, when desired quality outcomes are not met, nurses continue the QI process.

Communication of Results. The results of QI activities must be communicated to nurses and appropriate organizational departments. If findings are not communicated, changes in practice will likely not be followed by all staff. Regular discussion of QI activities in staff meetings, distribution of QI newsletters, and a mechanism for QI committee members to personally report to other nurses are good communication strategies. Often a QI study reveals information that applies to other nursing units or departments. In this case the organization must respond to support any necessary changes. Revision of policies and procedures, purchasing of new products, or modification of standards of care are examples of ways an organization may respond to quality issues.

A CQI program within a health care setting benefits the client, professional staff, and the institution. With a focus on client outcomes, QI activities will lead to a selection of interventions that improve client care. Professional staff learn from their own practice and gain satisfaction from seeing recommended changes improve client outcomes. An institution will benefit from an improved level of care delivery that reduces excessive use of resources and improves client satisfaction with services.

SUMMARY

The evaluation phase of the nursing process determines the effectiveness of the nursing care plan, offering nurses the information needed to ensure optimum client outcomes. A systematic process of evaluation requires the nurse to use critical thinking when comparing expected outcomes with the actual results of care. When client goals are achieved, the client has reached an improved level of health. If goals are unmet, the nurse analyzes the cause and reestablishes a more appropriate care plan.

The continuous quality improvement process serves to evaluate the quality of care within a health care organization. The active participation of care givers ensures that relevant practice issues are examined. QI activities provide opportunities for all health care professionals to elevate the level of care delivered to clients.

CRITICAL THINKING ACTIVITIES

1. Mrs. Wells is a 40-year-old woman who presented with acute low back pain that radiated down the left leg, with numbness in the left lateral calf. On a scale of 1 to 10, the client verbalized pain to be at a severity of 9. The client was unable to walk without limping. Pain is aggravated whenever the client sits. Lying in a supine position minimizes the discomfort. A nursing diagnosis of *decreased physical mobility related to pain* was made with the goal of "client will gain freedom of back movement without pain within 4 weeks." Identify expected outcomes to be incorporated into the plan of care. What evaluative measures would you use to judge the client's success in meeting outcomes?
2. Ms. Chevas works on a neurological nursing unit. As a member of the unit-based QI committee, Ms. Chevas reviews reports on the incidence of client falls. It appears that the number of falls for the unit increased over the last 3 months. What criteria for the indicator "incidence of client falls" might Ms. Chevas wish to measure?
3. Mr. Simpson has a nursing diagnosis, *high risk noncompliance related to knowledge deficit regarding medications.* Part of the nursing care plan is to provide Mr. Simpson with medication cards explaining the drugs newly prescribed for his condition. The nurse, Ms. Gray, enters the client's room and asks Mr. Simpson to describe the side effects of the new medications. Mr. Simpson is unable to do so. What actions must Ms. Gray take?

KEY CONCEPTS

Evaluation determines a client's response to nursing actions and the extent to which goals of care have been met.
During evaluation, the nurse compares the client's response to nursing actions with expected outcomes established during planning.
Evaluation may reveal new health care needs.
Evaluation measures are assessment skills used to collect data for evaluation.
Expected outcomes are stated in behavioral terms with time frames to describe the desired effect of nursing actions.
The nursing care plan is modified based on data obtained during evaluation.
When client goals are evaluated as having been achieved, that portion of the nursing care plan is discontinued.
When client goals are evaluated as having not been met, the entire nursing process sequence is reactivated until goals are met and problem resolution occurs.
Evaluation involves critical thinking because the nurse determines the optimal way to deliver nursing care.
Prevention is the focus for quality improvement activities.
Unit-based quality improvement committees involve staff in the monitoring of relevant practice issues in order to continuously improve the quality of nursing practice.
The three types of quality indicators are structure, process, and outcome.
Outcome indicators focus on the client.
Evaluation enables the nurse to determine the reason the nursing plan was successful or unsuccessful.
Quality improvement programs ensure excellent health care through evaluation of health care services and their impact on the health care consumer.
Quality improvement programs benefit the client and nurse.
A threshold is a standard for determining whether a problem with quality exists.
Quality improvement activities within organizations are focused on evaluating whether quality outcomes can be achieved at affordable costs.

References

Bleich MR: Clinical judgements: essential elements of the nursing process, *J Nurs QA* 4(4):1, 1990.
Benner P: *From novice to expert: excellence and power in clinical nursing practice,* Menlo Park, Calif., Addison-Wesley, 1984.
Fanucci D, Hammill M, et al.: Quantum leap into continuous quality improvement, *Nurs Manage* 24(6):28, 1993.
Hickey PW: *Nursing process handbook,* St. Louis, 1991, Mosby.
Joint Commission on Accreditation of Health Care Organizations: *Accreditation manual for hospitals,* Chicago, Ill., 1991, Joint Commission.
Joint Commission on Accreditation of Health Care Organizations: Proposed Assessment and Improvement of Organizational Performance Standards and Scoring Guidelines, 1994 *accreditation manual for hospitals field review,* Chicago, Ill., 1994, Joint Commission.
Marek KD: Outcome measurement in nursing, *J Nurs Qual Assurance* 4(1):1, 1989.
Schroeder P: Editorial, *J Nurs Care Qual* 6(1): viii, 1991.
Williams AD: Development and application of clinical indicators for nursing, *J Nurs Care Qual* 6(1):1, 1991.

Bibliography

Alfaro R: *Application of nursing process: a step-by-step guide,* Philadelphia, 1986, JB Lippincott.
Carpenito LJ: *Nursing diagnosis: application to clinical practice,* ed 4, Philadelphia, 1993, JB Lippincott.
Chwalek-Goldman R: Nursing process components as a framework for monitoring and evaluation activities, *J Nurs Qual Assur* 4(4):17, 1990.
Davis-Martin S: Outcome and accountability: getting into the consumer dimension, *Nurs Manage* 17(10):25, 1986.
Donabedian A: Evaluating the quality of medical care, *Milbank Q* 44:166, 1966.
Fogelsong D: Standards promote effective production, *Nurs Manage* 18(1):24, 1987.
Gillette B and Jenko M: Major clinical functions: a unifying framework for measuring outcomes, *J Nurs Care Qual* 6(1):20, 1991.
Green E and Katz J: A quality-assurance tool that works overtime, *RN* 30:18, 1989.
Maciorowski LF, Larson E, and Keane A: Quality assurance, evaluate thyself, *J Nurs Adm* 15(6):38, 1985.
Podgorny KL: Developing nursing-focused quality indicators: a professional challenge, *J Nurs Care Qual* 6(1):47, 1991.
Rew L: Intuitia in decision-making, *Image* 20(3):150, 1988.
Schroeder P: Editorial, *J Nurs Qual Assur* 4(4): viii, 1990.
Tucker SM, Cannobio MM, et al.: Patient care standards: nursing process, diagnosis, and outcome, ed 5, St. Louis, 1992, Mosby.
Valentine KL: Comprehensive assessment of caring and its relationship to outcome measures, *J Nurs Qual Assur* 5(2):59, 1991.

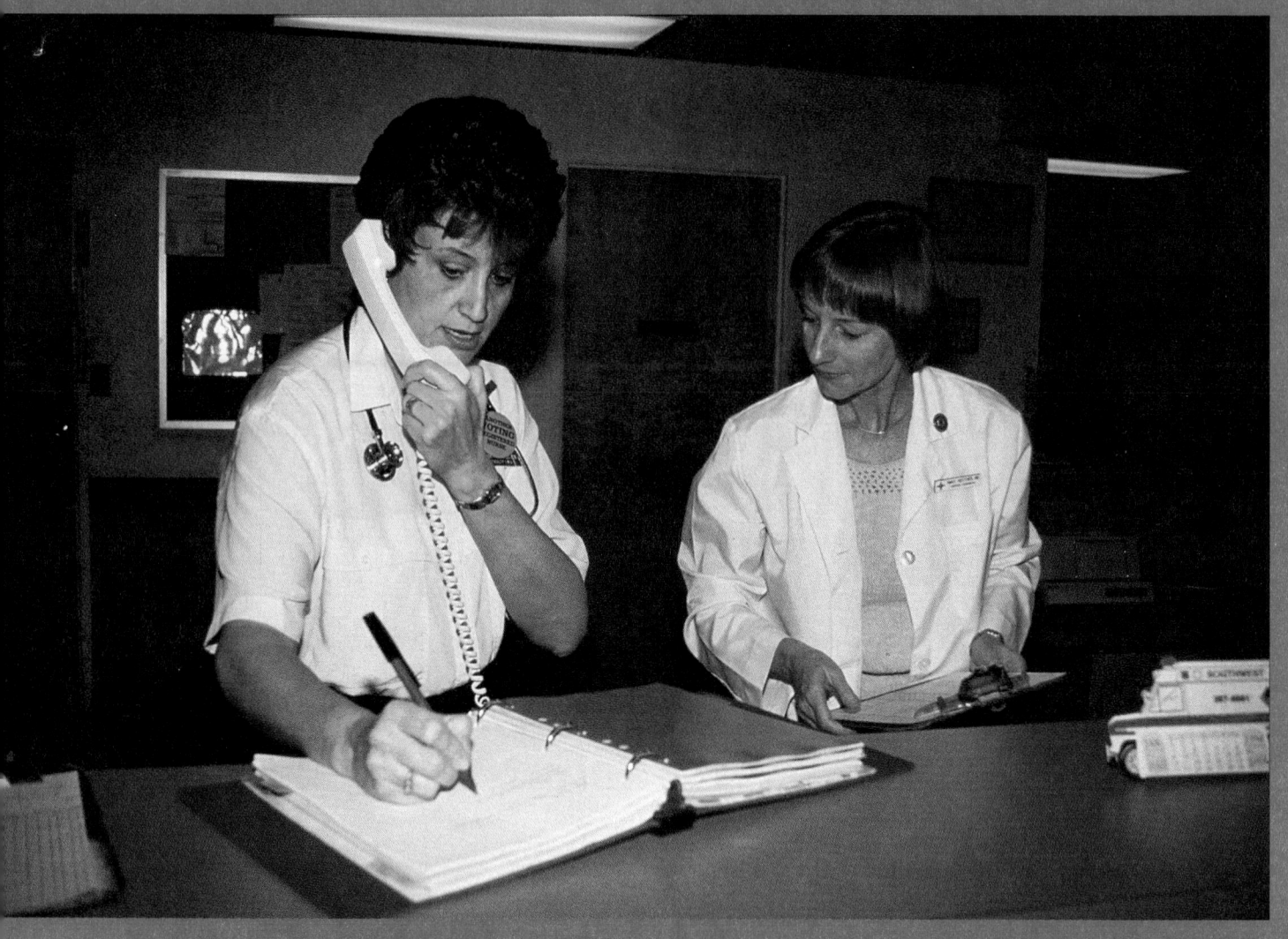

unit three

SKILLS BASIC TO NURSING PRACTICE

12 Recording and Reporting

OBJECTIVES

Mastery of content in this chapter will enable the student to:

- Define the key terms listed.
- Describe six guidelines for effectively communicating through reporting and recording.
- Discuss the relationship between documentation and reimbursement for health care.
- Identify ways to maintain confidentiality of records and reports.
- Describe the purpose of change-of-shift reports.
- Explain documentation relating to telephone use.
- Identify purposes of health care records.
- Discuss legal guidelines for recording.
- Describe different methods used in documentation.
- Discuss advantages and disadvantages of standardized documentation forms.
- Identify elements to include when documenting discharge plans.
- Identify computerized applications for documentation.

KEY TERMS

accreditation
change-of-shift reports
diagnosis-related group (DRG)
discharge summary
documentation
flow sheet
focus charting
incident report
Kardex
objective data
PIE note
problem-oriented medical record (POMR)
progress notes
record
report
SOAP note
standardized care plans
subjective data

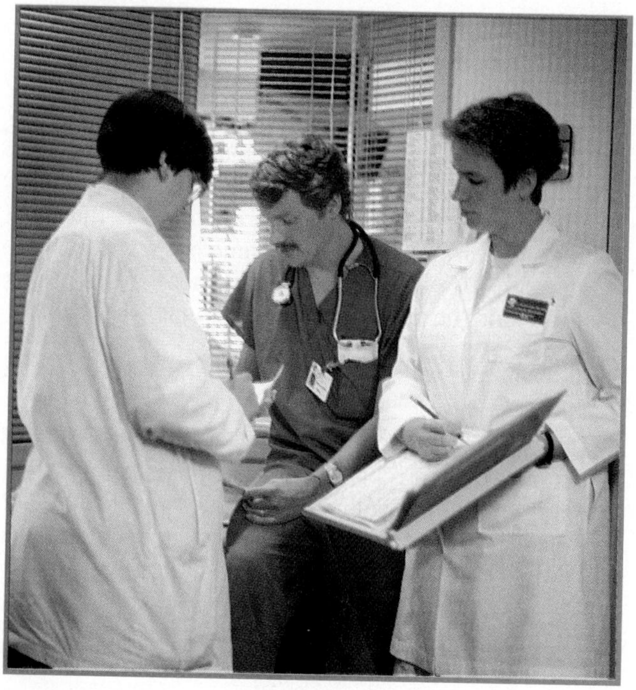

COMMUNICATION WITHIN THE HEALTH CARE TEAM

The more care givers know about a client, the better prepared they are to provide high-quality care. One of the major challenges facing nursing today is providing continuity of care for clients from shift to shift and day to day. A variety of methods are used to communicate information about clients.

Reports are oral or written exchanges of information shared between care givers. When nurses complete a shift, they give a verbal or tape-recorded report to nurses on the next shift.

Information about a client's health care is also communicated through formal or informal discussions among health team members, which may include nurses, physicians, social workers, dietitians, and others. Information about a client is shared to identify problems and desired outcomes and to recommend and plan solutions.

Nurses as members of the health care team must communicate information about clients accurately, completely, and effectively. All health care providers require the same information about clients so they can create and carry out a comprehensive plan of care.

The health care environment creates many challenges for documentation of care delivered to clients. Regulating agencies, which control licensing and reimbursement to hospitals, use information from clients' records to determine the quality of care administered. **Accreditation** agencies such as the Joint Commission on Accreditation of Health Care Organizations (JCAHO) specify guidelines for information to be documented. Under the prospective payment system, hospitals are reimbursed by Medicare for each **diagnosis-related group (DRG).**

The medical record is a legal document. During each hospitalization or clinic visit, or telephone contact, information about the reasons the client sought medical care, nursing care, diagnostic tests, the physician's diagnosis, choice of therapy, and client response is recorded. When the client returns to the hospital or clinic, the nurse or physician has the record available. It becomes a continuing account of the client's health care. Nurses are accountable for including information in the record that is clear and logical, describing accurately all care delivered. A well-documented clinical record is the nurse's best defense against any litigation when malpractice or negligence is alleged (Marrelli, 1992).

GUIDELINES FOR EFFECTIVE DOCUMENTATION AND REPORTING

The nurse is responsible for ensuring that all information needed for nursing care is successfully communicated. Seven important guidelines must be followed for quality recording and reporting.

Factual

Information documented about clients and their care must be factual. A record should contain descriptive, **objective** information about what a nurse sees, hears, feels, and smells (Bergerson, 1988). "Respirations 14 per minute, regular, with clear breath sounds bilaterally" is objective data resulting from direct observation and measurement. Avoid words only meaningful within a specific frame of reference, such as good, adequate, fair, or poor, which are subject to interpretation. **Inferences** are conclusions based on data. For example, an inference might be "Has a poor appetite." The factual data that needs to be documented is "Ate only two bites of dessert and the bread from the supper tray." Suppose in one case the client was nauseated, whereas in another case the client was hungry but did not like the food. If nurses document inferences or conclusions without supportive factual data, misinterpretations about the client's health status may occur.

Subjective data are clients' perceptions about their health problems. Documentation using the client's words within quotation marks, for example, "The client states she is nauseated" or "states she does not like the food choices" is factual and acceptable. In both cases it

EXAMPLES OF CRITERIA FOR REPORTING AND RECORDING

SUBJECTIVE DATA: Description of symptom (pain, nausea, headache, dizziness), including location, severity, onset, precipitating factors, frequency and duration, aggravating and relieving factors.

OBJECTIVE DATA: Description of sign (rash, abnormal or decreased breath sounds), including location, onset, aggravating and relieving factors. Example: Fine red raised rash noted under tape at IV site.

NURSING INTERVENTIONS Description of therapies administered such as planned ambulation, positioning, or dressing change: time administered, observations, and client's response. Example: 4×4 gauze dressing applied to incision; client denied pain during dressing change.

Client behavior (anxiety, confusion, anger), including onset, behaviors exhibited, precipitating factors, nursing action, client's response.

MEDICATION ADMINISTRATION: Time administered, preliminary observations (pulse and BP, or other assessment data), client's response. Example: Client reports pain reduced from 9 to 4 (scale 0-10) after Demerol 50 mg IM.

CLIENT TEACHING: Information presented, method of instruction (e.g., demonstration, discussion, resources used videotape, booklet), evidence that client understands instruction or needs more opportunity for learning.

DISCHARGE PLANNING: Client goals and involvement in care plan. Progress toward goals. Need for referrals or outside resources.

helps to document the actual food intake, as well as the subjective data.

Accuracy

Information must be reliable. Using precise measurements ensures accuracy as a means to determine whether a client's condition has changed. Charting that an "abdominal wound is 5 cm in length, without redness or edema" is more accurate and descriptive than "large abdominal wound is healing well."

Medical abbreviations and symbols help nurses reduce charting time. Most agencies have a list of approved abbreviations. To avoid misunderstandings, write out any abbreviations that may be confusing (e.g., o.d. [once daily] can be interpreted to mean OD [right eye]).

Correct spelling increases the accuracy of documentation. Consult a dictionary if necessary because terms can easily be misinterpreted (e.g., accept or except, and dysphagia or dysphasia).

An accurate entry reflects observations and care provided for assigned clients. Include observations reported to another care giver and interventions performed by someone else; for example, clearly indicate that "Surgical dressings removed by Dr. James. Pulse of 104 reported to J. Kemp, RN."

End any entry in a client's record with the care giver's signature including first name or first initial, last name, and title. Do not use nicknames. Nursing students include the approved abbreviation for their school and level.

Completeness

When records and reports are incomplete, communication is compromised and nurses are also unable to prove specific care was provided. Concise and thorough information is needed about the client's care. Consider the following example:

Mrs. Blake has recently been diagnosed with diabetes. She must learn to give herself insulin injections before going home. A nurse on the day shift fails to document or report the teaching session about giving insulin injections. During the evening shift, another nurse spends time assessing Mrs. Blake's learning needs because the previous teaching was not communicated. Valuable time is wasted, and Mrs. Blake becomes frustrated with the nurse's failure to know her needs.

Criteria for thorough communication exist for certain health problems or nursing activities (see box at left).

Conciseness

Keep all information concise and brief. Avoid any unnecessary words or irrelevant detail. A comparison of a concise and lengthy note follows:

Concise, factual entry	Lengthy entry using vague terms
L toes warm, color pink; capillary return within 2 sec; dorsalis pedis pulse strong 4+; client denies pain	The client's left toes are warm with color pink. There is no inflammation. There is good capillary return present. Dorsalis pedis pulse in left foot is strong. The client denies discomfort or pain.

Currentness

Ongoing decisions about care must be based on current, accurate information. Activities or findings to communicate at time of occurrence include the following:

1. Vital signs
2. Administration of medications and treatments
3. Preparation for diagnostic tests or surgery
4. Change in client status

table 12-1

COMPARISON OF MILITARY AND CIVILIAN TIMES

Military	Civilian	Military	Civilian
0100	1:00 AM	1420	2:20 PM
0200	2:00 AM	1800	6:00 PM
0415	4:15 AM	2400	midnight
1200	noon	0001	12:01 AM

5. Admission, transfer, discharge, or death of client
6. Treatment for sudden changes in client status
7. Client response to intervention

When describing an aspect of care, a nurse should refer to the client's problem, nursing intervention, and response as soon as possible. Timely information prevents errors in client therapy. Writing scratch notes at the time of an event helps ensure accuracy. Many agencies use military time, a 24-hour system that uses digit numbers to indicate morning, afternoon, and evening times. Table 12-1 gives examples of military and corresponding civilian times.

Organization

It is important to communicate information in a logical format or order. Disorganized notes do not clearly explain what happened first and can lead to confusion about whether proper care was given. The following compares a well-organized note with a disorganized note:

Organized Note

7/17/ 0630 Client reports sharp pain in left lower quadrant of abdomen, worsened by turning onto right side. Positioning on left side offers minimal relief. Abdomen is tender to touch and rigid. Bowel sounds are absent. Dr. Phillips notified; Demerol 75 mg IM given for pain. To x-ray for CT scan of abdomen. T. Reis, RN.

Disorganized Note

7/17 0630 Client experiencing sharp pain in lower quadrant of abdomen. MD notified. Abdomen tender to touch, rigid with bowel sounds absent. Demerol 75 mg IM ordered for pain. Positioning on left side offers minimal relief of pain. CT scan ordered of the abdomen. J. Adams, RN.

Confidentiality

Nurses should not disclose clients' status with other clients or staff not involved in their care. Nurses are legally and ethically obligated to keep information about clients confidential. When health care professionals have reason to use records for data gathering, research, or education, there is no break in confidentiality as long as the records are used with permission and according to established guidelines.

REPORTING

Information about clients is exchanged between health team members, the client, and family members. Reports offer a summary of activities seen, performed, or heard. Common types of reports given by nurses include change-of-shift reports, telephone reports, transfer reports, and incident reports.

Change-of-Shift Report

The **change-of-shift report** occurs 2 or 3 times a day in all types of nursing units. At the end of the shift, nurses report information about assigned clients to nurses working in the next shift. The purpose of the report is to provide better continuity of care. If a dressing is changed a certain way during the day shift, it should be changed the same way on the evening shift unless the client's condition changes or a physician's order changes the procedure. When a nurse finds a certain type of pain relief effective for a client, this information is relayed to the next nurse to continue effective pain control. A complete report establishes the nurse's accountability in providing uninterrupted, consistent care. A client who sees different nurses performing the same procedure in the same way will likely trust care givers more.

Change-of-shift reports are given orally in person, by audiotape recordings, or during rounds at the client's bedside (see box on p. 182). Oral reports given in person with staff members from both shifts participating permit nurses to ask questions and obtain immediate feedback. Audiotaped reports may be done before the end of the shift, which can increase efficiency and minimize social interactions. An opportunity for a last minute update on events that occur after taping and for clarification when there are questions is essential.

During rounds, two or more nurses may visit all clients to review their plan of care. When nurses make rounds, the client meets the staff providing care, activities to be expected during the shift are explained, and the nurse observes and meets the client and family members. Any information that might alarm the client is reported out of his or her hearing. The nurse giving the report ensures the client's privacy by speaking in a low voice to prevent others from overhearing. A disadvantage to rounds is the length of time it takes to complete for all clients.

The change-of-shift report should be given quickly and efficiently. A good report provides a baseline for

TIPS FOR CHANGE-OF-SHIFT REPORT

Provide only essential information about client (name, sex, age, diagnosis).
Identify nursing diagnosis.
Describe assessment relating to condition and response to health problem.
Share information about family members related to client's problems.
Review ongoing discharge plans and level of preparation to go home.
Describe instructions given, level of knowledge, and client's response to teaching.
Evaluate results of interventions.
Identify priorities to which oncoming staff must attend.

TELEPHONE TECHNIQUES

INCOMING CALLS

Cue yourself to smile before picking up the phone.
Identify the nursing division and yourself including title.
Use your natural voice, tone, and volume.
Treat each call as important.
Listen carefully, giving the caller your full attention.
Take notes as information is communicated.
Use courtesy and end the call graciously.
Let the caller hang up first.

OUTGOING CALLS

Have notes ready if necessary to organize your message clearly and concisely.
When the person answers, identify yourself and your title.
State the reason you are calling, using the other person's name.
Ask if there are any questions.
End the call graciously.

comparisons and indicates the kind of care to be anticipated for the next shift. An organized and comprehensive approach helps nurses anticipate client's needs and lessens the chance of overlooking important information. It is especially important to report any recent changes or priority situations concerning the client's condition. The following is an example of a change-of-shift report:

1. Background information: Cy Tolan, a 32-year-old client of Dr. Lang in Room 4, is scheduled for a colon resection today. He has had ulcerative colitis for 2 years. This is his first surgery, and he knows he may have a colostomy.
2. Mr. Tolan had trouble sleeping last night. He had several questions about surgery and expressed anxiety about changes in body function.
3. Nursing diagnosis: *Anxiety related to potential altered body function and inexperience with surgery.*
4. Nursing measures: He received a Dalmane 15 mg at bedtime. He slept well until 4 AM but has been awake off and on since then. I told him that if he has the colostomy, a nurse will help him learn how to care for it.
5. His wife is with him already this morning. She seems supportive and concerned.
6. Priority needs: Mr. Tolan is resting. The consent has been signed, and he is ready for surgery except for the preoperative medications on call.

When giving a report, the nurse discusses the client or family in a professional manner. It may be necessary to describe interactions in behavioral terms. A good report is objective, and the content of the report should be pertinent to the client's health care. Value-laden terms do not establish good working relationships. The nurse avoids using such judgmental labels as "uncooperative," "difficult," or "bad" when describing client behaviors. Any derogatory statements overheard by the client could lead to a lawsuit against the nurse. Staff members may unintentionally form a prejudicial opinion about the client.

Telephone Reports and Orders

It is important to be as courteous as possible when making or receiving telephone calls (see box above). Anyone calling a nursing unit should be treated as a consumer needing a service. Courtesy conveys a sense of caring and professionalism and promotes cooperation of all health team members.

Telephone reports are required when nurses need to inform others of changes in a client's condition or report the results of diagnostic tests. Persons involved with a telephone report or telephone orders should make sure the information given and received is clear, accurate, and concise. Critical facts about the information conveyed over the telephone are repeated back to the sender to verify accuracy.

Telephone orders from physicians are frequently given at night or during an emergency and should be used only when necessary. Information from a telephone report or orders should be documented in the client record. Include the time, who made the call, who was called, and the information given and received (Figure 12-1). An example would be "1020 Dr. Jones notified of potassium of 3.2. Orders for oral potassium supplement received. C. Towns, RN." Telephone orders involving a physician must be verified by repeating them

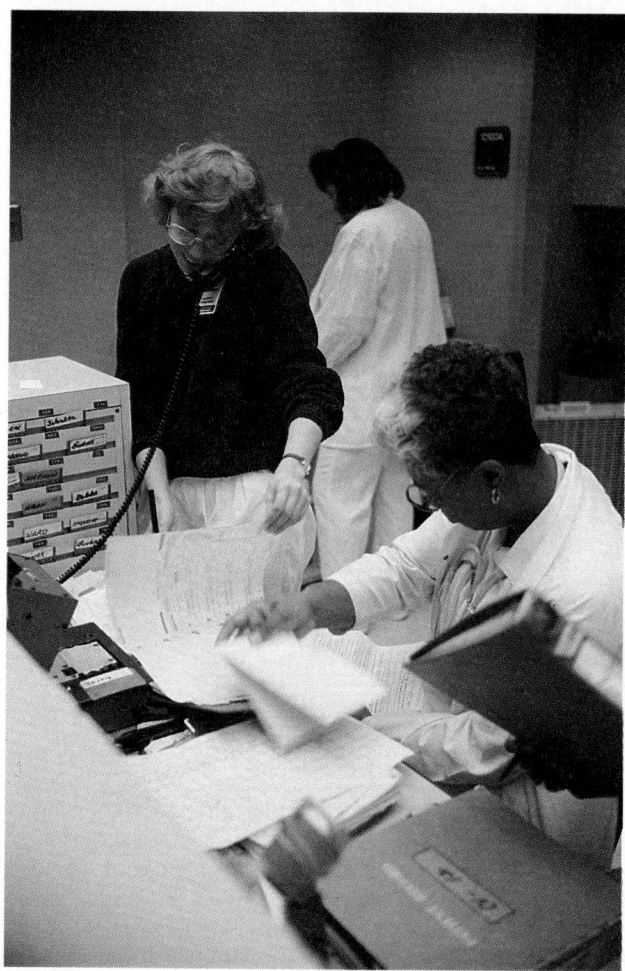

FIGURE 12-1 Telephone reports require the nurse's attention to ensure accurate information is conveyed.

clearly and then writing the order on the physician's order sheet in the client's permanent record and signed. The physician later verifies the telephone order legally by signing it within a set time. Student nurses in some states can have orders verified and co-signed by a registered nurse.

A transfer report involves communicating information about clients from the nurse on the sending unit to the nurse on the receiving unit. For example, the client may be transferred from the recovery room, an intensive care unit, or the emergency room to a standard nursing unit. The receiving nurse must know the most current information about clients and their progress. An accurate transfer report provides continuity of care. Transfer reports may be given by telephone or in person. Nurses document the client's status at the time of transfer, including assessments or interventions to be completed after transfer and any need for special equipment.

In some settings there is need for telephone contact with clients or their families following discharge. For example, the nurse may call to learn if a client has any questions concerning medications or activity restrictions. Whenever such contacts are made, they should be documented according to agency policy.

Incident Reports

An incident is any event not consistent with the routine operation of a health care unit or routine care of a client. Examples include client falls, needlestick injuries, a visitor becoming ill, and medication errors. When something that could have or did cause injury occurs, the nurse files an **incident report.** When the incident involves a client, the nurse documents in the medical record an objective description of what was actually observed. The nurse also records any follow-up care given in the medical record. The fact that an incident report was prepared is not included in the medical record. Incident reports are used for quality assurance and risk management. Incidents should trigger an investigation of the circumstances and changes needed to prevent recurrences. This could include educational programs, revised policies and procedures or improved equipment, or changes in client delivery systems (Iyer, Camp, 1991).

When a client is involved in an incident, the nurse documents the details in the incident report. A number of crucial elements must be described, including the date and time, how the nurse found the client, witness information, assessment of the client's injury, actions taken, and follow-up notations. The following example compares an accurate and inaccurate note.

Accurate Note

4/7/92 2200 Client found on floor alone in room, states he fell while getting out of bed. Alert and oriented x3. Noted external rotation of left leg. Complained of pain in left hip at an intensity of 4, (scale 0-10). Lifted back into bed with assistance from nursing assistant. BP, 142/88; P, 90, R, 22. Side rails up, call light within reach, instructed to remain in bed. Dr. Smith notified, portable x-ray ordered.

Inaccurate Note

4/7/92 Client fell out of bed, complained of pain in left hip. Noted external rotation of left leg. Dr. Smith notified.

DOCUMENTATION

Many types of records are used to convey information about the client's health status and care. (Edelstein 1990) defines **documentation** as anything written or printed that is relied on as a record of proof for authorized persons. Good documentation reflects quality of care and evidence of each health care member's accountability. Although each agency uses a different record format, all records contain the following types of information:

1. Demographic data
2. Informed consent for treatments and procedures
3. Admission nursing history
4. Nursing diagnoses or problems
5. Nursing care plan
6. Record of nursing care interventions and evaluation
7. Medical physical examination and history
8. Medical diagnosis
9. Therapeutic orders
10. Progress notes
11. Reports of diagnostic studies
12. Reports of operative procedures
13. Discharge plan and summary

Purpose of Records

The record is a valuable source of data used by all members of the health care team. Its purposes include communication of the nursing process, legal documentation, education, research, auditing and monitoring, and financial billing.

Communication of the Nursing Process. The record serves as a vehicle by which health team members communicate their contributions to the client's care. The record should explain measures needed for continuity and consistency of care. Information from the record supplements the nurse's observations and assessment. The record provides data that nurses use to identify and support nursing diagnoses and plan proper

table 12-2

LEGAL GUIDELINES FOR RECORDING

Guidelines	Rationale	Correct action
Do not erase, apply correction fluid, or scratch out errors made while recording.	Charting becomes illegible. It may appear as though you were attempting to hide information or deface record.	Draw single line through error, write word *error* above it, and sign your name or initials. Then record note correctly.
Do not write retaliatory or critical comments about client or care by other health care professionals.	Statements can be used as evidence for nonprofessional behavior or poor quality of care.	Enter only objective descriptions of client's behavior. Client comments should be quoted.
Correct all errors promptly.	Errors in recording can lead to errors in treatment.	Avoid rushing to complete charting. Be sure information is accurate.
Record only facts.	Record must be accurate and reliable.	Be certain entry is factual. Do not speculate or guess.
Do not leave blank spaces in nurse's notes.	Another person can add incorrect information in space.	Chart consecutively, line by line. If space is left, draw line horizontally through it and sign your name at end.
Record all entries legibly and in ink.	Illegible entries can be misinterpreted, causing errors and lawsuits. Ink cannot be erased. Records are photocopied and stored on microfilm.	Never erase entries or use correction fluid, and never use pencil.
If order is questioned, record that clarification was sought.	If you perform order known to be incorrect, you are just as liable for prosecution as physician.	Do not record "physician made error." Instead chart that "Dr. Smith was called to clarify order for—"
Chart only for yourself.	You are accountable for information you enter into chart.	Never chart for someone else (exception: if care giver has left unit for day and calls with information).
Avoid using generalized, empty phrases such as "status unchanged" or "had good day."	Specific information about client's condition or case can be accidentally deleted if information is too generalized.	Use complete, concise descriptions of care.
Begin each entry with time, and end with your signature and title.	This ensures that correct sequence of events is recorded. Signature documents who is accountable for care delivered.	Do not wait until end of shift to record important changes that occurred several hours earlier. Be sure to sign each entry.

interventions for care. It also includes the client's responses to interventions, allowing alterations in the plan of care as indicated by these responses. The record provides a total picture of the client's health status. Each observation is part of a larger puzzle, which helps explain and confirm interpretations and facilitate appropriate continuing nursing care.

Legal Documentation. The client's record is a legal document if it is used as evidence in a court of law. Contents of the record document the level of care provided for a client. In many agencies, clients have the right to review their records. However, the record is usually the property of the agency. Each agency has policies for controlling the manner in which records are shared. Table 12-2 lists legal guidelines for recording.

Financial Billing. In response to increasing health care costs, third-party payors, government, commercial, and others have increased their scrutiny and control of hospital resources (Marrelli, 1992). Detailed recording helps in establishing codable diagnoses used to determine a diagnosis-related group (DRG) (see box below). DRGs have become the basis for establishing reimbursement to hospitals. If a hospital treats a client for more than the price attached to the DRG, the hospital absorbs the loss.

Education. An effective way to learn the nature of an illness and the response to it is to read the medical record. Although no two clients have identical records, patterns of information can be identified in clients with similar medical problems. With this information, students learn patterns to look for and become better able to anticipate the type of care a client requires.

Research. Statistical data relating to the frequency of clinical disorders, complications, use of specific medical and nursing therapies, deaths, and recoveries from illness can be gathered from client records. Records are a valuable resource for describing characteristics of the client populations that use a specific health agency. A nurse may use a client's records during a research study to collect information that describes the client's health problem or response to variables studied.

Auditing and Monitoring. A regular review of client records is a basis for evaluating the quality of health care provided in an institution. The JCAHO requires hospitals to establish performance improvement programs. Performance improvement, also called quality improvement, suggests that nurses must continually look for ways to improve client care. Often the medical record helps to reveal ways to improve care. Investigation of new approaches are a never ending quest (Hurley, 1991). Nurses conduct objective ongoing and periodic reviews of client care based on identified standards. The box below lists examples of standards the JCAHO establishes for documentation. Nurses conduct audits regularly throughout the year to determine the degree to which quality improvement is progressing.

DIAGNOSIS-RELATED GROUPS (DRGs)

A DRG is a series of decision trees designed to cluster groups of clients together by diagnosis, surgical procedures, complications, comorbidities, preexisting illness, and age.

The statistical weight of a DRG is multiplied by a hospital's specific rate of reimbursement.

The hospital is reimbursed a fixed amount for every client grouped into the DRG, regardless of length of stay or cost of treatment.

An assigned DRG may change on the basis of documentation.

EXAMPLES OF JCAHO NURSING CARE STANDARDS (JCAHO, 1994)

1. Clients receive nursing care based on a documented assessment of their needs. Clients' needs for nursing care related to admission are assessed by a registered nurse. Needs are reassessed when warranted by clients' conditions.
2. Clients' assessment includes consideration of biophysical, psychosocial, environmental, self-care, educational, and discharge-planning factors. When appropriate, data from the client's significant others are included in the assessment.
3. Clients' nursing care is based on identified nursing diagnoses, client care needs, and care standards and is consistent with the therapies of other disciplines. The client and/or significant others are involved in the care as appropriate.
4. Throughout the client's stay, the client and his/her significant others (as appropriate) receive education specific to the client's health care needs. In preparation for discharge, continuing care needs are assessed and referrals for such care are documented in the medical records.
5. The client's medical records include documentation of the initial assessments and reassessments, the nursing diagnoses and client care needs, the interventions identified to meet the nursing care needs, the nursing care provided, the response to and outcome of care provided, and the abilities of the clients and families to manage continuing care needs after discharge.

Problems identified during monitoring are shared with all members of the nursing staff so that corrections in policy or practice can be made.

METHODS OF DOCUMENTATION

The documentation system selected by a nursing service should reflect the philosophy of the department and the way nursing care is given to clients. Professional care is reflected by professional charting, which proves what the nurse has done and effectively communicates the client's status and progress (Edelstein, 1990). Because the nursing process shapes a nurse's approach, good documentation reflects the steps of the nursing process from assessment to evaluation.

It is challenging to create a record-keeping system that ensures optimal communication and yet simplifies the charting process. The JCAHO (1994) requires documentation of nursing diagnoses or problems within the context of the nursing process, as well as evidence of client and family teaching and discharge planning. If members of more than one discipline regularly care for a client, the JCAHO also expects evidence of a multidisciplinary plan of care. The differences among the many methods used by health care institutions involve the organization of information.

Source Records. The traditional form of the medical record is a **source record,** in which the client's chart is organized so that each discipline (e.g., nursing, medicine, or social work) has a separate section in which to record data. The advantage of a source record is that care givers can easily locate the proper section of the record in which to make entries. All entries are made in chronological order, usually with the most recent nearest the front of the chart section. Components of a source record are summarized in Table 12-3.

A disadvantage of source records is fragmented data. Information is well organized but not according to the client's problems. Details about a particular problem may be distributed throughout the record. For example, in the case of a wound infection, the nurse describes the appearance of the wound in the nurse's notes. The physician notes in a separate section the progress of the wound's healing and the proposed course of therapy. The results of tests measuring growth of bacteria from the wound can be found in the laboratory test section. Thus any data relevant to a single problem may be difficult to locate.

In the source record, the nurse charts a narrative description of nursing care delivered. In a hospital, entries are made in the client's record each shift of duty. If a client is seen in a clinic or at home, the nurse documents the care provided during each visit or telephone contact.

table 12-3

ORGANIZATION OF TRADITIONAL SOURCE RECORD

Sections	Contents
Admission sheet	Specific demographic data about client: legal name, identification number, sex, age, birthdate, marital status, occupation and employer, health insurance, nearest relative to notify in an emergency, religious preference, name of attending physician, date and time of admission
Physician's order sheet	Record of physician's orders for treatment and medications, with date, time, and physician's signature
Nurse's admission assessment	Summary of nursing history and physical examination
Graphic sheet and flow sheet	Record of repeated observations and measurements such as vital signs, daily weights, and intake and output
Medical history and examination	Results of initial examination performed by physician, including findings, family history, confirmed diagnoses, and medical plan of care
Nurses' notes	Narrative record of nursing process: assessment, nursing diagnosis, planning, implementation, and evaluation of care
Medication records	Accurate documentation of all medications administered to client: date, time, dose, route, and nurse's signature
Physician's progress notes	Ongoing record of client's progress and response to medical therapy and review of disease process
Health care discipline's records	Entries made into record by all health-related disciplines: physical therapy, dietary, radiology, social work, and laboratories
Discharge summary	Summary of client's condition, progress, prognosis, rehabilitation, and teaching needs at time of dismissal from hospital or health care agency

SAMPLE NURSES' NOTE

4/6/93

1100 Client states "I'm having a hard time catching my breath." Respirations are labored at 28/min. P 96, BP 112/70. Breath sounds auscultated, crackles over both lower lobes. Chest excursion equal bilaterally. Elevated head of bed to Fowler's position. Obtained arterial blood gases at 1045 per order. Results are pH 7.34, $PaCO_2$ 45, PaO_2 80. Dr. Stein called. Applied O_2 at 2L/min per mask as ordered. Remained at bedside to calm client. P. Haake, RN.

The nurse's description summarizes important observations relating to the client's condition, nursing care, and evaluation of response (see box above).

Problem-oriented Medical Records. The **problem-oriented medical record (POMR)** is a structured method of documentation that emphasizes client problems (Figure 12-2). The method is based on the nursing process and facilitates communication of client needs. Data are organized by problem rather than by source of information. Each member of the health care team contributes to a single list of identified client problems.

In its classic format the POMR is composed of a data base, a numbered problem list, and progress notes referred to as **SOAP** notes (Marelli, 1992). The advantages of the POMR charting method include the following:

1. Gives emphasis to clients' perceptions of their problems.
2. Requires continuous evaluation and revision of care plan.
3. Provides greater continuity of care among health care team members.
4. Enhances effective communication among health care team members.
5. Increases efficiency in gathering data.
6. Provides easy-to-read information in chronological order.
7. Reinforces use of the nursing process.

With the POMR format, the list of problems is filed in an easily accessible location and referred to frequently. New problems are added as identified. After a problem has been resolved, the date of resolution is recorded and a line is drawn through the problem and its number on the problem sheet. The number for a resolved problem is not used again. This system keeps the problem list simple yet meaningful. After a problem list is developed, succeeding record entries (such as in the progress notes) are coded by the problem number.

Progress notes follow a SOAP format, which has evolved into a variety of forms including SOAPE, SOAPIE, and SOAPIER notes. These are acronyms for subjective data (S), objective data (O), assessment (A), and plan (P). Some organizations use intervention (I), evaluation (E), and response (R).

S—This section includes subjective data or information gathered from the client. For example, the client will describe a symptom such as pain or discuss an interest in learning about a medication. Whether the progress note includes subjective data depends on the acuteness of the client's illness or the nature of the problem.

O—Objective data consist of information that can be observed or measured. Physical findings, laboratory re-

Problem #	Date	Problem	Resolved
~~1.~~	~~4-7-XX~~	~~® Breast Mass~~	4-8-XX
2.	4-8-XX	Anxiety related to inexperience with postoperative routines.	
3.	4-9-XX	Pain related to incisional edema and movement of R. arm.	
4.	4-10-XX	Altered body image.	

FIGURE 12-2 POMR problem list.

sults, observations, or results of x-ray examinations are examples of objective data.

A—The individual who writes a SOAP note takes the subjective and objective data and forms conclusions. The assessment is an interpretation of the client's condition or level of progress. It is a statement of the status of the diagnosis or problem. The assessment determines whether the problem has been resolved or if further care is required.

P—Depending on the assessment of the situation, the health care member maintains or revises the previous plan of care. Plans may include specific orders or interventions designed to manage the client's problem, collection of additional data about the problem, individual or family education, and goals and expected outcomes of care.

PIE is an acronym for problem, intervention, and evaluation. The **PIE note** differs from SOAP notes because the narrative does not include assessment data. Instead, daily assessment information appears on special flow sheets, thus preventing duplication of information. PIE notes also differ from SOAP notes in that the format requires nurses to evaluate client outcomes.

P—Problem or nursing diagnosis applicable to client
I—Interventions or actions taken
E—Evaluation of outcomes of nursing interventions and client response to nursing therapies

Another version is the APIE format. The A represents assessment data, inclusive of objective findings made by nurses and subjective information from clients. Whether assessment data are duplicated elsewhere depends on the type of forms used by an agency. Figure 12-3 includes sample nurses' notes in SOAPE and PIE formats.

Charting by Exception. Recently an innovative approach has been created to streamline documentation by reducing repetition. Documenting normal findings and routine care is based on clearly defined standards of practice and predetermined criteria for nursing assessments and interventions (Murphy, Burke, 1990). The assumption with charting by exception is that all standards are met with a normal or expected response unless otherwise documented. With standards such as predefined normal assessment findings integrated into documentation forms, a nurse needs only to document abnormal findings or responses. The nurse writes a longhand note only when the standardized statement on the form is not met. Otherwise only a signature is needed. When nurses see written entries in the chart, they know that something out of the ordinary has been observed. This makes it easy to track changes in a client's condition as they develop.

Focus Charting. Focus charting (Lampe, 1988) structures **progress notes** according to the focus of the note. Examples include a sign or symptom, a condition, a nursing diagnosis, a behavior, a significant event, or an acute change in a client's condition. Each note includes data, actions, and client response (DAR) for the particular client situation. The following is an example of a focus charting entry for the following situation:

Ms. Worthy has developed a fever, 39° C, 2 days following surgery. The nurse has auscultated lung sounds and

S - "I'm worried about what it will be like after surgery."	**P** - Anxiety related to knowledge deficit of surgery manifested by frequent questions and first-time surgery.
O - Client asking frequent questions about surgery. First surgery experience. Wife present, expresses concern.	**I** - Explained normal preoperative preparations for surgery. Demonstrated TCDB exercises. Provided booklet to client on postoperative nursing care.
A - Anxiety related to knowledge deficit of surgery experience.	**E** - Able to demonstrate TCDB correctly. Needs review of postoperative nursing routines.
P - Explain routine preoperative preparation. Demonstrate and explain TCDB exercises. Provide explaination and booklet on postoperative care.	S. Lazarus, RN.
E - Expresses eagerness to learn as much as possible.	
S. Lazarus, RN.	

FIGURE 12-3 Examples of progress notes written in SOAPE and PIE formats.

found crackles in the right lower lobe. The client has difficulty coughing as a result of incisional pain. The nurse repositioned the client, began instruction on TCDB exercises, and ordered an incentive spirometer.

Focus Note

D—Temp 39° C, lungs auscultated with crackles over R lower lobe.

A—Repositioned client and instructed on TCDB. Ordered incentive spirometer for bedside.

R—Client has difficulty coughing as a result of incisional pain.

Computerized Documentation. The American Nurses Association's design criteria for computerized information systems identify the need for systems to support the nursing process (ANA, 1988). Additional criteria identify the need for systems that integrate elements of the client's automated record, permit electronic transport of data to other computer systems, and allow easy data retrieval (McLaughlin et al., 1990).

Information previously recorded on flow sheets, Kardexes, and nursing care plans can now be generated and communicated using computers. Nurse and physician plans of care can be integrated to provide comprehensive client data. Information is saved as part of a total history. Certain information, such as past illnesses or allergies, will appear in a client's record during all subsequent admissions.

Some legal risks are associated with computerized documentation. Passwords used to limit access to authorized users should not be shared with any other care giver. Data saved as a part of the record cannot be deleted. However, any incorrect entries not stored can be corrected (Collins, 1990). If incorrect information is accidentally stored, corrections entered indicate the error, including the date and time of the correction and who made the change.

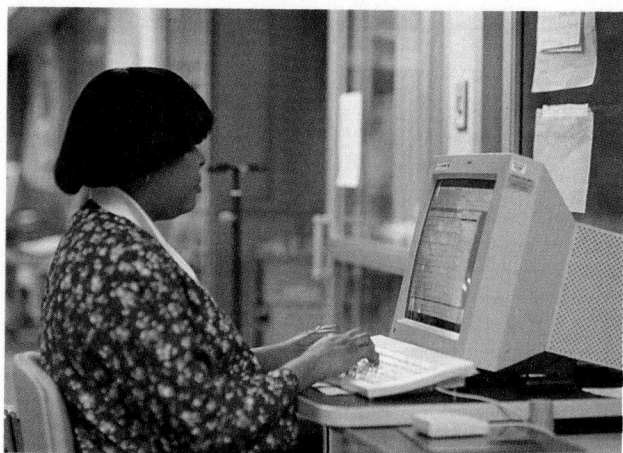

FIGURE 12-4 Computer terminal at nurses' station.

Nurses must be familiar with basic computer skills because most hospitals now have some form of automated system with a large mainframe computer system. A mainframe system consists of one centrally located computer with a large memory capacity to power a variety of programs throughout the hospital. Each nursing division has a computer screen with a keyboard attached to the main computer. Information may be entered or retrieved by using the keyboard or by pressing a light-sensitive pen directly onto the screen. Some hospitals have computers at each bedside (Figure 12-4). Nurses can enter assessment findings or document interventions that are quickly transmitted for storage. Documentation is timely, and fewer errors occur because the nurse does not have to leave the bedside to record information.

Well-designed computer systems reduce recording errors, save time, and make information readily available to nurses. This frees nurses to focus more directly on the delivery of professional nursing care.

Common Record Keeping Forms

Nurses use a variety of forms to make documentation easy, quick, and comprehensive. Duplication within the record should be avoided.

Admission Nursing History Forms. Admission nursing history forms provide baseline data for later comparisons with changes in the client's condition. The form allows the admitting nurse to make a thorough assessment to identify relevant nursing diagnoses. Each institution designs nursing history forms based on its standards of practice and philosophy of nursing care. Figure 12-5 is an example of an admission nursing history form.

Flow Sheets. Flow sheets allow documentation of certain routine observations or specific measurements made repeatedly. It is unnecessary to chart a narrative note each time a drug or bath is given or vital signs are checked. The flow sheets are a quicker and more efficient way to record information. Figure 12-6 is an example of a nursing assessment flow sheet.

The only time the nurse includes information from a flow sheet into a narrative or progress note is when a significant change or client response results in nursing intervention that must be reported. For example, if a client's blood pressure becomes dangerously high, the nurse may record the pressure and the medication administered to lower the pressure in the progress note. Subsequent evaluation of the client's blood pressure and additional interventions required should be included. Flow sheets provide a quick and easy reference for assessing changes in a client status. Critical care units commonly use flow sheets for many types of data.

Text continued on p. 196.

ST. JOHN'S HOSPITAL
Springfield, Illinois

ADMISSION PATIENT PROFILE

HEALTH PATTERNS ASSESSMENT (May be completed by RN or LPN)

Information Obtained From: ☒ Patient ☒ Family ☐ Friend ☐ Old Chart ☐ Transfer Sheet ☐ ER Record

Reason for Admission (as stated by patient): "I'VE HAD THIS SORE ON MY FOOT FOR 2 MOS AND IT WON'T HEAL." ADMITTED FOR RX OF VASCULAR DISEASE.

Previous Surgery(ies)/Hospitalizations: ____________________

Previous Transfusion(s)? ☐ Yes Date __________ ☒ No

Known Food, Drug, Contact Allergies: ☒ None *If yes, list and state reaction:* ____________________

MEDICTIONS: Patient is currently taking (include over-the-counter medications)

Name	Dose	Dosing Time	Day/Time of Last Dose	Brought to Hospital
INSULIN (NPH)	30 u	AC BKST		☐ No ☐ Yes Disposition:
INSULIN (REG)	8 u	AC BKST		☐ No ☐ Yes Disposition:
METAMUCIL	1 Tbsp	daily		☐ No ☐ Yes Disposition:
				☐ No ☐ Yes Disposition:
				☐ No ☐ Yes Disposition:
				☐ No ☐ Yes Disposition:
				☐ No ☐ Yes Disposition:
				☐ No ☐ Yes Disposition:
				☐ No ☐ Yes Disposition:
				☐ No ☐ Yes Disposition:
				☐ No ☐ Yes Disposition:
				☐ No ☐ Yes Disposition:

SYSTEMS ASSESSMENT (May be completed by RN or LPN)

NEURO/SENSORY	ADDITIONAL COMMENTS	Nursing Diagnosis must be completed by RN
☐ CVA ☐ Side affected: ☐ Rt ☐ Lt ☐ Head Injury ______ ☐ Headache ______ ☐ Hx of Seizures ______ ☐ Stiff Neck ☒ Alert ☒ Oriented ☐ Confused ☐ Comatose ☐ Cooperative ☐ Withdrawn ☐ Anxious ☐ Hearing Difficulty ☐ P.E.R.L. ☐ Unsteady Gait ☒ Vision Difficulty Cataracts: ☐ Rt ☐ Lt Blind: ☐ Rt ☐ Lt Glaucoma: ☐ Rt ☐ Lt ☐ Syncope ______ ☐ Speech impairment (describe) Pain/Discomfort: ☐ Yes ☐ No Describe ______ How is pain controlled: ______ ☒ All above areas addressed	c/o blurred vision. Wears glasses to read	☐ Sensory/Perceptual Alterations ☐ Impaired Communication ☐ Altered Thought Processes ☐ Potential for injury ☐ Pain ☐ Pain, chronic

#4678 (R 01/93)
(1 of 4)

ADMISSION PATIENT PROFILE

FIGURE 12-5 Nursing history form. (Courtesy St. John's Hospital, Springfield, Ill.)

PERFUSION

	ADDITIONAL COMMENTS	Nursing Diagnosis must be completed by RN
☐ Congenital Heart defects (describe) ______ ☐ CHF ☐ Anemia ☐ Heart Attack ______ ☐ Hypertension ☒ Peripheral Vascular Disease ☐ Pacemaker Check pt. I.D. Card for Model # ______ Manufacturer ______ ☐ Angina (describe): ______ ☐ Automatic Implantable Cardioverter Defibrillator (AICD) Apical Pulse: ☒ Reg. ☐ Irreg. KEY: P = Pulse Present by Palpation; D = Pulse Audible with Doppler; A = Absent Pulses: Radial ___ Rt. ___ Lt.; Posterior Tibial ___ Rt. ___ Lt.; Pedal D Rt. D Lt. ☒ All above areas addressed	Both feet cool to touch, capillary refill > 4 sec. c/o numbness & tingling both legs below knees	☐ Decreased Cardiac Output ☐ Fluid Volume Deficit ☐ Fluid Volume Excess ☒ Altered Tissue Perfusion ☐ Pain

OXYGENATION

	ADDITIONAL COMMENTS	Nursing Diagnosis must be completed by RN
Respiration History: ☐ Asthma ☐ COPD ☐ Pneumonia ☐ TB ☐ Other ______ Smoking History: Do you smoke? ☐ Yes ☒ No Packs/day: ___ # of years ___ Have you ever smoked? ☐ Yes ☐ No Packs/day: ___ # of years ___ When did you quit? ______ Oxygen Therapy/Resp. Therapy used at home? ☐ Yes ☐ No Describe: ______ Breathing: ☒ Deep and regular ☐ Shallow ☐ Irregular ☐ SOB (describe) ______ Breath Sounds: ☒ Clear bilaterally ☐ Abnormal (describe) ______ Describe Cough: ______ Describe Sputum: ______ ☒ All above areas addressed:		☐ Impaired Gas Exchange ☐ Ineffective Airway Clearance ☐ Ineffective Breathing Pattern ☐ Activity intolerance

SKIN CONDITION

	ADDITIONAL COMMENTS	Nursing Diagnosis must be completed by RN
Indicate locations of any of the following by number: 1. Abrasion 2. Burn 3. Contusion 4. Decubitis 5. Bruise 6. Laceration 7. Rash 8. Scars 9. Sutures 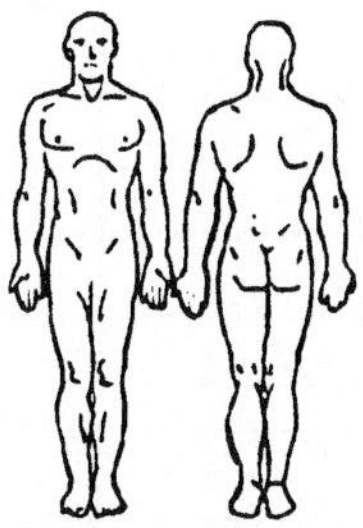 Skin color PINK Skin temperature ______ Skin moisture ______ ☒ Edema both feet ☒ All above areas addressed	3 cm open area over (L) metatarsal of (L) foot. Draining mod amt yellow thick drainage	☒ Impaired Skin Integrity ☐ Altered Oral Mucous Membrane

MUSCULO-SKELETAL/PHYSICAL MOBILITY

	ADDITIONAL COMMENTS	Nursing Diagnosis must be completed by RN
☐ Arthritis ☐ Gout ☐ Fracture ______ ☐ Deformity noted (describe) ☐ Contractures: ☐ Rt. Arm ☐ Lt. Arm ☐ Rt. Leg ☐ Lt. Leg ☐ Previous limitations in mobility (specify) ______ ☐ History of falls (indicate frequency and reason) ______ Gait: ☐ Steady ☐ Unsteady ☒ Independent ☐ Needs ___ # of persons assist Ambulatory devices: ☐ Cane ☐ Crutches ☐ Walker ☐ Other ______ ☐ Assistance needed with bathing ☐ Assistance needed with dressing ☐ Amputations ______ ☐ Prosthesis ______ ☐ Pain Location ______ Describe ______ ☒ All above areas addressed	DISCOMFORT WHEN BEARING WT ON L FOOT - MILD ACHING (4 on scale 1-10) UNABLE TO WALK REGULARLY EXCEPT AT HOME FOR 3 WKS	☐ Activity intolerance ☐ Self-care deficit ☒ Impaired Physical Mobility ☐ Potential for injury ☐ Pain

IMMUNE FUNCTION

	ADDITIONAL COMMENTS	Nursing Diagnosis must be completed by RN
☐ Fever in last 48° ☐ Transplant history ______ ☐ Radiation therapy (date) ______ ☐ Chemotherapy (date) ______ ☐ Venous access device ______ Site: ______ ☐ Central Catheter ______ Site: ______ Malignancy history ______ ☒ All above areas addressed	NO IDENTIFIED CONCERNS	☐ Potential for infection

#4678 (R 01/93)
(2 of 4)

Continued.

FIGURE 12-5, cont'd Nursing history form.

ST. JOHN'S HOSPITAL
Springfield, Illinois

ADMISSION PATIENT PROFILE

NUTRITIONAL/METABOLIC

☒ Current Diet 2000 cal ADA ☐ Assistance with eating needed (describe)
☐ Recent Weight Changes ☐ Increase ☐ Decrease (reason)
☐ Nausea and vomiting ☐ Heartburn ☐ Abdominal pain (describe)
☒ Diabetes ☒ Insulin Dependent
☐ Thyroid problems ☐ Hepatitis ☐ Alcohol use (Avg. number drinks/week)
☒ All above areas addressed.

ADDITIONAL COMMENTS: PT STATES "I FOLLOW MY DIET TO THE T"

Nursing Diagnosis must be completed by RN
☐ Altered Nutrition
☐ Noncompliance
☐ Self-Care Deficit, Feeding
☐ Pain

ELIMINATION

BOWEL: ☐ GI Bleed ☐ Colitis ☐ Diverticulitis ☐ Hemorrhoids Date of last BM 4/1
Bowel pattern (describe) QOD ☐ Stool changes (describe)
☒ Constipation ☐ Diarrhea Frequency ____ x/day ☐ Involuntary
Bowel Sounds: ☒ Present ☐ Absent ☐ Abdominal Distention
URINE: ☐ Burning ☐ Hematuria ☐ Urgency ☐ Retention ☐ Renal disease
☐ Dysuria ☐ Incontinence (describe)
☐ Nocturia (____ x/night) ☐ Stream initation difficulty
☐ Foley in place Date inserted/changed
☒ All above areas addressed

ADDITIONAL COMMENTS: OCCAS CONSTIPATION WORSE WHEN INACTIVE OR AWAY FROM HOME

Nursing Diagnosis must be completed by RN
☒ Constipation
☐ Diarrhea
☐ Bowel Incontinence
☐ Urinary Incontinence
☐ Urinary Retention
☐ Altered Patterns of Urinary Elimination

REPRODUCTIVE

MALE: ☐ Prostate Problem (describe)
☐ History of Sexually Transmitted Disease:
FEMALE: ☐ Menstrual changes/problems (describe)
☐ Breast changes/problems (describe)
☐ LMP YEARS AGO ☐ Pregnant
☐ History of Sexually Transmitted Disease:
☒ All above areas addressed

ADDITIONAL COMMENTS: POSTMENOPAUSE

Nursing Diagnosis must be completed by RN
☐ Sexual Dysfunction
☐ Body Image Disturbance

PSYCHO-SOCIAL-SPIRITUAL

☐ Lives with spouse ☒ Lives alone ☐ Lives with family
☐ Lives with friend ☐ Nursing Home ☐ Other
Do you have close family members or significant others that are supportive to you if you need help? ☐ No ☒ Yes ☐ Name ANN Relationship DAUGHTER
Are you the primary caregiver for someone at home? ☐ Yes ☒ No

ADDITIONAL COMMENTS:

Nursing Diagnosis must be completed by RN
☐ Ineffective Coping
☐ Altered Family Process
☐ Altered Health Maintenance
☐ Spiritual Distress

Do you have special religious requests during this hospitalization? ☐ Yes ☒ No
Describe

What concerns you most about your hospitalization? ☐ Yes ☐ No
Describe "I'M AFRAID THIS SORE WON'T HEAL AND THEY WILL HAVE TO AMPUTATE MY FOOT"

What concerns you most about your illness? ☐ Yes ☐ No
Describe "I JUST WANT TO GET BACK TO NORMAL."

Signature of Data Collector L. Reed RN Date: 4/2/XX Time: 1400

#4678 (R 01/93)
(3 of 4)

ADMISSION PATIENT PROFILE

FIGURE 12-5, cont'd Nursing history form.

TEACHING/DISCHARGE PLANNING (*Must* be completed by RN)

1. Patient/family have been identified, at this time, as having these educational needs: NEEDS REVIEW OF DIABETIC FOOT CARE AND WAYS TO IMPROVE CIRCULATION TO FEET & LEGS.

☒ Health Seeking Behavior
☐ Impaired Home Maintenance Management
☐ Knowledge Deficit

2. Teaching Record Initiated: (Indicate Title) DIABETIC FOOT CARE.

Does anyone from a community agency visit you at home?

☐ Yes ______

☒ No

4. Do you anticipate needing any assistance when you are discharged from the hospital? ☐ Yes ☒ No

Specify: Daughter is in process of divorce. Usually supportive but unable to help much now. Will be able to help in a few months.

5. Screening Referrals to:

	Date/Time
☐ Cardiac Rehabilitation (ext. 4448)	
☐ Clinical Dietitian (ext. 4880)	
☒ Home Health Services (ext. 5641)	4-9-XX 1000
☐ Lactation Nurse (ext. 3983)	
☐ Oncology Clinical Nurse Specialist (ext. 4547)	
☐ Oncology Pain Management Service (ext. 4547)	
☐ Pacemaker Clinic (ext. 5054)	
☐ Pastoral Care (ext. 4500)	
☐ Social Worker (ext. 4480)	
☐ Stoma Nurse (Ext. 4035)	
☐ Other	

6. What are your discharge plans?

☒ Home

☐ Home with Home Care Assistance

☐ Nursing Home

☐ Other (Specify) ______

Signature: L. Reed R.N. Date: 4-10-XX Time: 1000

#4678 (R 01/93)
(4 of 4)

FIGURE 12-5, cont'd Nursing history form.

ST. JOHN'S HOSPITAL
Springfield, Illinois
ROUTINE NURSING ASSESSMENT
Medical/Surgical

EDEMA: +1 = 0" - ¼"
+2 = ¼" - ½"
+3 = ½" - 1"

Ø = Negative/No
✓ = observed or positive response
Blank = no assessment at this time
NN = see nurses notes
LE = lower extremity
UE = upper extremity
OTA = open to air

PU = purulent
SS = serosanguinous
B = brown
R = red
Y = yellow
G = green
P = pink
A = amber
C = clear
CL = cloudy

Date		4-1-XX							
Time		1600							
MENTAL STATUS	Alert	✓							
	Oriented/Disoriented	✓ /							
	Lethargic								
	Unresponsive								
BEHAVIOR	Agitated								
	Anxious								
	Restless	✓							
MOTOR/SENSORY FUNCTION	Moves all extremities	✓							
	Weakness UE LT/RT	/							
	LE LT/RT	✓ / ✓							
	Paralysis UE LT/RT	/							
	LE LT/RT	/							
	Numbness/Tingling	✓ / ✓							
	location	both feet							
SKIN/MUCOUS MEMBRANE	Temperature: warm/cool	/ ✓							
	Moisture: dry/moist	✓ /							
	Skin: pink/pale	✓ /							
	flushed/cyanotic	/							
	jaundiced								
	Mucous Membrane: pink/pale	✓ /							
	flushed/cyanotic	/							
	Edema:	1+							
	location	feet							
CARDIO-VASCULAR	Apical rate: reg./irreg.	✓ /							
	Dorsalis pedis LT/RT	D (NN) / D							
	Posterior tibial LT/RT	/							

#4747 (R 10/91)
(1 of 2)

ROUTINE NURSING ASSESSMENT - Medical/Surgical

FIGURE 12-6 Nursing assessment flow sheet. (Courtesy St. John's Hospital, Springfield, Ill.)

Date		4-1-XX							
Time		1600							
RESPIRATORY	Quality: unlabored/labored	✓							
	deep/shallow	✓							
	O2 Therapy:	Ø							
	Sounds: clear LT/RT	✓ / ✓							
	diminished LT/RT								
	rales (crackles) LT/RT								
	rhonchi LT/RT								
	wheeze LT/RT								
	Cough: productive/nonproductive	Ø							
	Sputum: Color	Ø							
GASTROINTESTINAL ABDOMEN	Nondistended/Distended	✓							
	Sounds: present/absent	✓							
	Firm / Soft	✓ (Soft)							
	Hyperactive/Hypoactive								
	Expelling flatus	✓							
	Nausea	Ø							
WOUND	Location: (✓ = no redness or edema)								
	#1 (L) foot (toe)	NN							
	#2								
	#3								
DRESSING	Location: (✓ = clean & dry)								
	#1 dRy 4x4	✓							
	#2								
	#3								
DRAINAGE	Device and location:	description	description	description	description	description	description	description	description
	#1								
	#2								
	#3								
PAIN	Absent/Present	✓							
	Location:								
	#1								
	#2								
	Severity scale (0-10) #1/#2								
	Intervention								
PATIENT TEACHING	Description								
	#1 ORiented to shift	✓							
	#2 Routines								
	#3								
Signature		L. Reed RN							

#4747 (R 10/91)
(2 of 2)

FIGURE 12-6, cont'd Nursing assessment flow sheet.

Kardex and Client Care Summary. Traditionally, nursing information needed for the daily care of a client is readily accessible in a nursing **Kardex.** This is a flip-over card file usually kept at the nurse's station. The Kardex contains information concerning the client's current ongoing plan of care. The updated information in the Kardex eliminates the need for the nurse to refer continually to the client's chart. Many hospitals now have computerized systems that provide this same information in the form of a client care summary. This is printed for each client during each shift. Data are automatically updated as orders are entered and as nursing decisions are made. Figure 12-7 is a sample computerized client care summary.

Information commonly found in the Kardex or client care summary includes the following:

1. Basic demographic data (name, age, sex)
2. Primary medical diagnosis
3. Current physician's orders to be carried out by the nurse (diet, activity, vital signs, medications, diagnostic tests)
4. Nursing orders or nursing measures (intake and output, positioning, comfort measures, teaching)
5. Allergy history and safety precautions used in the client's care

Nursing Care Planning. Professional nurses are responsible for planning individualized nursing care for each client. Care planning should communicate a client's unique needs rather than standard routine information. When all nurses who have worked with the client collaborate to develop a plan of care, they achieve more improved continuity of care.

For example, a client may have a nursing diagnosis of fluid volume deficit related to severe sore throat and fever. A nursing intervention of "increase fluid intake" is relevant but not particularly individualized. However, if the nurse's assessment has revealed what beverages the client prefers, an entry of "offer orange juice and iced tea, 1000 ml per 7-3 shift, 700cc per 3-11 shift, and 100cc 11-7 shift" addresses the client's preferences and tailors the care plan to the client's needs. Nursing orders that concisely describe what needs to be done, how often, and how, most effectively achieve desired outcomes. Care planning clearly communicated makes individualized care possible.

Nursing computer systems today are developing care plans from a menu that can offer many options. These can be individualized by adding typed-in data. Computerizing documentation may decrease the time required for the documentation process by 40% to 50%, allowing professional nurses to spend more time at the bedside (Marrelli, 1992). Figure 12-8 is a sample computerized care plan generated in approximately 5 minutes.

Standardized Care Plans. Many institutions have attempted to make documentation easier for nurses with **standardized care plans.** The plans, based on the institution's standards of nursing practice, are preprinted established guidelines used to care for clients with similar health problems. After a nursing assessment is completed, the staff nurse identifies the standard care plans appropriate to the client. The care plans are placed in the client's record. Modifications can be made to individualize nursing activities. Most standardized plans also allow the nurse to insert specific desired outcomes and the dates when these outcomes should be achieved.

Standard care plans are usually generated by a group of people who use their collective expertise to develop more sophisticated plans. Standard care plans also educate nurses about the nursing care of a client with a particular nursing diagnosis. Part-time or float nurses find standard care plans useful for learning about the care of clients with unfamiliar problems (Iyer, Camp, 1991).

Controversy exists over the use of standardized care plans. The major disadvantage is the risk that they inhibit nurses' identification of unique, individualized interventions for clients. A second disadvantage is the need to formally update the plans routinely to ensure that content is current and appropriate. When standardized care plans are used in a health care facility, the nurse remains responsible for an individualized approach to care. Standardized care plans are not meant to replace the nurse's professional judgment and decision making.

Critical Pathways. With the arrival of managed care (see Chapter 1), documentation tools that integrate the standards of care of multiple disciplines have been developed. These tools or critical pathways allow staff from all disciplines to develop integrated care plans for a projected length of stay for clients of a specific case type. For example, the pathway for a total hip repair will recommend on a day-by-day basis the level of activity, pain control therapy, advancement in diet, and educational topics necessary for a client's normal recovery. The nurse and other team members use the pathway to monitor a client's progress and as a documentation tool. Charting by exception is frequently the method utilized with pathways. Staff only document when anticipated interventions are not provided as projected. The pathways eliminate other nursing forms such as nursing care plans.

Discharge Summary Forms. Much emphasis is placed on preparing a client for a timely discharge from a health care institution. Ideally, discharge planning begins at admission and in some cases even before admission as is necessary with same-day surgery admissions and childbirth. Nurses continue discharge planning as the client's condition changes. Clients and family should be involved in the discharge-planning process.

A **discharge summary** form (Figure 12-9) provides

Text continued on p. 200

CCHD -0410 ST. JOHNS DEVELOPMENT
03-26-XX 12:43 (QAB$$P) PAGE 001

DOE, JANE F W D 52
ACCT#: 93000775 MR#: 0895351 PATIENT CARE SUMMARY
SERV: MEDICAL CCHD ..CH09
DR: EDISON, THOMAS MD ADM: 03/26/XX
DR: DOB: 02/12/41

SUMMARY: 03/26 07:00 TO 15:15

PATIENT INFORMATION:
MEDICATION ALLERGIES:
03/26 MEDICATION ALLERGY: NONE KNOWN
OTHER NURSING INFORMATION:
03/26 ADMIT DX: DIABETIC ULCERS

ALL CURRENT MEDICAL ORDERS:

MD TO NURSE ORDERS:
03/26 8. BLOOD: ACCUCHECK AC AND HS, (0009)
03/26 9. VITAL SIGNS, T-P-R, BP BID, (0009)
03/26 10. DRESSINGS: CHANGE DRESSING --WET TO DRY --L FOOT ULCER, (0009)

DIET/I&O:
03/26 1. DIET: DIABETIC, 2000CAL, (0009)

LABORATORY:
03/26 2. CBC, TODAY, (03/26/XX), (0009)
03/26 3. GLUCOSE, TOMORROW, (03/27/XX), (0009)

ALL CURRENT PHARMACY/INFUSION ORDERS:

SCHEDULED MEDICATIONS:
03/26 5. INSULIN HUMAN REGULAR 100UNITS/ML INJ, 5 UNITS,SC, QAM,1/2HR AC/BKFST, (03/27/XX 0800-..), (0009)
03/26 6. INSULIN HUMAN REGULAR 100UNITS/ML INJ, 5 UNITS,SC, QPM,1/2HR AC/DINNR, (03/26/XX 1700-..), (0009)

UNSCHEDULED MEDICATIONS:
03/26 4. INSULIN HUMAN REGULAR 100UNITS/ML INJ, 5 UNITS,SC, TODAY(IF APPROPRIATE),,(03/26/XX) , (0009)

PRN MEDICATIONS:
03/26 7. DARVOCET-N PROPOXYPHENE N 50MG/ACETAMINOPHEN 325MG TAB, #2, PO, Q4H, PRN, (0009)

LASTPAGE

DOE, JANE 0895351 PATIENT CARE SUMMARY

FIGURE 12-7 Computerized patient care summary. (Courtesy St. John's Hospital, Springfield, Ill.)

ICUC -0284 ST. JOHNS DEVELOPMENT
04-01-XX 10:09 (QAY$$P) PAGE 001

PATIENT, JANE F W M 62
ACCT#: 93000811 MR#: 0895383
SERV: MEDICAL ICUC ..IC02
DR: TYLER, ANN MD ADM: 04/01/XX
DR: DOB: 10/06/30

PLAN OF CARE

ADMIT DX: DIABETIC ULCERS

CURRENT PROBLEMS:

04/01 IMPAIRED PHYSICAL MOBILITY
R/T:WEAKNESS & FATIGUE

EXPECTED OUTCOMES:		DATE:
04/01	PT WILL RESUME NORMAL ACTIVITIES	PRIOR TO DC

NURSING APPROACHES:

- 04/01 TURN & POSITION Q2HR
- 04/01 INSTRUCT IN PROPER BODY MECHANICS
- 04/01 INSTRUCT PT/S.O. IN PROPER TRANSFER TECHNIQUE
- 04/01 INVOLVE PT/S.O. IN DEVELOPING PLAN FOR INCREASING MOBILITY

04/01 ALTERED TISSUE PERFUSION: PERIPHERAL
R/T:DECREASED ARTERIAL FLOW

EXPECTED OUTCOMES:		DATE:
04/01	--IDENTIFY WAYS TO IMPROVE CIRCULATION TO FEET	PRIOR TO DC

NURSING APPROACHES:

- 04/01 ASSESS PERIPHERAL PULSES, SKIN TEMP, COLOR, SENSATION, & MOTION
- 04/01 DISCOURAGE PT FROM CROSSING LEGS
- 04/01 AVOID PRESSURE TO POSTERIOR KNEE AREA
- 04/01 AVOID PROLONGED SITTING OR STANDING
- 04/01 ENCOURAGE TO WIGGLE:....TOES
- 04/01 PERFORM ROM:....ACTIVE

04/01 FEAR
R/T: POSSIBILITY ULCER WON'T HEAL

EXPECTED OUTCOMES:		DATE:
04/01	PT WILL VERBALIZE &/OR DEMONSTRATE EFFECTIVE COPING MECHANISMS TO REDUCE OR ELIMINATE SOURCE OF FEAR	PRIOR TO DC

NURSING APPROACHES:

- 04/01 DISCUSS SITUATION & UNDERSTANDING OF SITUATION WITH PT & S.O.
- 04/01 BE ACTIVE LISTENER TO PT CONCERNS
- 04/01 ENCOURAGE EXPRESSION OF FEELINGS
- 04/01 --DESCRIBE EVIDENCE OF HEALING AS OBSERVED

NURSES: SIMMONS, TERRY AIS

LASTPAGE

PATIENT, JANE 0895383 PLAN OF CARE

FIGURE 12-8 Computerized nursing care plan. (Courtesy St. John's Hospital, Springfield, Ill.)

ST. JOHN'S HOSPITAL
Springfield, Illinois

DISCHARGE DOCUMENTATION - Part 1

KEY: NA = not applicable

ACTIVITY STATUS AT DISCHARGE

	Without Help	Uses A Device	Help of Another	Is Not Done	Comments	Patient/Family Indicates Understanding of Limitations
Walking	✓				Steady gait	☐ Yes ☐ No
Wheelchair				✓		☐ Yes ☐ No
Stair Climbing	✓				NO LIMITATION	☐ Yes ☐ No
Bathing	✓					☐ Yes ☐ No
Dressing	✓					☐ Yes ☐ No
Toileting	✓					☐ Yes ☐ No
Transferring	✓					☐ Yes ☐ No
Eating/Feeding	✓				1800 ADA Diet	☑ Yes ☐ No

MENTAL STATUS

Alert ☑ Yes ☐ No Oriented ☑ Yes ☐ No If no, Disoriented to ☐ Time ☐ Place ☐ Person

PATIENT CONDITION AT DISCHARGE (if no, explain variance)

Afebrile	☑ Yes	☐ No		
Vital signs stable	☑ Yes	☐ No		
Free of pain	☑ Yes	☐ No		Controlled with Tylenol q 4°
Appetite satisfactory	☑ Yes	☐ No		
Fluid intake satisfactory	☑ Yes	☐ No		
Voiding without difficulty	☑ Yes	☐ No		
Defecation without difficulty	☑ Yes	☐ No		Uses mom PRN
Skin in good condition	☑ Yes	☐ No		
No evidence of drainage from wound	☑ Yes	☐ No	☐ NA	
IV/Heparin lock removed	☑ Yes	☐ No	☐ NA	
IV/Heparin lock site without redness or swelling	☑ Yes	☐ No	☐ NA	

DISCHARGE INFORMATION

Date 10/18/XX Time 1000 Hrs. ☑ Home ☐ Alone ☑ With Family ☐ With Significant Other

☐ Health Care Facility (name) ______ ☐ Hospital (name) ______

☑ Ambulatory ☐ Wheelchair ☐ Ambulance (name) ______

Carried by: ______ Accompanied by: Jane Doe N.A. (staff member)

EXPIRATION INFORMATION

Date ______ Time ______ Hrs.

Notification of: Attending physician ☐ Yes ☐ No
Consultant(s) ☐ Yes ☐ No ☐ NA
Family ☐ Yes ☐ No
Coroner ☐ Yes ☐ No ☐ NA

Autopsy: ☐ Yes ☐ No Permit Signed: ☐ Yes ☐ No

Disposition of Body: ☐ Morgue Time ______ Hrs.
☐ Mortician Time ______ Hrs.

Mortician's Name ______

City, State ______

ORGAN/TISSUE DONATION INFORMATION

Organ Donation Requested ☐ Yes ☐ No

If NO, Reason ______

Tissue Donation Requested ☐ Yes ☐ No

If NO, Reason ______

If YES, Next of Kin consent: ☐ Yes ☐ No

Organ Procurement Coordinator or Enucleation Technician Contacted ☐ Yes ☐ No

DISCHARGE SIGNATURE

Martha E. Elkin R.N.

#325 (R 10/92) **DISCHARGE DOCUMENTATION** - *Part 1*

FIGURE 12-9 Discharge documentation form. (Courtesy St. John's Hospital, Springfield, Ill.)

TIPS ON WRITING DISCHARGE SUMMARY FORMS

INFORMATION FOR HOME HEALTH CARE NURSES

Describe nursing interventions (e.g., dressing changes and step-by-step wound care).
Describe information presented to client.
Describe client's ability to perform health care skills (e.g., administering medications and use of crutches).
Explain family members' involvement in care.
Describe resources needed in the home (e.g., Meals On Wheels and self-help devices).

INFORMATION FOR CLIENTS

Use clear concise descriptions in client's own language.
Provide step-by-step description of how to perform a procedure (e.g., home medication administration). Reinforce explanation with printed instructions.
Identify precautions to follow when performing self-care or administering medications.
Review signs and symptoms of complications that should be reported to physician.
List names and phone numbers of health care providers and community resources the client can contact.

important information pertaining to the client's continued health care after discharge. Information may include medication instructions, activity orders or restrictions, prescribed exercises, dietary instructions, and guidelines for calling a physician when problems arise. The client's status should be described in relation to planned outcomes or discharge criteria. The client or family member should receive a copy of the discharge summary form as a resource. Home health care agencies or extended nursing care facilities can also benefit from receiving information on the summary forms (see box at left) to ensure better continuity of care.

Home Care Documentation. The home health care business continues to grow as clients are discharged home earlier with significant health care problems. Medicare has specific guidelines for establishing eligibility for home care reimbursement. Documentation by home health care nurses must clearly describe the client's health status and nursing care required.

Clients need home health care if they have limited mobility, or are blind, senile, or otherwise unable to go out unassisted (Magliozzi, 1990). When clients require skilled care, specific descriptions of the required skills are entered into their medical records.

SUMMARY

Documentation and reporting are methods of communicating information related to a client's health care management. In any setting, the success of care planning depends on accurate and complete reporting and precise documentation. Effective reporting and documentation create a high level of communication that helps health team members share a common view of the client's needs. Nurses are the primary care providers and thus have the most contact with clients. Using basic principles for accurate and comprehensive documentation and reporting enhances the delivery of safe and effective nursing care.

CRITICAL THINKING ACTIVITIES

1. Locate a chart on a nursing division and find six examples of nursing documentation that follow guidelines for accuracy and currentness.
2. Describe criteria to use in charting client teaching, including subjective and objective data about a client and evaluation of responses.
3. Observe a change-of-shift report at your health care facility and discuss it in class or clinical conference.
4. Write a client's progress note using the SOAP and PIE formats using the following data:

Mrs. Brown is scheduled for surgery for the first time. The nurse instructed her on turning, coughing, and deep breathing. The nurse also explained routine postoperative monitoring procedures and pain management. The client asked questions and was able to demonstrate TCDB to the nurse. She stated "I think I know what to expect and I do not have any questions right now."

KEY CONCEPTS

A client's health care record is a written documentation of the care given.

Accurate record keeping requires an objective interpretation of data with precise measurements, correct spelling, and proper use of abbreviations.

The medical record is a legal document and requires information describing accurately the care delivered to a client.

A nurse's signature on an entry in a record designates accountability for the contents of that entry.

Any change in a client's condition warrants timely documentation to keep a record accurate.

An organized record presents information logically in order of the occurrence of events.

All information pertaining to a client's health care management gathered by examination, observation, conversation, or treatment is confidential.

The major purpose of the change-of-shift report is to maintain continuity of care.

The medical record is a financial record used as the basis for reimbursement to hospitals.

When information pertinent to care is communicated by telephone, the information must be verified.

Problem-oriented medical records are organized according to the client's health care problems.

Flow sheets eliminate the need to write narrative notes for repeated observations or measurements.

The logic of SOAP, SOAPE, or PIE narrative notes is to organize entries in the progress notes by the nursing process.

Computerized information systems provide information about clients in an organized and easily accessible fashion.

References

American Nurses Association: *Computer design criteria for systems that support the nursing process,* Kansas City, Mo., 1988, The Association.

Bergerson SR: Charting with a jury in mind, *Nurs 88* 18(4):51, 1988.

Collins HL: Legal risks of computer charting, *RN* 53(5):81, 1990.

Edelstein J: A study of nursing documentation, *Nurs Manage* 21(11): 40, 1990.

Hurley ML: What do the new JCAHO standards mean for you? *RN* 6:42, 1991.

Iyer P and Camp N: *Nursing documentation,* St. Louis, 1991, Mosby.

Joint Commission on Accreditation of Healthcare Organizations: *Accreditation manual for hospitals,* Chicago, 1994, The Commission.

Lampe S: *Focus charting: a patient centered approach,* ed 4, Minneapolis, 1988, Creative Nursing Management.

Magliozzi HM: Charting that makes it through the Medicare maze, *RN* 53(6):75, 1990.

Marrelli TM: *Nursing documentation handbook,* St. Louis, 1992, Mosby.

Murphy J, Burke LJ: Charting by exception, a more efficient way to document, *Nurs 90* 20(5):65, 1990.

McLaughlin K, et al.: Shaping the future, the marriage of theory and informatics, *Comput Nurs* 8(4):174, 1990.

Bibliography

Coles MC and Fullenwider SD: Documentation: managing the dilemma, *Nurs Manage* 19(12):65, 1988.

Feutz-Harter S: Documentation principles and pitfalls, *J Nurs Admin* 19(12):7, 1989.

Ford J: Computers and nursing possibilities for transforming nursing, *Comput Nurs* 8(4):160, 1990.

Fox-Unger E, et al.: Documentation: communicating professionalism, *Nurs Manage* 20:65, 1989.

Greve P: Documentation: every word counts, *RN* 55(7):56, 1992.

Hines GL: DRGs: nursing documentation contributes to the bottom line, *Nurs Clin North Am* 23(3):579, 1988.

Kerr SD: A comparison of four nursing documentation systems: *J Nurs Staff Develop* 8(1):26-31, 1992.

Kleiber C and Chase L: Solving documentation problems with a pediatric flow sheet, *Ped Nurs* 15(3):253, 1989.

Knapp-Spooner C, Brett J: Less is more: a med/surg flow sheet, *RN* 55(3):36-39, 1992.

Morrissey-Ross M: Documentation: if you haven't written it, you haven't done it, *Nurs Clin North Am* 23(2):363, 1988.

Potter P and Perry A: *Fundamentals of nursing: concepts, process, and practice,* ed 3, St. Louis, 1993, Mosby.

Schaffer CL: Documenting special legal situations: *Nurs* 22(5):32C-D, 1992.

Wright BA, Fishman N: Telephone reporting to physicians . . . what should you know before you pick up the phone? *Geriatr Nurs Am J Care Aging* 13(5):279-80, 1992.

13 Communication

OBJECTIVES

Mastery of content in this chapter will enable the student to:

- Define the key terms listed.
- Describe differences among the three levels of communication.
- Describe each element of the communication process.
- List factors influencing the communication process.
- Identify characteristics of verbal and nonverbal communication.
- Discuss the functions of communication in a nurse-client relationship.
- Describe the similarities and differences between social and informational interaction.
- Explain the role of communication in the nursing process.
- List and discuss the phases of a therapeutic helping relationship.
- Describe the role of communication in giving care.
- Identify factors that promote and inhibit effective communication.
- Explain techniques to promote communication with children of different ages.
- Discuss nursing care measures for clients with specific communication needs.

KEY TERMS

channels
communication
connotative
denotative
empathy
feedback
interpersonal communication
intimate zone
intonation
intrapersonal communication
message
metacommunication
nonverbal communication
personal zone
public communication
public zone
receiver
referent
sender
social zone
territoriality
therapeutic communication
verbal communication

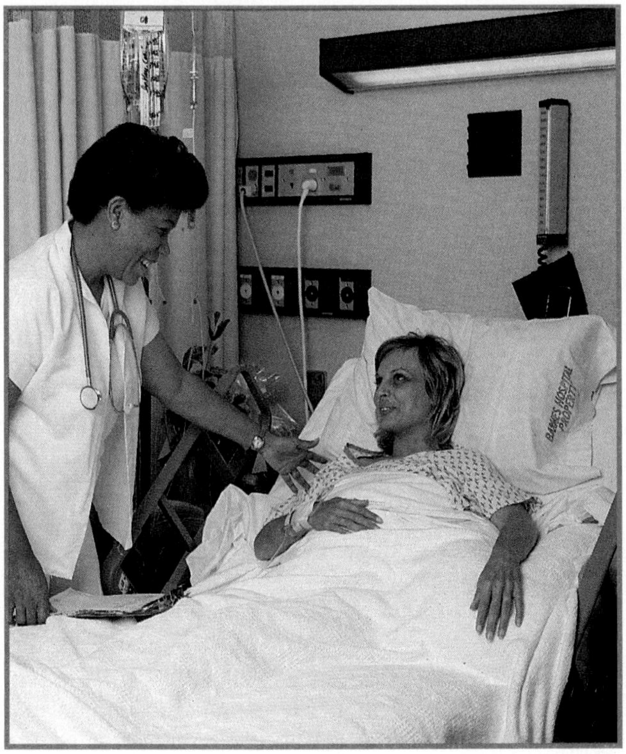

Communication is an important component of nursing practice. Several authors (Severtsen, 1990; Lindberg et al., 1990; Sarvimaki, 1988) describe nursing as communicative interaction and believe the foundation of nursing lies in the "communicative attitude." To communicate effectively with clients, nurses must develop skilled communication techniques in order to develop therapeutic or working relationships (Shives, 1990). Communication is ongoing and complex. It requires skill, practice, and conscious application of principles and techniques. These techniques enable the nurse to establish a working relationship with clients and eventually help them to meet their health care needs. Failure to communicate leads to serious problems and can threaten professional credibility. The nurse can also initiate change that promotes the client's well-being. Communication is the foundation of the relationships between the nurse and other members of the health care team. Knaus, et al. (1986) discovered that the lowest death rates in hospitals were related to coordinated interactions between nurses and physicians. Finally, the process of communication is not something a nurse simply memorizes and puts into practice. Communication is complex. It requires practice and a conscious application of principles.

Communication is the basic element of human interaction that allows people to establish, maintain, and improve contacts with others. Human communication is a complex process involving behaviors and relationships. It allows individuals to associate with others and the world around them. It is an ongoing, dynamic series of events in which meaning is generated and transmitted. Communication refers to nonverbal and verbal behavior within a social context and includes all symbols and clues used by people to give and receive meaning. An instructor's descriptions, a student's questions, and a nurse's gestures create responses in those who observe, listen, and interact. Meaning is not simply transferred from one person to another. It is mutually negotiated between the people communicating. Communication is thus an act of sharing. Many variables affect the meaning conveyed (e.g., the instructor's style of speech or the student's values placed on the subject). For communication to be effective, the meaning acquired by the person listening must be similar or identical to the message intended by the speaker.

LEVELS OF COMMUNICATION

Communication occurs at the intrapersonal, interpersonal, and public levels. **Intrapersonal communication** occurs within an individual. It is the way people consider their thoughts internally so they can express themselves appropriately to others. The goal of intrapersonal communication is self-awareness, which is influenced by self-concept and feelings of self-worth. For example, when a nurse walks into a client's room and thinks, "He looks uncomfortable, and I want to show him I'm concerned about his discomfort," the communication is intrapersonal.

Interpersonal communication is the interaction between two people or in a small group. Problem solving, sharing ideas, decision making, and personal growth are outcomes of effective interpersonal communication. Through interpersonal communication, nurses interact with clients, family members, physicians, fellow nurses, and other health care providers to develop strategies that bring about positive changes in a client's health status.

Public communication is interaction with large groups of people. Nurses often have opportunities to speak with groups of clients or consumers on health-related topics. Public communication requires special skills such as posture and voice inflection to communicate messages effectively.

ELEMENTS OF THE COMMUNICATION PROCESS

To understand communication, a person should examine the components of the communication process. A model can simply and graphically demonstrate the most complex of processes, but it can also make a process look simpler than it actually is. A communication model provides the nursing student with a framework for observing, understanding, and predicting the communication process.

Figure 13-1 depicts interpersonal communication as a simple process involving two people. The sender transmits a message to the receiver, who responds by giving feedback. However, the model fails to show all the levels of involvement between the people communicating. There may also be gestures, actions, or internal thinking occurring. As two people communicate, they mutually interact in sharing information.

The basic elements of communication are shown in Figure 13-2. Communication occurs on a social level, with the participants engaged in intrapersonal and interpersonal interactions. The process is dynamic, with the meaning of messages mutually negotiated by the participants. People communicating may or may not be consciously aware of each element of communication. During casual conversation, people do not bother to analyze the meaning of every gesture or word. The nurse, however, learns to be conscious of each element of the communication process to control interactions effectively with clients and to remain aware of the effects of communication on them. Each element can be considered from the perspectives of natural, uninhibited, and as appropriate, consciously manipulated communication.

The **referent** motivates one person to communicate with another. It may be an object, experience, emotion, idea, or act. A person who consciously considers the referent during an interaction can carefully develop and organize the message.

The **sender** is the person who initiates the interpersonal communication. This role may switch back and forth between the original sender and receiver.

The **message** is the information sent or expressed by the sender. The most effective message is clear and organized and is expressed in a manner familiar to the receiver. The message may be verbal or nonverbal.

The message is sent along a channel of communication. **Channels** are means of conveying messages, such as through the visual, auditory, and tactile senses. The sender's facial expression visually conveys a message to another person. The spoken word travels through auditory channels. Placing a hand on another person while communicating uses the channel of touch. Generally, the more channels the nurse uses to send a message, the better the client will understand it. To paraphrase Rogers (1986), a person remembers 5% of what he or she hears, 10% of what he or she reads, 30% of what he or she sees, 50% of what he or she discusses, 75% of what he or she does, and 90% of what he or she teaches others to do.

The **receiver** is the person to whom the message is sent. For communication to be effective, the receiver must perceive or become aware of the sender's message. The message then acts as one of the receiver's referents, prompting the receiver to respond to it. The nurse learns to engage in interpersonal communication while analyzing and interpreting the client's message. The more the sender and receiver have in common, the more likely the sender's meaning will be communicated.

The environment is the physical and emotional atmosphere present at the time of interaction. For effective communication to occur, the environment should be comfortable and suited to the needs of all participants. The more positive an environment the nurse can achieve with the client, the more successful the exchange.

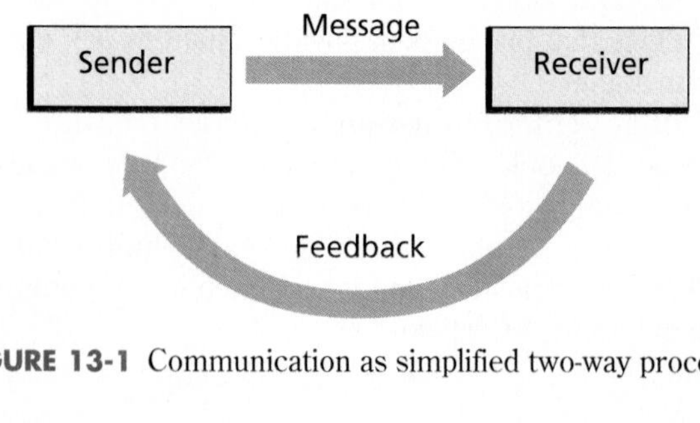

FIGURE 13-1 Communication as simplified two-way process.

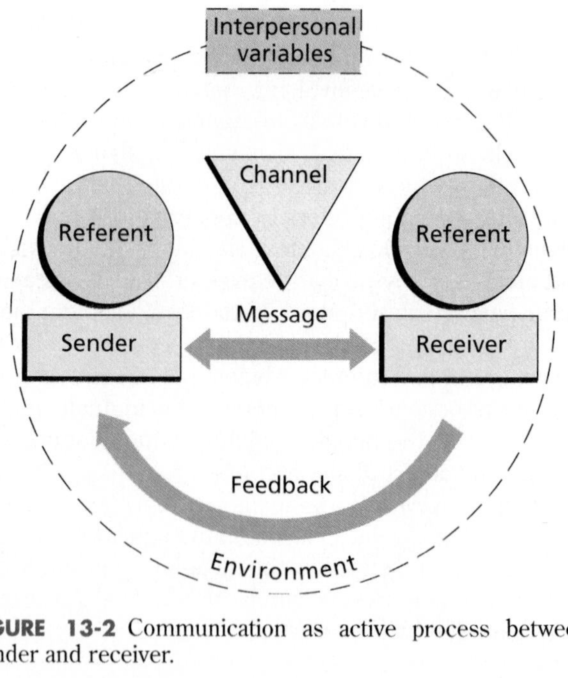

FIGURE 13-2 Communication as active process between sender and receiver.

The process of communication is ongoing. The receiver returns a message to the sender in the form of **feedback.** Feedback indicates whether the meaning of the sender's message was received. The mere intent to communicate is not enough to ensure accurate reception of a message. The receiver's verbal and nonverbal response sends feedback to the sender to reveal understanding of the message. The nurse must be open to feedback from a client to be sure the client understands the message.

The roles of sender and receiver change back and forth as two people interact. Because of this reciprocal relationship involved in communication, the model tends to oversimplify a complex process.

FACTORS INFLUENCING COMMUNICATION

Each person is unique and associates different things with messages and interprets them differently than any other person. A frown may convey unhappiness to one person and pain to another. The meaning that communication holds for one person can be influenced by many

FACTORS THAT INFLUENCE COMMUNICATION

PERCEPTIONS

Each person senses, interprets, and understands events differently. Perceptions are a person's personal view of events occurring in the environment. Perceptions are formed by goals and expectations. Differences can be obstacles to effective communication. Perceptions shaped from years of similar experiences are difficult to change.

VALUES

Values reflect the things a person considers important in life. Different experiences and expectations lead to the formation of different values. They influence the way a person expresses ideas and the way the ideas of others are interpreted.

DEVELOPMENT

The rate of speech development varies among children and is related to neurological competence and intellectual development.* Environment also affects speech and language development.

SPACE AND TERRITORIALITY

During social interaction, people consciously maintain a distance between themselves. When personal space becomes threatened, people respond defensively and communicate less effectively. Nurses often work very closely with clients. An intimate distance of 18 inches or less between nurse and client requires the nurse to be sensitive to the client's privacy and needs. A personal distance of 18 inches to 4 feet is ideal for sitting with a client during a conversation.

GENDER

Men and women have different communication styles. Be aware of cultural and ethnic influences that can influence communication. The nurse must be sensitive to how clients exhibit feelings and emotions, both of which can significantly influence the communication process.

EMOTIONS

Emotions are subjective feelings about events and influence the way a person communicates and relates to others. The nurse ensures that emotions do not interfere with providing optimal care. However, the nurse must be empathetic. Emotions can cause a person to misinterpret or not hear a message.

SOCIOCULTURAL BACKGROUND

Culture forms a person's generalizations and preconceptions about the world. Language, gestures, and attitudes reflect cultural origins. A nurse must accept a client's cultural background and frame of reference.

KNOWLEDGE

Different levels of knowledge make communication more difficult. A common language is essential. Knowledge is a product of development, education, environment, and sociocultural factors.

ROLES AND RELATIONSHIPS

Persons communicate with others in a style appropriate for the roles and relationships assumed with them. The formality or informality of communication depends on the roles and kinds of relationship one has with others. Effective communication is possible if the participants are aware of their roles. We feel more comfortable expressing ideas to people with whom we have developed a positive relationship.

ENVIRONMENTAL SETTING

Communication is more effective in a comfortable environment. Noise or lack of privacy or space may cause confusion, tension, or discomfort. Environmental distractions can distort communication.

*Modified from Whaley LF and Wong DL: *Nursing care of infants and children,* ed 4, St. Louis, 1991, Mosby.

factors (see box on p. 205). The role an individual plays in any exchange and the setting in which it occurs also affect the communication process.

MODES OF COMMUNICATION

Messages are conveyed verbally and nonverbally. These modes are closely related during interpersonal interaction. As people speak, they further express themselves through movements, tone of voice, facial expressions, and general appearance. These modes can convey the same or very different messages. The nurse masters the techniques of each mode.

Verbal Communication

Verbal communication involves the spoken or written word. **Language** is defined as the words, their pronunciation, and the method of combining them that is used and understood by a community (Boyle and Andrews, 1989). It is a code that conveys specific meaning. Adding a single word can change the entire meaning of a phrase or sentence. Language is effective only when the sender and receiver understand a message clearly.

A nurse meets clients of various cultures who speak many different languages. Also, some clients speak the same language as the nurse but use subcultural variations of certain words. For example, the word *dinner* may mean a midday meal to one person and the last meal of the day to another. Clear messages require using effective verbal communication techniques.

Vocabulary. Communication is unsuccessful if the receiver is unable to translate the sender's words and phrases. Nursing and medicine involve many technical terms. If the nurse often uses these terms, the client may become confused and unable to follow instructions or learn important information. Rather than telling the client, "Sit up while your lungs are auscultated," it might be better to say, "Sit up while I listen to your lungs." The first statement might make the client feel anxious. A message spoken in terms the client understands makes communication more effective.

Denotative and Connotative Meaning. A single word can have several meanings. A **denotative meaning** is one shared by individuals who use a common language. For example, the word *baseball* has the same meaning for all individuals who speak English, and the word *code* denotes cardiac arrest to nurses. The denotative meaning is what is used to define a word so it means about the same to everyone.

The **connotative** meaning of a word is the thought, feelings, or ideas people have about the word (Duldt, et al., 1984). Using the word *serious* to describe a client's condition may suggest to the family a nearness to death, but nurses may not consider this to be the case unless the word *critical* is used. Connotations are shades or interpretations of a word's meaning rather than different definitions.

When nurses communicate with clients they carefully select words that cannot be easily misinterpreted. This is important when explaining a client's condition, the therapy the client receives, or the purpose of treatments.

Pacing. Verbal communication is more successful when expressed at an appropriate speed or pace. Talking rapidly, using awkward pauses, or speaking slowly and deliberately can convey an unintended message. Consider the nurse who uses awkward pauses during this explanation to a client:

Client: Do you know if the doctor found anything wrong?
Nurse: No (pause), but I'm sure if he did (longer pause) he would have come to explain things to you. (then very rapidly) Now let's get back to where we were.

The long pauses and the rapid shift to another subject may give the client the impression the nurse is hiding the truth.

The speed with which a message is verbalized, in addition to the presence, absence, and length of pauses, can determine the degree to which communication satisfies the listener. The nurse should not talk so quickly that enunciation is unclear. Pauses should be used to accentuate or stress a particular point, giving the listener time to digest and comprehend the meaning of the speaker's words. A person achieves proper pacing by thinking before speaking. Looking for nonverbal cues from the listener that might suggest confusion or misunderstanding is also useful. Asking a listener whether the pace of a message is too fast or too slow helps to determine whether the pace is effective.

Intonation. The **intonation** (tone) of the speaker's voice can dramatically affect a message's meaning. Depending on the intonation, even a simple question or statement can express enthusiasm, anger, or concern. Emotions can directly influence tone of voice. Nurses must be aware of intonation so they do not send out unintended messages. If the client perceives or interprets the message as uncaring, condescending, or patronizing in nature, this could create barriers to the communication process. Also, a client's intonation may provide clues to emotional states or energy levels.

Humor. Humor can help promote well-being. The phrase, "laughter is the best medicine," applies when nurses use humor to help clients to adjust to stress imposed by illness. Dugan (1989) notes that laughter helps to relieve stress-related tension and pain, to increase the nurse's effectiveness in providing emotional support to clients, and to humanize the experience of illness. Laughter is a psychological and physical release. Studies show humor stimulates the production of catecholamines and hormones that enhance feelings of well-being, improve pain tolerance, reduce anxiety, make breathing easier, and enhance metabolism (Sullivan and Deane, 1988; Williams, 1986).

Nurses can appropriately use humor in conversations with clients through joke telling, sharing humorous incidents or situations, and using puns. A client who has become fearful or tense over events related to hospitalization can relax and become more open to interaction as a result of humor. When a client becomes withdrawn because of emotional grief, humor helps the client to release emotional tensions. Sullivan and Deane (1988) have found clients to become more self-disclosing and willing to share concerns of deeper significance. Humor should not become the only means of communication. However, it can be effective in helping clients to interact more openly and honestly.

Clarity and Brevity. Effective communication is simple, short, and to the point. Fewer words spoken result in less confusion. Because of the intrapersonal variables involved, human communication is often imprecise. Ambiguous phrases such as *you know* add little to the clarity of a message. Clarity is achieved by speaking slowly and enunciating clearly. Examples can make an explanation easier to understand. For example, instructing an arthritic client about self-care measures at home is more meaningful when the nurse provides specific examples of self-help techniques. Brevity is best achieved by using words that express an idea simply and directly.

Timing and Relevance. Timing is critical to the reception of a message. For example, the nurse should not explain the risks of surgery if a client is crying in pain. Even though a message is clear, poor timing can prevent it from being accurately received. Therefore the nurse must be sensitive to the appropriate time for discussions with clients. Often the best time for interaction is when a client expresses an interest in communicating. By asking a simple question such as, "Would you like to talk about your surgery?" the nurse can avoid wasting time and energy if the client does not feel like talking.

Furthermore, a person is more likely to communicate when a message is relevant. For example, when a client is facing open-heart surgery the next day, a discussion of the risks of cigarette smoking has less relevance than a review of preoperative procedures.

Nonverbal Communication

Nonverbal communication is the exchange of a message without using words. People communicate nonverbally in every face-to-face meeting. Nonverbal communication is considered a more accurate description of true feelings because one has less control over nonverbal reactions (Shives, 1990). Gestures impart meanings that are often more significant than words. Nonverbal messages help people judge the reliability of verbal messages. Nonverbal and verbal communication are interrelated. Nonverbal cues add meaning to the verbal communication (Table 13-1).

A nurse must be aware of verbal and nonverbal messages sent to clients. The perception and interpretation of a client's nonverbal cues require sensing the client's intentions while communicating. For example, a client who says she feels fine but grimaces with each movement and cradles her side communicates two different messages. Nonverbal messages are usually more subtle than verbal messages. Becoming an astute observer of nonverbal behavior requires time and practice.

Because nurses often interact with clients and families, they must be sure that nonverbal and verbal messages match. Any conflict arising from a mismatch can threaten the nurse-client relationship. For example, a nurse who says a client will feel better but simultaneously reveals an expression of doubt will not relieve the client's anxieties. The client's acceptance of the nurse as a professional may depend on the manner in which the nurse presents a professional and caring image.

Metacommunication. Metacommunication is a message within a message that conveys a sender's attitude toward the self and the message and the attitudes, feelings, and intentions toward the listener. It can be an explicit statement (verbal) or an implicit demonstration of feelings (nonverbal). For example, the client states to the nurse following reconstructive surgery to the face, "this scar does not look as bad as I thought it would look." The nurse notes the client is teary-eyed and appears apprehensive. The nurse should try to further explore with the client his/her feelings or concerns as appropriate.

Appearance. A person's appearance is one of the first things noticed during an interpersonal encounter. Physical characteristics, the manner of dress and grooming, and the presence of jewelry provide clues to physical well-being, personality, social status, occupation, religion, culture, and self-concept. Lalli-Ascosi (1990) found that 84% of a person's first impression of another is based on appearance. No established standards indicate good health for physical characteristics. However, nurses learn to observe weight, energy level, or physical deformity to assess general health status. Any sudden change in appearance can communicate onset of disease.

Physical appearance often leads to initial impressions about a person's self-concept. Unfortunately, stereo-

table 13-1

RELATIONSHIPS BETWEEN VERBAL AND NONVERBAL COMMUNICAITON

Relationship	Example
Repeating: verbal and nonverbal cues saying same thing but in different ways	When mother describes how tall her son is, she also holds her hands at some distance above floor equal to child's height.
Contradicting: verbal and nonverbal cues conveying different messages	Nurse tells client that obtaining blood specimen "won't hurt a bit," but sarcastic grin delivers different message.
Complementing: nonverbal messages adding to verbal messages	Client says she is afraid to be admitted to hospital, and her anxious expression and trembling hands leave little doubt of fear.
Accenting: nonverbal cues emphasizing verbal statements	Wave of hand while saying hello accentuates word spoken.
Relating and regulating statements: nonverbal cues indicating when to begin or stop talking	Client who continually opens and closes her mouth briefly as her physician is talking is seeking opportunity to speak.
Substituting: nonverbal cue being used instead of words	Nurse nods vigorously to show approval of client's decision.

typed views regarding the characteristics of the "perfect body" influence the image body features communicate. The nurse should assess the importance physical appearance holds for any client undergoing surgery or illness that threatens loss of body parts or body function.

The nurse's physical appearance influences the client's perception of care. Each client has a preconceived image of a nurse. Although the traditional white uniform is not a reflection of the nurse's abilities, it may become more difficult to establish a sense of trust and reliability if the nurse fails to meet the clients' image. Professional nurses today wear uniforms, scrubsuits, and laboratory coats, as well as street clothes, to perform duties. A professional appearance conveys competence.

Posture and Gait. The way people sit, stand, and move is a visible form of self-expression. Posture and gait reflect emotions, self-concept, and degree of health. An erect posture and a quick, purposeful gait communicate a sense of well-being and assuredness. A slumped posture and slow, shuffling gait may indicate depression or discomfort. Leaning forward or toward a person conveys attention. Leaning backward in a more relaxed manner may show less interest or caution.

Nurses can collect useful information by observing clients' posture and gait. Specific illnesses cause identifiable gaits, such as the shuffling gait in parkinsonism. Gait may be altered by factors such as pain, medications, fractures, and emotional depression. Gait and posture cannot be the sole basis for a diagnostic analysis, but they provide important clues regarding well-being.

Facial Expression. The face is a rich source of communication. As the most expressive part of the body, it supplies overt and subtle cues that assist in the interpretation of messages. Studies have shown the face reveals the six primary emotions of surprise, fear, anger, disgust, happiness, and sadness (Knapp, 1978).

Facial expressions often become the basis for important judgments by the listener. However, because of the diversity in facial expressions, the meaning may be difficult to judge. Such expressions may reveal, contradict, or suppress true emotions. People are often unaware of the messages their expressions convey. Providing clear feedback helps to lessen confusion created by conflicting messages and expressions. When facial expressions fail to reveal clear messages, verbal feedback should be sought to be sure of the speaker's intent. For example, nurses are frequently scrutinized by clients. Consider the impact a nurse's facial expression might have on a client who asks, "Am I going to die?" The slightest change of expression of the eyes, lips, or face can reveal the nurse's true feelings. It is difficult to control all facial expressions. However, the nurse should be aware of expressions revealed to a client.

Eye Contact. Eye contact ordinarily signals a willingness to communicate. By maintaining eye contact during a conversation, the people involved communicate respect for one another and a willingness to listen. Maintaining eye contact also allows one to become a close observer of another. A lack of eye contact indicates anxiety, defensiveness, and a discomfort and lack of confidence in communicating. In some cultures, eye contact is considered intrusive, a threat, or harmful in other ways and therefore avoided.

Eye contact is an important part of facial expressions. Eye movements communicate feelings and emotions. Wide eyes are associated with frankness, terror, and naivete, whereas downward glances reflect modesty.

Raised upper eyelids reveal displeasure, and a constant stare is frequently associated with hatred and coldness. Some suggest that the level at which eye contact occurs significantly influences communication. The nurse should avoid looking down at a client. The nurse appears less dominant and threatening when sitting across from the client at the same eye level.

Gestures. A salute, a thumb pointed up in the air, and the tapping of a foot are gestures. In gesturing, the hands and feet emphasize, punctuate, and clarify the spoken word.

Gestures alone may reveal specific meanings, or they may create messages with other communication cues. A finger pointed toward a person may communicate several meanings, but when the pointed finger is accompanied by a frown and a stern tone of voice, the gesture becomes a sign of accusation or threat. A nurse views gestures as a part of the total pattern of communication. A hand held lightly over the abdomen does not convey the same message that a grimace, bent posture, and hand on the abdomen do when expressing pain. Gestures combine with expressions and other nonverbal cues to create specific messages.

Touch. Touch is a personal form of communication. People must be in close proximity when touch is used. Because touch is more spontaneous than verbal communication, it generally seems more authentic. Many messages such as affection, emotional support, encouragement, tenderness, and personal attention are conveyed through touch. Touch is an important part of the nurse-client relationship, but it must be used with discrimination because strong social and cultural norms govern its use. Many people mistakenly perceive touch as having only sexual implications.

Nurses rely on touch when carrying out interventions. They can perform intentional, comforting touch during activities such as stroking a client's shoulder or holding a client's hands (Mulaik, et al., 1991). Touch may also occur during activities such as physical assessments, giving baths, turning, and assisting with dressing. The nurse unaccustomed to touching or being touched may feel uncomfortable when performing interventions.

Similarly, the client who assumes the sick role must permit closer physical contact than is normally tolerated. Illness places a client in a dependent role that calls for closer interpersonal contact. The nurse should remain sensitive to the client's feelings about touching. If the client shies away from touch or refuses to hold the nurse's hand during an episode of pain, the client is probably uncomfortable with being touched. Finally, touch can be a useful therapeutic tool. Holding the hand of a grieving client can often convey understanding better than words or other gestures. Nurses must be sure to use touch purposefully during interactions. Although touch can help a client, its use must always be clearly understood and accepted (Vortherms, 1991).

Sounds. Sighs, moans, or episodes of crying also communicate feelings and thoughts. Combined with other nonverbal forms of communication, sounds can help to send clear messages. Sounds can be interpreted in several ways. For example, moaning can convey pleasure or suffering. When communicating with clients, the nurse observes all nonverbal messages to interpret messages accurately.

Space and Territoriality. **Territoriality** is the drive to gain, maintain, and defend one's exclusive right to space (Pluckhan, 1978). During social interaction, people consciously maintain distance between themselves. Personal space is invisible, individual, and mobile; it goes with a person. Territory can be separated and made visible to others, such as a fenced-in yard, a towel on the beach, or the bed in a hospital room. Personal space threatened by intrusion elicits a defensive response, preventing effective communication. Nurses frequently work with clients in situations in which space and territory are important factors. As in the case of touch, the distance separating nurse from client must be judged by the nature of the situation. Giving mouth-to-mouth resuscitation, holding a crying infant, and helping an incontinent client with toileting require an intimate distance between nurse and client. Murray (1991) describes the **intimate zone** as 0 to 18 inches. The client receiving care is sensitive about how the nurse uses distance. The nurse must convey confidence and gentleness.

As the distance between them becomes greater, the client and nurse feel more at ease. Greater flexibility occurs when intimate contact is not required. Sitting with a client is an example of a nursing measure in which the **personal zone** (18 inches to 4 feet) provides the closeness needed in interpersonal relationships. Increasing the physical zone makes it easier for the client and nurse to communicate because the nurse's actions and appearance become less imposing. **Social zone** (4 to 12 feet) is needed when dealing with groups of people. Making rounds with physicians is an example of such a group interaction. Communication is less threatening than with intimate or personal zones because an intimate sharing of thoughts and feelings is generally not required.

Public zone is 12 feet and greater. It is primarily used for public speaking.

COMMUNICATION: THE ART OF NURSING

Communication is an art in action. Nursing is a process of social interaction whereby nurses bring about posi-

COMMUNICATION FUNCTIONS IN NURSING

INFORMATION

Gathering assessment information on which to base diagnosis and decision making
Using methods to provide information regarding medications, procedures, etc., that promote client understanding, retention, and comprehension

INFLUENCE

Using communication techniques when helping clients to change attitudes, beliefs, and actions

COMFORTING

Interacting with clients to provide reassurance, support, and comfort
Reducing a client's uncertainty during stressful times to alleviate or moderate emotional distress

RELATIONAL

Interacting to define, control, and modify the relationship between nurse and client
Establishing, maintaining, repairing, and ending relationships
Establishing a collaborative provider-client relationship*

IDENTITY

Establishing self-identities to present oneself in ways that build credibility and produce friendliness, respect, and nurturing
Presenting oneself in way that reflects competency

*Data from Barsky AJ et al: Evaluating the interview in primary care medicine, *Soc Sci Med* 14a:653, 1980; and Kim HS: Collaborative decision making in nursing practice: a theoretical framework. In Chinn PL, editor: *Advances in nursing theory development,* London, 1983, Aspen Publishers.

COMMUNICATION THROUGH THE NURSING PROCESS

ASSESSMENT

Interviewing and history taking
Giving a physical examination (use of visual, auditory, tactile channels)
Observing nonverbal behavior
Reviewing medical records, literature, and diagnostic tests

NURSING DIAGNOSIS

Analyzing assessment findings
Discussing health care needs and priorities with client and family

PLANNING

Writing care plans
Making health team referrals
Initiating health team planning sessions
Discussing methods of implementation with client and family

IMPLEMENTATION

Discussing care with other health professionals
Teaching therapies to client
Providing therapeutic support
Contacting other health resources
Recording client's progress in care plan and nurse's notes

EVALUATION

Acquiring verbal and nonverbal feedback
Writing results of expected outcomes
Updating written plan of care
Explaining revisions of plan to clients

tive changes in clients' health status as a result of therapeutic communication (Kasch, 1986). When caring for clients, nurses act intentionally and purposefully. Through communication a nurse and client come to an agreement about how to successfully meet the client's goals of care such as the ability to interact with family or to communicate more clearly. According to Kasch (1986), the nurse is a communication strategist who controls interpersonal behavior in ways to enhance the chances of accomplishing goals. A nurse strives to meet a client's communication needs through a variety of functions (see box above). These functions are a part of the ongoing nursing process. Communication skills are integrated throughout the nursing process (see box above, right).

Communication Through the Nursing Process

Assessment calls for collecting information from many sources and through several modes of communication. When making nursing diagnoses, the nurse uses communication skills to involve the client, family, and health care professionals in identifying health care needs and determining priorities of nursing care. When developing a care plan, the nurse interacts with clients to determine their preferences for the methods of delivering care. During implementation, communication skills are required so the nurse can attend to the client's physical and psychosocial needs. Nurses also communicate with clients to evaluate the outcomes of nursing care. Without communication the nurse is unable to determine whether implementation was successful. Evaluation

THERAPEUTIC COMMUNICATION TECHNIQUES

PROMOTING EFFECTIVE COMMUNICATION

Maintaining silence. Silence can help the nurse and client to organize thoughts. It also enables the nurse to observe the client more closely.

Listening attentively. Attentive listening allows a person to understand an entire message conveyed verbally and nonverbally. It also facilitates trust. To listen attentively, face the client, maintain eye contact, assume a relaxed posture, lean forward, and nod in acknowledgment to give feedback.

Conveying acceptance. Acceptance means not being judgmental. Acceptance is not synonymous with agreement. It is a willingness to hear a message. A person conveys acceptance through positive feedback, making sure verbal and nonverbal cues match, and avoiding argument.

Asking related questions. Questioning is a direct method of communicating. Asking related questions allows the client to give information logically. Open-ended questions are useful for eliciting more information about a subject. Such questions cannot be answered with "yes" or "no."

Paraphrasing. Paraphrasing or restating the client's message in the nurse's own words sends feedback to the client that information has been accurately received.

Clarifying. Clarifying helps to retain important information. Using examples can clarify abstract ideas. The nurse can try to repeat a message or ask the client to restate it.

Focusing. When a discussion becomes vague or ill-defined, focusing directs conversation to a specific topic or issue. It limits the area of discussion to which the client can respond. The nurse seeks meaning in the client's message.

Stating observations. Describing a client's observed behavior can provide feedback about whether an intended message was received. It can clarify conflicts between verbal and nonverbal cues.

Offering information. Offering information provides a client with relevant data and prevents one-sided conversations. It is useful for health teaching and helps in decision making.

Summarizing. Summarizing is a concise review of main ideas from a discussion. It sets the tone for further interactions. By reviewing a conversation, the participants can focus on key issues and add relevant information previously deleted.

Offering oneself. By expressing a willingness to be available, even though a client may not verbalize or state a need, the nurse shows a caring attitude.

Giving general leads. Prompting a client to continue a discussion in the direction it is taking shows the nurse's interest in hearing more. It indicates the nurse is following the discussion.

INHIBITING EFFECTIVE COMMUNICATION

Giving an opinion. Giving an opinion takes decision making away from the client. It inhibits spontaneity, stalls problem solving, and creates doubt. If offering suggestions, the nurse should stress that they are only options.

Offering false reassurance. Offering false reassurance can do more harm than good. False reassurance may allow the nurse to promise something that will not occur or is unrealistic.

Being defensive. Defensiveness in the face of criticism implies the client has no right to an opinion. The client's concerns often become ignored. Attentive listening helps the client to open up but does not imply agreement.

Showing approval or disapproval. Showing approval or disapproval is judgmental and may halt a conversation. It inhibits the ability to share ideas and make decisions independently. Disapproval can indicate rejection.

Asking why. Asking why may imply an accusation. It can cause resentment, insecurity, and mistrust. If additional information is needed, the nurse can phrase a question to avoid use of "why."

Changing the subject inappropriately. Changing the subject inappropriately is rude and shows a lack of empathy. It stalls communication. The client may then give incomplete or inadequate information.

Forming communication barriers. Forming communication barriers by inadvertently saying something that blocks a client's communication can break down communication. By acknowledging the mistake, the nurse can start the communication process anew.

may reveal the need to revise the care plan. The nurse also discusses with the client the rationale for any proposed therapeutic changes.

During all steps of the nursing process, the nurse uses communication skills, constantly gathering, analyzing, and transmitting information. The nursing process is a reliable framework for delivering comprehensive care, but the process does not work unless the nurse masters the art of therapeutic communication.

THERAPEUTIC COMMUNICATION

Beginning nursing students are frequently told to "get to know your clients" when they begin to care for them. This is not an easy task, and it frequently hinders effective relationships. A nurse cannot "get to know" clients without being able to appreciate their uniqueness. Without knowing these needs, a nurse is unable to effectively diagnose responses to illness and initiate actions.

Through **therapeutic communication** the nurse develops a working, functional relationship with clients and fulfills the purposes of the nursing process (see box on p. 211).

Social Interaction

The first attempt at communicating with a client usually results in a brief social interaction. The messages conveyed are superficial in that neither the nurse nor the client discusses deeply personal matters. Any interpersonal exchange tends to be based on intuitive, unthinking, and automatic responses. A superficial interaction makes the participants feel safe because the discussion holds no hidden intent for personal disclosures.

A nurse often uses the pattern of social interaction at the beginning of a conversation to establish a closer relationship of trust. For example, the nurse might greet a client by saying, "Good morning, Mrs. Sears, it's nice to see you today," or "Hi, Mr. Simpson, how do you like the great weather we're having?"

The skillful nurse does not allow social interaction to dominate a conversation but maintains a congenial and warm style of communicating to elicit the client's trust. The nurse's goal is to help the client to feel comfortable in sharing attitudes and feelings.

Informational Interaction

The nurse uses informational interaction to give information to and to gather information about clients. For example, briefly reviewing the contents of a teaching booklet, gathering a client's medical history, or reviewing hospital visitation rules are informational interactions. However, this approach can be dehumanizing if it is the only pattern of communication used. Informational interaction does not allow the nurse or client to establish a more meaningful relationship. The nurse may tend to ignore the client as a unique person.

Developing a Helping Relationship

The nurse-client relationship is more than a partnership. Travelbee (1971) calls it a human-to-human relationship. The titles of *nurse* and *client* disappear as each person tries to better understand one another. King (1971) calls the nurse-client relationship "learning experiences whereby two people interact to face an immediate health problem, to share, if possible, in resolving it, and to discover ways to adapt to the situation."

The nurse uses interpersonal communication skills to develop a relationship that will lead to understanding the client as a total person. The relationship is therapeutic, promoting a psychological climate that facilitates positive change and growth. The relationship also focuses on the primary goal of meeting the client's needs.

Creating a therapeutic environment depends on the nurse's ability to provide physical and psychosocial comfort for the client. The nurse should make sure the client's physiological needs are satisfied. For example, the nurse positions the client so that the client can breathe normally and sleep comfortably without interruption. The nurse's actions are not delivered without concern for the client's preferences. The nurse and client mutually determine how the client's needs will be met (see case study below).

A helping relationship between nurse and client does not just happen. It is built with care as the nurse logically uses therapeutic communication techniques.

CASE STUDY
Forming a Helping Relationship

Mrs. Greer is a 63-year-old widow hospitalized for cancer of the lung. She makes frequent requests for pain medication before a dose is due. When a nurse delivers the medication, Mrs. Greer criticizes her for being late. Nothing the nurses do seems to satisfy Mrs. Greer.

Ms. Edwards has cared for Mrs. Greer for 2 days. She could easily be tired of Mrs. Greer but chooses to be assigned to her for another day. Ms. Edwards enters her client's room and begins to straighten out the bed linen. Ms. Edwards asks, "Are you comfortable in that position, Mrs. Greer? Would you like pain medication now?" Mrs. Greer accepts the offer of the medication and begins to relax in Ms. Edwards' presence. The nurse helps Mrs. Greer to assume a more comfortable position on her side.

After the client's pain has diminished, Ms. Edwards sits by her bed and says, "I know you've been experiencing much discomfort. Over the past few days we have not always been able to help you feel better. Can you help me to know the best way to make you feel comfortable?" Mrs. Greer and Ms. Edwards decide on the following comfort measures:

1. When socializing with Mrs. Greer, help her to change positions.
2. At the beginning of each shift, talk to Mrs. Greer about her comfort measure for the next shift.
3. Spend extra time (10 to 15 minutes) in Mrs. Greer's room at mealtime, visiting hours, and before bedtime.

Ms. Edwards' efforts at improving Mrs. Greer's comfort make her more amenable to a discussion of her problems. Ms. Edwards learns of Mrs. Greer's great fear of death. She has made frequent requests of the nurses to avoid feeling lonely. By discussing the nature of Mrs. Greer's fears, both are able to find ways to minimize Mrs. Greer's loneliness. Ms. Edwards' endeavor to show a real concern for Mrs. Greer leads to helpful solutions to her problems.

Dimensions of the Helping Relationship. Characteristics of any helping relationship are trust, empathy, caring, and autonomy and mutuality (Sundeen, et al., 1989). These are essential if the nurse is to establish positive and supportive relationships with clients.

TRUST. Travelbee (1971) defines trust as "the assured belief that other individuals are capable of assisting in times of distress and will probably do so." Unless clients believe a nurse wishes to care for their needs, a trusting relationship cannot develop. Trust fosters open, therapeutic communication. Previous experiences may affect a client's willingness to trust a nurse. Lack of previous health care experience or a traumatic experience causes clients to hesitate in trusting care givers. To foster trust the nurse acts consistently, reliably, and competently. Honesty also builds trust. Without trust, a nurse-client relationship will not progress beyond social interaction and providing superficial care.

EMPATHY. **Empathy** is the ability to understand and accept the life of another person and to accurately perceive feelings. It is a fair, sensitive, and objective look at another person's experiences. In contrast, sympathy is the inclination to think or feel as another person does. Sympathy is a subjective look at another person's world that prevents a clear perspective of all sides of the issues confronting that person.

Empathy tends to depend on similarities of experiences between the persons communicating. A nurse can empathize more easily with the client in pain if the nurse has also experienced pain. Because it is difficult to empathize unless one has a similar experience or situation with which to relate, nurses cannot be empathetic in all situations. Nevertheless, empathy is a key to communicating concern and support for a client.

A nurse can accurately empathize by looking at the world from the client's perspective and getting a feeling for the client's world. The nurse communicates an understanding of the client's expressions about the self. A nurse who empathizes with another person avoids impulsive judgments about that person and is more likely to be sensitive and caring. Reflecting and restating are common communication skills used with empathy (see case study at right).

In contrast to empathy, sympathy is the concern, sorrow, or pity shown by the nurse for the client in which the needs of the client are seen as the nurse's needs. Sympathy has a place in human relationships. Sharing with another feels good, creates a bond, and minimizes differences. Sundeen, et al. (1989) claim this poses a difficulty in the helping relationship because helpers who share the needs of the client may be unable to help the client select realistic solutions for problems.

Social scientists and nurse researchers are examining the roles and uses of empathy in the nurse-client relationship. Empathy is still something of a controversial concept (Pike, 1990).

CARING. Caring is having a positive regard for another person. It is basic to a helping relationship. It is also the foundation of nursing as a human science (Watson, 1979). Gaut has identified three categories of meaning for the concept of caring: attention to or concern for the client; responsibility for the client; and regard, fondness, or attachment to a client (Chipman, 1991). Caring is more than simply having concern for another person. For caring to influence a nurse's practice, it must be integrated as a standard of performance in all care activities.

Most clients directly or indirectly express a need for care at some time. A nurse shows caring by accepting clients for themselves and respecting them as individuals. It must be applied to all persons in similar circumstances. When cared for, clients feel secure in threatening or anxiety-producing situations. Caring also promotes trust. Touching is an effective way for nurses to communicate care.

AUTONOMY AND MUTUALITY. Autonomy refers to an ability to be self-directed. Mutuality involves sharing with another. These are important in any helping relationship. The nurse and client work as a team. Both participate in the care process. Nurses offer clients opportunities to make decisions, even if it is as simple as choosing bath time. As a client becomes more indepen-

CASE STUDY
Empathy

Ms. Vincent has been caring for Mr. Pierce since his emergency admission to the hospital 2 days before. Mr. Pierce is scheduled to have open-heart surgery the next day. The nurse has learned that the 46-year-old client is a father with three teenage children and has never undergone surgery before. Ms. Vincent enters the client's room, makes eye contact with him, and sits in the chair beside his bed. The following conversation occurs:

Ms. Vincent: Hello, Mr. Pierce. You look as though you're rather deep in thought.

Mr. Pierce: Oh, I suppose I am. I just can't keep from worrying about tomorrow.

Ms. Vincent: You're worried about tomorrow's surgery? I imagine you have a lot of questions.

Mr. Pierce: Yes, I'd like to know more.

Ms. Vincent could easily have avoided Mr. Pierce's true concerns and even attempted to change the subject. An unhelpful remark would be, "Don't worry about tomorrow, Mr. Pierce. Would you like me to get you something to read?" Such a comment would ignore Mr. Pierce's fears about impending surgery and prevent the development of a meaningful relationship between nurse and client. Ms. Vincent moves the conversation forward to learn more about Mr. Pierce and his concerns.

dent, the nurse offers more opportunities for decision making. The nurse can also promote autonomy by acting as an advocate by keeping clients informed of health care alternatives and to give support in decision making. By advocacy and client teaching, the nurse works with the client to achieve and maintain an optimal level of wellness.

Phases of a Helping Relationship. The helping relationship is established and maintained by the professional nurse. The relationship is reciprocal. The nurse and the client relate to each other as they progress through the phases that eventually lead to therapeutic rapport. A helping relationship progresses over time as the nurse and client interact while the nurse carries out the nursing process, but the helping relationship is not the same as the nursing process. The nursing process is a series of steps the nurse takes to manage a client's health problems. A helping relationship is a bond between nurse and client that allows the nurse to be more effective in carrying out the nursing process. The nurse is responsible for directing the client through the phases of a helping relationship to ensure the client's needs are met.

Chapter 1 discusses the interview as a method for obtaining a nursing health history and identifying changes in level of wellness and living patterns. Although the phases of an interview and of a helping relationship are similar, the communication patterns are different. The interview can initiate a nurse-client relationship because it may be the first encounter between them. However, the interview is not the mechanism for maintaining a long-term therapeutic relationship. A helping relationship goes beyond the scope of an interview to establish a rapport between the nurse and client that is the basis for an ongoing resolution of the client's health problems. The case studies provide examples of therapeutic communication through all phases of the helping relationship.

PREINTERACTION PHASE. Before meeting a client, the nurse reviews information from the medical and nursing history, as well as data available from other care givers. During this review, the nurse thinks about concerns or issues that may arise during the nurse-client interaction. For example, before entering a relationship with a young cancer client, the nurse considers how the client is coping and whether death may be discussed. During the preinteraction phase, the nurse plans an approach and reviews personal values or attitudes. This process helps to avoid stereotyping clients.

The nurse also chooses a location and setting for the first meeting. A comfortable, private, quiet, and attractive setting fosters interpersonal interaction. In the home this may be the client's living room. In a clinic, it may be a quiet interview room. The nurse also plans enough time for the discussion.

ORIENTATION. The orientation phase begins when the nurse and client first meet. This phase sets the tone for the remainder of the nurse-client relationship. The relationship in the orientation phase is superficial and is often marked by uncertainty and exploration.

During any initial encounter, both participants closely observe each other. The nurse and client make inferences and form judgments about the content of messages and behaviors. Therapeutic communication is more effective if the nurse is empathetic, warm, and caring.

The nurse and client meet and identify each other by name. It is wise to address the client formally using the client's last name at first, for example, "Good morning, Mr. Spencer. My name is Ms. Tucker. I am a student nurse assigned to take care of you today." Later, the client may ask the nurse to be more informal.

Failure of the nurse to give a name can create uncertainty because the client often encounters many personnel from several agencies or departments when seeking health care. It can unintentionally convey lack of commitment or caring by the nurse.

At the beginning of the relationship, neither person is able to perceive the other's uniqueness. The nurse perceives a client who has come to the health care agency or institution as someone with a health problem. The client perceives the nurse as one of many health care professionals whose job is to help. Engaging in a social interaction initially helps the nurse and client to become relaxed in conversing (see box below).

TESTING. The client often tests the nurse during the orientation phase of a relationship because of the client's difficulty in acknowledging the need for help, fear of expressing true feelings, and anxiety over facing the need to change. The nurse who is aware of the client's doubts and concerns attempts to show confidence and

CASE STUDY

Placing the Client at Ease

Nurse: It certainly is a lovely day, Mrs. Spier.

Client: Yes, isn't it? If I were home and feeling better, I'd be planting my garden.

Nurse: You're a gardener? What types of plants do you enjoy growing?

Client: Oh, a little of everything. I like some tomatoes, lettuce, radishes, and maybe some squash.

The nurse directs the conversation so that she and Mrs. Spier feel at ease. No purpose would have been served if the nurse had rushed into a therapeutically oriented discussion with Mrs. Spier feeling uncomfortable. The nurse and Mrs. Spier can come to know one another better and begin to develop a meaningful relationship if the social interaction is directed properly.

CASE STUDY
Testing

Mr. Miles is a 52-year-old businessman who has been hospitalized for treatment of a bleeding stomach ulcer. He is very independent and is accustomed to making decisions for himself. Ms. Rains, the nurse, enters the client's room.

Ms. Rains: Good morning, Mr. Miles. My name is Ms. Rains and I will be caring for you today.

Mr. Miles: You will, huh? Tell me, how long have you been a nurse?

Ms. Rains: About 2 years. I've worked in this hospital since graduating from nursing school.

Mr. Miles: Well, you won't have to worry about me. I can take care of myself.

Ms. Rains: I can imagine it's frustrating to be very independent one minute and then suddenly become ill and feel as though everyone is telling you what to do.

Mr. Miles: You can say that again. I'm just not used to needing help.

Ms. Rains: Mr. Miles, I'm not here to take away your independence. There are a number of things I need to do for you, but there are also many things I want you to be able to do for yourself. Let me explain some of the procedures I will be doing.

Mr. Miles: OK, I appreciate that.

Ms. Rains recognizes Mr. Miles' attempt to test her competence. Mr. Miles is fearful of losing his independence. If Ms. Rains has had minimal experience in developing relationships with clients, she may feel the need to remain superficial and nondirective. The client will sense the nurse's superficiality during testing and avoid meaningful discussion. In Mr. Miles' case, Ms. Rains acknowledges concerns and acts to eliminate his fears.

competence. The nurse should not become defensive during testing but should be open and show a genuine interest in the client's concerns. The client may use silence to avoid communicating. The nurse can show a desire to help by explaining the actions taken and performing care smoothly (see box above).

Building trust. Trust is relying on someone without doubt or question. Confidence, dependability, and credibility are needed to build trust. It is not easy for a client to perceive the need for help or to ask for it. A client often trusts the nurse but is incapable of asking for assistance. Trust allows for effective communication as individuals become more open in expressing feelings and thoughts.

Trusting another person involves risk. The client who begins to share feelings and attitudes with the nurse becomes vulnerable. The client must be comfortable in revealing personal information. The nurse who is insecure with clients may choose superficial methods to build trust. These might include sharing secrets or encouraging the client to establish the relationship on a first name basis. Some clients accept such behaviors, but others may resent being treated differently. Instead of enjoying the nurse's extra attention, they become distrustful.

Genuine caring is a powerful method for acquiring

CASE STUDY
Building Trust

Mr. Squires: I've been home now for 4 days and I just don't know what to do.

Ms. Ramsey: You're obviously upset. Tell me what the problem is. I'd like to help.

Mr. Squires: The doctor put me on that new diet. It seemed easy in the hospital, but I'm afraid I'm not eating right.

Ms. Ramsey: You've improved so much since your hospitalization. Let's sit down together and see what kinds of foods you should eat. Then we'll look at the types of foods you like that are allowed in your new diet.

Mr. Squires begins to trust Ms. Ramsey who shows a willingness to help, not out of duty but out of a desire to meet his needs.

Mr. Squires: You shouldn't have to go to so much trouble for me.

Ms. Ramsey: You're not causing me trouble at all. An important part of my job is to help you stay healthy. If I can help you understand your diet better, I'll feel I did my job.

Mr. Squires: Well, if I can learn to fix and eat the right foods, my doctor says I may stay out of the hospital longer this time.

Ms. Ramsey: Your doctor is right. Now let's go over what you know so far.

Another element that helps establish trust is recognizing Mr. Squires' individuality. He realizes that Ms. Ramsey respects him as a unique person.

Mr. Squires: The doctor said I should eat more vegetables and fruits. I really don't like many vegetables.

Ms. Ramsey: Well, let's make a list of what you do like. You know there are different ways to prepare the same kinds of foods. If you're able to eat the things you like, you'll be able to follow the diet more easily.

Mr. Squires: That sounds good. Before I left the hospital, I didn't think I would have much choice in what I ate.

Ms. Ramsey: Sure you do. I'll show you that you can have a lot of variety in your diet and even enjoy it. It's important that the diet be planned for you and not someone else.

Trust develops on a foundation of caring. Ms. Ramsey's time, patience, and conscientiousness show her concern for Mr. Squires' welfare.

the client's trust. The nurse shows sensitivity and understanding of the client's needs. Expressing concern is one way to establish trust. By showing concern the nurse encourages the client's growth and progress (see box on p. 215).

Identifying problems and goals. During the initial encounter with the client, the nurse begins assessing the client's health status. Through observations and interaction, the nurse makes conclusions. The client's health problems may be simple, such as moving without discomfort, choosing foods that will be easily tolerated, or getting out of bed safely. The relationship with the client is strengthened if the nurse discovers what problems are important to the client (see box below). Also, the client may be unable to recognize problems. During the orientation phase, the nurse directs the client toward an awareness of problems, a focus on the nature of the problems, and exploring potential solutions. As problems are identified, the nurse and client mutually set goals. When the client is able to participate in goal setting and see the desired benefits, nursing interventions are more effective.

Identifying problems uses the techniques of attentive listening, open-ended questioning, paraphrasing, and clarifying. Initially the nurse avoids identifying a large number of actual or potential problems. Bombarding the client with too many questions can cause emotional and physical fatigue. Also, it makes the client less trusting and more suspicious of the nurse's intentions. Limiting problem identification facilitates the client's understanding of the client's and nurse's roles.

Clarifying roles. After a helping relationship is initiated, the roles of the nurse and client must be clarified. Clarification occurs through sharing information. This includes the nurse's assessment of the client's immediate needs, the client's perception of those needs, the times for nursing care measures, and ways the client can participate in this care. The helping relationship requires participation from both parties, but the nurse assumes leadership. Leadership does not mean control in the manipulative sense. Instead, the nurse takes the initiative in determining the client's point of view. The client assumes a role as receiver of care but also assumes an ongoing role as collaborator and participant in care.

Forming contracts. After goals and roles are clearly defined, the nurse establishes a contract with the client. Generally, this involves a brief verbal interchange, including location, frequency, and length of contacts and duration of the relationship. The nurse should not present the contract in an overly formal way but should outline a contractual agreement in a way that clarifies the client's and nurse's expectations. The nurse thus informs the client of measures to facilitate progress toward health (see box below).

The nurse should let the client know when the relationship will be terminated. If the relationship is successful, the nurse and client frequently share close bonds of respect and concern. The closer the nurse and client become in working together, the more difficult it is to end the relationship. If the client can anticipate the length of the relationship, termination will be less stressful. A student nurse often spends time with only one or two clients, often resulting in close relationships. Clients must be prepared for the end of the student's

CASE STUDY
Identifying Problems and Goals

Mr. Sachs is a 58-year-old man who has suffered a partial paralysis of his right side. Mr. Sachs needs to regain function in his right hand to retain his job as a telephone repairman. He is also fearful of damage to his self-image. He feels deformed and unable to live normally again.

Mr. Sachs: So much has happened to me. I know I may never again be able to do the things I once enjoyed.

Nurse: I know it's a difficult time for you now, but there are many things we can do to help you regain normal function.

Mr. Sachs: But there are so many things wrong with me.

Nurse: Let's take one at a time. What is most important to you?

Mr. Sachs: If only I could use my hand.

Nurse: Your doctor has ordered some exercises to increase the strength in your hand. I'll show you how to do each one. Are you willing to try them?

Mr. Sachs: You bet I am. If only I could use my hand again to work.

Nurse: Let's start with some simple goals. First we'll help you gain strength in your fingers so you can grasp eating utensils, a comb, or a razor. After that we'll try some more strenuous exercises.

Mr. Sachs: OK, that sounds reasonable. Show me what I need to do.

CASE STUDY
Forming a Contract

Nurse: Mr. Reed, I'll be seeing you each morning for the next 3 days. After we practice your exercises together, I'd like you to do them on your own. Practice the exercises as often as you can without feeling pain or fatigue. On Friday, I'll introduce you to the nurse who will work with you over the weekend. I'll be sure she knows the types of exercises you're doing.

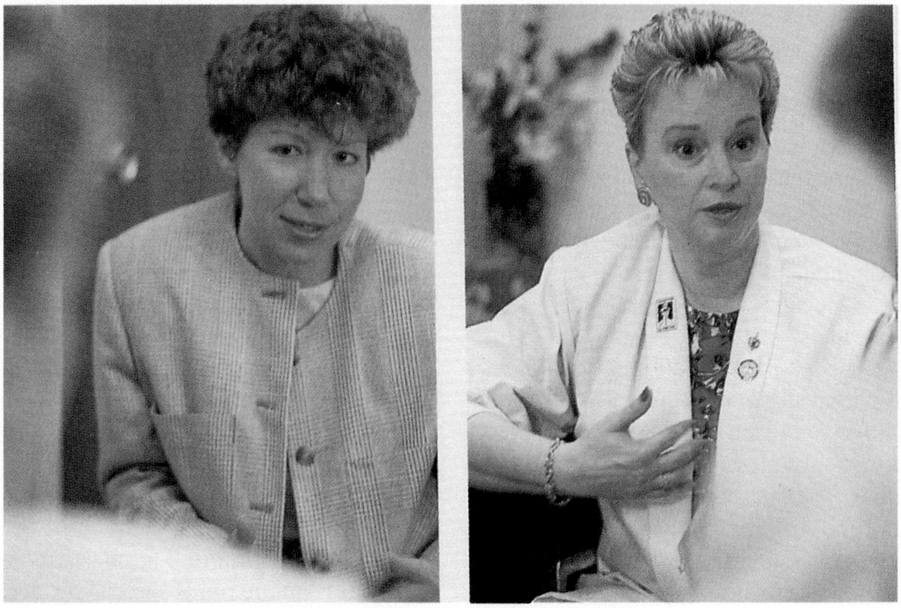

FIGURE 13-3 **A,** In a positive relationship, the client can communicate freely with the nurse. **B,** Nurse uses therapeutic communication skills to attend to the client's expressed needs.

clinical experience. Otherwise they may become angered or disappointed.

WORKING PHASE. During the working phase of a helping relationship, the nurse takes actions to meet the goals set with the client. The nurse uses therapeutic communication skills aimed at promoting successful interaction. The nurse and client work together. Changing a client's health status requires the nurse to perceive the client's personal goals and to help the client to set and attain goals.

In an effective nurse-client relationship, the client is able to openly express feelings about health status (Figure 13-3). The client participates in self-exploration and can discuss relevant issues. The nurse helps the client to understand changes in behavior or knowledge necessary to adapt to an improved level of health.

Sundeen, et al. (1989) describe three communication skills that help clients to gain better self-understanding (see box at right):

1. Confrontation. The nurse makes the client aware of inconsistencies in behavior or thoughts that interfere with self-understanding. The technique helps clients to recognize growth or deal with important issues.
2. Immediacy. The nurse focuses interaction on the present situation between nurse and client. The client learns to understand how interactions affect others. This involves drawing attention to the client's behavior or statements.
3. Self-disclosure. The nurse reveals personal experiences, thoughts, ideas, values, or feelings in con-

CASE STUDY

Communication Skills

CONFRONTATION

Ms. Perkins is a 60-year-old client with a history of obesity and high blood pressure. She has been returning to the clinic monthly for checkups:

Ms. Perkins: I feel frustrated and I'm tired of being fat.

Nurse: When I saw you last month you told me you had lost 10 pounds and your clothes fit better. I can tell the difference.

Ms. Perkins: You're right, but it takes so much time to lose weight. I just get down on myself.

IMMEDIACY

Nurse: As we've talked, you've seemed distant.

Client: Um-hm.

Nurse: Perhaps you are upset because I was not able to come talk with you as soon as I had promised.

SELF-DISCLOSURE

Ms. Wells' mother died just a month before. Since, she has had difficulty following her diet.

Nurse: This has been a difficult time for you.

Ms. Wells: It seems as though my world's collapsed.

Nurse: Three years ago I lost my mother. It was a very difficult time. I came to realize though that her death was a part of life and that she would want me to continue living life to its fullest.

text of the relationship. This is not therapy for the nurse. It shows the client that specific experiences can be understood.

If the working phase is successful, the client can act on ideas and feelings. This often requires risk, and the nurse must remain supportive. Clients must deal with success and failure as they make decisions and resolve problems. Any attempt at change should be within the client's abilities. Change becomes less threatening when clients express feelings about it and accept temporary setbacks. The nurse should encourage even the slightest progress.

Integrating communication with nursing actions. Nursing actions can generally be divided into physiological, psychological, and socioeconomic groups. Bradley and Edinberg (1990) categorize these three groups by their level of visibility. Physiological actions that attend to a client's physical needs, such as nutrition, elimination, and comfort, have high visibility. Most physiological actions are nonverbal and routinely performed. Traditionally, emphasis has been placed on a nurse's ability to perform physiological actions. The high visibility of such actions allows the client to recognize the nurse as an adept practitioner.

In contrast, psychological and socioeconomic nursing actions have low visibility. Psychological actions serve a client's emotional needs. Socioeconomic actions such as referring a client to a community health agency assist the client in adapting to a given environment. Low-visibility tasks are not readily observed or measured by others. Psychological and socioeconomic actions require cognitive and affective skills that are not routine and have traditionally led to less reward for the nurse.

Communication is important in performing high- and low-visibility tasks (Figure 13-4). Giving emotional support or educating the family requires effective communication as do basic nursing care procedures (see box below).

Termination. During the orientation phase, the nurse tells the client when to expect the conclusion of the relationship. The client should not be surprised by the termination. The nurse and client have remained aware of the goals of the relationship, and the client should be prepared to function effectively without the nurse's support. Termination can nonetheless be difficult and painful. The primary objective at the end of any helping relationship is a mutually planned and satisfying termination.

Evaluation of goal achievement. Vital to termination of a relationship is evaluating goals. The nurse encourages assessment of the appropriateness and out-

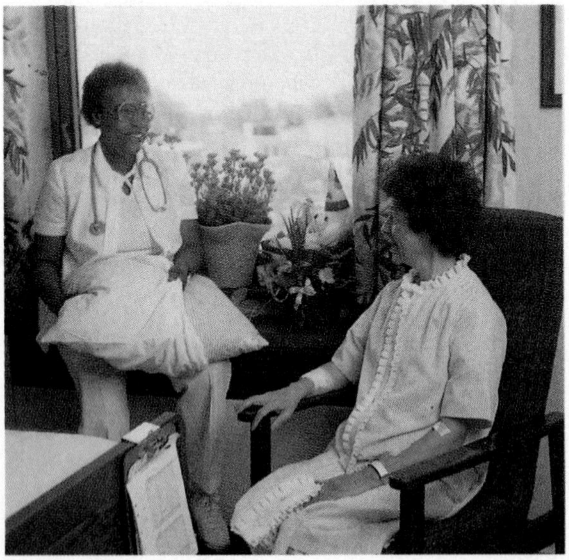

FIGURE 13-4 The nurse integrates therapeutic communication skills into all aspects of care.

CASE STUDY
Facilitating Nursing Care

The nurse, Ms. Thomas, silently enters Mr. Richards' room. She tells him, "It's time for your pain shot." He is mildly startled and grimaces as he turns to see Ms. Thomas. As Mr. Richards starts to ask a question, she quickly reaches for his arm and prepares to give the injection.

Another nurse, Mr. Ives, enters Mr. Richards' room and says, "I have that pain medication you requested. Are you still feeling uncomfortable?" He turns and replies, "Yes, my back feels like a knife went through it. Will the pain ever go away?" Mr. Ives lays the syringe on the table, sits down next to Mr. Richards, and says, "It's normal to have pain the first few days after surgery. Let me give you that shot and then I can show you how to move more carefully in bed to avoid worsening the pain."

Through communication, a nurse can convey the confidence, credibility, and knowledge that clients expect. In this example a few words of concern and reassurance (low-visibility communication skills) make receiving an injection more acceptable and encourage Mr. Richards to express his feelings.

Communication facilitates all nursing care measures. Integrating high- and low-visibility tasks allows Mr. Ives to accomplish several goals simultaneously. He quickly and efficiently assesses Mr. Richards' pain, provides a reassuring explanation, and demonstrates an alternative way of relieving pain. Therapeutic communication during high-visibility tasks increases the client's acceptance and understanding of procedures, lessens anxiety, and improves willingness to cooperate.

come of goals established (see case study below). Was there a mutual sense on the part of the nurse and client that goals of the relationship were met? Has the relationship facilitated achievement of goals within the nursing plan of care?

Separation. Depending on the nature of the relationship between nurse and client, the client may be anxious as termination nears. Ideally the client expresses feelings regarding termination. The nurse plans time to allow the client to share these concerns or fears.

If the client remains in the health care setting and the nurse is the one leaving, the client may feel abandoned. The nurse makes sure the client's care is uninterrupted, introducing the client to the new nurse who will be providing care. The nurse shares any information that might foster the development of a helping relationship between the new nurse and the client.

CASE STUDY
Evaluating Goals

Ms. Garner has worked with the client, Mr. Adams, during his 8-day stay in the hospital. Mr. Adams had surgery for the repair of a fractured leg. Together Ms. Garner and Mr. Adams set goals for his physical rehabilitation and eventual return home.

Ms. Garner: Well, Mr. Adams, your doctor has discharged you for tomorrow morning. How do you feel about going home?

Mr. Adams: Oh, I'll be glad to get out of here. My leg feels pretty good.

Ms. Garner: Do you feel comfortable walking with the crutches?

Mr. Adams: Yes, I do. As you suggested, I practiced climbing stairs quite a bit in physical therapy. As you know, I have five stairs to climb up to my front door. I can climb now without losing my balance.

Ms. Garner: You've also worked hard on learning to transfer from the bed and chair to a standing position with the crutches.

Mr. Adams: It's a lot easier now. All the practice you suggested helped. Because you've explained all of the right ways to hold the crutches, they feel like a natural part of me. I do hope I can get rid of them soon.

Ms. Garner: Well, it sounds like you're ready to leave. Continue your leg exercises as you've done them here and soon you won't need those crutches.

Mr. Adams: Thanks again for your help. I didn't think I'd ever be able to walk with these things, but now the crutches are no problem.

Ms. Garner and Mr. Adams experience satisfaction in meeting goals, particularly because the goals are mutually set. If goals are left unaccomplished, the reasons are examined and plans are made for attainment in the future. Mr. Adams has not achieved the ability to walk without his crutches. Ms. Garner encourages him to continue his exercise regimen so that he will become strong enough to walk independently.

NURSING PROCESS

Assessment

The assessment of a client's communication ability involves activities that systematically collect data, organize the data collected, and document the information that has been obtained. Information in this data base is obtained from the client and significant others. This information can be the first step in establishing a beneficial nurse/client relationship and the rapport needed for good communication (Doenges and Moorehouse, 1992). Assessment can begin with a review of factors that influence communication. The nurse must understand the client's developmental level, perceptions, emotions, cultural orientation, and knowledge before planning ways to promote communication. It may be difficult to assess all of these factors if a client has physical barriers to communication. Alternative communication methods such as a communication board, family, or friends may then become important for the nurse's assessment.

Physical and Psychological Barriers to Communication

A client may suffer physical or psychological alterations that impair communication. To speak spontaneously and clearly, a person must have an intact respiratory system, normal oral and nasal cavities, and a functioning

table 13-2

ASSESSMENT OF PHYSICAL COMMUNICATION BARRIERS

Speech and language mechanisms	Alterations affecting speech
Respiratory system	Extreme dyspnea (shortness of breath) Artificial airways: endotracheal tube or tracheostomy Laryngectomy (surgical removal of larynx)
Oral and nasal cavities	Cleft palate Loose-fitting dentures Neurological disease affecting articulation (parkinsonism)
Speech center	Aphasia related to cerebrovascular accident (stroke) or brain tumor
Auditory system	Conduction or nerve deafness

speech center. Normal reception of language requires an intact auditory system. The nurse assesses a child's ability to communicate, including the observation of sounds, gestures, and vocabulary. When an adult develops hearing problems, the ability to receive and understand messages is impaired. The medical history and physical assessment provide clues to the client's physical ability to communicate (Table 13-2).

The nurse should also consider whether clients are taking medications that impair speech or impair the ability to understand the message (such as antidepressants, neuroleptics, or sedatives). The nurse should be familiar with common side effects of such medications.

Some psychological illnesses such as psychosis or depression influence the ability to communicate. The client may demonstrate flight of ideas, constant verbalization of the same words or phrases, or a loose association of ideas. The nurse must isolate psychological causes of speech problems from possible neurological causes.

Nursing Diagnosis

The inability to communicate effectively influences a client's ability to express needs or react to the environment. Nursing diagnosis is a clinical judgement about individual, family, or community responses to actual and potential health problems/life problems. Success in accurately identifying the client's communication problem will ensure a correct nursing diagnosis. Defining characteristics must reveal the presence of a pattern. In the case of impaired verbal communication, the nurse must assess characteristics such as a client's inability to speak, find words, name words, identify objects, or speak in sentences. The diagnosis should focus on the cause of the communication disorder to provide the basis for selection of appropriate nursing interventions. The nurse may make additional diagnoses for clients who have difficulty in interacting with others. The client's difficulty of expression or change in communication patterns assists the nurse in formulating the diagnosis (see box above).

The nurse utilizes both objective and subjective information obtained from the assessment and clusters the identified findings to develop and support the nursing diagnosis. For example, the nurse may diagnose impaired verbal communication related to decreased circulation to the brain. To support this diagnosis, the nurse must verify certain assessment data such as history of a cerebrovascular accident, inability of the client to name words and identify objects. The correct related factor allows the selection and implementation of the correct nursing interventions. Decreased circulation to the brain implies the nurse will use therapies to assist a client with aphasia. If the nature of impaired communication is quite different and the related factor is cultural differences, the interventions are also very different.

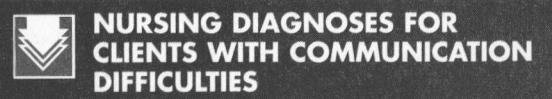

NURSING DIAGNOSES FOR CLIENTS WITH COMMUNICATION DIFFICULTIES

Communication, impaired verbal
Social interaction, impaired
Coping, family: potential for growth
Coping, ineffective family: compromised
Coping, ineffective individual
Powerlessness

Planning

As the nurse uses assessment data to formulate and support nursing diagnoses, the focus becomes directed to the appropriate actions that will effectively assist in addressing the identified problem or need. In planning, the nurse will begin to establish goals and expected outcomes of care and determine specific nursing interventions to assist in dealing with the client's communication difficulties. Consideration must be given to interventions and communication techniques appropriate for the client's age, cultural beliefs, and practices. Whenever possible, the nurse collaborates with the client, family, friends, other health care team members, and the discharge planning team. Often, the family can suggest ways that foster communication with the client. Goals of care established with the client and nurse are to be mutually set. The importance of collaboration allows the opportunity for all health care team members to have knowledge of the techniques that will best promote the client's ability to communicate.

Success in promoting a client's ability to communicate depends not only on the client's participation in goal setting but also on the nurse's style of communication and the ability to establish a therapeutic relationship. Therapeutic communication skills enable the nurse to perceive, react to, and respect the client's uniqueness. Successful interpersonal interaction meets the following objectives:

1. Gaining a sense of trust in the nurse as a care giver
2. Transmitting clear, concise, and understandable messages
3. Sending and receiving feedback

When developing the plan of care for the diagnosis *impaired verbal communication,* the nurse should consider the following client-centered goals and outcomes:

SAMPLE NURSING CARE PLAN
Impaired Verbal Communication

ASSESSMENT

Clinical scenario: Mr. Garcia is a 48-year-old client who just moved to the United States from Mexico. He *speaks very little English.* He was in a motor vehicle accident, suffering chest injuries that now cause him to be *intubated* and on a ventilator. The *presence of an endotracheal tube* makes it *impossible to speak or mouth words.* His hearing is normal and he has the ability to use his dominant hand.

NURSING DIAGNOSIS

Impaired verbal communication related to tracheal intubation and cultural differences.

PLANNING

Goal	Expected outcomes
Client will be able to express needs accurately while intubated by day 2 of hospitalization.	Client will use alternative communication system to make requests by day 1. Client will use own language to communicate to staff by day 2.

IMPLEMENTATION

Steps	Rationale
1. Develop communication board using Mexican words translated into English for client to make basic requests (e.g. pain medication, water, turning).	Simple, concise messages will reduce client's frustration in trying to communicate. Care givers use of client's language will help to build trust with client.
2. Speak to client in normal tone of voice.	Clients unable to speak are often treated as though they have a hearing problem as well. Normal voice tone is easier to understand and conveys a more calming message.
3. Set up a small bell at client's bedside for client to signal desire to communicate.	Enables client to initiate communication, giving more control in any interaction with staff.
4. Have a translater located and available when lengthier explanations or questions must be communicated to client.	Ensures client will be properly informed.

EVALUATION

Have family member or translator ask client if he perceives needs are met when using communication board.

Note client's nonverbal expressions when attempts are made to communicate.

Observe if client initiates communication.

Goal: Client transmits clear, concise, and understandable messages by day 3 of hospitalization.

Outcomes

Client communicates basic needs with nursing staff through use of eye blinks or movement of fingers for simple responses (e.g., yes or no) by day 2 of hospitalization

Client agrees verbal feedback from nurse is accurate interpretation of message intended by day 3 of hospitalization

Goal: Client responds to stimuli appropriately.

Outcomes

Client is oriented to time, person, and place within 24 hours of admission

Client is able to respond to stimuli, both verbal and nonverbal within 24 hours of admission

Goal: Client establishes effective communication with family and care givers by day 4 of hospitalization.

Outcomes

Client spontaneously interacts with family during problem solving by day 4 of hospitalization.

Goal: Client and family are able to communicate concerns and needs with all members of the health care team by day 6 of hospitalization.

Outcomes

Client freely questions nurses before planned procedures by day 4 of hospitalization.

Client and family openly discuss plans for discharge with social worker by day 5 of hospitalization.

The nurse develops goals and expected outcomes that are specific and realistic to the client, have a definitive time frame for which goals/expected outcomes are met, and include the client's needs and concerns (see care plan on p. 221).

The nurse must choose appropriate communication aids. The nurse also needs to identify other people who can help design the best communication strategies. Referrals might be necessary. They might include the speech therapist for a client with **aphasia,** an interpreter for a client who speaks a foreign language, or a psychiatric liaison nurse for an angry or highly anxious client. It is especially important to have the client make decisions about the care plan. The client must feel comfortable and willing to communicate.

Implementation

A helping therapeutic relationship will make clients more comfortable in communication interactions.

Developing Social Skills

In providing care for the client with impaired communication, it is important for the nurse to carry out interventions that assist the client in the following ways:

1. Express needs, feelings, and concerns
2. Develop interaction skills
3. Communicate thoughts and feelings clearly so needs can be met (both verbal and nonverbal)
4. Develop problem solving skills
5. Facilitate conversation with peers and staff
6. Increase the feeling of assertiveness

The nurse providing care for the client with impaired verbal communication may use communication boards, interpreters, or family to facilitate the communication process. The nurse's actions are directed at meeting the goals and expected outcomes identified in the plan of care. For example, the nurse caring for a client with impaired verbal communication related to cultural differences may leave at the client's bedside a table of simple words in the client's language. The nurses use the table to help the client communicate basic needs (e.g., need for food, water, toileting, rest, sleep, etc.)

The nurse may implement other methods to meet communication needs such as role playing. This allows clients to practice situations in which they have difficulty communicating. The following simple interventions can reinforce attempts at interaction:

1. Encourage the client to participate in normal social activities.
2. Discuss neutral topics or subjects in which clients have interests.
3. Utilize positive reinforcement for acceptable social interactions.
4. Help clients identify persons with whom they feel comfortable and encourage interactions with them.
5. Encourage socialization with other clients with the same interests.
6. Minimize the client's idle time.

Also important for the nurse in caring for the client with communication needs is to facilitate activities that provide the client with health promotion, maintenance, and restoration. The actions should be designed to maximize the client's ability to communicate. Health screenings or auditory testing and provision of sensory aids (see Chapter 38) are examples.

Controlling the Environment

An uncomfortable or distracting environment can inhibit communication. The nurse can control the environment to enhance interpersonal interactions in the following ways:

1. Regulating room temperature to a comfortable level
2. Eliminating or reducing loud noises in room
3. Making client comfortable
4. Asking other staff members or family (if appropriate) not to enter room during interaction
5. Reducing bright or glaring light

Communication With Health Care Team

During the implementation phase, it is important for the nurse to document the response to interventions carried out to meet the identified expected outcomes and goals for the client's plan of care. This method of communication ensures that all members of the health care team involved in the client's plan of care have knowledge of the client's response and progress. It also allows the opportunity for the health care team to modify or reevaluate the ongoing plan of care.

COMMUNICATING WITH CLIENTS HAVING SPECIAL NEEDS

It is sometimes necessary for nurses to use special communication techniques for successful nurse-client interactions. Clients with sensory and motor impairments, children, and older adult clients require individualized approaches to communication.

Providing Alternative Communication Methods

Clients with physical communication barriers (e.g., those with a laryngectomy or endotracheal tube) may be unable to speak, or the clarity of speech is so poor

COMMUNICATION AIDS

Pad and felt-tipped pen or magic slate
Communication board with words, letters, or pictures denoting basic needs (e.g., water, bedpan, pain medication)
Call bells or alarms
Sign language
Use of eye blinks or movement of fingers for simple responses (e.g., "yes" or "no")
Flash cards with common words or phrases the client may use
Language cards for non-English–speaking clients

that alternate methods of communication are needed (see box above). For these clients, the nurse should provide simple communication methods. Anything complicated can be frustrating and make communication more difficult. The nurse is patient as the client tries to communicate. The client must be able to physically use the method the nurse provides (such as communication boards or pencil and pad). A client who is unable to speak can be at risk for injury unless personal needs can be quickly communicated.

Communicating With Children

Communication with a child requires special considerations so the nurse can develop a working relationship with the child and family. The nurse receives much information about a child from parents. Because contact between parent and child is usually close, the information communicated by parents can be assumed to be reliable, although some parents may exaggerate. If the client is a young child, it helps to offer the child toys or materials so the parent can give full attention to the nurse. The nurse gives periodic attention to infants and younger children as they play to make them participants. An older child can be actively involved in communication.

To communicate effectively with children, the nurse must understand the influence of development on language and thought processes. Both factors affect the way a child communicates and the manner in which the nurse can successfully engage a child in an interaction (see box below).

Children, particularly the young, are especially responsive to nonverbal messages. Sudden movements or threatening gestures can frighten a child. The nurse walking into an examination room with a broad grin and animated hand movements will likely inhibit the formation of a relationship with a child. The nurse should remain calm and gentle. It helps to let the child make the first move in interpersonal contacts. A quiet, friendly, confident tone of voice is best when interacting with a child.

Children do not like people to stare at them. Adults looking down on them make them feel vulnerable. While communicating with a young child, the nurse should meet the child at eye level. The child feels helpless in most situations involving health care personnel.

TECHNIQUES FOR COMMUNICATING WITH CHILDREN

INFANT

The child communicates primarily nonverbally (coos, smiles, and cries) and seeks comfort. The nurse should avoid loud, harsh sounds and sudden movements. Gentle, close physical contact helps a child to become quiet. Keep the mother in view while holding and interacting with the child.

TODDLER OR PRESCHOOLER

The child communicates verbally and nonverbally. The child is egocentric with all activities focused on the *self.* Speech and thought processes are concrete. The nurse should focus discussion on the child's personal needs and concerns. Tell the child specifically what to do and how he or she will feel. Allow the child to explore the environment (handle a stethoscope or play with a tongue blade). Use simple, short sentences, familiar words, and concrete explanations. Avoid ambiguous phrases the child cannot interpret, such as "the shot will just feel like a bee-sting" or "take this medicine for your tummy ache."

SCHOOL-AGE CHILD

Speech is primarily verbal. The child seeks explanations of the world and is interested in functional aspects of objects and events. The child is concerned about body integrity. The nurse should give simple explanations. Demonstrate how equipment works. Allow the child to manipulate equipment (hold a percussion hammer or wear a stethoscope). Allow the child to express fears or concerns.

ADOLESCENT

An adolescent thinks more abstractly, fluctuates between childish and adult thinking behavior, and likes talking with adults outside of the family. The nurse should avoid imposing values or judgments. Allow the adolescent time to talk. Be attentive and avoid interrupting or showing gestures of disapproval. Avoid embarrassing questions or the impulse to give advice. Adolescents frequently use a language of their own. Clarify your terms.

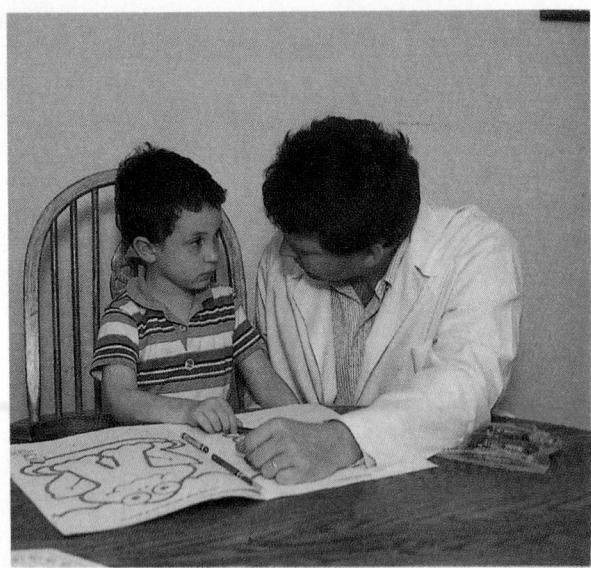

FIGURE 13-5 Drawing helps children to communicate.

When it is necessary to give explanations or directions, the nurse uses simple, direct language. The nurse must be honest. Deceiving a child into thinking a painful procedure is painless will only make the child angry. To minimize fear and anxiety immediately before a procedure begins, a child should always be told what to expect.

Drawing and play are two effective ways of communicating with young children (Figure 13-5). Drawing allows the child to communicate nonverbally (by making the drawing) and verbally (by explaining the picture). The nurse can use a child's drawing as a basis for beginning a conversation.

Communicating With Older Adult Clients

Because of sensory disturbances and motor disabilities, older adults often have communication problems. Sensory alterations prevent them from receiving messages clearly. Motor disturbances such as dysarthria interfere with speech clarity. Many older adults adapt to sensory losses (see Chapter 38) and can learn to communicate effectively. When obvious deficits exist, the nurse maximizes existing motor and sensory function so the client can communicate more effectively (see box above).

Ebersole (1990) indicates that older adults also may suffer from other sensory deprivations (elimination of order or meaning and restricting the environment to dull monotony) and sensory overload (see gerontological box, p. 225). The nurse identifies these challenges and works with the client accordingly to enhance effective communication.

COMMUNICATING WITH SENSORIALLY OR MOTOR-IMPAIRED CLIENTS

HEARING IMPAIRED

Be sure the hearing aid is clean, is inserted properly, and has a functioning battery.
Adjust the volume of the hearing aid to a comfortable level.
Speak slowly and articulate clearly. Use simple sentences.
Stand in front of the client to provide an opportunity for lip reading.
Talk toward the client's best ear.
Reduce background noise.

VISUALLY IMPAIRED

Announce yourself when entering the client's room.
Orient the client to sounds in the environment.
Keep eyeglasses clean and intact (allows client to see nonverbal communication).
Inform the blind client of when conversation is over and when you are leaving the room.

APHASIA

Ask simple questions that require "yes" or "no" answers.
Allow time for understanding and a response.
Use visual cues (e.g., words, pictures, and objects) when possible.
Only one person should talk at a time.
Do not shout or speak too loudly.

DYSARTHRIA

Listen attentively, be patient, and do not interrupt.
Encourage the client to converse.
Refer the client to a speech therapist as needed.

Evaluation

Evaluating whether communication has been therapeutic is determined by the client's progress or lack of progress toward goals and expected outcomes. The nurse evaluates if nursing interventions met established outcomes to determine if goals were achieved. If so, interventions were effective. For example, the nurse delivering care to the client with impaired verbal communication related to cerebral dysfunction may have established the goal "client is able to communicate basic needs" (water, food, toileting, etc.). The outcome was "client uses communication board to request water, food, and assistance with toileting." While caring for the client, the nurse observes if the client uses the communication board easily and effectively. Was the client able

GERONTOLOGIC NURSING PRACTICE FOR COMMUNICATION

In dealing with impaired communication with older persons, Matteson and McConnell (1988) indicates that the primary goal is to establish a reliable communication system that is easily understood by all health care team members since nursing care of the older person is ideally delivered by an interdisciplinary model. Communication with older adults requires special attention. The nurse must be aware of the physical, psychological, and social changes of aging.

The nurse can utilize the following interventions to assist with impaired communication with older persons:

1. During conversation, maintain a quiet environment that is free from background noise.
2. Avoid shifting from subject to subject; allow time for conversation.
3. Be an attentive listener. Use explorative questions to facilitate conversation (e.g., "How do you feel?").
4. Avoid long sentences to explain the subject. Try to keep it short, simple, and to the point of subject.
5. Allow the older adult the opportunity to reminisce. Reminiscing has therapeutic properties that increase the sense of well-being.
6. If you are experiencing problems understanding the client (e.g., dysarthria), let the client know and facilitate methods that help the client speak more clearly. The nurse may need to consult with a speech therapist.
7. Include the client's family and friends in conversations, particularly in known subjects to the client.
8. Be aware of cultural differences among clients.

to communicate basic needs with the staff and thus were the needs met? The nurse might question the client about whether needs were adequately met. If the goal was met, interventions were appropriate for the client. If not, the plan of care should be modified in order to achieve the goal and outcome. This modification process is ongoing and continues until the time of discharge.

For clients with actual communication alterations, a variety of approaches can be used to evaluate success of the plan of care. Goals, outcomes, and corresponding evaluative measures for the problem of impaired communication include:

Goal: Client transmits clear, concise, and understandable messages by day 3 of hospitalization.

Outcome

Client communicates basic needs with nursing staff through use of eye blinks or movement of fingers for simple responses (e.g., yes or no) by day 2 of hospitalization

Evaluative measures

Observe client's response when you ask if a need exists

When a routine voiding schedule is established, observe client's response when asked if there is a need to void

Goal: Client responds to stimuli appropriately.

Outcome

Client is oriented to time, person, and place within 24 hours of admission

Evaluative measure

Ask client to identify time of day, name, and location. Compare client's response to current time, place and client's name

Outcome

Client is able to respond to stimuli, both verbal and nonverbal within 24 hours of admission

Evaluative measure

Watch client's nonverbal expressions when conversation is dircted toward him or her. Do nonverbal and verbal responses match with intent of message?

Goal: Client establishes effective communication with family and care giver by day 4 of hospitalization.

Outcome

Client spontaneously interacts with family during problem solving by day 4 of hospitalization

Evaluative measure

Conduct a discussion with client and family regarding plans for client's return home from hospital and observe interaction

Goal: Client and family communicate concerns and needs with all members of the health care team by day 6 of hospitalization.

Outcome

Client freely questions nurses before planned procedures

Evaluative measures

Ask if client has questions about an activity or procedure

Observe client and family during conference with social worker

The nurse evaluates success of the care plan but also determines the level of trust established with the client. Evaluative measures for determining that a client trusts the nurse include:

Observing client's willingness to be open about personal feelings

Observing client expressing feelings about care and treatment

SUMMARY

Communication is one of the most important skills for a nurse to master. Through communication a nurse establishes a relationship with clients to help them acquire healthy behaviors. A nurse's competence depends on the ability to convey meaningful messages as effectively and intelligently as the client's needs dictate and on the ability to understand the client's communications. Communication is a complex process that includes verbal and nonverbal communication. The nurse communicates more effectively when conscious of all the factors influencing the sending and receiving of messages and when receptive to the client's feedback.

Communication skills are essential throughout the nursing process. Therapeutic communication with the client involves planned, deliberate interactions that foster a helping relationship. Throughout the relationship the nurse uses the specific skills that promote effective communication and avoids words and actions that inhibit communication. Effective communication is necessary for the nurse's role in helping the client to adapt to the changes resulting from health alterations.

KEY CONCEPTS

Effective communication allows nurses to establish working relationships with clients.

Successful communication requires the message intended by the speaker to be similar or identical to the meaning acquired by the receiver.

The manner in which a message is communicated depends on the perceptions, values, emotions, knowledge, sociocultural background, and roles of the sender and receiver.

Words that have different connotative meanings can be easily misinterpreted by the person receiving the message.

Effective verbal communication requires appropriate voice intonation, clear and concise phrasing of words, proper pacing of statements, and proper timing and relevance of a message.

When the sender's verbal and nonverbal communications complement each other, a receiver is unlikely to misinterpret a message.

Nursing action is a process of social interaction whereby nurses bring about positive changes in a client's health status through therapeutic communication.

Social or informational interaction should not dominate a conversation with a client.

Therapeutic communication through a helping relationship requires the nurse to establish trust, empathy, caring, autonomy, and mutuality.

Communication helps the nurse perform nursing care effectively and efficiently.

Communication is a means for the nurse to help clients to adjust to changes imposed by illness.

Client teaching is an effective way of enhancing the nurse-client relationship and helps achieve a client's optimal level of wellness.

During the orientation phase of a helping relationship, the client may test the nurse before trust is established and goals are set.

During the working phase of a nurse-client relationship, the nurse uses therapeutic communication techniques.

Ineffective communication skills tend to inhibit the client's willingness to express ideas or concerns openly.

Effective communication allows a nurse to perform routine nursing care procedures more skillfully.

Methods that facilitate communication with children include sitting at eye level, using simple direct language, and incorporating play into discussion.

Older adult clients with sensory losses require communication techniques that maximize existing sensory and motor functions.

CRITICAL THINKING ACTIVITIES

1. Walter is a 34 year old brought to the emergency room with complaints of crushing chest pain, shortness of breath, and exercise intolerance. His wife is at his side, in tears, moaning that "He's dying." What elements of the communication process are needed to develop a helping relationship with Walter and his wife?
2. The nurse grabs the wife's arm to drag her away. She reacts violently. What should the nurse do differently?
3. The couple's child (a 4-year-old boy) is in the emergency room. His eyes are wide open, his skin is pale, and his eyes are tearing. How would you explain to him what is happening with his dad?

4. Their 16-year-old daughter is also present and is wringing her hands. Construct a way to explain the situation to her.
5. The 60-year-old mother of Walter is there and walking in circles. How would you develop a helping relationship with her?
6. Walter is admitted to the coronary care unit. Develop a plan for winning his trust and conducting a therapeutic communication with him.

References

Barsky AJ, et al.: Evaluating the interview in primary care medicine, *Soc Sci Med* 14a:653, 1980.

Boyle JS and Andrews MA: *Transcultural concepts in nursing care,* Glenview Ill., 1989, Scott, Foresman.

Bradley J and Edinberg MA: *Communication in the nursing context,* New York, 1990, Appleton and Lange.

Chipman Y: Caring: its meaning and place in the practice of nursing, *J Nurs Educ* 30(4):171-175, 1991.

Doenges ME, Moorhouse MF: Watch your language, *Nurs* 22(11):29, 1992.

Dugan DO: Laughter and tears: best medicine for stress, *Nurs Forum* 24(1):18, 1989.

Duldt BW, et al.: *Interpersonal communication in nursing,* Philadelphia, 1984, FA Davis.

Ebersole P and Hess P: *Toward healthy aging,* ed 4, St. Louis, 1990, Mosby.

Kasch CR: Toward a theory of nursing action: skills and competency in nurse-patient interaction, *Nurs Res* 35(4):226, 1986.

Kim HS: Collaborative decision making in nursing practice: a theoretical framework. In Chinn PL, editor: *Advances in nursing theory development,* London, 1983, Aspen Publishers.

King I: *Toward a theory for nursing,* New York, 1971, John Wiley & Sons.

Knapp M: *Nonverbal communication in human interaction,* New York, ed 2, 1978, Holt, Rinehardt & Winston.

Knaus WA, et al.: An evaluation of outcome from intensive care in major medical centers, *Ann Intern Med* 104(3):410, 1986.

Lalli-Ascosi S: Polishing your self-image, *Health Trends Transition* 1(2):15, 1990.

Lindberg B, Hunter ML, Kruszewski AZ: *Introduction to nursing: concepts, issues, and opportunities,* Philadelphia, 1990, JB Lippincott.

Matteson MA, McConnell ES: *Gerontological nursing: concepts and practice,* Philadelphia, 1988, WB Saunders.

Mulaik JS, et al.: Patients' perceptions of nurses' use of touch, *West J Nurs Res* 13(3):306-323, 1991.

Murray RB: Therapeutic communication for emotional care. In Murray RB and Huelskoetter MM: *Psychiatric and mental health nursing: giving emotional care,* New York, 1991, Appleton & Lange.

Pike AW: On the nature and place of empathy in clinical nursing practice, *J Prof Nurs* 6:235, 1990.

Pluckhan ML: *Human communication: the matrix of nursing,* New York, 1978, McGraw-Hill.

Rogers A: *Teaching adults,* Philadelphia, 1986, University Press.

Sarvimaki A: Nursing care as moral, practical, communicative and creative activity, *J Adv Nurs* 13:462, 1988.

Severtsen BM: Therapeutic communication demystified, *J Nurs Educ* 29(4):190, 1990.

Shives LR: *Basic concepts of psychiatric–mental health nursing,* ed 2, Philadelphia, 1990, JB Lippincott.

Sullivan JL and Deane DM: Humor and health, *J Gerontol Nurs* 14(1):20, 1988.

Sundeen SJ, et al.: *Nurse-client interaction: implementing the nursing process,* ed 4, St. Louis, 1989, Mosby.

Travelbee J: *Interpersonal aspects of nursing,* ed 2, Philadelphia, 1971, FA Davis.

Vortherms RC: Clinically improving communication through touch, *J Gerontol Nurs* 17(5):6, 1991.

Watson J: *Nursing: the philosophy and science of caring,* Boston, 1979, Little, Brown & Co.

Whaley LF and Wong DL: *Nursing care of infants and children,* ed 4, St. Louis, 1991, Mosby.

Williams H: Humor and healing: therapeutic effects in geriatrics, *Geronton* 1(3):14, 1986.

Bibliography

Anderson C: *Patient teaching and communication in an information age,* New York, 1990, Delmar Publishing.

Arnold E and Bogg K: *Interpersonal relationships/professional communication skills for nurses,* Philadelphia, 1989, WB Saunders.

Beck C, Rawlins R, and Williams S: *Mental health-psychiatric nursing: a holistic life-cycle approach,* St. Louis, 1988, Mosby.

Estabrooks CA and Morse JM: Toward a theory of touch: the touching process and acquiring a touching style, *J Adv Nurs* 17:448-456, 1992.

Egan G: *The skilled helper,* ed 3, Monterey, Calif., 1985, Brooks/Cole Publishing Co.

Enelow A and Scott S: *Interviewing and patient care,* ed 3, New York, 1985, Oxford University Press.

Farrell J: *Nursing care of the older person,* Philadelphia, 1990, JB Lippincott.

Kasch CR: Interpersonal competence and communication in the delivery of nursing care, *ANS* 6(2):1984.

Stanhope M and Lancaster J: *Community health nursing: process and practice for promoting health,* ed 2, St. Louis, 1988, Mosby.

14

Teaching and Learning

OBJECTIVES

Mastery of content in this chapter will enable the student to:

- Define the key terms listed.
- Describe the similarities and differences between teaching and learning.
- Identify the purposes of client teaching.
- Compare the communication and teaching processes.
- Describe the domains of learning.
- Differentiate factors that determine readiness to learn from those that determine ability to learn.
- Compare the nursing and teaching processes.
- Write a learning objective.
- Describe characteristics of a good learning environment.
- Identify principles of effective teaching.
- Describe ways to adapt teaching for different kinds of clients.
- Describe ways to incorporate teaching with routine nursing care.
- Identify methods for evaluating learning.

KEY TERMS

affective learning
attentional set
cognitive learning
compliance
health belief
learning
learning objective
motivation
psychomotor learning
reinforcement
teaching

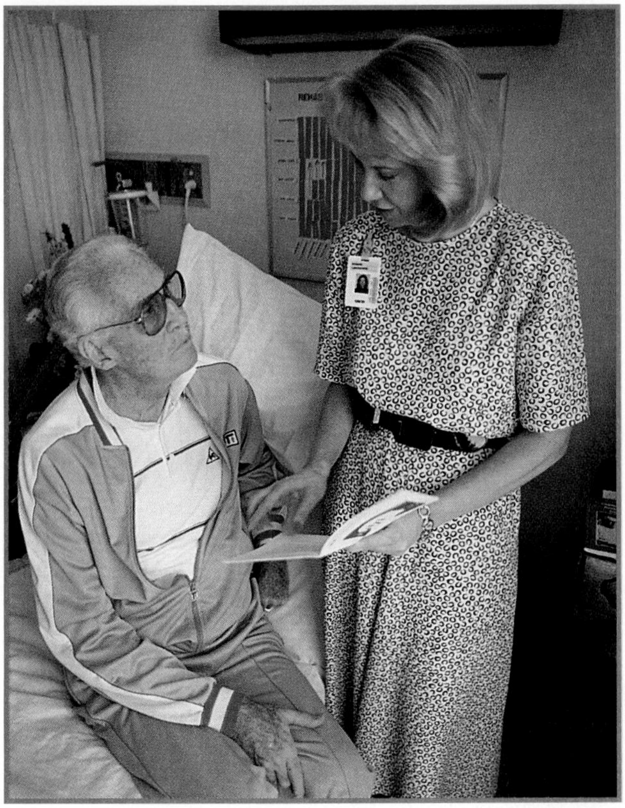

Client education has become one of the more important roles for nurses. Shorter hospital stays, increased demands on nurses' time, and the need to give seriously ill clients complex information as soon as possible emphasize the importance of quality client education (Bull, 1992). As nurses try to find the best way to educate clients, the general public has become more assertive in seeking knowledge and understanding of personal health and the resources available within the health care system (Kruger, 1991). Providing clients with needed information for self-care is necessary to ensure continuity of care from the hospital to the home (Bull, 1992). A well-designed, comprehensive teaching plan that fits a client's learning needs can reduce health care costs, improve the quality of care, and help clients to gain optimum wellness and more independence.

STANDARDS FOR CLIENT EDUCATION

Accrediting agencies in the United States and Canada set guidelines for providing client education in health care institutions (Barnes, 1993; American Association of Diabetes Educators, 1992). The guidelines ensure that clients and their families receive information necessary to maintain the client's optimal level of health. In the United States, the JCAHO (1994) describes the following standards for client/family education:

1. The client/family are provided with education that can enhance knowledge, skills, and behaviors that are necessary to benefit fully from the health care interventions provided by the organization.
2. The organization plans and supports the provision and coordination of client/family education activities and resources.
3. Clients/families have their learning needs, capabilities, and readiness to learn assessed.
4. The client/family educational process is interdisciplinary, as appropriate to the plan of care.
5. The client/family receive education specific to the client's assessed needs, capabilities, and readiness. Such education includes medication administration, use of medical equipment, knowledge about food/drug interactions and diet modification, rehabilitation, and how to obtain further treatment.
6. Information about any discharge instructions given to the client/family is provided to the organization or individual responsible for the continuing care of the client.

The successful completion of these standards is based on nursing assessments, implementation, and evaluation. Evidence of successful client education is noted in the client's medical record.

In 1986 the Alberta Association of Registered Nurses developed a set of client education standards (see box on p. 230) that addresses the educational process related to adult clients. The standards help to direct nurses in client education.

PURPOSES OF CLIENT TEACHING

Nursing's Agenda for Healthcare Reform (ANA, 1991) recommends restructuring of the health care system. The focus should be on wellness and care rather than on illness and cure. The emphasis is on maintaining health. Clients now know more about health and want to be involved in health maintenance. Nursing needs to provide education so clients receive information about care in more convenient and familiar places (ANA, 1991). Comprehensive client education includes three important purposes, each involving a separate phase of health care.

Maintenance and Promotion of Health and Illness Prevention

The public has recently become more health conscious. Participation in fitness clubs, diet programs, regular ex-

CLIENT EDUCATION STANDARDS

STRUCTURE

Standards in regard to structure relate to human and material resources, including administration and management of the health care agency. Nurses in both staff and administrative roles should contribute to their development and implementation.

Standard 1

The health care agency has a philosophy, goals, and objectives that reflect its mandate and provide direction for client education.

Standard 2

Client education is integrated into all areas of nursing practice in the health care system.

Standard 3

The nursing department of the health care agency is active in developing a comprehensive plan for client education.

Standard 4

An individual/department is responsible for facilitating and coordinating matters of client education.

PROCESS

Process standards outline criteria by which client education is delivered. The educational process includes the same steps as the nursing process.

Standard 1

The primary focus of the educational process is the client.

Standard 2

An educational assessment is done by the nurse in collaboration with the client.

Standard 3

The nurse demonstrates planning in the educational process.

Standard 4

The nurse applies principles of the educational process in implementation of client education.

Standard 5

A written outline of the educational process is available as a communication tool, a resource to health professionals, and as a record.

OUTCOME

Outcome standards are the criteria to measure results of the educational process.

Standard 1

The nurse evaluates the educational process.

Standard 2

The client participates in evaluating the educational process.

From the Alberta Association of Registered Nurses: *Client education: position statement and guidelines,* 1985, Edmonton, Alberta, Canada, 1986, The Association.

ercise activities, and health-screening programs are examples of ways people pay more attention to their health.

The nurse is a convenient resource for health-minded clients who want to learn to improve physical and psychological well-being. The nurse provides clients with information and skills that will allow them to assume healthier behaviors (see box on p. 231). For example, in childbearing classes, nurses teach expectant parents about physical and psychological changes in the woman and about fetal development. After learning about normal childbearing, the mother is more likely to eat healthy foods, engage in physical exercise, and avoid substances that might harm the fetus. Promoting healthy behavior through education increases self-esteem by allowing clients to assume more responsibility for health. When clients become more health conscious, they are more likely to seek early diagnosis of health problems.

Restoration of Health

Injured or ill clients need information or skills that will help them to regain improved levels of health (see box on p. 231). Clients recovering from the initial stress of illness or injury and adapting to the changes that result seek information about their conditions. However, clients who find it difficult to adapt to illness may become passive and uninterested in learning. The nurse learns to identify clients' willingness to learn and helps to motivate interest.

The family is a vital part of a client's return to health and may need to know as much as the client. If the nurse excludes the family from a client's teaching plan, conflicts may arise. For example, if the family does not understand a client's need to regain independent function, their efforts may cause the client to become unnecessarily dependent and slow the client's recovery. The nurse should not assume the family should be involved and must first assess the client-family relationship.

TOPICS FOR HEALTH EDUCATION

HEALTH MAINTENANCE AND PROMOTION AND ILLNESS PREVENTION

First aid
Avoidance of risk factors (smoking, alcohol)
Growth and development
Hygiene
Immunizations
Normal childbearing
Nutrition
Exercise
Safety (in home and hospital)
Screening (blood pressure, vision, cholesterol level)

RESTORATION OF HEALTH

- Client's disease or condition
  - Anatomy and physiology of body system affected
  - Cause of disease
  - Origin of symptoms
  - Expected effects on other body systems
  - Prognosis
    - Limitations on function
    - Rationale for treatment
    - Medications
    - Tests and therapies
    - Nursing measures
    - Surgical intervention
- Expected duration of care
- Hospital or clinic environment
- Hospital or clinic staff
- Long-term care
- Methods for client participation in care
- Limitations posed by disease or surgery

COPING WITH IMPAIRED FUNCTIONS

- Home care
  - Medications
  - Diet
  - Activity
  - Self-help devices
- Rehabilitation of remaining function
  - Physical therapy
  - Occupational therapy
  - Speech therapy
- Prevention of complications
  - Knowledge of risk factors
  - Implications of noncompliance with therapy
  - Environmental alterations

Coping With Impaired Functioning

Not all clients fully recover from illness or injury. Many must learn to cope with permanent health changes. New knowledge and skills are often needed for clients to continue activities of daily living (see box above). For example, the client whose ability to speak is lost after surgery of the larynx learns new ways of communicating, and the client with severe heart disease learns to avoid physical activities that might cause further heart damage. In the case of serious disability, the client's family role may change. Family members thus need to be understanding and accepting. The family's ability to provide support results from education, which begins as soon as the client's needs are identified and the family displays a willingness to help. The nurse teaches family members to assist clients with health care management. This includes, for example, giving medications and baths and applying dressings. Families of clients with alcoholism, mental retardation, or drug dependence also learn to adapt to the additional emotional effects.

A nurse learns to recognize what information to teach at different levels of wellness by assessing clients' needs and abilities. Learning occurs when information is practical and useful to the learner. Comparing the desired level of health with the actual state enables the nurse to plan effective teaching programs.

TEACHING AND LEARNING

It is impossible to separate teaching from learning. **Teaching** is an interactive process that promotes learning. It consists of a conscious and deliberate set of actions that helps individuals gain new knowledge or perform new skills (Redman, 1992). A teacher provides information that prompts the learner to engage in activities that lead to a desired change.

Learning is the acquisition of new knowledge or skills through reinforced practice and experience. A diabetic client demonstrates the technique for preparing insulin in a syringe. Before surgery, a surgical client discusses ways to relieve postoperative pain. Generally, teaching and learning begin when a person identifies a need for knowing or acquiring an ability to do something. Teaching is most effective when it responds to a learner's needs. The teacher identifies these needs by asking questions and determining the learner's interests. Interpersonal communication is essential for successful teaching.

Role of the Nurse in Teaching and Learning

Clients and their families often ask nurses for health information. If they do not, then the need for teaching may not be obvious. The nurse should try to anticipate client's needs for information based on their physical conditions or treatment plans. The nurse needs to teach information that the clients and their families need. The nurse clarifies information provided by physicians and becomes the primary source of information for adjusting to health problems.

To be an effective educator, the nurse must engage the client in learning and not merely pass on facts. The nurse must carefully determine what clients need to know and find the time when they are ready to learn. Kruger (1991) noted three areas for nurse responsibility in patient education: (1) preparation of clients receiving care (e.g., preoperative teaching, self-injection of insulin); (2) preparation of clients being discharged from a health care facility (e.g., discharge medications and procedures, potential complications that require the client to return to the physician or hospital); and (3) documentation of client education activities (e.g., noting the specific education within the client's health record, educational flow sheet, or discharge summary).

When nurses value client education and are able to implement it, clients are better prepared to assume health care responsibilities. The relationship between client education and favorable client outcomes is important and needs to be researched further.

TEACHING AS COMMUNICATION

The teaching process closely parallels the communication process (see Chapter 13). Effective teaching is a form of interpersonal communication. A teacher applies each element of the communication process while giving information to learners. Thus the teacher and student become involved in a teaching process that increases the student's knowledge and skills.

The steps of the teaching process can be compared to those of the communication process (Table 14-1). In teaching, the referent is the need to provide the client with information. The client may request information, or the nurse may perceive a need for information. The nurse then identifies specific learning objectives. A **learning objective** describes what the learner will be able to do after successful instruction.

The nurse is the sender who wants to convey a mes-

table 14-1

COMPARISON OF TERMS USED IN TEACHING AND COMMUNICATION

Communication	Teaching
REFERENT	
Idea that initates reason for communication	Perceives need to provide person with information, establishment of relevant learning objectives by teacher
SENDER	
Person who conveys message to another	Teacher who performs activities aimed at assisting other person to learn
INTRAPERSONAL VARIABLES (SENDER)	
Knowledge, values, emotions, and sociocultural influences that affect sender's thoughts	Teacher's philosophy of education (based on learning therapy); knowledge of teaching content; teaching approach; experiences in teaching; teacher's emotions and values
MESSAGE	
Information expressed or transmitted by sender	Content or information taught
CHANNELS	
Methods used to transmit message (visual, auditory, touch)	Methods used to present content (visual and auditory materials, touch, taste, smell)
RECEIVER	
Person to whom message is transmitted	Learner
INTRAPERSONAL VARIABLES (RECEIVER)	
Knowledge, values, emotions, and sociocultural influences that affect receiver's thoughts	Willingness and ability to learn (physical and emotional health, education, experience, developmental level)
FEEDBACK	
Information revealing that true meaning of message was received	Determination of whether learning objectives were achieved

sage to the client. The nurse promotes learning by communicating in a language recognized by the learner. Many intrapersonal variables influence the nurse's style and approach. Attitudes, values, emotions, and knowledge influence the way the nurse sends messages. Past experiences with teaching help the nurse to choose the best way to present information.

The message or content to be taught is delivered clearly and precisely. The nurse organizes information in a logical sequence so the client will more easily understand the skills or ideas. Each lesson progresses from the simple to the more complex skills or ideas.

The nurse may use a variety of ways to present teaching content. All the senses are channels for presenting information. The auditory channel is the simplest, as in a lecture or discussion. The learning process becomes more active and stimulating, however, when several sensory channels are used together.

The receiver in the teaching-learning process is the learner. Intrapersonal variables affect a client's motivation and ability to learn. Clients are ready to learn when they express a desire to do so and are more likely to receive the message when they understand the content. Attitudes, anxiety, and values influence the ability to understand a message. The ability to learn depends on emotional and physical health, education, stage of development, and previous knowledge.

An effective teacher provides a mechanism for evaluating the success of a teaching plan. Return demonstration is a good form of feedback. The learner restates the received information, which allows the teacher to assess the success of learning.

DOMAINS OF LEARNING

Learning occurs in the cognitive (understandings), affective (values), and psychomotor (motor skills) domains. Any topic to be learned may involve all domains or only one. The nurse often works with clients who need to learn in each domain. The characteristics of learning within each domain affect the teaching and evaluation methods the nurse selects.

Cognitive learning includes all intellectual behaviors such as the acquisition of knowledge, comprehension (ability to understand), application (using abstract ideas in concrete situations), analysis (relating ideas in an organized way), synthesis (recognizing parts as a whole), and evaluation (judging the worth of a body of information).

Affective learning deals with the expression of feelings related to attitudes, opinions, or values. The learner receives information, responds to the teacher, values the worth of the teachers and the information, organizes values, and characterizes by acting and responding with a consistent value system.

Psychomotor learning involves acquiring skills that require the integration of mental and muscular activity such as the ability to walk, use an eating utensil, or climb stairs. The learner perceives objects or information through sensory organs. Then the learner demonstrates readiness to take an action through mental, physical, and emotional acts. The teacher guides the learner's response, leading to the confidence to perform the desired behavior in gradually more complex ways. Adaptation is the next step, involving responses to changes and problems. This results in organization, which involves creating new patterns of behavior.

Teaching the client a specific behavior often involves incorporating behaviors from all three learning domains. A client being taught the proper method of giving an injection must first understand the reasons injections are needed and then must know the proper location for administering the injection and the importance of using sterile technique **(cognitive).** The techniques of locating an acceptable area on the skin and introducing the needle use the senses of touch and vision **(psychomotor).** In addition, the client must be willing to accept the need of injections and must overcome any fear or distaste for injections **(affective).**

BASIC LEARNING PRINCIPLES

To teach effectively and efficiently, the nurse must first understand how people learn. Learning depends on the motivation to learn, the ability to learn, and the learning environment. Motivation addresses a person's desire to learn (Redman, 1992). Previous knowledge and successful learning, attitudes, and sociocultural factors influence motivation.

The ability to learn depends on physical and cognitive attributes, developmental level, physical wellness, and intellectual thought processes. If learning ability is impaired, such as with a client in pain, a teacher postpones teaching activities or modifies strategies to better meet the learner's needs.

The environment also affects the ability to learn. For example, when the environment is noisy, the teacher should modify conditions to enhance learning.

Motivation to Learn

Attentional Set. People often use mental pictures to visualize ideas. While a teacher explains how to give support to a dying client, students might envision themselves grasping the fragile hand of a dying person. Before learning anything, students must give attention to, or concentrate on, the information to be learned. An **attentional set** is the mental state that allows the learner to focus on and comprehend the material. Physical discomfort, anxiety, and environmental distractions can influence the ability to attend.

Any physical condition that impairs the ability to concentrate (e.g., pain, fatigue, or hunger) interferes with learning. Therefore the nurse determines the client's level of comfort and energy before beginning a teaching plan and makes sure the client is comfortable enough for discussion. Nonverbal cues can also reveal that a client is not ready to learn.

Anxiety may increase or decrease the ability of a person to pay attention. Anxiety is uneasiness or uncertainty resulting from anticipating a threat or danger. When faced with change or the need to act differently, a person feels anxious. Learning requires a change in behavior and thus produces anxiety. A mild level of anxiety may motivate learning. However, a high level of anxiety prevents learning from taking place. It incapacitates a person, making it impossible for the person to attend to anything other than to relieve the anxiety.

Environmental distractions, which interfere with the ability to attend, will be discussed later.

Motivation. **Motivation** is an internal impulse (e.g., an idea, an emotion, or a physical need) that causes a person to take action. If a person does not want to learn, it is unlikely that learning will occur.

Social task mastery and physical motives stimulate a person to learn. Social motives are a need for connection, social approval, or self-esteem. Task mastery motives are based on needs such as achievement and competence. After a person succeeds at a task, they are usually motivated to achieve more.

Often client motives are physical. A client with a physical change in function may be motivated to learn strategies to help adapt to the functional change. According to Tanner (1989) knowledge that is necessary for survival creates a stronger stimulus for learning than knowledge that merely promotes health. Teaching strategies reflect the relative importance of each kind of physical motive.

Not all persons are interested in maintaining health. A client with lung disease may continue to smoke. An obese client may worsen a heart condition by refusing to follow a low-fat diet. No therapy will have an effect unless a client is motivated to comply by the belief that health is important. The trend in health care is to treat clients in their own homes after they recover from the acute phase of illness. Such treatment can be successful only if clients follow with the recommendations of the care givers. **Compliance** is the client's fulfillment of the prescribed course of therapy. The nurse must assess the client's motivation to learn and what the client needs to know in order to adhere to the prescribed therapy.

A client's **health beliefs** can be powerful motivators, and they are influenced by a number of variables (see Chapters 2 and 17). Knowledge of a client's health beliefs helps to determine the factors that will motivate learning. However, there is no standard method for motivating a person with a given health belief. Health teaching often involves changing attitudes and values that cannot be altered by teaching facts. Therefore the nurse gives attention to ideas or beliefs that motivate a person to learn and applies the motivating factor to the teaching plan. For example, when a client is a busy executive with high blood pressure, the nurse can use the following factors to motivate a client to learn new health habits: the client's desire to succeed and the concern that illness will impair work.

Psychosocial Adaptation to Illness. A temporary or permanent loss of health is difficult for clients to accept. Clients require time to grieve. Grieving gives them time to adapt psychologically to the emotional and physical implications of illness. The stages of grieving (see Chapter 21) also encompass a series of responses clients also experience during illness. Clients experience these stages at different rates and sequences. Readiness to learn thus significantly relates to the stage of grieving (Table 14-2). When unwilling or unable to accept the reality of illness, clients cannot learn. The nurse identifies the client's stage of grieving on the basis of typically displayed behaviors. When the client enters the stage of acceptance, which is compatible with learning, the nurse begins to introduce the teaching plan. Continuous assessment of clients' behaviors determines their progress through the stages of grieving. Teaching continues as long as the client remains in a stage conducive to learning.

Active Participation. A client's involvement in learning implies an eagerness to acquire knowledge or skills

REQUIRED FOR PARTICULAR LEARNING SITUATIONS

MATH CALCULATION

Computing drug doses
Measuring liquid or solid food portions
Reading a thermometer or syringe calibrations

READING

Reading directions and instructions in teaching booklets and on medication labels

PROBLEM SOLVING

Learning to regulate insulin doses on the basis of signs and symptoms

COMPREHENSION AND APPLICATION

Knowing physical restrictions imposed by illness
Following directions when performing self-care in accordance with limitations

table 14-2

RELATIONSHIP BETWEEN PSYCHOSOCIAL ADAPTATION TO ILLNESS AND LEARNING

Stage	Client's behavior	Learning implications	Rationale
Denial or disbelief	Client avoids discussion of illness ("There's nothing wrong with me"), withdraws from others, and disregards physical restrictions. Client suppresses and distorts information that has not been presented clearly.	Provide support, empathy, and careful explanations of all procedures while they are being done. Let client know you are available for discussion. Explain situation to family. Teach in present tense (explain current therapy).	Client is not prepared to deal with problem. Any attempt to convince or tell client about illness will result in further anger or withdrawal. Provide only information client pursues or absolutely requires.
Anger	Client blames and complains and often directs anger toward nurse.	Do not argue with client, but listen to concerns. Teach in present tense. Reassure family of client's normality.	Client needs opportunity to express feelings and anger. Client is still not prepared to face future.
Bargaining	Client offers to live better life in exchange for promise of better health ("if God lets me live, I promise to be more careful").	Continue to introduce only reality. Teach only in present tense.	Client is still unwilling to accept limitations.
Resolution	Client begins to express emotions openly, realizes that illness has created changes, and begins to ask questions.	Encourage expression of feelings. Begin to share information needed for future, and set aside formal times for discussion.	Client begins to perceive need for assistance and is ready to accept responsibility for learning.
Acceptance	Client recognizes reality of condition, actively pursues information, and strives for independence.	Focus teaching on future skills and knowledge required. Continue to teach about present occurrences. Involve family in teaching information for discharge.	Client is more easily motivated to learn. Acceptance of illness reflects willingness to deal with its implications.

and improves the opportunity for the client to make decisions during teaching sessions. For example, a client with diabetes learns to monitor blood glucose levels to gain control of the disease. The nurse helps the client learn to adapt a successful monitoring system and schedule.

Ability to Learn

Developmental Capability. Cognitive development influences the ability to learn. A nurse can be a competent teacher, but if the client's intellectual abilities are not considered, teaching is unsuccessful. Sometimes a nurse has shared teaching booklets and brochures and then discovered that the client cannot read. Learning, like developmental growth, is an evolving process. The nurse must know the client's level of knowledge and intellectual skills before beginning a teaching plan. The box on p. 234 shows the types of learning problems clients may have when their intellectual skills are not fully developed.

A requisite level of maturation and cognitive development must exist before an individual is capable of learning new information. It is wrong to assume that a client has a certain level of knowledge; instead, the nurse should assess the client's level of knowledge. Learning occurs more readily when new information complements existing knowledge.

Age-Group. Age reflects the developmental capability for learning and learning behaviors that can be acquired (Table 14-3). Without proper biological, motor, language, and personal-social development, many types of learning cannot take place. Learning occurs when be-

table 14-3

DEVELOPMENTAL CAPACITIES FOR LEARNING

Learning capacity	Teaching methods
INFANT	
Infant relies on parents for basic needs. Infant learns to trust adults when they convey love and compassion. Infant explores environment through senses.	Keep routines (feeding, bathing) consistent. Hold infant firmly while smiling and speaking softly to convey sense of trust.
TODDLER	
Toddler learns to understand words and express feelings verbally. Toddler learns by associating words with objects. Toddler likes to explore environment through play.	Use play to teach procedure or activity (handling examination equipment, applying bandage to doll). Offer picture books that describe story of children in hospital or clinic. Use simple words such as *cut* instead of *laceration* to promote understanding.
PRESCHOOLER	
Vocabulary grows. Preschooler uses language without comprehending meaning of words, especially concepts (right or left, time). During play, child expresses feelings more through actions than words. Preschooler asks questions and imitates adults.	Use role playing, imitation, and play to make it fun for preschoolers to learn. Encourage questions and offer explanations. Use simple explanations and demonstrations. Encourage children to learn together through pictures and short stories of how to perform hygiene.
SCHOOL-AGE CHILD	
Child interacts with adults and peers outside immediate family. Child begins to acquire ability to relate series of events and actions to mental representations that can be expressed verbally and symbolically. Child is able to make judgments. Child matures physically. Play becomes more formal and imaginative. Child is inquisitive and asks many questions about health.	Teach psychomotor skills needed to maintain health. (Complicated skills, such as learning to use a syringe, may take considerable practice.) Offer opportunities to discuss health problems and answer questions.
ADOLESCENT	
Adolescent struggles between childlike feelings of dependence and independence of adults. Teenager wants to be in control but, during illness, fears loss of self-concept or body image. Adolescent is able to solve abstract problems. Teenager learns best when immediate benefit is gained.	Help adolescent learn about feelings and need for self-expression. Use teaching as collaborative activity. Allow adolescents to make decisions about health and health promotion (safety, sex education, substance abuse). Use problem solving to help adolescents make choices.
YOUNG OR MIDDLE ADULT	
Adult complies with health teaching because client fears the results, is trying to gain approval, is responding to nurse's attitude, or knows it is in best interest.* Learning occurs when adult values information being taught.	Encourage participation in teaching plan by setting mutual goals. Encourage independent learning. Offer information so that adult can understand effects of health problem.

*Data from Woodward S: *Preoperative patient education seminar presentation,* Denver, 1983, Resource Applications.

table 14-3—cont'd

DEVELOPMENTAL CAPACITIES FOR LEARNING

Learning capacity	Teaching methods
OLDER ADULT	
Often, there is decline in visual and auditory acuity, which impairs perception of stimuli. Sensory alterations, mobility limitations, and physical coordination problems affect capacity to learn. Sleep-wake cycles are more fragemented. Older adult takes pride in being independent and caring for self. There is no decline in intelligence with age.	Teach when client is alert and rested. Involve adult in discussion or activity. Focus on wellness and the person's strength. Use approaches that enhance sensorially impaired client's reception of stimuli (see Chapter 38). Keep teaching sessions short.

havior changes as a result of experience or growth (Whaley and Wong, 1991).

Physical Capability. The ability to learn often depends on a person's level of physical development and overall physical health. To learn psychomotor skills, a client must have the necessary level of strength, coordination, and sensory acuity. For example, it would be useless to teach a client to transfer from a bed to a wheelchair if the client does not have enough upper body strength. An older adult cannot learn to apply an elastic bandage if he has poor eyesight or cannot grasp the bandage tightly. Therefore the nurse should not overestimate the client's physical development. The following physical attributes are required to learn psychomotor skills:

1. Size (height and weight match the task to perform or the equipment to use [e.g., crutch walking])
2. Strength (ability of client to follow strenuous exercise program)
3. Coordination (dexterity needed for complicated motor skills such as using utensils or changing a bandage)
4. Sensory acuity (visual, auditory, tactile, gustatory, and olfactory: sensory resources needed to receive and respond to messages taught)

Any condition that depletes a person's energy will also impair the ability to learn. If a client spends the entire morning undergoing a rigorous schedule of diagnostic tests, it is unlikely that he or she will be capable of the effort needed for any learning discussion. When a client's illness is aggravated by complications such as a high fever or respiratory difficulty, teaching should be postponed. After working with a client, the nurse can assess the energy level by the willingness to communicate, amount of activity initiated, and responsiveness toward questions. The nurse may halt teaching temporarily if a client needs rest. The nurse achieves greater teaching success when the client is an active participant.

Learning Environment

Factors in the physical environment where teaching takes place make learning a pleasant or difficult experience. The nurse chooses a setting that helps the client to focus attention on the learning task. The number of persons being taught, need for privacy, room temperature, room lighting, noise, room ventilation, and room furniture are important when choosing the setting.

The ideal environment for promoting learning is a room that is well lit and has good ventilation, appropriate furniture, and a comfortable temperature (Figure 14-1). A darkened room interferes with the client's ability to watch the nurse's actions, especially when demon-

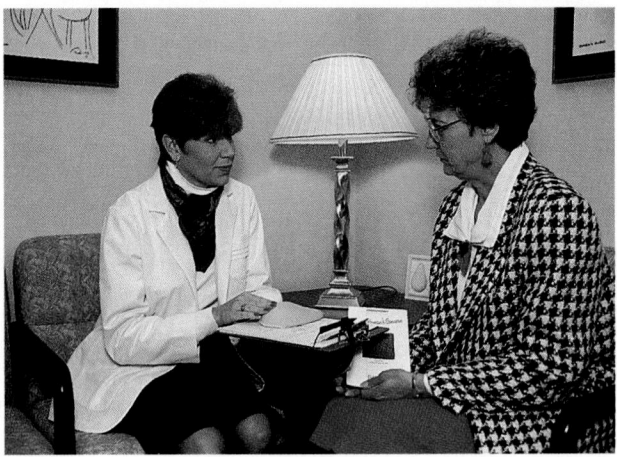

FIGURE 14-1 Choosing comfortable, pleasant environments enhances the learning experience. This nurse is explaining health care principles to the client.

strating a skill or using visual aids such as posters or pamphlets. A room that is too cold, hot, or stuffy will make the client too uncomfortable to attend to the nurse's activities. Comfortable furniture helps to eliminate distractions such as the need to change position or shift body weight.

It is also important to choose a quiet setting. When a nurse is working with a client, a quiet setting where frequent interruptions are unlikely to occur offers privacy that is best. If the client desires, family members might share in discussions. However, a client is often reluctant to discuss the nature of the illness when other persons, even family members, are in the room.

Teaching a group of clients requires a room that allows all persons to be seated comfortably and within hearing distance of the teacher. The size of the room should not overwhelm the group, tempting participants to sit outside the group along the perimeter. Arranging the group to allow participants to observe one another further enhances learning. More effective communication occurs as learners observe others' verbal and nonverbal interactions.

NURSING PROCESS IN TEACHING

A relationship exists between the nursing and teaching processes. With the nursing process, assessment reveals the client's health care needs. The nursing diagnoses identified are unique to the client's situation. A care plan is individualized and evaluation determines the level of success in meeting goals of care.

During the diagnosis phase the nurse may also identify the need for education. When education becomes a part of the care plan, the teaching process begins. Like the nursing process, the teaching process requires assessment. In this case the nurse analyzes the client's need, motivation, and ability to learn (Table 14-4). A diagnostic statement specifies the information or skills the client requires. The nurse sets specific learning objectives and implements the teaching plan using learning and teaching principles to ensure that the client acquires knowledge and skills. Finally, the teaching process requires an evaluation of learning based on learning objectives.

The nursing and teaching processes are not the same. The nursing process requires assessment of all sources of data to determine a client's total health care needs. The teaching process focuses on the client's learning needs and willingness and capability to learn. Table 14-4 compares the teaching and nursing processes.

Assessment

Success in teaching a client requires the nurse to assess all factors influencing the content to be taught, the client's ability to learn, and the resources for instruction. The client's learning needs determine the choice of teaching content.

table 14-4

COMPARISON OF THE NURSING AND TEACHING PROCESSES

Basic steps	Nursing process	Teaching process
Assessment	Collect data about client's physical, psychological, social, cultural, developmental, and spiritual needs from client, family, diagnostic tests, medical record, nursing history, and literature.	Gather data about client's learning needs, motivation, ability to learn, and teaching resources from client, family, learning environment, medical record, nursing history, and literature.
Nursing diagnosis	Identify appropriate nursing diagnoses.	Identify client's learning needs on basis of three domains of learning.
Planning	Develop individualized care plan. Set diagnosis priorities based on client's immediate needs. Collaborate with client on care plan.	Establish learning objectives, stated in behavioral terms. Identify priorities regarding learning needs. Collaborate with client on teaching plan. Identify type of teaching method to use.
Implementation	Perform nursing care therapies. Include client as active participant in care. Involve family in care as appropriate.	Implement teaching methods. Actively involve client in learning activities. Include family participation as appropriate.
Evaluation	Identify success in meeting desired outcomes and goals of nursing care.	Determine outcomes of teaching-learning process. Measure client's ability to achieve learning objectives. Re-teach as needed.

LEARNING NEEDS

The nurse determines the information critical for the client to learn, which determines the choice of teaching content. Learning needs change depending on where the client is in the recovery process. Assessment is thus an ongoing activity. An effective assessment is the basis by which instruction can be individualized to each client (Redman, 1992). Some examples of key assessment concerns are observation of the client's behavior, client's response to direct questions, and simple tests of capabilities (e.g., reading level or ability to manipulate equipment). The nurse can assess attention span, memory, and ability to concentrate by noting reactions to questions during the nursing history. If the client seems uninterested in a discussion topic or is unable to recall significant events, learning may be difficult. A short attention span may be caused by poor physical health, anxiety, fatigue, or inability to understand questions and concepts.

MOTIVATION TO LEARN

Nurses use several tools to assess the client's motivation to learn. In the absence of such tools the nurse can ask questions that define the client's motivation. These questions help to determine whether the client is prepared and willing to learn. They include asking the client about learning behaviors, health beliefs, attitudes about health care providers, knowledge of information to be learned, and physical symptoms that interfere with learning, client's sociocultural background, and preferences for formats for learning.

ABILITY TO LEARN

The nurse determines the client's physical and cognitive levels. Many factors can impair the ability to learn. The nurse needs to assess the client's physical strength and coordination, any sensory deficits, the client's reading and developmental level (see Table 14-3, p. 236), and the client's level of cognitive functioning.

TEACHING ENVIRONMENT

The environment for a teaching session must be conducive to learning. The nurse assesses for distractions, noise, comfort level, and availability of rooms and equipment.

RESOURCES FOR LEARNING

A final assessment involves an inventory of available teaching resources, including brochures, audiovisual materials, or posters. The nurse should also be sure that such materials are available when needed (Figure 14-2). The nurse also assesses the readiness of family and friends to learn any information necessary to help care for the client. The nurse assesses family perceptions, the client's willingness to involve family members, the family's willingness to help provide care, resources available in the home, and needed teaching tools.

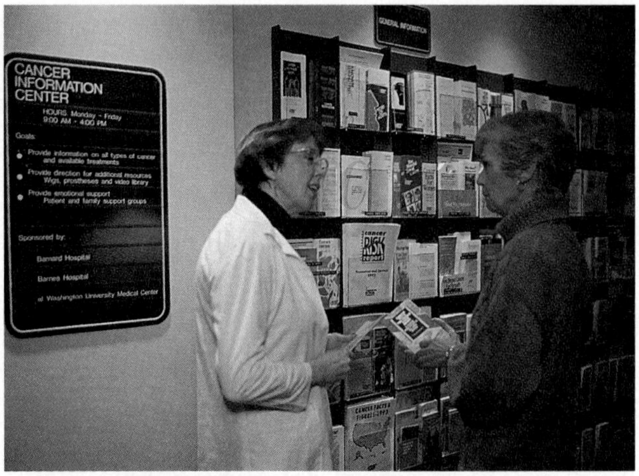

FIGURE 14-2 At this cancer information center the nurse has a wide array of resources for patient education.

The assessment phase brings the scope of a teaching plan into focus. A thorough assessment helps the nurse to choose the best teaching methods and ensures a more individualized approach toward client education.

Nursing Diagnosis

After assessing information related to the client's ability and need to learn, the nurse interprets the data to form diagnoses that reflect the client's specific learning needs (see box on p. 240). This ensures that the nurse's teaching efforts will be adequately goal directed and individualized. If a client appears to have several learning needs, nursing diagnoses allow for priority setting.

Several nursing diagnoses apply to learning needs. Each diagnostic statement describes the specific type of learning need and its cause. Classifying diagnoses by the three learning domains helps the nurse to focus specifically on subject matter and teaching methods. Some health care problems can be managed or eliminated through education. In these situations the related factor of the diagnostic statement is knowledge deficit. For example, a client may have difficulty in interacting socially because of a lack of effective communication skills.

Some nursing diagnoses also indicate that teaching may be inappropriate. The nurse may identify condi-

NURSING DIAGNOSES RELATED TO LEARNING NEEDS

ALTERED HEALTH MAINTENANCE related to:

Lack of knowledge about health practices
Lack of fine motor skills

KNOWLEDGE DEFICIT (AFFECTIVE) related to:

Misunderstanding of prognosis

KNOWLEDGE DEFICIT (COGNITIVE) related to:

Newly diagnosed disease
Newly prescribed therapy

KNOWLEDGE DEFICIT (PSYCHOMOTOR) related to:

Inexperience with skill
Lack of interest in learning

NONCOMPLIANCE WITH MEDICATIONS related to:

Poor understanding of therapies
Disbelief of health risk

BATHING/HYGIENE SELF-CARE DEFICIT related to:

Neuromuscular impairment
Unfamiliarity with preventive care measures

IMPAIRED SOCIAL INTERACTION related to:

Poor communication skills

tions that can cause barriers to effective learning (e.g., pain or activity intolerance).

Planning

After determining the nursing diagnoses that identify a client's learning needs, the nurse develops a teaching plan, determines goals and expected outcomes, and involves the client in selecting learning experiences (see teaching plan). Expected outcomes guide the choice of teaching strategies and approaches with a client. Client participation ensures a more relevant and meaningful plan.

A learning objective identifies the expected outcome of a learning experience. Objectives are short or long term. The nurse and client develop learning objectives together. Each objective is a statement of a singular behavior that identifies the client's ability to do something after a learning experience. The objective contains an active verb describing what the client will do after the objective is met, such as *to perform* a crutch gait, *to administer* an injection, or *to identify* drug doses. The verb should have few interpretations and be stated in terms of how the client is to demonstrate learning, rather than what or how the teacher is to teach (Redman, 1992).

Behavioral objectives are measurable and observable, indicating how learning is evidenced (e.g., to perform the *three-point crutch gait*). If content is missing, the objective cannot guide teaching and learning. The precise behaviors and content set the standard for feedback that reflects learning and forms the basis for evaluation of the teaching plan.

An objective is more precise when it also describes the conditions or timing under which the behavior occurs. Conditions or time frames should be realistic and designed for the learner's needs. It also helps to consider the conditions under which the client or family will typically perform the learned behavior (e.g., to walk from bedroom to bath using crutches).

Criteria for acceptable performance set a standard by which achievement is measured. A teacher sets criteria on the basis of a desired level of accuracy, success, or satisfaction. For example, a client undergoing therapy for a fractured leg will walk on crutches *to the end of the hall within 3 days.* Criteria are more acceptable when established by the teacher and learner. However, the nurse serves as a resource in setting the minimal criteria for success. Criteria on which the client and nurse agree help to define the expected behaviors and the quality of performance. The client also uses these criteria for self-evaluation, which is a powerful motivator of behavior.

After formulating objectives, the nurse and client work to establish a teaching plan. During planning the nurse integrates basic teaching principles, and develops and prioritizes a well-timed, organized teaching plan.

INTEGRATING BASIC TEACHING PRINCIPLES

Teaching priorities should reflect the priorities of the nursing diagnoses. Teaching, or instruction, is the process of leading someone to learn. Just as there are basic principles that promote learning, there are also principles that enhance a teacher's effectiveness. The realm of teaching deals with the teacher's behavior, the reason teachers behave the way they do, and effects of their behavior on learners. There is no single correct way to teach since each learning situation determines the best way to teach. The principles of teaching are, in effect, techniques that incorporate the principles of learning.

Setting Priorities

Priorities for teaching are based on nursing diagnoses and the learning objectives established for the client. A client's learning needs must be set in order of priority to conserve the client's and nurse's time and energy. For example, a client with a permanent leg injury has a knowledge deficit regarding the nature of the injury and its implications, as well as the types of skills needed to resume a normal life at home. The client will benefit most from first learning about the injury and the resultant physical changes before learning to cope with the disability.

Timing

When is the right time to teach? When a client first enters a clinic or hospital? At discharge? At home? Each may be appropriate because clients continue to have learning needs and opportunities as long as they stay in the health care system. The nurse determines the client's readiness to learn. Timing can be difficult because emphasis is placed on a client's early discharge from a hospital. For example, it may take several days after surgery for a client to become free of discomfort so that attention can be given to learning. By the time the client feels ready to learn, discharge may already be scheduled. The nurse should plan teaching activities for a time when the client is most attentive, receptive, and alert. Many hospitals provide information to clients before admission. The client's activities should be organized to provide time for rest and teaching-learning interactions.

The length of teaching sessions also influences learning ability. Prolonged sessions cause clients to lose concentration and attentiveness. Frequent sessions lasting 20 to 30 minutes are more easily tolerated and retain the client's interest in the material. The nurse can assess a client's loss of concentration by observing for nonverbal cues such as poor eye contact or slumped posture. After loss of concentration is noted, the session should be stopped. However, teaching sessions should not be too brief. The client needs time to comprehend the information and to give feedback.

Teaching sessions should be held frequently enough to document the client's learning. The frequency of sessions depends on the learner's abilities and the complexity of the material. Intervals between teaching sessions should not be so long that the client might forget information. For clients discharged home early, home health nurses must reinforce learning.

Organizing Teaching Material

A good teacher gives careful consideration to the order of information presented. Usually an outline of content helps to organize information into a logical sequence. Material should progress from simple to complex ideas because a person must learn simple facts and concepts before learning how to make associations or complex interpretations of ideas. For example, to teach a client with diabetes how to calculate a 1200-calorie diet, the nurse first teaches the client about calories, proteins, and carbohydrates and then uses simple mathematical problems to help the client to learn to calculate amounts.

The nurse begins any instruction with essential content. Clients are most likely to remember information presented during the first third of a teaching session (Miller, 1985). For example, after surgical removal of a cancerous lung tumor, the client's predisposition to cancer recurrence makes learning about the warning signs of cancer crucial. The nurse starts with essential information and completes the teaching session with informative but less critical content. Finally, it helps to summarize important points. Repetition reinforces learning. A concise summary of key topics will help the learner to know the most important information.

Maintaining Learner Attention and Participation

Active participation is key to learning. Persons learn better when more than one of the body's senses are stimulated. Audiovisual aids and role playing are good teaching strategies. By actively experiencing a learning event, the person will be more likely to retain the knowledge gained.

A teacher's actions can also increase learner attention and interest. When conducting a discussion with a learner, the teacher should stay active by changing tone and intensity of voice, making eye contact, and using gestures that accentuate key points of discussion. An effective teacher often uses as much energy as the learner, talking and moving among a group rather than remaining stationary behind a lectern or table. A learner remains interested in a teacher who is actively enthusiastic about the subject under discussion.

Building on Existing Knowledge

A client learns best on the basis of preexisting cognitive abilities and knowledge. Thus a teacher is more effective by presenting information that builds on a learner's existing knowledge. The key is assessing the learner's level of knowledge by finding out how much is known about the topic.

Speaking the Client's Language

It is important to use words a client can understand. The nurse defines unfamiliar medical or nursing terms and uses them consistently throughout a teaching session. Medical jargon can be confusing.

Byrne and Edeani (1984) found that clients understand fewer medical words than health professionals predict. The problem of functional illiteracy is also real. Kozol (1985) reports that 44% of black adults, 33% of Hispanic adults, and 16% of white adults in the United States are functionally or marginally illiterate.

The nurse uses simple terminology to enhance clients' understanding. Frequently asking clients for feedback determines whether clients comprehend.

Matching Teaching Methods With Learners' Needs

The efficiency of a teaching method depends in part on the client's learning need (see box below). Clients with psychomotor deficits learn best through demonstrations and supervised practice. The client masters skills by handling equipment and practicing manual skills. Discussions, question-and-answer sessions, and formal lectures are effective methods for promoting cognitive learning. Clients with intellectual deficits are given the opportunity to explore new ideas, recognize new relationships, and apply knowledge to their unique needs. A highly effective method for stimulating affective learning is group discussion. Clients learn to share ideas and values with one another, realizing that there are alternative ways to view the world. The method should complement the client's needs.

Implementation

Implementation of a teaching plan (see the case study on pp. 243-244) involves applying all teaching and learning principles. Assessment of the client reveals his or her learning needs. Implementation involves believing that each interaction with a client is an opportunity to teach. The nurse acts on these opportunities for effective learning and uses a variety of approaches to create an active learning environment.

TEACHING APPROACHES

A nurse's approach in teaching is different from teaching methods. Approach involves the nurse's task and re-

TEACHING METHODS

COGNITIVE

Discussion (one-on-one or group)

May involve nurse and client or nurse with several clients
Promotes active participation and focuses on topics of interest to client
Allows peer support
Enhances application and analysis of new information

Lecture

Is more formal method of instruction because it is controlled by teacher
Helps learner acquire new knowledge and gain comprehension

Question-and-answer session

Is designed specifically to address client's concerns
Assists client in applying knowledge

Role play, discovery

Allows client to actively apply knowledge in controlled situation
Promotes synthesis of information and problem solving

Independent project (computer-assisted instruction), field experience

Allows client to assume responsibility for completing learning activities at own pace
Promotes analysis, synthesis, and evaluation of new information and skills

AFFECTIVE

Role play

Allows expression of values, feelings, and attitudes

Discussion (group)

Allows client to acquire support from others in group
Permits client to learn from other experiences
Promotes responding, valuing, and organization

Discussion (one-on-one)

Allows discussion of personal, sensitive topics of interest or concern

PSYCHOMOTOR

Demonstration

Provides presentation of procedures or skills by nurse
Permits client to incorporate modeling of nurse's behavior
Allows nurse to control questioning during demonstration

Practice

Gives client opportunity to perform skills using equipment
Provides repetition

Return demonstration

Permits client to perform skill as nurse observes
Is excellent source of feedback and reinforcement

Independent projects, games

Require teaching method that promotes adaptation and origination of psychomotor learning
Permit learner to use new skills

CASE STUDY AND TEACHING PLAN

Mrs. Clemmons is a 58-year-old woman seen in the clinic for treatment of arthritis. She repeatedly returns to the clinic as a result of her poor compliance with therapy. The nurse, Ms. Bingham, decides that Mrs. Clemmons might benefit from a teaching program directed toward improving her ability to cope with her disease. (Relevant data are in italic and in parentheses.)

ASSESSMENT AND RELEVANT DATA

The nurse's assessment reveals that Mrs. Clemmons weighs 158 pounds (71 kg) and is 5 feet, 1 inch (153 cm) tall. Her arthritis affects primarily the joints of her hands and knees. (*Obesity adds stress to affected joints.*)

She has difficulty picking up small objects such as a pen or a safety pin. Her grasp is also quite weak. Because of the knee involvement, Mrs. Clemmons has difficulty rising from a sitting to a standing position. (*Physical deficits.*)

When discussing Mrs. Clemmons' condition, the nurse learns that her client knows only that arthritis is a "disease of the joints." However, the client does not understand how obesity can increase stress on her joints. She is also unaware of measures that can help her to perform activities of daily living without added discomfort and of how various medications act to relieve the symptoms of arthritis. (*Knowledge deficit.*)

Ms. Bingham is concerned that if Mrs. Clemmons has a history of poor compliance, she may not benefit from a teaching plan. However, she learns that Mrs. Clemmons has an interest in learning more because she asks the nurse several questions. (*Readiness to learn.*)

The client is unfamiliar with many of the terms Ms. Bingham uses to describe arthritis. (*Cognitive capability.*)

Mrs. Clemmons is married to a carpenter. She tells the nurse that her husband becomes distressed over her inability to feel better: "It's hard for him to understand why I can't do more. He doesn't know how arthritis can cripple you." When asked if Mr. Clemmons would be interested in attending a teaching session, Mrs. Clemmons says, "Yes, I know he will come if I ask." (*Family support.*)

The nurse reserves a conference room for the first teaching session. She also arranges to use a film on arthritis and locates pamphlets on self-care devices and medications for arthritis. (*Teaching resources.*)

NURSING DIAGNOSES

Assessment reveals a number of diagnoses:

Impaired physical mobility related to:

- Joint inflammation

Knowledge deficit: cognitive regarding illness related to:

- Poor understanding of interaction of obesity and arthritis

Knowledge deficit: cognitive regarding illness related to:

- Poor understanding of how medications control disease

PLANNING

On the basis of the diagnoses, Ms. Bingham sets specific learning objectives. After proper instruction, Mrs. Clemmons will be able to:

1. Perform fine motor skills with activities of daily living in the home within 1 month
2. Stand from a sitting position without assistance within 2 months
3. Describe how arthritis affects the joints of the body within 1 month
4. Develop a low-calorie meal plan for a week
5. Describe the actions and side effects of arthritic medications within 2 months

The nurse does not plan to cover all topics in one teaching session. Mrs. Clemmons expresses interest in first learning about arthritis and beginning to use some of the motor skills Ms. Bingham has proposed. The nurse and client decide that the best time to have the teaching session is on a Tuesday evening when Mr. Clemmons can come to the clinic with his wife.

IMPLEMENTATION

Ms. Bingham begins the session by getting to know Mr. Clemmons and observing how he and Mrs. Clemmons interact. She recognizes that Mr. Clemmons is interested in helping his wife if he can. The client and her husband are attentive and responsive to Ms. Bingham's questions.

The nurse shows the film to give Mr. and Mrs. Clemmons a thorough introduction to arthritis. After the film the nurse and her clients discuss aspects of the film relevant to Mrs. Clemmons' condition, and the nurse answers the couple's questions. Then they discuss how arthritis has affected Mrs. Clemmons' ability to perform activities of daily living. The nurse asks questions designed to help Mr. Clemmons to gain an understanding of the long-term impact of his wife's disease. Throughout the discussion Ms. Bingham uses simple terms to explain key concepts. When the Clemmonses show confusion, Ms. Bingham clarifies information with illustrations on the blackboard.

Ms. Bingham uses the remaining class time to demonstrate some simple exercises to maintain Mrs. Clemmons' joint mobility and muscle strength. This is a type of teaching strategy that gets Mr. and Mrs. Clemmons actively involved. The nurse shows Mrs. Clemmons how to do the exercises and then assists Mr. Clemmons in learning how to direct his wife appropriately. The nurse also discusses types of self-help devices with the Clemmonses. Mr. Clemmons' carpentry skill can be put to use to build several of the devices. One device is wooden blocks or platforms to elevate chairs and the bed so that Mrs. Clemmons will not have to raise herself up so far from a sitting position.

Continued.

CASE STUDY—cont'd

EVALUATION

The nurse asks the Clemmonses to briefly explain the nature of arthritis. After viewing the film they are able to give a simple but complete description of how joints are injured. The nurse knows that it is easy to forget information unless it is reinforced. She gives the Clemmonses a pamphlet to review before the next class and asks them to write down any questions they might have.

It is too early to evaluate Mrs. Clemmons' joint mobility or muscle strength. The client is given an exercise plan to follow for a week. Ms. Bingham asks Mr. Clemmons to come to the next class with ideas on types of self-help devices he might be able to construct for his wife. Thus the nurse has begun a constructive teaching plan that will enable Mrs. Clemmons and her husband to cope more effectively with her disease. As the teaching process continues, Ms. Bingham will work with Mr. and Mrs. Clemmons to reach all the objectives based on the nursing diagnoses.

lationship behaviors (Paulish, 1987). Some situations require the teacher to be directive. Others may require a nondirective approach. An effective teacher concentrates on the task and uses teaching approaches according to client needs.

Telling

The telling approach is useful when limited information must be taught (e.g., when preparing the client for an emergent diagnostic procedure). When using telling, the nurse outlines the task to be done by the client and gives explicit instructions. There is no time for feedback with this method.

Selling

The selling approach uses two-way communication. The nurse paces instruction based on the client's response. Specific feedback is given to the client who shows success at learning. For example, the clients learns a step-by-step procedure for changing a dressing. The nurse uses information from the client to adapt the teaching approach.

Participating

The participating approach involves the nurse and client in setting objectives and participating in the learning process together. The client helps decide content, and the nurse guides and counsels the client. For example, a client with diabetes works with the nurse to menu plan or self-administer insulin. In this method there is opportunity for discussion, feedback, and revision of the teaching plan.

Entrusting

The entrusting approach provides the client the opportunity to manage self-care. The client accepts responsibilities and performs the tasks well. The nurse observes the client's progress (e.g., a diabetic client who has correctly administered injections for 3 months). The nurse instructs the client about a new prescribed dose of insulin and allows the client to perform the injection.

Reinforcing

The principle of reinforcement applies to the process of learning; however, the teacher must often be the source of reinforcement. **Reinforcement** is using a stimulus that increases the probability of a response. A learner who receives reinforcement before or after a desired learning behavior will likely repeat the behavior. Feedback is a common form of reinforcement.

Reinforcers are positive or negative. Positive reinforcement such as a smile or praise and approval produces the desired responses. Negative reinforcement such as frowning or complaining produces the desired behavior when the reinforcers are removed. People usually respond better to positive reinforcement.

Three types of reinforcers are social, material, and activity. When a nurse works with a client, most reinforcers are social—a smile, a compliment, a word of encouragement, or physical contact, which are used to acknowledge a learned behavior. Examples of material reinforcers are food, toys, and music. These work best with young children. Activity reinforcers rely on the principle that a person is motivated to engage in an activity if promised that, after its completion, the opportunity to engage in more desirable activity will be available. For example, a client will more likely perform a painful exercise if given the chance to take a nap afterward.

Choosing the right reinforcer involves careful thought and attention to individual preferences. Reinforcers should never be used as threats. Reinforcement is not always effective with every client.

Incorporating Teaching With Nursing Care

Many nurses find that they can teach more effectively while delivering nursing care. An informal unstructured style relies on the positive therapeutic relationship between nurse and client, which fosters a spontaneity in the teaching-learning process. This does not suggest that teaching should occur without a formal plan. When the nurse follows a teaching plan informally, the client feels less pressure to perform, and learning becomes more of a shared activity. Teaching during routine care is efficient and cost effective.

Instructional Methods

Instructional methods chosen depend on the client's learning needs. There are a variety of methods appropriate for clients (see box on p. 242). Skilled teachers are flexible and combine more than one method into a teaching plan.

Preparatory Instruction

Clients frequently face unfamiliar tests or procedures that create anxiety. Information helps the client to form a realistic image of procedures. When the experience coincides with expectations, the client is more likely to attend to future explanations. A nurse gains respect when preparatory explanations are useful. The following are guidelines for giving preparatory explanations:

1. Physical sensations during the procedure are described but not evaluated. For example, before drawing a blood specimen, the nurse explains that the client will feel a sticking sensation as the needle punctures the skin.
2. The cause of the sensation is described, preventing misinterpretation of the experience. For example, the nurse explains that a needle insertion burns because alcohol used to cleanse the skin enters the puncture site.
3. Clients are prepared only for aspects of the experience that have commonly been noticed by other clients. For example, the nurse explains that it is normal for a tight tourniquet to cause a person's hand to tingle and feel numb.

The client finds comfort in knowing what to expect. When the nurse's descriptions accurately portray the actual experience, the client is able to cope more effectively with the stress from procedures and therapies.

Demonstrations

Demonstrations are useful methods for teaching psychomotor skills. An effective demonstration requires advanced planning, including the following:

1. Review the rationale and steps of the procedure.
2. Assemble and organize equipment.
3. Perform each step in sequence while analyzing the knowledge and skills involved.
4. Determine when explanations need to be given, considering the client's learning needs.
5. Judge the proper speed and timing of the demonstration.

The nurse demonstrates a procedure or skill in the same order in which the client will perform it. In addition, the nurse encourages the client to ask questions so that each step is clearly understood. To enable the client to easily observe each step of the procedure, demonstrations should be performed slowly. The nurse gives an opportunity to practice the procedure under supervision after the client has practiced handling equipment. Ultimately the client demonstrates the procedure independently to ensure acquisition of the skill. This demonstration should occur under the same conditions the client will experience at home.

Special Needs of Children and Older Adults

A nurse's choice of instructional methods may be based on a client's age. Children, adults, and older adults learn differently. The nurse adapts teaching strategies to each learner.

Children pass through several developmental stages (see Chapter 19). In each stage, children acquire new cognitive and psychomotor abilities that respond to different types of learning. Parental input and participation are needed in planning health education for children.

Older adults go through many physical and psychological changes as they age. These changes can create barriers to learning. Sensory changes require teaching methods that enhance the client's functioning. Research shows that older adults learn and remember effectively if the learning is paced properly and the material is relevant to the learner's needs and abilities (Weinrich, 1989; Heese, 1984; Whitman, 1986). The box below provides an example of educational strategies for gerontological nursing practice.

EDUCATIONAL STRATEGIES FOR GERONTOLOGICAL NURSING PRACTICE

Use a slow pace of presentation
Give information in short frequent sessions
Repeat information frequently
Reinforce teaching with audiovisual material, written exercises, and practice
Use examples
Allow more time for learners to express themselves, demonstrate learning, and ask questions
Establish reachable short-term goals
Apply teaching to present situations
Base new information on clients' previous level of learning

Modified from Weinrich SP, Boyd M, et al.: *J Gerontol Nurs* 15 (11):17, 1989.

BARNES

C-33

DIABETIC INSTRUCTION RECORD

TI = TEACHING INITIATED
D/V = DEMONSTRATES/VERBALIZES UNDERSTANDING
FI = FAMILY INCLUDED

ADDRESSOGRAPH PLATE

ASSESSMENT

1. HIGHEST LEVEL OF FORMALIZED EDUCATION ATTAINED: High School
2. VISION: Glasses required for reading
3. LITERACY: Able to read and explain information in teaching booklet
4. IDENTIFIED BARRIERS TO LEARNING

	DATE & INITIAL			
	TI	D/V	FI	COMMENTS
A) DISEASE OVERVIEW 1. DEFINITION OF DIABETES	P.L. 3/28	R.K. 3/29	P.L. 3/28	Wife included in teaching session
2. LONGTERM COMPLICATIONS (MICROVASCULAR/MACROVASCULAR/NEUROPATHY)	P.L. 3/28	R.K. 3/29	P.L. 3/28	
3. 3 FACTORS OF CONTROL (DIET, EXERCISE, MEDICATION)	P.L. 3/28	R.K. 3/29	P.L. 3/28	
B) DIET 1. TYPE 1800 Cal. ADA	R.K. 3/29			
SNACK TIMES 8:00 pM	3/29 R.K.			
2. MEAL TIMING 8am 12N 6pM	3/29 R.K.			
3. FOOD TYPES TO AVOID (FRIED FATTY FOODS, SIMPLE SUGARS)				
4. IMPORTANCE OF WEIGHT CONTROL				
C) EXERCISE 1. TYPE				
2. FREQUENCY				
3. DURATION				
4. EFFECTS ON BLOOD SUGAR CONTROL & INSULIN UTILIZATION				
D) MEDICATION 1. NAME/DOSAGE				
2. ORAL AGENT				
a. WHEN TO TAKE				
b. ACTION OF MEDICATION				
3. INSULIN				
a. ACTION, KINDS, STORAGE				
b. PREPARATION, ADMINISTRATION				
c. SITE SELECTION/ROTATION				

FIGURE 14-3 Documentation tool for client teaching. (Courtesy Barnes Hospital, St. Louis.).

Evaluation

Client education is not complete until the nurse evaluates the outcomes of the teaching-learning process. Did the client learn what was intended? The nurse evaluates success by observing the client's performance of each expected behavior. Success depends on the client's ability to meet the established performance criteria.

Return demonstrations, use of questions, observation of client behaviors, role playing, and discussions can be used to evaluate clients. For example, the client who will use a three-point crutch gait while walking to the end of the hall must demonstrate the actual crutch-walking technique. A client who is to identify five signs and symptoms of hypertension must be able to do so when questioned or during a discussion of the disease.

If evaluation indicates a knowledge or skill deficit, the nurse repeats or modifies the teaching plan. Alternative teaching methods often help to clarify information or strengthen skills the client was unable to comprehend or perform originally.

Evaluation may also reveal new learning needs or new factors that may interfere with the client's ability to learn. The nurse reassesses those factors to update the teaching plan and make it relevant to client needs. Like the nursing process, the teaching process is continuous and ever changing.

Because client teaching often occurs informally between nurse and client (e.g., during medication administration or physical examination), it is difficult to document client education consistently. Nurses often fail to take the time to write down information they have taught. However, because a nurse is legally responsible for providing accurate and timely information to clients, quality documentation is essential. Barron (1987) suggests the following for documenting client education:

1. Specific content. Specifically describe subject matter so that other nurses can follow up and reinforce teaching (e.g., "insulin injection demonstrated" or "explained side effects of Inderal"). Avoid generalizations such as "medications taught" that leave staff uninformed about what content has been taught.
2. Evaluation of learning. Document evidence of learning (e.g., a return demonstration or the attempt to evaluate learning). This informs staff about the client's progress and determines matters that still need to be taught.
3. Method of teaching. Describe how the subject was taught. Knowing methods used in instruction (e.g., demonstrations or discussion) helps staff to follow up more efficiently or offer alternate teaching methods if learning does not occur. When resources such as pamphlets or audiovisual materials are used, the nurse documents it in the client's record. Many institutions have special forms that allow easy documentation. For instance, teaching flow sheets (Fig. 14-3) are excellent records that document the plan, implementation, and evaluation of client teaching.

SUMMARY

More than ever, an emphasis in health care today is to provide clients and families with information about health and management of health problems. During interaction with a client, the nurse can teach something about health. The nurse teaches clients to function more independently. Client education focuses on the client's unique needs and capacity for learning. The most effective teaching plan is one in which the nurse and client work together to define the type of information and skills the client needs to learn.

A nurse cannot teach effectively without understanding the basic learning domains: cognitive, affective, and psychomotor. Each involves acquisition of different types of behaviors. The characteristics of each domain affect the selection of teaching methods and the manner in which learning is evaluated. A good teacher uses basic teaching principles to promote a student's participation in learning. Teaching sessions convene when the learner is most receptive. A teacher organizes teaching material in a format that progresses from simple to more complex ideas. The teacher's actions and use of instructional resources help to stimulate interest in learning.

The nursing process provides a useful framework for organizing the teaching process. Nursing diagnoses focus on specific types of learning needs. The teaching plan involves the nurse and client in a collaborative effort, setting realistic learning objectives. During implementation the nurse uses a variety of teaching methods to engage the client in active learning. To determine whether a client has gained the necessary knowledge or skills, the nurse evaluates the success of the plan on the basis of expected learning outcomes.

KEY CONCEPTS

Teaching is most effective when it is responsive to the learner's needs.
Teaching is a form of interpersonal communication, with teacher and student actively involved in a process that increases the student's knowledge and skills.
Teaching a client a specific behavior can involve incorporation of behaviors from all three learning domains.
The client's ability to attend to the learning process depends on physical comfort and anxiety level and the presence of environmental distraction.
A person's health beliefs influence the willingness to gain knowledge and skills necessary to maintain health.
Clients of different age-groups require different teaching strategies as a result of developmental capabilities.
Presentation of teaching content should progress from simple to more complex ideas.
Instructional resources promote active learner participation.
A combination of teaching methods improves the learner's attentiveness and involvement.
A teacher is more effective when presenting information that builds on a learner's existing knowledge.
Teaching methodologies should match the client's learning need.
Learning objectives describe what a person is to learn in behavioral terms.

CRITICAL THINKING ACTIVITIES

1. Mr. Clifford is a 75-year-old widower admitted with newly diagnosed insulin-dependent diabetes mellitus. He is hard of hearing, has poor eyesight, and lives alone. Design a teaching plan, including appropriate resources and modifications, for Mr. Clifford to monitor his blood glucose and administer his insulin.
2. Amy Smith is a 17 year old with rheumatoid arthritis. She is angry about taking medications and having activity restrictions. She complains about her nurses, parents, and friends. What resources does Amy require before you can begin to teach her how to be independent?
3. Mrs. Jones, 38 years old, is scheduled for a breast biopsy. Her mother and sister have a history of breast cancer. They are both currently in remission and are in their sixth and seventh year post initial diagnoses. Mrs. Jones has never had surgery. She is nervous and "scared of the diagnosis." List your teaching priorities for this client.
4. Joey Carter is a 6 year old who was recently hospitalized for bronchial asthma. This was his first admission and initial diagnosis of asthma. He is being sent home on inhaled and nebulized bronchodilators and is to return to the clinic in 1 week. Design teaching plans for both Joey and his parents.

References

Alberta Association of Registered Nurses: *Client education: position statement and guidelines, 1985,* Edmonton, Alberta, Canada, 1986, The Association.

American Association of Diabetes Educators: The scope of practice for diabetes educators and the standards of practice for diabetes educators, *Diabetes Educator* 18(1):52, 1992.

American Nurses Association: *Nursing's agenda for health care reform,* Washington, DC, 1991, The Association.

Barnes LP: Patient education standards, *MCN Am J Matern Child Nurs* 18(1):45, 1993.

Barron S: Documentation of patient education, *Patient Educ Couns* 9:81, 1987.

Bull MJ: Managing the transition from hospital to home, *Qual Health Res* 2(1):27, 1992.

Byrne TJ and Edeani D: Knowledge of medical terminology among hospitalized patients, *Nurs Res* 33:178, 1984.

Heese H: How elders view learning, *Geriatr Nurs* 5(1): 37, 1984.

Joint Commission on Accreditation of Healthcare Organizations: *Accreditation manual of hospitals,* Chicago, 1993, The Commission.

Kozol J: *Illiterate America,* Garden City, NY, 1985, Doubleday & Co.

Kruger S: The patient educator role in nursing, *Appl Nurs Res* 4(1):19, 1991.

Miller A: When is the time ripe for teaching, *Am J Nurs* 85: 801, 1985.

Paulish C: A model for situational patient teaching. *J Contin Educ Nurs* 18: 163, 1987.

Redman BK: *The process of patient education,* ed 7, St. Louis, 1992, Mosby.

Tanner G: A need to know, *Nurs Times* 85(31):54, 1989.

Weinrich SP, Boyd M, Nussbaum J: Continuing education adapting strategies to teach the elderly, *J Gerontol Nurs* 15(11):17, 1989.

Whaley LW and Wong DL: *Nursing care of infants and children,* ed 4, St. Louis, 1991, Mosby.

Whitman NI: Age-related factors influencing selection of teaching strategies. In Whitman NI, et al., editors: *Teaching in nursing practice: a professional approach.* Norwalk, Conn., 1986, Appleton & Lange.

Woodward S: *Preoperative patient education seminar presentation,* Denver, 1983, Resource Applications.

Bibliography

Bartlett EE: Assessing benefits of patient education under prospective pricing, *Patient Education Newsletter,* University of Alabama, 1984.

Bennett HL: Why patients don't follow instructions, *RN* 49:45, 1986.

Bille DA: Educational strategies for teaching the elderly patient, *Nurs Health Care* 5:256, 1980.

Bille DA: *Practical approaches to patient teaching,* Boston, 1981, Little, Brown & Co.

Close A: Patient education: a literature review, *J Adv Nurs* 88:203, 1988.

Cushing M: Legal lessons on patient teaching, *Am J Nurs* 84:721, 1984.

Huckabay LMD: *Conditions of learning and instruction in nursing,* St. Louis, 1980, Mosby.

Joint Commission on Accreditation of Healthcare Organizations: *Accreditation manual of hospitals,* Chicago, Ill., 1989, The Commission.

Joyce B and Weil M: *Models of teaching,* ed 2, Englewood Cliffs, NJ, 1980, Prentice-Hall.

McHatton M: A theory for timely teaching, *Am J Nurs* 85:798, 1985.

McHugh NG, Christman NJ, and Johnson JE: Preparatory information: what helps and why, *Am J Nurs* 82:780, 1982.

Miller A: When is the time ripe for teaching? *Am J Nurs* 85:801, 1985.

Morrison JL: The special needs of the special patient, *RN* 49:49 1986.

Pohl ML: *The teaching function of the nursing practitioner,* ed 2, Dubuque, Iowa, 1973, William C. Brown.

Streiff LD: Can clients understand our instructions? *Image* 18(2):48, 1986.

Ward DB: Why patient teaching fails, *RN* 49:45, 1986.

15 Vital Signs

OBJECTIVES

Mastery of content in this chapter will enable the student to:

- Define the key terms listed.
- Explain the principles and mechanisms of thermoregulation.
- Describe nursing measures that promote heat loss and heat conservation.
- Discuss physiological changes associated with fever.
- Accurately assess body temperature.
- Accurately assess pulse, respirations, oxygen saturation, and blood pressure.
- Explain physiological activities for the normal regulation of blood pressure, pulse, oxygen saturation, and respirations.
- Describe factors that cause variations in body temperature, pulse, oxygen saturation, respirations, and blood pressure.
- Identify normal vital sign values for an adult, child, and infant.
- Explain variations in technique used to assess an infant's, child's, and adult's vital signs.

KEY TERMS

afebrile
antipyretic
apical pulse
apnea
auscultatory gap
basal metabolic rate (BMR)
bradycardia
bradypnea
calorie
cardiac output
Centigrade
core temperature
diaphoresis
diaphragmatic breathing
diastole
dysrhythmia
eupnea
Fahrenheit
febrile
fever
frostbite
heat stroke
hematocrit
hypercarbia
hypercapnia
hypertension
hyperthermia
hyperventilation
hypotension
hypothermia
hypoxemia
Korotkoff sounds
malignant hyperthermia
nonshivering thermogenesis
orthostatic hypotension
oximetry
oxygen saturation
perfusion
postural hypotension
pulse deficit
pulse pressure
pyrexia
pyrogens
radiation
sphygmomanometer
stroke volume
systole
tachycardia
tachypnea
thermoregulation
vasoconstriction
vasodilation
ventilation
vital signs

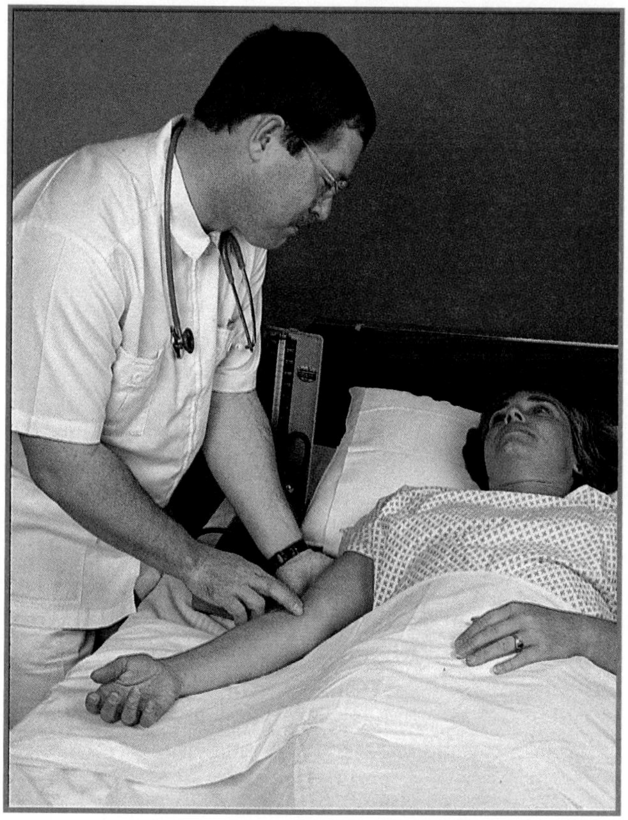

The **vital signs**—temperature, pulse, respiration, blood pressure, and oxygen saturation—indicate health status. Many factors such as the temperature of the environment, physical exertion, and the effects of illness cause vital signs to change, sometimes outside normal range. Measurement of vital signs provides data to determine a client's usual state of health (baseline data), as well as response to physical and psychological stress and medical and nursing therapy. A change in vital signs can indicate a change in physiologic functioning. An alteration in vital signs may signal the need for medical or nursing intervention.

Vital signs are a quick and efficient way of monitoring a client's condition or identifying problems and evaluating the client's response to intervention. The basic skills required to measure vital signs are simple but should not be taken for granted. Vital signs and other physiological measurements are the basis for clinical problem solving. Assessment of vital signs allows the nurse to identify nursing diagnoses, implement planned interventions, and evaluate success when vital signs have returned to acceptable values. When the nurse learns the physiological variables influencing vital signs and recognizes the relationship of vital sign changes to other physical assessment findings, precise determinations of the client's health problems can be made. Careful measurement techniques ensure accurate findings.

GUIDELINES FOR TAKING VITAL SIGNS

The nurse assesses vital signs whenever a client enters a health care agency. Vital signs are included in a complete physical assessment (see Chapter 16) or obtained individually to assess a client's condition. The client's needs and condition determine when, where, and how vital signs are measured. The nurse must be able to measure vital signs correctly, understand and interpret the values, communicate findings appropriately, and begin interventions as needed. The following guidelines assist the nurse to incorporate vital sign measurement into nursing practice:

1. The nurse caring for the client is responsible for vital signs. The nurse should obtain the vital signs, interpret their significance, and make decisions about interventions.
2. Equipment should be functional and appropriate. Equipment used to measure vital signs (e.g., a thermometer) must work properly to ensure accurate findings.
3. Equipment should be selected based on the client's condition and characteristics (e.g., an adult-size blood pressure cuff is not used for a child).
4. The nurse knows the client's normal range of vital signs. A client's normal values may differ from the standard range for that age or physical state. The client's normal values serve as a baseline for comparison with findings taken later. Thus a nurse can detect a change in condition over time. Changes in vital signs help the nurse detect deviations from normal.
5. The nurse knows the client's medical history, therapies, and prescribed medications. Some illnesses or treatments cause predictable vital sign changes. Most medications affect at least one of the vital signs.
6. The nurse controls or minimizes environmental factors that may affect vital signs. Measuring the pulse after the client exercises may yield a value that is not a true indicator of the client's condition.
7. The nurse uses an organized, systematic approach when taking vital signs. Each procedure requires following a step-by-step approach to ensure accuracy. Organization facilitates efficiency.
8. Based on the client's condition, the nurse collaborates with the physician to decide the frequency

of vital sign assessment. In the hospital the physician orders a minimum frequency of vital sign measurements for each client. Following surgery or treatment intervention, vital signs are measured frequently to detect complications. The nurse may use vital sign assessment to determine indications for medication administration. The physician may order certain cardiac drugs to be given only within a range of pulse or blood pressure. The nurse does not administer these drugs if vital sign assessment is outside of these limits. Outside of the hospital vital sign assessment occurs whenever the client seeks care from a health care provider. In either environment the nurse is responsible for judging whether more frequent assessments are needed (see box below). Taking vital signs to determine clinical changes and trends is useful in making therapeutic decisions. As a client's physical condition worsens, it may be necessary to monitor vital signs as often as every 5 to 10 minutes.

9. The nurse analyzes the results of vital sign measurement. The nurse is often in the best position to assess all clinical findings about a client. Vital signs are not interpreted in isolation. The nurse must also know other physical signs or symptoms and be aware of the client's ongoing health status.
10. The nurse verifies and communicates significant changes in vital signs. Baseline measurements allow a nurse to identify changes in vital signs. When vital signs appear abnormal, it may help to have another nurse or a physician repeat the measurement. The nurse informs the physician of abnormal vital signs and documents and reports vital sign changes to nurses working the next shift.

Vital signs provide physiological data the nurse uses in practice and are the most frequently collected form of assessment data. Vital signs assist the nurse in performing routine care measures, such as judging a client's exercise tolerance or determining interventions for client problems such as administering analgesics.

WHEN TO TAKE VITAL SIGNS

When the client is admitted to a health care facility
In a hospital on a routine schedule according to a physician's order or hospital standards of practice
Before and after a surgical procedure
Before and after an invasive diagnostic procedure
Before and after the administration of medications that affect cardiovascular, respiratory, and temperature-control function
When the client's general physical condition changes (as with loss of consciousness or increased intensity of pain)
Before and after nursing interventions influencing a vital sign (such as before a client previously on bed rest ambulates or before a client performs range of motion exercises)
When the client reports nonspecific symptoms of physical distress (such as feeling "funny" or "different")

BODY TEMPERATURE

The body temperature is the difference between the amount of heat produced by body processes and the amount of heat lost to the external environment.

Heat produced − Heat lost = Body temperature

Despite extremes in environmental conditions and physical activity, temperature-control mechanisms of human beings keep the body's **core temperature** or temperature of deep tissues relatively constant (Figure 15-1). However, surface temperature fluctuates depending on blood flow to the skin and the amount of heat lost to the external environment. Because of these surface temperature fluctuations the acceptable temperature of human beings ranges from 36° C to 38° C (96.8° F to 100.4° F). The body's tissues and cells function best within the relatively narrow temperature range.

The site of temperature measurement (oral, rectal, axillary, tympanic membrane, esophageal, pulmonary artery, or even urinary bladder) is one factor that determines the client's temperature within this narrow range. For healthy young adults the average oral temperature is 37° C (98.6° F). In clinical practice, nurses learn the temperature range of individual clients. No single temperature is normal for all people.

The measurement of body temperature is aimed at obtaining a representative average temperature of core body tissues. Average normal temperatures vary depending on the measurement site. Sites reflecting core temperatures are more reliable indicators of body temperature than sites reflecting surface temperatures (see box below). The pulmonary artery offers accurate read-

CORE AND SURFACE TEMPERATURE MEASUREMENT SITES

CORE	SURFACE
Rectal	Skin
Tympanic membrane	Axillary
Esophageal	Oral
Pulmonary artery	
Urinary bladder	

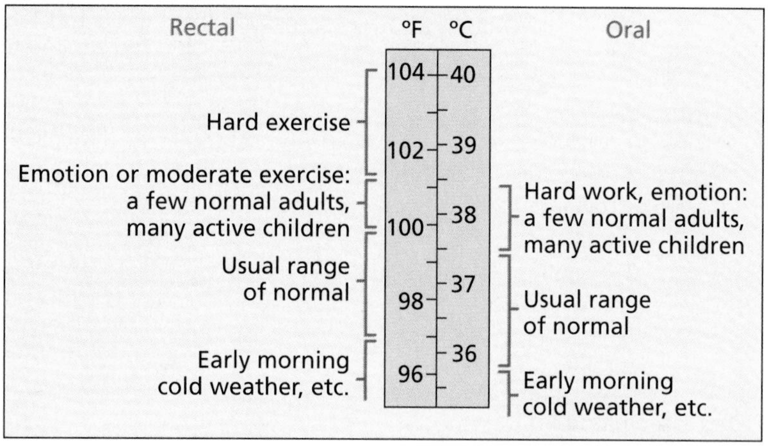

FIGURE 15-1 Ranges of rectal and oral temperatures found in normal persons. (Redrawn from Mountcastle VB: *Medical physiology,* vol 2, ed 14, St. Louis, 1980, Mosby; based on Dubois EF: *Fever and regulation of body temperature,* Springfield, Ill. 1948, Charles C Thomas.)

ings because of the blood mix from all regions of the body. Measurement of the pulmonary artery temperature is the standard against which all other sites are judged for accuracy. The accuracy of body sites depends on the relationship to core temperature.

Body Temperature Regulation

Body temperature is precisely regulated by physiological and behavioral mechanisms. For the body temperature to stay constant, and within the normal range, the relationship between heat production and heat loss must be maintained. This relationship is regulated by neurological and cardiovascular mechanisms. A nurse applies knowledge of temperature control mechanisms to promote temperature regulation.

Neural and Vascular Control. The hypothalamus, located between the cerebral hemispheres, controls body temperature the same way a thermostat works in the home. A comfortable temperature is the "set point" at which a heating system operates. In the home a fall in environmental temperature activates the furnace, whereas a rise in temperature shuts the system down. The hypothalamus senses minor changes in body temperature. The anterior hypothalamus controls heat loss, and the posterior hypothalamus controls heat production.

When nerve cells in the hypothalamus become heated beyond the set point, impulses are sent out to reduce body temperature (Figure 15-2). Mechanisms of heat loss include sweating, **vasodilation** (widening of blood vessels), and inhibition of heat production. If the hypothalamus senses the body's temperature lower than set point, signals are sent out to increase heat production by muscle shivering or heat conservation by **vasoconstriction** (narrowing) of surface blood vessels. Lesions or trauma to the hypothalamus or spinal cord, which carries hypothalamic messages, can cause serious alterations in temperature control.

Heat Production. Thermoregulation requires the normal function of heat-production processes. Heat is produced as a by-product of metabolism. Cellular chemical reactions require energy in the form of ATP. The amount of energy used for metabolism is the metabolic rate. Activities requiring additional chemical reactions increase the metabolic rate. As metabolism increases, additional heat is produced. When metabolism decreases, less heat is produced. Heat production occurs during rest, voluntary movements, involuntary shivering, and nonshivering thermogenesis.

1. Basal metabolism accounts for the heat produced by the body at absolute rest. The average **basal metabolic rate** (BMR) depends on the body surface area. Thyroid hormones also affect the BMR. By promoting the breakdown of body glucose and fat, thyroid hormones increase the rate of chemical reactions in almost all cells of the body. When large amounts of thyroid hormones are secreted, the BMR can increase 100% above normal. Absence of thyroid hormones can cut the BMR in half, causing a decrease in heat production. Stimulation of the sympathetic nervous system by norepinephrine and epinephrine also increases the metabolic rate of body tissues by causing blood glucose levels to fall, which stimulates cells to manufacture glucose. The male sex hormone testosterone increases BMR. Men have a higher BMR than women.
2. Voluntary movements such as muscular activity during exercise require additional energy. The

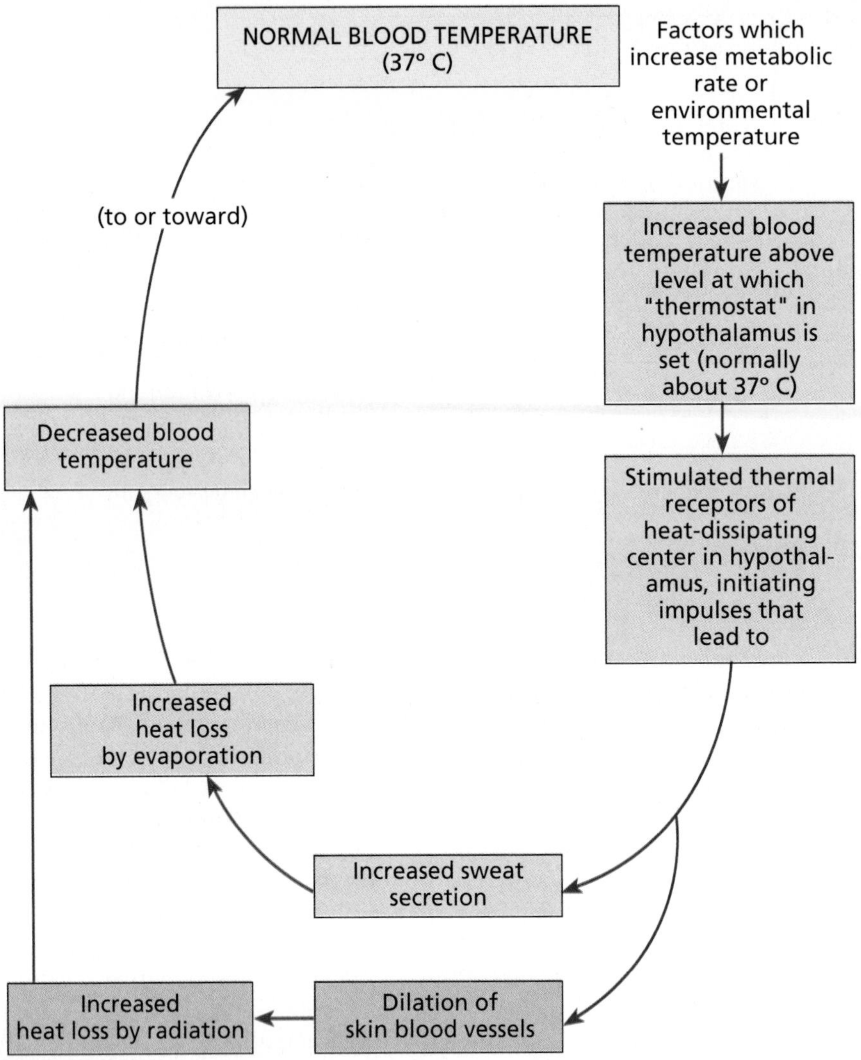

FIGURE 15-2 Heat loss mechanisms to maintain normal body temperature. (From Thibodeau GA: *Anatomy and physiology,* St. Louis, 1987, Mosby.)

metabolic rate can increase up to 2000 times normal. Heat production can increase up to 50 times normal.

3. Shivering is an involuntary body response to temperature differences in the body. The skeletal muscle movement during shivering requires significant energy. Shivering can increase heat production 4 to 5 times greater than normal. Heat is produced to equalize body temperature.
4. **Nonshivering thermogenesis** occurs primarily in neonates. Vascular brown adipose tissue present at birth is metabolized for heat production.

Heat Loss. Heat loss and heat production occur simultaneously. The skin's structure and exposure to the environment result in constant, normal heat loss through radiation, conduction, convection, and evaporation (Figure 15-2).

Radiation is the transfer of heat between two objects by electromagnetic waves. Objects radiate heat to one another without physical contact. Blood flows from the core internal organs carrying heat to skin and surface blood vessels. The amount of heat carried to the surface depends on the extent of vasoconstriction and vasodilation regulated by the hypothalamus. Heat radiates from the skin to any surrounding cooler object. Radiation increases as the temperature difference between the objects increases.

Peripheral vasodilation increases blood flow to the skin to increase radiant heat loss. Peripheral vasoconstriction minimizes radiant heat loss. Up to 85% of the human body's surface area radiates heat to the environment. However, if the surroundings are warmer than the skin, the body absorbs heat through radiation.

The nurse increases heat loss through radiation by removing clothing or blankets. The client's position enhances radiation heat loss (e.g., standing exposes a greater radiating surface area and lying in a fetal position minimizes heat radiation). Covering the body with dark, closely woven clothing also reduces the amount of radiation heat lost.

Conduction is the transfer of heat from one object to another with direct contact. When the warm skin touches a cooler object, heat is lost. When the temperatures of the two objects are the same, conductive heat loss stops. Heat conducts through solids, gases, and liquids. Conduction normally accounts for a small amount of heat loss. The nurse increases conductive heat loss when applying an ice pack or bathing a client with cool water. Applying several layers of clothing reduces conductive loss. The body gains heat by conduction when contact is made with materials warmer than skin temperature.

Convection is the transfer of heat away by air movement. Heat is first transferred to air molecules directly in contact with the skin. Air currents carry away the warmed air. As the air current velocity increases, convective heat loss increases. An electric fan promotes heat loss through convection. Convective heat loss increases when moistened skin comes into contact with slightly moving air.

Evaporation is the transfer of heat energy when a liquid is changed to a gas. During evaporation, approximately 0.6 **calorie** of heat is lost for each gram of water that evaporates (Guyton, 1991). The body continuously loses heat by evaporation. About 600 to 900 ml a day evaporates from the skin and lungs, resulting in water and heat loss.

By regulating perspiration or sweating, the body promotes additional evaporative heat loss. Millions of sweat glands located in the dermis of the skin secrete sweat through tiny ducts on the skin's surface. When body temperature rises, the anterior hypothalamus signals the sweat glands to release sweat. During exercise and emotional or mental stress, sweating is one way to lose excessive heat produced by the increased metabolic rate.

People who lack sweat gland function are unable to tolerate warm temperatures because they cannot cool themselves adequately. **Diaphoresis** is visual perspiration of the forehead and upper thorax. When diaphoresis occurs, the body temperature is reduced. A lowered body temperature inhibits sweat gland secretion.

Behavioral Control. Humans voluntarily act to maintain comfortable body temperature when exposed to temperature extremes. When the environmental temperature falls, a person can add clothing, move to a warmer place, raise the thermostat setting on a furnace, increase muscular activity by running in place, or sit with arms and legs tightly wrapped together. In contrast, when the temperature becomes hot, a person can remove clothing, stop activity, lower the thermostat setting on an air conditioner, seek a cooler place, or take a cool shower. The ability of a person to control body temperature depends on (1) the degree of temperature extreme, (2) the person's ability to sense feeling comfortable or uncomfortable, (3) thought processes or emotions, and (4) the person's mobility or ability to remove or add clothes. Body temperature control is difficult if any of these abilities are absent or lost. Infants can sense uncomfortable warm conditions but need assistance in changing their environment. Older adults may need help in detecting cold environments and minimizing heat loss. Illness, a decreased level of consciousness, or impaired thought process result in an inability to recognize the need to change behavior for temperature control. When temperatures become extremely hot or cold, health promoting behaviors have a limited effect on controlling temperature. The nurse assesses for variables that place clients at high risk for ineffective thermoregulation.

Factors Affecting Body Temperature

Many factors affect the body temperature (see box on p. 256). Changes in body temperature occur when the relationship between heat production and heat loss is altered by physiological or behavioral variables. The nurse must be aware of these factors when assessing temperature variations and evaluating deviations from normal.

Temperature Alterations

Changes in body temperature outside the normal range affect the set point. These changes can be related to excess heat production, excessive heat loss, minimal heat production, minimal heat loss, or any combination of these alterations. The nature of the change affects the type of clinical problems a client experiences.

Fever. Hyperpyrexia or **fever** occurs because heat loss mechanisms are unable to keep pace with excess heat production, resulting in an abnormal rise in body temperature. The level at which a fever threatens health is often a source of disagreement among health care providers. A fever is usually not harmful if it stays below 39° C (102° F). A single temperature reading may not indicate a fever. Davis and Lentz (1989) recommend determining a fever based on several temperature readings at different times of the day compared to the normal for that person at that time, in addition to physical signs and symptoms of infection.

A true fever results from an alteration in the hypothalamic set point. **Pyrogens** such as bacteria cause a rise in body temperature. When they enter the body, pyrogens act as antigens, triggering the immune system. Hormone-like substances are released to promote the body's defense against infection. These hormones also

FACTORS AFFECTING BODY TEMPERATURE

AGE

The newborn's temperature normally ranges from 36.5° to 37° C (97.9° to 98° F) Axillary.

Temperature regulation is labile during infancy because of immature physiological mechanisms. This can continue until puberty.

With aging the normal mean temperature is lower. Thus a temperature that seems normal in a young adult may represent a fever in an older adult.

The older adult has a narrower range of body temperature than the younger adult.

With aging, control mechanisms deteriorate and sensitivity to temperature extremes increases.

EXERCISE

Any form of exercise can increase body temperature.

Prolonged, strenuous exercise can temporarily raise body temperatures up to 41° C (105° F).

HORMONAL INFLUENCES

Females generally have greater variations in body temperature than males.

Hormone changes during ovulation and menstruation cause body temperature fluctuations.

DAILY VARIATIONS

Body temperatures normally change 0.5° to 1° C (0.8° to 1.8° F) over 24 hours. Temperature drops between 1 and 4 AM (Figure 15-3) and peaks between 4 and 7 PM in clients who work days and sleep nights.

In general the circadian cycle does not change with age. Research, however, indicates an earlier timing of circadian temperature peak in older adults.†

STRESS

Physical or emotional stress, such as anxiety, can raise body temperature.

ENVIRONMENT

Environmental temperature extremes can raise or lower body temperature. The changes depend on the extent of exposure, air humidity, and the presence of convection currents.

INGESTION OF HOT/COLD LIQUIDS

Drinking hot or cold liquids can cause slight variations in actual oral temperature readings (0.2° F to 1.6° F)

SMOKING

Smoking cigarettes or cigars can increase body temperature measurement.

*Data from Lobban M and Tredre B: Diurnal rhythms of renal excretion and of body temperature in aged subjects, *Proc Phys Soc* 188:48P, 1988.

†Data from Lentz M: Circadian phase relationships of sleep-wake cycle and body temperature rhythm in aging, unpublished doctoral dissertation, Seattle, 1984, University of Washington.

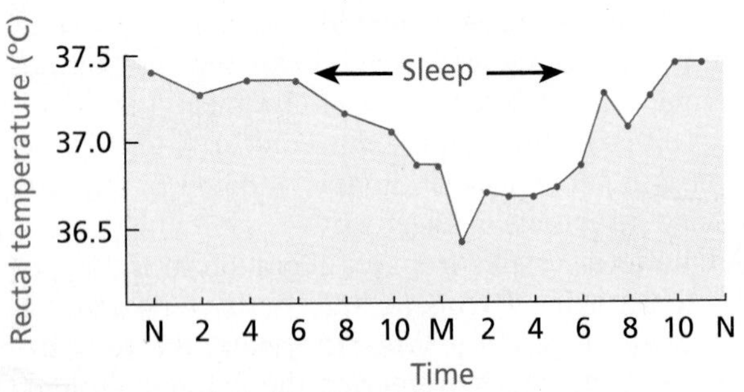

FIGURE 15-3 Temperature cycle for 24 hours. (From Mountcastle VB: *Medical physiology,* vol 2, ed 14, St. Louis, 1980, Mosby.)

trigger the hypothalamus to raise the set point. To meet the new higher set point, the body produces and conserves heat. Several hours may pass before the body temperature reaches the new set point. During this period the person experiences chills, shivers, and feels cold, even though the body temperature is rising. The chill phase resolves when the new set point, a higher temperature, is achieved. During the next phase, the plateau, the chills subside and a person feels warm and dry. If the new set point has been "over shot" or the pyrogens are removed, the third phase of a **febrile** episode occurs. The skin becomes warm and flushed because of vasodilation. **Diaphoresis** assists in evaporative heat loss. When the fever "breaks," the client becomes **afebrile** (Figure 15-4).

Fever is an important defense mechanism. Mild temperature elevations up to 39° C enhance the body's immune system. During a febrile episode, white blood cell production is stimulated. Increased temperature reduces the concentration of iron in the blood plasma, suppressing the growth of bacteria. Fever also fights viral infections by stimulating interferon, the body's natural virus-fighting substance.

Fevers also serve a diagnostic purpose. Fever patterns differ depending on the causative pyrogen (see box below). The increase or decrease in the amount of pyrogens results in fever spikes and declines at different times of the day. The duration and degree of fever depends on the pyrogen's strength and the ability of the individual to respond. The term **fever of unknown origin** (FUO) refers to a fever whose **etiology** (cause) cannot be determined.

During a fever, cellular metabolism increases and oxygen consumption rises. Heart and respiratory rates increase to meet the body's metabolic needs. The increased metabolism uses energy that produces additional heat. A prolonged fever can weaken a client by exhausting energy stores. Increased metabolism requires additional oxygen. If the demand for additional oxygen cannot be met, cellular **hypoxia** (inadequate oxygen) occurs. Cerebral hypoxia produces confusion. Interventions during a fever may include oxygen therapy. The regulatory mechanism used to compensate for fever places a client at risk for fluid volume deficit. Water loss through increased respiration and diaphoresis can be excessive. Dehydration can be a serious problem for older adults and children with low body weights. Maintaining optimum fluid volume status is an important nursing action (see Chapter 35).

Heat exhaustion occurs when profuse diaphoresis results in excess water and electrolyte loss. Caused by environmental heat exposure, the signs and symptoms of fluid volume deficit are common during heat exhaustion (see Chapter 35). First aid includes transporting the client to a cooler environment and restoring fluid and electrolyte balance.

Hyperthermia. An elevated body temperature related to the body's inability to promote heat loss or reduce heat production is **hyperthermia.** Any disease or trauma to the hypothalamus can impair heat loss mechanisms. **Malignant hyperthermia** is a hereditary condition of uncontrolled heat production. Malignant hyperthermia occurs when susceptible persons receive certain anesthetic drugs.

Prolonged exposure to the sun or high environmental temperatures can overwhelm the body's heat loss mechanisms. Heat also depresses hypothalamic function. These conditions cause **heat stroke,** a dangerous heat emergency. Clients at risk include those who are very young or very old, or have cardiovascular disease, hypothyroidism, diabetes, or alcoholism. Also at risk are those who take medications that decrease the body's ability to lose heat (e.g., phenothiazines, anticholinergics, diuretics, amphetamines, and beta-adrenergic receptor antagonists), or who exercise or work strenuously (e.g., athletes, construction workers, and farmers). Signs and symptoms of heat stroke include giddiness, confusion, delirium, excess thirst, nausea, muscle cramps, visual disturbances, and even incontinence. The most important sign of heat stroke is hot, dry skin.

Victims of heat stroke do not sweat because of severe electrolyte loss and hypothalamic malfunction. Vital signs reveal a body temperature sometimes as high as 45° C (113° F), tachycardia, and hypotension. As the condition progresses, a client becomes unconscious with fixed, unreactive pupils. Permanent neurological

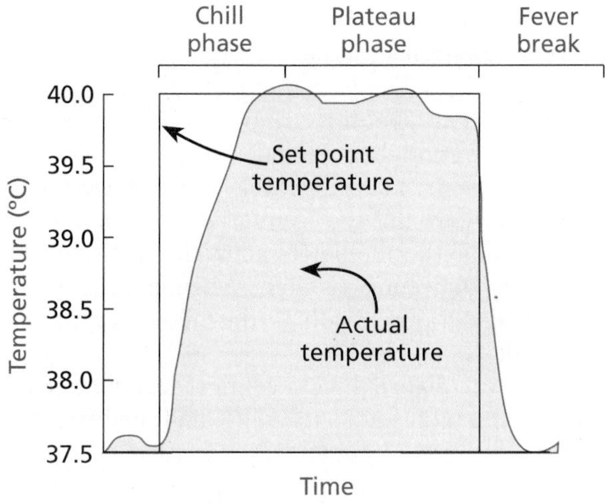

FIGURE 15-4 Stages of a febrile episode. (Modified from Holtzclaw B: The febrile response in critical care: state of the science, *Heart Lung* 21(5):482, 1992.)

PATTERNS OF FEVER

Sustained	Persistent elevation over 24 hours varying by 1 C° to 2 C°
Intermittent	Fever spikes interspersed with normal temperature levels. Temperature returns to normal at least once in 24 hours.
Remittent	Fever spikes and falls without a return to normal temperature levels.
Relapsing	Periods of febrile episodes interspersed with normal temperature levels. Febrile episodes and periods of normothermia may be longer than 24 hours.

table 15-1

CLASSIFICATION OF HYPOTHERMIA

	C	F
Mild	33.1° – 36°	91.5° – 96.8°
Moderate	30.1° – 33°	86.1° – 91.4°
Severe	27° – 30°	80.6° – 86.0°
Profound	<27°	<80.6°

damage occurs unless cooling measures are rapidly started.

Hypothermia. Heat loss during prolonged exposure to cold overwhelms the body's ability to produce heat, causing **hypothermia.** Hypothermia is classified by core temperature measurements (Table 15-1). It can be accidental or unintentional, such as falling through the ice of a frozen lake. Hypothermia may be intentionally induced during surgical procedures to reduce metabolic demand and the body's need for oxygen.

Accidental hypothermia develops gradually and may go unnoticed for several hours. A client suffers uncontrolled shivering, loss of memory, depression, and poor judgment. As the body temperature falls below 34.4° C (94° F), heart and respiratory rates and blood pressure fall. The skin becomes cyanotic. If hypothermia progresses, a client experiences cardiac dysrhythmias, loss of consciousness, and becomes unresponsive to painful stimuli. The assessment of core temperature is critical when hypothermia is suspected. A special low-reading thermometer may be required because standard devices do not register below 35° C (95° F).

Frostbite occurs when the body is exposed to subnormal temperatures. Ice crystals forming inside the cell can result in permanent circulatory and tissue damage. Areas susceptible to frostbite are the earlobes, tip of the nose, and fingers and toes. The injured area appears white, waxy, and firm to touch. The client loses sensation in the affected area. Intervention includes warming measures, analgesia, and protection of the injured area.

NURSING PROCESS AND THERMOREGULATION

Knowledge of the physiology of body temperature regulation helps a nurse to assess the client's response to temperature alterations and to intervene safely. Independent measures can be implemented to increase or minimize heat loss, promote heat conservation, and increase client comfort. These measures add to the effects of medically ordered therapies during illness. Many measures can also be taught to family members, parents of children, or other care givers.

Assessment of Body Temperature

Sites. There are several sites for measuring core and surface body temperature. The core temperatures of the pulmonary artery, esophagus, and urinary bladder are often used in intensive care settings. These measurements require the use of continuous invasive devices placed in body cavities or organs. The temperature devices obtain accurate readings quickly and continually display readings on an electronic monitor.

The sites used most commonly may be invasive but are used intermittently. These include the tympanic membrane, mouth, rectum, and axillary sites. Special chemically prepared thermometer patches can also be applied to the skin. Oral, rectal, axillary, and skin temperatures rely on effective blood circulation at the measurement site. The heat of the blood is conducted to the thermometer probe. Tympanic temperature relies on the radiation of body heat to an infrared sensor. Because the tympanic membrane shares the same arterial blood supply as the hypothalamus, tympanic temperature is considered a core temperature.

To ensure accurate temperature readings, each site must be measured correctly (Procedure 15-1). The temperature obtained varies depending on the site used but should be between 36.0° C (96.8° F) and 38.0° C (100.4° F). Rectal temperatures are usually 0.5° C (0.9° F) higher than oral temperatures. Axillary temperatures are usually 0.5° C (0.9° F) lower than oral temperatures. Each of the common temperature measurement sites has advantages and disadvantages (Table 15-2). The nurse chooses the safest and most accurate site for the client. The same site should be used when repeated measurements are necessary.

Thermometers. The three types of thermometers used for measuring body temperature are mercury-in-glass, electronic, and disposable. Each device measures temperature in the centigrade or Fahrenheit scale. Electronic thermometers allow the nurse to convert scales by activating a switch. When it is necessary to convert temperature readings, the following formulas can be used:

1. To convert Fahrenheit to centigrade, subtract 32° from the Fahrenheit reading and multiply the result by 5/9.

$$(F - 32°) \times 5/9 = C$$

Example: $(104° F - 32° F) \times 5/9 = 40° C$

2. To convert centigrade to Fahrenheit, multiply

table 15-2

ADVANTAGES AND DISADVANTAGES OF SELECT TEMPERATURE MEASUREMENT SITES AND METHODS

TYMPANIC MEMBRANE SENSOR

Advantages

Easily accessible site
Minimal client repositioning required
Provides accurate core reading (Castles, et al., 1992)
Very rapid measurement (2 to 5 seconds)
Can be obtained without disturbing or waking client
Eardrum close to hypothalamus; sensitive to core temperature changes

Disadvantages

Hearing aids must be removed before measurement
Should not be used with clients who have had surgery of the ear or tympanic membrane
Requires disposable probe cover
Expensive

ELECTRONIC THERMOMETER

Advantages

Plastic sheath unbreakable; ideal for children
Quick readings

Disadvantages

May be less accurate by axillary route

RECTAL

Advantages

Argued to be more reliable when oral temperature cannot be obtained

Disadvantages

May lag behind core temperature during rapid temperature changes
Should not be used with clients who have had rectal surgery, a rectal disorder, bleeding tendencies, and heart disease
Requires positioning and may be source of client embarrassment and anxiety
Risk of body fluid exposure
Requires lubrication
Contraindicated in newborns

ORAL

Advantages

Accessible—requires no position change
Comfortable for client
Provides accurate surface temperature reading
Indicates rapid chage in core temperature

Disadvantages

Affected by ingestion of fluids or foods, smoke, and oxygen delivery (Neff J, et al., 1992)
Should not be used with clients who have had oral surgery, trauma, history of epilepsy, or shaking chills
Should not be used with infants, small children, or confused, unconscious, or uncooperative clients
Risk of body fluid exposure

AXILLA

Advantages

Safe and noninvasive
Can be used with newborns and uncooperative clients

Disadvantages

Long measurement time
Requires continuous positioning by nurse
Measurement lag behind core temperature during rapid temperature changes
Requires exposure of thorax

SKIN

Advantages

Inexpensive
Provides continuous reading
Safe and noninvasive

Disadvantages

Lags behind other sites during temperature changes, especially during hyperthermia
Diaphoresis or sweat can impair adhesion

---

the centigrade reading by $\frac{9}{5}$ and add 32° to the product.

$$(\tfrac{9}{5} \times C) + 32° = F$$

$$\text{Example: } (\tfrac{9}{5} \times 40°\ C) + 32° = 104°\ F$$

GLASS THERMOMETER. The mercury-in-glass thermometer is the most familiar. It is a glass tube sealed at one end with a mercury-filled bulb at the other. Exposure of the bulb to heat causes the mercury to expand and rise in the enclosed tube. The length of the thermometer is marked with Fahrenheit or centigrade calibrations. The farthest point reached by the mercury in the tube is the temperature reading. The mercury will not fluctuate or fall unless the thermometer is shaken vigorously.

The nurse reads a mercury thermometer by holding it with the fingertips horizontally at eye level, with the bulb pointed to the left. By rotating the thermometer

Text continued on p. 265.

procedure 15-1

MEASURING BODY TEMPERATURE

Steps	Rationale
1. Assess for signs and symptoms of temperature alterations and for factors that influence body temperature.	Physical signs and symptoms may indicate abnormal temperature. Nurse can accurately assess nature of variations.
2. Explain way temperature will be taken and importance of maintaining proper position until reading is complete.	Clients are often curious about such measurements and should be cautioned against prematurely removing thermometer to read results.
3. When taking oral temperature, wait 20 to 30 minutes before measuring temperature if client has smoked or ingested hot or cold liquids or foods.	Smoking and hot or cold substances can cause false temperature readings in oral cavity (Terndrup TE, Allegra JR, et al. 1987).
4. Prepare equipment and supplies:	
a. Appropriate thermometer	Chosen on basis of preferred site for temperature measurement.
b. Soft tissues	
c. Lubricant (for rectal only)	
d. Pen, vital signs flowsheet or record form	
e. Disposable gloves, plastic sleeve, or disposable probe cover.	Maintains universal precautions.
5. **Measure oral temperature with glass thermometer:**	
a. Wash hands.	Reduces transmission of microorganisms.
b. Assist client in assuming comfortable position that provides easy access to mouth.	Ensures comfort and accuracy of temperature reading.
c. Don disposable gloves.	Maintains universal precautions when exposed to items soiled with body fluids (for example, saliva) (CDC, 1988).
d. Hold end (if color-coded, tip will be blue) of glass thermometer with fingertips.	Reduces contamination of thermometer bulb.
e. Read mercury level while holding thermometer at eye level and gently rotating it.	Mercury should be below 35.5° C (96° F). Thermometer reading must be below client's actual temperature before use.
f. If mercury is above desired level (35.5° C [96° F]) shake thermometer. Grasp tip securely and stand away from solid objects. Sharply flick wrist downward as though cracking a whip. Continue shaking until reading is below 35.5° C (96° F).	Brisk shaking lowers mercury level in glass tube. Standing in open spot avoids breakage of thermometer.
g. Insert thermometer into plastic sleeve.	Protects nurse from contact with saliva.
h. Ask client to open mouth and gently place thermometer under tongue in posterior sublingual pocket lateral to center of lower jaw (see illustration).	Heat from superficial blood vessels in sublingual pocket produces temperature reading.

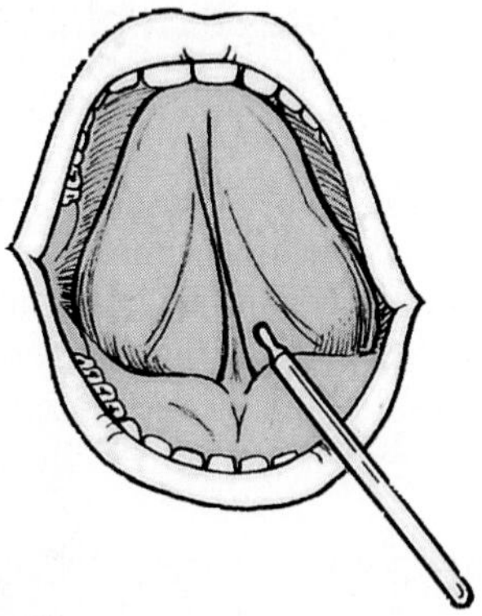

Step 5h

Steps	Rationale
i. Ask client to hold thermometer with lips closed. Caution against biting down on the thermometer.	Maintains proper position of thermometer during recording. Breakage of thermometer may injure mucosa and cause mercury poisoning.
j. Leave thermometer in place for 3 minutes or according to agency policy.	Studies as to proper length of time for recording vary. Holtzclaw (1992) recommends 3 minutes.
k. Carefully remove thermometer, remove and discard plastic sleeve or cover in appropriate receptacle. Read thermometer at eye level.	Prevents cross contamination. Ensures accurate reading.
l. Inform client of reading.	Promotes participation in care and understanding of health status.
m. Cleanse any additional secretions on thermometer by wiping with clean soft tissue. Wipe in rotating fashion from fingers toward bulb. Dispose of tissue in appropriate receptacle. Store thermometer at bedside in protective storage container.	Wipe from area of least contamination to area of most contamination. Glass thermometers should not be shared between clients unless terminal disinfection is performed between each measurement. Storage container prevents breakage and reduces risk of mercury spill.
n. Remove and dispose of gloves in appropriate receptacle. Wash hands.	Reduces transmission of microorganisms.
6. **Measure oral temperature with electronic thermometer:** Follow steps 5a, b.	
a. Don disposable gloves (optional).	Worn for handling items soiled with body fluids (for example, saliva) (CDC, 1988). Use of oral probe cover, which can be removed without physical contact, minimizes need to wear gloves.
b. Remove thermometer pack from charging unit. Be sure oral probe (blue tip) is attached to thermometer unit. Remove probe from storage well of recording unit. Grasp top of stem, being careful not to apply pressure to ejection button.	Charging provides battery power. Removal of probe from recording unit prepares it to measure temperature. Ejection button releases plastic cover from probe.
c. Slide disposable plastic probe cover over thermometer probe until it locks in place.	Soft, plastic cover will not break in mouth, and prevents transmission of microorganisms between clients.
d. Ask client to open mouth and gently place probe under tongue in posterior sublingual pocket lateral to center of lower jaw.	Heat from superficial blood vessels in sublingual pocket produces temperature reading. With electronic thermometer, temperatures in right and left posterior sublingual pocket are significantly higher than in area under front of tongue.
e. Ask client to hold thermometer with lips closed.	Maintains proper position of thermometer during recording.
f. Leave probe in place until audible signal occurs. Temperature appears on digital display.	Probe must stay in place until signal occurs to ensure an accurate reading.
g. Remove probe from under tongue and inform client of reading.	Promotes participation in care and understanding of health status.
h. Push ejection button on probe to discard plastic probe cover into appropriate receptacle.	Reduces transmission of microorganisms.
i. Return probe to storage well of recording unit.	Protects probe from damage. Automatically causes digital reading to disappear.
j. Remove and dispose of gloves if worn. Wash hands.	Reduces transmission of microorganisms.
k. Return thermometer to charger.	Maintains battery charge.
7. **Measure rectal temperature with glass thermometer:**	
a. Wash hands.	Reduces transmission of microorganisms.

Continued.

procedure 15-1—cont'd

MEASURING BODY TEMPERATURE

Steps	Rationale
b. Draw curtain around bed and/or close room door. Keep client's upper body and lower extremities covered with sheet or blanket.	Maintains privacy, minimizes embarrassment, and promotes comfort.
c. Assist client in assuming Sims' position with upper leg flexed. Move aside bed linen to expose only anal area.	Exposes anal area for correct thermometer placement. Maintains universal precautions when exposed to items soiled with body fluids (for example, feces) (CDC, 1988).
d. Don disposable gloves.	Reduces contamination of thermometer bulb.
e. Hold end (if color-coded, it will be red) of glass thermometer with fingertips.	Mercury should be below 35.5° C (96° F). Thermometer reading must be below client's actual temperature before use.
f. Read mercury level while holding thermometer at eye level and gently rotating it.	Brisk shaking lowers mercury level in glass tube. Standing in open spot avoids breakage of thermometer.
g. If mercury is above desired level, shake thermometer. Grasp tip securely and stand away from solid objects. Sharply flick wrist downward as though cracking a whip. Continue shaking until reading is below 35.5° C (96° F).	Lubrication minimizes trauma to rectal mucosa during insertion. Tissue avoids contamination of remaining lubricant in container.
h. Squeeze liberal portion of lubricant onto tissue. Dip thermometer's blunt end into lubricant, covering 2.5 to 3.5 cm (1 to 1½ in).	Fully expose anus for thermometer insertion.
i. With nondominant hand, separate buttocks to expose anus.	Relaxes anal sphincter for easier thermometer insertion. Ensures adequate exposure against blood vessels in rectal wall.
j. Ask client to breathe slowly and relax.	
k. Gently insert thermometer (bulb tip) into anus in direction of umbilicus 3.5 cm (1½ in) for adult. Do not force thermometer.	Prevents trauma to mucosa. Glass thermometers can break.
l. If resistance is felt during insertion, withdraw thermometer immediately. Never force thermometer.	Prevents injury to client. Recommended times vary among institutions. Studies as to exact length of time for recording vary. Holtzclaw (1992) recommends 2 mintues.
m. Hold thermometer in place for 2 minutes or according to agency policy.	Avoids nurse's contact with microorganisms. Wipe from area of least contamination to area of most contamination.
n. Carefully remove thermometer from anus and wipe off remaining secretions with clean tissue. Wipe in rotating fashion from fingers toward bulb. Dispose of tissue in appropriate receptacle.	Ensures accurate reading.
o. Read thermometer at eye level.	Provides participation in care and understanding of status.
p. Inform client of reading.	Provides for comfort and hygiene.
q. Wipe anal area to remove lubricant or feces.	Restores comfort.
r. Assist client in assuming a comfortable position.	Mechanically removes organic material that can harbor microorganisms and hinder action of disinfectant. Storage container prevents breakage.
s. Wash thermometer in lukewarm, soapy water, rinse in cool water, dry, and replace in protective storage container at bedside.	Reduces transmission of microorganisms.
t. Remove and dispose of gloves in appropriate receptacle. Wash hands.	

Steps	Rationale
8. **Measure rectal temperature with electronic thermometer:** Follow steps 7a, b, c, & d.	
e. Remove thermometer pack from charging unit. Be sure rectal probe (red tip) is attached to thermometer unit. Remove probe from storage well of recording unit. Grasp top of stem, being careful not to apply pressure to ejection button.	Charging provides battery power. Removal of probe from recording unit prepares it to measure temperature. Ejection button releases plastic cover from probe.
f. Slide disposable plastic cover over thermometer probe until it locks in place.	Probe cover prevents transmission of microorganisms between clients.
g. Continue as for 7h, i, j, k & l.	
h. Hold electronic probe until audible signal occurs. Read temperature on digital display.	Probe must stay in place until signal occurs to ensure accurate reading.
i. Carefully remove probe from rectum and inform client of reading.	Promotes participation in care and understanding of health status.
j. Push ejection button to discard plastic probe cover into appropriate receptacle.	Reduces transmission of microorganisms.
k. Return probe to storage well of recording unit.	Protects probe from damage. Automatically causes digital reading to disappear.
l. Wipe anal area to remove lubricant or feces. Remove and dispose of gloves.	Provides for comfort and hygiene. Reduces transmission of microorganisms.
m. Assist client in assuming a comfortable position.	Restores comfort.
n. Wash hands.	Reduces transmission of microorganisms.
9. **Measure axillary temperature with glass thermometer:**	
a. Wash hands.	Reduces transmission of microorganisms.
b. Draw curtain around bed and/or close door.	Provides privacy and minimizes embarrassment.
c. Assist client to supine or sitting position.	Provides easy access to axilla.
d. Move clothing or gown away from shoulder and arm.	Exposes axilla.
e. Prepare glass thermometer following Steps 5d to 5f.	Mercury must be below client's temperature level before insertion.
f. Insert thermometer into center of axilla, lower arm over thermometer, and place arm across chest (see illustration).	Maintains proper position of thermometer against blood vessels in axilla.

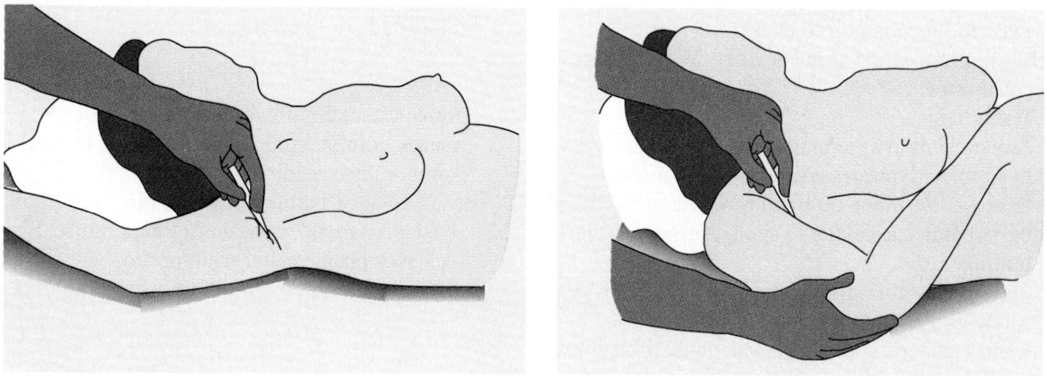

Step 9f

Continued.

procedure 15-1—cont'd

MEASURING BODY TEMPERATURE

Steps	Rationale
g. Hold thermometer in place for 3 minutes or according to agency policy.	Studies as to proper length of time for recording vary. Stephen and Sexton (1987) concluded that changes after 3 minutes had little clinical significance.
h. Remove thermometer, remove plastic sleeve, and wipe off remaining secretions with tissue. Wipe in rotating fashion from fingers toward bulb. Dispose of sleeve and tissue in appropriate receptacle.	Avoids nurse's contact with microorganisms. Wipe from area of least contamination to area of most contamination.
i. Read thermometer at eye level.	Ensures accurate reading.
j. Inform client of reading.	Promotes participation in care and understanding of health status.
k. Store thermometer at bedside in protective storage container.	Glass thermometers should not be shared between clients unless terminal disinfection is performed between each measurement. Storage container prevents breakage and reduces risk of mercury spill.
l. Assist client in replacing clothing or gown.	Restores sense of well-being.
m. Wash hands.	Reduces transmission of microorganisms.
10. **Measure axillary temperature with electronic thermometer:**	
a. Wash hands.	Reduces transmission of microorganisms.
b. Draw curtain around bed and/or close room door.	Provides privacy and minimizes embarrassment.
c. Assist client to supine or sitting position.	Provides easy access to axilla.
d. Move clothing or gown away from shoulder and arm.	Exposes axilla.
e. Prepare electronic thermometer following steps 6b and 6c.	
f. Insert probe into center of axilla, lower arm over thermometer, and place arm across client's chest.	Maintains proper position of thermometer against blood vessels in axilla.
g. Hold electronic probe until audible signal occurs. Temperature appears on digital display.	Probe must stay in place until signal occurs to ensure accurate reading.
h. Remove probe from axilla and inform client of reading.	Promotes participation in care and understanding of health status.
i. Push ejection button to discard plastic probe into appropriate receptacle.	Reduces transmission of microorganisms.
j. Return electronic probe to storage well of recording unit.	Protects probe from damage. Automatically causes digital reading to disappear.
k. Assist client in replacing clothing or gown.	Restores comfort.
l. Wash hands.	Reduces transmission of microorganisms.
m. Return thermometer to charger.	Maintains battery charge.
11. **Measure tympanic temperature with electronic thermometer.**	
a. Wash hands.	Reduces transmission of microorganisms.
b. Assist client in assuming comfortable position with head turned toward side, away from nurse.	Ensures comfort and exposes auditory canal for accurate temperature reading.
c. Remove thermometer handheld unit from charging base, being careful not to apply pressure to ejection button.	Base provides battery power. Removal of hand unit from base prepares it to measure temperature. Ejection button releases plastic cover from probe.
d. Slide disposable plastic speculum cover over otoscope-like tip until it locks in place.	Reduces transmission of microorganisms.
e. Follow manufacturer's instructions for tympanic probe positioning.	

Steps	Rationale
(1) Pull ear pinna upward and back for an adult. (2) Pull ear pinna down and back for a child. (3) Move thermometer in a figure-eight pattern. (4) Fit probe snug into canal. Do not move.	Correct positioning of the probe with respect to ear canal ensures accurate readings. The ear tug straightens the external auditory canal allowing maximum exposure of the tympanic membrane.
(5) Point toward nose, following manufacturer's positioning recommendations.	Ensures accurate readings.
f. Depress scan button on hand unit. Temperature appears on digital display.	Depression of scan button causes infrared energy to be measured. Probe must stay in place until signal occurs to ensure accurate reading.
g. Carefully remove sensor from auditory meatus and inform client of reading.	Promotes participation in care and understanding of health status.
h. Push release button to eject plastic probe cover. Discard into appropriate receptacle.	Reduces transmission of microorganisms.
i. Return hand unit to charging base.	Protects probe from damage. Automatically causes digital reading to disappear.
j. Assist client in assuming a comfortable position.	Restores comfort.
k. Wash hands.	Reduces transmission of microorganisms.
12. Compare temperature reading with baseline and normal temperaure range for client's age-group.	Normal body temperature fluctuates within narrow range. Comparison reveals presence of abnormality
13. If temperature is abnormal, repeat measurement. If indicated, select an alternative site or instrument.	Improper placement or movement of thermometer can cause inaccuracies. Second reading confirms initial finding of abnormal body temperature.
14. Record temperature on vital sign flow sheet or nurses' notes and report abnormal findings to nurse in charge or physician.	Vital sign measurements should be recorded promptly on flow sheets to avoid omissions from record. Abnormalities may require immediate therapy.

slowly, the column of silver mercury appears. The calibrated line at the end of the mercury column is the temperature reading. The bulb should not be touched. Touching it might affect the temperature reading or bring the fingers into contact with the client's body secretions. Disposable plastic sleeves may be available to cover the body of the thermometer. Observe universal precautions, including gloves, when using a glass thermometer because of potential contact with body fluids.

Three types of glass thermometers are the oral, the stubby, and the rectal (Figure 15-5). The oral thermometer is slender, allowing for greater exposure of the bulb against the blood vessels in the mouth. An oral thermometer usually has a blue tip. The stubby thermometer is shorter and thicker than the oral type. It can be used to measure temperature at any site. The rectal thermometer has a blunt end designed to prevent trauma to the rectal tissues during insertion. It is usually recognized by a red tip.

The time delay for recordings and the easy breakability are disadvantages of mercury-in-glass thermometers. Advantages are the low price, wide availability, and reliable accuracy.

Electronic thermometer. The electronic thermometer consists of a rechargeable battery-powered display unit, a thin wire cord, and a temperature-processing probe covered by a disposable plastic sheath (Figure 15-6). One form of electric thermometer uses a pencil-like probe. Separate nonbreakable probes are available for oral and rectal use. The oral probe can also be used

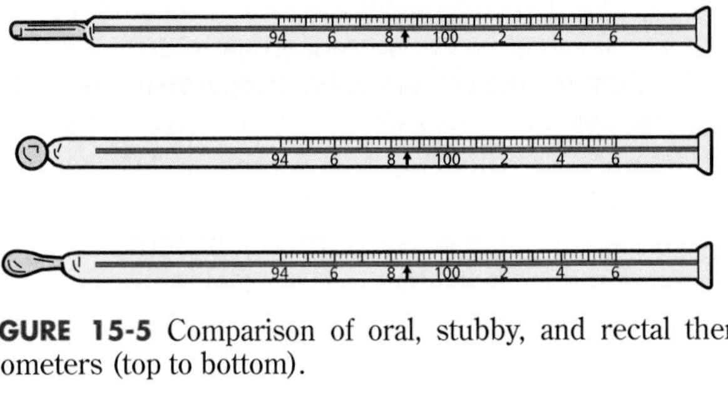

FIGURE 15-5 Comparison of oral, stubby, and rectal thermometers (top to bottom).

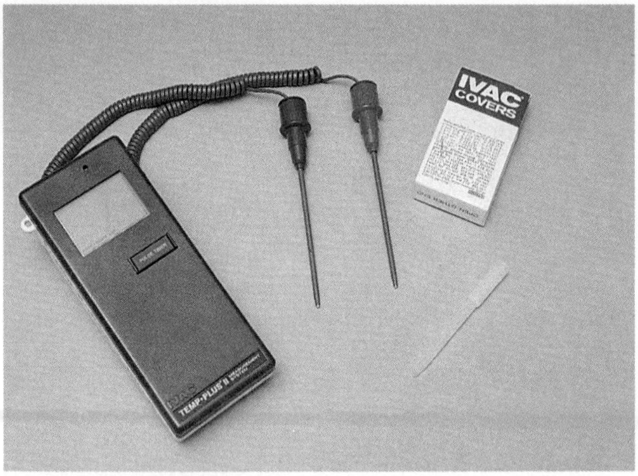

FIGURE 15-6 Electronic thermometer used for oral, rectal, or axillary measurements.

for axillary temperature measurement. Within 20 to 50 seconds of insertion, a reading appears on the display unit. A sound signals when the peak temperature reading has been measured.

Another form of electronic thermometer is used exclusively for tympanic temperature (Figure 15-7). An otoscope-like speculum with an infrared sensor tip detects heat radiated from the tympanic membrane. Within 2 to 5 seconds of placement in the auditory canal, a reading appears on the display unit. A sound signals when the peak temperature reading has been measured.

An electronic thermometer using an oral probe is not necessarily more accurate than a glass thermometer. For example, variables that alter oral temperature measurements affect all types of thermometers. The greatest advantages of electronic thermometers are that they can be inserted immediately, their readings appear within seconds, and they are easy to read. Their expense is a major disadvantage.

DISPOSABLE THERMOMETERS. Disposable, single-use thermometers are thin strips of plastic with chemically impregnated paper. They are used for oral or axillary temperatures, particularly with children (Figure 15-8). They are inserted the same way as an oral thermometer and used only once. Chemical dots on the thermometer change color to reflect the temperature reading. Only 45 seconds are needed to record a temperature.

Another form of disposable thermometer is a temperature-sensitive patch or tape. Applied to the forehead or abdomen, the patch changes color at different temperatures.

Both forms of disposable thermometers are useful for screening temperatures, especially with newborns. Glass or electronic thermometers are preferred for their accuracy.

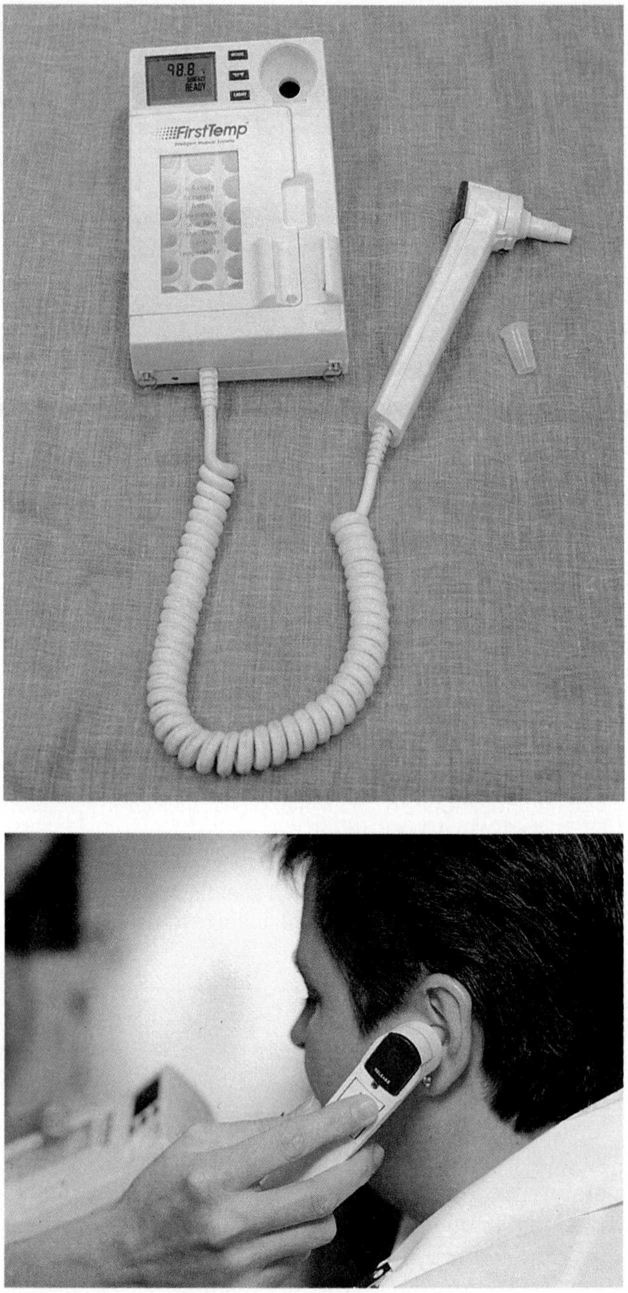

A

B

FIGURE 15-7 **A,** Electronic tympanic thermometer. **B,** Tympanic thermometer inserted in auditory canal.

Nursing Diagnosis Related to Body Temperature

The nurse identifies assessment findings and clusters defining characteristics to form a nursing diagnosis. For example, an increase in body temperature, flushed skin, skin warm to touch, and tachycardia indicate the diagnosis, hyperthermia. The nursing diagnosis identifies the client's risk for altered body temperature or an ac-

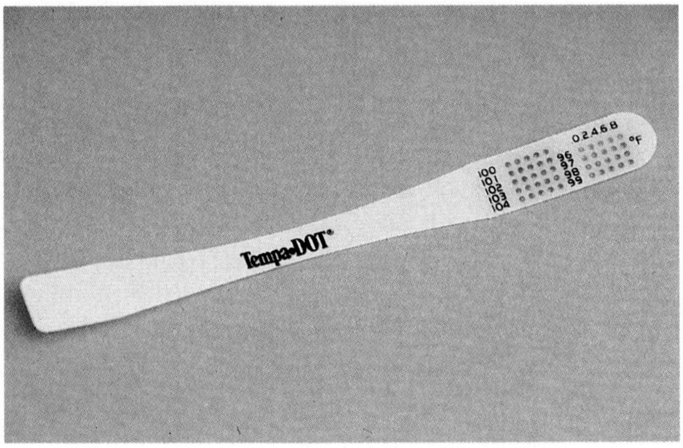

FIGURE 15-8 Disposable, single-use thermometer strip.

> **NURSING DIAGNOSES FOR BODY TEMPERATURE ALTERATIONS**
>
> High risk for altered body temperature
> Ineffective thermoregulation
> Hypothermia
> Hyperthermia

tual temperature alteration. If the client possesses risk factors, the nurse minimizes or eliminates factors promoting temperature alterations. Assessment of temperature alterations outside the normal range lead to nursing diagnoses (see box above).

Once a diagnosis is determined, the nurse must accurately select the related factor or etiology. The related factor allows the nurse to select appropriate nursing interventions. In the example of hyperthermia, a related factor of vigorous activity will result in much different interventions than a related factor of febrile illness.

Planning Interventions Related to Body Temperature

Clients at high risk for alterations in body temperature require an individualized care plan directed at maintaining normothermia and reducing risk factors. Education is important so clients can participate in maintaining normothermia. This is particularly the case for parents who need to know how to take action at home when an infant or child develops a temperature alteration. The care plan for clients with actual temperature alterations focuses on restoring normothermia, minimizing complications, and promoting comfort. The severity of a temperature alteration will influence the nurse's priorities in the care of a client. The nurse's care plan supports the client's goals:

Goal: Restore and maintain normothermia.

Outcome

- Temperature maintained within normal range (36° C and 38° C) during environmental temperature changes

Goal: Minimize complications of altered body temperature.

Outcomes

- Client's blood pressure, pulse, and respirations are within normal limits
- Client's urine output over 30 cc per hour
- Client's skin integrity maintained
- Client's nutritional intake meets body needs
- Client's mucous membranes are moist
- Client is able to participate in ADL activities
- Client's skin is warm and pink
- Client reports sense of rest and comfort

Goal: Reduce risk of altered body temperature.

Outcomes

- Client identifies risk factors for altered body temperature
- Client practices measures to prevent body temperature alteration

Implementing Interventions Related to Body Temperature

Hyperthermia. The procedures used to intervene and treat an elevated temperature depend on the fever's cause, any adverse effects, and the strength, intensity, and duration of the fever. The physician may try to determine the cause of the fever by isolating the causative pyrogen. The nurse obtains necessary culture specimens for laboratory analysis, such as urine, blood, sputum, and wound sites. Collecting these specimens requires strict aseptic technique to avoid introducing any outside organisms that might affect culture results. The physician will order antibiotics to be given after the cultures have been obtained. Administering antibiotics destroys pyrogenic bacteria and eliminates the body's stimulus for fever. The nurse administers antibiotics promptly. The nurse educates the client regarding the importance of taking and continuing the antibiotic as directed until the course of treatment is completed.

Viral infections cannot be identified by cultures. Most fevers in children are of a viral origin, last only briefly, and have limited effects. However, children still have undeveloped temperature control mechanisms and temperatures can rise rapidly. Dehydration and febrile seizures occur in rapidly rising temperatures of children younger than 5 years of age. Some researchers believe the rate of rise is more important than absolute temperature in precipitating a seizure (Leung and Robson, 1991). Children are at risk for fluid volume deficit because they can quickly lose large amounts of fluids in proportion to their body weight. The nurse maintains accurate intake and output records and encourages fluids.

The temperature of older adults is normally at the lower end of the temperature range. However, they are very sensitive to slight changes in temperature. The nurse must be aware that fever in an older adult may mean a temperature within the normal range.

Overall physical condition influences a client's ability to tolerate the increased heart rate, increased respiratory rate, decreased fluid volume, and metabolic oxygen demands. Debilitated clients and clients with severe burns, neoplastic disease, or a compromised immune system are at high risk for fever-induced complications. Temperatures higher than 39° C (102° F) serve little physiological purpose. As core temperature approaches 40° C (104° F), intervention is essential to avoid irreversible damage to cells.

A fever may be a hypersensitivity response to a drug. Drug fevers can be accompanied by other allergy symptoms such as rash or **pruritis** (itching). Treatment involves withdrawing the medication.

Fever therapy reduces heat production, increases heat loss, and prevents complications. **Antipyretics,** drugs that reduce fever, include corticosteroids and nonsteroidal compounds. Corticosteriods reduce heat production by interfering with the hypothalamus response. These drugs mask signs of infection by suppressing the immune system. Corticosteriods are not used to treat a fever. However, the nurse must be aware of their effect on the ability of the client to develop a fever in response to a pyrogen. Nonsteroidal drugs such as acetaminophen, salicylates, indomethacin, ibuprophen, and ketoralac reduce fever by increasing heat loss.

Nonpharmacological therapy of fever uses methods that increase heat loss by evaporation, conduction, convection, or radiation. Traditionally nurses have used tepid sponge bathes, bathing with alcohol-water solutions, applying ice packs to axillae and groin areas, and cooling fans. Recent research has not demonstrated any advantage of these methods over antipyretic medications (Morgan, 1990). Blankets cooled by circulating water delivered by motorized units increase conductive heat loss. The nurse must follow manufacturer's instructions for applying these hypothermia blankets because of the risk for skin breakdown and "freeze burns." Placing a bath blanket between the client and the hypothermia blanket and wrapping distal extremities (fingers, toes, genitalia) is recommended (Holtzclaw, 1990).

Nursing measures to enhance body cooling must

NURSING MEASURES FOR CLIENTS WITH A FEVER

ASSESSMENT

Obtain core temperature during each phase of febrile episode.
Assess for contributing factors such as dehydration, infection, or environmental temperature.
Identify physiological response to temperature.
- Obtain all vital signs.
- Observe skin color.
- Assess skin temperature.
- Observe for shivering and diaphoresis.
- Assess client comfort and well-being.

Determine phase of fever—chill, plateau, fever break.

INTERVENTION

Obtain blood cultures when ordered. Blood specimens are obtained to coincide with temperature spikes when the antigen-producing organism is most prevalent.
Initiate therapies to minimize heat production.
- Reduce the frequency of activities that increase oxygen demand such as excessive turning and ambulation. Allow rest periods.
- Limit physical activity.

Initiate therapies to maximize heat loss.
- Reduce external covering on client's body to promote heat loss through radiation and conduction. Do not induce shivering.
- Keep clothing and bed linen dry to increase heat loss through conduction and convection.

Initiate therapies to meet requirements for increased metabolic rate.
- Provide supplemental oxygen therapy as ordered to improve oxygen delivery to body cells.
- Provide measures to stimulate appetite, and offer well-balanced meals.
- Provide fluids (at least 3 liters per day for client with normal cardiac and renal function) to replace fluids lost through insensible water loss and sweating.

Initiate therapies to promote client comfort.
- Encourage oral hygiene because oral mucous membranes dry easily from dehydration.
- Control temperature of the environment without inducing shivering.

Identify onset and duration of febrile episode phases.
Examine previous temperature measurements for trends.
Initiate health teaching as indicated.

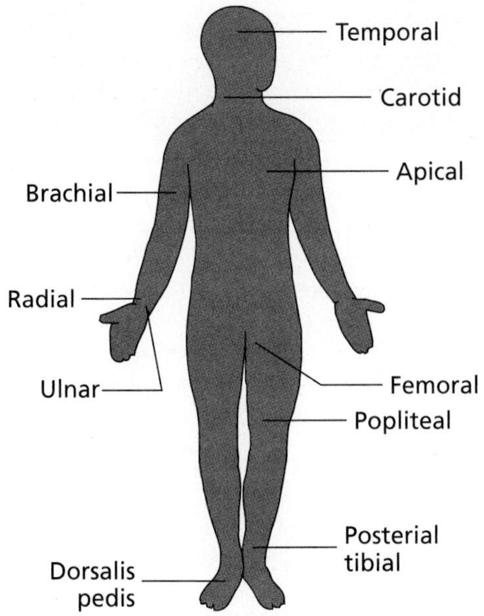

FIGURE 15-9 Location of pulse points.

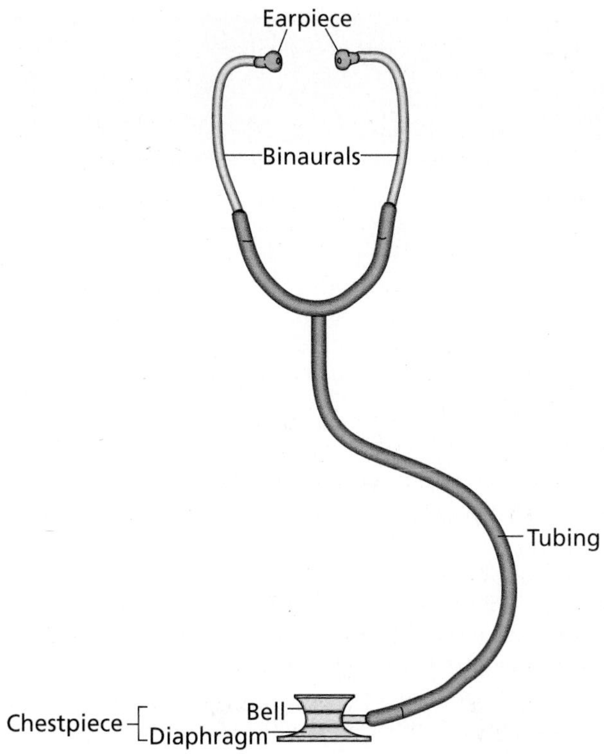

FIGURE 15-10 Parts of a stethoscope.

parts of the stethoscope are the earpieces, binaurals, tubing, and chestpiece.

The plastic or rubber earpieces should fit snugly and comfortably in the nurse's ears. The binaurals should be angled and strong enough so the earpieces stay firmly in the ears without causing discomfort. To ensure the best reception of sound, the earpieces follow the contour of the ear canal pointing toward the face when the stethoscope is in place.

The polyvinyl tubing should be flexible and 30 to 40 cm (12 to 18 inches) in length. Longer tubing decreases the transmission of sound waves. The tubing should be thick walled and moderately rigid to eliminate transmission of environmental noise and prevent the tubing from kinking, which distorts sound wave transmission. Stethoscopes can have single or dual tubes.

The chestpiece consists of a bell and a diaphragm. The diaphragm is the circular, flat-surfaced portion of the chestpiece covered with a thin plastic disk. It transmits high-pitched sounds created by the high velocity movement of air and blood. Bowel, lung, and heart sounds are auscultated using the diaphragm. The nurse positions the diaphragm to make a tight seal against the client's skin (Figure 15-11). Pressure is exerted enough to leave a temporary red ring on the client's skin when the diaphragm is removed.

The bell is the bowl-shaped chestpiece usually surrounded by a rubber ring. The ring avoids chilling the patient with cold metal when placed on the skin. The bell transmits low-pitched sounds created by the low velocity movement of blood. Heart and vascular sounds are auscultated using the bell. The nurse applies the bell lightly, resting the chestpiece on the skin (Figure 15-12). Compressing the bell against the skin reduces low-pitch sound amplification and creates a "diaphragm of skin." The bell and diaphragm are rotated into position on the chestpiece, depending on which part the nurse chooses to use. The diaphragm or bell must be in proper position during use for the nurse to hear sounds through the stethoscope. To test, lightly tap to determine which side is functioning.

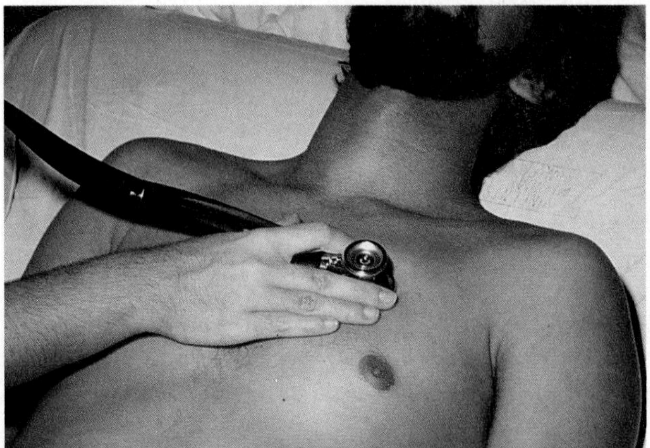
FIGURE 15-11 Positioning the diaphragm of the stethoscope.

Text continued on p. 275.

procedure 15-2

ASSESSING PULSE RATE

Steps	Rationale
1. Before measuring pulse, consider factors that normally influence pulse character (for example, age, exercise, and postural changes).	Allows nurse to accurately assess presence and significance of pulse alterations.
2. Explain that pulse or heart rate is to be assessed. Encourage client to relax and not speak. (If client has been active, wait 5 to 10 minutes.)	Activity and anxiety can elevate the heart rate. Client's voice interferes with nurse's ability to hear sound when apical pulse is measured.
3. Prepare equipment and supplies:	
a. Stethoscope, alcohol swab	Stethoscope used for apical rate assessment. Alcohol swab used as needed to cleanse earpieces and diaphragm.
b. Pen, pencil, vital signs flow sheet or record form	
c. Wristwatch with second hand or digital display	
4. Wash hands.	Reduces transmission of microorganisms.
5. Measure radial pulse:	
a. If client is supine, place forearm across lower chest or alongside torso with wrist extended and palm facing down. If client is sitting, bend elbow 90 degrees and support lower arm on chair or on nurse's arm. Slightly extend wrist with palm facing down (see illustration).	Permits full exposure of artery to palpation.
b. Place tips of first two fingers of hand over groove along radial or thumb side of client's inner wrist (see illustration).	Fingertips are most sensitive parts of hand to palpate arterial pulsation. Nurse's thumb has pulsation that may interfere with accuracy.
c. Lightly compress against radius, obliterate pulse initially, and then relax pressure so that pulse becomes easily palpable.	Pulse is more accurately assessed with moderate pressure. Too much pressure occludes pulse and impairs blood flow.
d. After pulse can be felt regularly, look at watch's second hand and begin to count rate: when sweep hand hits number on dial, start counting with *zero,* then *one,* and so on (see illustration).	Rate is determined accurately only after assessor is assured pulse can be palpated. Timing begins with zero. Count of one is first beat palpated after timing begins.

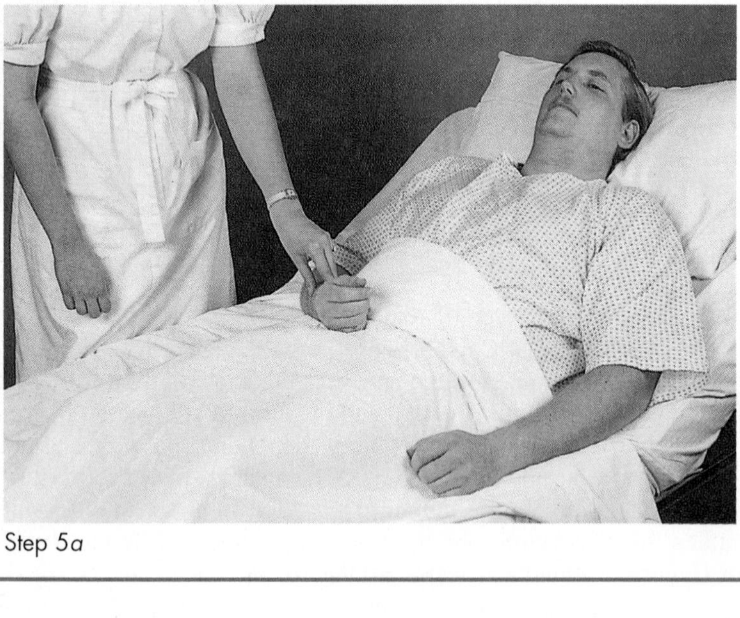

Step 5*a*

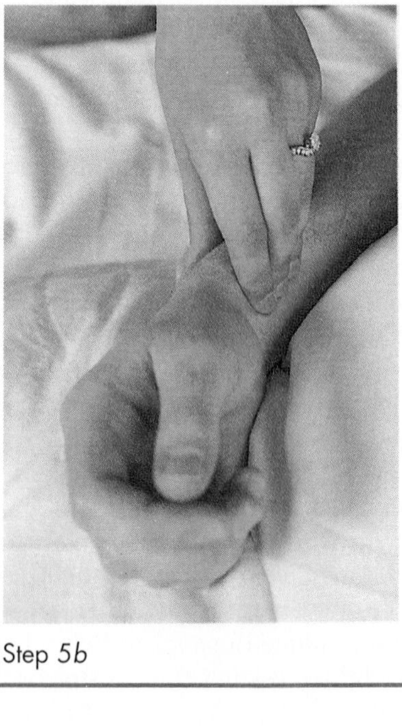

Step 5*b*

Steps	Rationale
e. If pulse is regular, count rate for 30 seconds and multiply total by two.	A 30-second check is adequate for rapid, slow, or regular heart rates.
f. If pulse is irregular, count rate for 60 seconds. Assess frequency and pattern of irregularity.	Inefficient contraction of heart fails to transmit pulse wave, interfering with cardiac output, resulting in irregular pulse. Longer time period ensures accurate count. Irregular pulse necessitates assessment for pulse deficit.
g. Determine strength of pulse. Note thrust of vessel against fingertips (see Chapter 16)	Strength reflects volume of blood ejected against arterial wall with each heart contraction.
h. Assist client in returning to comfortable position.	Promotes senses of well-being.
i. Discuss findings with client.	Promotes participation in care and understanding of health status.
j. Wash hands.	Reduces transmission of microorganisms.
6. Measure apical rate:	
a. Clean earpieces and diaphragm of stethoscope with alcohol swab as needed.	Ensures clean instrument and promotes auscultation.
b. With client in supine or sitting position, turn down bed linen and raise gown to expose sternum and left side of chest.	Exposes portion of chest wall for selection of auscultatory site.
c. Palpate angle of Louis, located just below suprasternal notch at point where horizontal ridge is felt along body of sternum. Place finger just to left of client's sternum and palpate second intercostal space. Place next finger in intercostal space below and proceed downward until fifth intercostal space is located. Move finger horizontally along fifth intercostal space to left midclavicular line (see illustration). Palpate point of maximal impulse (PMI).	Use of anatomical landmarks allows nurse to place stethoscope over apex of heart, which lies just under fifth intercostal space along left midclavicular line. This position enhances ability to hear heart sounds clearly. PMI is over apex of heart.

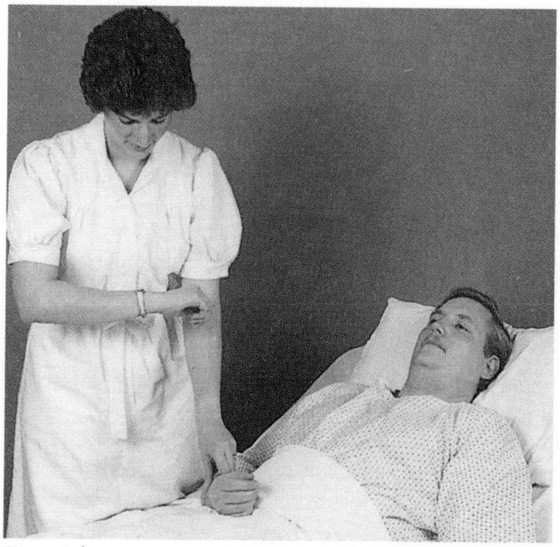
Step 5*d*

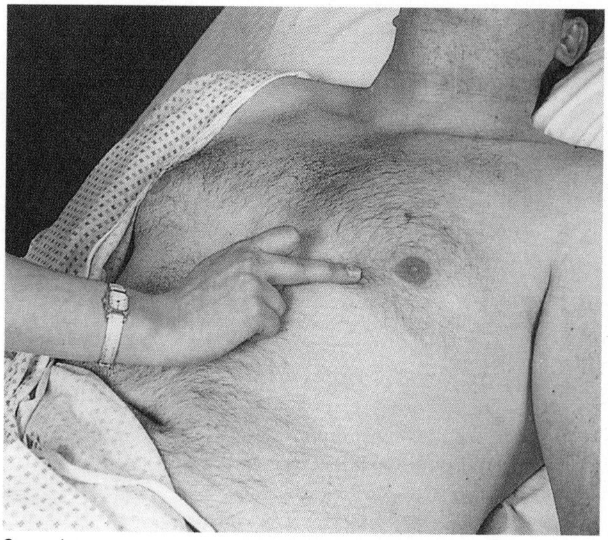
Step 6*c*

Continued.

procedure 15-2—cont'd

ASSESSING PULSE RATE

Steps	Rationale
d. Place diaphragm of stethoscope in palm of hand for 5 to 10 seconds.	Warming of diaphragm prevents client from being startled and promotes comfort.
e. Place diaphragm over PMI and auscultate for normal S_1 and S_2 heart sounds (heard as "lub-dub") (see illustration).	Heart sounds are caused by movement of blood through heart valves.

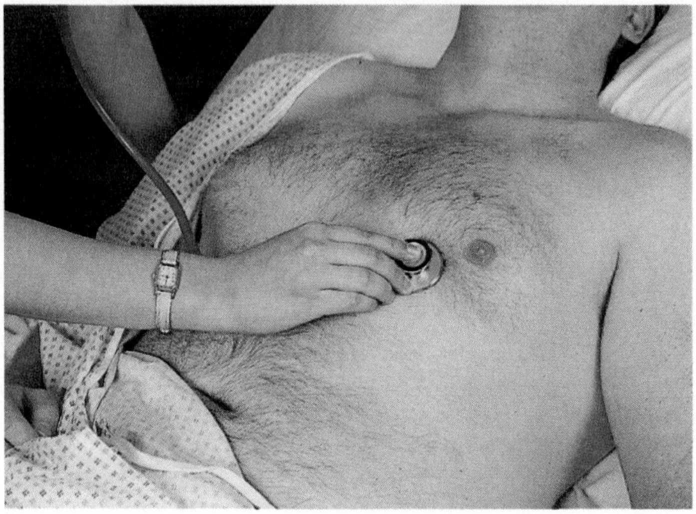

Step 6e

Steps	Rationale
f. After occurrence of S_1 and S_2 can be heard with regularity, use watch's second hand and begin to count rate: when sweep hand hits number on dial, start counting with *zero,* then *one,* and so on. Each "lub-dub" equals one heartbeat.	Rate is determined accurately only after nurse is able to auscultate sounds clearly.
g. If heart rate is regular, count for 30 seconds and multiply by two.	Regular apical rate can be assessed within 30 seconds.
h. If heart rate is irregular, count for 60 seconds. Assess frequency and pattern of irregularity.	Regular occurrence of irregularity may precipitate compromised cardiac output. Longer time period ensures more accurate count.
i. Replace gown and bed linen. Assist client in returning to comfortable position.	Maintains comfort.
j. Discuss findings with client.	Promotes participation in care and understanding of health status.
k. Wash hands, clean diaphragm with alcohol swab.	Reduces transmission of microorganisms.
7. Compare peripheral pulse rate with apical rate and note discrepancy.	Differences between measurements indicates pulse deficit and may warn of cardiovascular compromise.
8. Record pulse characteristics on vital signs flow sheet or nurses' notes and report abnormal findings.	Immediate documentation ensures accuracy in medical record. Abnormalities may require therapy.

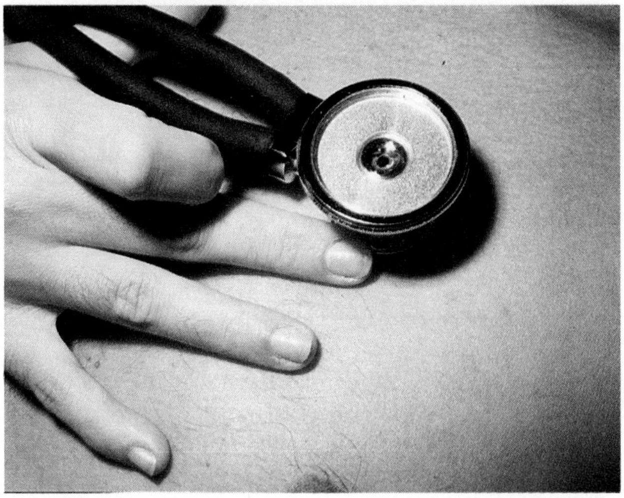

FIGURE 15-12 Positioning the bell of the stethoscope.

table 15-4
NORMAL HEART RATES

Age	Heart rate (beats/min)
Infants	120-160/min
Toddlers	90-140/min
Preschoolers	80-110/min
School agers	75-100/min
Adolescent	60-90/min
Adult	60-100/min

Modified from Hazinski MF: Children are different. In Hazinski MF, editor: *Nursing care of the critically ill child,* St. Louis, 1984, Mosby; and Kinney MR, et al.: *AACN's clinical reference for critical care nursing,* ed 3, St. Louis, 1993, Mosby.

The stethoscope is a delicate instrument and requires proper care for optimal function. The earpieces should be removed regularly and cleaned of cerumen (ear wax). The bell and diaphragm are cleaned of dust lint and body oils. The tubing should be kept away from the nurse's body oils. Avoid draping the stethoscope around the neck next to the skin. Cleaning the tubing with alcohol can dry and crack the material and is not recommended. Mild soap and water are preferred.

Pulse Rate. Before measuring a pulse, the nurse reviews the client's baseline rate for comparison (Table 15-4). Some practitioners prefer to make baseline measurements of the pulse rate as the client assumes a sitting, standing, and lying position. Postural changes cause changes in pulse rate because of alterations in blood volume and sympathetic activity. The heart rate temporarily increases when a person changes from a lying to a sitting or standing position.

When assessing the pulse, the nurse must consider the variety of factors influencing pulse rate (Table 15-5). A combination of these factors may cause significant changes. If the nurse detects an abnormal rate while palpating a peripheral pulse, the next step is to assess the apical rate. The apical rate provides a more accurate assessment of cardiac contraction.

The nurse assesses the apical rate by listening for heart sounds (see Chapter 16). The nurse tries to identify the first and second heart sounds (S_1 and S_2). At normal slow rates, S_1 is low pitched and dull in quality, sounding like a "lub." S_2 is a higher pitched and shorter sound and creates the sound, "dub." Each set of "lub-dub" is counted as one heartbeat. Using the diaphragm or bell of the stethoscope, the nurse counts the number of "lub-dubs" occurring in 1 minute.

Peripheral and apical pulse rate assessment may re-

table 15-5
FACTORS INFLUENCING PULSE RATES

Factor	Increase pulse rate	Decrease pulse rate
Exercise	Short-term exercise	Long-term exercise conditions the heart, resulting in lower rate at rest and quicker return to resting level
Temperature	Fever and heat	Hypothermia
Emotions	Acute pain and anxiety increase sympathetic stimulation, affecting heart rate	Unrelieved severe pain increases parasympathetic stimulation, affecting heart rate; relaxation
Drugs	Positive chronotropic drugs such as atropine	Negative chronotropic drugs such as digitalis
Hemorrhage	Loss of blood increases sympathetic stimulation	
Postural changes	Standing or sitting	Lying down
Pulmonary conditions	Diseases causing poor oxygenation	

veal variations in heart rate. Two common abnormalities in pulse rate are tachycardia and bradycardia. **Tachycardia** is an abnormally elevated heart rate, above 100 beats per minute in adults. **Bradycardia** is a slow rate, below 60 beats per minute in adults.

Pulse Rhythm. Normally a regular interval of time occurs between each pulse or heart beat. An interval interrupted by an early or late beat or a missed beat indicates an abnormal rhythm or **dysrhythmia.** A dysrhythmia may alter cardiac output, particularly if it occurs repetitively. The nurse identifies a dysrhythmia by palpating an interruption in successive pulse waves or auscultating an interruption between heart sounds. If a dysrhythmia is present, the regularity of its occurrence should be assessed. Dysrhythmias may be described as regularly irregular or irregularly irregular. To document dysrhythmia, a physician may order an electrocardiogram or a Holter monitor. An electrocardiogram records the electrical activity of the heart for a 12-second interval. The Holter monitor records 24 hours of electrical activity.

An inefficient contraction of the heart that fails to transmit a pulse wave to the peripheral pulse site creates a **pulse deficit.** To assess a pulse deficit the nurse and a colleague assess radial and apical rates simultaneously and then compare rates. The difference between the apical and radial pulse rates is the **pulse deficit.** Pulse deficits are frequently associated with dysrhythmias.

Strength. The strength or amplitude of a pulse reflects the volume of blood ejected against the arterial wall with each heart contraction and the condition of the arterial vascular system leading to the pulse site. Normally the pulse strength remains the same with each heartbeat. Pulse strength may be graded or described as strong, weak, thready, or bounding. It is included during assessment of the vascular system (see Chapter 16).

NURSING PROCESS AND PULSE DETERMINATION

Pulse assessment evaluates the general state of cardiovascular health and the response to other system imbalances. Tachycardia, bradycardia, and dysrhythmias are defining characteristics of many nursing diagnoses and are considered along with other assessment data. For example, the defining characteristics of abnormal heart rate, exertional dyspnea, and a client's verbal report of fatigue lead to a diagnosis of activity intolerance (see box above). The nursing care plan includes interventions based on the nursing diagnosis identified and the related factor. The nurse evaluates client outcomes by assessing the pulse rate following each intervention.

NURSING DIAGNOSES FOR PULSE DETERMINATION

Activity intolerance
Altered tissue perfusion
Decreased cardiac output
Fluid volume deficit
Fluid volume excess
Impaired gas exchange

RESPIRATION

Human survival depends on the ability of oxygen (O_2) to reach body cells and for carbon dioxide (CO_2) to be removed from the cells. Respiration is the mechanism the body uses to exchange gases between the atmosphere and the blood and the cells. Respiration involves **ventilation** (the movement of gases in and out of the lungs), **diffusion** (the movement of oxygen and carbon dioxide between the alveoli and the red blood cells), and **perfusion** (the distribution of red blood cells to and from the pulmonary capillaries). They can be assessed independently. However, analyzing respiratory efficiency requires integrating assessment data from all three processes. The processes are interdependent. Ventilatory adequacy can affect diffusion and perfusion, which in turn will affect ventilation. Respiration can be affected by various factors (see box on p. 277).

Assessment of Ventilation

The nurse assesses ventilation by determining the rate, depth, and rhythm of breathing. Adults normally breathe in a smooth, uninterrupted pattern of 12 to 20 breaths per minute. Ventilation is regulated by levels of CO_2, and O_2 in the arterial blood. The most important factor in the control of ventilation is the level of $CO_{2\ (carbia)}$ in the arterial blood. **Hypercarbia** causes the respiratory control system in the brain to increase rate and depth of breathing. The increased ventilatory effort removes excess CO_2 during exhalation.

Chemoreceptors in the carotid artery and aorta are sensitive to **hypoxemia,** or low levels of arterial O_2. If arterial oxygen levels fall, these receptors signal the brain to increase the rate and depth of ventilation. Hypoxemia helps to control ventilation in clients with chronic lung disease. Hypercarbia is constant in clients with chronic lung disease. Once an elevated CO_2 level fails to increase the rate and depth of breathing, hypoxemia, also present in these clients, becomes the stimulus to increase ventilation. Because low levels of arterial

FACTORS INFLUENCING CHARACTER OF RESPIRATIONS

EXERCISE

Exercise increases rate and depth to meet the body's need for additional oxygen.

ACUTE PAIN

Acute pain increases rate and depth as a result of sympathetic stimulation.

Client may inhibit or splint chest wall movement when pain is in area of chest or abdomen.

ANXIETY

Anxiety increases rate and depth as a result of sympathetic stimulation.

SMOKING

Chronic smoking changes the lung's airways, resulting in an increased rate.

BODY POSITION

A straight, erect posture promotes full chest expansion.

A stooped or slumped position impairs ventilatory movement.

MEDICATIONS

Narcotic analgesics and sedatives depress rate and depth.

Amphetamines and cocaine may increase rate and depth.

BRAIN STEM INJURY

Injury to the brain stem impairs the respiratory center and inhibits respiratory rate and rhythm.

O_2 provide the stimulus that allows the client to breathe, administration of high oxygen levels can be fatal for clients with chronic lung disease.

In normal breathing, muscular work is involved in moving the lungs and chest wall. Inspiration is an active process. During inspiration the diaphragm contracts and abdominal organs move downward and forward to move air into the lungs. The diaphragm moves approximately 1 cm ($\frac{4}{10}$ inch), and the ribs retract upward from the body's midline approximately 1.2 to 2.5 cm ($\frac{1}{2}$ to 1 inch). During a normal relaxed breath a person inhales 500 ml of air. This amount is referred to as the tidal volume. During expiration the diaphragm relaxes and the abdominal organs return to their original positions. The lung and chest wall return to a relaxed position. Expiration is a passive process. The normal rate and depth of ventilation, **eupnea,** is interrupted by sighing. The sigh, a prolonged deeper breath, is a protective physiological mechanism for expanding small airways and alveoli not ventilated during a normal breath.

The accurate assessment of respirations depends on the nurse's recognition of normal thoracic and abdominal movements. During quiet breathing the chest wall gently rises and falls. Contraction of the intercostal muscles between the ribs or contraction of the muscles in the neck and shoulders, the accessory muscles of breathing, is not visible. During normal quiet breathing, diaphragmatic movement causes the abdominal cavity to rise and fall slowly.

When breathing requires greater effort, the intercostal and accessory muscles work actively to move air in and out. The shoulders may rise and fall, and the accessory muscles of ventilation in the neck visibly contract. Diaphragmatic movement becomes less noticeable as costal breathing increases.

Measurement of Respirations

Respirations are the easiest of all vital signs to assess, but they are often the most haphazardly measured. A nurse must not estimate respirations. Accurate measurement requires observation and palpation of chest wall movement.

A sudden change in the character of respirations may be important. Because respiration is tied to the function of numerous body systems, the nurse must consider all variables when changes occur. For example, a drop in respirations occurring in a client after head trauma may signify injury to the brain stem.

A skillful nurse does not let a client know that respirations are being assessed. A client aware of the nurse's intentions may consciously alter the rate and depth of breathing. Assessment can best be done immediately after measuring pulse rate, with the nurse's hand still on the client's wrist as it rests over the chest or abdomen. When assessing a client's respirations, the nurse should keep in mind the client's normal ventilatory rate and pattern, the influence any disease or illness has on respiratory function, the relationship between respiratory and cardiovascular function, and the influence of therapies on respirations. The objective measurements of an assessment of respiratory status include the rate and depth of breathing and the rhythm of ventilatory movements (Procedure 15-3).

Respiratory Rate. The nurse observes a full inspiration and expiration when counting ventilation or respiration rate. The respiratory rate varies with age (Table 15-6). The normal respiratory rate declines throughout life.

Ventilatory Depth. The depth of respirations is assessed by observing the degree of excursion or move-

procedure 15-3

ASSESSING RESPIRATIONS

Steps	Rationale
1. Assess for factors that normally influence character of respirations.	Allows nurse to accurately assess for presence and significance of respiratory alterations.
2. If client has been active, wait 5 to 10 minutes.	Exercise increases respiratory rate and depth.
3. Be sure client is in comfortable position, preferably sitting or lying with head of bed elevated 45 to 60 degrees.	Discomfort causes client to breathe more rapidly. Erect, sitting position promotes full ventilation.
4. Prepare needed equipment and supplies: a. Watch with second hand or digital display. b. Pen, vital sign flow sheet or record form	
5. Draw curtain or close door. Wash hands.	Maintains privacy. Prevents transmission of microorganisms.
6. Be sure client's chest is visible. If necessary, move bed linen or gown.	Ensures clear view of chest wall and abdominal movements.
7. Place client's arm in relaxed position across abdomen or lower chest, or place nurse's hand directly over client's upper abdomen (see illustration).	A similar position is used during pulse assessment, allowing respiratory rate assessment to be inconspicuous. A client aware of respiratory assesment may intentionally or unintentionally alter rate and depth of breathing.

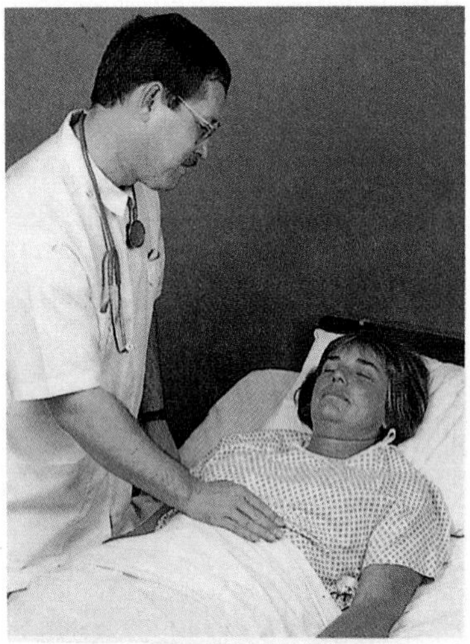

Step 7

Steps	Rationale
8. Observe complete respiratory cycle (one inspiration and one expiration).	Rate is accurately determined only after nurse has viewed respiratory cycle.
9. After observing cycle, look at second hand and count rate: when sweep hand hits dial, begin counting *one* with first full respiratory cycle.	Timing begins with count of *one*. Respirations occur more slowly than pulse; thus timing does not begin with *zero*.
10. If rhythmn is regular in adult, count number of respirations in 30 seconds and multiply by 2. In infant or young child, count respirations for full minute	Respiratory rate is equivalent to number of respiratory cycles per minute. Young infants and children normally breathe irregularly.
11. In an adult, if rhythm is irregular or rate is less than 12 or more than 20, count for 60 seconds.	Suspected irregularities require assessment for at least 1 minute.
12. Note depth, assessed subjectively by observing degree of chest wall movement while counting rate. Objectively assess depth by palpating chest wall excursion (see Chapter 16) after rate is counted.	Character of ventilatory movements may reveal specific alterations or disease status.
13. Note rhythmn of ventilatory cycle.	Character of ventilations can reveal specific types of alterations. Normal breathing is regular and uninterrupted.

Steps	Rationale
14. Replace gown and cover with bed linen.	Restores comfort.
15. Wash hands.	Reduces transmission of microorganisms.
16. Discuss findings with client as needed.	Promotes participation and understanding of health status.
17. Compare respirations to baseline and/or normal respiratory rate for age-group.	Allows nurse to assess for change in condition and for respiratory alterations.
18. Record respiratory rate and character on vital sign flow sheet and report abnormal findings.	Vital signs should be recorded immediately for accuracy. Abnormalities may require intervention.

table 15-6

NORMAL AVERAGE RESPIRATORY RATES BY AGE

Age	Rate
Newborn	35-40
Infant (6 months)	30-50
Toddler (2 years)	25-32
Child	20-30
Adolescent	16-19
Adult	12-20

ment in the chest wall. The nurse subjectively describes ventilatory movements as deep, normal, or shallow. A deep respiration involves a full expansion of the lungs with full exhalation. Respirations are shallow when only a small quantity of air passes through the lungs and ventilatory movement is difficult to see. More objective techniques are used if the nurse observes that chest excursion is unusually shallow (see Chapter 16). Table 15-7 summarizes types of respiratory alterations.

Ventilatory Rhythm. With normal breathing a regular interval occurs after each respiratory cycle. Infants tend to breathe less regularly. The young child may breathe slowly for a few seconds and then suddenly breathe more rapidly. While assessing respirations, the nurse estimates the time interval after each respiratory cycle. Respiration is regular or irregular in rhythm.

table 15-7

ALTERATIONS IN BREATHING PATTERN

Alteration	Description
Bradypnea	Rate of breathing is regular but abnormally slow (less than 12 breaths per minute).
Tachypnea	Rate of breathing is regular but abnormally rapid (greater than 20 breaths per minute).
Hyperpnea	Respirations are increased in depth. Occurs normally during exercise.
Apnea	Respirations cease for several seconds. Persistent cessation results in respiratory arrest.
Hyperventilation	Rate and depth of respirations increases. Hypocarbia may occur.
Hypoventilation	Respiratory rate is abnormally low, and depth of ventilation may be depressed. Hypercarbia may occur.
Cheyne-Stokes respiration	Respiratory rate and depth are irregular, characterized by alternating periods of apnea and hyperventilation. Respiratory cycle begins with slow, shallow breaths that gradually increase to abnormal rate and depth. The pattern reverses, breathing slows and becomes shallow, climaxing in apnea before respiration resumes.
Kussmaul respiration	Respirations are abnormally deep but regular.
Biot's respiration	Respirations are abnormally shallow for two to three breaths followed by irregular period of apnea.

procedure 15-4

ASSESSMENT OF OXYGEN SATURATION WITH PULSE OXIMETER

Steps	Rationale
1. Assess for signs and symptoms of alterations in respiratory status, hypoxia, and factors that influence Spo_2.	Physical signs and symptoms may indicate abnormal arterial saturation. Early identification of clients at risk for unstable oxygen status prevents complications. Nurse can accurately assess nature of variations.
2. Assess factors that influence client's respiratory status (e.g., oxygen therapy, hemoglobin level, temperature).	Factors may influence Spo_2 evaluation.
3. Review client's medical record for physician's order for pulse oximetry.	Medical order is required to assess oxygen saturation.
4. Prepare equipment and supplies and make sure they are in working order: a. Oximeter b. Oximeter probe appropriate for client and recommended by manufacturer c. Pen, vital sign flow sheet or record form d. Acetone or nail polish remover	Mixing probes from different manufacturers can result in burn injury to client. Clip-on probes are convenient, quicker to apply but more susceptible to movement interference. Adhesive probes suitable for pediatric use are less susceptible to motion artifact and can be taped to the skin.
5. Explain that Spo_2 is to be assessed; instruct client to breathe normally.	Clients are often curious about measurements. Prevents large fluctuations in minute ventilation and possible error in Spo_2 measurement.
6. Assess best site for obtaining Spo_2 measurement (e.g., finger, toe, earlobe, nose, palm or foot).	Site selected must include a pulsating vascular bed. Changes in Spo_2 are reflected in the circulation of finger capillary bed within 30 seconds and the capillary bed of earlobe within 5 to 10 seconds. Peripheral vasoconstriction can interfere with Spo_2 determination.
7. Assist client in assuming a comfortable sitting or supine position that provides easy access to measurement site.	Ensures comfort and accuracy of Spo_2 measurement. Movement can interfere with signal transmission between LED and photodetector.
8. If necessary, remove nail polish with acetone from digit to be assessed.	Ensures accurate readings. Opaque coatings decrease light transmission; nail polish containing blue pigment can absorb light emissions.
7. Measure Spo_2 a. Apply oximeter probe and turn on oximeter by activating power. Observe pulse waveform/intensity display and audible beep. Correlate oximeter pulse rate with client's radial pulse.	Pulse waveform/intensity display enables detection of valid pulse or presence of interfering signal. Pitch of audible beep is proportional to Spo_2. Double checking pulse rate ensures oximeter accuracy.
b. Leave probe in place until oximeter readout reaches constant value and pulse display reaches full strength during each cardiac cycle.	Reading may take 10 to 30 seconds depending on site selected.
c. Read Spo_2 on digital display and inform client of reading.	Promotes participation in care and understanding of health status.
d. Remove probe and turn oximeter power off.	Batteries can be depleted if oximeter left on.
e. Assist client in returning to comfortable position.	Restores comfort, promotes sense of well-being.
f. Wash hands.	Reduces transmission of microorganisms.
8. Compare Spo_2 readings with baseline.	Comparison reveals presence of abnormality.
9. Record Spo_2 on vital sign flow sheet or nurses notes and report abnormal findings to nurse in charge or physician.	Vital sign measurement should be recorded promptly on flow sheet to avoid omissions from record. Abnormalities may require immediate intervention.

Assessment of Diffusion and Perfusion

The respiratory processes of diffusion and perfusion can be assessed by measuring the oxygen saturation of the blood. After oxygen diffuses from the alveoli into the pulmonary blood, most of the oxygen attaches to hemoglobin molecules in red blood cells. Blood flow through the pulmonary capillaries provides red blood cells for oxygen attachment. Red blood cells carry the oxygenated hemoglobin molecules to the peripheral capillaries, where the oxygen detaches depending on the needs of the tissues.

The percent of hemoglobin that is bound with oxygen in the arteries is the percent saturation of hemoglobin (or Sao_2). It is normally between 95% and 100%. Sao_2 is affected by factors that interfere with ventilation, perfusion, or diffusion (see Chapter 34). The saturation of venous blood (Svo_2) is lower because the tissues have removed some of the oxygen from the hemoglobin molecules. A normal value for Svo_2 is 70%. Svo_2 is affected by factors that interfere or increase the tissue's need for oxygen.

Measurement of Arterial Oxygen Saturation

The recent development of a reliable device, a pulse oximeter, allows for the indirect measurement of oxygen saturation in the client's vital sign data base (Procedure 15-4). The pulse oximeter is a probe with a light-emitting diode (LED) and photodectetor connected by cable to an oximeter (Figure 15-13). The LED emits light wavelengths that are absorbed by the oxygenated and deoxygenated hemoglobin molecules. The light reflected back from the hemoglobin molecules is processed by the oximeter, which calculates **pulse saturation** (Spo_2). Spo_2 is a reliable estimate of Sao_2.

The measurement of Spo_2 is affected by factors that affect light transmission or peripheral arterial pulsations. An awareness of these factors allows the nurse to interpret abnormal Spo_2 measurements accurately (see box on p. 282).

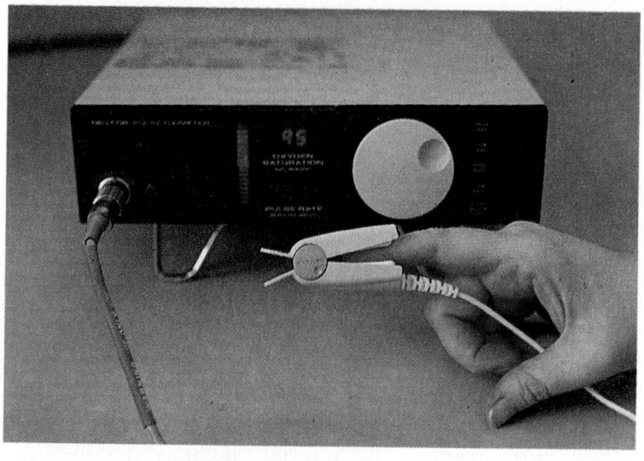

FIGURE 15-13 Pulse oximeter.

NURSING PROCESS AND RESPIRATORY VITAL SIGNS

Vital sign measurement of respiratory rate, pattern, and depth, along with Spo_2, allows the nurse to assess ventilation, diffusion, and perfusion. The nurse may also conduct other assessments to measure respiratory status (see Chapter 16). Each measurement gives clues in determining the nature of a client's problem. The nursing care plan and appropriate interventions are chosen on the basis of the nursing diagnosis identified (see box below). The nurse evaluates the plan by assessing the respiratory vital signs following each intervention.

BLOOD PRESSURE

Blood pressure is the lateral force on the walls of an artery by the pulsing blood under pressure from the heart. Systemic or arterial blood pressure, the blood pressure in the system of arteries in the body, is a good indicator of cardiovascular health. Blood flows throughout the circulatory system because of pressure changes. It moves from an area of high pressure to an area of low pressure. The heart's contraction forces blood under high pressure into the aorta. The peak of maximum pressure when ejection occurs is the **systolic** blood pressure. When the ventricles relax, the blood remaining in the arteries exerts a minimum or **diastolic** pressure. Diastolic pressure is the minimal pressure exerted against the arterial walls at all times.

The standard unit for measuring blood pressure is millimeters of mercury (mm Hg). The measurement indicates the height to which the blood pressure can raise a column of mercury. Blood pressure is recorded with the systolic reading before the diastolic (e.g., 120/80).

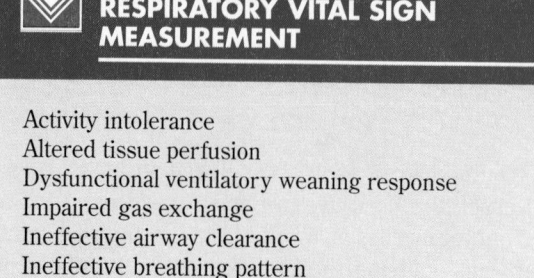

NURSING DIAGNOSES FOR RESPIRATORY VITAL SIGN MEASUREMENT

Activity intolerance
Altered tissue perfusion
Dysfunctional ventilatory weaning response
Impaired gas exchange
Ineffective airway clearance
Ineffective breathing pattern

FACTORS AFFECTING DETERMINATION OF PULSE OXYGEN SATURATION

INTERFERENCE WITH LIGHT TRANSMISSION

Outside light sources can interfere with the oximeter's ability to process reflected light
Carbon monoxide (caused by smoke inhalation or poisoning) artificially elevates Spo_2 by absorbing light similar to oxygen
Client motion can interfere with the oximeter's ability to process reflected light
Jaundice may interfere with the oximeter's ability to process reflected light
Intravascular dyes (methylene blue) absorb light similar to deoxyhemoglobin and artificially lowers saturation

REDUCTION OF ARTERIAL PULSATIONS

Peripheral vascular disease (Raynaud's, atherosclerosis) can reduce pulse volume
Hypothermia at assessment site decreases peripheral blood flow
Pharmacological vasoconstrictors (epinephrine, neosynephrine, dopamine) will decrease peripheral pulse volume
Low cardiac output and hypotension decrease blood flow to peripheral arteries
Peripheral edema can obscure arterial pulsation

The difference between systolic and diastolic pressure is the **pulse pressure.** For a blood pressure of 120/80, the pulse pressure is 40.

Physiology of Arterial Blood Pressure

Blood pressure reflects the interrelationships of cardiac output, peripheral vascular resistance, blood volume, blood viscosity, and artery elasticity.

Cardiac Output. A person's **cardiac output** is the volume of blood pumped by the heart (stroke volume) during 1 minute (heart rate):

$$CO = HR \times SV$$

The blood pressure (BP) depends on the cardiac output (CO) and peripheral vascular resistance (R):

$$BP = CO \times R$$

When volume increases in an enclosed space such as a blood vessel, the pressure in that space rises. Thus as cardiac output increases, more blood is pumped against arterial walls, causing the blood pressure to rise. Cardiac output can increase as a result of greater heart muscle contractility, an increase in heart rate, or an increase in blood volume.

Peripheral Resistance. Blood circulates through a network of arteries, arterioles, capillaries, venules, and veins. Arteries and arterioles are surrounded by smooth muscle that contracts or relaxes to change the size of the lumen. The size of arteries and arterioles changes to adjust blood flow to the needs of local tissues. For example, when more blood is needed by a major organ the peripheral arteries constrict, decreasing their supply of blood. More blood becomes available to the major organ because of the resistance change in the periphery. Normally, arteries and arterioles remain partially constricted to maintain a constant flow of blood. Peripheral vascular resistance is the resistance to blood flow determined by the tone of vascular musculature and diameter of blood vessels. The smaller the lumen of a vessel, the greater peripheral vascular resistance to blood flow. As resistance rises, arterial blood pressure rises. As vessels dilate and resistance falls, blood pressure drops.

Blood Volume. The volume of blood circulating within the vascular system affects blood pressure. Most adults have a circulating blood volume of 5000 ml. Normally the blood volume remains constant. However, if volume increases, more pressure is exerted against arterial walls. For example, the rapid, uncontrolled infusion of intravenous fluids elevates blood pressure. When circulating blood volume falls, as in the case of hemorrhage or dehydration, blood pressure falls.

Viscosity. The thickness or viscosity of blood affects the ease with which blood flows through small vessels. The **hematocrit,** or percentage of red blood cells in the blood, determines blood viscosity. When the hematocrit rises and blood flow slows, arterial blood pressure increases. The heart must contract more forcefully to move the viscous blood through the circulatory system.

Elasticity. Normally the walls of an artery are elastic and easily distensible. As pressure within the arteries increases, the diameter of vessel walls increases to accommodate the pressure change. Arterial distensibility prevents wide fluctuations in blood pressure. With a reduced elasticity there is greater resistance to blood flow. As a result, when the left ventricle ejects its stroke volume, the vessels no longer yield to pressure. Instead, a given volume of blood is forced through the rigid arterial walls, and the systemic pressure rises. Systolic pressure is more significantly elevated than diastolic pressure as a result of reduced arterial elasticity.

Each hemodynamic factor significantly affects the others. For example, as arterial elasticity declines peripheral vascular resistance increases. The complex

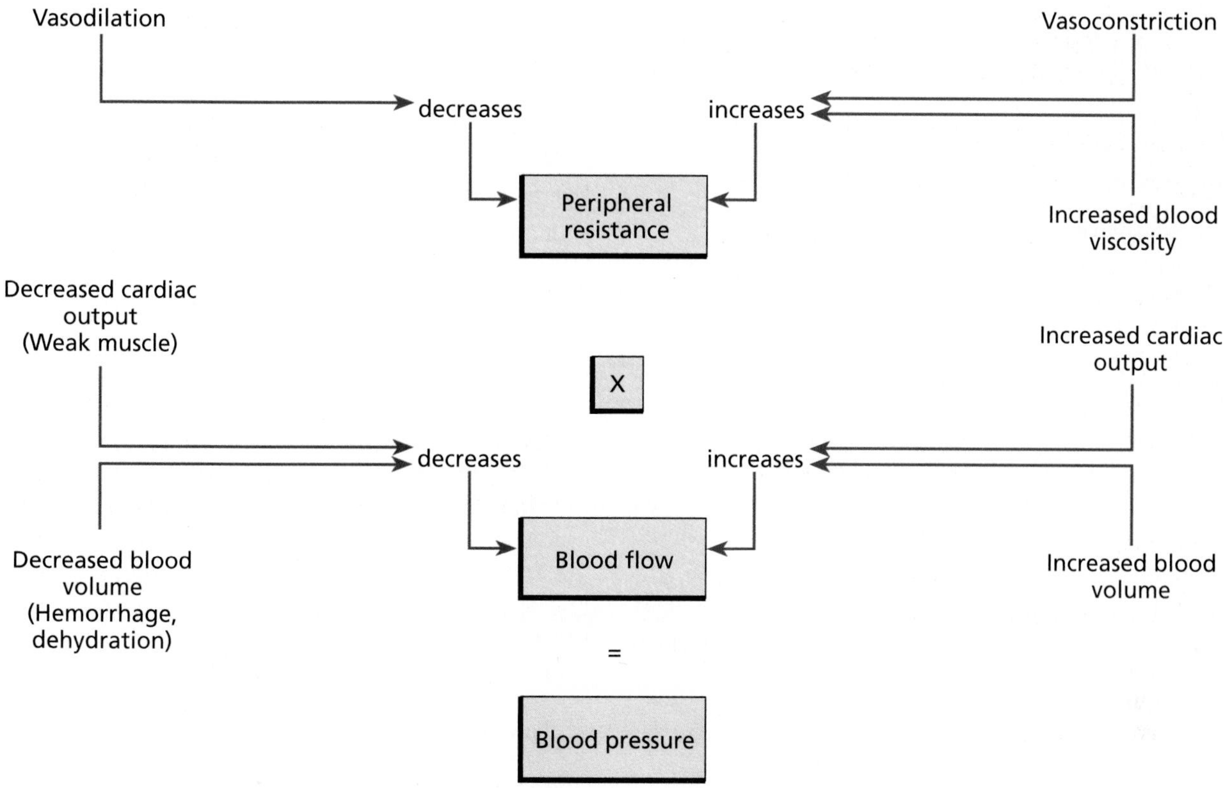

FIGURE 15-14 Hemodynamic factors that affect blood pressure.

control of the cardiovascular system normally prevents any single factor from permanently changing the blood pressure. For example, if the blood volume falls, the body compensates with an increased vascular resistance. Figure 15-14 illustrates how hemodynamic variables can affect blood pressure.

Blood Pressure Variations

Blood pressure is not constant but is continually influenced by many factors during the day. Understanding these factors ensures a more accurate interpretation of blood pressure readings. The box on p. 284 summarizes factors affecting blood pressure.

Hypertension. The most common alteration in blood pressure is **hypertension,** an often asymptomatic disorder characterized by persistently elevated blood pressure. The diagnosis of hypertension in adults is made when an average of two or more diastolic readings on at least two subsequent visits is 90 mm Hg or higher or when the average of two or more systolic readings on at least two subsequent visits is consistently higher than 140 mm Hg. Categories of hypertension have been developed and determine medical intervention (Table 15-8).

One elevated blood pressure measurement does not qualify as a diagnosis of hypertension. However, if the nurse assesses a high reading during the first blood pressure measurement (for example, 150/90 mm Hg), the client should be encouraged to return for another checkup at least within 2 months (Table 15-9).

Hypertension is associated with the thickening and loss of elasticity in the arterial walls. Peripheral vascular resistance increases within thick and inelastic vessels. The heart must continually pump against greater resistance. As a result, blood flow to vital organs such as the heart, brain, and kidney decreases.

Persons with a family history of hypertension are at significant risk. Obesity, cigarette smoking, heavy alcohol consumption, high blood cholesterol levels, and continued exposure to stress are also linked to hypertension. The incidence of hypertension is greater in older persons and in blacks. When clients are diagnosed with hypertension, the nurse helps to educate them about blood pressure values, long-term follow-up care and therapy, the usual lack of symptoms (the fact that it may not be "felt"), therapy's ability to control but not cure hypertension, and a consistently followed treatment plan that can ensure a relatively normal life-style (Joint National Committee on Detection, Evaluation, and Treatment of High Blood Pressure, 1993).

FACTORS INFLUENCING BLOOD PRESSURE

AGE

Blood pressure tends to rise with advancing age:

Age	Arterial pressure (mm Hg)
Newborn (3000 g [6.6 lb])	40 (mean)
1 month	85/54
1 year	95/65
6 years	105/65
10-13 years	110/65
14-17 years	120/75
Middle adult	120/80
Older adult	140-160/80-90

Level of a child's or adolescent's blood pressure is assessed with respect to body size and age.* Larger children have higher blood pressures than smaller children of the same age. Older adults have a rise in systolic pressure related to decreased elasticity.

STRESS

Anxiety, fear, and pain can initially increase blood pressure because of increased heart rate and increased peripheral vascular resistance. (If stress is not relieved, the blood pressure falls.)

GENDER

There is no clinically significant difference in blood pressure levels between boys and girls.
After puberty, males have higher readings.
With menopause women tend to have higher levels of blood pressure than men of the same age.

RACE

The incidence of hypertension is greater in urban black Americans than white Americans because of genetic and environmental influences.

DAILY VARIATION

Variations may include a lower blood pressure in the morning, rising throughout the day, peaking in late afternoon or evening, and lowering at night.

MEDICATIONS

Some medications directly or indirectly affect blood pressure. Antihypertensive medications including diuretics, beta-adrenergic blockers, vasodilators, ace inhibitors, and calcium channel blockers lower blood pressure.

EATING

The elderly often experience a fall in blood pressure after eating.

Data from Baines EM: *J Community Health Nurs* 3(4):225, 1986.
*Data from Task Force on Blood Pressure Control in Children: *Pediatrics* 79:1, 1987.

Blood Pressure Equipment

Before assessing blood pressure the nurse must be comfortable in using a sphygmomanometer and stethoscope. A **sphygmomanometer** includes a pressure manometer, an occlusive cuff that encloses an inflatable rubber bladder, and a pressure bulb with a release valve to inflate the cuff. The two types of sphygmomanometers are the aneroid and the mercury (Figure 15-15). The aneroid manometer has a glass-enclosed circular gauge containing a needle that registers millimeter calibrations. A metal bellows within the gauge expands and collapses in response to pressure variations in the inflated cuff.

Aneroid manometers have the advantages of being lightweight, portable, and compact. Because metal parts in the aneroid model are subject to temperature expansion or contraction, the aneroid instrument is less reliable than the mercury type. Aneroid sphygmomanometers require biomedical calibration at routine intervals to verify their accuracy.

table 15-8

CLASSIFICATION OF BLOOD PRESSURE FOR ADULTS AGE 18 YEARS AND OLDER*

Category	Systolic (mm Hg)	Diastolic (mm Hg)
Normal†	<130	<85
High normal	130-139	85-89
Hypertension‡		
STAGE 1 (Mild)	140-159	90-99
STAGE 2 (Moderate)	160-179	100-109
STAGE 3 (Severe)	180-209	110-119
STAGE 4 (Very Severe)	≥210	≥120

From National High Blood Pressure Education Program; National Heart, Lung and Blood Institute; National Institutes of Health: *The fifth report of the Joint National Committee on Detection, Evaluation and Treatment of High Blood Pressure.* NIH Pub No 93-1088, Bethesda, Md., NIH, January 1993.

*Not taking antihypertensive drugs and not acutely ill. When systolic and diastolic pressures fall into different categories, the higher category should be selected to classify the individual's blood pressure status. For instance, 160/92 mm Hg should be classified as Stage 2, and 180/120 mm Hg should be classified as Stage 4. Isolated systolic hypertension (ISH) is defiend as SBE ≥ 140 mm Hg and DBP <90 mm Hg and staged appropriately (e.g., 170/85 mm Hg is defined as Stage 2 ISH).

†Optimal blood pressure with respect to cardiovascular risk is SBP <120 mm Hg and DBP <80 mm Hg. However, unusually low readings should be evaluated for clinical significance.

‡Based on the average of two or more readings taken at each of two or more visits following an initial screening.

Note: In addition to classifying stages of hypertension based on average blood pressure levels, the clinician should specify presence or absence of target-organ disease and additional risk factors. For example, a patient with diabetes and a blood pressure of 142/94 mm Hg plus left ventricular hypertrophy should be classified as "Stage 1 hypertension with target-organ disease (left ventricular hypertrophy) and with another major risk factor (diabetes)." The specificity is important for risk classification and management.

Mercury manometers are more accurate than aneroid manometers. Repeated calibrations are not necessary. The mercury manometer is an upright tube containing mercury. Pressure created by the inflation of the compression cuff moves the column of mercury upward against the force of gravity. Millimeter calibrations mark the height of the mercury column. To ensure accurate readings, the mercury column should fall freely as pressure is released and should always be at zero when the cuff is deflated. Mercury manometers may be wall mounted or portable. Accurate readings are obtained by looking at the meniscus of the mercury at eye level. Looking up or down at the mercury results in distorted readings.

Cloth or disposable vinyl compression cuffs used with the sphygmomanometer come in several sizes. The size selected is proportional to the circumference of the limb being assessed. Ideally, the width of the cuff should be 40% of the circumference (or 20% wider than

Text continued on p. 290.

table 15-9

RECOMMENDATIONS FOR FOLLOW-UP BASED ON INITIAL SET OF BLOOD PRESSURE MEASUREMENTS FOR ADULTS AGE 18 AND OLDER

Initial screening blood pressure (mm Hg)*		
Systolic	**Diastolic**	**Follow-up recommended†**
<130	<85	Recheck in 2 years
130-139	85-89	Recheck in 1 year ‡
140-159	90-99	Confirm within 2 months
160-179	100-109	Evaluate or refer to source of care within 1 month
180-209	110-119	Evaluate or refer to source of care within 1 week
≥210	≥120	Evaluate or refer to source of care immediately

*If the systolic and diastolic categories are different, follow recommendations for the shorter time follow-up (e.g., 160/85 mm Hg should be evaluated or referred to source of care within 1 month)

†The scheduling of follow-up should be modified by reliable information about past blood pressure measurements, other cardiovascular risk factors, or target-organ disease.

‡Consider providing advice about life-style modifications (see Chapter III).

From National High Blood Pressure Education Program; National Heart, Lung and Blood Institute; National Institutes of Health: *The fifth report of the Joint National Committee on Detection, Evaluation and Treatment of High Blood Pressure.* NIH Pub No 93-1088, Bethesda, Md., NIH, January 1993.

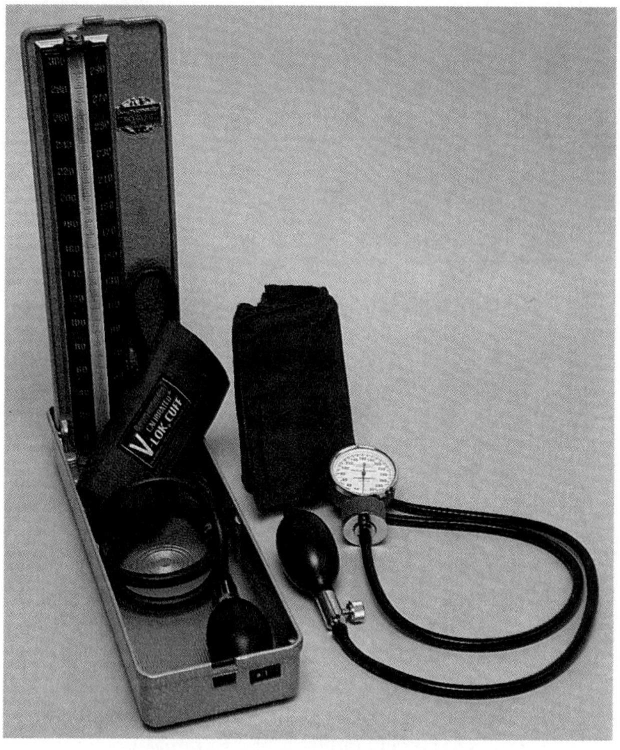

FIGURE 15-15 Sphygmomanometers.

procedure 15-5

ASSESSING BLOOD PRESSURE BY AUSCULTATION

Steps	Rationale
1. Assess for factors that influence blood pressure.	Allows nurse to assess blood pressure accurately and the significance of pressure changes.
2. Assess best site for obtaining blood pressure measurement. Avoid applying cuff to arm when intravenous catheter is in antecubital fossa and intravenous fluids are infusing; when client has arteriovenous shunt (a surgically created vessel for hemodialysis); when breast or axillary surgery has been performed on that side; when arm or hand has been traumatized or diseased; when client has lower arm cast or bulky bandage.	Inappropriate site selection may result in poor amplification of sounds, causing inaccurate readings. Application of pressure from inflated bladder can temporarily impair and compromise blood flow in extremity that already has impaired circulation.
3. Prepare equipment and supplies and make sure they are in working order:	
a. Sphygmomanometer: control valve should be clear and freely adjustable; when closed, valve should hold mercury constant; when released, valve allows controlled fall in mercury level; air vent at top of mercury manometer should be patent; rubber tubing connecting bladder to manometer should be at least 80 cm (32 in) long and with airtight connections.	Used to measure arterial blood pressure indirectly. Accurate measurements depend on functional equipment.

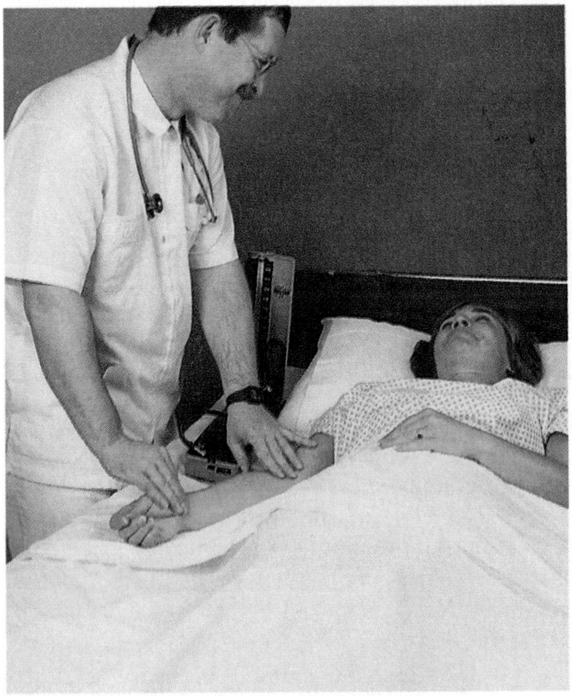

Step 8

Steps	Rationale
b. Bladder and cuff: bladder should completely encircle arm without overlapping; cuff should be long enough to encircle arm several times.	Secure cuff and proper-sized bladder are needed to exert equal pressure around artery being auscultated. Bladder too narrow causes false high reading.
c. Stethoscope	Auscultates arterial pressure waves.
d. Pen, vital sign flowsheet or record form	Provide for timely documentation of findings.
4. Encourage client to avoid caffeine and smoking for 30 minutes before assessment (Joint National Committee on Detection, Evaluation, and Treatment of High Blood Pressure, 1988).	Can cause false elevations in blood pressure.
5. Have client assume sitting or lying position. Be sure room is warm and quiet.	Maintains comfort.

Steps	Rationale
6. Explain procedure to client and have client rest at least 5 minutes before measurement.	Reduces anxiety that can falsely elevate readings. Blood pressure readings taken at different times can be objectively compared when assessed with client at rest.
7. Wash hands.	Reduces transmission of microorganisms.
8. With client sitting or lying, position client's bare upper arm (support if needed) at heart level with palm turned up (see illustration, p. 286).	If arm is unsupported, client may perform isometric exercise that can increase diastolic pressure 10%. Placement of arm above heart causes false low reading.
9. Expose upper arm fully by removing any constricting clothing.	Ensures proper cuff application.
10. Palpate brachial artery (see illustration). Position cuff 2.5 cm (1 in) above site of brachial pulsation (antecubital space). Center bladder of cuff above artery (see illustration).	Inflating bladder directly over brachial artery ensures proper pressure is applied during inflation.
11. With cuff fully deflated, wrap cuff evenly and snugly around upper arm (see illustration, p. 288).	Loose-fitting cuff causes false high readings.
12. Be sure manometer is positioned vertically at eye level. Observer should be no further than 1 m (approximately 1 yd) away.	Ensures accurate reading of mercury level.
13. Palpate brachial or radial artery with fingertips of one hand while inflating cuff rapidly to pressure 30 mm Hg above point at which pulse disappears. Slowly deflate cuff and note point when pulse reappears.	Identifies approximate systolic pressure and determines maximal inflation point for accurate reading. Prevents auscultatory gap.

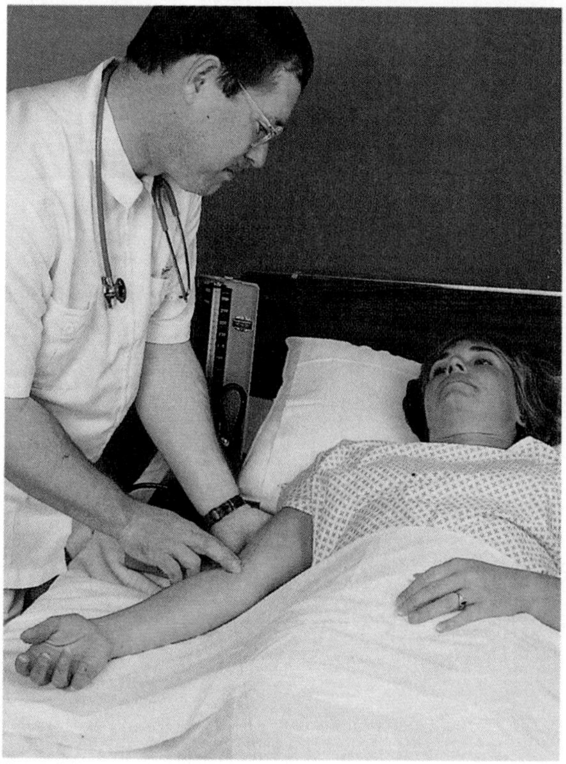
Step 10

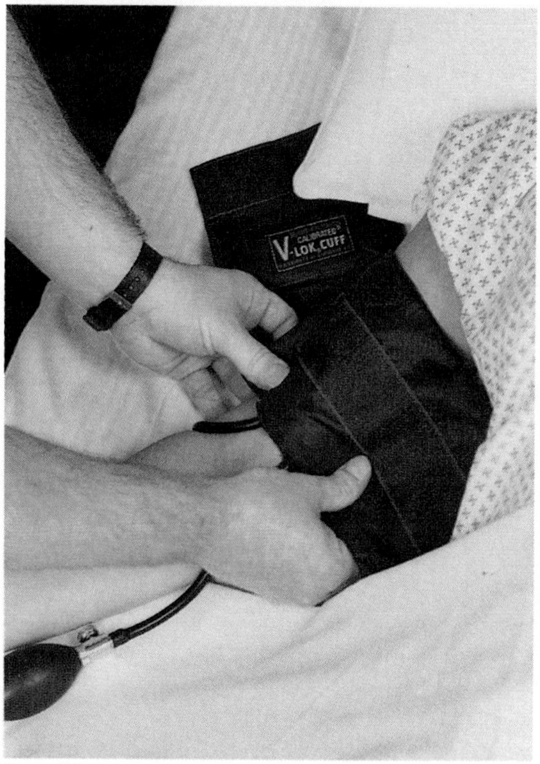

Step 10

Continued.

procedure 15-5—cont'd

ASSESSING BLOOD PRESSURE BY AUSCULTATION

Steps	Rationale
14. Deflate cuff fully and wait 30 seconds.	Prevents venous congestion and false high readings.
15. Place stethoscope earpieces in ears and be sure sounds are clear, not muffled.	Each earpiece should follow angle of ear canal to facilitate hearing.
16. Relocate brachial artery and place bell or diaphragm chestpiece over it. Do not allow chestpiece to touch cuff or client's clothing (see illustration).	Ensures optimal sound reception. Stethoscope improperly positioned causes muffled sounds that often result in false low systolic and false high diastolic readings.
17. Close valve of pressure bulb clockwise until tight.	Prevents air leak during inflation.
18. Inflate cuff to 30 mm Hg above palpated systolic pressure (see illustration).	Ensures accurate measurement of systolic pressure.
19. Slowly release valve and allow mercury to fall at rate of 2 to 3 mm Hg per sec.	Too rapid or slow a decline in mercury level can cause inaccurate readings.
20. Note point on manometer when first clear sound is heard.	**First Korotkoff sound indicates systolic pressure.**
21. Continue to deflate cuff, noting point at which muffled or dampened sound appears.	Fourth Korotkoff sound involves distinct muffling of sounds and is recommended by AHA as indication of diastolic pressure in children.

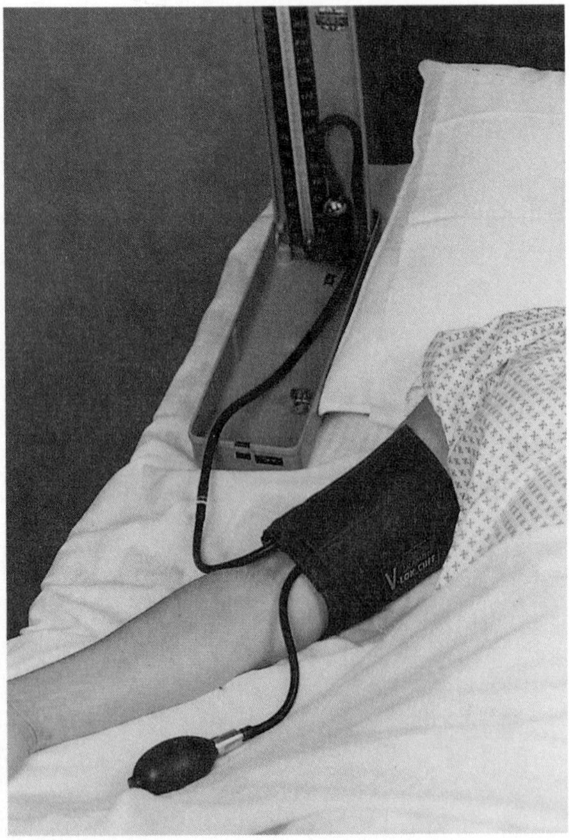

Step 11

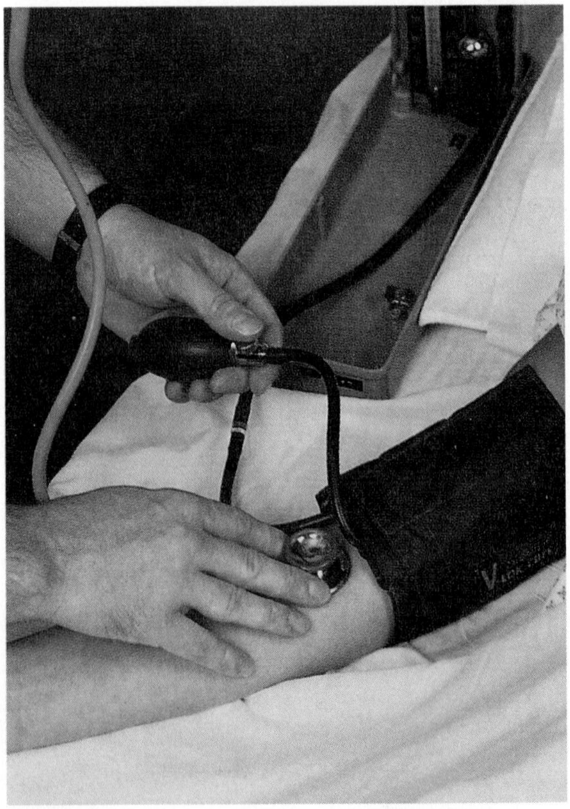

Step 16

Steps	Rationale
22. Continue cuff deflation, noting point on manometer to nearest 2 mm Hg at which sound disappears.	American Heart Association recommends recording fifth Korotkoff sound as diastolic pressure in adults.
23. Deflate cuff rapidly and completely. Remove from arm unless planning to repeat.	Continuous cuff inflation causes arterial occlusion, resulting in numbness and tingling of arm.
24. If this is first assessment of client, repeat procedure on other arm.	Comparison of pressure in both arms serves to detect any circulatory problems. Normal systolic difference of 5 to 10 mm Hg exists between arms.
25. Assist client in returning to comfortable position and cover upper arm.	Restores comfort.
26. Inform client of reading.	Promotes participation in care and understanding of health status.
27. Wash hands.	Prevents transmission of microorganisms.
28. Compare reading with previous baseline and/or normal average pressure for client's age.	Evaluates for change in condition and alterations.
29. Inform client of value and need for periodic reassessment.	Makes client accountable for follow-up assessment.
30. Record blood pressure in nurses' notes or vital sign flow sheet and report abnormal findings immediately.	Vital signs should be recorded immediately to ensure accuracy.

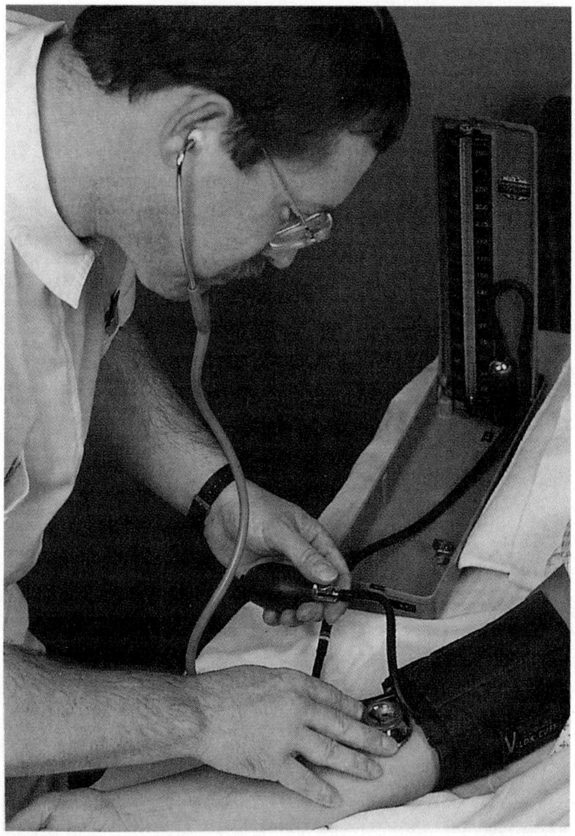

Step 18

the diameter) of the midpoint of the limb on which the cuff is to be used (American Heart Association, 1987). The bladder, enclosed by the cuff, should encircle at least two thirds of the arm of an adult and the entire arm of a child (Joint National Committee on Detection, Evaluation and Treatment of High Blood Pressure, 1988). In children the lower edge of the cuff should be above the antecubital fossa, allowing room for placement of the stethoscope. An improperly fitting cuff causes inaccurate blood pressure measurement.

Assessment of Blood Pressure

Arterial blood pressure may be measured either directly (invasively) or indirectly (noninvasively). The direct method requires the insertion of a thin catheter into an artery. Tubing connects the catheter with electronic monitoring equipment. The monitor displays a constant arterial pressure waveform and reading. Because of the risk of sudden blood loss from an artery, invasive blood pressure monitoring is used only in intensive care settings. The more common noninvasive method requires use of the sphygmomanometer and stethoscope. The nurse measures blood pressure indirectly by auscultation or palpation. Auscultation is the most widely used technique (Procedure 15-5).

Auscultation. The best environment for blood pressure measurement by auscultation is a quiet room at a comfortable temperature. Although the client may lie or stand, sitting is the preferred position. In most cases blood pressure readings obtained with the client in the supine, sitting, and standing positions are similar. In some clients, however, blood pressure changes with position. The nurse may compare sitting and standing blood pressure readings to determine whether a change occurs. **Orthostatic** or **postural hypotension,** or the lowering of blood pressure when the client moves from a sitting to a standing position is frequently accompanied by dizziness, light-headedness, and even syncope (fainting). Orthostatic hypotension may be a symptom of fluid volume deficit or inadequate neurovascular control. Antihypertensive medications may cause orthostatic blood pressure changes. Blood pressure should always be measured before administering such medications. When recording orthostatic blood pressure measurements, the nurse records the client's position in addition to the blood pressure measurement. For example: 140/80 supine, 132/72 sitting, 108/60 standing. The readings are obtained 1 to 3 minutes after the client changes position.

The client's position should be the same during each blood pressure measurement to permit a meaningful comparison of values. Before assessment the nurse should attempt to control factors responsible for artificially high readings such as pain, anxiety, or exertion.

During the initial assessment the nurse should obtain and record the blood pressure in both arms. Normally there is a difference of 5 to 10 mm Hg between the arms. In subsequent assessments the blood pressure should be measured in the arm with the higher pressure. Pressure differences greater than 10 mm Hg indicate problems in the arm with the lower pressure.

The nurse asks the client to state his or her normal blood pressure. If the client does not know, the nurse informs him or her after measuring and recording the blood pressure. This is a good opportunity to educate a client about normal blood pressure, the risk factors for developing hypertension, and dangers of hypertension.

Indirect measurement of arterial blood pressure works on a basic principle of pressure. Blood flows freely through an artery until an inflated cuff applies pressure to tissues and causes the artery to collapse. After the cuff pressure is released, the point at which blood flow returns and sound appears through auscultation is the systolic pressure.

Korotkoff, a Russian surgeon, first described the sounds heard over an artery during cuff deflation in

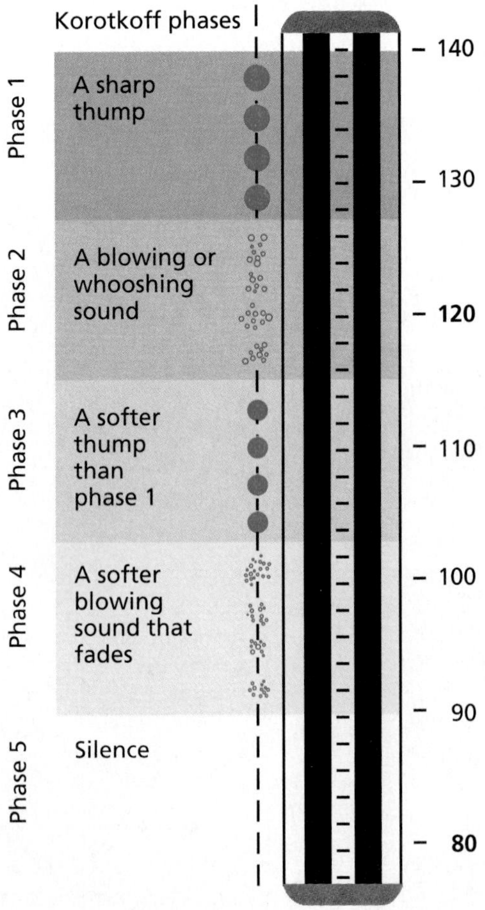

FIGURE 15-16 The sounds auscultated during blood pressure measurement can be differentiated into five Korotkoff phases. In this example, the blood pressure is 140/90.

1905. The first Korotkoff sound is a clear rhythmical tapping corresponding to the pulse rate that gradually increases in intensity. Onset of the sound corresponds to the systolic pressure. A murmur or swishing sound appears as the cuff continues to deflate, the second Korotkoff sound. As the artery distends, there is a turbulence in blood flow. The third Korotkoff sound is a crisper and more intense tapping. The fourth Korotkoff sound becomes muffled and low pitched as the cuff is further deflated. Cuff pressure falls below the pressure within the vessel walls; this sound is the diastolic pressure in infants and children. The fifth Korotkoff sound is an absence of sound; in adolescents and adults, this sound corresponds with the diastolic pressure (Figure 15-16).

The American Heart Association (1987) recommends recording two numbers for a blood pressure measurement: the point on the manometer when the first sound is heard for systolic and the point on the manometer when the fifth sound is heard for diastolic. Some institutions recommend recording the point when the fourth sound is heard as well, especially for clients with hypertension. The numbers are divided by slashed lines (for example, 120/80 or 120/100/80), and the arm used to measure the blood pressure is noted (for example, RA 130/70).

There are several possibilities for error if the auscultation procedure is not followed correctly. Table 15-10 summarizes common mistakes in measurement.

Assessment in Children. The nurse should include blood pressure measurement in the routine assessment of any child. The Task Force on Blood Pressure Control in Children (1987) recommends that all children age 3 through adolescence should have blood pressures checked at least yearly. The nurse can help parents to understand the importance of this routine screening to detect children who may be at risk for hypertension. The measurement and interpretation of blood pressure in infants and children is difficult for several reasons.

1. Different arm size requires careful and appropriate cuff size selection.
2. Readings are difficult to obtain in restless or anxious infants and children.
3. Placing stethoscope too firmly on the antecubital fossa can cause errors in auscultation of Korotkoff sounds.
4. Korotkoff sounds are difficult to hear in children because of low frequency and amplitude.
5. Blood pressure in children changes with growth and development.

The same auscultation method used with adults is appropriate for children. An infant or child under 5 years of age should lie supine with the arms supported at heart level. Older children may sit. It is important to have the child relaxed and calm. A delay of at least 15 minutes before taking a reading is recommended to allow the child to recover from recent activity or apprehension. Those 15 minutes can be used for other quiet nursing activities. It may help to have a parent nearby. The nurse should prepare the child for the blood pressure cuff's unusual sensation during inflation. Most children understand the analogy of a "tight hug on your arm" and will be more cooperative.

table 15-10

COMMON MISTAKES IN BLOOD PRESSURE ASSESSMENT

Error	Effect
Bladder or cuff too wide	False low reading
Bladder or cuff too narrow	False high reading
Cuff wrapped too loosely	False high reading
Deflating cuff too slowly	False high diastolic reading
Deflating cuff too quickly	False low systolic and false high diastolic reading
Stethoscope that fits poorly or impariment of the examiner's hearing, causing sounds to be muffled	False low systolic and false high diastolic reading
Inaccurate inflation level	False low systolic reading
Multiple examiners using different Korotkoff sounds for diastolic readings	Inaccurate interpretation of systolic and diastolic readings

Ultrasonic Stethoscope. If a nurse is unable to auscultate sounds because of a weakened arterial pulse, an ultrasonic stethoscope can be used (see Chapter 16). This stethoscope allows the nurse to hear low-frequency systolic sounds and is commonly used when measuring the blood pressure of infants, children, and low blood pressure in adults.

Palpation. Indirect palpation is useful for clients whose arterial pulsations are too weak to create Korotkoff sounds. Severe blood loss and weakened heart contractility are examples of conditions that result in blood pressures too low to auscultate accurately. Only the systolic blood pressure can be assessed by palpation (see box on p. 292). The diastolic pressure is difficult to determine by palpation. A subtle change in sensation, usually in the form of a thin, snapping vibration, marks the diastolic level. When the palpation technique is used, the systolic value and the manner in which it was measured are recorded (e.g., RA 90/-, palpated).

The palpation technique is used along with auscultation in some instances. In some hypertensive clients, the sounds usually heard over the brachial artery when the cuff pressure is high disappear as pressure is re-

PALPATING THE SYSTOLIC BLOOD PRESSURE

1. Apply blood pressure cuff to the upper arm in the same manner as the auscultation method.
2. Palpate the radial artery.
3. Inflate blood pressure cuff 30 mm Hg above the point at which the radial pulse can no longer be palpated.
4. Release valve and allow mercury to fall 2 mm Hg per second.
5. As soon as the radial pulse is palpable, note the manometer reading.

duced and then reappear at a lower level. This temporary disappearance of sound is the **auscultatory gap.** It typically occurs between the first and second Korotkoff sounds. The gap in sound may cover a range of 40 mm Hg and thus may cause an underestimation of systolic pressure or overestimation of diastolic pressure. The examiner must be certain to inflate the cuff high enough to hear the true systolic pressure before the auscultatory gap. Palpation of the radial artery helps to determine how high to inflate the cuff. The examiner inflates the cuff 30 mm Hg above the pressure at which the radial pulse was palpated. The range of pressures in which the auscultatory gap occurs is recorded (e.g., "BP RA 180/94 with an auscultatory gap from 180 to 160").

Assessment of Lower Extremities. Dressings, casts, intravenous catheters, or arteriovenous fistulas or shunts can make the upper extremities inaccessible. Blood pressure must then be measured in the lower extremities. Comparing upper extremity blood pressure with that in the legs is also necessary for clients with certain blood pressure abnormalities. The popliteal artery, palpable behind the knee in the popliteal space, is the site for auscultation. The cuff is positioned with the bladder over the posterior aspect of the midthigh. The cuff must be wide and long enough to allow for the larger girth of the thigh. Placing the client in a prone position is best. If such a position is impossible, the client should be asked to flex the knee slightly for easier access to the artery. The procedure is identical to brachial artery auscultation. Systolic pressure in the legs is usually higher by 10 to 40 mm Hg than in the brachial artery, but the diastolic pressure is the same.

AUTOMATIC BLOOD PRESSURE DEVICES

Many electronic devices can determine blood pressure automatically (Figure 15-17). Once the blood pressure cuff is applied, the nurse can program the device to obtain and record blood pressure readings at preset intervals. Alarm limits can be programmed to alert the nurse if the blood pressure measurement is outside desired parameters. The system includes either a microphone or a pressure sensor built into the inflatable cuff. The microphone or acoustic system hears Korotkoff sounds and registers diastolic and systolic readings. The pressure sensor or ultrasonic system responds to the pressure waves generated by the movement of blood through the artery. The advantages of automatic devices are the ease of use and efficiency when repeated or when frequent measurements are indicated. The ability to use a stethoscope is not required. However, automatic devices are more sensitive to outside interference and are susceptible to error.

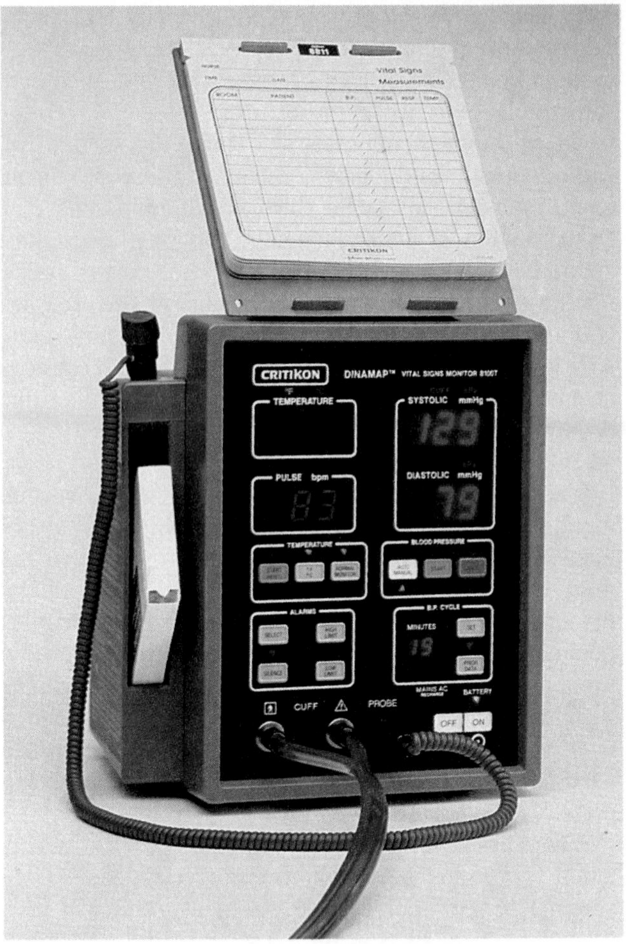

FIGURE 15-17 The Dinamap* automatic blood pressure monitor reports systolic, diastolic, and mean blood pressure. (Dinamapp* Vital Signs Monitor is a trademark of Critikon, Inc. Photo courtesy Critikon, Inc., Tampa, Fla.)

NURSING DIAGNOSES FOR BLOOD PRESSURE ASSESSMENT

Activity intolerance
Altered tissue perfusion
Decreased cardiac output
Fluid volume deficit
High risk for injury

NURSING PROCESS AND BLOOD PRESSURE DETERMINATION

The assessment of blood pressure along with pulse assessment is used to evaluate the general state of cardiovascular health and its response to other system imbalances. Hypotension, hypertension, and narrow or wide pulse pressures are defining characteristics of many nursing diagnoses and are considered along with other assessment data (see box above). The nursing care plan and appropriate interventions are related to the nursing diagnosis identified. The nurse evaluates the plan by assessing the blood pressure following each intervention.

SUMMARY

Vital sign measurements are a basic series of physiological assessments that reflect a client's health status. The nurse uses these data when making clinical decisions. Many physical and psychological factors can change vital signs. The nurse is often the one who determines the need for and frequency of vital sign assessment. Assessment of vital signs is not simply a routine task but rather an integral part of the nursing process.

The nurse should understand the physiological controls for vital signs before obtaining measurements. Each physiological control is influenced by variables such as age, physical activity, or hormonal changes. The nurse who understands the effects of these variables is better prepared to anticipate normal variations in vital signs. A nurse cannot recognize abnormalities without first knowing normal values.

Basic principles apply in the procedures for assessing vital signs accurately. Aseptic technique following the principles of universal precautions should be used. The client should be placed in the most comfortable, suitable position for measurements. Procedures should be explained to the client to reduce anxiety. The nurse should not rush through vital sign assessment and should not estimate values. All characteristics of a vital sign are assessed. Results are recorded promptly and accurately.

KEY CONCEPTS

- Vital signs include the physiological measurement of temperature, pulse, blood pressure, respirations, and oxygen saturation.
- Vital signs are measured as part of a complete physical examination or in a review of a client's condition.
- The nurse assesses vital sign changes with other physical assessment findings using clinical judgment to determine measurement frequency.
- Knowledge of the factors influencing vital signs assists the nurse in determining and evaluating abnormal values.
- Vital signs provide a basis for evaluating response to nursing interventions.
- Vital signs are best measured when the client is inactive and the environment is controlled for comfort.
- The nurse assists the client in maintaining body temperature by initiating interventions that promote heat loss, production, or conservation.
- A fever is one of the body's normal defense mechanisms.
- The tympanic route is the most accessible and acceptable site for core temperature measurement.
- To assess cardiac function, pulse rate and rhythm are most easily measured using the radial or apical pulse.
- Respiratory assessment includes determining the effectiveness of ventilation, perfusion, and diffusion.
- Assessment of respirations involves observing ventilatory movements throughout the respiratory cycle.
- Oxygen saturation is influenced by variables affecting ventilation, perfusion, and diffusion.
- Several hemodynamic variables contribute to blood pressure determination.
- Hypertension is diagnosed only after an average of readings made during two or more subsequent visits reveals an elevated blood pressure.
- Errors in blood pressure measurement can be made by selecting and applying the cuff improperly.
- Changes in one vital sign can influence characteristics of the other vital signs.

CRITICAL THINKING ACTIVITIES

1. An 18-year-old healthy college student arrives at the clinic complaining of sunburn. He just returned from 12 hours on the beach playing volleyball. What alterations in vital signs would you expect? What nursing interventions are indicated?
2. A 69-year-old homeless person has been brought into the emergency department by police who report she was found wandering incoherently in the middle of the street. The temperature outside is −21.0° F and it has been snowing for 2 hours. In what order should the nurse obtain vital signs? What method should be used to obtain each vital sign? What factors place this client at risk for impaired temperature regulation?
3. At a blood pressure screening clinic a client is worried that the blood pressure reading you measured, 140/60, is very different from the one he obtained using "one of those machines" in the neighborhood mall. Explain to the client the possible reasons for the discrepancy.
4. A hospitalized client, admitted for pneumonia, has a tympanic temperature of 100.2° F, pulse of 84, blood pressure of 130/84, respirations of 22, Sao_2 of 98%. Explain the rationale for your anticipated interventions for this client.
5. A 22-year-old client sustained a fractured mandible, fractured right radius, and fractured left humerus during a motorcycle accident. He is admitted postoperatively with an intravenous line in an unaffected extremity. What are the most effective methods for obtaining this client's vital signs?

References

American Heart Association: *Recommendations for human blood pressure determination by sphygmomanometers,* Pub no. 701005, Dallas, 1987, The Association.

Baines EM: *J Community Health Nurs* 3(4):225, 1986.

Centers for Disease Control: Update: universal precautions for prevention of transmission of human immunodeficiency virus, hepatitis B virus, and other bloodborne pathogens in health care settings, *MMWR* 37(24):377, 1988.

Davis C and Lentz MJ: Circadian rhythms; charting oral temperatures to spot abnormalities, *J Gerontol Nurs* 15(4):34, 1989.

Guiffre M, et al.: Rewarming postoperative patient: lights, blankets or forced warm air, *JOPAN* 6(6):387, 1991.

Guyton AC: *Textbook of medical physiology,* ed 8, Philadelphia, 1991, WB Saunders.

Holtzclaw B: Effects of extremity wraps to control drug induced shivering: a pilot study, *Nurs Res* 39:280, 1990.

Holtzclaw B: The febrile response in critical care: State of the science, *Heart Lung* 21(5):482, 1992.

Joint National Committee on Detection, Evaluation, and Treatment of High Blood Pressure: The 1988 report of the Joint National Committee on Detection, Evaluation, and Treatment of High Blood Pressure, *Arch Intern Med* 148:1023, 1988.

Lentz M: Circadian phase relationships of sleep-wake cycle and body temperature rhythm in aging, unpublished doctoral dissertation, Seattle, 1984, University of Washington.

Leung AK and Robson WL: Febrile convulsions: how dangerous are they? *Postgrad Med* 89(5):217, 1991.

Lobban M, Tredre B: Diurnal rhythms of renal excretion and of body temperature in aged subjects, *Proc Phys Soc* 188:48P, 1988.

Morgan SP: Comparison of three methods of managing fever in the neurologic patient, *J Neuro Sci Nurs* 132:19, 1990.

Mountcastle VB: *Medical physiology,* vol 2, ed 14, St. Louis, 1980, Mosby.

Neff J, et al.: Effect of respiratory rate, respiratory depth and open versus closed mouth breathing on sublingual temperature, *Res Nurs Health,* 12:195, 1992.

Neff T: Routine oximetry: a fifth vital sign? *Chest* 94:227, 1988.

Stephen SB, Sexton PR: Neonatal axillary temperatures: increases in readings over time, *Neonatal Network* 5:25, 1987.

Task Force on Blood Pressure Control in Children: Report of Second Task Force on Blood Pressure Control in Children—1987, *Pediatrics* 79:1, 1987.

Terndrup TE, Allegra JR, Kealy JA: A comparison of oral, rectal, and tympanic membrane-derived temperature changes after ingestion of liquids and smoking, *Amer J Emerg Med* 7:150, 1987.

Thibodeau GA: *Anatomy and physiology,* St. Louis, 1987, Mosby.

Vogelsang J and Hayes S: Butorphanol tartrate relieves postanesthesia shaking more effectively than meperidine or morphine, *J Post Anethesia Nurs* 7(2):94, 1992.

Bibliography

Alexander C, et al.: Principles of pulse oximetry: theoretical and practical considerations, *Anesth Analg* 68:368, 1989.

Anderson F, Cunningham S, Maloney J: Indirect blood pressure measurement: a need to reassess, *Amer J Critical Care* 2(4):272, 1993.

Castle S, et al.: Equivalency of infrared tympanic membrane thermometry with standard thermometry in nursing home residents, *JAGS* 40(12):1212, 1992.

Enhright T and Hill MG: Treatment of fever, *Focus Crit Care* 16(2):96, 1989.

Erickson R and Yount S: Comparison of tympanic and oral temperatures in surgical patients, *Nurs Res* 40(2):90, 1991.

Fontana SA: Update on high blood pressure: highlights from the 1988 National Report, *Nurse Pract* 13:8, 1998.

Guiffre M, et al.: The relationship between axillary and core body temperatures, *Appl Nurs Res* 3(2):52, 1990.

Hanson M: Drug fever: remember to consider in it diagnosis, *Post Grad Med* 89(5):67, 1991.

Hay W, et al.: Neonatal pulse oximetry: accuracy and reliability, *Pediatrics* 83(5):717, 1989.

Hill M and Grim C: How to take a precise blood pressure, *AJN* 91(2):38, 1991.

Hollerbach AD and Sneed NV: Accuracy of radial pulse assessment by length of counting interval., *Heart Lung* 19(3):258, 1990.

Holtzclaw B: Monitoring body temperature, *Clin Issue CCN* 4(1):44, 1990.

Hunter L: Measurement of axillary temperatures in neonates, *Wes Jnl Nurs Res* 13(3):324, 1991.

Longman A, et al.: Research utilization: an evaluation and critique if research related to oral temperature measurement, *App Nurs Res* 3(1):14, 1990.

Rebenson-Piano M, et al.: An evaluation of two indirect methods of blood pressure measurements in ill patients, *Nurs Res* 39:42, 1989.

Root R and Petersdorf RC: Alteration in body temperature. In Wilson, JD, et al., editors: *Harrison's principles of internal medicine,* ed 12, New York, 1991, McGraw-Hill.

Schnapp L and Cohen N: Pulse oximetry: uses and abuses, *Chest* 98:1244, 1990.

Severinghaus J and Kelleher J: Recent developments in pulse oximetry, *Anesthesiology* 76(6):1018, 1992.

Stevens S and Becker KL: How to perform picture-perfect respiratory assessment, *Nurs 88* 19:57, 1988.

The National High Blood Pressure Education Program Coordination Committee: National high blood pressure education program working group report on ambulatory blood pressure monitoring, *Arch Intern Med* 150:2270, 1990.

Webster H and Chellis M: Physiologic monitoring of infants and children, *Clinical Issues CCN* 4(1):180, 1993.

Whaley LF and Wong DL: *Nursing care of infants and children,* ed 4, St. Louis, 1991, Mosby.

White H, et al.: Body temperature in elderly surgical patients, *Res Nurs Health* 10:317, 1987.

16

Health Assessment and Physical Examination

OBJECTIVES

Mastery of content in this chapter will enable the student to:

- Define the key terms listed.
- Discuss the purposes and techniques of physical examination.
- List techniques to promote a client's physical and psychological comfort during a physical examination.
- Describe the proper position for the client during each phase of a physical examination.
- Use physical assessment skills during routine nursing care.
- Identify information to collect from the nursing history before an examination.
- Conduct properly organized physical examinations.
- Discuss normal physical findings in a young and middle-age adult compared with an older adult.
- Discuss ways to incorporate health teaching into the examination process.
- Describe physical measurements made in assessing each body system.
- Identify common self-screening examinations for clients.

KEY TERMS

adventitious sounds
aphasia
brachial pulse
bruit
carotid pulse
cerumen
crackles
diplopia
dorsalis pedis pulse
dysmenorrhea
dyspnea
dysrhythmia
edema
exophthalmos
femoral pulse
gingiva
gurgles
hernias
hematemesis
induration
integument
leukoplakia
melena
murmurs
nystagmus
orthopnea
pallor
palpitations
phlebitis
photophobia
pigmentation
pleural friction rub
point of maximal impulse (PMI)
postural hypotension
ptosis
reactive hyperemia
rhonchi
strabismus
striae
tactile fremitus
turgor
varicosities
ventricular gallop
vertigo
vocal fremitus
wheezes

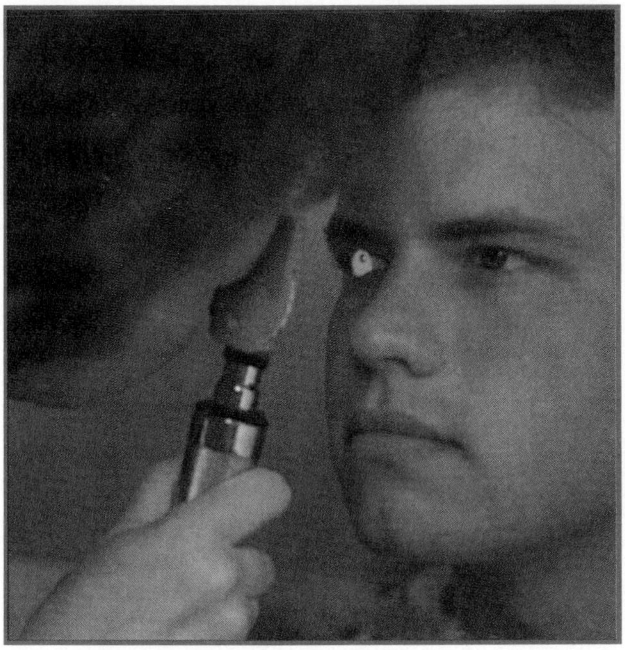

Nurses work in many settings, seeking information about clients' health status. The nurse conducts health assessments at health fairs, clinics, in physicians' offices, a client's home, or in hospitals. Health screenings focus on a specific physical problem. If a screening determines that a client has a risk for a disease, the client is referred for a more complete physical examination. A complete health assessment involves a health history and behavioral and physical examination. The health history involves a lengthy client interview to gather subjective data about the client's condition. A physical examination is a head-to-toe review of each body system that offers objective information about the client. In contrast, a health screening helps to determine whether a person has a high probability of having a characteristic for a disease (Larson, 1986). An example is a blood pressure screening.

The nurse uses physical assessment skills during an examination to make clinical judgments. The client's condition and response affect the extent of the examination. The accuracy of the nurse's assessment influences the choice of therapies a client receives and the evaluation of response to those therapies. Continuity of health care improves when the nurse makes ongoing objective and comprehensive assessments.

PURPOSES OF PHYSICAL EXAMINATION

An examination should be designed for the client's needs. If a client is acutely ill, the nurse may assess only the involved body systems. A more comprehensive examination is conducted when the client feels more at ease, and the nurse then learns about the client's total health status. A complete physical examination is performed for routine screening to promote wellness behaviors and preventive health care measures, to determine eligibility for health insurance, military service, or a new job, and to admit a client to a hospital setting or long-term care facility.

The nurse uses physical examination to:

1. Gather baseline data about the client's health status.
2. Supplement, confirm, or refute data obtained in the nursing history.
3. Confirm and identify nursing diagnoses.
4. Make clinical judgments about a client's changing health status and management.
5. Evaluate the physiological outcomes of care.

Gathering a Data Base

The nurse initially gathers thorough and detailed information about the client's health status from the client's health history (see Chapter 7). However, a client may be unaware of a physical problem, so a thorough assessment of physical status is necessary. Even if a history is complete, physical examination reveals information that refutes, confirms, or supplements the existing data base. One assessment finding usually cannot conclusively reveal the nature of an abnormality. A complete assessment is needed for a definitive diagnosis. The nurse groups significant findings into patterns of data that reveal actual or high-risk nursing diagnoses (Figure 16-1). Each abnormal finding also directs the nurse to gather additional information. Information gathered during an initial physical examination provides a baseline of the client's functional abilities. The baseline is not the normal range of physical findings but the pattern of findings identified when the client was first assessed. This baseline is used as a comparison for future assessment findings. During a subsequent examination the nurse can determine whether changes in the client's condition have occurred.

Developing Nursing Diagnoses and a Care Plan

The accuracy of the data base allows the nurse to develop individualized nursing diagnoses. Physical examination findings help determine diagnoses so the nurse can select the correct type of interventions. Physical as-

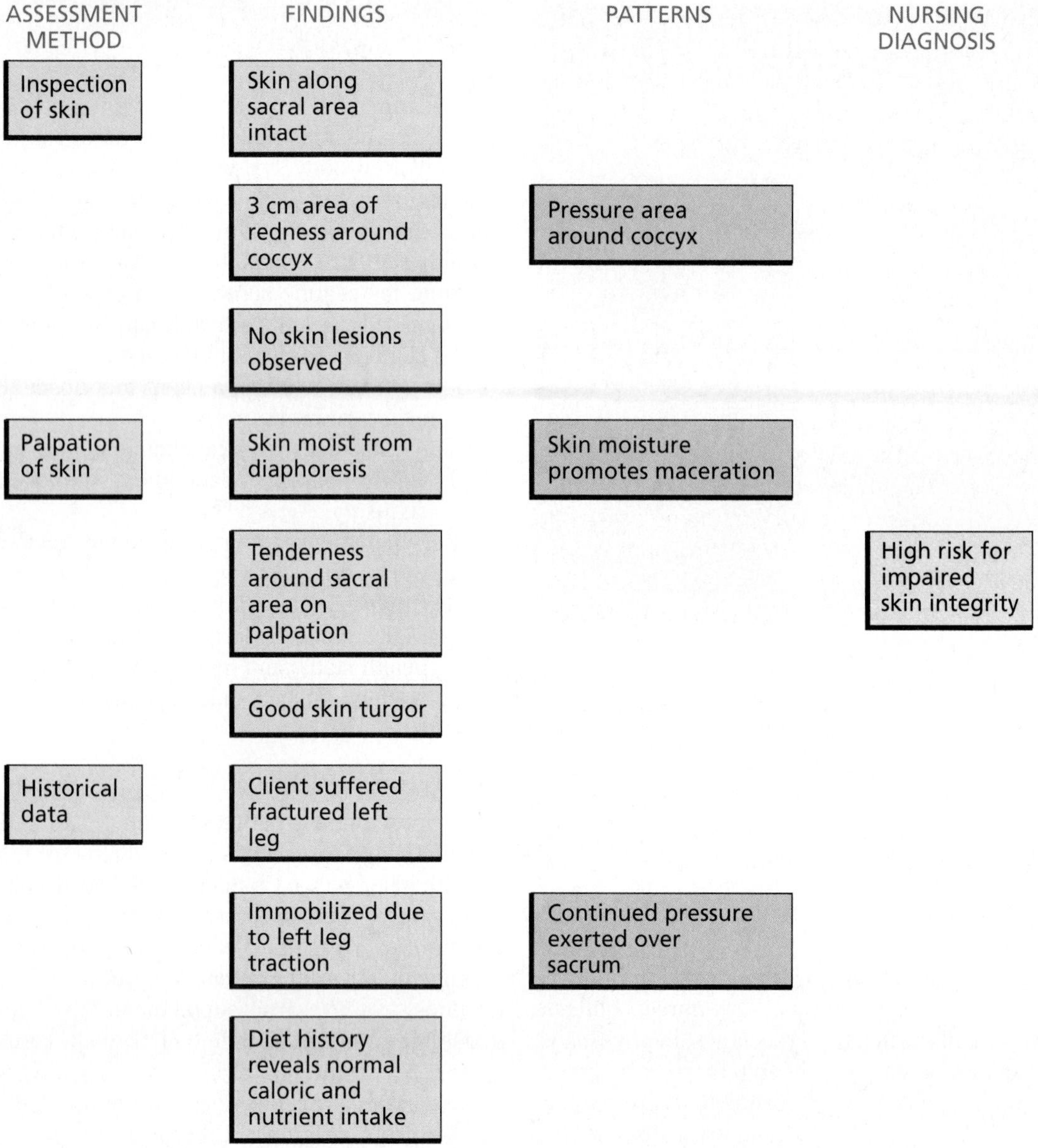

FIGURE 16-1 Application of health assessment data in nursing diagnosis.

sessment is ongoing. The care plan changes with the client's condition. The nurse monitors the client's progress and responses to therapies to review existing diagnoses and identify new problems.

Managing Client Problems

When caring for clients, the nurse makes many observations and performs many therapies. Yet the nurse's success in giving care depends on the ability to recognize change in status and to modify therapies for the most desirable client outcome. Physical assessment skills allow the nurse to judge the status of the client's health and to direct care. For example, during a bath the nurse notices a client's skin to be dry. The nurse revises the care plan to recommend application of body lotion to the skin and elimination of soap during bathing. The mechanics of physical assessment are relatively simple. The challenge is in using findings to make decisions.

Evaluating Nursing Care

Nurses become accountable by evaluating the results of nursing interventions. Physical assessment skills enhance evaluation of nursing measures through monitoring physiological and behavioral outcomes of care. The same physical assessment skill used to assess a condition (e.g., palpation of the client's pulse) can be used as an evaluative measure after care is administered (e.g., checking a client's pulse after exercise).

Physical assessment skills allow a nurse to make accurate, detailed, objective measurements to determine whether the expected outcomes of care are met.

INTEGRATION OF PHYSICAL EXAMINATION WITH NURSING CARE

An examination should be integrated into routine care. For example, the nurse can assess the condition of body parts during a bed bath. The nurse observes a client's gait and muscle strength while assisting with ambulation down a hallway. This practice makes more efficient use of time. The nurse also learns that physical assessment should become automatic when the nurse and client interact. The result is the nurse's ability to gather more comprehensive and relevant assessment findings.

SKILLS OF PHYSICAL ASSESSMENT

Chapter 7 briefly describes the skills of inspection, palpation, percussion, and auscultation. This chapter provides a more detailed description of those skills and their use in the physical examination.

Inspection

Inspection is the use of vision, hearing, and smell to detect normal characteristics or significant physical signs of body parts and function. It helps to know normal physical characteristics before trying to distinguish abnormal findings. It is also important to know normal characteristics of clients of different ages. Experience is needed to recognize normal variations among clients. Inspection is a simple technique, but it is often underused. The quality of an inspection depends on the nurse's willingness to spend time to be thorough and systematic. If hurried, a nurse may overlook significant findings or make incorrect conclusions. To inspect body parts accurately, the nurse follows these principles:

1. Good lighting and exposure are essential.
2. Inspect each area for size, shape, color, symmetry, and position and compare with the opposite side of the body. Look for the presence of abnormalities.
3. Use additional light (e.g., a penlight) to inspect body cavities.
4. Inspection is considered a visual skill but should include olfaction, since the sense of smell can sometimes detect abnormalities that may not be seen.
5. Ask a colleague to confirm the assessment if you are unsure about an odor.

After inspection of a body part, findings may indicate further examination. Palpation is often used with or after visual inspection.

Palpation

Further assessment of body parts is made through palpation, which uses the hands to touch body parts in order to make sensitive measurements of specific physical signs. Palpation is used to examine all accessible parts of the body. For example, the skin is palpated for temperature, moisture, texture, turgor, tenderness, and thickness. The organs such as the liver are palpated for size, shape, tenderness, and absence of masses. The nurse uses different parts of the hand to detect characteristics such as texture, temperature, and perception of movement.

The client should be relaxed and comfortable because muscle tension during palpation impairs effective assessment. Requesting a client to take slow deep breaths enhances muscle relaxation. Tender areas are palpated last. The nurse asks the client to point out the more sensitive areas and notes any nonverbal signs of discomfort.

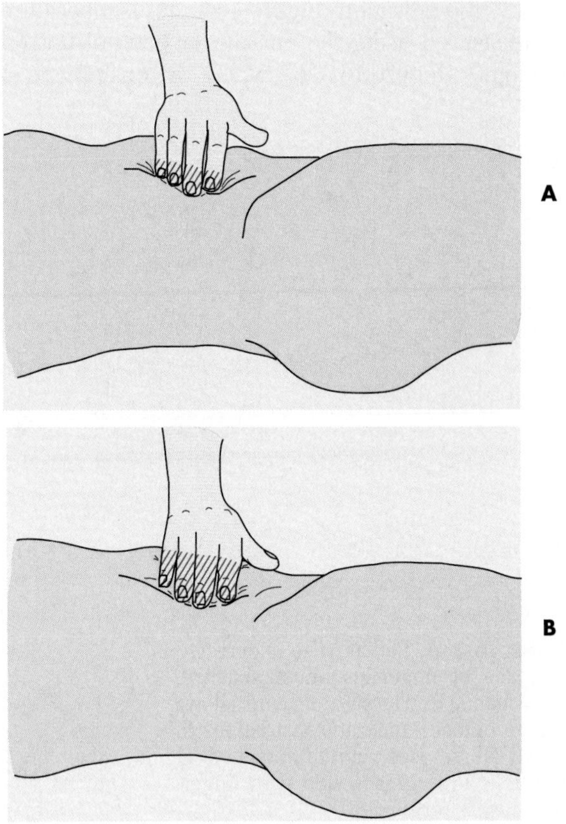

FIGURE 16-2 A, During light palpation, gentle pressure against underlying skin and tissues can detect areas of irregularity and tenderness. **B,** During deep palpation, nurse depresses tissue to assess condition of underlying organs.

The client appreciates warm hands, short fingernails, and a gentle approach. The nurse applies palpation slowly, gently, and deliberately. Light palpation of structures such as the abdomen determines areas of tenderness (Figure 16-2, *A*). The nurse's hand is placed on the part to be examined and depressed about 1 cm (½ inch). Tender areas are examined further for potentially serious abnormalities. The sensation of touch is best preserved with a light intermittent pressure. Heavy, prolonged pressure causes loss of sensitivity in the nurse's hand.

After light palpation, deeper palpation is used to examine the condition of organs such as those in the abdomen (Figure 16-2, *B*). The nurse depresses the area being examined approximately 2.5 cm (1 inch). Caution is the rule. A student should not attempt deep palpation without clinical supervision to avoid injuring a client. Deep palpation may be applied with one hand or both hands (bimanually). When the nurse uses bimanual palpation, one hand (sensing hand) is relaxed and placed lightly over the client's skin. The other hand (active hand) applies pressure to the sensing hand. The lower hand does not exert pressure directly and thus retains the sensitivity needed to detect organ characteristics.

The most sensitive parts of the hand, the pads of the fingertips, are used to assess texture, shape, size, consistency, and pulsation (Figure 16-3, *A*). Temperature is best measured using the dorsum or back of the hand and fingers (Figure 16-3, *B*), where the examiner's skin is thinnest. The palm of the hand (Figure 16-3, *C*) is more sensitive to vibration. The nurse measures position, consistency, and turgor by lightly grasping the body part with the fingertips (Figure 16-3, *D*).

The nurse must not palpate without considering the client's condition. For example, if the client has a fractured rib, extra care is used to locate the painful area. A vital artery is not palpated with pressure that obstructs blood flow. The nurse also considers the body area being palpated and the reason for using palpation and must be able to discriminate and interpret the significance of what is sensed.

Percussion

Percussion is striking the body's surface with a finger to produce a vibration that travels through body tissues. The character of sound determines the location, size, and density of underlying structures to verify abnormalities assessed by palpation and auscultation. This vibration is transmitted through the body tissues, and the character of the sound heard depends on the density of the underlying tissue. By knowing the way various densities influence sound, the nurse can locate organs or masses, map their boundaries, and determine their size. An abnormal sound suggests a mass or substance such as air or fluid within an organ or body cavity. The skill of percussion requires dexterity.

Direct percussion involves striking the body surface

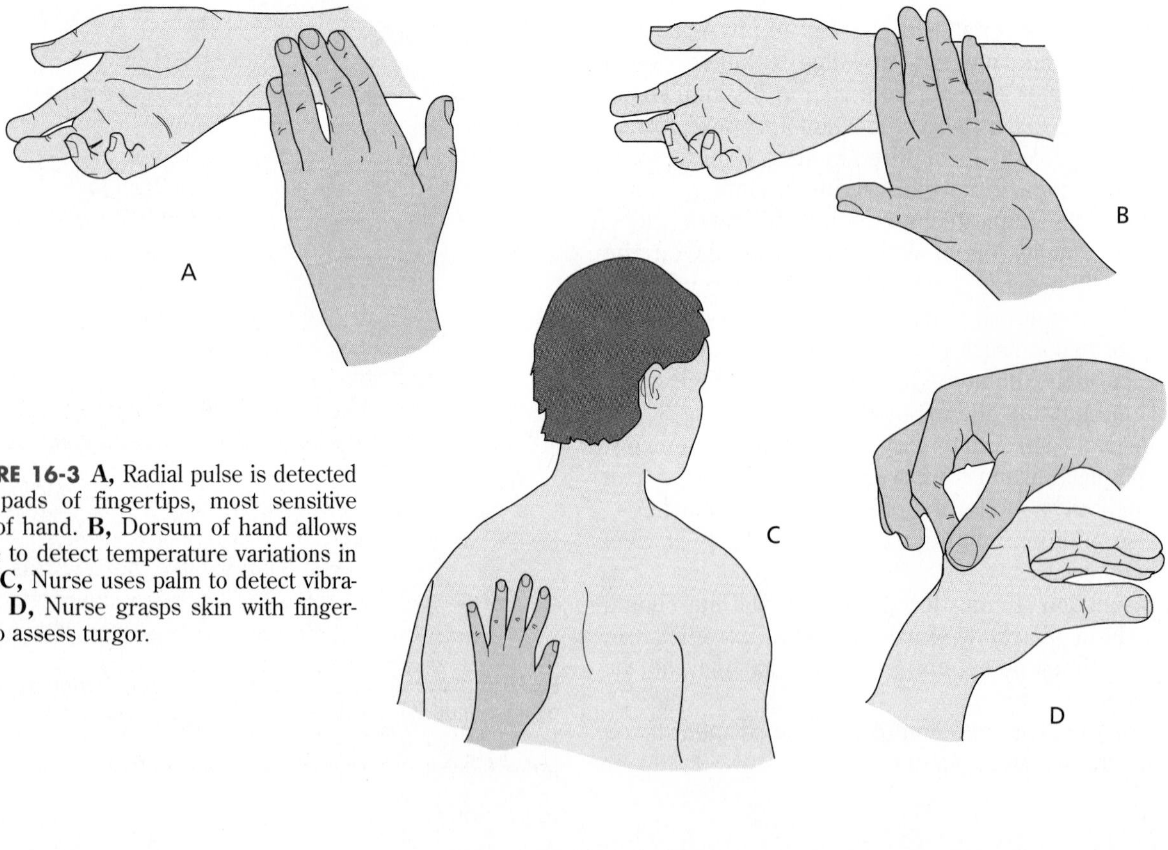

FIGURE 16-3 A, Radial pulse is detected with pads of fingertips, most sensitive part of hand. **B,** Dorsum of hand allows nurse to detect temperature variations in skin. **C,** Nurse uses palm to detect vibrations. **D,** Nurse grasps skin with fingertips to assess turgor.

table 16-1
SOUNDS PRODUCED BY PERCUSSION

Sound	Intensity	Pitch	Duration	Quality	Anatomic Finding
Tympany	Loud	High	Moderate	Drumlike	Enclosed, air-containing space; gastric air bubble, puffed-out cheek
Resonance	Moderate to loud	Low	Long	Hollow	Normal lung
Hyperresonance	Very loud	Very low	Longer than resonance	Booming	Emphysematous lung
Dullness	Soft to moderate	High	Moderate	Thudlike	Liver
Flatness	Soft	High	Short	Flat	Muscle

directly with one or two fingers. Indirect percussion is performed by placing the middle finger of the nondominant hand (pleximeter) firmly against the body surface (Figure 16-4). With palm and fingers remaining off the skin, the tip of the middle finger of the dominant hand (plexor) strikes the base of the distal joint of the pleximeter. The nurse uses a quick, light stroke with the plexor finger, keeping the forearm stationary. The wrist must remain relaxed to deliver the proper blow. If the blow is not sharp, if the pleximeter is held loosely, or if the palm rests on the body surface, the sound is dampened or softened. This prevents transmission of sound to underlying structures. The same force must be applied to each area of the body. Parrino (1987) cautions that variations in percussion findings often occur between two different examiners. For this reason, percussion may screen for gross abnormalities, but more in-depth examination, such as by x-ray examination, will be needed.

Percussion produces five types of sounds: tympany, resonance, hyperresonance, dullness, and flatness. Each sound is typically created by certain types of underlying tissues. Each sound is judged by its intensity, pitch, duration, and quality (Table 16-1).

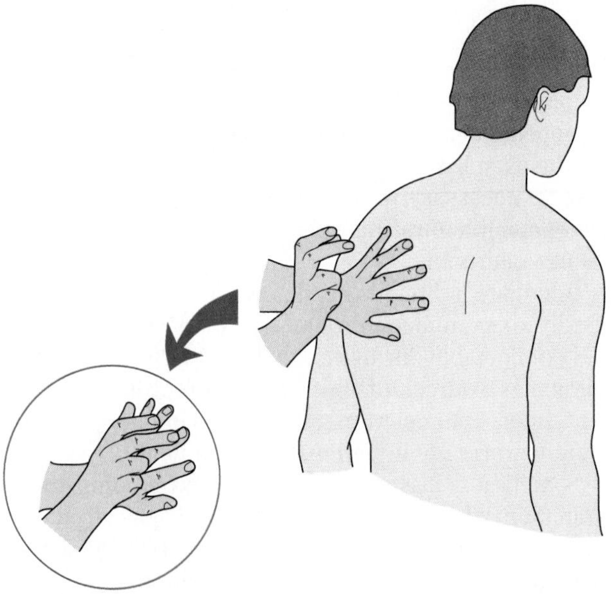

FIGURE 16-4 To perform indirect percussion, nurse places middle finger of nondominant hand against body's surface. Tip of middle finger of dominant hand strikes top of middle finger of nondominant hand.

Auscultation

Auscultation is listening to sounds created in body organs to detect variations from normal. Some sounds can be heard with the unassisted ear, although most sounds can be heard only through a stethoscope. A student must first become familiar with the normal sounds created by the cardiovascular, respiratory, and gastrointestinal systems. Abnormal sounds can be recognized only after learning normal variations. The nurse becomes more successful in auscultation by knowing the types of sounds arising from each body structure and the location in which they can most easily be heard. Likewise, the nurse learns the areas that normally do not emit sounds.

To auscultate correctly the nurse needs to hear well, have a good stethoscope, and know how to use the stethoscope properly. Nurses with hearing disorders should use stethoscopes with greater sound amplification or ask colleagues to check findings.

Chapter 15 describes the parts of the acoustic stethoscope and the general use of the bell and diaphragm. The bell is best for low-pitched sounds, and the diaphragm is best for high-pitched sounds.

EXERCISES TO INCREASE FAMILIARITY WITH THE STETHOSCOPE

Ensure that the earpieces follow the contour of the ear canals. Learn what fit is best for you by comparing amplification of sounds with the earpieces in both directions.

Place the earpieces in your ears with the tips of the earpieces turned toward the face. *Lightly* blow into the diaphragm. Again place the earpieces in your ears, this time with the ends turned toward the back of the head. *Lightly* blow into the diaphragm. After you have learned the right fit for the loudest amplification, wear the stethoscope the same way each time.

Put on the stethoscope and *lightly* blow into the diaphragm. If the sound is barely audible, *lightly* blow into the bell. Sound is carried through only one part of the chestpiece at a time. If the sound is greatly amplified through the diaphragm, the diaphragm is in position for use. If the sound is barely audible through the diaphragm, the bell is in position for use. Rotation of the diaphragm and bell places the chestpiece in the desired position. Leave the diaphragm in position for the next exercise.

Place the diaphragm over the anterior part of your chest. Ask a friend to speak in a normal conversational tone. Environmental noise seriously detracts from hearing the noise created by body organs. When a stethoscope is used, the client and the examiner should remain quiet.

Put the stethoscope on and gently tap the tubing. It is often difficult to avoid stretching or movement of the stethoscope's tubing. The examiner should be in a position so that the tubing hangs free. Moving or touching the tubing creates extraneous sounds.

A nurse must be familiar with the stethoscope before attempting to use it with a client. It helps to practice using the stethoscope with a friend. Extraneous sounds created by movement of the tubing or chestpiece can interfere with auscultation of body organ sounds. By deliberately producing these sounds, the nurse can learn to recognize and disregard them during the actual examination (see box above). Through auscultation, the nurse notes the following characteristics of sounds:

1. Frequency, or the number of sound wave cycles generated per second by a vibrating object. The higher the frequency, the higher the pitch of a sound and vice versa.
2. Loudness of a sound wave. Auscultated sounds are described as *loud* or *soft*.
3. Quality, or the sounds of similar frequency and loudness from different sources. Terms such as *blowing* or *gurgling* describe the quality of sound.
4. Duration, or the length of time sound vibrations last. The duration of sound is short, medium, or long. Layers of soft tissue dampen the duration of sounds from deep internal organs.

Auscultation requires concentration and practice. The nurse considers the part of the body auscultated and the causes of the sounds. For example, the sounds heard over the abdomen are caused by intestinal peristalsis. The nurse identifies where the sound is best heard and how the sound is heard normally. Peristalsis is heard over all four abdominal quadrants as intermittent "tinkling" sounds. After understanding the cause and character of normal auscultated sounds, it becomes easier to recognize abnormal sounds and their origins.

Olfaction

While assessing a client, the nurse should be familiar with the nature and source of body odors (Table 16-2). Olfaction helps to detect abnormalities not recognized by other means. For example, a client's cast should not have a sweet, heavy, thick odor indicative of an underlying infection. Findings from olfaction and other assessment skills allow the nurse to detect serious abnormalities.

PREPARATION FOR EXAMINATION

A disorganized approach when preparing for a physical examination can cause errors and incomplete findings. Proper preparation of the environment, equipment, and client ensures a smooth examination with few interruptions.

Environment

A physical examination requires privacy. A well-equipped examination room is preferable. However, often the examination occurs in the client's room, where it may be necessary to use room dividers or curtains. In the home, the nurse may perform an examination in the client's bedroom.

Adequate lighting is needed to illuminate body parts. Ideally an examination room is soundproofed so clients feel comfortable discussing their conditions. The nurse eliminates sources of noise, takes precautions to prevent interruptions from others, and makes sure the room is warm enough to maintain comfort.

Sometimes, it is difficult to perform a complete examination when clients are in beds or on stretchers. Special examination tables make clients easily accessible and help them assume special positions. The tables are high and narrow. The nurse must carefully assist clients so they do not fall while getting on and off them. A confused, combative, or uncooperative client should not be left on an examination table unsupervised.

table 16-2

ASSESSMENT OF CHARACTERISTIC ODORS

Odor	Site or Source	Potential Causes
Alcohol	Oral cavity	Ingestion of alcohol
Ammonia	Urine	Urinary tract infection
Body odor	Skin, particularly in areas where body parts rub together (e.g., under arms and breasts)	Poor hygiene, excess perspiration (hyperhidrosis), foul-smelling perspiration (bromidrosis)
Feces	Wound site	Wound abscess
	Vomitus	Bowel obstruction
	Rectal area	Fecal incontinence
Foul-smelling stools in infant	Stool	Malabsorption syndrome
Halitosis	Oral cavity	Poor dental and oral hygiene, gum disease
Sweet, fruity ketones	Oral cavity	Diabetic acidosis
Stale urine	Skin	Uremic acidosis
Sweet, heavy, thick odor	Draining wound	*Pseudomonas* (bacterial) infection
Musty odor	Casted body part	Infection inside cast
Fetid, sweet odor	Tracheostomy or mucous secretions	Infection of bronchial tree (*Pseudomonas* bacteria)

Examination tables are often hard and uncomfortable. When the client lies supine, the head of the table can be raised about 30 degrees. The client may also use a small pillow. When examining a client in bed, the nurse can raise the bed to reach the client's body parts more easily.

Equipment

Handwashing is done before equipment preparation and the examination to reduce the transmission of microorganisms. The equipment should be readily available and arranged in order for easy use (Figure 16-5). It should be kept warm as appropriate. For example, the diaphragm of the stethoscope may be briskly rubbed between the hands before it is applied to the skin. All equipment must be checked to see that it functions properly.

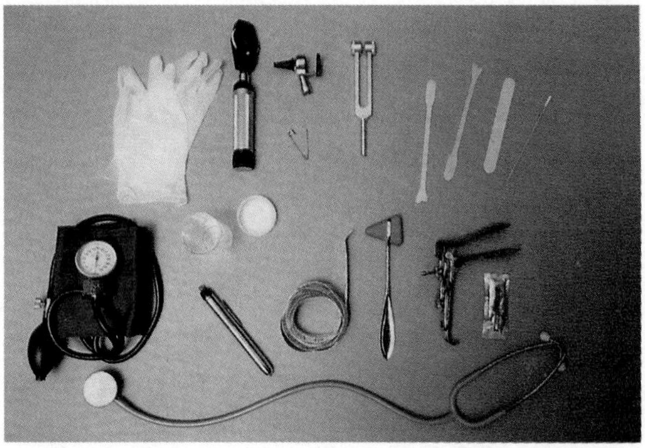

FIGURE 16-5 Types of equipment used during physical examination *(clockwise from upper left):* Disposable gloves, ophthalmoscope, otoscope attachment, sterile safety pin, tuning fork, cervical spatulas, tongue depressor, cotton-tip swab, lubricant, vaginal speculum, reflex hammer, tape measure, penlight, specimen cup, sphygmomanometer, and stethoscope *(bottom).*

Client

Physical Preparation. The client's physical comfort is vital for a successful examination. Before starting, the nurse asks if the client needs to use the toilet. An empty bladder and bowel facilitate examination of the abdomen, genitalia, and rectum. The nurse collects urine or fecal specimens at this time after explaining the proper method for collecting specimens. Each specimen is properly labeled.

Physical preparation involves being sure the client is dressed and draped properly. The client in the hospital will likely be wearing a simple gown. An outpatient will have to undress. If the examination is limited to certain body systems, it may not be necessary for the client to undress completely. The client should have privacy during undressing and plenty of time to finish. Walking into the room as the client undresses causes embarrassment. Drapes and gowns are made of linen or disposable paper. After clients have undressed and donned the gown, they should sit or lie down on the examination table with the drape over the lap or lower trunk. The ex-

table 16-3

POSITIONS FOR EXAMINATION

Position	Areas assessed	Rationale	Limitations
Sitting 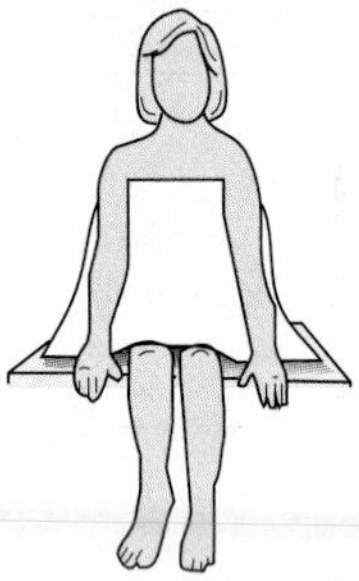	Head and neck, back, posterior thorax and lungs, anterior thorax and lungs, breasts, axillae, heart, vital signs, and upper extremities	Sitting upright provides full expansion of lungs and provides better visualization of symmetry of upper body parts.	Physically weakened client may be unable to sit. Examiner should use supine position with head of bed elevated instead.
Supine 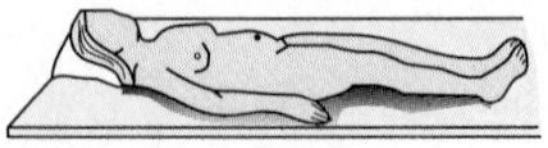	Head and neck, anterior thorax and lungs, breasts, axillae, heart, abdomen, extremities, pulses	This is most normally relaxed position. It provides easy access to pulse sites.	If client becomes short of breath easily, examiner may need to raise head of bed.
Dorsal recumbent 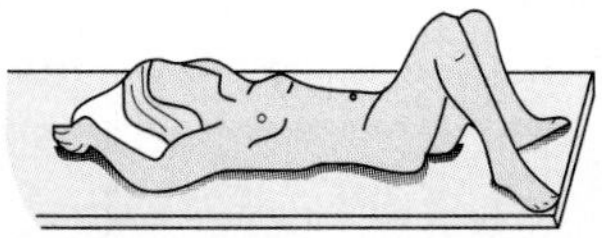	Head and neck, anterior thorax and lungs, breasts, axillae, heart, abdomen	Position is used for abdominal assessment because it promotes relaxation of abdominal muscles.	Clients with painful disorders are more comfortable with knees flexed.
Lithotomy* 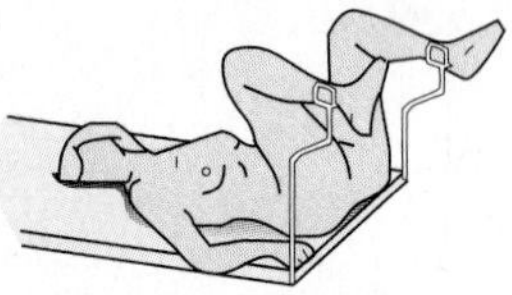	Female genitalia and genital tract	This position provides maximal exposure of genitalia and facilitates insertion of vaginal speculum.	Lithotomy position is embarrassing and uncomfortable, so examiner minimizes time that client spends in it. Client is kept well draped.
Sims' 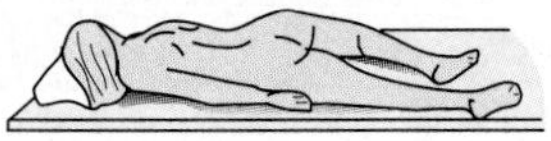	Rectum and vagina	Flexion of hip and knee improves exposure of rectal area.	Joint deformities may hinder client's ability to bend hip and knee.
Prone 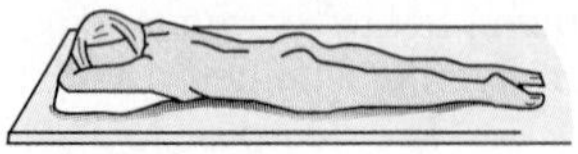	Musculoskeletal system	This position is used only to assess extension of hip joint.	This position is poorly tolerated in clients with respiratory difficulties.
Lateral recumbent 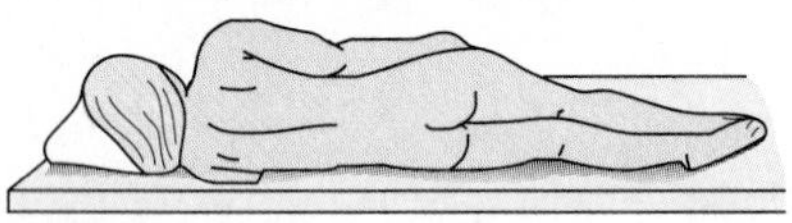	Heart	This position aids in detecting murmurs.	This position is poorly tolerated in clients with respiratory difficulties.
Knee-chest* 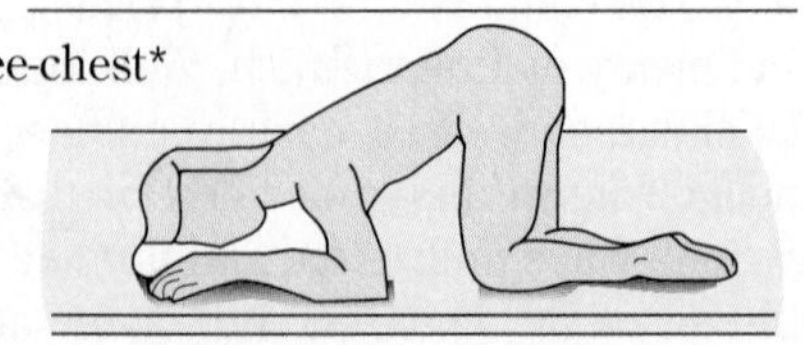	Rectum	This position provides maximal exposure of rectal area.	This position is embarassing and uncomfortable.

*Clients with arthritis or other joint deformities may be unable to assume this position.

aminer makes sure the client stays warm by eliminating drafts, controlling room temperature, and providing warm blankets. A seriously ill client or older adult is susceptible to chilling. The nurse should routinely ask if the client is comfortable.

POSITIONING. During the examination, the nurse asks clients to assume proper positions so body parts are accessible and clients stay comfortable. Table 16-3 lists the preferred positions for each part of the examination and contains figures illustrating these positions. Clients' abilities to assume positions will depend on their physical strength and degree of wellness. Many positions, such as the lithotomy and knee-chest, are embarrassing and uncomfortable. Therefore clients should be kept in these positions no longer than necessary. The examiner explains the positions and assists clients in assuming them. The drapes are adjusted to be sure the area to be examined is accessible and that no body part is unnecessarily exposed. More than one position can be assumed for the same part of an examination. If clients are too weak or are physically unable to assume a position, the nurse may choose an alternative position. The nurse uses extra care to position older adults to avoid having them look into the source of light, which can cause discomfort from glare.

Psychological Preparation. Because many clients find a physical examination tiring, stressful, or experience anxiety about possible assessment findings, the examiner should psychologically prepare the client beforehand. A thorough explanation of the purpose and steps of each assessment lets clients know what to expect and what to do so they can cooperate. The nurse explains the examination in simple, understandable terms. Clients should feel free to ask questions and mention any discomfort. As the nurse examines each body system, a more detailed explanation is given.

The nurse's manner should be professional yet relaxed. When the client and nurse are of opposite gender, it may help to have a third person of the client's gender in the room. The presence of a third person assures the client the examiner will behave ethically, and the third person is a witness to the examiner's and client's conduct.

During the examination the nurse watches the client's emotional responses. The nurse observes whether the client's facial expression shows fear or concern and if body movements show anxiety. The nurse remains calm and explains each step clearly. It may be necessary to temporarily stop the examination and ask how the client feels. The client should not be forced to continue. Postponing the examination may be best because the findings may be more accurate when the client can cooperate and relax. If the fears result from misconceptions, the nurse clarifies the purpose of the examination and how it is to be performed.

Assessment of Age-Groups

The nurse will use different approaches when interviewing clients of different age-groups. The following are useful guidelines:

1. Gather an infant's or child's health history from parents or guardians.
2. Because parents may think they are being tested by the nurse, offer support and do not pass judgment.
3. Call children by their first name. Address the parents by their surname (e.g., "Mr. and Mrs. Brown").
4. Use open-ended questions to encourage parents to share more information. Example: Describe for me what caused your child's injury.
5. Interview older children to observe parent-child interactions. They also can provide details about their history and symptoms.
6. Treat adolescents as adults and individuals.
7. Adolescents have the right to confidentiality. After talking with parents, speak alone with adolescents.
8. Do not stereotype older adults. Most are able to provide reliable histories.
9. Give the older adult time to answer questions.
10. Be sure the older adult can see and hear you clearly before beginning an interview.

EXAMINATION

A physical examination, using the skills of physical assessment, is composed of assessments for each body system. The extent of an examination depends on its purpose and the client's condition. Clients with specific symptoms or needs require only portions of an examination. When a client is first admitted to a health care center, however, a total examination is usually performed. A complete health assessment follows the format of the health history (see Chapter 7). The nurse uses information from the history to focus attention on specific parts of the physical examination. For example, if the history shows that the client experiences difficulty in breathing, the nurse examines the thorax and lungs more carefully. The physical examination supplements information from the history to confirm or refute the data.

The examination should be systematic and well organized so important assessments are not deleted. A head-to-toe approach includes all body systems and helps the nurse anticipate each step. In an adult, the nurse begins by assessing the head and neck, progressing methodically down the body to include all body systems. Both sides of the body are inspected and compared for symmetry. If a client is seriously ill, the body system most at risk for being abnormal is examined first. If a client becomes fatigued, rest periods are provided. Painful procedures should be performed near the end of the examination. Assessments are recorded in specific terms on a physical assessment form or in the nurse's notes. The use of common and accepted medical abbreviations help to keep notes brief and concise.

GENERAL SURVEY

Assessment begins when the nurse first meets the client. The nurse determines the reason for the client seeking health care. Initial data from the general survey begins with a review of the client's primary health problems. The nurse makes mental notes of the client's behavior and appearance. The examination begins with a general survey that includes observing general appearance and measuring behavior, vital signs, height, and weight. The survey provides information about characteristics of an illness, a client's hygiene and body image, emotional state, recent changes in weight, and the client's developmental status. If any abnormalities or problems are found, the affected body system is closely assessed later.

General Appearance and Behavior

Assessment of appearance and behavior can be conducted while the nurse prepares the client for the physical examination. The review of appearance and behavior includes the following:

1. Gender and race. A person's gender affects the type of examination performed and the manner in which assessments are made. Different physical features are related to gender and race. Certain illnesses more likely affect a specific gender or race; for example skin cancer is 10 times higher in whites than blacks, whereas cancer of the larynx is more common in men (American Cancer Society, 1993).
2. Age. Age influences normal physical characteristics. The ability to participate in some parts of the examination is also influenced by age.
3. Signs of distress. There may be obvious signs or symptoms indicating pain, difficulty in breathing, or anxiety. These signs help to establish priorities regarding what to examine first.
4. Body type. The nurse observes if a client appears trim and muscular, obese, or excessively thin. Body type can reflect level of health, age, and life-style.
5. Posture. Normal standing posture is an upright stance with parallel alignment of hips and shoulders. Normal sitting involves some degree of rounding of the shoulders. Observe whether the client has a slumped, erect, or bent posture. Posture may reflect mood or pain. Many older adults have a stooped, forward-bent posture, with hips and knees somewhat flexed and arms bent at the elbows, raising the level of the arms.
6. Gait. Observe the client walk into the room or along the bedside (if ambulatory). Note if movements are coordinated or uncoordinated. A person normally walks with arms swinging freely at the sides, with the head and face leading the body.
7. Body movements. Observe whether movements are purposeful. Note any tremors involving the extremities. Determine if any body parts are immobile.
8. Hygiene and grooming. Note the client's level of cleanliness by observing the appearance of the hair, skin, and fingernails. Note if the client's clothes are clean. Grooming may depend on the activities being performed just before the examination as well as the client's occupation. Also note amount and type of cosmetics used.
9. Dress. Culture, life-style, socioeconomic level, and personal preference affect the type of clothes worn. Note if the type of clothing worn is appropriate for temperature and weather conditions. Depressed or mentally ill persons may be unable to choose proper clothing. An older adult tends to wear extra clothing because of sensitivity to cold.
10. Body odor. An unpleasant body odor may result from physical exercise, poor hygiene, or certain disease pathologies. Poor oral hygiene may cause bad breath.
11. Mood and affect. Affect is a person's feelings as they appear to others. Mood or emotional state is expressed verbally and nonverbally. Note if verbal expressions match nonverbal behavior. Observe if mood is appropriate for the situation. Observe facial expressions while asking questions.
12. Speech. Normal speech is understandable and moderately paced. It shows an association with the person's thoughts. Note if the client talks rapidly or slowly. An abnormal pace may be caused by emotions or neurological impairment. Observe if the client speaks in a normal tone with clear inflection of words.
13. Client abuse. Abuse of children, women, and older adults is a growing health problem. It may be first suspected in clients who have suffered obvious physical injury or neglect. Assess for the client's fear of the spouse or partner, care giver, parent, or child. Note if the partner or care giver has a history of violence, alcoholism, or drug abuse. Is the person unemployed, ill, or frustrated in caring for the client (Elder Abuse, 1987)? Many states mandate a report to a social service center or abuse hotline of any suspected abuse or neglect.

Vital Signs

Most nurses prefer measuring vital signs (see Chapter 15) before the physical examination because positioning or moving the client can interfere with obtaining accurate values. The nurse can also measure specific vital signs during individual body system assessments. For example, respirations may be assessed during examination of the thorax.

Height and Weight

A person's general level of health can be reflected by his or her height and weight. Weight is a routine measure during health screenings and visits to physicians' offices or clinics. Both height and weight are routine during admission to a health care setting. A nurse measures an infant's or child's height and weight to assess growth and development. (Note: more detailed assessment of infants and children require measurement of circumference of head, chest, and abdomen).

A client's weight normally will vary daily because of fluid loss or retention. The assessment screens for abnormal weight changes. Before measurement, the nurse asks clients their current height and weight. The nurse also assesses if clients have had recent weight gains or losses. A weight gain of 5 pounds or 2.3 kilograms in a day may indicate fluid retention problems. If a change exists, the nurse assesses the amount, the period of time over which the change occurred, and a change in diet habits, appetite, prescription or over-the-counter drugs, or physical symptoms. It is also helpful to note if a client has a concern with weight loss or body shape (e.g., never feeling thin enough). An unusually strict caloric intake, laxative abuse, or excessive exercise could be warning signs for anorexia or bulimia.

Clients should be weighed at the same time of day, on the same scale, and in the same clothes to allow for an objective comparison of subsequent weights. While body weight may seem routine, care should be taken to be certain of accuracy since significant medical and nursing decisions are made on weight changes. Clients capable of bearing their own weight use a standing scale. The nurse calibrates a standard platform scale by moving the large and small weights to zero. The balance beam should be made level and steady by adjusting the calibrating knob (Figure 16-6). Electronic scales are automatically calibrated each time they are used. The client stands on the scale platform and remains still (Figure 16-7). The nurse moves the largest weight to the 50-lb or 22.5-kg increment under the client's weight. Then the smaller weight is adjusted to balance the scale at the nearest $\frac{1}{4}$ lb or 0.1 kg (Seidel et al., 1991). Electronic scales automatically display weight within seconds.

Stretcher and chair scales are available for clients unable to bear weight. After being transferred to the scale, the client is lifted above the bed by a hydraulic device and the weight is measured on a balance beam or digital display. Caution must be used when transferring clients to and from the scales.

Infants can be weighed in baskets or on platform scales. The nurse removes clothing and weighs infants

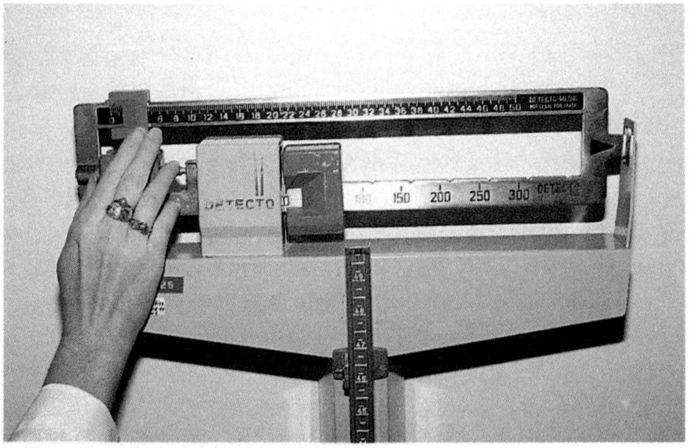

FIGURE 16-6 Adjusting calibrating knob (just below small weight) on scale.

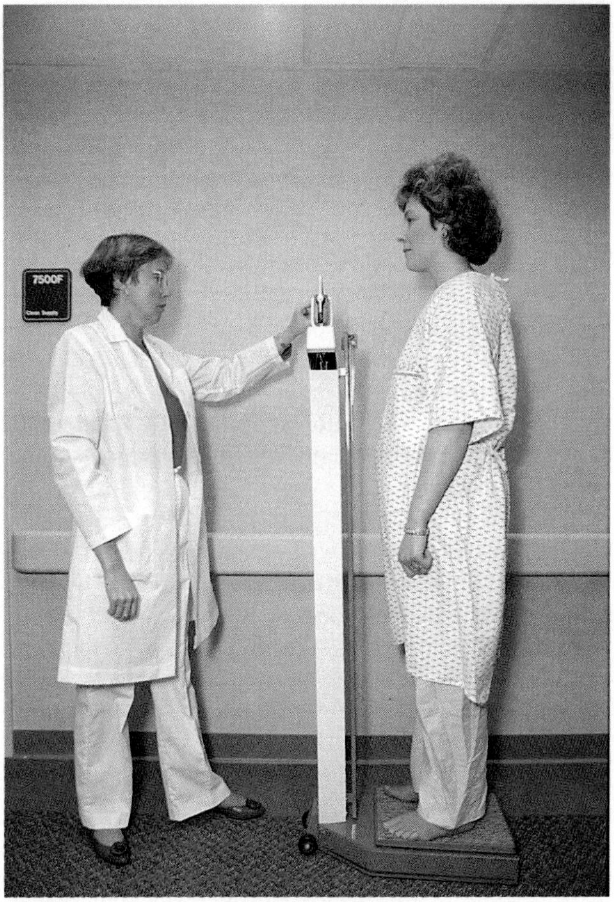

FIGURE 16-7 Client stands on scale as nurse adjusts balance.

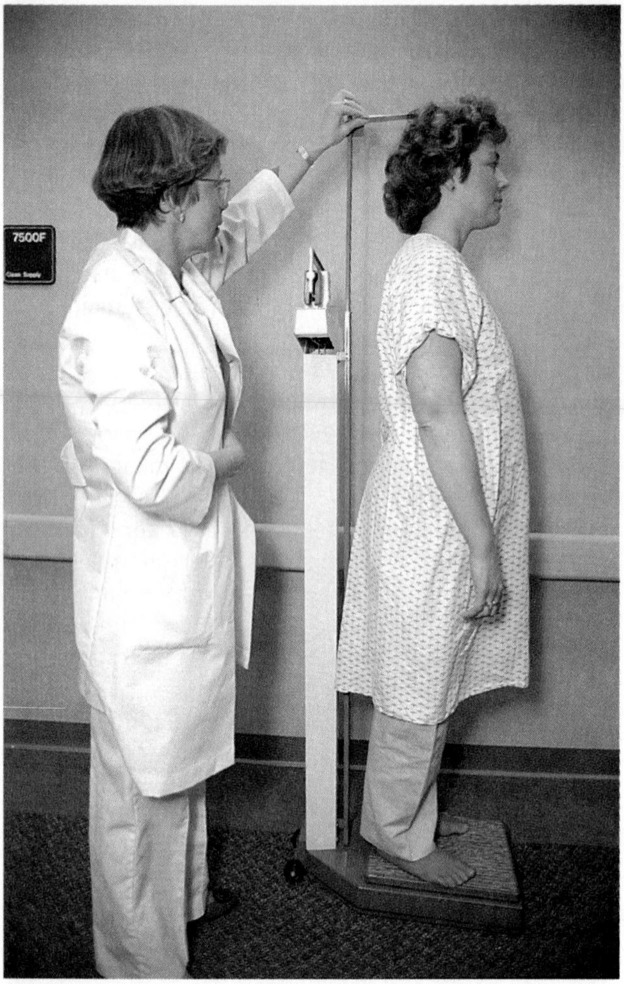

FIGURE 16-8 Client stands erect to permit accurate measurement of height.

in dry, disposable diapers to ensure accurate readings. The weight can later be adjusted for the weight of the diaper. The room should be warm to prevent chills. A light cloth or paper placed on the scale's surface prevents cross-infection from urine or feces. The nurse places infants in baskets or on platforms and holds a hand lightly above to prevent accidental falls. Weight is measured in ounces and grams.

There are different ways to measure the height of weight-bearing and non–weight-bearing clients. Clients able to stand remove their shoes. A paper towel is placed on the scale platform or floor so clients' feet remain clean. A measuring stick or tape is attached vertically to the weight scales or wall. The nurse asks the client to stand erect, exercising good posture. On a platform scale, a metal rod, attached to the back of the scale, swings out and over the crown of the client's head (Figure 16-8). A measuring stick or flat book can be placed on the client's head when a scale is unavailable. With the rod or stick placed level horizontally at a 90-degree angle to the measuring stick, the nurse measures height in inches or centimeters.

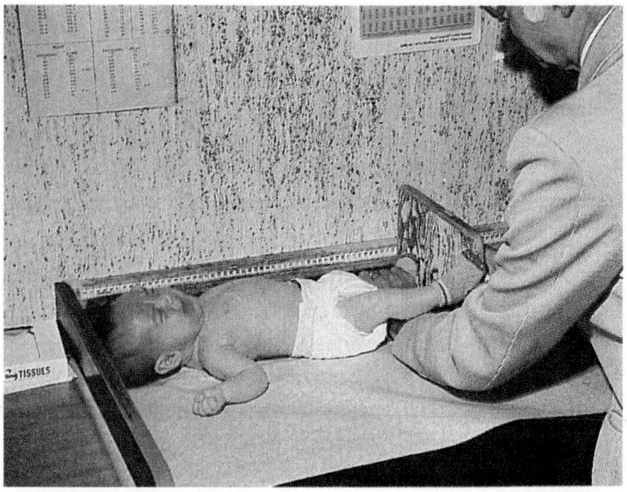

FIGURE 16-9 Measurement of infant length. (From Seidel HM, et al.: *Mosby's guide to physical examination,* ed 2, St. Louis, 1991, Mosby.)

A non–weight-bearing client (such as an infant) is positioned supine on a firm surface. The legs are extended straight with the soles of the feet supported upright. The nurse places a tape measure from the soles of the feet to the vertex of the head to measure the recumbent length (Figure 16-9).

INTEGUMENT

The **integument,** consisting of the skin, nails, hair and scalp, provides the body's external protection, regulates body temperature, and acts as a sensory organ for pain, temperature, and touch. The nurse may first inspect all skin surfaces or may assess the skin gradually as other body systems are examined. The physical assessment skills of inspection, palpation, and olfaction are used to assess the integument's function and integrity.

Skin

The skin is a window for the nurse to detect a variety of conditions affecting a client. Changes in oxygenation, circulation, nutrition, local tissue damage, and hydration are just a few. In a hospital setting the majority of clients are older adults, debilitated clients, or young but seriously ill. They are at risk for skin lesions caused by trauma to the skin while administering care, from exposure to pressure during immobilization, or from reaction to medications. Pressure ulcers are a major health problem (Chapter 24). Clients most at risk are the neurologically impaired, chronically ill, the orthopedic client, and clients with diminished mental status, poor tissue oxygenation, low cardiac output, and inadequate nutrition. An assessment of the skin prevents pressure ulcers from developing or leads to early treatment. In addition the assessment helps to determine the type of hygiene measures required by a client and the need for nutritional or hydration therapy.

Adequate illumination of the skin is required during assessment. If moist or draining skin lesions are present, disposable gloves are needed for palpation. Because the nurse inspects all skin surfaces, the client must assume several positions. The examination includes inspecting the skin's color, moisture, temperature, texture, and turgor. Vascular changes, edema, and lesions are also noted. Abnormalities are carefully palpated. Skin odors are usually noted in skin folds, such as the axilla.

HEALTH HISTORY. Before assessing the skin, the nurse asks the client about the presence of lesions, rashes, or bruises. Can the alterations be linked to heat, cold, stress, exposure to toxic material or the sun, or new skin care products? The nurse determines if there has been a recent change in skin color or trauma to the skin. If a client has been out in the sun, it is useful to know if a sunscreen has been worn. If not, the client will require education on ways to safeguard the skin. The nurse also assesses for history of allergies, use of topical medications, and a family history of serious skin disorders. The nurse uses assessment findings to determine abnormalities and the type of hygiene measures needed to maintain integrity of the integument.

Color. Skin color varies from body part to body part and from person to person. Despite individual variations, skin color is usually uniform over the body. Normal skin **pigmentation** ranges from ivory or light pink to ruddy pink in white skin; light to deep brown or olive in dark skin. Assessment of color first involves areas of the skin not exposed to the sun, such as the palms. The nurse notes if the skin is unusually pale or dark. Exposed areas such as the face will be darker. It is more difficult to note changes such as **pallor** or **cyanosis** in clients with dark skin. Usually they have lighter areas of pigmentation in the palms, soles of feet, lips, and nail beds.

The nurse focuses inspection on sites where abnormalities are more easily identified. For example, **pallor** is more easily seen in the face, buccal mucosa, conjunctivae, and nail beds. Cyanosis is best observed in the lips, skin, and nail beds. Normal reactive **hyperemia,** or redness, is most often seen in regions exposed to pressure such as the sacrum, heels, and greater trochanter.

The nurse inspects for any patches or areas of skin color variation. With sun exposure, some areas are more pigmented. Localized skin changes, such as pallor or **erythema,** may indicate circulatory changes. Areas of redness with scaling, flaking, and cracking may indicate dry skin (Hardy, 1990). It is important to ask a client if changes in skin coloring have been noticed (see box above). The client usually knows whether a change has occurred.

CLIENT TEACHING DURING SKIN ASSESSMENT

Instruct client to conduct a monthly self-examination of the skin, noting moles, blemishes, and birthmarks. Tell client to inspect all skin surfaces. Cancerous melanomas start as small, mole-like growths that increase in size, change color, become ulcerated, and bleed. A simple **ABCD** rule (American Cancer Society, 1993) outlines warning signals:

- **A** is for **asymmetry.**
- **B** is for **border** irregularity, edges are ragged, notched, or blurred.
- **C** is for **color;** pigmentation is not uniform.
- **D** is for **diameter,** greater than 6 millimeters.

Tell client to report to a physician changes in skin lesions or a sore that does not heal.

Instruct client to prevent skin cancer by avoiding overexposure to the sun: wear wide-brimmed hat and long sleeves; apply sunscreens with SPF greater than or equal to 15 approximately 15 minutes before going into the sun and after swimming or perspiring; avoid tanning under direct sun between 10 AM and 3 PM; and do not use indoor sunlamps, tanning parlors, or tanning pills.

Older adults and clients with certain chronic diseases tend to have delayed wound healing. Instruct client to report any lesion that bleeds or fails to heal to a physician.

To treat "winter itch" or excessively dry skin, tell client to avoid hot water, use a superfatted (Dove) soap, pat rather than rub the skin dry after bathing, apply mineral oil to body parts, and wear cotton clothing (Hardy, 1990).

Moisture. The hydration of skin and mucous membranes helps to reveal body fluid imbalances, changes in the skin's environment, and regulation of body temperature. Moisture refers to wetness and oiliness. Skinfolds such as the axillae are normally moist. After exercise or exposure to warm temperatures, the skin may be moist from perspiration. The nurse uses ungloved fingertips to palpate skin surfaces to feel the skin's moisture. The skin is normally dry. Flaking is the appearance of dandruff-like flakes when the skin surface is lightly rubbed. Scaling are fish-like scales that are easily rubbed off the skin's surface. Both flaking and scaling are believed to be valid indicators for abnormally dry skin (Hardy, 1990). If there are skin lesions oozing fluid, the nurse must apply gloves and assess the color, odor, amount, and consistency. Gloves prevent exposure to infectious drainage during palpations of oozing lesions.

Temperature. The temperature of the skin depends on the amount of blood circulating through the dermis. Increased or decreased skin temperature reflects an increase or decrease in blood flow. Localized erythema or redness of the skin often may be accompanied by an increase in skin temperature. A reduction in skin temperature reflects a decrease in blood flow. It is good to remember that if an examination room is cold, the client's skin temperature and color can be affected.

Temperature is more accurately assessed by palpating the skin with the dorsum or back of the hand. The nurse compares symmetric body parts. Normally the skin is warm. Skin temperature may be the same throughout the body or may vary in one area. Skin temperature is a basic assessment when the client is at risk of having impaired circulation, such as after a cast application. In addition, a nurse can identify a stage I pressure ulcer early when noting warmth and erythema. After a reduction in blood flow to tissues, the skin can undergo one of two types of changes. Normal **reactive hyperemia** is the redness of local vasodilation, the body's normal response to lack of blood flow. If an area of redness is noted, the nurse places a fingertip over the area, applies gentle pressure, and then releases. Areas of skin affected by normal reactive hyperemia will blanch with fingertip pressure, and the condition lasts less than 1 hour (Pires and Muller, 1991). Abnormal reactive hyperemia is an excessive vasodilation and **induration.** It can last more than 1 hour up to 2 weeks.

Texture. The character of the skin's surface and the feel of deeper portions are its texture. The nurse determines if the client's skin is smooth or rough, thin or thick, tight or supple by stroking it lightly with the fingertips. The texture of the skin is normally smooth, soft, and flexible in children and adults. However, the texture is usually not uniform. The palms of the hand and soles of the feet tend to be thicker. In older adults the skin becomes wrinkled and leathery because of a decrease in collagen, subcutaneous fat, and sweat glands.

Localized changes may result from trauma, surgical wounds, or lesions. When irregularities in texture such as scars or hardening are found, the nurse asks whether the client has had a recent injury to the skin. Deeper palpation may reveal irregularities such as tenderness or areas of induration, localized edema under the skin.

Turgor. Turgor is the skin's elasticity, which can be diminished by edema or dehydration. Normally the skin loses its elasticity with age. To assess skin turgor, a fold of skin on the back of the hand or forearm is grasped with the fingertips and released (Figure 16-10). Normally the skin lifts easily and snaps back immediately to its resting position. The skin stays pinched when turgor is poor. The client with poor turgor does not have a resilience to the normal wear and tear on the skin. A decrease in turgor predisposes the client to skin breakdown.

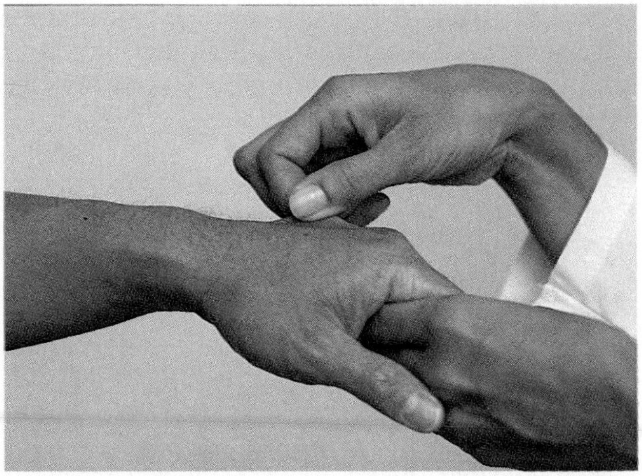

FIGURE 16-10 Assessment for skin turgor. (From Canobbio MM: *Cardiovascular disorders,* St. Louis, 1990, Mosby.)

Vascularity. The circulation of the skin affects color in localized areas and the appearance of superficial blood vessels. With aging, capillaries become fragile. Localized pressure areas, found after a client has laid or sat in one position, appear reddened, pink, or pale (see Chapter 24). Petechiae are tiny, pinpoint-sized, red or purple spots on the skin caused by small hemorrhages in the skin layers. Petechiae may indicate serious blood-clotting disorders, drug reactions, or liver disease.

Edema. Areas of the skin become swollen or edematous from fluid buildup in the tissues. Direct trauma and impairment of venous return are two common causes for **edema.** The nurse inspects edematous areas for location, color, and shape. The formation of edema separates the skin's surface from the pigmented and vascular layers, masking skin color. Edematous skin also appears stretched and shiny. The nurse palpates areas of edema to determine mobility, consistency, and tenderness. When pressure from the nurse's finger leaves an indentation in the edematous area, it is called *pitting edema.* To assess pitting edema, the nurse presses the edematous area firmly with the thumb for 5 seconds and releases. The depth of pitting, recorded in millimeters (Seidel et al., 1991) determines the degree of edema. For example, 1+ edema equals 2 mm depth.

Lesions. The skin is normally free of lesions, except common freckles or age-related changes such as skin tags or **senile keratosis.** When a lesion is detected, it is inspected for color, location, size, type (see box on p. 311), grouping (e.g., clustered or linear), and distrib-

TYPES OF SKIN LESIONS

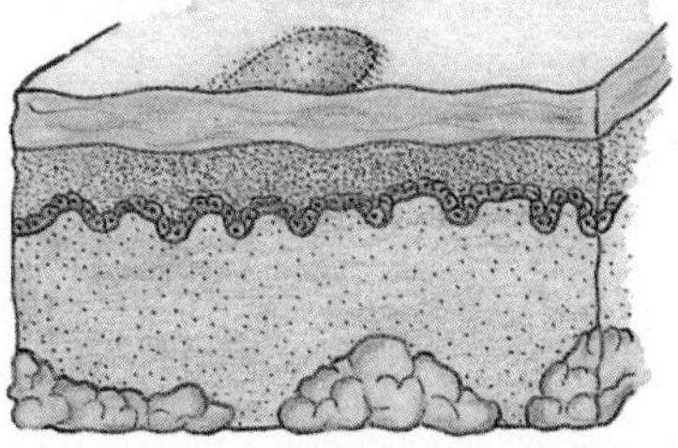

Macule: flat, nonpalpable, change in skin color, smaller than 1 cm (e.g., freckle or petechia)

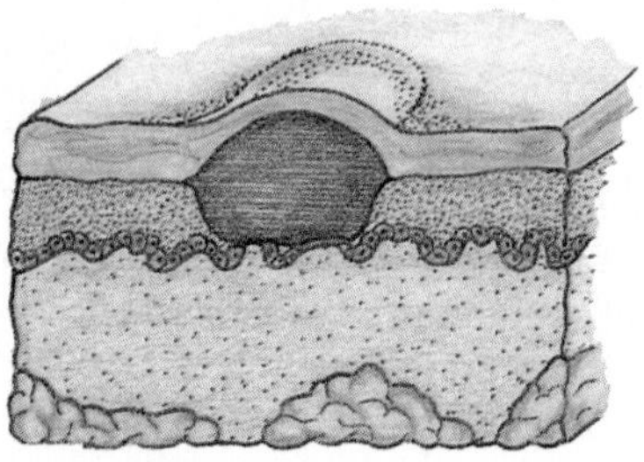

Papule: palpable, circumscribed, solid elevation in skin, smaller than 0.5 cm (e.g., elevated nevus)

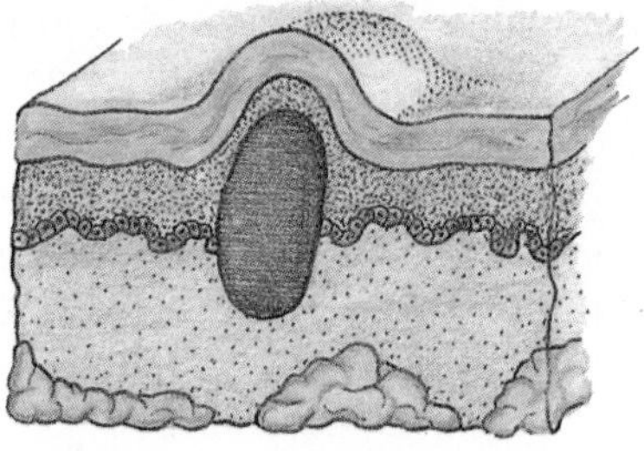

Nodule: elevated solid mass, deeper and firmer than papule, 0.5 to 2.0 cm (e.g., wart)

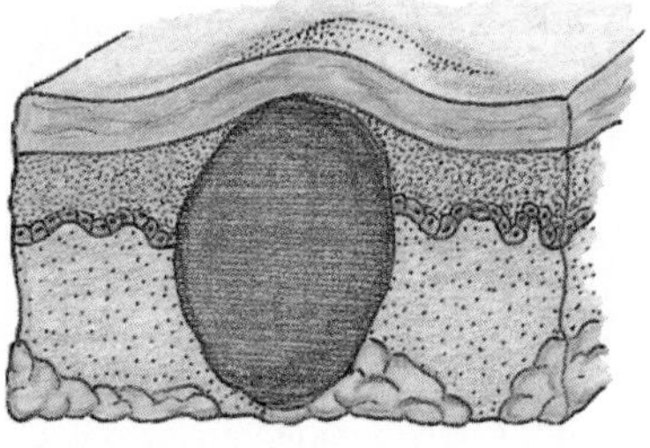

Tumor: solid mass that may extend deep through subcutaneous tissue, larger than 1 to 2 cm (e.g., epithelioma)

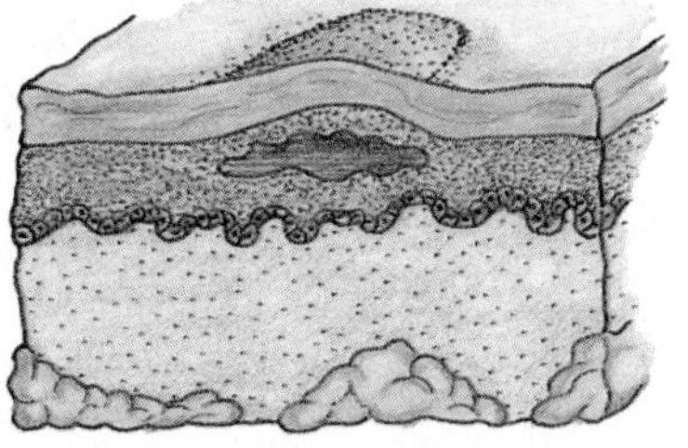

Wheal: irregularly shaped, elevated area or superficial localized edema, varies in size (e.g., hive or mosquito bite)

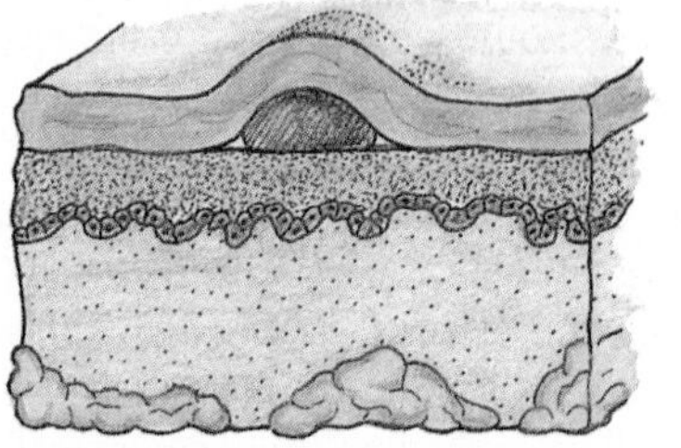

Vesicle: circumscribed elevation of skin filled with serous fluid, smaller than 0.5 cm (e.g., herpes simplex or chickenpox)

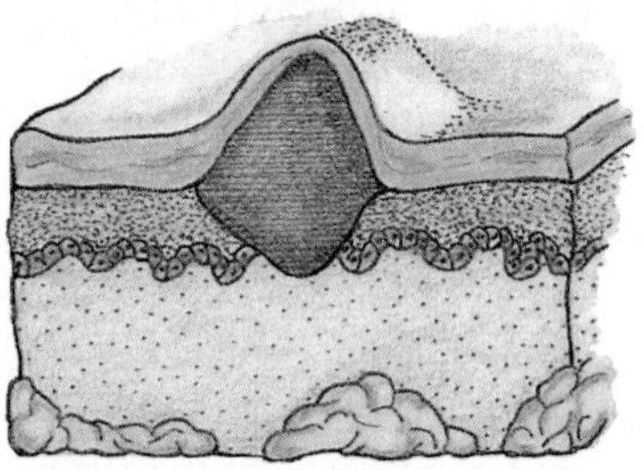

Pustule: circumscribed elevation of skin similar to vesicle but filled with pus, varies in size (e.g., acne or staphylococcal infection)

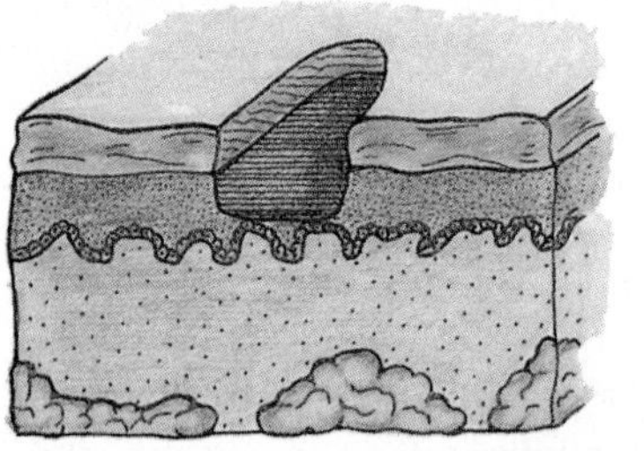

Ulcer: deep loss of skin surface that may extend to dermis and frequently bleeds and scars, varies in size (e.g., venous stasis ulcer)

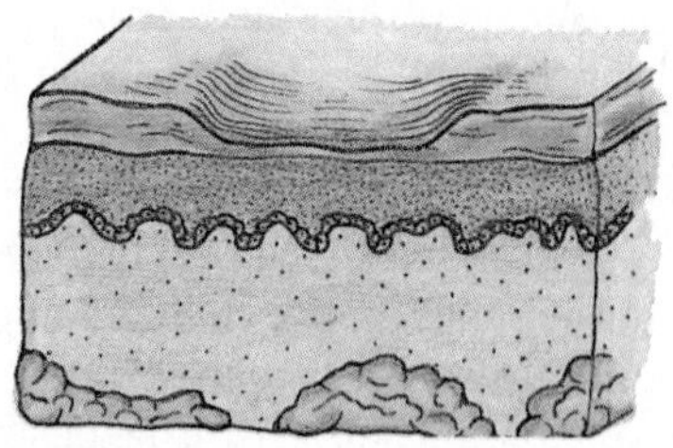

Atrophy: thinning of skin with loss of normal skin furrow with skin appearing shiny and translucent, varies in size (e.g., arterial insufficiency)

ution (localized or generalized). Palpation determines the lesion's mobility, contour (flat, raised, or depressed), and consistency (soft or hard). After a lesion is identified, it is closely inspected with good illumination. It is palpated gently, covering its entire area. If the lesion is moist or has draining fluid, gloves are worn during palpation. The nurse notes if the client complains of tenderness during palpation. Any abnormalities, especially lesions that have changed in character (e.g., color or size), are reported to a physician because further examination may be needed. Precancerous lesions frequently undergo changes in color and size.

Hair and Scalp

The following types of hair cover the body: terminal hair (long, coarse, thick hair easily visible on the scalp, axillae, and pubic areas) and vellus hair (small, soft, tiny hairs covering the whole body except for the palms and soles). Good lighting allows the nurse to inspect the condition and distribution of hair and integrity of the scalp. Assessment of the hair occurs during all portions of the examination. The nurse assesses the distribution, thickness, texture, and lubrication of hair. In addition, the nurse inspects for infection or infestation of the scalp.

HEALTH HISTORY. The nurse should ask questions such as the following: Has the client noted change in growth or loss of hair? What types of hair care products are used? Has the client recently been on chemotherapy (drugs that can cause hair loss)? If a client has a hairpiece, it should be removed if inspection of the scalp is essential.

Inspection. During inspection explain that it may be necessary to separate parts of the hair to detect abnormalities. First inspect the distribution, thickness, texture, and lubrication of body hair. Hair is normally distributed evenly, is neither excessively dry nor oily, and is pliant. While separating sections of scalp hair the nurse observes characteristics of color and coarseness. Normal terminal hair is black, brown, red, yellow, or variations in shades of these colors. The hair is coarse or fine and shiny. Normal variations exist in the shape of hair fibers. Clients' hair may be straight, curly, spiral, or wavy. The hair of African Americans is usually thicker and drier than the hair of European Americans.

In older adults, the hair becomes dull gray, white, or yellow. It also thins over the scalp, axillae, and pubic areas. Older men lose facial hair, whereas older women may develop hair on the chin and upper lip.

Changes may occur in the thickness, texture, and lubrication of scalp hair. Disturbances such as a febrile illness or scalp disease can result in hair loss. Conditions such as thyroid disease can alter the condition of the hair, making it fine and brittle. Baldness **(alopecia)** or thinning of the hair is usually related to genetic tendencies and endocrine disorders such as diabetes and even menopause (DeWitt, 1990). Poor nutrition can cause stringy, dull, dry, and thin hair. The hair is lubricated from the oil of sebaceous glands. Excessively oily hair is associated with androgen hormone stimulation. Dry, brittle hair occurs with aging and excessive use of chemical agents.

The nurse inspects the scalp for lesions, which can easily go unnoticed in thick hair. The scalp is normally smooth and inelastic, with even coloration. Moles are common. Careful inspection of hair follicles on the scalp and pubic areas may reveal lice or other parasites. The three types of lice are *Pediculus humanus capitis* (head lice), *Pediculus humanus corporis* (body lice), and *Pediculus pubis* (crab lice). Lice attach their eggs to hair. The head and body lice are tiny and have grayish white bodies. Crab lice have red legs. Lice eggs look like oval particles of dandruff. The lice themselves are hard to see. The nurse looks for bites or pustular eruptions in the follicles and in areas where skin surfaces meet, such as behind the ears and in the groin. The discovery of lice requires immediate treatment (see box above).

CLIENT TEACHING DURING HAIR AND SCALP ASSESSMENT

Clients may require instruction about basic hygiene measures, including shampooing and combing of the hair (see Chapter 30).

Instruct clients who have head lice to shampoo thoroughly with pediculicide (shampoo available at drug stores) in cold water, comb thoroughly with fine-tooth comb (following product directions), and discard comb.

After combing remove any detectable nits or nit cases with tweezers or between the fingernails. A dilute solution of vinegar and water may help loosen nits.

Instruct clients and parents about ways to reduce transmission of lice:

- Do not share personal care items with others.
- Vacuum all rugs, car seats, pillows, furniture, and flooring thoroughly and discard vacuum bag.
- Seal nonwashable items in plastic bags for 14 days if parents are unable to afford dry cleaning and do not have vacuum (Clore, 1989).
- Use thorough handwashing.
- Launder all clothing, linen, and bedding in hot soap and water and dry in hot dryer for at least 20 minutes. Dry-clean nonwashable items (Whaley and Wong, 1991).
- Instruct the client that his or her partner must be notified if lice were sexually transmitted.

Nails

The condition of the nails can reflect general health, state of nutrition, and a person's occupation. The most visible portion of the nails is the nail plate, the transparent layer of epithelial cells covering the nail bed. The vascularity of the nail bed creates the nail's underlying color. The semilunar, whitish area at the base of the nail bed from which the nail plate develops is the lunula.

HEALTH HISTORY. Before assessing the nails the nurse asks if the client has had any recent trauma. A blow to the nail can change the shape and growth of the nail as well as loss of all or part of the nail plate. The nurse also asks the client to describe nail care practices.

ABNORMALITIES OF THE NAIL BED

160 degrees

Normal nail

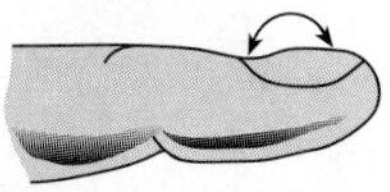

Normal nail: Approximately 160-degree angle between nail plate and nail

180 degrees

Clubbing

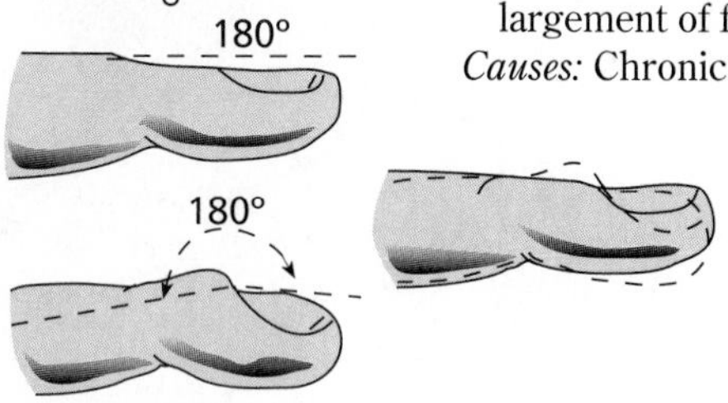

Clubbing: Change in angle between nail and nail base (eventually larger than 180 degrees); nail bed softening, with nail flattening; often enlargement of fingertips
Causes: Chronic lack of oxygen: heart or pulmonary disease

Beau's lines

180 degrees

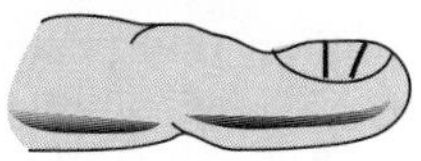

Beau's lines: Transverse depressions in nails indicating temporary disturbance of nail growth (Nail grows out over several months.)
Causes: Systemic illness such as severe infection, nail injury

Koilonychia (spoon nail)

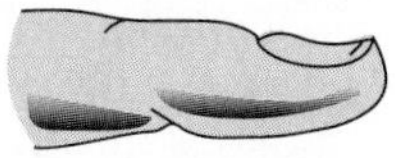

Koilonychia (spoon nail): Concave curves
Causes: Iron deficiency anemia, syphilis, use of strong detergents

Splinter hemorrhages

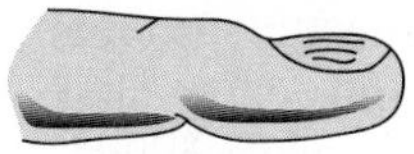

Splinter hemorrhages: Red or brown linear streaks in nail bed
Causes: Minor trauma, subacute bacterial endocarditis, trichinosis

Paronychia

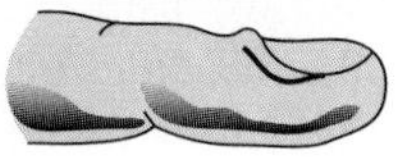

Paronychia: Inflammation of skin at base of nail
Causes: Local infection, trauma

Improper care can damage nails and cuticles. It is helpful to know if the client has noticed changes in nail appearance or growth. Alterations may occur slowly over time. Knowing if the client has risks for nail or foot problems (e.g., diabetes, peripheral vascular disease, older adulthood) will influence the level of hygienic care recommended.

Inspection and Palpation. The nurse inspects the nail bed color, the thickness and shape of the nail, the texture of the nail, and the condition of tissue around the nail. The nails are normally transparent, smooth, and convex, with surrounding cuticles smooth, intact, and without inflammation. In European Americans, nail beds are pink with translucent white tips. In African Americans, a brown or black pigmentation is normal with longitudinal streaks. Splinter hemorrhages can be caused by trauma, cirrhosis, diabetes mellitus, and hypertension (Kpea, 1987). Vitamin, protein, and electrolyte changes can cause various lines or bands to form on nail beds.

Nails normally grow at a constant rate, but direct injury or generalized disease can slow growth. With aging, the nails of the fingers and toes develop longitudinal striations. The rate of nail growth also slows. The cuticles may appear inflamed, swollen, rough, or dry. This is the result of chronic nail biting.

Inspection of the angle between the nail and nail bed normally reveals an angle of 160 degrees (see box above). A larger angle and softening of the nail bed can indicate chronic oxygenation problems. The nurse palpates the nail base to determine firmness and condition of circulation. The nail base is normally firm. To palpate, the nurse gently grasps the client's finger and observes the color of the nail bed. Next, gentle, firm, quick pressure is applied with the thumb to the nail bed and re-

CLIENT TEACHING DURING NAIL ASSESSMENT

Instruct clients to cut nails only after soaking them about 10 minutes in warm water.

Instruct client to avoid using over-the-counter preparations to treat corns, calluses, or ingrown toenails.

Tell client to cut nails straight across and even with the tops of the fingers or toes. If client has diabetes, tell client to file, not cut, nails.

Instruct client to shape nails with a file or emery board.

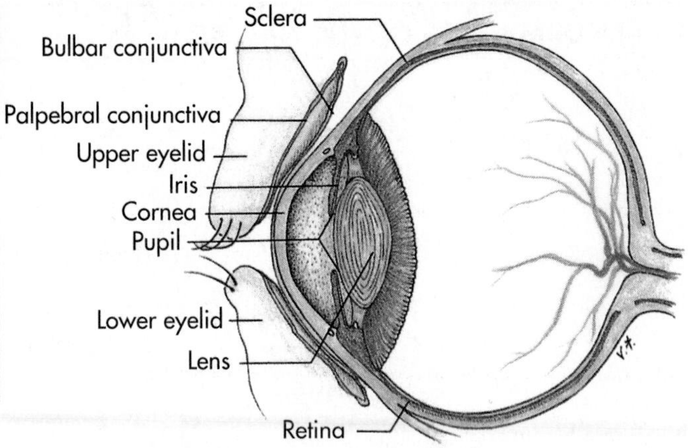

FIGURE 16-11 Cross section of eye.

leased. As the pressure is applied, the nail bed appears white or blanched; however, the pink color should return immediately on release of pressure. Failure of the pinkness to return promptly indicates circulatory insufficiency. An ongoing bluish or purplish cast to the nail bed occurs with cyanosis. A white cast or pallor results from anemia.

Calluses and corns are often found on the toes or fingers. A callus is flat and painless, resulting from thickening of the epidermis. Corns are caused by friction and pressure from shoes and are usually seen over bony prominences. During the examination, the nurse instructs clients on proper nail care (see box above).

HEAD AND NECK

An examination of the head and neck reviews the integrity of anatomical structures including the head, eyes, ears, nose, mouth, pharynx, and neck (lymph nodes, carotid arteries, thyroid gland, and trachea). The carotid arteries can also be assessed during the assessment of peripheral arteries. The nurse needs to understand each anatomical area and its normal function. Assessment of the head and neck uses inspection, palpation, and auscultation.

Head

HEALTH HISTORY. The history allows the nurse to determine a client's risk for intracranial injury. The nurse asks whether the client experienced recent trauma to the head or if neurological symptoms such as headache, dizziness, seizures, blurred vision, or loss of consciousness have been noticed. The history also includes a review of the client's occupation, focusing on those clients who should wear safety helmets. In addition, the nurse learns if the client participates in contact sports or cycling.

Inspection and Palpation. The nurse inspects the client's head, noting the position, size, shape, and contour. The head is normally held upright and midline to the trunk. A horizontal jerking or bobbing may indicate a tremor. Tilting the head to one side to favor a good eye or ear is common with unilateral hearing or vision loss (Seidel et al., 1991). The skull is generally round with prominences in the frontal area anteriorly and the occipital area posteriorly. Local skull deformities are typically caused by trauma. In infants, a large head may result from congenital anomalies or the accumulation of cerebrospinal fluid in the ventricles (hydrocephalus). Adults may have enlarged jaws and facial bones resulting from **acromegaly.** The nurse palpates the skull for nodules or masses. Gentle rotation of the fingertips down the midline of the scalp and then along the sides of the head reveals abnormalities.

Eyes

Examination of the eye includes assessment of visual acuity, visual fields, extraocular movements, and external and internal eye structures. Figure 16-11 shows a cross section of the eye. The assessment detects visual alterations and determines the level of assistance clients require when ambulating or performing self-care activities.

HEALTH HISTORY. The nurse determines if the client is at risk for partial or complete visual loss by reviewing history of eye disease (e.g., glaucoma, cataracts), eye trauma, diabetes, or hypertension. Assessment for common symptoms of eye disease such as eye pain, **photophobia,** burning, itching, excess tearing or crusting, **diplopia,** blurred vision, awareness of a "film" or "curtain" over the field of vision, floaters, flashing lights, or halos around lights is critical. The nurse also reviews the client's occupational history, use of glasses or contact lenses, use of safety glasses during hobbies, and regularity of visits to an opthalmologist or optometrist. Last, the nurse assesses medications the client is taking, including eye drops.

Visual Acuity. The assessment of visual acuity, the ability to see small details, tests central vision. The easiest way to assess visual acuity is to ask the client to read printed material under adequate lighting. If clients wear glasses or contact lenses, they should wear them. The nurse should know the language a client speaks and if the client is literate. Asking the client to read aloud tests literacy. If the client has difficulty reading, move to the next step.

A more accurate assessment of visual acuity uses a Snellen chart (paper chart or projection screen). The chart should be well lighted. Always test vision without corrective lenses first. The nurse has the client sit or stand 20 feet (6.1 m) away from the chart and try to read all of the letters beginning at any line—once with both eyes open and then with each eye separately (with opposite eye covered). The nurse notes the smallest line in which the client can read all of the letters correctly and records the visual acuity for that line. Repeat the test with the client wearing corrective lenses.

If a client is unable to read, the nurse uses an "E" chart or one with pictures of familiar objects. Instead of reading letters, clients tell the nurse which direction each E is pointing or the name of the object. The visual acuity score is recorded for each eye and both eyes.

The Snellen chart has standardized numbers at the end of each line of the chart. The numerator is the number 20 or the distance the client stands from the chart. The denominator is the distance from which the normal eye can read the chart. Normal vision is 20/20. The larger the denominator, the poorer the client's visual acuity. The nurse records acuity as sc (without correction) and cc (with correction), depending on whether the client wears glasses or contacts.

If clients cannot read even the largest letters or figures of a Snellen chart, the nurse tests their ability to count upraised fingers or distinguish light. The nurse holds a hand 30 cm (1 foot) from the face and instructs the client to count the upraised fingers. To check light perception, the nurse shines a penlight into the eye and then turns the light off. If the client notes when the light is turned on or off, light perception is intact.

Visual Fields. As a person looks straight ahead, all objects in the periphery can normally be seen. To assess visual fields, the nurse has the client stand or sit 2 feet (60 cm) away, facing the nurse at eye level. The client gently closes or covers one eye (such as the left) and looks at the nurse's eye directly opposite (client's left eye, nurse's right eye). The nurse closes the opposite eye so that the field of vision is superimposed on that of the client. The nurse moves a finger equidistant at arm's length from the nurse and client outside the field of vision, then slowly brings it back into the visual field. The client is asked to tell when the nurse's finger is seen. If the nurse sees the finger before the client does, this reveals that a portion of the client's visual field is reduced. The procedure is repeated for each field of vision. The examination is only approximate and presumes the nurse's visual fields are normal. If there is any concern, a more extensive medical examination is needed to confirm presence of alterations.

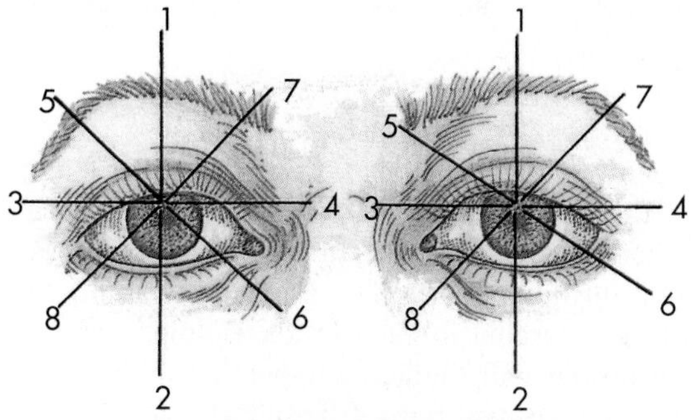

FIGURE 16-12 Eight directions of gaze. Nurse directs client to follow finger movement through each gaze.

Extraocular Movements. Six small muscles guide the movement of each eye. Both eyes move parallel to each other in each of the eight directions of gaze (Figure 16-12). The client sits or stands 2 feet away, facing the nurse. The nurse holds a finger at a comfortable distance (6 to 12 in or 15 to 30 cm) in front of the client's eyes. The client keeps the head in a fixed position facing the nurse and follows the movement of the finger with the eyes only. The client looks to the right, to the left, up, down, and diagonally up and down to the left and right. The nurse's finger moves smoothly and slowly within the normal field of vision.

As the client gazes in each direction, the nurse observes for parallel eye movement, the position of the upper eyelid in relation to the iris, and the presence of abnormal movements such as **nystagmus.** With nystagmus a fine, rhythmical oscillation of the eyes is present. The nurse can initiate nystagmus in clients with normal eye movement by having them gaze to the far left or right. As the eyes move through each direction of gaze, the upper eyelid only covers the iris slightly. Disturbances in eye movement reflect local injury to eye muscles and supporting structures or a disorder of the cranial nerves.

To assess for alignment of the eyes, the nurse shines a penlight onto the bridge of the client's nose from 60 to 90 cm (2 to 3 ft) away in a darkened room. The client looks straight ahead. Normally light reflects on the cornea in the same spot on both eyes. If there is an abnormality, the light shines on a different spot on each eye.

External Eye Structures. To assess external eye structures, the nurse stands in front of the client at eye level and asks the client to look at the nurse's face.

POSITION AND ALIGNMENT. The nurse assesses the position of the eyes in relation to one another. Normally they are parallel to each other. Bulging eyes **(exophthalmos)** usually indicates hyperthyroidism. The crossing of eyes **(strabismus)** results from neuromuscular injury or inherited abnormalities. Tumors or inflammation of the orbit can cause abnormal eye protrusion.

EYEBROWS. For the remainder of the eye exam the client removes contact lenses. The nurse inspects the eyebrows for size, extension, and hair texture. Coarseness of hair and failure to extend beyond the temporal canthus may reveal hypothyroidism. If the brows are thinned, the client may pluck or wax the hair. The nurse has the client raise and lower the eyebrows. The brows should raise and lower symmetrically. An inability to move the eyebrows may indicate a facial nerve paralysis.

EYELIDS. The nurse inspects the eyelids for position, color, condition of surface, condition and direction of lashes, and the ability to close and blink. When the eyes are open, normally the lids do not cover the pupil and sclera cannot be seen above the iris. The lids are also close to the eyeball. An abnormal drooping of the lid over the pupil is called **ptosis,** caused by edema or impairment of the third cranial nerve. Defects in the position of the lid margins may be observed. If the lid turns in or away from the eyeball, this may irritate the conjunctiva.

To inspect the surface of the upper lids, the nurse has the client close the eyes and then raises both eyebrows gently with the thumb and index finger. This stretches the skin. The lids are usually smooth and the same color as the skin. Redness indicates inflammation or infection. Lid edema may be due to allergies or heart and kidney failure. If lesions are present, the nurse observes the size, shape, and distribution. Gloves should be worn if drainage is present.

While inspecting the position of the eyelashes, the nurse looks for evenly distributed lashes that curve outward away from the eye. While inspecting the lower lids, the nurse asks the client to open the eyes and observes the blink reflex. Normally a client blinks involuntarily and bilaterally as many as 20 times a minute.

LACRIMAL APPARATUS. The nurse asks the client to close the eyes. Failure of the lids to close can cause corneal drying. This condition is common in unconscious clients or those with facial nerve paralysis. The anterior surface of the eye, composed of the sensitive cornea and conjunctiva, is moistened by tears secreted from the lacrimal gland (Figure 16-13). The gland is located in the upper, outer wall of the anterior part of the orbit. Tears flow from the gland across the eye's surface to the lacrimal duct, which is located in the nasal corner or inner canthus of the eye. The lacrimal gland can be the site of tumors or infection. The area of the gland is inspected for edema and redness and palpated gently to detect tenderness. Normally the gland cannot be felt. The nasolacrimal duct may become obstructed, blocking the flow of tears. The nurse looks for evidence of excess tearing or edema in the inner canthus. Gentle palpation of the duct at the lower eyelid just inside the orbital rim may cause a regurgitation of tears.

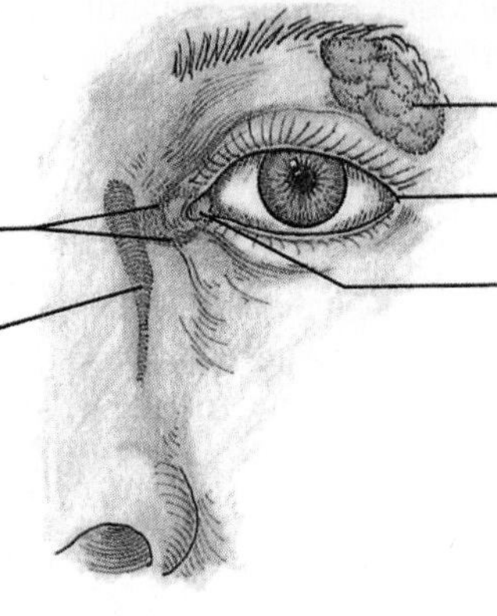

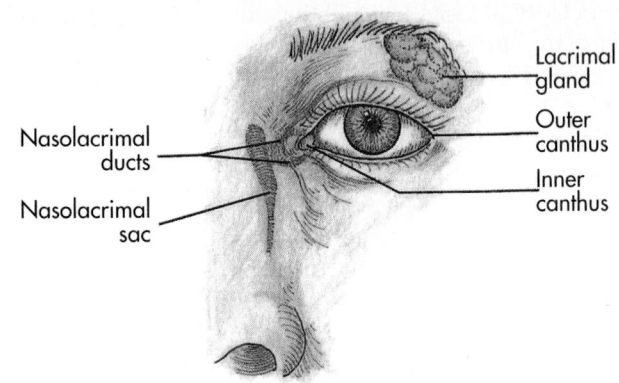

FIGURE 16-13 Lacrimal apparatus.

CONJUNCTIVA AND SCLERA. The bulbar conjunctiva covers the exposed surface of the eyeball up to the outer edge of the cornea. The sclera is seen under the bulbar conjunctiva and normally has the color of white porcelain in white-skinned clients and light yellow in black-skinned clients. To view both structures, the nurse gently retracts both lids simultaneously with thumb and index finger pressed against the lower and upper bony orbits. If there is crusty drainage on eyelid margins, the nurse should wear gloves. A pair of new gloves should be worn to examine each eye so as to prevent cross-contamination. For adequate exposure the eyelids must be retracted without placing pressure directly on the eyeball. The client is asked to look up, down, and side to side. Many clients begin to blink, making the examination difficult.

The palpebral conjunctiva is the delicate membrane lining the eyelids. Normally the conjunctiva is transparent, enabling the nurse to view the tiny underlying blood vessels that give it a pink color. To inspect the palpebral conjunctiva the nurse gently depresses the lower lid (Figure 16-14). Often the client can depress the eyelid to facilitate examination. The conjunctiva's color and the presence of edema or lesions are noted. A pale conjunctiva results from anemia, whereas a fiery red appearance is the result of inflammation (conjunctivitis).

A special technique (Figure 16-15) is used to inspect the upper palpebral conjunctiva and should not be tried

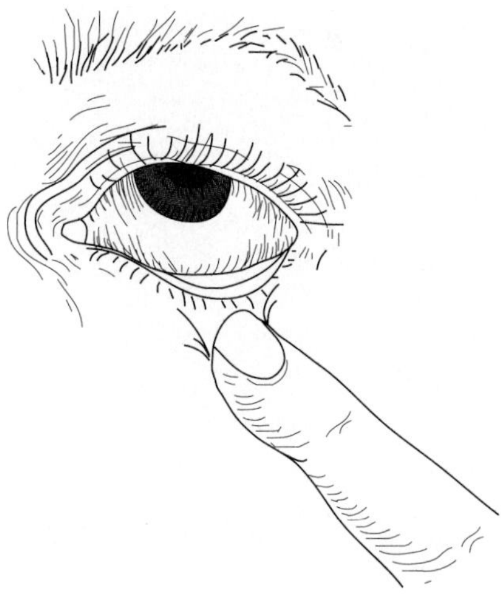

FIGURE 16-14 Technique for retracting lower eyelid.

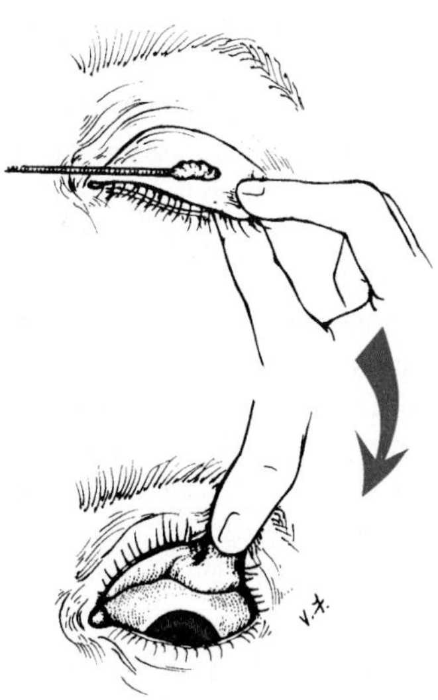

FIGURE 16-15 Technique for inspecting upper palpebral conjunctiva.

the first time without qualified assistance. The client is asked to look down, relax the eyes, and avoid sudden movement. The upper lid is gently grasped with a gloved hand and the lashes are pulled down and forward. The end of a cotton applicator is placed 1 cm (½ inch) above the lid margin. The nurse pushes down on the upper eyelid, turning it inside out. A light grasp on the upper lashes keeps the lid inverted. After inspection the eyelashes are gently pulled forward and the client is instructed to look up. The eyelid will return to its normal position. If a foreign body appears to be embedded in the eye, the nurse *must not attempt to remove it.* A physician should be notified immediately.

Cornea. The cornea is the transparent, colorless portion of the eye covering the pupil and iris. It looks like the crystal of a wrist watch. While standing at the client's side, the nurse inspects the cornea for clarity and texture while shining a penlight obliquely across the cornea's surface. The cornea is normally shiny, transparent, and smooth. In older adults, the cornea loses its luster. Any irregularity in the surface may indicate an abrasion or tear that warrants further examination by a physician. Both conditions are quite painful. To test for the corneal blink reflex, see the cranial nerve test section of this chapter.

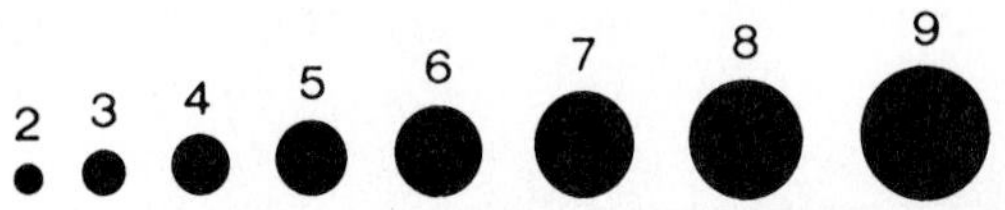

FIGURE 16-16 Chart depicting pupillary size in millimeters.

Pupils and Irises. The nurse observes the pupils for size, shape, equality, accommodation, and reaction to light. The pupils are normally black, round, regular, and equal in size (3 to 7 mm in diameter, see Figure 16-16). Cloudy pupils indicate cataracts. Dilated or constricted pupils can result from neurological disorders or the effect of ophthalmic or certain systemic drugs. When a beam of light is shined through the pupil and onto the retina, the third cranial nerve is stimulated and causes the muscles of the iris to constrict. Any abnormality along the nerve pathways from the retina to the iris alters the ability of the pupils to react to light. Changes in intracranial pressure, lesions along the nerve pathways, locally applied eye drugs, and direct trauma to the eye may alter pupillary reaction.

Pupillary reflexes (to light and accommodation) should be tested in a dimly lit room. As the client looks straight ahead, the nurse brings a penlight from the side of the client's face, directing the light onto the pupil (Figure 16-17). If the client looks at the light, there will be a false reaction to accommodation. A directly illuminated pupil constricts, and the opposite pupil constricts consensually. The nurse observes the quickness and equality of the reflex. The exam is repeated for the opposite eye.

To test accommodation, the client is asked to gaze at a distant object (the far wall) and then at a test object (finger or pencil) held by the nurse approximately 10 cm (4 inches) from the bridge of the client's nose. The pupils normally converge and accommodate by constricting when looking at close objects. The pupil responses are equal. If assessment of pupillary reaction is normal in all tests, the nurse records the abbreviation, PERRLA (pupils equal, round, reactive to light, and accommodation).

Internal Eye Structures. The examination of internal eye structures is beyond the scope of a new gradu-

A

B

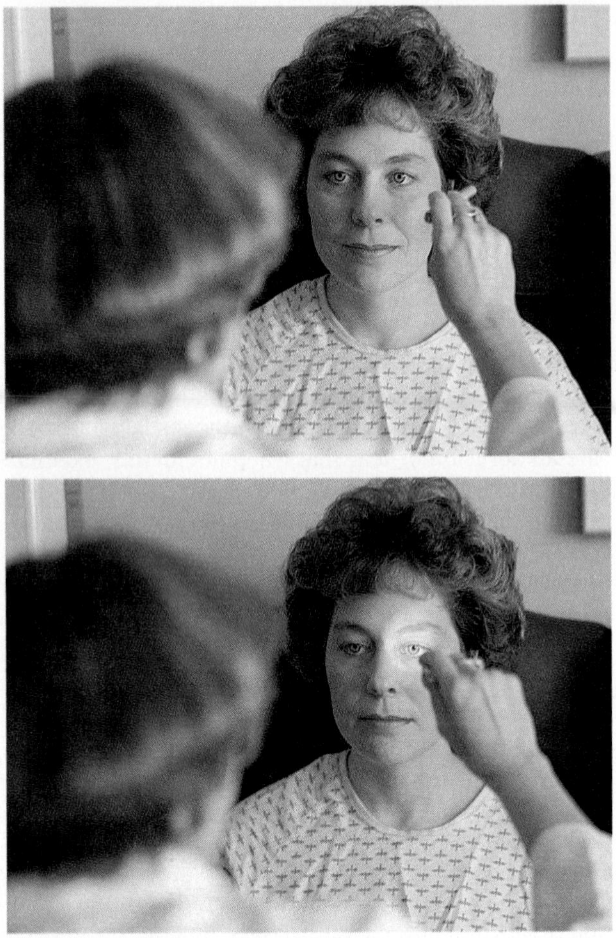

FIGURE 16-17 **A,** To check pupil reflexes, nurse first holds penlight to side of client's face. **B,** Illumination of pupil causes pupillary constriction.

CLIENT TEACHING DURING EYE ASSESSMENT

Tell client that people under age 40 should have complete eye examinations every 3 to 5 years (or more often if family histories reveal risks such as diabetes or hypertension).

Tell client that people over age 40 should have eye examinations every 2 years to screen for conditions that may develop without client awareness (e.g., glaucoma).

Tell clients that people over age 65 should have yearly eye examinations.

Describe the typical symptoms of eye disease.

Instruct older adults to take the following precautions because of normal visual changes: avoid driving at night, increase lighting in home to reduce risk of falls, and paint the first and last steps of a staircase and the edge of each step in between a bright color to aid depth perception.

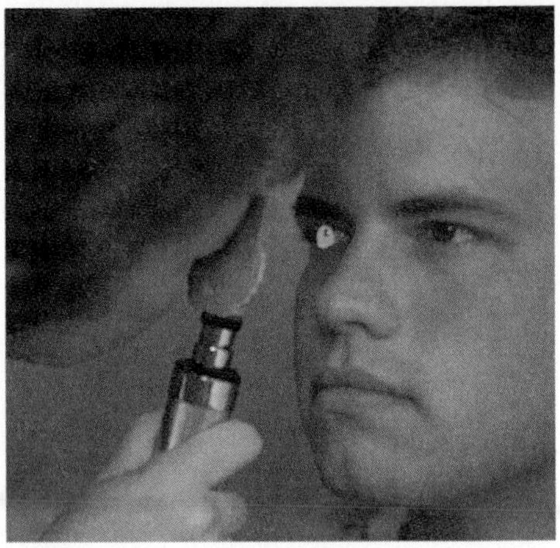

FIGURE 16-18 Opthalmoscopic examination.

ate nurse's practice. However, it is important to understand its purpose and the significance of findings. Clients in greatest need of the examination are those with diabetes, hypertension, and intracranial disorders. By illuminating the internal eye structures with an **opthalmoscope,** an examiner is able to view the optic disc, macula, and fovea centralis.

The opthalmoscope consists of a battery tube light source, two dials or disks, and a keyhole viewer. The examination is done in a darkened room. The examiner and client sit in comfortable positions facing each other with their eyes at the same height. As the client gazes straight ahead, the light of the opthalmoscope is shined onto the pupil (Figure 16-18). A bright, orange glow in the pupil called the *red reflex* is normally seen. The light from the opthalmoscope is very bright, causing the pupil to constrict. The examiner keeps focused on the red reflex while moving the opthalmoscope toward the pupil. Rotation of the lenses allows the examiner to focus on internal eye structures. Direct visualization of the internal eye allows the examiner to inspect the size, color, and clarity of the optic disc, the integrity of retinal vessels, the presence of retinal lesions, and the appearance of the macula and fovea. The presence of abnormalities should result in a referral to an opthalmologist (see box at left).

The client's fundus should not be illuminated for extended periods. The bright light is irritating and can cause discomfort and tearing. During the examination the nurse assesses the client for discomfort.

Ears

The ear assessment determines the integrity of ear structures and hearing acuity. The nurse inspects and palpates external ear structures, inspects middle ear

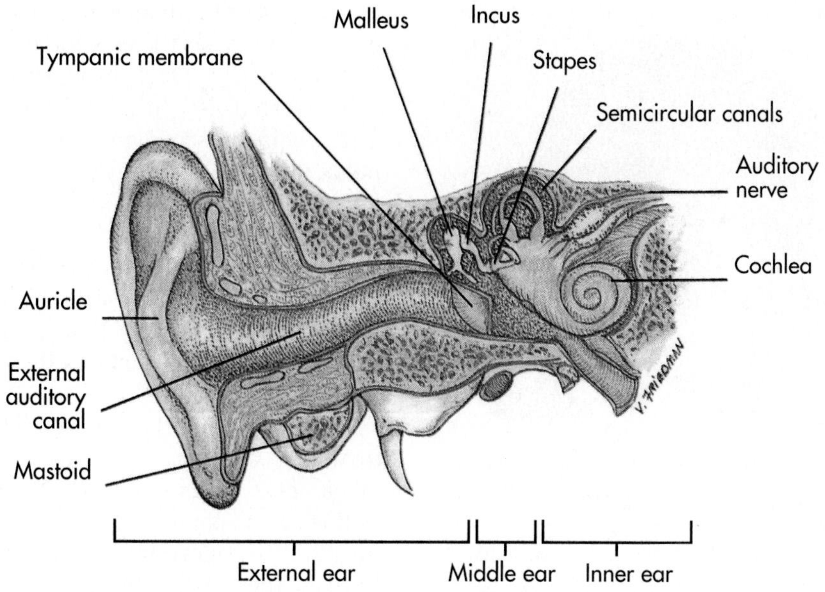

FIGURE 16-19 Structures of external, middle, and inner ear.

structures with the otoscope, and tests the client's hearing acuity (Figure 16-19). Assessment of clients with hearing impairment provides useful data for the nurse in planning effective communication techniques.

HEALTH HISTORY. The client's health history includes a review of risks for hearing problems (e.g., hypoxia at birth, meningitis, intake of aspirin or other ototoxic drugs, and exposure to noise), a history of ear surgery or trauma, and the client's current exposure to high noise levels. The nurse determines if the client has ear pain, itching, discharge, tinnitus, **vertigo,** or change in hearing. If the client has had a recent hearing problem, the nurse determines the onset, contributing factors, and effect on activities of daily living. The nurse also assesses if the client wears a hearing aid and how the client normally cleans the ears.

Auricles. With the client sitting, the nurse inspects the auricle's position, color, size, shape, and symmetry. It is important to examine lateral and medial surfaces and surrounding tissue. The auricles are normally of equal size and level with each other. The upper point of attachment to the head is in a straight line with the outer canthus or corner of the eye. The color is the same as the face. Low-set ears are a sign of congenital abnormality. Redness is a sign of inflammation or fever. Pallor can indicate frostbite.

The nurse palpates the auricles for texture, tenderness, swelling, and nodules. The auricle is normally smooth, firm, mobile, and without nodules. If folded forward, the auricle returns to its normal position upon release. The nurse also palpates the mastoid process for tenderness, swelling, and nodules.

Normally the mastoid is smooth, without nodules, and nontender. If the client complains of pain, the nurse gently pulls the lobule of the auricle and presses on the tragus and behind the ear. If palpating the external ear increases the pain, an external ear infection is likely. If palpation of the auricle and tragus cause no pain, the client may have a middle ear infection.

The nurse inspects the opening of the ear canal for size and presence of discharge. If discharge is present, gloves should be worn during the examination. The meatus should not be swollen or occluded. A yellow, waxy substance called **cerumen** is common. A purulent, foul-smelling discharge is associated with infection or a foreign body.

Ear Canals and Eardrums. The deeper structures of the external and middle ear can be observed only with the use of an otoscope. A special ear speculum attaches to the battery tube of the ophthalmoscope. The nurse selects the largest speculum that fits comfortably in the client's ear. Before inserting the speculum, the examiner checks for foreign bodies in the opening of the auditory canal.

The client must avoid moving the head during the examination to avoid damage to the canal and tympanic membrane. Infants and young children often need to be restrained. Infants should lie supine with their heads turned to one side and their arms held securely at their sides. Young children can sit on their parents' laps with their legs held between the parents' knees.

To insert the speculum properly, the nurse asks the client to tip the head slightly to the opposite shoulder. The nurse holds the handle of the otoscope in the space

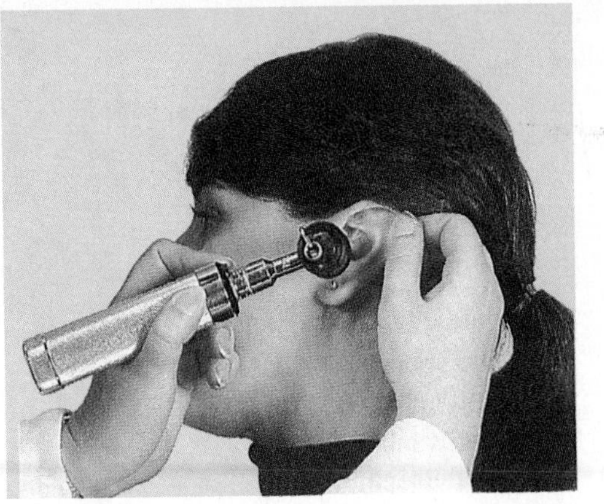

FIGURE 16-20 Otoscopic examination. (From Seidel HM, et al.: *Mosby's guide to physical examination,* ed 2, St. Louis, 1991, Mosby.)

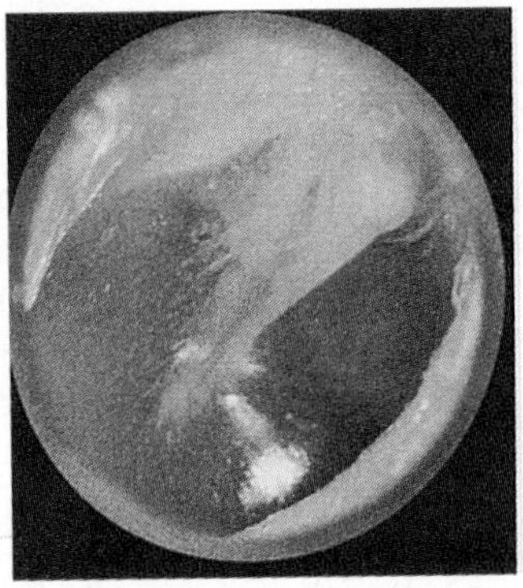

FIGURE 16-21 Normal tympanic membrane. (Courtesy Dr. Richard A. Buckingham, Abraham Lincoln School of Medicine, University of Illinois, Chicago; from Malasanos L, et al., 1990.)

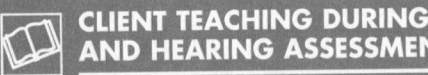

CLIENT TEACHING DURING EAR AND HEARING ASSESSMENT

Instruct client about the proper way to clean outer ear (Chapter 30), avoiding use of cotton-tipped applicators and sharp objects such as hairpins.

To remove cerumen, instruct client to use 5 gtts of an over-the-counter ceruminolytic agent in the affected ear three times daily for 4 to 7 days before irrigation. Irrigate gently with approximately 60 ml of tepid water (Mahoney, 1987).

Tell client to avoid inserting objects into the ear canal.

Encourage clients over 65 to have regular hearing checks.

Instruct family members of clients with hearing losses to avoid shouting and instead speak in low tones, and to be sure client can see the speaker's face.

between the thumb and index finger, supported on the middle finger. This leaves the ulnar side of the hand to rest against the client's head, stabilizing the otoscope as it is inserted into the canal (Seidel et al., 1991). Two grips on the otoscope may be used. In one, the examiner holds the battery tube along the client's neck with the fingers against the neck. In the other grip, the inverted otoscope is lightly braced against the side of the client's head or cheek. The nurse inserts the scope while pulling the auricle upward and backward in the adult and older child (Figure 16-20). This maneuver straightens the ear canal. In infants the auricle is pulled backward and downward.

The nurse inserts the speculum slightly down and forward, 1.0 or 1.5 cm (0.5 in) into the ear canal. Care is taken not to abrade the sensitive lining of the ear canal, as this can be painful. The canal normally has little cerumen and is uniformly pink with tiny hairs in the outer third of the canal. The nurse observes for color, discharge, scaling, lesions, foreign bodies, and cerumen. A reddened canal is a sign of inflammation. In older adults, accumulated cerumen is a common problem. Buildup of cerumen can create a mild hearing loss. During the examination the nurse asks the client how the ear canal is normally cleaned (see box at left). The nurse should caution the client on the danger of inserting pointed objects into the canal. The use of cotton-tipped applicators to clean the ears should be avoided because this causes impaction of cerumen deep in the ear canal.

The light from the otoscope allows visualization of the eardrum (tympanic membrane). The nurse must be familiar with the common anatomical landmarks and their appearance (Figure 16-21). The nurse moves the auricle to see the entire drum and its periphery. Because the eardrum is angled away from the ear canal, the light from the otoscope appears as a cone shape rather than a circle. The umbo is near the center of the drum, behind which is the attachment of the malleus. A knoblike structure at the top of the drum is created by the underlying short process of the malleus. The examiner should check carefully to be sure there are no tears or breaks in the eardrum's membrane. The normal eardrum is translucent, shiny, and pearly gray. It is free from tears or breaks. A pink or red bulging membrane indicates inflammation. If the tympanic membrane is blocked by cerumen, a warm water irrigation will safely remove the wax. An irrigation may require a physician's order.

Hearing Acuity. The nurse can often tell if the client has a hearing loss from a response to conversation. The three types of hearing loss are conduction, sensorineural, and mixed. A conduction loss involves an interruption of sound waves as they travel from the outer ear to the cochlea of the inner ear because they are not transmitted through the outer and middle ear structures. A sensorineural loss involves the inner ear, the auditory nerve, or the hearing center of the brain. Sound is conducted through the outer and middle ear structures, but the continued transmission of sound becomes interrupted at some point beyond the bony ossicles. A mixed loss involves a combination of conduction and sensorineural loss. Clients most at risk for hearing loss are those who spend time around loud noises. Older adults lose the ability to hear high-frequency sounds and consonants.

To begin a hearing assessment, the nurse has the client remove any hearing aid that is worn. The nurse notes the client's response to questions. Normally the client should respond without excess requests to have the nurse repeat questions. If hearing loss is suspected, the nurse checks the client's response to the whispered voice. One ear is tested at a time while the client occludes the other ear with a finger. The nurse asks the client to gently move the finger up and down during the test. While standing 1 foot (30 cm) from the ear being tested, the nurse covers the mouth so the client is unable to read lips. After exhaling fully, the nurse whispers softly toward the unoccluded ear, reciting random numbers with equally accented syllables such as "nine-four-ten." If necessary, the nurse gradually increases voice intensity until the client correctly repeats the numbers. The other ear is then tested for comparison. Seidel et al. (1991) report that clients normally hear numbers clearly when whispered. A ticking watch may be used to test hearing acuity, but the spoken word allows for more accuracy and control in testing.

If a hearing loss is present, there are tests that can be performed utilizing a tuning fork or audiometry. Both tests are best performed by either experienced practitioners or specially trained audiometry technicians.

Nose and Sinuses

The integrity of the nose and sinuses is assessed by inspection and palpation. The client sits during the examination. A penlight allows for gross examination of each naris. A more detailed examination requires using a nasal speculum to inspect deeper nasal turbinates. A student should not use a speculum unless a qualified practitioner is present.

Health History. It is useful to know whether the client's health history indicates exposure to dust or pollutants, allergies, nasal obstruction, recent trauma, discharge, frequent infections, headaches, or postnasal drip. An assessment for a history of nosebleed **(epistaxis)** should include review of frequency, amount of bleeding, and predisposing factors. The nurse also determines whether the client has a history of using nasal spray or drops, including the amount, frequency, and duration of use (see box at right). The nurse also asks if the client has been told he or she snores or has difficulty breathing.

Nose. When inspecting the external nose the nurse observes for shape, size, skin color, and presence of deformity or inflammation. The nose is normally smooth and symmetric with the same color as the face. Recent trauma may have caused edema and discoloration. If swelling or deformities exist, the nurse gently palpates the ridge and soft tissue of the nose by placing one finger on each side of the nasal arch and gently moving fingers from the nasal bridge to the tip. The nurse notes any tenderness, masses, and underlying deviations. Nasal structures are usually firm and stable.

Air normally passes freely through the nose as a person breathes. To assess patency of the nares, the nurse places a finger on the side of the client's nose and occludes one naris. The client is asked to breathe with the mouth closed. The nurse repeats the procedure for the other naris.

As the nurse illuminates the anterior nares, the mucosa is inspected for color, lesions, discharge, swelling, and evidence of bleeding. If discharge is present, gloves should be applied. Normal mucosa is pink and moist without lesions. Pale mucosa with clear discharge indicates allergy. A mucoid discharge indicates rhinitis. A sinus infection results in yellowish or greenish discharge. For the client with a nasogastric tube, the nurse checks for local excoriation of the naris, characterized by redness and skin sloughing.

To view the septum and turbinates, the client tips the head back slightly to give the nurse a clearer view. Advanced clinicians may use a nasal speculum. The septum is inspected for alignment, perforation, or bleeding. Normally the septum is close to midline, thicker anteriorly than posteriorly. The mucosa is pink and moist, with clear mucus. A deviated septum can obstruct breathing and interfere with passage of a nasogastric tube.

CLIENT TEACHING DURING NOSE AND SINUS ASSESSMENT

Caution clients against overuse of over-the-counter nasal sprays, which can lead to "rebound," causing nasal inflammation and congestion.

Instruct parents on care of children with nose bleeds: have child sit up and lean forward to avoid aspiration of blood; apply pressure to anterior nose with thumb and forefinger as child breathes through mouth; apply ice or a cold cloth to bridge of nose if pressure fails to stop bleeding.

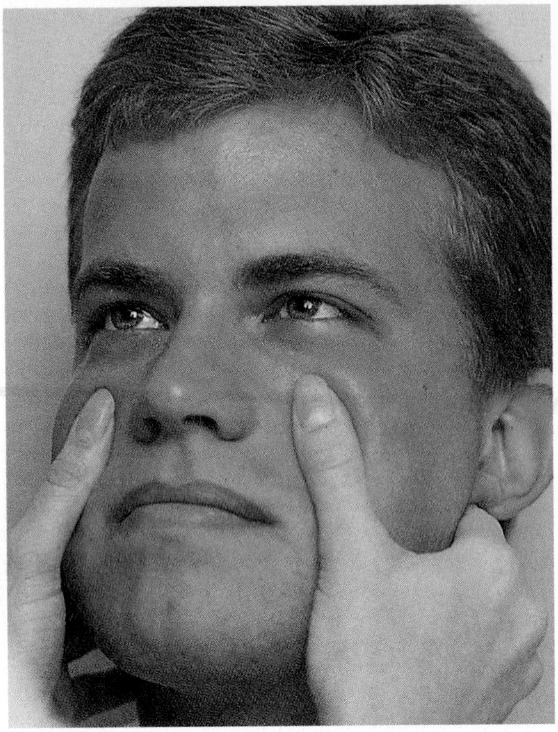

FIGURE 16-22 Palpation of maxillary sinuses.

Sinuses. The examination of the sinuses is limited to palpation. In cases of allergies or infection, the interior of the sinuses becomes inflamed and swollen. The most effective way to assess for tenderness is by externally palpating the frontal and maxillary facial areas (Figure 16-22). The frontal sinus is palpated by exerting pressure with the thumb up and under the client's eyebrow. Gentle upward pressure elicits tenderness easily if sinus irritation is present. Do not apply pressure to the eyes. If tenderness of sinuses is present, the nurse transilluminates the sinuses. This procedure, however, requires advanced experience.

Mouth and Pharynx

The nurse assesses the mouth and pharynx to detect signs of overall health, determine oral hygiene needs, and develop nursing therapies for clients with dehydration, restricted intake, oral trauma, or oral airway obstruction. To assess the oral cavity the nurse uses a penlight and tongue depressor or single gauze square. Gloves should be worn when contacting mucous membranes. The client may sit or lie during the examination. The nurse may assess the oral cavity while administering oral hygiene.

HISTORY. The nurse determines if the client wears dentures or retainers and if they comfortably fit. An assessment of a recent change in appetite or weight may point to a problem with chewing or swallowing. The nurse assesses the client's dental hygiene practices and when the client last visited a dentist. To rule out risks for mouth and throat cancer, the nurse asks if the client smokes or chews tobacco or smokes a pipe. The nurse also assesses for a history of pain or lesions of the mouth and pain with chewing. It can be helpful to know if the client has a history of tonsillectomy or adenoidectomy.

Lips. The lips are inspected for color, texture, hydration, contour, and lesions. As the client opens the mouth, the nurse views the lips from end to end. Normally the lips are pink, moist, symmetrical, and smooth with the surface free from lesions.

Mucosa. To view the inner oral mucosa, the nurse has the client open the mouth slightly and gently pulls the lower lip away from the teeth (Figure 16-23, *A*). This process is repeated for the upper lip. The mucosa is inspected for color, hydration, texture, and lesions such as ulcers, abrasions, or cysts. Normally the mucosa is a glistening pink. Hyperpigmentation is normal in 10% of European Americans and 90% of African Americans over 50 years of age. Any lesions are palpated with a gloved hand for tenderness, size, and consistency.

To inspect the buccal mucosa, the nurse asks the client to open the mouth and then gently retracts the cheeks with a tongue depressor or gloved finger covered with gauze (Figure 16-23, *B*). A penlight illuminates the posterior mucosa. The surface of the mucosa must be viewed from right to left and top to bottom. Normal mucosa is glistening, pink, soft, moist, and smooth. For clients with normal pigmentation the buccal mucosa is a good site to inspect for jaundice and pallor. In older adults, the mucosa is normally dry because of reduced salivation. Thick white patches **(leukoplakia)** are often a precancerous lesion seen in heavy smokers and alcoholics. The nurse palpates for any buccal lesions by placing the index finger within the buccal cavity and the thumb on the outer surface of the cheek.

Gums and Teeth. The gums or **gingivae** are examined for color, edema, retraction, bleeding, and lesions. If a client wears dentures, irregularity or lesions of the gums can create discomfort and significantly impair the ability to chew. The nurse asks the client to remove dentures for a complete assessment. Healthy gums are pink, moist, smooth, and tightly fit around each tooth. African Americans may have patchy pigmentation. Older adults may have pale gums. The nurse assesses firmness of the gums by palpation with a tongue depressor. Spongy gums that bleed easily indicate periodontal disease or vitamin C deficiency.

The nurse asks the client to clench the teeth and smile to observe teeth occlusion. The upper molars

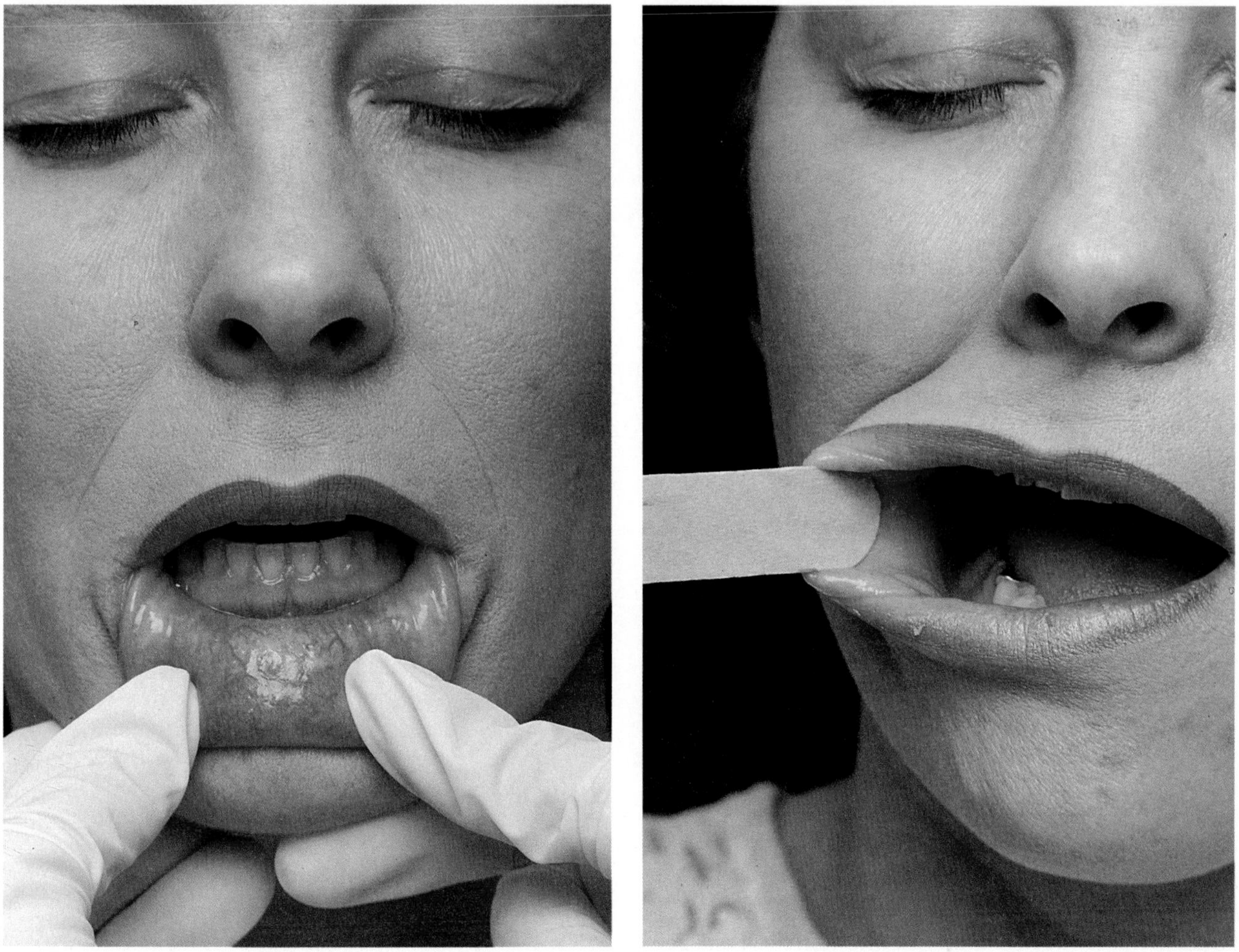

FIGURE 16-23 **A,** Inspection of inner oral mucosa of lower lip. **B,** Retraction allows for clear view of buccal mucosa.

should rest directly on the lower molar, and upper incisors slightly override the lower incisors. The position and alignment of teeth are noted. The nurse probes each tooth gently with a tongue blade when the client complains of any localized discomfort. The teeth are normally firmly set.

The quality of a client's dental hygiene is easily determined by inspecting the teeth (see box on p. 324). To examine the posterior surface of the teeth, the nurse has the client open the mouth with lips relaxed. A tongue depressor may be needed to retract the lips and cheeks, especially when one is viewing the molars. The nurse notes the color of teeth and the presence of dental caries, tartar, and extraction sites. Normal healthy teeth are smooth, white, and shiny. A chalky white discoloration of the enamel is an early indication that caries are forming. Brown or black discolorations indicate advanced caries. A stained yellow color is from tobacco use while coffee and tea cause a brown stain. In older adults, teeth become loose, rough, yellowed, or darkened.

Tongue and Floor of Mouth. The tongue is carefully inspected on all sides, and the floor of the mouth is checked. The client first relaxes the mouth and sticks the tongue out halfway. If the client protrudes the tongue too far, the gag reflex may be elicited. Using the penlight, the nurse examines the tongue for color, size, position, texture, movement, and coating or lesions. The tongue should appear medium or dull red in color, moist, slightly rough on the top surface and smooth along the lateral margins. The tongue remains at midline. The nurse asks the client to raise the tongue and move it side to side. The tongue should move freely.

The undersurface of the tongue and floor of the mouth is highly vascular. Extra care is taken to inspect this area, a common site of origin for oral cancer lesions. The client lifts the tongue by placing its tip on the palate

CLIENT TEACHING DURING MOUTH AND PHARYNX ASSESSMENT

Discuss proper techniques for oral hygiene, including brushing and flossing.

Explain the early warning signs of oral cancer, including a sore that bleeds easily and does not heal, a lump or thickening, and a persistent red or white patch on the mucosa.

Encourage regular dental examinations every 6 months for children and adults.

Older adults may need to eat soft foods and cut food into small pieces because of difficulty in chewing and changes in the teeth.

behind the upper incisors. The nurse inspects for color, swelling, and lesions such as cysts. The ventral surface of the tongue is pink and smooth with large veins between the frenulum folds. To palpate the tongue the nurse asks the client to protrude the tongue and gently grasps its tip with a gauze square. While gently pulling the tongue to one side at a time, the nurse palpates its full length and base or floor of the mouth, noting any hardening or ulceration. The tongue should have a smooth, even texture and be free of lesions.

Palate. The client should extend the head backward, holding the mouth open so that the nurse can inspect the hard and soft palates. The hard palate or roof of the mouth is located anteriorly. The soft palate extends posteriorly toward the pharynx. The palates are observed for color, shape, texture, and extra bony prominences or defects. It is common to visualize a bony growth or exostosis between the two palates. Normal palates are light pink.

Pharynx. An examination of the pharyngeal structures is performed to rule out infection, inflammation, or lesions. The client tips the head back slightly, opens the mouth wide, and says "ah." The nurse places the tip of a tongue depressor on the middle third of the tongue, taking care not to press the lower lip against the teeth (Figure 16-24). If the tongue depressor is placed too far anteriorly, the posterior part of the tongue mounds up, obstructing the view. Placing the tongue depressor on the posterior tongue elicits the gag reflex.

With a penlight, the nurse first inspects the uvula and soft palate. Both structures, which are innervated by the tenth cranial nerve (vagus), should rise centrally as the client says "ah." The anterior and posterior tonsillar pillars are examined, and the presence or absence of tonsillar tissue is noted. The posterior pharynx is the last structure to view. Normally pharyngeal structures are smooth, glistening pink, and well hydrated. Small irregular spots of lymphatic tissue and small blood vessels are normal. Edema, petechiae (small hemorrhages), lesions, or exudate should be noted. Clients with chronic sinus problems frequently exhibit a clear exudate that drains along the wall of the posterior pharynx. Yellow or green exudate indicates infection. A client with a typical sore throat has a reddened and edematous uvula and tonsillar pillars with possible yellow exudate.

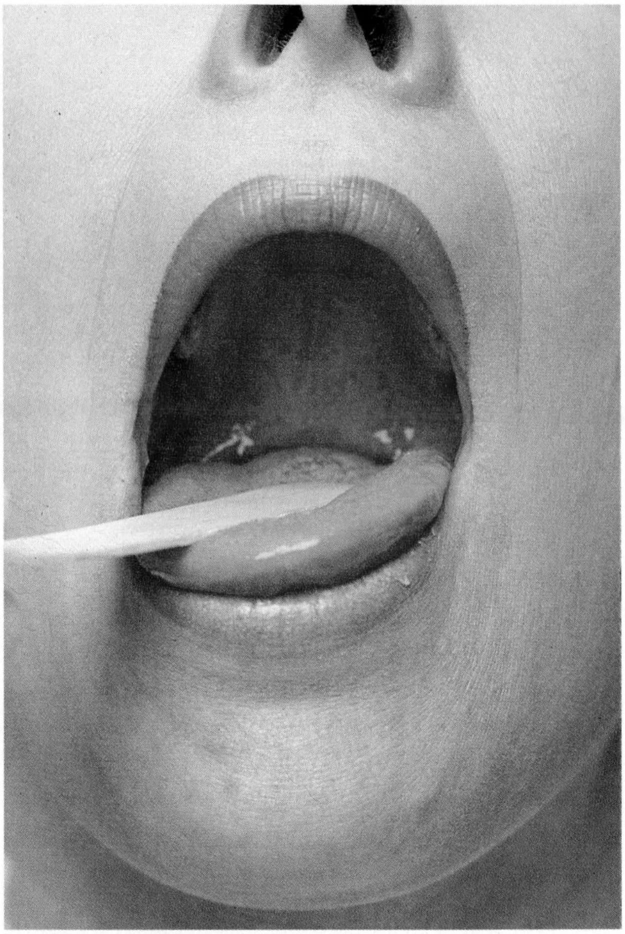

FIGURE 16-24 Tongue depressor allows nurse to view uvula and posterior soft palate.

Neck

Assessment of the neck includes assessing the neck muscles, lymph nodes of the head, carotid arteries, jugular veins, thyroid gland, and trachea (Figure 16-25). An examination of the carotid arteries and jugular veins can be deferred until conducting assessment of the vascular system. The nurse inspects the neck to determine the integrity of neck structures and to examine the lymphatic system. An abnormality of superficial lymph nodes may reveal the presence of infection or malig-

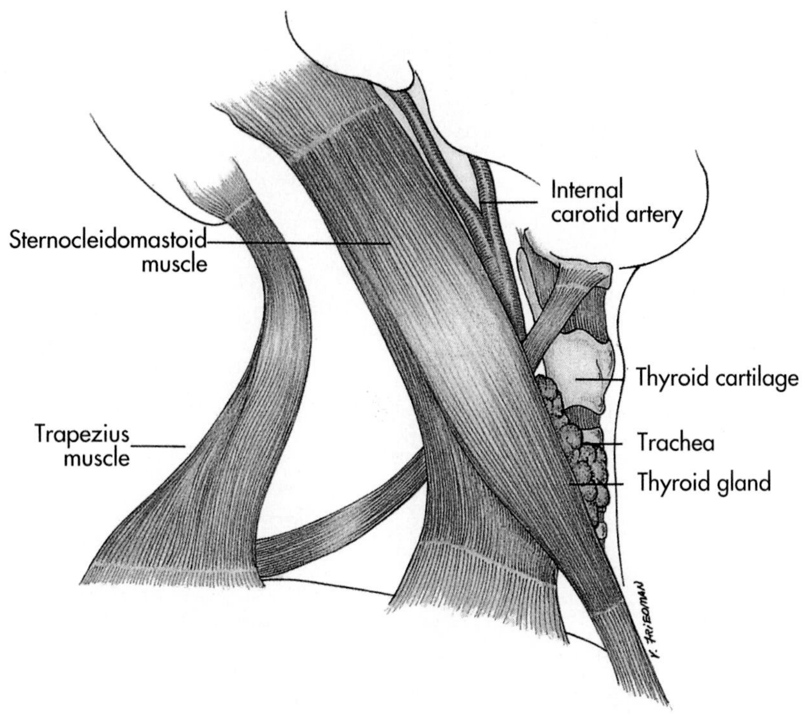

FIGURE 16-25 Anatomical position of major neck structures.

nancy. Examination of the thyroid gland and trachea also aids in ruling out malignancies. Examination is best performed with the client sitting.

Health History. The nurse determines if the client has had a recent cold or infection or feels weak or fatigued. Screening for hypothyroidism and hyperthyroidism and risk factors for HIV infection may be necessary. The nurse also assesses if the client has been exposed to radiation, toxic chemicals, or infection. The client is asked to describe any history of thyroid problems, neck or head injury, or pain of head and neck structures. Finally, the nurse asks if the client is taking thyroid medication or has a family history of thyroid disease.

Neck Muscles. With the client sitting and facing the nurse, an inspection of gross neck structures is made. The nurse observes for symmetry of neck muscles, alignment of the trachea, and any subtle fullness at the neck. Any distention or prominence of jugular veins and carotid arteries is abnormal. The nurse asks the client to flex the neck with the chin to the chest, hyperextend the neck backward, and move the head laterally to each side and then sideways with the ear moving toward the shoulder. This tests the sternocleidomastoid and trapezius muscles. The neck should move freely without discomfort.

Lymph Nodes. An extensive system of lymph nodes collects lymph from the head, ears, nose, cheeks, and lips (Figure 16-26). With the client's chin raised and head tilted slightly back, the nurse first inspects the area where lymph nodes are distributed and compares both sides. This position stretches the skin slightly over any possible enlarged nodes. Visible nodes are inspected for edema, erythema, or red streaks. Nodes are not normally visible.

A methodical approach is used to palpate the lymph nodes to avoid overlooking any single node or chain. The client relaxes muscles and tissues by keeping the neck flexed slightly forward and, if needed, toward the side of the nurse. Both sides of the neck are palpated for comparison. During palpation the nurse faces or stands to the side of the client for easy access to all nodes. Using the pads of the middle three fingers of each hand, the nurse palpates gently in a rotary motion over the nodes. Each node is checked methodically in the following sequence; occipital nodes at base of skull, postauricular nodes over the mastoid, preauricular nodes just in front of the ear, retropharyngeal nodes at angle of the mandible, submaxillary nodes, and submental nodes in the midline behind the mandibular tip. The nurse avoids applying excessive pressure; otherwise small nodes are missed or obliterated. Both sides are compared for size, shape, delineation, mobility, consistency, and tenderness.

To palpate supraclavicular nodes the nurse asks the client to bend the head forward and relax the shoulders. The nurse may have to hook the index and third finger

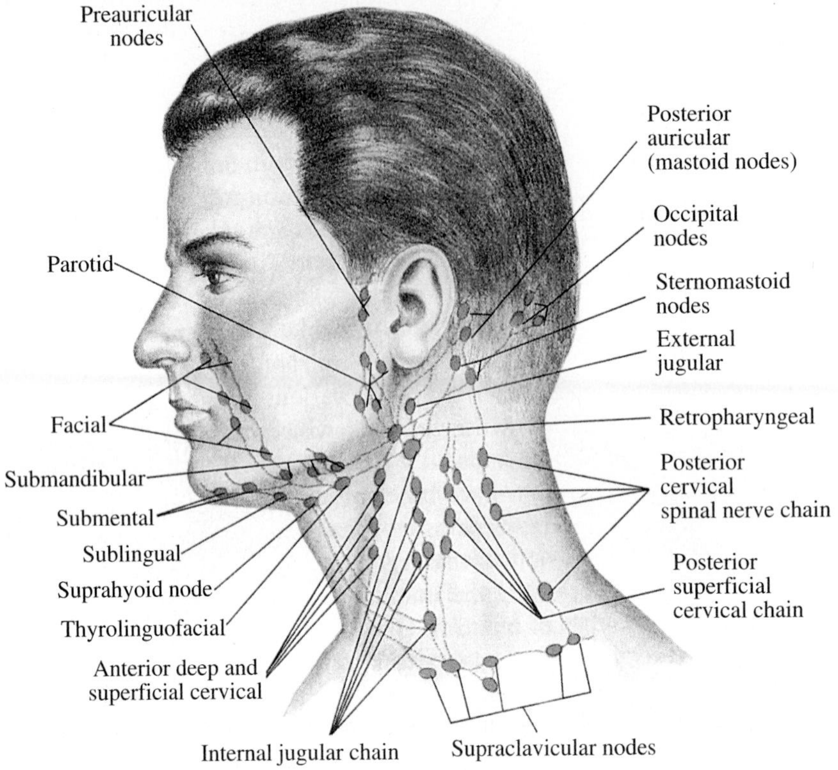

FIGURE 16-26 Lymphatic drainage system of head and neck. (From Seidel HM, et al.: *Mosby's guide to physical examination,* ed 2, St. Louis, 1991, Mosby.)

over the clavicle, lateral to the sternocleidomastoid muscle, to palpate these nodes. The deep cervical nodes can be palpated only with the nurse's fingers hooked around the sternocleidomastoid muscle.

Normally lymph nodes are not easily palpable. Large, fixed, inflamed, or tender lymph nodes indicate problems such as local infection, systemic disease, or neoplasm (McConnell, 1988). Tenderness almost always indicates inflammation (see box below). A problem involving a lymph node of the head and neck may mean an abnormality in either the mouth, throat, abdomen, breasts, thorax, or arms. These are the areas drained by the head and neck nodes.

CLIENT TEACHING DURING NECK ASSESSMENT

Stress the importance of regular compliance with medication schedule to clients with thyroid disease.

Instruct client to call the physician when a lump or mass is noted in the neck.

Thyroid Gland. The thyroid gland lies in the anterior lower neck, in front of and to both sides of the trachea. The gland is fixed to the trachea with the isthmus overlying the trachea and connecting the two irregular, cone-shaped lobes (Figure 16-27). The nurse inspects the lower neck over the thyroid gland for obvious masses and symmetry.

More experienced nurses can examine the thyroid by palpating for more subtle masses. Gentle palpation as the client swallows allows an examiner to feel movement of the thyroid. Displacement of the gland during swallowing allows the nurse to palpate each lobe. Thin clients often have palpable glands that should be small, smooth, and free from nodules. Enlargement of the thyroid may indicate gland dysfunction or tumor. An enlarged tender thyroid indicates thyroiditis.

Trachea. The trachea is a part of the upper airway that can be directly palpated. It is normally located in the midline above the suprasternal notch. Masses in the neck or mediastinum and pulmonary abnormalities can cause displacement laterally. The client may sit or lie down during palpation. The position of the trachea is determined by palpating at the suprasternal notch, slipping the thumb and index fingers to each side. The nurse notes if the finger and thumb are shifted laterally.

Forceful pressure must not be applied to the trachea because this may elicit a cough.

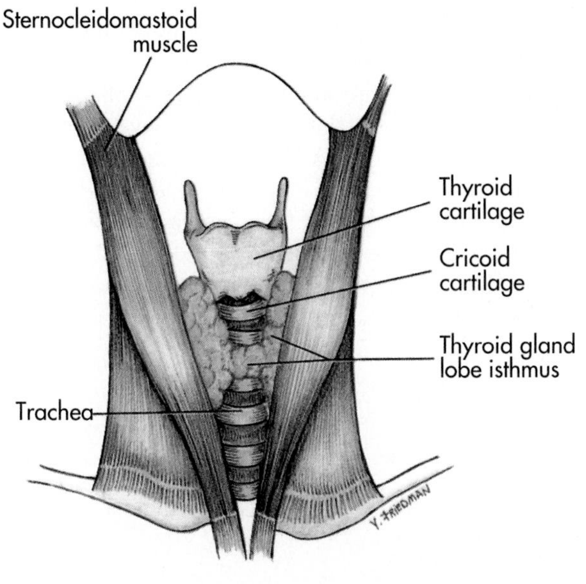

FIGURE 16-27 Thyroid gland.

THORAX AND LUNGS

Physical assessment of the thorax and lungs includes an in-depth look at ventilatory and respiratory functions of the lungs. If the lungs are affected by disease, other body systems are also affected. For example, reduced oxygenation can cause changes in mental alertness because of the brain's sensitivity to lowered oxygen levels. The nurse uses data from all body systems to determine the nature of pulmonary alterations.

Before assessing the thorax and lungs, the nurse must be familiar with chest landmarks (Figure 16-28). These help the nurse locate findings and use assessment skills correctly. The client's nipples, angle of Louis, suprasternal notch, costal angle, clavicles, and vertebrae are key landmarks. The nurse keeps a mental image of the location of the lobes of the lung and the position of each rib (Figure 16-29). The proper orientation to anatomic structures ensures a thorough assessment of the anterior, lateral, and posterior thorax.

Locating the position of each rib is critical to visualizing the lobe of the lung being assessed. The angle of

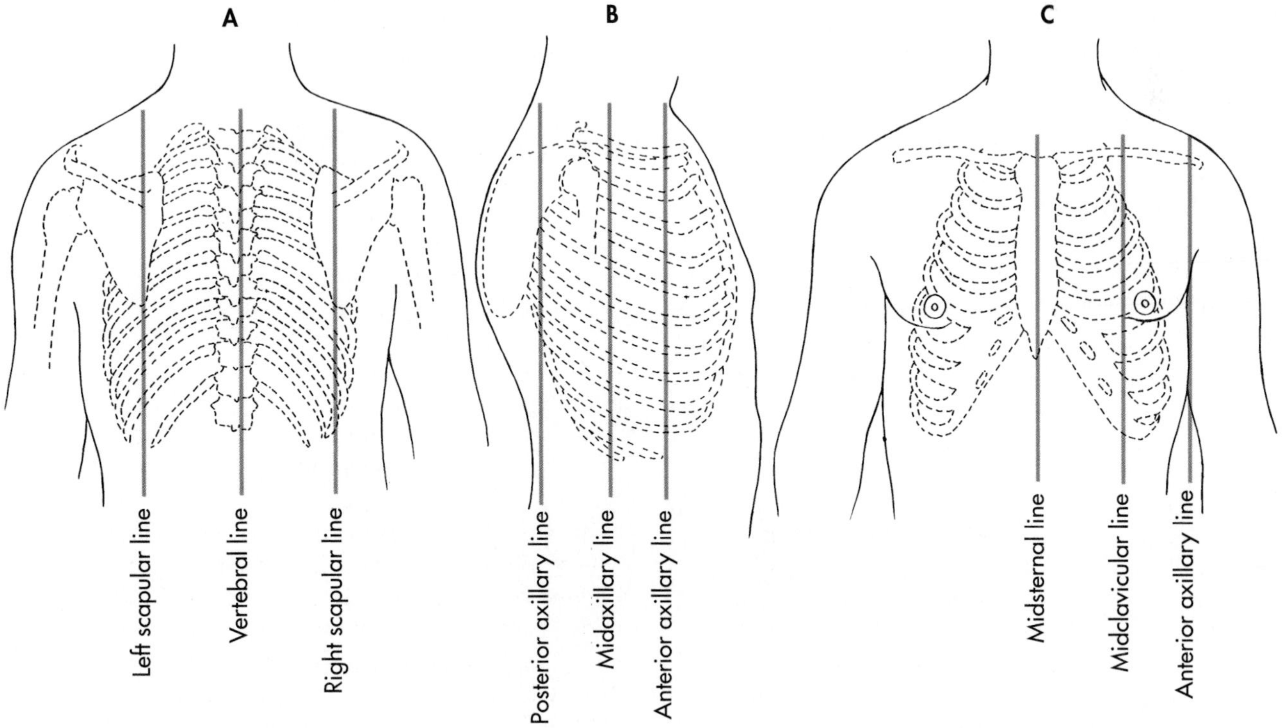

FIGURE 16-28 Anatomical chest wall landmarks. **A,** Posterior chest. **B,** Lateral chest. **C,** Anterior chest.

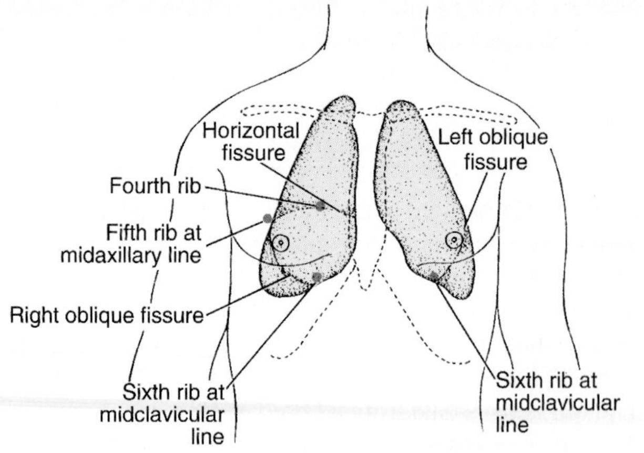

FIGURE 16-29 Anterior position of lung lobes in relation to anatomical landmarks.

Louis, at the junction between the manubrium and the body of the sternum, is the starting point for locating the ribs anteriorly. Knowing that the second rib extends from the angle makes it easy to locate and palpate the intercostal spaces (between the ribs) in succession. The spinous process of the third thoracic vertebra and the fourth, fifth, and sixth ribs serve to locate the lung's lobes laterally (Figure 16-30). The lower lobes project laterally and anteriorly.

Posteriorly the tip or inferior margin of the scapula lies approximately at the level of the seventh rib. After the seventh rib is identified, the examiner can count upward to locate the third thoracic vertebra and align it with the inner borders of the scapula to locate the posterior lobes (Figure 16-31).

Examination requires the client to be undressed to

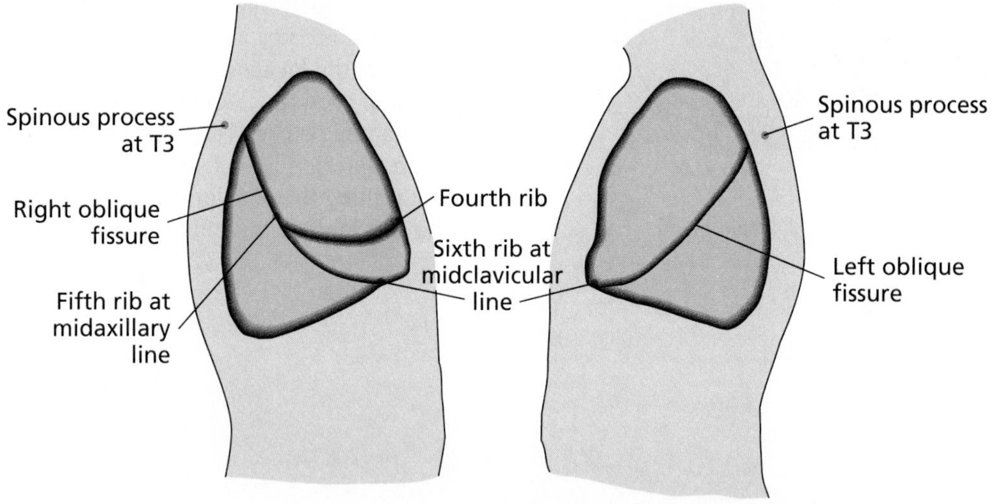

FIGURE 16-30 Lateral position of lung lobes in relation to anatomical landmarks.

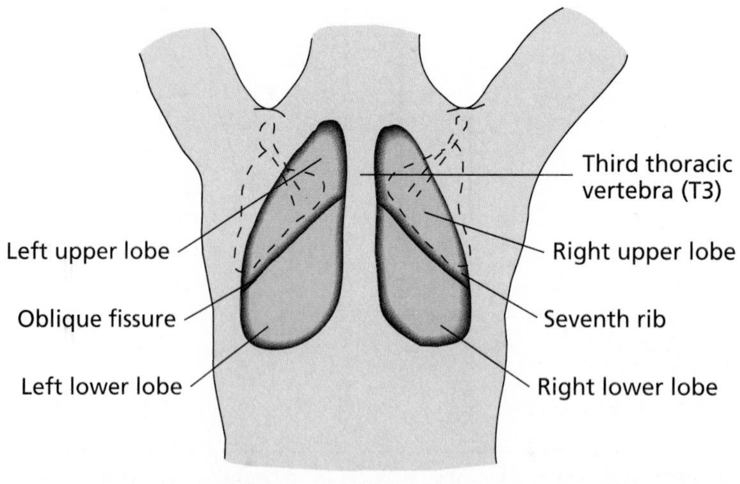

FIGURE 16-31 Posterior position of lung lobes in relation to anatomical landmarks.

the waist. Good lighting is needed. The examination begins with the client sitting for assessment of the posterior and lateral chest. The client may sit or lie for assessment of the anterior chest.

Health History. A complete health history includes determining if the client has a history of tobacco or marijuana use, including number of years smoked, age started, number of cigarettes or cigars daily, and length of time since smoking stopped. To screen for warning signals of lung cancer, the nurse asks if the client has a persistent cough, sputum production, chest pain or recurrent attacks of pneumonia or bronchitis. Asking the client about symptoms of **orthopnea,** shortness of breath, **dyspnea** during exertion or at rest, and poor activity tolerance can reveal other pulmonary problems. A client's risk for having lung disease is further assessed by reviewing presence of pollutants in the work environment or at home, and reviewing the client's family history.

Tuberculosis is on the increase in the United States. Nurses should be alert for clients at risk, including persons with HIV infection, substance abusers, residents of nursing homes, and low-income individuals (ATS, 1992). Clients who present symptoms of cough, hemoptysis, weight loss, fatigue, night sweats, and fever should be evaluated for tuberculosis.

The nursing history also includes assessment of allergies to airborne irritants, foods, drugs, or chemical substances. It is important to learn if a client has had a pneumonia or influenza vaccine and a tuberculosis test.

Posterior Thorax

The examination begins with observing for any signs or symptoms in other body systems that may indicate pulmonary problems. Reduced mental alertness, nasal flaring, somnolence, and cyanosis are examples of signs assessed during other portions of the examination that can indicate oxygenation problems. The nurse begins inspecting the posterior thorax by observing the shape and symmetry of the chest from the back and front. The anteroposterior diameter is noted. The shape of the chest or the client's posture can impair ventilation. Normally chest contour is symmetrical with the anteroposterior diameter ⅓ to ½ of the transverse or side-to-side diameter. Aging and chronic lung disease are characterized by a barrel-shaped chest (anteroposterior diameter equals transverse). A client may lean over a table or splint the side of the chest because of a breathing problem. Splinting or holding the chest wall because of pain causes a client to bend toward the affected side. This impairs ventilation.

Standing at a midline position behind the client, the nurse looks for deformities, position of the spine, slope of the ribs, retraction of the intercostal spaces during inspiration, and bulging of the intercostal spaces during expiration. The spine is normally straight, and scapulae normally are symmetrical and closely attached to the chest wall. The spine normally is straight without lateral deviation. Posteriorly, the ribs tend to slope across and down. The ribs and intercostal spaces are easier to see in a thin person. Normally no bulging or active movement occurs within the intercostal spaces during breathing. Bulging indicates that the client is using great effort to breathe.

The nurse may also assess the rate and rhythm of breathing at this time (see Chapter 15). The thorax as a whole is observed. The thorax normally expands and relaxes with equality of movement bilaterally.

Palpation of the posterior thorax assesses further characteristics. The thoracic muscles and skeleton are palpated for lumps, masses, pulsations, and unusual movement. If pain or tenderness is noted, the nurse avoids deep palpation. Fractured rib fragments could be displaced against vital organs. Normally the chest wall is not tender.

To measure chest excursion or depth of breathing, the nurse stands behind the client and places the thumbs along the spinal processes at the 10th rib, with the palms lightly contacting the posterolateral surfaces. The nurse's thumbs should be about 2 inches (5 cm) apart, pointing toward the spine and fingers pointing laterally. The hands are pressed toward the spine so that a small skinfold appears between the thumbs. The nurse does not slide the hands over the skin. The nurse instructs the client to take a deep breath after exhaling. The nurse notes movement of the thumbs. Chest excursion should be symmetric, separating the thumbs 1¼ to 2 inches (3 to 5 cm). Reduced chest excursion may be caused by pain, postural deformity, or fatigue. In older adults, chest excursion normally declines.

During speech the sound created by the vocal cords is transmitted through the lung to the chest wall. The sound waves create vibrations that can be palpated externally. These vibrations are called **tactile** or **vocal fremitus.** The buildup of mucous secretions, the collapse of lung tissue, or the presence of lung lesions can block the vibrations from reaching the chest wall.

To palpate for fremitus, the nurse places the ball or lower palm of the hand over symmetric intercostal spaces, beginning at the lung apex. A firm light touch is best. The client is asked to say "99." Normally there is a faint vibration as the client speaks. Both sides of the thorax are compared, moving from top to bottom (Figure 16-32). Only one hand is used to ensure accuracy. If the fremitus is faint, it may be necessary to ask the client to speak louder or lower the tone of voice. Tactile fremitus is symmetrical and strongest at the top near the level of the tracheal bifurcation. It is easy to assess for fremitus in a crying infant because strong vibrations can be felt through the chest wall.

Percussion of the chest wall determines whether un-

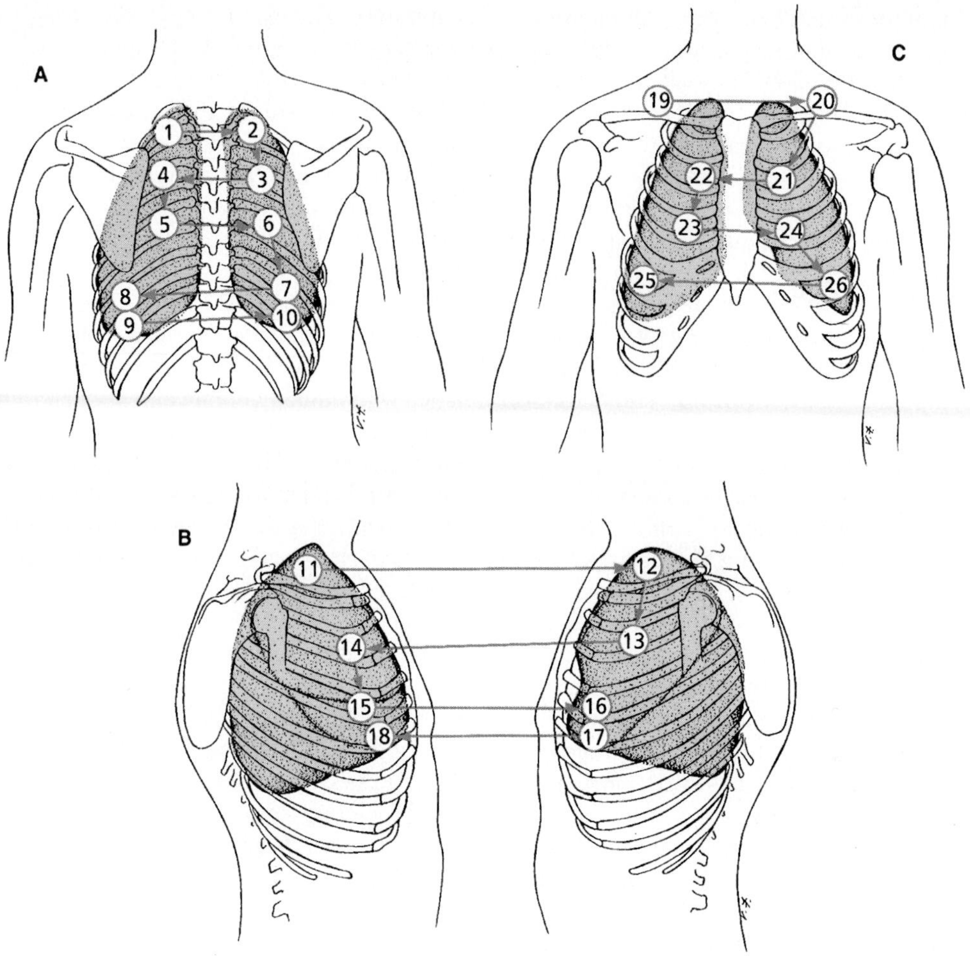

FIGURE 16-32 Nurse follows systematic pattern (posterior- lateral-anterior) when comparing palpation, auscultation, and percussion across the thorax.

derlying lung tissue is air filled, fluid filled, or solid. The client folds the arms forward across the chest with head bent forward. This position separates the scapulae further to expose more lung to assessment. Using the indirect technique, the nurse percusses in the intercostal spaces over symmetrical areas of the lung. Figure 16-32 shows how following a systematic pattern starting posteriorly and then moving laterally and anteriorly allows the nurse to compare percussion notes for all lung lobes. Resonance, the sound created by air-filled lungs, is normally heard over the posterior thorax. Percussion over the scapula, ribs, or spine is dull. The chest is normally more resonant in the child than in the adult. A lung mass causes a flat sound.

Auscultation assesses the movement of air through the tracheobronchial tree and detects mucus or obstructed airways. Normally air flows through the airways in an unobstructed pattern. Recognizing the sounds created by normal airflow allows the nurse to detect sounds caused by airway obstruction.

The nurse places the diaphragm of the stethoscope over the posterior chest wall between the ribs. The client folds arms in front of the chest and keeps the head bent forward while taking slow deep breaths with the mouth slightly open. The nurse listens to an entire inspiration and expiration at each position of the stethoscope. If sounds are faint, as with an obese client, the client should be asked to breathe harder and faster temporarily. Breath sounds are much louder in children because of their thin chest wall. The same systematic pattern used in percussion should be used when comparing the right and left sides. The nurse compares the sounds in one region on one side of the body with sounds in the same region on the opposite side.

The nurse auscultates for normal breath sounds and abnormal **(adventitious)** sounds. Normal breath sounds differ in character, depending on the area being auscultated. Sounds normally heard over the posterior thorax include bronchovesicular and vesicular sounds. Bronchovesicular sounds are medium-pitched blowing

table 16-4

ADVENTITIOUS SOUNDS

Sound	Site auscultated	Cause	Character
Crackles (also called *rales*) 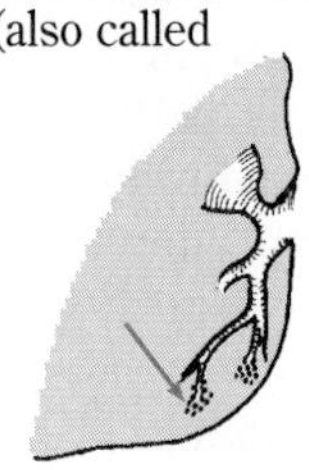	Are most commonly heard in dependent lobes: right and left lung bases	Random, sudden reinflation of groups of alveoli*	Are fine, short, interrupted crackling sounds heard during inspiration, expiration, or both; vary in pitch: high or low; may or may not change with coughing*
Rhonchi (also called *gurgles*) 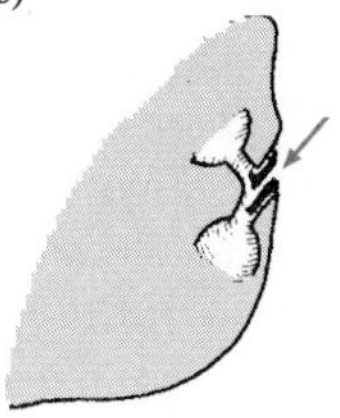	Are primarily heard over trachea and bronchi; if loud enough, can be heard over most lung fields	Fluid or mucus in larger airways, causing turbulence	Are low-pitched, continuous musical sounds heard more during expiration; may be cleared by coughing
Wheezes 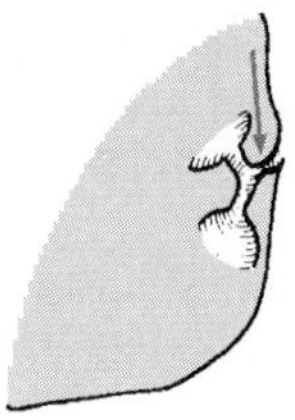	Can be heard over all lung fields	Severely narrowed bronchus	Are high-pitched, continuous musical sounds heard during inspiration or expiration; do not clear with coughing†
Pleural friction rub 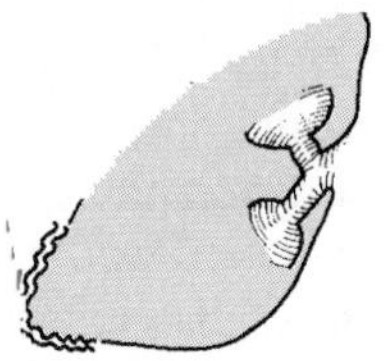	Is heard best over anterior lateral lung field (if client is sitting upright)	Inflamed pleura, parietal pleura rubbing against visceral pleura	Has grating quality heard best during inspiration; does not clear with coughing

*Data from Forgacs P: *Chest* 73:399, 1978.
†Data from Wilkins RL, Hodgkin JE, Lopez B: *Lung sounds: a practical guide,* St. Louis, 1988, Mosby.

sounds normally heard posteriorly between the scapulae. The sounds have equal inspiratory and expiratory phases. The character of bronchovesicular sounds is related to the larger underlying airways. Vesicular sounds are heard over the lungs' periphery. The sounds are created by air moving through the smaller airways. Vesicular sounds are soft, breezy, and low pitched, and the inspiratory phase is about three times longer than the expiratory phase.

Abnormal sounds result from air passing through moisture, mucus, or narrowed airways. They can also result from alveoli suddenly reinflating or from an inflammation between the lung's pleural linings. Adventitious sounds are superimposed over normal sounds. The four types of adventitious sounds include **crackles** (also called rales), **rhonchi** (also called gurgles), **wheezes,** and **pleural friction rub.** Each sound is caused by a specific entity and is characterized by typical auditory features (Table 16-4). The location and characteristics of the sounds should be noted, as should the absence of breath sounds (found in clients with collapsed or surgically removed lobes).

Lateral Thorax

The client sits during the lateral chest examination. Usually the nurse extends the assessment of the posterior thorax to the lateral sides of the chest (see Figure 16-32, *B*). The client is asked to raise the arms, which improves access to lateral thoracic structures. The nurse uses all four assessment skills. Excursion cannot be assessed laterally. Normally, percussion notes are resonant, and breath sounds are vesicular.

Anterior Thorax

The anterior thorax is inspected for the same features as the posterior thorax. The client sits or lies down with head elevated. The nurse observes the accessory muscles of breathing: sternocleidomastoid, trapezius, and abdominal muscles. The accessory muscles move little with normal passive breathing. When a client requires effort to breathe as a result of strenuous exercise or disease (see box below), the accessory muscles and abdominal muscles contract. Some clients may produce a grunting sound.

The nurse observes the width of the costal angle. It is usually larger than 90 degrees between the two costal margins. Respiratory rate and rhythm are more often assessed anteriorly (Chapter 15). The male client's respirations are usually diaphragmatic, whereas the female's are more costal.

The nurse palpates anterior thoracic muscles and skeleton for lumps, masses, tenderness, or unusual movement. The sternum and xiphoid are relatively inflexible. To measure chest excursion anteriorly, the nurse places the thumbs along the costal margin parallel $2\frac{1}{2}$ inches (6 cm) apart with the palms touching the anterolateral chest (Figure 16-33, *A*). The thumbs are pushed toward the midline to create a skinfold. As the client inhales deeply, the thumbs should normally separate approximately 3 to 5 cm ($1\frac{1}{4}$ to 2 inches), with each side expanding equally (Figure 16-33, *B*).

Tactile fremitus is assessed over the chest wall. Anterior findings differ from posterior findings because of the heart and female breast tissue. Fremitus is best felt next to the sternum at the second intercostal space, at the level of the bronchial bifurcation. It is decreased over the heart, lower thorax, and breast tissue. The nurse will not be able to sense vibrations over breast tissue and thus must retract the breasts gently during palpation. If the breasts are large, this portion of the examination may be omitted.

Percussion of the anterior thorax again follows a systematic pattern. The nurse should imagine the location of all internal organs anteriorly accessible to examination. The underlying liver, heart, and stomach create percussion notes different from those of the lung. Percussion may be conducted with the client in a sitting or lying position; however, the procedure is easier if the client lies down. The nurse starts above the clavicles and moves across and then down. The female's breasts are displaced as needed. The normal lung is resonant. The percussion notes over the heart and liver are dull. The gastric air bubble is tympanic.

Auscultation of the anterior thorax follows the same pattern as percussion. The client should sit, if possible, to maximize chest expansion. Special attention should be paid to the lower lobes, where mucous secretions commonly gather. Bronchovesicular and vesicular sounds are heard above and below the clavicles and along the lung periphery. An additional normal breath sound, bronchial sound, can be heard over the trachea. Bronchial sounds are loud, high pitched, and hollow sounding, with expiration lasting longer than inspiration (3:2 ratio).

CLIENT TEACHING DURING LUNG ASSESSMENT

Explain the risk factors for chronic lung disease and lung cancer, including cigarette smoking, history of smoking for over 20 years, exposure to environmental pollution, and radiation exposure from occupational, medical and environmental sources. Residential radon exposure may also increase risk, especially for cigarette smokers. Exposure to sidestream cigarette smoke increases risk for nonsmokers.

Discuss the warning signs of lung cancer, such as a persistent cough, sputum streaked with blood, chest pains, and recurrent attacks of pneumonia or bronchitis.

The older adult may benefit from receiving influenza and pneumonia vaccinations because of a greater susceptibility to respiratory infection.

Persons at risk for TB and who visit clinics or health care centers should be referred for skin testing.

HEART

Assessment of heart function is closely compared with findings from the vascular examination. Alterations in either system may be manifested as changes in the other. A client with signs and symptoms of heart problems may have a life-threatening condition requiring immediate attention. In this case, the nurse acts quickly and conducts only portions of an examination that are absolutely necessary. When a client is more stable, a nurse conducts a more thorough examination.

Assessment of cardiac function is performed through the anterior thorax. The nurse forms a mental image of the heart's exact location (Figure 16-34). In the adult the heart is located in the center of the chest (precordium)

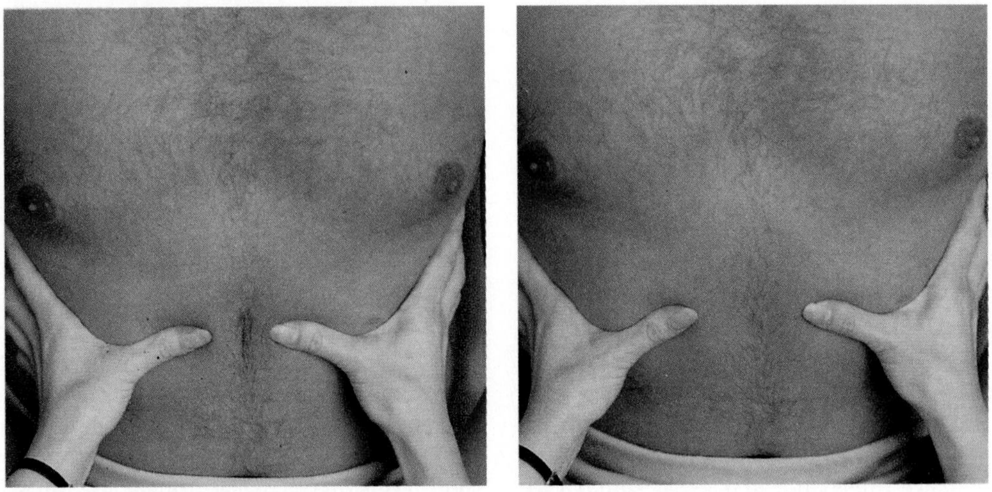

FIGURE 16-33 **A,** Position of nurse's hands before excursion. **B,** As client inhales, nurse's hands normally separate 3 to 5 cm (1½ to 2 inches).

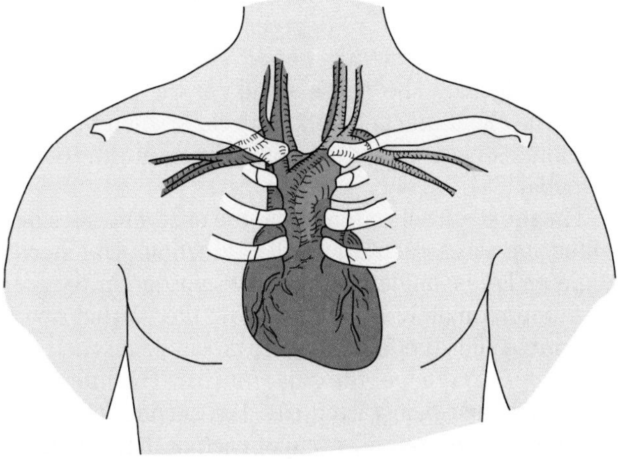

FIGURE 16-34 Anatomical position of heart.

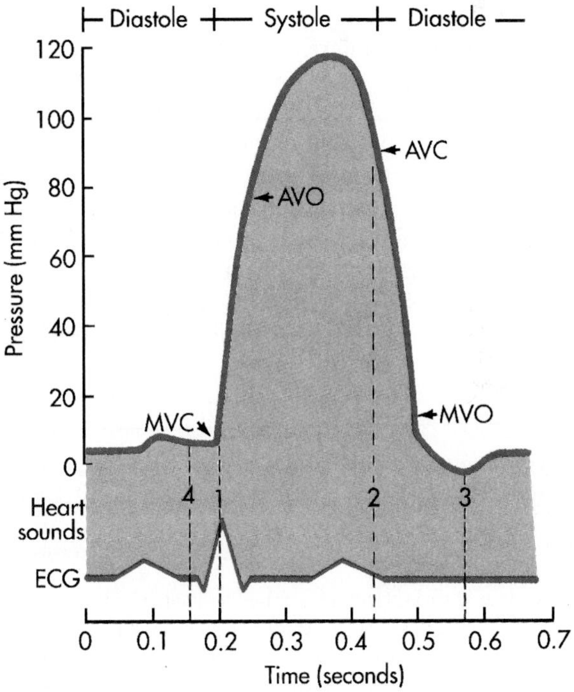

FIGURE 16-35 Cardiac cycle. *MVC,* Mitral valve closes; *AVO,* aortic valve opens; *AVC,* aortic valve closes; *MVO,* mitral valve opens.

behind and to the left of the sternum, with a small section of the right atrium extending to the sternum's right. The base of the heart is the upper portion, and the apex is the bottom tip. The surface of the right ventricle comprises most of the heart's anterior surface. A section of the left ventricle shapes the left anterior side of the apex. The apex actually touches the anterior chest wall at approximately the fourth to fifth intercostal space along the midclavicular line. This is known as the **point of maximal impulse (PMI).**

An infant's heart is positioned more horizontally. The apex of the heart is at the third or fourth intercostal space, just to the left of the midclavicular line. By the age of 7 a child's PMI is in the same location as the adult's. In tall slender persons the heart hangs more vertically and is positioned more centrally. With increased stockiness and shortness, the heart tends to lie more to the left and horizontally (Seidel, et al., 1991).

To assess heart function, the nurse must understand the cardiac cycle and the physiological signs of each event (Figure 16-35). The heart normally pumps blood through its four chambers in a methodical, even sequence. Events on the left side occur just before those on the right. As the blood flows through each chamber, valves open and close, pressures within chambers rise and fall, and chambers contract. Each event creates a physiological sign. Both sides of the heart function in a coordinated fashion.

There are two phases to the cardiac cycle: **systole** and **diastole.** During systole the ventricles contract and eject blood from the left ventricle into the aorta and from the right ventricle into the pulmonary artery. During diastole the ventricles relax and the atria contract to move blood into the ventricles and fill the coronary arteries.

Heart sounds occur in relation to physiological events in the cardiac cycle. As systole begins, ventricular pressure rises and closes the mitral and tricuspid valves. Valve closure causes the first heart sound (S_1), often described as "lub." The ventricles then contract and blood flows through the aorta and pulmonary circulation. After the ventricles empty, ventricular pressure falls below that in the aorta and pulmonary artery. This allows the aortic and pulmonary valves to close, causing the second heart sound (S_2), described as "dub." As ventricular pressure continues to fall, it drops below that of the atria. The mitral and tricuspid valves reopen to allow ventricular filling. Rapid ventricular filling may create a third heart sound (S_3). This is heard more often in children and young adults. An S_3 can also be heard as an abnormality in adults over 30 years of age. A fourth heart sound (S_4) may be heard when the atria contract to enhance ventricular filling. The S_4 is not normally heard in adults but may be heard in healthy older adults, children, and athletes. Because it may also indicate an abnormal condition, it should be reported to a physician.

CLIENT TEACHING DURING HEART ASSESSMENT

Explain the risk factors for heart disease, including high dietary intake of saturated fat or cholesterol, lack of regular aerobic exercise, smoking, excess weight, stressful life-style, hypertension, and family history of heart disease.

Refer client (if appropriate) to resources available for controlling or reducing risks (e.g., nutritional counseling and exercise class).

Recommend reduction in dietary intake of cholesterol and saturated fats. The National Institutes of Health recommends a daily intake of total fat less than 30% of calories, saturated fatty acids less than 10% of calories, and cholesterol less than 300mg/100ml (Ernst, 1989).

Encourage clients to have regular measurements of blood cholesterol and triglycerides.

HEALTH HISTORY. The health history should focus on risk factors for heart disease. The nurse assesses the client's history of smoking, alcohol intake, caffeine intake, use of prescriptive and recreational drugs, exercise habits, and dietary patterns including fat and sodium intake. Does the client have a stressful life-style? It is important to know if the client takes medication for cardiac function or hypertension. The nurse also assesses for signs and symptoms suggestive of heart problems, including chest pain or discomfort, palpitations, excess fatigue, dyspnea, edema of the feet, cyanosis, fainting, or orthopnea. If the client reports chest pain, the nurse determines if it is cardiac in nature (Rossi and Leary, 1992); anginal pain is usually a deep pressure or ache that is substernal and diffuse, radiating to one or both arms, neck, or jaw. Finally, the nurse assesses the client's personal and family history for heart disease (see box below).

Inspection and Palpation

The examination begins with the client supine and the upper body elevated 45 degrees, because clients with heart disease frequently suffer shortness of breath while lying flat. The nurse stands at the client's right side. The client must not talk, especially when the nurse auscultates heart sounds. Good lighting in the room is essential.

The nurse directs attention to the anatomic sites best suited for assessment of cardiac function. The sternal angle or Louis' angle can be felt as a ridge in the sternum approximately 2 inches below the sternal notch. The nurse slips the fingers along the angle on each side of the sternum to feel the adjacent ribs. The intercostal spaces are just below each rib. The second intercostal space allows for identification of each of the 6 anatomic landmarks (Figure 16-36, dots *1* and *2*). The second intercostal space on the right is the aortic area *(dot 1),* and the left second intercostal space is the pulmonic area *(dot 2).* Deeper palpation is needed to feel the spaces in obese or heavily muscled clients. After the pulmonic area is located, the nurse moves the fingers along the client's sternal border to the third intercostal space, called *Erb's point (dot 3).* The tricuspid area *(dot 4)* is located at the fifth intercostal space along the sternum. To find the apical area the nurse locates the fifth intercostal space just to the left of the sternum and moves the fingers laterally to the left midclavicular line *(dot 5).* Some can locate the apical area with the palm of the hand, but others use the fingertips. Normally at the point of maximal impulse (PMI) the apical pulse is a light tap felt in an area 1 to 2 cm ($\frac{1}{2}$ in) in diameter at the apex. The final landmark is the epigastric area at the tip of the sternum *(dot 6).*

As the nurse locates the six anatomic landmarks of the heart, each area is inspected and palpated. The

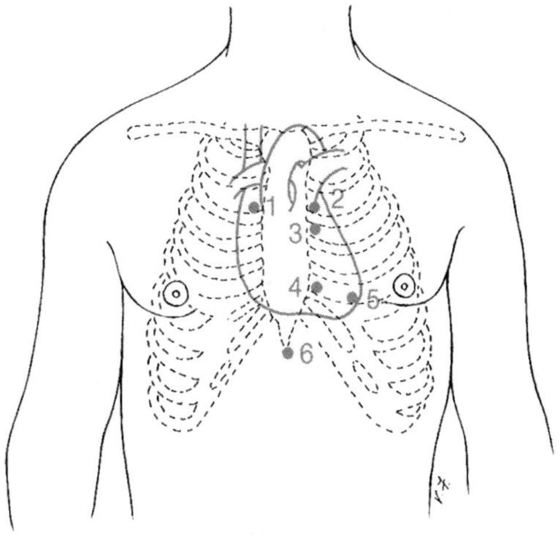

FIGURE 16-36 Anatomical sites for assessment of cardiac function.

nurse looks for the appearance of pulsations, viewing each area over the chest at an angle to the side. Normally, no pulsations can be seen except perhaps at the PMI in thin clients or at the epigastric area as a result of abdominal aorta pulsation. Palpation for pulsations is best done using the proximal halves of the four fingers together and then alternating with the ball of the hand. The nurse touches the areas gently to allow movements to lift the hand. Normally no pulsations or vibrations can be felt in the aortic, pulmonic, Erb's point, or tricuspid area.

The apical impulse should be felt easily. If not, the nurse has the client turn onto the left side, moving the heart closer to the chest wall. The PMI may be difficult to find in older adults because the chest deepens in its anteroposterior diameters. It may also be difficult to find in muscular or overweight clients. An infant's PMI is usually found near the third or fourth intercostal space. It is easy to palpate because of the child's thin chest wall.

Auscultation

Auscultation of the heart detects normal heart sounds, extra heart sounds, and murmurs. Concentration is needed to detect the low-intensity sounds caused by valve closure. To begin auscultation the nurse eliminates all sources of room noise and explains the procedure to relieve the client's anxiety. The nurse follows a systematic pattern beginning with the aortic area and inching the stethoscope along each of the six landmarks. The nurse must be sure to hear heart sounds clearly at each location. Then the sequence is repeated using the bell of the stethoscope. The client may be asked to assume three different positions during the examination (Figure 16-37):

Sitting up and leaning forward (good for all areas and to hear high-pitched murmurs)
Supine (good for all areas)
Left lateral recumbent (good for all areas and is best position to hear low-pitched sounds in diastole)

The nurse learns to identify the first and second heart sounds (S_1 and S_2). At normal rates, S_1 occurs after the long diastolic pause and preceding the short systolic pause. S_1 is high pitched, dull in quality, and heard best at the apex. If the nurse has difficulty hearing S_1, it can be timed in relation to the carotid pulse. It occurs just before the carotid pulsation. S_2 follows the short systolic phase and precedes the long diastolic phase. It is heard best at the aortic area.

The nurse auscultates for rate and rhythm after both sounds can be heard clearly (see Chapter 15). Each combination of S_1 and S_2 or "lub-dub" counts as one heartbeat. The nurse counts the rate for 1 minute and listens for the interval between S_1 and S_2 and then the

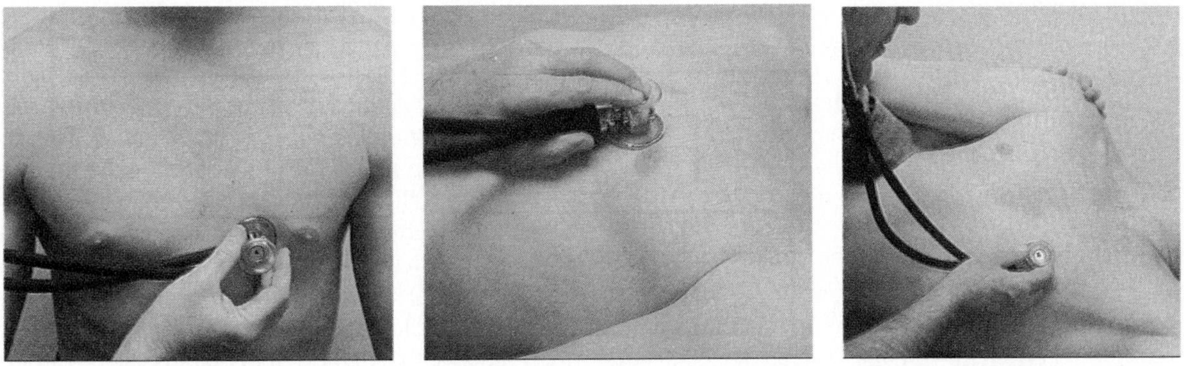

A **B** **C**

FIGURE 16-37 Sequence of client positions for auscultation. **A,** Sitting up and leaning slightly forward. **B,** Supine. **C,** Left lateral recumbent. (From Seidel HM, et al.: *Mosby's guide to physical examination,* ed 2, St. Louis, 1991, Mosby.)

time between S_2 and the next S_1. A regular rhythm involves regular intervals of time between each sequence of beats. There is a distinct silent pause between S_1 and S_2. Failure of the heart to beat at regular successive intervals is a **dysrhythmia.** Some dysrhythmias can be life threatening (see Chapter 34).

When the heart rhythm is irregular, the nurse compares apical and radial pulse rates to determine if a pulse deficit exists. The nurse auscultates the apical pulse first and then immediately assesses the radial pulse (one examiner technique). When two examiners are available, the apical and radial rates are assessed at the same time. Compare the two rates. When a client has a *pulse deficit,* the radial pulse is slower than the apical because ineffective contractions fail to send pulse waves to the periphery. A difference in pulse rates is reported to the physician immediately.

The nurse also learns to assess for extra heart sounds at each auscultatory site. Using the bell of the stethoscope, the nurse listens for low-pitched sounds such as S_3 and S_4 gallops, clicks, and rubs. S_3 or a *ventricular gallop* occurs just after S_2 at the end of ventricular diastole. Some examiners describe the combination of S_1, S_2, and S_3 as sounding like "Ken-tuc-ky." It can be a sign of heart failure in adults.

S_4 or an *atrial gallop* occurs just before S_1 or ventricular systole. The sound of an S_4 is similar to that of "Tennessee." It may indicate hypertension. One can often hear extra sounds more easily with the client on the left side and the stethoscope at the apical site.

The final portion of the examination includes assessment for heart murmurs. **Murmurs** are sustained swishing or blowing sounds heard at the beginning, middle, or end of the systolic or diastolic pause. They are caused by an increased blood flow through a normal valve, forward flow through a stenotic valve or a dilated vessel or heart chamber, or backward flow through a valve that fails to close. A murmur can be asymptomatic or a sign of heart disease. Murmurs are common in children. Murmurs that occur between S_1 and S_2 are systolic, whereas murmurs that occur between S_2 and the next S_1 are diastolic. The nurse notes the intensity or loudness of murmurs, with grade I murmurs being barely audible and grade VI murmurs being loud enough to be heard without a stethoscope.

VASCULAR SYSTEM

Examination of the vascular system includes measuring the blood pressure (see Chapter 15) and assessing the integrity of the peripheral vascular system. The skills of inspection, palpation, and auscultation are used. The nurse notes the condition of extremities perfused by the vascular system. Disturbances in arterial perfusion or venous return cause skin and tissue changes in affected extremities. The nurse may perform portions of the vascular examination during other body system assessments.

Health History. The health history includes determining if the client has leg cramps, numbness or tingling in the extremities, or the sensation of cold hands or feet. These signs and symptoms indicate vascular disease. The nurse also learns if the client has noted swelling or cyanosis of the feet, ankles, or hand, or pain in the feet or legs. If the client has leg pain or cramps, the nurse asks if symptoms are aggravated by walking or standing for long periods or during sleep. This question helps to clarify if the problem is musculoskeletal or vascular in nature. For example, arterial occlusion can create muscle ischemia or **claudication.** This particular type of pain is a dull ache and cramping, usually appearing during sustained exercise and disappearing after a short rest. Musculoskeletal pain is not generally relieved when exercise ends. The nurse also asks if clients wear tight-fitting garters or hosiery and sit or lie in bed with their legs crossed. These activities can impair venous return. The history includes a review of the client's medical history for heart disease, hypertension, phlebitis, diabetes, or varicose veins. Finally, risk factors assessed earlier for smoking, exercise, and nutritional problems are important when assessing the vascular system.

Carotid Arteries

When the left ventricle pumps blood into the aorta, pressure waves are transmitted throughout the arterial system. The carotid artery reflects heart function better than peripheral arteries because its pressure correlates with that of the aorta. The carotid artery supplies oxygenated blood to the head and neck (Figure 16-38) and is protected by the overlying sternocleidomastoid muscle.

To examine the carotid arteries, the nurse has the client sit or lie supine with the head of the bed elevated 15 to 30 degrees. *One carotid artery is examined at a time.* If both arteries were to be occluded during palpation, the client could lose consciousness as a result of inadequate circulation to the brain. *The carotid arteries must not be vigorously palpated or massaged.* The carotid sinus is in the upper third of the neck. Its stimulation can cause a reflex drop in heart rate and blood pressure.

To inspect the right common carotid, the nurse has the client turn the head slightly to the left. Then the nurse looks at the medial border of the sternocleidomastoid muscle. The neck is inspected for obvious, forceful pulsation of the artery. Repeat the procedure for the left common carotid with the client's head turned slightly to the right (Durham, 1988). Sometimes, the wave of the pulse can actually be seen.

To palpate the pulse, ask the client to look straight

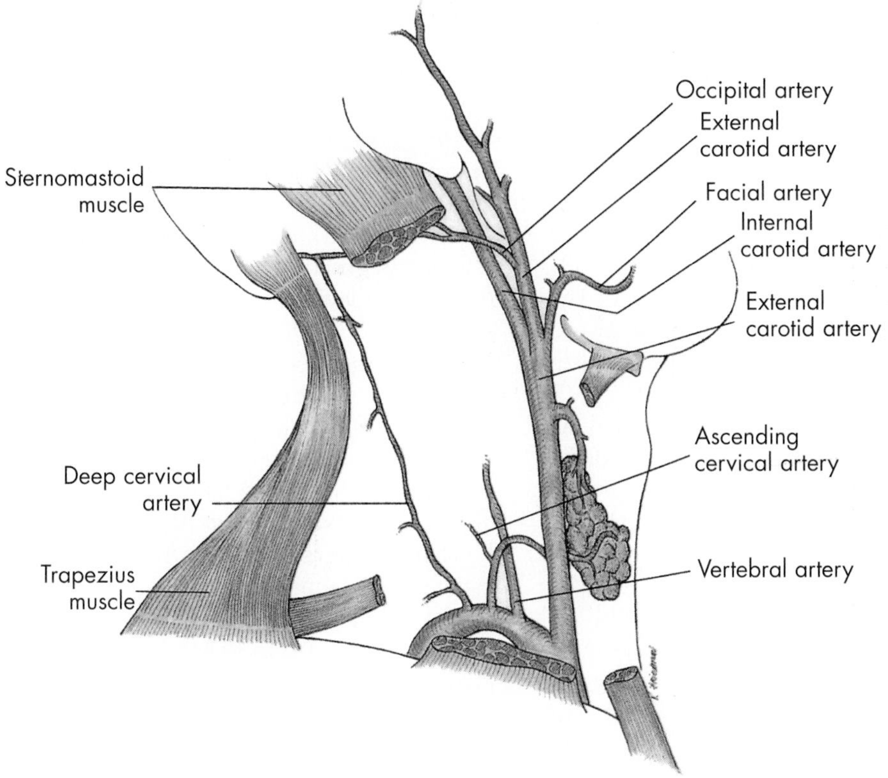

FIGURE 16-38 Anatomical position of carotid artery.

ahead or turn the head slightly to the side being examined. Turning relaxes the sternocleidomastoid muscle. The nurse slides the index and middle fingers around the medial edge of the sternocleidomastoid muscle. The nurse palpates gently to avoid occlusion of circulation (Figure 16-39).

The normal **carotid pulse** is localized rather than diffuse. As a strong pulse, the carotid has a thrusting quality. As the client breathes, no change occurs. Rotation of the neck or a shift from a sitting to a supine position should not change the carotid's quality. Both carotid arteries should be equal in pulse rate, rhythm, and strength and should be equally elastic. If the nurse palpates diminished or unequal carotid pulsations, the client may have atherosclerosis or other forms of arterial disease.

The carotid is the only pulse that is auscultated. Auscultation is especially important for middle-age or older adults or clients suspected of having cerebrovascular disease. When the lumen of a blood vessel is narrowed, its blood flow is disturbed. As blood passes through the narrowed section, a turbulence is created, causing a blowing or swishing sound. The blowing sound is called a **bruit** (pronounced "brew-ee"). The bell of the stethoscope is placed over the carotid artery at the base of the neck and moved gradually toward the jaw. The nurse

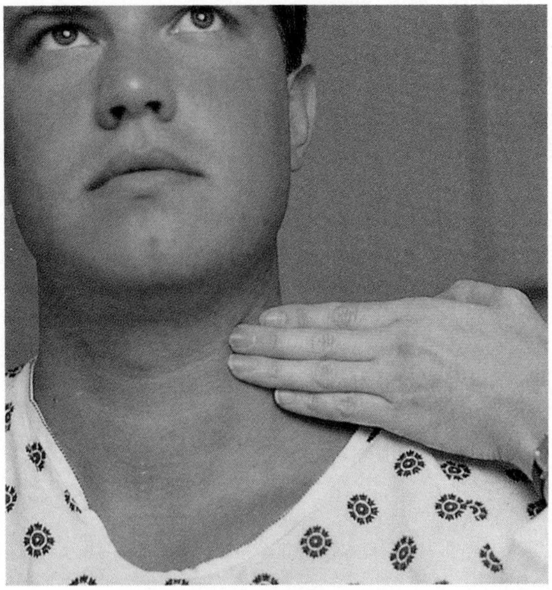

FIGURE 16-39 Palpation of internal carotid artery.

asks the client to hold the breath. Normally, no sound is heard. If a bruit is heard, the nurse notes its pitch, loudness, location, and timing in relation to the cardiac cycle and reports it to a physician.

Jugular Veins

The most accessible veins are the internal and external jugular veins in the neck. Both veins drain bilaterally from the head and neck into the superior vena cava. The external jugular lies superficially and can be seen just above the clavicle. The internal jugular lies deeper, along the carotid artery.

It is best to examine the right internal jugular because it follows a more direct anatomical path to the right atrium of the heart. The column of blood inside the internal jugular reflects pressure in the right atrium. The higher the column, the greater the venous pressure. Raised venous pressure indicates right-sided heart failure.

When a client lies supine, the external jugular commonly distends and becomes easily visible. The jugular veins normally flatten when the client is sitting. A client with right-sided heart disease may have distended jugular veins when sitting.

The jugular veins are inspected to assess for elevations in venous pressures, which can be caused by increased blood volume, the reduced capacity of the right atrium to receive blood and send it to the right ventricle, and the reduced ability of the right ventricle to contract and force blood into the pulmonary artery. Any factor resulting in greater blood volume within the venous system causes elevated venous pressure.

The nurse first has the client sit upright at a 90 degree angle and inspects the jugular veins. Normal veins are flat and pulsations are not evident. Then the nurse asks the client to lie supine with the head elevated 30 to 45 degrees. The neck and upper thorax should be visible. A pillow can be used to align the head (Figure 16-40). Hyperextension or flexion may stretch or kink the vein. The nurse looks for the usual position of the internal jugular vein, just visible 2 to 3 cm (1 in) above the sternal angle or suprasternal notch. Next, the nurse places a palm over the client's right upper abdominal quadrant. Moderately firm pressure is applied 30 to 60 seconds. If jugular venous pressure increases, the vein

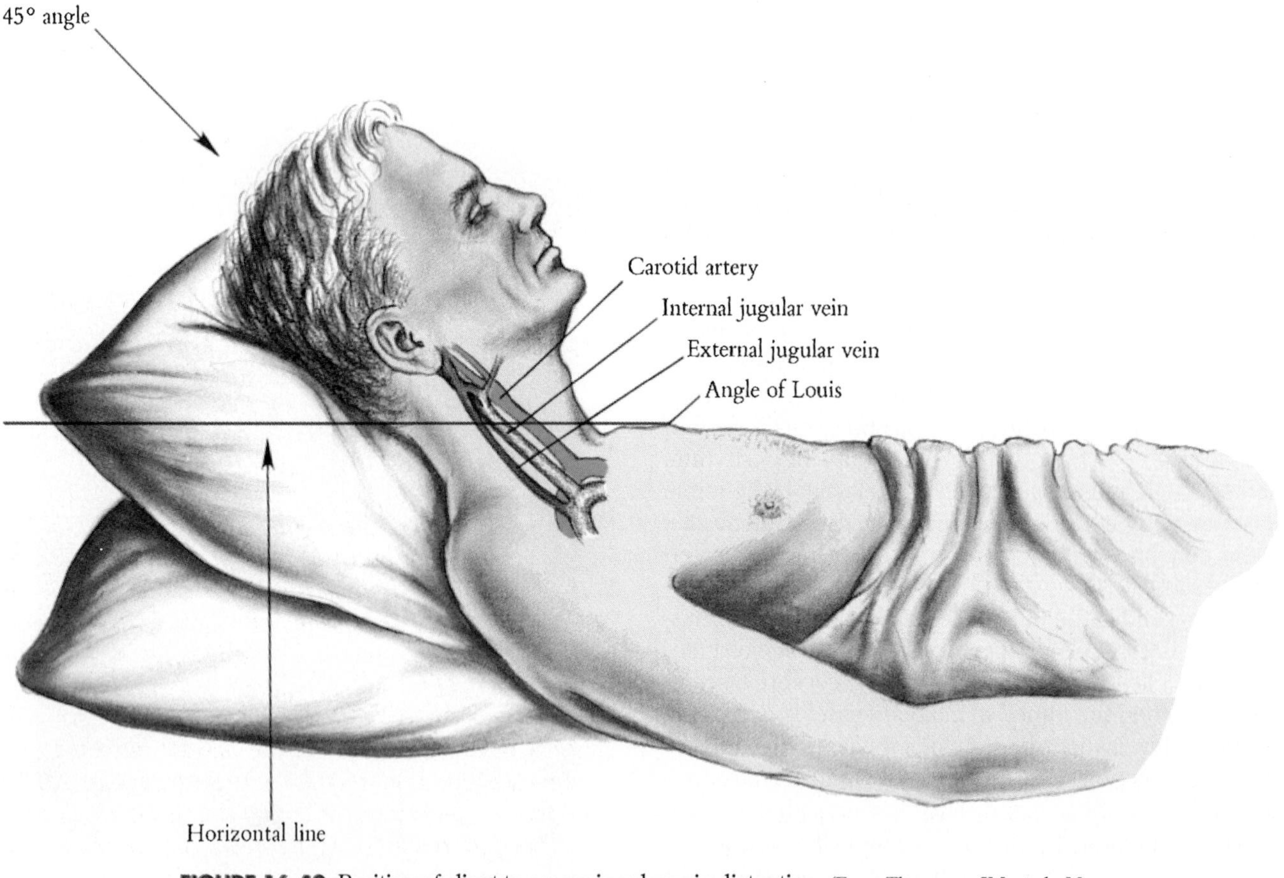

FIGURE 16-40 Position of client to assess jugular vein distention. (From Thompson JM, et al.: *Mosby's manual of clinical nursing,* ed 3, St. Louis, 1993, Mosby.)

will appear more prominent. This response is called the *hepatojugular reflux* and should be reported to a physician immediately.

Peripheral Arteries

The most accurate assessment of peripheral arteries involves palpation over arteries that are close to the body surface and lie over bones. An arterial pulsation is a bounding wave of blood that diminishes in intensity with increasing distance from the heart (Seidel, et al., 1991).

The nurse assesses the arterial pulses in the extremities to determine sufficiency of the entire arterial circulation. Factors such as coagulation disorders, local trauma or surgery, constricting casts or bandages, and systemic disease such as diabetes or arteriosclerosis can impair circulation to the extremities. The nurse should discuss with the client the risk for circulatory problems (see box below).

The nurse examines each peripheral artery using the distal pads of the second and third fingers. The thumb may help anchor the brachial and femoral artery. The nurse applies firm pressure but avoids occluding the pulse. When it is difficult to find a pulse, it is helpful to vary pressure and feel all around the pulse site. The nurse must be sure not to palpate his or her own pulse.

Routine vital signs usually include assessment of the rate and rhythm of the radial artery because it is easily accessible (see Chapter 15). The pulse is counted for either 30 seconds or a full minute, depending on the character of the pulse. With palpation the nurse normally feels the pulse wave at regular intervals. When an interval is interrupted by an early, late, or missed beat, the pulse rhythm is irregular. In emergencies, the carotid artery is chosen because it is accessible and closest to the heart and thus most useful in evaluating heart activity. To check local circulatory status of tissues, the nurse palpates peripheral arteries long enough to note that a pulse is present.

The nurse assesses each peripheral pulse site for elasticity, contour of the pulse wave, amplitude or strength, and equality. The arterial wall is normally elastic, making it easily palpable. After the artery is depressed, it will spring back to shape when pressure is released. An abnormal artery may be described as hard, inelastic, or calcified.

The contour of a pulse wave in a healthy artery is smooth, rounded, or domed in shape. An experienced nurse can feel the ascending contour, peak, and descending part of the wave. The nurse compares each pulse wave with the next to determine cyclic differences. Normally pulse waves are equal. A weak or thready pulse is slower to rise, has a sustained peak, and falls more slowly than normal.

The strength of a pulse is a measurement of the force in which blood is ejected against the arterial wall. Some examiners use a rating from 0 (zero) to 4+ (Seidel, et al., 1991):

0 Absent, not palpable
1+ Pulse is diminished, barely palpable
2+ Easily palpable, normal pulse
3+ Full, increased pulse
4+ Bounding, cannot be obliterated.

All peripheral pulses are measured for equality and symmetry. The left radial pulse is compared with that of the right, the left brachial pulse is compared with the left radial, and so on. Lack of symmetry may indicate impaired circulation such as a localized obstruction or an abnormally positioned artery.

In the upper extremities the brachial artery channels blood to the radial and ulnar arteries of the forearm and hand. If circulation in this artery becomes blocked, the hands will not receive adequate blood flow. If circulation in the radial or ulnar arteries becomes impaired, the hand will still receive adequate perfusion. An interconnection between the radial and ulnar arteries guards against arterial occlusion (Figure 16-41).

To locate pulses in the arm, the nurse has the client sit or lie down. The **radial pulse** is found along the radial side of the forearm at the wrist. In a thin individual a groove is formed lateral to the flexor tendon of the wrist. The radial pulse can be felt with light palpation in the groove (Figure 16-42). The **ulnar pulse** is on the opposite side of the wrist and feels less prominent (Figure 16-43). An examiner palpates the ulnar pulse only when arterial insufficiency to the hand is expected.

If a client has a weak radial or ulnar pulse, the Allen's test can be performed to assess collateral circulation. The client makes a fist as the ulnar and radial arteries are compressed simultaneously. The client then opens the hand, and the nurse releases the ulnar artery. The

CLIENT TEACHING DURING VASCULAR ASSESSMENT

Tell clients their blood pressure readings. Explain the normal reading for a client's age. Discuss implications of abnormalities.

Instruct clients with risk or evidence of vascular insufficiency in the lower extremities to avoid tight clothing over the lower body or legs, to avoid sitting or standing for long periods, to walk regularly, and to elevate the feet when sitting.

Advise client to avoid cigarette smoking because nicotine causes vasoconstriction.

Older adults with hypertension may benefit from regular self-monitoring of blood pressure (daily, weekly, or monthly). Consult with physician regarding device to use.

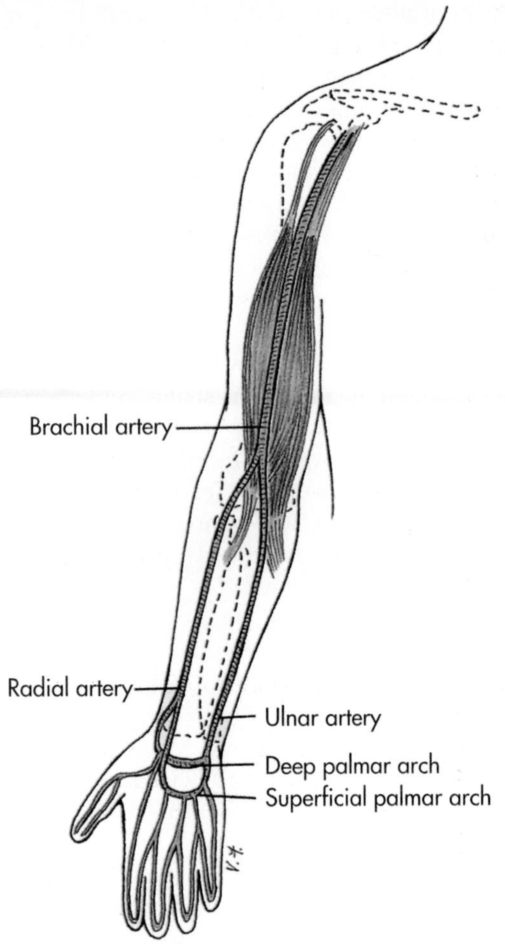

FIGURE 16-41 Anatomical positions of brachial, radial, and ulnar arteries.

hand should quickly turn pink if the ulnar artery is patent. The test may be repeated by releasing only the radial artery.

To palpate the **brachial pulse,** the nurse finds the groove between the biceps and triceps muscle above the elbow at the antecubital fossa (Figure 16-44). The artery runs along the medial side of the extended arm. The nurse palpates the artery with the fingertips of the first three fingers in the muscle groove.

The femoral artery is the primary artery in the leg, delivering blood to the popliteal, posterior tibial, and dorsalis pedis arteries (Figure 16-45). An interconnection between the posterior tibial and dorsalis pedis arteries guards against local arterial occlusion.

The **femoral pulse** is found best with the client lying down with the inguinal area exposed (Figure 16-46). The femoral artery runs below the inguinal ligament, midway between the symphysis pubis and the anterosuperior iliac spine. Deep palpation may be required to feel the pulse. Bimanual palpation is effective in obese clients. The nurse places the fingertips of both hands on opposite sides of the pulse site. A pulsatile sensation can be felt as the fingertips are pushed apart by the arterial pulsation.

The **popliteal pulse** is found behind the knee (Figure 16-47). The client should slightly flex the knee with the foot resting on the examination table. The client may also assume a prone position with the knee slightly flexed. The client is instructed to keep leg muscles relaxed. The nurse palpates with the fingers of both hands deeply into the popliteal fossa, just lateral to the midline. The popliteal pulse is one of the more difficult pulses to locate.

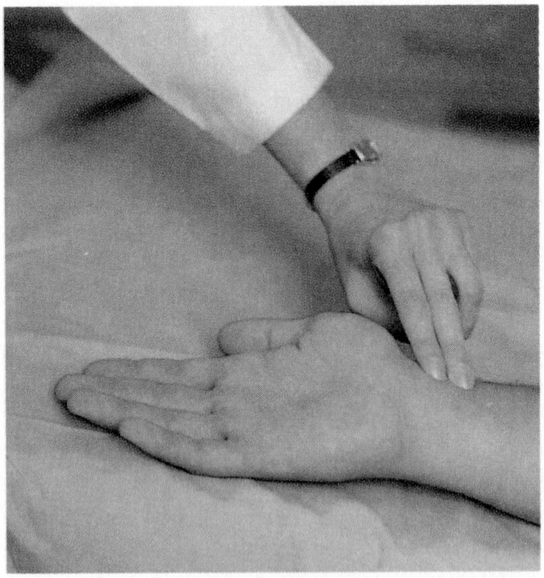

FIGURE 16-42 Palpation of radial pulse.

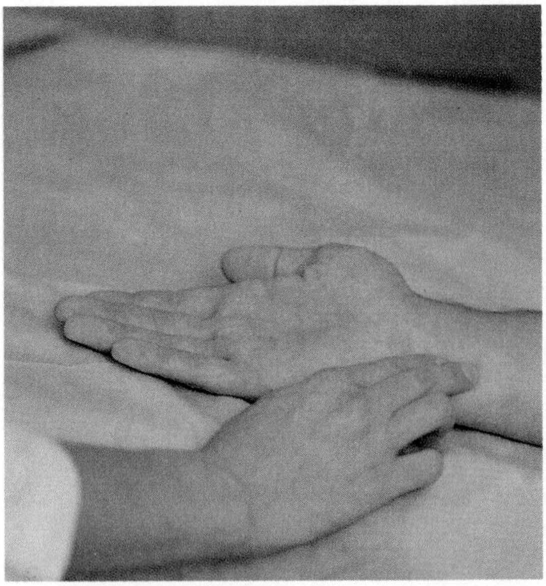

FIGURE 16-43 Palpation of ulnar pulse.

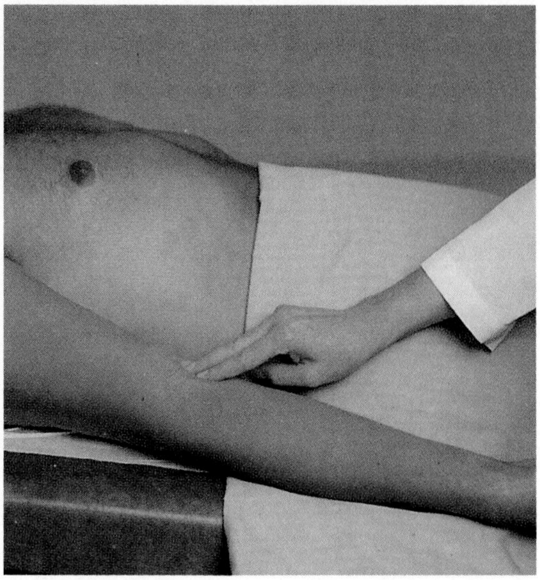

FIGURE 16-44 Palpation of brachial pulse.

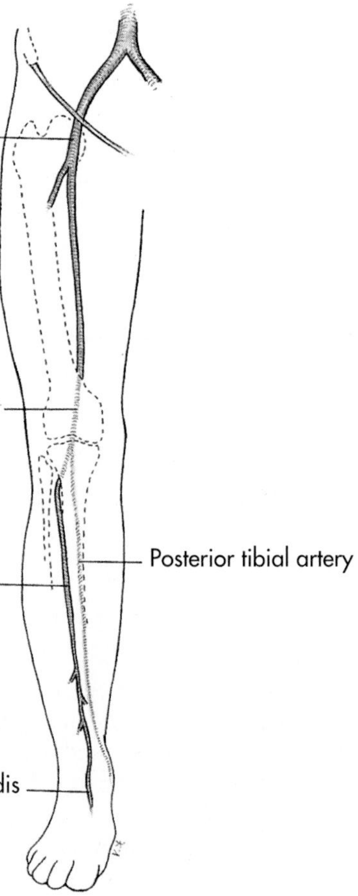

FIGURE 16-45 Anatomical position of femoral, popliteal, dorsalis pedis, and posterior tibial arteries.

With the client's foot relaxed the nurse locates the **dorsalis pedis pulse.** The artery runs along the top of the foot in a line with the groove between the extensor tendons of the great toe and first toe (Figure 16-48). Often an examiner finds the pulse by placing the fingertips between the great and first toe and slowly inching up the foot. This pulse may be congenitally absent.

The **posterior tibial pulse** is found on the inner side of each ankle (Figure 16-49). The nurse places the fingers behind and below the client's medial malleolus (an-

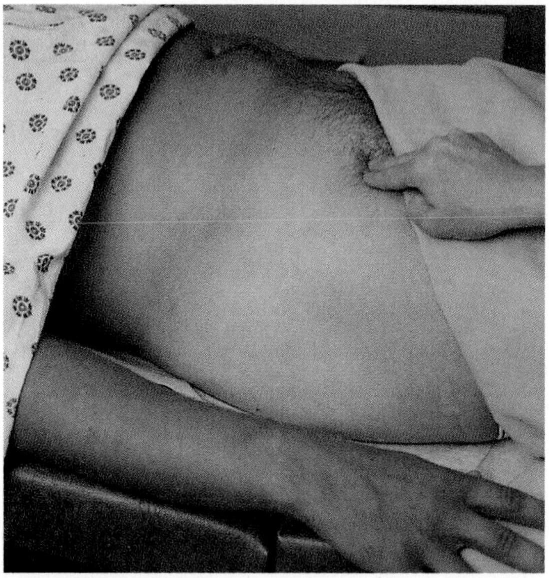

FIGURE 16-46 Palpation of femoral pulse.

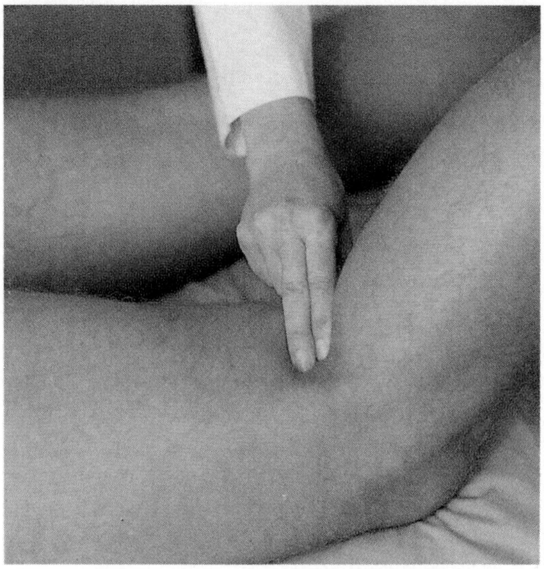

FIGURE 16-47 Palpation of popliteal pulse.

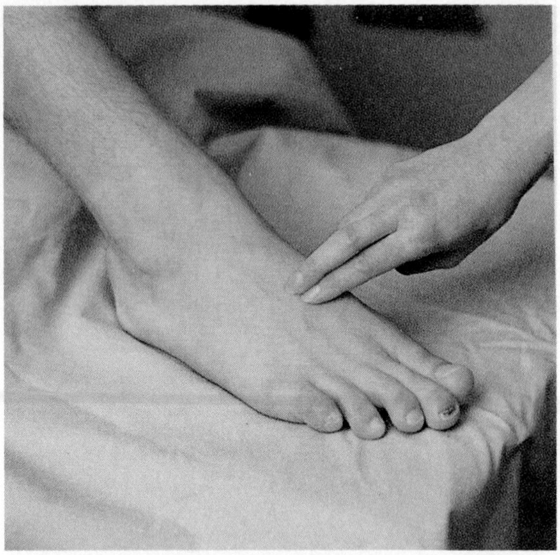

FIGURE 16-48 Palpation of dorsalis pedis pulse.

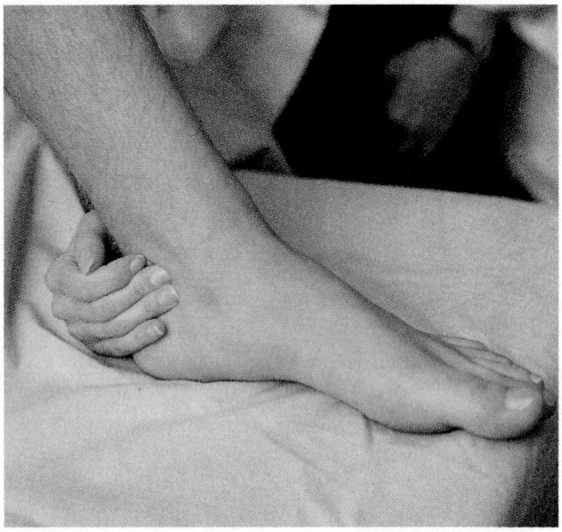

FIGURE 16-49 Palpation of posterior tibial pulse.

kle bone). The artery is easily located with the client's foot relaxed and slightly extended.

Ultrasound Stethoscopes

If a nurse has difficulty palpating a pulse, an ultrasound stethoscope is a useful tool that can amplify sounds of a pulse wave. A thin layer of transmission gel is first applied to the client's skin at the pulse site or directly onto the transducer tip of the probe. The nurse then turns the volume control to "on" and places the tip of the probe at a 45- to 90-degree angle on the skin. The nurse moves the probe until hearing a pulsating "whooshing" sound that indicates that arterial blood flow is present.

table 16-5

SIGNS OF VENOUS AND ARTERIAL INSUFFICIENCY

Assessment criterion	Venous	Arterial
Color	Normal or cyanotic	Pale; worsened by elevation of extremity; dusky red when extremity lowered
Temperature	Normal	Cool (blood flow blocked to extremity)
Pulse	Normal	Decreased or absent
Edema	Often marked	Absent or mild
Skin changes	Brown pigmentation around ankles	Thin, shiny skin; decreased hair growth; thickened nails

Peripheral Veins

The nurse assesses the status of the peripheral veins by asking the client to assume sitting and standing positions. Assessment includes inspection and palpation of the skin, nail beds, and extremities for signs of venous insufficiency versus arterial insufficiency (Table 16-5). If an arterial occlusion is present, the client has signs resulting from an absence in blood flow. Venous congestion causes tissue changes, indicating an inadequate circulatory flow back to the heart.

The nurse inspects the lower extremities for varicosities, peripheral edema, and phlebitis. Varicosities are superficial veins that become dilated. They are common in older adults because the veins normally fibrose, dilate, and stretch. They are also common in people who stand for prolonged periods. Varicosities in the anterior or medial part of the thigh and the posterolateral part of the calf are abnormal.

Dependent edema around the feet and ankles can be a sign of venous insufficiency or right-sided heart failure. To assess for pitting edema the nurse uses a thumb to press firmly over the medial malleolus or the shins. A depression left in the skin indicates edema. The severity of the edema is characterized by grading 1+ through 4+ (Figure 16-50).

Phlebitis is an inflammation of a vein that occurs commonly after trauma to the vessel wall, infection, immobilization, and after prolonged insertion of intravenous catheters (see Chapter 35). Phlebitis promotes clot formation, a potentially dangerous situation be-

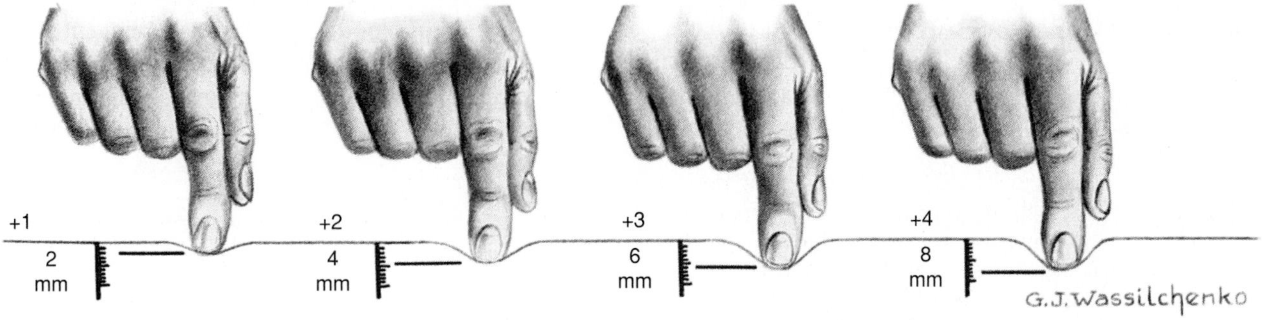

FIGURE 16-50 Assessing for pitting edema. (From Seidel HM, et al.: *Mosby's guide to physical examination,* ed 2, St. Louis, 1991, Mosby.)

cause a clot within a deep vein of the leg can become dislodged and travel through the heart, causing a pulmonary embolus. The nurse inspects superficial veins for redness and thickening, and palpates gently for tenderness. The color should be the same as normal skin and there should be no tenderness. If veins in the calves appear reddened or swollen, the nurse gently palpates the calf muscles, noting tenderness or firmness of muscle. The nurse may also check for Homans' sign by supporting the leg while dorsiflexing the foot. If phlebitis is present in the lower leg, forced dorsiflexion causes pain in the calf. The nurse refers a client who is complaining of calf pain to a physician immediately.

Lymphatic System

The legs are drained by superficial and deep lymph nodes, but only two groups of superficial nodes are palpable. With the client supine, the nurse palpates the area of the superior superficial nodes in the groin area (Figure 16-51). Then the nurse moves the fingertips toward the inner thigh, feeling for any palpable inferior nodes. Palpable superior nodes are not usually significant (McConnell, 1988). Enlarged inferior nodes may result from penile and scrotal lesions.

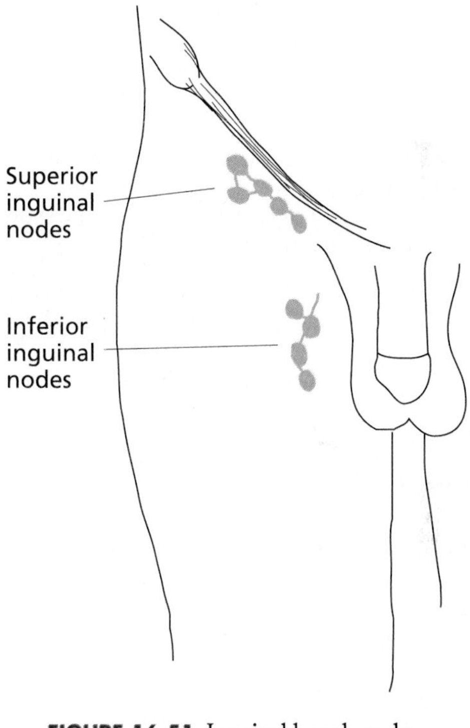

FIGURE 16-51 Inguinal lymph nodes.

BREASTS

It is important to examine the breasts of female and male clients. A small amount of glandular tissue, a potential site for the growth of cancer cells, is located in the male breast. In contrast, the majority of the female breast is glandular tissue.

Female Breasts

Breast cancer is the second leading cause of death among women. Approximately one of every nine women will develop breast cancer by age 85 (American Cancer Society, 1993). Early detection is the key to cure. A major responsibility for nurses is to teach clients health behaviors such as breast self-examination (BSE) (see box on p. 344). Studies suggest a minority of women actually perform BSE. Nurses should know factors that increase the likelihood of a woman performing BSE. Champion (1989) found that knowledge and individualized teaching with return demonstration correlated significantly with a woman's intent to practice BSE and with proficiency in examination.

If the client already performs self-examinations, the

BREAST SELF-EXAMINATION

Instruct client on BSE. All women 20 years of age and older should perform this self-examination monthly using the following steps:

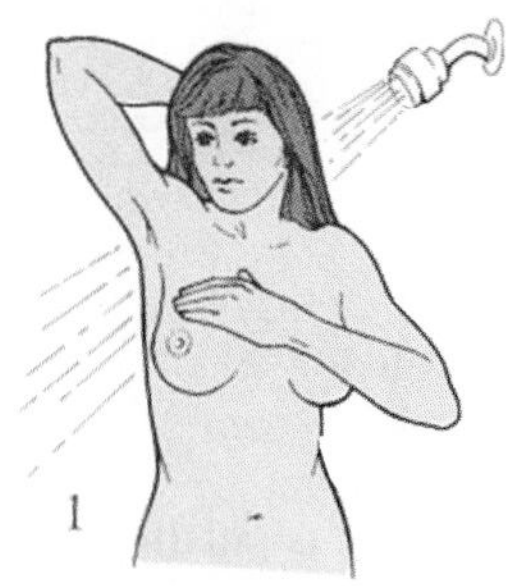

1. Stand before a mirror. Look at both breasts for anything unusual, such as discharge from the nipples, puckering, dimpling, or scaling of the skin.
2. To note changes in the shape of the breasts, perform the following measures (see figure 2):

   Watch in the mirror while raising the arms above the head.

   Press hands firmly on the hips and bow slightly toward the mirror when pulling the shoulders and elbows forward.

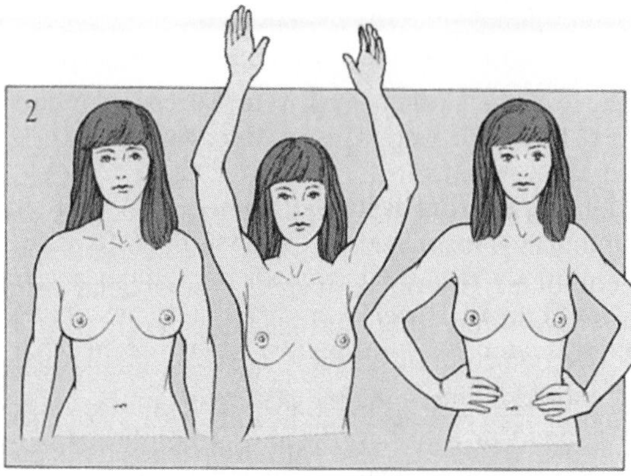

3. In the shower or in front of the mirror, palpate each breast. Raise the left arm and use three or four fingers of the right hand to explore the breast carefully (see figure 1). Then start at the outer edge, pressing the flat part of the fingers in small circles, moving the circles slowly around the breast, gradually working toward the nipple. Pay close attention to the area between the breast and armpit and feel for unusual lumps or masses. Repeat the process for the right breast (see figure 3).

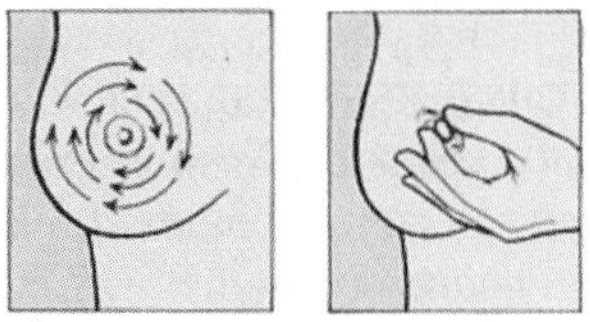

3

4. Gently squeeze each nipple, looking for discharge (see figure 3).
5. Repeat the third and fourth steps lying down. Lie flat on the back with the left arm over the head and a small pillow under the left shoulder. Palpate the left breast. Repeat the process on the right breast.
6. Call your physician if you find a lump.

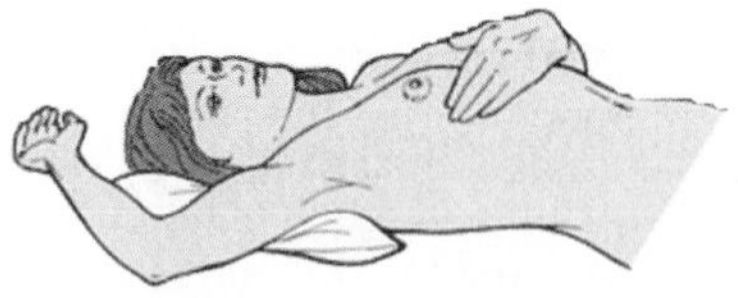

Illustrations from Payne WA, Hahn DB: *Understanding your health,* ed 2, St. Louis, 1989, Mosby.

nurse determines the method she uses and the time she does the examination in relation to her menstrual cycle. The best time for a self-examination is on the last day of the menstrual period, when the breast is no longer swollen or tender from hormone elevations. If the woman is postmenopausal, she should check her breasts the same time each month. The pregnant woman also must check her breasts on a monthly basis.

Older women may require special assistance when learning BSE. Many older women ignore changes in their breasts, assuming they are a part of aging. Normal physiological changes of aging that affect the breast can mimic breast cancer (Williams, et al., 1987). Many older adults have fixed incomes that prohibit regular clinical examinations and mammography. The physiological factors of aging can affect the ease in which older women can perform BSE. Musculoskeletal limitations, diminished peripheral sensation, reduced eyesight, and changes in joint range of motion can limit palpation and inspection abilities. The nurse should find resources such as family members or free screening programs for older clients.

The American Cancer Society (1993) recommends the following guidelines for the early detection of breast cancer:

1. Breast self-examination (BSE) should be performed monthly by women 20 years of age and older.

2. An examination by a physician should be performed every 3 years from ages 20 to 40, and yearly for women over 40. Women with a family history of breast cancer should have a yearly examination.
3. A screening mammogram is a low-dose x-ray examination that can detect breast cancer early. There has been recent controversy over its efficacy (especially in women ages 40 to 50). However, the ACS recommends it should be performed by age 40. Thereafter, women 40 to 49 should have a mammogram every 1 to 2 years; asymptomatic women age 50 and over should have a mammogram yearly. Women age 40 or over with a family history of breast cancer should have a yearly mammogram.

Health History. A health history can reveal risk factors for breast cancer, including clients over age 40, women with a personal or family history of breast cancer, women with early onset menarche or late age menopause, and women who have never had children, who gave birth to their first child after age 30, or who have not breastfed their infants. A health history should also determine whether a woman has a history of signs and symptoms of breast cancer such as a lump, thickening, pain or tenderness of the breast; discharge, distortion, retraction, or scaling of the nipple; or change in breast size. The client's use of medications such as oral contraceptives, digitalis, diuretics, steroids, estrogen, or foods high in fat is also assessed. The nurse assesses the client's caffeine intake to review risk factors for fibrocystic disease. Finally, the nurse determines the date of the first day of the client's last menstrual period and reviews the typical onset, course, and associated problems.

Inspection. The client is asked to remove the top gown or drape to allow simultaneous visualization of both breasts. The client may stand or sit with her arms hanging loosely at her sides. If possible, the nurse places a mirror in front of the client during inspection so she can see what to look for when performing a self-examination. To recognize abnormalities, the client must be familiar with the normal appearance of her breasts.

The nurse describes observations or findings in relation to imaginary lines that divide the breast into four quadrants and a tail. The lines cross at the center of the nipple. Each tail extends outward from the upper outer quadrant (Figure 16-52).

Both breasts are inspected for size and symmetry. Normally, the breasts extend from the third to the sixth ribs, with the nipple at the level of the fourth intercostal space. It is common for one breast to be smaller. However, a difference in size may be caused by inflammation or a mass. As the woman becomes older, the ligaments supporting the breast tissue weaken, causing the breasts to sag and the nipples to lower.

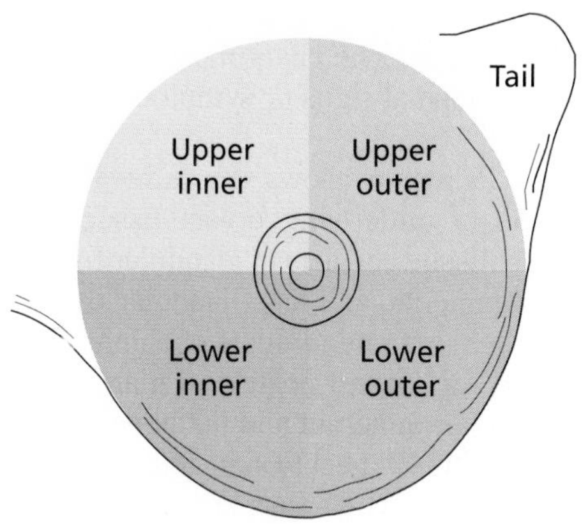

FIGURE 16-52 Breast divided into four quadrants and an axillary tail.

The nurse observes the contour or shape of the breasts and notes masses, flattening, retraction, or dimpling. Breasts vary in shape from convex to pendulous or conical. Retraction or dimpling results from invasion of underlying ligaments by tumors. The ligaments fibrose and pull the overlying skin inward toward the tumor. Edema also changes the breasts' contour. To bring out the presence of retraction or changes in the shape of breasts, the nurse asks the client to assume three positions: raise arms above the head, press hands against the hips, and extend arms straight ahead while sitting and leaning forward. Each maneuver causes a contraction of the pectoral muscles, which will accentuate the presence of any retraction.

The overlying skin is carefully inspected for color, venous pattern, and presence of edema, lesions, or inflammation. The nurse lifts each breast when necessary to observe lower and lateral aspects for color and texture changes. The breasts are the color of neighboring skin and venous patterns are the same bilaterally. Venous patterns are more easily seen in thin clients or pregnant women. Women with large breasts often have redness and excoriation of the undersurface caused by rubbing of skin surfaces.

The nurse inspects the nipple and areola for size, color, shape, discharge, and the direction the nipples point. The normal areolae are round or oval and nearly equal bilaterally. Color ranges from pink to brown. In light-skinned women the areola turns brown during pregnancy and remains dark. In dark-skinned women the areola is brown before pregnancy (Seidel, et al., 1991). Normally the nipples point in symmetrical directions, they are everted, and without drainage. If the nipples are inverted, the nurse asks if this has been a lifetime history. A recent inversion or inward turning of the nipple may indicate an underlying growth. Rashes or ulcerations are not normal on the breast or nipples. Bleeding or discharge from the nipple is noted. Clear yellow discharge 2 days after childbirth is common.

While inspecting the breasts the nurse explains the characteristics seen. The client must be taught the significance of abnormal signs or symptoms.

Palpation. Palpation allows the nurse to determine the condition of underlying breast tissue and lymph nodes. Breast tissue consists of glandular tissue, fibrous supportive ligaments, and fat. Glandular tissue is organized into lobes that end in ducts opening onto the nipple's surface. The largest portion of glandular tissue is in the upper outer quadrant and tail of each breast. Suspensory ligaments connect to skin and fascia underlying the breast to support the breast and maintain its upright position. Fatty tissue is located superficially to and to the sides of the breast.

A large proportion of lymph from the breasts drains into axillary lymph nodes. If cancerous lesions metastasize or spread, the nodes commonly become involved. The nurse learns the location of supraclavicular, infraclavicular, and axillary nodes (Figure 16-53). A tumor of one breast may involve nodes on the opposite side, as well as those on the same side.

To palpate lymph nodes the nurse has the client sit with arms at her sides and muscles relaxed. While facing the client and standing on the side being examined, the nurse supports the client's arm in a flexed position and abducts the arm from the chest wall. The nurse places the free hand against the client's chest wall and high in the axillary hollow. With the fingertips the nurse presses gently down over the surface of the ribs and muscles. The axillary nodes are palpated with the fingertips gently rolling soft tissue. Four areas of the axilla are palpated: at the edge of the pectoralis major muscle along the anterior axillary line, the chest wall in the mid-axillary area, the upper part of the humerus, and the anterior edge of the latissimus dorsi muscle along the posterior axillary line. Normally lymph nodes are not palpable. A palpable node feels like a small mass that may be hard, tender, and immobile. The nurse also palpates along the upper and lower clavicular ridges. The procedure is reversed for the client's other side.

It may be difficult for the client to learn to palpate for lymph nodes. Lying down with the arm abducted makes the area more accessible. The client is instructed to use her left hand for the right axillary and clavicular areas and vice versa. The nurse can take the client's fingertips and move them in the proper circular fashion.

Palpation of breast tissue is best performed with the client lying supine and hands behind the neck. The supine position allows the breast tissue to flatten evenly against the chest wall. Often the examiner places a small pillow or towel under the client's shoulder blade to further position breast tissue.

The consistency of normal breast tissue varies widely. The breasts of a young client are firm and elastic. In an older client the tissue may feel stringy and nodular. The client's familiarity with the texture of her own breasts is most important; this is gained through monthly self-examination.

If the client complains of a mass, the nurse examines the opposite breast first to ensure an objective comparison of normal and abnormal tissue. The inframammary ridge at the lower edge of the breast is normally firm or hard but should not be confused with a tumor. The nurse uses the pads of the first three fingers to compress breast tissue gently against the chest wall, noting tissue consistency. Palpation is performed systematically in one of two ways: clockwise or counterclockwise, forming small circles with the fingers along each quadrant and the tail, or a back-and-forth technique with the fingers moving up and down each quadrant (Figure 16-54). Whatever approach is used, all surfaces of the breast must be palpated. The tail of Spence is where tumors develop most frequently. The nurse gives special attention to any areas of tenderness. After light palpation, the nurse repeats the examination with deeper palpation (Seidel, et al., 1991).

When palpating large pendulous breasts, the nurse uses a bimanual technique. The inferior portion of the breast is supported in one hand while the nurse uses the other hand to palpate breast tissue against the supporting hand.

Breast tissue normally feels dense, firm, and elastic. In fibrocystic disease, a common problem in women, tissue feels lumpy, but it is found bilaterally. With menopause, breast tissue shrinks and becomes softer. Older adults have elongated breasts that become flaccid. It may help to move the client's hand so she can feel normal tissue variations. Abnormal masses are palpated to determine location in relation to quadrants, diameter in centimeters, shape (e.g., round or discoid), consistency (soft, firm, or hard), tenderness, mobility, and discreteness (clear or unclear borders). Cancerous lesions are hard, fixed, nontender, and irregular in shape.

Special attention is given to palpating the nipple and areola. The entire surface is gently palpated. The thumb and index finger compress the nipple, and the nurse notes any discharge. As the nurse examines the nipple and areola, the nipple may become erect with wrinkling of the areola. These changes are normal.

After the nurse has completed the examination, the client can demonstrate self-palpation (see box on p. 347). Observing the client's technique helps the nurse to emphasize the importance of a systematic approach. The client is urged to see her physician if she discovers an abnormal mass during monthly self-examination. She also should know all signs and symptoms of breast cancer.

Male Breasts

Examination of the male breast is relatively easy. The nipple and areola are inspected for nodules, edema, and ulceration. An enlarged male breast may result from obesity or glandular enlargement. Breast enlargement in young males may be indicative of steroid use. Fatty tissue feels soft, whereas glandular tissue is firm. Masses are palpated for the same characteristics as in the female breast. Because male breast cancer is relatively rare, routine self-examinations are unnecessary.

CLIENT TEACHING DURING FEMALE BREAST ASSESSMENT

Have client perform return demonstration of BSE and offer the opportunity to ask questions.

Explain recommended frequency of mammography and BSE.

Discuss signs and symptoms of breast cancer.

Discuss signs and symptoms of fibrocystic disease.

Encourage client to reduce intake of caffeine. Although controversial, decreasing caffeine intake is believed to reduce symptoms of fibrocystic disease.

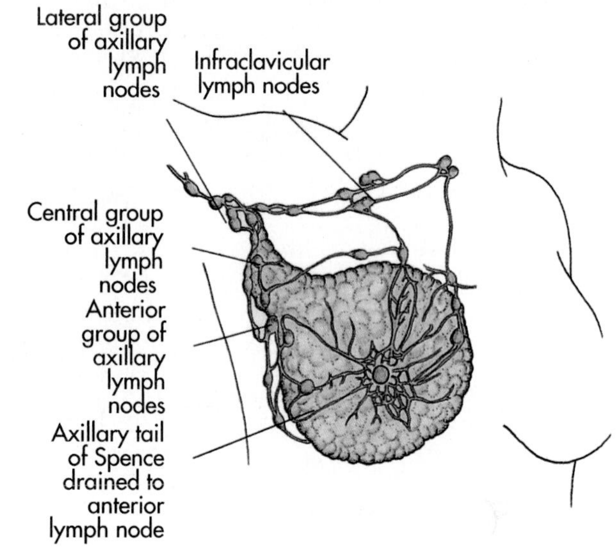

FIGURE 16-53 Anatomical position of axillary and clavicular lymph nodes.

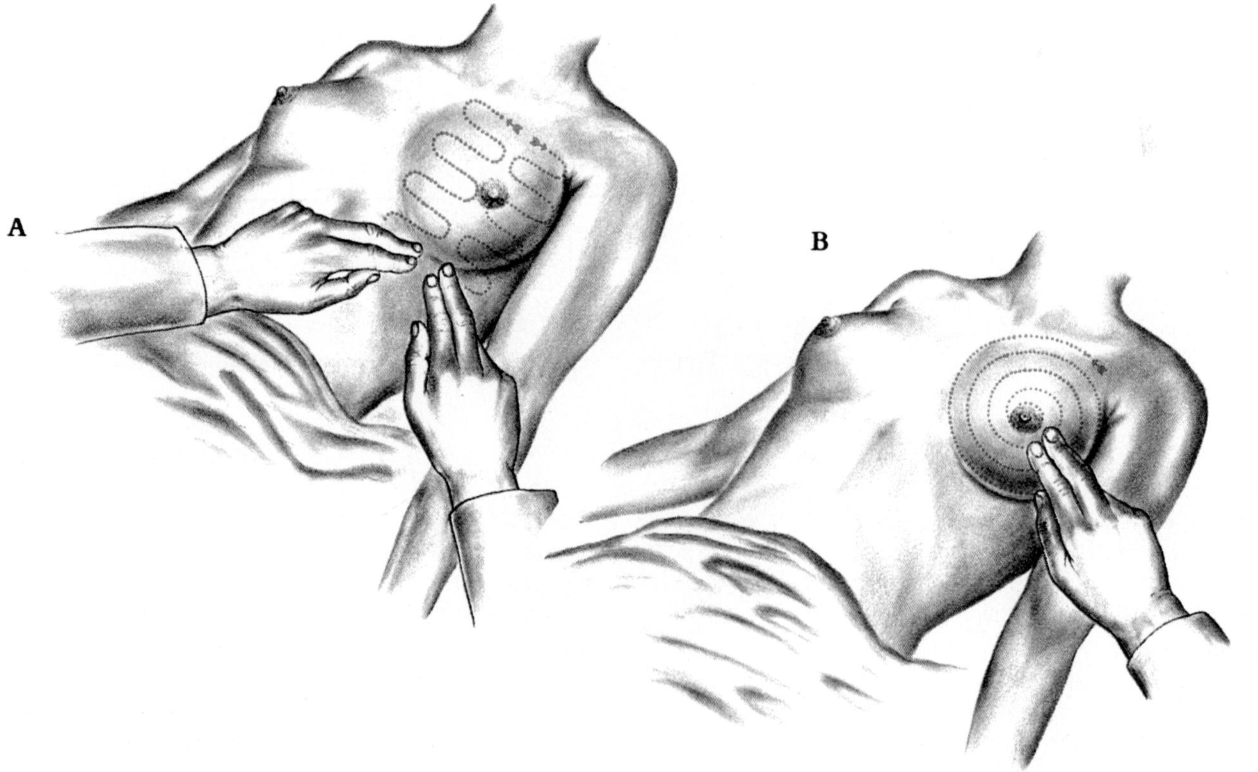

FIGURE 16-54 Methods for breast palpation. **A,** Back and forth. **B,** Concentric circles. (From Seidel HM, et al.: *Mosby's guide to physical examination,* ed 2, St. Louis, 1991, Mosby.)

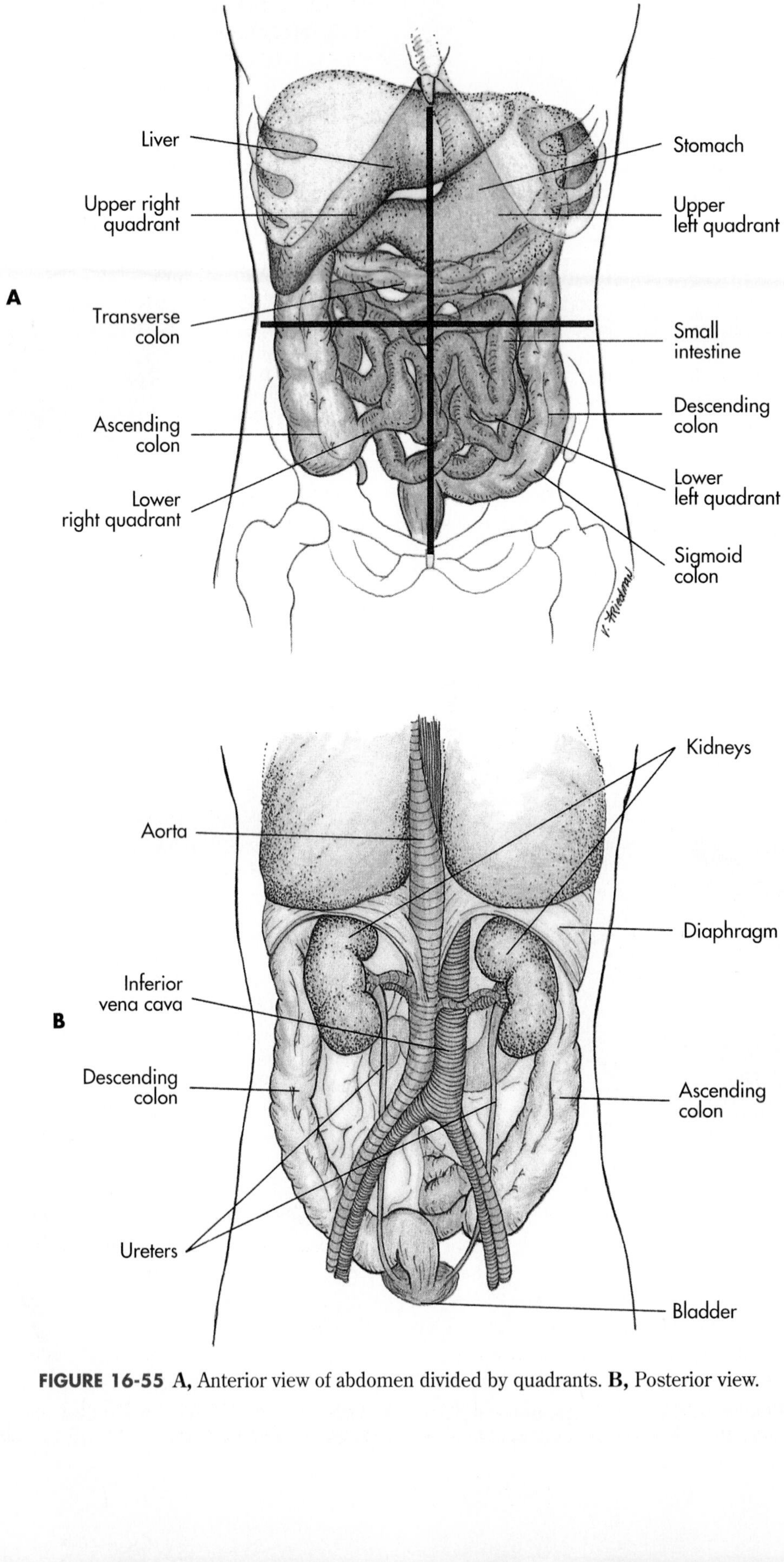

FIGURE 16-55 **A,** Anterior view of abdomen divided by quadrants. **B,** Posterior view.

ABDOMEN

The abdominal examination can be complex because of the organs located within and near the abdominal cavity (Figure 16-55, *A* and *B*). The examiner assesses abdominal organs anteriorly and posteriorly.

A system of landmarks helps to map out the abdominal region. The xiphoid process (tip of the sternum) is the upper boundary of the anterior abdominal region. The symphysis pubis is the lowermost boundary. By dividing the abdomen into four imaginary quadrants (Figure 16-55, *A*), the nurse can refer to assessment findings and record them in relation to each quadrant. Posteriorly the kidneys, located from the T12 to L3 vertebrae, are protected by the lower ribs and heavy back muscles. The costovertebral angle formed by the last rib and vertebral column is a landmark used during palpation of the kidney.

The examination includes an assessment of structures of the lower gastrointestinal (GI) tract in addition to the liver, stomach, kidneys, and bladder. Abdominal pain is one of the most common symptoms clients will report when seeking medical care. An accurate assessment requires matching client history data with a careful assessment of the location of physical symptoms.

During the abdominal examination, the client should be relaxed. A tightening of abdominal muscles hinders palpation. The nurse asks the client to void before beginning. The room should be warm and the client's upper chest and legs draped. The client lies supine or in a dorsal recumbent position with the arms at the sides and knees slightly bent. Small pillows can be placed beneath the knees (McConnell, 1990). If the client places the arms under the head, the abdominal muscles may tighten. The examiner proceeds calmly and slowly, being sure there is adequate lighting. The abdomen is exposed from just above the xiphoid process down to the symphysis pubis. The client is asked to report pain and point out areas of tenderness. Tender areas are assessed last.

The order for an abdominal examination differs slightly from previous assessments. The nurse begins with inspection and then auscultation. By using auscultation before palpation and percussion, there is less chance of altering the frequency and character of bowel sounds. During the examination the nurse uses a tape measure.

Health History. The nurse asks whether the client has abdominal or low back pain and assesses the pain in detail (Chapter 28). The client's normal bowel habits and stool character are also reviewed, with the nurse asking if the client uses laxatives. The nurse also determines if the client has had abdominal surgery, trauma, or diagnostic tests. Signs and symptoms of belching, difficulty swallowing, flatulence, bloody emesis **(hematemesis), melena,** heartburn, diarrhea, or constipation may reveal a pattern of a problem. The nurse also asks if the client has had a recent weight change or intolerance to diet. If the client takes antiinflammatories (e.g., aspirin, ibu-prophen, or steroids) and antibiotics, there may be risk for GI upset or bleeding. Finally, the nurse asks the client to locate tender areas before beginning the examination.

Inspection

The nurse may be able to observe the client during routine care activities. The nurse notes the client's posture and looks for evidence of abdominal splinting, lying with the knees drawn up, or moving restlessly in bed. A client free from abdominal pain will not stoop or splint the abdomen. To inspect the abdomen for abnormal movement or shadows, the nurse stands on the client's right side and inspects from above the abdomen. By sitting down to look across the abdomen, the nurse assesses contour.

The nurse inspects the skin over the abdomen for color, scars, venous patterns, lesions, and **striae,** or stretch marks. The skin is subject to the same color variations as the rest of the body. Venous patterns are normally faint, except in thin clients. Artificial openings may indicate drainage sites resulting from surgery or an ostomy (see Chapters 32 and 33). Scars reveal evidence of past trauma or surgery that may have created permanent changes in underlying organ anatomy. Lesions are observed for characteristics. Striae result from stretching of tissue by obesity or pregnancy.

Inspection continues with the umbilicus. The nurse notes the position, shape, color, and presence of inflammation or discharge. A normal umbilicus is flat or concave with the color the same as surrounding skin.

The nurse inspects for contour, symmetry, and surface motion of the abdomen, noting any masses, bulging, or distention. If the abdomen appears distended, ask the client to roll onto a side and inspect for a bulging flank. Does the client report tightness? Normally a flat abdomen forms a horizontal plane from the xiphoid process to the symphysis pubis. A round abdomen is evenly convex, with maximum height at the umbilicus. A concave abdomen appears to sink into the muscular wall. A concave abdomen is common in thin adults.

Generalized symmetric distention can be caused by a heavy meal, obesity, or gas. In obesity there are rolls of adipose tissue along the flanks and clients deny tightness. **Hernias,** or protrusions of abdominal organs through the muscle wall, cause upward protrusion of the umbilicus.

If abdominal distention is expected, the nurse measures the abdomen's girth by placing a tape measure around the abdomen at the umbilicus. A marking pen is used to indicate where the tape measure was applied.

Consecutive measurements will show any change in girth.

Masses on only one side or asymmetry is abnormal and can indicate an underlying pathological condition. The nurse observes the abdomen's contour while asking the client to take a deep breath. Then as the client raises the head, the nurse looks for bulging. No bulges should appear.

The abdomen is next inspected for movement. Normally men breathe abdominally, and women breathe more costally. If the client has severe pain, respiratory movement is diminished, and the client tightens abdominal muscles to guard against the pain. The nurse also observes for peristaltic movement or aortic pulsation by looking across the abdomen from the side. These movements may be seen in thin clients; otherwise no movement is present.

CLIENT TEACHING DURING ABDOMINAL ASSESSMENT

- Explain factors such as diet, regular exercise, and fluid intake that promote normal bowel elimination (see Chapter 33).
- Caution clients about dangers of excessive use of laxatives or enemas.
- If client has chronic pain, explain measures used for pain relief (e.g., relaxation exercises [see Chapter 28]).
- Instruct client about warning signs of colon cancer, including bleeding from the rectum, blood in the stool, and a change in bowel habits.

Auscultation

The nurse auscultates the abdomen to listen to the bowel sounds of intestinal motility and to detect vascular sounds. Clients with gastrointestinal tubes connected to suction must have them temporarily turned off before beginning the examination. First the warmed diaphragm of the stethoscope is placed lightly over the lower left quadrant. The nurse asks the client not to speak. Normally, air and fluid move through the intestines, creating soft gurgling or bubbling sounds 5 to 35 times per minute in each quadrant. The sounds do not occur with regularity. It normally takes 5 to 20 seconds to hear a bowel sound. It may take 5 minutes of continuous listening before determining bowel sounds are absent. The best time to auscultate is between meals. Sounds are generally described as normal or audible, absent, hyperactive, or hypoactive. If bowel sounds are not easily audible, the nurse proceeds systematically over each abdominal quadrant.

Silen (1992) reports that auscultation of bowel sounds is not useful when ruling out causes for abdominal pain, as sounds may be absent one moment and present the next. Absent sounds indicate cessation of gastrointestinal motility. Hyperactive sounds are loud, growling-type sounds called **borborygmi,** which indicate increased gastrointestinal motility. Inflammation of the bowel, excess ingestion of laxatives, and reaction of the intestines to certain foods cause increased motility (see box above).

Bruits indicate narrowing of major blood vessels and disruption of blood flow. Presence of bruits in the abdominal area can reveal aneurysms or stenotic vessels. The nurse uses the stethoscope's bell to auscultate in the epigastric region and each of the four quadrants. Normally there are no vascular sounds over the aorta (midline through the abdomen), renal (costovertebral angle), or femoral arteries (lower quadrants). If bruits are present the nurse avoids palpation of the abdomen and consults a physician immediately.

Percussion

Percussion of the abdomen maps out underlying organs and masses and reveals the presence of air in the stomach and intestines. The nurse percusses each of the four quadrants to discriminate between the sounds of dullness and tympany. Potentially painful areas are percussed last. Tympany predominates because of air existing within the stomach and intestines. A dull percussion note can be heard over the liver, spleen, pancreas, kidneys, and a distended bladder. In addition, a dull percussion note may indicate a tumor.

Percussion allows the nurse to identify borders of the liver to detect organ enlargement. The nurse starts at the client's right iliac crest and percusses upward along the midclavicular line. The percussion note changes from tympanic to dull at the liver's lower border, which is usually at the right costal margin. Extension beyond the right costal margin is an abnormality that should be reported immediately. The nurse marks the border with a marking pen. The upper border is found by percussing down from the clavicle along the intercostal spaces. This time the note changes from resonant to dull. The liver's upper border is usually found in the fifth, sixth, or seventh intercostal space. The nurse measures the distance from the upper to lower border. The distance between the points where dullness is percussed should be 6 to 12 cm (2½ to 5 inches). With liver disease the liver enlarges.

The kidneys are percussed posteriorly to rule out inflammation. The client may sit or stand upright. The nurse may use direct or indirect percussion. The nurse strikes the client firmly with the ulnar surface of the partially closed fist along each costovertebral angle at the scapular lines. Normal percussion is painless. If the kid-

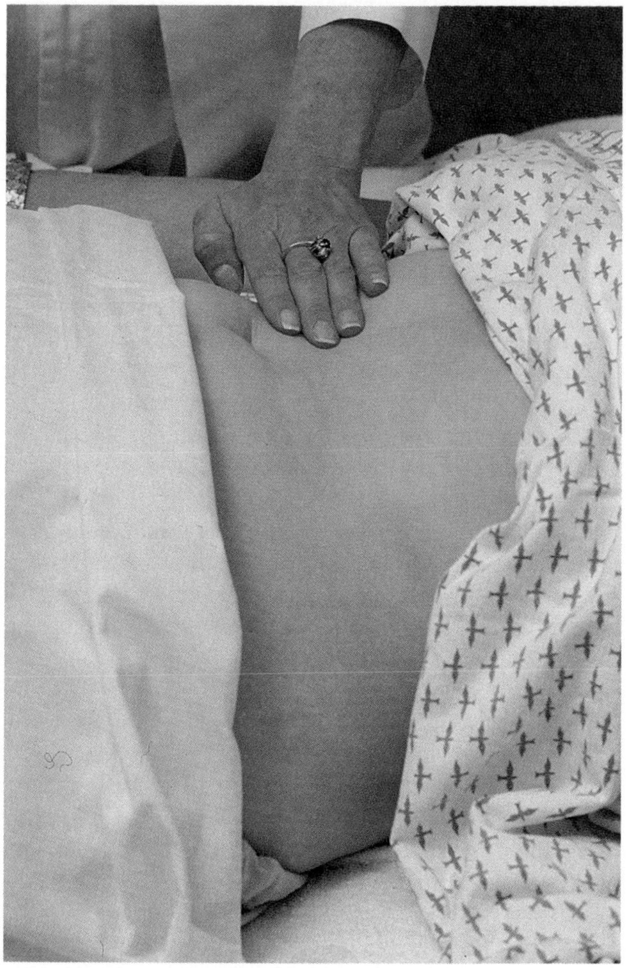

FIGURE 16-56 Light palpation of the abdomen.

neys are inflamed, tenderness is easily elicited during percussion.

Palpation

Palpation primarily detects areas of abdominal tenderness, abnormal distention, or masses. As students become more skilled, they learn to palpate for specific organs such as the liver. Light and deep palpation are used.

The nurse performs light palpation over each abdominal quadrant. Areas previously identified as problem spots are avoided. The nurse lays the palm of the hand with fingers extended and approximated lightly on the abdomen. With the palmar surface of the fingers the nurse depresses ½ inch (1.3 cm) in a gentle dipping motion (Figure 16-56). The nurse avoids quick jabs and uses smooth coordinated movements. For ticklish clients, the nurse first places the hand under the client's until palpation is tolerated. The nurse feels for muscular resistance, tenderness, and superficial organs or masses. While palpating, the nurse observes the client's face for signs of discomfort. The abdomen is normally smooth with consistent softness and nontender without masses. One organ the nurse can detect with light palpation is the distended bladder, just above the symphisis pubis.

With experience the nurse can perform deep palpation to delineate abdominal organs and to detect less obvious masses. A qualified examiner must assist until the nurse becomes skilled in the technique. It is important for the client to be relaxed as the nurse's hands are depressed approximately 2.5 to 7.5 cm (1 to 3 inches) into the abdomen. Deep palpation is never used over a surgical incision or over extremely tender organs. It is also unwise to use deep palpation on abnormal masses. Deep pressure may cause tenderness in the healthy client over the cecum, sigmoid colon, aorta, and in the midline near the xiphoid process (Seidel, et al., 1991).

Each quadrant is surveyed systematically. The nurse palpates masses for size, location, shape, consistency, tenderness, pulsation, and mobility. If tenderness is found, the examiner checks for rebound tenderness. This test may be performed by having the examiner press a hand slowly and deeply into the involved area and then letting go quickly. If pain is elicited with the release of the hand, the test is positive. Rebound tenderness occurs in clients with inflammation of the abdominal cavity (peritonitis).

A maneuver that reveals abdominal masses requires the client to lift the head from the examining table. This causes contraction of abdominal muscles. Masses in the abdominal wall will continue to be palpable.

FEMALE GENITALIA

Examination of the female genitalia including external and internal sex organs can be embarrassing to the client unless the nurse uses a calm relaxed approach. The exam is one of the most difficult experiences for adolescents. Cultural background may further add to apprehension (Chapter 18). The lithotomy position is also embarrassing. Comfort is achieved through correct client positioning and draping. The nurse explains each portion of the examination in advance so clients can anticipate actions. Adolescents may choose to have parents present.

A client may require a complete examination, including assessing external genitalia and performing a vaginal examination or the nurse may examine external genitalia while performing routine hygiene measures or preparing to insert a urinary catheter. An examination should be a part of each woman's preventive health care because uterine and vaginal cancers have a high incidence rate. Adolescents and young adults should be examined because of the growing incidence of sexually transmitted diseases (STDs). Rectal and anal assessments are easily combined with this examination because the client can assume a lithotomy or dorsal recumbent position.

Health History. The nursing history reviews the client's previous illnesses or surgeries involving reproductive organs, including sexually transmitted disease. A review of the menstrual history includes age at menarche, frequency and duration of cycle, character of flow, presence of **dysmenorrhea,** date of last menstrual period, and premenstrual symptoms. The nurse also assesses for signs of bleeding, vaginal discharge, or pain outside the normal menstrual period or after menopause. A review of the client's obstetric history is also valuable. The nurse also asks if clients have symptoms of genitourinary problems such as burning on urination, frequency, urgency, nocturia, hematuria, or signs of vaginal discharge and lesions of genitalia.

It is important to determine if the client uses safe sex practices. The nurse asks the client to describe current and past contraceptive practices or problems and identifies risk of STDs and HIV infection.

Preparing the Client

The following equipment will be needed for a complete examination: examination table with stirrups, vaginal speculum of correct size, adjustable light source, sink, clean disposable gloves, glass microscopic slides, plastic spatula and/or cytobrush, and specimen bottles with fixative spray.

Equipment must be ready before the examination begins. The client is asked to empty her bladder so that urine is not accidentally expelled during the examination. Often it is necessary to collect a urine specimen. Assist the client to the lithotomy position, in bed or on an examination table for an external genitalia assessment. Assist the client into stirrups if a speculum examination is to be performed. Have the woman stabilize each foot in a stirrup and then have her slide the buttocks down to the edge of the examining table. The nurse places a hand at the edge of the table and instructs the client to move until touching the hand. The client's arms should be at her sides or folded across the chest to prevent tightening of abdominal muscles.

A woman suffering pain or deformity of the joints may be unable to assume a lithotomy position. In this situation, it may be necessary to have the client abduct only one leg or to have another nurse assist in separating the client's thighs. The side-lying position may also be used with the client on the left side and right thigh and knee drawn up to her chest.

A square drape or sheet is given to the client. She holds one corner over her sternum, the adjacent corners fall over each knee, and the fourth falls over the perineum. After the examination begins, the drape over the perineum is lifted. The male examiner should always have a female in attendance during the examination. A female examiner may prefer to work alone but should have a female attendant if the client is particularly anxious or emotionally unstable.

External Genitalia

The perineal area must be well illuminated. The nurse gloves both hands. The perineum is extremely sensitive and tender; the area is not touched suddenly without warning the client. It is best to touch the neighboring thigh first before advancing to the perineum.

While sitting at the end of the examination table or bed the nurse inspects the quantity and distribution of hair growth. Preadolescents have no pubic hair. During adolescence, hair grows along the labia, becoming darker, coarser, and curlier. In an adult, hair grows in a triangle over the female perineum and along the medial surface of the thighs. Hair should be free of nits and lice.

The nurse inspects surface characteristics of the labia majora. The skin of the perineum is smooth, clean, and slightly darker than other skin. The mucous membranes appear dark pink and moist. The labia majora may be gaping or closed and appear dry or moist. They are usually symmetric. After childbirth the labia majora are separated, causing the labia minora to become more prominent. When a woman reaches menopause, the labia majora become thinned. With advancing age they become atrophied. The labia majora are normally without inflammation, edema, lesions, or lacerations.

To inspect the remaining external structures, the nurse, with the nondominant hand, gently places the thumb and index finger inside the labia minora and retracts the tissues outward (Figure 16-57). The nurse should be sure to have a firm hold to avoid repeated retraction against the sensitive tissues. The nurse uses the other hand to palpate the labia minora between the thumb and second finger. On inspection the labia minora are normally thinner than the labia majora and one side may be larger. The tissue should feel soft on palpation and without tenderness. The size of the clitoris is variable, but it normally does not exceed 2 cm in length and 0.5 cm in diameter. If inflamed, the clitoris will be a bright cherry red. In young women it is a common site for syphilitic lesions or chancres, which appear as small open ulcers that drain serous material. Older women may have malignant changes that result in dry, scaly, nodular lesions.

The nurse inspects the urethral orifice carefully for color and position. It is normally intact without inflammation. The urethral meatus is anterior to the vaginal orifice and is pink. It often appears as an irregular slit or opening in the midline. The nurse notes any discharge, polyps, or fistulas.

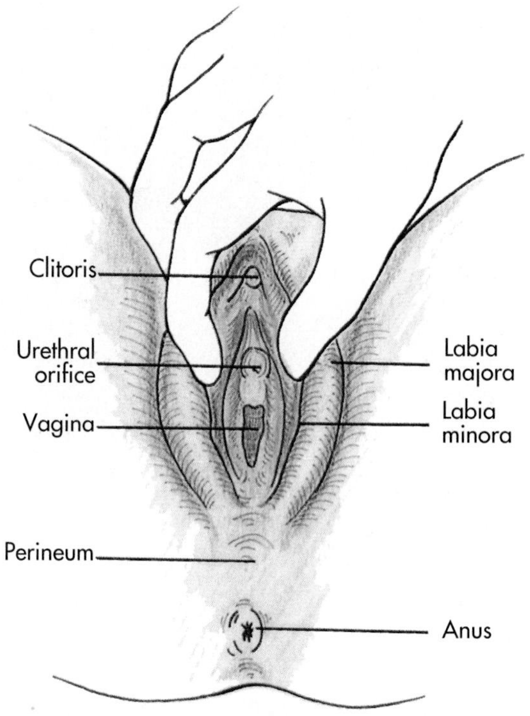

FIGURE 16-57 Female external genitalia.

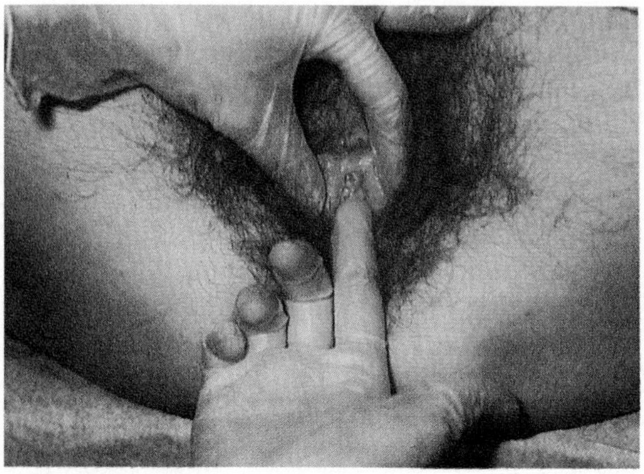

FIGURE 16-58 Milking the urethra and paraurethral glands. (From Seidel HM, et al.: *Mosby's guide to physical examination,* ed 2, St. Louis, 1991, Mosby.)

The vaginal introitus is next inspected for inflammation, edema, discoloration, discharge, and lesions. Normally the introitus is a thin vertical slit or a large orifice. The tissue is moist. In women who have had several children, the opening to the vaginal canal may extend upward, blocking the view of the urethra.

With the labia retracted, the nurse examines the Skene and Bartholin glands. Tell the client you are going to insert one finger in her vagina and that she will feel pressure. With the palm facing upward, the nurse inserts an index finger of the examining hand into the vagina as far as the second joint. Exerting upward pressure, the nurse milks the Skene glands by moving the finger outward. Discharge and tenderness are abnormal. The exam is done on both sides of the urethra and then directly on the urethra (Figure 16-58). This technique may cause discharge to appear. If so, the nurse notes the color, odor, and consistency and obtains a culture. The nurse next changes to a clean pair of gloves.

While inspecting the vaginal orifice or introitus, the examiner notices the condition of the hymen, which is just inside the introitus. In the virgin the hymen may restrict the opening of the vagina. Only remnants of the hymen remain after sexual intercourse.

If inflammation and edema are found near the posterior end of the introitus, Bartholin's glands may be infected. The glands cannot normally be palpated. To attempt palpation the nurse places a thumb and index finger between the labia majora and introitus and palpates one side at a time.

Often there is a loss of muscle tone of the vaginal outlet. A portion of the vaginal wall and bladder may prolapse or fall into the introitus. The client is asked to strain downward around the nurse's finger, as if she were voiding or having a bowel movement. If the client lacks adequate muscular support, the vaginal walls will bulge, blocking the introitus opening. Normally when a client is asked to close the vaginal orifice, the nurse will palpate tension in the muscles.

The nurse may also inspect the anus at this time, looking for lesions and hemorrhoids (see rectal examination).

Speculum Examination of Internal Genitalia

An examination of internal genitalia requires much skill and practice. Usually it is performed only by advanced nurse practitioners. Beginning students will more than likely only observe the procedure or assist the examiner.

The examination involves use of a plastic or metal speculum. Consisting of two blades and an adjustable thumbscrew, the speculum is inserted into the vagina to assess the internal genitalia for cancerous lesions and other abnormalities. During the examination a Papanicolaou (Pap) smear is collected to test for cervical and vaginal cancer.

To assist an examiner, the nurse makes sure the client is comfortably positioned in the stirrups. A variety of speculum sizes (small, medium, large) should be available so that the examiner may select the appropriate size for the client. In addition, the nurse will have

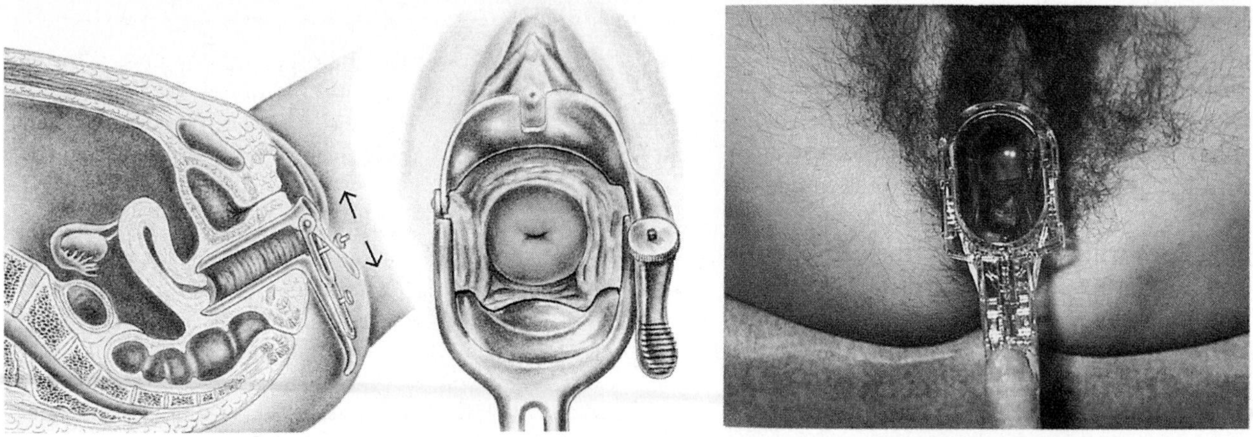

A B C

FIGURE 16-59 **A,** Angle of speculum insertion. **B,** View of cervix. **C,** Vaginal speculum in place with cervix in full view. (From Seidel HM, et al.: *Mosby's guide to physical examination,* ed 2, St. Louis, 1991, Mosby.)

CLIENT TEACHING DURING FEMALE GENITALIA ASSESSMENT

Instruct client about recommended frequency of Pap smears. The test is painless and has no side effects. The American Cancer Society (Facts and Figures, 1993) has recommended women who are or have been sexually active and women who are 18 or older and do not have symptoms of disease to have annual tests until three smears are negative. Thereafter tests may be done at physician discretion; however in practice most physicians advise annual Pap smears.

Counsel clients with sexually transmitted diseases about diagnosis and treatment. Teach preventive measures (e.g., male partner's use of condoms, restricting number of sexual partners, avoiding sex with persons who have several other partners, and perineal hygiene measures).

Tell clients with sexually transmitted diseases that they must inform sexual partners of the need for an examination.

Reinforce the importance of perineal hygiene (as appropriate).

table 16-6

METHODS FOR OBTAINING PAP SMEARS

Location	Technique
Outer cervix	Use plastic spatula. Place tip of longer arm in os. Rotate spatula, scraping outer surface of cervix. Apply cells to glass slide. Apply fixative solution and label slide. 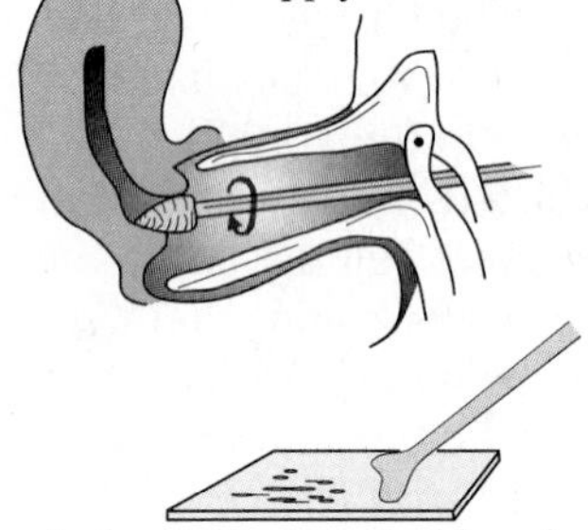
Endocervical	Use cervical brush (cytobrush). Gently insert brush through os. Rotate brush 180-360 degrees. Apply cells by rolling and twisting brush on glass slide. Apply fixative solution and label slide. WARNING: Do *not* use on pregnant clients. 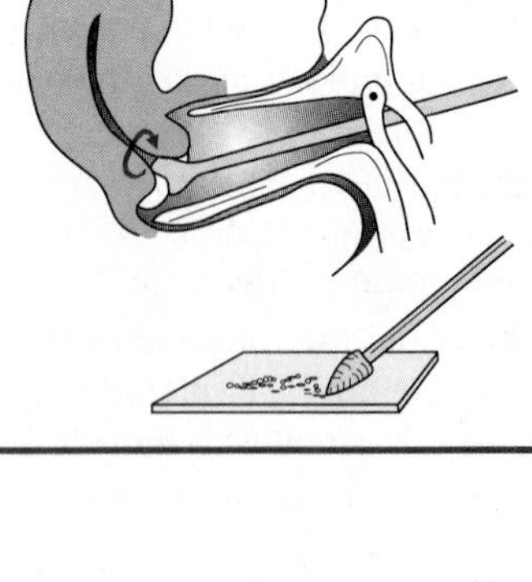

gloves, specimen slides, and a spatula and/or cytobrush close at hand. Water-soluble lubricant is only used when specimens are not being collected. Most examiners lubricate the speculum with warm water.

The first portion of the examination involves careful insertion of the speculum until the examiner can fully visualize the cervix (Figure 16-59). The cervix is examined for color, appearance of the os or opening, position, size, surface characteristics, and discharge. The normal cervix is glistening pink, smooth, and round. Its diameter is about 1 inch (2.5 to 3 cm) in a young woman and smaller in an older adult. The cervix should be midline and without lesions.

The surface of the cervix, at the cervical canal opening, is lined with layers of vaginal squamous cells. The cells meet a different group of cells, columnar cells. The columnar cells secrete mucus and line the passageway that leads up into the central cavity of the uterus. A Pap smear is a painless screening test for cervical cancer (see box on p. 354). Specimens are taken from the endocervix and ectocervix (Table 16-6). The examiner first collects a sample of the outer cervix or ectocervix. A plastic spatula is rotated 360 degrees against the cervical surface. Once the spatula is withdrawn, the examiner spreads the specimen lightly over a glass slide. The nurse assisting sprays the specimen with cytologic fixative and labels the slide. The examiner next uses a cytobrush to collect endocervical cells. The cytobrush is inserted into the cervical os and rotated one full turn. The specimen is then spread across the slide by rolling the brush with moderate pressure. Again the specimen is sprayed and the slide is labeled. At the end of the procedure the nurse warns the client that blood spotting is normal for a few hours.

There is also a paintbrush device (Cervex-brush) that can be used to collect both specimens at the same time. It reportedly causes less spotting (Seidel, et al., 1991).

Once specimens are collected, the examiner will view the vaginal walls as the speculum is slowly withdrawn. The examiner notes the color, surface characteristics, and secretions. The vaginal walls are normally pink throughout and free from discharge and lesions. The surface should be moist and smooth or rugated. Normal secretions are thin, clear or cloudy, and odorless. Women commonly acquire yeast infection, causing thick, white, patchy, malodorous, curdlike discharge.

After speculum withdrawal, the nurse assists the client to a sitting position and allows the client to redress and perform hygiene. In a hospital setting, the client may need assistance with perineal hygiene. The nurse makes sure gloves, speculum, and other disposable equipment are appropriately discarded in a receptacle. The client is informed that Pap smear results will be available in 3 to 4 days (check agency policy).

MALE GENITALIA

An examination of the male genitalia assesses the integrity of the external genitalia, the inguinal ring, and canal. Because the incidence of sexually transmitted disease (STDs) in adolescents and young adults is high, an assessment of the genitalia should be a routine part of any health maintenance examination for this age-group. The nurse uses a calm and gentle approach to lessen the client's anxiety. The position and exposure obtained during the examination can be embarrassing. It often helps to minimize the client's anxiety by offering explanations of each step of the examination so the client can anticipate all actions. The genitalia are gently manipulated to avoid causing erection or discomfort. The nurse examines the genitalia carefully and completely but also briskly.

Health History. The nurse assesses the client's normal urinary pattern, including frequency of voiding, character and volume of urine, daily fluid intake, symptoms of burning, urgency and frequency, difficulty starting stream, and hematuria. The history also includes a review of previous surgery or illness involving urinary or reproductive organs, including STDs. The client's sexual history and use of safe sex habits alert the nurse to any risks for HIV or other STDs. A client's sexual performance can be influenced by a number of disorders; thus the nurse asks if the client has difficulty achieving erection or ejaculation. The nurse also reviews medications that might influence sexual performance, including diuretics, sedatives, antihypertensives, and tranquilizers. Finally, the nurse asks if the client has noted penile pain or swelling, lesions of the genitalia, or urethral discharge. The client's knowledge of testicular self-examination will guide the nurse in health teaching (see box on p. 356).

Sexual Maturity

The examination begins by having the client void. The examination room should be warm. The client lies supine with the chest, abdomen, and lower legs draped or the client may also stand during the examination. The nurse applies disposable gloves.

First, the nurse notes the sexual maturity of the client by observing the size and shape of the penis and testes, the size, color, and texture of scrotal skin, and the character and distribution of pubic hair. The testes first increase in size in preadolescence. During this time there is no pubic hair. By the end of puberty, testes and penis enlarge to adult size and shape and scrotal skin darkens and becomes wrinkled. With puberty, hair is coarse and abundant in the pubic area. The penis has no hair, and the scrotum has scant amounts. The nurse also inspects

CLIENT TEACHING DURING MALE GENITALIA ASSESSMENT

Instruct client on testicular self-examination. All men 15 years and older should perform this self-examination monthly using the following steps:

- Perform the examination after a warm bath or shower when the scrotal skin is relaxed.
- Stand naked in front of a mirror and look for swelling or lumps in the skin of the scrotum.
- Use both hands, placing the index and middle fingers under the testicles and the thumbs on top.
- Gently roll the testicle, feeling for lumps, thickening, or a change in consistency (hardening).
- Find the epididymis (a cordlike structure on the top and back of the testicle). This is *not* a lump.
- Feel for small, pea-sized lumps on the front and side of the testicle. The lumps are usually painless and are abnormal.
- Call your doctor if you find a lump.

Counsel clients with sexually transmitted diseases about diagnosis and treatment. Teach preventive measures (e.g., using condoms, restricting the number of sexual partners, avoiding sex with persons who have several other partners, and using perineal hygiene).

Tell clients with sexually transmitted diseases that they must inform sexual partners of the need for an examination.

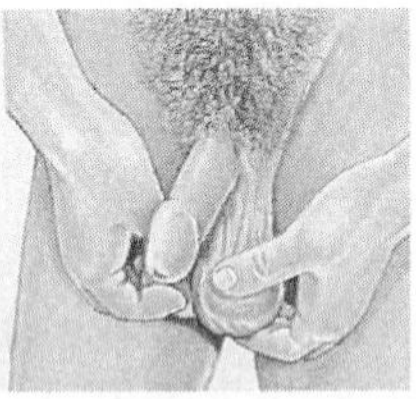

Illustration from Payne WA and Hahn DB: *Understanding your health,* ed 2, St. Louis, 1989, Mosby.

the skin covering the genitalia for lice, rashes, excoriations, or lesions. Normally the skin is clear without lesions.

Penis

To inspect penile surfaces thoroughly the nurse must manipulate the genitalia or have the client assist. The nurse inspects the corona, prepuce (foreskin), glans, urethral meatus, and shaft (Figure 16-60). In uncircumcised males the foreskin is retracted to reveal the glans and urethral meatus. The nurse inspects for discharge, lesions, edema, and inflammation. The foreskin should retract easily. A bit of white cheesy smegma may be seen over the glans. If the client is circumcised, the glans is exposed and appears erythematous and is dry. The meatus is slit-like and normally positioned at the tip of the glans. The glans is smooth and pink along all surfaces. In some congenital conditions the meatus is displaced along the penile shaft. The area between the foreskin and glans is a common site for venereal lesions.

Gentle compression of the glans between the nurse's thumb and index finger opens the meatus to allow inspection for discharge, lesions, and edema. (The client may perform this maneuver.) Normally the opening is glistening and pink without discharge. Any lesion is palpated gently to note tenderness, size, consistency, and shape. When inspection of the glans is completed, the foreskin is pulled down to its original position.

The nurse continues by inspecting the entire shaft of the penis, including the undersurface, looking for any lesions, scars, or areas of edema. The shaft is palpated between the thumb and first two fingers to detect localized areas of hardness or tenderness. A client who has laid in bed for a prolonged time may develop dependent edema in the penile shaft.

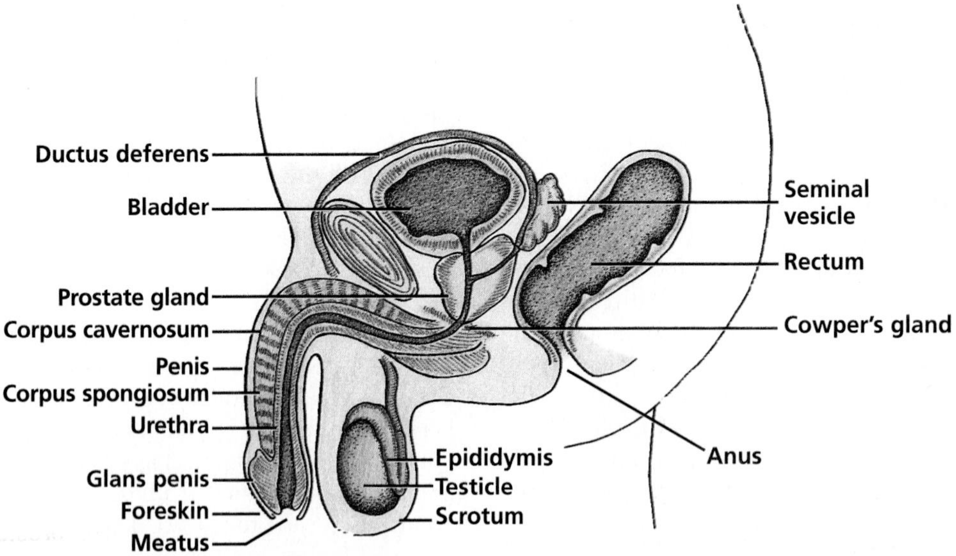

FIGURE 16-60 External and internal male sex organs.

Scrotum

The nurse is especially cautious while inspecting and palpating the scrotum because the structures that lie within the scrotal sac are very sensitive. The scrotum is a saclike structure divided internally into halves. Each half contains a testicle, epididymis, and the vas deferens, which travels upward into the inguinal ring. The left testicle is normally lower than the right. The nurse inspects the scrotum's size, color, shape, and symmetry while observing for lesions or edema.

The scrotum is gently lifted to view the posterior surface. The scrotal skin is usually loose and the surface is coarse. The skin color is often more deeply pigmented than body skin. Tightening or loss of wrinkling may reveal edema. The scrotum's size normally changes with temperature variations as its dartos muscle contracts in cold and relaxes in warm temperature. Lumps in the scrotal skin are commonly sebaceous cysts.

Testicular cancer is a solid tumor commonly found in young men. Early detection is critical. Clients must learn to perform testicular self-examinations (TSE) (see box on p. 356). The nurse can explain the technique while examining the client. While the client retracts the penis upward, the nurse gently palpates the testes and epididymis between the thumb and first two fingers (Figure 16-61). The nurse notes the size, shape, and consistency of tissue and asks if the client feels any tenderness. The testes should be sensitive but not tender. The underlying testicles are normally ovoid and approximately 2 by 4 cm ($\frac{4}{5}$ by $1\frac{3}{5}$ inches) in size. The testes feel smooth, rubbery, and are free from nodules. The epididymis is resilient. In the older adult the testicles decrease in size and are less firm during palpation. The most common symptoms of testicular cancer are a painless enlargement of one testis and appearance of a palpable small, hard lump about the size of a pea on the front or side of the testicle.

The nurse continues to palpate the vas deferens separately as it forms the spermatic cord toward the inguinal ring, noting nodules or swelling. It normally feels smooth and discrete.

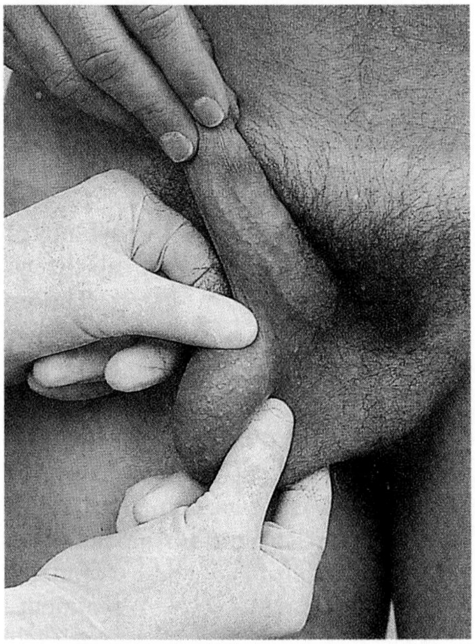

FIGURE 16-61 Palpating contents of scrotal sac. (From Seidel HM, et al.: *Mosby's guide to physical examination,* ed 2, St Louis, 1991, Mosby.)

Inguinal Ring and Canal

The external inguinal ring provides the opening for the spermatic cord to pass into the inguinal canal. The canal forms a passage through the abdominal wall, a potential site for hernia formation. A hernia is a protrusion of a portion of intestine through the inguinal wall or canal. An intestinal loop may even enter the scrotum. The client stands during this portion of the examination.

During inspection the client is asked to strain or bear down. The maneuver will help to make a hernia more visible. The nurse looks for obvious bulging. The nurse next palpates the inguinal ring and canal to be sure a hernia is not present. Standing on the right side of the client, the nurse places the index finger of the examining hand against the scrotal skin low on the right side. Gently the nurse moves the finger toward the inguinal canal with the folds of scrotal tissue covering the finger. Carrying the index finger upward along the vas deferens into the inguinal canal, the nurse follows the spermatic cord. It is important not to force the finger into the canal. When the finger reaches the farthest point along the canal, the nurse asks the client to cough and strain down. The maneuver is repeated on the left side. As the client strains, no bulging pressure will be felt. A tightening around the finger is normal.

The nurse completes the examination by palpating for inguinal lymph nodes. Small, nontender, mobile horizontal nodes may normally be found. Any abnormality may indicate local or systemic infection or malignant disease.

Rectum and Anus

A good time to perform the rectal examination is after the genital examination. The procedure can be uncomfortable, so the nurse helps the client to relax by explaining all steps. Usually the examination is not performed in young children or adolescents. The exam can detect colorectal cancer in its early stages. In men the rectal examination can also detect prostatic tumors.

HEALTH HISTORY. The nursing history includes review of the client's personal history of colorectal cancer,

CLIENT TEACHING DURING RECTAL ASSESSMENT

Discuss the American Cancer Society's (1993) guidelines for early detection of colorectal cancer:

- Digital rectal examination performed yearly after age 40
- Stool blood slide test (guaiac test) performed yearly after age 50
- Proctosigmoidoscopy, involving visual inspection of the rectum and lower colon with a hollow, lighted tube, performed by a physician every 3 to 5 years after age 50, on the advice of a physician
- Know warning signs of colorectal cancer
- Discuss dietary planning to reduce fat and increase fiber content

Warn clients against problems caused by overuse of laxatives, cathartic medications, codeine, or enemas

Discuss with male client the American Cancer Society's guidelines for early detection of prostatic cancer:

- Digital rectal exam performed annually after 40
- Possible prostate ultrasound testing for men at high risk
- Screening test for prostate-specific antigen (PSA)
- Know warning signs of prostate cancer

polyps, or inflammatory bowel disease. If the client is over 40, the nurse asks if the client has ever had a rectal examination or proctosigmoidoscopy. The client is asked about symtoms of bleeding from the rectum, black or tarry stools (melena), rectal pain, or change in bowel habits, all of which are indicative of colorectal cancer. The client's dietary habits including intake of high-fat foods or deficient fiber content may be linked to colon cancer. To screen male clients for possible prostate cancer the nurse asks if clients have experienced weak or interrupted urine flow, an inability to urinate, difficulty in starting or stopping urinary stream, polyuria, nocturia, hematuria, dysuria, and continuing pain in the lower back, pelvis, or upper thighs. The nurse also reviews the client's use of laxatives, cathartics, codeine, or iron preparations, which can cause elimination problems (see box above).

Inspection

Female clients may remain in the dorsal recumbent position following genitalia examination or they may assume a sidelying (Sims) position. Men are best examined by having the client bend over forward with the hips flexed and upper body resting across the examination table. A nonambulatory client can be examined in the Sims position. The nurse uses disposable gloves.

Using the nondominant hand the nurse gently retracts the buttocks to view the perianal and sacrococcygeal areas. Perianal skin is smooth and more pigmented and coarser than skin overlying the buttocks. The nurse inspects anal tissue for skin characteristics, lesions, external hemorrhoids (dilated veins that appear as reddened skin protrusions), ulcers, inflammation, rashes, or excoriations. Anal tissues are moist and hairless, and the anus is held closed by the voluntary sphincter. Next, the nurse asks the client to bear down as though having a bowel movement. Any internal hemorrhoids or fissures will appear at this time. Clock referents (e.g., 12 o'clock or 5 o'clock) are used to describe findings. There normally is no protrusion of tissue.

Digital Palpation

Many institutions prohibit nurses from performing digital examinations, so check agency policy. After lubricating the index finger of the gloved hand the nurse presses the finger pad against the anal opening and asks the client to bear down. As the anal sphincter relaxes, the nurse inserts the fingertip gently into the anal canal in a direction toward the umbilicus (Figure 16-62). Normally the client feels as though stool is being passed. The nurse never forces digital insertion.

The nurse has the client tighten the external sphincter around the finger and notes the muscle tone. Muscles normally close snugly without client discomfort. The nurse rotates the examination finger to palpate the muscular anal ring, noting any tissue irregularities. The anal ring should be smooth. To examine the rectal wall, the nurse inserts the finger farther and carefully palpates each side of the wall, noting nodules, lesions, hemorrhoids, or irregularities. Ask if the client feels any tenderness. The finger can examine about 6 to 10 cm into the rectum. After the finger is advanced fully the client is asked to bear down again. High lesions within the rectum will descend against the fingertip.

In male clients, the nurse turns the index finger to palpate the anterior rectal wall. Warn the client that he may feel the urge to urinate but that he will not do so. The nurse palpates the prostate gland to determine size, shape, firmness, tenderness, or lesions (Figure 16-63). The gland is round and heart shaped, 1 to $1\frac{1}{2}$ inches (2.5 to 4 cm) in diameter, divided into two lobes by a small groove. It is firm and nontender and is often described as feeling like a pencil eraser. Normally the gland protrudes less than 1 cm into the rectum (Seidel, et al., 1991).

After palpation the nurse gently withdraws the finger and observes for feces. Feces are normally brown. The presence of mucus, blood, or black tarry stool should be reported. A sample of the feces is tested for occult blood (see Chapter 33). For women suspected of having sexually transmitted disease, a rectal culture is taken to rule out cross infection from vaginal discharge. The nurse

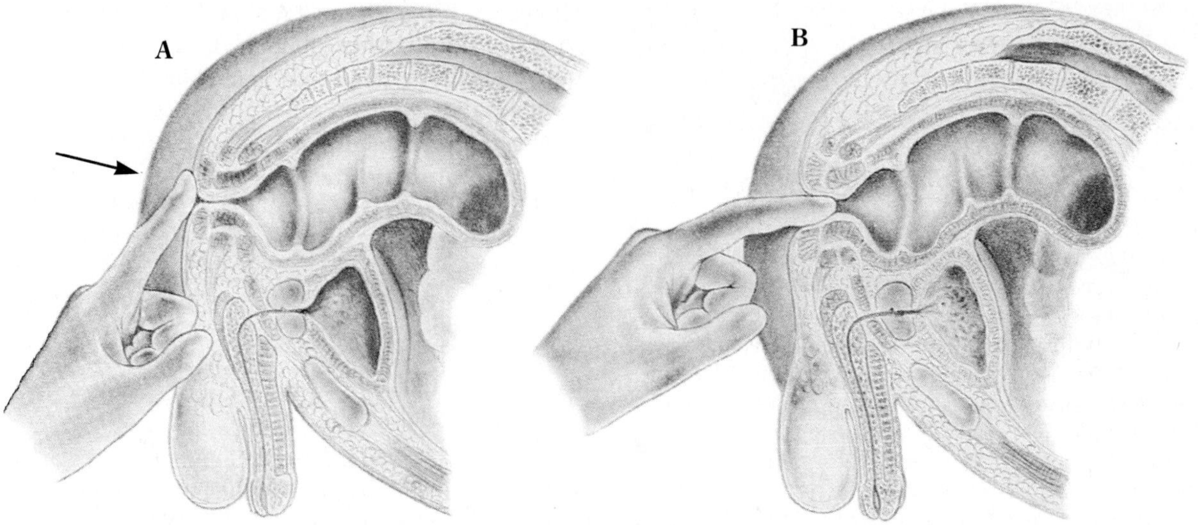

FIGURE 16-62 **A,** Correct procedure for introducing finger into male rectum. **B,** As external sphincter relaxes, advance fingertip into canal. (From Seidel HM, et al.: *Mosby's guide to physical examination,* ed 2, St. Louis, 1991, Mosby.)

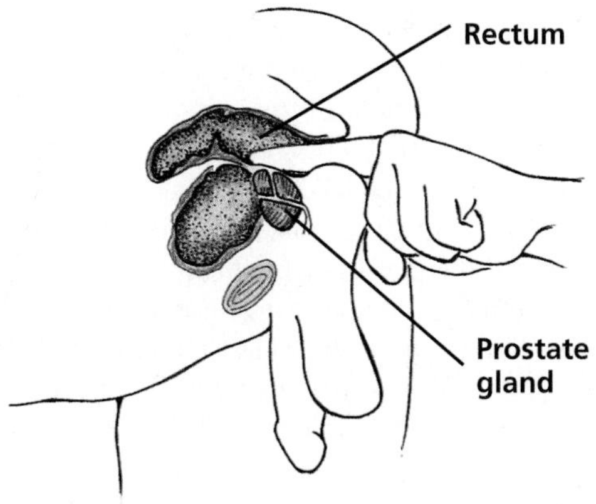

FIGURE 16-63 Palpation of prostate gland.

cleans the perianal area before continuing to the next part of the examination.

MUSCULOSKELETAL SYSTEM

The musculoskeletal assessment can be done as a separate examination or integrated with other parts of the total physical exam. The nurse can also assess while performing other nursing care measures such as bathing or positioning. The assessment of musculoskeletal integrity is especially important when the client reports pain or loss of function in a joint or muscle. Frequently, muscular disorders are the result of neurological disease. For this reason a neurological assessment is often conducted simultaneously.

While examining the client's musculoskeletal function, the nurse visualizes the anatomy of bone and muscle placement and joint structure. Joints vary in their degree of mobility. Some, as in the knee, are freely movable. The spinal vertebrae are examples of slightly movable joints. For a complete examination the muscles and joints should be exposed and free to move. Depending on the muscle groups being assessed, the client assumes a sitting, supine, prone, or standing position.

HEALTH HISTORY. A health history includes the client's description of any problems in bone, muscle, or joint function including history of recent falls, trauma, lifting heavy objects, and bone or joint disease. The nurse asks the client to point out locations of any alterations. It is useful to assess the client's normal activity pattern, including the type of exercise routinely performed (see box on p. 360). The nurse also assesses the nature and extent of pain or stiffness and determines if a musculoskeletal problem affects the client's ability to perform ADLs and participate in social activities. In women the nurse assesses diet history, focusing especially on calcium intake. An assessment of height loss in women over age 50 may predict osteoporosis (Reed and Birge, 1988). (Subtract current height from recall of maximum adult height).

General Inspection

The nurse observes the client's gait and posture when entering the examination room. When a client is unaware of the nurse's observation, gait is more natural. Later a more formal test has the client walk in a straight line away from the nurse. The nurse notes how the

CLIENT TEACHING DURING MUSCULOSKELETAL SYSTEM ASSESSMENT

Instruct client about correct postural alignment. Consult with physical therapist to provide client with exercises for improving posture.

To reduce bone demineralization, instruct older adult about a proper exercise program (e.g., walking) to be followed three or more times a week. Also encourage intake of calcium to meet the recommended daily allowance. Increased vitamin D will aid calcium absorption. Recommendations for calcium supplements are 1000 mg before and 1500 mg after menopause.

Instruct client on use of assistive devices (e.g., zippers on clothing instead of buttons and elevation of chairs to minimize bending of knees and hips) when he or she is unable to perform ADLs.

Instruct older adults and those with osteoporosis on proper body mechanics and ROM and moderate weight bearing exercises (swimming and walking) to minimize trauma and subsequent bone fractures.

client walks, sits, and rises from a sitting position. Normally clients walk with arms swinging freely at the sides and the head leading the body. Older adults walk with smaller steps and a wider base of support. Foot dragging, limping, shuffling, and the position of the trunk in relation to the legs are noted.

The nurse observes the client from the side in a standing position. The normal standing posture is an upright stance with parallel alignment of the hips and shoulders. The nurse can note the normal cervical, thoracic, and lumbar curves. The head is held erect. As the client sits, some degree of rounding of the shoulders is normal. Common postural abnormalities include kyphosis, lordosis, and scoliosis. Kyphosis, or hunchback, is an exaggeration of the posterior curvature of the thoracic spine. Lordosis or swayback is an increased lumbar curvature. A lateral spinal curvature is called scoliosis.

During inspection, the nurse looks at skin and subcutaneous tissues overlying muscles, bones, and joints. Discoloration, swelling, or masses are noted. The tissues normally conform to the shape of body parts. The nurse also observes extremities for overall size, gross deformity, bony enlargement, alignment, and symmetry. Usually there is bilateral symmetry in length, circumference, and alignment.

Range of Joint Motion

The nurse asks the client to put each major joint and its muscle groups through full range of motion (ROM) (Table 16-7). The examination includes comparison of both active and passive ROM. To assess range of motion passively, the nurse asks the client to relax and then passively moves the joints until the end of range is felt. The same body parts are compared for equality in movement. The nurse does not force a joint into a painful position. The nurse must know each joint's normal range and the extent to which the client's joints can be moved. Ideally, the client's normal range is assessed to determine a baseline for assessing later change (see Chapter 22). Joints should be free from stiffness, instability, swelling, or inflammation. There should be no discomfort when the nurse applies pressure to bones and

table 16-7

TERMINOLOGY FOR NORMAL RANGE OF MOTION POSITIONS

Term	Range of motion	Examples of joints
Flexion	Movement decreasing angle between two adjoining bones; bending of limb	Elbow, fingers, knee
Extension	Movement increasing angle between two adjoining bones	Elbow, knee, fingers
Hyperextension	Movement of body part beyond its normal resting extended position	Head
Pronation	Movement of body part so that front or ventral surface faces downward	Hand, forearm
Supination	Movement of body part so that front or ventral surface faces upward	Hand, forearm
Abduction	Movement of extremity away from midline of body	Leg, arm, fingers
Adduction	Movement of extremity toward midline of body	Leg, arm, fingers
Internal rotation	Rotation of joint inward	Knee, hip
External rotation	Rotation of joint outward	Knee, hip
Eversion	Turning of body part away from midline	Foot
Inversion	Turning of body part toward midline	Foot
Dorsiflexion	Flexion of toes and foot upward	Foot
Plantar flexion	Bending of toes and foot downward	Foot

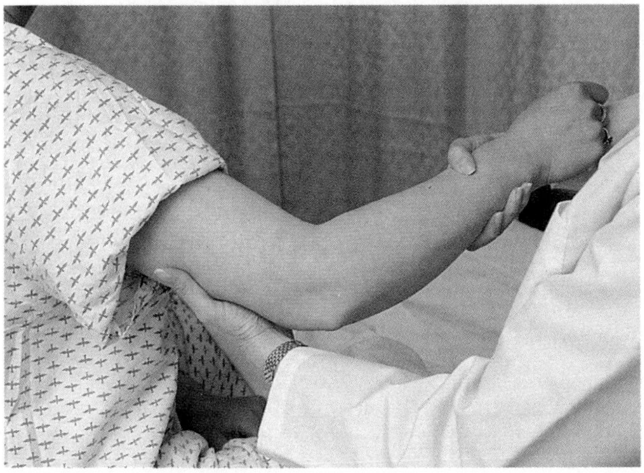

FIGURE 16-64 Nurse assesses muscle tone when moving the extremity passively.

joints. In older adults, joints often become swollen and stiff, with reduced range of motion. If a joint appears swollen and inflamed, the nurse palpates for warmth.

Muscle Tone and Strength

The nurse assesses muscle strength and tone during the measurement of range of motion. Tone is the slight muscular resistance felt by the examiner as the relaxed extremity is passively moved through its range of motion. The client is asked to allow an extremity to relax or hang limp. This is often difficult, particularly if the client feels pain in the extremity. The extremity is supported, and each limb grasped, moving it through the normal range of motion (Figure 16-64). Normal tone causes a mild, even resistance to passive movement through the entire range.

If a muscle has increased tone or hypertonicity, sudden passive movement of a joint is met with considerable resistance. Continued movement eventually causes the muscle to relax. A hypotonic muscle that has little tone feels flabby. The involved extremity hangs loosely in a position determined by gravity.

To assess muscle strength, the client must assume a stable position. The nurse asks the client to flex the muscle being tested (e.g., biceps flexing forearm) and then to resist as the nurse applies an opposing force (pulling down on forearm) against flexion. Symmetrical muscle pairs are compared. Muscle strength is bilaterally symmetrical with resistance to opposition. The dominant arm may be slightly stronger than the nondominant arm. If a weakness is identified, the muscle's size is compared with its opposite counterpart by measuring the muscle body's circumference with a tape measure. A muscle that has atrophied or become reduced in size may feel soft and boggy when palpated.

NEUROLOGICAL SYSTEM

An assessment of neurological function alone can be quite time consuming. An efficient nurse integrates neurological measurements with other parts of the physical examination. Cranial nerve function can be tested during the survey of the head and neck. Mental and emotional status is observed during the nursing history.

Many variables must be considered when deciding the extent of the examination. A client's level of consciousness influences the ability to follow directions. General physical status influences tolerance to assessment. The client's chief complaint also helps to determine the need for a thorough neurological assessment. If the client complains of headache or a recent loss of function in an extremity, a complete neurological review is needed. The nurse will require use of special equipment including reading material, vials of aromatic substances (vanilla extract or coffee), sterile needle, Snellen eye chart, penlight, vials of sugar or salt, tongue blade, two test tubes (one containing hot water, the other containing cold), cotton balls or cotton-tipped applicators, tuning fork, and reflex hammer.

HEALTH HISTORY. The nurse gathers a health history that includes a screening for symptoms of headache, seizures, tremors, dizziness, vertigo, numbness or tingling of body parts, visual changes, weakness, pain, or changes in speech. The presence of any symptom then requires a more detailed review (e.g., onset, severity, precipitating factors or sequence of events). The client's use of analgesics, sedatives, hypnotics, antipsychotics, antidepressants, or nervous system stimulants is reviewed. The nurse also assesses if the client's family has noticed any recent changes in the client's behavior (e.g., mood swings or memory loss). The nurse asks about any noticeable changes in vision, hearing, smell, taste, and touch. A history of head or spinal cord trauma, meningitis, congenital anomalies, neurological disease, or psychiatric counseling will focus the nurse's assessment of select findings.

Mental and Emotional Status

A great deal can be learned about mental capacities and emotional state by interacting with the client. A nurse can ask questions during an examination to gather data and observe the appropriateness of emotions and thoughts. To ensure an objective assessment the nurse considers the client's cultural and educational background, values, beliefs, previous experiences, and current level of coping. Such factors influence response to questions. The cerebral cortex controls and integrates functions measured in the assessment.

Level of Consciousness. The level of consciousness exists along a continuum from full awakeness, alert-

table 16-8
GLASGOW COMA SCALE

Action	Response	Score
Eyes open	Spontaneously	④
	To speech	3
	To pain	2
	None	1
Best verbal response	Oriented	⑤
	Confused	4
	Inappropriate words	3
	Incomprehensible sounds	2
	None	1
Best motor response	Obeys commands	⑥
	Localized pain	5
	Flexion withdrawal	4
	Abnormal flexion	3
	Abnormal extension	2
	Flaccid	1
	Total Score	⑮

ness, and cooperation to unresponsiveness to any form of external stimuli. The nurse converses with a client, asking questions about events involving the client or concerns about any health problem. A fully conscious client responds to questions quickly, and ideas are expressed logically. With a lowering of the client's consciousness, the nurse uses the Glasgow coma scale (GCS) for an objective measurement of consciousness on a numerical scale (Table 16-8). The client must be as alert as possible before testing. Caution is needed in using the scale if a client has sensory losses (e.g., vision or hearing).

The GSC allows the nurse to evaluate a client's neurological status over time. The higher the score, the better the client's neurological function. The nurse asks short simple questions such as "What is your name?" or "Where are you?". The nurse also asks the client to follow simple commands such as "move your toes."

If the client's consciousness is lowered to the point of being unable to follow commands, the nurse tries to elicit a response by applying firm pressure with a thumb over the root of the client's fingernail. The normal response to painful stimuli is withdrawal of the body part from the stimulus.

Behavior and Appearance. Behaviors, moods, hygiene, grooming, and choice of dress reveal pertinent information about mental status. The nurse remains perceptive of the client's mannerisms and actions during the entire physical assessment. The nurse notes nonverbal as well as verbal behaviors. Does the client respond appropriately to directions? Does the client's mood vary with no apparent cause? Does the client show concern about appearance? Is the client's hair clean, neatly groomed, and are the nails trim and clean? The client should behave in a manner expressing concern and interest in the examination. The client should make eye contact with the nurse and express appropriate feelings that correspond to the situation. Normally the client will show some degree of personal hygiene.

Choice and fit of clothing may reflect socioeconomic background or personal taste rather than deficiency in self-concept or self-care. The nurse avoids being judgmental and focuses assessment on the appropriateness of clothing for the weather. Older adults may neglect their appearance because of a lack of energy, finances, or reduced vision.

Language. Normal cerebral function allows a person to understand spoken or written words and to express the self through writing words or gestures. The nurse observes the client's voice inflection, tone, and manner of speech. The client's voice should have inflections, be clear and strong, and increase in volume appropriately. Speech should be fluent. When communication is clearly ineffective (e.g., omission or addition of letters and words, misuse of words, hesitations), the nurse assesses for **aphasia.** Injury to the cerebral cortex may result in aphasia.

The two types of aphasia are sensory (or receptive) and motor (or expressive). With receptive aphasia a person cannot understand written or verbal speech. With expressive aphasia a person understands written and verbal speech but cannot write or speak appropriately when attempting to communicate. A client may suffer a combination of receptive and expressive aphasia. Assessment requires the nurse to ask the client to name familiar objects when the nurse points at them. The client may also be asked to respond to simple verbal commands such as "stand up." Finally, the nurse may ask the client to read a simple sentence out loud. Normally a client names objects correctly, follows commands, and reads sentences correctly.

Intellectual Function

Intellectual function includes memory, knowledge, abstract thinking, association, and judgment. Each aspect of function is tested with a specific technique. However, because cultural and educational background influences the ability to respond to test questions, the nurse does not ask questions related to concepts or ideas with which the client is unfamiliar.

Memory. The nurse assesses immediate recall and recent and remote memory. Immediate recall is reflected in the ability of the client to repeat a series of numbers in the order they are presented, or in reverse order. Clients can normally recall five to eight digits forward or four to six digits backward.

The nurse asks if the client's memory can be tested. Then the nurse says clearly and slowly the name of three unrelated objects. After the nurse says all three, the client is asked to repeat each. This is continued until the client is successful. Then, later in the assessment, the nurse asks the client to repeat the three words again. The client should be able to identify the three words. Another test for recent memory involves asking the client to recall events occurring during the same day (e.g., what was eaten for breakfast). Information may need to be validated with a family member.

To assess past memory, the nurse can ask the client to recall the mother's maiden name, a birthday, or special date in history. It is best to ask open-ended questions rather than simple yes/no questions. A client should have immediate recall of such information. With older adults, a nurse should not interpret a hearing loss as confusion. Older adults commonly show symptoms of confusion and forgetfulness because of normal neurological changes. Sudden confusion, however, is usually not related to age.

Knowledge. The nurse can assess the client's knowledge by asking how much is known about the illness or the reason for hospitalization. By assessing a client's knowledge, the nurse determines the client's ability to learn or understand. If there is an opportunity to teach information, the nurse can test the client's mental status by asking for feedback during a follow-up visit.

Abstract Thinking. Interpreting abstract ideas or concepts reflects the capacity for abstract thinking. A higher level of intellectual functioning is required for an individual to explain common sayings such as "A stitch in time saves nine" or "Don't count your chickens before they're hatched." The nurse notes whether the client's explanations are relevant and concrete. The client with altered mentation will probably interpret the phrase literally or will merely rephrase the words.

Association. Another higher level of intellectual function involves finding similarities or associations between concepts: a dog is to a beagle as a cat is to a Siamese. The nurse names related concepts and asks the client to identify their associations. Questions should be appropriate to the client's level of intelligence.

Judgment. Judgment requires a comparison and evaluation of facts and ideas to understand their relationships and to form appropriate conclusions. The nurse attempts to measure the client's ability to make logical decisions with questions such as "Why did you decide to seek health care?" or "What would you do if you suddenly became ill at home?". Normally a client can make logical decisions.

Cranial Nerve Function

The nurse may assess all 12 cranial nerves or test a single nerve or related group of nerves. A dysfunction in one nerve reflects an alteration at some point along the cranial nerve's distribution. Measurements used to assess the integrity of organs within the head and neck also assess cranial nerve function. A complete assessment involves testing the twelve cranial nerves in order of their number. To remember the order of the nerves, this simple phrase can be used: "On old Olympus' towering tops a Finn and German viewed some hops." The first letter of each word in the phrase is the same as the first letter of the names of the cranial nerves listed in order (Table 16-9).

Sensory Function

The sensory pathways of the central nervous system conduct the sensations of pain, temperature, position, vibration, and crude and finely localized touch. Different nerve pathways relay the various types of sensations. Most clients require only a quick screening of sensory function, unless there are symptoms of reduced sensation, motor impairment, or paralysis.

Normally a client has sensory responses to all stimuli tested. Sensations are felt equally on both sides of the body in all areas. All sensory testing is performed with the client's eyes closed so that the client is unable to see when or where a stimulus strikes the skin (Table 16-10). Stimuli are then applied in a random, unpredictable order to maintain the client's attention and to prevent detection of a predictable pattern. The client tells the nurse when, what, and where each stimulus is felt. The nurse compares symmetrical areas of the body while applying stimuli to the arms, trunk, and legs.

Motor Function

An assessment of motor function includes measurements made during the musculoskeletal examination. In addition, cerebellar function is determined. The cerebellum coordinates muscular activity, maintains balance and equilibrium, and helps to control posture.

Balance. The nurse assesses balance by asking the client to stand, feet together and arms at the sides with eyes open and closed. Standing close to the client prevents an accidental fall. Slight swaying of the body is expected in the Romberg test. A loss of balance (positive Romberg) causes a client to fall to the side.

Another test for balance involves asking the client to stand on one foot while eyes are closed with arms held

table 16-9
CRANIAL NERVE FUNCTION AND ASSESSMENT

Number	Name	Type	Function	Method
I	Olfactory	Sensory	Sense of smell	Ask client to identify different non-irritating aromas such as coffee and vanilla.
II	Optic	Sensory	Visual acuity	Use Snellen chart or ask client to read printed material while wearing corrective lenses.
III	Oculomotor	Motor	Extraocular eye movement	Assess directions of gaze.
			Pupil constriction and dilation	Measure pupil reaction to light reflex and accommodation.
IV	Trochlear	Motor	Upward and downward movement of eyeball	Assess directions of gaze.
V	Trigeminal	Sensory and motor	Sensory nerve to skin of face	Lightly touch cornea with wisp of cotton. Assess corneal reflex. Measure sensation of light pain and touch across skin of face.
			Motor nerve to muscles of jaw	Palpate temples as client clenches teeth.
VI	Abducens	Motor	Lateral movement of eyeballs	Assess directions of gaze.
VII	Facial	Sensory and motor	Facial expression	As client smiles, frowns, puffs out cheeks, and raises and lowers eyebrows, look for asymmetry.
			Taste	Have client identify salty or sweet taste on front of tongue.
VIII	Auditory	Sensory	Hearing	Assess ability to hear spoken word.
IX	Glossopharyngeal	Sensory and motor	Taste	Ask client to identify sour or sweet taste on back of tongue.
			Ability to swallow	Use tongue blade to elicit gag reflex.
X	Vagus	Sensory and motor	Sensation and pharynx	Ask client to say "ah." Observe palate and pharynx movement.
			Ability to swallow	Use tongue blade to elicit gag reflex.
			Movement of vocal cords	Assess speech for hoarseness.
XI	Spinal accessory	Motor	Movement of head and shoulders	Ask client to shrug shoulders and turn head against passive resistance.
XII	Hypoglossal	Motor	Position of tongue	Ask client to stick out tongue to midline and move it from side to side.

CLIENT TEACHING DURING NEUROLOGICAL SYSTEM ASSESSMENT

Explain to family or friends the implications of any behavioral or mental impairment shown by the client.

If the client has sensory or motor impairments, explain measures to ensure safety (e.g., use of ambulation aids or use of safety bars in bathrooms or stairways).

Teach older adults to plan enough time to complete tasks because reaction time is slowed.

Teach older adults to observe skin surfaces for areas of trauma because their perception of pain is reduced.

straight at the sides. The test is repeated on the opposite foot. Normally balance is maintained for 5 seconds with slight swaying.

Coordination. To avoid confusion, the nurse demonstrates each assessment maneuver and then has clients repeat them while observing for smoothness and balance in the client's movement (see box at left). In older adults normally slow reaction time may cause movements to be less rhythmical.

To assess fine motor function, the nurse has the client extend the arms out to the sides and touch each forefinger alternately to the nose (first with eyes open, then with eyes closed). Normally the client alternately touches the nose smoothly. Performing rapid, rhythmical, alternating movements demonstrates coordination

table 16-10

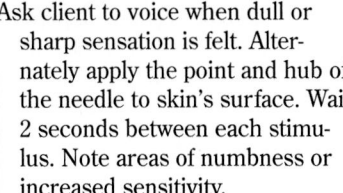

ASSESSMENT OF SENSORY NERVE FUNCTION

Function	Equipment	Method	Precautions
Superficial pain	Sterile needle	Ask client to voice when dull or sharp sensation is felt. Alternately apply the point and hub of the needle to skin's surface. Wait 2 seconds between each stimulus. Note areas of numbness or increased sensitivity.	Areas where skin is thickened, such as heel or sole of foot, may be less sensitive to pain.

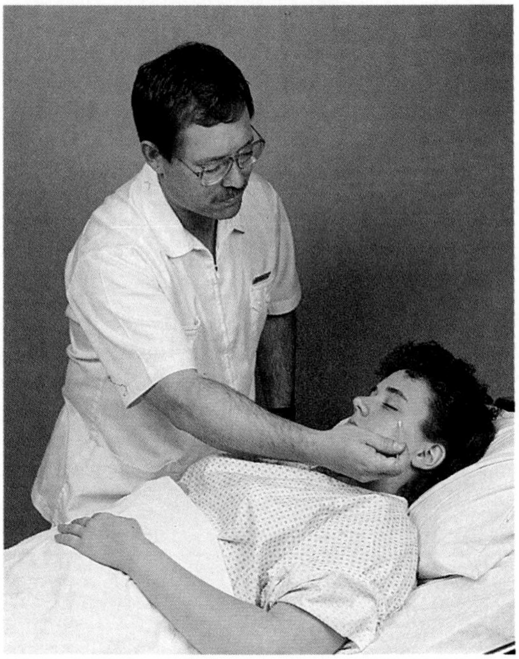

Function	Equipment	Method	Precautions
Temperature	Two test tubes, one filled with hot water and other with cold	Touch skin with tube. Ask client to identify hot or cold sensation and where it is felt.	Omit test if pain sensation is normal.
Light touch	Cotton ball or cotton-tip applicator	Apply light wisp of cotton to different points along skin's surface. Ask client to voice when sensation is felt.	Apply at areas where skin is thin or more sensitive (e.g., face, neck, inner aspect of arms, top of feet and hands). Do not depress the skin; avoid stroking area hard.

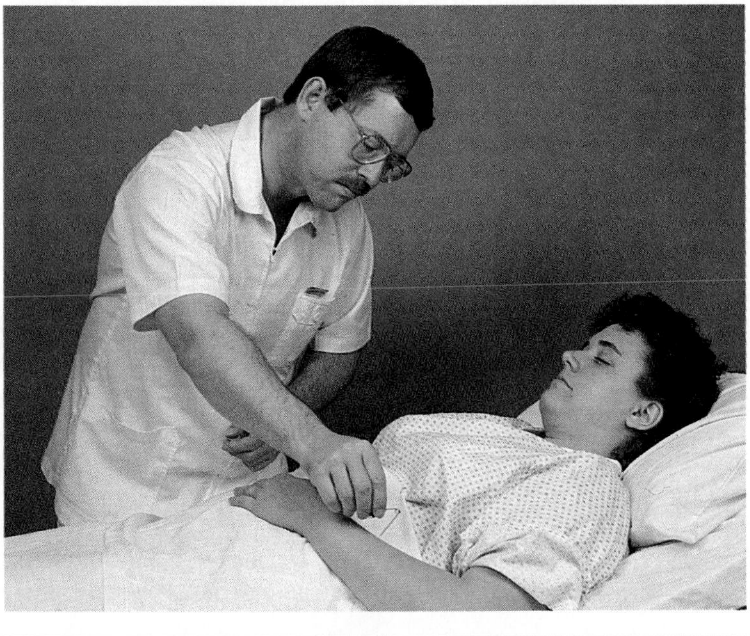

Continued.

table 16-10—cont'd

ASSESSMENT OF SENSORY NERVE FUNCTION

Function	Equipment	Method	Precautions
Vibration	Tuning fork	Apply stem of vibrating fork to distal interphalangeal joint of fingers and interphalangeal joint of great toe, elbow, and wrist. Have client voice when and where the vibration is felt.	Be sure client feels vibration and not merely pressure.
Position		Grasp finger or toe, holding it by its sides with thumb and index finger. Alternate moving finger or toe up and down. Ask client to state when finger is up or down. Repeat with toes.	Avoid rubbing adjacent appendages as finger or toe is moved. Do not move joint laterally; return to neutral position before moving again.
Two-point discrimination	Two needles	Lightly apply one or both points of needles simultaneously to skin's surface. Ask client if one or two pinpricks are felt. Find the distance at which client can no longer distinguish 2 points.	Apply pins to same anatomical site (e.g., fingertips, palm of hand, or upper arms). Minimum distance at which client can discriminate two points varies (2 to 8 mm on fingertips).

in the upper extremities. While sitting, the client begins by patting the knees with both hands. Then the client alternately turns up the palm and back of the hands while continuously patting. The maneuver should be done smoothly and regularly with increasing speed.

An additional maneuver for upper extremity coordination involves touching each finger with the thumb of the same hand in rapid sequence. The client moves from the index finger to the little finger and back with one hand tested at a time. The client's dominant hand is slightly less awkward when performing this movement. Movement should be smooth and in succession.

Lower extremity coordination is tested with the client lying supine, legs extended. The nurse places a hand at the ball of the client's foot. The client taps the nurse's hand with the foot as quickly as possible. Each foot is tested for speed and smoothness. The feet do not normally move as rapidly or evenly as the hands.

Reflexes

Reflex testing assesses the integrity of sensory and motor pathways of the reflex arc and specific spinal cord segments. When a muscle and tendon are stretched, nerve impulses travel along afferent nerve pathways to the dorsal horn of the spinal cord segment. Impulses synapse and travel to the efferent motor neuron in the spinal cord. A motor nerve then sends the impulses back to the muscle, causing the reflex response. Experience is needed to test reflexes accurately.

The two categories of normal reflexes are deep tendon reflexes, elicited by mildly stretching a muscle and tapping a tendon, and cutaneous reflexes, elicited by stimulating the skin superficially.

When reflexes are being assessed, the client relaxes as much as possible to avoid voluntary movement or muscle tensing. The nurse positions the limbs to slightly stretch the muscle being tested. The reflex hammer is held loosely between the nurse's thumb and fingers so it can swing freely and tap the tendon briskly (Figure 16-65). The nurse compares the symmetry of the reflex from one side of the body to the other. Reflexes are graded based on the degree of response. Table 16-11 summarizes common deep tendon and cutaneous reflexes. In older adults, reflexes are normally less brisk or even absent.

AFTER THE EXAMINATION

The nurse may record findings from the physical assessment during the examination or at the end. Special forms are available to record data. The nurse reviews all findings before assisting the client with dressing in case of a need to recheck any information or gather additional data. Physical assessment findings are integrated into the care plan.

After completing the assessment, the nurse gives the client time to dress. The hospitalized client may need help with hygiene and returning to bed. When the client

table 16-11
ASSESSMENT OF COMMON REFLEXES

Type	Procedure	Normal reflex
DEEP TENDON REFLEXES		
Biceps	Flex client's arm up to 45 degrees at elbow with palms down. Place your thumb in antecubital fossa at base of biceps tendon and your fingers over the biceps muscle. Strike triceps tendon with reflex hamer.	Flexion of arm at elbow
Triceps	Flex client's arm at the elbow, holding arm across chest, or hold upper arm horizontally and allow lower arm to go limp. Strike triceps tendon just above elbow.	Extension at elbow
Patellar	Have client sit with legs hanging freely over side of table or chair or have client lie supine and support knee in a flexed 90-degree position. Briskly tap patellar tendon just below patella.	Extension of lower leg
Achilles	Have client assume same position as for patellar reflex. Slightly dorsiflex client's ankle by grasping toes in palm of your hand. Strike Archilles tendon just above heel at the ankle malleolus.	Plantar flexion of foot
Plantar (Babinski's)	Have client lie supine with legs straight and feet relaxed. Take handle end of reflex hammer and stroke lateral aspect of sole from heel to ball of foot, curving across ball of foot toward big toe.	Bending of toes downward
CUTANEOUS REFLEXES		
Gluteal	Have client assume side-lying position. Spread buttocks apart and lightly stimulate perineal area with cotton applicator.	Contraction of anal sphincter
Abdominal	Have client stand or lie supine. Stroke abdominal skin with base of cotton applicator over lateral borders of rectus abdominus muscle toward midline. Repeat test in each abdominal quadrant.	Contraction of rectus abdominis muscle with pulling of umbilicus toward stimulated side

is comfortable, it helps to share a summary of the assessment findings. If the findings have revealed serious abnormalities such as a highly irregular heart rate, the client's physician should be consulted before any findings are revealed. The physician must make definitive medical diagnoses. The nurse can explain the type of abnormality found and the need for the physician to conduct an additional examination.

The nurse may delegate support staff to clean the examination area. Infection control practices are used in removing materials or instruments soiled with potentially infectious wastes (Chapter 25). If the client's bedside was the site for the examination, the nurse clears away soiled items from the bedside table and makes sure the bed linen is dry and clean. The client may appreciate a clean gown and the opportunity to wash the face and hands. Afterward, the nurse washes hands.

The nurse checks to be sure the recording of the as-

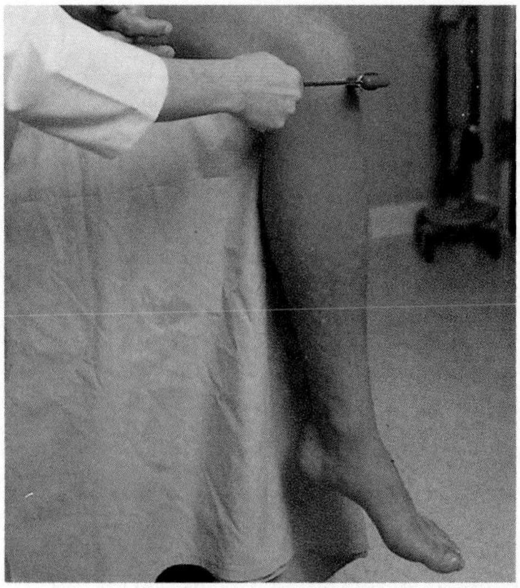

FIGURE 16-65 Position for testing patellar tendon reflex. Lower leg will normally extend.

sessment is complete. If entry of items into the assessment form was delayed, the nurse enters them at this time to avoid forgetting important information. If entries were made periodically during the examination, they are reviewed for accuracy and thoroughness. Significant findings are communicated to appropriate medical and nursing personnel, either verbally or in the client's written care plan.

The client often needs a number of other examinations such as x-ray or laboratory tests after a physical examination. The tests provide additional screening information to rule out and to help diagnose specific abnormalities found during the examination.

SUMMARY

Through physical assessment, the nurse makes insightful clinical decisions about the best approaches to client care. Before an examination begins, the nurse prepares the client and setting. Measures are taken to ensure privacy and psychological and physical comfort. The client becomes an active participant as the nurse carefully explains each step of the examination. Each body system is reviewed through history taking and a methodical sequence of observations and measurements. Physical examination findings supplement data obtained in the health history and from ongoing nurse-client interactions.

The examination must be organized. Each system review entails numerous observations. Basic principles for a thorough examination include comparing both sides of the body for symmetry, completing each system before moving to the next, using each skill as appropriate, and recognizing the observations that have priority for a client. The nurse uses time during an examination to teach clients ways to improve or maintain their health.

As a result of a thorough physical examination, the nurse can make nursing diagnoses with greater accuracy. Therefore the client's plan of care becomes more individualized and comprehensive. Physical assessment findings also reveal if nursing measures were successful and if the client's level of health is improving.

KEY CONCEPTS

- Baseline assessment findings reflect the client's functional abilities when the nurse first assesses the client and serve as the basis for comparison with subsequent assessment findings.
- Assessment data are used to make nursing diagnoses, select appropriate nursing interventions, and measure outcomes of nursing care.
- When assessing older adults the nurse learns to recognize how the normal process of aging affects physical findings.
- Client teaching should be integrated throughout the examination to help clients learn about health promotion and disease prevention.
- The nurse can use time more efficiently by integrating physical assessment with routine nursing care.
- Inspection requires good lighting, full exposure of the body part, and a careful comparison of the part with its counterpart on the opposite side of the body.
- Palpation involves the use of parts of the hand to detect different types of physical characteristics.
- Percussion is the detection of differences in density of underlying tissues by listening to sounds produced while striking the body's surface.
- Through auscultation the nurse assesses the character of sounds created in various body organs.
- A physical examination should be performed only after proper preparation of the environment and equipment and after preparing the client physically and psychologically.
- Throughout the examination the nurse should keep the client warm, comfortable, and informed of each step of the assessment process.
- The nurse should use a systematic approach when conducting a physical assessment.
- Information from the health history helps the nurse to focus on body systems likely to be affected.
- During physical examinations the nurse can demonstrate self-examination techniques for clients.
- The client assumes various positions during the physical examination to provide greater accessibility of body parts and increase accuracy in assessment.
- A competent examiner learns to combine assessments of different body systems simultaneously.
- At the end of the examination the nurse provides for the client's comfort and then completes a detailed review of physical assessment findings.

CRITICAL THINKING ACTIVITIES

1. You palpate a mass while examining a client's neck. Describe any additional assessments you would make.
2. When turning a client from the supine to side lying position, identify two body systems you might assess.
3. Mr. Leonard enters the clinic with a history of weight loss and general fatigue. Describe three body systems that may be involved. What questions might you ask the client to discover the primary system involved?

4. What physical examination measures might you use to evaluate abdominal pain, oral hygiene, and application of a cast to the arm.
5. Mrs. Jones is 48 years old and enters the physician's office for a routine annual checkup. What screening examinations are necessary for a client this age?
6. Explain the different findings you might gather when assessing coordination in a 40 year old versus an 80 year old.

References

American Cancer Society: *Cancer facts and figures 1993,* Atlanta, 1993, The Society.
American Thoracic Society: Control of tuberculosis in the United States, *Am Rev Resp Disease* 146(6):1623-1633, 1992.
Champion VL: Effect of knowledge, teaching method, confidence and social influence on breast self-examination behavior, *Image J Nurs Sch* 21(2):76, 1989.
Clore ER: Dispelling the common myths about pediculosis, *J Pediatr Health Care* 3:28-33, 1989.
DeWitt S: Nursing assessment of the skin and dermatologic lesions, *Nurs Clin North Am,* 25(1):235, 1990.
Durham CF: The no fault way to assess carotid arteries, *Nursing 88* 18:65-67, Nov. 1988.
Elder abuse: common clues help identify high-risk patients, *Geriatrics* 42:26, 1987.
Ernst ND: The national cholesterol education program's recommendations for treatment of high blood cholesterol, *Fam Community Health* 12(1): 23,1989.
Hardy MA: A pilot study of the diagnosis and treatment of impaired skin integrity: dry skin in older persons, *Nurs Diag* 1(2):57-63, 1990.
Kpea NT: Easily observed signs of systemic disease, *Consultant* 27(8):47, 1987.
Larson E: Evaluating validity of screening tests, *Nurs Res* 35:186, 1986.
Mahoney D: One simple solution to hearing impairment, *Geriatr Nurs* 8(5):242, 1987.
Mettlin C, et al.: Defining and updating the American Cancer Society guidelines for the cancer-related checkup: prostate and endometrial cancers, CA *Cancer J Clin* 43(1):42-46, Jan/Feb 1993.
McConnell EA: Getting the feel of lymph node assessment, *Nurs 88* 18:55-57, Aug. 1988.
McConnell EA: Auscultating bowel sounds, *Nurs 90,* 20:106, 1990.
Parrino TA: The art and science of percussion, *Hosp Pract* 15:25, 1987.
Pires M, Muller A: Detection and management of early tissue pressure indicators: a pictorial essay, *Progressions* 3(3):3, 1991.
Reed AT, Birge SJ: Screening for osteoporosis, *J Gerontol Nurs* 14(7):18, 1988.
Rossi L and Leary E: Evaluating the patient with coronary artery disease, *Nurs Clin North Am* 27 (1):171, March 1992.
Seidel HM, et al.: *Mosby's guide to physical examination,* St. Louis, 1991, Mosby.
Silen W: Pitfalls to avoid when evaluating severe abdominal pain, *J Crit Illness* 7(5):685-689, 1992.
Whaley LF, Wong DL: Nursing care of infants and children, ed 4, St. Louis, 1991, Mosby.
Wilkins RL, Hodgkin JE, Lopez B: *Lung sounds: a practical guide,* St. Louis, 1988, Mosby.
Williams ED, et al.: Barriers to breast cancer screening in older women, *Fam Community Health* 10(3):51, 1987.

Bibliography

Andersen GP: A fresh look at assessing the elderly, *RN* p. 28, June 1989.
Becker KL, Stevens SA: Performing in-depth abdominal assessment, *Nurs 88* 18(6):59, 1988.
Berman R, et al.: Physiology of aging. II. Clinical implications, *Patient Care* 23:39, 1989.
Burkhart C: Guidelines for rapid assessment of abdominal pain indicative of acute surgical abdomen, *Nurs Prac* 17(6):39-46, 1992.
Casey MP: Testicular cancer: the worst disease at the worst time, *RN* 50:36, 1987.
Centers for Disease Control: Update: universal precautions for prevention of transmission of HIV, HBV, and other blood borne pathogens in the healthcare setting, *MMWR* 37:377, 1988.
Dennison R: Cardiopulmonary assessment, *Nurs 86* 16:34, 1986.
Ebersole P and Hess P: Toward healthy aging, ed 3, St. Louis, 1990, Mosby.
Erickson BA: Detecting abnormal heart sounds, *Nurs 86* 16:58, 1986
Flory C: Skin assessment, *RN* 55:22, June 1992.
Garnick MB: Prostate cancer: screening, diagnosis and management, *Ann Intern Med* 118(10):804-818, May 15, 1993.
Gehring PE: Vascular assessment, *RN* 55:40, Jan. 1992.
Hollerbach AD, Sneed NV: Accuracy of radial pulse assessment by length of counting interval, *Heart Lung* 19(3):258, 1990.
Lindsey M: Abdominal assessment, *Orthop Nurs* 8(4):34, 1989.
Maklebust J: Impact of AHCPR pressure ulcer guidelines on nursing practice, *Decubitus* 4(2):46, 1991a.
McConnell E: Auscultating bowel sounds, *Nurs 90* 20:106, 1990.
Malasanos L, Barkauskas V, and Stoltenberg-Allen K: Health assessment, St. Louis, 1990, Mosby.
McHugh J, McHugh W: How to assess deep tendon reflexes, *Nurs 90,* 20:62, 1990.
Moore S, et al.: Screening for prostate cancer: PSA blood test, rectal examination, and ultrasound, *Urol Nurs* 12(3):106-107, 1992.
Prigel CLB: How to spot melanoma, *Nurs 87* 17:60, June 1987.
Pugliese G and Lampinen T: Prevention of human immunodeficiency virus infection: our responsibilities as health care professionals, *Am J Infect Control* 17(1):1, 1989.
Rutledge DN: Factors related to women's practice of breast self-examination, *Nurs Res* 36:117, 1987.
Smith C: Assessing bowel sounds: more than just listening, *Nurs 88* 18:42, 1988.
Stanford J: Testicular self-examination teaching: learning, and practice by nurses, *J Adv Nurs* 12:13-19, 1987.
United States Department of Health and Human Services: *Pressure ulcers in adults: prediction and prevention,* Pub No 92-0047, 92-0050, Rockville, Md., 1992, Public Health Service, Agency for Health Care Policy and Research.
Weinrich SP, et al.: Timely detection of colorectal cancer in the elderly: implications of the aging process, *Cancer Nurs* 12(3):170, 1989.
Whaley LF and Wong DL: Nursing care of infants and children, ed 4, St. Louis, 1991, Mosby.
Wilkins RL: Lung sounds: a practical guide, St. Louis, 1988, Mosby.

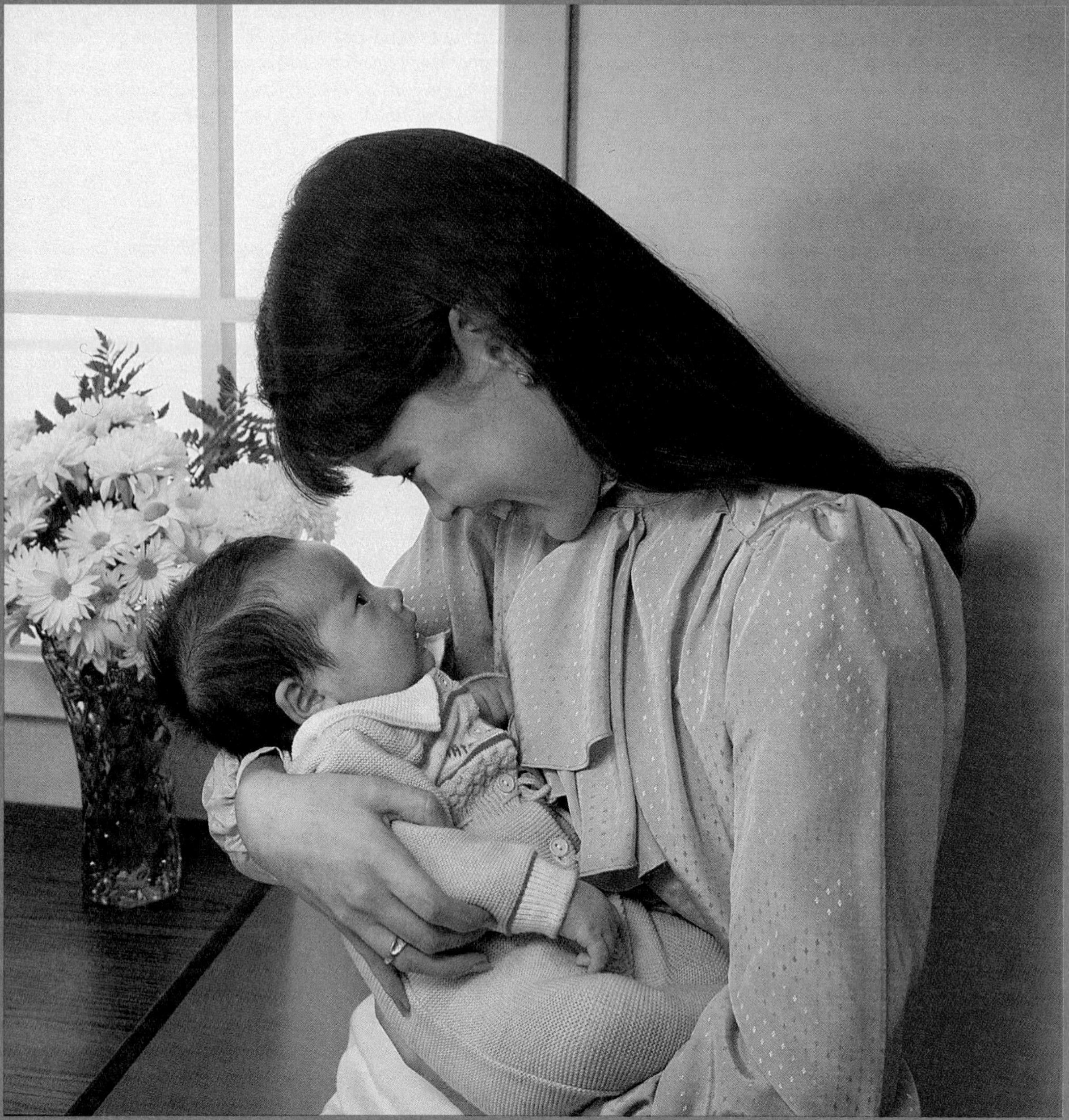

unit four

PSYCHOSOCIAL AND DEVELOPMENTAL NEEDS

17 Psychosocial Factors in Health

OBJECTIVES

Mastery of content in this chapter will enable the student to:

- Define the key terms listed.
- Discuss factors that influence the following components of self-concept: body image, self-esteem, roles, and identity.
- Identify stressors that affect each of the four components of self-concept.
- Discuss ways in which the nurse's self-concept and nursing activities can affect the client's self-concept.
- Discuss the nurse's role in maintaining or enhancing a client's sexual health.
- Define sexuality as a component of personality.
- Describe key concepts of sexual development during infancy, childhood, adolescence, and adulthood.
- Discuss the relationship of spiritual health to physiological and psychosocial health.
- Describe the signs of unmet spiritual needs.
- Apply the nursing process to assess, diagnose, plan, implement, and evaluate interventions to promote a client's self-concept, sexual health, and spirituality.

KEY TERMS

body image
gender identity
gender role
identity
religious
role
self-concept
self-esteem
sexual dysfunction
sexual orientation
sexual response cycle
sexuality
socialization
spiritual
spiritual distress
spiritual health
spirituality

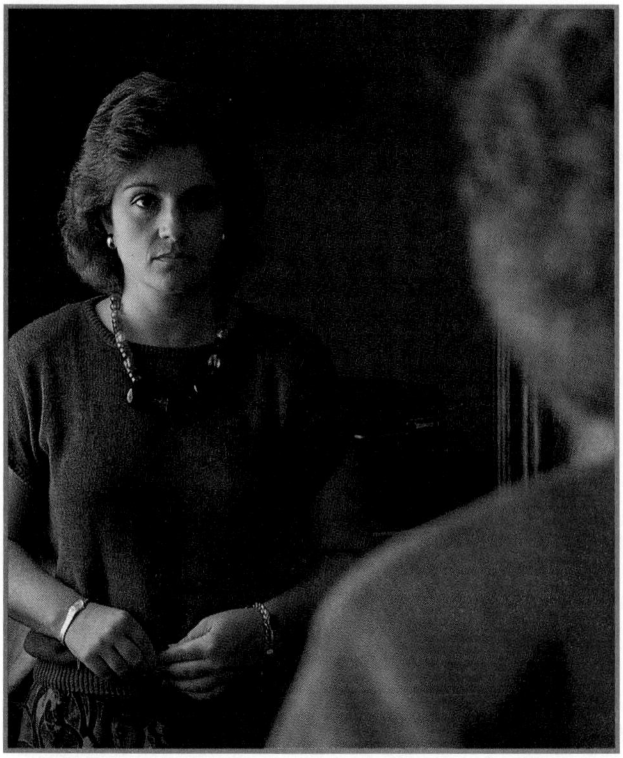

Self-concept, sexuality, and spirituality affect the health status of an individual. They are intimately connected to our sense of who we are in the world. Changes in health status may create stressors in self-concept, sexuality, and spirituality that the nurse needs to identify. The nurse needs to possess the skills to intervene and then assist the client in reestablishing healthy functioning.

SELF-CONCEPT AND HEALTH

The self is one of the most important aspects of human experience, yet it is one of the most difficult to define. What we think of ourselves affects the care we give ourselves both physically and emotionally. If our sense of self is poor, we feel we do not deserve care and consideration. If we do not feel worthy of care, we will not seek care. Thus clients with poor self-concept often have difficulty taking care of the "self," physically and emotionally.

A person's **self-concept** represents a subjective image of the self. It is a complex integration of conscious and unconscious feelings, attitudes, and perceptions. The self-concept is a frame of reference affecting self-image, behaviors, and relationships with others. Self-concept is resistant to change; often even though the self may have undergone great change, changes take time to be incorporated into the self-concept. Discrepancies between the self and self-concept may become a source of stress or conflict.

Sexuality reflects a person's sense of femaleness or maleness. This dynamic and diverse function of the total personality involves the biological, psychological, sociological, spiritual, and cultural dimensions and affects values, attitudes, behaviors, and relationships with others. Sexuality shapes and is shaped by life experiences.

Spirituality generally refers to a person's awareness of a larger meaning of life, a divine being, and the internal forces that motivate people toward goodness, beauty, and health. A person's concept of spirituality can reflect on or be reflected by self-concept and other psychosocial aspects such as sexuality.

Development of Self-Concept

The development of a self-concept is a complex process involving many variables. Of the major theories concerned with how self-concept develops, Piaget's and Erikson's are perhaps most useful. Piaget's consists of three stages that find completion at adulthood; Erikson describes eight stages that end with senescence. In both theories, each stage builds on the tasks of the former stage (Erikson, 1963 and Piaget and Inhelder, 1969).

Piaget was concerned with the development of thinking processes by children. His theory described the five stages of cognitive development, progressing from a reflexive infant to an abstractly thinking adolescent (Piaget and Inhelder, 1969). All stages progress through a schematic restructuring of thinking to get to the next stage. To Piaget, *schema* were organized forms of behavior that had a definite purpose associated with a particular image of an experience or an event. The child internalized these various events. The cognitive process of accommodation involves developing new schemata from old ones to solve new problems. Piaget proposed that all people develop cognitively in a similar pattern.

Whereas Piaget was concerned with thinking, Erikson was concerned with behaviors. In each stage of Erikson's psychosocial development, an individual faces certain tasks that, if not positively completed, may lead to psychological problems. Through social and cultural reinforcement, an individual spends a lifetime learning the relevance of, cultural connotations of, and emotional significance of concepts. Erikson's theory demonstrates the influence of society and the environment on the development of self-concept. A person who does not develop a sense of trust as an infant may have difficulty with later stages of psychosocial development. For example, illness could lead to a sense of physical and psychosocial vulnerability and a distrust of the environment, especially a hospital environment. By using Erikson's theory, nurses can identify the phase of psychosocial development a client is experiencing and direct care toward the appropriate stage of development.

A new dimension in the area of self-concept is the field of gender differences. It is one of the most important contributions to understanding the differences between male and female thinking. Formerly, females fell short on measures of maturity that had been developed by male theorists. It is now believed that the differences do not reflect deficiency, but different values. Beginning in 1982, with research done by Carol Gilligan (1982), some developmental theorists began to feel that female moral development (which influences how males and females make decisions) may be different from that of males.

Females in our culture are allowed to display a full range of emotions and are taught to value relationships and care about others. Males in our culture are allowed only a very narrow range of emotionality and are taught to display leadership, be aggressive, and become accomplished (Bly, 1990; Farrell, 1986; Fine, 1988; Goldberg, 1977; Shapiro, 1984). Females are socialized in our culture to value caring as the highest form of development; males are socialized to value justice and fairness (Chaney, 1993). Developmental theorists no longer believe females are deficient, merely different from males. Gender research is validating this thinking (Davenport and Yurich, 1991; Frank, 1986; Mellor, 1989; Pratt, Dressner, et al., 1991; Shreve and Kankel, 1991). This important difference is now being associated with the high rate of male stress disorders in mid-life (Cooper, 1982; Benson, 1984; Breo, 1989).

Components of Self-Concept

A person's self-concept involves body image, self-esteem, roles, and identity. Each aspect develops from birth onward and reflects the changes that take place throughout life. Although they can be considered as separate aspects, they overlap and are interrelated.

The body is the container for the self. **Body image** is an individual's psychological experience of his or her body; it includes feelings and attitudes. It is the most visible manifestation of who we are; it is with us from birth to death. Body image is affected by cognitive growth and physical development. Normal developmental changes such as growth and aging have more apparent effects on body image than on other aspects of self-concept. The body is submitted to comparisons of what is considered valuable in society. What is emphasized in a particular culture often is the measuring stick to which we compare our bodies. If we deviate markedly from what is valued, our self-concept is lowered. For example, Stein (1987) found in studying obese adolescents in our culture, that those who saw themselves as obese had lower self-esteem scores and elevated neurosis scores.

What our culture and society value influences body image. For example, youth, beauty, and wholeness are emphasized in American society. Because a person's body image depends only partly on the reality of the body, people generally do not adapt quickly to physical changes. As with the total self-concept, a physical change may not be incorporated into the image one has of one's body. It may take someone who has lost a great deal of weight a long time to incorporate the thin self into the self-concept. Formerly obese people will tell you there is still a "fat person" inside. Conversely, people who have had a large weight gain frequently say the gain was easy to repress because they still perceive themselves as thin.

Like body image, self-esteem is based on many internal and external factors. **Self-esteem** is derived from two sources: the self and others. In its most basic form it hinges on love and approval. When love and approval are not given, the child incorporates a low sense of self-esteem. Self-esteem is often related to how a child evaluates himself or herself at school, at work, and within the family. Self-worth is a basic human need; everyone has a need to feel competent and worthy of living. Self-esteem is innately involved in the enhancement and maintenance of self-concept.

Self-esteem, although dependent on many factors, can be understood in terms of the relationship of a person's self-concept to the ideal self. The ideal self consists of the aspirations, goals, values, and standards of behavior that the person considers ideal and strives to attain. The ideal self originates in early childhood and develops throughout life. In general, a person whose self-concept comes close to matching the ideal self has a high level of self-esteem. In contrast, when self-concept varies widely from the ideal self, a low level of self-esteem results (Figure 17-1).

A **role** is a set of behaviors by which a person participates in a social group. Each individual may have many roles. Roles involve expectations or standards of behavior that have been accepted by the social group in which one participates. Fulfillment of these expectations leads to rewards; failure to fulfill the perceived role expectations can result in lowered self-esteem. Behavior is based on patterns established through the process of socialization. **Socialization** is the "acquisition of the requisite orientation for satisfactory functioning in a role" (Parsons, 1951). The process of socialization begins just after birth, when an infant responds to an adult and the adult responds to the behavior of the infant. During socialization, a person generally develops the skills necessary for satisfactory functioning in many different roles. Unsuccessful socialization may lead to an inability to function acceptably according to society's values.

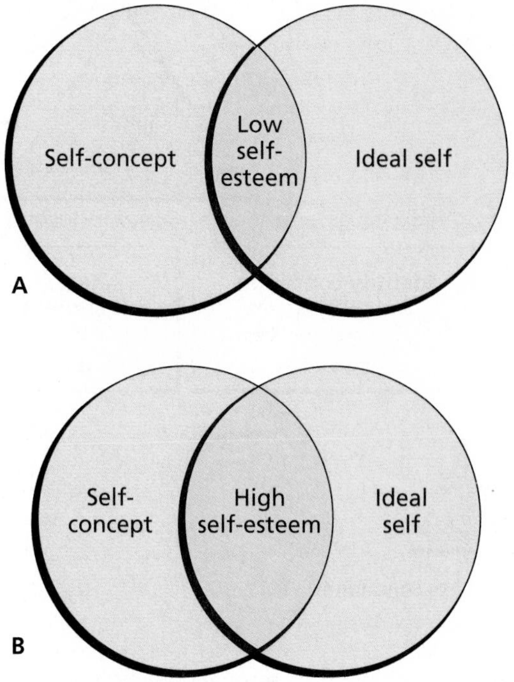

FIGURE 17-1 A, Individual with low level of self-esteem; discrepancy between self-concept and ideal self. **B,** Person with greater conformity between self-concept and ideal self; high level of self-esteem. (Modified from Sundeen SG, et al.: *Nurse-client interaction,* ed 3, St. Louis, 1986, Mosby.)

Identity is derived from the Latin word *idem,* which means "the same." Identity involves the persistent individuality and sameness of a person over time and in various circumstances. It implies a consciousness of being oneself, distinct and separate from others.

Adolescence, Erikson's fifth stage of development, is a particularly crucial time for the development of identity. The child identifies with those around him, incorporating various aspects of others into himself. Identity includes a conscious sense of individuality, an unconscious striving for consistency in personal character, and maintenance of solidarity with the ideals of one's social group. A person with a sense of identity will feel integrated rather than diffused. However, a person's sense of identity continually evolves and is influenced by circumstances throughout life.

Stressors Affecting Self-Concept

A self-concept stressor is any factor or change, whether real or perceived, that threatens body image, self-esteem, roles, or sense of identity. Stressors challenge the adaptive capacities of a person. Individuals react to the same situation differently. A variety of responses including anxiety, frustration, anger, inability to adjust, difficulty in making decisions, and tension may be observed. An individual's perception of the stress is the most important factor that influences the response. Each person has learned a pattern of behavior enabling him or her to cope with or adapt to stressors. For example, some people apply problem-solving methods to stressful situations. However, some people are immobilized by perceived threats and require help from other people.

Stressors can affect self-concept in any or all of its components. Hospitalization, illness, and surgery are common stressors that can have interrelated effects on self-concept. A physical change in the body leads to an altered body image, but self-esteem and identity may also be affected. Certain chronic illnesses often alter roles, which may change self-esteem and identity (Figure 17-2).

Body-Image Stressors. When a body part changes in appearance or function, the body image may change. Changes in the appearance of the body, such as an amputation, an ostomy, a mastectomy, or facial alterations, are examples of stressors affecting body image. Depending on their severity, cause, or perception by the client, they can be destructive to social functioning or actually change social functioning for the better (e.g., war injuries and heroic rehabilitation efforts that are models for others). Changes such as cardiac disease or renal failure that affect the body's capacity to function at optimum levels also affect body image, although the body may not have outwardly changed. Pregnancy, often viewed as a normal event, can have very negative effects on women whose body image is closely tied to their self-concept.

The significance of a loss of function or a change in appearance is affected by the individual's perception of the alteration (e.g., an ideal image of femininity could be altered by a mastectomy). Body image consists of both real and ideal elements. Another consideration is the importance of body image within self-concept. The greater the importance of body image, the greater the threat that a change in body image may alter perception of self (e.g., severe burn scars that may affect socialization).

Self-help groups are available in most communities for persons who have had ostomies (United Ostomy Association), mastectomies (Reach to Recovery), or laryngectomies (Laryngectomy Club). These groups provide a special kind of support to persons coping with a particular type of physical impairment. Someone who has experienced a particular stressor and who has adapted to it can be instrumental in helping a hospitalized client adapt to a body-image change.

Self-Esteem Stressors. Self-esteem begins in infancy, with perceived acceptance or rejection by parents. Persons with high self-esteem are generally happier and more able to cope with demands and stressors than per-

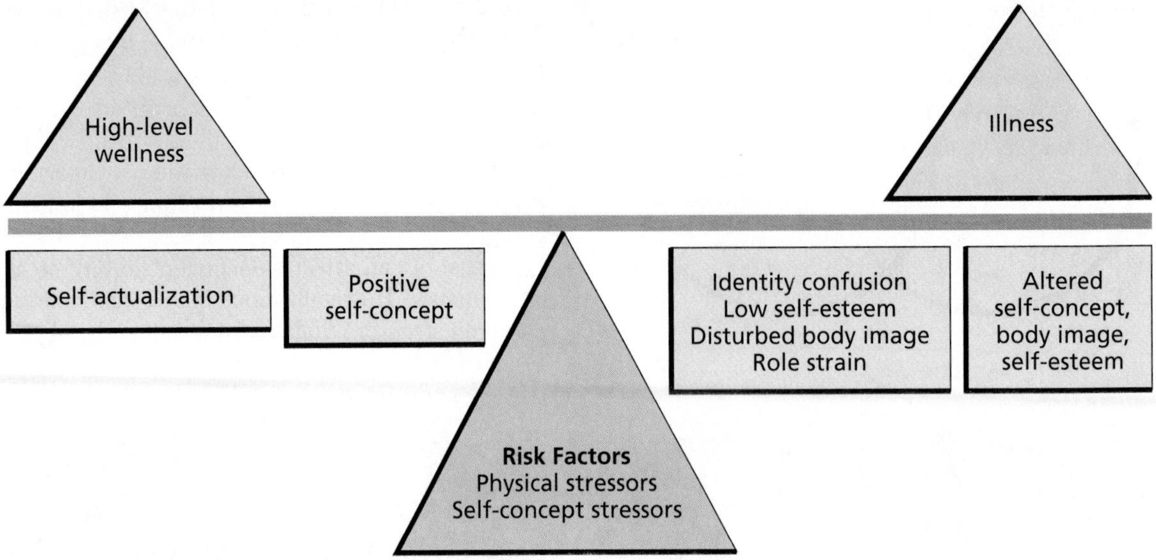

FIGURE 17-2 Self-concept health-illness continuum.

sons with low self-esteem (Gibson, 1980). Persons with low self-esteem tend to feel unloved and often experience depression and anxiety. Many stressors may affect the self-esteem of children. Inability to meet parental expectations, harsh criticism, or repeated defeats may reduce the level of self-worth. Examples of stressors affecting the self-esteem of adults include failures in relationships, divorce, and loss of a job.

Illness, surgery, or accidents that interrupt or change life patterns may also decrease the feeling of self-worth. Chronic illnesses such as diabetes, arthritis, and cardiac dysfunction require changes in behavioral patterns. Chronic illness, surgery, or severe trauma may necessitate a change in a person's life work, affecting one's self-esteem (see box below).

Role Stressors. Throughout life, a person undergoes many role changes. Change within the same role and the adoption of new roles require the incorporation of new expectations and standards for behavior. Meleis (1975) identifies the following categories of role transition: developmental, situational, and health-illness. Normal changes associated with growth and maturation result in developmental transitions. Situational transitions occur when a person loses a parent, spouse, or close friend, or moves, marries, or changes jobs. A health-illness transition is a movement from a state of health or well-being to one of illness. Any of these types of role transitions may threaten self-concept. They may result in role conflict, role ambiguity, or role strain.

Role conflict occurs when a person tries to assume two or more roles that have contradictory expectations. The role of wife and employee can conflict if the husband expects his wife to be home each night by 6:00, and the job expectation is that the employee finish the task at hand (writing a report) that cannot be done without office data, which can only be retrieved after 5:30. Role overload may happen if the role is simply too complex. The individual does not possess the intellectual, economic, emotional, or physical resources to perform the role.

Role ambiguity, common among adolescents and in job situations, involves unclear role expectations. Persons can become unsure of others' expectations of them. A role strain, which incorporates role conflict and role ambiguity, is the sense of frustration that occurs when a person feels inadequate for a role.

EXAMPLES OF BEHAVIORS ASSOCIATED WITH LOW SELF-ESTEEM

Feels guilty, punishes self for not meeting ideal self
Sets unrealistic goals, feels worthless when goals not attained
Has disturbed interpersonal relationships
Exaggerates self-importance

Identity Stressors. Although identity is challenged throughout the lifespan, adolescence is clearly one of the most critical periods for identity stress. Adolescence is a time of change, insecurity, and anxiety. The changes in body and emotion, peer pressure, and the unclear role of adolescents in our society cause much anxiety. An adult generally has a more stable identity and a more firmly held image of self. Once the identity is more se-

IDENTITY CONFUSION

Withdraws from activities because of underlying feelings of not belonging
Is prejudiced against others to strengthen own identity
Uses escape behavior (e.g., drugs, alcohol, or hard physical exercise)

cure, the adult can weather stressors such as marriage, divorce, menopause, aging, and retirement.

Identity is closely tied to physical appearance or physical actions. As these decline, the individual may become highly stressed. These physical changes necessitate adaptation by the individual.

Retirement often brings about social isolation and decreased feelings of worth. If investment in other areas such as travel, community, church, and volunteerism are not made, the individual may succumb to the stressor with depression. Often a grieving spouse relates that they had invested their identity in the roles of the dead spouse, leaving them with no remaining personal identity.

Stressors that can affect self-concept are also risk factors to health. If a person is unable to adapt to such stressors, the level of health may be lowered, and illness may result if the subsequent identity confusion, low self-esteem, disturbed body image, role conflict, strain, or ambiguity are not relieved (see box above).

Effects of Health Care

The nurse can have profound influence in the health care of clients experiencing alterations in self-concept. Often the nurse is the first health care provider to see the client.

The nurse accepts the client through verbal and nonverbal means. Recognizing the alteration and prioritizing the care plan to include self-concept problems can be the most meaningful nursing judgment of the treatment plan. Clients respond much better to physical alterations in health when their emotional status is stable, adaptable, and motivated.

The nurse's impact is most visible to the client in the area of body image. A client who must adapt to a changed body image caused by illness or surgery needs support, as does the family. If the nurse feels, for example, that an ostomy or a mastectomy is a horrible, disfiguring event, the nurse should talk with someone who has more experience in the care and rehabilitation of such clients. Clients watch nurses' reactions to the body change to extract their perceptions of their altered status.

It is critical that the nurse recognize any feelings of revulsion, shock, horror, lack of compassion, or anger toward clients or their illness. If such feelings arise within the nurse, she can often convey these feelings to other nurses experienced in dealing with such issues. The nurse tries to convey compassion in a nonjudgmental manner to help clients adapt despite an alteration in body, role, identity, or self-esteem.

The very issue of an alteration in health puts the client in a dependent position, often in a controlled setting (hospital) in which the client must eat, sleep, dress, and socialize at the appropriate times. In addition, physical examination of the body, drawing blood samples for laboratory analysis, and many other "routine" actions threaten the client's perception of body privacy. A health care environment often makes a client feel isolated and vulnerable. Encouraging visits by family members helps the client to maintain the usual role within the family. Discussing all procedures with the client and encouraging participation in the nursing care plan are examples of ways in which a nurse can respect the client's identity as a person capable of making decisions. In general, the nurse's goal is to assist the client in carrying on as usual, as much as possible, with activities and relationships that support self-concept.

Each client is an individual, and the nurse's role differs with each client. An often primary, but hidden role, is as a role model. The nurse provides an example for the client and family; acceptance of the client as a human being who has ideas, feelings, and values and who is worthy and whole despite illness or physical alterations is important. Feelings of insecurity, fears of rejection, or loss of self-worth can be lessened through sensitive, knowledgeable care.

NURSING PROCESS

Assessment

The nursing assessment should focus on actual and potential self-concept stressors and on behaviors associated with an altered self-concept. The following are examples of stressors that may affect self-concept:

Component	Examples
Body image	Altered functioning after cerebrovascular accident Incontinence Arthritis Alteration or loss of body part (amputation, mastectomy, or colostomy) Normal growth and developmental changes (aging or pregnancy)

Component	Examples
Self-esteem	Loss of job Divorce or separation Repeated failures Unrealistic self-ideal Dependency on others Homelessness
Roles	Incompatible role expectations Unclear role expectations Inability to adequately perform and cope with multiple roles
Identity	Tasks of adolescence Peer pressure Parent-child conflicts Sexual concerns Relationship concerns

The nursing assessment should include consideration of previous coping behaviors, the nature, number, and intensity of the stressors, and the client's internal and external resources. Many times the nurse neglects to assess how the client has dealt with prior stressors. This knowledge can often give the nurse valuable information as to what the client's style of coping may be. Coping may be through avoidance of the problem, information gathering, deferring decisions about themselves to the significant other to make, denial, and so on. Not all issues are addressed in the same way by clients, but many times one uses a significant coping pattern.

Are the stressors many, or just several pressing ones? Are they urgent, or are they something that can be resolved in stages? Resources and strengths such as helpful significant others should also be an important part of the nursing assessment.

Nursing Diagnosis

The assessment should reveal the presence of defining characteristics and client behaviors that lead to a nursing diagnosis (see box below). The nurse assesses the four primary areas of self-concept: body image, role, self-esteem, and identity.

Alterations in **body image** are indicated by nonverbal display of shame or embarrassment of the body part and verbal statements such as "I'm not whole anymore, no one wants to look at this." Personal **identity** problems are manifested by children and adolescents as behaviors that are markedly different from their usual patterns of behavior. Adults often verbalize confusion as to who they are now that this event has happened to them. Nonverbally they often display a decrease in **self-esteem** by slovenly dress. An example might involve a client refusing to dress for the day, remaining in a pajama top and everyday trousers, following retirement. If one's role has been to provide meals, a clean home, and socialization for one's husband, with his death the role dissolves.

Finally, if one has engaged in any activity (no matter how small) that provides a sense of accomplishment and that activity is extinguished, self-esteem suffers. For example, a widowed client, although retired, kept bees on his property, read about them, and informed others about them. He had no children or close relatives. His **body image** had been altered by the diabetes (leg ulcers), his **role** as a beekeeper dissolved and, along with it, his sense of **self-esteem.** When his diabetes became so severe that he could not take care of the bees anymore, he suffered a severe loss of **self-concept.** Three of the four primary areas had been markedly affected.

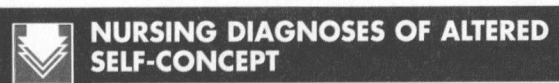

NURSING DIAGNOSES OF ALTERED SELF-CONCEPT

Altered role performance
Body-image disturbance
Self-esteem disturbance
Personal identity disturbance

Planning

Planning to enhance the self-concept is done initially by the nurse from the assessment information. The client should be consulted as an active participant in goal-setting.

Planning interventions for clients with altered self-concept involves goal-setting with expected outcomes that are measurable by the nurse, family, and client. Clients with altered self-concepts require nursing care plans directed at meeting actual or potential self-concept needs in the areas of body image, self-esteem, role, and identity. The plans are based on one or more of the following goals and expected outcomes:

Goal: Client's self-awareness and body image are improved within 1 week.

Outcome

- Client verbalizes improved body image
- Client's posture and appearance are improved

Goal: Client's statements reflect improved self-worth.

Outcome

- Client verbalizes increasing self-worth
- Client attempts new tasks
- Client independently seeks out social activities

Goal: Client adjusts to new role within 2 months.

Outcome

- Client establishes realistic short-term, role-related goals by 1 month

Client modifies role expectations

Goal: Client adapts to changes in body image and role within 1 month

Outcome

Client actively socializes with family and friends

Client posture and appearance are consistent with positive self-image

When planning interventions, the nurse considers the client's present level of adaptation. The level of adaptation can be located on a continuum in each of the following five areas (Bernstein and Cope, 1976):

Active coping ↔ Passive surrender

Leading and co-managing treatment ↔ Resisting treatment

Loving exchange ↔ Rage

Awareness ↔ Denial

Adaptive defenses ↔ Maladaptive defenses

Planning should therefore take into account the client's position on each continuum. The nursing care plan should include understanding and support as the client explores self-concept and should permit expression of feelings (crying, anger, or depression). Clients need time to adapt to changes, and they need manageable, sequential steps to follow.

Implementation

The nurse should provide a therapeutic environment that supports the client emotionally as well as physically. The client who must adapt to an altered body image as a result of surgery or other physical change often finds a visit by a rehabilitated person helpful. However, the timing of such a visit is important because the client may still be denying that the problem exists. Each client must be individually evaluated for such a visit, and "rules of thumb" often must go out the window. Forcing an issue has the potential to be harmful to the client who simply needs more acceptance time.

When providing care to a client experiencing stressors affecting self-worth and identity, the nurse should include activities in which the client will achieve success. Tasks should be realistic; success is best achieved when tasks are sequential in difficulty. The nurse needs to keep other nurses and other health care professionals up to date on the client's progress; others can be involved in offering support and reinforcement for the client if they are aware of the current status. Supporting the client's healthy coping mechanisms strengthens the client's self-esteem and self-identity.

Promoting the Healthy Self-Concept

Interventions designed to help a client reach the goal of adapting to changes in self-concept or attaining a positive self-concept are based on the premise that the client first develops insight and self-awareness concerning problems and stressors and then acts to solve the problems and cope with the stressors. This approach, established by Stuart and Sundeen (1991), involves the following levels of intervention: expanded self-awareness, self-exploration, self-evaluation, planning realistic goals, and commitment to action.

Increasing the client's self-awareness is achieved through establishing a trusting relationship that allows the client to participate fully in health care. This makes the situation less threatening for the client and encourages behaviors that expand self-awareness. The nurse facilitates this relationship by being open, direct, and honest and by conveying to the client a sense of positive identity. The sensitive nurse will encourage the client to make decisions that affect health care, reinforcing the client's sense of control in the environment and strengthening self-worth.

Encouraging the client's self-exploration is achieved by accepting the client's feelings and thoughts, by helping the client to clarify interactions with others, and by

GERONTOLOGIC NURSING PRACTICE

Life review is a technique that can be used to help clients nearing the end of life view their lifespan in a positive way. Strengths and accomplishments are emphasized in this process.

PRINCIPLES OF LIFE REVIEW

1. Expression of feelings is elicited
2. Review cannot be forced, the client must be willing
3. Is best when done in a group, where mutual support and sharing can occur, but can be done individually as well
4. May be written and shared (as in an autobiography) or done orally
5. The nurse and the group make no judgmental statements
6. Life review should move from one event to another without dwelling on one time period

ADVANTAGES OF LIFE REVIEW

Past difficulties may take action to resolve past difficulties

Client may come to an acceptance of past events

Through acceptance and resolution, further coping strength is developed

DISADVANTAGES OF LIFE REVIEW

May become sad and depressed, if one cannot come to resolution or acceptance

May dwell on negative aspects if nurse does not emphasize strengths

being empathetic. This encouragement reinforces the client's self-concept, reduces anxiety, and shows that the client has self-control. The nurse encourages self-expression and stresses the client's self-responsibility.

Assisting the client in self-evaluation involves helping the client to define problems clearly and identifying positive and negative coping mechanisms. The nurse works closely with the client to help to analyze adaptive and maladaptive responses, contract different alternatives, and discuss outcomes. Self-evaluation in a geriatric client often encompasses a form of life-review (see box on p. 379).

Assisting the client to establish realistic goals involves helping the client to identify alternative solutions and develop realistic goals based on them. This facilitates real change and encourages further goal-setting behaviors. The nurse designs opportunities that result in success, reinforces the client's skills and strengths, and assists the client in getting needed assistance.

Assisting the client to become committed to decision and actions to achieve goals involves teaching the client to reject ineffective coping mechanisms and develop successful coping strategies. The nurse designs opportunities that result in success, reinforcing the client'kills and strengths. The client who becomes successful at achieving even the smallest of goals is working toward health. Supporting attempts that are health promoting is essential, because with each success another attempt can be made. Supporting adaptive, flexible coping is critical to intervening in self-concept alterations.

Evaluation

Alterations in self-concept are highly individual. The nurse evaluates whether interventions successfully strengthened the client's body image, self-esteem, role, or identiy. Evaluation must involve family members since they may be the best to judge significant changes in client behavior. The following are examples of goals and corresponding outcomes and evaluative measures:

Goal: Client's self-awareness and body image are improved within 1 week.

- **Outcome**
  - Client verbalizes improved body image
- **Evaluative measures**
  - Talk to client about appearance
  - Ask client's family about client's self-perception
- **Outcome**
  - Client's posture and appearance are improved
- **Evaluative measure**
  - Observe client's posture and appearance

Goal: Client's statements reflect improved self-worth.

- **Outcome**
  - Client verbalizes increasing self-worth
- **Evaluative measure**
  - Ask family and friends about how client talks about self
- **Outcome**
  - Client attempts new tasks
- **Evaluative measure**
  - Ask client about attendance at social activities
- **Outcome**
  - Client independently seeks out social activities
- **Evaluative measure**
  - Ask client about participation in new and familiar activities

Goal: Client adjusts to new role within 2 months.

- **Outcome**
  - Client establishes realistic short-term, role-related goals by 1 month
- **Evaluative measure**
  - Ask client about success or failure of short-term, role-related goals
- **Outcome**
  - Client modifies role expectations
- **Evaluative measure**
  - Observe client in new role

Goal: Client adapts to changes in body image and role within 1 month.

- **Outcome**
  - Client works with family to establish new roles and relationships
- **Evaluative measure**
  - Observe client-family/friend interactions
- **Outcome**
  - Client posture and appearance are consistent with positive self-image
- **Evaluative measure**
  - Observe client's posture and appearance

Not all goals may be achieved; some may have more progress than others. New goals may need to be set as previous goals are accomplished, or previous goals may need to be approached in a different way. Just as the "self" is the most individualized aspect of the human being, so must be those interventions that intercede in one's self-concept.

SEXUALITY AND HEALTH

Sexuality is an integral component of the psychosocial human being. It affects life experiences from conception through death. Sexuality is expressed through one's concept of self, through functioning in response to giving and receiving physical pleasure, and through relationships with others (Woods, 1987).

Since the 1940s, studies have added to knowledge of human sexual function and dysfunction. In the 1970s, health care professionals began to recognize, learn about, and assess sexuality as a component of health. Even in light of this knowledge and openness, sexuality remains controversial in society.

Regardless of controversies and societal trends, sexuality remains a part of one's being. As such, sexual wellness is a relevant area for nursing assessment and intervention. The intimacy of the nurse-client relationship during bathing, toileting, and support of other ADLs provides a unique opportunity to educate, discuss concerns, and promote sexual health.

Concepts of Sexuality

The process by which people come to know themselves as females or males is not clearly understood. The fact that a person is born with female or male genitalia and subsequently learns female or male social roles seems to be a key ingredient yet does not explain all variations of sexuality and sexual behavior. The Sex Information and Education Council of the United States (1980) has defined *sexuality* in holistic terms as

> a function of the total personality . . . concerned with the biological, psychological, sociological, spiritual and cultural variables of life which, by their effects on personality development and interpersonal relations, can in turn affect social structure.

Biological differences between men and women are determined at conception. The X or Y chromosome, with hormonal influences at about the seventh week of conception, produce a male or female fetus. Genital differences are visible at about 16 weeks of gestation.

Gender identity, the sense of being masculine or feminine, begins prenatally under genetic and hormonal influences (Hogan, 1989). As children begin to explore and understand their own bodies, they combine this information with the way society treats them to create an image of themselves as girls or boys. By the age of 3, children are aware that they will remain girls or boys and that changes in outward appearance will not alter their gender.

Gender role is the way people act as women or men. Biological, sociological, and cultural theories have been proposed. Hormones and parental and societal influences that reward or sanction various behaviors may play roles in the development of gender roles. Cultural factors, such as advertising and societal trends, add to definitions of gender-appropriate behaviors. The level of role flexibility, however, varies with culture, peer group, and over time.

Sexual orientation is a clear, persistent sexual preference for persons of one sex. Human sexual attraction is on a continuum between heterosexual and homosexual orientations. Based on Kinsey's studies (1948, 1953), most people cluster toward the heterosexual end of the continuum; a smaller percentage are at the homosexual end. Other individuals are bisexual. The percentage of individuals in each category is unknown.

The origins of sexual orientation are not understood. Biological determinants proposed include genetic, hormonal, and fetal brain "programming" as potential causes of sexual orientation. Psychosocial determinants based on life experiences and cultural influences may also contribute to sexual orientation. Social-learning approaches also focus on peer and parental relationships and childhood opportunities and experiences. No theory will probably ever fully explain the roots of sexual orientation.

Attitudes Toward Sexuality

Nurses' and clients' attitudes toward sexuality and sexual behavior can significantly affect health care. Attitudes can be reflected openly and dramatically through comments and actions or, more subtly, through a lack of regard for a client's need for time alone with a sexual partner. Because good health includes sexual health, a client's sexuality should be a part of a health care program. Yet sexual assessment and interventions are not always included in health care. The area of sexuality can be emotionally loaded for nurses and clients. Lack of information, conflicting value systems, anxiety, or the client's or nurse's guilt may cancel out the best intentions to promote sexual health.

The most common concern of people about sexuality is whether their sexual attitudes, feelings, and actions are normal. Given that society has not encouraged open talk about sexuality, such anxiety is understandable. Religion, society, the media, family, peers, and experience send messages about "normal" and "right" sexuality and behavior.

Clients may be concerned about how illness, hospitalization, and nursing care will affect their independence, self-care abilities, and sexual expression. Cultural or societal expectations about illness or aging may heavily influence the client's beliefs and actions.

Diverse sexual attitudes and behaviors are understandable and expected among health care professionals. Professional behavior need not compromise the personal sexual ethics of nurse or client. Nor should the provider place personal values and judgment upon the client's choices. Professional behavior must guarantee that the client is provided with the best health care possible without diminishing self-worth.

Nurses may find it difficult to be nonjudgmental about a client's sexuality when the client's orientation or values are different from their own. This is the result of the diversity of cultural and societal norms with which we live. Attempting to change a client's sexual attitudes and behaviors ignores the fundamental differences in attitudes of people. Promotion of sex education and honest examination of one's own sexual values and beliefs can help in reducing sexual bias.

As the nurse provides care for the whole person, assessment of sexuality is addressed as one component. Diagnosis of problems will then lead to appropriate interventions such as providing information, support, or referral. As in other aspects of nursing, this should be approached in a factual, scientific, and therapeutic manner.

Sexual Development

Infancy. At birth, the infant is given a gender assignment of female or male. Psychologically the infant is developing trust in parents, the environment, and himself or herself (Erikson, 1963). This trust is established when needs are promptly and predictably met by the care giver. The infant also learns to trust his or her own body to respond in predictable ways (e.g., "if I move these muscles, I will turn over" and "if I am cuddled, it feels good").

The learning process involves exploration and experimentation to define body limits, actions and responses, and pleasant from unpleasant sensations. Exploration includes the discovery of self-soothing behaviors such as thumb sucking and other pleasant forms of self-stimulation such as touching the genital area.

Parental response to these exploratory behaviors may set the tone for the child's sexual development, education, and comfort for dealing with sexuality in the home. Parents should be encouraged to accept the infant's exploratory behavior as a positive step toward development of a positive self-identity. Providing other forms of tactile stimulation through sucking, cuddling, and touching or stroking aids the infant in defining pleasant and comforting experiences through human interaction and from body contact.

Preschool. The child from ages 1 to 5 or 6 continues to solidify the sense of gender identity and to differentiate socially defined, gender-appropriate behaviors. This learning process occurs in the course of normal adult-child interactions, from the toys given to the child, clothing worn, games played, and responses encouraged. Children also observe adult behavior, begin to imitate actions of the same-sex parent, and maintain or modify behavior based on parental feedback.

Body exploration continues at this age. Exploration may include self-stroking, genital manipulation, cuddling of dolls, pets, or people, and other sensual experimentation. Concepts of pleasant and unpleasant are thus reinforced. During this stage, the child may extend exploration to others. Children may role play games of doctor or mommy and daddy and explore each other's bodies in various stages of undress. Questions regarding anatomical differences between female and male and where babies come from are opportunities for parents to continue sex education in an open manner.

Childhood. Children from 6 to 10 years of age, or prepuberty, expand their horizons from home to include school and the community. Learning and reinforcement of gender-appropriate behavior come from parents and teachers but more significantly from the peer group. North American society today defines a broad range of behavior acceptable for girls and boys (e.g., both sexes participate in cooking and sports).

Cultural, religious, and peer influences may more narrowly define appropriate behaviors. Parents should encourage socially acceptable behaviors without applying labels of feminine or masculine. Health care personnel must take their cues from the child, family, and community and should remain nonjudgmental in labeling behavior unless it is overtly gender inappropriate.

School-age children will probably continue self-stimulating behavior. Again, cultural and religious values become more strongly ingrained and must be respected. Parents and children can be informed that masturbation does not have any harmful physical or emotional effects. Acceptance of this behavior may, however, be contrary to the family's religious beliefs.

Children at this age continue to have questions about sex and will assert their independence by testing the limits of appropriate behavior. Limit testing may be displayed by using "dirty words" or telling jokes with sexual connotations while watching adult reaction. Limit testing is an important part of developing a sense of independence from the family. The testing of sexual limits is also a means of identifying appropriate expressions of sexuality and an opportunity the parents should use to explore questions and concerns.

Children also have a desire and need for privacy. As the body begins to prepare for puberty, the child will experience an increased sense of modesty. Questions about sex may or may not be asked of parents, depending on communication patterns established earlier. Education regarding those physical changes to anticipate during puberty may more comfortably be provided and received at this age before these dramatic, personal bodily changes.

Puberty and Adolescence. The onset of puberty in girls is usually signaled by development of the breasts. This process, which in part is controlled by heredity, may begin as early as 8 and may not be complete until the late teen years. The age of menarche varies widely but usually occurs at about 12 years of age. Although the menstrual cycle is initially irregular and ovulation may not occur at first, fertility should always be assumed unless proved otherwise.

Ejaculation in boys does not occur until the sex organs begin to mature, around the age of 12 or 14. Ejaculation may first occur during sleep (nocturnal emission). This may be interpreted as an episode of bed-wetting and even in knowledgeable boys can be very embarrassing. Boys must understand that, although they may not produce sperm with their first ejaculations, they will soon be fertile.

The emotional changes during puberty and adolescence are as dramatic as the physical ones. The adolescent confronts a powerful peer group with the almost constant anxiety of "Am I normal?" and "Will I be accepted?" Same-sex peers remain influential in defining appropriate behavior, but the task of establishing a relationship with the opposite sex begins. Adolescence is a very self-centered, egocentric stage. The degree of introspection is probably necessary to establish a sense of self within the context of family, community, and emotional relationships. Assurance of normalcy in physical and emotional development should be given honestly and often. Because of the concerns of normalcy, body changes and normal introspection of adolescents' modesty and privacy become increasingly important.

The adolescent is faced with many decisions and thus needs accurate information on topics such as body changes, sexual relationships and activity, sexually transmitted diseases (STDs), and pregnancy. Pressure from peers may encourage the adolescent to demonstrate "maturity" through sexual relations. Education that includes information on sexuality, disease prevention, and resistance (say no) skills has demonstrated decreased numbers of sexual partners and increased condom use in an adolescent male population (Ku, Sonenstein, and Pleck, 1992). Health education must be based on providing factual information within a developmentally appropriate format with consideration of societal and cultural values.

More significant than the factual content is guidance in establishing a personal value or beliefs system to use as a framework for decision making. Much of this guidance has already been conveyed by parents in the course of child-rearing. Parents must accept the responsibility to provide information, share their values, and promote sound decision-making styles, but they must be aware that the ultimate decision can be made only by the adolescent.

If not recognized earlier, this may be the age of identifying a same sex sexual orientation. Many adolescents will have at least one homosexual experience with an individual or in a group. Adolescents may fear that this experience defines their total sexuality as homosexual. This is not true, because many individuals continue with a strictly heterosexual orientation after such experiences. However, some teens may recognize their preference as distinctly homosexual. This can be a frightening and confusing recognition for the adolescent and family and may require a great deal of support. Support may come from a variety of sources such as school counselors, clergy, family, or health professionals.

Adulthood. The adult has gained physical maturation but is continuing to explore and define emotional maturation in relationships. Intimacy and sexuality are issues for all adults including those who choose to abstain from sex, remain single by choice, are homosexual, widowed, and so on.

Sexual health has been defined as "the integration of the somatic, emotional, intellectual, and social aspects of sexual being, in ways that are positively enriching and that enhance personality, communication, and love" (World Health Organization, 1975). All adults can and should strive for sexual health regardless of how they choose to express their sexuality. Although sexual activity is often defined as a basic need, it can be denied and channeled into other forms of intimacy throughout a lifetime.

All sexually active adults, as they develop intimate relationships, should learn techniques of stimulation and sexual response that are satisfying to themselves and their sexual partners. Some adults only may need permission to experiment with alternative behaviors or assurance that sexual expression other than penile-vaginal intercourse is normal. Other individuals may require significant education or therapy to achieve mutually satisfying sexual relationships.

Later in the adult years, the individual adjusts to social and emotional changes as children move away from home. Renewed intimacy may be possible or needed between partners. A potential problem may be the threat to self-image one may experience as the body ages. Couples can be helped to find novelty and new excitement in a long-standing, monogamous relationship through experimentation with sexual positions, techniques, and use of fantasy.

Actual physical changes occur in the course of aging. With decreased estrogen, the postmenopausal woman often experiences diminished vaginal lubrication and elasticity and possible changes in her desire for and enjoyment of sex. The aging man experiences an increase in the postejaculatory refractory period, delayed ejaculation, and other changes. The reasons for these changes should be explained before they occur to prevent fears of performance failure. Aging adults also need to adjust sexual action and response to chronic illness, medications, aches and pains, or other health concerns. The health care professional can again provide guidance on stimulation techniques to enhance sexual enjoyment.

Older Adulthood. The capacity for sexuality is lifelong. Theoretically, people can engage in sex as far into old age as they choose. The best indicator for continued sexual satisfaction with aging is a regularly active sex life during adulthood and into later life (Masters and Johnson, 1970). However, older people face health concerns and societal attitudes that may make it difficult for them to continue sexual activity. Although declining physical abilities may make sex as they knew it painful or impossible, with sympathetic intervention they can experiment with and learn alternative ways of sexual expression. The decreasing vaginal lubrication that occurs with aging may make a supplemental lubricant necessary. Erectile difficulties become common with advancing age (Buczny, 1992). An erect penis is not necessary for sexual pleasure. Men can be encouraged to continue to express their sexual feelings through touch.

Aging individuals, particularly women, face a real concern over lack of sexual partners. Another obstacle for some older adults is the myth that sex is for the young. Some older adults may stop having sexual activity because they feel it is inappropriate for their age-group. Hospitals, nursing homes, and other health care institutions may discourage sexual behavior among clients, although some nursing homes now give clients the opportunity and privacy to meet their needs for intimacy. The need to touch and be touched and be sexual must be considered when dealing with all ages.

Sexual Response Cycle

Masters and Johnson (1970) have defined a **sexual response cycle** as the following phases: excitement, plateau, orgasm, and resolution. Kaplan (1979) identified three phases: desire, arousal, and orgasm. These phases are the result of vasocongestion and myotonia, the basic physiological responses of sexual arousal. In women this reaction leads to vaginal lubrication, tumescence of the clitoris and the labia minora and majora, and engorgement of the outer third of the vagina (orgasmic platform). In men, vasocongestion leads to erection of the penis. Myotonia, or neuromuscular tension, gradually increases throughout the body during the excitement and plateau phases. Myotonia peaks during orgasm, resulting in involuntary contractions of the woman's vagina and the man's vas deferens and urethra. Women and men may experience contractions of the arm and leg muscles, facial muscles, and gluteal muscles. After orgasm, vasocongestion and myotonia return to prearousal levels.

The phases described are not absolute. Although phases vary in duration, intensity, and timing, the female and male response patterns are more similar than different. They are strongly influenced by psychological and environmental factors such as fatigue or alcohol intake.

Developmental Issues

Pregnancy and Menstruation. Many cultures have placed taboos against sexual intercourse or even male-female contact during menstruation and pregnancy. There is no physiological contraindication to intercourse during menstruation or during most pregnancies. Because of increased pelvic venous congestion, pregnancy may be a time of heightened sexual desire and arousal. Emotional overtones (e.g., dealing with blood during menstruation or fear of injury to fetus or mother during pregnancy) may need to be resolved to promote mutual sexual satisfaction.

Aging. As discussed earlier, aging causes changes in male and female sexual response. Education can minimize fears in both sexes that these biological changes result in an end to sexual functioning. Couples who are informed and encouraged to explore variations in sexual response may achieve a more satisfying relationship because of mutual gratification, decreased parental responsibility, and no fear of pregnancy. Aging may also result in negative changes in self-image. A decreased sense of worth can affect perceived sexual desirability and therefore interfere with interpersonal relationships.

Decisional Issues

Contraception. The ability to prevent a pregnancy or to plan the time between pregnancies should be part of a client's health care plan. An unwanted pregnancy can affect health on many levels. The health of the parent, child, and community in which they live depends on the presence of adequate physical, emotional, and financial resources to care for the child.

Ways of preventing unwanted pregnancy have been developed. Each woman's right to choose if and when to become pregnant is generally acknowledged. It would seem that it should be simple to match the desire to control pregnancy with an appropriate method of contraception. Yet the number of pregnancies among teenagers, abortions in all age-groups, and unwanted children indicate that many sexually active people are not using contraceptive measures. The nurse should consider the following factors when exploring why a client is not using contraception effectively: the client, client's environment, and appropriateness of the contraception technique (Fogel and Woods, 1981).

Adolescents may fail to use contraceptives because of lack of awareness that pregnancy can occur with first intercourse, lack of knowledge about contraceptive availability, fear of rejection from sexual partner, lack of planning for sexual interaction, view of planning as unromantic, and unclear partner communication about who is to assume responsibility for contraception (Zelnik and Kantner, 1979).

A second factor influencing the effective use of contraception is the client's environment. The client's family, community, or religion may disapprove of or prohibit contraception. The client may have been reared in an environment in which he or she was taught that sex for pleasure is wrong. Good contraception requires health care and educational systems that can deliver accurate information to the community.

Finally, the method of contraception must be appropriate for the client. The effectiveness of contraception is related to its safety, comfort, expense, availability, and ease of use. When discussing contraception with clients, the nurse should remember that each method has a theoretical effectiveness and an actual effectiveness. The former is based on the ideal circumstances under which the method could be used. Actual effectiveness may be considerably lower based on techniques and frequency of use. Contraceptive failure rates are generally higher among younger women who are unmarried, poor, and from racial/ethnic minority groups. Poverty is the most critical of these variables (Jones and Forrest, 1992).

The decision to use or not use a contraceptive method must be made by the client. The nurse can play an effective role in the decision-making process by providing accurate information and helping the client weigh risks against benefits. Some factors include cost, effectiveness of pregnancy and STD prevention, risks of unplanned pregnancy, inconvenience, and long-term health consequences (Kost, et al., 1991; Lichtman and Papera, 1990).

Some contraception methods do not require the help of a health care provider. Refraining from sexual intercourse is 100% effective. Over-the-counter spermicidal products such as creams, jellies, foams, and sponges are put into the vagina before intercourse. Because of the effect of nonoxynol 9, they create a spermicide barrier between the uterus and ejaculated sperm. A rubber or condom is a thin rubber sheath that fits over the penis. Vaginal spermicides and condoms are most effective when instructions are carefully followed; their combined use has been found to be more effective in preventing pregnancy than the use of either alone. Effectiveness rates are from 99% to 85% (Lichtman and Papera, 1990; Jones and Forrest, 1992).

Contraceptive methods based on the menstrual cycle include the mucus method and the basal body temperature method. Such methods are popular among clients who reject the idea of putting anything foreign into their bodies or whose religious beliefs prohibit the use of contraceptive agents. Both methods require that the client thoroughly understand the reproductive cycle of her body and be aware of the subtle signs and signals her body gives during the cycle. These methods also require that both partners abstain from sexual intercourse during designated fertile periods. The mucus method is based on changes in the cervical mucus during menstruation. In the basal body temperature method, the client records her body temperature to determine the rise in temperature after ovulation. Education by trained individuals is essential for optimal effectiveness. The symptothermal method using these parameters has been reported to have a success rate in the range of 80% to 99.6% (Scalone, 1990).

Contraception methods that require the intervention of a health care provider include oral contraception (the "pill"), the intrauterine device (IUD), the diaphragm, and sterilization. Oral contraceptives alter the hormonal environment to prevent ovulation and thicken cervical mucus. IUDs are plastic devices inserted by a health care provider into the uterus through the cervical opening. They vary in shape and may contain copper or may be impregnated with progesterone. They have an increased risk of pelvic infection and possibly result in sterility in some groups of women. The diaphragm is a round, rubber dome that has a flexible spring around the edge. It must be used with a contraceptive cream or jelly and is inserted in the vagina so that it provides a contraceptive barrier over the cervical opening. The cervical cap functions like the diaphragm; however, it covers only the cervix. It may be left in place longer and may be perceived as more comfortable than the diaphragm. Effectiveness rates are reported as follows: oral contraceptives 92% to 99.9%, IUDs from 90% to 99%, diaphragm from 70% to 98.5%, and the cervical cap from 50% to 92% (Lichtman and Papera, 1990; Jones and Forrest, 1992).

Sterilization is the most effective contraception method other than abstinence. It should be considered permanent. Female sterilization, or tubal ligation, involves cutting, tying, or otherwise ligating the fallopian tubes. In male sterilization, or vasectomy, the vas deferens that carries the sperm away from the testicles is cut and tied.

Among the least effective methods are withdrawal and douching. Withdrawal is pulling the penis out of the vagina just before ejaculation. Because sperm may be present in the urethra even when there is no ejaculation, this method is not very effective. In addition, sperm can be carried into the vagina by the fingers, and thus even an ejaculation outside the vagina can impregnate. Douching is also ineffective for contraception because sperm move rapidly into the cervix after ejaculation and are quickly beyond the reach of the water from douching.

Abortion. Abortion remains an issue that stimulates heated discussions of morality, women's rights to body control, and the beginning of life. Abortions have been performed since ancient times. The Supreme Court decision, *Roe v. Wade,* 1973, permitted legal abortions in the United States. The availability of abortions, however, may change because individual states have increased control over abortion regulations based on a 1989 Supreme Court ruling, *Webster v. Reproductive Health Services of St. Louis.*

Abortions are safer and less costly when performed in the early weeks of pregnancy. This is possible with improved pregnancy testing and more accurate early diagnosis.

Reasons for selecting an abortion vary and may include a decision to terminate an untimely pregnancy or a choice to abort a fetus known to have a defect incompatible with life. The woman who has an abortion experiences a sense of loss and should be prepared for and supported through the necessary grief. The partner may also experience this loss and grief. Clients who decide to abort a pregnancy may experience guilt. The guilt may surface immediately or may be more covert and manifest by sexual dysfunction or inappropriate perceptions.

Health care providers must sort out personal values related to abortion. The health care provider is entitled to personal opinions and should not be forced to participate in procedures or counseling contrary to beliefs and values. Nurses should choose specialties or places of employment so their personal values are not compromised and the care of a client in need of health care is not jeopardized.

Alterations in Sexual Health

Infertility. When one thinks of family planning, it is generally in terms of pregnancy prevention. A group with special needs are adults who want to conceive but cannot. Infertility is defined as the inability to conceive after 1 year of unprotected intercourse. The couple may experience a sense of failure and may feel that their bodies are somehow defective. They may direct every waking moment toward creating the right timing for conception. With advances in reproductive technology, infertile couples face many dilemmas that involve religious and ethical values and financial constraints.

The decision to pursue adoption or medical assistance with fertilization or to adapt to the probability of remaining childless are options a couple must weigh. Organizations such as RESOLVE or international adoption groups may provide the couple with much needed support.

STDs. STDs are discussed widely in professional literature and periodically receive wide media attention. AIDS continues to receive wide public attention; however, other STDs and their potential health consequences need to be included in educational programs. Prevalent STDs include syphilis, gonorrhea, chlamydia, genital warts, and the human papillomavirus (HPV) and herpes simplex virus (HSV) type II.

STDs may go untreated because of lack of symptoms, embarrassment, or unawareness of clinics. If untreated, these diseases continue to spread and cause devastating health effects, such as sterility, newborn illnesses, or death. Nursing care should include education of symptoms, consequences of inadequate treatment, and safer sex practices.

Sexual abuse. Sexual abuse occurs far more often than reported. The known cases of rape, incest, or child molestation probably represent only the tip of an iceberg. Incidents such as these have a traumatic effect on the victim; they may cause psychological problems and later sexual dysfunction. Physical injury, STD, and pregnancy may be the result of sexual abuse. The covert nature of some forms of abuse is one rationale for assessing sexuality in all ages.

Evidence of sexual abuse in children may be uncovered during history taking or physical examination. In children under 6 years of age, the child may exhibit behavioral changes such as excessive nail biting, thumb sucking, or excessively clinging to parent or others. School-age children may display similar behaviors or symptoms with excessive fears and anxieties such as tics, phobias, and truancy. The adolescent older than 12 years of age may exhibit antisocial or socially unacceptable behavior (e.g., sexual promiscuity, drug abuse, or running away from home). Low self-esteem and depression may be present. Often the child may avoid close contact with others, especially adults. Specific symptoms raising questions of abuse include a child showing an early, exaggerated awareness of sex or exhibiting seductive behavior toward adults; swelling or bruising of the external genitalia, anus, breasts, or buttocks; lacerations of or foreign substance in vagina or anus; and STD in a child under 15 years of age.

Abuse of women by husbands, boyfriends, and others is a problem of great magnitude; 8.5% to 35% of couples may be involved (Plichta, 1992; Sampselle, 1991). This abuse may begin, continue, or even intensify during pregnancy. In many cases, the abuse may include forced sexual relations. Women may show signs of bruises on the neck, black eyes, chronic headaches, abdominal pain, or attempt suicide. Spouse abuse crosses all socioeconomic and ethnic groups. The abuser may not fit any classic description; however, he may be extremely jealous or refuse to leave the woman's side. The overall appearance may be of the very concerned and caring husband or boyfriend. Rape is another prevalent crime that is increasing in frequency, yet as many as 50% of cases may go unreported (Becker, 1990).

When abuse is recognized, support needs to be mobilized for the victim and the family. All family members may require therapy in situations of incest to promote healthy interactions and relationships. Rape victims may need to work through the crisis before feeling comfortable with intimate expressions of affection. The partner may need support in understanding this process and ways to assist the victim. Children who have been sexually molested need to understand that they are not at fault for the incident. The parents must understand that their response is critical to how the child reacts and adapts. The nurse may come in contact with clients confronting these stressors. They are in an ideal role to assess occurrences in all clients and to educate individual clients of community services. Nurses should be aware of sources for referral and support in the community and refrain from applying personal values to the individuals and families.

Personal and Emotional Conflicts. Ideally, sex is a natural, spontaneous act that passes easily through a number of recognizable physiological stages and culminates in one or more orgasms. In reality, this sequence of events is more the exception than the rule. Nurses encounter clients who have problems with one or more of the stages of sexual behavior, including the feeling of wanting sex, the physiological processes and emotions of having sex, and the feelings experienced after sex.

Sexual desire varies among individuals. Sexual desire becomes an issue if the client simply wants to feel sexier more often, if the client believes it is necessary to measure up to some imagined cultural norm, or if there is a discrepancy in the sexual desires of the partners in a relationship. The client should be assured that almost any change in environment or sense of self may lead to sexual changes ranging from mild, transient emotional discomfort to a sexual dysfunction that requires professional counseling or therapy. Physical reasons why a client may experience a decrease in sexual desire include pain, fatigue, the side effects of drugs, or an altered sense of body image. Issues in a relationship can also distract a person from wanting sex. Couples often find that after the initial glow of the relationship has faded, they are faced with major differences in their values or life-styles. The degree to which they still feel close to each other and interact on an intimate level will depend on their ability to negotiate and compromise. Life-style factors such as the use or abuse of alcohol and the lack of time to devote to a relationship can also influence sexual desire. Lowered sexual self-esteem can result from lack of adequate sex education, negative role models, attempts to live up to unrealistic personal or cultural expectations, and rape, incest, or abuse.

Illness. Healthy sexuality involves all human dimensions, and illness can directly or indirectly influence any or all of these dimensions. The nurse must help the client to integrate the physical, psychological, and social systems during the illness. The degree to which any nursing intervention involving sex is successful depends on the attitudes and beliefs of nurse and client and their understanding of the effects of the illness and its treatment on sexual functioning.

The media's treatment of sexuality suggests that only the young and fit are sexual. Chronic pain and limited range of movement present obstacles to sexual activity. To adjust to these limitations, the client must learn effective communication skills and be willing to experiment with new positions for sexual activity. Changes in body functions and structures as a result of illness may not directly influence sexuality but may affect feelings of desirability and arousal. In this case the client's perception of self as sexually capable and desirable is being influenced.

The nurse has an essential role in facilitating adjustment in sexual expression, particularly when the client's background does not encourage open discussion of personal matters. Nursing has a responsibility to educate clients regarding potential alterations in sexuality related to surgery, medical treatment such as radiation or chemotherapy, medications such as antihypertensives, and emotional strains of chronic or terminal illness affecting all family members. The nurse may intervene in a manner as simple as allowing a hospitalized client a specific period of guaranteed uninterrupted privacy. Intervention may often include referral to more advanced practitioners to provide more comprehensive assessment and intervention.

Sexual Dysfunction. The causes of **sexual dysfunction** may be physiological or psychological. Sometimes the cause of a dysfunction cannot be identified or is a combination of several factors. An estimated 10% to 20% of sexual dysfunctions are caused by physiological factors (Kolodny, Masters, and Johnson, 1979). In another 15% of cases, physiological problems contribute to the sexual dysfunction but are not its sole cause (Masters, Johnson, and Kolodny, 1982). Sexual dysfunction may stem from simple issues such as lack of knowledge to much more complex issues including guilt over previous sexual behavior. In most cases, sexual dysfunction requires thorough assessment and interventions beyond basic nursing practice.

The distinction between physiological and psychological causes of sexual dysfunction is not always clear. Physiological interventions sometimes clear up the problem. At other times, psychological concerns are masked by a physiological condition. These issues must be closely evaluated during treatment by an advanced practitioner.

NURSING PROCESS

Assessment

Sexuality involves physical, psychological, social, and cultural variables. The nurse must assess all relevant factors to determine sexual well-being.

Many nurses find that they are uncomfortable talking about sexuality with clients, but they can reduce discomfort with several methods. First the nurse must learn the skills of communication and establishing the nurse-client relationship, which are essential before the nurse assesses sensitive health issues. The nurse should build a sound knowledge base and understanding of healthy sexuality and the most common sexual dysfunctions. The nurse must understand how sexual orientation, culture, and religious beliefs influence sexuality. This understanding must include a personal assessment of comfort level and limitations when discussing sexuality and sexual functioning. Finally, it is imperative that the nurse recognize sexual problems that require the expertise of other health care providers and refer the client to appropriate resources for help (Shuman and Bohachick, 1987).

Clients may use a variety of terms to describe their sexuality and sexual experiences. Nurses must be prepared to ask for explanations and clarifications if the terms used are unfamiliar. Nurses need to acknowledge their own values and belief systems concerning sexual functioning and not impose them on clients. The goal is to be nonjudgmental, caring, and supportive.

Sexual Health History

The nursing history is the first step in assessment. Every nursing history, whether taken in a clinic or hospital, should include a few questions related to sexual functioning to determine whether the client has any sexual concerns. An opening statement such as "Sex is an important part of life and can be affected by our health status or vice versa. To better understand your health, it is useful to know. . . ." is a good example to use. Other questions for adults are the following:

1. How do you feel about the sexual part of your life?
2. How has your illness, medication, or impending surgery affected your sex life?
3. It is not unusual for people with your condition to experience some sexual problems. Has that been a concern to you at all?

In light of the prevalence of domestic violence and sexual abuse, two questions a nurse should consider asking all female clients are:

1. Are you in a relationship in which someone is hurting you?
2. Have you ever been forced to have sex when you didn't want to?

These questions avoid using the emotionally laden and sometimes confusing terms of abuse or rape.

Questions that may be addressed to a child's parents include the following:

1. Have you noticed your child exploring his or her body (e.g., touching his penis or her labia)?
2. Has your child begun to ask questions about where babies come from?
3. Have you talked with your child about sex, pregnancy, or contraception?

Adolescents may best respond to a question such as:

1. Many adolescents have questions about STDs or whether their bodies are developing at the right rate. Do you have any questions about sex or other things?

Physical Factors

Sexual desire and function may be influenced, positively or negatively, by a variety of physical factors. Sexual intercourse may result in pain or discomfort from arthritis, angina, endometriosis, or lack of vaginal lubrication. Even imagining that sex may hurt, such as postpartum or postoperatively, can lessen sexual desire. Minor illnesses and fatigue are reasons a person may not feel sexually aroused. Medications may affect sexual desire, but the effect is not always predictable. Poor body image, especially when magnified by fear of rejection or body altering surgery, may inhibit sexual desire and/or function. Illness may also separate sex partners during short-term hospitalization or permanently in some cases of nursing home placement.

Relationship Factors

Sexual appetite varies by individual and with circumstances. These desires may not be the same for both partners in a relationship. In beginning a relationship the initial glow may obscure value and life-style differences. These may later create major disagreement that may hinder sexual compatibility. Communication skills play a critical role in partners' sexual compatibility. Decreased sexual activity can result from anxiety regarding telling a partner about pleasurable versus uncomfortable sexual behavior. Relationships may be very fragile.

Life-Style Factors

Factors such as use or abuse of alcohol or lack of time to devote to a relationship may influence sexuality. The depressant effects of alcohol usually inhibit sexual function. Ingestion of alcohol or drugs may also cloud judgment and contribute to ill-considered acts that may lead to STD's or pregnancy.

The life-style patterns of dual career families or a woman caring for teenagers and aged parents and other obligations leave little time for other pursuits. Sex may be viewed as another demand or obligation when what is desired is time alone or sleep. Aging women may find

BRIEF SEXUAL HISTORY

Purpose: To provide format or guidelines for nurses to obtain sexual information with minimal questioning.

1. What does the client perceive as sexual concerns?
2. When did these concerns begin and how have they changed over time?
3. What does the client see as the cause of these concerns?
4. What treatments has the client sought to alleviate concerns?
5. How would the client like this concern resolved?

Anon, 1975.

themselves widowed and without available, acceptable sex partners.

Self-Esteem Factors

Perceptions of self may lead to personal and emotional conflict involving sexuality. Rape, incest, and physical or emotional abuse may leave deep scars. Lowered sexual self-esteem can result from inadequate knowledge of sexual functioning, negative role models, and attempts to live up to unrealistic personal or cultural expectations.

Sexual Dysfunction

If the client brings up sexual concerns, the nurse may want to take a more detailed sexual health history or may refer the client for further evaluation. By including sexuality in the discussion, the nurse indicates that the client's sexual health is an important component of total health care (see box above).

Some clients may be too embarrassed or not know how to directly ask questions about sex. Thus they may be very subtle when asking for information. The nurse must be aware of cues such as flushing or inappropriate laughter that may indicate a question or problem in the area of sexuality.

Nursing Diagnosis

Altered sexuality patterns and *sexual dysfunction* are approved nursing diagnoses (Kim, et al., 1993). The difference in diagnosing sexual dysfunction or altered patterns of sexuality depends on whether the client perceives problems in achieving sexual satisfaction or expresses concern regarding sexuality. When making diagnoses of sexual problems, the nurse must assess anatomical, physiological, sociocultural, ethical, and situational issues that may be related factors. Factors that may exist and should signal a possible diagnosis related to sexuality may include surgery of reproductive organs or changes in appearance, past or current physical abuse, chronic illness, and developmental milestones such as puberty or menopause (see box for examples of nursing diagnoses above).

NURSING DIAGNOSES FOR ALTERATIONS IN SEXUAL HEALTH

Altered sexuality patterns
Sexual dysfunction
Rape-trauma syndrome

The critical factor for a diagnosis of altered sexual patterns is the identification of sexual difficulties, limitations, or changes. Sexual dysfunction is characterized by expression of sexual function problems or reports of limitations of function following disease or therapy. Additional factors may include misinformation, values conflict, or feared future limitations in sexual performance (Carpenito, 1993).

Interventions are contingent upon selecting the correct related factor. Sexual dysfunction may be related to antihypertensive medication, fear of sudden death during future sexual intercourse, or fatigue evidenced by poor exercise tolerance. In the case of medication the nurse may suggest discussion with the physician to prescribe an alternative medication. A fear of future dysfunction may best be addressed in a cardiac rehabilitation program that involves professionals and peers. Sexual dysfunction related to fatigue may require a physical rehabilitation program to increase exercise tolerance and suggested altered sexual behaviors or positions to conserve energy.

Planning

When planning interventions, the nurse should involve the client and, with permission, the sex partner. The client must select goals. Because of the interpersonal nature of sexuality, goals must be regularly reevaluated to determine whether they remain realistic and of mutual interest.

Referrals may be necessary to physicians such as gynecologists or urologists for physical impediments to sexual functioning (for example, severe pelvic discomfort with intercourse or the inability to obtain an erection). Sexual problems related to illness may also be addressed by clinical nurse specialists in the field such as cardiology or women's health. Sexual conflict in marriage or trauma over past sexual assault or incest requires intensive treatment with mental health professionals or a certified sex therapist.

Any plan should include referral to resources to promote achievement of goals after contact with the health care provider is discontinued. Many community resource groups exist for self-help or peer support. The client experiencing diabetes, respiratory problems, cancer, or rape crisis may benefit from interaction with individuals with the same problem. They can share concerns and successes related to all aspects of coping with the disease/trauma, including sexual consequences. Self-help centers and shelters support women who experience abuse. Parents without partners and single-adult groups appropriately deal with issues of sexuality such as STDs. Groups for older adults or community residents may be a source of help in confirming continuing sexual desires, issues of limited male partners, and raising concerns of safer sex for those again beginning sexual contact after widowhood. All plans should consider this type of community involvement.

After a diagnosis is established and goals are set, expected outcomes should be established to serve as guidelines for care and evaluation.

Goal: Adapt to new post-mastectomy body image.

Outcomes

Client views scar

Client discusses feelings regarding altered view of self.

Client resumes self-grooming and enhancing behaviors such as hair styling, make-up, and selection of clothing modifications

Goal: Client returns to mutually pleasurable sexual relations postpartum.

Outcomes

Client and husband verbalize concerns regarding change in routine such as sleeplessness or interruptions of baby crying

Client and husband understand postpartum physiological changes

Client and husband express satisfaction with current sexual relationship

Goal: Client achieves sexual satisfaction in light of diabetic vascular changes.

Outcomes

Client and wife will discuss beliefs and preferences regarding various sexual behaviors

Client describes nonintercourse stimulation that has resulted in pleasurable relations

Client and wife understand physiological changes of delayed or absent erection because of vascular changes

Goal: Adolescent utilizes safer sex behaviors to minimize STD risks.

Outcomes

Client understands behaviors that place him at risk for STD

Client demonstrates appropriate method of condom use

A sample care plan for altered sexuality patterns post-myocardial infarction is included on p. 391.

Implementation

Nursing interventions that address sexual problems generally provide the client with information and thus raise the client's awareness, assisting him or her to clarify issues or concerns. Nurses who have pursued specialized education in sexual functioning and counseling may provide more intensive sex therapy. As in any area of practice, nurses should recognize when a client's needs exceed their levels of expertise and provide appropriate referral. Most clients seen in clinics or hospitals may benefit from the discussion and teaching provided by the nurse generalist.

Health Promotion/Restoration

Preschool. Questions should be addressed openly, honestly, and simply. If children wish more information than the answer provided, they should be encouraged to ask and a more detailed response given. Even if questions are not asked, learning opportunities should be offered through pointing out pregnant women, animal behavior at the zoo, or discussions of sexuality as a follow-up to stories or television programs that touch on these topics. Information should not be forced on the child, but through presenting opportunities for discussion, the adult gives the child permission to question.

Childhood. By early school age, the child should also be given information to guard against sexual abuse potential. Very young children can be taught the differences between good touch and bad touch and that certain body parts are not ordinarily touched by adults except at bath time or during physical examination. Children should be told that if they feel uncomfortable about how they are touched, they should say "no" and tell a trusted adult about the incident.

The child should receive accurate information from home and school about the changes that will occur during puberty. This timing for education allows the child to gain information and ask questions before these become personal concerns regarding normalcy and therefore too threatening to ask.

SAMPLE NURSING CARE PLAN

Altered Sexuality Patterns

ASSESSMENT

Clinical Scenario: Mr Clark is a 39-year-old business executive who is 2 weeks post *myocardial infarction.* He has successfully completed 1 week of cardiac rehabilitation and is tolerating activity. Both he and his wife have expressed *fears* about *resuming their sexual relationship.* Their fears include a *recurrence of chest pain, re-infarction,* or *cardiac death.*

NURSING DIAGNOSIS

Altered sexuality patterns related to fear of MI or death with intercourse

Definition: Altered sexuality patterns is the state in which an individual expresses concern regarding his/her sexuality (Kim, et al., 1993).

PLANNING

Goals	Expected outcomes
Client and spouse will resume intimate expression of affection after myocardial infarction by discharge home.	Spouse will touch client. Client and spouse will progress to hand holding, hugging, or previous level of nonsexual affection by discharge home.
Client and spouse will regain positive adult level interaction by 5 weeks.	Client and spouse will speak in terms of their abilities in positive gender-appropriate terms. Spouse will describe fears of loss and proceed to acceptance of necessary life-style changes for heart health.
Client will resume physical relationship by 8 weeks.	Client and spouse will express satisfaction of sexual activity.

IMPLEMENTATION

Steps	Rationale
1. Involve spouse in care (e.g., bathing, showering, and hair care). 2. Invite spouse to hug or kiss client goodbye. 3. Schedule periods of ambulation to coincide with visiting hours (McCann, 1989).	Touch is basic form of communication and is basis of affection and sexual expression. Promoting intimacy while improving activity tolerance reinforces client's capacity.
4. Guide client in imagery exercise to visualize self as healthy and performing daily routines and sexual function (McCann, 1989). 5. Discuss grief-adaptation process and allow privacy and permission to share fears and tears.	Client can verbalize fears and recognition that others experience same feelings.
6. Refer to myocardial infarction support group for spouse and client.	Support group provides contact with similar clients to provide evidence of progress.
7. Discuss alternative sexual expression, (e.g., fondling, cuddling) as satisfying, not just as foreplay. Define realistic low-pressure expectation for gradual return to intercourse.	Sexual expression in continuum and sensate exercise provide low-stress, positive sexual experience (McCann, 1989).

EVALUATION

Observe interaction between client and spouse.

Observe client's nonverbal behavior (e.g., use of personal clothing, personal toiletries, and grooming aids).

Listen to client's description of self, abilities, discharge plans, and interactions with visitors.

Observe for signs of cheerfulness, description of self in positive terms, and talk of future plans. Ask spouse in privacy about feelings regarding MI and life-style and role changes required.

Ask client and spouse about expression of intimacy and feelings related to these behaviors.

Adolescence. Adolescence may be the first time the child seeks health care without parental accompaniment. The health care provider establishes an environment of trust and a willingness to listen. Issues of confidentiality must be clarified and respected. Nurses need to sort out personal values regarding teen sexuality before they can be effective. Whether an adolescent may be given contraceptives or an abortion without parental consent may be a legal issue in some states, but it is always an ethical issue. Persons providing adolescent or reproductive health care must deal with their own ethical concerns and know the legal concerns and have an in-depth knowledge of adolescent development.

Health care should include suggestions for good health maintenance practices (e.g., self-breast and testicular examination [Chapter 16] and more general issues such as nutrition and hygiene). Care providers should encourage discussion of fears and concerns and should ease communication between the adolescent and parents regarding issues such as contraception, STDs, or pregnancy. If the health care provider believes confidentiality must be breached for the welfare of the adolescent, this information should be shared with the teen. The teen should be informed out of respect for the client relationship and safety concerns. This decision cannot be taken lightly however; it may be necessary, for example, to prevent a suicide, but the decision must be weighed against possible perceptions of mistrust of the health care system that may remain throughout adulthood.

Adulthood and Older Adulthood. Major developmental (e.g., puberty or climacteric) and situational crises should prompt education about effects on sexuality. A life change such as pregnancy, illness, extreme financial stress, placement of a spouse in a nursing home, or loss and grief affects sexuality and anticipatory information should be provided.

Discussions of healthy sex should always include contraception when talking with women and men of childbearing age. Men should not be excluded from discussions of contraception. The discussion may include future desires for children, usual sexual practices, and acceptable methods of contraception. All methods of contraception should be reviewed to provide necessary data for an informed client choice.

Older adults deserve a thorough explanation of age-related changes in physical appearance, physiology, and sexual response. Adequate time is needed to answer questions. Discussion should include past methods of sexual expression and options available to enhance current levels of satisfaction.

All individuals having more than one sex partner or whose partner has other sexual experiences should learn more about safer-sex practices. Information should be provided about STD transmission and symptoms, use of condoms, and risky sexual activities (for example, the trauma of penile-anal sex). Safe sex may also consider the client's emotional risks in a relationship.

Altered Sexuality in Illness

Illness and surgery are situational stressors. Clients may experience major physical changes, effects of drugs or treatments, and the emotional stress related to prognosis, future functioning, and separation and hospitalization. Sexuality, as a component of personality, may be affected by all components of illness. The nurse should never assume that sexual functioning is not a concern merely because of an individual's age or severity of prognosis. After concerns are assessed and identified, they can be addressed in the context of the individual's value system.

In response to identified concerns, the nurse may initiate discussion of methods of sexual stimulation, the sexual response cycle, or the use of creativity and fantasy in sexual relations. It may be appropriate to discuss sexual practices such as oral-genital sex or mutual masturbation as methods of expressing intimate affection when penile-vaginal intercourse is contraindicated. A partner experiencing joint pain may appreciate a discussion of various positions for intercourse. Use of fantasy or a sense of playfulness may add new romance or stimulation to a long-term relationship. A couple may need confirmation or assurance that these thoughts and the acting out of nonharmful fantasy is normal and healthy.

When sexual dysfunctions are identified as ongoing premature ejaculation, vaginismus, or concerns over transsexual dressing, the nurse should provide appropriate referral. Clients may still require support to follow through with a referral and reinforcement of explanations of procedures, treatments, or exercises. To be effective with any intervention, the nurse must be comfortable with sexuality and aware of personal values and biases. Referral may also be necessary when a client's values or needs conflict with those of the nurse.

Evaluation

Individuals have a right to understand how their bodies function and to predict developmental changes. Clients should understand development of the body, the manner of male and female sexual response, and changes that normally occur with aging and life stresses.

Sexuality is dynamic and requires frequent reevaluation of the client's desired outcomes. As goals are changed, the interventions must be modified.

Examples of evaluative measures are:

Goal: Client adapts to postmastectomy body image.

Outcome

Client views scar

Evaluative measure

Observe client looking at scar

Outcome

Client discusses feelings regarding altered view of self

Evaluative measure

Ask client to discuss feelings about body changes; may include sense of mutilation, humorous comments about being lopsided

Goal: Adolescent utilizes safer sex behaviors.

Outcome

Client understands behaviors that place him at risk for STD

Evaluative measure

Have client describe STD prevention/risk reduction techniques including limiting number of sex partners, knowing and communicating with sex partners, and use of condom before any penile-vaginal contact

Outcome

Client demonstrates appropriate method of condom use

Evaluative measure

Have client demonstrate on a model the correct technique for condom application, including leaving a reservoir at tip

Resolution of sexual concerns must meet the client's perceptions of improvement. Sexuality is not an absolute. An individual must define what is acceptable and satisfying. The partner's level of sexual satisfaction must also be considered. To effectively resolve concerns, the client must also have a positive sense of self.

SPIRITUALITY AND HEALTH

Spiritual health or distress can be critical to the healing process of the client. Nightingale (1969) recognized this when she stated in *Notes on Nursing:* "It is a matter of painful wonder to the sick themselves, how much painful ideas predominate over pleasurable ones in the impressions; they reason with themselves; they think themselves ungrateful; it is all of no use." Nightengale went on to speak of the importance of food for the spirit and the lack of it as a "craving, desperation." She suggested flowers, color, and a view of nature for the patient. Such suggestions highlight the importance of a spiritual component in our lives; that was clear to Nightingale. The spiritual dimension was not clearly recognized until holism became popular in the 1960s.

In the early day of psychological thought, spirituality was not promoted as it had been in pre-Victorian times. Freud, who was a neurologist, led the belief that formal religion was punitive and should be outmoded by his "talking cure" (Butler, 1990). Carl Jung, who had been a student of Freud, was the lone challenger to Freud's pathologizing of the spiritual. Not until the 1960s, except for Carl Jung, did anyone support the concept of healthy spirituality.

In the 1960s, psychologist and theorist Abraham Maslow gave legitimacy to the spiritual by considering spiritual longings to be legitimate in their own right and not a reflection of unresolved emotional conflict. His hierarchy of needs placed longings for transcendent experiences and moral values at the top of the ladder, saying that all people would seek them after more basic needs for food, love, and self respect were met (Butler, 1990). He believed self-actualization concerned something "beyond oneself" and urged those who sought it "to find some challenging work to do."

Spirituality is now undergoing a surge of interest both in and out of hospital settings for a variety of reasons. With the focus on cost containment, any measure that saves the client, the insurance company, or the government money, and is documented, is a focus for attention. Spiritual care is just beginning to document itself as such a cost-containing measure.

The similarities of the issues between the once ominous diagnosis of cancer with the new diagnosis of HIV infection are many (Carson et al., 1990). Both diseases are life threatening, with often extended courses of highly technical treatment. Recently, interest in spirituality research has accelerated. With the explosion of a relatively young population infected with the HIV virus, a young population of large proportion is facing impending disability and death.

Terminal, chronic, traumatic, and acute illness often bring with them issues of spirituality. Nurses struggle to help their clients with issues of life, death, trauma, and chronicity, and in doing so are forced to confront their own feelings and beliefs about such issues. Spiritual pain (suffering) is a loss of one's sense of personal integrity, a fragmenting of one's sense of internal togetherness. The human spirit does not need judgment, advice, or exhortation to change. It needs acceptance, listening, and the opportunity to be heard and understood: compassionate human contact (Dugan, 1987).

Terminal Illness and Spirituality

Miller (1991) and Reed (1987) discovered that terminally ill hospitalized clients exhibited a far more spiritual perspective than did non–terminally ill or healthy adults. Dugan (1987) has identified several expectations that our society has for the dying client. He says "there is a subtle yet widespread social expectation that fatally ill persons make the most of the time they have left. Terminally ill clients, according to this expectation, ought to be heroic. If they are not heroic, they ought to be noble. If they are neither heroic nor noble, they ought to put on a good act. If they are neither heroic nor noble, and they do not even pretend to be, social reprisals, like lectures of avoidance behaviors, may be quick to follow. In general, we do not tolerate the angry dying client, we expect the acceptance of suffering. The spirit does not need judgements, advice or exhortations; what it needs is acceptance, and the opportunity to be heard and understood with compassion."

We have very similar expectations of clients with chronic illnesses. We expect them to bear their chronicity with acceptance and valor without displays of anger or frustration. Often when such displays are evidenced, we distance ourselves from such clients at the time when their needs are greatest. The spiritual needs of such clients incorporate the key elements of the meaning and purpose of life—the need for love and relatedness and the problems of guilt and forgiveness.

Often nurses practice a type of subtle avoidance of clients who do not share their beliefs, or share the common spirituality practices of the culture. Belief systems that are foreign to health care providers often distance them because they do not understand the meanings or practices. Care of the agnostic or atheist client often forces the nurse to examine one's own beliefs. Kindness, support, and compassion are central elements in caring for all clients regardless of beliefs. Every client is entitled to dignity in health, illness, and death. A humanistic stance that asserts the basic dignity and worth of man enables the nurse to give compassionate care to all clients.

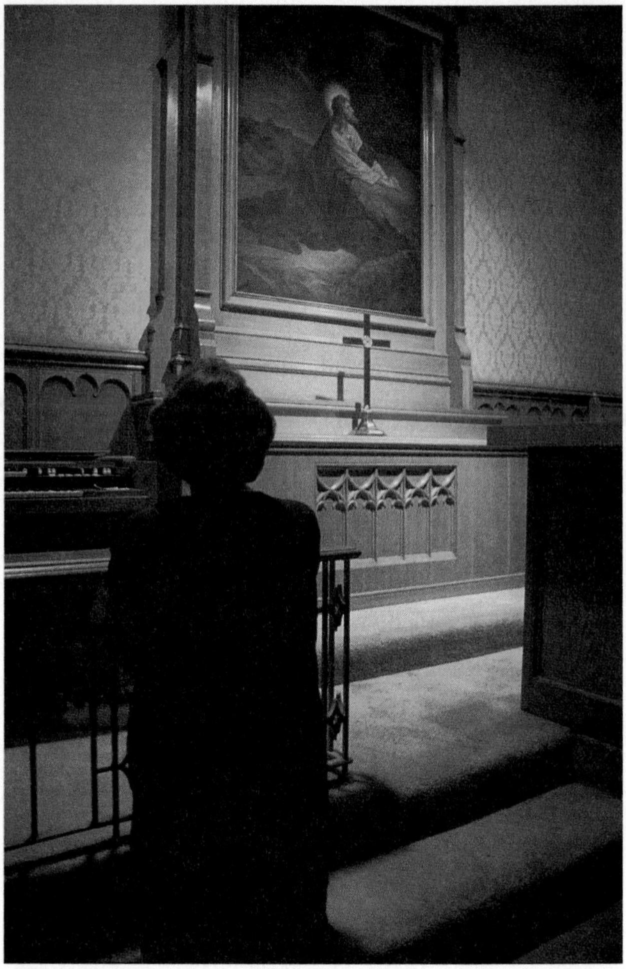

FIGURE 17-3 Clients of all faiths can find comfort in a chapel or a quiet area of a hospital.

Basic Concepts of Spirituality

Spiritual health often changes as other dimensions of health fluctuate. Spirituality is a dimension that pervades the entire being and encompasses the human need to search for meaningful answers to questions about life, illness, and death. At its core is a person's deepest relationships with others, self, and a supreme being. Agnostic or atheist clients simply believe there is not afterlife, heightening the importance of this life.

In many belief systems, disease is viewed as part of a divine plan to test the individual's faith in a supreme being or to make him or her an example of patience or restitution. Thus one can find meaning in suffering. Suffering is often one of the most difficult issues for nurses and for families. Exploring with clients what is symbolic and spiritually supportive to them, providing the spiritual resources they request, and suggesting alternatives or sharing beliefs without imposing values are ways nurses can help clients to find significance in suffering (Figure 17-3).

Practitioners of holistic health care believe that each person has a spirit that coexists with the physical body and that this spirit is the life spark that energizes the body. The nurse's goal in holistic health care is not simply to help a client to be physically well but to help the client to achieve a balanced, dynamic integration of body, mind, and spirit.

Spiritual and Religious Practices Related to Health. Every person has a spiritual dimension. In this sense, spirituality includes but is not limited to religion. The word **religious** refers to the specific practices, rites, and rituals of a person's professed religion. Rites and rituals may enhance spirituality but may not be essential to the relationship with a supreme being. The nurse should be aware of the client's general spiritual needs, which may be manifested in ways other than through specific religious practices, and should make it possible for the client to engage in chosen practices. The following sections describe Hindu, Buddhist, Moslem, Jewish, and Christian beliefs and practices regarding birth, dietary restrictions, procedures in health crises, and death.

HEALTH BELIEFS. Hindus believe that praying for health is the lowest form of prayer; thus they tend to dismiss or to be unconcerned about bodily ills. Various branches and sects of Buddhism emphasize different practices; for example, the Theravada branch uses an intellectual approach, the Mahayana branch emphasizes involvement with humanity, and the Zen sect practices austerity. Followers of Hinduism and Buddhism usually accept modern medical science.

In Islam, the believer is considered to be a unique individual with an eternal soul. Older or more conservative Moslems may have a fatalistic view and may resist compliance with medical treatment.

Jews tend to believe in long life as a reward for fidelity to God and may observe Sabbath regulations, which may interfere with scheduled therapeutic procedures. The procedures should be scheduled around the client's belief system whenever possible. Christians generally regard themselves as children of God, redeemed by Christ and destined for eternal life. They seek to discern the will of God in life and suffering, but their beliefs generally do not conflict with modern medical practice.

BIRTH. No special birth ritual is required by Hinduism. Buddhist rites, which are infant presentation, affirmation, confirmation, or ordination, are performed in late childhood. According to Islamic doctrine, if abortion occurs after 130 days, the fetus is treated as a fully developed human being. Ritual circumcision by a rabbi is required by Orthodox and Conservative Jews on the eighth day after birth. Reform Jews favor ritual circumcision but do not consider it a religious imperative. Among Jews a fetus is buried, not discarded.

Various forms of baptism are practiced by Christians. Episcopalians and Roman Catholics require infant baptism; the former do not baptize aborted fetuses and stillborn infants but the latter do. Baptists, Seventh-Day Adventists, Bahái followers, and Mennonites are some of the religious groups that do not practice infant baptism. The form of baptism differs from sect to sect; for example, sprinkling is customary for Orthodox Presbyterians, whereas Pentacostals, Mormons, and Baptists perform immersion.

DIET. Hindus have many dietary restrictions. Some sects are vegetarian, believing meat and intoxicants to be too stimulating to the senses. Some Buddhists also are vegetarians. Most members of the Buddhist religion practice moderation and do not use alcohol, tobacco, or drugs.

Eating pork is prohibited by Islam, and Ramadan, the ninth month of the Muhammedan or Moslem year (around June and July), is a period of daylight fasting. Orthodox and Conservative Jews may observe kosher dietary laws, which prohibit eating pork and shellfish and eating any meat with milk or milk products. Jews also have regulations about food preparation. Reform Jews often do not observe kosher dietary laws.

Many Christian traditions have no dietary proscriptions. Some groups such as Seventh-Day Adventists, Baptists, and Mormons prohibit the use of alcohol, coffee, and tea, and certain groups include tobacco with these prohibitions. Roman Catholics fast and abstain from meat on Ash Wednesday and Good Friday. Armenian Catholics fast during Lent, and members of several branches of Christianity fast 1 to 6 hours before communion.

HEALTH CRISES. Hindus may view illness as the result of misuse of the body or as a consequence of sins committed in a previous life. However, they generally do not oppose medical treatment. Buddhist clients or their families may ask to have a Buddhist priest for counseling during illness. A family member usually remains with the sick person to care for physical and emotional needs.

Moslems use faith healing to provide psychological support rather than to treat the pathological condition. Family members are a great comfort to a Moslem, and group prayer without a leader is often used.

In Judaism the sick must seek medical care. Rabbinical consultation is necessary before donation or transplantation of organs. Visiting the ill is considered a religious obligation for Jews.

Christians may want to receive communion from their minister or priest during illness; Roman Catholics may wish to receive several sacraments: reconciliation, the Eucharist, and anointing of the ill. Jehovah's Witnesses are generally opposed to blood transfusions and some dialysis. Some religious sects believe in faith healing and some in laying on of hands.

DEATH. To Hindus, death and rebirth are nearly synonymous. After death, certain rites are prescribed. The family of a Buddhist may wish to have a priest called at the time of death; and last rite chanting is often practiced at the bedside.

Before death, the Islamic client confesses sins and asks the family for forgiveness. After death the family washes the body, then turns toward Mecca. As with Hindus, only relatives and friends touch the body. There is no autopsy unless required by law.

All Orthodox Jews and some Conservative and Reform Jews also oppose autopsy and cremation. Human remains may be ritually cleansed, and burial is carried out as soon as possible.

Among Christians, no rituals are required before or after death by Christian Scientists, Baptists, Presbyterians, Church of Christ members, and Jehovah's Witnesses. Last rites are optional for Episcopalians and

Lutherans but mandatory for Eastern Orthodox Christians and Roman Catholics. Additional restrictions may apply to cremation, autopsy, and burial of amputated parts or burial in consecrated ground.

NURSING PROCESS

Assessment

The nurse comes into contact with the client more than any other health care professional. This accessibility enables the nurse to assess for spirituality needs in both the nursing assessment and in day-to-day verbal and nonverbal communication with the client. One's spiritual or humanistic beliefs about the meaning of health and illness are critical in resolving issues of chronic, traumatic, or terminal illness.

The spiritual assessment of the client is often included in the initial nursing assessment. If it is not included, the spiritual assessment may need to be done separately, particularly if the clients indicate increasing anxiety or fear about their physical condition, as indicated by statements and behaviors.

A spiritual assessment may be as structured as specific questions provided on a nursing assessment form, or it may be as unstructured as the nurse taking notice of the presence of religious items (a Bible, crucifix, religious jewelry, or books) in the hospital or home setting. Conversing about the religious practices of the client gives the nurse an indication of what may be helpful during illness. However, the participation of the client may be limited because of the impact of the illness (Peterson, 1987). Often, just noticing whether the client is appreciative of visitors from the religious affiliation of choice is helpful.

Often, just getting the client to talk about his or her spirituality can give the nurse much useful information. Inquiry about religious preference may also bring about revealing spiritual information. Verbal indicators of wanting to talk about spirituality may be asking for the chaplain or pastor to visit, or questions about suffering, pain, or dying. Some clients display a great deal of anger and will verbalize such anger to the nursing staff about anything and everything in their environment.

Often the client may display distress nonverbally. Behaviors may vary from touching and reaching out for others to crying and withdrawing in silence. One particularly angry client kept dumping over his pitchers of water, until an observant nurse sat down beside him and asked him what he was angry about. He then began to cry and tell of his extreme anger at this diagnosis.

McSherry (1988) has developed one of the more widely used spiritual assessment tools. It contains three sections of scores: assessing stressors, religiosity, and values. The following nine points are taken from the religiosity tool that was adapted by McSherry from Westberg. The tool closely resembles the Holmes Life Change Scale. The focus is to be on events that have taken place in the past 2 years (see box above).

A nurse wanting to do a spiritual assessment needs to include these nine points considered salient to spirituality. These elements are checked by the client and then scored. Negative responses have higher scores, indicating increased distress in spirituality. However, a formal test such as McSherry's need not be given; simply discussing such issues with the client will lend spirituality information.

Spiritually healthy persons are generally aware of their limitations as human beings but strive to act in accordance with their beliefs. They assume life's responsibilities with joy and cheerfulness. They relate in a loving manner to others. They act justly and peacefully in their relationships. They exert a positive influence through their spiritual awareness of a larger meaningfulness in their lives and in the world.

As the nurse observes and analyzes the behaviors that demonstrate the client's level of spiritual health, it becomes obvious that the client's attitudes toward a supreme being, self, and others demonstrate the value the client places on spiritual health. Reactions to adversity, setbacks, delays in plans, aging, sickness, and suffering give clues to spiritual values that can assist the nurse in assessing spiritual health.

If the client demonstrates an incongruity between professed beliefs and actions, a nursing diagnosis of **spiritual distress** may be indicated. The client may express anger at a supreme being, a member of the pastoral care team, or the nurse. Verbalizations about internal conflicts concerning beliefs, the meaning of life, and required treatment may demonstrate a spiritual need.

SPIRITUAL ASSESSMENT

In the past 2 years, have you experienced:

1. A lack of meaningfulness in life
2. A lack of purpose in life
3. A major change in your world view or your philosophy of life
4. A new set of values or priorities in life
5. A change in your relationship with your spiritual being or God
6. A change in your church activity or prayer life
7. A significant spiritual experience
8. Spiritual emptiness
9. Constant feelings of guilt

From McSherry E: Modern clinical science of the spiritual dimension in chaplaincy and the parish, *JCHCC,* 1988.

The nurse should bear in mind that the moral and ethical implications of the diagnosis or treatment may conflict with the client's religious or spiritual values. Also the etiology, diagnosis, and sometimes the treatment of the disease may possibly conflict with the client's spiritual beliefs.

Nursing Diagnosis

After assessing the client's spiritual needs, the nurse may find evidence of spiritual distress. Indicators for the diagnosis of spiritual distress are questioning the meaning of life and death ("what is this all for, anyway?"), anger at God ("even God has forsaken me, what have I done?"), questioning suffering ("why does He let me suffer like this?"), conflicts about beliefs ("I used to believe the people who suffered, deserved it, what have I done?"), concern about the relationship with the deity ("God doesn't answer any of my prayers"), and the meaning for one's existence ("I can't do anything anymore but be a burden to everyone"). These are only a few examples of statements nurses will hear clients verbalize when they are in spiritual distress.

A diagnosis of spiritual distress related to anger at his terminal illness would be appropriate for the client who was continually overturning his water pitcher. Because the nurse had assessed this continuing behavior as inappropriate to the situation, the nurse would follow up on the assessment, spend some time alone with the client and assess the client's anger. "Mr. Smith, tell me how you feel about how things are going" would be an opening statement that could be interpreted by the client in many ways, giving him the freedom to discuss something in depth or something superficial. The nurse has introduced time for discussion and may corroborate a diagnosis with the client, or if the diagnosis is unfounded, the nurse must reassess for the correct diagnosis (see box below).

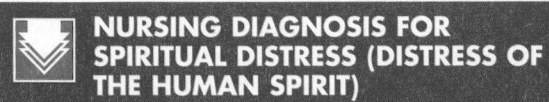

NURSING DIAGNOSIS FOR SPIRITUAL DISTRESS (DISTRESS OF THE HUMAN SPIRIT)

Spiritual distress can be related to every facet of human life. It may encompass:

- Separation from religious or cultural ties as evidenced by anxiety, insomnia, guilt, or questioning the meaning of life's events
- Unresolved guilt or anger
- Feelings of powerlessness

Planning

If the client agrees with the diagnosis after validation, the nurse and client plan steps to meet this spiritual need. In planning nursing interventions for spiritual distress, the nurse and the client must work together. This collaboration between the nurse and the client initiates the client into an active participatory role in spiritual well-being. The nurse may propose alternative interventions such as a visit from the hospital pastoral care department, or if the client is not comfortable with this, a visit by the community pastor.

If the nurse has doubts about the client's ability to recognize spiritual needs, consultation with the family may confirm the nursing diagnosis. If the client and family deny the existence of a spiritual need, the nurse should accept their decision. Possibly the client's minister, priest, or other spiritual adviser may have already recognized and ministered to the client's spiritual needs without the nurse's knowledge, or the client and the family may have their own plan in mind. Often families will call on one special clergy member with whom they have a history.

The plan should be prioritized with the client. The highly distressed client may feel like a burden to loved ones. This question must always be asked: "Have you ever felt like hurting yourself?" If the answer is positive, the physician and the family must be informed of this statement. This statement should be recorded verbatim onto the chart. However, as long as the client is competent, the wish to limit or deter treatment is with the client.

If the client is not competent, decisions are made by the family. In many states, advanced treatment directives are signed by all Medicare clients or their families before receiving treatment in a facility, so that the staff know exactly what the client and the family want done in an emergency (see Chapter 5).

The plan should be collaborative. It may involve friends, relatives, pastoral care, community clergy, reading materials, phone conversations, family members, and so forth. It is important that it be flexible and meet actual or potential needs the client and nurse identify. The plan is based on one or more of the following goals:

Goal: Client will verbalize acceptance of self with decreasing self-blame.

Outcome

Client will make statements of self-acceptance

Client will decrease self-blaming statements

Goal: Client will demonstrate anger in an appropriate manner.

Outcome

Client will verbalize anger about illness and suffering to staff and clergy

Client will not physically discharge anger on

staff or equipment (water pitchers, trays, plates, etc.)

Goal: Client will verbalize spiritual needs to staff and family.

Outcome

Client will verbalize the need to see clergy to staff and family

Note: The client without religious base may verbalize humanistic needs to staff and family:

Wish to be visited by family members

Desire to hear favorite music

Wants reading materials that give comfort

Goal: Client will verbalize a greater sense of strength, peace, or calmness.

Outcome

Client will demonstrate nonverbally or verbally state a greater sense of strength, peace, or calmness

Implementation

Implementing the plan of care consists of pulling together the resources that the client and the nurse identify as helpful. The nurse has the opportunity, more than any other health care professional to be emotionally accessible to the client, to listen, and to support the client as they begin to accept and problem solve their particular situations. The key to spiritual support is open communication, sharing the pain of another during loss and suffering and supporting the family of the client.

Spiritual Health Promotion

In addition to spiritual issues, the client's view of the self is another area for intervention. If the nurse consistently treats the client as a unique individual with significant value and unlimited potential, the client's self-concept will be enhanced. Strong self-concept aids one when considering issues of such significance in one's life.

Some clients need time for quiet and reflection but will not ask for this. It is up to the nurse to open this subject for the client, so that the client's needs may be met. Meeting such a small need for the client assists the client in feeling valued and worthwhile. Holistic care encompasses helping the client meet needs that will promote the body and spirit toward health.

Relationships with others often sustain a person's belief system. However, painful relationships may require the help of a mental health professional to help those involved repair the relationship. A psychiatric clinical specialist with family training or experience might be consulted, or the local mental health department often will make hospital or house visits. Many home health or community health departments have psychiatric clinical specialists on their staffs. Intervening in painful relationships promotes a sense of family strength and adaptability and can be preventive in the future.

The nurse should ask clients if they would like to have their minister, priest, rabbi, or spiritual adviser notified of their hospitalization. Ministers and pastors should be made welcome in nursing units. Keeping ministers informed of physiological, psychosocial, and spiritual concerns, when requested by the client or family, helps in providing holistic health care. A willingness to cooperate with and facilitate the administration of sacraments, rites, and rituals of the client's religion shows respect for spiritual values and needs.

The nurse should value the relationship with the client. Montgomery (1991) researched those nurses regarded by their peers as excellent care givers. What she found in her interviews with these nurses suggested that in a caring encounter, "the caregiver and the client experience a union of spirit, beyond the level of the self." Opening oneself to caring about another elevates one beyond the level of oneself.

Evaluation

Nurse self-evaluation is important. The nurse must assess how it will feel to give support to someone outside one's belief system. It is imperative to meet the client's needs, not the nurse's. If the nurse cannot give compassionate care to one whose beliefs differ greatly from the nurse, then the nurse should remove oneself from the care of that client. Such issues are evident to the client; we unconsciously give verbal and nonverbal indications about how we feel without meaning to reveal our feelings. The client will benefit from an honest self-assessment by the nurse.

The client's responses to the interventions must be evaluated. Has the client responded to the collaborated nursing interventions that were constructed? If not, the plan should now be restructured, perhaps by breaking down the goals into smaller components. Perhaps the goals need to be changed altogether, and the client was not verbalizing what the need really was. In actuality, attainment of spiritual health can be considered a lifelong goal. Evaluation of the spirituality consists of looking at each behavior for either improvement or maintenance of the behaviors given. Often the most helpful changes are those suggested by the client, as clients know best how they go about resolving issues. The nurse should consider the client the expert on himself or herself and construct new ways of meeting the goals collaborating once again with client.

SUMMARY

The self-concept is a complex, dynamic entity. Many variables including self-worth, body image, identity, and roles can affect any or all of the components of self-concept. A person's self-concept is a combination of the real and ideal selves. The ideal self is based on social and cultural standards an individual accepts and attempts to incorporate into self-concept. A discrepancy between the real and ideal can be a source of stress. A positive self-concept is important to developmental and cognitive growth. The nurse's role in providing care for a client with a self-concept change depends on the severity of the alteration.

The nurse who provides care for a client with sexual concerns needs knowledge about sexuality, communication skills, and an understanding of the interaction between personal and cultural value systems. Knowledge about sexuality includes the effects of illness and treatment on sexual desire and sexual functioning. The client's sense of self as attractive, desirable, and sexual can be affected by illness and body changes resulting from surgery or disease. Aging, changes in life-style, and alterations in value system also affect sexuality. Nurses can learn to apply all stages of the nursing process to maintain or improve sexual health. Sexuality is an integral component of personhood and therefore may have an impact on or be affected by health states. The nurse, as provider of care and education, continually confronts issues related to client sexuality. With sensitivity and insight, the nurse can assist clients in assuming responsibility for decisions about sexuality, thus enhancing their total health.

Individualized nursing care also involves the spiritual dimension. To provide spiritual care, the nurse must understand spiritual health and be able to recognize the spiritually healthy person. If spiritual needs are identified during assessment, plans are made to intervene appropriately. When implementing the plan for spiritual care, nursing interventions are individualized according to the client's specific needs. The family's involvement and the ministrations of spiritual counsel are sought when indicated. Resources for facilitating spiritual care and providing support for nurses are used as necessary.

KEY CONCEPTS

The self-concept is an integrated set of conscious and unconscious feelings, attitudes, and perceptions about oneself.

Components of self-concept are body image, self-esteem, roles, and identity.

Roles are learned through socialization; they involve the expectations of other about behavior in particular positions (for example, family member and employee).

The nurse should be aware of how his or her self-concept and nursing actions can affect a client's self-concept.

Sexuality is related to all dimensions of health; therefore sexual concerns or problems should be addressed as a part of nursing care.

Attitudes toward sexuality vary widely and are influenced by spirituality, society's values, the media, family, and other factors. A nurse should not judge a client's sexual preferences and needs.

Sexual development begins in infancy and involves some kind of sexual behavior or growth in all developmental stages.

Sexual health involves physical and psychosocial aspects and contributes to an individual's sense of self-worth and positive interpersonal relationships.

A client's sexuality is affected by development and life changes, ethical decisional issues, fertility, personal and emotional conflicts, illness, and hospitalization, and the nurse helps the client to adapt to situations and maintain healthy sexuality.

When making a spiritual assessment, the nurse includes questions about the client's concept of a supreme being, source of strength and hope, significance of religious practices and rituals, and perceived relationships between spiritual beliefs and health.

To be attuned to spiritual aspects of care, the nurse should be aware of his or her own spiritual dimension and be comfortable in discussing spiritual matters.

The nurse should use available resources such as family members, clergy, and other members of the health care team to help the client to maintain or regain spiritual health.

CRITICAL THINKING ACTIVITIES

1. Relate the differences between role and identity. How do these relate to self-concept?
2. What are the four components of self-concept? How do they differ?
3. Would an obese client who has recently lost a great deal of weight necessarily envision himself as thinner? Why or why not? Defend your position.
4. Mrs. Smith is 48 years old and is scheduled for a hysterectomy tomorrow. She expresses concern regarding whether this is the right choice and how she will adjust to the loss of femininity. What issues may be influencing Mrs. Smith? How do you proceed with care for Mrs. Smith?
5. Mr. Jackson is 65 years old and admitted post-diabetic ketoacidosis. During his stay you notice great intimacy (hand holding, kissing, massage, affectionate names) expressed between Mr. and Mrs. Jackson. How might you approach the topic of sexuality? What is relevant information to provide regarding age and disease state?
6. Mrs. Jones has given birth to her third child. In assisting her with ADLs you notice bruises on her neck and both arms. Mr. Jones seems to be in constant attendance and very resistant to leave the room. You suspect that some form of domestic abuse may be occurring. How do you approach validating this suspicion without putting Mrs. Jones at risk? What referrals, education, and support materials can you provide Mrs. Jones during this brief 24-hour stay? What are your further obligations?

References

Becker JV, Coleman E: Sexual abuse. In Lichtman R, Papera S, editors: *Gynecology: well woman care,* Norwalk, Conn., 1990, Appleton-Lange.

Benson H: *Beyond the relaxation response,* New York, 1984, Times Books.

Bernstein NR, Cope O: *Emotional care of the facially burned and disfigured,* Boston, 1976, Little, Brown, & Co.

Bly R: *Iron John: a book about men,* New York, 1990, Vintage Book.

Breo D, Eliot R: *Is it worth dying for? A self-assessment program to make stress work for you, not against you,* New York, 1989, Banton Books.

Buczny B: Impotence in older men: a newly recognized problem, *J Gerontol Nurs* 18(5):25, 1992.

Butler K: Spirituality reconsidered, *The Family Therapy Network* 14(5):1, 1990.

Carpenito LJ: *Nursing diagnosis: application to clinical practice,* ed 4, Philadelphia, 1993, JB Lippincott.

Carson V, et al.: Hope and well-being: essentials for living with AIDS, *Perspectives in Psychiatric Care,* 26(2):28-34, 1990.

Chaney J: *Sex role identification: psychological type and caring in male therapists,* doctoral dissertation, St. Louis, 1993, St. Louis University.

Cooper K: *The aerobics program for total well-being,* New York, 1982, M. Evans and Co.

Davenport D and Yurich J: Multicultural gender issues, *J Counsel Develop* 70(1):25, 1991.

Dugan D: Death and dying: emotional, spiritual, and ethical support for patients and families, *J Psychosoc Nurs* 25(7), 1987.

Erikson EH: *Childhood and society,* New York, ed 2, 1963, WW Norton & Co.

Farrell W: *Why men are the way they are,* New York, 1986, McGraw Hill.

Fine R: *Troubled men: the psychology, emotional conflicts and therapy of men,* San Francisco, 1988, Jossey-Bass.

Fogel C and Woods NF: *Health care of women,* St. Louis, 1981, Mosby.

Frank D: Androgyny, sexual satisfaction, and women, *J Psychosoc Nurs Ment Health Serv* 24(7), 1986.

Givson DE: Reminiscence, self-esteem, and self-other satisfaction in adult male alcoholics, *J Psychiatr Nurs* 18:7, 1930.

Gilligan C: *In a different voice,* Cambridge, Mass., 1982, Harvard University Press.

Goldberg H: *The hazards of being male,* New York, 1977, New American Library.

Hogan R: Family sexuality. In Bomar PJ: *Nurses and family health promotion,* Baltimore, 1989, Williams & Wilkins.

Jones EF, Forrest JD: Contraceptive failure rates based on the 1988 NSFG, *Fam Plann Perpect* 24(1):12, 1992.

Kaplan J: *Disorders of sexual desire,* New York, 1979, Simon & Schuster.

Kim MJ, et al.: *Pocket guide to nursing diagnoses,* ed 5, St. Louis, 1993, Mosby.

Kinsey AC, et al.: *Sexual behavior in the human male,* Philadelphia, 1948, WB Saunders.

Kinsey AC, et al.: *Sexual behavior in the human female,* Philadelphia, 1953, WB Saunders.

Kolodny R, et al.: *Textbook of sexual medicine,* Boston, 1979, Little, Brown & Co.

Ku LC, Sonenstein FL, and Pleck JH: The association of AIDS education and sex education with sexual behavior and condom use among teenage men, *Fam Plann Perspect* 24(93):100, 1992.

Lichtman R and Papera S: *Gynecology: well woman care,* Norwalk, Conn., 1990, Appleton-Lange.

Masters W, Johnson V, Kolodny R: *Human sexuality,* Boston, 1992, Little, Brown & Co.

McCann ME: Sexual healing after heart attack, *Am J Nurs* 89(9):1132, 1989.

Meleis A: Role insufficiency and role supplementation: a conceptual framework, *Nurs Res* 24:264, 1975.

Mellor S: Gender differences in identity formation as a function of self-other relationship, *J Youth and Adolescence* 18(4), 1989.

Miller J: Developing and maintaining hope in families of the critically ill, *AACN Clin Iss Crit Care* 2(2):307, 1991.

McSherry E: Modern clinical science of the spiritual dimension in chaplaincy and in the parish, *JCHCC,* 1988.

Montgomery C: The care-giving relationship: paradoxical and transcendent aspects, *J Transpersonal Psych* 23(2), 1991.

Nightengale F: *Notes on nursing,* New York, 1969, Dover Publications.

Parsons T: Illness and the role of physician: a sociological perspective, *Am J Orthopsychiatry* 21:452, 1951.

Peterson E: How to meet your client's spiritual needs, *J Psych Nurs Mental Health Servs* 25(5):34-40, 1987.

Piaget J and Inhelder B: *The psychology of the child,* New York, 1969, Basic Books.

Plichta S: The effects of woman abuse on health care utilization and health status: a literature review, *Woman's Health Issues* 2(3):154, 1992.

Pratt M, Dressner R, et al.: Four pathways in the analysis of adult development and aging: comparing analyses of reasoning about personal life dilemmas, *Psychology and Aging* 6(4):12, 1991.

Reed PG: Spirituality and well-being in terminally ill hospitalized adults, *Res Nurs Health* 10:335, 1987.

Scalone, MRC: Natural family planning and fertility awareness. In Lichtman R and Papera S, editors: *Gynecology: well woman care,* Norwalk, Conn., 1990, Appleton-Lange.

Sex Information and Education Council of the United States: The SIECUS/New York University/Uppsala principles basic to education for sexuality, *SIECUS Report* 8:8, 1980.

Shapiro S: *Manhood,* New York, 1984, G.P. Putnam.

Shreve B and Kankel M: Self-psychology, shame, and adolescent suicide: theoretical and practical considerations, *J Counsel Develop* 69(4), 1991.

Shuman NA and Bohachick P: Nurses' attitudes towards sexual counseling, *DCCN* 6(2):75 1987.

Stein R: Comparison of self-concept of non-obese and obese university junior female nursing students, *Adolescence,* 22(85), 1987.

Stuart GW and Sundeen SJ: *Principles and practice of psychiatric nursing,* ed 4, St. Louis, 1991, Mosby.

Woods NF: *Human sexuality in health and illness,* ed 4, St. Louis, 1987, Mosby.

World Health Organization: Education and treatment in human sexuality: the training of health professionals, *WHO Tech Rep Ser,* 572, Geneva, 1975, WHO.

Zelnik M and Kantner JF: Reasons for nonuse of contraception by sexually active women aged 15-19, *Fam Plann Perspect* 11(3):289, 1979.

Bibliography

Billy JOG, Tranfer K, et al.: The sexual behavior of men in the United States, *Fam Plann Perspect* 25(2):52, 1993.

Boyle CA, Berkowitz GS, and Kelsey JL: Epidemiology of premenstrual symptoms, *Am J Public Health* 77(3):349, 1987.

Bunting S and Campbell JC: Feminism and nursing: historical perspectives, *ANS* 12(4):11, 1990.

Carson V: *Spiritual dimensions of nursing practice,* Philadelphia, 1989, WB Saunders.

Covey L and Feltz D: Physical activity and adolescent female psychological development, *J Youth and Adolescence,* 20(4), 1991.

Dunn ME: Sexual health. In Lichtman R and Papers S, editors: *Gynecology: well woman care,* Norwalk, Conn., 1990, Appleton-Lange.

Flick LH: Paths to adolescent parenthood: implications for prevention, *Public Health Rep* 101(2):132, 1986.

Howard M and McCabe JB: Helping teenagers postpone sexual involvement, *Fam Plann Perspect* 22(1):21, 1990.

Jain H, Shamoian CA and Mobarak A: Sexual disorders in the elderly: *Med Aspects Human Sexuality* (special issue) 21(3):14, 1987.

Katsin L: Chronic illness and sexuality, *Am J Nurs* 90(1):54, 1990.

Mayer RA and Boggio NT: The adolescent rape victim, *Emerg Med* 24(93):98, 1992.

McCracken AL: Sexual practices by elders, *J Gerontol Nurs* 14(10):13, 1988.

Muscari ME: Obtaining the adolescent sexual history, *Pediatr Nurs* 13(5):307, 1987.

Rankin SH: Psychosocial adjustments of coronary artery disease patients and their spouses: nursing implications, *Nurs Clin North Am* 27(1):271, 1992.

Rieve JE: Sexuality and the adult with acquired physical disability, *Nurs Clin North Am* 24(1):265, 1989.

Sampsell CM: The role of nursing in preventing violence against women, *J Ob Gyn Neonatal Nurs* 20(6):481, 1991.

Stokes K: *Faith is a verb,* Mystic, Conn., 1989, Twenty-Third Publications.

Volden C et al.: The relationship of age, gender, and exercise practice to health, lifestyle, and self-esteem, *Appl Nurs Res* 3(1):20, 1990.

18

Multicultural Nursing

OBJECTIVES

Mastery of content in this chapter will enable the student to:

- Define the key terms listed.
- Describe ways in which culture influences an individual and family.
- Describe the relationship of sociocultural background to health and illness beliefs and practices.
- Compare concepts of traditional and modern health and illness beliefs and practices.
- List examples of traditional health and illness beliefs and practices from selected ethnic groups.
- Describe communication and economic sociocultural barriers to health care.
- Perform a cultural assessment using heritage consistency.
- List potential nursing diagnoses related to a client's ethnocultural background.
- Design nursing interventions appropriate to client's ethnocultural background.

KEY TERMS

acculturation
assimilation
culture
demography
ethnicity
ethnocentrism
healing
heritage consistency
metacommunication system
modern approach
multicultural nursing
Raza-Latina
religion
socialization
territoriality
time orientation
traditional approach

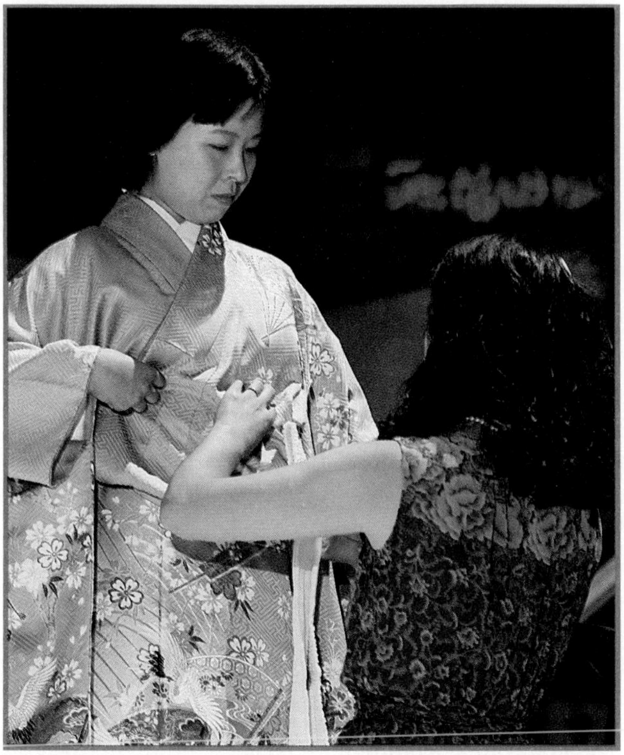

As we enter the twenty-first century, nurses are perched on the cutting edge of enormous demographic, social, and cultural change. Many of these changes will play a dramatic role in the delivery of nursing care to a given client and family. Multicultural nursing provides a practice framework for broadening nurses' understanding of health-related beliefs, practices, and issues that are part of the experiences of people from diverse cultural backgrounds. In addition, multicultural nursing provides the nurse the opportunity to explore, understand, and learn from the background of clients and fellow workers, including their unique perspectives on health and health care as well as their perspective on community and social issues. With a basic knowledge and understanding of multicultural nursing, the nurse can appreciate the total diversity of our society.

It is predicted that in the United States the percentage of people of European origin, which was 80.3% in 1990 (U.S. Bureau of the Census, 1991), will be only 54% by the year 2020 (Hodgkinson, 1988). Nurses must be aware of this demographic reality so they can address the future nursing care needs of the changing population. A nurse must have a basic understanding of and sensitivity to the unique health and illness beliefs and practices found among the culturally diverse populations in the United States and Canada.

Nurses also come from diverse ethnic, cultural, and religious backgrounds, and rapport is established when nurses are able to convey to the client and family that they are aware of and sensitive to their unique health and illness beliefs and practices. This rapport facilitates the delivery of safe and effective multicultural nursing care.

A person's cultural background primarily involves internal standards of behavior and shared values and attitudes. The standards of a given group, however, are not clearly defined or expressed and vary among and between group members (Figure 18-1). Many members of a given group do not follow all behaviors and standards, and others assume that all people share the same behaviors, values, and attitudes.

A broad range of health and illness beliefs exists among cultural groups in North America. Many of these beliefs have roots in the cultural, ethnic, religious, or social background of a person, family, or community. When people anticipate, fear, or experience an illness or crisis, they may use a **modern approach** (present-day beliefs and practices of the providers within the American, or Western, health care delivery system) or a **traditional approach** (ancient ethnocultural or religious beliefs and practices that have been handed down through generations) toward prevention or healing. The traditional approaches may be derived from heritage. These beliefs and practices may be internal or personal, and the person may be able to define and describe them. However, they may result from external social forces out of the person's control. Examples of these forces include communication barriers such as language differences or economic barriers causing limited access to modern health care facilities.

For a nurse to provide care for a client of a different cultural or ethnic background, effective intercultural communication must take place. The demographic profile of the North American population is changing rapidly, and the need for intercultural awareness and understanding is escalating. Because nurses deal with clients on a one-to-one basis, they must interact and relate to all peoples.

HERITAGE CONSISTENCY

One way of analyzing belief systems is through the "melting pot" theory, whereby people have been acculturated into the dominant culture through schools, television, radio, and motion pictures (McLemore, 1980). Another theory is **heritage consistency,** which looks at **acculturation** as a continuum. Using this theory, the nurse not only analyzes the degree to which a person identifies with the dominant culture but also how he or she identifies with a traditional culture. It is possible to assess health beliefs by determining a person's ties to

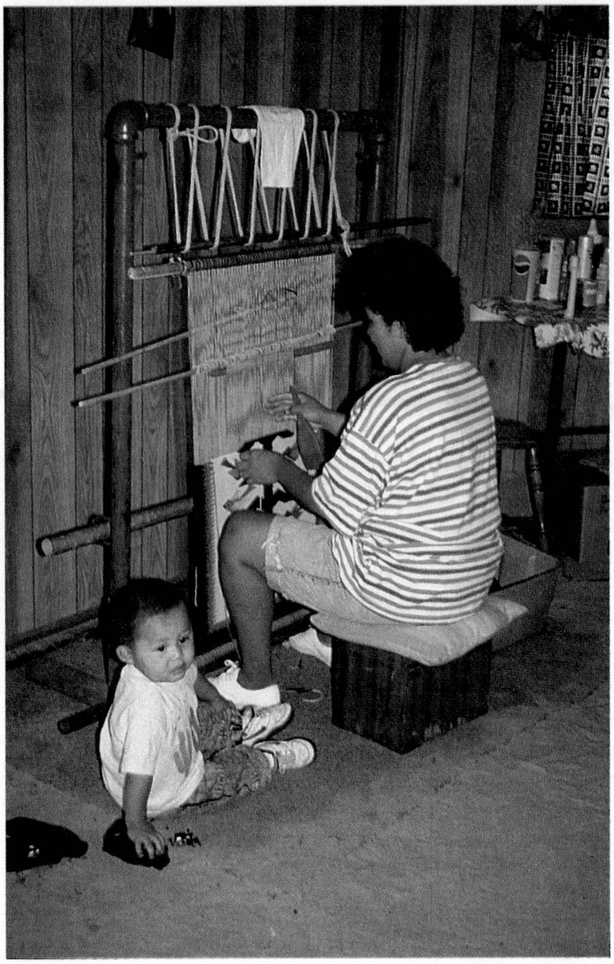

FIGURE 18-1 Traditional artforms are one method of demonstrating a person's cultural heritage. (Courtesy Michael S. Clement, MD, Mesa, Ariz.).

traditional beliefs and his or her stage of acculturation.

Heritage consistency was developed in 1980 by Estes and Zitzow to assess and counsel Native American alcoholics within a cultural context. It describes "the degree to which one's life-style reflects his/her tribal culture" (Estes and Zitzow, 1980). The theory has now been expanded in an attempt to study the degree to which any person's life-style reflects the traditional culture, whether it is European, Asian, African, or Spanish. For the same person, some aspects of life-style may reflect cultural heritage, whereas other aspects are inconsistent with that heritage because the person has undergone acculturation (Spector, 1991).

The degree of heritage consistency is evaluated by determining the importance of culture, ethnicity, and religion to a person, although it is difficult to isolate the specific aspects of these factors that shape a person's world view. Figure 18-2 illustrates the way these variables intertwine in the socialization of the person. When religion is discussed, culture and ethnicity must also be included. It is possible to describe and compare diverse health and illness beliefs and practices within North American society.

Culture

Culture is the socially inherited characteristics of a human group that are transmitted from one generation to the next (Fejos, 1959). These include world view, values, beliefs, and patterns of social conduct. In addition, culture is learned and serves as the framework of our individuality and personhood, of social relationships, and a series of symbols. Culture occurs simultaneously in a person's cognitive and behavioral development (Bohannan, 1992). Culture shapes a person's way of experiencing health and illness. Such beliefs are an integral part of life.

Ethnicity

Ethnicity is a cultural group's sense of identification associated with its common social and cultural heritage. It is the characteristics a group may have in common. These characteristics include nationality, race, language, religious faith, food preferences, and folklore and many traits relevant to physical appearance. There are more than 106 ethnic groups and 170 Native American tribes in North America (Thernstrom, 1980).

Religion

Religion is the belief in a divine or superhuman power or powers to be obeyed and worshipped as the creators and rulers of the universe (see Chapter 17). Ethical values and religion, a system of beliefs and practices, further clarify ethnicity (Abramson, 1980) by providing a frame of reference and perspective within which to organize information. The major religions in North America are Protestant, Catholic, Jewish, Eastern Orthodox, Muslim, Hindu, Baha'i, and Buddhist. Countless religious beliefs and practices are related to health and illness.

HERITAGE ASSESSMENT

Heritage consistency occurs on an ever-changing continuum. This concept does not stereotype or diagnose; it is a way to understand a client's or family's sociocultural background and how it creates a framework within which the client can view and interpret life events. The client and family may interpret events through a traditional or modern viewpoint.

The box on p. 406 is a sample assessment tool of the

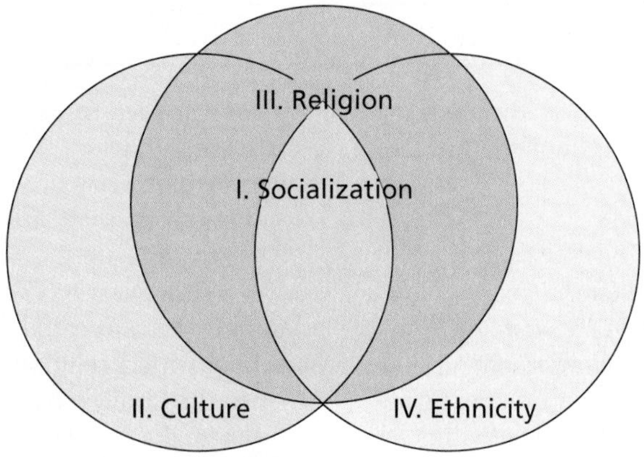

I. Socialization — Extended family
Place reared
Visits home
Raised with extended family
Name

II. Culture — Extended family
Participation in folk ways
Language

III. Religion — Extended family
Church membership and participation
Historic beliefs

IV. Ethnicity — Extended family
Residence in ethnic community
Participation in folk ways
Socialization with members of same ethnic group
Identification as ethnic American

FIGURE 18-2 Model of heritage consistency. (From Spector R: *Cultural diversity in health and illness,* ed 3, Norwalk, Conn., 1991, Appleton-Lange.)

factors comprising heritage consistency and some sample questions that may be asked to determine a family's circumstances. Before these questions are asked of a client or family, the nurse should first assess and understand personal ethnoreligious heritage. By using this tool, the nurse can determine the degree to which a client identifies with his or her heritage. A person who deeply identifies with a traditional heritage is more likely to maintain the traditional health beliefs of the group.

ETHNOCULTURAL GROUPS IN NORTH AMERICA

The populations of the United States and Canada consist largely of the descendants of immigrants. The only true natives are American Indians, Aleuts, and Eskimos because they settled here thousands of years before the Europeans, Asians, Hispanics, and African Americans. People have come to North America from every nation in the world and continue to immigrate in large numbers.

Table 18-1 presents an overview of the nationalities of the North American population, themes of traditional ethnocultural health and illness beliefs and practices, samples of traditional remedies, and some examples of pathological conditions that occur more frequently among people of specific ethnic backgrounds.

HEALTH TRADITIONS

When discussing health beliefs and practices as they stem from a cultural, ethnic, and religious framework, the word *may* should be used to prevent stereotyping. The range of health and illness definitions, beliefs, and practices is infinite, and there are differences within and between groups. However, some recognizable commonalities exist. The nurse must remember that it is important to constantly assess and communicate with clients to clarify their beliefs about health and illness.

HERITAGE ASSESSMENT

- Childhood development occurred in the country of origin or in an immigrant neighborhood of like ethnic group.
  Where were you born?
  Where did you grow up?
  What was your neighborhood like?
  Are you and your parents from the same or different ethnoreligious or racial background?
- Extended family members encourage participation in traditional religious or cultural activities.
  Do you and your family celebrate holidays and festivals together at home and in the community?
  Do you participate in other church or fraternal events with family members?
- Client and family members frequently visit the country of origin or the "old neighborhood."
  How often do you return to the neighborhood in which you grew up?
- Client's and family members' homes are within an "ethnic" community.
  What ethnic group or groups live in your neighborhood?
- Client and family members participate in ethnic cultural events such as religious festivals or holidays, sometimes with singing, dancing, and national costumes.
  Do you now participate in ethnic or religious events?
- Client was reared in an extended family setting.
  Who lived in your home when you were young?
  Did you live with grandparents, aunts, uncles, and cousins?
  What are the present circumstances?
- Client and family members maintain regular contact with the extended family.
  How often do you visit family members?
  Do you keep in close contact with those at a distance?
- Family name has not been "Americanized."
  What was your family's name when it immigrated?
  Have the members kept or changed their name?
- Client was educated in a parochial (nonpublic) school with a religious or ethnic philosophy similar to the family's background.
  Where did you go to school?
  What kind of a school is it?
- Client and family members engage primarily in social activities with others of the same ethnic or religious background.
  What are the ethnic and religious backgrounds of your friends?
  Are they from your same ethnoreligious background?
- Client and family members have a knowledge of the culture and language of origin.
  Have you studied the history of the people from the nation from which you come?
  Do you speak your native language?
  What language did you learn first?
  What language do you speak at home?
- Client and family members possess elements of personal pride about their heritage.
  How do you identify yourself?
  With which group, if parents are from the different groups?
- Client and family members incorporate elements of historical beliefs and practices into the present philosophy.
  What is your history?
  What can you tell me about your specific health and illness beliefs?

Health and Illness Beliefs

A person's beliefs about health and illness and the causes or treatments of illness are that person's health beliefs. Modern beliefs are "established, scientific" health beliefs (for example, bacteria or viruses cause communicable diseases and antibiotics are effective treatment for bacterial infections).

When a person thinks the "evil eye" or "envy" is the cause of illness and that disease is best treated by removing the "source of evil or envy," he or she has traditional beliefs. A religious or ethnic background may produce these beliefs. Another traditional theme is that of balance; for example, the Chinese believe that factors such as yin (feminine, negative, dark, and cold forces) and yang (masculine, positive, light, and warm forces) must be in balance, and the Spanish believe that "hot" and "cold" must be balanced.

Health and Illness Practices

Health practices are actions one performs to prevent or treat illness. Modern health practices are recognized by contemporary health care workers as established, scientific ways of preventing illness (e.g., immunizations)

table 18-1

CULTURAL GROUPS: HEALTH AND ILLNESS BELIEFS, PRACTICES, AND MORBIDITY PROBLEMS

Origin	Health beliefs	Health practices	Illness beliefs	Illness practices	Traditional remedies	High morbidity incidence
ASIAN AMERICAN						
China Hawaii Philippines Korea Japan Southeast Asia Laos Cambodia Vietnam	Balance of yin and yang	Prevent imbalances of yin and yang and changes in climate	Imbalance of yin and yang	Restore balance of yin and yang; use herbal remedies and acupuncture	*Huo li jian mei su* *Jen shen lu jung wan* Ginseng root Tiger balm White flower	Liver cancer Stomach cancer Coccidioidomycosis Hypertension Parasites
AFRICAN AMERICAN						
West coast of Africa (as slaves) Many African countries West Indian islands Dominican Republic Haiti Jamaica	Harmony with nature	Prevent disharmony; respect cleanliness and religion; avoid sick people	Disharmony	Use folk remedies and healers	Bangles Talisman *Asafoetida* Voodoo candles	Cancer of the esophagus Stomach cancer Coccidioidomycosis Hypertension Sickle cell anemia
EUROPEAN						
England France Germany Other European countries	Physical and emotional well-being; feeling OK	Respect proper nutrition, exercise, cleanliness, faith in God	Absence of well-being; feeling bad	Use home remedies, liniments, poultices, and medical care	Amulets Syrup of Black Draught Father John's Medicine Swamp root *Olbas*	Breast cancer Thalassemia
NAI/AN (North American Indians/Alaska Natives)						
170 Native American tribes Western part of United States Reservations Tribal homelands	Living in harmony with nature	Respect nature; avoid evil spirits	Disharmony with nature	Use medicine man and traditional herbal remedies	Masks Sweet grass Thunderbird Sand paintings	Accidents Heart disease Cirrhosis of the liver Diabetes mellitus Lung cancer
SPANISH AND CENTRAL AMERICAN						
Spain Cuba Central and South America Mexico Puerto Rico	Reward for good behavior; balance of "hot and cold" humors	Wear amulets; use proper diet to maintain balance of "hot and cold"; pray	Punishment for wrong-doing; imbalance of hot and cold	Restore body's balance; use folk healers and remedies	Amulets: *Mano Negro* Special soaps Candles *Manzanilla* *Anis*	Diabetes mellitus Parasites Coccidioidomycosis

and treating illness (e.g., medication and surgery). Traditional health practices are those in which a person wears amulets to ward off "evil," eats select foods to prevent illness, and uses folk medicine or healers to treat illness.

Traditional Remedies

The admitted use of folk or traditional medicine is increasing, and the practice may be observed among people from all walks of life and cultural and ethnic backgrounds. Among people who are heritage consistent, this is not a new practice, and many of the remedies have been used and passed on for generations. The pharmaceutical properties of vegetation—plants, roots, stems, flowers, seeds, and herbs—have been studied, tested, catalogued, and used for many centuries. Many of these plants are used by specific communities; others cross ethnic-community lines and are used geographically. These remedies are generally purchased in special stores or markets that serve the members of the community (Figure 18-3), or they may be purchased in the person's country of origin. Frequently, the active ingredients of these traditional remedies are unknown. When clients do not adhere to a pharmacological regimen, an effort must be made to determine whether they are taking traditional remedies. If a nurse believes a client is taking these remedies, the nurse must make an effort to determine the active ingredients of the remedy. These ingredients can often be antagonistic or synergistic to the prescribed medications. When this is the situation, the medication may have no effect, or a severe overdose may occur. Figure 18-4 presents an array of available remedies from African, Asian, European, Native, and Raza/Latina sources.

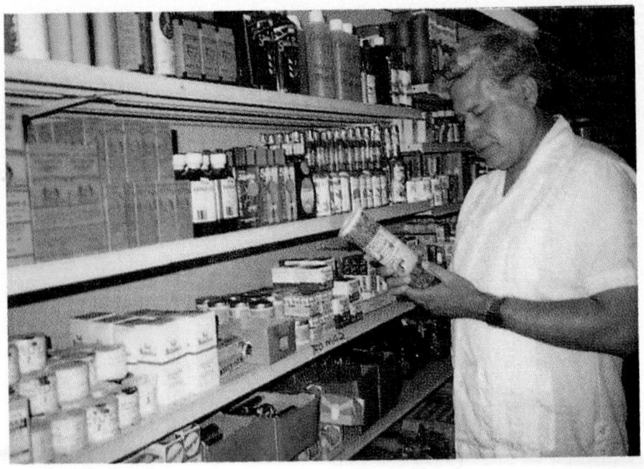

FIGURE 18-3 Traditional remedies are often purchased in specialty stores in a community. (Photograph by Rachel E. Spector, Boston College School of Nursing, Chestnut Hill, Mass.)

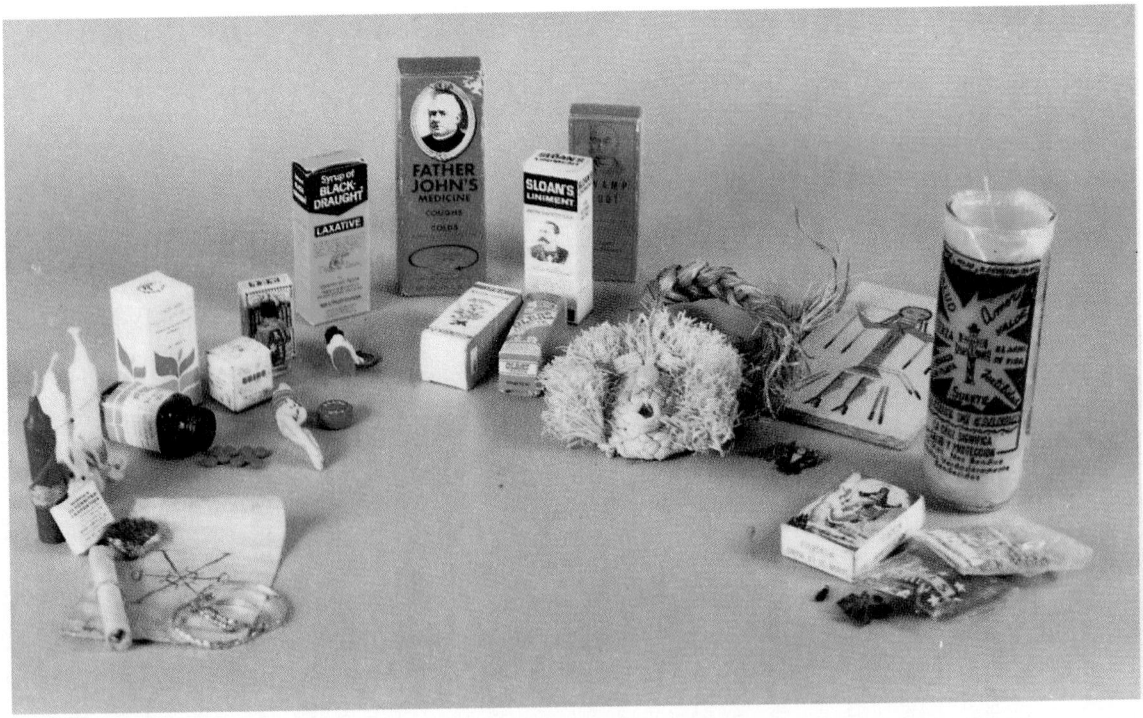

FIGURE 18-4 A variety of remedies are used by many cultural groups in United States. See text for description of origins, names, and uses of these remedies. (Photograph by Lucy Rozier, Boston College Audio Visual Services, Boston College, Chestnut Hill, Mass.)

African Americans. Bangles in the folk tradition are silver bracelets worn by people originating in the West Indies. They are open to let out evil and closed to prevent evil from entering the body. They are worn from infancy, but as the child grows, they are replaced with larger bracelets. These bracelets tend to tarnish and leave a black ring on the skin when a child becomes ill. When this occurs, the parent knows that the child must rest, improve the diet, and be wary of any other sources of harm. Some individuals wear several bangles; when they move, the bracelets jingle to frighten away evil spirits. Many people believe that they are extremely vulnerable to evil, even to death, when such bracelets are removed. Nurses must realize that the child and parents experience a great deal of anxiety when these bracelets are removed.

Talismans are sacred pieces of parchment believed to protect the wearer from all illness when worn on a string around the waist or carried in a pocket. *Asafoetida* is a foul-smelling, gummy substance from a plant resin that is worn to ward off colds and evil. It is known as "the incense of the devil." Voodoo candles are said to have a peculiar spiritualistic character and are used for sacred rituals and rites. Their colors are significant; for example, pink corresponds to love, white to peace, and blue to success and protection from harm.

Asian Americans. *Huo li jian mei su* are small, brown, round pills taken twice a day for prevention of senility, relief of fatigue, and maintenance of youth, health, and beauty. *Jen shen lu jung wan* is a brown liquid used as a general tonic to brace the whole system or as an aid to improve digestion; it may be taken before elective surgery. Tiger balm is a clear, smooth salve used for temporary relief of minor aches and pains. White flower is a colorless liquid used to treat colds, influenza, headache, and coughs.

Ginseng root is the most famous of Chinese medicines. It has universal medicinal usage and is used to "build the blood," especially after childbirth. The legend states that the more the root looks like the human form, the more effective it is. Ginseng is also native to the United States, where it is used as a restorative tonic.

European Americans. An example of an amulet is the *Malocchio,* an Italian horn worn with the *Gobo,* a hunchbacked man, to ward off the "evil eye." The *Gobo* is holding a horseshoe for luck in his left hand and is pointing the first and fourth digits of his right hand to ward off the evil spirit.

Syrup of Black Draught is used as an "over-the-counter" laxative. Father John's Medicine is a medicine used for colds and coughs since 1855. Sloan's Liniment aids in the temporary relief of minor pains from arthritis and other ailments. *Swamp root* is a liquid used as a diuretic. Olbas and Magentropfen are medicines purchased in Germany to treat sore throats and lack of appetite.

Native Americans. Masks are worn to hide from the devil or evil spirits. Sweet grass is burned as rite of purification by the medicine man. The thunderbird is an amulet worn for good luck and protection. Sand painting is executed by the Navajo medicine man to guide the diagnosis of an ailment.

Raza/Latinas. *Mano Negro* (Puerto Rican) is an amulet, a black hand in the shape of a fist with a coral bead on top, that is pinned on a baby's shirt to protect it from evil. *Jabon de la Mano Milagrosa* is a soap used to cleanse a person and protect him or her. Candles are burned to ward off evil. *Manzanilla* is a herb taken as a tea; it is used to treat stomach and intestinal pain, uterine cramps, anxiety, and insomnia. *Anis* is a star-shaped seed used to treat painful gas, upset stomach, colic, and anorexia and to increase breast milk.

Traditional Healers

In the traditional context, **healing** is the restoration of the person to a state of harmony between the body, mind, and spirit—the restoration of holistic health. Within a community, there are specific people who have the power to heal. The healer may be a man or woman and is most often a person thought to have received the gift of healing from a divine source.

In many instances, a person who is heritage consistent may consult a traditional healer before, instead of, or concurrent with the use of a Western health care provider. The relationship between the person and healer is quite often much closer than that of the person and the health care professional. The healer understands the problem within a cultural context, speaks the same language, and shares a similar world view. The following are some examples of traditional healers:

1. Medicine man: The traditional healer of the Native Americans
2. *Senora:* A Puerto Rican woman knowledgeable in the treatment of illness
3. *Esperitista:* A person who possesses more sophisticated skills than the *Senora*
4. *Curandero:* A person with a god-given ability to heal using a religious approach
5. *Partera:* A Mexican-American midwife
6. Root-worker: An African American who is able to determine the cause of an illness and the treatment

The nurse must remember that traditional healers have been a part of human cultures for as long as they have existed. The methods used to heal have been developed over generations by trial and error, with religious beliefs and social circumstances contributing to

table 18-2
COMPARISONS: TRADITIONAL HEALER VERSUS PHYSICIAN

Healer	Physician
Maintains an informal, friendly, effective relationship with the entire family.	Business-like and formal, dealing primarily with the client.
Comes to the house day or night.	Client must go to the physician's office or clinic. Home visits are rarely, if ever, made.
Consults with head of house, creates a mood of awe, talks to all family members, is not authoritarian, has social rapport, builds expectation of cure.	Deals primarily with the ill person, may address only person's illness. Authoritarian manner can create fear.
Less expensive than the physician.	More expensive than the healer.
Has ties to the "world of the sacred"; has rapport with the symbolic, spiritual, creative, or holy force.	Primarily secular, pays less attention to the religious beliefs of a client or meanings of an illness.
Shares the world view of the client; that is, speaks the same language, lives in the same neighborhood or in the same similar socioeconomic conditions, may know the same people, understands the life-style of the client.	Generally does not share the world view of the client; that is, may not speak the same language, live in the same neighborhood or in the same socioeconomic conditions, may not understand the life-style of the client.

Modified from Spector RE: *Cultural diversity in health and illness,* ed 3, Norwalk, Conn., 1991, Appleton and Lange.

the methods. The effective methods have been preserved and adapted to meet the needs of the time. There are several differences between the Western health care provider and the traditional healer; Table 18-2 compares the two.

DIFFERENCES AND SIMILARITIES AMONG ETHNIC GROUPS

Health and illness beliefs and practices vary among ethnic groups. These differences occur not only among groups but also among the nurse, client, and family. In addition to these health and illness beliefs and practices, the nurse must be sensitive to other factors, such as communication, physiological susceptibility to disease, and emotional and mental health differences, to practice safely and effectively.

Communication

Communication is an integral part of culture, since culture can be called a metacommunication system. Communication, like culture, influences and reflects how feelings are expressed and what verbal and nonverbal languages mean. Nurses must be sensitive to several factors related to communication. These include both nonverbal and verbal communication/language, space, and time (Table 18-3).

Language. Language differences are possibly the most important factor when providing nursing care to

SUGGESTIONS FOR COMMUNICATING WITH CLIENTS WHO SPEAK OTHER LANGUAGES

Respect clients as individuals, regardless of differences in language skills and values. Avoid judging clients' intellectual abilities or emotional states on the basis of how they use language.

Avoid treating emerging majority group members differently from other clients because such "special" treatment may be interpreted as patronizing.

Take care not to assume that clients are angry, aggressive, or hostile if they speak more loudly or emotionally than most European Americans.

Use titles such as "Mr." or "Ms." unless you have established a first-name basis for the relationship.

Never attempt to use ethnic dialects with clients. This may be interpreted as making fun of clients or as condescension.

Avoid attempting to impress clients by saying you have friends of the same ethnic or racial background.

Be attentive to clients' nonverbal communications, which can help to clarify seemingly confusing verbal communications.

Make use of ethnic group preferences when giving care. Involve the extended family in communication, for example, or focus on oral rather than written teaching methods.

Explain medical and nursing terms in simple, everyday words and be sure that clients truly understand.

If you do not understand what a client is saying, ask for clarification. Do not let embarrassment at not understanding lead to the risks of misinformation.

table 18-3

CROSS-CULTURAL EXAMPLES OF SELECTED COMMUNICATION PHENOMENA AFFECTING NURSING CARE

Nations of origin	Communication	Space	Time orientation
ASIAN ORIGIN	National and local languages	Noncontact	Present
China	Cantonese		
Hawaii			
Philippines	Tagalog		
Korea	Korean		
Japan	Haragei†		
Southeast Asia	French and national languages		
Laos			
Cambodia			
Vietnam			
AFRICAN ORIGIN	National languages	Close personal space	Present over future
West Coast (as slaves)	Dialect		
Many African countries			
West Indian Islands	Creole		
Dominican Republic	Spanish		
Haiti	French		
Jamaica			
EUROPEAN ORIGIN	National languages	Noncontact people	Future over present
Germany	Many learn English immediately	Aloof	
England		Distant	
Italy		Southern countries—closer contact and touch	
Ireland			
Other European countries			
NAI/AN*	Tribal languages	Space is very important and has no boundaries	Present
170 North American Tribes	Use of silence and body language		
Aluets			
Eskimoes			
HISPANIC ORIGIN	Spanish and Portuguese primary languages	Tactile relationships	Present
Spain and Portugal		Touch	
Cuba	Native languages and dialects	Handshakes	
Mexico		Embracing	
Central and South America		Values physical presence	

From Spector R: Culture, ethnicity, and nursing. In Potter P and Perry A: *Fundamentals of nursing*, ed 3, St. Louis. 1992, Mosby.
**NAI/AN*, North American Indian/Alaska Native.
†*Haragei*, the Japanese art or practice of using nonverbal communication. (From Matsumoto M: *The unspoken way,* Tokyo, 1988, Kodansha International.)

ethnic group clients because these differences can affect all stages of the nursing process. Clear and effective communication is important when dealing with any client and is crucial if language differences create a cultural barrier (see box on p. 410). If the client and nurse do not speak the same language, a translator is necessary. More often, however, the client speaks the nurse's language with limited ability or uses language with denotative or connotative meanings different from the nurse's meanings. For example, a client with limited language ability might know customary greetings such as "How are you?" or "Hello" but not understand health terms such as "inflammation" or "temperature" that are usually understood by lay persons in the dominant cultural group. Failure to communicate effectively with the client may not only cause unnecessary and costly delays in diagnosis and treatment but also may lead to tragic consequences.

Nurses need the ability to communicate with clients limited in the use of the nurse's language because, when deprived of the most common medium of interaction with clients (the spoken word), nurses often become frustrated and ineffective in interventions. Some nurses avoid clients with whom they cannot communicate. Unfortunately, this creates a vicious circle of cultural misunderstandings between the nurse and client. All too often, the nurse might behave toward the client in ways that could be misconstrued by the client (for example, shouting, focusing on the task instead of the client, or doing things for the client without speaking) or using body language, such as arms folded across the chest, which might be read by the client as anger or hostility.

Language differences can be overcome, however. Differences in denotative and connotative meanings may exist between members of two cultures, causing miscommunication. The health institution must provide an interpreter. Medical terms must be clearly explained to all clients. Hospital jargon (for example, "force fluids") or abbreviations (for example, qid) should be eliminated. Another linguistic block to communication between ethnic groups comes from differences in connotative meanings for certain words, even when the denotative meanings are the same. For example, the word *hospital* may mean a facility for health care to one client, but it may represent death or a threat to life for another.

By giving special attention to the communication process, nurses can overcome language barriers. Observing nonverbal behaviors, for example, can help to clarify a client's communication, although nonverbal communication is also influenced by culture. Nurses can also learn to phrase questions and statements to elicit information from clients whose ethnic background shapes their response.

Time Orientation. **Time orientation** varies among cultural groups, and a nurse who has an ethnocentric attitude toward time may find it difficult to understand and to plan care for clients with a different time orientation. For example, certain cultural groups see a value in taking steps early to prevent the occurrence of illness in the future. Other cultural groups may see little value in planning for the future and thus fail to make appointments or to try to stop habits that place them at risk for disease. This time orientation difference may become important in health care measures such as long-term planning and explanations about when medications should be taken.

Personal Space and Territoriality. **Territoriality** is an attitude toward an area a person has claimed and defends or reacts emotionally about when another encroaches on it. Personal space involves a person's set of behaviors and attitudes toward the space around the self. Territoriality and personal space are influenced by culture, and thus different ethnic groups have varying norms related to the use of space.

Staff members and other clients frequently encroach on a client's territory in the hospital. The client's territory includes the room, bed, closet, and belongings. The nurse should try to respect the client's territory as much as possible, especially when performing nursing procedures. Even routine procedures should be explained to all clients to indicate to them that the nurse accepts them as persons. If a client has no critical problems, the nurse should encourage visits from members of the extended family, which can remind the client of home and thus lessen the effects of isolation and shock from hospitalization.

Personal space is involved in many nursing activities, and the nurse should be sensitive about the client's attitudes toward space. For example, certain nursing measures involve touching clients, an action that may be threatening to members of certain cultural groups. Standards of behavior vary also in terms of who, male or female, can touch the client and where. The meaning of personal space also varies among cultures. Hall (1963) studied the meaning of space and identified the following zones:

1. Intimate zone (up to 1½ feet)
2. Personal distance (1½ to 4 feet)
3. Social distance (4 to 12 feet)
4. Public distance (12 feet or more)

Use of personal space varies among individuals and ethnic groups. The extreme modesty practiced by members of some groups may prevent members from seeking preventive health care. For example, women who are shy about physical exposure may avoid being examined by male physicians.

Physiological Differences

Countless differences regarding susceptibility to disease, dermatological conditions, and food and eating habits exist among ethnic groups. The nurse should assess family history carefully.

Susceptibility to Disease. Because of genetic or life-style differences, some ethnic groups are more susceptible to certain diseases than others. In general, ethnic groups with lower socioeconomic status are more susceptible to acquired diseases and conditions such as malnutrition and infections. Refer to Table 18-1 for selected diseases and the ethnic groups with high occurrences.

Dermatological Conditions. For all ethnic groups, skin color is an important factor in physiological assessment, but assessment of skin color depends more on the individual than on racial or genetic factors because individuals within a race vary widely in skin color. Color changes in dark-skinned clients must be determined differently from those in whites. For instance, in a dark-skinned person, pallor is the absence of the underlying red tones that normally give brown and black skin its glow. The skin of a black person will appear ashen gray, and an individual with brown skin will become yellow brown (Geiger and Davidhizar, 1991).

Keloid formation, an exaggerated skin healing process after trauma to the skin, is more common among blacks, as are conditions that cause hypopigmentation and hyperpigmentation. A mongolian spot, a blue pigmentation found in sacral and gluteal areas of some Raza/Latina and other ethnic minority group infants, is normal and harmless and usually fades and disappears in weeks or months.

Food and Eating Habits. Food and eating habits vary widely among cultural groups, but these customs usually carry emotional and social significance. Therefore it helps for nurses to have a general understanding of the food habits of ethnic clients. In many cases, family members can be permitted to bring special foods to hospitalized clients unhappy about hospital food. When teaching a client about dietary requirements related to specific illnesses, the nurse should be sensitive to cultural meanings of eating and food preferences.

Nurses should also be aware of their own cultural values related to food and eating because these values influence their attitudes toward eating, including determinations about the best foods, preferable methods of preparation, appropriate times for eating, and ways in which illness affects these factors. Nurses can be aware of a client's differences only when they identify their own cultural values related to food.

Psychological Differences

Differences may exist between the nurse's expectations and client's perceptions of emotional and mental health, emotional expression and reactions to pain, gender role behaviors, and attitudes toward family.

Emotional and Mental Health. People from all cultural groups undergo emotional and mental stresses and conflicts. An additional stressor, however, is the prejudice and discrimination by the dominant group toward members of the other ethnic group. Clients may form defense mechanisms for relating to others from the dominant culture. The following patterns of behavior are linked to these defense mechanisms: acceptance, aggression, obsessive sensitivity, efforts of ego enhancement, self-hatred, and assimilation. A person might use more than one of these mechanisms when attempting to cope with a situation.

Acceptance occurs when group members accommodate themselves to the prejudice of the dominant group. This apparently good-natured behavior can block genuine communication and often causes a client to accept unpleasant symptoms and situations without alerting a nurse.

Aggression occurs when group members strike out with hostile acts against members of the dominant group. Sullenness and stubbornness are effective ways of expressing frustration with the nurse. When interacting with members of the dominant group, the person may be hypersensitive to signs of bigotry. Clients who detect bigotry may fail to seek health care because of prejudices seen in health care workers.

As a defense mechanism, a person may also seek to enhance self-concept through ego enhancement. An example might involve a client who requests a private duty nurse for their personal care.

Acceptance of the dominant group's evaluation might also lead a person to develop unconscious self-hatred, usually accompanied by ambivalent feelings of inferiority. For example, a client may be quick to criticize behaviors of his or her own family during visitation in the hospital.

Finally, another reaction of a person is assimilation. In this case, the person acquires behaviors or attitudes similar to the dominant culture.

Reactions to Pain. To determine a client's emotional state, the nurse needs to understand how patterns of emotional expression vary among ethnic groups. Reaction to pain is influenced by cultural background, and it is important for the nurse to objectively evaluate pain. To do so, nurses should be aware that their own attitudes about pain are culturally influenced.

Gender Role Behaviors. Accepted norms for traditional gender role behaviors vary among cultures. Certain roles for men and certain roles for women may be stressed. For example, in matriarchal cultures, the wife or mother is responsible for many family decisions, including when to seek health care. When providing family health care and involving family members in the client's care, the nurse needs to know variables in gender role behaviors to understand the client's behaviors. Understanding multicultural behavioral differences is also crucial when the nurse provides client care involving emotional and social dimensions.

Attitudes Toward the Family. Many chapters in this book discuss the importance of involving the client's family or significant others in all stages of the nursing process. Family behavior patterns vary among cultural groups, however, and the nurse must be aware of such variations when involving the family in care. The nurse should also be aware of specific differences in attitudes toward the family among ethnic groups.

MULTICULTURAL NURSING ASSESSMENT

CULTURAL

What customs and values of the client may influence health behaviors and the provision of care?
Could the client's communication process or language affect the provision of care? How?
What health care beliefs and practices of the client may influence acceptance of and response to illness?
Could nutritional variables and preferences or restrictions affect the provision of care?

SOCIOLOGICAL

Could the client's economic status affect the provision of care?
Could educational status affect the provision of care?
How does the client's social network affect the provision of care?
What family structural variables may influence the provision of care?
Are community support systems available and do they help to fight against institutional racism?

PSYCHOLOGICAL

Could self-concept and identity factors affect the provision of care?
What are the client's defense mechanisms, and are they adaptive or maladaptive?
Could religious or cultural considerations affect the provision of care?

BIOLOGICAL AND PHYSIOLOGICAL

Does the nurse need to take racial or anatomical characteristics or factors into account when providing care?
Do growth and development patterns influence physical assessment findings?
What variations in body systems are present?
Does the nurse need to take skin pigmentation or other skin conditions into account?
Are there any culturally specific diseases to note? Are there any diseases to which the client has increased (decreased) resistance?

CULTURAL FACTORS AND THE NURSING PROCESS

When caring for clients, the nurse uses the nursing process. Because nurses are frequently from a cultural group other than that of the client, they must consider their client's cultural values, behaviors, and attitudes during all stages of the nursing process. This consideration involves two kinds of awareness of self and cultural needs of others.

Assessment

The nurse must be aware of his or her own ethnocultural heritage, both as a person and as a nurse. In addition, the nurse must be aware of and sensitive to the health beliefs and practices of a client's heritage. This sensitivity and awareness can be developed through careful assessment of a client's heritage and cultural beliefs. The box above describes the factors that must be explored during a multicultural nursing assessment.

Data gathered relating to providing care for a particular client are divided into the following sections: cultural, sociological, psychological, and biological/physiological. Not all areas apply to all ethnic groups or to all individuals within a group; the nurse addresses the applicability of each factor for each client. This information can be gathered with standard nursing history data during the interview.

Cultural data to be gathered include ethnic origin, race, place of birth, relocations, habits and customs, valued behaviors, cultural sanctions and restrictions, language and communication processes, healing belief practices, nutritional variables, and food practices. Sociological data include economic status, educational status, social networks, family support networks, community support systems, and the influence of institutional racism. Psychological data include self-concept and identity factors, cognitive and behavioral processes, religious influences, and psychological-cultural responses to stress and illness. Biological and physiological data include racial and physical findings, growth and development patterns, variations in body systems, diseases more prevalent in an ethnic group, and diseases to which an ethnic group might be more resistant.

Nursing Diagnosis

Nursing diagnoses for an ethnic client are the same as those for any client; however, there are diagnoses specifically related to cultural differences. A diagnosis might involve problem areas during the client's interaction with the health care delivery system or the principal complaint for which the client is seeking health care (see box on p. 415). When determining nursing diagnoses for a client, the nurse should be as specific as possible when identifying cultural variables so individualized interventions can be planned.

> **NURSING DIAGNOSES FOR CULTURALLY RELATED HEALTH PROBLEMS**
>
> **SOCIOCULTURAL DISSONANCE WITHIN FAMILY**
>
> *Impaired communication*
> *Ineffective family coping: compromised*
> *Altered health maintenance*
> *Impaired social interaction*
>
> **INSUFFICIENT FINANCIAL RESOURCES**
>
> *Noncompliance*
>
> **CULTURAL VALUES**
>
> *Spiritual distress*

The nurse also identifies clusters of defining characteristics that support the diagnostic label. For example, the nurse may diagnose *impaired verbal communication related to language differences.* The nurse verifies certain assessment data such as the client's inability to speak dominant language, frustration in not making needs known, and client speaks only in native language. The related factor must be accurate to ensure that the correct interventions are used.

Planning

When establishing the goals and expected outcomes of care and planning interventions, the nurse again considers cultural variables. The extended family should be involved in care, for example, if the family is the client's strongest support group. Cultural beliefs and practices can be incorporated into therapy to help the nurse to achieve realistic outcomes of care. This is especially important if interventions will eventually be directed toward changing the client's behavior. When cultural factors influence the planning of care, the client and key family members must become active participants in the plan. Although a plan of care must contain specific client-centered goals, the nurse must consider the following goals when cultural variables are involved:

Goal: Client maintains cultural health practices as appropriate.

Outcomes

Client can select foods consistent with cultural heritage

Client can practice cultural/religious rituals

Goal: Client expresses health care needs to family and care giver.

Outcomes

Client is able to communicate needs through interpreter and "sign board" for basic needs of food, hygiene, pain, and so on with nursing staff

Client's facial expression is free from frustration when making needs known

Goal: Client and family understand the implications that health care beliefs have on health status.

Outcomes

Client/family is able to modify cultural and health practices to achieve an optimal level of health

As with all other needs, the client's cultural needs must be included when establishing the goal and expected outcomes of care. For example, the newly diagnosed diabetic client may need to know that his diet modification can be coordinated with cultural food preferences. To creatively blend a client's cultural food preferences with a 1500-calorie diet may take creative multidisciplinary planning, coordination, and collaboration among nursing, nutritionists, physicians, community support groups, and the client/family.

Implementation

Client education and effective communication are important interventions when a client's ethnic or cultural heritage is a factor in the plan of care. An explanation of all aspects of care ensures a client's understanding of the therapeutic plan. If a client's language skills inhibit communication, the nurse may use interpreters, word signs, or charts. Nurses may have to alter usual ways of interacting with clients to avoid offending or alienating a client and family members with different attitudes toward social interaction and etiquette. For example, a client who is modest and self-conscious about the body will need psychological preparation before some procedures and tests.

The client and family should be involved in all aspects of the care. This should occur in every case, even if nursing care cannot be modified because of the client's condition. Discussing with the client and family any cultural questions related to care ensures individualization of interventions because the client will understand the way cultural variables relate to health beliefs and practices.

Communication and open-mindedness are keys to successful interventions with clients. In almost all cases the nurse will be able to adapt nursing interventions to avoid cultural conflicts after the client understands that the nurse maintains respect for ethnicity and individuality.

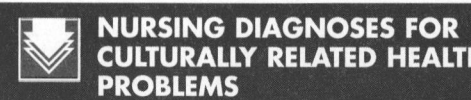

Evaluation

The nurse evaluates the results of nursing care, determining the extent to which the goals of care have been met. Evaluation continues throughout the nursing process and should include clear feedback from the client and family. Clear, concise communication is critical to evaluate the progress of the client's care fairly. The nurse's self-evaluation is also crucial as he or she increases skills for interacting with clients. The nurse should consider the following questions:

1. Am I open to understanding ways in which the client's values differ from mine?
2. Have I given sufficient attention to communicating with the client with limited language skills?
3. Have I successfully involved the client's family in the nursing process?
4. Am I incorporating the client's traditional beliefs and practices into nursing therapies?
5. Is my therapeutic relationship with the client respectful, regardless of cultural differences?

Nurses should evaluate their attitudes toward multicultural nursing care. Some nurses may believe that they should treat all clients the same and simply act naturally, but this attitude fails to acknowledge that cultural differences exist and that there is no "natural" human behavior. The nurse cannot act the same with all clients and still hope to deliver effective, individualized, holistic care. Sometimes inexperienced nurses are so self-conscious about cultural differences and so afraid of making a mistake that they impede the nursing process by not asking questions about areas of difference or by asking so many questions that they seem to pry into the client's personal life.

Self-evaluation can help the nurse to become more comfortable when providing care to clients. To determine whether goals that incorporate cultural needs are met, the nurse uses specific evaluative measures.

Examples of goals, outcomes, and corresponding evaluative measures include:

Goal: Client maintains cultural health practices as appropriate.

Outcome

Client is able to select foods consistent with cultural heritage

Evaluative measure

Ask client if he or she is able to get appropriate dietary requests

Outcome

Client is able to practice cultural/religious rituals

Evaluative measures

Ask the client to describe how he or she will follow prescribed therapies (e.g., diet and medications)

Review the client's preferences for follow-up health care

Goal: Client expresses health care needs to family and care giver.

Outcome

Client is able to communicate needs through interpreter and "sign board' for basic needs of food, hygiene, pain, and so on with nursing staff

Evaluative measures

Ask for client feedback while using the client's language

Ask family members to determine whether the client understands all communication between care givers

Outcome

Client's facial expression is free from frustration when making needs known

Evaluative measure

Observe the client's ability to follow instructions after giving explanations of care

Goal: A client understands the implications that health care beliefs have on health status.

Outcome

Client/family able to modify cultural and health practices to achieve an optimal level of health

Evaluative measures

Have the client explain how he or she plans to adjust to restrictions posed by health problems

Ask the client how health care beliefs will influence self-care at home

SUMMARY

The need for nurses to be sensitive toward culturally different clients is growing. Nurses are challenged to learn about different cultures because they practice in a multicultural society. Multicultural nursing care is the effective integration of the client's ethnocultural background into nursing care, which is based on the nursing process. Awareness of ways in which clients with varying cultural backgrounds differ is important if the nurse is to provide safe and effective individualized nursing care to all clients.

KEY CONCEPTS

Cultural background and heritage consistency affect health in all dimensions; therefore the nurse should consider the client's background when planning care.

Many ethnic groups in North America retain the traditional heritage of their original culture.

The way in which traditional beliefs influence behaviors, attitudes, and values depends on many factors and thus is not the same for different members of a cultural group.

Stereotyping ethnic group members can lead to mistaken assumptions about a client and family.

Cultural groups vary widely in health and illness beliefs and practices; areas of verbal and nonverbal communication; time orientation; use of personal space and territoriality; susceptibility to disease; emotional and mental health; emotional expression and pain reactions; gender role behaviors; and attitudes toward the family.

Before assessing the heritage and cultural background of a client, the nurse should assess personal influences of his or her own culture.

The nursing diagnosis for a traditional client should include problems involving the effects of cultural conflict.

The planning and implementation of nursing interventions should be adapted as much as possible to the client's cultural background.

CRITICAL THINKING ACTIVITIES

1. Discuss the problems that ethnic stereotyping and ethnocentrism may cause for the nurse. Suggest some ways nurses can learn to recognize such tendencies in themselves.
2. Discuss modifications in the health care system that can discourage members of ethnic and cultural groups to access and continue with health care programs.
3. Discuss the different illnesses and their susceptibility to different ethnic and cultural groups.

References

Abramson HJ: Religion. In Thermstrom S, editor: The *Harvard encyclopedia of American ethnic groups,* Cambridge, Mass., 1980, Harvard University Press.

Bohannon P: *We, the alien,* Prospects Heights Ill., 1992, Waveland Press.

Estes G and Zitzow D: Heritage consistency as a consideration in counseling Native Americans. Paper presented at the convention of the National Indian Education Association, Dallas, 1980.

Fejos P: Man, magic, and medicine. In Goldstone I, editor: *Medicine and anthropology,* New York, 1959, International Universities Press.

Geiger JN and Davidhizar RE: *Transcultural nursing intervention,* St. Louis, 1991, Mosby.

Hall ET: Proxemics: the study of man's spatial relations. In Goldstein I, editor: *Man's image in medicine and anthropology,* New York, 1963, International Universities Press.

Hodgkinson H: The changing demographics of minority populations and their effects on American higher education: trends, projections, and larger implications. Address delivered at the conference on Developing Multi-Cultural Leadership for the Twenty-First Century, Boston, Mass., June 15, 1988, Boston College.

McLemore SD: *Racial and ethnic relations in America,* Newton, Mass., 1980, Allyn & Bacon.

Spector RE: Culture, ethnicity, and nursing. In Potter PA and Perry AG: *Fundamentals of nursing,* ed 3, St. Louis, 1993, Mosby.

Spector RE: *Cultural diversity in health and illness,* ed 3, Norwalk, Conn., 1991, Appleton-Lange.

Thernstrom S, editor: *The Harvard encyclopedia of American ethnic groups,* Cambridge, Mass., 1980, Harvard University Press.

U.S. Bureau of the Census, Current Population Reports, 1990 Census of Population and Housing, Summary Population and Housing Characteristics, United States, Washington, DC, 1991, U.S. Government Printing Office.

Bibliography

Airhihenbuwa CO: Health education for African Americans: a neglected task, *Health Educ* 20:9-14, 1989.

Barringer F: Census shows profound change in racial makeup of nation, *The New York Times* March 11, p. 1, 1991.

Bartlett EE: Learning from special populations, *Patient Educ Counsel* 13(2):87-89, 1989.

Bernal H and Forman R: The confidence of community health nurses in caring for ethnically diverse populations, *Image* 19(4):201, 1987.

Bushy A: Cultural considerations for primary health care, *Holistic Nurs Prac* 6(3):10-18, 1992.

DeSantis L and Thomas J: The immigrant Haitian mother: transcultural nursing perspective on preventive health care for children, *J Transcult Nurs* 2:2-10, 1990.

DeSantis L and Thomas JT: Health education and the immigrant Haitian mother: cultural insights for community health nurses, *Public Health Nurse* 9(2):87-96, 1992.

Dinnerstein L and Reimers DM: *Ethnic americans,* ed 3, New York, 1988, Harper & Row.

Douglass T: A real case for non-verbal communication in nursing practice, *Washington Nurse* 19(10):12-14, 1989.

Fleming J: Meeting the challenge of culturally diverse populations, *Ped Nurs* 15(6):566, 634, 648, 1989.

Frye BA: The Cambodian refugee patient: providing culturally sensitive rehabilitation nursing care, *Rehab Nurs* 15(3):156-158, 1990.

Gibbs JT, et al.: *Children of color,* San Francisco, 1989, Jossey-Bass.

Gorrie M: Reaching clients through cross cultural education, *J Gerontol Nurs* 15(10):29, 1989.

Herndon TR: Cultural factors play a role in pediatric assessment, *Florida Nurse* 38:11, 1990.

Hirsch ED: *Cultural literacy: what every American needs to know,* Boston, 1987, Houghton Mifflin.

Hobus R: Living in two worlds: A Lakota transcultural nursing experience, *J Transcult Nurs* 2(Summer):33-36, 1990.

Hodgkinson HL: *A demographic look at tomorrow,* Washington, DC, 1992, Institute for Demographic Policy.

Holtz C and Bairan A: Personal contact: a method of teaching cultural empathy, *Nurse Educ* 15(3):13, 24, 28, 1990.

Horn B: Cultural concepts and postpartal care, *J Transcult Nurs* 2(Summer):48-51, 1990.

Huttlinger K and Wiebe P: Transcultural nursing care: achieving understanding in a practice setting, *J Transcult Nurs* 1(Winter):17-21, 1989.

Kavanagh K and Kennedy PH: *Promoting cultural diversity: strategies for the health care professionals,* New York, 1992, Sage.

Lawson LV: Culturally sensitive support for grieving parents, *Am J Maternal Child Nurs* 15(2):76-79, 1990.

Leininger M: The significance of cultural concepts in nursing, *J Transcult Nurs* 2(Summer):52-59, 1990.

Leininger M: The transcultural nurse specialist: imperative in today's world, *Nurs Health Care* 10(5):250-256, 1989.

Luna L: Transcultural nursing care of Arab Muslims, *J Transcult Nurs* 1(Winter):22-26, 1989.

McNall MCC: Healing we cannot explain, *Am J Nurs* 89(9):1162, 1989.

Muecke MA: Nursing research with refugees: a review and guide, *Western J Nurs Res* 14(6):703-720, 1992.

Parfitt BA: Cultural assessment in the intensive care unit, *Intensive Care Nurs* 4(3):124, 1988.

Ray M: Transcultural caring: political and economic visions, *J Transcult Nurs* 1(Summer):17-21, 1990.

Reizian A and Meleis AI: Arab-Americans' perceptions of and responses to pain, *Crit Care Nurse* 6(6):30, 1986.

Rosenbaum JN: Depression: viewed from a transcultural nursing theoretical perspective, *J Adv Nurs* 14(1):7-12, 1989.

Russell K and Jewell N: Cultural impact of health-care access: challenges for improving the health of African-Americans, *J Community Health Nurs* 9(3):161-169, 1992.

Shadick KM: Development of a transcultural health education program, *Clin Nurs Special* 7(2):48-53, 1993.

Spector RE: Heritage consistency: a predictor of health beliefs and practices, *Rec Adv Nurs* 23:23, 1989.

Tripp-Reimer T: Cross-cultural perspectives on patient teaching, *Nurs Clin North Am* 24(3):613-619, 1989.

Wenger AF: Transcultural nursing and health care issues in urban and rural contexts, *J Transcult Nurs* 4(2)(Winter):4-10, 1992.

Wilson DA: My trips over the language barrier, *Am J Nurs* 89:1718, 1989.

19

Family Context in Nursing

OBJECTIVES

Mastery of content in this chapter will enable the student to:

- Define the key terms listed.
- Discuss the way family members influence one another's health.
- Describe current trends in the American family.
- Define the family in terms applicable to all family forms.
- Describe common family forms and their health implications.
- Explain the way family structure and pattern of functioning affect the health of family members and the family as a whole.
- Compare family as context to family as client, and explain the way these perspectives influence nursing practice.
- Describe the family nursing process in terms of assessment, nursing diagnosis, planning, intervention, and evaluation.
- Describe both external and internal factors that promote family health.

KEY TERMS

family
family as client
family as context
family functioning
family health
family structure

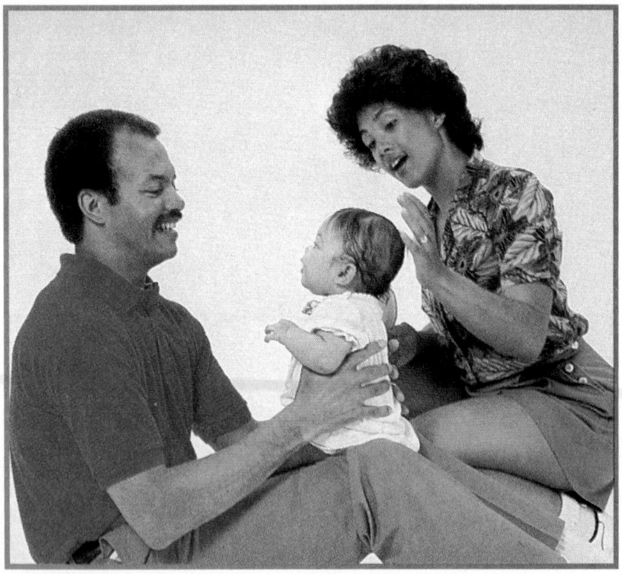

"Others may change us, but we all start and end with the family," Anthony Brandt. A few decades ago some family scholars predicted that the family was in a state of decline with lessening influence on its individual members. These scholars anticipated that rapid social change and an increasingly mobile population would cause psychological and physical distancing of family members. However, optimistic social scientists felt that family members would remain committed to each other and close family ties would continue. Major changes have occurred in the family since these predictions were made, but it is clear that the family remains the central institution in American society. The current general assumption is that although the family is in transition and may look very different from the family of the 1950s, it is here to stay. Although contemporary families have their share of problems and challenges, they are characterized by three important attributes (i.e., durability, resiliency, and diversity) (Fine, 1992).

The influence of the family is important in American society, and this must always be considered in interactions with clients. The family shapes early health beliefs and values, and family members affect one another's health practices and status. The nurse views the client as an individual and as a person who is an integral part of a family. All members need to be incorporated into the nursing process when possible because the family environment significantly influences health outcomes.

CONCEPT OF FAMILY

A popular notion exists about what the family is or at least what it should be. This "ideal" model suggests that the family is a nuclear unit, consists of a mother, father, and at least one child, and exhibits a traditional sexual division of labor (i.e., the father is the bread-winner and the mother stays home, cooks, cleans, and is responsible for rearing the children). "Family" evokes a visual image of adults and children living together in a satisfying, harmonious fashion (Zinn, Eitzen, 1993). Families are, however, as diverse as the individuals that compose them, and clients have deeply ingrained values about their families that deserve respect. Thus, the nurse must think of family as defined by each individual. In other words, the nurse can think of the family as a set of relationships that the *client* identifies as family or as a network of individuals who influence each other's lives.

FAMILY FORMS

Family forms are patterns of people considered by family members to be included in the family. Although all families have some things in common, each family form has unique problems and strengths. The nurse needs to have an open mind about what constitutes a family so that potential resources and concerns are not overlooked. Several family forms are displayed in the box on p. 421.

Current Trends and New Family Forms

Although the institution of the family remains strong, the "typical" family has become a rarity. Married couples with at least one child make up only 26% of contemporary families (U.S. Bureau of the Census, 1991). The diversity in life-style and living arrangements is an outgrowth of economic and social trends. The increase in alternatives is associated with new patterns of divorce and remarriage and new expectations about individual fulfillment (Zinn, Eitzen, 1993).

Families are smaller today. People are marrying later, women are delaying childbirth, and couples are choosing to have fewer children or none at all. Divorce rates have tripled since the 1950s and, although the rate appears to have stabilized, it is estimated that two out of every three new marriages will end in divorce or separation (Price, 1990). Although divorce occurs often, marriage is valued. Ninety percent of young Americans are likely to marry, and about three fourths of those who divorce remarry. In fact, remarriage has become as common as first marriages (Bumpass, Sweet, Martin, 1990), which often results in a complex set of relationships between step-parents and step-children and half-brothers and half-sisters.

FAMILY FORMS

NUCLEAR FAMILY

This family consists of husband and wife and perhaps one or more children.

The presence of children affects family's time and economic resources.

The absence of children may lead husband and wife to seek counseling and health care.

EXTENDED FAMILY

This family includes relatives (aunts, uncles, grandparents, and cousins) in addition to nuclear family.

The closer the extended family, the more influence it has on health care.

This family can provide a diverse support base for members needing health care.

SINGLE-PARENT FAMILY

Formed when one parent leaves the nuclear family because of death, divorce, or desertion, or when a single person decides to have or adopt a child.

Circumstances of separation influence its impact on the family; it is most commonly the result of divorce today.

Reduced financial and emotional resources affect the health of single-parent families.

BLENDED FAMILY

This family is formed when parents bring unrelated children from prior relationships into a new joint living situation.

The nature of prior living situations and rate of adapting to the change affect health.

Stress of newly formed family patterns can affect the mental health of family members.

ALTERNATE PATTERNS OF RELATIONSHIPS

Multi-adult households

"Skip-generation" families (grandparents caring for grandchildren)

Communal groups with children

"Non-families" (adults living alone)

Cohabitating partners

Homosexual couples

Health concerns focus on the specific needs integral to each form but may include the stability of the relationships, child-rearing practices, and availability of community resources.

The majority (approximately 56%) of women work outside the home, and about 57% of this work force have at least one child under the age of 6 (Eshleman, 1991). Although there appear to be few direct effects on the mother-child relationship (see for example, Barling, 1990), the need for consistent substitute child care is growing. The number of people living alone is expanding rapidly and represents approximately 25% of all households (U.S. Bureau of Census, 1991). Although some people choose a single life-style, being single is not always a matter of choice. Demography and culture have created a "marriage squeeze" or shortage of men in the prime marrying ages (Zinn, Eitzen, 1993).

Many individuals structure their lives differently from their parents. Glick (1990) estimates that between 1970 and 1988 the number of cohabitating couples increased from 500,000 to 2.5 million. Some who choose to cohabit view it as an alternative to marriage, whereas others view it as a pretrial marriage. This "pretrial," however, does not guarantee a successful marriage. The number of single-parent families has increased dramatically since the 1970s, as has the number of babies born to unwed mothers. Although 90% of single-parent families are headed by mothers, father-only families are on the rise (Meyer, Garaskey, 1993). "Children having children" (adolescent pregnancy) is an ever-increasing concern. The Children's Defense Fund (1990) notes that every 67 seconds a U.S. teenager gives birth. The majority of these adolescents (between 65% to 85%) continue to live with their families. A teen pregnancy tends to have long-term consequences for the mother and often severely stresses family relationships and resources (Hanson, et al., 1992).

Although unable to marry by law, many homosexual couples define their relationship in family terms. Approximately half of all gay male couples live together, compared to three fourths of lesbian couples. They have become more open about their sexual preference and more vocal about their legal rights.

The fastest growing age-group is 65 and older. For the first time in history, the average American has more living parents than children, and children are more likely to have living grandparents and even great-grandparents. This "graying" of America has affected the family life-cycle, perhaps most significantly for middle-age adults. This generation is finding that they must balance the needs of their offspring and the needs of their aging parents, sometimes at the expense of their own well-being and resources. Caring for a frail or chronically ill relative is a primary concern for a growing number of families.

In addition to family challenges related to divorce, changing structures and roles, and the aging of its older members, there are three additional trends that social scientists (Schvaneveldt and Young, 1992) identify as threats or concerns facing the family: (1) changing economic status, (2) family violence, and (3) acquired immunodeficiency syndrome (AIDS).

Making ends meet is a daily concern for many people because of the declining economic status of families. Even though two-income families have become the norm, real family income has not increased since 1973 (Levy, Michel, 1991). Families at the lower end of the income scale have been particularly affected, and single-parent families are especially vulnerable. Basic necessities such as food and shelter are not taken for granted for an increasing number of our country's youth. In fact, families with children are the fastest growing group within our nation's homeless population (Schvaneveldt, Young, 1991; Wisendale, 1991).

The statistics regarding family violence are even more disturbing. The inflicting of emotional and physical pain on family members occurs in more than half of all households in the United States; approximately 50 million people are victimized a year (Henslin, 1990). Emotional, physical, and sexual abuse occurs toward spouses, children, the elderly, and across all social classes. Two decades of research have demonstrated that the cause of family violence is complex and multidimensional. Factors associated with violence include stress, poverty, social isolation, psychopathology, and the cycle of violence—the intergenerational transmission of violence (Gelles, Maynard, 1987).

The statistics regarding AIDS are becoming more alarming every day. It is estimated that between 1 and 1.5 million people in the United States are currently infected with the human immunodeficiency virus (HIV) (Jurich, Adams, Schlenberg, 1992). Finding that one is HIV-positive is not only devastating for the individual, but for the family as well. As with all terminal illnesses, caring for a family member with AIDS is emotionally and financially devastating. Unfortunately, an AIDS diagnosis often carries the additional burdens of guilt, social stigma, and isolation that affects all family members (Macklin, 1988).

STRUCTURE AND FUNCTION

Families have a structure and a way of functioning. Structure and function are closely related and continually interact with one another. **Family structure** is based on organization (i.e., the ongoing membership of the family and the pattern of relationships). Relationships can be numerous and complex. For example, a woman's relationships may include wife-husband, mother-son, and mother-daughter, each with different demands, roles, and expectations.

Although the definitions of structure vary, the nurse asks the following questions: "Who is included in the family?" "Who performs which tasks?" and "Who makes which decisions?" Structure may enhance or detract from the family's ability to respond to the expected and unexpected stressors that are realities of daily life. Very rigid or very flexible structures can be detrimental to the functioning of the family. A rigid structure specifically dictates persons permitted to accomplish a task and may also limit the number of persons outside the immediate family allowed to assume these tasks. For example, the mother might be considered the only acceptable person to provide emotional support for the children or the husband the only one to provide financial support. A change in the health status of the person responsible for a task places a burden on the family because no other person is available or considered acceptable to assume that task. An extremely open structure can also present problems for the family. An underlying stability that otherwise leads to automatic action during a crisis or rapid change is often absent.

Friedman (1986) describes functioning as what the family does. **Family functioning** involves the processes used by the family to achieve its goals. These processes include communication among family members, goal setting, conflict resolution, nurturing, and use of internal and external resources. The reproductive, sexual, economic, and educational goals once considered central family goals no longer apply to all families. Although many families pursue these goals at various times during their development, the provision of psychological support remains an important goal throughout the life span.

Goals are more easily achieved when communication is clear and direct. Clear communication enhances problem solving and resolution of conflict. Another family process facilitating goal achievement is the ability to nurture and promote growth. Families need to have available internal and external resources and must be able to use them. A social network is useful as an external support system. Social relationships act as buffers, particularly during times of stress, and reduce a family's vulnerability.

DEVELOPMENTAL STAGES

Families, like individuals, change and grow over time. Although families are far from identical to one another, they have a basic pattern and similarity in experiences resulting in predictable stages. Each of these developmental stages has its own challenges, needs, and resources and includes tasks that need to be completed before the family can successfully move on to the next stage. McGoldrick and Carter (1985) have developed a model of family life stages based on expansion, contraction, and realignment of family relationships that support the entry, exit, and development of members. This

table 19-1

STAGES OF THE FAMILY LIFE CYCLE

Family life cycle stage	Emotional process of transition: key principles	Changes in family status required to proceed developmentally
Between families: unattached young adult	Accepting parent-offspring separation	Differentiation of self in relation to family of origin Development of intimate peer relationships Establishment of self in work
Joining of families through marriage: newly married couple	Commitment to new system	Formation of marital system Realignment of relationships with extended families and friends to include spouse
Family with young children	Accepting new generation of members into system	Adjusting marital system to make space for children Taking on parenting roles Realignment of relationships with extended family to include parenting and grandparenting roles
Family with adolescents	Increasing flexibility of family boundaries to include children's independence	Shifting of parent-child relationships to permit adolescents to move in and out of system Refocus on midlife marital and career issues Beginning shift toward concerns for older generation
Launching children and moving on	Accepting multitude of exits from and entries into family system	Renegotiation of marital system as dyad Development of adult-to-adult relationships between grown children and their parents Realignment of relationships to include in-laws and grandchildren Dealing with disabilities and death of parents (grandparents)
Family in later life	Accepting shifting of generational roles	Maintaining own or couple functioning and interests in face of physiological decline; exploration of new familial and social role options Support for more central role for middle generation Making room in system for wisdom and experience of older adults; supporting older generation without overfunctioning for them Dealing with loss of spouse, siblings, and other peers, and preparation for own death; life review and integration

From McGoldrick M and Carter E: The stages of the family life cycle. In Henslin J, editor: *Marriage and family in a changing society,* New York, 1985, The Free Press; In Walsh F: *Normal family processes,* New York, 1982, The Guilford Press.

model provides the nurse with the emotional aspects of transition, as well as the changes and tasks necessary for the family to proceed developmentally (Table 19-1). Consequently, the nurse can promote behaviors consistent with achievement of the essential tasks and help families to prepare for later transitions. This model does not take into account diverse family forms. However, other researchers suggest alternative models. For example, Aldous, as reported in McCubbin and Dahl (1990), has devised a six-stage system for single-mother families resulting from divorce. The initial stage is the establishment of the single-parent family, and the final stage is retirement of women from their work-life or from the responsibilities of parenthood.

FAMILY AND HEALTH

Family health influences family functioning, and family functioning, in turn, influences its own and society's perceptions of its health. When the family satisfactorily meets its goals through adequate functioning, its members tend to feel positive about themselves and their family. Conversely, when they do not meet goals, families view themselves as ineffective. Constant stress resulting from inadequate functioning can also adversely affect an individual family member's health. Constant stress may disrupt cardiovascular function, blood pressure, and circulating neuroendocrine substances, and these disruptions are suspected precursors of poor health (see Chapter 4). Maladaptive behaviors within the family have a negative impact on the health of members and the overall ability of the family to meet its goals. A lack of communication or poor communication inhibits the family's ability to make decisions and solve problems. Good health may not be highly valued, and, in fact, detrimental practices may be accepted. In some cases, a family member may provide mixed messages about health. For example, a parent may continue to smoke while telling children that smoking is bad for them. Family environment is crucial because health behavior reinforced in early life has a strong influence on later health practices.

Rueben Hill (1958) noted more than 30 years ago that it is possible to explain the reactions of crisis-proof and crisis-prone families by the factors of integration and adaptability. The crisis-proof or effective family is able to integrate the need for stability with the need for growth and change and has a flexible structure allowing adaptable performance of tasks and acceptance of help from outside the family unit. Recently, health promotion research has started to focus on the stress-moderating effect of "hardiness" as a factor that contributes to long-term health (Bigbee, 1992). Danielson, Hamell-Bissell, et al. (1993) define family hardiness as "the internal strengths and durability of the family unit; characterized by a sense of control over the outcome of life events and hardships, a view of change as beneficial and growth-producing, and as an active rather than passive orientation in responding to stressful life events."

The health of the family is influenced by its relative position in society. Although American families exist within the same culture, they live in very different ways. The structure, function, and health of any family is a reflection and a result of its social class, economic resources, and racial and ethnic background. For some minority groups and the poor, patterned differences in family living are consequences of inequalities deeply rooted in society. Class and ethnicity can produce differences in the access of families to society's resources and rewards, and this access creates differences in family life and most significantly in different life changes for its members (Zinn and Eitzen, 1990). Economic stability increases a family's access to adequate health care, creates more opportunity for education, sound nutrition, rest, and decreases in stress. The higher infant mortality rates and shortened life span of the poor and some minority groups demonstrate how inequality affects health status (see Chapter 18).

FAMILY NURSING: FAMILY AS ENVIRONMENT AND AS CLIENT

The goal of the family nurse is to help the family and its individual members reach and maintain maximum health in any given situation. Hanson, Helms, et al. (1992) contends that the health care focus is starting to shift from the individual to the family and that family nurses are at the forefront of this movement. Currently, however, the American health care system can make it difficult to provide effective nursing care to the family as a whole since the emphasis has generally been on the individual. The nurse must always be aware that clients are affected by their families whether their members are present or not and that clients, in turn, affect their families. A family nursing focus includes both family as context and family as client (Figure 19-1). Although theoretical and practical distinctions can be made between the two approaches, they are not necessarily mutually exclusive. Both approaches recognize that a nursing intervention for one member influences all members and affects family functioning.

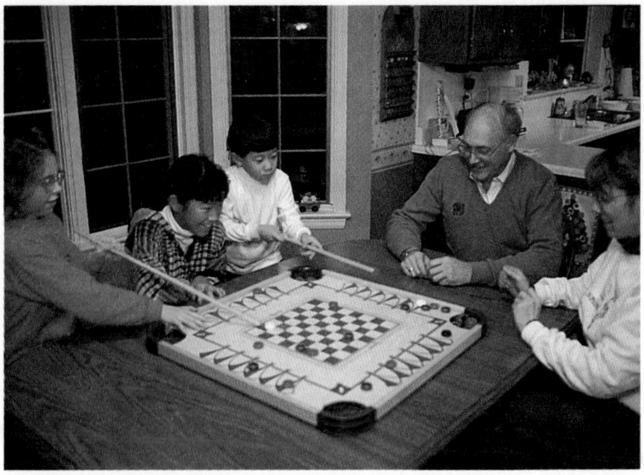

FIGURE 19-1 Observing family interactions assists in understanding family functioning.

Family as Context

With this approach the primary focus is the health and development of an individual member existing within a specific environment (i.e., the family). Although assessment, nursing diagnosis, planning, implementation, and evaluation concentrate on the individual's health status, the nurse assesses the extent to which the family provides for the individual's basic needs. Families provide more than just material essentials, so their ability to help the client reach psychological needs and strive for optimal health must also be considered.

Family as Client

With this approach the family is the primary focus of nursing care. Family patterns and processes are studied. The nursing process concentrates on the extent to which these patterns and processes are consistent with reaching and maintaining family and individual health. To better understand the distinction between the two approaches, consider the following situation.

A single, 25-year-old man lives at home with his parents and two younger siblings. He requests the assistance of the nurse in altering his diet and developing stress management techniques to help him to cope with his borderline hypertension, which is thought to be related to high sodium intake, a stressful job, and continuing expectations by his family for participation in their activities. If the family is viewed as context, the nurse focuses on the client as an individual. The nurse might assess the client's knowledge of high-sodium foods, strategies for reducing the number of high-sodium foods in the diet, realistic opportunities to reduce the number and extent of perceived stressors in work and family environments, and knowledge and skill in stress management such as relaxation or biofeedback techniques. If the family is viewed as client, the nurse would assess the family's current dietary patterns and its desire and resources for changing the patterns. The nurse also determines the demands placed on the hypertensive family member and explores the potential for redistribution of the demands among other family members. The family's capabilities to support the hypertensive member's development and use of stress management are also assessed.

NURSING PROCESS FOR THE FAMILY

Family nursing process is the same, whether the focus is family as client or family as context. It is also the same as that used with individuals.

Assessment

Family assessment is an essential component of the nursing process (see box on p. 426). Although the family as a whole differs from individual members, the measure of family health must be more than a summation of the health of all members. Areas included in family assessment are the form, structure, and function of the family, its developmental stage, and its progress toward or accomplishment of developmental tasks. Cultural background is an important variable when assessing the family because race and ethnicity have an impact on structure and function and influence health beliefs and values. The nurse begins assessment by considering family members and the client's attitude toward family. The nurse also incorporates family needs into the nursing process. To determine the family form and membership, the nurse can ask the client, "Whom do you consider your family?" or ask with whom the client shares strong emotional feelings. If the client is unable to express a concept of family, the nurse can ask with whom the client lives, spends time, and shares confidences and then ask the client to validate this observation: "Do you consider this person to be family or like family to you?" To further assess the family structure, the nurse asks questions that determine the power structure and patterning of roles and tasks. For example, "How are the tasks divided in your family?" "Who does the laundry?" "Who mows the lawn?" "Who decides on where to go on vacation?" Because a moderately flexible structure is generally most beneficial to the family, nursing interventions therefore may involve modulating the family patterns away from extremely rigid or flexible structures if either extreme causes problems related to the health of an individual or the family as a whole. In general, however, the nurse attempts to work within the family structure when providing care and does not attempt to change the structure.

The nurse assesses family functions such as the ability to provide emotional support for members, the ability to cope with its current health problem or situation, the appropriateness of its goal setting, and progress toward achievement of tasks of the developmental stage. Although families' goals vary, measures of family health care must be flexible. The nurse also assesses whether the family can provide and allocate sufficient economic resources and if its social network is extensive enough to provide support.

To illustrate the nursing process using a family approach, consider the following clinical scenario.

Mr. and Mrs. Smith are in their mid 70s, have recently celebrated their 50th wedding anniversary, and have been living in Florida since Mr. Smith retired 10 years ago. They have two married sons living in Minnesota and Michigan. Mr. and Mrs. Smith's marriage has been a very traditional one, with Mrs. Smith performing all the household tasks and willingly catering to all of Mr. Smith's needs. They have a wide circle of friends and have been active in various church groups. Both have been comparatively healthy until 3 weeks ago when Mrs. Smith suffered a stroke that has left her with a fair amount of left-sided weakness. Mrs. Smith has rehabilitation therapy daily, demonstrates a great deal of determination, and is making good progress. Her therapist expects her to be discharged in about a month to the care of her husband. Although Mr. Smith is anxious to take her home, his behavior suggests that he has unrealistic expectations of her current and future abilities. For example, he becomes impatient with her slowness at performing activities such as feeding herself and has stated that he expects her to "be her old self" as soon as he gets her home. Mrs. Smith has stated that their rela-

ASSESSMENT TOOL

The family assessment tool is used when the beginning student interviews family members and observes family interaction. It is a guideline only and is not meant to be all inclusive. The student must also ensure that individual health histories accompany this assessment.

FAMILY FORM AND STRUCTURE

Names of adults Ages

___

Relationship ___
(Single, married, divorced, separated, cohabiting)

Names of children Ages

___

___

___

Others living in home (include age, sex, relationship)

___

Cultural background (include pertinent health beliefs, child-rearing practices, related health concerns)

___

Developmental stage ___

Progress toward accomplishment of developmental tasks ___

Concerns related to developmental stage ___

RESOURCES

Significant relatives and friends not occupying immediate residence ___

Strengths and coping skills ___

How does the family obtain health services? ___

Membership in community groups (e.g., church affiliation) ___

Education (formal and informal) ___

Finances (ability to meet current and future needs) ___

FAMILY PATTERNS

Persons working outside the home ___

Type of work ___ Number of hours ___

Satisfaction with work ___

How are the housekeeping tasks accomplished? ___

Are family members satisfied with the way tasks are divided? ___

How are child-rearing responsibilities divided? ___

Who makes the major decisions in the family? ___

Who makes day-to-day decisions? ___

Are family members satisfied with the way decisions are made? ___

FAMILY FUNCTION

Goals

Long term ___

Short term ___

Individual family member's goals ___

Are individual and family goals appropriate, considering their current health problem and status? ___

How are individual family members and the family as a whole coping with their current health problem and status?

___

Communication

Do husband and wife communicate regularly and effectively with each other? ___

Are family members able to communicate openly and honestly with each other? ___

Is conflict openly expressed and discussed? ___

Do family members respect one another's point of view? ___

Do family members offer emotional support to each other? ___

tionship is "strained" and that her husband often tells her that she is "just not trying hard enough to get well." This older couple exemplifies a very common case; the need for one member of the family to take on the role of care giver. The most common care givers for older adults are their spouses (Chappell, 1991). Every health care decision has profound implications for both of their lives (Phillips, 1989). This case also points out how an illness can disrupt the well-established patterns in a family and the necessity of both short-term and long-term planning.

NANDA APPROVED NURSING DIAGNOSES

- Altered family processes
- Altered parenting
- Altered role performance
- Family coping: potential for growth
- High risk for care giver role strain
- Ineffective family coping: compromised
- Ineffective family coping: disabled
- Parental role conflict

Nursing Diagnosis

Nursing assessment results in clustering pertinent data that support the nursing diagnosis and identifying cases in which functioning is inadequate or deficient and intervention is needed. The diagnostic label may include the family's health needs, current and potential health problems, level of wellness, or a combination of the above. In addition, the diagnostic statement should indicate possible causes and etiologies.

The nursing diagnosis often focuses on the family's ability to cope with its current situation, whether it is an acute illness, an anticipated developmental transition, or negative behaviors that are threatening short-term or long-term health (see box above). Appropriate use of internal and external resources can allow the family to cope with day-to-day challenges and with unexpected occurrences that threaten health and equilibrium. Coping strategies can be adaptive or maladaptive. During times of acute illness the family can become extremely distressed and focuses solely on the ill member, neglecting the needs of the other family members (McClowery, 1992). The needs of other family members can be easily overlooked unless the nurse consistently employs a family nursing perspective. The diagnosis of high risk for care giver role strain, for example, should always be considered a possibility when long-term care of a family member is necessary.

"Nursing diagnosis involves a data base regulated by the family and the nurse's identification and evaluation of potential stressors that pose a threat to the stability of the family unit" (Berkey, Hanson, 1993). Identifying the correct related factor or factors is essential to choosing the appropriate plan of action. In the aforementioned clinical situation, during the assessment phase the nurse concluded that Mr. Smith was not providing Mrs. Smith with adequate emotional and physical support, thus threatening Mrs. Smith's well-being, their relationship, and their overall family functioning. Without intervention it was unlikely that this family would be able to reach their optimal level of wellness. The nurse also concluded that inadequate support was related to Mr. Smith's lack of understanding of his wife's physical limitations. This allowed the nurse to plan interventions directed at the underlying cause.

Planning

After nursing diagnoses are developed, the next step is to plan a course of action with the family. Planning includes goal setting, identification of potential internal and external resources, choosing effective approaches, and setting priorities. It is imperative that the plan of care be clearly understood and agreed on by the family. Goal setting must be a mutual endeavor, and the goals must be concrete, realistic, compatible with the developmental stage, and acceptable to the family.

Collaboration with family members is an essential component during this stage (Figure 19-2). A positive collaborative relationship is based on mutual respect and trust (Danielson, Hamell-Bissell, et al., 1993) and is facilitated by allowing the family to feel as "in control" as possible. For example, offering alternative actions and asking family members for their own ideas and suggestions can reduce feelings of powerlessness. Collaboration also extends to other health care professionals. As Danielson, Hamell-Bissell, et al. (1993) point out, it is impossible to be all things to all families. Collaborating with other disciplines increases the likelihood of a comprehensive care plan and can provide for continuity of care. Using other disciplines is particularly important for discharge planning since referrals are often necessary to ensure that long-term goals will be attained.

Goals for a care plan that incorporate a family approach may include those that view the family as client or the family as context or a combination of the two. The client situation and availability of family members dictate the type of goals that are feasible. The following are examples of general family-oriented goals and outcomes.

Examples of **family as client** goals and expected outcomes includes:

Goal: The family functions at its optimal level.

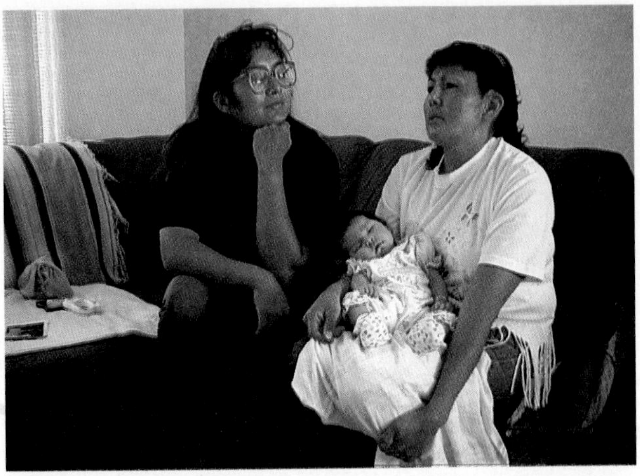

FIGURE 19-2 Family members assisting one another in caring for a newborn. (Courtesy Michael S. Clement, MD, Mesa, Ariz.).

Outcomes

Communication between family members is appropriate, direct, and clear

Family members are able to confront and resolve conflict in a healthy way

Goal: The family understands and copes with the health problems of its members.

Outcomes

Family members use external and internal resources as needed

The family is able to meet the needs of all its individual members

Examples of **family as context** goals and expected outcomes include:

Goal: The client functions at optimal level within the family context.

Outcomes:

The client uses external and internal resources as appropriate

Goal: The client accomplishes appropriate developmental tasks within the family context.

Outcome

The client communicates needs and goals appropriately to family members

In Mr. and Mrs. Smith's case, short-term planning must include actions that will help Mr. Smith better understand the effects of stroke and to recognize his wife's limitations. Long-term planning must focus on new adaptive patterns in order for this couple to reach their maximum individual health and family functioning. Mr. Smith will have to assume the majority of household tasks and essentially change roles with Mrs. Smith. This may very well be difficult for both of them, and comprehensive discharge planning is critical. Collaboration with a social worker and/or a family therapist could provide additional perspectives and suggestions. During the planning stage the nurse must keep in mind this couple's long marital history, their developmental stage, and the limitations and strengths inherent in both. The care plan box on p. 429 provides a sample nursing care plan for the short-term goal.

Implementation

After goals and actions have been defined, implementation begins. Interventions are strategies that help families adjust goals or are the processes by which the family attains them. Family interventions include nursing actions that increase members' abilities in a certain area, remove barriers to health care, and do things that the family cannot do for itself (Friedman, 1986). The nurse guides family members in problem solving and provides practical service and concrete aid. In the above example, one of the roles the nurse will need to adopt is that of educator. Providing accurate health information about diagnosis and prognosis helps the care giver not to "blame" the client and to interpret behavior correctly (Phillips, 1989). As a general framework, effective interventions for Mr. and Mrs. Smith will focus on the elder–care giver unit, plus the needs of the care giver and the elder. As Phillips (1989) states, "Caregivers are not born with the knowledge of how to be caregivers and elders are not born with the knowledge of how to accept dependency."

Health Promotion

Identifying attributes that contribute to healthy and resilient families has been a focus of ongoing research for at least three decades. "Strong" families that adapt to expected transitions and unexpected crises and change tend to be characterized by clear communication, problem-solving skills, a commitment to each other and to the family unit, and a sense of cohesiveness and spirituality. Prevention programs aimed at enhancing or developing these attributes are available for families and children in many communities. The nurse needs to be aware of family-oriented offerings so that clients can be referred as needed. Often, health promotion behaviors that the nurse needs to encourage are tied to the developmental stage of the family (for example, effective prenatal care for the child-bearing family and adherence to immunization schedules for the child-rearing family) see box on p. 429.

One approach for meeting goals and promoting health is the use of family strengths. Families are not accustomed to looking at their own system as one that has inherent positive components. The nurse can help the family become aware of its own unique strengths,

SAMPLE NURSING CARE PLAN
Ineffective Family Coping: Compromised

NURSING DIAGNOSIS (see discussion on p. 425)

Ineffective family coping: compromised related to husband's inadequate understanding of wife's physical limitations

DEFINITION:

Ineffective family coping: compromised is insufficient, ineffective, or compromised support, comfort, or assistance—usually by a supportive primary person (family member or close friend); client may need it to manage or master adaptive tasks related to his/her health challenge (Kim, et al., 1991).

PLANNING

Goals	Expected outcomes
Husband will gain improved understanding of wife's physical limitations (3/25).	Husband will be able to identify activities appropriate for his wife to perform and activities with which he will have to assist her (3/24).
Husband will accept wife's physical limitations (3/30).	Husband will not demonstrate impatient behavior (such as telling his wife to "hurry up") while she performs activities (3/27).

IMPLEMENTATION

Steps	Rationale
1. Discuss with husband effects of stroke and reasons it occurs, and provide reading material designed for family members of clients with strokes.	Accurate information will assist husband in interpreting wife's limitations (Phillips, 1989).
2. Provide list of care giver support groups.	Group support allows care giver to share experiences, stresses, and coping methods (Reissman, Gartner, 1987).

EVALUATION

Ask husband to describe activities wife will be able to perform and activities that will require assistance.

Observe husband interacting with wife during home visit.

CLIENT AND FAMILY TEACHING FOR HEALTH PROMOTION

Instruct client and family members about medication, treatment, and future appointments.

Provide specific strategies for modification in family's nutritional, exercise, and coping patterns.

Provide new parents with immunization schedules and community resources for obtaining necessary immunization.

GERONTOLOGIC NURSING PRACTICE

Members in later life families may have more difficulty with role reversal and/or taking on new tasks since roles were learned during a more traditional era.

Nurse must consider care giver strain; care givers are usually either spouses who are also an older adult who may have declining physical stamina, or middle-aged daughters who often have other responsibilities.

Later life families may have a different social network than younger families since friends and same-generation family members may have died or be ill themselves. May need to look for social support within the community and church affiliation.

As in the other stages of life, members of later life families need to be working on developmental tasks (see Chapter 20).

thereby increasing its potentials and capabilities. Family strengths include clear communication, adaptability, healthy child-rearing practices, support and nurturing among family members, active community participation, and the use of crisis for growth. The nurse can help the family focus on its strengths instead of its problems and weaknesses. For example, the nurse can point out to the Smiths that their 50-year marriage must have endured many life crises and transitions. Therefore they are likely to have the capabilities to adapt to this latest challenge (see box on p. 429).

Evaluation

When the client's family functions as context, evaluation focuses on attainment of client needs. Thus evaluation is client centered, although nursing measures may have involved assisting the client to adapt to the family environment. The response of the client is compared with predetermined outcomes.

When the family receives care as the client, the measure of family health must be more than a summation of the health of all family members. For example, the family's attainment of family developmental tasks may be a useful criterion. The nurse evaluates the family's change in functioning and its satisfaction with the new level of functioning.

Evaluation is an ongoing process. Goals and interventions are modified as needed. Examples of goals, outcomes, and corresponding evaluative measures include:

Goal: The family functions at optimal level.

Outcome

Communication between family members is appropriate, direct, and clear

Evaluative measure

Observe family members performing care-centered activities

Outcome

Family members are able to confront and resolve conflict in a healthy way

Evaluative measures

Ask the client to identify ways to include family members in care

Observe family's communication patterns

Goal: The family understands and copes with the client's health problem.

Outcome

Family members use external and internal resources as needed

Evaluative measure

Asking family members about the nature and implications of the client's illness

Outcome

The family is able to meet the needs of all of its individual members

Evaluative measure

Observe the family members' abilities to perform care measures correctly

Goal: Client returns to a functional state within the family context.

Outcome

The client uses external and internal resources as appropriate

Evaluative measures

Observing the client perform self-care activities at home

Observing the client discuss ways that care measures have been adapted to the home

Goal: Client accomplishes appropriate developmental tasks within the family.

Outcome

The client communicates needs and goals appropriately to family members

Evaluative measures

Observe client's interaction with family

Ask client how health care needs and practices are incorporated within family life-style.

SUMMARY

Although the structure and form of the American family are changing, the institution remains central in American society and strongly influences the client's health practices, beliefs, and values. The family's impact on health is as significant now as ever, and each family member can influence the health of other family members, as well as the health of the family as a unit. Because the concept of family varies, the nurse begins family assessment by determining the client's definition of and attitude toward family.

Different family forms often have many health concerns and resources for resolving those concerns. When the family faces health problems, the nurse assesses its structure and function to plan effective interventions. At times, family structure and functioning may require alteration before a specific health problem is managed.

The nurse can apply the nursing process, whether the family is viewed as a highly significant context within which the client seeks to maintain health or whether it is viewed as the client itself. If the family is viewed as the client's environment, the nursing focus is on the individual member's health. If the family as a whole is viewed as the client, the nurse focuses on the family's health, which is more than a summation of the health of its individual members. Using either perspective, the nurse maximizes therapeutic effectiveness by recognizing the family's influence and using its resources to promote individual and family health.

KEY CONCEPTS

The family has a significant impact on the lives of its members.

Family members mutually influence one another's health beliefs, practices, and status.

Because the concept of family is highly individualized, the nurse should base care on the client's attitude toward family rather than on an inflexible definition of it.

Specific family forms tend to have typical family health problems with which the nurse should be familiar.

The family's structure and functioning significantly influence its health and ability to respond to health problems.

The nurse can view the family as an important context for the individual family member or can view the family unit as the client. The approach for any family depends in part on the situation.

Measures of family health involve more than a summation of individual members' health.

The family's health is influenced by its social class, economic stability, and racial and ethnic background.

CRITICAL THINKING ACTIVITIES

1.. Discuss the concept of the family as client. Suggest ways the nurse can focus on family development and assess family health.
2. Describe how the concept of the family as client differs from the concept of the family as context. In what situations would each be a more appropriate focus?
3. Imagine one of your clients is a young child with a contagious illness. List some suggestions you might give the parents to deal with the care of the child and to provide a positive family life for the client's siblings. How would your approach differ if the child was from a single-parent family?
4. Describe societal factors that influence a family's health status.
5. Discuss the attributes of healthy family functioning.
6. Describe ways in which families of today differ from the "ideal" model of the family.
7. Think of the family in which you grew up. Describe the values and attitudes you learned in this environment and the influence they may have on how you view your client's family and health practices.

References

Barling J: Employment, *Stress and family functioning,* Chichester, England, 1990, John Wiley.

Berkey KM and Hanson SM: *Family assessment and intervention,* St. Louis, 1993, Mosby.

Bigbee JL: Family stress, hardiness, and illness: a pilot study, *Family Relations* 41(2):212, 1992.

Bumpass L, Sweet J, and Martin TC: Changing patterns of remarriage, *J Marriage Family* 52(3):747, 1990.

Chappell NM: Living arrangements and sources of caregiving, *J Gerontol* 46(1):11, 1991.

Danielson DB, Hamell-Bissell B, and Winstead-Fry P: *Family, health and illness,* St. Louis, 1993, Mosby.

Eshleman JR: *The family,* ed 6, Boston, 1991, Allyn & Bacon.

Fine MA: Families in the United States: their current status and future prospects, *Family Relations* 41(4):430, 1992.

Friedman M: *Family nursing: theory and assessment,* ed 2, New York, 1986, Appleton-Century-Crofts.

Gelles R and Maynard P: A structural approach to intervention in cases of family violence, *Family Relations* 36(3):270, 1987.

Glick P: Divorce, *NCFR presidential report 2001: preparing families for the future,* Minneapolis, 2-3, 1990.

Hanson S, Helms M, and Julian D: Education for family health care professionals: nursing as a paradigm, *Family Relations* 41(1):49, 1992.

Henslin JM: *Social problems,* ed 2, New Jersey, 1990, Prentice Hall.

Jurich JA, Adams RA, and Schlenberg JE: Factors related to behavior change in response to AIDS, *Family Relations* 41(1):97, 1992.

Levy F and Michel R: *The economic future of American families,* Washington DC, 1991, The Urban Institute Press.

Macklin ED: AIDS: Implications for families, *Family Relations* 37(2):141, 1988.

McClowery SG: Family functioning during a critical illness, *Crit Care Nurs Clin Am* 4(4):559, 1992.

McCubbin H and Dahl B: *Marriage and family: individuals and life cycles,* ed 2, New York, 1990, The Free Press.

McGoldrick M and Carter E: The stage of the family life cycle. In Henslin J, editor: *Marriage and family in a changing society,* New York, 1985, The Free Press.

Meyer DR and Garasky S: Custodial fathers: myths, realities and child support policy, *J Marriage Family* 55(1):73, 1993.

Phillips LR: Elder-family caregiver relationships, *Nurs Clin North Am* 24(24):795, 1989.

Price S: Divorce, *NCFR presidential report 2001: preparing families for the future,* Minneapolis, 30-31, 1990.

Reissman F and Gartner A: The Surgeon General and the self-help ethos, *Social Policy* 18(2):23, 1987.

Schvaneveldt JD and Young MH: Strengthening families: new horizons in family life education, *Family Relations* 41(4):385, 1992.

U.S. Bureau of the Census: *Statistical abstracts of the United States: 1991,* ed 111, Washington DC, 1991, U.S. Government Printing Office.

Wisendale SK: Toward the 21st Century: family change and public policy, *Family Relations* 41(4):417, 1992.

Zinn MB and Eitzen DS: *Diversity in A rican families,* ed 2, New York, 1990, Harper & Row.

Bibliography

Bahr S and Peterson E: *Aging and the family,* Lexington, Mass., 1989, Lexington Books.

Bowen G: *Navigating the marital journey,* New York, 1991, Praeger.

Campbell J and Humphreys J: *Nursing care of survivors of family violence,* St. Louis, 1993, Mosby.

Glenn N and Coleman M: *Family relations: a reader,* Belmont, Calif., 1988, Wadsworth.

Hanson S: Involving families in programs for pregnant teens: consequences for teens and their families, *Family Relations* 41(4):303, 1992.

Rosenheim M and Testa F, editors: *Early parenthood and coming of age in the 1990s,* New Brunswick, NJ, 1992, Rutgers University Press.

Simon R, Beaman J, et al.: Determinants of emotional well-being and parenting, *J Marriage and Family* 55(2):385, 1993.

Skolnick A: *Embattled paradise: the American family in an age of uncertainty,* 1991, Basic Books.

20

Growth and Development

OBJECTIVES

Mastery of content in this chapter will enable the student to:

- Define the key terms listed.
- Compare the frameworks for growth and development as described by major developmental theorists.
- Describe the characteristics of growth and physiological change from conception to old age.
- Identify the principles of development and maturation across the lifespan.
- Identify factors that can facilitate or hinder the growth and development of individuals of every age-group.
- Describe the physical and psychosocial changes and health concerns facing the pregnant woman and childbearing family.
- Describe the evolution of an individual's definition of health and perception of health status.
- Specify the physical and psychosocial health concerns of infants, children, adolescents, and adults.
- Use the nursing process and principles of growth and development when providing nursing care for individuals across the life span.
- Identify specific nursing interventions for the health concerns of clients across the lifespan.

KEY TERMS

adolescence
Alzheimer's disease
Apgar score
assimilation
associative play
attachment
bonding
climacteric (andropause)
concrete operations
dementia
development
differentiation principle
egocentricity
fertilization
infancy
infertility
lactation
menstrual cycle
menarche
menopause
middle adulthood
neonate
older adulthood
organic brain syndrome
parallel play
parturition
preadolescence
prenatal care
preoperational thought
puberty
puerperium
reality orientation
regression
reminiscence
respite care
school-age
sensorimotor period
sexual response cycle
social isolation
teratogens
toddler
trimester
young adulthood
zygote

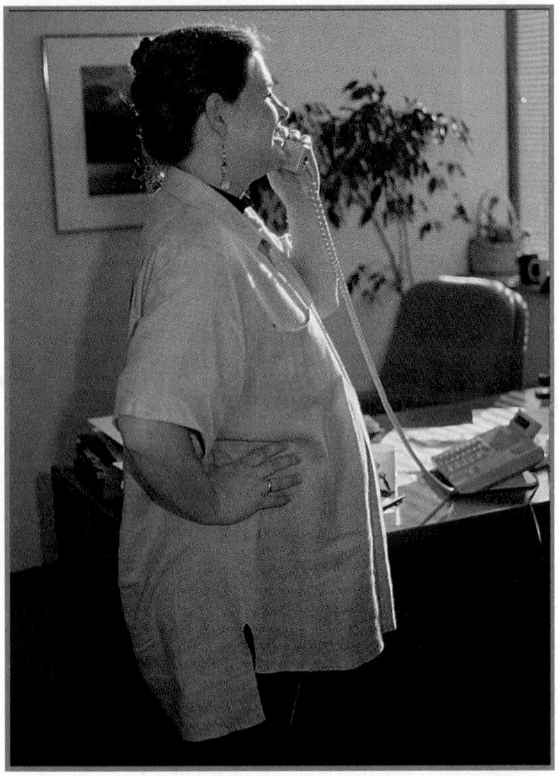

Human growth and development are orderly, predictable processes that begin with conception and continue until death. All persons progress through definite phases of growth and development, but the pace and behaviors of their progression are highly individual. An individual's ability to progress through each developmental phase influences the level of health. Because nursing promotes the health of individuals of all ages, the nurse must (1) understand the theories and principles of the growth and development process, (2) identify the stages of the process and the factors that influence progress, and (3) assess an individual's ability to respond in a healthy manner to the process. A developmental perspective helps the nurse to provide care in a manner that takes into consideration the unique needs and level of development of each individual.

GROWTH AND DEVELOPMENT THEORY

Growth and development are synchronous processes that are interdependent in the healthy individual and experienced as quantitative and qualitative changes. Physical growth is the quantitative or measurable aspect of an individual's increase in physical measurements (Whaley and Wong, 1991). Measurable growth indicators include height, weight, and dental, skeletal, and sexual age. Increases in these indicators demonstrate growth. Physical growth occurs in a predictable sequence and pattern with certain growth events expected at certain ages. Patterns or events that are out of sequence (e.g., late menarche) should alert the nurse to the need for further assessment.

Development is the qualitative or behavioral aspect of an individual's progressive adaptation to the environment (e.g., increased functioning capability resulting from mastering several smaller skills) (Table 20-1). Maturation is the process of becoming fully developed and grown. It involves the individual's biological ability, physiological condition, and desire to learn more mature behaviors. To mature, the individual may have to give up previous behaviors and learning, integrate new patterns into existing behaviors, or both. Maturation influences the sequence and timing of the qualitative and quantitative changes associated with growth and development.

The stages of growth and development involve the concept of critical periods of development, specific spans of time during which the environment has its greatest impact on the individual (Papalia and Olds, 1989). During these critical periods, some form of sensory stimulation is necessary for developmental progression. Without stimulation, task completion is difficult or unattainable. For example, the toddler who has not been encouraged to walk during a set time may have difficulty learning to walk at another time. Therefore developmental progression depends on the timing and degree of stimulation and on the readiness to be stimulated by the environment. A stimulus provided too early may not be useful. For example, an 18-month-old child cannot learn to write regardless of the intensity of the stimuli.

PRINCIPLES OF GROWTH AND DEVELOPMENT

Growth and development involve the following concepts:

1. Individuals have adaptive potential for qualitative and quantitative changes by receiving stimuli from and giving stimuli to the environment.
2. Individuals gain uniqueness from the interaction of heredity, environment, and human relationships.
3. The primary goal of development is achievement of potential (self-realization or self-actualization).

table 20-1

CHRONOLOGY OF GROWTH AND DEVELOPMENT

Stage	Age span	Significant behavioral milestones
Prenatal	Conception to birth	Maternal physical and psychosocial adjustment and progression through pregnancy Health and growth of fetus
Neonatal	Birth to 1 month	Physical: infant attachment behaviors: rooting, sucking, grasping, clinging Visual fixation: objects, face Equality of body movements
Infancy	1 month to 1 year	Physical: lifts head, rolls, sits, crawls, pulls to stand, walks, grasps, rakes, transfers hand objects, uses pincer grasp Psychosocial: smiles, vocalizes, laughs, feeds self finger foods, says "Da-Da" and "Ma-Ma," plays peek-a-boo and pat-a-cake
Toddler	1 to 3 years	Physical: walks well forward and backward, stoops and recovers, climbs, runs, jumps in place, throws overhand, voluntarily releases hand, uses spoon, drinks from cup, scribbles, builds two- then four-block tower Psychosocial: indicates wants by behaviors other than crying, increases vocabulary, imitates, helps with household chores, points to body parts, recognizes animals, engages in solitary play
Preschool	3 to 6 years	Physical: rides tricycle, walks up then down stairs alternating feet, hops on one foot, tandem walks, draws circle then cross then triangle, dresses with assistance then with supervision then alone Psychosocial: knows first name then age then last name, engages in parallel play progressing to interaction play, uses plurals and three-word sentences progressing to complex sentences, follows directions, counts
School age	6 to 11 years	Physical: skips, skates, tumbles, tandem walks backward, prints progressing to script, ties knots then bows Psychosocial: engages in interactive play with rules progressing to organized sports or activities, has significant peer relationships, enjoys hobbies, assumes complete responsibility for personal care
Adolescence	11 to 21 years	Physical: undergoes cognitive growth spurt, develops secondary sex characteristics, increases cognitive ability and formal operational thought Psychosocial: develops sense of identity and sex role, establishes independence, develops peer relationships with both sexes, develops life philosophy (values, beliefs), makes occupational decisions
Young and middle adult	21 to 65 years	Physical/cognitive: has established physical growth state and functioning, undergoes menopause, begins physical/physiological degeneration, refines formal operational abilities Psychosocial: develops self-sufficiency, pursues vocation/occupation, has intense interpersonal relationships (most frequently marriage and children)
Older adult	65 years to death	Physical cognitive: has general slowing of physical and cognitive functioning Psychosocial: needs to establish highest degree of independence (self-sufficiency) physically possible by adapting environment to ability, continues interpersonal relationships, reflects on life accomplishments, events, and experiences

The basic principles of growth and development are as follows:

1. Development is orderly and follows an established sequence.
2. Development is directional and proceeds along the following body axes:
   a. **Cephalocaudal**—development proceeds from the head to the lower extremities.
   b. **Proximodistal**—development proceeds from the central parts (proximal) of the body to the outer parts (peripheral).
   c. **Differentiation**—development proceeds from the simple to the complex.
3. Development is complex yet predictable, occurring with a consistent pattern and chronology.
4. Development is unique to individuals and their genetic potential. Most individuals strive for the highest level of development possible.

table 20-2

MAJOR FACTORS INFLUENCING GROWTH AND DEVELOPMENT

Factors	Relevant influences
FORCES OF NATURE	
Heredity	Genetic endowment determines sex, race, hair and eye color, physical growth, stature, and to some extent psychological uniqueness.
Temperament	Temperament is characteristic psychological mood with which the child is born and includes behavioral styles of easy, slow-to-warm, and difficult. It influences interactions between the individual and environment.
EXTERNAL FORCES	
Family	Family purpose is to protect and nurture its members. Family functions include means for survival, security, assistance with emotional and social development, assistance with maintenance of relationships, instruction about society and world, and assistance in learning roles and behaviors. Family influences through its values, beliefs, customs, and specific patterns of interaction and communication. Ordinal position and sex influence individual's interaction and communication in family.
Peer group	Peer group provides new and different learning environment. Peer group provides different patterns and structures of interaction and communication, necessitating different style of behavior. Functions of peer group include allowing individual to learn about success and failure; to validate and challenge thoughts, feelings, and concepts; to receive acceptance, support, and rejection as unique person apart from family; and to achieve group purposes by meeting demands, pressures, and expectations.
Life experiences	Life experiences and learning processes allow individual to develop by applying what has been learned to what needs to be learned. Learning process involves series of steps: recognition of need to know task; mastery of skills to perform task; mastery of task; expertise in performing task, which expands capabilities; integration into whole functioning; and use of accumulated skills and experiences to develop repertoire of effective behavior.
Health environment	Level of health affects individual's responsiveness to environment and responsiveness of others to the individual.
Prenatal health	Preconception (e.g., genetic and chromosomal factors, maternal age, health) and postconception (e.g., nutrition, weight gain, use of tobacco and alcohol, medical problems, use of prenatal services) factors affect fetal growth and development.
Nutrition	Growth is regulated by dietary factors. Adequacy of nutrients influences whether and how physiological needs, as well as subsequent growth and development needs, are met.
Rest, sleep, and exercise	Balance between rest or sleep and exercise is essential to rejuvenating body. Disturbances diminish growth, whereas equilibrium reinforces physiological and psychological health.
State of health	Illness or injury potentially hampers growth and development. Nature and duration of health problem influence its impact. Prolonged injury or illness may leave one unable to cope and respond to demands and tasks of developmental stages.
Living environment	Factors affecting growth and development include season, climate, home life, and socioeconomic status.

5. Development occurs through conflict and adaptation, with different aspects developing at different rates, creating periods of equilibrium and disequilibrium.
6. Development presents challenges to individuals in the form of tasks specific to age and ability.
7. Developmental tasks require practice and energy, the focus of which varies with each developmental stage and task accomplished.

MAJOR FACTORS INFLUENCING GROWTH AND DEVELOPMENT

The human being is a complex, open system influenced by natural forces from within and by external forces from the environment (Table 20-2). Interaction between these forces affects development. In general, natural factors set limits for development, whereas external factors present opportunities for achieving potential. The most

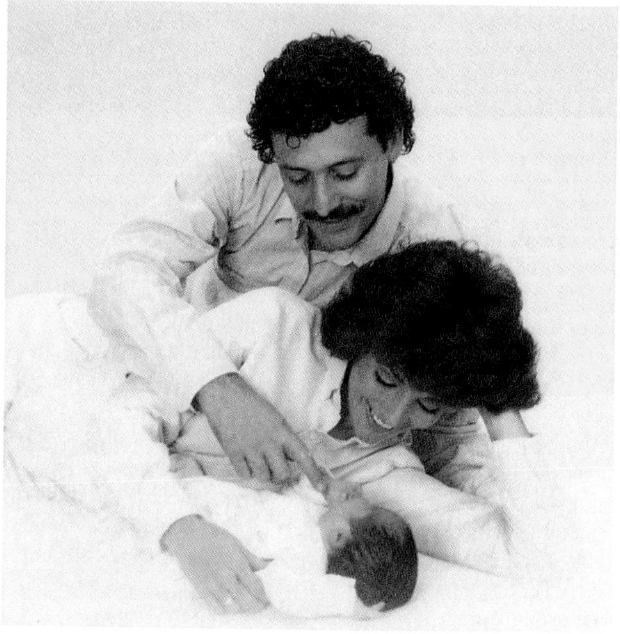

FIGURE 20-1 Healthy family relationships promote the growth potential of the newborn and other family members. (From Dickason EJ, Silverman BL, Schult MO: *Maternal-infant nursing care*, ed 2, St. Louis, 1994, Mosby.)

influential forces of nature are heredity and temperament. Family and peer relationships are the primary external forces (Figure 20-1).

Research has identified factors that place children at risk for developmental delays. Established risk is related to disorders such as Down's syndrome. Biological risk occurs as a result of damage to the central nervous system during intrauterine and neonatal periods. Limited early life experiences, resulting from parental inability or knowledge deficit, comprise environmental risk (King et al., 1992).

THEORIES OF HUMAN DEVELOPMENT

Research into human growth and development has led to a number of developmental theories (Table 20-3). These theories vary in the way humans are viewed and in the aspect of development emphasized. Some theories view development as a continuous process, moving from the simple to the more complex. Others consider it as discontinuous, with alternating periods of relative equilibrium and disequilibrium. To communicate effectively with other health professionals when providing coordinated health care, the nurse must be familiar with the common theories of growth and development. No one framework addresses all developmental concerns.

Freud's Psychosexual Theory

Sigmund Freud's (1969) theory of life development is the psychoanalytic theory. According to Freud, the personality is composed of the id, ego, and superego. The id directs behaviors toward the goal of immediate gratification of needs. Newborns, ruled by the id, cry until they feel pleasure (e.g., through feeding or being held). The superego is the conscience, formed as the result of internalizing societal restrictions and demands. For example, parental demands for a child to conform to certain expectations, such as telling the truth, lead to automatic learned behaviors on the part of the child. The ego represents the conscious self, which has a compromising capacity. Dealing with the real world forces the individual to make a compromise between the permissiveness of the id and the restrictions of the superego.

Freud's theory of life development is based on a series of psychosexual stages, with pleasure shifting from one bodily erogenous zone to another. Specific developmental accomplishments must be attained in each stage. Gratification that is too much or too little can have a significant impact on development and result in the individual becoming emotionally fixated at a particular stage. For example, infants who have cleft lips have trouble satisfying instinctual sucking needs and achieving oral gratification because they cannot feed and suck effectively. Freudian theory highlights the importance of certain life experiences and early interactions that may have implications for later development.

Erikson's Psychosocial Development Theory

Erikson (1963) bases his theory of psychosocial development on the process of socialization. He views life development as a continuous struggle for an emotional-social equilibrium. Personality development is affected by genetic, societal, and cultural influences including family and peer relationships, neighborhood, and school.

Erikson defines eight stages of development during which specific tasks must be achieved. The stages each have a personality crisis involving a major conflict critical at that time. The successful mastery of each conflict is based on achieving specific developmental tasks and is built on satisfactorily completing the previous core conflict. A positive outcome of each crisis includes developing a particular virtue such as hope and purpose.

When using Erikson's theory in nursing practice, the nurse needs to recognize that achievement in a stage is not absolute. Also, a wide spectrum of behavioral patterns is available to the individual in achieving the positive portion of the stage. The key to progression through the stages is a balance between two major conflicting behaviors of the stage. The nurse's role is to help the individual to recognize assets and liabilities and to build on the assets.

table 20-3

OVERVIEW OF DEVELOPMENT THEORIES

Stage	Characteristics	Strengths	Limitations
FREUDIAN PSYCHOSEXUAL THEORY			
Five age-related fixed stages: oral-sensory, anal-muscular, phallic-locomotion, latency, and genital	Basis of inner drives; psychosexual focus	Recognizes importance of instinctual needs Defines id, ego, super-ego as personality	Heavy emphasis on sexual behaviors Does not deal with adult development Based on data from psychiatric clients
ERIKSON'S PSYCHOSOCIAL DEVELOPMENT THEORY			
Eight interdependent stages: trust vs. mistrust, autonomy vs. doubt and shame, initiative vs. inferiority, identity vs. role confusion, intimacy vs. isolation, genarativity vs. self-absorption, ego integrity vs. despair	Socialization focus; ongoing process throughout life directed toward balance Positive and negative components that individual must balance	Recognizes role of social, biological, and environmental factors in development Relates specific tasks to appropriate age Well organized Includes all ages	Broad age ranges Does not include cognitive or moral development Tasks within stages are not absolute
MASLOW'S THEORY OF HUMAN NEED			
Six overlapping and variable need achievement levels: Physiologic well being, safety, belongingness, love, self-esteem, and self-actualization	Human need focus Ongoing process directed toward homeostasis	Identifies human needs Recognizes physical and psychosocial aspects of person	Does not identify age chronologically, making assessment difficult Last stage/goal not generally attainable in absolute sense Does not fully explain complex nature of human beings
PIAGET'S THEORY OF COGNITIVE DEVELOPMENT			
Four major fixed stages: Sensorimotor, preoperational, concrete operations, formal operations	Cognitive focus Defines process in terms of assimilation, accommodation, and adaptation	Accounts for heredity and environmental interaction Well defined Incorporates language concepts	Does not deal with psychosocial aspects Does not account for individual differences and variability in progression Strict hierarchical progress questionable
KOHLBERG'S THEORY OF MORAL DEVELOPMENT			
Three levels and six stages that are overlapping and variable in regard to age: Premoral, conventional morality, and postconventional morality	Follows a sequence corresponding to cognition Morality developed when cognitively prepared	Assigns order and definition to moral code development Serves as basis for assessment of morality	Levels and stages are not absolute Variability probably does exist Final level difficult to achieve Does not address psychosocial issues

Maslow's Theory of Human Needs

Maslow (1970) developed a theory of growth and development based on a set of human needs. The order of needs flows upward from basic human needs for physiological well-being and stability to self-actualization and fulfillment.

Maslow's theory is useful to the nurse because it focuses on basic physical and psychosocial needs essential to human life. Recognizing the importance of these needs at certain times in the individual's life enables the nurse to facilitate their satisfaction.

Piaget's Theory of Cognitive Development

Piaget's (1952) theory focuses on the development of cognition. Cognitive processes such as abstract reasoning, problem solving, and intellectual growth develop gradually through childhood and reach a stable operational phase in adolescence that is subsequently refined through the adult years.

Piaget views the development of the mind as occurring through adaptation to the environment via **assimilation** and **accommodation.** Assimilation is the process in which a person incorporates new experiences into existing cognitive structures (schema) and thus adapts experiences for repeated use. For example, the toddler seeing a horse for the first time fits it into the current scheme of four-legged animals and calls it a "doggie." The experience and the environment are thus adapted by the child. Accommodation is the process of responding to the environment through new activity and thinking, changing schema to deal with the new information. For example, the toddler who wants a cookie asks for one because simply taking one earlier led to punishment. The child thus changes to fit the experience and the environment. The combination of these two processes allows the individual to organize the world by ordering and classifying experiences, which results in adaptation or the balance between the organism and the outside environment. Cognitive development within and between stages is a function of maturation, experience, social interaction, and balancing. Piaget emphasizes genetics and interaction. He stresses that the environment provides "food for thought" with humans in an active learning role.

Piaget's theory provides a well-defined framework for understanding intellectual abilities. The stages offer insight into how interactions are processed and interpreted based on the individual's skill. This theory assists nurses in understanding how children of various ages view and interpret health and health care measures. The nurse should consider Piaget's principles when providing instructions, explanations, and health teaching, especially to children.

Kohlberg's Theory of Moral Development

According to Kohlberg (1964, 1969), moral development is one component of psychosocial development. It involves the individual's establishment of a moral code consistent with society. Moral development depends on the child's ability to accept social responsibility and to integrate personal principles of justice and fairness. In addition, the child's knowledge of right and wrong and behavioral expression of this knowledge must be founded on respect and regard for the integrity and rights of others. Cognitive development underlies the progression of a person's morality from level to level. These stages occur in the same order regardless of culture, though individuals differ as to how quickly and how far they progress through these stages.

Kohlberg's theory provides the basis on which to assess an individual's moral development. By assessing the extent to which the individual has completed a level or stage, the nurse can help to guide the individual, particularly a child, toward a productive, wholesome life. If the individual encounters difficulty in a developmental stage, this theory may help the individual and nurse to understand the conflict.

CONCEPTION AND FETAL DEVELOPMENT

From the moment of conception, human development proceeds rapidly. The ovum and sperm each carry half the genetic material that guides biochemical processes essential to the developing organism. Abnormalities in the genes or chromosomes can alter health. Other health problems result from environmental factors, such as fetal alcohol syndrome, which is induced by maternal alcoholism.

Physical Development

Intrauterine life generally lasts 9 calendar or 10 lunar months. The organism's life begins when the ovum is penetrated by one sperm. **Fertilization** most often takes place in the fallopian tube, usually within 12 to 24 hours after the ovum is released from the ovary (Figure 20-2). The ovum and sperm fuse, and the materials from both cell nuclei unite. The organism then has its full genetic complement in one pair of sex chromosomes and 22 pairs of autosomal chromosomes. The ovum and the sperm each contribute one chromosome to each pair. The fertilized ovum, or **zygote,** passes through the fallopian tube to the uterus within 4 days. During this time the zygote continues to divide. By the third day a solid ball of cells, the morula, has formed. This solid ball soon develops a central cavity, or blastocyst. Even at this early

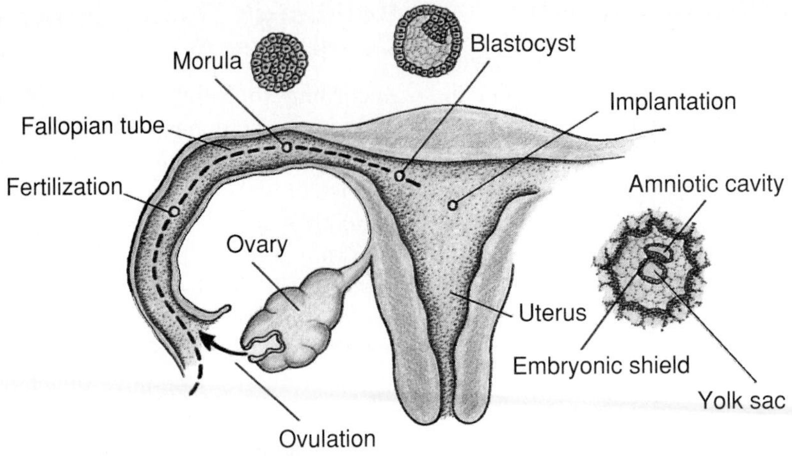

FIGURE 20-2 Fertilization cycle.

stage the cells begin to differentiate in structure and function. Cells at one end of the blastocyst develop into the embryo, and those at the opposite end form the placenta. By day 4 the embryo has traveled through the fallopian tube into the uterus and is implanted in the uterine wall.

The first **trimester** is the first 3 calendar months. After implantation the fetal cells continue to differentiate and develop into essential organ systems (Figure 20-3). These processes occur at different rates and times. Because several organ systems are developing during the same time, disruption of one system is often associated with disruption of others.

The second trimester is the period from the third to the sixth prenatal months of life. Some organ systems continue basic development during this time, and the functional capabilities of others are refined. By the end of the second trimester most organ systems are complete and can function. The fetus weighs about 0.7 kg (1½ pounds) and is approximately 30 cm (12 inches) long.

During the last 3 months of intrauterine life, the fetus grows to approximately 50 cm (19 to 20 inches) in length. Subcutaneous fat is stored, and weight increases to approximately 3.2 to 3.4 kg (7 to 7½ pounds). The skin thickens, lanugo begins to disappear, and the fetal body becomes rounder and fuller. A tremendous spurt in brain growth begins during this trimester and lasts well into the first few years of life. The central nervous system has established its total number of neurons and connections between neurons, and myelination of nerve fibers progresses rapidly. Damage to the central nervous system during the third trimester can potentially alter later, higher-level cognitive functions. Exposure to noxious agents and the absence of essential nutrients are the most common causes of damage during this trimester. The nurse can teach the woman about these factors in prenatal education. At the end of the third trimester the normal fetus is physically able to make the transition from intrauterine to extrauterine life.

Cognitive and Psychosocial Development

Relationships between prenatal events and cognitive development are difficult to establish. However, periods of diminished oxygen (anoxia) during fetal life are associated with deficits in later cognitive functioning (Westwood et al., 1983). Some research shows an association between severely inadequate prenatal nutrition and subsequent lower brain weight, head circumference, and specific cognitive abilities. Until more is known, the nurse intervenes to support adequate prenatal nutrition and prevent fetal anoxia.

Little is known about the relationship between prenatal experiences and the child's later psychosocial development. Some believe the biochemical environment of the uterus can significantly influence later psychosocial development. Because the biochemical environment is influenced by the mother's emotional state, maternal emotional and physical states may have significant psychosocial consequences for the unborn child. Furthermore, the mother's emotional state may influence her behavior after childbirth, which in turn influences the child's psychosocial development.

Health Concerns

Before implantation, the embryo is relatively safe from the external environment. However, the organism is sensitive to changes in the environment of the fallopian tube and uterus through which it travels. With implantation the embryo is connected to the larger maternal environment via the placenta. Materials essential for

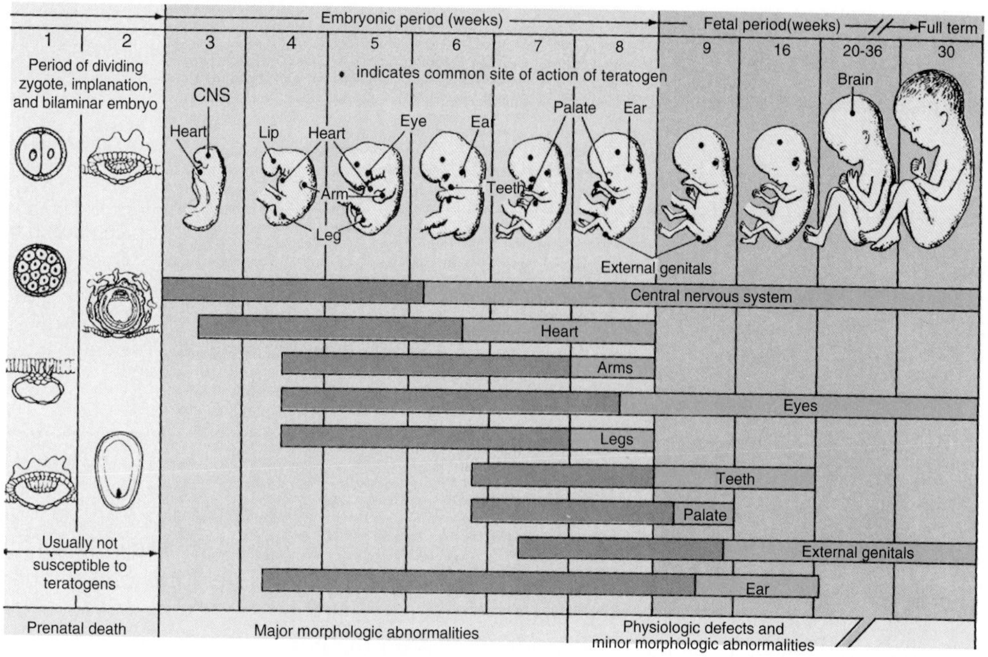

FIGURE 20-3 Periods of organ differentiation.

healthy growth and development (oxygen and nutrients) are received, and waste products and carbon dioxide are excreted. Because the placenta is extremely porous, **teratogens** (agents capable of having adverse effects on the fetus) such as viruses, drugs, alcohol, and environmental pollutants can also pass from mother to fetus. The fetal effect of these harmful agents depends on the developmental stage in which exposure takes place. Some teratogens produce defects only if the fetus is exposed to the agent at a critical time when the vulnerable organ is developing. One such teratogen is the rubella or measles virus, which can cause spontaneous abortion, stillbirth, or defects of the eyes, ears, and heart, primarily when exposure is in the first trimester.

Many drugs are teratogenic during the period of rapid organ growth in the first trimester. Barbiturates, alcohol, anticonvulsants, and anticoagulants are associated with fetal abnormalities. The benefits of prescribed medications must be weighed against potentially harmful fetal effects. In addition, there is evidence that mothers who smoke deliver infants with lower birth weights than nonsmoking mothers.

Nurses should explore life-style changes that can help women abstain from tobacco, alcohol, and drugs, not only during pregnancy but also while thinking about pregnancy. Preconception counseling is a growing trend in health care. The goal is to facilitate an optimal outcome for mother, fetus, and significant others. Health guidance during pregnancy should include nutrient requirements, balanced rest and activity, and stress management. A discussion of physiological events, fetal development, and family adaptation to pregnancy is critical. In the third trimester, nurses assist in developing birth plans and encourage participation in childbirth preparation classes.

Transition from Intrauterine to Extrauterine Life

The transition from intrauterine to extrauterine life at birth requires rapid changes in the **neonate.** The nurse assesses the neonate's ability to make these changes and intervenes as needed to ensure success. Gestational age, exposure to depressant drugs before or during labor, and the neonate's own behavioral style influence adjustment to the external environment. The initial nursing assessment includes physical and psychosocial elements. The nurse assesses the neonate's current functioning, supports transition, and provides opportunities for parents and child to develop close emotional ties.

Because the nurse's first concern is the physiological functioning of the neonate's major organ systems, an immediate assessment of the neonate's condition is performed. Care is then directed toward maintaining an open airway, stabilizing body temperature, and protecting the neonate from infection.

Patency of the neonate's airway is best ensured by removing nasoorpharyngeal secretions with suction or a bulb syringe. After the airway is open, the nurse acts

table 20-4

APGAR NEWBORN SCORING SYSTEM*

	Score		
Sign	**0**	**1**	**2**
Heart rate	Not detectable	Below 100 beats/min	Above 100 beats/min
Respiratory effort	Absent	Slow or irregular	Good strong cry
Muscle tone	Flaccid, limp	Some flexion of extremities	Well flexed, active motion
Reflex irritability	No response	Grimace, some motion	Cough, sneeze, or cry
Color	Blue or pale	Body pink; extremities blue (acrocyanosis)	Completely pink undertone

From Dickason EJ, Schultz MO, et al.: *Maternal-infant nursing care,* ed 2, St. Louis, 1994, Mosby.

to stabilize body temperature. Wrapping the neonate in small, soft blankets usually provides adequate heat preservation. Isolettes, incubators, and radiant heat warmers, which supply radiant heat, can also be used, especially for neonates unable to sustain body temperature.

Prevention of infection is a major concern in the care of the neonate, whose immune system is immature. Gloves are worn to handle the neonate in the delivery room and later when handling other body fluids. Good handwashing technique is essential to protect the neonate and the nurse from infection. Although it is not required by the Centers for Disease Control and Prevention (CDC), some nurses also wear gloves during diaper changes.

The most commonly used prophylactic treatment against ophthalmia conjunctivitis is erythromycin (0.5%) because it prevents *Neisseria gonorrhoea* and other infections such as *Chlamydia,* which can be transmitted during passage through an infected vaginal canal. The traditional use of 1% silver nitrate solution is uncommon today because of chemical irritation to the eyes and its more narrow action against bacteria.

The stump of the umbilical cord is an excellent medium for bacterial growth and should be swabbed with an antibacterial agent such as triple dye shortly after birth. Stump drying is quickened by applying alcohol at each diaper change and folding the diaper away from the cord.

The nurse is often responsible for assessing the neonate's physiological functioning. A widely used assessment tool is the **Apgar score,** which rates five physiological characteristics. The newborn's heart rate, respiratory effort, muscle tone, reflex irritability, and color are rated at 1 and 5 minutes after birth to determine overall status. Table 20-4 outlines the scoring criteria of physiological functioning. A total score of 0 to 3 signifies severe distress, a score of 4 to 6 represents moderate difficulty, and a score of 7 to 10 indicates little difficulty in adjusting to extrauterine life. In addition, the nurse monitors body temperature and vital signs until the neonate is stable.

After the immediate physical evaluation the nurse assesses the parents' and newborn's needs for close physical contact. Early parent-child interaction encourages close parent-child **attachment.** Physical factors, such as parental fatigue and hunger, and emotional factors, such as happiness about the birth and needs to touch, see, and be close to the infant, are assessed. Parent and neonate must be capable and desirous of exploring and responding to the other. Most healthy neonates are awake and alert for the first half hour after birth, and if the parents are receptive, this is a good time for parent-child acquaintance to begin. Close body contact, often including breast feeding, is a satisfying way for most families to start.

If immediate contact is not possible, the nurse incorporates such contact into the care plan as early as possible for parents and neonate. **Bonding** occurs when parents and newborn elicit reciprocal and complementary behaviors (Figure 20-4). Parental bonding behaviors include attentiveness and physical contact with the newborn. Neonate bonding behavior involves maintaining eye contact with the parents. Preterm and ill neonates and their parents have greater difficulty forming this bond if separation is prolonged.

NEONATE

The neonatal period is the first 28 days of life. The nurse performs an assessment as soon as the neonate's physiological functioning is stable, generally within a few hours after birth. At this time the nurse measures length, weight, head circumference, temperature, pulse, and respirations and observes general appearance, body functions, sensory capabilities, and responsiveness. The nurse also coordinates screening tests and other labora-

A

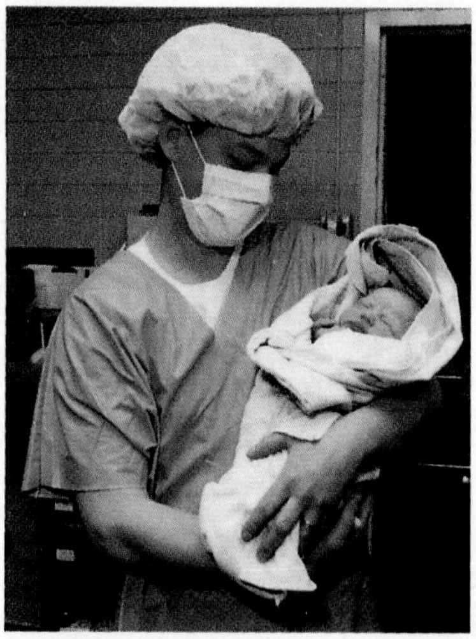

B

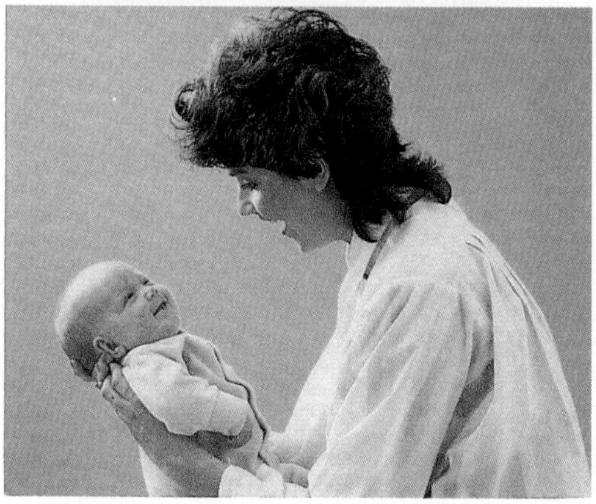

FIGURE 20-4 A, Father-infant bonding. (Courtesy St John's Mercy Medical Center, St Louis, Mo.). B, Mother-infant bonding. (Courtesy Ross Laboratories, Columbus, Ohio.)

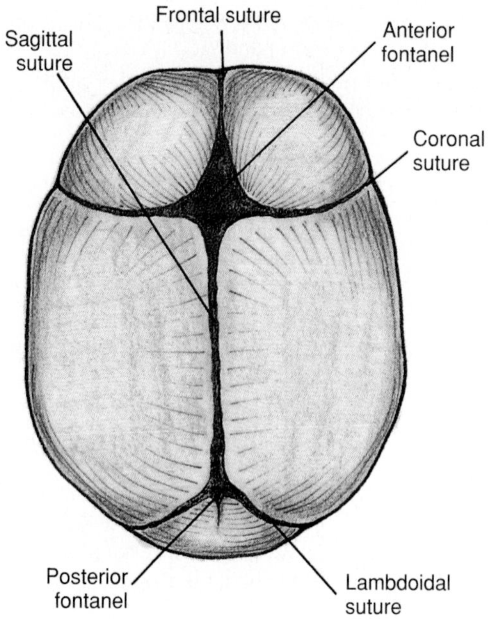

FIGURE 20-5 Fontanels and suture lines.

tory tests as indicated by the neonate's state of health. Blood tests, such as those for hypothyroidism and phenylketonuria (PKU), are eventually performed on all neonates and allow early detection and treatment. This prevents permanent central nervous system damage. These and other screening tests are required by law in many states. A comprehensive neonatal assessment must also include the psychosocial status of the family and the manner in which family processes are affected by the birth. The data provide baseline information and may reveal the need for nursing interventions. Sharing assessment knowledge with parents allows them to recognize and respond appropriately to the neonate's cues.

Physical Development

The primary physical developmental goal for the neonate is to stabilize major body systems. This is characterized by functioning and behavior that are predominantly reflexive.

The average newborn weighs 3200 g (7 pounds, 1 ounce), is 50 cm (20 inches) in length, and has a head circumference of 35 cm (14 inches). Up to 10% of birth weight is lost in the first few days of life, primarily through fluid losses by respiration, urination, defecation, and decreased intake. Birth weight is usually regained by the second week of life, and a gradual pattern of increase in weight (4 to 8 ounces a week), length (0.6 to 2.5 cm), and head circumference (2 cm) is evident by 1 month.

The neonate's heart rate gradually decreases from the fetal rate of 120 to 160 beats per minute to 120 to 140 beats per minute. The average blood pressure is 70/55 mm Hg. Neonates are nasal breathers. Their respiratory movements are primarily abdominal and vary in rate and rhythm. The average rate is 35 to 40 respirations per minute. The axillary temperature ranges from 36.5 to 378 C (97.9 to 98.68 F) and generally stabilizes within 24 hours after birth.

Normal physical characteristics include the continued presence of lanugo on the skin of the back, cyanosis of the hands and feet (acrocyanosis), especially during activity, and a soft, protuberant abdomen. Skin color variations according to racial and genetic heritage occur gradually during infancy. Molding, or overlapping of the soft skull bones, is common during birth. The bones readjust in a few weeks, producing a more rounded appearance. Suture lines and fontanels are palpable between the unfused skull bones (Figure 20-5). The anterior (diamond-shaped) and posterior (triangular-shaped) fontanels are usually palpable at birth and will feel flat and firm when the neonate is at rest.

table 20-5

INFANT REFLEXES

Reflex	Stimulus	Response
Babinski	Using blunt object, stroke lateral aspect of plantar surface of foot from heel to toes.	Hyperextension or fanning of toes occurs. As myelinization is completed, normal response is flexion (downward curling) of all toes; positive (pathological) sign is hyperextension (dorsiflexion) of great toe, with or without fanning of remaining toes.
Blinking	Shine light suddenly at infant's open eyes.	Eyelids close in response to light (disappears after first year).
Landau	Suspend infant carefully in prone position by supporting infant's abdomen with hand.	By 3 months, expected response consists of extension of head, trunk, and hips. Head is slightly above horizontal plane. (Reflex disappears by 2 years).
Moro	With infant in supine position, gently support head and lift it a few centimeters off surface. As soon as neck relaxes, suddenly release head and let it drop back to surface. OR Produce sudden, loud noise or jar table or crib suddenly.	Normal response is present at birth. Arms extend outward and hands open and then are brought together in midline. Legs flex slightly. Infant may cry. (Reflex usually disappears by 3 to 4 months.)
Neck righting	With infant in supine position, turn head to one side.	Infant's trunk rotates in direction in which head is turned (appears at 4 to 6 months and disappears at 24 months).
Palmar grasp	With infant's head positioned in midline, place index fingers from ulnar side into infant's palm and press against palm.	Normal response is flexion of all fingers around examiner's fingers (present at birth and disappears by 4 months when infant is ready to reach).
Placing	Hold infant erect, with dorsum of one foot touching undersurface of examining table top.	Infant flexes hip and knee and places stimulated foot on top of table (present at birth and disappears by 6 weeks or variable).
Plantar grasp	Place finger firmly across base of infant's toes.	Toes curl downward (present at birth and disappears by 10 to 12 months).
Rooting	Hold infant in supine position with head in midline and hands against chest. Stroke perioral skin at corner of mouth or cheek.	Infant opens mouth and turns head toward stimulated side (present at birth and disappears by 3 to 4 months [awake]; by 7 months [asleep]).

Modified from Chow M et al.: *Handbook of pediatric primary care,* ed 2, Somerset, NJ, 1984, John Wiley & Sons.

Normal behavioral characteristics of the newborn include periods of sucking, crying, sleeping, and activity. Movements are generally sporadic, but they are symmetrical and involve all four extremities. Newborns respond to sensory stimuli, particularly the care giver's face, voice, and touch.

Neurological function is assessed by observing the neonate's level of activity, alertness, irritability, responsiveness to stimuli, and the presence and strength of reflexes. Normal reflexes include blinking in response to bright lights and startling in response to sudden, loud noises. Table 20-5 lists other commonly evaluated neonatal reflexes. Their absence indicates possible trauma or central nervous system complications. Because the newborn depends largely on reflexes for response to the environment, assessment of these response characteristics is vital as an indicator of neuromuscular integrity.

Cognitive and Psychosocial Development

Early cognitive development begins with innate behaviors, reflexes, and sensory functions. During this time newborns initiate reflex activities, add new objects into behavior, and accommodate these behaviors to achieve their desires. For example, neonates learn to turn to the nipple. Newborns can focus on objects 8 to 10 inches from their faces and respond to auditory stimuli. Therefore parents should be taught the importance of talking to their babies and providing appropriate visual stimuli.

Whether infant crying leads to refined language is debatable. However, crying elicits a response and care givers discriminate among cry patterns. Crying therefore has significance to newborns and parents. For neonates, crying is a means of communication. They cry for a reason, although at times this reason is difficult to determine. Crying may be frustrating for parents if

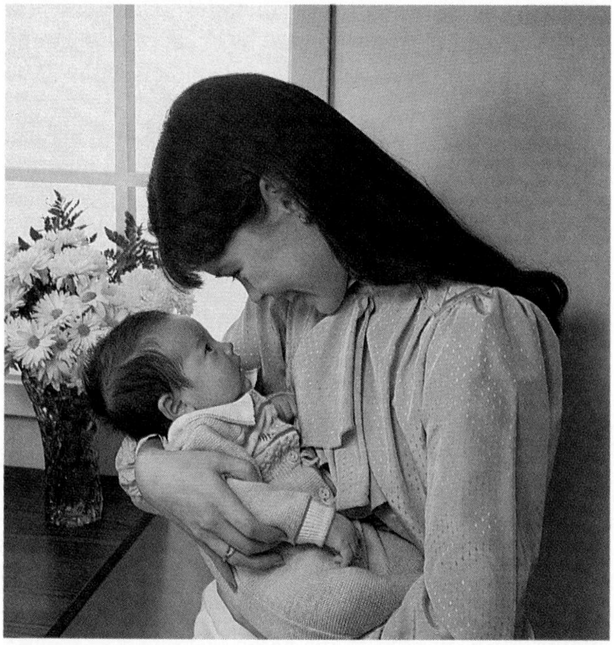

FIGURE 20-6 During the first months of life parents and newborns normally develop a strong bond that grows to a deep attachment. (From Dickason EJ, Silverman BL, Schult MO: *Maternal-infant nursing care,* ed 2, St. Louis, 1994, Mosby.)

they cannot see an apparent cause. With the nurse's help, parents can learn to define their infant's cry patterns and take appropriate action.

Health Concerns

During the first month of life parents and newborns normally develop a strong bond that grows to a deep attachment (Figure 20-6). Feeding, hygiene, comfort measures, and brief periods of play are interactive experiences that provide a foundation from which later attachments form (Figure 20-7). Nurses assist parents to attain the knowledge and skills required to foster the newborn's physical, psychosocial, and cognitive well-being and development (see box on p. 446).

If parents or the newborn experience health complications after the birth, bonding may be compromised. Neonatal behavioral cues may be weak or absent. Care and care giving are less mutually satisfying. A tired, ill parent may have difficulty interpreting cues and responding to the newborn. Neonates who have congenital anomalies, who are too weak to be responsive to parental cues, or who require special care need supportive nursing measures. For example, infants born with heart defects may tire easily during feeding. They may rest frequently after several bursts of sucking and may awaken hungry after 1½ hours. Parents, not understanding the physiological reason for the behavior, may

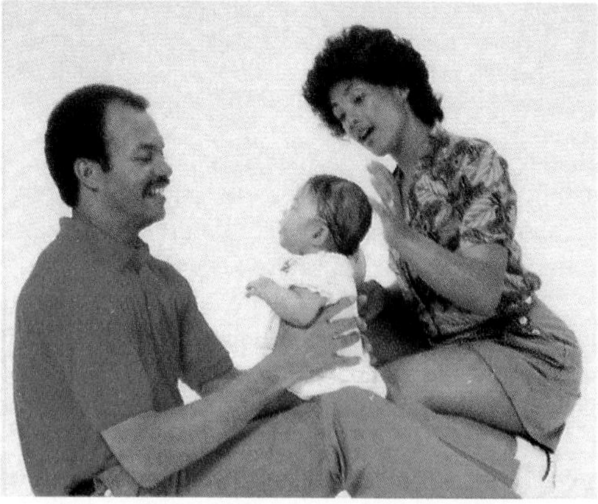

FIGURE 20-7 Desire to hold infant and participate in care giving activities provides foundation for bonding and later attachments. (Courtesy Ross Laboratories, Columbus, Ohio.)

think the infant is being fussy or that they are inadequate as parents. The attachment process is not enhanced and may even be hindered without nursing intervention.

INFANT

Infancy is the period from 1 month to 1 year of age. Rapid physical, cognitive, and psychosocial growth and development characterize this stage.

Physical Development

Steady and proportional growth of the infant is more important than absolute growth values. Infants usually double their birth weight by 5 months and triple it by 12 months. Infants grow at a rate of 1 inch per month during their first 6 months and then ½ inch per month to the end of their first year. Charts of normal age- and sex-related growth measurements enable the nurse to compare growth with norms for a child's age. Using growth charts, the nurse evaluates growth patterns by recording measurements of weight, length, and head circumference at intervals. Measurements recorded over time are the best way to monitor growth and identify problems.

By the end of the first year, the heart rate is 90 to 140 beats per minute and the blood pressure is 72 to 95 mm Hg systolic and 33 to 65 mm Hg diastolic. The respiratory rate is 30 to 35 per minute. Patterns of body functions such as sleep, elimination, and feeding are more stabilized.

The quality and quantity of nutrition influence the infant's growth and development. Breast feeding is recommended for infants because human milk contains an

> **TEACHING TOPICS FOR PARENTS OF NEWBORNS**
>
> Expected physiological newborn behaviors
> Variability of behavioral cycles (sleep-awake states)
> Principles and techniques for feeding method chosen
> Feeding patterns and behaviors
> Care measures including hygiene, dressing, comfort
> Protective measures including asepsis, safety, CPR, thermoregulation
> Sensory capabilities and appropriate stimulation techniques
> Signs and symptoms requiring evaluation of the newborn by a health care professional
> Recommended health care guidance

appropriate balance of protein, fat, and carbohydrate essential for growth during the first few months. Immunoreactive proteins are also present to build resistance to infection. Commercially prepared formulas fortified with vitamins and minerals can be used successfully. The nurse supports the parents' choice of feeding method and helps them feed their infant successfully. Cow's milk is not recommended in the first year because the amounts of proteins, fats, and carbohydrates are out of balance for human infants.

The 1-month-old infant takes approximately 28 ounces of milk per day. This increases slightly during the first 6 months and drops to about 24 ounces per day by the end of the first year. Usually between 6 and 12 months of age, the infant is started on solid foods and gradually progresses to a diet that includes cereal, fruits and vegetables, meat, fish, poultry, eggs, and cheese. After 6 months of age, iron supplements with fortified cereal are recommended. Infants may also need fluoride supplements.

Cognitive and Psychosocial Development

The infant learns by experiencing and manipulating the environment. Developing motor skills and increasing mobility expand an infant's environment and, with developing visual and auditory skills, enhance cognitive development. According to Piaget, the child is in the **sensorimotor period** and is gradually moving from reflexive to symbolic behavior.

Speech is an important part of cognition that develops during the first year. Infants proceed from crying, cooing, and laughing to imitating sounds, comprehending the meaning of simple commands, and repeating words with knowledge of their meaning. By 1 year of age, infants not only recognize their own names but also have two- or three-word vocabularies. The nurse can promote language development by encouraging parents to name objects on which the infant's attention is focused.

Infants need opportunities to develop and use the senses. Nurses evaluate the appropriateness and adequacy of these opportunities. For example, ill or hospitalized infants may lack the energy to interact with their environments, thereby slowing cognitive development. On the other hand, continuous stimulation can overwhelm and confuse infants. They need to be stimulated according to their temperament, energy, and age. Stimulation strategies maximize the development of infants while conserving their energy and orientation.

During the first year, infants begin to differentiate themselves from others as separate beings capable of acting on their own. This process is slow, and infants occasionally experience brief frustrations with more frequent and consistent satisfactions. When determining physical boundaries, infants begin to respond to others. Infants 2 to 3 months of age begin to smile responsively rather than reflexively. Similarly, they can recognize differences in people when their sensory and cognitive capabilities improve. By 8 months of age most infants can differentiate a stranger from a familiar person and respond differently to the two. Close attachment to the primary care givers, most often parents, is usually established by this age. Infants seek out these persons for support and comfort during times of stress. Finally, the ability to distinguish self from others allows infants to interact and socialize more within their environment.

The nurse assesses the availability and appropriateness of experiences contributing to psychosocial development. Hospitalized infants may have difficulty establishing physical boundaries because of repeated bodily intrusions and painful sensations. Limiting these negative experiences and providing pleasurable sensations support early psychosocial development. Extended separations from parents complicate the attachment process and increase the number of care givers with whom the infant must interact. Ideally, parents should provide most of the routine daily care during hospitalization. When this is impossible, an attempt should be made to limit the number of care givers who have contact with the infant and to follow the parents' direction for care, thus fostering the infant's continuing development of trust.

Health Concerns

The foundation for children's perceptions of their health status is laid early in life. Internal body sensations and experiences with the outside world affect self-perceptions. The nature of this influence and the value of nursing interventions to alter later perceptions are unknown. It is known, however, that parents tend to label infants

TEACHING TOPICS FOR PARENTS OF INFANTS AND TODDLERS

Expected growth and developmental norms
Play activities to stimulate gross and fine motor development
Techniques to encourage development of speech and language
Appropriate methods for toilet training, discipline, exercise, and rest
Nutrition including weaning, addition of solids, appropriate types and amount of foods and fluids to meet growth and activity needs
Safety measures including childproofing the home environment, car seats, pool and water precautions, toy selection, limit setting
Criteria to use when choosing day care
Recommended health care including immunizations and their scheduling, developmental assessments, gross evaluation of visual and auditory capabilities, dental care
Signs of illness, measures for assessment (temperature taking), and appropriate action

who are ill in early life as vulnerable and this labeling may later affect children's perceptions of their own health. In addition, because infants and children depend on others for health care, care givers influence children's health attitudes and behaviors. The nurse educates parents and other care givers about health promotion behaviors that will positively affect the child's perception of health and self (see box above).

TODDLER

The toddler period ranges from the time when children begin to walk independently until they walk and run with ease, which is approximately from 12 to 36 months of age. A **toddler** is characterized by increasing independence bolstered by greater physical mobility and cognitive abilities. Toddlers are increasingly aware of their abilities to control and are pleased with their successful efforts with this new skill. Unsuccessful attempts at control may result in undesirable behaviors and temper tantrums. Parents need support in finding ways to set consistent, firm limits for a toddler while also promoting the child's independence.

Physical Development

The rapid development of motor skills allows the child to participate in self-care activities such as feeding, dressing, and toileting. Toddlers walk in an upright position with a broad-stanced gait, protuberant abdomen, and arms flung out to the sides for balance. Soon the child begins to navigate stairs, run, jump, stand on one foot for several seconds, and kick a ball. Most toddlers can ride a tricycle, climb ladders, and run well by their third birthday. Fine motor capabilities move from scribbling spontaneously to drawing circles and crosses accurately. Improved mobility, the ability to undress, and development of sphincter control allow toilet training if the toddler has the necessary cognitive abilities.

The cardiopulmonary system becomes stable in the toddler years. The heart and respiratory rates slow to 110 beats and 25 to 30 breaths per minute. The blood pressure rises slightly to an average of 92/56 mm Hg. The anterior fontanel closes between 12 and 18 months of age, ending the period of most rapid growth of the skull and brain. Routine measurement of head circumference is usually not continued past this age. The rate of increase in weight and height slows. By 2 years of age, the child weighs four times the birth weight. Height during toddlerhood increases 3 to 5 inches a year, mainly as a result of increases in leg length.

Cognitive and Psychosocial Development

According to Piaget (1952), toddlers move from the sensorimotor stage of cognitive development to the **preoperational thought** stage. In this stage children learn the permanency of objects, develop a memory of events, begin to understand cause and effect, and put their thoughts into words. Toddlers recognize they are separate beings from their mothers but they are unable to assume the view of another, because their thought has an egocentric focus. The toddler becomes increasingly capable of symbolic interaction and frequently expresses fantasy and magical thinking.

Because moral development is closely associated with cognitive ability, the moral development of toddlers is only beginning and is also **egocentric.** Toddlers do not understand concepts of right and wrong. However, they do grasp that some behaviors bring pleasant results (positive reinforcement) and others elicit unpleasant results (negative reinforcement).

The 18-month-old child uses approximately 10 words. The 24-month-old child has a vocabulary of up to 300 words and is generally able to speak in short sentences. By 36 months of age, most toddlers talk incessantly.

According to Erikson (1963), a sense of autonomy emerges during toddlerhood. Although toddlers are moving out to explore their immediate environment, they continue to return at periodic intervals for encouragement and the emotional support of parents (called refueling). Toddlers begin to participate in **parallel play** with others, playing next to rather than with one another. Toddlers, who are just learning what belongs to them, are often possessive of their toys. They begin to learn that sharing is a desirable behavior when they offer parents toys to hold and the parents express pleasure.

Because a toddler is extremely active and curious yet unable to limit behaviors, parents must set limits. Firm, consistent limit setting, patience, and support allow the toddler to develop socially acceptable behavior. Limiting is important for safety (e.g., car seats, water safety, and poisons kept out of reach). Limit setting causes conflict between the parent and child, often leading to a child's temper tantrums. Parents appreciate reassurance that this conflict lessens as the child grows older and internalizes behavior limits. Parents also need to provide toddlers with graded independence, allowing them to do things that do not harm themselves or others. Liller, Kent, and McDermott (1991) found that postpartum mothers lacked knowledge concerning certain childhood injuries, their cause, and prevention. They recommend that prenatal education programs include topics related to the cause and prevention of common young childhood injuries.

Health Concerns

Slower growth rates are accompanied by a decrease in caloric needs and a smaller food intake. Confirming the child's pattern of growth with charts can be reassuring to parents concerned about their toddler's decreased appetite (physiological anorexia). Daily food intake is usually 3 to 4 servings of milk, 2 to 3 servings of meat, 4 servings of vegetables and fruits, and 4 or more servings of cereals and breads. Food jags (desire to eat one food repeatedly) and mealtime rituals frustrate parents but are expressions of a toddler's need for autonomy and control. Parents are encouraged to offer a variety of nutritious foods, in reasonable servings, for mealtime and snacks. Special dietary considerations are made for the toddler who is ill, is going to have surgery, or is on a vegetarian diet.

Toddlers' perceptions of health are limited by cognitive capabilities. Children increasingly recognize internal body sensations but have difficulty pinpointing their location. Therefore they often associate generalized responses with illness. Children who deviate radically from their usual patterns of eating, sleeping, or playing require assessment to determine whether these alterations result from illness.

Toddlers begin to internalize the labels that parents or health care professionals give to the somatic states. That is, if the parents label particular sensations, such as abdominal discomfort, an "illness," children begin to label related sensations similarly. At the same time children observe and mimic parents' health care practices. When providing health care to toddlers, nurses apply principles of growth and development to help toddlers establish trust with health care providers.

PRESCHOOL CHILD

The preschool years are a transition between toddlerhood and the school-age years. The period spans the ages between 3 and 6. Many people consider these the most intriguing years of parenting because children are more cooperative, can share thoughts with greater accuracy, and can interact and communicate more effectively (Figure 20-8). Physical development continues to slow, whereas cognitive and psychosocial development are rapid.

Physical Development

Several aspects of physical development stabilize in the preschool years. Heart and respiratory rates decrease only slightly to approximately 90 beats and 22 to 24

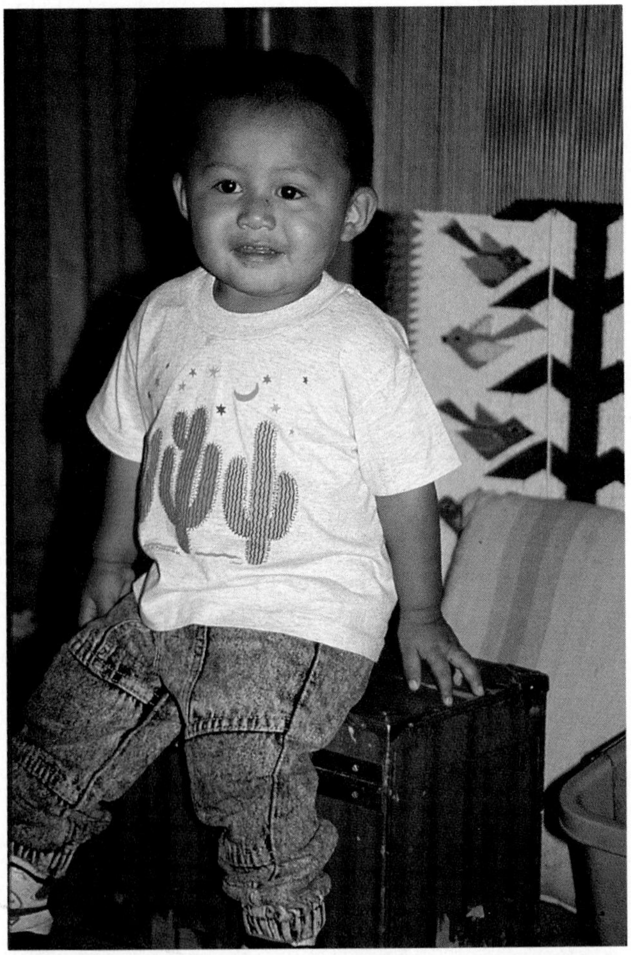

FIGURE 20-8 Many people consider the preschool years the most intriguing years of parenting. (Courtesy Michael S. Clement, MD, Mesa, Ariz.).

breaths per minute. Blood pressure rises slightly to an average of 95/58 mm Hg. Weight increases about 5 pounds per year, making the average weight about 42 pounds (6 times the birth weight) by age 5. Height increases 2 to 3 inches per year. Birth length is generally doubled by age 4, making the average height 42 inches. The elongation of the legs results in the preschooler's more slender appearance.

Large and fine muscle coordination improves. Preschoolers run well, walk up and down steps with ease, and learn to hop. By 6 years of age, they can usually skip and throw and catch balls. Improving fine motor skills allows intricate manipulations such as drawing circles and triangles as well as printing letters and numbers. Children need to learn and practice these physical skills. Nursing care of healthy and ill children includes assessing the availability of these opportunities. Children who have chronic conditions or who have been hospitalized for long periods need ongoing exposure to developmental opportunities.

Cognitive and Psychosocial Development

Preschoolers continue to master the preoperational stage of cognition. The continued egocentricity of early thinking makes it difficult to suggest acceptable alternatives to the preschooler. With maturation, experience, and the increasing use of symbolic thinking, the child is more able to take the view of another and is capable of social interactions.

Around 4 years of age, the intuitive phase of preoperational thought develops. Preschoolers can increasingly solve problems intuitively on the basis of one aspect of a situation. For example, they can classify objects according to size or color but not both. The preschooler's knowledge of the world remains closely linked to concrete experiences. The mixing of fantasy and reality can lead to many childhood fears and may be misinterpreted by adults as lying when children are actually presenting reality from their perspective. The greatest fear of this age-group appears to be of bodily harm.

Early causal thinking is evident in preschoolers' transductive thoughts (reasoning occurs from one particular to another). If two events are related in time or space, children link them causally. The hospitalized child, for example, may reason, "I cried last night, and that's why the nurse gave me the shot." As children near age 5, they begin to use or can be taught to use rules to understand causation. They then begin to reason from the general to the particular. This forms the basis for more formal logical thought.

The preschooler's moral development expands to include a beginning understanding of behaviors considered socially right or wrong. The child continues to be motivated, however, by the wish to avoid punishment or the desire to obtain a reward. The preschooler is better able than the toddler to identify behaviors that elicit rewards or punishment and begins to label these behaviors as right or wrong.

Preschoolers' vocabularies increase rapidly. By 5 years of age children use more than 2000 words. They identify colors and body parts and define familiar objects. Language is more social and questions expand to "Why?" and "How come?" The child may confuse phonetically similar words such as "die" and "dye." Because of this limitation and a literal interpretation of words, the preschooler may misunderstand things. The nurse should avoid such words and assess comprehension of explanations when preparing children for procedures.

Preschoolers continue to rely heavily on the support of parents or primary care givers for security but increasingly venture out to initiate contact with other children and adults. Their curiosity and developing initiative lead to actively exploring the environment, developing new skills, and making new friends. Preschoolers have a surplus of energy, permitting them to attempt many activities that may be beyond their capabilities. Guilt arises when they overstep limits and feel they have misbehaved. Erikson (1963) recommends that parents allow children to do things on their own while setting firm limits and providing guidance.

Socially interactive play begins during preschool. Parallel play progresses to **associative play.** By the third birthday, children play with others in similar activity, without organization or division of responsibility. By age 4, children play in groups of two or three, and by age 5 the group has a temporary leader for each activity with pretend (sociodramatic) play becoming more dominant. With play, children learn sex role identification, express questions, fears, anger, and frustration, and develop skills in solving problems and interacting with others. Play also helps the nurse to learn about children and to teach them about health.

Health Concerns

During times of stress or illness, the preschool child returns to a greater reliance on parents for care and comfort. This return to an earlier pattern of behavior, called **regression,** is not limited to the preschool years. It occurs most often when people experience stress they are unable to relieve with current coping behaviors. Regression involves stepping back to a more comfortable behavior. Parents need reassurance of the normality of this behavior.

Parental beliefs about health, children's bodily sensations, and their ability to perform usual daily activities help children develop attitudes about their own health. Preschoolers are usually quite independent in washing, dressing, and feeding. Alterations in this independence can influence feelings about their health.

TEACHING TOPICS FOR PARENTS OF PRESCHOOL CHILDREN

- Expected growth parameters and developmental tasks
- Nutritional requirements for optimal growth
- Methods to stimulate continued progress in the development of motor, language, cognitive, and social skills
- Signs of common childhood communicable diseases and measures to reduce their risk and spread
- Safety measures including limit setting, choosing developmentally appropriate toys, environmental adjustments
- Criteria to use when evaluating preschool education programs
- Teaching methods used to help preschoolers learn about their health, including nutrition, exercise, rest, and safety
- Child abuse, including how to protect children, identifiable signs of abuse, and community agencies available for assistance

Families have a major effect on the health status of their children. Keltner (1992) found that children had higher health levels if their families followed a routine for daily life activities and created a stimulating home environment. Parents often require and seek guidance from the nurse as they strive to facilitate optimal growth and development of their preschoolers (see box on left).

SCHOOL-AGE CHILD

During the **"middle years"** of childhood (ages 6 to 12), the foundation for adult roles in work, recreation, and social interaction is laid. Great developmental strides are made in physical, cognitive, and psychosocial skills (Table 20-6). Children become "better" at things. For example, they can run faster and farther as proficiency and endurance develop.

The school or educational experience expands the child's world and is a transition from a life of relatively free play to a life of structured play, learning, and work. The school and home influence growth and develop-

table 20-6

DEVELOPMENTAL BEHAVIORS OF SCHOOL-AGE CHILDREN AND ADOLESCENTS

School-Age children	Adolescents
RELATIONSHIPS WITH PARENTS	
Children learn that parents are less than perfect; they can be disillusioned with them and wish that friends' parents were their own. They rely on parents for unconditional love, security, guidance, and nurturing.	Adolescents' desire for increasing independence and autonomy and continuing need for dependence and limit setting by parents place strain on their relationship. Effective communication and democratic parenting are critical.
RELATIONSHIPS WITH SIBLINGS	
School-agers seem to be at odds with one another at home; yet they are each others' best defenders away from home. Younger children often idolize older siblings, leading to competition. Older children may envy attention that younger siblings require and be quite bossy or abusive.	Younger siblings rarely understand their adolescent siblings' need for privacy to think, dream, and talk with peers. Adolescents often enjoy interacting with and guiding younger brothers and sisters when timing is convenient for them and they can remain in control.
RELATIONSHIPS WITH PEERS	
During ages 6 to 7, children of both sexes play together, depending on who is available and interested. Around age 8, social groupings of same-sex peers form. These "gangs" allow children to declare independence from parental rules and establish secret codes or languages and rules of membership and behavior. Period is often referred to as *secret society* of childhood. Preadolescent (10-12 years) friendships are characterized by having best friend of same sex. These relationships may be transient, but they are intense and allow discussion of all areas of life. Some interest in heterosexual relationships develop, but usually are not reciprocal.	Peer group is critical to adolescents, who have increasing need for recognition and acceptance. Companionship of peer groups provides secure environment for individuals to try out new ideas and share similar feelings and attitudes. Adolescents often form cliques with peers from same socioeconomic group with similar interests. Cliques, which are highly exclusive, help their members, who have strong emotional bonds, develop their identities. The crowd, which is more impersonal than a clique, offers opportunities for heterosexual interaction and social activities. The crowd also maintains rigid membership requirements.

table 20-6

DEVELOPMENTAL BEHAVIORS OF SCHOOL-AGE CHILDREN

School-Age children	Adolescents
SELF-CONCEPT	
Children's feelings of competence in mastery of tasks are key elements in forming self-esteem. Children need positive feedback from teachers and parents for their efforts. It is important for children to develop skills in at least one area such as reading or swimming. Pets that require children's care and attention reward them with unconditional love and promote feelings of self-worth.	Formal and informal peer groups shape self-concept of group members. Popularity and recognition within peer group enhance self-esteem and reinforce self-concept. Total involvement in peer group may make it seem that adolescents have no original thoughts and are not able to make decisions. Adolescents who withdraw from peers into isolation struggle with developing identity.
FEARS	
There is decline in fears related to body safety such as storms, dogs, darkness, and scratches. Fears of supernatural such as ghosts persist and decline slowly. New fears are related to school and family. They fear ridicule from teachers and friends and disapproval and rejection of parents. They also become frightened about death and items that they hear on news such as war.	Fears in this age-group center around peer group acceptance, body changes, loss of self-control, and emerging sexual urges. Adolescents often examine their bodies for changes and signs of imperfection. Any defect, real or imagined, is cause of endless worry. Adolescents' developing awareness of economic and political problems may result in fear of going to war.
COPING PATTERNS	
To deal with stress, school-agers use problem solving and defense mechanisms including regression, denial, and aggression. Coping behaviors of hospitalized school-agers include inactivity (total silence, lack of activity, and apathy), orientation or precoping (looking and listening, and asking questions), cooperation, resistance (attempt to get away by turning away or making physical or verbal attacks), and controlling (assuming responsibility for self-care and suggesting how things could be done).	Coping behaviors expand with experiences adolescents have gained from life and from cognitive maturity. By age 15, most use full range of defense mechanisms, including rationalization and intellectualization. Adolescents' problem solving abilities have matured. They can reason through philosophical discussions as well as complex situations. Some adolescents use avoidance coping strategies and attempt to reduce tension by engaging in chemical abuse or avoiding people.
MORALS	
Children learn rules from parents, but their understanding of rules or reasons for them is limited until about 10 years. Before that, they are concerned with own needs first and may cheat to win. After 10, justice is based on "eye for an eye," and punishment should correct situation (e.g., children pay for what they break).	Adolescents begin to internalize expectations of their family and society. Initially, there is much comformity to rules to win praise or approval from others and to avoid social disapproval or rejection; later, they seek to avoid criticism from persons of authority in institutions.
DIVERSIONAL ACTIVITY	
School-agers play cooperatively in group activities such as jumping rope, soccer, and baseball. Play becomes competitive, and children often have difficulty learning to lose. Teasing, insults, dares, and increased sensitivity are common.	Teenagers develop special interests in certain sports and concentrate on developing maximal skills. Recreational activities are determined by what is popular with peers and what can provide independence from parents (e.g., computers, cars).
NUTRITION	
Children have definite likes and dislikes. Few nutritional deficiencies occur in this age-group. Children have voracious appetites after school and need quality snacks such as fruit and sandwiches to avoid empty calorie foods such as chips and candy.	Total nutritional needs become greater during adolescence. Girls' caloric needs decrease, and their need for protein increases slightly. Iron needed by adolescents is almost twice that of adult men, and growth spurt increases calcium demand.

ment. For optimal development to occur, the child must learn to cope with the rules and expectations of school and peers. Parents should learn to allow their child to make decisions, accept responsibility, and learn from life's experiences.

Physical Development

The rate of growth during these early school years is slower than at any time since birth but continues steadily. Growth accelerates at different times for different children. Height increases approximately 2 inches per year. Weight, which is more variable, increases by 4 to 7 pounds per year. Muscle tissue represents an increased percentage of the body weight. Children lose their baby-like contours and appear slimmer as fat decreases and its distribution pattern changes (Whaley and Wong, 1991).

School gives children the opportunity to compare themselves with other children of the same age. Regular measurement of height and weight may reveal alterations in growth that are signs of a variety of childhood diseases. Boys are slightly taller and heavier than girls during these early school years. Approximately 2 years before puberty, they experience a rapid acceleration in skeletal growth, and girls, who reach puberty first, begin to surpass boys in height and weight, which often causes embarrassment to both sexes. These changes may begin as early as 9 years of age in girls and 12 years of age in boys.

Cardiovascular functioning is refined and stabilized. The heart rate averages 75 to 100 beats per minute, the blood pressure normalizes to approximately 110/65 mm Hg, and the respiratory rate stabilizes to 19 to 21 breaths per minute. Lung growth is minimal. However, by the end of this period the heart has generally reached its adult size.

School-age children become more graceful as they gain increasing control over their bodies. Strength doubles, and large muscle coordination improves. Participation in the basic gross motor skills of running, jumping, balancing, throwing, and catching refines neuromuscular function and skills.

Fine motor coordination improves. Most 6-year-old children can hold a pencil adeptly and print letters and words. By age 12 the child can make detailed drawings and write sentences in script. Assessment of neurological development is often based on fine motor coordination. Teachers frequently ask school nurses to conduct fine motor assessment of children with questionable ability. Nurses need to know the items that constitute normal fine motor functioning and should refer the child with deviations for more comprehensive assessments.

Other physical changes take place during the school-age years. A steady skeletal growth in the trunk and extremities occurs, and small and long bone ossification is present but not complete by age 12. Facial bones grow and remodel as indicated by the presence of frontal sinuses by age 8 or 9. Dental growth is prominent. By 12 years of age, all primary teeth have been shed and the majority of permanent teeth have erupted. As skeletal growth progresses, overall body appearance and posture change. Earlier posture, which was characterized by a stoop-shouldered, slightly lordotic stance and prominent abdomen, changes to a more erect posture. Eye shape alters as a result of skeletal growth. This improves visual acuity, and normal adult 20/20 vision is achievable. Screening for vision and hearing problems is easier, and results are more reliable because school-age children can more fully understand and cooperate with test directions. The school nurse typically assesses the dental, visual, and auditory status of school-age children biannually and refers any problems to a pediatrician.

Cognitive Development

Cognitive changes provide the school-age child with the ability to think logically about the here and now but not about abstraction. The thoughts of school-agers are no longer dominated by their perceptions, and thus their ability to understand the world greatly expands. Around 7 years of age, children enter Piaget's third stage of cognitive development, known as **concrete operations,** in which they are able to use symbols to carry out operations (mental activities) in thought rather than in action. They begin to use logical thought processes and concrete materials (objects, people, and events they can touch and see).

Children in this stage are much less egocentric than younger children and develop the ability to decenter (concentrate on more than one aspect of a situation). They also develop reversibility (ability to trace a line of thinking back to its origin). Both of these cognitive skills allow the child to use conservation (ability to recognize that the amount or quantity of a substance remains the same even when its shape or appearance changes). By age 7 or 8, the child can place objects in order according to their increasing or decreasing size. The mental process of classification becomes more complex as the child develops the ability to separate objects into groups according to more than one aspect or quality (e.g., shape, color, and size). During the school-age years, children refine their understanding of spatial relationships. This is reflected in their ability to move around their neighborhood and read simple maps.

Middle childhood youngsters can use their newly developed cognitive skills to solve problems. Some are better than others at problem solving because of native intelligence, education, and experience, but all children can improve these skills. Middle school-agers who are good problem solvers demonstrate a positive attitude.

They see the problem can be solved with persistence, a concern for accuracy, and the ability to avoid guessing while searching for facts. Problem solving can be improved by helping children to define the problem and its nature, plan their solution carefully, and evaluate their plan and the solution (Dacey and Travers, 1991). Nurses can use these strategies to help school-agers assume responsibility for their general health and understand an illness and its treatment.

Language growth is so rapid it is no longer possible to match age with language achievements. The average 6-year-old child has a vocabulary of 8000 words that quickly expands with exposure to peers, adults, and reading materials. These children are less bound by the restrictions of their family's language and, by the end of this period, their language is similar to adults. They become more aware of the rules of syntax. School-age children can identify generalizations and exceptions to rules. They accept language as a means for representing the world subjectively and realize that words have arbitrary, rather than absolute, meanings. They can use different words for the same object or concept, and they understand a single word may have multiple meanings. "Bad language" may be used to gain status among their peers and to shock adults.

Psychosocial Development

During the school-age years the child's psychosocial development is influenced by physical and cognitive skill development. Most school-age children demand independence in activities of daily living because of their improved fine motor skills. They develop strong preferences for how their needs are met. An adult's introduction or suggestion of new practices, styles of clothing, or food can meet strong resistance. The nurse who tries to change the activities of daily living of children needs to consider their need for independence. School-age children should be involved in any decisions about changes and the specific actions for implementing them. Children who are ill or hospitalized should be allowed to participate in their care and maintain as much independence and control as possible.

Group and personal achievements become important to the school-age child, stimulating a sense of achievement. Success is important in physical and cognitive activities. Play involves peers and the pursuit of group goals (Figure 20-9). Although solitary activities are not eliminated, they are overshadowed by group play. Learning to contribute, collaborate, and work cooperatively toward a common goal becomes a measure of a success.

The school-age child prefers same-sex peers to opposite-sex peers. In general, girls and boys view the opposite sex negatively. Peer influence becomes diverse during this stage. Conformity is evidenced in mannerisms, clothing styles, and speech patterns that are reinforced and influenced by peer contact. Group identity increases as adolescence approaches.

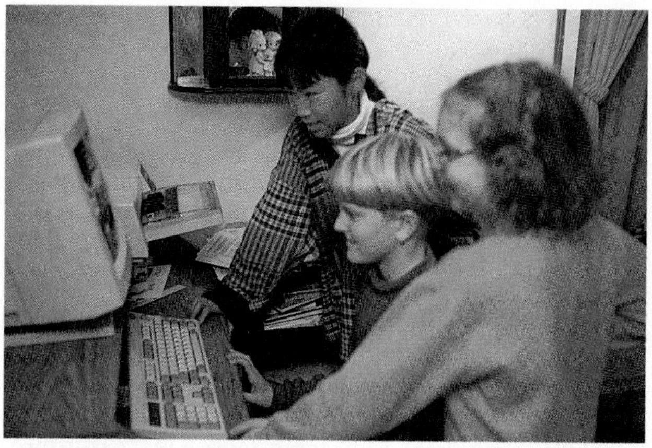

FIGURE 20-9 School-age children gain a sense of achievement when playing with peers.

Many researchers believe school-agers have a great deal of interest in their sexuality and engage in sex play and masturbation. Children hide it, however, because of adult disapproval. During the school-age years children also begin to develop a moral code. Between 6 and 9 years of age they recognize and label behaviors as right or wrong, good or bad. This labeling is influenced by their family and culture. Gradually children apply these labels to personal behavior based on the pleasurable or unpleasurable results of an action. As they progress through the school-age years, children become more concerned with activities that maintain and support society's norms. Peers, school, and society begin to influence behavior labeling. Children between 9 and 12 years of age are concerned with conformity, loyalty, and behavior. This concern not only gains approval but also helps others.

The need for a moral code and social rules increases as school-age children's cognitive abilities and social experiences increase. Children view rules as necessary principles of life, not just dictates from authorities. In the early school years, children strictly interpret and adhere to rules. As they develop, they make more flexible judgments and evaluate how rules apply to a given situation. Late school-age children consider motivations and actual behavior when making judgments about the way their behavior will affect themselves and others. The ability to be flexible when applying rules and to understand the perspective of others is essential in developing moral judgments.

Health Concerns

During the school-age years, identity and self-concept become stronger and more individualized. Perception of wellness is based on facts such as the presence or absence of illness and the adequacy of eating or sleeping. Functional ability is the standard for personal health and the health of others. Promotion of good health practices is a nursing responsibility. Programs directed at health education are frequently organized and conducted in school. During these programs, the nurse discusses developing behaviors that positively affect children's health status. Nurses use health assessment tools such as the questionnaire developed by Antwerp and Spaniolo (1991) to increase children's and parents' awareness of activities that promote health and prevent injury. Children's developing cognitive and psychomotor skills allow them to become more involved in promoting their own health and managing chronic illness (see box below).

A school-age child's nutritional requirements remain relatively stable. Nutritional problems such as obesity and deficits of vitamin A, iron, or calcium can develop. A balanced diet that includes a variety of nutritious foods for meals and snacks ensures nutritional intake to support growth and provide energy for activities. Children can learn about the principles of good nutrition and put them into practice by helping to plan and prepare their own lunches and snacks. In addition, the physical examination for the first grade is an excellent time for the nurse to discuss with the child and parents the influences of genetics, nutrition, and exercise on height and weight.

TEACHING TOPICS FOR SCHOOL-AGERS AND THEIR PARENTS

- Expected growth parameters and developmental tasks including the middle childhood growth spurt and puberty
- Measures to enhance adjustment to school and reduce school-related stressors
- Influence and importance of peers
- Development and expression of sexuality including sex play
- Recreational safety including helmets for sports and bicycling
- Substance abuse (tobacco, alcohol, drugs) including dangers, signs of use, and available community agency support
- Measures to facilitate development of cognitive skills (reading out loud, appropriate use of television, family discussions regarding school performance and homework), and decision-making skills including weighing the consequences of actions taken
- Responsibility for health promoting activities including nutrition, exercise, safety

Accidents and injuries are major health problems affecting school-age children. Motor vehicle accidents and accidents related to recreational activities or equipment are the leading causes of death or injury for these children. According to the U.S. Preventive Services Task Force, safety belt use by children older than age 5 could reduce fatalities by 50% and injuries by 65%. School-age children are also significantly affected by cancer, birth defects, homicide, and heart disease (Department of Health and Human Services, 1989). In this age-group these problems have a relatively low mortality but a high morbidity as compared with accidents. Infections, especially respiratory, account for nearly 80% of all childhood illnesses. Colds are the most common illnesses of childhood. Certain groups of children are more prone to disease, often because they cannot get proper health care. These include homeless children, children who were low–birth-weight infants, foreign-born adopted children, and children who are homeless or suffer chronic illness (Bell et al., 1989). Involvement with social and health care reform is necessary if the nurse wants to positively influence the health of children.

Children often require an assessment of their health status before entering school. Nurses can assess the child's readiness for school by using a variety of developmental screening tools. For example, the Denver Developmental Screening Test (DDST), Pediatric Examination of Educational Readiness (PEER), and Early Screening Inventory (ESI) can be useful. Parents can learn to help their children get ready for and succeed in school. Referral can be made as appropriate to deal with identified risk factors or delays (Wilson and Knudtson, 1992). Speech, hearing, and vision must also be evaluated periodically because problems can affect the child's academic performance.

It is important to know potential school-related stressors, and the nurse should help parents to plan for minimizing them. These stressors include adjusting to teachers' expectations and disciplinary actions, maintaining self-concept, competing with peers, testing new behaviors, assuming responsibility, and setting behavioral standards.

PREADOLESCENT

Today children experience more emotional and social pressures than youngsters 30 years ago. As a result, children 10 to 12 years of age are now having experiences that were once unique to 13- and 14-year-old youths. This transitional period between childhood and adolescence is often referred to as **preadolescence.** Some refer to this period as late childhood, early adolescence, pubescence, and transescence. Physically it refers to the beginning of the second skeletal growth spurt, when the physical changes such as the development of pubic hair and female breasts begin. Children also become more social, and their behavioral patterns become much less predictable. This preparatory period often includes experimentation with makeup by girls and an interest in music and performers popular among older adolescents. Both sexes usually develop "best friends" with whom they share intimate feelings. New interest in the opposite sex develops, but little activity other than talk usually occurs. Youths of both sexes often develop a friendship with adults other than their parents (ego ideal), which allows them to acquire information about adults.

ADOLESCENT

Adolescence is the transition from childhood to adulthood, usually between 13 and 18 years of age. The term **adolescence** refers to the psychological maturation of the individual, whereas **puberty** refers to the point when reproduction is possible. This period is characterized by a steady progression of physical, social, cognitive, psychological, and moral changes. The adaptations required by these changes push adolescents to develop individualized coping mechanisms and styles of behaviors, which they will continue to use or adapt throughout life. Most teenagers successfully meet the challenges of this period (see Table 20-6).

During this stage of development an adolescent must establish an identity, make major decisions regarding life and a vocation, develop and refine adult cognitive skills, and establish a code of morality by which all of these tasks are ordered. The nurse's understanding of adolescents' developmental tasks provides a unique perspective for helping teenagers and their parents anticipate and cope with the stresses of adolescence. Nursing activities, particularly education, can promote healthy development. These activities occur in a variety of settings and are directed toward the adolescent, parents, or both.

Physical Development

Although timing varies greatly, physical changes occur rapidly during adolescence. Sexual maturation occurs with the development of primary and secondary sexual characteristics. Primary characteristics are physical and hormonal changes necessary for reproduction. Secondary characteristics externally differentiate males from females.

Height and weight increases usually occur during the prepubertal growth spurt. The growth spurt for girls generally begins between 8 and 14 years of age, with height increases of 2 to 8 inches and weight increases of 15 to 55 pounds. The male growth spurt usually takes place between 10 and 16 years of age, with height increases of approximately 4 to 12 inches and weight increases of 15 to 65 pounds. Personal growth curves continue to be meaningful in assessing physical development. The individual's sustained progression along the curve, however, is more important than how closely measurements correspond to the norm.

Girls attain 90% to 95% of their adult height by **menarche** (the onset of menstruation) and reach their full height by 16 to 17 years of age. Boys continue to grow taller until 18 to 20 years of age. Fat is redistributed into adult proportions as height and weight increase, and gradually the adolescent torso takes on an adult appearance.

Adolescents are sensitive about physical changes that make them different from peers. Thus they are generally interested in the normal pattern of growth, as well as in their personal growth curves. The nurse may share this information to reassure adolescents their own patterns are normal. If an adolescent deviates radically from the usual pattern, further assessment is necessary. Weight extremes resulting from excessive or inadequate caloric intake are common during the adolescent years. Allowing the adolescent to see weight curve changes can be a first step in identifying the problem and implementing dietary changes.

Puberty

A wide variation exists between the sexes and within the same sex as to when the physical changes of puberty begin. This variation is more pronounced in boys (Tanner and Whitehouse, 1982). Boys who mature early have been shown by some research to be more poised, relaxed, good-natured, skilled in athletic activities, and more likely to be school leaders than boys who mature late. In contrast, girls who mature early have been found to be less sociable and more shy and introverted, perhaps from feeling so conspicuous (Papalia and Olds, 1989). The sequence of pubertal growth changes is the same in most individuals (Table 20-7). Ranges of normal should be used when assessing progress of growth. As with increases in height and weight, the pattern of sexual changes is more significant than their time of onset. Large deviations from normal time frames require attention.

Being like one's peers is very important for adolescents. Any deviation in the timing of the physical changes can be extremely difficult to accept. Therefore the nurse should provide emotional support for adolescents undergoing assessment of early or delayed puberty. Even adolescents experiencing normal pubertal growth may seek confirmation and reassurance.

Visible and invisible changes take place during puberty as a result of hormonal change. The hypothalamus begins to produce gonadotropin releasing factors

table 20-7

AVERAGE SEQUENCE OF PHYSIOLOGICAL CHANGES IN ADOLESCENCE

Age range for girls	Characteristics	Age range for boys
8–14½ (peak: 12)	Beginning of skeletal growth spurt	10½–16 (peak: 14)
8–13	Beginning of breast development	
	Enlargement of testes and scrotal sac	10–13½
8–14	Appearance of straight, pigmented pubic hair, which gradually becomes curly	10–15
	Early voice changes (cracks)	11–14½
	Enlargement of penis and prostate gland	11–14½
10.5–15.5 (average:12¼)	Menarche	
	Spermatogenesis (ejaculation of sperm)	11–17 (average: 13½)
11–18	Ovulation and completion of breast development	
	Appearance of downy facial hair	12–17
10–16	Appearance of axillary (underarm) hair and increased output of oil and sweat-producing glands, which may lead to acne	12–17
10–18	Widening and deepening of female pelvis, with deposition of subcutaneous fat that gives rounded appearance to body	
	Increase in shoulder width	11–21
	Deepening of voice, appearance of coarse and pigmented facial hair, and appearance of chest hair	16–21

that signal the pituitary to secrete gonadotropic hormones. Gonadotropic hormones stimulate the ovarian cells to produce estrogen and the testicular cells to produce testosterone. These hormones contribute to the development of secondary sex characteristics such as pubic hair growth and voice changes and play an essential role in reproduction. Changing hormonal levels are also linked to acne and body odor. Understanding these hormonal changes enables the nurse to reassure adolescents and educate them about body care and needs.

Cognitive Development

The adolescent's social environment and progressive mental changes result in **formal operations,** the highest level of intellectual development, according to Piaget. Young persons with sufficient neurological development to reach this stage may not attain it if they do not have an appropriate cultural and educational environment. Those who are guided toward rational thinking may reach this stage early.

During this period of cognitive development, teenagers develop the ability to solve problems through logical operations. They can think abstractly and deal effectively with hypothetical problems. When confronted with a problem, the teenager can consider an infinite variety of causes and solutions. For the first time the young person can move beyond the physical or concrete properties of a situation and use reasoning powers to understand the abstract. School-agers think about what is, whereas adolescents imagine what might be. They can solve problems that require simultaneously manipulating several abstract concepts. Cognitive development is important in the adolescent's pursuit of identity. For example, the teenager becomes able to define appropriate, effective, and comfortable sex role behaviors and considers their potential impact on peers, family, and society. A higher level of cognition makes the adolescent receptive to more detailed and diverse information about sexuality and sexual behaviors. The complex development of thought also leads adolescents to question society and its values. Although teenagers have the capability to think as well as an adult, they do not have the experiences on which to build. Teenagers commonly consider their parents too narrow minded or too materialistic.

Cognitive abilities and performance vary greatly among adolescents. An adolescent may perform at different cognitive levels in different situations based on past experiences and formal education.

Language development is fairly complete by adolescence, although vocabulary continues to expand. The primary focus becomes developing diverse communication skills that can be used effectively in many situations and refined later in life. Adolescents need to communicate thoughts, feelings, and facts to peers, parents, teachers, and other persons of authority. The skills used in these diverse communication situations are varied. Adolescents must select the person with whom to communicate, decide on the exact message, and choose the way to transmit the message. They develop different skills and styles of communication and learn how and when to use them most effectively.

Psychosocial Development

The search for personal identity is the major task of adolescent psychosocial development. Teenagers must establish close peer relationships or remain socially isolated. Erikson (1968) sees identity (or role) confusion as the prime danger of this stage. Teenagers must become emotionally independent from their parents and yet retain family ties. They also need to develop their own ethical systems based on personal values. Teenagers must make choices about vocation, future education, and lifestyle. The various components of total identity evolve from the accomplishment of these tasks and comprise an adult personal identity unique to the individual.

According to Erikson (1968), the period of adolescence provides a "time-out period" when society allows the physically mature teenager to delay assuming adult responsibilities. This provides time for adolescents to try a variety of ideological and vocational roles before making a commitment. It ends in the selection of values and a consolidation of identity.

Achievement of sexual identity is enhanced by the physical changes of puberty. The physical evidence of maturity encourages the development of masculine and feminine behaviors. If these physical changes involve deviations, the person has more difficulty developing a comfortable sexual identity. Adolescents depend on these physical clues because they want assurance of maleness or femaleness and because they do not wish to be different from peers (Figure 20-10). Sexual identity is also influenced by cultural attitudes and expectations of sex role behavior and available role models. The masculine and feminine behaviors teenagers see and the expectations they perceive for behaving as a man or woman affect how they express sexuality. Adolescents master age-appropriate sexuality when they feel comfortable with sexual behaviors, choices, and relationships.

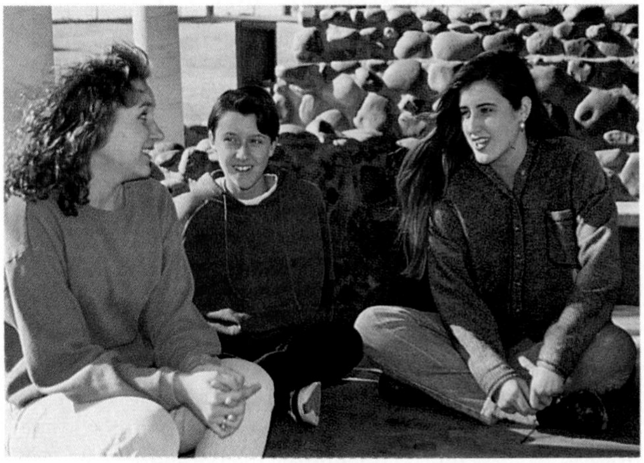

FIGURE 20-10 Adolescents acquire sexual identity from interacting with peers. (Courtesy Michael S. Clement, MD, Mesa, Ariz.).

Adolescents seek a group identity because they need approval, support, and acceptance. Similarity in dress, speech, or recreational activities is common among teenagers as a means of providing security, self-esteem, and confidence. Belonging is a major concern (Whaley and Wong, 1991). Being popular with opposite and same-sex peers is also very important to teenagers. Conforming to group activities, being friendly, being oneself, and having a good personality are considered by teenagers to be the most important factors in gaining popularity (Padin, Lerner, and Spiro, 1981). The strong need for group identity seems to conflict at times with the search for personal identity. It is as though adolescents require close bonds with peers so they can later redefine themselves against this group identity.

The movement toward stronger peer relationships is contrasted with the movement away from parents. Although financial independence for adolescents is not the norm in American society, many adolescents work part-time, using their income to bolster their independence. When adolescents cannot have a part-time job because of studies, school-related activities, and other factors, parents can provide allowances for clothing and incidentals, which encourage adolescents to develop decision-making and budgeting skills.

Some adolescents and families have more difficulty during these years than others. The differences can result from the number, extent, and nature of the movements from periods of independence to relative dependence. Adolescents need to make choices, act independently, and experience the consequences of their actions. This testing is best done against a firm, supportive, family foundation. The family needs to allow independence while providing a haven in which adolescents can contemplate their actions. Families unable to provide this support complicate movement toward identity formation. Nurses can provide essential support by assisting families to consider ways appropriate for them to foster the independence of their adolescent while maintaining the family structure.

One goal for adolescents is to select an occupation or vocational direction in life. Because of society's changing needs, adolescents must be future-oriented when making these choices. However, because the jobs that will be available or that adolescents will find rewarding 10 or 20 years in the future are not clear, selecting a career is complicated. The nurse should provide emotional support during this process and should help adolescent clients consider courses of action that promote self-satisfaction, identity, and continued opportunity for growth.

Developing moral judgment depends heavily on cognitive and communication skills and peer interaction. Although moral development begins in early childhood, it is consolidated more fully in adolescence. Adolescents learn to understand that rules are cooperative agreements that can be modified to fit the situation, rather than absolutes. Adolescents learn to apply rules by using their own judgment rather than simply to avoid punishment as in the earlier years. Adolescents judge themselves by internalized ideals, which often leads to conflict between personal and group values. Group values become less significant in later adolescence. Not all adolescents attain the same level of moral development. However, there is a general forward movement through the stages of moral development, and the sequence of the stages is similar for all individuals.

TEACHING TOPICS FOR ADOLESCENTS AND THEIR PARENTS

Expectations regarding growth and development including sexual maturation

Decision-making skills, communication skills, and coping mechanisms for dealing with peer pressures, parental and adult authority, school-related stressors, college, and career-related goals

Automobile safety including seatbelts, avoidance of alcohol and drugs

Appropriate measures to prevent sexually transmitted diseases and pregnancy including available community agencies for care

Signs and symptoms of depression and substance abuse

Measures to promote and maintain health

Health Concerns

A component of personal identity is perception of health. Healthy adolescents evaluate their own health according to feelings of well-being, ability to function normally, and absence of symptoms. Health problems causing severe or long-term alteration of these factors may permanently alter self-identity. Nurses can assist adolescents to take responsibility for their own health status and practices (see box above).

Physical injuries remain the leading cause of death in adolescence. Between the ages of 15 to 24, 61% of deaths in boys and 39% of deaths in girls are caused by accidental injuries (Whaley and Wong, 1991). Motor vehicle accidents are the most common cause of death (Rivara, 1988). Such accidents are often associated with alcohol intoxication or drug abuse. Other frequent causes of accidental death are drowning, shootings, and poisoning. Feelings of being indestructible lead to risk-taking behaviors. Nurses can help prevent accidental deaths by supporting organizations that promote responsible behavior, including Mothers Against Drunk Driving (MADD) and Drug Abuse Resistance Education (DARE), and encouraging students to participate in Students Against Drunk Driving (SADD).

Substance abuse is a major concern to those who work with teenagers. All adolescents are at risk for experimental or recreational substance use. Those who have unconventional values or come from unstable homes are at greater risk for chronic use and physical dependency. Some adolescents believe substance use makes them more mature, will create a sense of well-being, and improves their level of performance. The nurse can identify those at risk, educate them to prevent accidents related to substance abuse, and counsel those in rehabilitation.

Suicide is the third leading cause of death in persons between 15 and 24 years of age (Valente and Saunders, 1987; Hawton, 1990). Depression and social isolation commonly precede a suicide attempt, but suicide most likely results from a combination of several factors. Nurses should be alert to the following warning signs, which often occur for at least 1 month before a suicide attempt (Mattsson, 1992):

1. Decrease in school performance
2. Withdrawal
3. Loss of initiative
4. Loneliness, sadness, and crying
5. Appetite and sleep disturbances
6. Expressing suicidal thoughts

Immediate referrals to mental health professionals need to be made when assessment suggests an adolescent may be considering suicide. Guidance can help focus on the positive aspects of life and strengthen coping abilities.

Another area of concern is the formation of healthy habits of daily living. Emphasis on exercise, sleep, nutrition, and stress reduction habits is increasing. The nurse must recognize the importance of these habits and identify ways to adapt them to each adolescent.

Sexual experimentation is common among adolescents. Peer pressure, physiological and emotional changes, and societal expectations contribute to heterosexual and homosexual relations. According to Hofferth, et al. (1987), 25% of girls are sexually active by 16 years of age, and most girls and boys are sexually active by 19 years of age. Data collected by the Centers for Disease Control and Prevention (1991) reveal that 22% of teenagers report having had at least four sex partners. The nurse must provide adolescents and their families with sex education and counseling. The degree of sexual activity among teenagers may not change, but the degree of informed, consenting participation can. Adolescent sexual activity can lead to sexually transmitted diseases (STDs) and pregnancy.

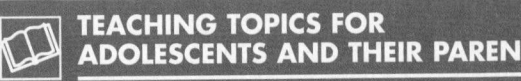

Reports indicate that 63% of all cases of STDs occur in persons younger than 24 years of age (Tyre, Rothbart, et al., 1990). This high degree of incidence requires sexually active adolescents to be screened regularly for STDs. Early identification of such problems as condylomata acuminata (genital warts), chlamydia, gonorrhea, and syphilis through physical examination and diagnostic testing is critical to preserve optimal reproductive health and fertility. Adolescents are also at risk for acquired immunodeficiency syndrome (AIDS) and may need to be tested for the human immunodeficiency virus (HIV). Extensive educational efforts to prevent the spread of AIDS and other STDs should include responsible safer-sex practices, genital-self examination techniques, and the importance of regular physical examinations by a health care professional.

Adolescent pregnancy is common in the United States. One of every 10 adolescent girls (approximately 1 million females under 20 years of age) becomes pregnant. More than 50% of these pregnancies result in birth with most teenage mothers choosing to keep their babies (McAnarney and Hender, 1989; Whaley and Wong, 1991). Pregnancy does not pose a major physical risk to teenagers over 16 years of age as long as they receive comprehensive prenatal care that begins early in their pregnancy and continues throughout. Adolescent mothers, and to a lesser degree fathers, face many social, educational, and economic problems as a result of pregnancy. Nurses can counsel teenagers concerning appropriate measures to use to avoid pregnancy. If teenagers become pregnant, the nurse can guide them in decision-making and help them to obtain needed assistance.

YOUNG ADULT

Adult development involves orderly and sequential changes in characteristics and attitudes. Developmental changes are based on earlier characteristics that help shape subsequent behavior and characteristics (Rawlins, Williams and Beck, 1993). The changes experienced by young adults include the natural processes of maturation and socialization.

Young adulthood is the period between the late teens and the middle to late thirties (Edelman and Mandle, 1990). Young adults increasingly separate from their families, establish career goals, and decide whether to marry and begin families or remain single. They are active and must adapt to new experiences. The transition into middle age occurs when young persons become aware that changes in reproductive and physical abilities signify the beginning of another stage in life. During this transition period, life goals must be reassessed and new goals added.

Maturity involves attaining a balance of growth physiologically, psychologically, cognitively, and socially. Mature individuals are open minded, acknowledge accomplishments and shortcomings, set realistic long-term goals, and learn to cope with stressors. They are open to suggestions and can accept constructive criticism without loss of self-esteem. Tasks are confronted openly, and decision-making techniques are used to solve problems. Mature adults are accountable and responsible for their actions (Schuster and Ashburn, 1986). Young adults pass through alternating periods of stability and change. During periods of stability they make choices and build a structure around them. In periods of change they reevaluate these choices and consider new alternatives (Erikson, 1968, 1982).

Many theorists have attempted to describe the phases of young adulthood and related developmental tasks. These theories provide nurses with a basis for understanding the life events and developmental tasks of the young adult. Levinson (1978) has identified the following phases of young and middle adult development:

Early adult transition (ages 18 to 20), when the person separates from the family and desires independence; entrance into the adult world (ages 21 to 27), when the person tries out careers and life-styles; transition (ages 28 to 32), when the person may modify life activities greatly; settling down (ages 33 to 44), when the person experiences greater stability; and the pay-off years (ages 45 to 65), a time for maximal influence, self-direction, and self-appraisal.

Another theory for young adult development has been proposed by Diekelmann (1976). Diekelmann theorizes that young adults experience the following developmental tasks:

1. Independence from parental controls
2. Development of strong friendships and intimate relationships outside the family
3. Establishment of a personal set of values
4. Development of a sense of personal identity
5. Preparation for life work and the capacity for intimacy

According to Gilligan (1982), women struggle with the issues of care and responsibility, and in turn their relationships progress toward interdependence. As women progress toward adulthood the moral dilemma changes from how to exercise their rights without interfering in the rights of others to "how to lead a moral life," which includes obligations to themselves, their families, and people in general.

Women hope to develop caring and nurturing roles in their male colleagues (Gordon, 1991). Women have long recognized that, without caring, the perceived quality of life is changed. As a result women maintain caring in the home and in educational and work environments. Women become frustrated in their development when the responsibility of caring has not been shared (Benner and Wrubel, 1989).

Physical Development

The young adult completes physical growth by age 20. An exception to this is the pregnant or lactating woman. The physical, cognitive, and psychosocial changes and the health concerns of the pregnant woman and the childbearing family are detailed in a later section.

Young adults are usually quite active, experience severe illnesses less commonly than older adults, tend to ignore physical symptoms, and often postpone seeking health care. The physical characteristics of young adults begin to change as middle age approaches.

Cognitive Development

Rational thinking habits increase steadily through the adult years. Formal and informal educational experiences, general life experiences, and occupational opportunities dramatically increase conceptual, problem-solving, and motor skills. A rich, stimulating environment for the growing and maturing adult encourages the development of full creative potential.

Identifying preferred occupational areas is a major task of young adults. When individuals know their skills, talents, and personality characteristics, occupational choices are easier, and they are generally more satisfied with their choices. In the young and middle adult years, job satisfaction has been found to be a major factor in achievement and responsibility.

An understanding of how adults learn assists the nurse in developing teaching plans for them. Adults come to the teaching-learning situation with a background of unique life experiences. Therefore the nurse should view adults as unique individuals. Their compliance with regimens such as medications, treatments, or life-style changes involves a decision-making process. The nurse should present as much information as the adult needs to make decisions about the prescribed course of treatment.

Because young adults are continually evolving and adjusting to changes in home, workplace, and personal life, their decision-making processes need to be flexible. The more secure young adults are in their roles, the more flexible and open they are to change. Insecure persons tend to be more rigid in making decisions.

Decision making may be proactive or reactive. In proactive decision making the choices made are goal directed. In reactive decision making the choices are made in response to the influence of others (Rawlins, Williams and Beck, 1993). When secure in role, values, knowledge, and beliefs, a person tends to make more proactive decisions. The nurse encourages open-minded, flexible, proactive decision making by helping young adults cope with stressors that may affect their sense of security.

Psychosocial Development

The emotional health of young adults is related to their ability to effectively address personal and social tasks. Certain patterns or trends are relatively predictable. Between the ages of 23 and 28 the person refines self-perception and the ability for intimacy. From 29 to 34 years of age the person directs great energy toward achievement and mastery of the world. The years from ages 35 to 43 are a time of vigorous examination of life goals and relationships. Alterations are made in personal, social, and occupational lives. Often the stresses of this reexamination result in a "midlife crisis," in which marital partner, life-style, and occupation may change.

During the young adult years individuals generally give more attention to occupational and social pursuits. They attempt to improve socioeconomic status through career choices. Career and personal counseling can help individuals to make choices and set realistic goals. The nurse can make appropriate referrals when problems involving socioeconomic status and career or educational issues become apparent.

Ethnic and gender factors have a sociological and psychological influence in an adult's life. An understanding of ethnicity, race, and gender differences enables the nurse to provide individualized care.

Many adults devote a major portion of their energy and interest to their chosen careers. Therefore successful vocational adjustment is important in the lives of most men and women. Successful employment not only ensures economic security but also leads to friendships, social activities, and support from co-workers. The women's movement and the cost of living have made two-career marriages increasingly common. The two-career marriage has both benefits and liabilities. It can increase the family's financial base, and a person who works outside the home is able to expand friendships, activities, and interests. However, stresses may occur as a result of relocations, increased expenditures of physical, mental, or emotional energy, child care demands, household needs, or failure of partners to share responsibilities.

Health Concerns

Physiological Concerns. Young adults are generally active and have no major health problems. However, their fast-paced life-styles may put them at risk for illnesses or disabilities during their middle or older adult years. Risk factors for the young adult's health originate in the community, life-style, and family history. Stanhope and Lancaster (1992) have identified the following risk factors: violent injury and death, substance abuse, unplanned pregnancies, STDs, and environmental or occupational factors. Young adults may benefit from a personal life-style assessment to help them and the nurse identify habits such as smoking, stress, lack of exercise, and poor personal hygiene that increase the risk for cancer, as well as cardiac, pulmonary, renal or other chronic diseases. Research shows that changing unhealthy life-style behaviors reduces selected risk factors.

Violence is the greatest cause of morbidity and mortality in the young adult population. In the 20- to 48-year-old age-group, homicides account for approximately 10% of deaths, motor vehicle accidents for 48.7% of deaths, and suicides for 32.5% of deaths (Stanhope and Lancaster, 1992).

Substance abuse directly or indirectly contributes to morbidity and mortality in young adults. Intoxicated young adults may be severely injured in motor vehicle accidents that also may result in death or permanent disability to others. Dependence on stimulant or depressant drugs can result in overdose and death. It is a misconception that drug abuse occurs only among adolescents. Cocaine is increasingly used by young adults who have families and responsible jobs. A young adult who has recovered from substance abuse is still at risk for long-term effects that surface in middle or older adult years. These include liver disease, cardiovascular and pulmonary disease, chromosome damage, and recurrent infections (Stanhope and Lancaster, 1992).

Unplanned pregnancies, although more common among adolescents, can also have long-term physical and emotional effects if they occur in the young adult years. Such pregnancies can interrupt educational and career goals and affect future relationships, including those formed with the child.

STDs may occur in any sexually active person. Recently, sexual activity with multiple partners has decreased. Many young adults are seeking to establish meaningful relationships before engaging in sexual activity. In addition, partners are encouraged to know one another's previous sexual history and sexual practices (Hayes, Sharp, and Miner, 1989; Khabbaz et al., 1990). STDs have immediate effects such as infection, discharge, and discomfort. They can lead to chronic disorders, infertility, or even death.

A common environmental or occupational risk factor is exposure to airborne particles, which may cause lung diseases and cancer. Such lung diseases include silicosis from inhaling talcum and silicon dust, and emphysema from inhaling smoke. Cancers resulting from occupational exposures may involve a variety of organs.

Life-style habits, particularly those that activate the stress response, increase the risk of illness. Smoking is a well-documented risk factor for pulmonary, cardiac, and vascular diseases in smokers and those exposed to secondhand smoke. Prolonged stress increases wear and tear on the body's adaptive capacities. Stress-related diseases such as ulcers, emotional disorders, and infections can occur. Exercise patterns can affect present and future health status. Research has indicated that exercise producing a sustained increase in pulse rate for 15 to 20 minutes 3 times a week improves cardiopulmonary function by decreasing blood pressure and heart rate. Exercise also decreases fatigability, insomnia, tension, and irritability.

Poor personal hygiene habits can be risk factors. Sharing eating utensils with a person who has a contagious illness increases the risk of illness. Poor dental hygiene increases the risk of periodontal disease. A familial history of a disease may put a young adult at risk for developing the disease in the middle or older adult years. Certain chronic illnesses in the family increase the family members' risk of developing a disease. This family risk is distinct from hereditary disease.

Poor adherence to routine screening schedules can put the client at risk for severe illnesses because of failed early detection. Clients should be encouraged to perform monthly breast self-examination (BSE), testicular self-examination (TSE), and regular genital self-examination. Women should be informed of the benefits and suggested schedule for routine mammography, and men should be informed about the need for regular prostate gland examinations (Chapter 16).

Infertility is defined as the inability to conceive after 1 year or more of regular sexual intercourse (Bobak and Jensen, 1993). An estimated 10% to 15% of all couples are infertile. However, about half of the couples who are evaluated and treated in infertility clinics become pregnant. In about 10% to 20% of couples the cause of infertility is unknown and they remain infertile. In the remaining 30% the cause for infertility is diagnosed but they remain infertile because treatment measures are unavailable or ineffective.

Infertility occurs in both men and women. Infertility in women can result from endocrine or nutritional imbalances, ovulation failure, congenital abnormalities, or infections. In men infertility results from interference with the development of sperm, decreased sperm motility, obstruction in transport of sperm from the testicles to the urethra, and interference with ejaculation of sperm.

For some infertile couples, the nurse may be the first resource identified. In a community or clinic setting where the nurse-client relationship has developed over time, the couple may feel more comfortable expressing their fears and concerns. When fertility problems exist, couples frequently experience a variety of "stages" including disbelief, denial, and anger in trying to deal with the stress (Blenner, 1990). To intervene effectively, the nurse should be familiar with the fertility problem, the couple's stage of coping, and fertility centers for referral.

HALLMARKS OF EMOTIONAL HEALTH

A sense of meaning and direction in life
Successful negotiation through transitions
Absence of feelings of being cheated or disappointed by life
Attainment of several long-term goals
Satisfaction with personal growth and development
When in a stable intimate relationship, feelings of mutual love for partner; when single, satisfaction with social interactions
Satisfaction with friendships
Generally cheerful attitude
Ability to view self realistically
No unrealistic fears

Modified from Stanhope M and Lancaster J: *Community health nursing: process and practice for promoting health,* ed 3, St. Louis, 1992, Mosby.

Psychosocial Concerns. Most young adults have the physical and emotional resources to meet challenges, tasks, and responsibilities. During a psychosocial assessment the nurse can assess for the hallmarks of emotional health (see box above).

The psychosocial health concerns of the young adult are often related to stress involving job or family. Stress can motivate a client to change. However, if the stress is prolonged and the client is unable to adapt to the stressor, health problems can develop.

Job stress can occur every day or from time to time. Most young adults are able to handle day-to-day crises. Situational job stress may occur when a new boss enters the workplace, a deadline is approaching, or the worker is given new responsibilities. Job stress also occurs when a person becomes dissatisfied with the job or responsibilities. Because individuals perceive jobs differently, the types of job stressors vary from client to client.

Family stressors can occur at any time. Family life has peaks, when everyone in the family works together, and valleys, when everyone appears to pull apart. Situational stressors occur during events such as births, deaths, illnesses, marriages, divorces, job losses, and holidays. In some situations, family stressors are the result of marital dissatisfaction, which can have many causes. As with other stressors, some marital stressors can be resolved but others cannot.

Family stress may also occur in the step-family. The high number of divorces and remarriages has greatly increased the number of new family units. These new family groups require the attention of the nurse who is concerned with health maintenance and health promotion. A nurse's anticipatory guidance to step-family members reduces feelings of isolation, fear, and stress. The nurse teaches the family members that feelings of grief and loss are to be expected and are actually a healthy response to a major life transition. Bargaining with a supreme being, self, and other family members can be expected as new family ties and traditions are established. Bargaining is a difficult process, and the individual reaches out for strength from others. Step-family members develop new community and friendship networks and a unique family identity.

Stress is also common in single-parent families. The single parent often experiences stress related to being the sole wage earner, disciplinarian, problem solver, and decision maker. The single parent needs a support system that can provide advice, financial support, and a respite from day-to-day decision making.

Adult Sexuality

Physical development is accompanied by the ability to perform sexual acts. Young adults usually have the emotional maturity to complement their physical ability and therefore are able to form mature sexual relationships. For young adults, the psychodynamic aspect of sexual activity is as important as the type or frequency of sexual intercourse. To maintain total wellness, adults should be encouraged to explore various aspects of their sexuality and be aware that their sexual needs and concerns evolve.

The nurse should be able to recognize the normal anatomical and physiological features of the adult sexual organs. This is important in assessing health alterations and in assisting clients to understand abnormalities in sexual response.

Female Sex Organs. The female genitalia comprise external and internal sex organs (see Chapter 16). The external sex organs consist of the mons veneris, labia majora, labia minora, and vaginal opening. The vagina, uterus, fallopian tubes, and ovaries constitute the internal sex organs. The breasts are not a part of the external or internal sex organs but rather are considered secondary sex characteristics (physical characteristics other than genitals that distinguish females from males).

MENSTRUAL CYCLE. The **menstrual cycle** is the process by which the ovaries develop an ovum for fertilization and the uterus prepares its lining (endometrium) for implantation of a zygote (fertilized ovum). This cycle lasts an average of 28 days. **Menarche,** the onset of a girl's first menstruation, usually occurs between 11 and 15 years of age. **Menopause,** the cessation of menstruation, usually takes place between the ages of 45 and 50.

The menstrual cycle is a dynamic process involving the hypothalamus and pituitary gland (located in the brain), ovaries, and uterus (Figure 20-11). Hormones travel through the bloodstream to chemically regulate the menstrual cycle. The hypothalamus secretes go-

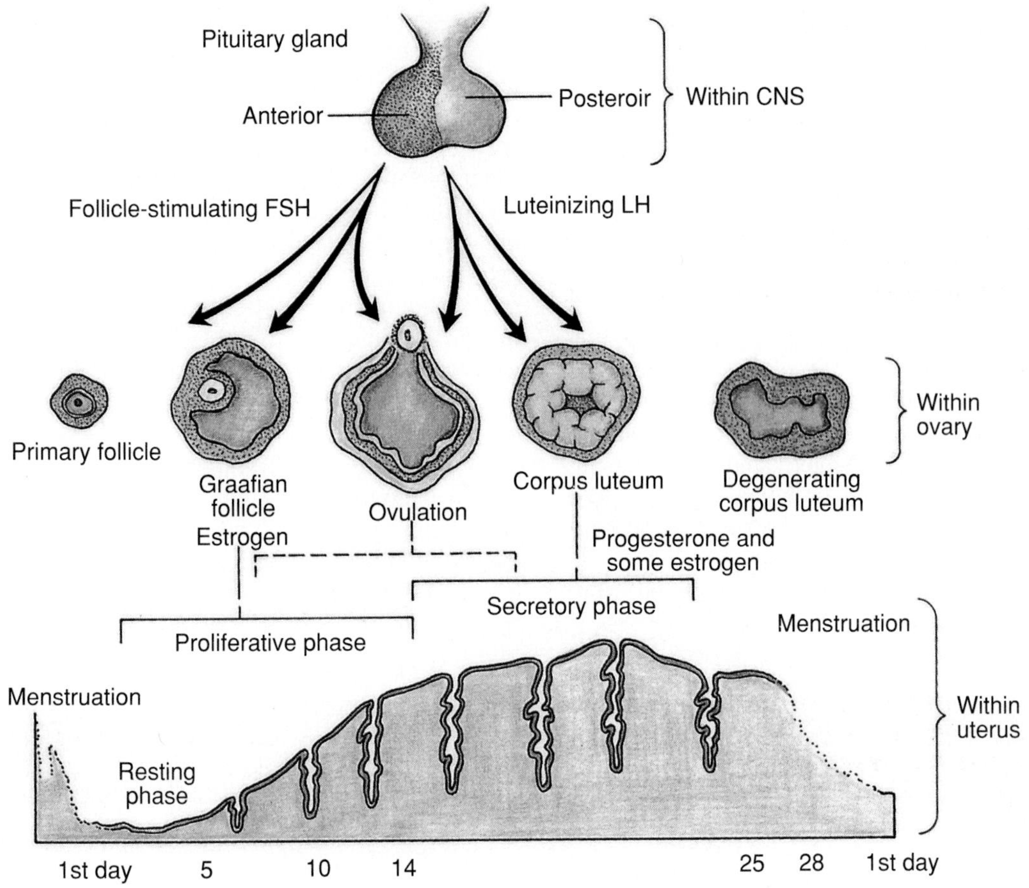

FIGURE 20-11 Hormonal control of menstrual cycle.

nadotropin-releasing hormone, which signals the pituitary gland to produce two hormones that act on the ovaries. Follicle-stimulating hormone (FSH) stimulates the ovaries to prepare for ovulation. Luteinizing hormone (LH) stimulates the release of an egg from an ovarian follicle and the development of the leftover follicle into the corpus luteum. The corpus luteum in turn produces the hormone progesterone.

The menstrual cycle includes three phases: the follicular phase, ovulation, and the luteal phase. During the follicular phase the pituitary gland releases FSH that stimulates the growth of ovarian follicles, clusters of cells around an egg.

Ovulation occurs about 14 days before the beginning of the next menstrual period. A mature follicle ruptures under the influence of the LH. The released egg begins its journey into and down the fallopian tube. At the mouth of the uterus, the cervical mucus becomes more receptive to sperm by responding to increased estrogen levels.

The last phase of the menstrual cycle is the development of the corpus luteum from the follicle left behind after ovulation. The corpus luteum produces large amounts of the hormones estrogen and progesterone. The progesterone causes thickening or proliferation of the endometrium as the uterus prepares to receive a zygote. If fertilization does not occur, the corpus luteum degenerates and the estrogen and progesterone levels fall, leading to the shedding of the lining of the uterus during menstruation. The lower levels of estrogen and progesterone stimulate the hypothalamus to increase the secretion of gonadotropin-releasing hormone and the cycle begins again.

Male Sex Organs. The male sex organs (see Chapter 16) produce sperm and hormones and provide a system for conveying sperm from the testicles to outside the body. The external male genitalia are the penis and scrotum. The male internal sex organs include the testicles (which produce hormones and sperm), the epididymis and vas deferens (a system of ducts that transport sperm), and the prostate gland, seminal vesicles, and Cowper's glands (whose secretions become part of the ejaculated semen).

Sexual Response Cycle. Masters and Johnson (1970) have defined a **sexual response cycle** with four phases: excitement, plateau, orgasm, and resolution.

These phases are not absolute. They are strongly influenced by psychological and environmental factors, and their timing and intensity vary from individual to individual (see Chapter 17).

PREGNANT WOMAN AND CHILDBEARING FAMILY

Physiological Adaptations

Conception, pregnancy, birth, and lactation are the major phases of the childbearing cycle. The changes during these phases are complex. The nurse can assist clients to prepare for this cycle through health teaching in nutrition, anatomy, and physiology and by discussing feelings and attitudes toward childbearing and child rearing. Education such as Lamaze classes can prepare the clients to participate in the birthing process.

Women who are anticipating pregnancy benefit from health and risk assessment along with initiating good health practices before becoming pregnant. Life-style adjustments should include a balanced diet, exercise, dental checkups, avoidance of alcohol, and cessation of smoking. Preconception education classes can address the implication of medical, family, and genetic histories, the danger of using drugs, alcohol, and tobacco, and being exposed to environmental teratogens. The role prospective parents play in ensuring a healthy pregnancy and outcome is stressed (Frede, 1993). The physiological changes and needs of the pregnant woman vary with each **trimester** (Table 20-8). The nurse needs to be familiar with these changes, their causes, and appropriate interventions.

First Trimester All women experience some physiological changes in the first trimester. These changes vary from woman to woman. The changes of this trimester are usually subjective. However, if a woman has frequent morning sickness, her family, friends, and

table 20-8

MAJOR PHYSIOLOGICAL CHANGES DURING PREGNANCY

Signs and symptoms	Causes	Appropriate nursing interventions
FIRST TRIMESTER		
Amenorrhea (missed periods)	Fertilization of egg by sperm	Advise client to have pregnancy test.
Positive pregnancy test done at home or in laboratory	Presence of human chorionic gonadotropin (HCG) in urine	Instruct client to obtain prenatal care, avoid all medications not approved by physician, avoid alcohol intake, maintain good nutritional habits, stop smoking.
Morning sickness (nausea and vomiting from sixth week to end of fourth month, which occurs in morning, evening, or all day)	Increased serum hormone levels Psychological response to pregnancy: ambivalence, pride, rejection	Suggest client eat dry crackers on awakening; avoid irritating foods, and have small, frequent meals with fluids between meals. Have client inform physician if intractable vomiting occurs.
Breast enlargement and tenderness, and enlarged nipples	Increased estrogen levels cause hypertrophy of glandular tissue and increased circulation	Advise client to wear supportive bra at all times, even while asleep. Tell client that application of ice packs decreases tenderness.
Urinary frequency and urgency	Pressure of uterus on bladder decreases capacity	Reassure client that frequency decreases as enlarging uterus moves from pelvis up to abdominal region, teach Kegal exercises, recommend to limit fluid at hour of sleep, wear peri pad. Have client inform physician if burning or pain occurs.
Fatigue, lack of energy	Increases in hormone levels Increased nutritional demands Decreased nutritional intake resulting from morning sickness Psychological response	Ensure that client has adequate nutrition, sleep, and rest periods to help decrease fatigue. Instruct client to take prenatal vitamins as prescribed.

Data from Bobak IM, Jensen MD: *Maternity and gynecologic care,* ed 5, St. Louis, 1993, Mosby.

co-workers may suspect she is pregnant. Limited intake resulting from morning sickness may result in a weight gain for this trimester of only a few pounds. Routine prenatal care should begin early.

Second Trimester During the second trimester, the growing uterus and fetus result in both objective and subjective physiological changes. Morning sickness has usually disappeared and the pregnant woman's energy level is restored if her nutritional intake has caught up with the metabolic demands imposed by pregnancy. Weight gain now progresses at approximately 1 pound per week until the end of pregnancy for a total of 26 to 35 pounds. Urinary frequency ceases, allowing the pregnant woman to sleep through the night more easily. The pregnant woman may begin to "show," especially if she is a multiparous woman (experienced two or more pregnancies), and may feel "life" (quickening). In general, the second trimester is relatively free of pregnancy-re-

table 20-8—cont'd

MAJOR PHYSIOLOGICAL CHANGES DURING PREGNANCY

Signs and symptoms	Causes	Appropriate nursing interventions
SECOND TRIMESTER		
Pigmented nipple and areola, hyperpigmentation of abdominal line (linea nigra), mottling of cheeks or forehead (chloasma or "mask of pregnancy"), local or generalized pruritus	Increased levels of melanocyte-stimulating hormone	Reassure client that skin changes are normal and temporary. Instruct client to avoid hot baths and use of soap or lotions, which can dry skin and increase itching.
Hypertrophy of gums (pregnancy epulis), causing gingival swelling and bleeding	Proliferation of interdental papillary blood vessels, resulting in local inflammation and hyperplasia	Teach client good flossing technique, use soft bristle brush. Instruct client to get routine dental checkups and eat well-balanced meals.
Increasing size of uterine fundus: at level of symphysis pubis at 9 weeks, at intraabdominal organs at 12 weeks, between symphysis pubis and umbilicus at 16 weeks, at umbilicus at 20-22 weeks	Growth of fetus	Reinforce nutrition teaching. Advise client to sleep in a lateral position, move slowly, elevate legs at end of day.
Sensation of movement (quickening)	Fetal motion	Instruct client to notify physician if movements are absent or decline. Begin daily fetal movement counts at 27th week.
Braxton Hicks contractions	Expanding uterus and preparation of uterus for labor	Explain that they are irregular, short contractions, not early labor, and that they will continue throughout pregnancy. Instruct client to notify physician if contractions become regular and increase in frequency and duration. Discuss signs of impending labor.
THIRD TRIMESTER		
Increased colostrum (precursor of true milk)	Preparation of breasts for lactation by hormones	Instruct client to wear absorbant breast pads and cleanse with warm water.
Increasing size of fundus: at xiphoid process at 36 weeks; downward position of baby's head by month 9 as determined by palpation (Mother may feel that baby has "dropped" and that pressure on xiphoid process, diaphragm, and stomach is relieved	Descent of baby's head into pelvis (engagement), which may occur at any point from week 36 to onset of labor	Reassure client of baby's growth. Reassure client that baby can be safely repositioned in utero if needed. Reassure client that pregnancy is ending.
Increased urinary frequency, constipation	Pressure on bladder from enlarged fetus; pressure and displacement of colon and decreased gastric motility	Instruct client to reduce fluid intake after 8 PM, increase roughage and fluids in diet, and practice moderate exercise. Avoid laxatives, enemas, and mineral oil.

lated discomforts, allowing the woman and her family time and energy to anticipate the addition of a new member.

Third Trimester During the third trimester, pregnancy related discomforts return, with an increase in Braxton Hicks contractions (irregular, short uterine contractions that are the basis of false labor), fatigue, urinary frequency, constipation, and hemorrhoids. As the uterus enlarges, mobility is impaired and the woman may find it hard to sleep because of nocturia and more vigorous fetal movements. Close to the onset of labor, the woman may have a burst of energy. This period is called nesting, believed by many to signal a rapidly approaching time of delivery.

Parturition The onset of the process of childbirth occurs at approximately 40 weeks' gestation (term) as a result of interrelated maternal and fetal stimuli. The pregnant woman and her partner generally approach labor and birth with both anticipation and anxiety. Uterine contractions begin to occur and progress in duration, frequency, and intensity. They accomplish the cervical changes required to allow fetal passage, fetal descent and placental separation, and prevent postpartum hemorrhage. Uterine contractions are also stressors for both the mother and fetus, causing maternal pain and temporarily interfering with fetal exchange of oxygen and carbon dioxide.

Puerperium The puerperium is a period of approximately 6 to 8 weeks after delivery. During this time the uterus returns to its approximate prepregnancy condition. The uterine lining regenerates. The top layer of lining is sloughed off, and the endometrium re-forms. The sloughed-off layer, referred to as lochia, is excreted through the vagina. Lochial discharge is present in all women who have delivered a fetus, whether the delivery is vaginal or via caesarean section. Lochia changes in character from rubra (bright red) to serosa (pink or brownish) and, finally, to alba (white or yellow). It may continue for 4 to 8 weeks, although the quantity steadily decreases. Body system adaptations including weight gain regress gradually during this period.

Breast changes occur about the third or fourth postpartum day in preparation for **lactation.** The breast becomes firm and tender (engorgement), indicating that milk is available for the infant. The tenderness is relieved by nursing. The mother is encouraged to begin nursing as soon as possible after delivery and to feed using both breasts. She should begin each nursing period using a different breast because the infant sucks more vigorously at the beginning of the nursing period. Alternating holding positions, correct latch on and removal techniques, and breast care measures are critical to preserving the integrity of the nipples and areola.

The greater the quantity of milk consumed, the greater the quantity of milk produced. When the mother decides to decrease the number of breast feedings or the infant's needs decrease, the quantity of milk production decreases. Unfortunately, the demand and supply of lactation is not foolproof, and the woman's breasts may become engorged and painful. Aspirin, if not contraindicated, may decrease the pain. Warm, moist compresses on the breast increase circulation to the breast and reduce engorgement. Manual expression of the milk also relieves engorgement.

The nursing mother must care for her breasts. She should wear a supportive bra, which may be needed continuously if her breasts are tender. She should be instructed to cleanse her nipples and areola only with water and to apply breast milk after a feeding for its lubricating and bacteriostatic qualities. After nursing, the nipples should be exposed to the air to dry thoroughly. If it is impractical for the mother to expose her breasts to the air for 10 to 15 minutes after every nursing, she can dry her breasts with a blow dryer set on cool and held 12 inches from the breast. If the mother notices nipple cracking, she can use nipple shields for the first few minutes of nursing when the infant's suck is the strongest.

Finally, the nursing mother requires a balanced diet, with an additional 500 to 750 calories, depending on the infant's milk requirements. Fluid intake should be increased by 2500 to 3000 ml, with further increases during the hot summer months.

Cognitive Development

Cognitive changes during pregnancy affect both parents and primarily involve sensory perception and needs for education. The pregnant woman generally experiences changes in sensory perception. Temporary changes occur in visual and hearing acuity, taste, and smell. Many pregnant women frequently stroke the abdomen, possibly because of a change in the sensation of touch or other sensory need. She may be using the sensation of touch to initiate bonding with her child (Bobak and Jensen, 1993).

The entire childbearing family needs education about pregnancy, labor, delivery, breast feeding, and integration of the newborn into the family structure (see box on p. 467). Teaching plans should meet the unique learning needs of each trimester and of each family member. Family-centered perinatal education programs address the learning needs of every family member as they arise throughout the childbearing experience (Peterson and Peterson, 1993). Childbirth classes such as Lamaze are scheduled for the third trimester when the pregnant woman and her partner are most motivated to plan for the birth of their baby. Such classes focus on the normal physiological and psychological changes that occur with labor and birth, methods to cope with the stressors of childbirth, and newborn care measures. Many health care centers also offer sibling and grandparent classes. Sibling preparation classes not only reduce the degree of sibling rivalry exhibited by participants but

TEACHING TOPICS FOR THE CHILDBEARING FAMILY

- Expected physiological and psychological adaptations that accompany pregnancy and birth
- Family adjustments to pregnancy and birth, including appropriate techniques to cope with altered family processes and role changes
- Warning signs of pregnancy and birth-related complications
- Signs of impending labor
- Required life-style adjustments including nutrition, work and recreational activity, rest, and stress reduction
- Importance of avoiding use of drugs (unless prescribed by physician), alcohol, and tobacco
- Discomforts that accompany pregnancy, their physiological basis, and effective relief measures
- Sexuality during pregnancy and after birth including changes that can occur, alternative approaches for sexual expression, and postpartum birth control measures
- Birth plan and childbirth options
- Formal education classes available such as Early Bird, Lamaze, Refresher, Sibling Preparation, Grandparent
- Parenting needs, techniques, and child care options
- Healing and recovery following birth including measures to enhance its progress

also enhance parents' ability to cope with the responses of their children to the newborn (Fortier et al., 1991).

Psychosocial Development

Psychosocial changes occur at various times during the 9 months of pregnancy and in the puerperium. The major categories of psychosocial changes involve body image, role, sexuality, coping mechanisms, and stresses during the puerperium.

Although the physical changes of pregnancy are not obvious to others until the second trimester, the woman generally perceives changes in her body during the first 3 months. One change some women consider positive is an increase in breast size, which may make the woman feel more feminine and sexually appealing. Also, because she is pregnant, the woman may take extra time with her hygiene and grooming. The woman having difficulty with morning sickness and fatigue may also have a poor body image. She may be too tired and ill to care about her appearance. Her major goal is often just coping with the effects of morning sickness and fatigue.

Most women, particularly those who are pregnant for the first time, enjoy the second trimester. They are beginning to "show" and start planning their maternity wardrobe. Their energy level has returned to normal, and they have a general feeling of well-being. Because they are able to feel the baby move and hear the heart beat, the baby becomes real to them and they are able to fantasize about the infant's features.

During the third trimester the fetus grows more rapidly. Toward the end of the pregnancy the woman may feel big, awkward, and unattractive. It is important that her family and support group help her to feel more attractive. She should be counseled not to anticipate wearing her prepregnancy clothes home from the hospital. Because the uterus takes time to involute completely, she will need to wear loose clothing for a bit longer.

Pregnancy does not alter a woman's basic sexual response, and sexual activity is not harmful to a normally developing fetus. Often the pregnant woman and her partner need to be reassured about these facts. However, the woman's perception of her body image influences her desire for sexual activity. Some women may feel more attractive and sexually desirable. Others perceive the changes in their bodies as unattractive. A woman may desire cuddling and holding rather than sexual intercourse. Her partner's sexual response may also be affected by her changing body shape and the perception of the fetus as an intruder during sexual activity.

Pregnancy requires many adjustments that the pregnant woman and her partner need to remember. Although childbirth and child rearing are natural, positive experiences, they can also be stressful. The partners may have difficulty coping with a particular stressor such as taking on new roles, juggling financial demands, altering family processes to accommodate the newborn, selecting child care, or participating in childbirth classes. Nurses should keep in mind that such stressors can affect the health of the expectant parents and that methods used to cope with these stressors may be unhealthy. Disturbing data are now revealing that the risk of battering against women appears to increase during pregnancy. Some surveys indicate an even greater risk among pregnant adolescents. Nurses may use assessment tools to detect the signs of abuse before dangerous consequences, such as abortion, stillbirth, preterm birth, and low birth weight occur (Parker and McFarland, 1991; Noel and Yam, 1992). The nurse can help parents overcome these stresses by assisting them to use appropriate measures to reduce stress and to cope with situational crises. A strong social support system that includes family and friends can be a valuable resource for expectant parents.

Health Concerns

Prenatal care is the routine examination of the pregnant woman by a physician (obstetrician, family practitioner), nurse practitioner or certified nurse midwife. Research studies now indicate a strong link between early and ongoing prenatal care and a positive pregnancy outcome, including a reduced incidence of low birth weight (Arnold and Grad, 1992; Willis and Fullerton, 1991).

During the prenatal visit the pregnant woman's weight and blood pressure are monitored, her urine is checked for glucose, acetone, and protein, the fundal height is measured, and the fetal heart patterns and movements are evaluated. Ongoing risk assessments help to identify the potential for developing complications of pregnancy such as pregnancy induced hypertension (PIH), gestational diabetes, anemia, and intrauterine growth retardation (IUGR). Risk factors include age, poor nutritional intake, under or over weight, and preexisting chronic health problems such as diabetes and heart disease.

As part of prenatal care, the pregnant woman should receive guidance concerning nutrition, rest and exercise patterns, stress management, sexuality, and child care. Prenatal care should assist the childbearing family to adjust to the pregnancy by providing opportunities to ask questions, discuss feelings, and experience the developing fetus by hearing its heart beat.

Commonly the new mother will return home feeling helpless, particularly with the current trend toward discharge of low-risk postpartum women and newborns within 12 to 24 hours of birth. Fatigue can add to the new mother's stress and should not only be assessed but also addressed in a nurse's care plan (Gardner and Campbell, 1991). A visiting nurse, as well as supportive family members and friends, can help the new parents, during the transition from hospital to home, to meet physical, emotional, and learning needs. Many childcare books designed to prepare parents for their baby's needs and for their own emotional and social adjustments are available. Nurses should be prepared to recommend those books that are accurate and clear in their presentation.

The mother's return to work can be an added stressor during the puerperium. She may feel guilt, anxiety, relief, or a sense of freedom. Whether a return to work is necessary or desired, the mother may have mixed emotions about leaving her child.

MIDDLE-AGE ADULT

In **middle adulthood,** the adult generally makes lasting contributions through involvement with others. The middle adult years begin around age 35 and last through the late sixties (Edelman and Mandle, 1990). Personal and career achievements have often already been experienced along with socioeconomic stability. Many find particular joy in assisting their children and other young people to become productive and responsible adults. During this period they may also begin to help aging parents. Using leisure time in satisfying and creative ways is a challenge that, if met satisfactorily, will enable middle adults to prepare for retirement.

According to Erikson (1968, 1982), the primary developmental task of the middle adult years is to achieve **generativity,** which is the willingness to care for and guide others. Failure to achieve generativity leads to stagnation, which is manifested by excessive concern for self or destructive behavior toward children and the community.

Havighurst (1972) identifies the following seven developmental tasks for the middle adult:

1. Achieving adult civic social responsibility
2. Establishing and maintaining a standard of living
3. Helping teenage children become responsible and happy adults
4. Developing leisure activities
5. Relating to one's spouse as a person
6. Accepting and adjusting to the physiological changes of middle age
7. Adjusting to aging parents

Men and women must adjust to biological changes of middle adulthood. As in adolescence, middle adults use much energy to adapt self-concept and body image to physiological realities and changes in physical appearance. High self-esteem, a favorable body image, and a positive attitude toward physiological changes are fostered when the adult engages in positive health behaviors. Physical exercise, balanced diets, adequate sleep, and good hygiene practices promote a vigorous, healthy body. Such health habits also support the body during the time when stressors place the individual at risk for acute and chronic illness.

Physical Development

Major physiological changes occur between the ages of 40 and 65. The box on p. 469 summarizes these normal developmental changes. The most visible changes are graying hair, wrinkling skin, and a thickening waist. In men, balding commonly begins during the middle years but may also occur in young adults. Often these physiological changes affect self-concept and body image. The most significant physiological changes during middle age are menopause in women and the climacteric in men.

Menstruation and ovulation occur in a cyclical rhythm in women from adolescence into middle adulthood. **Menopause** is the cessation of menstruation. The ovaries no longer produce estrogen and progesterone, and the blood level of these hormones drops markedly. Menopause typically occurs between 45 and 60 years of age.

The **climacteric** or **andropause,** so named because of the decreased level of androgens, occurs in men in their late forties or early fifties. Throughout this period

PHYSICAL ASSESSMENT FINDINGS IN THE MIDDLE ADULT

INTEGUMENT

Intact
Appropriate distribution of pigmentation
Slow progressive decrease in skin turgor
Graying and loss of hair (Baldness patterns in males established by age 55; hair loss after this time might have other causes)

HEAD AND NECK

Symmetry of scalp, skull, and face
Normal accessory organs of vision

EYES

Visual acuity by Snellen chart <20/50
Pupillary reaction to light and accommodation
Normal visual fields and extraocular movements
Normal retinal structures

EARS

Normal auditory structures and acuity

NOSE, SINUSES, AND THROAT

Patent nares and intact sinuses, mouth, and pharynx
Trachea at midline
Lateral thyroid lobes nonpalpable

THORAX AND LUNGS

Anterior-posterior diameter increased
Respiratory rate 16 to 21 breaths per minute and regular
Ratio of respiratory rate to heart rate 1:4
Normal tactile fremitus, resonance, and breath sounds heard throughout

HEART AND VASCULAR SYSTEM

Normal heart sounds
- Systole: S_1 softer than S_2 at base; diastole: S_1 louder than S_2 at apex
- PMI at fifth intercostal space in the midclavicular line and 2 cm or less in diameter

HEART AND VASCULAR SYSTEM—cont'd

Vital signs
- Temperature 36.7° to 37.6° C (97° to 99.6° F)
- Pulse 60 to 100 (conditioned athlete ≅ 50)
- Blood pressure: systolic, 95 to 140 mm Hg; diastolic, 60 to 90 mm Hg

All pulses palpable

BREASTS

Decreased size owing to decreased muscle mass
Normal nipples

ABDOMEN

No tenderness or organomegaly
Decreased strength of abdominal muscles

FEMALE REPRODUCTIVE SYSTEM

Change in menstrual cycle and in duration and quantity of menstrual flow
"Hot flashes"
Changes in cervical mucosa

MALE REPRODUCTIVE SYSTEM

Normal penis and scrotum
Prostatic enlargement in some individuals

MUSCULOSKELETAL SYSTEM

Decreased muscle mass
Pathological fractures related to osteoporosis
Decreased range of joint motion

NEUROLOGICAL SYSTEM

Appropriate affect, appearance, and behavior, lucidity and appropriate level of cognitive ability
Intact cranial nerves
Adequate motor responses
Responsive sensory system

and thereafter, a man is still capable of producing fertile sperm and fathering a child. After the male climacteric, however, penile erection is less firm, ejaculation is less frequent, and the refractory period is longer (Rawlins, Williams and Beck, 1993).

Cognitive Development

Changes in the cognitive function of middle adults are rare except with illness or trauma. Middle adults can learn new skills and information. Some middle adults use educational or vocational programs to prepare for entering the job market or changing jobs. When caring for middle adults, the nurse should remember that the level of cognitive function is usually unchanged and they are able to participate fully in health education or health promotion programs.

Psychosocial Development

The psychosocial changes in the middle adult may involve expected events such as children moving away from home or unexpected events such as a marital separation or the death of a spouse. These changes may result in stress that can affect the middle adult's overall level of health.

Career changes may occur by choice or as a result of changes in the workplace or society as a whole. In recent decades, middle adults more often change occupations because they find themselves less satisfied with their present employment. In some cases, technological advances or changes in the direction of industry force middle adults to change work situations. Such changes, especially when unanticipated, may result in stress that affects family relationships, self-concept, and financial security for the later years.

The onset of menopause can affect the middle-aged woman's sexual health. With the cessation of ovulation and the inability to conceive, the woman may desire more sexual activity with her partner because pregnancy is no longer possible. Often sexual activity becomes more enjoyable. On the other hand, although menopause does not decrease sexual response, the menopausal woman may feel less sexually attractive and may not be eager to participate in regular sexual intercourse or may feel stress in her sexual relationship with her partner. Menopause centers assist women through this period by providing information, clarifying misconceptions, and establishing a forum for women to share information and provide support for one another (Wilton et al., 1991). The middle-aged man may notice changes in the strength of his erection and a decrease in his ability to experience repeated orgasm. Both men and women may experience stresses related to sexual changes or a conflict between their sexual needs, social attitudes, or expectations.

Marital changes that may occur during middle age include death of a spouse, separation, divorce, and the choice of remarrying or remaining single. A widowed, separated, or divorced client goes through a period of loss and grief in which it is necessary to adapt to the change in marital status. If the single middle adult decides to marry, the stressors of marriage are similar to those for the young adult. In addition, the couple may have to cope with the social expectations and pressures related to middle-aged marriage.

The departure of the last child from the home of the middle-aged parents may be a stressor. Many parents welcome freedom from child-rearing responsibilities, whereas others feel lonely or without direction. Parents may need to reassess relationships, resolve conflicts, and plan for the future.

The increasing life span in the United States and Canada has led to increased numbers of older adults in the population. Therefore greater numbers of middle adults must address the personal and social issues confronting their aging parents (Scharlach, 1990). Housing, employment, health, and economic realities have altered the traditional social expectations between generations in families. The middle adult and the older adult parent may have conflicting relationship priorities. Negotiations and compromises are useful in defining and resolving such problems. The nurse can help identify the health needs of both groups and can assist the multigenerational family in finding health and community resources needed.

Health Concerns

Physiological Concerns. Because middle adults experience physiological changes and face certain health realities, their perceptions of health and health behaviors are often important factors in maintaining health. Individuals today are more prone to stress-related illnesses such as heart attacks, hypertension, migraine headaches, ulcers, backache, arthritis, and cancer.

When middle adults seek health care, the nurse focuses on the goal of wellness to evaluate health behaviors, life-style, and environment. More middle adults are interested in health promotion activities. Exercise and fitness clubs, for example, give adults the opportunity to participate in many physical activities (Figure 20-12). Attention to risk factors that can be altered to improve the client's health can add years to the client's life and increase its quality.

The nurse acts as teacher and facilitator in helping the client form positive health habits. By providing information about how the body functions and how habits are formed and changed, the nurse raises the client's level of knowledge regarding the potential impact of behaviors on health. The nurse can help an adult client adjust through the changes imposed during middle adulthood, including the effects of aging and altered family processes. Those who have a realistic vision of these changes, positive strategies planned for dealing with them, and supportive relationships are more likely to meet the challenges of the transition effectively (Frank, 1991).

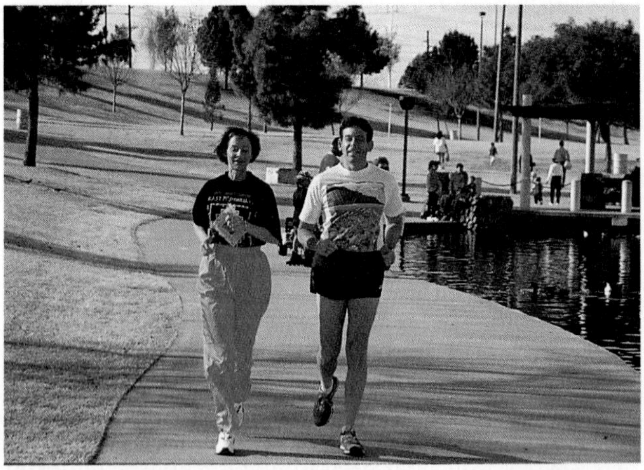

FIGURE 20-12 Jogging is a favorite activity of many middle adults. (Courtesy Michael S. Clement, MD, Mesa, Ariz.).

Psychosocial Concerns. Two common psychosocial health concerns of the middle adult are anxiety and depression. Adults are often anxious about the physiological and psychosocial changes they experience as they enter middle age. Such anxiety can motivate the adult to rethink life goals and can stimulate productivity. For some adults, however, this anxiety precipitates psychosomatic illness and preoccupation with death. In this case the middle adult views life as half or more over and thinks in terms of the time left to live (Rawlins, Williams and Beck, 1993). A life-threatening illness, marital transition, or job stressor increases the anxiety of the client and family. The nurse may need to use crisis intervention or stress management techniques to help the client to adapt to these changes positively to foster continued growth.

Depression is common among adults in the middle years and may have many causes. The risk factors for depression include social isolation, losses, and a family history of depression. Depression during the middle years, often referred to as agitated depression, is characterized by moderate to high anxiety, bizarre physical complaints, and paranoid thoughts. Depression may be worsened by the abuse of alcohol or other substances. The nurse should refer a severely depressed client to a mental health care professional.

Health Promotion. Community health programs for young and middle adults are designed to prevent illness and promote health, as well as to detect disease in the early stages. Nurses can contribute to community health by planning screening and teaching programs. Family planning, birthing, and parenting skills are program topics in which adults might be interested. Screening for diabetes, hypertension, eye disease, and cancer is a good opportunity for the nurse to perform assessment and provide health teaching and counseling. Increasingly, employers are expressing interest in the health of their employees. This interest has resulted in workplace health promotion and fitness programs (Pencak, 1991).

Health education programs can promote changes in behavior and life-style. The nurse as health teacher offers clients information that will enable them to make informed decisions regarding health practices. With health counseling the nurse and client design a plan of action that promotes the client's health and well-being.

Regardless of the age of family members and the structure of the family, adults face certain health tasks. The nurse understands the autonomy of the family and supports it while promoting family health.

OLDER ADULT

Older adulthood traditionally begins after retirement, usually between 65 and 75 years of age. The number of people in this age-group is increasing dramatically, and demographers project a continuing increase in the older adult population well into the next century (Table 20-9). Health professionals are spending increasing time with older persons in all health care settings. Therefore they must focus on identifying and meeting their special needs. Older adults are seeking greater participation in identifying, defining, and resolving issues affecting them. A greater incidence of chronic health problems, technological advances, and contemporary economic, social, ethical, and health issues has prompted health care professionals to focus on improving the duration and quality of life (Stanhope and Lancaster, 1992).

Increased life expectancy and decreased birth rate have contributed to this "graying" population. The number of persons age 85 and older is expected to steadily increase. The life expectancy at birth for men born in the urban United States is 71 years. For women it is 79 years (Ebersole and Hess, 1990). The older adult population is expanding in all cultural and ethnic groups in the United States and Canada. In the United States, blacks comprise approximately 8% of persons 65 years and older. This is expected to increase to 11% by 2000 (Stanhope and Lancaster, 1992). Older adults are distributed among the states in the same pattern as the total population. However, concentrations are found in some larger states, as well as the Northeast and North Central regions (Yurick et al., 1989).

Nursing care of older adults poses special challenges because of diversity in clients' physical, cognitive, and psychosocial health. Older adults vary in level of function and productivity. Before making a health assessment, the nurse should be aware of the normal expected findings of physical and psychosocial assessment for an

table 20-9

POPULATION GROWTH AND PROJECTIONS FOR OLDER ADULTS

Year	Number*	Total population†
1960	16.6	5.8
1970	20.1	7.1
1980	25.7	8.3
1990	31.5	10.3
2000	34.8	13.3
2010	38.3	15.5
2020	52.0	12.5
2030	85.6	17.4
2040	85.1	18.0

From U.S. Bureau of the Census: *Statistical abstract of the United States,* Washington, DC, 1990, The Bureau.
*In millions.
†Percentage.

older adult and should consider the normal changes of aging.

Geriatrics is the branch of health care dealing with the physiology and psychology of aging and with the diagnosis and treatment of diseases affecting older adults. Gerontology is the study of all aspects of the aging process and its consequences. Although research concerning the health needs of older adults has increased greatly, many myths and stereotypes about this age-group persist. Some of these stereotypes depict older adults as people who lack understanding, have difficulty remembering, are rigid, spend most of their time drowsing, and are unpleasant to others. Many people believe that most older adults are institutionalized. In fact, only about 5% are in institutions (Ebersole and Hess, 1990). Most older adults are physically active, intelligent, and socially engaging.

The incomes of most older adults are fixed or do not rise as quickly as inflationary increases. Many people incorrectly believe that older adults have decreased learning ability. As a result, health care professionals often fail to provide health education opportunities for older adults (Stanhope and Lancaster, 1992). Many nurses will find that older adult clients often become the teachers because of their wealth of experiences.

Many misconceptions exist concerning older adults and sex. Older adults are thought to be without sexual desire for a variety of reasons (see box above). In reality, the older adult still experiences sexual drive and activity, although these may be altered because of physiological changes, sociocultural expectations, health problems, and medications.

The concept of ageism, discrimination against people because of increasing age, has developed because of a cultural emphasis on youth. However, ageists are usually dimly aware that someday they too will be old. Unfortunately, when we allow a youthful image to dominate society, we lose touch with the most diversified segment of our population. Older adults have a unique perspective on many social, economic, and technological developments.

A nurse may enter the profession with certain preconceptions about older adults. To provide correct and individualized care for these clients, a nurse may first need to clarify values. The nurse must learn to distinguish between myth and reality and be able to identify clients' strengths and weaknesses.

COMMON MYTHS AND MISCONCEPTIONS ABOUT SEX AND AGING

Sex does not matter. The later years are supposed to be (and usually are) sexless.
Interest in sex is abnormal for older people.
After a spouse dies, the surviving spouse is not interested in sex.
It is all right for older men to seek younger women as sex partners, but it is ridiculous for older women to be sexually involved with younger men.
In institutions, older people should be separated according to sex to avoid problems for the staff and criticism by families and the community.
Emission of semen during sexual activity weakens men and therefore should be avoided in old age.
Masturbation should not continue after adolescence.

Theories of Aging

Biological theories of aging are classified as genetic and nongenetic. Genetic theories include gene theory, error theory, somatic mutation theory, programmed theory, and immunological theory.

Gene theory suggests that harmful genes are activated by aging, resulting in death. The error theory proposes that an error occurs at some point in the molecular development of a cell. As subsequent faulty cells reproduce, the organism's ability to maintain function is adversely affected. Somatic mutation theory suggests that randomly occurring genetic cell mutations result in a decrease in organ efficiency and eventual death. The premise of the programmed theory is that aging may be caused by the cell's loss of ability to exchange genetic information, resulting in cell death.

Nongenetic theories include the immunological, free radical, and cross-link theories of aging. Immunological or autoimmune theory suggests that erratic cellular mechanisms attack body tissues through autoaggression. Some believe that chronic diseases characteristic of old age, such as diabetes and cancer, may be explained by this type of immune dysfunction. The free radical theory stresses the use of oxygen at the cellular level. Oxidation of fat, protein, and carbohydrate produces free radicals, molecules with an extracellular charge. These free radicals attach to other molecules and alter cellular structure and function. The cross-link or connective tissue theory asserts that the molecules of collagen, elastin, and connective tissue form bonds as a result of chemical reactions. These bonds then increase cell rigidity and instability.

The psychosocial theories of disengagement, activity, and continuity attempt to explain psychological development. The development theory states that aging people withdraw from customary roles and engage in more introspective, self-focused activities. In contrast, activity theory holds that the continuation of middle adult activities is the criterion for successful aging. According to this perspective, maintaining optimal physical, mental, and social activity is necessary for successful aging

(Havighurst, 1972). The continuity theory states personality remains the same and behavior becomes more predictable as people age.

All of these theories provide possible explanations to aging, but they raise as many questions as they attempt to answer. Knowledge of these theories helps the nurse understand some of the manifestations of aging from a variety of perspectives.

Developmental Tasks

As in the other stages of life, the older adult has specific developmental tasks. These are described by Burnside (1988), Duvall (1977), and Havighurst (1953) and include seven major categories.

The older adult must adjust to the physical changes of aging. These changes are not associated with a disease state but are the normal changes anticipated with aging. The older adult is also commonly retired from full-time employment and therefore may need to adjust to decreased socialization and reduced income. However, because retirement is usually anticipated, the person may be able to plan ahead to participate in consultation or volunteer activities.

The majority of older adults experience the death of their spouses, friends, and in some instances children. These losses are often difficult to resolve. When the grieving process has ended, the surviving spouse, friend, or parent may need help in identifying other resources to fill the void left by the deceased.

Although aging is inevitable, it is often difficult for older adults to perceive themselves as aging. They may attempt tasks beyond their physical capabilities. The inability to accept the realities of aging is different from merely remaining active and can pose a threat to the client's level of health if physical limitations are exceeded.

An older adult may need to change living arrangements. A change in an older client's living arrangements may require an extended period of adjustment during which assistance and support will be needed from health care professionals and the client's family.

Older adults often need to redefine their relationships with adult children. The issues of role reversal, dependence, conflict, guilt, and loss require recognition and resolution. Often adult children need help understanding that the behaviors of older adults are symptoms rather than inherent meanness, stubbornness, or cantankerousness.

The older adult must also learn to acquire new activities and interests to maintain the quality of life. People vary in their ability to adjust to new circumstances brought on by aging. Persons who have not acquired social and communication skills and who have needed to make new social contacts will have more difficulty in adjusting.

These seven developmental tasks are common to many older adults. The way in which an older adult adjusts to the changes of aging, however, depends on the individual. For some, adaptation and adjustment are easy and without stress. For others, each developmental task presents a major stress for which nursing intervention is needed.

Physical Development

The physiological changes that occur with advancing age vary with each client. Table 20-10 describes the general types of physiological changes that can be expected with older adults. These changes are not pathological processes. They occur in all persons but take place at different rates and depend on accompanying circumstances in an individual's life. The nurse assessing the older adult client should also consider the potential for sensory changes that may influence data gathering.

Cognitive Development

Much of the psychological and emotional trauma of old age arises from the misconception that older adults always have cognitive impairments, that all older adults suffer from memory loss and confusion. Gerontologists have documented that the structural and physiological changes occurring in the brain during the aging process do not necessarily affect the older adult's adaptive and functional abilities (Ebersole and Hess, 1990). Older adults often remain alert and highly perceptive until the time of their death.

Neurophysiological cellular changes vary among individuals, and even with obvious cellular loss some older adults do not have mental deterioration. Furthermore, some clients with significant cerebral cell loss respond well to therapy and regain function. But since cognitive impairment can occur in this age-group, nurses must be aware of the nature and type of these impairments.

Dementia is an irreversible syndrome involving progressive impairment of memory, thinking, judgment, and personality change, which can have a variety of causes. Dementia has three basic components (Ebersole and Hess, 1990). First, cognitive impairments may include memory loss (usually involving recent events), personality changes, and decreased problem-solving ability. Second, neuropathological impairments may result in changes in body functioning, such as ambulation, hygiene activities, elimination, and other activities of daily living. Third, the cognitive and neuropathological changes may lead to immobility, infection, or trauma. Alzheimer's disease is the most frequent cause of irreversible dementia, afflicting 10% to 13% of persons over 75 years of age.

Organic brain syndrome, also referred to as *or-*

table 20-10

NORMAL PHYSICAL CHANGES OF AGING

System	Normal findings
Integumentary	
Skin color	Spotty pigmentation in areas exposed to sun; pallor even in absence of anemia
Moisture	Dry, scaly
Temperature	Extremities cooler; perspiration decreased
Texture	Decreased elasticity; wrinkles; folding, sagging
Fat distribution	Decreased on extremities; increased on abdomen
Hair	Thinning and graying on scalp; axillary and pubic hair and hair on extremities may be decreased; facial hair in men decreased; chin and upper lip hair may be present in women
Nails	Decreased growth rate
Head and neck	
Head	Nasal and facial bones sharp and angular; loss of eyebrow hair in women; men's eyebrows become bushier
Eyes	Decreased visual acuity; decreased accommodation; reduced adaptation to darkness; sensitivity to glare
Ears	Decreased pitch discrimination; diminished light reflex; diminished hearing acuity
Nose and sinuses	Increased nasal hair; decreased sense of smell
Mouth and pharynx	Use of bridges or dentures; decreased sense of taste; atrophy of papillae of lateral edges of tongue; occasionally change in voice pitch
Neck	Thyroid gland nodular; slight tracheal deviation resulting from muscle atrophy
Thorax and lungs	Increased anterior-posterior diameter; increased chest rigidity; increased respiratory rate with decreased lung expansion
Heart and vascular	Significant increase in systolic pressure with slight increase in diastolic pressure; peripheral pulses easily palpated; pedal pulses weaker and lower extremities colder, especially at night
Breasts	Diminished breast tissue; pendulous, flabby condition
Gastrointestinal	Decreased salivary secretions, which make swallowing more difficult; decreased peristalsis; decreased production of digestive enzymes: hydrochloric acid, pepsin, and pancreatic enzymes; constipation
Reproductive	
Female	Decreased estrogen; decreased uterine size; decreased secretions; atrophy of epithelial lining of the vagina; vaginal dryness
Male	Decreased testosterone; decreased sperm count; decreased testicular size
Urinary	Decreased renal filtration and renal efficiency; subsequent loss of protein from kidney; nocturia
Female	Urgency and stress incontinence from decrease in perineal muscle tone
Male	Frequent urination resulting from prostatic enlargement
Musculoskeletal	Decreased muscle mass and strength; bone demineralization (more pronounced in women); shortening of trunk from intervertebral space narrowing; decreased joint mobility; decreased range of joint motion; kyphosis (usually in women)
Neurological	Decreased rate of voluntary or automatic reflexes; decreased ability to respond to multiple stimuli; insomnia; shorter sleeping periods

Modified from Ebersole P and Hess P: *Toward healthy aging: human needs and nursing response,* ed 3, St. Louis, 1990, Mosby.

ganic mental disorder, is any psychological or behavioral abnormality associated with transient or permanent brain dysfunction caused by a disturbance of the physiological functioning of brain tissue. Some organic brain syndromes are acute and potentially reversible, whereas others are chronic with irreversible cerebral impairments. All clients with organic brain syndromes have impairments in attention span, learning, and memory. In addition, some clients have hallucinations, delusions, aphasias, emotional lability, and depression. Acute disorders of organic brain syndrome are potentially reversible. Acute disorders have many causes, including toxins such as lead, diseases, metabolic imbalances, drugs, malnutrition, trauma (especially head injuries), infections, neoplasms, overwhelming stress such as that caused by abrupt translocation or loss, and severe depression. According to Ebersole and Hess (1990), at least 21% of cases of acute organic brain syndrome are misdiagnosed as chronic organic brain disorders. Chronic brain disorders are irreversible and usually progressive. However, with careful and supportive nursing management, clients with chronic brain disorders can remain in their homes.

Alzheimer's disease affects the brain parenchyma. The disease has a gradual course with a progressive decline in cognitive and physical functioning. Nursing management of clients with Alzheimer's disease is complex. The mental and physical changes these clients experience increase their risk of injury. This continually challenges the nurse to identify ways to meet the client's needs. Confusion usually increases at night, and the client may wander through the home. As the disease progresses, communication becomes increasingly difficult. The client may easily misperceive the environment and feel threatened. The typical behavioral responses of the client with Alzheimer's disease who feels threatened include aggressive gestures or acts, increased voice volume, restlessness, agitation, and hostility.

Vascular brain disorders result from arteriosclerotic changes in the brain that impair cerebral circulation and ultimately affect its functioning. Arteriosclerotic dementia has several distinguishing characteristics: periods of remission, preservation of personality, insight, lability of emotion, and epileptoid attacks. The client with cognitive impairment resulting from a vascular disorder may have a history of hypertension, diabetes mellitus, blackouts, falls, or seizures. Some physical impairment such as hemiplegia or hemiparesis is also usually present.

Long-term abuse of alcohol and drugs can affect cognitive functioning. After 15 to 20 years of alcohol abuse, tolerance for drinking declines. Prolonged use of large amounts of alcohol creates central and peripheral nervous system damage. With chronic alcoholism many clients also have vitamin B_1 deficiency. A prolonged deficiency can cause neuropathy, myopathy, and encephalopathy. The exact effects of prolonged drug abuse on the older adult have not been clearly described, but cognitive impairments may occur that are similar to those associated with alcohol abuse. In addition, a drug overdose may cause cerebral impairment. In this case, cognitive impairment may be the result of decreases in oxygen supply and its delivery to the brain.

Psychosocial Development

The older adult must adapt to many psychosocial changes that occur with aging. Although these changes vary among clients, some psychosocial changes are common to most older adults (see box above).

TEACHING TOPICS FOR THE OLDER ADULT

Inform the client about preretirement planning to ease the transition from a full-time work schedule.

Discuss housing alternatives to help the older adult to make a decision regarding the sale of the home, relocation to another area of the country, or retirement communities.

Instruct client about health maintenance programs such as exercise activities, which are designed to increase exercise tolerance, flexibility, and socialization.

Teach client that the need for influenza immunizations increase, especially with chronic illness

Teach client about safe and appropriate administration of prescribed drugs: purpose, effect, possible other prescription, over-the-counter, or dietary interactions, and reportable side effects.

Instruct client regarding environmental safety issues (e.g., lighting, floor coverings, stairs, shoes, electrical cords) to reduce the risk of falling.

Discuss changes in sleep patterns with age and methods to promote adequate rest and energy.

Instruct client about nutritional aspects related to disease (e.g., a low-fat diet with hypertension, or the need for a balanced diet with reduced total calories because of aging changes and lower energy expenditures).

Teach an individual exercise program based on an assessment of the client's overall health status and lifestyle.

Retirement. Retirement in our society often carries associations of passivity and seclusion and thus often leads to psychosocial stresses. These stresses include role changes with the spouse or family and the problems of social isolation. Retirement age varies depending on the individual's occupation and circumstance. An increasing number of companies are developing early retirement plans to provide opportunities for advancement of younger employees. One popular program is the "30 and out" plan, which allows workers to retire with full pension, and in some cases large bonuses, after 30 years. The most powerful factors that influence the retired person's satisfaction with life are health status, the option to continue working, and sufficient income. Those who retire unwillingly are at risk for alcoholism, depression, and suicide (Ebersole and Hess, 1990).

The nurse can help clients and their families prepare for retirement. The counseling of older adults for retirement should focus on six issues (Diekelmann, 1978). First, what provisions have the client and family made for retirement income? Older adults need resources to adequately meet housing, food, clothing, and health care expenses. Second, what postretirement activities are available? It is important to assess clients' abilities, skills, and interests. Third, what living arrangements may be needed? Many older adults decide to relocate into smaller living quarters for easier maintenance. Fourth, what preparations have been made for role changes? Sharing of household tasks and spending more time with grandchildren or community work are options. Fifth, what provisions have been made to meet health care needs? With increasing health care costs, this can be a serious concern. Sixth, how will the retired person attend to legal affairs? Older adults should understand the importance of estate planning.

Social Isolation. Many older adults experience **social isolation,** which increases as they age. The four types of social isolation are attitudinal, presentational, behavioral, and geographical. Some older adults may be affected by all four types, and others may be affected by only one (Ebersole and Hess, 1990).

Attitudinal isolation occurs because of personal and cultural values. Ageism is a negative bias against and rejection of people of advanced age. Therefore attitudinal social isolation occurs when the older adult is not as easily accepted into social interactions or relationships because of ageist bias.

Presentational isolation results from an unacceptable appearance or other factors involved in how a person presents the self to others. Factors contributing to presentation isolation are body image, hygiene, or visible signs of illness or functional loss (Ebersole and Hess, 1990). The person becomes isolated because of the rejection of others or because little interaction is sought because of self-consciousness.

Behavioral isolation results from unacceptable behaviors. Socially unacceptable behaviors cause other people to withdraw. Behaviors commonly associated with behavioral isolation of the older adult include confusion, behaviors associated with organic brain syndrome, alcoholism, eccentricity, and incontinence.

Geographical isolation occurs because of distance from family, urban crime, and institutional barriers such as the absence of wheelchair ramps and safety-equipped bathrooms. A client who is alone is not necessarily lonely. Many people enjoy being alone. Nurses need to determine whether these clients are lonely or have merely chosen to be alone. The effects of loneliness and social isolation vary, depending on ways the person is

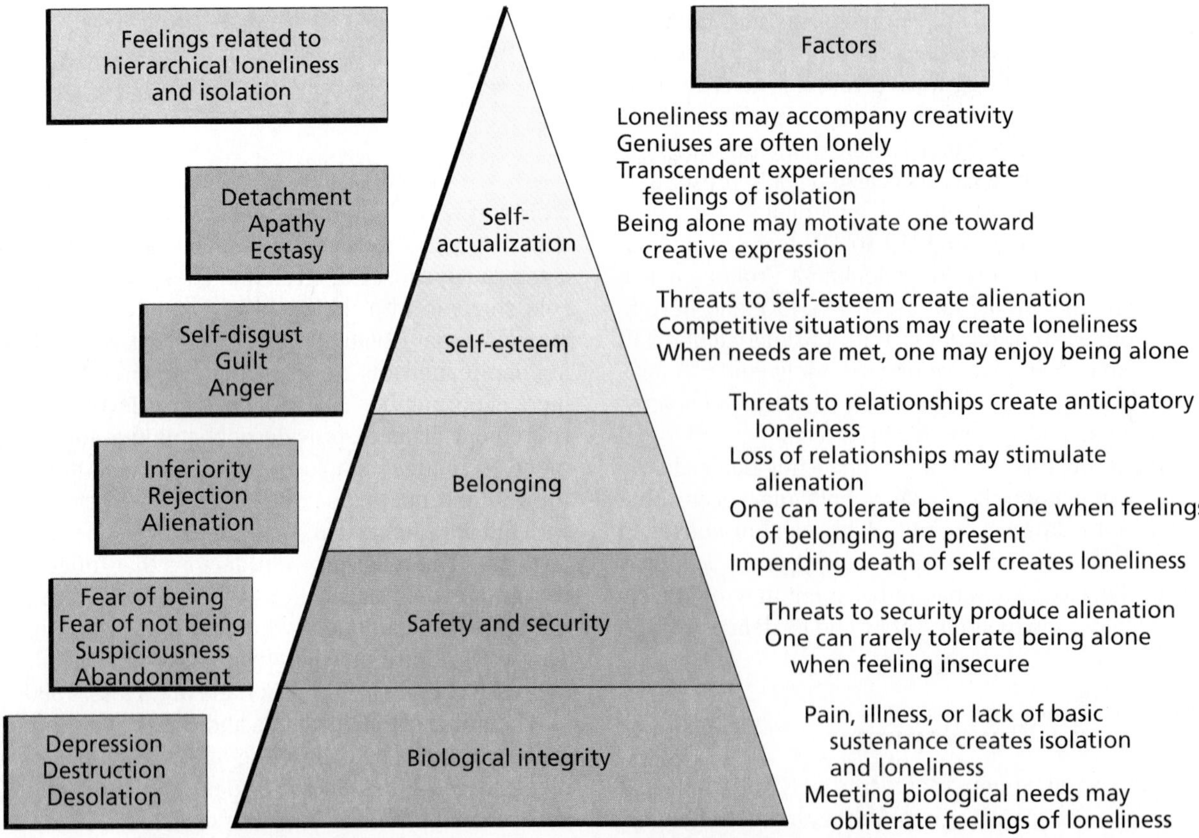

FIGURE 20-13 Loneliness in relation to Maslow's hierarchy of needs. (Modified from Ebersole P and Hess P: *Toward healthy aging: human needs and nursing response,* ed 3, St. Louis, 1990, Mosby.)

able to meet basic human needs. Figure 20-13 shows the relationship of basic human needs to loneliness and social isolation. Loneliness is often associated with poor health, dissatisfaction with housing and other environmental factors, and the loss of a spouse.

The nurse can assist the lonely older adult in rebuilding a social network through outreach programs designed to make contact with isolated older adults. The program may be planned to meet the nutritional needs of older adults (such as Meals on Wheels), socialization needs (such as daily telephone calls by volunteers), or need for activities (such as outings to a play or park).

Sexuality. Changes in the structure and function of the reproductive system occur as the result of hormonal alterations. The changes in reproductive structure and function do not affect libido. The older adult, whether healthy and active or frail, needs to express sexual feelings. Sexuality is linked with identity and validates a person's belief that he or she can give to others and have the gift appreciated. Sexuality involves love, warmth, sharing, and touching between people, not just the physical act of intercourse.

When caring for the older adult, the nurse must ensure that nursing care is also directed toward helping the client maintain sexual health. Sexual health is the integration of somatic, emotional, intellectual, and social aspects of sexual being in positively enriching ways that enhance personality, communication, and love. To help the older adult achieve or maintain sexual health, the nurse needs to understand the physical changes in sexual response. The knowledge of sexual changes described in Table 20-11 and the physical changes in male and female genitalia enables the nurse to educate the older adult client about actual or anticipated changes in sexual functioning.

table 20-11

PHYSICAL CHANGES IN SEXUAL RESPONSE IN THE OLDER ADULT

Female	Male
EXCITATION	
Diminished vaginal lubrication (1 to 3 minutes may be required for adequate amounts to appear) Diminished flattening and separation of labia majora Disappearance of elevation of labia majora Decreased vasocongestion of labia minora Decreased elastic expansion of vagina (depth and breadth) Slower and less prominent uterine elevation or tenting Decreased muscle tension	Less intense and slower erection (but can be maintained longer without ejaculation) Less vasocongestion of scrotal sac Less pronounced elevation and congestion of testicles Decreased muscle tension
PLATEAU	
Decreased capacity for vasocongestion Decreased areolar engorgement Labial color change less evident Less intense swelling of orgasmic platform Decreased secretions of Bartholin's glands	Nipple erection and sexual flush less often No color change at coronal ridge of penis Decrease or absence of secretory activity (lubrication) by Cowper's gland before ejaculation
ORGASM	
Fewer contractions of orgasmic platform Rectal sphincter contractions with severe tension only	Fewer penile contractions Fewer rectal sphincter contractions Decreased force of ejaculation with decreased amount of semen (if long ejaculation, seepage of semen occurs)
RESOLUTION	
Observably slower subsidence of nipple erection Quicker subsidence of vasocongestion of clitoris and orgasmic platform	Slow subsidence of vasocongestion of nipples and scrotum Loss of erection and descent of testicles shortly after ejaculation Refractory time extended (time required before another erection ranges from several to 24 hours, occasionally longer)

Modified from Ebersole P and Hess P: *Toward healthy aging: human needs and nursing response,* ed 3, St. Louis, 1990, Mosby.

Housing and Environment. Changes in social roles, family responsibilities, and health status influence the older client's choice of living arrangements. Some older adults choose to live in a multigenerational household with family members. Others prefer to live in their own homes or apartments in multigenerational neighborhoods or communities. Leisure or retirement communities can provide the older person with living and social opportunities in a one-generational setting.

Housing and the environment as a whole are important because they can have a major impact on the health of the older adult. The environment can support or hinder physical and social functioning, enhance or drain the individual's energy, and complement or tax existing physical changes such as vision and hearing.

Dying Process. Birth and death are universal yet individually unique events in the human life span. Death of a young or middle-aged person is often viewed as tragic because life goals are uncompleted. A common misconception is that the death of an older adult is always a blessing and the culmination of a full and rich life. Many dying older adults still have life goals, and they are not emotionally prepared to die. Families and friends are often unable to cope with the process of dying and the subsequent loss of a loved one. With appropriate knowledge and skills the nurse can help to make the dying process a time of fulfillment and growth and a completion of life governed by clients with the support, understanding, and assistance of those around them (see Chapter 21).

Health Concerns

Older adults particularly value good health. A state of wellness provides energy, vitality, and a zest for life. The nurse can establish health maintenance programs that promote the older adult's wellness. Senior citizens' centers, churches, schools, shopping malls, supermarkets, libraries, and hospital lobbies can be used to conduct screening tests and present information to older adults on specific health topics.

Physiological Concerns. Approximately 80% of adults over 65 years of age have at least one chronic health problem. The effect of the chronic health problem on mobility and independence depends on the individual.

Hypertension is diagnosed when repeated blood pressure measurements over 90 mm Hg diastolic and 140 mm Hg systolic are present (see Chapter 15). Risk factors for hypertension include smoking, obesity, lack of exercise, and stress. Blacks are at greater risk than whites, and men are at greater risk than women. Treatment of hypertension includes weight reduction, decreased salt intake, exercise, stress management, and medications (Stanhope and Lancaster, 1992).

Angina pectoris is a coronary artery disease in which chest pain is usually induced by exercise or stress. The risk factors for angina include family history of heart disease, obesity, hyperlipidemia, smoking, and stress. Treatment varies but usually includes vasodilator therapy, an exercise program, smoking cessation, weight reduction, and stress management.

Myocardial infarction (heart attack) is a disease in which one portion of a coronary artery or the entire artery becomes occluded, thus depriving the myocardium of its oxygen and blood supply. Myocardial necrosis and ischemia then occurs. Risk factors include a family history of cardiac disease, angina pectoris, diabetes mellitus, smoking, obesity, hypertension, hyperlipidemia, lack of exercise, and stress. Treatment of a myocardial infarction involves hospitalization, followed by a rehabilitation period in which habits are modified. These modifications include weight reduction, exercise, smoking cessation, dietary changes, and stress management.

Cerebrovascular accident (stroke) occurs when the vessels supplying blood to a certain portion of the brain become occluded or vessels rupture to cause bleeding into the brain, resulting in decreased circulation to that area. Risk factors for cerebrovascular accident include hypertension, hyperlipidemia, diabetes mellitus, and family history of cardiovascular disease.

Malignant neoplasms are the second most common cause of death among older adults. Early detection and treatment are important. The nurse can also develop programs to decrease the older adult's risk for cancer, including encouraging smoking cessation, teaching clients to perform breast self-examinations (see Chapter 16), encouraging clients to have routine Pap smears, and educating clients about the warning signs of cancer.

Arthritis affects approximately 44% of older adults. It is more common in women than in men (Stanhope and Lancaster, 1992). The degree to which the mobility of the older adult with arthritis is affected depends on the extent of the disease and the joints affected. At the present time there is no known cure for arthritis, but recently developed pharmacological agents can decrease joint pain and swelling and therefore increase range of joint motion.

Sensory impairments such as changes in vision, hearing, taste, and smell are common in the older adult. These changes are frequently the result of the normal aging process. The nurse can aid the older adult in identifying resources to help to correct visual and auditory problems (see Chapter 38).

Dental problems are common in older adults. They can lead to changes in taste and a decrease in nutritional intake. Because of missing teeth or poorly fitting dentures, the older adult may restrict the diet to soft foods.

The nurse can help to prevent dental and gum disease through health education. In addition to teaching the older adult to maintain routine dental care, the nurse can teach specific measures to reduce the risk of gum disease. The nurse can help the client with ill-fitting dentures or other dental problems by identifying resources in the community that provide dental services to older adults at reduced rates.

As a group, adults over 65 years of age are the greatest users of prescription drugs. The most frequently prescribed drugs are for heart and vascular disease, hypertension, depression, diabetes mellitus, respiratory diseases, chronic skin disorders, and gastrointestinal disorders (Ebersole and Hess, 1990). Many drugs may interact with one another, potentiating or negating the effect of another drug. Some drugs cause confusion, affect balance, cause dizziness, nausea, or vomiting, or promote constipation or urinary frequency.

Sedatives and tranquilizers may cause an acute confusional state. Ironically, these drugs are frequently given to confused older clients. Confusion that varies with time is known as sundown syndrome and occurs most frequently in institutions. Older clients with clear mental status by day suddenly become disoriented at night. Drugs used to manage this behavior should be carefully administered, taking into account age-related changes in body systems that can affect the drugs' activity. The goal of all drug therapy with the older client is to ensure the greatest therapeutic benefit with the least amount of harm.

Minimal nutritional needs for the older adult are the same as those of younger adults, except that greater amounts of calcium, vitamin C, and vitamin A are required. Total caloric intake usually declines in response to illness and changes in metabolic rate and physical activity. Nutritional needs of the older adult are described in Chapter 31.

The older adult should be encouraged to maintain a pattern of physical exercise and activity. Before beginning an exercise program, the client should have a complete physical examination, which may include a stress cardiogram or stress test. This provides information about cardiovascular function during periods of sustained exercise. Before the older adult begins an exercise program, the nurse should assess activity tolerance and plan a program that meets physical needs while allowing for physical impairments.

Psychosocial Concerns. Psychosocial health concerns vary widely among older adults. Many role transitions occur between middle age and older adulthood. Because of these changes, the cognitive and social changes, and the physical effects of aging, many older adults require nursing assistance to maintain psychosocial health.

NURSING PROCESS FOR CLIENTS ACROSS THE LIFESPAN

Assessment

Assessment of clients' developmental level provides information about the ability to understand, cooperate with, and possibly assume responsibility for immediate and long-term care needs for themselves or family members. Nursing assessment focuses on the physiological, cognitive, psychosocial, and health concerns of clients.

From infancy through adolescence, illness and hospitalization are stressful experiences. The selection of coping behaviors for a client is limited. A child's reaction to illness and hospitalization is based on developmental age, previous experiences with hospitalization, available

STRATEGIES FOR ASSESSMENT OF THE OLDER ADULT

Focus on the older adult's degree of function, noting structural alterations as function is assessed.

Be aware of one's stereotypes and attitudes related to aging and older persons since they affect nurse-client communication.

Remember that sensory-perceptual deficits, anxiety, reduced energy level, pain, the multiplicity and interrelatedness of health problems, and the tendency to reminisce are the major client factors requiring the nurse's special consideration when obtaining a health assessment.

Include any alternate sources (family, friends, health records) to supplement the older adult's own health history if necessary.

Conduct all steps of the nursing process at a slower pace, depending on the older adult's degree of functional ability.

Consider financial and social resources, and the older person's own goals, desires, and coping skills when planning nursing care.

Be alert to the typically altered presentation of signs and symptoms of illness in older adults because of the aging process.

Pay attention to environmental factors as sources of difficulty for the older adult in any setting. Interventions should always include consideration of how such factors affect function and health status at all levels.

Be alert to the altered pharmacology of drugs in older adults; carefully monitor the dosage and response of all drug therapy.

Implement rehabilitative and restorative nursing techniques with the goal of maximizing functional independence.

Consider the impact of ethnicity on the older adult's responses to aging, illness, disease, and development.

support persons, coping skills, and the seriousness of the diagnosis (Whaley and Wong, 1991).

The young and middle-aged adult's ability to cope with illness and hospitalization is also affected by developmental level, coping skills, previous experiences with illnesses, and the availability of support resources. The middle-aged client is also faced with situational crises and the potential need to modify habits.

The older adult's ability to cope with the adjustments of retirement, illnesses, hospitalization, and normal physiological changes is affected by developmental level, availability of support resources, coping skills, previous experiences with illnesses and stressors, and the number of actual or potential life-style changes. The older adult must frequently adjust to the death of loved ones. Adjustments are also associated with retirement, relocation, and living alone. The nurse's assessment approach with older adults (see box on p. 479) must incorporate strategies that will provide an accurate and thorough data base.

Nursing Diagnosis

Nursing assessment of the client reveals clusters of data that provide defining characteristics. These assist in identifying nursing diagnoses. Such defining characteristics support the diagnostic statement and provide the rationale for the diagnosis. They are found in pertinent assessment data obtained during the nursing history, physical examination, and review of laboratory information. Skill in critical thinking allows the nurse to analyze data systematically to develop nursing diagnoses. Defining characteristics for the nursing diagnosis of altered sexuality patterns would include factors such as the following:

- Difficulties or limitations in sexual functioning
- Expressions of concern about sexuality
- Inappropriate verbal and nonverbal sexual behavior
- Changes in physical appearance or functioning, or psychosocial roles or functioning

The box below includes examples of nursing diagnoses for clients with developmental health problems.

The nursing diagnostic statement should include expected causes for the identified problem to enable the nurse to target specific goals and interventions as they relate to causative factors. For example, the nursing diagnosis of altered sexuality patterns can be related to the stress of an impaired relationship with a significant other, fear of pregnancy and birth, or lack of a significant other. The causal factors for a specific nursing diagnosis can vary and necessitate different nursing approaches.

NURSING DIAGNOSES FOR CLIENTS ACROSS THE LIFE SPAN

- Altered family processes
- Altered growth and development
- Altered parenting or high risk for altered parenting
- Altered sexuality patterns
- Body-image disturbance
- Care giver role strain or high risk for care giver role strain
- Decisional conflict
- Dysfunctional grieving
- Effective breast feeding or ineffective breast feeding
- Family coping: potential for growth
- High risk for injury
- High risk for poisoning
- Hopelessness
- Impaired adjustment
- Impaired social interaction or social isolation
- Ineffective family coping: compromised or disabled
- Ineffective individual coping
- Ineffective infant feeding pattern
- Parental role conflict
- Sexual dysfunction

Planning

The nursing care plan (see the nursing care plan on p. 481) is a further application of the nursing process for the client with developmental needs. The plan is based on the nurse's assessment of the client's physiological and pathophysiological conditions, psychosocial factors, and human growth and development. Assessment of the family or support system should also be considered. The degree of participation in planning depends on the client's developmental status, as well as physiological and psychological condition. For example, because young children may be unable to articulate feelings and needs, their parents must become involved in establishing goals.

Nursing diagnoses are chosen and addressed in order of priority, with the most pressing problems receiving immediate attention. Prioritizing nursing diagnoses is based on such factors as the nature of the problem (e.g., is it life threatening, does it interfere with activities of daily living, or does it affect level of comfort?) and the degree of importance attributed to the problem by the client or family. Maslow's theory of human need is often used as a guide when arranging nursing diagnoses in order of priority.

Shorter hospital stays require early and close attention to discharge planning, which should involve the health care team, the client, and the client's support system. Nursing interventions need to be individualized for the client and modified accordingly for home- or hospital-based nursing care. Needed referrals to community

SAMPLE NURSING CARE PLAN
Client with Developmental Needs

ASSESSMENT

Clinical scenario: Cathy and Joe Moeller, both age 48, have been married for 18 years. They have *three girls, ages, 9, 12, and 15.* Cathy's parents are deceased. Joe's *father,* age 80, *was recently diagnosed with Alzheimer's disease. His mother,* age 76, had a stroke 5 years before with some *residual left-sided weakness.*

The *physician has discussed placement of Joe's father into a nursing home. Joe's mother is unable to accept this alternative.* She has agreed to move closer to Cathy and Joe's neighborhood. However, she wants to live in a ranch-style home and care for her husband in the house. Joe's *mother views an apartment life-style as "one step away from a nursing home."*

Cathy and Joe are committed to helping his parents. However, they realize that their daughters' needs are increasing. These needs are financial, as well as time demands. *Cathy and Joe express frustration about feeling squeezed between two generations of love and commitment.* Their frustrations do not originate from a lack of commitment, desire, or willingness but rather from a lack of time and *lack of knowledge about available health care resources.*

Their daughters love their grandparents but want to have Cathy and Joe available for thier activities. *The three daughters help with their grandparents.* The *declining mental status of their grandfather has made this more difficult.* In addition, it is difficult for the girls to understand that their grandfather's unwillingness to participate in hygiene and his argumentative behavior are part of Alzheimer's disease.

NURSING DIAGNOSIS

Altered family processes related to demands of caring for chronically ill grandparents.

PLANNING

Goal	Expected outcomes
Family will communicate and solve problems regarding grandparents health care needs within 1 month.	Parents and daughters are able to set time priorities within 1 week. Parents and daughters have 2 hours to themselves and together each week. Parents investigate realistic alternatives to care for grandparents within 4 weeks.

IMPLEMENTATION

Steps	Rationale
1. Family meets at least once a week to determine needs for each member and the estimated time to meet these needs.	Time management is effective approach to reducing stress, when there are many demands on clients' financial and time resources (Pender, 1987).
2. Alternative plan for maintaining grandparents' needs is planned for at least 2 hours each week.	Anticipatory planning assists in maintaining activities for nuclear family while assuring safe care for grandparents.
3. Refer family to respite care resource in community.	Respite care provides time for care givers to be freed of direct care-giving activities.

EVALUATIVE MEASURES

Talk with parents and daughters about their ability to meet priorities.
Observe family interaction in home or clinic.
Ask whether parents have located and used respite care agency.

*Defining characteristics are in italic type.

agencies should be made to coincide with the client's arrival home.

The nursing care plan may include the following basic goals:

Goal: Client learns health concerns for developmental status.

Outcomes

Client describes impact of risk factors on level of health

Client discusses physiological basis for illness

Client describes rationale for treatment

Goal: Client acquires healthy psychosocial behaviors by 2 months.

Outcomes

Client participates in health-promotion activities within 6 weeks

Client demonstrates problem-solving skills within 1 month

Client communicates family communication patterns within 2 weeks

Goal: Client progresses through normal growth and development levels.

Outcomes

Client accomplishes age-appropriate developmental tasks

Client displays coping mechanisms when dealing with developmental changes

Client develops along accepted norms and progress levels

Implementation

Interventions are performed by nurses, the client, and the family or significant others. The goal is to keep the client as active a participant as possible. Interventions are designed to take into consideration the uniqueness of clients and their developmental status. Collaboration with other team members is important in providing optimal care for clients at every developmental level. Each hospital and health care agency has its own guidelines for recording and exchanging information about clients. It is always important to include the following:

1. Assessments and nursing actions related to nursing diagnoses
2. Client and family response to teaching
3. Questions and concerns expressed by the client and family along with the nurse's response
4. Evaluation of goals in terms of expected outcomes

Conception Through Preschool

Minimizing Separation Anxiety. Being separated from family in an unfamiliar environment when not feeling well is possibly the greatest stress a child faces in the hospital. Parents are more likely to remain with their young child when the nurse and active members of the health care team make them feel comfortable. When parents cannot continuously be with the child at the hospital, the nurse and parents need to plan together to make this situation more tolerable for the child. Appropriate interventions include the following:

1. Parents should tell the child when they are leaving and when they will return in terms the child can understand. The nurse should be present when they leave to provide distraction and support. Parents should understand that protest is normal and demonstrates a strong parent-child relationship.
2. The child should bring favorite toys and familiar objects from home to provide comfort and security. Parents can also tape pictures of family members where the child can easily see them.
3. Telephone calls and cassette tapes from family members can provide a link between home and hospital. Hearing the family singing, talking, or telling a story can comfort the child.

Establishing Trust. The nurse's establishment of a trusting relationship with the child and family requires careful planning. The nurse who is friendly and informative, listens well to the concerns of the family, and is not threatening to the child has laid the foundations for a positive relationship. The parents' trust of the nurse will be enhanced by the efforts made to make their child feel comfortable. Taking the time to discover the child's daily routine, keeping parents informed, and providing them with frequent opportunities to ask questions assure parents of the nurse's interest and concern.

Reducing Fear. Fear reduction begins with understanding the origins of fear as it varies according to the child's cognitive and perceptual development. According to Servonsky and Opas (1987) the common fears according to selected age-groups are the following:

1. Infants from birth to 3 months: sudden movements, loud noises, and loss of physical support
2. Infants from 4 to 12 months: strangers, strange objects, heights, and anticipation of previous uncomfortable situations
3. Toddlers from 1 to 3 years: the dark, being alone, separation from parent, some animals such as barking dogs, and loud machines
4. Preschoolers from 3 to 6 years: body mutilation, supernatural beings, monsters, ghosts, separation from trusted adults and familiar routines, and abandonment

Some fears are associated with health care, including being stuck with needles, taking bad-tasting medicine, invasive procedures, being forced to lie down, and being subjected to the unknown. Measures to reduce fears should be included when planning interventions. Such measures can include allowing the child to sit up for assessments and procedures when possible, demonstrating the procedure on another person or doll, allowing the child to see and handle equipment, encouraging the parents to be present, allowing the child to assist with the procedure as appropriate, and leaving the room door open at night.

Minimizing Physical Discomfort. Children of all ages, including newborns, experience pain. The nurse is often unable to prevent pain but can do much to reduce the physical discomfort. The expression of pain is influenced by the children's culture and parents' child-rearing practices. Children's perception of pain varies according to their pain threshold and their degree of anxiety.

Pain in infants can be differentiated from other sensations by crying that does not decrease with comfort measures, increased restlessness, and increased random movements. Toddlers cannot clearly identify where pain is felt and often find anything intrusive or causing pressure as painful. Preschoolers can point to the painful area but have difficulty describing or discussing it. They may experience fear and anxiety with pain and may perceive it as punishment for a misdeed or "bad" thought. Restraint and being forced to lie down are difficult for most children because their sense of control is threatened and their mobility is inhibited. Nurses can reduce the physical discomfort experienced by keeping periods of restraint or immobility to a minimum. They can also limit invasive procedures, comfort with a soft voice and physical contact, provide items that represent security and comfort, allow acceptable choices, encourage participation, give pain medication, and use a developmentally appropriate pain assessment tool to determine effectiveness of pain relief measures (Chapter 28).

Promoting Growth and Development. Illness and hospitalization disrupt children's developmental progress. When illness is mild and hospitalization is short, the effect may be minimal. A serious illness can have a more significant impact, requiring a formalized plan to facilitate developmental progress (Lipsi et al., 1991). Adding to the disruption of development is the feeling of loss of control that may result from separation, physical restriction, interruption of daily routines, enforced dependency, magical thinking, and altered roles (Whaley and Wong, 1991). Regression to earlier behaviors that provide security is the most common defense mechanism used by young children to cope with these stresses. The nurse can implement many interventions to promote growth and development (see box below).

FOSTERING NORMAL GROWTH AND DEVELOPMENT IN THE ILL CHILD

- Provide an environment of acceptance for regressive behavior and teach parents how to handle regressive behavior with a firm, kind, consistent approach.
- Encourage participation in self-care activities such as bathing, dressing, and feeding. Incorporate usual activities of daily living into hospital care.
- Provide intermittent auditory and visual stimulation by such activities as rides in a wheelchair or wagon, playing records or tapes from home, and reading stories.
- Provide opportunities for social interaction with other children in a playroom and encourage sibling visits.
- Provide toys and play equipment that promote development of fine and gross motor activities. Provide favorite toys from home.
- Encourage development of new vocabulary by learning names for hospital items and personnel. Explain routines, procedures, and therapies in age-appropriate language.
- Encourage participation in assessment and procedures, allowing the child to make choices when possible.
- Discuss the effects of hospitalization on growth and development with parents and other team members. Explain how they can help children regain and attain optimal levels of growth and development.

Incorporation of Play and Diversional Activity into Care

For children, play is work. It can be one of the most effective tools for managing the care of hospitalized children. Play in the hospital allows the child to work out fears, release frustrations, and meet the developmental need for stimulation. It brings a sense of normality to the strange and sometimes seemingly hostile environment. Diversional play allows children to focus attention on pleasurable experiences. Play can also be an effective communication technique and teaching tool.

Play helps children deal with the strains and stresses of illness and hospitalization, develop their capacities, and strengthen their defenses (Servonsky and Opas, 1987). Because it is vital to development, interventions should be implemented to provide play and diversional activities (see box on p. 484).

School-Age Child and Adolescent

The care plan must be highly individualized. As the child matures, there is an increased need to participate in care. There is also, however, an increased need to make independent decisions, which can result in conflicts between the child and parents and the child and the health care team.

Limit Setting. The nurse may need to establish interventions to set boundaries. Thus the client is able to

INCORPORATION OF PLAY AND DIVERSIONAL ACTIVITIES INTO THE CARE OF THE ILL CHILD

Incorporate play into the daily activities of bathing, dressing, feeding, and measuring of vital signs.
Keep the playroom as a "safe" area by prohibiting the administration of medications or performance of any procedures.
Allow children to play with other children.
Provide materials that encourage creativity such as paper, paint, paste, clay, and crayons.
Provide sense-pleasure play that allows infants and young children to enjoy sound, movement, smells, tastes, touch, and color through such activities as water play, mobiles, and stuffed toys.
Promote motor development through skill play such as putting objects in a container and dumping them out.
Promote cognitive development through activities such as reading, hiding and seeking objects, and counting games.
Plan special activities for children whose activities are limited (e.g., provide a sense of mobility for a child in traction by playing a game of ring toss).
Prepare children for procedures through play with hospital equipment. Consider cognitive level of the child.
Provide for judicious television and video watching.

DYNAMICS OF BEHAVIOR AND HABITS

Habits are frequently repeated behaviors.
The more often a behavior is repeated, the more likely it will be repeated thereafter.
Habits can be a stress-reduction mechanism for the individual (e.g., nail biting) but may be simultaneously detrimental to health (e.g., alcohol consumption).
Habits often meet some basic need for the person involved.
Changing a habit requires a significant motivation by the client. Changing the habit must provide greater pleasure or satisfaction than the habit itself provides.
Any change in habits or behavior patterns creates stress.

make some independent decisions within the health care plan. Within the limits set, the client is able to assume some responsibility for care. For example, an older child wants privacy when using an inhalant or administering an injection.

Providing Accurate Knowledge. The nurse may be the initial source of education for the school-age child or adolescent. The nurse has the opportunity to teach the client about the illness, positive health care practices, and treatment. The nurse may also counsel the young client who has an illness and may affect the client's motivation to change negative health behaviors.

Young and Middle Adult

Changing Health Habits. Health teaching and health counseling are often directed at improving health habits (see box above, right). The more fully the nurse understands the dynamics of behavior and habits (see box on p. 485), the more likely interventions will help the client to bring about or reinforce health-promoting behaviors.

To help clients form positive health habits, the nurse becomes a teacher and facilitator. By providing information about body functions and how habits are formed and changed, the nurse raises the client's level of knowledge regarding the potential impact of behavior on health. A nurse cannot change clients' habits. Clients have control of and are responsible for their own behaviors. The nurse can explain psychological principles of changing habits, offer information about health risks, and provide positive reinforcement of health-directed behaviors and decisions. Barriers to change, such as lack of facilities, special support, knowledge, or motivation, need to be minimized or eliminated to bring about change.

Health Promotion. Community health programs for young and middle adults are designed to prevent illness, promote health, and detect disease in the early stages. Nurses can contribute to community health by actively planning screening and teaching programs. Family planning, birthing, and parenting skills are program topics in which adults might be interested. Health screening is a good opportunity for the nurse to perform assessment and provide health teaching and health counseling.

Health education programs can promote changes in behavior and life-style. The nurse offers information for the client to make wise decisions about health practices. During health counseling the nurse and client design a plan of action that addresses the client's health and well-being. Through objective problem solving, the nurse assists the client to grow and change. Regardless of age and family structure, family members face certain health tasks. The nurse understands the autonomy of the family and supports it while promoting family health.

Stress Reduction. Throughout life, people are exposed to many stressors (see Chapter 4). After identifying these stressors, the client and nurse can work to modify the stress response. Specific interventions for stress reduction can fall into three categories (Pender, 1987). First, the frequency of stress-producing situa-

CLIENT TEACHING FOR POSITIVE HEALTH HABITS

INTERVENTIONS

Instruct client on benefit of regular exercise (e.g., walking) three times a week
Review with client the daily work schedule and identify potential times for exercise.
Inform client about the effect of exercise on weight control and improved cardiac function.
Demonstrate how to calculate target heart rate and assess pulse correctly.
Provide warm-up and cool-down exercises and demonstrate how to do them.
Instruct client about supportive shoes for walking exercises.

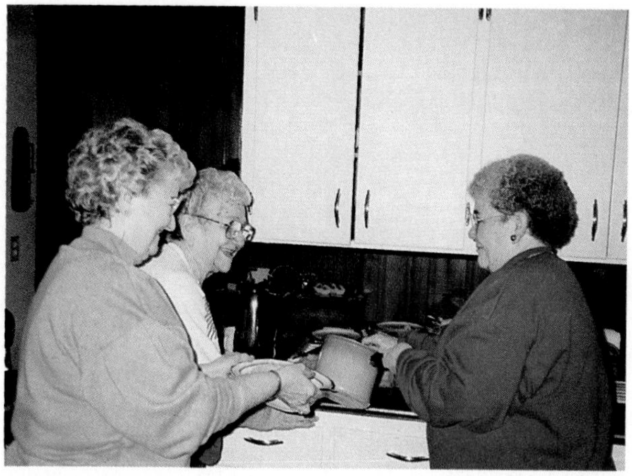

FIGURE 20-14 Socialization with family is important for an older adult.

tions is minimized. Together the nurse and client identify ways to prevent stressful situations, such as habituation, change avoidance, time blocking, time management, and environmental modification (Pender, 1987). Second, psychophysiological preparation, such as increasing self-esteem, improving assertiveness, redirecting goal alternatives, and reorienting cognitive appraisal increases stress resistance (Pender, 1987). Third, the physiological response to stress is avoided. The nurse uses relaxation techniques, imagery (see Chapter 4), and biofeedback to recondition the client's response to stress.

Older Adult

Increasing Socialization. The older adult needs assistance in increasing social outlets (see box on p. 486) (Figure 20-14). Frequently these clients have experienced the death of a spouse, sibling, or close friend. They feel their social circle is diminishing. In some instances older adults have relocated to smaller residences and must reacquaint themselves with churches, stores, and health care services.

The nurse can help the older adult to form secondary relationships with peers by holding discussions of topics of mutual interest at day-care centers, nutrition program sites, or long-term care centers. The older adult appreciates information that is accurate, logically organized, and relevant to health needs. The following are some guidelines for conducting discussion sessions:

1. Select a small, quiet room that is well lit and has comfortable furniture. Be sure to consider visual, hearing, or musculoskeletal impairments.
2. Keep meeting short enough to promote learning while not becoming exhausting (20 minutes).
3. Choose participants who are able to learn and participate in discussions.
4. Consider the older adults' sensory deficits when choosing content and visual aids (e.g., brightly colored posters with large print).
5. Present only one topic for discussion at each meeting.
6. Make it clear to clients that participation in the group is voluntary.

Establishing peer group meetings for the older adult allows participants to develop secondary relationships independently. The older adult learns to share ideas and solve problems without dwelling on physical ailments or feelings of hopelessness.

Therapeutic Communication. With therapeutic communication the nurse perceives, reacts to, and respects the client's uniqueness. The nurse who communicates effectively with an older adult will be accepted as one who shares a genuine concern for the client's welfare. The nurse cannot simply walk into a client's environment and immediately establish a therapeutic relationship. He or she must first be knowledgeable and skilled in different communication techniques (see Chapter 13).

Touch. Throughout the life span, the sense of touch provides knowledge about others. In all cultures, gently touching another person conveys affection and friendliness. Older adults who are victims of social isolation are often deprived of the touching and holding that were important parts of their earlier lives. Touch is a therapeutic tool that nurses can use to help to meet the comfort needs of the older adult. Touch can provide sensory stimulation, reduce anxiety, orient the person to reality,

FORMAL AND INFORMAL CONTACTS INCREASING SOCIAL NETWORKS OF THE OLDER ADULT

FORMAL

Church
Grandparenting
Foster grandparents
Vista
Peace Corps
Retired Senior Volunteer Program
Unions
Friends of the Library
Volunteers
Public school
Senior centers
Title VII nutrition sites
Social issues for seniors

INFORMAL

Neighbors
Maids, waitresses in small hotels
Beauty salons, restaurants, bars, service personnel, shops
Fiction kin: soap operas
Interest in celebrities
Laundromats
Sports
Bus for the elderly
Special tours
Education, arts and crafts courses
Trailer courts
Retirement communities
Pets
Plants
Dancing
Physicians' office
Clinics
Lobby gazers
Vicarious participation
Surrogate families: nurses, aides
Nursing home: social corridor
General social touching
Radio shows
Nostalgia
Phone lines

From Ebersole P and Hess P: *Toward healthy aging: human needs and nursing response,* ed 3, St. Louis, 1990, Mosby.

relieve physiological and emotional pain, and give comfort during the dying process.

Reality Orientation. Reality orientation was first described by Taulbee and Folsom in 1966. It is a communication modality used for making the client aware of time, place, and person. The major purposes of reality orientation include restoring the client's sense of reality, improving level of awareness, promoting socialization, elevating the client to a maximal level of independent functioning, and minimizing confusion, disorientation, and physical regression.

The nurse can use reality orientation techniques in any setting. When an older adult experiences a change in environment, surgery, illness, or emotional stress, such as the death of a spouse or a friend, he or she is at risk for becoming disoriented. Environmental changes such as the bright lights and lack of windows in intensive care and specialized units in a hospital often lead to disorientation and confusion. The client's environment and the nursing personnel are constantly changing in the hospital, and the immediate environment is unstable, making coping and adaptation difficult. The problem is compounded by tranquilizers, sleeping pills, anesthesia, and restraints that immobilize and take away dignity. The nurse should anticipate disorientation and confusion as a consequence of hospitalization, relocation, surgery, loss, or illness and incorporate reality orientation interventions into the nursing care plan. These interventions are based on seven principles (see box on p. 487). Consistent use of the techniques of reality orientation helps to reorient the older adult to the surroundings.

Reminiscence. Reminiscence is recalling the past for the purpose of assigning new meaning to past experiences. Reminiscing is an adaptive function of the older adult. As a therapeutic technique, reminiscence is an elaboration of the natural way older adults revive their past in an attempt to make order and meaning and reconcile conflicts and disappointments as they prepare for death (Butler, 1963). Reminiscence can be used for cognitively impaired, psychologically disturbed, or depressed older adults. The nurse organizes the group and selects strategies for reminiscence by adapting the size of the group; the group's structure, process, and goals; and personal activities to meet the needs of group members.

Body Image Interventions. The way older adults present themselves significantly affects their body image and feelings of isolation. Certain physical characteristics of old age are socially desirable, such as slimness and distinguished-looking gray hair. Other features, such as a lined face that displays character or wrinkled hands that convey a lifetime of hard work, are also impressive. Too often, however, society envisions older adults as incapacitated, deaf, obese, or shrunken in stature. When an older adult is hospitalized or has an acute or chronic illness, the related physical dependence makes it difficult for the person to maintain body image. A nurse who has stereotyped views about the

GUIDELINES FOR REALITY ORIENTATION

REALISM

Use reality information such as time, date, place, and name in conversation.
Refer to clocks and other reality orientation props when necessary.
Do not reinforce delusions or hallucinations.
Direct them back to reality-oriented endeavors if they ramble in conversation or talk unrealistically.
If erratic behavior such as picking at clothes is shown, give purposeful things to do.

INDEPENDENCE

Express confidence in the person's ability to be self-directing.
Encourage him or her to perform tasks and make decisions, assisting only when necessary.
Make sure the person has needed aids such as glasses, dentures, and hearing aids and that they work.
Provide bowel and bladder training when necessary.
Provide speech or physical therapy when necessary.
Reduce medication to a minimum.

INDIVIDUALIZATION

Keep reality orientation classes small to permit individual attention.
Allow the person to keep treasures and objects.
Encourage meaningful object relationships.

REINFORCEMENT

Watch for small changes in behavior that indicate progress, and reward them.
Reward correct behavior with verbal praise, touch, or smiles.
Reinforce achievement with increased responsibility.
Encourage special talents or interests.

REPETITION

Repeat information, directions, statements, and questions as necessary.
Be patient and allow time for a response or reply.
Give clues to the answer when asking a question; if a client is unable to answer, provide the correct response and let him or her repeat it.

CLARITY

Enunciate clearly and speak slowly.
Reword statements and questions if necessary.
Give directions in clear, simple, short statements.

CONSISTENCY

Maintain continuity of care.
Adhere to scheduling.
Use the same personnel when possible.

From Rawlins RP, Williams SR, and Beck CM: *Mental health—psychiatric nursing: a holistic life-cycle approach,* ed 3, St. Louis, 1993, Mosby.

appearance of older adults may give little attention to grooming or hygiene activities.

Consequences of illness and aging that can threaten the older adult's body image include invasive diagnostic procedures, pain, surgery, prostheses, loss of sensation in a body part, skin changes, dependence on life-sustaining drugs, denture odor, loss of scalp hair, and incontinence. The nurse has a direct influence on the older adult client's appearance. The nurse must consider the importance of maintaining a pleasant appearance and presenting a socially acceptable image. It takes little effort for the nurse to assist the client in combing matted hair, cleaning stained dentures, shaving an unkempt beard, or changing urine-stained clothing. The older adult does not choose to have an objectionable appearance. The nurse should also be sensitive to odors in the client's environment. Nurses commonly lose awareness of objectionable odors after constant exposure to them. By controlling sources of offending odors, the nurse may prevent family members and friends from shortening their visits or not coming at all because of these factors.

Health Care Services. A variety of health care services are generally available to the population. There are, however, five types of services used more frequently by the older population than by others. Home health care services and homemaker services prevent or delay institutionalization for older adults who need assistance with self-care and activities of daily living. These agencies may be governmental, private, or voluntary.

The **hospice** is a community resource for the terminally ill. A hospice can be an independent unit within the community or may be contained within an institutional setting. Clients seeking hospice care include those with cancer; end-stage renal, cardiovascular, or pulmonary disease; or degenerative neuromuscular disease. The hospice program focuses on meeting the needs of the dying client and the family (see Chapter 21). The hospice provides pain control and maintains the client's quality of life. The hospice does not institute life support or other measures to prolong the life of the terminally ill.

Day care is a program that provides an alternative to

institutionalization. A day-care center offers health services for a client able to remain at home during the evening and night. In addition, day care often enables the client's family or other care giver to maintain employment and other activities (Stanhope and Lancaster, 1992).

Respite care is a form of short-term health service provided to the dependent older adult in the home or institution. Respite care enables the permanent care giver to be away from the home (e.g., to go on vacation or just to have a rest from the responsibilities of caring for a dependent older adult). Respite care can be a valuable resource for a person whose ill or dependent parent lives with the family. With such services the adult child is able to care for the parent but can also have time alone with the spouse and children.

Situations of declining health, decreased physical and human resources, and increased dependence may necessitate the older adult's institutionalization in a long-term care facility. Such a facility provides extended residential, intermediate, or skilled nursing care, medical care, and personal and psychosocial services. The decision for institutional care is not easy to make, and the family requires a great deal of support. In addition, the family may need the nurse's help in locating the proper facility to meet the needs of the client. When possible, the facility chosen should be close to the client's and family's home to provide accessibility for visits.

Evaluative Measures

Evaluation measures the degree to which the planned interventions were effective in meeting the expected outcomes. The nurse evaluates the client's behavioral and physical response to the interventions and thus determines the success or failure of the nursing action. The nurse also evaluates the client's response within the family or community. The interventions and subsequent evaluation of growth and developmental needs usually include the family or significant others. When outcomes are not met, client, nurse, and family collaborate with a revised plan of care. Evaluative measures for the goals of care include:

Goal: Client learns health concerns for developmental status.

Outcome

Client describes impact of risk factors on level of health

Evaluative measure

Ask client or parent to identify risk factors specific for developmental level

Outcome

Client describes physiological basis for illness

Evaluative measure

Have client explain relationship between disease symptoms and physiological cause

Outcome

Client describes rationale for treatment

Evaluative measure

Have client identify purpose for each prescribed medication

Goal: Client acquires healthy psychosocial behaviors within 2 months.

Outcome

Client participates in health-promotion activities within 6 weeks

Evaluative measure

Interview family regarding client's regular exercise habits and schedule

Outcome

Client demonstrates problem-solving skills within 1 month

Evaluative measure

Ask client to describe the proper response in the event of a change in health

Outcome

Client communicates family communication patterns within 2 weeks

Evaluative measure

Have client discuss manner in which family members talk about health problems

Goal: Client progresses through normal growth and development levels.

Outcome

Client accomplishes age-appropriate developmental tasks

Evaluative measure

Complete Denver Developmental Screening for toddler

Outcome

Client displays coping mechanisms when dealing with developmental changes

Evaluative measure

Have adolescent client describe interaction with parents when independence is threatened

Outcome

Client develops along accepted norms and progress levels

Evaluative measure

Conduct physical examination of select body systems

SUMMARY

This chapter has discussed the complexities of growth and development as interrelated processes influenced by many factors. Physiological and psychological theories that account for each stage of growth and development aid the nurse in understanding how to best plan nursing interventions. All stages of growth and development, from intrauterine life to old age, have unique features and present unique nursing care problems. All five human components are involved in each stage.

A person's level of health depends on many factors and influences. The nurse considers these interrelationships to provide optimal care and to help clients to achieve optimal health and well-being.

KEY CONCEPTS

Growth and development are orderly, predictable, interdependent processes that continue throughout the life span.

People progress through similar stages of growth and development but at an individual pace and with individual behaviors.

A psychosocial health concern that begins at childbirth is establishing parent-child attachment.

Physiological, cognitive, and psychosocial development continues throughout the neonate, infant, and toddler periods, and the nurse must be familiar with normal parameters to determine potential problems and promote normal development.

The nurse educates the parents about risk factors and the child's health needs, provides emotional support to the parents in the prenatal period, and helps the parents to understand the changes and needs of the developing child.

Changes in a child's growth pattern may indicate the onset of disease.

The extent to which the school-age child develops physically and cognitively will influence psychosocial development.

The school-age child learns to develop cognitively and psychosocially through peer relationships.

The adolescent must adapt to significant stressors to gain a sense of identity and achieve psychological maturity.

The adolescent is capable of abstract thought and deductive reasoning.

Adult development involves orderly and sequential changes in characteristics and attitudes that adults experience over time.

Cognitive development continues throughout the young and middle adult years.

The pregnant woman needs to understand the physiological changes occurring in each trimester.

The cognitive and psychosocial changes and health concerns during pregnancy and the puerperium affect the parents, siblings, and often the extended family.

Psychosocial changes for the middle adult may be related to career transition, sexuality, marital changes, family transition, and care of the aging parent.

The health concerns of the middle adult commonly involve stress-related illnesses, health assessment, and adopting of positive health habits.

The older adult must adjust to normal physical changes in all body systems.

Structural and physiological changes that occur in the brain during the aging process do not necessarily impair the older adult's adaptation and functional ability.

Psychosocial changes affecting the older adult include retirement, social isolation, change in housing, sexual changes, and death.

CRITICAL THINKING ACTIVITIES

1. Sara is a 1-week-old newborn hospitalized for low birth weight status. What measures can the nurse use to help develop attachment between Sara and her family (mother, father, and 4-year-old brother)?
2. Steven is a 4-year-old boy admitted for open heart surgery in 2 days. Describe the approach the nurse should use to prepare him for the procedures and care measures involved with the surgery and to help him to cope with the required separation from his family and home environment.
3. Andrew, a 16-year-old adolescent, confides to the school nurse, "All my friends are having sex but I am not sure I am ready especially since I read about a teenage boy who died from AIDS." How should the nurse counsel him?
4. During a routine prenatal visit, Suzanne, a 23-year-old primigravida woman (pregnant for the first time) asks the nurse, "Why do I need to come in every month, especially since I feel fine and no one in my family has ever experienced any pregnancy problems? I just cannot find the time, since I have a full-time job and we are in the process of building a new home." Describe how the nurse should respond to her question.
5. You suspect your older adult client is having difficulty adjusting to his impending retirement. What do you need to know about his developmental task achievement before you develop a nursing care plan aimed at assisting him with this transition?
6. You are conducting a health history on a 77-year-old man who tells you he is having an increasingly more difficult time with constipation. What normal, age-related physical changes are likely to be contributing to his constipation?

References

Antwerp CV and Spaniolo AM: Checking out children's lifestyles, *MCN* 16(3):144, 1991.

Arnold LS and Grad RK: Low birth weight and infant mortality: a health policy perspective, *NAACOG's Clinical Issues in Perinatal and Women's Health Nursing* 3(1), 1992.

Bell D, et al.: Illness associated with child day care: a study of incidence and cost, *Am J Pub Health* 79(4):479, 1989.

Benner P and Wrubel J: *The primacy of caring: stress and coping in health and illness,* Menlo Park, Calif., 1989, Addison-Wesley.

Blenner J: Passage through infertility treatment: stage theory, *Image* 22(3):153, 1990.

Bobak IM and Jensen MD: *Maternity and gynecologic care,* ed 5, St. Louis, 1993, Mosby.

Burnside IM: *Nursing and the aged,* ed 3, New York, 1988, McGraw-Hill.

Butler R: Life review: an interpretation of reminiscence in the aged, *Psychiatry* 26:65, 1963.

Chow MP et al.: *Handbook of pediatric primary care,* ed 2, New York, 1984, John Wiley & Sons.

Centers for Disease Control and Prevention: *Survey: teen health and sex habits,* Atlanta, 1991, The Centers.

Dacey J and Travers J: *Human development across the lifespan,* Dubuque, Iowa, 1991, Wm C Brown.

Department of Health and Human Services: *Health, United States, 1989 and prevention profile,* DHHS Pub No (PHS) 89-1232, Hyattsville, Md., 1989, U.S. Department of Human Services, National Center for Health Statistics, 1989.

Diekelmann N: Staying well while growing old: pre-retirement counseling, *Am J Nurs* 78:1337, 1978.

Diekelmann NL: The young adult: the choice is health or illness, *AJN* 76:1276, 1976.

Duvall EM: *Family development,* ed 5, Philadelphia, 1977, JB Lippincott.

Ebersole P and Hess P: *Toward healthy aging: human needs and nursing response,* ed 3, St. Louis, 1990, Mosby.

Edelman CL and Mandle CL: *Health promotion throughout the lifespan,* ed 2, St. Louis, 1990, Mosby.

Erikson E: *Childhood and society,* ed 2, New York, 1963, WW Norton & Co.

Erikson E: *Identity: youth and crisis,* New York, 1968, WW Norton & Co.

Erikson E: *The life cycle completed: a review,* New York, 1982, WW Norton & Co.

Fortier JC, et al.: Adjustment to a newborn: sibling preparation makes a difference, *JOGNN* 20(1):73, 1991.

Frank ME: Transition into midlife, *NAACOG's Clinical Issues in Perinatal and Women's Health Nursing* 2(4):421, 1991.

Frede DJ: Preconceptional education, *AWHONN's Clinical Issues in Perinatal and Women's Health Nursing* 4(1):60, 1993.

Freud S: *A general introduction into psychoanalysis,* New York, 1969, Pocket Books.

Gardner DL and Campbell B: Assessing Postpartum Fatigue, *MCN* 16(5):264, 1991.

Gilligan C: *In a different voice,* Cambridge, Mass., 1982, Harvard University Press.

Gordon S: *Prisoners of men's dreams: striking out for a new feminine future,* Boston, 1991, Little Brown.

Havighurst RJ: Successful aging. In Williams RH, et al., editors: *Process of aging,* vol 1, New York, 1972, Atherton Press.

Havighurst RJ: *Human development and education,* New York, 1953, David McKay Co.

Hawton K: *Suicide and attempted suicide among children and adolescents,* Beverly Hills, Calif., 1990, Sage Publishers.

Hayes C, et al.: Knowledge, attitudes, and beliefs of HIV seronegative women about AIDS, *J Nurse Midwifery* 34(5):318, 1989.

Hofferth SL, et al.: Premarital sexual activity among U.S teenage women over the past three decades, *Family Planning Perspectives* 19:46, 1987.

Keltner BR: Family influences on child health status, *Ped Nurs* 18(2):128, 1992.

Khabbaz R, et al.: Seroprevalence and risk factors for HTLV-I/II infection among female prostitutes in the United States, *JAMA,* 263(1): 60, 1990.

King EH, et al.: Risk factors for developmental delay among infants and toddlers, *Child Health Care* 21(1):39, 1992.

Kohlberg L: Development of moral character and moral ideology. In Hoffman ML and Hoffman LNW, editors: *Review of child development research,* vol 1, New York, 1964, Russell Sage Foundation.

Kohlberg L: Stages and sequence: the cognitive-developmental approach to socialization. In Goslin DA, editor: *Handbook of socialization theory and research,* Chicago, 1969, Rand McNally & Co.

Levinson D, et al.: *The seasons of a man's life,* New York, 1978, Alfred A Knopf.

Liller KD, et al.: Postpartum patient's knowledge, risk perceptions, and behaviors pertaining to childhood injuries, *J Nurse-Midwifery,* 38(6):355, 1991.

Lipsi K, et al.: Developmental rounds: an intervention strategy for hospitalized infants, *Ped Nurs* 17(5):433, 1991.

Maslow AH: *Motivation and personality,* ed 2, New York, 1970, Harper & Row.

Masters WH and Johnson VE: *Human sexual response,* Boston, 1970, Little, Brown & Co.

Mattsson A: Adolescent depression and suicide. In Hoekelmann R, Friedman SB, et al., editors: *Primary pediatric care,* ed 2, St. Louis, 1992, Mosby.

McAnarney ER and Hender R: Adolescent pregnancy and its consequences, *JAMA,* 262(53):74-77, 1989.

McFarland GK and McFarlane ED: *Nursing diagnosis and intervention: planning for patient care,* ed 2, St. Louis, 1993, Mosby.

National Cancer Institute, Breast Cancer Screening Consortium: Screening mammography: a missed clinical opportunity? Results of the NCI breast cancer screening consortium and National Health interview survey studies, *JAMA* 264(1):54, 1990.

Noel NL and Yam ML: Domestic violence—the pregnant battered woman, *Nurs Clin North Am* 27(4):871, 1992.

Padin M, et al.: Stability of body attitudes and self-esteem in late adolescence, *Adolescence* 61:371, 1981.

Papalia DC and Olds SW: *Human development,* ed 4, St. Louis, 1989, McGraw-Hill.

Parker B and McFarland J: Identifying and helping battered pregnant women, *MCN* 16(3):161, 1991.

Pencak M: Workplace health promotion programs: an overview, *Nurs Clin North Am* 26(1):233, 1991.

Pender NJ: *Health promotion in nursing practice,* ed 2, Norwalk, Conn., 1987, Appleton & Lange.

Peterson KJ and Peterson FL: Family-centered perinatal education, *AWHONN'S Clinical Issues in Perinatal and Women's Health Nursing* 4(1):1, 1993.

Piaget J: *The origins of intelligence in children,* New York, 1952, International Universities Press.

Rawlins RP, Williams SR, and Beck CK: *Mental health—psychiatric nursing: a holistic life-cycle approach,* ed 3, St. Louis, 1993, Mosby.

Rivara FP: Motor vehicle injuries during adolescence, *Pediatric Annual* 17:107, 1988.

Scharlach A: A comparison of employed caregivers of cognitively and physically impaired elderly persons, *Res Aging* 11(2):225, 1989.

Schuster CS and Ashburn SS: *The process of human development: a holistic approach,* ed 2, Boston, 1986, Little Brown.

Servonsky J and Opas SR: *Nursing management of children,* Monterey, Calif., 1987, Jones & Bartlett.
Stanhope M and Lancaster J: *Community health nursing: process and practice for promoting health,* ed 3, St. Louis, 1992, Mosby.
Tanner JM: Sequence and tempo in the somatic changes of puberty. In Grumbach MM, et al., editors: *Control of the onset of puberty,* New York, 1974, John Wiley & Sons.
Tanner JM and Whitehouse RH: *Atlas of children's growth: normal variation and growth diseases,* New York, 1982, Academic Press.
Taulbee LR and Folsom JC: Reality orientation for geriatric patients, *Hosp Community Psychiatry* 17:133, 1966.
Tyre L, Rothbart B, and Anderson K: Helping adolescents make the right contraceptive choice, *Contemporary OB/GYN* 35(3):37, 1990.
U.S. Bureau of the Census: *Statistical abstract of the United States,* Washington, DC, 1984, 1990, The Bureau.
U.S. Preventive Services Task Force: Counseling to prevent household and environmental injuries, *Ann Fam Prac* 42(1):136, 1990.
Valente S and Saunders JM: High school suicide prevention programs, *Ped Nurs* 13(2):108, 1987.
Westwood M, et al.: Growth and development of full term nonasphyxiated small-for-gestational-age newborns: follow-up through adolescence, *Pediatrics* 71:376, 1983.
Whaley LD and Wong DL: *Nursing care of infants and children,* ed 4, St. Louis, 1991, Mosby.
Willis WO and Fullerton JT: Prevention of infant mortality: an agenda for nurse-midwifery, J *Nurse-Midwifery* 36(6):343, 1991.
Wilson DA and Knudtson MD: Assessing school readiness through school entry screening exam, *Nurse Pract* 17(9):24, 1992.
Wilton J, et al.: A menopause center: bridging the midlife gap, *NAACOG's Clinical Issues in Perinatal and Women's Health Nursing* 2(4):527, 1991.
Yurick AG, et al.: *The aged person and the nursing process,* ed 3, Norwalk, Conn., 1989, Appleton-Century-Crofts.

Bibliography

Alexander D, et al.: Anxiety levels of rooming-in and non-rooming-in parents of young hospitalized children, *Maternal Child Nurs J* 12(2):79, 1988.
Ali NS: Promoting safe use of multiple medications by elderly persons, *Geriatr Nurs* 13(3):157-159, 1992.
American College of Obstetricians and Gynecologists: *ACOG Guide to planning for pregnancy, birth, and beyond,* Washington, DC, 1990, ACOG.
Bailey DB: Issues and perspectives on family assessment, *Infants and Young Children* 4(1):26, 1991.
Beverly L and Travis I: Constipation: proposed natural laxative mixtures, *J Gerontol Nurs* 18(10):5-12, 1992.
Bezon J: Approaching drug regiments with a therapeutic dose of suspicion, *Geriatr Nurs* 12(4):180-182, 1991.
Biasella S: A comprehensive perinatal education program, *AWHONN's Clinical Issues in Perinatal and Women's Health Nursing* 4(1):5, 1993.
Bonheur B and Young S: Exercise as health-promoting lifestyle choice, *Applied Nurs Res* 4(1):2, 1991.
Casby MW: Symbolic play: development and assessment considerations, *Infants and Young Children* 4(3):43, 1992.
Dixon SD and Stein MT: *Encounters with children,* St. Louis, 1992, Mosby.
Donaher-Wagner BM and Braun DH: Infant cardiopulmonary resuscitation for expectant and new parents, *MCN,* 17(1):27, 1989.
Fielo S and Warren S: Medication usage by the elderly, *Geriatr Nurs* 14(1):47-51, 1993.
Fontaine KL: The conspiracy of culture: women's issues in body size, *Nurs Clin North Am* 26(3):669, 1991.
Garner CH: Midlife women's health, *NAACOG's Clinical Issues in Perinatal and Women's Health Nursing* 2(4):473, 1991.
Glascoe FP: Developmental screening: rational, methods, and application, *Infants and Young Children* 4(1):1, 1991.
Green CP: Clinical considerations: midlife daughters and their aging parents, *J Gerontol Nurs* 17(11):6-12, 1991.
Hauenstein CJ: Young women and depression: origin, outcome, and nursing care, *Nurs Clin North Am* 26(3):12, 1991.
Heiney SP: Helping children through painful procedures, *AJN* 91(11): 20, 1991.
Jones NE: Childhood injuries: an epidemiological approach, *Ped Nurs* 18(3):235, 1992.
Kelly GL: Childhood depression and suicide, *Nurs Clin North Am* 26(3):545, 1991.
Kennedy CM, Gyr PM, and Garst KF: A nursing tool to assess children upon hospital admission, *MCN* 16(2):78, 1991.
Kizilay PE: Predictors of depression in women, *Nurs Clin North Am* 27(4):983, 1992.
Kramer NA: Comparison of therapeutic touch and causal touch in stress reduction of hospitalized children, *Ped Nurs* 16(5):483, 1990.
Malloy C: Children and poverty: America's future at risk, *Ped Nurs* 18(6):553, 1992.
Mangino MW: Hypertension in elders: clinical diagnosis and treatment considerations, *J Gerontol Nurs* 17(12):14-22, 1991.
Martin DA: Children in peril: a mandate for change in health care policies for low-income children, *Family and Community Health* 15(1): 75, 1992.
McClowry SG: Temperament Theory and Research, *Image* 24(4):319, 1992.
Mitford J: *The American way of birth,* New York, 1992, Dutton.
Nagley SJ: Predicting and preventing confusion in your patients, *J Gerontol Nurs* 12:27, 1986.
National Center for Health Statistics: *Advance report of final mortality statistics (1987),* Monthly vital statistics report 138 (suppl 5), DHHS Pub No (PHS) 89-1120, 1989.
Oehler JM: How to target infants at highest risk for developmental delay, *MCN* 18(1):20, 1993.
Pridham KF: Anticipatory guidance of parents of new infants: potential contribution of the internal working model construct, *Image* 25(1):49, 1993.
Riesch SK: Effects of communication training on parents and young adolescents, *Nurs Res* 42(1):10, 1993.
Sadler LS: Depression in adolescents, *Nurs Clin North Am* 26(3):559, 1991.
Schepp KG: Factors influencing the coping effort of mothers of hospitalized children, *Nurs Res* 40(1):42, 1991.
Sheehy G: *The silent passage—menopause,* New York, 1992, Random House.
Smith DP: *Comprehensive child and family nursing skills,* St. Louis, 1991, Mosby.
Spero D: Sibling preparation classes, *AWHONN's Clinical Issues in Perinatal and Women's Health Nursing* 4(1):122, 1993.
Vance CJ: *Preventing adolescent injury: roles for the health professionals,* Newton, Mass., 1989, Education Development Center.
York R and Brooten D: Prevention of low birth weight, *NAACOG's Clinical Issues in Perinatal and Women's Health Nursing* 3(1):13, 1992.

21 Loss, Death, and Grief

OBJECTIVES

Mastery of content in this chapter will enable the student to:

- Define the key terms listed.
- Identify the nurse's role in assisting clients with problems related to loss, death, and grief.
- Describe and compare the phases of grieving from Engel, Kübler-Ross, and Martocchio.
- List and discuss five basic categories of loss.
- Describe six dimensions of hope.
- Describe characteristics of a person experiencing grief.
- Discuss variables that influence a person's response to grief.
- Develop a care plan for a client or family experiencing grief.
- Describe effective therapeutic communication interventions for grieving clients.
- Select interventions aimed at maintaining a dying client's independence and self-esteem.
- Describe how the nurse provides comfort to a dying client.
- Explain ways for the nurse to assist a family in caring for a dying client.
- Describe the procedure for care of the body after death.
- Discuss the nurse's own loss experience as it influences care of grieving clients.
- Identify two ways nurses can meet their own needs related to loss.

KEY TERMS

anticipatory loss
autopsy
bereavement
death
grieving process
hope
hospice
loss
maturational loss
mourning
palliative
situational loss

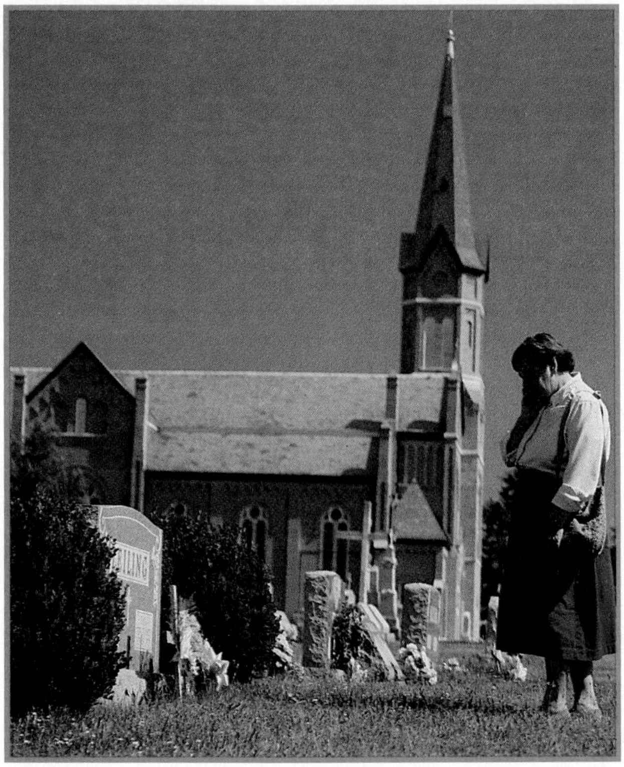

Loss and death are universal and individually unique events of the human experience. Life is a series of losses and gains. A child beginning to walk gains independence with mobility. An older person with visual and hearing changes may lose self-reliance. Illness and hospitalization frequently cause losses.

A nurse works with many clients who experience different types of loss. Coping mechanisms a person learns have much to do with that person's ability to face and accept loss and grief. The nurse's role is to assist clients in understanding and accepting loss so that quality of life can continue. When clients do not do grief work after a profound loss, emotional, mental, and social problems can occur.

Death in our culture is often difficult for the dying person, as well as for the person's family, friends, and care givers. When a person becomes terminally ill, people are reminded of their own mortality. Feelings of guilt, anger, and fear can cause family members and care givers to withdraw at a time when the dying person needs love, reassurance, and support. The style of dying reflects a person's style of living, and a person's attitudes about death depend on the systems of beliefs and emotional strengths that person brings to the task of dying.

CONCEPT OF LOSS, DEATH, GRIEF, AND NURSING

Death is a frequent reality in many nursing care settings. Most nurses interact daily with clients and families experiencing loss and grief. While caring for clients and their families, nurses also experience personal loss as client-family-nurse relationships end through transfer, discharge, recovery, or death. Many nurses find that it is easy to relieve physical symptoms associated with illness and death but difficult to become involved in a meaningful interpersonal relationship to support a person who is suffering or dying. Personal feelings, values, and experiences influence the extent to which nurses can support clients and families during loss or death. Self-assessment—exploring personal attitudes, feelings, and values—is necessary before nurses can use a sensitive, therapeutic approach with others. Developing the art of being with the grieving and dying requires an inner strength that arises from knowledge of and a positive belief in self. Formulation of a philosophy of life helps nurses function during difficult times. Knowledge of the concepts of loss and the grieving process enables nurses to use creative interventions to promote health, prevent illness, and support dying clients.

A person experiences **loss** in the absence of an object, person, body part or function, or emotion or idea that was formerly present. Losses may be actual or perceived. An actual loss is easily identified as with a child whose playmate moves away or an adult who loses a partner. A perceived loss is less tangible, such as the loss of confidence, and is easily misunderstood. Loss may be maturational, situational, or both. The client may experience **maturational loss** (loss resulting from normal life transitions such as a child going off to school for the first time), **situational loss** (loss occurring in response to a specific external event such as the sudden death of a loved one), or both. The child learning to walk loses the infant-like body image, the woman experiencing menopause loses the ability to bear children, and the unemployed person may lose self-esteem.

Loss requires adaptation through the grieving process. The type of loss and the perception of the loss influence the degree of stress. One might assume that the loss of an object would not generate the same stress as loss of a loved one. The more important the object to the person, the more intense the feelings of loss will likely be. However, each individual responds to loss differently. The death of a person's pet that has been a constant companion would likely cause more stress than the loss of a relative not seen for years.

Five types of losses (Table 21-1) include loss of external objects, loss of a known environment, loss of a significant other, loss of an aspect of self, and loss of life. Nurses may care for clients who have experienced more

table 21-1

TYPES OF LOSS

Definition	Implications of loss
Loss of external objects (for example, loss, misplacement, deterioration, theft, or destruction by natural causes)	Extent of grieving depends on object's value, sentiment attached to it, and its usefulness
Loss of a known environment (for example, moving from a neighborhood, hospitalization, a new job, moving out of ICU)	Loss occurs through maturational or situational events and through injury or illness. Loneliness or newness of unfamiliar setting threatens self-esteem and makes grieving difficult
Loss of a significant other (for example, being promoted, moving, or running away, loss of a family member, friend, trusted nurse, acquaintance, and animal companion)	Significant other typically fulfills another person's need for psychological safety, love and belonging, and self-esteem
Loss of an aspect of self (for example, body part or psychological or physiological function)	Illness, injury, or developmental changes result in loss of aspect of self that causes grief and permanent changes in body image and self-concept
Loss of life (for example, death of family member, friend, acquaintance, or own death)	Loss of life creates grief for those left behind. Person facing death often fears pain, loss of control, and dependency on others

than one type of loss, either from family crises, chronic illness, hospitalization, or occupational crises for example. Lewis (1983) describes several potential permanent losses that accompany chronic illness (see box at left). Losses may threaten a client's self-concept, self-esteem, and sense of worth. The nurse needs to assess the meaning loss has for a client and its effect on the client's health status.

POTENTIAL LOSSES FACED BY THE CHRONICALLY ILL

Former good health
Independence
Sense of control over life
Privacy
Modesty
Body image
Relationships
Established roles inside and outside the home
Social status
Sense of self-confidence
Possessions
Financial security
Means of productivity and self-fulfillment in a job or at home
Life-style
Plans or fantasies for the future
Fantasy of immortality
Familiar daily routine
Sleep
Sexual functioning
Leisure activities

Modified from Lewis K: *J Rehabil* 49:8, 1983.

GRIEVING PROCESS

The terms *grief, mourning,* and *bereavement* are often used interchangeably. **Bereavement** is the state of thought, feeling, and activity that follows loss. It includes grief and mourning. **Grief** is a form of sorrow that follows the perception or anticipation of a loss of one or more valued or significant objects. These responses often include helplessness, loneliness, hopelessness, sadness, guilt, and anger. **Mourning** is the process that follows a loss and includes working through grief. The processes of grief and mourning can be intense, internal, painful, and lengthy.

Grief is a normal response to a loss. Grief is a process, not an event. Behaviors and feelings associated with the **grieving process** occur in individuals experiencing the loss of anything important to them. These same feelings and behaviors can occur when individuals face their own death. Grief not only occurs in the persons experiencing the loss but also in family or friends.

There is no one "right" way to grieve. The concept

table 21-2

COMPARISON OF THREE THEORIES OF THE GRIEVING PROCESS

Engel (1964)	Kübler-Ross (1969)	Martocchio (1985)
Shock and disbelief	Denial	Shock and disbelief
	Anger	Yearning and protest
Developing awareness	Bargaining	Anguish, disorganization, and despair
	Depression	Identification in bereavement
Reorganization and restitution	Acceptance	Reorganization and restitution

and theories of grief are only tools that can be used to anticipate the emotional needs of clients and families and plan interventions to help them understand and deal with their grief. The nurse's role in assisting the client is to assess grieving behaviors, recognize the influence of grief on behavior, and provide empathetic support.

The classic works of Engel (1964) and Kübler-Ross (1969), as well as the more recent work of Martocchio (1985), provide frameworks for understanding the concept and dynamics of the grieving process. Each theory includes phases or stages a person experiences while resolving grief.

Engel's Theory

Engel's framework is process oriented and incorporates the following phases: shock and disbelief, development of awareness, and reorganization and restitution (Table 21-2). In the first step, the individual denies the reality of the loss and protects himself or herself from the effects of stress by withdrawing from family and friends or sometimes wandering aimlessly. Initial physical reactions may include fainting, diaphoresis, nausea, diarrhea, rapid heart rate, restlessness, insomnia, and fatigue. In the second step, the individual begins to feel the loss acutely and may experience desperation. Suddenly the emotions of anger, guilt, frustration, depression, and emptiness occur. Crying is common as a person becomes preoccupied with the loss. In the third step, the individual experiences the work of mourning when the loss is acknowledged. This involves resolving the loss in some way (e.g., the individual is able to put the loss into a larger perspective). Feelings of guilt and remorse are common. The individual begins to reorganize his/her life and a new self-awareness develops.

Kübler-Ross' Stages of Dying

The framework provided by Kübler-Ross (1969) is behavior oriented and includes five stages (see Table 21-2). In the denial stage, the individual acts as though nothing has happened and may refuse to believe or understand that a loss has occurred. In the anger stage, the individual resists the loss and may strike out at everyone and everything in the environment. In the bargaining stage, there is postponement of the reality of the loss; the individual may try to deal in a subtle or overt way to prevent the loss from occurring. The depression stage occurs when the loss is realized and the full impact of its significance is apparent; the grieving person may feel overwhelmingly lonely and withdraw from interpersonal interactions. In the fifth stage, acceptance, the individual finally accepts the loss.

Martocchio's Phases of Grieving

Martocchio (1985) describes five phases of grief that have overlapping boundaries and no expected order (see Table 21-2). It is important to remember that while a client passes through phases of grief, family and friends also experience grief in their way and at their pace. A person progresses and then regresses until the loss is finally resolved. The duration of grief is variable and depends on the factors influencing the grief response. Intense reactions of grief usually subside within 6 to 12 months, but active mourning may continue 3 to 5 years, according to Martocchio's theory. Table 21-3 shows nursing implications related to Martocchio's phases of grief.

HOPE

Hope is a multidimensional, changing life force, characterized by a confident yet uncertain expectation of achieving a future goal (Dufault and Martocchio, 1985). Hope is not a single act but a complex series of thoughts, feelings, and actions that change often. Clients dealing with loss and the families of these clients may experience different dimensions of hope. Dufault and Martocchio define the concept of hope as having the following dimensions:

1. Affective. Sensations and emotions (for example, feelings of confidence or an attraction to the desired outcome) that are part of hoping
2. Cognitive. The processes by which persons wish, imagine, perceive, think, learn, or judge in relation to hope
3. Behavioral. The actions, including those that are physiological, psychological, spiritual, cultural, or developmental, a person takes to achieve hope
4. Affiliative. A person's sense of involvement be-

table 21-3

NURSING IMPLICATIONS OF MARTOCCHIO'S PHASES OF GRIEF AND KÜBLER-ROSS' STAGES OF DYING

Behaviors	Nursing Implications
SHOCK AND DISBELIEF (Martocchio) **Denial (Kübler-Ross)**	
Denial is immediate response to news of loss or impending loss. Physiological responses may include muscular weakness, tremors, deep sighs, flushed or cold and clammy skin, diaphoresis, anorexia, and discomfort. Individuals avoid accepting reality of situation by not making decisions; they may attempt activities that they are no longer able to do, fail to comply with treatment, search for evidence that loss has not or will not occur, and appear artificially happy. Mood swings are common. Individuals isolate themselves from sources of accurate information or reject offers of comfort and support.	Support emotional needs without reinforcing denial. Offer to remain with clients without discussing reasons for behavior or need to cope unless they bring it up. Offer supportive care such as food, drink, and safety.
YEARNING AND PROTEST (Martocchio) **Anger (Kübler-Ross)**	
Individuals may express anger and retaliate against family, staff, physicians, or supreme being. Bereaved may express anger toward deceased. Individuals become demanding and accusing. Anger may precipitate guilt and lead to anxiety and lowered self-esteem. Individuals may feel resentful and jealous of others who still have lost object or loved one. Individuals may be reluctant to share feelings and thoughts.	Provide anticipatory guidance about feelings and their intensity experienced as part of grief; focus especially on anger. Do not take anger personally. Meet needs that cause angry response.
ANGUISH, DISORGANIZATION, AND DESPAIR (Martocchio) **Bargaining (Kübler-Ross)**	
Individuals are willing to do anything to avoid loss or change prognosis or fate. Individuals make bargains with supreme being. Individuals accept new forms of therapy.	Provide information needed for decision making.
IDENTIFICATION IN BEREAVEMENT (Martocchio) **Depression (Kübler-Ross)**	
Reality and permanence of loss become recognized.	Provide support and empathy. Support crying by offering touch that communicates caring.
Confusion, lack of motivation, disinterest, indecision, and crying are common.	Listen attentively.
Withdrawal from relationships and activities occurs. Individuals may become quiet and noncommunicative. Feelings of loneliness surface. Reminiscence about past and lost object begins. Individuals may lose interest in appearance. Individuals may become suicidal or cope by beginning unhealthy behaviors such as excessive drug use.	Assess risk of harm to self and refer to mental health professional if needed.
REORGANIZATION AND RESTITUTION (Martocchio) **Acceptance (Kübler-Ross)**	
Individuals accept terms of loss and death and begin plans for it. Individuals can share feelings about loss. Reminiscence about past occurs. Periods of depression and well-being occur. Good times begin to outweigh bad. Life begins to stabilize.	Offer opportunities to share feelings verbally, in writing or art, or by tape recordings. Allow and encourage review as often as clients want to talk. Show acceptance of labile emotions. Assist in discussing future plans.

yond self, including social interaction, attachment, and intimacy with others
5. Temporal. The person's experience of past, present, and future time in relation to hoping
6. Contextual. A person perceiving and interpreting hope within the context of life (Life situations influence and are part of hope. Hope may arise with an actual or potential loss.)

Awareness of the dimensions of hope helps a nurse to support a client's hope and assists him or her through the grieving process. It is important to include the family.

NURSING PROCESS IN GRIEF, LOSS, AND DEATH

Assessment

During assessment the nurse should not hold a preconceived expectation of grief on the client or family. The nurse also should not assume that a particular behavior indicates grief. Adequate information is needed to make accurate conclusions and diagnoses.

Assessment of the client and family begins by exploring the meaning of loss to them. This is done by collecting objective and subjective data. The nurse interviews the client and family, observes their responses and behaviors, and uses open communication, emphasizing listening skills. The nurse should be alert for nonverbal cues. Initial impressions are validated with the client and family so that nursing diagnoses and effective interventions can be developed.

The nurse must assess not *how* the client *should be* reacting but how the client *is* reacting. Sequences of behavior or phases may occur in order, they may be skipped, or they may recur. Many variables affect grief. Assessment of these variables gives the nurse a broad data base from which to individualize care (see box on pp. 498-499).

Grief Behaviors

Assessment of the client and family includes consideration of the stages of grief. By observing behavior, the nurse can make an assessment regarding the effects of loss. The nurse carefully assesses the existence of unique individual, family, and situational characteristics such as the relationship of spouses or events leading to the loss. It may be possible on the basis of careful observations and nurse-client interactions to predict the nature of grief resolution.

No two people grieve in exactly the same way. However, grieving patterns have been researched and documented and are observable in persons experiencing loss. A person in Engel's shock stage of grief will display different behaviors than a person experiencing the stage of developing awareness (Table 21-4). A client moves back and forth among the stages of grief until final reorganization occurs.

A client experiences a variety of emotions, depending on the stage of the Kubler-Ross model of dying or grief (Table 21-5). The nurse must recognize that each emotion serves a purpose in helping the client to cope with loss. The nurse must not focus on a single behavior or emotion displayed in an effort to label the grief stage. However, the client's behaviors guide the interventions used by the nurse to assist the client.

A client's death takes place in a social context. Even during the dying phase the family begins to reorganize itself; the client is no longer available to fulfill the same number and types of roles. The nurse assesses the family's grief process, recognizing that family members may be dealing with different aspects of grief than the client.

table 21-4

BEHAVIORS COMMON TO ENGEL'S STAGES OF GRIEVING

Stage of grief	Behaviors
Shock and disbelief	Emotionally denies loss occurred; intellectually can accept loss but does not comprehend implications; withdraws from social interactions; is preoccupied with image of lost object or person; seems to stare or move about aimlessly; has difficulty carrying out normal daily activities; has somatic complaints, including shortness of breath, choking, sighing, chills, anorexia, fatigue, faintness
Developing awareness	Begins to realize loss is real; experiences guilt, anger, frustration, depression, frequently cries
Reorganization and resolution	Involves the work of mourning, including the steps of resolving the loss and idealization; accepts loss; desires to renew life and looks to the future; becomes interested in new objects and relationships; seeks pleasurable experiences; is able to talk about loss realistically

FACTORS INFLUENCING A GRIEF REACTION

AGE

Infant

It is assumed that an infant is not able to understand concepts of loss and death until he or she is able to recognize familiar persons or form an attachment to a care giver. After trust forms with parents, even temporary loss can cause anxiety.

Toddler

Self-centeredness and confusion of fact and fantasy prevent an understanding of death. The toddler feels anxiety over loss of objects and separation from parents.

Preschooler

The preschooler perceives death as a kind of sleep or temporary absence. Unfamiliarity with the concept of time prevents understanding the finality of death. The toddler may react to less significant loss (e.g., a pet) with more outward grief.

School-age child

This age child experiences grief over the loss of a body part or function. He or she associates misdeeds with causing death and may feel guilty about the loss of significant others. The school-age child equates death with destruction.

Adolescent

The adolescent usually feels acute grief over the loss of a body part or function. He or she fears peer rejection. The teenager has an adult comprehension of the concept of death but is the least likely of any age-group to accept the loss of life because of the developmental task of establishing identity and purpose in life.

Young adult

The young adult relates loss to its significance for status, roles, and life-style. The loss of economic well-being, divorce, or health causes much grief. The concept of death is greatly influenced by religious and cultural beliefs.

Middle-aged adult

This adult usually begins to reexamine life and is sensitive to physical changes. The loss of others poses a significant threat to life-style. He or she considers how death will occur.

Older adult

The older adult experiences anticipatory grief because of aging and the possible loss of capabilities for self-care. He or she often fears loss of independence. Acceptance of death depends on many personal factors. This adult may fear events surrounding death more than death itself.

CULTURAL AND SPIRITUAL BELIEFS

Cultural

Values, attitudes, beliefs, and customs influence reactions to loss, grief, and death. Each individual is influenced by them in many ways. Chapter 18 explores aspects of culture and ethnic background.

Spiritual

Spiritual reactions include practices, rites, and rituals involving loss and grieving. People turn to religion for solace and support. Loss can sometimes cause internal conflicts about spiritual values and the meaning of life.

SEX ROLES

Men

It is often socially and culturally more difficult for men to express grief openly because they are expected to be strong and supportive.

Women

It is often socially and culturally more acceptable for women to express grief openly because they are expected to need support.

SOCIOECONOMIC STATUS

All levels

The family's financial resources often determine options.

SOCIAL SUPPORT

The support that clients receive is based on their value to the members of the social system and the manner and circumstances of their loss.

NATURE OF LOSS

Circumstances

Sudden, unanticipated death frequently leads to slower resolution from grief. Deaths by violence are generally more difficult to accept.

DYING PERSON'S GRIEF

The intensity and rate of grieving are influenced by the time between the client's first awareness that he or she will die and the moment of death. In intensive care units, death is frequently sudden, and clients and family have little time for grief.

NATURE OF RELATIONSHIPS

Spouse

Impact of the death of a spouse is usually greater than that with the death of a parent because of the effect on life-style. The loss of a sexual partner threatens perception of sexuality and desire for sex. It can be difficult to establish new friendships.

FACTORS INFLUENCING A GRIEF REACTION—cont'd

Child

The death of a child is generally perceived as premature (i.e., out of sync with usual development). Parents often feel guilt and blame.

Significant other

The death of a significant other involves many needs for the survivor, including a need for support and a need to express emotions. Many relationships common in today's society are unacceptable to others, often leaving these grievers disenfranchised (e.g., gay couples) (Doka, 1989).

GOALS

The more goals a person has, the more likely the person will be able to adapt to a loss of only one goal. The more central to one's life the goal is, the more intense the grief. An example would be if a person's whole life was dedicated to the goal of becoming a dancer and then that person lost the use of their legs, their life goal would be lost.

table 21-5

BEHAVIORS REPRESENTATIVE OF KÜBLER-ROSS' STAGES OF DYING

Stage	Behaviors
Denial	Avoids reality; cannot deal with decisions about treatment; may attempt activities of which he/she is no longer physically capable; isolates self from sources of accurate information; fails to comply with medical therapy; uses considerable emotional energy to deny truth; may appear artificially happy.
Anger	May retaliate against family members, nursing staff, or physicians; becomes demanding and accusing; anger may arouse guilt because client knows he/she depends on care givers; guilt may foster feelings of anxiety and low self-esteem.
Bargaining	Fears losing body functions, experiencing uncontrollable pain, and losing control; is willing to do anything to change prognosis or fate; accepts new forms of therapies.
Depression	Recognizes potential loss; may withdraw from important relationships to avoid painful feelings; may become quiet and noncommunicative when feeling loss of control; may express feelings of loneliness; does little to maintain appearance; may become suicidal when unrealistic hopes of a cure fade.
Acceptance	Accepts terms of death; begins to make plans for death (for example, writes a will, completes financial arrangements for the family, gives up personal possessions); is able to discuss feelings about death; reminisces about past.

When assessing the client's or family members' responses to loss, the nurse will find it helpful to have a framework for collecting data. Subjective data collected allow the nurse to determine relationships between the family and client that may affect responses to loss. The focus is on individual family members, their experiences with grief, their understanding of loss, and their knowledge of grief reactions. Objectively, the nurse also observes the level of communication between the client and family members. Expressions of anger, guilt, or other emotions reflecting the stages of grief can help in identifying individual needs.

The nurse observes behaviors that may indicate grief, such as difficulty sleeping or eating. Gastrointestinal disturbances such as indigestion, nausea and vomiting, anorexia, or a recent change in weight may indicate grieving. Fatigue and a reduced activity level may also be present. The presence of a single physical symptom does not necessarily lead to a nursing diagnosis related to grief.

Nurse's Grief

Nurses may also experience grief when working with clients, especially with dying clients. As a result, nurses' roles in supporting grieving clients and family can become complicated. However, nurses should avoid imposing their own grief on clients and families. This is not to say one should not share in the grief experience when appropriate. The nurse needs to be aware of the relationship he/she has with the client and family and how his/her grief can affect them. Nurses who are not aware of their own grief issues usually have more difficulty in relating to clients as unique individuals; for example, a dying client may remind the nurse of a beloved grandparent, and the nurse may become overly emotionally involved. Other requisites for working with dying clients include coming to grips with one's own mortality, understanding the grief process and appreciating the experience of the dying client, using effective listening skills, acknowledging personal limits, and knowing when there is a need to get away and take care of self.

Nursing Diagnosis

The nurse gathers subjective and objective data to identify a pattern of defining characteristics that lead to a definitive nursing diagnosis (see box below). For example, a client's impending move to a new town, the behaviors of anger and sorrow, and a history of poor sleep can indicate the diagnosis of dysfunctional grieving. A diagnosis related to grieving indicates that patterns of grieving or responses to loss have been identified and validated. Identifying specific related factors such as loss of spouse or a move away from home helps the nurse to develop interventions appropriate to the client's needs. When the related factor is loss of a spouse, the nurse will focus on helping the client express thoughts and feelings and develop strategies for resocialization. When the related factor is a move away from home, the nurse helps the client look to the future home and the positive experiences it will bring. An inaccurately identified related factor will prevent the nurse from choosing successful therapies.

The phenomenon of **anticipatory grief** refers to the process of accomplishing part of the grief work before an actual loss. For example, a woman who anticipates losing a breast because of cancer may have begun to grieve the moment the breast mass was first discovered. Nurses feel anticipatory grief while watching clients experience the stages of dying. Anticipatory grief can be beneficial if it helps a person to progress to a healthier emotional state after the loss has occurred.

Complicated grief and mourning is characterized by emotional expressions of unresolved grief that interfere with life functioning. The nurse must recognize that recurring feelings of sorrow may occur while a person normally moves through the grieving process to resolution of a loss. A person with complicated grief may not move through the grieving process but instead experience serious mental regression. If resolution does not occur in a reasonable time, unresolved grief may become chronic and be complicated by depression (Werner-Beland, 1980).

Behavioral manifestations of unresolved or complicated grief include the following:

1. Overactivity without a sense of loss
2. Alteration in relationships with friends and family
3. Hostilities against specific persons
4. Agitated depression with tension, agitation, insomnia, feelings of worthlessness, extreme guilt, and even suicidal tendencies
5. Diminished participation in religious and ritual activities related to the client's culture
6. Inability to discuss the loss without crying (particularly more than a year after the loss)
7. False euphoria

In addition to a diagnosis of grief, the nurse may also diagnose other health problems common to grieving, such as sleep disturbance or altered nutrition. In these situations, the nurse's interventions must focus on resolving grief before the problems are solved. For example, simply introducing sleep therapies will do little if the client continues to be depressed.

The dying client requires special consideration when nursing diagnoses are formulated. A client with a terminal illness that may cause deformity or physical disabilities is likely to undergo alterations in body image or self-concept. An example of this is a client with leukemia who receives chemotherapeutic drugs that cause loss of hair. As a dying client's condition worsens, the nurse makes diagnoses relevant to basic needs such as comfort, nutrition, or sensory/perceptual status. Because of the nature and severity of terminal illness, physical assessment data are collected frequently to validate diagnoses.

NURSING DIAGNOSES RELATED TO LOSS, DEATH, AND GRIEF

Anticipatory grieving
Impaired adjustment
Altered nutrition: less than body requirements
Ineffective family coping: compromised
Altered family processes
Hopelessness
Social isolation
Spiritual distress
Sleep pattern disturbance

Planning

Grieving is the natural response to loss. Grieving has a therapeutic value, enabling people to think through loss, recollect their thoughts, and resume life with new insights and direction. Nursing care is planned to meet the physiological, emotional, developmental, and spiritual needs of the grieving client. The nurse develops a plan of care (see care plan on p. 501) based on nursing diagnoses and designed to meet goals set with the client. Goals for clients and family members may include:

Goal: Client resolves grief within 2 months.

Outcomes

Client expresses thoughts and feelings related to loss within 3 weeks

SAMPLE NURSING CARE PLAN
Dysfunctional Grieving

ASSESSMENT

Clinical scenario: Mr. Knowles is a 79-year-old client seen in the local community health clinic. Two years ago Mr. Knowles' *wife of 45 years died.* Since then, he has reported *difficulty falling and remaining asleep.* As a result, he feels exhausted all the time. His son and daughter live close by and report that Mr. Knowles has *difficulty discussing his loss,* that he continues to talk *as though his wife is still alive,* and that he experiences *frequent crying* episodes in public, causing him embarrassment. Consequently, he doesn't want to go anywhere. He is spending increasing time isolating himself.

NURSING DIAGNOSIS

Dysfunctional grieving related to difficulty expressing feelings over loss of spouse

PLANNING

Goals	Expected outcomes
Client will experience resolution of complicated grief and mourning within 3 months.	Client will discuss feelings related to wife's death with nurse and family within 2 months. Client expresses emotions through crying openly. Client is able to reminisce about positive past experiences involving his wife within 3 months. Acknowledges the reality of his wife's death and uses past tense when referring to her at 3 months.

IMPLEMENTATION

Steps	Rationale
1. Acknowledge client's grief, be empathetic, and encourage open expression of feelings.	Allows client to recognize feelings are normal and demonstrates staff's understanding (Mulhern, 1986). Expression of feelings is unique to individual. Listening to client without judgment promotes development of therapeutic relationship that will support further trust and sharing (Rando, 1984).
2. Listen attentively and use nonverbal cues that display interest in conversation.	Grieving client needs to know staff cares about him (Stockdale and Hutzenbiler, 1986).
3. Give client chance to talk about goals for remainder of life and to reminisce or reflect on meaning of life and death.	Client focuses on reality, promoting eventual acceptance of death (Dufault and Martocchio, 1985).
4. Arrange meetings with others who share same experience as client.	

EVALUATION

Observe client discussing loss with nurse, son, or daughter.
Observe client's nonverbal behaviors.
Ask client to talk about feelings about loss.

Defining characteristics are shown in italic type.

Client participates in decision making and cooperates with recommended treatments within 1 month.

Goal: Client regains sense of self-esteem within 2 weeks.

Outcomes

Client resumes rest and sleep habits and leisure activities within 2 weeks

Client will maintain well-groomed appearance in 1 week

Goal: Client renews normal activities or relationships within 2 months.

Outcomes

Client resumes participation in church activities within 1 month

Client returns to work within 1 week

When caring for dying clients, the nurse's responsibilities extend to the dying clients' physical needs and unique psychological and social problems. The three most crucial needs of the dying client are control of pain, preservation of dignity and self-worth, and love and affection (Rando, 1984). Additional goals for dying clients may include:

Goal: Client achieves comfort within 1 week.

Outcome

Client perceives a reduction in pain severity within 3 days

Goal: Client maintains independence in daily activities within 1 week.

Outcome

Client dresses and feeds self within 3 days

Goal: Client maintains hope.

Outcome

Client verbalizes finding meaning in life

Goal: Client achieves spiritual comfort.

Outcome

Client expresses satisfaction with belief system

Goal: Client gains relief from loneliness and isolation within 1 month.

Outcomes

Client verbalizes feelings about loneliness and isolation in 2 weeks

Client invites friend for regular visit to the home within 1 month

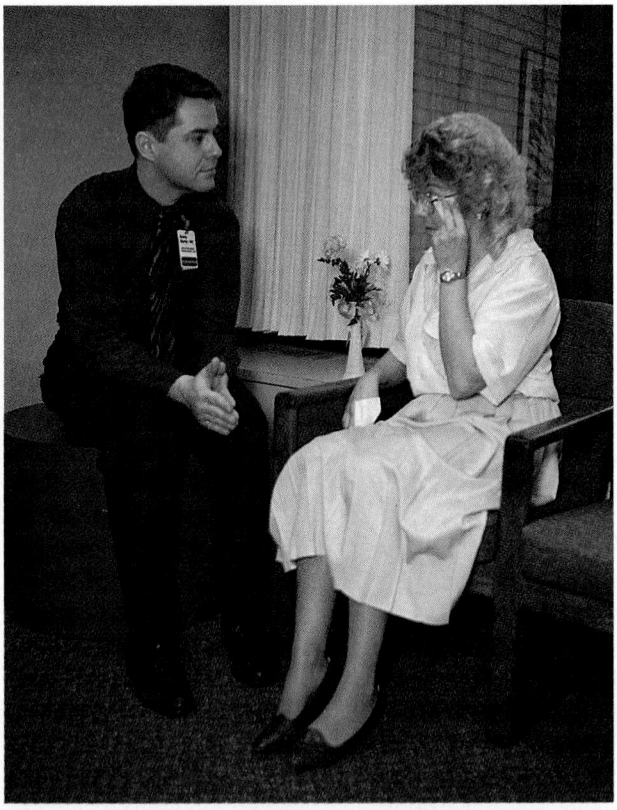

FIGURE 21-1 Nurses assist family members in finding resources to help with the grieving process.

Whatever loss a client has experienced or is facing, the nurse can utilize resources for the plan of care. Friends, family, clergy, support groups, and even legal consultants can assist (Figure 21-1). In the case of a terminally ill client, the nurse also supports the grieving family and provides opportunities for them to support the client. Each client and family should be treated as unique, with recognition that their needs, fears, hopes, expectations, and concerns will change throughout the illness. Once a plan is implemented, continuing reevaluation will be necessary.

Nurses are in a unique position to address client goals. Their presence can bring comfort and reduce anxiety for the client. Nurses can structure schedules and surroundings so that the client has a sense of security and control over life and the environment. Nurses support the client's self-esteem by asking for opinions regarding care. Nurses encourage families to make decisions with the client, not for the client. This may help prepare the family for when the client may not be able to make choices. As circumstances and the illness change, the client changes as well.

Implementation

Therapeutic Communication

Nursing care of the grieving client begins with trying to understand the significance of the loss to the client. This may be difficult if the client is unwilling to express feelings or is in shock or denial. The nurse observes the response to the loss and then attempts to identify the client's strengths in dealing with it. To identify client strengths, the nurse uses open-ended questions and reflective statements such as "You appear concerned about your brother's condition" or "When the doctor informed you about the test results, you appeared frightened" or "What were you thinking?". The nurse schedules adequate time with the client and family to promote open communication and, where possible, provides a private location for a discussion regarding the loss situation. The nurse's words and actions convey acceptance of the client's and family's grief reactions. For example, if a client begins to cry, the nurse quietly remains ready to offer support, rather than abandoning the client when comfort needs are the greatest. Acknowledging grief through touching the client and expressing concern may evoke the client's trust. Clients have differing needs regarding touch. It is important to be sensitive to the client's reactions to closeness and touch.

If a client chooses not to share feelings or concerns, the nurse conveys a willingness to be available when needed. When the nurse is reassuring and acknowledges the client's beliefs and values, a therapeutic relationship may evolve. Sometimes clients need to begin resolving the grief before they can discuss the loss.

It is also important to recognize clients' normal styles of dealing with difficult situations. If they do not normally talk about their feelings, they are unlikely to discuss feelings regarding loss.

When considering reactions to loss, the nurse is alert to the possibility of expressions of denial, anger, depression, or guilt. An initial denial of the loss is normal. If the nurse encourages the client to face the reality of the loss before the client is ready, the nurse may become the target of the client's anger or fear after denial is resolved. Because it is difficult not to take anger personally, the nurse may avoid a client who expresses anger or guilt. The nurse needs to understand his/her own personal feelings before encouraging the client's expression of anger. The nurse remains supportive by letting the client and family know that feelings of anger are normal. For example, the nurse might say "You are obviously upset. I just want to let you know I'm available to talk if you'd like."

It is important for the nurse to avoid erecting barriers to communication (see Chapter 13) by denying the client's grief, providing false reassurance, or avoiding discussion of the problem. For example, when a client expresses anger about a terminal illness, the nurse avoids making statements such as "Don't worry; you'll probably outlive us all" or "Since you're upset, why don't we discuss something else?"

When a client demonstrates a readiness to deal with grief, the nurse can discuss the recognized grief reactions. Effective listening techniques and communication of concern and understanding also help the client to move through the grieving process.

No topic that a dying client wishes to discuss should be avoided. The client will be more likely to discuss impending death with a person willing to listen. The client may initially test the nurse by offering a statement that does not explicitly express true concerns. For example, the client may make an open-ended statement such as "My doctor talked with me today . . . .," hoping the nurse will respond.

If the nurse senses the client's desire to begin a discussion, it is important to let the client discuss his or her concerns. The nurse responds to questions as honestly and positively as possible without giving false reassurance. Strategies to support a client's or family member's hope depend on the dimension of hope (Dufault and Martocchio, 1985) and include the following:

1. Showing an empathetic understanding of the client's and family member's strengths such as patience and courage (affective)
2. Clarifying or modifying the hoping person's reality perceptions by offering information about an illness or treatment and correcting misinformation (cognitive)
3. Assisting the client to use personal resources and those of others by balancing levels of independence, interdependence, and dependence (behavioral)
4. Strengthening or fostering relationships with others that are consistent with hope so that client knows he or she is cared for and important (affiliative)
5. Attending to a client's experience of time, using client's insights from past experience and applying them to the present (temporal)
6. Giving the client the opportunity to discuss life situations that have an influence on hope and encouraging discussion about desired goals and reminiscing (contextual)

The nurse can help the client to develop a hopeful attitude while the client is still physically strong. A dying client easily can become depressed. If the nursing staff can encourage feelings of hope when the client is still receiving active treatment, the client will be better able to participate in the treatment. The refusal to die or accept the feeling of helplessness serves as a motivator. Clients who remain confident and determined despite severe illness may be better able to tolerate side effects of treatment, make fewer demands on staff, serve as models for other clients, and often live longer than predicted. By teaching clients and families the early signs of hopelessness and despair (such as asking few questions about treatment, avoiding discussions of the client's condition, refusing to eat, or ignoring efforts to maintain personal hygiene), the nurse can help the client to assume healthier behaviors.

As the grieving client moves toward resolution, the nurse can encourage discussion of effects of the loss on the client. The nurse may discuss signs of resolution with the client and family. The nurse encourages efforts to loosen ties with the past and begin to look to the future.

The nurse needs to recognize limitations in being able to provide appropriate interventions for a grieving client. When the expertise of other professionals is needed, the nurse explores alternatives in selecting appropriate resource persons, community agencies, or groups to enhance grief work. Some groups available in communities are self-help groups, bereavement groups, widow-to-widow groups, and parent groups. Signs of unresolved grief and complicated grieving reactions may require referral to a psychologist, psychiatrist, or counselor.

Maintenance of Self-Esteem

Nursing interventions focus on promoting the client's sense of identity, dignity, and self-esteem. The nurse can help by listening, responding quickly and positively to requests, maintaining confidentiality and privacy, and providing comfort and support. The quality and quantity of time spent with the client are important in creating a therapeutic environment for the grieving process. Davitz and Davitz (1980) explored the characteristics of nurses who demonstrate a "highly refined" empathetic response to clients. These nurses identified their relationship with the client as the very core of nursing. Measures that provide comfort and support should be implemented in a caring, unhurried manner to reinforce the client's feelings of self-worth and dignity and to decrease the fear of rejection, isolation, and the sense of hopelessness.

Self-esteem and dignity complement each other. Dignity is the person's ability to maintain a self-concept as a person. Disabilities experienced by the client may threaten dignity. Care givers often take control of the client's life. Taking away the client's right to make decisions about care fosters hopelessness and feelings of despair. The client may lose the will to live. To maintain self-esteem, the client must believe that his or her opinions are valuable in decisions that will affect the course of his or her life.

The nurse can maintain and promote self-esteem by giving attention to the client's appearance. Cleanliness, a lack of body odors, attractive clothing, and personal grooming (e.g., shaving or wearing ribbons in the hair) are some ways to promote a sense of worth. It is important for the nurse, who assumes management of the client's body functions, to show an attitude of respect and helpfulness rather than encourage dependence or feelings of guilt.

THE DYING PERSON'S BILL OF RIGHTS

I have the right to be treated as a living human being until I die.

I have the right to maintain a sense of hopefulness, however changing its focus may be.

I have the right to be cared for by those who can maintain a sense of hopefulness, however changing this might be.

I have the right to express my feelings and emotions about my approaching death in my own way.

I have the right to participate in decisions concerning my care.

I have the right to expect continuing medical and nursing attention even though "cure" goals must be changed to "comfort" goals.

I have the right not to die alone.

I have the right to be free from pain.

I have the right to have my questions answered honestly.

I have the right not to be deceived.

I have the right to have help from and for my family in accepting my death.

I have the right to die in peace and dignity.

I have the right to retain my individuality and not be judged for my decisions that may be contrary to beliefs of others.

I have the right to discuss and enlarge my religious and/or spiritual experiences, whatever these may mean to others.

I have the right to expect that the sanctity of the human body will be respected after death.

I have the right to be cared for by caring, sensitive, knowledgeable people who will attempt to understand my needs and will be able to gain some satisfaction in helping me face my death.

From Barbus AJ: The dying person's bill of rights, *Am J Nurs* 75:99, 1975.

Promotion of Return to Daily Activities

As clients begin to work through their losses, the nurse encourages a resumption of their usual daily activities. If clients and families are able to express grief openly and progress through the grief process with support and understanding, the resolution of grief is easier. Depending on the nature of a client's loss, many demands may be placed on the client's and family members' resources.

The nurse can help by encouraging clients to participate in decisions about their care, relationships with others, and resources for the future. The identification of usual life-style practices helps to bring a sense of closure to the loss. For example, if a woman has begun to accept the loss from a mastectomy, the nurse introduces the client to a member of Reach for Recovery who shows the client breast prostheses, talks about clothing and grooming, and discusses ways to resume normal activities.

CARE OF DYING CLIENTS AND THEIR FAMILIES

Special Needs of the Dying

Nursing care of the terminally ill client can be demanding and stressful. However, helping a dying person retain dignity can be one of nursing's greatest rewards. A client may experience symptoms of grief for months before death occurs. The nurse can share the dying client's grief and intervene in a way that improves the quality of life. A dying client has a right to be cared for with respect and concern. The dying person's bill of rights (see box at left) ensures comprehensive and compassionate care.

Promotion of Comfort. Comfort for a dying client includes pain control and control of symptoms of dis-

table 21-6
PROMOTING COMFORT IN THE TERMINALLY ILL CLIENT

Symptoms	Characteristics or causes	Nursing implications
Pain	Pain can be acute or chronic.	Individualize pharmacologic therapies for each patient. Administer narcotic analgesics on a regular schedule to prevent pain recurrence (see Chapter 28).
	Pain from progressive cancer is usually chronic and constant.	Cutaneous stimulation, including application of heat and cold, massage, pressure or vibration, relieves pain of muscle tension or spasm.** Relaxation and guided imagery relieve pain through distraction. Oral route for narcotics is preferred, but choose route with fewest risks and greatest benefit.** Introduce psychosocial intervention early.**
Discomfort	Any source of physical irritation may worsen pain.	Provide thorough skin care, including daily baths, lubrication of skin, and dry, clean bed linens to reduce irritants.
	As client approaches death, mouth remains open, tongue becomes dry and edematous, and lips become dry and cracked.	Provide oral care at least every 2 to 4 hours. Use soft toothbrushes or foam swabs for frequent mouth care. Apply a light film of petroleum jelly to lips and tongue (see Chapter 30).
	Blinking reflexes diminish near death, causing drying of cornea.	Eye care removes crusts from eyelid margins. Artificial tears reduce corneal drying.
Nausea and vomiting	Nausea and vomiting result from disease process (for example, gastric cancer), complications (for example, bowel obstruction), or medications.	Confer with physician about changing medications when possible. Administer antiemetics before meals. Bowel decompression with a nasogastric tube may relieve obstruction. Give mouth care and quickly clean up emesis.
Fatigue	Metabolic demands of a cancerous tumor cause weakness and fatigue.	Help client to identify valued or desired tasks; then help client to conserve energy for only those tasks. Promote frequent rest periods in a quiet environment.
	Exhaustion phase of the general adaptation syndrome causes energy depletion.	Time and pace nursing care activities.
Constipation	Narcotic medications and immobility slow peristalsis.	Give preventive care, which is most effective: increase fluid intake; include bran, whole grain products, and frest vegetables in diet; and encourage exercise.
	Lack of bulk in diet or reduced fluid intake may occur with appetite changes.	
	Constipation can add to discomfort.	Administer prophylactic stool softeners.
Diarrhea	Results from disease process (for example, colon cancer) and complications of treatment or medications.	Assess for fecal impaction. Confer with physician to change medication if possible. Provide low-residue diet.
Urinary incontinence	Incontinence results from progressive disease (for example, involvement of spinal cord or reduced level of consciousness).	Protect skin from irritation or breakdown. Indwelling urinary catheter or condom catheters may be used.
Inadequate nutrition	Nausea and vomiting can decrease appetite.	Serve smaller portions and bland foods, which may be more palatable.*
	Depression from grieving may cause anorexia.	Allow home-cooked meals, which may be preferred by client and gives the family a chance to participate.
Dehydration	As disease progresses, client is less willing or able to maintain oral fluid intake.	Remove factors causing decreased intake; give antiemetics, apply topical analgesics to oral lesions. Reduce discomfort from dehydration; give mouth care minimum of every 4 hours; offer ice chips or moist cloth to lips.

*Data from Jacox A, Carr DB, Payne R, et al.: Management of cancer pain. *Clinical Practice Guideline No. 9,* AHCPR Pub. No. 94-0592, Rockville, Md., Agency for Health Care and Policy Research, Public Health Service, U.S. Department of Health and Human Services, March, 1994.
**Data from Marino L: *Cancer nursing,* St. Louis, 1981, Mosby.

Continued.

table 21-6—cont'd

PROMOTING COMFORT IN THE TERMINALLY ILL CLIENT

Symptoms	Characteristics or causes	Nursing implications
Ineffective breathing patterns	Causes include disease progression involving lung tissue capacity, pneumonia, and pulmonary edema.	Position upright to improve breathing capacity. Administer supplemental oxygen as ordered. Administer bronchodilator as ordered.
	Clients may also be severely anemic, causing reduced oxygen carrying capacity.	Narcotics can suppress cough and ease breathing and apprehension. Suction secretions from mouth and nose.

ease or therapies (Table 21-6). Fear of pain is common in many clients and may heighten perception of discomfort. The nurse assesses the character of the client's pain and carefully individualizes interventions (see Chapter 28). Once a dying client gains pain relief, more energy is available to maintain quality life activities.

Personal hygiene is a routine part of keeping the terminally ill comfortable. The client eventually depends on the nurse or family for basic needs. To avoid a client's embarrassment over dependence on others, the nurse encourages clients to make decisions about their care whenever possible.

Maintenance of Independence. Most dying clients gain satisfaction from being independent as long as possible. Allowing the client to perform simple tasks such as washing the face, putting on eyeglasses, or eating maintains dignity and sense of worth. When a client becomes physically unable to perform self-care, the nurse still encourages participation and decision making to give a sense of control. The nurse looks for nonverbal cues that suggest unwillingness to participate in care. The nurse should not force the client to participate, particularly if physical limitations make it difficult.

A dying client has the right to choose the location of care. An acute care hospital is not the only option. Hospice care offers comprehensive care in the home.

Prevention of Loneliness and Isolation. When the nurse caring for the dying person is detached by directing attention to physical care and avoiding discussion of the emotional aspects of the situation, the client may experience an overwhelming loneliness. It usually takes time and experience for a nurse to react positively toward dying clients. Nurses are oriented to the cure of clients and may find it difficult to provide the necessary support for them. For many health care providers, death symbolizes failure. Furthermore, the process of dying may cause a client to be unpleasant. If the client's condition causes offensive odors, incontinence, confusion, or combativeness, nurses may avoid the client.

To prevent loneliness and sensory deprivation, the nurse intervenes to improve the quality of the client's immediate environment. Dying clients should not be routinely placed in private rooms in out-of-the-way locations. Clients feel a sense of involvement when sharing a room and watching the nurse's activities. The client can then also share conversation and companionship with roommates and visitors. When the client dies, however, the nurse should give attention to the client's roommate, because watching a person die can be frightening.

Providing meaningful environmental stimulation comforts the client. Rooms should be well lit, attractively decorated, and offer a stimulating view. Pictures, cherished objects, cards or letters from family members, and live plants and flowers console the client. Familiar objects provide security in an alien environment.

Perhaps the most important factor in preventing loneliness is visits by family members or significant others. Visitors should be allowed to remain with dying clients at any time, if the client wants them. If the client shares a semiprivate room, however, the nurse should be sure that the visitors do not disturb the client's roommate. If several family members visit, it may be necessary to provide a private room. Older adults often become particularly lonely at night and may feel more secure if someone stays at the bedside during the night. The nurse should know how to contact family members at any time if the client requests a visit or the client's condition worsens.

It is very important for the dying person to have someone who can be with them and support them in the dying experience. Nurses should not feel guilty if they cannot provide this support. The nurse cares for the client's bodily needs. This may require long intervals of time with the client. The nurse has the responsibility to stay with dying clients when needed and to show concern and compassion.

Promotion of Spiritual Comfort. Providing a client with spiritual comfort means much more than asking clergy to visit. The nurse must support the client in the expression of a philosophy of life. As death approaches, the client often seeks comfort by analyzing values and beliefs related to life and death. A dying client seeks to find purpose and meaning to life before surrendering to death (Conrad, 1985). A dying client often feels guilty if life is perceived as unfulfilled. Therefore the client will often ask for forgiveness from God or people around him or her. Additional spiritual needs are hope and love (Conrad, 1985). The nurse and family can assist in understanding and expressing hope. Love can best be expressed through kind, compassionate care.

Ways in which the nurse or family can provide spiritual comfort include therapeutic communication skills, expressing empathy, praying with the client, reading inspirational literature, and playing music. Prayer should not be used to avoid the client or the dying process. Reciting prayers or praying as a means to close a discussion does not address the client's feelings (Conrad, 1985). Attentive listening encourages the client to express feelings, clarify them, and accept death. When clients seek clergy and do not have their own, the nurse makes referrals.

Support for the Grieving Family. Nurses support family members through the dying and death of the client and simultaneously encourage support of the client. In an institutional setting, the family may have difficulty in carrying out supportive activities. It is important for the nurse to recognize the value of family members as resources and assist them in working with the dying person.

To use family members as resources, the nurse assesses family relationships to determine the family's desired role: observer, comforter, or care giver (see box at right). Identifying how family roles are influenced by the client's condition is crucial. Family members have their own need to express their feelings, and they must also deal directly with the client's expressions of anger, denial, and fear. Sometimes the family refuses to care for the client or shows excessive concern. Benoliel (1985) describes circumstances including a lengthy period of dying, symptoms difficult to control, unpleasant sights and smells, limited coping resources, poor relationships with care givers, and a dying child that make it difficult for families to cope with terminal illness.

The nurse can most effectively help families and clients by showing kindness, respect, and courtesy. The box on p. 508 provides guidelines for supporting families in their grief and helping them support the client.

SUGGESTIONS FOR INVOLVING THE FAMILY IN THE CARE OF A DYING CLIENT

Assist in planning a visitation schedule for family members to prevent client and family from becoming fatigued.

Allow young children to visit a dying parent when the client is able to communicate.

Be willing to listen to family complaints about the client's care, as well as positive or negative feelings about the client.

Help family members learn to interact with the dying person (for example, using attentive listening, avoiding false reassurances, conducting conversations about normal family activities or problems).

When the family becomes fatigued with care activities, relieve them from their duties so they can acquire needed rest and support. Refer them to resources for meals and lodging.

Support grieving between client and family. Provide privacy when preferred. Do not discourage open expression of grief between family and client.

Provide information daily with regard to the client's condition. Prepare the family for sudden changes in appearance and behavior.

Communicate news of impending death when the family is together if possible. Members can provide support for one another. Convey the news in a private area and be willing to stay with the family.

At the time of death, help the family to stay in communication with the dying person through short visits, caring silence, touch, and telling the client of their love for him or her.

After death, assist the family with decision making such as selection of a mortician, transportation of family members, and collection of the client's belongings.

Special Considerations for Children. A child's reaction to and understanding of death and dying depends on the developmental stage of the child, parental values and beliefs, culture, and religious orientation. The nurse helps children to develop positive attitudes toward death by first counseling parents regarding a child's age-specific understanding of death and the normal reactions of a child to death (Whaley and Wong, 1991). Parents learn to use "small deaths" of a pet, for example, to help children become familiar and comfortable with a loss.

When death in a family occurs, parents often try to shield children from the loss. They fear the child will not be able to cope with the grief. However, allowing children to feel emotions prepares them for more traumatic experiences later in life (Whaley and Wong, 1991). The child's developmental level determines the amount and type of detailed information that needs to be discussed

CLIENT TEACHING FOR THE DYING CLIENT'S FAMILY

Describe and demonstrate feeding techniques and selection of foods to facilitate ease of chewing and swallowing.
Demonstrate bathing, mouth care, and other hygiene measures and allow family to perform return demonstration.
Show video on simple transfer techniques to prevent injury to themselves and the client; help family to practice.
Describe ways the family can promote the client's comfort, such as frequent rest periods and repositioning.
Teach family to recognize signs and symptoms to expect as the client approaches death and information on whom to call in an emergency.
Discuss ways to support the dying person and listen to needs and fears.
Solicit questions from family and provide information as needed.

with the child. It is important to know the child's thoughts; the parents must be honest.

When a child is dying, parents and siblings can feel considerable anger and resentment. The death of a child is usually seen as unfair. Parents may prefer to withhold information about the illness from the child. It is believed that even young children, however, can perceive that something is wrong with them because of the changes in behavior they see in parents. Nursing implications include planning the child's care with parents to determine the level of participation they desire. A nurse should not usurp parents' roles or relinquish important nursing responsibilities (Whaley and Wong, 1991). Parents and children need to know specifics about the plan of therapy and the normalcy of their reaction to the loss. It is common for friends and relatives to avoid contact with the dying child and family because of fear over the child's illness. Parents must decide whether they wish to maintain contact with significant others. Such a resource can prove valuable.

Hospice Care. **Hospice** care is an alternative for terminally ill clients. It is not a facility but a concept for family-centered care designed to assist the terminally ill to be comfortable and maintain a satisfactory life-style until death. There are several hospice programs. Acute care hospitals and long-term care facilities often have separate units or dedicated beds for hospice care. A trained interdisciplinary team works with clients and families. The home care component of a hospice is operated by a hospital or separate home health agency. Independent hospices also care only for the terminally ill. Home health agencies and skilled nursing facilities also operate hospice programs. Pitorak (1985) describes the following components of hospice care:

1. Coordinated home care with available inpatient beds under hospital administration
2. Control of symptoms (physical, sociological, psychological, and spiritual)
3. Physician-directed services
4. Provision of an interdisciplinary care team composed of physicians, nurses, clergy, social workers, and counselors
5. Medical and nursing services available at all times
6. Client and family as the unit of care
7. Bereavement follow-up after a death
8. Use of trained volunteers as a part of the team
9. Clients accepted into the program on the basis of health care needs rather than ability to pay.

A hospice program emphasizes **palliative** treatment and the control of symptoms rather than curative treatment of disease (Aroskar, 1985). The client and family participate in care. Client care is well coordinated between the home and inpatient setting. Efforts are directed at keeping the client at home as much as possible. The family becomes the care giver, administering medication and treatment, whereas the interdisciplinary team provides psychological and physical resources needed for family support.

Care After Death. The nurse who has cared for a client is often the best person to provide **postmortem** care because of the nurse-client relationship. The client's body should be cared for with dignity and sensitivity. At the time of a client's death, the following procedural activities must be completed (see agency policy):

1. Pronouncement of death. The physician records in the medical record the time of the client's death and a description of any therapies or actions taken before death.
2. Death certificate. This certificate is recorded by the health care agency or physician. It documents the time and cause of death.
3. Request for postmortem examinations **(autopsy).** The physician or nurse (at the request of the physician) asks for written consent of legal (next-of-kin) permission. Consent is usually not required when the circumstances of the death are such that the law requires an autopsy.
4. Request for organ or tissue donation. A nurse, physician, or appropriately trained requestor asks the next of kin or guardian for organ or tissue donation if the client is medically judged to be a suitable donor.
5. Determination of funeral home. The family selects the **mortician** to **embalm** or **cremate** the body.

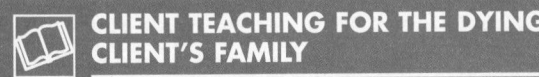

> **TISSUES AND ORGANS USED FOR TRANSPLANT**
>
> **NONVITAL TISSUES**
>
> Corneas
> Skin
> Long bones
> Middle ear bones
>
> **VITAL ORGANS***
>
> Heart
> Liver
> Lungs
> Kidneys
> Pancreas
>
> *These organs are recovered after a client is pronounced clinically dead or brain dead; circulatory and ventilatory support is maintained to perfuse the organs before removal.

Federal legislation requires hospitals to formulate policies and procedures for the identification and referral of potential donors to procurement agencies or tissue banks (see box above). Hospital policies are meant to ensure that families of appropriate potential donors are provided the option of organ, eye, or tissue donation. Discussions of donations should be performed in a sensitive and caring manner. A trained staff member, often a nurse, discusses donation with families or guardians, making certain that they understand that donation is an option and that it is all right not to donate.

After death, the body undergoes many physical changes. The body should be cared for as soon as possible after death to prevent tissue damage or disfigurement of body parts.

The nurse offers the family the opportunity to view the body. It may help to suggest that this is an opportunity to say "good-bye" especially if they were not present at the time of death. If the family hesitates, the nurse gives them time to think about it. If they decide not to view the body, the nurse accepts their decision without judgment. If the family decides to view the body, they are assured that they need not be alone and that the nurse will accompany them or will request whomever they would like. The nurse spends time assisting the grieving family and offers to contact other support services such as social services and a spiritual adviser. The family becomes the client.

The nurse prepares the body by making it look as natural and comfortable as possible. If it is placed in a supine position with arms at the sides, palms down, or across the abdomen, a mortician can better prepare the body for interment. The nurse places a small pillow or folded towel under the head to prevent discoloration from blood pooling. The eyelids usually remain closed, if gently held down for a few seconds. If this does not work, moistened cotton balls hold the eyelids in place. If the family wishes to view the body, the cotton balls can be temporarily removed. Later, if the eyelids remain open, the nurse may reapply the cotton balls.

The nurse inserts the client's dentures to maintain normal facial features. A rolled-up towel under the chin helps to keep the mouth closed. Agency policy dictates whether tubes (e.g., endotracheal tubes) can be removed.

The nurse washes soiled body parts, dresses the body in a clean gown, combs or brushes the hair, and covers the body to the shoulders with clean linen. Most shroud kits or body bags contain absorbent pads that are placed under the perineal and rectal area to collect oozing feces or urine from relaxed sphincter muscles. The nurse removes jewelry and presents it and other valuables to the family. In some agencies a single wedding band may be left in place as long as it is taped securely to the finger. After the body is prepared, the family is allowed into the room. The nurse or another family member can be there to provide emotional support. It is important not to rush the family while they spend time with the deceased.

After the family leaves, the nurse places tags containing name and other information on the client's wrist and ankle or toe. The gown is removed, and the body is wrapped completely in a body bag or shroud, a large rectangular piece of plastic or cotton material. Another identification tag is placed on the bag or shroud. If the client had a known transmissible infection, special labeling may be used to alert those who move and store the remains. The body is then transported to the morgue, or the mortician picks it up from the client's room. Although methods for transporting the body through hallways vary among institutions, the nurse should be certain that this procedure is as unobtrusive as possible. Such action protects the privacy of the deceased and respects the needs of the other clients.

Nursing personnel are also responsible for disposition of the deceased's personal belongings and noting this in the medical record. The nurse can check with the client's family about taking the belongings or ensure that the belongings are transported with the deceased. If the family or friends have left, the supervisor is usually contacted.

CARE FOR THE NURSE

Nurses working with critically or terminally ill clients also experience grief. Grief is the natural response to loss, and each loss needs to be grieved. When nurses experience multiple losses and fail to adequately process them, they can experience bereavement over

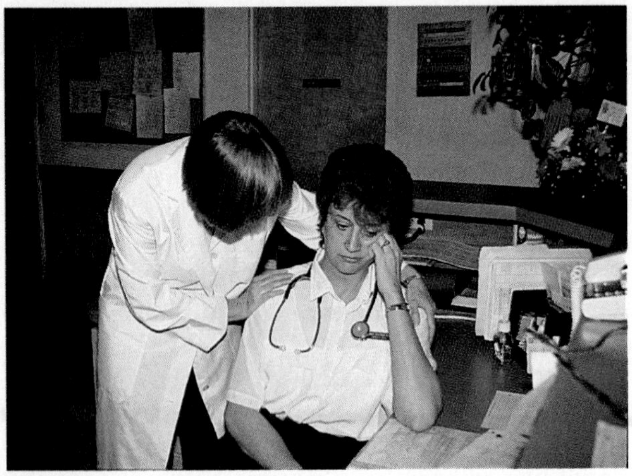

FIGURE 21-2 Nurses benefit from support of colleagues during their time of loss. (Courtesy Michael S. Clement, MD, Mesa, Ariz.).

load. They experience frustration, anger, guilt, sadness, helplessness, anxiety, depression, and feelings of being overwhelmed.

Self-care is critical to survival. Nurses need to do for themselves what they do for their clients and families. They need to mourn their losses (Figure 21-2). This is done on an individual basis and as part of a larger group caring for the client. Nurses need to develop personal support systems that allow time away from the care-giving setting, opportunities to share feelings in nonjudgmental, open relationships, and use of stress-management techniques that restore energy. Some institutions provide opportunities for staff to get together for mutual support and for closure and grieving over the loss of a client.

Nurses' roles in the care of the dying and bereaved are filled with experiences that bring grief and stress. Nurses must be attuned to the need for relief from these demands. Unrelieved grief and stress can lead to diminished well-being and inability to care for others.

Evaluation

Although resolution of grief may require months or years, the majority of clients are often under the care of a nurse for only a short time. The nurse may become frustrated when, just as the client and family begin to express grief, the client leaves the health care institution or dies. It helps to remember that grieving is an individualized process, and resolution of loss does not proceed according to a set schedule.

To evaluate the effectiveness of nursing interventions in meeting the goals of care, the nurse uses evaluative measures to identify actual outcomes. These outcomes are compared with expected outcomes to determine the client's health status and the need for revising the plan of care. Examples of goals, outcomes, and evaluative measures include:

Goal: Client resolves dysfunctional grieving within 2 months.

Outcome

Client expresses thoughts and feelings related to loss within 3 weeks

Evaluative measures

Observe client discuss loss with significant other

Ask client to talk about feelings of loss

Outcome

Client participates in decision making and cooperates with recommended treatments within 1 month

Evaluative measures

Have family member keep log of treatment schedule followed

Ask client about choices made in therapy

Goal: Client regains sense of self-esteem within 2 weeks.

Outcome

Client resumes rest and sleep habits and leisure activities within 2 weeks

Evaluative measure

Have client keep sleep log

Ask family about type of activities client has participated in since last visit

Outcome

Client will maintain well-groomed appearance within 1 week

Evaluative measure

Observe client's appearance

Ask family to report on client's appearance

Goal: Client renews normal activities or relationships within 2 months.

Outcome

Client resumes participation in church activities within 1 month

Evaluative measure

Evaluate client's level of participation in church activities with family

Outcome

Client returns to work within 1 week

Evaluative measure

Have client report on return to work

Care of the dying client requires that the nurse evaluate whether the client has accepted the loss and whether the nurse was able to promote quality of life. The success of the nurse's evaluation depends on the bond formed with the client. Unless the client has learned to trust the nurse, he or she will be unlikely to share true feelings and concerns. Examples of goals, outcomes, and evaluative measures for dying clients follows:

Goal: Client achieves comfort within 1 week.

Outcome

Client perceives a reduction in pain severity within 3 days

Evaluative measure

Have client report on a 10-point visual analog scale, the perceived level of pain

Note the number of requests made by the client for analgesics or other pain relief measures

Goal: Client maintains independence in daily activities within 1 week.

Outcome

Client dresses and feeds self within 3 days

Evaluative measure

Observe client during meal time. Observe the client verbalize decisions regarding care

Goal: Client maintains hope.

Outcome

Client verbalizes finding meaning in life

Evaluative measure

Ask the client to describe actions taken to achieve hope (for example, praying or renewing relationships with friends)

Goal: Client achieves spiritual comfort.

Outcome

Client expresses satisfaction with belief system

Evaluative measures

Discuss with client values and beliefs regarding life and death

Observe the client engaging in prayer or other religious practices

Goal: Client gains relief from loneliness and isolation within 1 month.

Outcome

Client verbalizes feelings about loneliness and isolation in 2 weeks

Evaluative measure

Ask the client to discuss feelings about loneliness and isolation

Outcome

Client invites friend for regular visit to home within 1 month

Evaluative measure

Ask client or family to report visits by friends

SUMMARY

Categories of loss include loss of an aspect of self, of external objects, of a significant other, of a known environment, and of life. Nurses interact daily with clients and families experiencing loss. Knowledge of the concepts and theories concerning loss, death, and the grieving process provides a framework for the nursing process. The nurse's responses and interactions with the grieving client and family create the climate for openness in expressing grief. The nurse explores the strengths of the client and support systems available through listening, being with the client when needed, and conveying respect for the client's values and beliefs. A trust relationship creates a therapeutic environment that enhances grief work and fosters the client's dignity and self-esteem. The nurse's understanding promotes growth and paves the way for effective nursing care of grieving or dying clients and their families.

CRITICAL THINKING ACTIVITIES

1. Jim Jones, a 19-year-old victim of a traumatic injury, has become increasingly angry and noncooperative. He refuses all treatments. When approached, he yells "Stay away from me. I just want to die." Describe how you would approach Jim and what you think you need to assess.
2. Mrs. Franks has been admitted for the third time for complaints of chest pain and difficulty breathing. Her tests continue to reveal no physical cause for the symptoms. A review of the chart notes that she lost her husband of 40 years, 3 months ago. He died of a heart attack. What do you think is happening and how would you approach Mrs. Franks?
3. Jane is in the final phase of her terminal illness. It is clear she will die soon. Her family has asked you what they can do. Identify four needs of Jane and discuss what her family can do to help her.
4. Mrs. James has been in the hospital for 4 months. You have taken care of her the last 4 weeks. You spend every free moment you have with her. When not at the hospital you worry about her and are concerned that no one else can give her as good care as you. Your supervisor has commented on your apparent over-involvement with Mrs. James. What could some of the factors be that are influencing your reactions to Mrs. James?
5. The Smith family has decided to take their father home and care for him in his last days. Discuss what you need to teach the family before they take him home.

KEY CONCEPTS

A loss is the absence of an object, person, body part or function, emotion, or idea.

The grieving process involves emotional, cognitive, and behavioral responses to an actual or perceived loss.

Individuals experience different aspects of the grieving process at different times.

Dying may lead to a grief response similar to that with other kinds of losses.

A nurse's support of a client's hope can help promote an effective grieving process associated with a loss.

The individual's reaction is influenced by many factors, including developmental stage, beliefs, roles, culture, relationships, and socioeconomic status.

Assessment of the grieving client considers behavioral characteristics that suggest the client's stage of grieving.

Nursing diagnoses focus on the type of grief experienced by clients or health-related problems common to grieving clients.

Therapeutic communication is an important nursing intervention to assist the grieving and the dying client in coping with loss.

Nursing care of the grieving and dying client should promote the client's sense of identity, dignity, and self-esteem.

Nursing care of the terminally ill focuses on promoting comfort and improving the quality of remaining life.

As death approaches, a client reviews and analyzes values and beliefs pertinent to the meaning of life and death.

A nurse must assess whether family members are willing to be involved in a dying client's care before using them as resources.

Care after death involves caring for the body with dignity and sensitivity.

The evaluation of nursing care for the grieving and dying client is ongoing and is based on identifiable behavioral changes through the grieving process.

The nurse's own loss history influences responses to client losses.

Nurses who work with critically or terminally ill clients experience loss and grief.

Nurses need to be aware of and mourn their own losses on an ongoing basis to avoid bereavement overload.

References

Aroskar MA: Access to hospice—ethical dimensions, *Nurs Clin North Am* 20:299, 1985.

Barbus AJ: The dying person's bill of rights, *Am J Nurs* 75:99, 1975.

Benoliel JQ: Loss and terminal illness, *Nurs Clin North Am* 20:439, 1985.

Conrad NL: Spiritual support for the dying, *Nurs Clin North Am* 20:415, 1985.

Davitz L and Davitz J: *Nurses' responses to patients' suffering,* New York, 1980, Springer.

Doka KJ: *Disenfranchised grief: recognizing hidden sorrow,* New York, 1989, Lexington Books.

Dufault K and Martocchio BC: Hope: its spheres and dimensions, *Nurs Clin North Am* 20:379, 1985.

Engel GL: Grief and grieving, *Am J Nurs* 64:93, 1964.

Kubler-Ross E: *On death and dying,* New York, 1969, Macmillan.

Lewis K: Grief in chronic illness and disability, *J Rehabil* 49:8, 1983.

Marino L: *Cancer nursing,* St. Louis, 1981, Mosby.

Martocchio BC: Grief and bereavement: healing through hurt, *Nurs Clin North Am* 20:327, 1985.

Mulhern RM: When there's no treatment left but the truth, *RN* 49:26, 1986.

Pitorak, EF: Establishing a medicare-certified inpatient unit, *Nurs Clin North Am* 20:311, 1985.

Rando TA: *Grief, dying and death,* Champaign, Ill., 1984, Research Press.

Stockdale L and Hutzenbiler T: How you can comfort a grieving family, *Nurs Life* 6:23, 1986.

U.S. Bureau of the Census: *Statistical abstract of the United States,* Washington, DC, 1990, The Bureau.

Werner-Beland JA: *Grief response of long term illness and disability,* Reston, Va., 1980, Reston.

Whaley LF and Wong DL: *Nursing care of infants and children,* ed 4, St. Louis, 1991, Mosby.

Bibliography

Anderson J: Nursing management of the cancer patient in pain: a review of the literature, *Cancer Nurs* 5:33, 1982.

Brown P and Chekryn J: The dying patient and dehydration, *Can Nurse* 85:14, May 1989.

DeSpelder LA, Strickland AL: *The last dance: encountering death and dying,* ed 2, Mountain View, Calif., 1991, Mayfield.

Ebersole P and Hess P: *Toward healthy aging: human needs and nursing responses,* ed 3, St. Louis, 1990, CV Mosby.

Engel GL: *Psychological development in health and disease,* Philadelphia, 1962, WB Saunders.

Grollman EA: *Straight talk about death for teenagers: How to cope when losing someone you love,* Boston, 1993, Beacon Press.

Hainsworth M: Women in grief, *Perspect Psychiatr Care* 23(3/4):85, 1988.

Kalish RA: *Death, grief, and caring relationships,* ed 2, Monterey, Calif., 1985, Brooks/Cole.

Kastenbaum RJ: *Death, society and human experience,* ed 2, New York, 1991, Macmillan.

Kim MJ, et al.: *Pocket guide to nursing diagnoses,* ed 5, St. Louis, 1993, Mosby.

Leavitt PF, et al.: The patient who is dying. In Lewis S, et al., editors: *Manual of psychosocial nursing interventions: promoting mental health in medical-surgical settings,* Philadelphia, 1989, WB Saunders.

Moseley JR: Alterations in comfort, *Nurs Clin North Am* 20:427, 1985.

Musgrave CF: The ethical and legal implications of hospice care: an international overview, *Cancer Nurs* 10:183, 1987.

Redmond LM: *Surviving when someone you loved was murdered: a professional guide to group therapy for families and friends of murder victims,* Clearwater, Fla., 1989, Psychological Consultation and Education Services.

Reed PG: Religiousness among terminally ill and healthy adults, *Res Nurs Health* 9:35, 1986.

Stickney SK and Gardner ER: Companions in suffering, *Am J Nurs* 84:1491, 1984.

Wegmann JA: Hospice home death, hospital death, and coping abilities of widows, *Cancer Nurs* 10:148, 1987.

Zach MV: Loneliness: a concept relevant to the care of dying persons, *Nurs Clin North Am* 20:403, 1985.

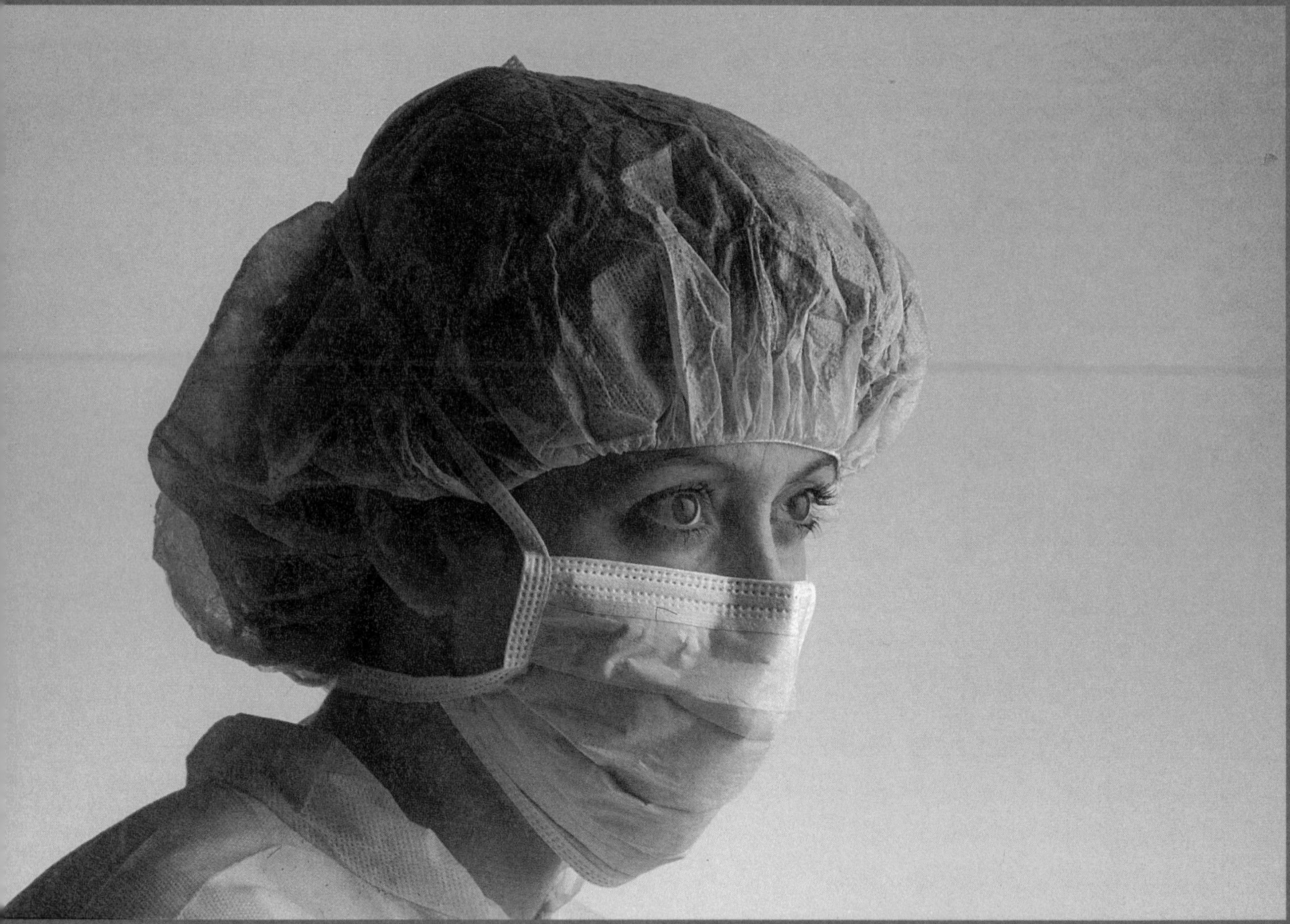

unit five

PROTECTION, SAFETY, AND COMFORT NEEDS

22 Body Mechanics

OBJECTIVES

Mastery of content in this chapter will enable the student to:

- Define the key terms listed.
- Describe the roles of the skeleton, skeletal muscles, and nervous system in the regulation of movement.
- Discuss physiological and pathological influences on body alignment and joint mobility.
- Identify changes in physiological and psychosocial function associated with immobility.
- Assess for impaired body alignment and mobility.
- State correct nursing diagnoses for problems related to impaired body alignment and mobility.
- Write nursing care plans for impaired body alignment and mobility.
- Describe the intervention for maintaining proper alignment, assisting a client to move up in bed, repositioning a helpless client, and transferring a client from a bed to a chair.
- Evaluate the nursing plan for maintaining body alignment and mobility.

KEY TERMS

abduction
active ROM
activity tolerance
adduction
balance
bed boards
body mechanics
center of gravity
crutch gait
dorsiflexion
eversion
extension
flexion
foot boot
footdrop
fracture
friction
gait
hand rolls
hand-wrist splints
hyperextension
inversion
isometric contraction
isotonic contraction
joints
joint contracture
muscle tone
passive range of motion exercises
plantar flexion
pronation
range of motion
restraints
side rails
supination
trapeze bar
trochanter roll

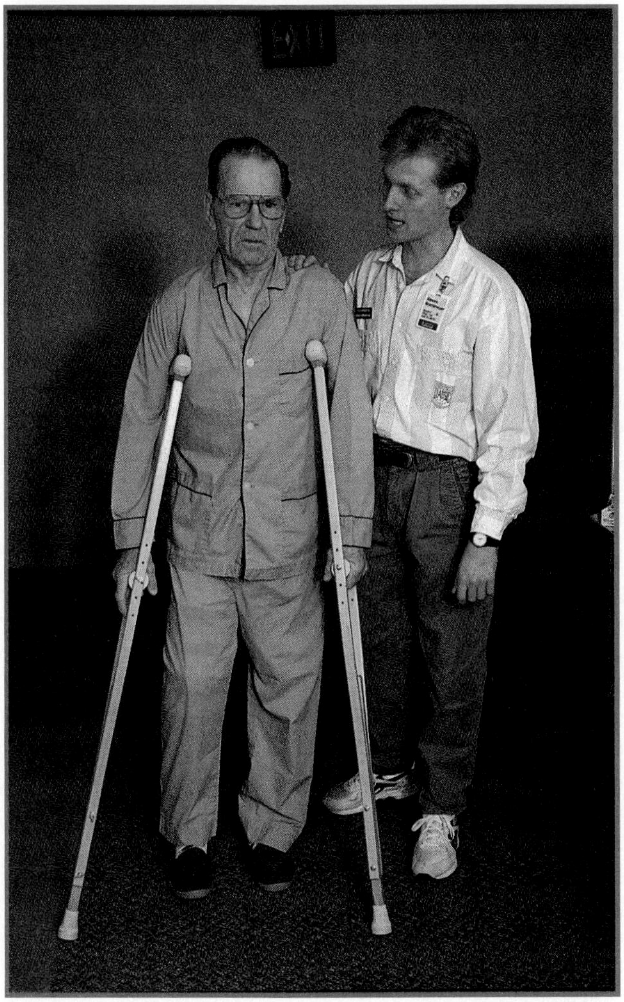

Clinical nursing requires the nurse to incorporate knowledge and skills into practice. One such component of knowledge and skill is body mechanics, a broad term used to describe coordinated efforts of the musculoskeletal and nervous systems.

Many nursing activities require muscle exertion by the nurse. To reduce the risk of injury to the client and nurse when transferring a client, the nurse must know and practice proper body mechanics. Body mechanics includes knowing how and why certain muscle groups are used. The nurse also needs to understand how coordinated body movement involves integrated functioning of the skeletal system, skeletal muscle, and nervous system.

OVERVIEW OF BODY MECHANICS

Body mechanics is the coordinated effort of the musculoskeletal and nervous systems to maintain balance, posture, and body alignment during lifting, bending, moving, and performing activities of daily living. Use of proper body mechanics reduces the risk of injury to the musculoskeletal system. Proper body mechanics also facilitates body movement that allows physical mobility without muscle strain and excessive use of muscle energy.

Body Alignment

Body alignment refers to the relationship of one body part to another. Correct body alignment reduces strain on musculoskeletal structures, maintains adequate muscle tone, and contributes to balance.

Body Balance

Body balance is achieved when a relatively low center of gravity is balanced over a wide, stable base of support, and a vertical line falls from the center of gravity through the base of support. When the vertical line from the center of gravity does not fall through the base of support, the body loses balance and a fall or muscle strain (in an effort to maintain balance) could result.

Body balance is also enhanced by posture. The nurse maintains proper body alignment and posture by using two simple techniques. First, the base of support can easily be widened by separating the feet to a comfortable distance. Second, balance is increased by bringing the center of gravity closer to the base of support. This is achieved by bending the knees and flexing the hips until the person is squatting and still maintaining proper back alignment by keeping the trunk erect.

Coordinated Body Movement

Weight is the force exerted on a body by gravity. When an object is lifted, the lifter must overcome the object's weight and be aware of its center of gravity. In symmetrical objects the center of gravity is located at the exact center of the object. Because people are not geometrically perfect, their centers of gravity are usually at 55% to 57% of standing height and are located in the midline. The force of weight is always directed downward, which is why an unbalanced object falls. Clients who are unsteady fall because, as their centers of gravity become unbalanced, the gravitational force of their weight eventually causes them to fall. Therefore the nurse needs to design interventions that protect such clients from falling and ensure their safety (see Chapter 29).

Friction is a force that occurs in a direction to oppose movement. As the nurse turns, transfers, or moves a client up in bed, friction must be overcome. A nurse can reduce friction by following some basic principles.

The greater the surface area of the object to be moved, the greater the friction. If a client is unable to assist in moving up in bed, the client's arms should be placed across the chest. This decreases surface area and reduces friction.

A passive or immobilized client produces greater friction to movement. Thus, when possible, the nurse should use some of the client's strength and mobility when lifting, transferring, or moving the client up in bed. This can be done by explaining the procedure and telling the client when to move. The client can then participate, and friction is decreased. For instance, friction is decreased if the client can bend his or her knees as the nurse assists him or her to move up in the bed.

Friction can be reduced by lifting rather than pushing a client. Lifting has an upward component and decreases the pressure between the client and the bed or the chair. The use of a pull sheet reduces friction because the client is more easily moved along the bed's surface.

REGULATION OF MOVEMENT

Coordinated body movement involves integrated functioning of the bones, skeletal muscle, and nervous system. Because these three systems cooperate so closely in mechanical support of the body, they can be considered as a single functional unit.

Skeletal System

The skeleton is the body's supporting framework and comprises four types of bones: long, short, flat, and irregular.

Long bones contribute to height (e.g., the femur, fibula, and tibia in the leg) and length (e.g., the phalanges of the fingers and toes). **Short bones** occur in clusters and, when combined with ligaments and cartilage, permit movement of the extremities. **Flat bones** provide structural contour, such as bones in the skull and the ribs in the thorax. **Irregular bones** make up the vertebral column and some bones of the skull, such as the mandible.

The skeleton provides attachments for muscles and ligaments. These attachments allow movement of parts of the skeleton, such as opening and closing the mouth or extending an arm or a leg. It also protects vital organs; for example, the skull protects the brain and the ribs protect the heart and lungs. Bones assist in regulation of calcium balance. Bones can store calcium and release it into the circulation as needed. In addition, the internal structure of the bones contains bone marrow, participates in red blood cell production, and acts as a reservoir for blood.

Clients with altered calcium regulation and metabolism are at risk for developing osteoporosis and pathological fractures, which can occur in all types of bone but are most commonly found in the ribs and weight-bearing bones. Clients with altered bone marrow function or diminished red blood cell production are usually weakened and fatigued. This decreases mobility and places clients at risk of falling.

Bone. The characteristics of bone include firmness, rigidity, and elasticity. A mature bone is a rigid connective tissue, consisting of cells, fibers, and gelatinous material called *ground substance.* Bone also contains blood vessels and nerves. Bone tissue is nourished by a network of capillaries and major vessels (McCance and Huether, 1990).

The functional activities of the bone include modeling, remodeling, and repairing. **Modeling** involves the growth process that allows the bones of the newborn to develop into the large, identically shaped bones of the adult, and depends on dietary and physiological factors. **Remodeling** is the process in which existing bone is resorbed and new bone is laid down to replace it (McCance and Huether, 1990). The remodeling process occurs in the growing and full-grown skeleton. **Repair** is the cellular process that occurs in response to a fracture (Gröer and Shekleton, 1989). The speed in which bone heals depends on the severity of the injury, the type and amount of bone tissue needing repair, the blood supply to the site, the presence of infection, and the extent of the aging process (McCance and Huether, 1990).

The composition of the skeleton changes throughout life. This change begins in fetal development with the formation of cartilage. At birth, the newborn has a large amount of cartilage and is highly flexible but is unable to support weight. The toddler's bones are more pliable than those of an older adult and are able to withstand some falls better. As a result of aging, bones become porous and brittle, increasing the risk of fractures.

Joints. Joints are the connection between bones. Each joint is classified according to its structure and degree of mobility. The four classifications of joints are synostotic, cartilaginous, fibrous, and synovial.

The **synostotic joint** occurs when bones are joined by bones. No movement is associated with this type of joint, and the bony tissue that forms between the bones provides strength and stability. The classic example of this type of joint is the sacrum, in which vertebrae are joined together (Figure 22-1, *A*).

The **cartilaginous** or synchondrodial **joint** has little movement but is elastic and uses cartilage to unite body surfaces. Cartilaginous joints are found when bones are exposed to a constant pressure, such as the costosternal joints between the sternum and the ribs (Figure 22-1, *B*).

The **fibrous** or syndesmodial **joint** has a tough layer

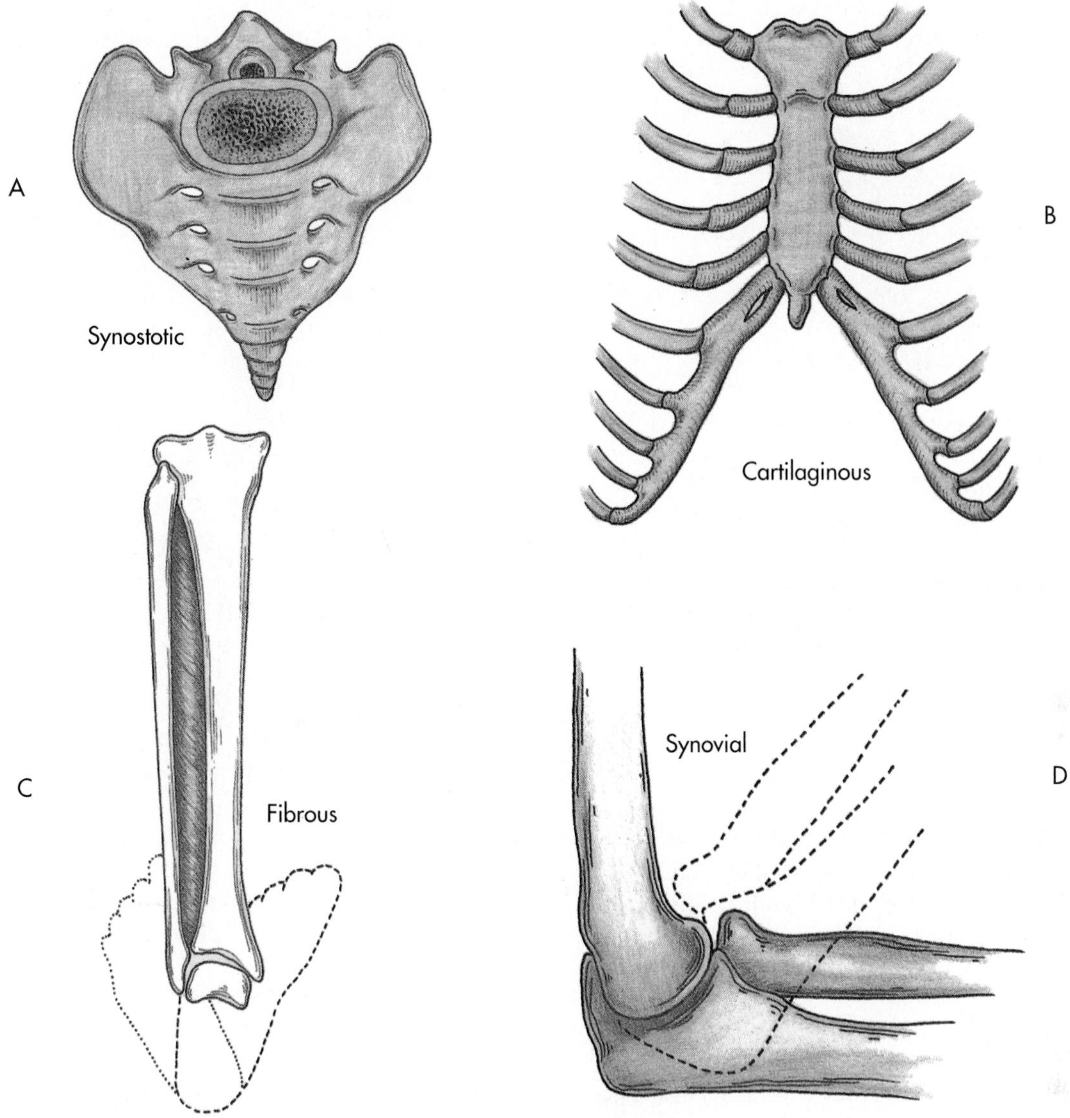

FIGURE 22-1 Joint types.

of fibrous connective tissue that binds bones firmly together. Because of the flexibility of connective tissue, some movement of the joint is permitted. For example, the tibia, fibia, and talar bones and their connective tissues form the ankle joint, which permits plantar and dorsal flexion of the foot (Figure 22-1, *C*).

The **synovial** or true **joint** is a freely movable joint in which contiguous bony surfaces are covered by articular cartilage and are connected by ligaments lined with a synovial membrane. The joining of the humeral radius and ulna by cartilage and ligaments forms a pivotal joint (Figure 22-1, *D*). Other types of synovial joints are the ball-and-socket joints, such as the hip joint, and the hinge joints, such as the interphalangeal joints of the fingers.

Ligaments. Ligaments are white, shiny, flexible bands of fibrous tissue that bind joints and connect bones and cartilages. Ligaments are elastic and aid joint flexibility and support (Figure 22-2). Some areas of the body ligaments also have a protective function. For example, ligaments between vertebral bodies prevent damage to the spinal cord during back movement.

Tendons. Tendons are white, glistening, fibrous bands of tissue that connect muscle to bone. Tendons are strong, flexible, and inelastic, and occur in various lengths and thicknesses. The Achilles tendon is the thickest and strongest tendon in the body. It begins near the middle of the posterior of the leg and attaches the gastrocnemius and soleus muscles in the calf to the calcaneal bone in the back of the foot (Figure 22-3).

Cartilage. Cartilage is nonvascular, supporting connective tissue located chiefly in the joints and in the thorax, trachea, larynx, nose, and ear. Permanent cartilage

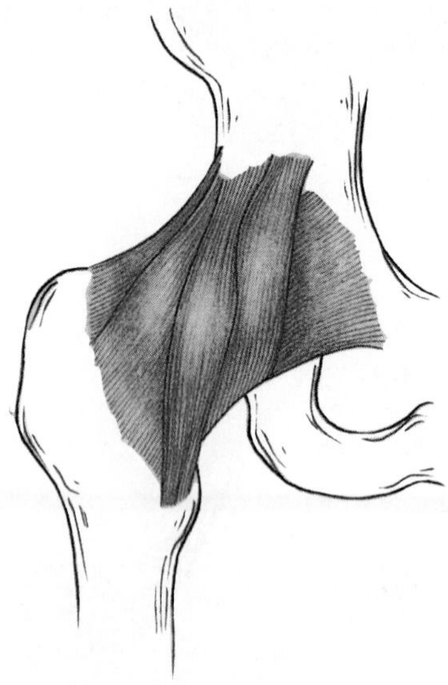

FIGURE 22-2 Ligaments of hip joint.

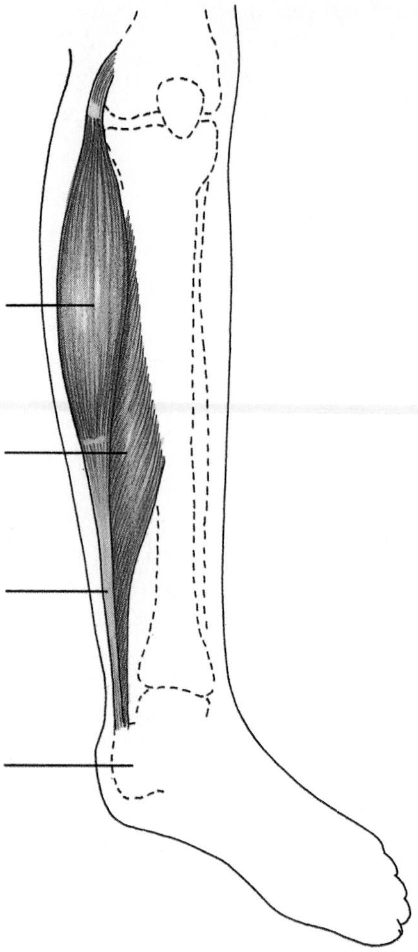

FIGURE 22-3 Achilles tendon.

is unossified except in advanced age and certain diseases such as osteoarthritis.

Joints, ligaments, tendons, and cartilage permit strength and flexibility of the skeleton. Strength enables the skeletal system to support the body. A person's flexibility is demonstrated through range of motion (ROM). However, strength and flexibility do not result entirely from these four structures; adequate skeletal muscle is also necessary.

Skeletal Muscle

Movement of bones and joints involves active processes that must be carefully integrated to achieve coordination. Skeletal muscles, because of their ability to contract and relax alternately, are the working elements of movement. Contractile elements of the skeletal muscle are enhanced by its anatomical structure and attachment to the skeleton.

Muscle contraction is stimulated by an electrochemical impulse that travels from the nerve to the muscle across the myoneural junction. The electrochemical impulse causes the thin actin-containing filaments to shorten, thus contracting the muscle. Removal of the stimulus results in muscle relaxation.

The two types of muscle contractions are isotonic and isometric. In **isotonic contraction,** increased muscle tension results in muscle shortening. **Isometric contraction** causes an increase in muscle tension or muscle work but no shortening of the muscle. Voluntary movement is a combination of isotonic and isometric contractions.

Although isometric contractions do not result in muscle shortening, energy expenditure is increased. The nurse should recognize the energy expenditure associated with isometric exercises because they may be contraindicated in cardiopulmonary and other illnesses. Each skeletal muscle is capable of isometric and isotonic contractions. Some skeletal muscles are concerned primarily with movement, whereas others are concerned primarily with posture.

Muscles Concerned With Movement

Muscles concerned primarily with movement are located near the skeletal region where movement is caused by leverage. Leverage occurs when specific bones, such as the humerus, ulna, and radius, and the associated joints, such as the elbow, act as a lever. Thus the force applied to one end of the bone to lift a weight at another point tends to rotate the bone in the direction opposite that of the applied force. Muscles that attach to bones of leverage provide the necessary strength to move the object.

Leverage is characteristic of the movements of the upper extremities. Arm muscles are parallel to one another and extend the full length of the bones. The long parallel muscles provide strength and work together with bones and joints to enable lifting an object with the arms.

Muscles Concerned With Posture

Muscles concerned primarily with maintaining posture are short and featherlike in appearance because they converge obliquely at a common tendon. Muscles of the lower extremities and of the trunk, the neck, and the back are concerned primarily with posture. These muscle groups work together to stabilize and support body weight. These muscles allow an individual to maintain a sitting or standing posture.

Muscle Regulation of Posture and Movement. Posture and movement can reflect personality and mood. For example, an outgoing individual gestures with the hands, and a fatigued person may slouch. Posture and movement also depend on the skeleton and the shape and development of the skeletal muscles. Coordination and regulation of different muscle groups depend on muscle tone and the activity of antagonistic, synergistic, and antigravity muscles.

Muscle tone or tonus is the normal state of balanced muscle tension. Tension is achieved by alternate contraction and relaxation of neighboring fibers of a specific muscle group. Muscle tone enables a body part to be maintained in a functioning position without muscle fatigue. In addition, muscle tone promotes venous return to the heart, as is the case with leg muscles.

Muscle tone is maintained through continual use of the muscles. Activities of daily living require muscle action and help maintain muscle tone. As a result of immobility or prolonged bed rest, activity level and muscle tone decrease.

MUSCLE GROUPS. The antagonistic, synergistic, and antigravity muscle groups are coordinated by the nervous system and maintain posture and initiate movement. **Antagonistic muscles** bring about movement at the joint. During movement, the active mover muscle contracts while its antagonist relaxes. For example, when flexing the arm, the active mover, the biceps brachii, contracts and its antagonist, the triceps brachii, relaxes. During extension of the arm the active mover, now the triceps brachii, contracts and the new antagonist, the biceps brachii, relaxes.

Synergistic muscles contract to accomplish the same movement. When the arm is flexed, the strength of the contraction of the biceps brachii is increased by contraction of the synergistic muscle, the brachialis. Thus with synergistic muscle activity there are now two active movers, the biceps brachii and the brachialis, which contract while the antagonistic muscle, the triceps brachii, relaxes.

Antigravity muscles are involved with joint stabilization. These muscles continuously oppose the effect of gravity on the body and permit a person to maintain an upright or sitting posture. In an adult the antigravity muscles are the extensors of the leg, the gluteus maximus, the quadriceps femoris, the soleus muscles, and the muscles of the back.

Skeletal muscles support posture and carry out voluntary movement. The muscles are attached to the skeleton by tendons, which provide strength and permit motion. The movement of the extremities is voluntary and requires coordination from the nervous system.

Nervous System. Movement and posture are regulated by the nervous system. The major voluntary motor area, located in the cerebral cortex, is the precentral gyrus or motor strip. A majority of motor fibers descend from the motor strip and cross at the level of the medulla. Thus the motor fibers from the right motor strip initiate voluntary movement for the left side of the body, and motor fibers from the left motor strip initiate voluntary movement for the right side of the body.

During voluntary movement, impulses descend from the motor strip to the spinal cord. An impulse leaves the spinal cord through efferent motor nerves and travels through nerves to the muscles, where movement occurs. The impulse is controlled by synapses, which keep the impulse traveling in one direction.

Transmission of the impulse from the nervous system to the musculoskeletal system is an electrochemical event and requires a neurotransmitter. Basically, neurotransmitters are chemicals such as acetylcholine that transfer the electric impulse from the nerve across the myoneural junction to the muscle. The neurotransmitter reaches a muscle and stimulates it, causing movement.

Movement can be impaired by disorders that alter neurotransmitter production, transfer from the neurotransmitter to the muscle, or activation of muscle activity. Posture is also regulated by the nervous system and requires coordination of proprioception and balance.

PROPRIOCEPTION. Proprioception is the sensation of spatial position and muscular activity. Proprioception is monitored by **proprioceptors,** nerve endings in muscles, tendons, and joints.

As a person carries out activities of daily living, proprioceptors monitor muscle activity and body position. For example, the proprioceptors on the soles of the foot contribute to correct posture while standing or walking. In standing, pressure is continuous on the bottom of the feet. The proprioceptors monitor the pressure, communicating this information through the nervous system to the antigravity muscles. The standing person remains upright until deciding to change position. As a person walks, the proprioceptors on the bottom of the feet monitor pressure changes. Thus, when the bottom of the moving foot comes in contact with the walking surface, the individual automatically moves the stationary foot forward. The proprioceptors allow people to walk without having to watch their feet.

Balance

When standing, running, lifting, or performing activities of daily living, a person must have adequate balance. Balance is assisted through control by the nervous system, specifically by the cerebellum and the inner ear. The major function of the cerebellum is to coordinate all voluntary movement, particularly highly skilled movements, such as those required in skiing. In addition, the cerebellum assists in balance, such as permitting a person to stand on one foot with eyes closed (Romberg test; see Chapter 16).

Within the inner ear are the semicircular canals, three fluid-filled structures that assist in maintaining balance. Fluid within the canals has a certain inertia, and when the head is suddenly rotated in one direction, the fluid remains stationary for a moment while the canal turns with the head. This allows a person to change position suddenly without losing balance.

PRINCIPLES OF BODY MECHANICS

Proper body mechanics is as important to the nurse and client as proper nutrition. It can affect the nurse's and client's level of wellness. Correct body mechanics is necessary to promote health and to prevent disability.

Health promotion activities that involve physical exercise use basic principles of body mechanics. Proper exercise increases the work and strength of certain muscle groups.

Using principles of body mechanics during routine activities also prevents disability. The nurse teaches colleagues and clients' families to lift, transfer, or position clients properly. A nurse teaching a client's family to transfer the client from bed to chair can increase and reinforce the family's knowledge by consistently demonstrating proper body mechanics.

Whether the nurse is moving an immobilized client, assisting a client from the bed to the chair, or teaching a client to carry out activities of daily living efficiently, knowledge of basic principles of body mechanics is crucial. The nurse also incorporates knowledge of physiological and pathological influences on body alignment and mobility. The box above lists principles useful for a variety of nursing settings and all clients.

PRINCIPLES OF BODY MECHANICS

The wider the base of support, the greater the stability of the nurse.
The lower the center of gravity, the greater the stability of the nurse.
The equilibrium of an object is maintained as long as the line of gravity passes through its base of support.
The stronger the muscle group, the greater amount of work that can be safely done by it.
Facing the direction of movement prevents abnormal twisting of the spine.
Dividing balanced activity between arms and legs reduces the risk of back injury.
Leverage, rolling, turning, or pivoting requires less work than lifting.
When friction is reduced between the object to be moved and the surface on which it is moved, less force is required to move it.
Reducing the force of work reduces the risk of injury.
Maintaining good body mechanics reduces fatigue of the muscle groups.
Alternating periods of rest and activity helps to reduce fatigue.

Modified from McAbee RR: Nurses and back injuries: a literature review, *AAOHN J* 36(5):221, 1988; and Marchette L: Back injury: a preventable occupational hazard, *Orthop Nurs* 4(6):25, 1985.

DEVELOPMENTAL CHANGES

Throughout life, the body's appearance and functioning undergo change. The greatest variations are observed in childhood and old age.

Infants

The newborn infant's spine is flexed and lacks the anteroposterior curves of the adult. The first spinal curve occurs when the infant extends the neck from the prone position. As stability increases and growth continues, the thoracic spine straightens and the lumbar spinal curve appears, which allows sitting and standing. The infant's musculoskeletal system is flexible.

The extremities are flexed, and joints have complete range of motion. As the newborn matures, the musculoskeletal system becomes stronger, and the infant is able to resist movement and reach out and grasp objects.

As the baby grows, musculoskeletal development permits support of weight for standing and walking. Posture is awkward because the head and trunk are carried forward. Because body weight is not evenly distributed along a line of gravity, posture is off balance and falls.

Toddlers

The toddler's posture is awkward, slightly swaybacked with a protruding abdomen. As the child walks, the legs and feet are usually far apart and the feet are slightly everted. Toward the end of toddlerhood the posture appears less awkward, the curves in the cervical and lumbar vertebrae are accentuated, and foot eversion disappears.

Preschool and School-Age Children

By the third year the body is slimmer, taller, and better balanced. Abdominal protrusion is decreased, the feet are not as far apart, and the arms and legs have increased in length. The child also appears more coordinated. From the third year through beginning adolescence the musculoskeletal system continues to develop. Long bones in the arms and legs grow. Muscles, ligaments, and tendons become stronger, resulting in improved posture and increased muscle strength. Greater coordination enables the child to perform tasks that require fine motor skills.

Adolescents

Adolescence is usually initiated by a tremendous growth spurt. Growth is frequently uneven. As a result, the adolescent may appear awkward and uncoordinated. Adolescent girls usually grow and develop earlier than boys. Hips widen, and fat is deposited in the upper arms, thighs, and buttocks. The boy's changes in shape are usually the result of long bone growth and increased muscle mass. Legs become longer and hips narrower. Muscular development increases in the chest, arms, shoulders, and upper legs.

Adults

An adult who has correct posture and body alignment feels good, looks good, and generally appears self-confident. The healthy adult also has the necessary musculoskeletal development and coordination to carry out activities of daily living.

In men there is an increase in muscle strength, which peaks in the mid 30s and is maintained into the 50s. This increase in muscle strength is correlated with testosterone levels. The decline in the muscle strength of men is not usually evident until the 70s (McCance and Huether, 1990).

Older Adults

The aging process can result in musculoskeletal changes. Degenerative joint changes may decrease ROM. Skeletal muscle mass and strength may be reduced. Changes in the structure of the bone matrix may result in fragile, brittle bones (Holm, 1989; Holm and Walker, 1990).

Older adults may walk more slowly and appear less coordinated. They may also take smaller steps, keeping the feet closer together, which decreases the base of support. Thus body balance is unstable, and they are at greater risk for falls and injuries.

PATHOLOGICAL INFLUENCES ON BODY MECHANICS

Many pathological conditions affect body alignment and mobility. These pathological influences are broken down into six categories: postural abnormalities, impaired bone formation, altered joint mobility, impaired muscle development, central nervous system damage, and musculoskeletal trauma.

Postural Abnormalities

Congenital or acquired postural abnormalities affect the efficiency of the musculoskeletal system. They also affect alignment, balance, and appearance. Postural abnormalities impair alignment, mobility, or both.

The nurse needs to know about the characteristics, causes, and treatment of common postural abnormalities (Table 22-1). The nurse uses this baseline knowledge to improve the client's body alignment during lifting, transfer, and positioning. Because some postural abnormalities affect range of motion, the nurse also maintains range of motion in the affected joint and uses the client's range in the remaining joints. In addition, the nurse can design interventions to strengthen affected muscle and joint groups, improve the client's posture, and adequately use the affected and the unaffected muscle groups.

Altered Joint Mobility

Joint mobility can be altered by inflammatory and noninflammatory joint diseases and by articular disruption. Inflammatory joint disease (e.g., arthritis) is characterized by inflammation or destruction of the synovial membrane, articular cartilage, and systemic signs of inflammation. Noninflammatory diseases have none of these characteristics, and the synovial fluid is normal (McCance and Huether, 1990).

Joint degeneration, which can occur with inflammatory and noninflammatory disease, is marked by changes in articular cartilage combined with overgrowth of bone at the articular ends (Gröer and Shekleton, 1989). Degenerative changes commonly affect weight-bearing joints.

Articular disruption may be as mild as a sprain or as severe as dislocation. Articular disruption involves trauma to the articular capsules, such as a tear in a sprain or a separation in a dislocation. Articular disruption usually results from trauma but can also be congenital, as with congenital hip dysplasia.

Inflammation, degeneration, or articular disruption alters the degree of joint mobility of the affected joints. Nurses must know the cause of limited joint mobility and ways to assess joint mobility and design interventions directed toward maintaining and improving range of joint motion.

table 22-1

POSTURAL ABNORMALITIES

Abnormality	Description	Cause	Treatment
Torticollis	Head is inclined to affected side, in which sternocleidomastoid muscle is contracted	Congenital or acquired	Surgery, heat, support, or immobilization, depending on cause and severity
Lordosis	Exaggeration of anterior convex curve of lumbar spine	Congenital Temporary as with pregnancy	Based on cause; frequently treated with spine-stretching exercises
Kyphosis	Increased convexity in curvature of thoracic spine	Congenital Rickets Tuberculosis of spine	Based on cause and severity; includes spine-stretching exercises, sleeping without pillows, using bed board, bracing, and spinal fusion
Kypholordosis	Combination of kyphosis and lordosis	Congenital	Based on cause; similar to methods used in kyphosis or lordosis
Scoliosis	Lateral curvature of spine, unequal heights of hips and shoulders	Congenital Poliomyelitis Spastic paralysis Unequal leg length	Based on cause and severity; includes immobilization and surgery
Kyphoscoliosis	Abnormal anteroposterior and lateral curvature of spine	Congenital Poliomyelitis Cor pulmonale	Based on cause and severity; includes immobilization and surgery
Congenital hip dysplasia	Hip instability with limited abduction of hips and, occasionally, adduction contractures; head of femur does not articulate with acetabulum because of abnormal shallowness of the acetabulum	Congenital; more common with breech deliveries	Maintaining continuous abduction of thigh so that head of femur presses into center of acetabulum Abduction splints, casting, or surgery
Knock-knee (genu valgum)	Legs curved inward so that knees knock together as person walks	Congenital Rickets	Knee braces and surgery if not corrected by growth
Bowlegs (genu varum)	One or both legs bent outward at knee; normal until 2 to 3 years of age	Congenital Rickets	Slowing rate of curving if not corrected by growth With rickets, vitamin D, calcium, and phosphorus intake increased to normal ranges
Clubfoot	95%: medial deviation and plantar flexion of foot (equinovarus) 5%: lateral deviation and dorsiflexion (calcaneovalgus)	Congenital	Based on degree and rigidity of deformity; includes casts, splints such as Denis Browne splint, and surgery
Footdrop	Characterized by plantar flexion, inability to invert foot because of peroneal nerve damage	Congenital Trauma Improper position of immobilized client	Cannot be corrected May be prevented through physical therapy
Pigeon-toes	Internal rotation of forefoot or entire foot, common in infants	Congenital Habitual	Corrected by growth or by wearing reversed shoes

Data from McCance KL and Huether SE: *Pathophysiology: the biologic basis for disease in adults and children*, St. Louis, 1990, Mosby.

Impaired Muscle Development

Inadequate development of the skeletal muscles affects body alignment, balance, and mobility. Muscular dystrophies are the most common developmental impairments of skeletal muscles. They are a group of genetically transmitted diseases characterized by progressive pathological changes in the skeletal muscles, resulting in muscle wasting and weakness. Muscular dystrophies can affect single muscle groups (e.g., extraocular muscles in ocular myopathy) or large muscle groups (e.g., the entire trunk in Duchenne's dystrophy).

Central Nervous System Damage

Damage to any component of the central nervous system that regulates voluntary movement results in impaired body alignment and mobility. For example, the motor strip in the cerebrum can be damaged by trauma from a head injury. The amount of voluntary motor impairment is directly related to the amount of destruction of the motor strip. A client with a right-sided cerebral hemorrhage with complete necrosis shows destruction of the right motor strip with left-sided hemiplegia. However, a client with a right-sided head injury may only have cerebral edema (but not destruction) of the motor strip. With extensive physical therapy, voluntary movement gradually returns to the left side.

Because voluntary motor fibers descend from the motor strip in the cerebrum down the spinal cord, trauma to the spinal cord also impairs mobility. The most common trauma is transection of the spinal cord in which motor fibers are cut and a complete bilateral loss of voluntary motor control occurs below the level of the trauma.

Musculoskeletal Trauma

Musculoskeletal trauma can result in bruises, contusions, sprains, and fractures. A **fracture** is a disruption of bone tissue continuity. Fractures most commonly result from direct external trauma. They can also occur because of some deformity of the bone, as with pathological fractures of osteoporosis.

As the fracture heals, the bone undergoes repair. During repair the fractured bone begins a cellular process that results in bone formation. Young children are able to form new bone more easily than adults and thus have fewer complications after a bone fracture. Treatment includes positioning the fractured bone in proper alignment and immobilizing it to promote the normal healing process and to restore function. Immobilization results in a certain amount of muscle atrophy, loss of tone, and joint stiffness. The nurse designs a program of exercises to restore full joint mobility and muscle strength gradually to the affected area.

Any acquired or congenital condition that affects the structure of the musculoskeletal or nervous system impairs to some degree body alignment or joint mobility. The impairment can be temporary or permanent. Regardless of the duration of the impairment, the nursing care plan includes interventions that maintain the present level of alignment and joint mobility and increase the level of motor function.

NURSING PROCESS FOR IMPAIRED BODY ALIGNMENT

Assessment

Assessment of body alignment can be carried out with the client standing, sitting, or lying down. This assessment has the following objectives:

1. Determining normal physiological changes in body alignment resulting from growth and development
2. Identifying deviations in body alignment caused by poor posture
3. Providing opportunities for clients to observe their posture
4. Identifying learning needs of clients for maintaining correct body alignment
5. Identifying trauma, muscle damage, or nerve dysfunction
6. Obtaining information about other factors that contribute to poor alignment, such as fatigue, malnutrition, and psychological problems

The first step in assessing body alignment is to put the client at ease so unnatural or rigid positions are not assumed. When assessing body alignment of an immobilized or unconscious client, pillows and positioning supports should be removed from the bed if not contraindicated and the client placed in the supine position.

Standing. The nurse should focus assessment of body alignment for the standing client on the following points:

1. The head is erect and midline.
2. When observed posteriorly, the shoulders and hips are straight and parallel.
3. When observed posteriorly, the vertebral column is straight.
4. When the client is observed laterally, the head is erect and the spinal curves are aligned in a reversed S pattern. The cervical vertebrae are anteriorly convex, the thoracic vertebrae are posteriorly convex, and the lumbar vertebrae are anteriorly convex.
5. When observed laterally, the abdomen is comfortably tucked in and the knees and ankles are

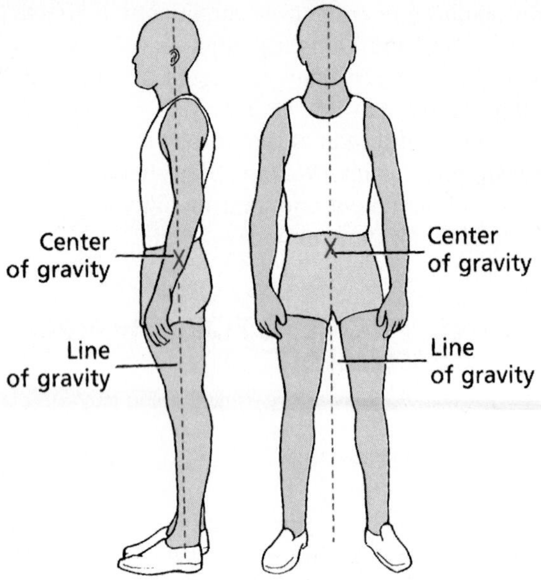

FIGURE 22-4 Correct body alignment when standing.

slightly flexed. The person appears comfortable and does not seem conscious of the flexion of knees or ankles.
6. The client's arms are comfortably at the sides.
7. The feet are placed slightly apart to achieve a base of support, and the toes are pointed forward.
8. When the client is viewed anteriorly, the center of gravity is in the midline, and the line of gravity is from the middle of the forehead to a midpoint between the feet. Laterally, the line of gravity runs vertically from the middle of the skull to the posterior third of the foot (Figure 22-4).

Sitting. The nurse assesses the alignment of the sitting client by the following observations:

1. The head is erect, and the neck and vertebral column are in straight alignment.
2. The body weight is distributed on the buttocks and thighs.
3. The thighs are parallel and in a horizontal plane.
4. Both feet are supported on the floor. With short clients, a footstool is used and the ankles are comfortably flexed.
5. A 2.5- to 5-cm (1- to 2-inch) space is maintained between the edge of the seat and the popliteal space on the posterior surface of the knee. This space ensures there is no pressure on the popliteal artery or nerve to decrease circulation or impair nerve function.
6. The forearms are supported on the armrest, in the lap, or on a table in front of the chair.

Assessing alignment is particularly important when the client is sitting if there is muscle weakness, muscle paralysis, or nerve damage. A client with these alterations has diminished sensation in affected areas and is unable to perceive pressure or decreased circulation. Proper sitting alignment reduces the risk of musculoskeletal system damage in such a client.

Recumbent. People who are conscious have voluntary muscle control and normal perception of pressure. As a result, they usually assume a position of comfort when lying down. Because their range of motion, sensation, and circulation are within normal limits, they change positions when they perceive muscle strain and decreased circulation.

Assessment of body alignment while the client is recumbent requires that the client be placed in the lateral position with all but one pillow and all positioning supports removed from the bed. The body should be supported by an adequate mattress. The vertebrae should be in straight alignment without observable curves. This assessment provides baseline data concerning the client's body alignment.

Conditions that create a risk of damage to the musculoskeletal system when lying down include impaired mobility (e.g., traction), decreased sensation (e.g., hemiparesis from a stroke), impaired circulation (e.g., diabetes), and lack of voluntary muscle control (e.g., spinal cord injuries).

When a client is unable to change position voluntarily, the nurse assesses the position of body parts while the client is lying down. The vertebrae should be in straight alignment without any observable curves. The extremities should be in alignment and not crossed over one another. The head and neck should be aligned without excessive flexion or extension.

When assessment predicts a client is at risk for damage to the musculoskeletal system while lying down, nursing interventions are directed toward maintaining proper body alignment while positioning the client.

Mobility

Assessment of mobility enables the nurse to determine the client's coordination and balance while walking, the ability to carry out activities of daily living, and the ability to participate in an exercise program. The assessment of mobility has three components: range of joint motion, gait, and exercise.

Range of Motion. Range of motion (ROM) is the maximal amount of movement possible at a joint in one of the three planes of the body: sagittal, frontal, and transverse (Figure 22-5). The **sagittal plane** is a line that passes through the body from front to back, dividing the body into a left and a right side. The **frontal plane** passes through the body from side to side and divides the body into front and back. The **transverse**

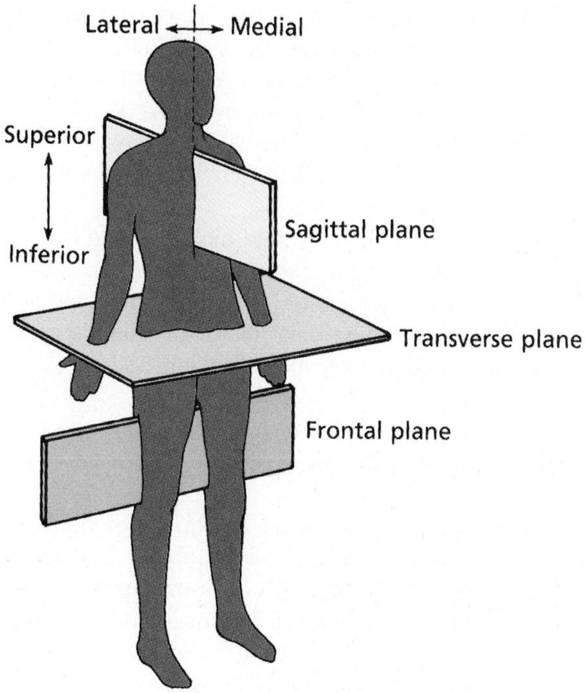

FIGURE 22-5 Planes of body.

plane is a horizontal line that divides the body into upper and lower portions.

Joint mobility in each of the planes is limited in direction by ligaments, muscles, and the construction of the joint. However, some joint movements are specific to each plane. In the sagittal plane, the movements are flexion and extension (fingers and elbow) and hyperextension (hip). In the frontal plane, the movements are abduction and adduction (arms and legs) and eversion and inversion (feet). In the transverse plane, the movements are pronation and supination (hands), internal and external rotation (knees), and dorsiflexion and plantar flexion (feet).

The nurse assesses ROM to collect data to answer questions about joint stiffness, swelling, pain, limited movement, and unequal movement. Clients whose joint mobility is restricted because of illness, disability, or trauma require exercise of their joints to reduce the hazards of immobility. These exercises, performed by the nurse, are called *passive range of joint motion exercises.* The nurse takes each affected joint through its complete range of motion.

Gait. Gait is the manner or style of walking, including rhythm, cadence, and speed. Assessing gait allows the nurse to draw conclusions about balance, posture, and ability to walk without assistance. Initially the nurse observes the overall appearance of the walking client. The adult posture is normally well aligned. Walking is smooth, coordinated with the trunk, head, and neck properly aligned.

EFFECTS OF EXERCISE

CARDIOVASCULAR SYSTEM

Increased cardiac output
Improved myocardial contraction, thereby strengthening cardiac muscle
Decreased resting heart rate
Improved venous return

PULMONARY SYSTEM

Increased respiratory rate and depth followed by a quicker return to resting state
Improved alveolar ventilation
Decreased work of breathing
Improved diaphragmatic excursion

METABOLIC SYSTEM

Increased basal metabolic rate
Increased use of glucose and fatty acids
Increased triglyceride breakdown
Increased gastric motility
Increased production of body heat

MUSCULOSKELETAL SYSTEM

Improved muscle tone
Increased joint mobility
Improved muscle tolerance to physical exercise
Possible increase in muscle mass
Reduced bone loss

ACTIVITY TOLERANCE

Improved tolerance
Decreased fatigue

PSYCHOSOCIAL FACTORS

Improved tolerance to stress
Reports of "feeling better"
Reports of decrease in illness (e.g., colds and influenza viruses)

Modified from Gröer MW and Shekleton ME: *Basic pathophysiology: a conceptual approach,* ed 3, St. Louis, 1989, Mosby; and McCance KL and Huether SE: *Pathophysiology: the biologic basis for disease in adults and children,* St. Louis, 1990, Mosby.

Exercise. Exercise is physical activity for conditioning the body, improving health, maintaining fitness, or providing therapy for correcting a deformity or restoring the overall body to a maximal state of health. When a person exercises, physiological changes occur in body systems (see box above).

To sustain increased skeletal muscle activity during exercise, the blood supply delivered to the muscles must increase. Initially the heart rate speeds up during exercise. The contractile force of the cardiac muscle of the left ventricle increases, as does the volume of blood ejected (stroke volume). Increases in heart rate and stroke volume increase the cardiac output. Dilation of the arterioles within the skeletal muscles increases delivery of blood and oxygen to muscle tissue. The person's body surface becomes warm and red as the result of the localized hyperemia from arteriolar dilation.

The increased physiological activity during exercise requires an increased supply of oxygen for delivery to body tissues. To have an increased amount of oxygen available for delivery, the person must increase the amount of oxygen inhaled. The body increases the depth of respiration, resulting in an increased tidal volume and more oxygen inhaled. Then the respiratory rate quickens. Finally, the increased tidal volumes and respiratory rate cause increased alveolar ventilation.

Exercise affects the functioning and strength of the musculoskeletal system. During exercise the muscle tone, size, and strength increase. As a result the person is able to exercise longer with each strengthening of the muscles. Joint mobility is also maintained because the exercise itself requires movement of body parts. The overall effect of exercise on physiological functioning is improvement.

Activity Tolerance. The nurse's assessment of the client's energy level includes the physiological effects of exercise and activity tolerance. **Activity tolerance** is the kind and amount of exercise or work a person is able to perform. Assessment of activity tolerance is necessary when planning physical activity for clients with acute or chronic illness.

Activity tolerance assessment includes data from the client's physiological, emotional, and developmental domains (see box below, left). This assessment provides the nurse with baseline data about the client's activity patterns and activity tolerance (Gordon, 1976).

Nursing Diagnosis

Nursing diagnoses identifying actual or potential alterations in body alignment and joint mobility are based on data collected during the nursing assessment (see nursing diagnoses box below). Alterations in body alignment and joint mobility can result from developmental changes, postural abnormalities, abnormalities in bone formation, impaired muscle development, damage to the central nervous system, and direct trauma to the musculoskeletal system. Assessment data should contain appropriate defining characteristics to support the diagnostic label.

Nursing diagnoses often focus on the individual's ability to move. The diagnostic label is supported by the defining characteristics, identified in the assessment, and the related-to factor should direct nursing interventions (Carpenito, 1993). For example, in the nursing care plan the diagnostic label *impaired physical mobility* is supported by the characteristics: difficulty in extending shoulder during activities of daily living and reduced

FACTORS INFLUENCING ACTIVITY TOLERANCE

PHYSIOLOGICAL FACTORS

Skeletal abnormalities
Muscular impairments
Endocrine or metabolic illnesses (e.g., diabetes mellitus or thyroid disease)
Hypoxemia
Decreased cardiac function
Decreased endurance
Impaired physical stability
Pain
Sleep pattern disturbance
Prior exercise patterns
Infectious processes and fever

EMOTIONAL FACTORS

Anxiety
Depression
Chemical addictions
Motivation

DEVELOPMENTAL FACTORS

Age
Sex
Pregnancy
Physical growth and development of muscle and skeletal support

Physiological data from Gröer MW and Shekleton ME: *Basic pathophysiology: a conceptual approach*, ed 3, St. Louis, 1989, Mosby.

NURSING DIAGNOSES FOR IMPROPER BODY MECHANICS AND IMPAIRED JOINT MOBILITY

- Activity intolerance
- High risk for injury
- Impaired physical mobility
- Ineffective airway clearance
- Ineffective breathing pattern
- Impaired gas exchange
- Impaired skin integrity
- Altered patterns of urinary elimination
- High risk for infection
- Total incontinence
- High risk for fluid volume deficit
- Ineffective individual coping
- Sleep pattern disturbance

range of joint motion. The related-to factor is supported by the assessment of pain on movement.

Planning

The nurse plans therapeutic interventions according to severity of risks to the client. Then the plan is individualized based on the client's developmental stage, level of health, and life-style. It is important to consider the client's home environment when planning therapies to maintain or improve body alignment and mobility. Planning care also involves an understanding of the client's need to maintain motor function and independence. The nurse, client, and other members of the health care team collaborate to establish ways of maintaining optimal body alignment and mobility. The nurse individualizes a plan of care directed at meeting the actual or potential needs of the client (see nursing care plan below). The plan is based on one or more of the following client-centered goals:

Goal: Client remains free of musculoskeletal problems.

Outcomes

Proper body alignment is maintained
Contractures are prevented
All joints are moveable

Goal: Client performs locomotion activities independently or with assistive devices, as appropriate.

Outcomes

Client ambulates twice daily
Transfers to and from chair

Goal: Client increases activity tolerance.

Outcomes

Verbalizes less fatigue
Increases participation in self-care activities

SAMPLE NURSING CARE PLAN
Impaired Physical Mobility

ASSESSMENT

Clinical scenario: Mr. Carr, a 56-year-old client hospitalized with multiple orthopedic traumas, reports pain in left shoulder during movement. He reports *difficulty extending his shoulder joint in carrying out activities of daily living.* Nurses observe that he limits motion in his left arm. *Range of motion is reduced* 30 degrees during abduction of arm.

NURSING DIAGNOSIS

Impaired physical mobility related to left shoulder pain

PLANNING

Goals	Expected outcomes
Client will gain optimal range of motion of left shoulder within 4 months.	Client reports decreased pain. Client will increase range of joint motion in upper extremity joints by 20 degrees. Client will perform self-care activities using left arm within 2 days. Client will follow a regular exercise program by discharge.

IMPLEMENTATION

Steps	Rationale
1. Offer analgesic 30 minutes before range of joint motion exercises.	Peak action of analgesic will occur as client begins exercises.
2. Schedule active range of joint motion exercises between meals and hygiene activities.	This promotes frequent exercise to affected joints and reduces risk of contracture development (Lehmkuhl, et al., 1990).
3. Teach client specific range of joint motion exercises for left shoulder and arm.	Teaching provides the client with opportunity and knowledge to maintain and increase range of joint motion (Lehmkuhl, et al., 1990).

EVALUATION MEASURES

1. Ask client to report changes in perception of left shoulder joint pain.
2. Observe client do ROM exercises in upper extremities and while doing self-care.
3. Measure range of joint motion.

Goal: Client remains free of bodily injury.
Outcomes
Identifies factors that increase the potential for injury

Implementation

To maintain proper body alignment the nurse correctly lifts the client, uses proper positioning techniques, and safely transfers the client from bed to chair or bed to stretcher. Procedures described in this section incorporate principles of body mechanics needed to maintain or restore body alignment.

Lifting Techniques. The rate of injuries in occupational settings has increased in recent years, and more than one half are back injuries directly resulting from improper lifting and bending techniques (Owen, 1980; Owen, Garg, 1991; Owen, 1993). The most common back injury is strain on the lumbar muscle group, which includes the muscles around the lumbar vertebrae (Owen, Garg, 1991). Muscle injury to these areas affects the ability to bend forward, backward, and side to side. The ability to rotate the hips and lower back is also decreased (see teaching box below).

The nurse is at risk for injury to the lumbar muscles during lifting, transferring, or positioning the immobilized client (Jensen, 1987). Before lifting, the nurse should assess the ability to lift the client or object by determining the following basic lifting criteria:

1. Position of weight. The weight to be lifted should be as close to the lifter as possible. Positioning the object in such a manner uses the lifting force of the nurse because the object is in the same plane (Stamps, 1989).
2. Height of the object. The best height for lifting vertically is slightly above the level of the middle finger of a person with the arm hanging at the side (Owen, 1980; Owen, Garg, 1991). This is approximately 2 feet off the ground and is close to the lifter's center of gravity.
3. Body position. When the lifter's body position varies with different lifting tasks, the following general rule is applicable to most lifting situations: the body is positioned with the trunk erect so that multiple muscle groups work together in a synchronized manner.
4. Maximum weight. Each nurse should know the maximum weight that is safe to carry. A nurse who weighs 130 pounds should not try independently to lift an immobilized 100-pound client. Although the nurse may be able to do it, there is a risk of injury to the client or nurse.

When lifting, the nurse should follow a procedure designed to protect the musculoskeletal system (Procedure 22-1).

Lifting an object from a high shelf increases risks to the lifter because it is more difficult to maintain body balance. To reach an object overhead, people frequently stand on tiptoe with the feet together, thereby decreasing the base of support, elevating the center of gravity, and ultimately decreasing balance.

The nurse who must lift an object from a high shelf should use a safe, stable step stool or ladder for elevation. While standing as close to the shelf as possible the nurse quickly transfers the weight of the object from the shelf to the arms and over the base of support. These principles maintain the nurse's base of support and align the weight of the object close to the nurse's center of gravity.

CLIENT TEACHING FOR BODY MECHANICS

Instruct client to exercise joints only as ordered by the physician. Increases in discomfort should be reported immediately and not attributed to the exercise activity.

Teach family members to safely use adaptive aids (e.g., transfer belts and lifts) because not all clients or family members will be able to transfer a dependent client in the home.

Instruct clients and family members to assess and stabilize their centers of gravity so that they can safely lift and position objects.

Positioning Techniques. Clients with impaired nervous, skeletal, or muscular system functioning and increased weakness and fatigability frequently require assistance from the nurse to attain proper body alignment while lying in bed or sitting. Several devices are available for the nurse to use in maintaining good body alignment for clients while clients are being positioned (Table 22-2).

Pillows are readily available in most hospitals or extended care facilities, as well as when the client is at home. Before using any pillow, the nurse should determine if it is the proper size. A thick pillow under the client's head may increase cervical flexion. A thin pillow under body prominences may be inadequate to protect the underlying skin and tissue from damage caused by pressure. When additional pillows are unavailable or if pillows are an improper size, the nurse can fold sheets, blankets, or towels for positioning aids.

procedure 22-1

PROPER LIFTING

Steps	Rationale
1. Assess four lifting measures: position of weight, height of object, body position, and maximum weight.	Determines whether person is able to do it alone or needs assistance.
2. Lift object correctly from below center of gravity:	
a. Come close to object to be moved.	Increases body balance during lift.
b. Enlarge base of support by placing feet slightly apart.	Maintains better body balance, thus reducing risk of falling.
c. Lower center of gravity to object to be lifted (see illustration).	Increases body balance and enables muscle groups to work together in synchronized manner.
d. Maintain proper alignment of head and neck with vertebrae.	Reduces risk of injury to lumbar vertebrae and muscle groups.

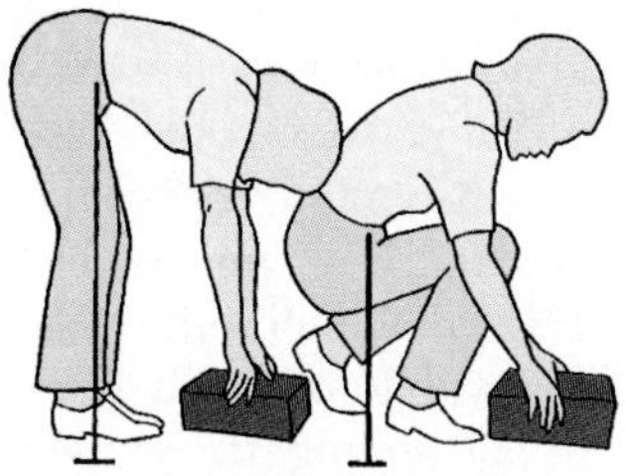

Step 2c

Steps	Rationale
3. Lift object correctly from shelf above center of gravity.	
a. Use safe, stable step stool.	Raises center of gravity closer to object.
b. Stand as close to shelf as possible.	Moves center of gravity closer to object.
c. Quickly transfer weight of object from shelf to arms and over base of support.	Reduces danger of falling by moving lifted object close to center of gravity over base of support.

table 22-2

DEVICES USED FOR PROPER POSITIONING

Device	Uses
Pillow	Provides support of body or extremity; elevates body part; splints incisional area to reduce postoperative pain during activity or coughing and deep breathing
Foot boot	Maintains feet in dorsiflexion
Trochanter roll	Prevents external rotation of legs when client is in supine position
Sandbag	Provides support and shape to body contours; immobilizes extremity; maintains specific body alignment
Hand roll	Maintains thumb slightly adducted and in opposition to fingers; maintains fingers in slightly flexed position
Hand-wrist splint	Are individually molded for client to maintain proper alignment of thumb; are slightly adducted in opposition to fingers; maintains wrist in slight dorsiflexion
Trapeze bar	Enables client to raise trunk from bed; enables client to transfer from bed to wheelchair; allows client to perform exercises that strengthen upper arms
Side rail	Allows weak client to roll from side to side or to sit up in bed
Bed board	Provides additional support to mattress and improves vertebral alignment

A **foot boot** is a device used to maintain the foot in dorsiflexion. The boot is made of rigid plastic or heavy foam, thus supporting the foot while keeping it flexed at the proper angle. The nurse should remove the foot boots 2 or 3 times a day to assess skin integrity and joint mobility.

The **trochanter roll** is used to prevent external rotation of the hips when the client is in the supine position. To form a trochanter roll, a cotton bath blanket or a sheet is folded lengthwise to a width that will extend from the greater trochanter of the femur to the lower border of the popliteal space (Figure 22-6). The blanket is placed under the buttocks and then rolled away from the client until the thigh is in the neutral position or in inward rotation. When the correct alignment of the hip is achieved, the patella faces directly upward.

Sandbags are sand-filled plastic tubes that can be shaped to body contours. Sandbags can be used in place of or in addition to trochanter rolls. They immobilize an extremity or maintain body alignment.

Hand rolls place the thumb in slight adduction and in opposition to the fingers. The hand roll maintains the hand, thumb, and fingers in a functional position. Hand rolls can be made by folding a washcloth in half, rolling it lengthwise, and securing the roll with tape. The roll is placed against the palmar surface of the hand. The nurse evaluates the position of the hand roll to make sure the hand is indeed in a functional position. If washcloths are in short supply, a hand roll can be made by placing a roll of gauze against the palmar surface of the hand.

Hand-wrist splints are individually molded for the client to maintain proper alignment of the thumb (slight adduction) and the wrist (slight dorsiflexion). These splints should be used only for the client for whom the splint was made.

The **trapeze bar** descends from a securely fastened overhead bar that is attached to the bed frame (Figure 22-7). The trapeze allows the client to use upper extremities to raise the trunk off the bed, to assist in transfer from bed to wheelchair, or to perform upper arm strengthening exercises.

Side rails, bars positioned along the sides of the length of the bed, ensure client safety (see Chapter 29) and are also useful for increasing mobility. In addition, they allow the weak client to roll from side to side or sit up in bed.

Bed boards are plywood boards placed under the entire surface area of a mattress. They are useful for increasing back support and alignment, especially with a soft mattress.

All of these devices, except the hand and wrist splints, are readily available for use in a hospital or community setting. Hand-wrist splints are especially designed to mold to the contour of the hand and are most commonly used to increase function in a client with limited mobility related to nervous system dysfunction, such as the client with hemiplegia after a stroke.

During client positioning, the nurse must also determine the presence of pressure points. When actual or potential pressure areas exist, nursing interventions in-

Text continued on p. 537.

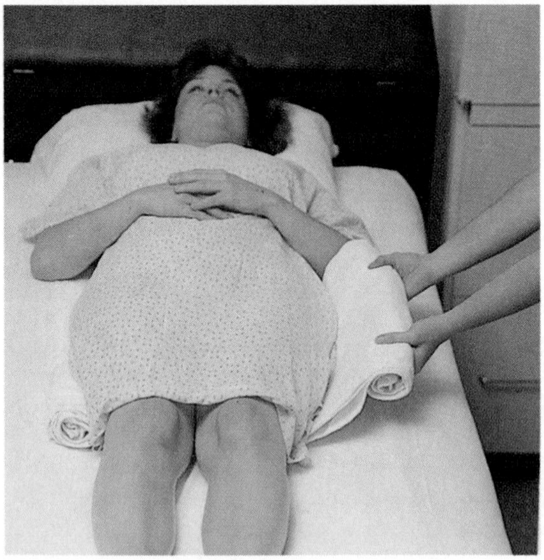

FIGURE 22-6 Trochanter roll.

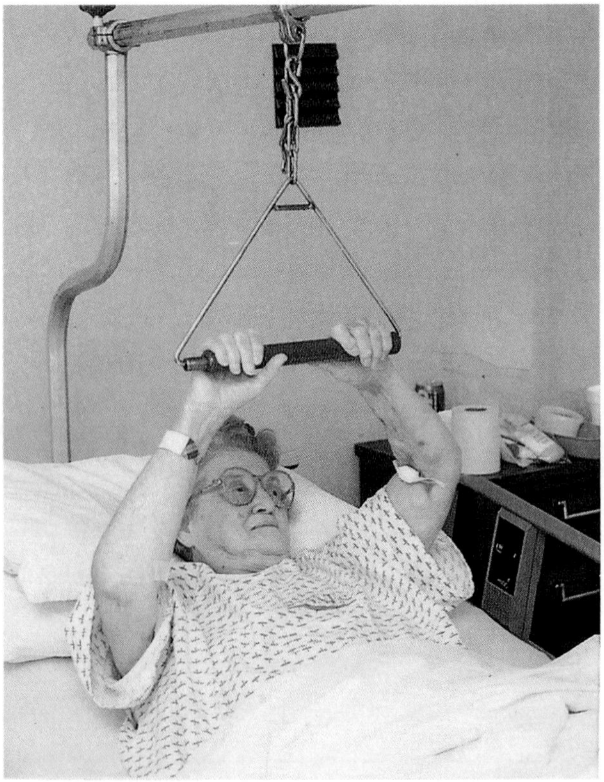

FIGURE 22-7 Client using a trapeze bar.

procedure 22-2

POSITIONING CLIENTS IN BED

Steps	Rationale
1. Assess client's body alignment and comfort level while client is lying down.	Provides baseline data concerning body alignment and comfort level. Determines ways to improve position and alignment.
2. Prepare equipment and supplies: a. Pillows b. Footboot c. Trochanter d. Sandbags e. Hand rolls f. Restraints g. Side rails	Provides easy access to equipment necessary for proper positioning.
3. Raise level of bed to comfortable working height.	Raises level of work toward nurse's center of gravity.
4. Remove pillows and devices used in previous position.	Reduces interference from bedding during positioning procedure.
5. Get help as needed.	Provides for safety.
6. Explain procedure to client.	Helps to decrease anxiety and increase cooperation.
7. Wash hands	Reduces transmission of infection.
8. Provide for privacy.	Client's mental comfort is as important as physical comfort.
9. Put bed in flat position and lower side rail closest to nurse.	Provides easy access to client and allows nurses to reposition client without working against gravity.
10. Move client to head of bed.	Maintains comfort. Allows room for proper positioning. Helps to maintain proper body alignment.
11. Position client in **supported Fowler's position:**	
a. Elevate head of bed 45 degrees to 60 degrees.	Increases comfort, improves ventilation, and increases client's opportunity to socialize or relax.
b. Rest head against mattress or on small pillow.	Prevents flexion contractures of cervical vertebrae.
c. Use pillows to support arms and hand if client does not have voluntary control or use of hands and arms (see illustration).	Prevents shoulder dislocation from effect of downward gravitational pull of unsupported arms, promotes circulation by preventing venous pooling, prevents flexion contractures of arms and wrists.
d. Position pillow at lower back.	Supports lumbar vertebrae and decreases flexion of vertebrae.
e. Place small pillow or roll under thigh.	Prevents hyperextension of knee and occlusion of popliteal artery from pressure from body weight.
f. Place small pillow or roll under ankles.	Prevents prolonged pressure on heels from mattress.
g. Place foot boots on client's feet.	Maintains dorsiflexion and prevents footdrop.

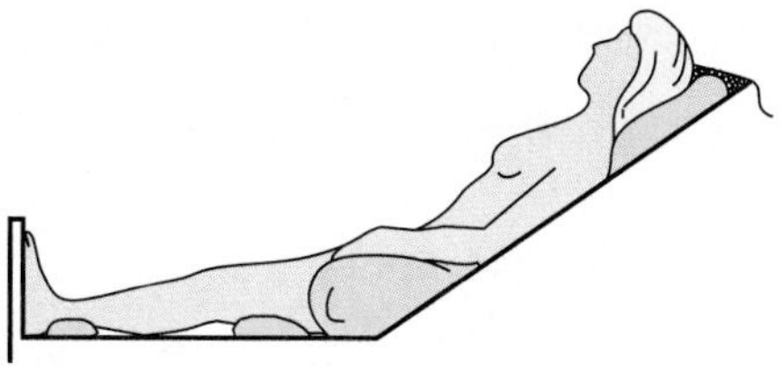

Step 11c

Steps	Rationale
12. Position **hemiplegic client in supported Fowler's position:**	
a. Elevate head of bed 45 degrees to 60 degrees.	Increases comfort, improves ventilation, increases client's opportunity to relax.
b. Sit client up as straight as possible.	Counteracts tendency to slump toward affected side. Improves ventilation and cardiac output; decreases intracranial pressure. Improves client's ability to swallow and helps to prevent aspiration of food, liquids, or gastric secretions.

Continued.

procedure 22-2—cont'd

POSITIONING CLIENTS IN BED

Steps	Rationale
c. Position head with chin slightly forward.	Reduces risk of joint dislocation. When muscle tone is decreased and muscles do not actively respond, limbs are subject to injury.
d. Provide support for involved arm and hand on pillow or overbed table in front of client; place arm away from client's side and support elbow with pillow.	Paralyzed muscles do not automatically resist pull of gravity as they do normally. As a result, shoulder subluxation, pain, or edema may occur.
e. Position *flaccid* hand in normal resting position with wrist slightly extended, arches of hand maintained, and fingers partially flexed. Use one section of a rubber ball cut in half; place client's hand around rubber ball.	Maintains hand in functional position. Prevents contractures.
f. Position *spastic* hand with wrist in neutral position or slightly extended; fingers should be extended with the palm down or may be left in relaxed position with palm up.	Maintains hand in functional position. Inhibits flexor spasticity.
g. Flex knees and hips by using small pillow or folded blanket under lower thighs.	Ensures proper alignment. Flexion prevents prolonged hyperextension, which could impair joint mobility.
h. Support feet in dorsiflexion with soft pillow or foot boot.	Prevents footdrop. Stimulation of ball of foot by hard surface has tendency to increase muscle tone in client with extensor spasticity of lower extremity.
13. Position client in **supine position:**	
a. Place client on back with head of bed flat.	Necessary for positioning in supine position.
b. Place small rolled towel under lumbar area of back.	Provides support for lumbar spine.
c. Place thin pillow under neck and head.	Maintains correct alignment and prevents flexion contractures of cervical vertebrae.
d. Place trochanter rolls or sandbags parallel to lateral surface of thighs.	Reduces external rotation of hip.
e. Place small pillow or roll under ankle to elevate heels.	Reduces pressure on heels, helping to prevent pressure sores.
f. Place foot boot or soft pillows against bottom of feet.	Maintains feet in dorsiflexion. Prevents footdrop.
g. Place pillows under pronated forearms, maintaining upper arms parallel to client's body (see illustration).	Reduces internal rotation of shoulder and prevents extension of elbows. Maintains correct body alignment.
h. Place hand rolls in hands.	Reduces extension of fingers and abduction of thumb. Maintains thumb slightly adducted and in opposition to fingers.

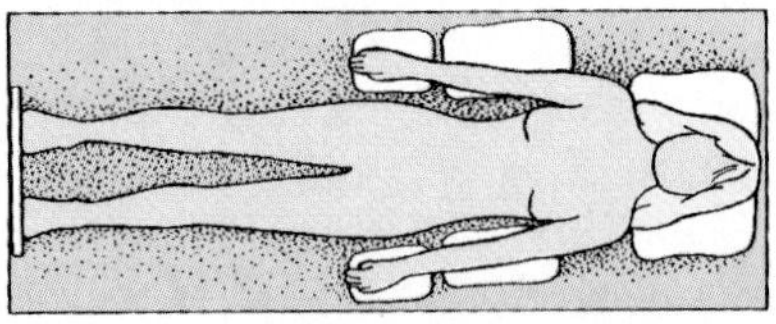

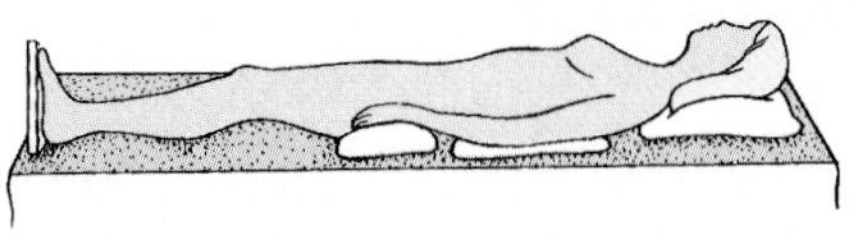

Step 13g

Steps	Rationale
14. Position **hemiplegic client in supine position:**	
a. Place head of bed flat.	Necessary for positioning in supine position.
b. Place folded towel or pillow under shoulder of affected side.	Decreases possibility of pain, joint contracture, or subluxation. Maintains mobility in muscles around shoulder to permit normal movement patterns.

Steps	**Rationale**
c. Keep affected arm away from body with elbow extended and palm up. (Alternative is to place arm out to side with elbow bent and hand toward head of bed.)	Maintains mobility in arm, joints, and muscles around shoulder to permit normal movement pattens. (Alternative position counteracts limitation of ability of arm to rotate outward at shoulder [external rotation]. External rotation must be present to raise arm overhead without pain.)
d. Position affected hand in one of recommended positions for flaccid or spastic hand (Step 11e or 11f).	Maintains hand in functional position.
e. Place folded towel under hip of involved side.	Diminishes effect of spasticity in entire leg by controlling hip position.
f. Flex affected knee 30 degrees by supporting it on pillow or folded blanket.	Slight flexion breaks up abnormal extension pattern of leg. Extensor spasticity is most severe when client is supine.
g. Support feet with soft pillows at right angle to leg.	Maintains foot in dorsiflexion and prevents footdrop. Soft pillows prevent stimulation to ball of foot by hard surface, which has tendency to increase muscle tone in client with extensor spasticity of lower extremity.
15. Position client in **prone position:**	
a. Place small pillow on abdomen below level of diaphragm.	Positions client correctly so that alignment can be maintained.
b. Roll client over arm positioned close to body with elbow straight and hand under hip. Position on abdomen in center of bed with bed flat.	Reduces flexion or hyperextension of cervical vertebrae.
c. Turn client's head to one side and support with small pillow (see illustration). 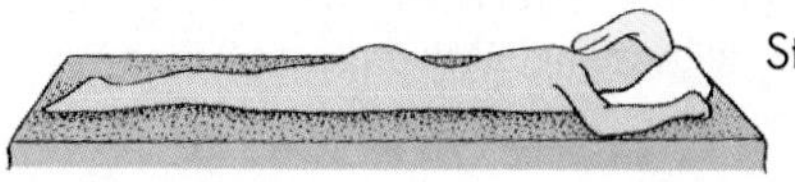 Step 15c	Reduces pressure on breasts of some female clients, decreases hyperextension of lumbar vertebrae and strain on lower back. Improves breathing by reducing mattress pressure on diaphragm.
d. Support arms in flexed position level at shoulders.	Maintains proper body alignment. Support reduces risk of joint dislocation.
e. Support lower legs with pillow to elevate toes (see illustration).	Prevents footdrop. Reduces external rotation of legs. Reduces mattress pressure on toes. 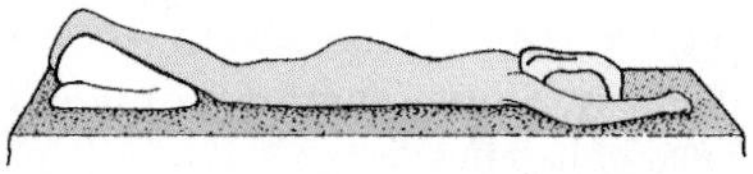 Step 15e
16. Position **hemiplegic client in prone position:**	
a. With head of bed flat, move client toward unaffected side.	Moving client to one side of bed ensures proper client alignment in center of bed when rolled onto abdomen.
b. Roll client onto side.	
c. Place pillow on abdomen.	Prevents sagging of abdomen when client is rolled over. Decreases hyperextension of lumbar vertebrae and strain on lower back.
d. Roll client onto abdomen by positioning involved arm close to body with elbow straight and hand under hip. Roll client carefully over arm.	Prevents injury to affected side.
e. Turn head toward involved side.	Promotes development of neck and trunk extension, which is necessary for standing and walking.
f. Position involved arm out to side with elbow bent and hand toward head of bed, fingers extended if possible. Keep uninvolved arm as in 15d.	Counteracts limitation of arm's ability to rotate outward at shoulder (external rotation). External rotation must be present to raise arm over head without pain.
g. Flex both knees slightly by placing pillow under legs from knees to ankles.	Flexion prevents prolonged hyperextension, which could impair joint mobility.

Continued.

procedure 22-2—cont'd

POSITIONING CLIENTS IN BED

Steps	Rationale
h. Keep feet at right angles to legs by using pillow high enough to keep toes off mattress.	Maintains feet in dorsiflexion.
17. Position client in **lateral (side-lying) position:**	
a. Lower head of bed completely or as low as client can tolerate.	Position of comfort for client, removes pressure from bony prominences on back.
b. Position client to side of bed. Nurse stands on same side of bed that the client is to be turned.	Provides room for client to turn to side.
c. Turn client onto side:	
(1) To turn helpless client onto side, flex client's knee that will not be next to mattress. Place one hand on hip and one hand on shoulder.	Prevents injury to joints as client is rolled to the side. Client is positioned so that leverage on hip makes turning easy.
(2) Roll client onto side.	Rolling client toward nurse causes less trauma to client's tissues.
d. Place pillow under head and neck, being sure ear is not folded back.	Maintains alignment. Reduces lateral neck flexion. Decreases strain on sternocleidomastoid muscle.
e. Bring shoulder blade forward.	Prevents client's weight from resting directly on shoulder joint.
f. Position arms in slightly flexed position. Uppermost arm is supported by pillow level with shoulder, other arm by mattress.	Decreases internal rotation and adduction of shoulder. Supporting both arms in slightly flexed position protects joint. Ventilation is improved because chest is able to expand more easily.
g. Place tuck-back pillow lengthwise behind back. (Make tuck-back pillow by folding pillow lengthwise. Smooth area is slightly tucked under back.)	Provides support to maintain client on side.
h. Place pillow under semiflexed upper leg level at hip from groin to foot (see illustration). Step 17h 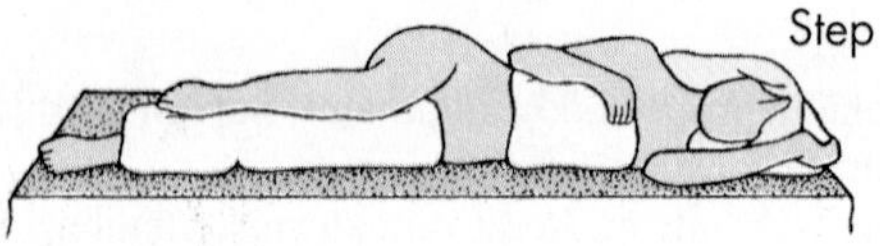	Flexion prevents hyperextension of leg. Maintains leg in proper alignment. Prevents pressure on bony prominence.
i. Place sandbag parallel to plantar surface of dependent foot.	Maintains dorsiflexion of foot. Prevents footdrop.
18. Position **client in Sims' (semiprone) position:**	
a. Place head of bed flat.	Provides for proper body alignment while client is lying down.
b. Place client in supine position (see Step 13).	Prepares client for Sims' position.
c. Position client in lateral position lying partially on abdomen (see Step 17).	Client is rolled only partially on abdomen.
d. Place small pillow under head, being sure ear is not folded back.	Maintains proper alignment and prevents lateral neck flexion.
e. Place pillow under flexed upper arm, supporting arm level with shoulder.	Prevents internal rotation of shoulder. Maintains proper alignment.
f. Place pillow under flexed upper leg, supporting leg level with hip (see illustration).	Prevents internal rotation of hip and adduction of leg. Flexion prevents hyperextension of leg. Reduces mattress pressure on knees and ankle.
g. Place sandbags parallel to plantar surface of foot.	Maintains foot in dorsiflexion. Prevents footdrop.
19. Wash hands.	Reduces transmission of infection.
20. Lower bed and raise siderails.	Provides for client safety.

Steps	Rationale
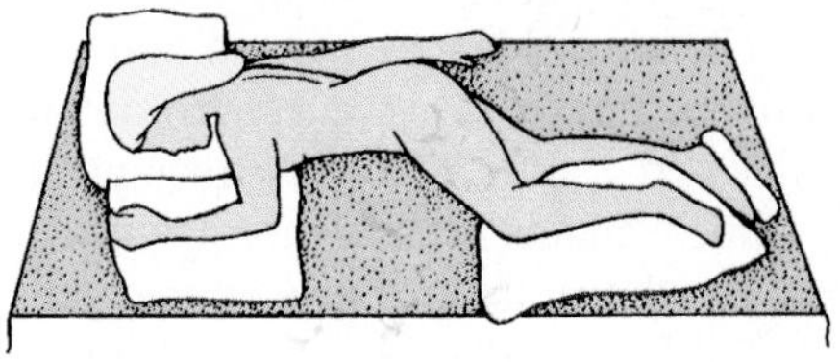 Step 18f	
21. Observe client's body alignment position, level of comfort, and potential pressure points.	Determines effectiveness of positioning, maintenance of body alignment, and protection from pressure. Reduces risk of musculoskeletal injury related to improper positioning.
22. Record procedure in nurse's notes, including position assumed, frequency of turning, condition of skin, joint movement, use of supports or splints, client's ability to assist with repositioning, number of staff needed to complete procedure, and client comfort.	Documents effectiveness of nursing care. Provides for consistency among nursing staff.

volve removing the pressure and changing the position. These interventions are aimed at decreasing the risk of pressure sores and further trauma to the musculoskeletal system.

Various positions are described in the following paragraphs. The methods of positioning clients in bed are all described in Procedure 22-2.

Supported Fowler's position. In the supported Fowler's position, the head of the client's bed is elevated 45 to 60 degrees and the client's knees are slightly elevated without pressure to restrict circulation to the lower legs. Proper alignment of the body when the client is in this position requires support that maintains comfort and reduces the risk of damage to body systems. The angle of head and knee elevation and the length of time the client should remain in the Fowler's position are influenced by the type of illness and the client's overall condition. The supports must permit flexion of the hips and proper alignment of the normal curves in the cervical, thoracic, and lumbar vertebrae. The following are common trouble areas for the client in the Fowler's position:

1. Increased cervical flexion because the pillow at the head is too thick and the client's head thrusts forward
2. Extension of knees, allowing the client to slide to the foot of the bed
3. Pressure on the posterior aspect of the knee, decreasing circulation to the feet
4. External rotation of hips
5. Arms hanging unsupported at the client's sides
6. Feet unsupported without use of footboard or footdrop prevention aids (e.g., foot boots)
7. Unprotected pressure points at the sacrum and heels

Supine position. The supine position is when the client rests on the back. In the supine position the relationship of body parts is essentially the same as in good standing alignment except that the body is in the horizontal plane. Pillows, trochanter rolls, and hand rolls or arm splints are used to increase comfort and reduce injury to the skin or musculoskeletal system.

The mattress should be firm enough to support the cervical, thoracic, and lumbar vertebrae. The shoulders are supported and the elbows are slightly flexed to control shoulder rotation. A foot support is used to prevent footdrop, maintain proper alignment, and provide freedom of movement for the feet.

The following are some common trouble areas for the supine position:

1. Pillow at the head too thick, increasing cervical flexion
2. Head flat on the mattress
3. Shoulders unsupported and internally rotated
4. Elbows extended
5. Thumb not in opposition to the fingers
6. Hips externally rotated
7. Unsupported feet

8. Unprotected pressure points at the occiput, lumbar vertebrae, elbows, and heels

PRONE POSITION. The client assuming the prone position is lying face down. The pillow under the head should be thin enough to prevent cervical flexion or extension and maintain alignment of the lumbar spine. Placing a pillow under the lower leg permits dorsiflexion of the ankles and some knee flexion, which promotes relaxation. If a pillow is unavailable, the client's ankles should be in dorsiflexion over the end of the mattress. Body alignment is poor when the ankles are continuously in plantar flexion and the lumbar spine remains in hyperextension. As with other positions the nurse should assess for and correct any of the following trouble points:

1. Neck hyperextension
2. Hyperextension of lumbar spine
3. Plantar flexion
4. Unprotected pressure points at the chin, hips, and knees

SIDE-LYING POSITION. In the side-lying (or lateral) position the client rests on the side, with the major portion of body weight on the dependent hip and shoulder. When the client is in the side-lying position, the trunk alignment should be the same as in good standing position. For example, the structural curves of the spine should be maintained, the head should be supported in line with the midline of the trunk, and rotation of the spine should be avoided, especially in the helpless client (McConnell, 1990.). The following trouble points are commonly observed in clients in the side-lying position:

1. Lateral flexion of the neck
2. Spinal curves out of normal alignment
3. Shoulder and hip joints internally rotated, adducted, or unsupported
4. Lack of support for feet
5. Lack of protection for pressure points at the ear, ilium, knees, and ankles

SIMS' POSITION. The Sims' position differs from the side-lying position in the distribution of the client's weight. In the Sims' position the client's weight is placed on the anterior ilium, humerus, and clavicle. Trouble points commonly observed in clients in the Sims' position include the following:

1. Lateral flexion of the neck
2. Internal rotation, adduction, or lack of support to shoulders and hips
3. Lack of support for the feet
4. Lack of protection for pressure points at the ilium, humerus, clavicle, knees, and ankles

CHANGING THE CLIENT'S POSITION. Correct positioning of clients is crucial for maintaining proper body alignment. A client whose mobility is decreased is at risk for developing contractures, postural abnormalities, and pressure sores. The nurse must minimize these risks by positioning clients in one of the positions presented here at least every 2 hours. However, assessment may indicate the need for more frequent positioning.

Transfer Techniques. Nurses often provide care for immobilized clients whose position must be changed, who must be moved up in bed, or who must be transferred from a bed to a chair or a bed to a stretcher. Proper use of body mechanics enables the nurse to move, lift, or transfer clients safely and also protects the nurse from injury to the musculoskeletal system.

Nurses use many transfer techniques. The following general guidelines should be followed in any transfer procedure:

1. Think through the transfer steps before beginning to ensure the safety of both the client and the nurse.
2. Assess the client's mobility and strength to determine the assistance he or she can offer during transfer.
3. Determine the amount and type of assistance required of the nurse.
4. Explain the procedure and describe what is expected of the client.
5. Raise the side rail on the side of the bed opposite the nurse to prevent the client from falling out of bed on that side.
6. Position the level of the bed to a comfortable and safe height.
7. Assess for correct body alignment and pressure areas after the transfer.

Clients experiencing pain may require analgesia before movement to minimize discomfort and promote relaxation. The nurse who is attempting transfer or moving techniques for the first time should request help to reduce the risk of injury to client and nurse. The nurse should also recognize personal strength and its limits. Moving a completely immobilized client alone is difficult and dangerous.

MOVING CLIENTS. Clients require various levels of assistance to move up in bed or to the side-lying position, or to sit up at the side of the bed. To determine what the client is able to do alone and how many people are needed to help move the client, the nurse assesses how the client tolerates exertion, as with cardiovascular disease. Next, the nurse determines whether the client comprehends what is expected of him or her. Then the nurse determines the comfort level of the client. The nurse also evaluates personal strengths and knowledge of the procedure. Finally the nurse determines whether the client is too heavy or too immobile for the nurse to complete the procedure alone. In doubtful cases the nurse should always request some assistance from another person. Procedures 22-3 and 22-4 describe the methods nurses most commonly use when moving clients in bed.

procedure 22-3

MOVING A CLIENT UP IN BED

Steps	Rationale
1. Wash hands.	Reduces transmission of microorganisms.
2. Assess client's comfort level, activity tolerance, muscle strength, and mobility.	Provides baseline data to determine ability of client to assist in moving.
3. Raise level of bed to comfortable working height.	Raises level of work toward nurse's center of gravity.
4. Remove all pillows and devices used in previous position.	Reduces interference from bedding during positioning procedure.
5. Get extra help as needed.	Provides for safety.
6. Explain procedure to client.	Helps to decrease anxiety and increase cooperation.
7. Provide for privacy.	Ensuring client's mental comfort is as important as ensuring physical comfort.
8. Put bed in flat position and lower siderails.	Provides easy access to client and allows nursing personnel to reposition client without having to work against gravity.
9. Move helpless client up in bed (one nurse):	
a. Place client on back.	Enables nurse to assess body alignment. Reduces gravitational pull on client's upper body.
b. Place pillow at head of bed.	Prevents striking client's head against bed.
c. Begin at client's feet. Face foot of bed at 45-degree angle. Place feet apart with foot nearest head of bed behind other foot (forward-backward stance). Flex knees and hips as needed to bring arms level with client's legs. Shift weight from front to back leg and slide client's legs diagonally toward head of bed.	Legs are lighter and easier to move. Facing direction of movement ensures proper balance. Shifting nurse's weight reduces force needed to move load. Diagonal motion permits pull in direction of force. Flexing knees lowers nurse's center of gravity and uses thigh muscles rather than back muscles.
d. Move parallel to client's hips. Flex knees and hips as needed to bring arms level with client's hips.	Maintains nurse's proper body alignment. Brings nurse closest to object to be moved and lowers center of gravity. Uses thigh muscles rather than back muscles.
e. Slide client's hips diagonally toward head of bed.	Aligns client's hips and feet.
f. Move parallel to client's head and shoulders. Flex knees and hips as needed to bring arms level with client's body.	Maintains nurse's proper body alignment. Brings nurse closest to object to be moved and lowers center of gravity. Uses thigh muscles rather than back muscles.
g. Slide arm closest to head of bed under client's neck, with hand reaching under and supporting client's shoulder.	Supports client's head and neck, maintaining proper alignment and preventing injury during movement.
h. Place other arm under client's chest.	Supports client's body weight and reduces friction during movement.
i. Slide client's trunk, shoulders, head, and neck diagonally toward head of bed.	Realigns client's body on one side of bed.
j. Elevate side rail. Move to other side of bed and lower side rail.	Protects client from falling out of bed.
k. Repeat procedure, switching sides until client reaches desired height in bed.	
l. Center client in middle of bed, moving body in same three sections.	Maintains proper body alignment. Provides ample room for turning, positioning, or other nursing activities.
10. Assist a client to move up in bed (one or two nurses):	
a. Place client on back.	Enables nurse to assess body alignment. Reduces gravitational pull on client's upper body.
b. Place pillow at head of bed.	Prevents striking client's head against bed.

Continued.

procedure 22-3—cont'd

MOVING A CLIENT UP IN BED

Steps	Rationale
c. Face head of bed.	
(1) If two nurses assist client, each nurse should have one arm under client's shoulders and one arm under client's thighs.	Facing direction of movement prevents twisting nurse's body while moving client.
(2) Alternate position. Position one nurse at client's upper body. Nurse's arm nearest head of bed should be under client's head and opposite shoulder. Other arm should be under client's closest arm and shoulder. Position other nurse at client's lower torso. This nurse's arms should be under client's lower back and torso.	Prevents trauma to client's musculoskeletal system by supporting shoulder and hip joints and evenly distributing client's weight.
d. Place feet apart with foot nearest head of bed behind other foot (forward-backward stance).	Wide base of support increases nurse's balance. Stance enables nurse to shift body weight as client is moved up in bed, thereby reducing force needed to move load.
e. Ask client to flex knees with feet flat on bed.	Enables client to use femoral muscles during movement.
f. Instruct client to flex neck, tilting chin toward chest.	Prevents hyperextension of neck.
g. Instruct client to assist moving by pushing with feet on bed surface.	Reduces friction. Increases client's mobility. Decreases nurse's workload.
h. Flex knees and hips, bringing forearms closer to level of bed.	Increases balance and strength by bringing nurse's center of gravity closer to client. Uses thigh muscles instead of back muscles.
i. Instruct client to push with heels and elevate trunk while breathing out, thus moving toward head of bed on count of 3.	Prepares client for actual move. Reinforces client's assistance in moving up in bed. Increases client cooperation. Breathing out avoids Valsalva maneuver.
j. On count of 3, rock and shift weight from the front to back leg. At the same time, client pushes with heels and elevates trunk.	Rocking enables nurse to improve balance and overcome inertia. Shifting nurse's weight counteracts client's weight and reduces force needed to move load. Client's assistance reduces friction and nurse's workload.
11. Realign client in supported Fowler's supine, prone, lateral, or Sims' position. Raise siderails.	Maintains client's proper body alignment, preventing injury to skin and musculoskeletal system.
12. Wash hands.	Reduces transmission of microorganisms.
13. Observe client's body alignment, position, level of comfort, and potential pressure points.	Maintains support to musculoskeletal system and reduces risk of injury related to improper movement or positioning.
14. Record procedure in nurse's notes, including position assumed, frequency of turning, condition of skin, joint movement, use of supports or splints, client's ability to assist with moving and positioning.	Documents effectiveness of nursing care. Provides for consistency of care.

TRANSFERRING A CLIENT FROM A BED TO A CHAIR. Transfer of a client from bed to chair by one nurse requires assistance from the client and should not be attempted with clients unable to assist or comprehend instructions (see Procedure 22-4). The nurse explains the procedure to the client before attempting transfer. The environment is also prepared by moving obstacles out of the way. The chair is placed next to the bed with the chair back parallel to the head of the bed. This placement allows the nurse to pivot with the client and to transfer the client's weight quickly to the chair.

A safe transfer is the first priority. The nurse who is doubtful about personal strength or the client's ability to help should request assistance. The client should sit and dangle their feet at the side of the bed for a minute before standing. Then the client should stand at the side of the bed for another minute so that the client can quickly be lowered back into it in case of dizziness or fainting.

TRANSFERRING A CLIENT FROM A BED TO A STRETCHER. An immobilized client who must be transferred from bed to stretcher or bed to bed requires a three-person carry (see Procedure 22-4). This technique is best im-

procedure 22-4

TRANSFER TECHNIQUES

Steps	Rationale
1. Assess the following: a. Muscle strength b. Joint mobility c. Presence of paralysis or paresis d. Orthostatic hypotension e. Activity tolerance f. Level of consciousness g. Level of comfort h. Ability to follow instructions	Determines client's physiological and cognitive level for participating in transfer technique.
2. Prepare equipment and supplies:	
a. Transfer belt (if needed)	Reduces risk of injury. Transfer belts should be used with all clients who require moderate to maximum assistance or have high risk of falling or injury.
b. If transferring to wheelchair, position chair at 45-degree angle to bed and lock brakes; remove foot rests and lock bed brakes	Position of wheelchair or stretcher facilitates quick transfer from bed to wheelchair or bed to stretcher.
c. If using stretcher, position at right angle (90 degrees) to bed; lock brakes on stretcher and bed.	
d. If using hydralic lift, use frame, canvas strips or chains, and hammock or canvas strips.	Lifts safely transfer large, immobile clients unable to maintain weight bearing.
3. Explain procedure to client. Close door or curtain.	Promotes cooperation and understanding of procedure and benefits of mobilization. Ensures privacy.
4. Wash hands.	Reduces transfer of infection.
5. **Assist client to sitting position in a regular bed in the home:**	
a. Place client in supine position.	Enables nurse to continually assess client's body alignment and to administer additional care, such as suctioning or hygiene needs.
b. Remove pillows from bed.	Decreases interference while sitting client up in bed.
c. Face head of bed.	Reduces twisting of nurse's body when moving client.
d. Place feet apart with foot nearer bed behind other foot.	Improves nurse's balance and allows for transfer of body weight as client is moved to sitting position.
e. Place hand farther from client under shoulders, supporting head and cervical vertebrae.	Maintains alignment of head and cervical vertebrae and allows for even lifting of client's upper trunk.
f. Place other hand on bed surface.	Provides support and balance.
g. Raise client to sitting position by shifting weight from front leg to back leg.	Improves nurse's balance, overcomes inertia, and transfers weight in direction in which client is moved.
h. Push against bed using arm that was placed on bed surface.	Divides activity of raising client to sitting position between nurse's arms and legs and protects back from strain. By bracing hand against mattress and pushing against it as client is lifted, part of weight that would be lifted by back muscles is transferred through arms onto mattress.
6. **Assist client to sitting position on side of bed:**	
a. Place client in side-lying position, facing nurse on side of bed on which client will be sitting.	Prepares client to move to side of bed and protects client from falling.
b. Raise head of bed to highest level client is able to tolerate.	Decreases amount of work needed by client and nurse to raise client to sitting position.
c. Stand opposite client's hips.	Places nurse's center of gravity nearer client.
d. Turn on diagonal so that nurse faces client and far corner of foot or bed.	Reduces twisting of nurse's body because nurse is facing direction of movement.
e. Place feet apart with foot closer to head of bed in front of other foot.	Increases balance and allows nurse to transfer weight as client is brought to sitting position at side of bed.

Continued.

procedure 22-4—cont'd

TRANSFER TECHNIQUES

Steps	Rationale
f. Place arm nearer head of bed under client's shoulders, supporting the head and neck.	Maintains alignment of head and neck as nurse brings client to sitting position.
g. Place other arm over client's thighs (see illustration).	Supports hip and prevents client from falling backward during procedure.
h. Move client's lower legs and feet over side of bed.	Decreases friction and resistance.
i. Pivot toward rear leg, allowing client's upper legs to swing downward.	Allows gravity to lower client's legs.
j. At same time, shift weight to rear leg and elevate client (see illustration).	Allows nurse to transfer weight in direction of motion.
k. Remain in front of client until he or she regains balance.	Reduces risk of falling.
l. Lower level of bed until client's feet touch floor.	Supports client's feet in dorsiflexion and allows client to easily stand at side of bed.

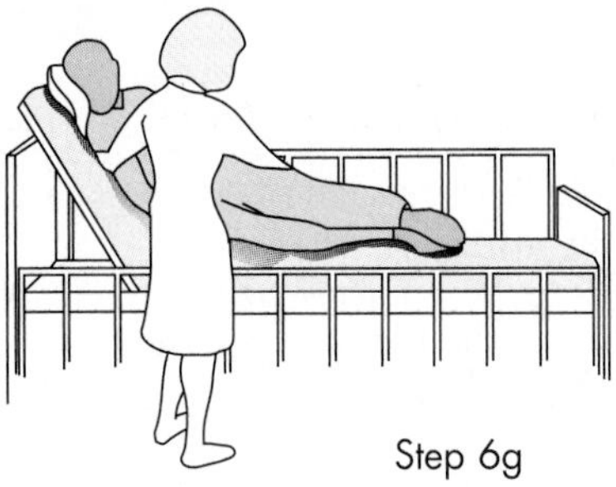

Step 6g

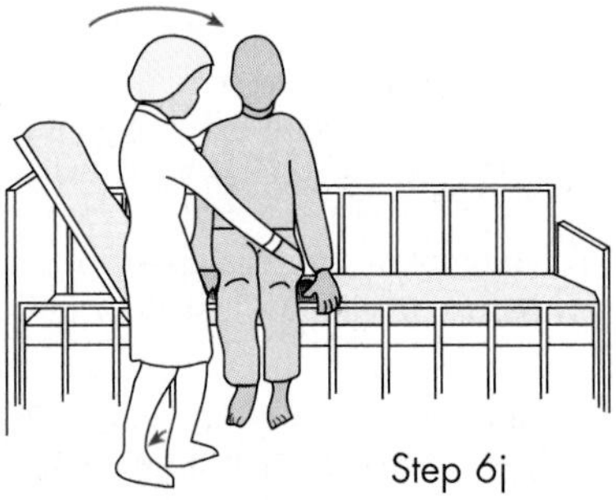

Step 6j

Steps	Rationale
7. **Transfer client from bed to chair:**	
a. Assist client to sitting position on side of bed. Have chair in position at 45-degree angle to bed.	Positions chair within easy access for transfer.
b. Apply transfer belt if necessary.	Allows nurse to maintain stability of client during transfer, reducing risk of falling.
c. Ensure client has stable nonskid shoes.	Decreases risk of slipping during transfer.
d. Spread feet apart.	Ensures balance with wide base of support.
e. Flex hips and knees, aligning your knees with client's.	Lowers nurse's center of gravity to object to be raised and allows for stabilization of knees when client stands.

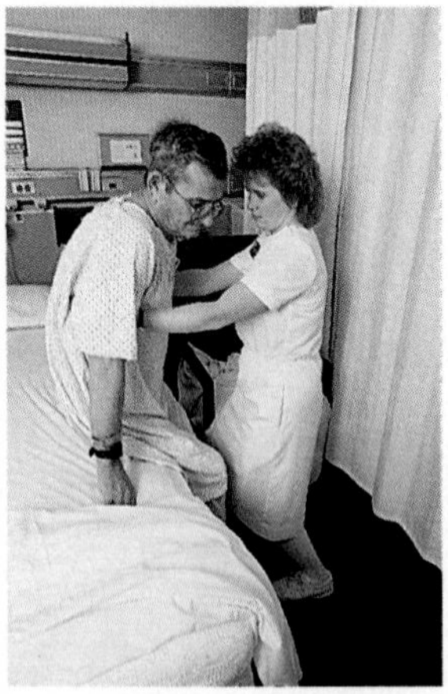

Step 7f

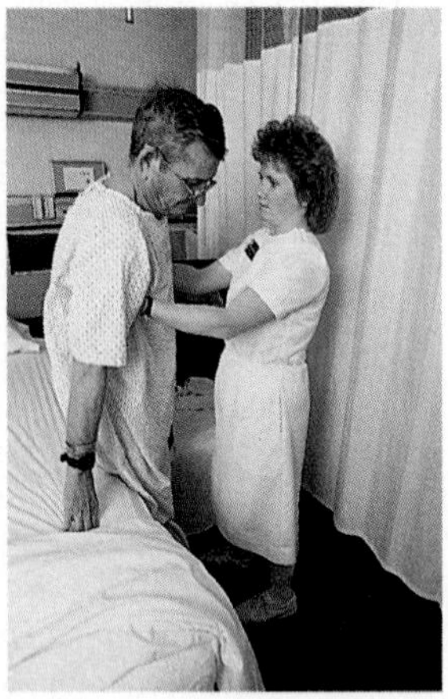

Step 7g

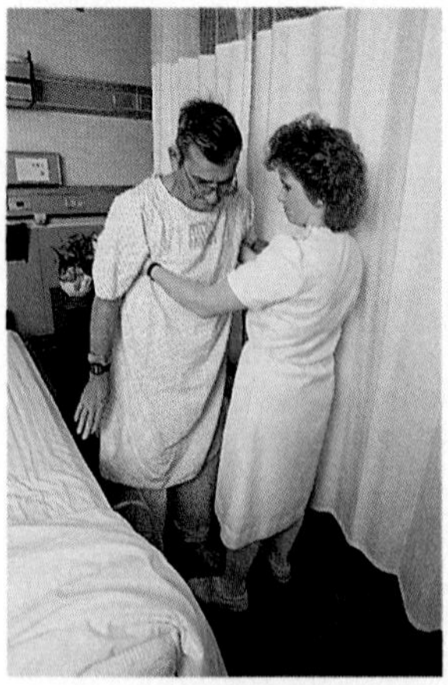

Step 7i

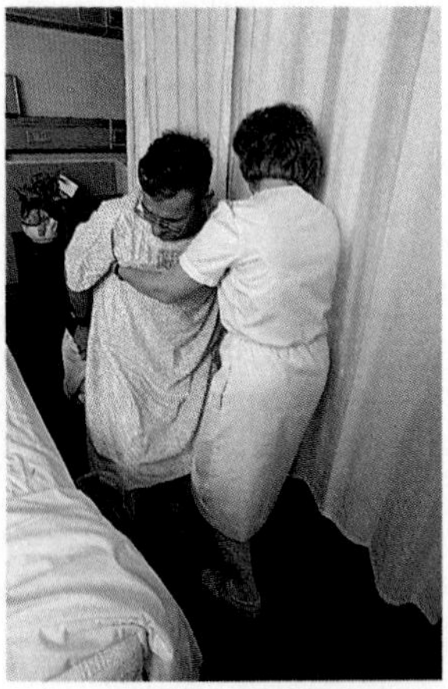

Step 7k

Steps	Rationale
f. Grasp transfer belt from underneath or reach under client's axillae and place hands on client's scapulae (see illustration).	Reduces pressure on axillae and maintains client stability.
g. Rock client up to standing on count of 3 while straightening hips and legs, keeping knees slightly flexed (see illustration).	Rocking motion gives client's body momentum and requires less muscular effort to lift client. Uses correct body mechanics to raise client to standing position.
h. Maintain stability of weak or paralyzed leg with knee.	Ability to stand can often be maintained in a paralyzed or weak limb with support of knee to stabilize.
i. Pivot on foot that is farther from chair (see illustration).	Maintains support of client while allowing adequate space for client to move.
j. Instruct client to use arm rests on chair for support.	Increases client's stability.
k. Flex hips and knees while lowering client into chair (see illustration).	Prevents injury to nurse resulting from poor body mechanics.
l. Assess client for proper alignment for sitting position.	Prevents injury to client from poor body alignment.
8. **Perform three-person carry:**	
a. Three nurses stand side by side facing side of client's bed. These people should be nearly equal height.	Prevents twisting of nurses' bodies. Maintains client's alignment.
b. Each person assumes responsibility for one of three areas: head and shoulders, hips, or thighs and ankles.	Distributes client's body weight.
c. Each assumes wide base of support, with foot closer to stretcher in front, knees slightly flexed.	Increases balance and lowers nurses' center of gravity.
d. Nurses' arms are placed under client's head and shoulders, hips, and thighs and lower legs, with their fingers securely around other side of client's body (see illustration).	Distributes client's weight over nurses' forearms. 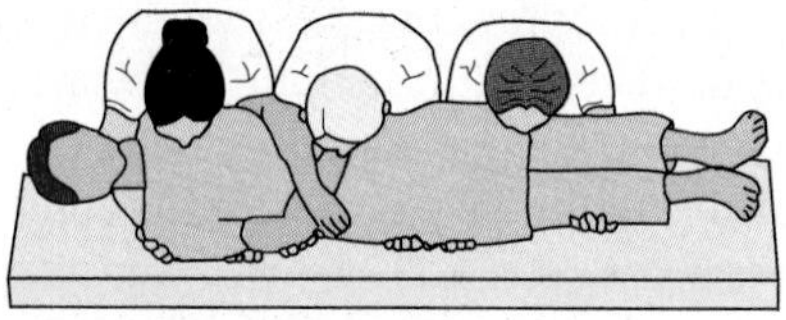 Step 8d
e. Nurses roll client toward their chests.	Moves workload over nurses' base of support.
f. On count of 3, client is lifted and held against nurses' chests.	Enables nurses to work together and safely lift client.
g. On second count of 3, nurses step back and pivot toward stretcher, moving forward if needed.	Transfers weight toward stretcher.
h. Nurses gently lower client onto center of stretcher by flexing their knees and hips until their elbows are level with edge of stretcher.	Maintains nurses' alignment during transfer.
i. Nurses assess client's body alignment, place safety straps across him or her, and raise side rails.	Reduces risk of injury from poor alignment or falling.
9. Position client in selected position.	Reduces risk of injury to musculoskeletal system from improper positioning.
10. Wash hands.	Reduces transmission of infection.
11. Observe client to determine the response to transfer. Observe for correct body alignment and pressure points.	Reduces risk of injury from subsequent transfers and positioning.
12. Record procedure in nurses' notes, including client's tolerance and length of time out of bed and if transferred to another area for diagnostic test, including specific test and time client returned.	Documents effectiveness of nursing care. Provides for consistency among nursing staff.

plemented when personnel are of a similar height. If their centers of gravity are within the same plane, they can lift as a team.

Caution is used when the client has spinal cord trauma. If the client must be moved, the three-person carry is used and spinal alignment is maintained during the transfer.

The client should be prepared for the transfer and asked to help (e.g., by folding the arms over the chest). The environment should be free from obstacles, and unnecessary equipment should be removed from the bed. The stretcher should be placed at a right angle to the bed so the lifters can pivot toward the stretcher and transfer the client quickly.

As with all procedures, safety is the priority. Safety is increased in the three-person carry if all the lifters work together. Therefore one person should assume the leadership role and direct the other two.

Joint Mobility

Range of motion exercises may be active (the client is able to move all joints through their range of motion unassisted), passive (the client is unable to move independently, and the nurse moves each joint through its range of motion), or somewhere in between. The nurse first assesses the client's ability to engage in active range of motion exercises and the need for joint support from the nurse. As a general principle, exercises should be as active as the client's health and mobility allow.

Gerontologic nursing practice for the client with impaired physical mobility might include an awareness of the following (see box at right for additional principles):

- A general decline in physical activity comes with aging.
- Falls are experienced more frequently by the older adult.
- Glare causing visual difficulty is often responsible for falls in the older adult.
- Changes in joints because of age cause a decrease in flexibility and impair flexion and extension movements.

GERONTOLOGIC NURSING PRACTICE

- Encourage the older adult client to avoid prolonged sitting; get up and stretch. Frequent stretching decreases joint contractures.
- Be sure client maintains proper body alignment when sitting. Proper alignment minimizes joint and muscle stress.
- Teach clients how to use stronger joints or larger muscle groups to manipulate spray cans, container lids, and so on. Efficient distribution of workload decreases joint stress and pain.
- Provide resources for planned exercise programs. Proper exercise activities slow further bone loss and prevent fractures in the older adult with osteoporosis.
- Encourage older adults to assess the home environment for fall hazards. Changes in client's mobility, vision, cardiovascular status, and so on increase the risk of falls in the home. Since prevention of falls is a key factor, older adults and their families need to routinely assess their environments for potential hazards and make necessary modifications.

From Carnevali DL, Patrick: *Nursing management for the elderly,* ed 3, Philadelphia, 1993, JB Lippincott.

Range of Motion Exercises. Clients with restricted mobility are unable to perform some or all range of motion exercises independently. This limitation can be identified in clients who have limited movement in one extremity or in completely immobilized clients. When caring for clients with an actual or potential impaired mobility, the nurse designs interventions directed toward maintaining maximal joint mobility. One such nursing intervention is ROM exercises.

To ensure that clients routinely receive these exercises, the nurse should schedule them at specific times, perhaps along with another nursing activity such as a bath. This enables the nurse to systematically assess and improve the client's range of motion.

To ensure adequate joint mobility the nurse can teach the client about range of motion exercises. When the client does not have voluntary motor control, the nurse uses passive range of motion exercises. Joint mobility is also increased by walking. Occasionally clients need to use mechanical devices such as crutches to increase the ability to walk.

Contractures may develop in joints that are not moved periodically through their range of motion. A **contracture** is a permanent shortening of a muscle and the eventual shortening of associated ligaments and tendons. If a contracture occurs because the joint is immobilized for a long time, the client will not be able to use the joint normally and it may become fixed in one position.

Unless contraindicated, the nursing plan should include moving the extremities through as nearly full range of motion as possible. The nurse should move joints to the point of discomfort, tension, or spasm but not beyond. Passive range of motion exercises should be initiated as soon as the client loses the ability to move the extremity or joint. Movements are carried out slowly and smoothly and should not cause pain. Each movement should be repeated five times during the exercise period.

table 22-3

RANGE OF JOINT MOTION EXERCISES

Body part	Type of joint		Type of movement
Neck and cervical spine	Pivotal	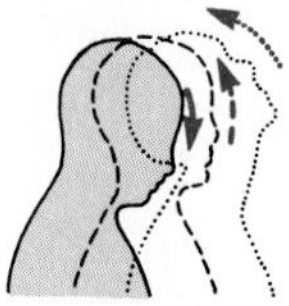	Flexion: bring chin to rest on chest Extension: return head to erect position Hyperextension: bend head back as far as possible
		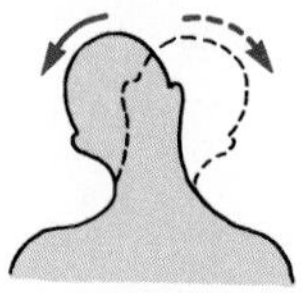	Lateral flexion: tilt head as far as possible toward each shoulder
		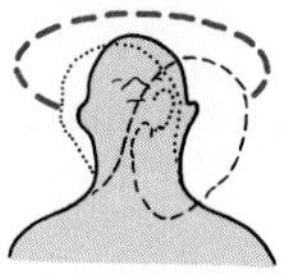	Rotation: turn head as far as possible to right and left
Shoulder	Ball and socket	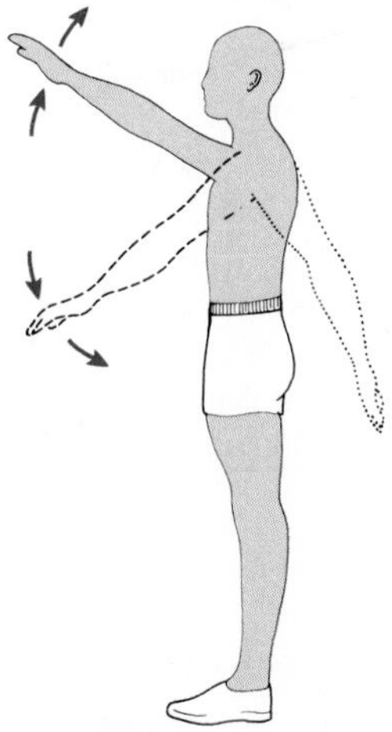	Flexion: raise arm from side position forward to position above head Extension: return arm to position at side of the body Hyperextension: move arm behind body, keeping elbow straight
		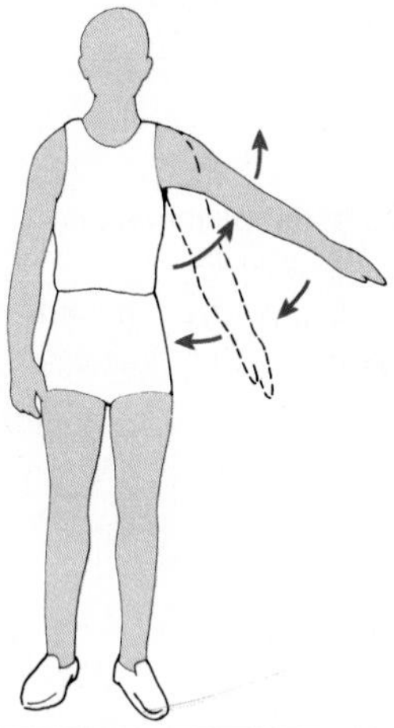	Abduction: raise arm to side to position above head with palm away from head Adduction: lower arm sideways and across body as far as possible
		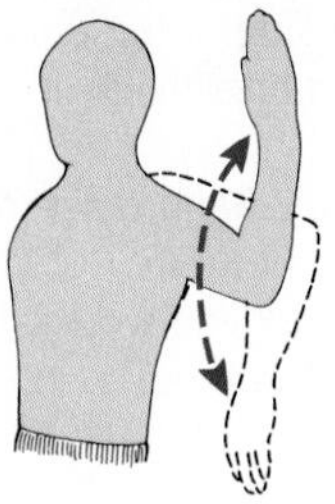	Internal rotation: with elbow flexed, rotate shoulder by moving arm until thumb is turned inward and toward back External rotation: with elbow flexed, move arm until thumb is upward and lateral to head
		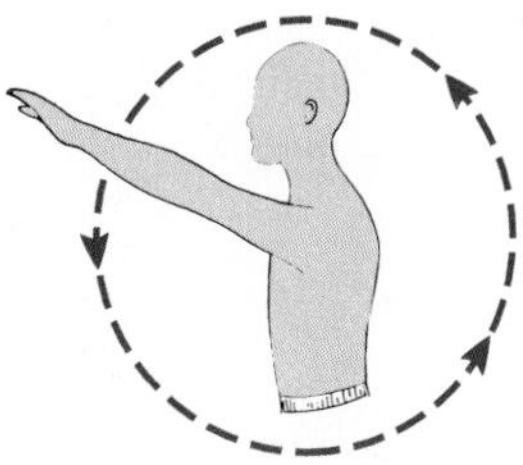	Circumduction: move arm in full circle. Circumduction is combination of all movements of ball-and-socket joint
Elbow	Hinge	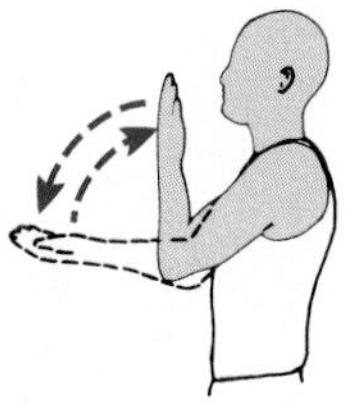	Flexion: bend elbow so that lower arm moves toward its shoulder joint and hand is level with shoulder Extension: straighten elbow by lowering hand Hyperextension: bend lower arm back as far as possible
Forearm	Pivotal	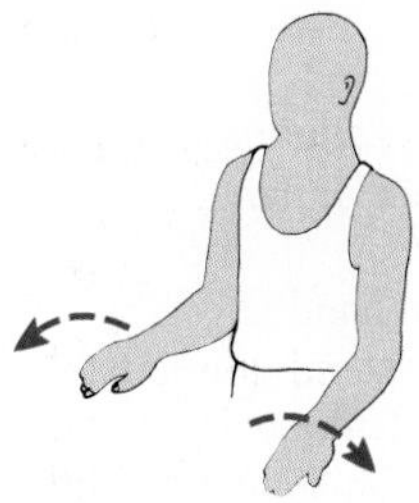	Supination: turn lower arm and hand so that palm is up Pronation: turn lower arm so that palm is down
Wrist	Condyloid	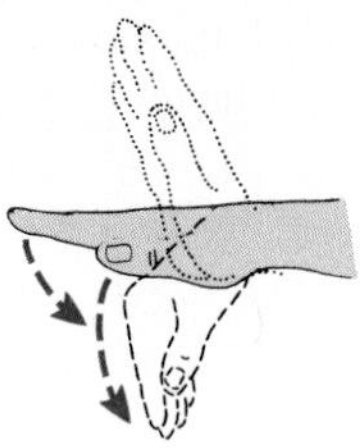	Flexion: move palm toward inner aspect of the forearm Extension: move fingers so that fingers, hands, and forearm are in same plane

Continued.

table 22-3—cont'd

RANGE OF JOINT MOTION EXERCISES

Body part	Type of joint	Type of movement
	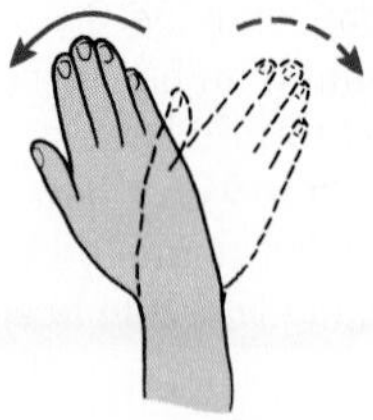	Hyperextension: bring dorsal surface to hand back as far as possible Radial flexion: bend wrist medially toward thumb Ulnar flexion: bend wrist laterally toward fifth finger
Fingers	Condyloid hinge 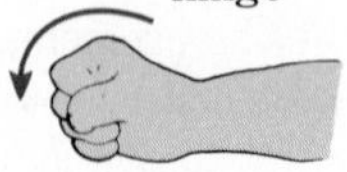 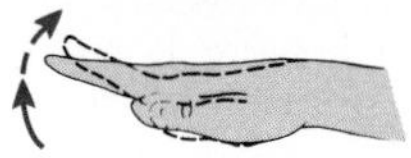	Flexion: make fist Extension: straighten fingers Hyperextension: bend fingers back as far as possible
	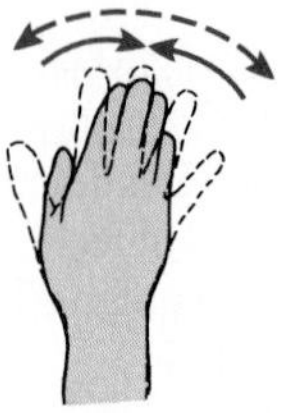	Abduction: spread fingers apart Adduction: bring fingers together
Thumb	Saddle 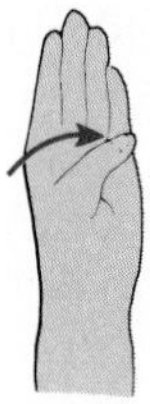 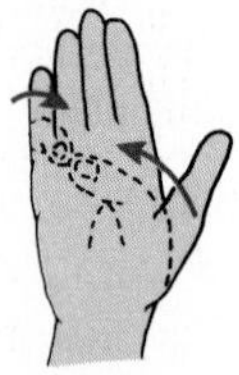	Flexion: move thumb across palmar surface of hand Extension: move thumb straight away from hand Abduction: extend thumb laterally (usually done when placing fingers in abduction and adduction) Adduction: move thumb back toward hand Opposition: touch thumb to each finger of same hand

Body part	Type of joint	Type of movement
Hip	Ball and socket 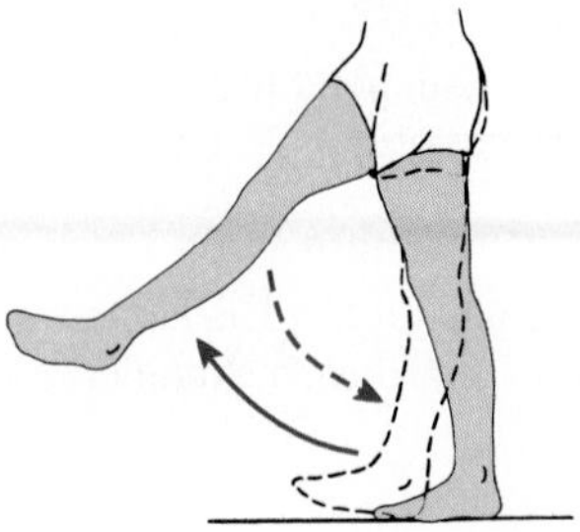	Flexion: move leg forward and up Extension: move leg back beside other leg
	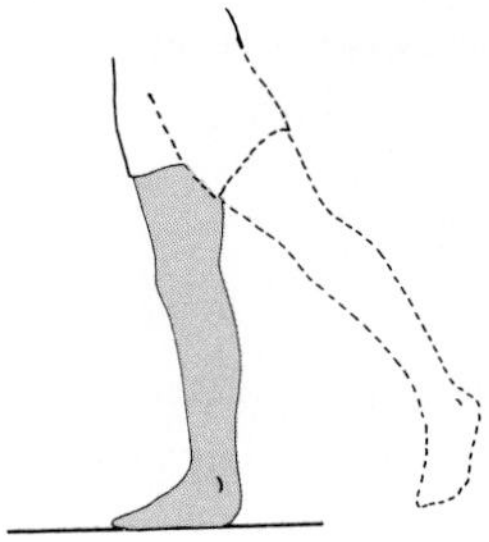	Hyperextension: move leg behind body
	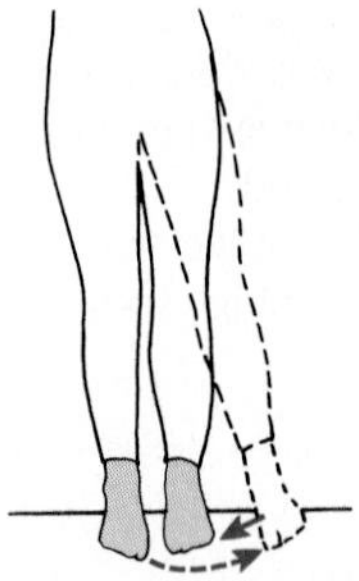	Abduction: move leg laterally away from body Adduction: move leg back toward medial position and beyond if possible
	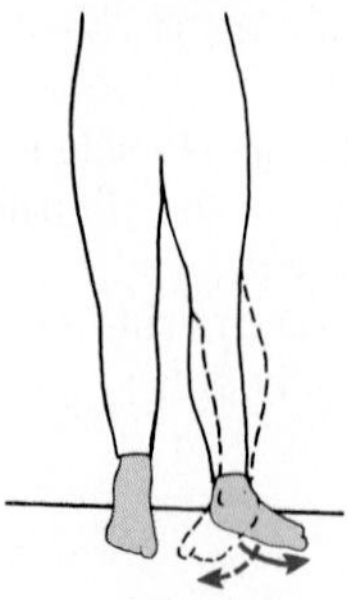	Internal rotation: turn foot and leg toward other leg External rotation: turn foot and leg away from other leg

[redacted]

Body part	Type of joint	Type of movement
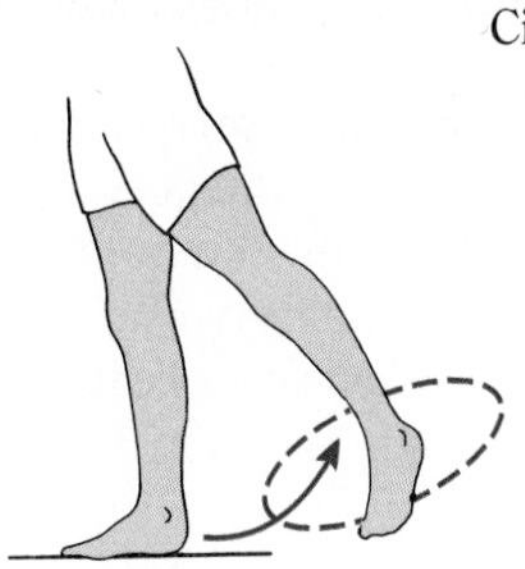		Circumduction: move leg in circle
Knee 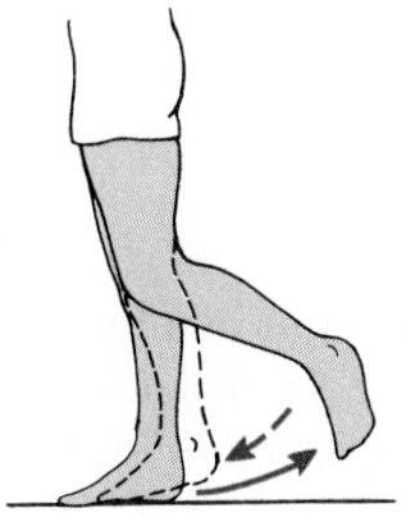	Hinge	Flexion: bring heel back toward back of thigh Extension: return heel to floor
Ankle 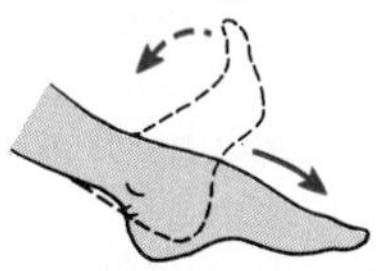	Hinge	Dorsal flexion: move foot so that toes are pointed upward Plantar flexion: move foot so that toes are pointed downward
Foot 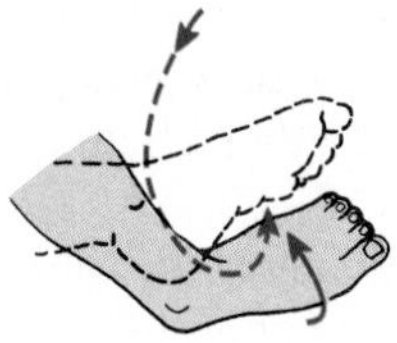	Gliding	Inversion: turn sole of foot medially Eversion: turn sole of foot laterally
Toes 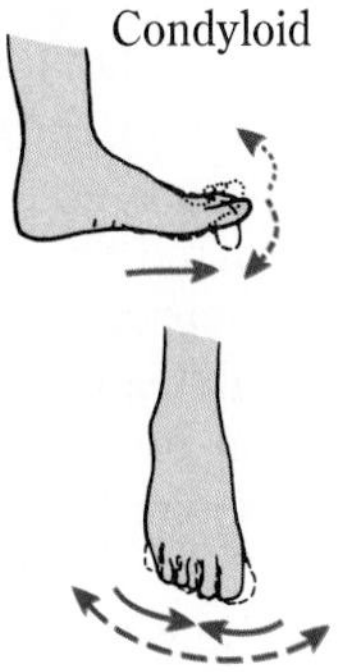	Condyloid	Flexion: curl toes downward Extension: straighten toes Abduction: spread toes apart Adduction: bring toes together

When performing **passive range of motion exercises,** the nurse stands at the side of the bed closest to the joint being exercised. If an extremity is to be moved or lifted, the nurse places a cupped hand under the joint to support it, supports the joint by holding the adjacent distal and proximal areas, or supports the joint with one hand and cradles the distal portion of the extremity with the remaining arm.

The following sections describe the specific movements for the major joints in the body. Table 22-3 details range of motion for each area and illustrates the motion of each joint.

NECK. Range of motion for the neck is permitted by the flexibility of the cervical vertebrae and the pivotal connection between the head and neck. Unless contraindicated because of central nervous system trauma, range of joint motion exercises should be performed by clients with limited neck mobility. When flexion contracture of the neck occurs, the client's neck is permanently flexed with the chin close to or actually touching the chest. Ultimately, the client's total body alignment is altered, the visual field is changed, and the overall level of independent functioning is decreased.

SHOULDER. One feature of the shoulder that sets it apart from other joints in the body is that the strongest muscle controlling it, the deltoid, is in complete elongation in the normal position of rest. No other muscle exerts its full strength if it begins a movement when in complete elongation. Thus exercising the shoulder effectively increases the power of the deltoid and range of motion; to accomplish this, the shoulder must first be abducted.

The goal of action in the shoulder is full range of motion. Shoulder movements include flexion, extension, hyperextension, abduction, adduction, internal and external rotation, and circumduction. The full range of motion in the shoulder must be maintained or regained to avoid pain.

When caring for a client with limited voluntary control of the shoulder, the nurse should design interventions to place and support the shoulder in the adducted position. This can be achieved with slings when the client is standing or sitting, or with pillows when the client is in bed. Supporting and positioning the shoulder prevent pain, joint dislocation, and further changes in body alignment.

ELBOW. The elbow functions optimally at an angle of approximately 90 degrees. An elbow fixed in full extension is very disabling and limits the client's independence. The normal elbow joint movements include flexion, extension, and hyperextension. The nurse should not force the elbow beyond its capacity. This joint is particularly likely to develop pain because of limited mobility, and unlike the shoulder joint, increasing the range of motion will not relieve the pain.

FOREARM. Most functions of the hand are best carried out with the forearm in moderate pronation. When the forearm is fixed in a position of full supination, the client is quite disabled. For optimal functioning, the forearm must be able to rotate from supination to pronation.

WRIST. The primary function of the wrist is to place the hand in slight dorsiflexion, the position of functioning. Therefore full range of joint motion in the wrist is not as great a priority as maintaining the wrist in a functional position. When the wrist is fixed in even a slightly flexed position, the client's grasp is weakened. In the immobilized client the functional position of the wrist can be achieved by using hand and splint rolls.

FINGERS AND THUMB. The range of motion in the fingers and the thumb enables the client to perform activities of daily living and activities requiring fine motor skills, such as carpentry, needlework, drawing, or painting. The functional position of the fingers and thumb is slight flexion of the thumb in opposition to the fingers. In clients with restricted mobility, hand rolls help to maintain this functional position.

HIP. Because the lower extremities are concerned chiefly with locomotion and weight bearing, the stability of the hip joint may be more important than its overall mobility. For example, if one hip has no mobility but is fixed in a neutral position and fully extended, it is possible for the client to walk without a significant limp.

However, contractures often fix the hip in positions of deformity. Excessive abduction makes the affected leg appear too long, whereas excessive adduction makes the affected leg appear too short; in either case the client has limited locomotion and walks with an obvious limp. Flexion contractures result in lordosis when the person is standing. Internal and external rotation contractures cause an unacceptable, unbalanced gait.

KNEE. A primary function of the knee is stability, which is achieved by a combination of the skeletal bones, joint motion, ligaments, and muscles. However, the knees cannot remain stable under weight-bearing conditions unless there is adequate quadriceps power, which maintains the knee in full extension. Range of joint motion exercises should include pulling the knee into full extension.

An immobile knee joint can result in serious disability. If the knee is fixed in full extension, the person must sit with leg thrust straight out in front. When the knee is flexed, the person limps while walking. The greater the flexion, the greater the limp. Complete flexion contractures prevent the person from walking without a walker or crutches.

ANKLE AND FOOT. During walking, movement of the ankle joint is minimal; however, the joint must be stabilized and able to bear weight, or the person will fall. If joint mobility is diminished, the nurse should maintain the joint in a position in which walking can be carried out with a forward rolling motion from the heel onto the forefoot.

When the person relaxes as in sleep or in a coma, the foot relaxes and assumes a position of plantar flexion. This results from relaxation of the gastrocnemius and soleus muscles, which maintain dorsiflexion. If the foot remains in plantar flexion without support, these two muscles shorten and the dorsiflexion muscles try to compensate by overstretching. As a result the foot becomes fixed in plantar flexion (footdrop), which impairs the client's ability to walk.

Inversion and eversion must also be avoided to allow the foot to rest flat on the floor (see Table 22-2). The foot must be flat on the floor to allow weight bearing and proper walking.

TOES. Excessive flexion of the toes results in a clawing. When this is a permanent deformity, the foot is unable to rest flat on the floor. Flexion contractures are the most common foot deformity associated with reduced joint mobility. Adequate range of joint motion gives the client the necessary mobility to carry out activities of daily living, to exercise, and to engage in relaxing activities. In addition, adequate range of motion in the lower extremities allows the client to walk.

Walking. In the normal walking posture the head is erect, the cervical, thoracic, and lumbar vertebrae are aligned, the hips and knees have appropriate flexion, and the arms swing freely in alternation with the legs. Illness or trauma can reduce activity tolerance so that assistance in walking is required. In addition, damage to the musculoskeletal and nervous systems may necessitate use of a mechanical device for walking.

ASSISTING A CLIENT TO WALK. Like the other procedures, assisting the client to walk requires preparation. The nurse assesses the client's activity tolerance, strength, presence of pain, coordination, and balance to determine the exact type of assistance needed. The client should be wearing supportive, non-slipping shoes.

Then the nurse explains the distance the client should try to walk, the list of helpers, the time the walk will take place, and the reasons walking is important. In addition, the nurse and client determine the amount of independence that the client can assume.

Then the nurse double-checks the environment to be sure no obstacles are in the client's path—that the chairs, over-the-bed table, and wheelchair are out of the way so that the client does not need to expend energy walking an obstacle course. Before the client begins to walk, resting points should be established in case the client's activity tolerance is less than was estimated or the client becomes dizzy.

Finally, the client should be assisted to a position of sitting at the side of the bed and should rest for 1 to 2 minutes before standing up. Likewise, after standing, the client should remain stationary for a minute or two before moving. It is important to allow the client to stabilize before walking; if the client becomes dizzy, the bed is still nearby and the nurse can quickly ease him or her back to bed. The longer the period of immobility, the greater the physiological changes, especially the changes in circulation; when the person stands, blood pressure may drop (see Chapter 23). Several methods are used for walking a client.

The nurse should provide support at the waist so that the client's center of gravity remains midline. This can be achieved when the nurse places both hands at the client's waist or uses a walking belt. A walking belt is a leather belt that encircles the client's waist and has handles attached for the nurse to hold while the client walks. Clients should not lean to one side because their center of gravity is no longer midline, distorting their balance, and their risk of falling is increased.

The client who appears unsteady or complains of dizziness should be returned to the closest bed or a chair. If the client faints or begins to fall, the nurse should assume a wide base of support with one foot in front of the other, thus supporting the client's body weight. Then the nurse gently lowers the client to the floor, protecting the head. Although lowering a client to the floor is not difficult, the student should practice this technique with a friend or classmate before attempting it in a clinical setting.

Clients with hemiplegia (one-sided paralysis) or hemiparesis (one-sided weakness) need assistance to walk. The nurse always stands by the client's affected side and supports the client by holding one arm around the client's waist and the other arm around the inferior aspect of the client's upper arm so that the nurse's hand is supporting the client's axilla. Providing support by holding the client's arm is incorrect because, if the client should faint or fall, the nurse cannot easily support the weight and lower the client to the floor. In addition, if the client falls with the nurse holding the arm, the shoulder joint may be dislocated.

A nurse who has even the slightest doubt about his or her strength and ability to ambulate a client alone should request help. The two-nurse method helps to distribute the client's weight evenly. The two nurses stand on either side of the client. Each nurse's near arm is around the client's waist, and the other arm is around the inferior aspect of the client's arm so that both nurses' hands are supporting the client's axillae.

A second method requires that the nurses and client be of similar height. The nurses stand by either side of the client with their near arms slipped under the client's arms toward the back. The nurses then grasp each other's arms. The client's arms are placed over the nurses' shoulders, and the nurses stabilize the client's hands with their free hands. This technique is very effective with weakened or heavy clients.

ASSISTIVE DEVICES FOR WALKING. Walkers are extremely light, movable devices, about waist high and made of metal tubing (Figure 22-8). They have four widely placed, sturdy legs. The client holds the handgrips on the upper bars, takes a step, moves the walker forward, and takes another step.

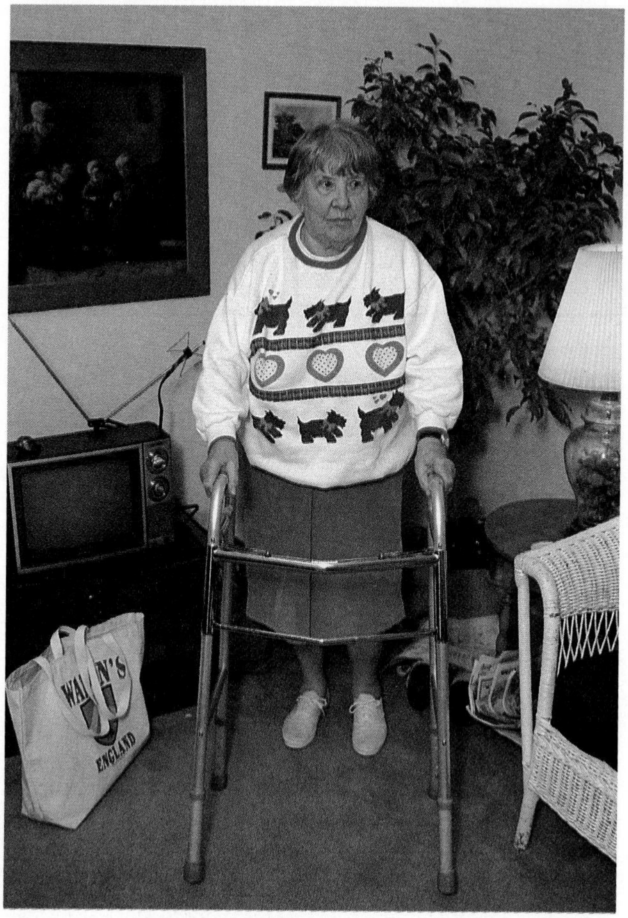

FIGURE 22-8 Client using a walker.

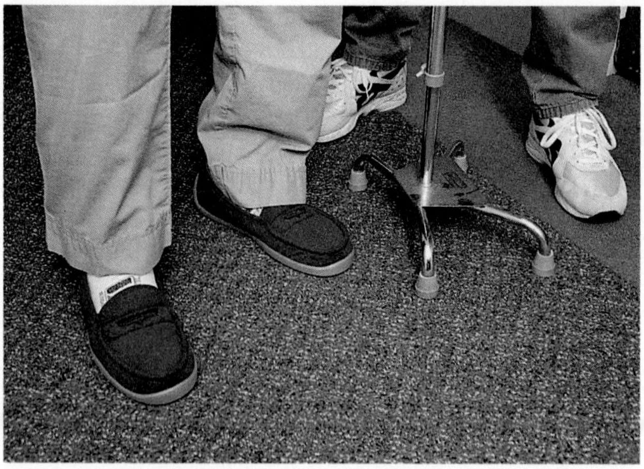

FIGURE 22-9 Quad cane.

Canes are lightweight, easily movable devices about waist high, made of wood or metal. Two common types of canes are the single straight-legged cane and the quad cane. The single straight-legged cane is more common and is used to support and balance a client with decreased leg strength. This cane should be kept on the stronger side of the body. For maximum support when walking, the client places the cane forward 15 to 25 cm (6 to 10 inches), keeping body weight on both legs. The weaker leg is moved forward to the cane so that body weight is divided between the cane and the stronger leg. The stronger leg is then advanced past the cane so the weaker leg and the body weight are supported by the cane and weaker leg. During walking, the client continually repeats these three steps. The client must be taught that two points of support, such as both feet or one foot and the cane, are present at all times.

The quad cane provides the most support and is used when there is partial or complete leg paralysis or some hemiplegia (Figure 22-9). The same three steps used with the straight-legged cane are taught to the client.

Crutches are often needed to increase mobility. The use of crutches may be temporary, such as after ligament damage to the knee. However, crutches may be needed permanently by a client with paralysis of the lower extremities. A crutch is a wooden or metal staff. The two types of crutches are the double adjustable Lofstrand or forearm crutch (Figure 22-10) and the axillary wooden or metal crutch. The forearm crutch has a handgrip and a metal band that fits around the client's forearm. The metal band and the handgrip are adjusted to fit the client's height. The axillary crutch has a padded curved surface at the top, which fits under the axilla. A handgrip in the form of a crossbar is held at the level of the palms to support the body. It is important that crutches be measured for the appropriate length and that clients be taught to use their crutches safely, to achieve a stable gait, to ascend and descend stairs, and to rise from a sitting position.

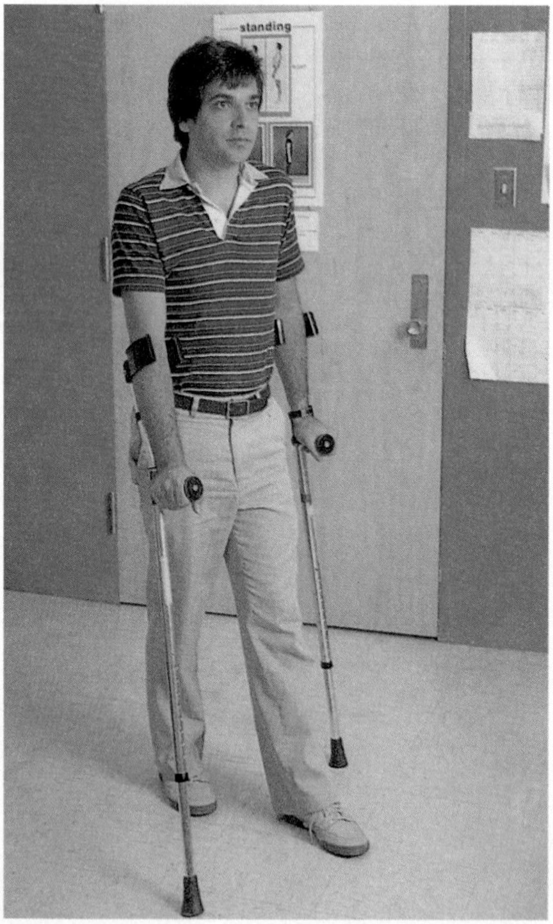

FIGURE 22-10 Double adjustable Lofstrand or forearm crutch.

MEASURING FOR CRUTCHES. The axillary crutch is the more common crutch used. Measurements include the client's height, the angle of elbow flexion, and the distance between the crutch pad and the axilla. When crutches are fitted, the length of the crutch should be from three to four finger widths from the axilla to a point 15 cm (6 inches) lateral to the client's heel (Sine et al., 1981) (Figure 22-11).

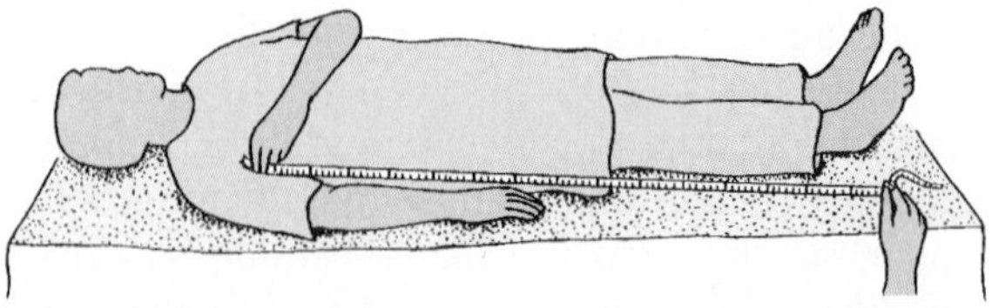

FIGURE 22-11 Measuring crutch length.

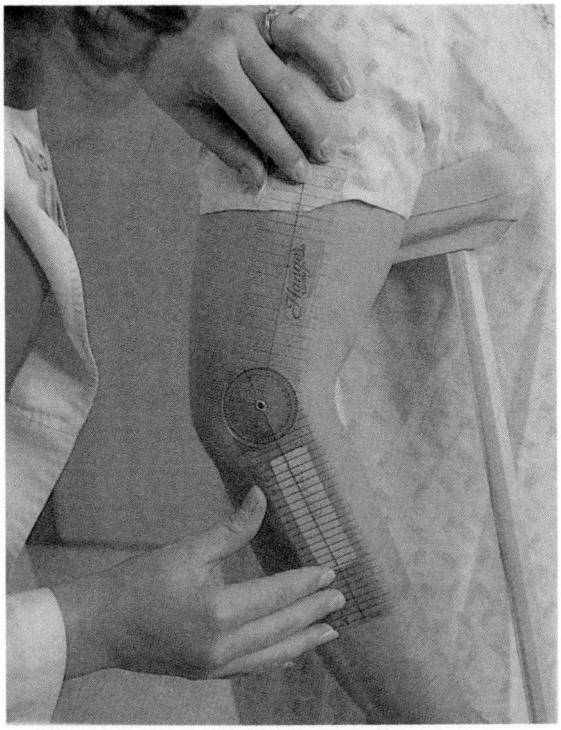

FIGURE 22-12 Verifying correct elbow flexion with crutches. Measurement obtained with goniometer.

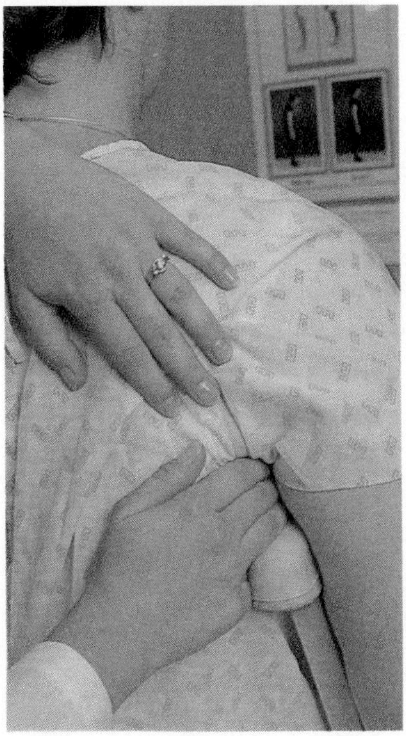

FIGURE 22-13 Verifying correct distance between crutch pads and axilla.

The handgrips should be positioned so the client's body weight is not supported by the axillae. Pressure on the axillae increases risk to underlying nerves, which could result in partial paralysis of the arm. Correct position of the handgrips is determined with the client upright, supporting weight by the handgrips with the elbows slightly flexed (20 to 25 degrees). Elbow flexion is verified with a goniometer (Figure 22-12). When the height and placement of the handgrips have been determined, the nurse should again verify that the distance between the crutch pad and the client's axilla is three to four finger widths (Figure 22-13).

Crutch safety. Before being allowed to walk independently with crutches, the client should be taught the following safety guidelines:

1. Clients with axillary crutches must be aware of the dangers of pressure on the axilla. Therefore they must not use crutches that fit improperly or lean on their crutches to support body weight.
2. Crutch-dependent clients should be taught to inspect the crutch tips routinely. The rubber tips should be securely attached to the crutches. When the tips are worn, they should be replaced immediately. Rubber crutch tips increase surface friction and prevent the crutches from slipping.
3. Crutch tips should remain dry. If the tips become wet, the client should dry them. Water decreases surface friction and increases the risk that the crutches will slip.
4. The structure of the crutches should also be routinely inspected. Cracks in a wooden crutch decrease the crutch's ability to support weight. Bends in aluminum crutches can alter body alignment, increasing the risk of further damage to the musculoskeletal system.
5. Clients should be given a list of medical suppliers in their community. This allows the clients to ob-

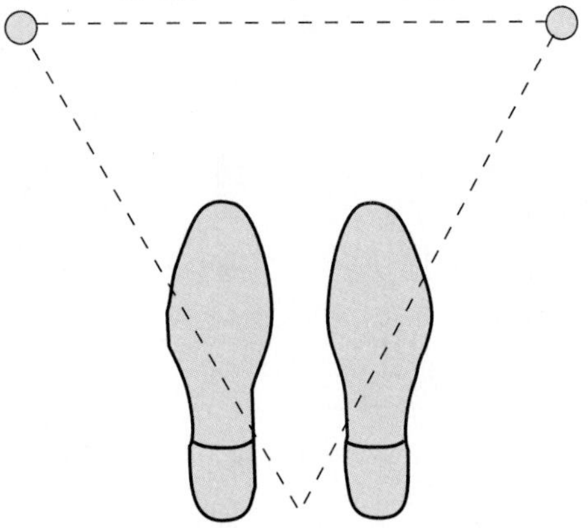

FIGURE 22-14 Tripod position, basic crutch stance.

tain repairs, new rubber tips, handgrips, and crutch pads.

6. Crutch-dependent clients should always have spare crutches and tips on hand.

Crutch gait. The **crutch gait** is assumed by alternately bearing weight on one or both legs and on the crutches. The gait selected by the physician is determined by assessing the client's physical and functional abilities and the disease or injury that resulted in the need for crutches. This section summarizes the basic crutch stance and the four standard gaits: four-point alternating gait, three-point alternating gait, two-point gait, and swing-through gait.

The basic crutch stance is the *tripod position*, formed when the crutches are placed 15 cm (6 inches) in front of and 15 cm to the side of each foot (Figure 22-14). This position improves the client's balance by providing a wider base of support. The body alignment of the client in the tripod position includes erect head and neck, straight vertebrae, and extended hips and knees. No weight should be borne by the axillae. The tripod position is used before crutch walking.

Four-point alternating or *four-point gait* gives stability to the client but requires weight bearing on both legs. Each leg is moved alternately with each opposing crutch so that three points of support are on the floor at all times (Figure 22-15).

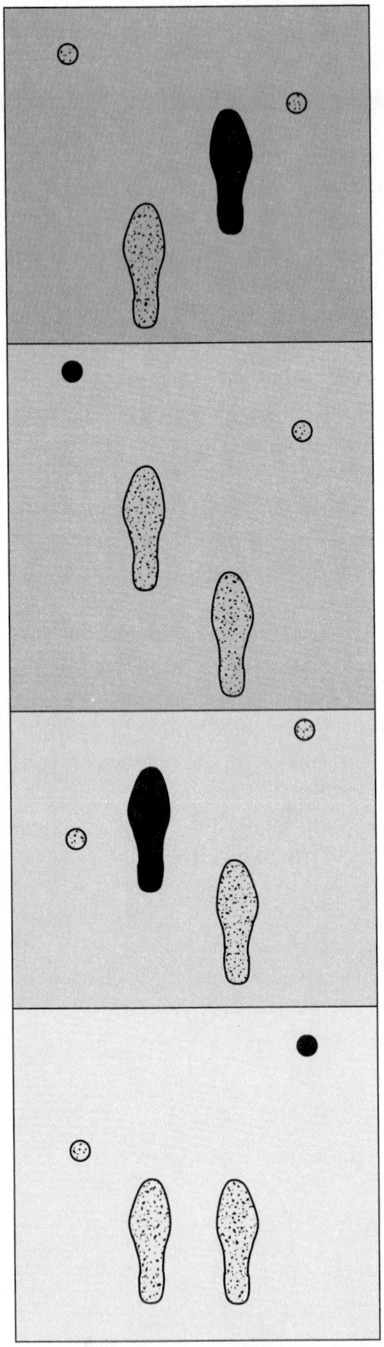

FIGURE 22-15 Four-point alternating gait. Solid feet and crutch tips show foot and crutch tip moved in each of the four phases.

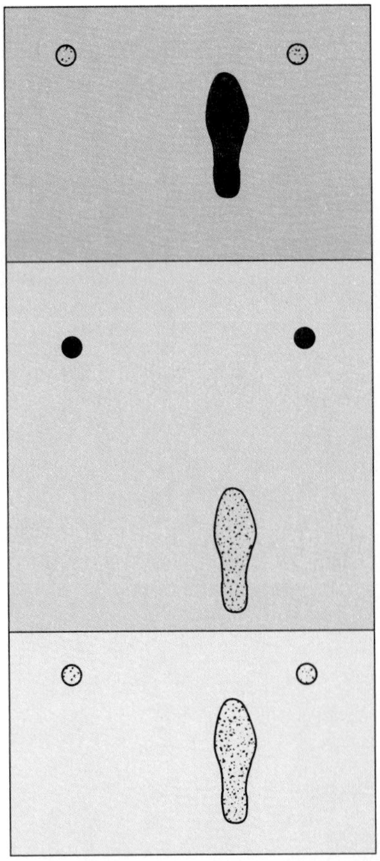

FIGURE 22-16 Three-point gait with weight borne on unaffected leg. Solid foot and crutch tips show weight-bearing in each phase.

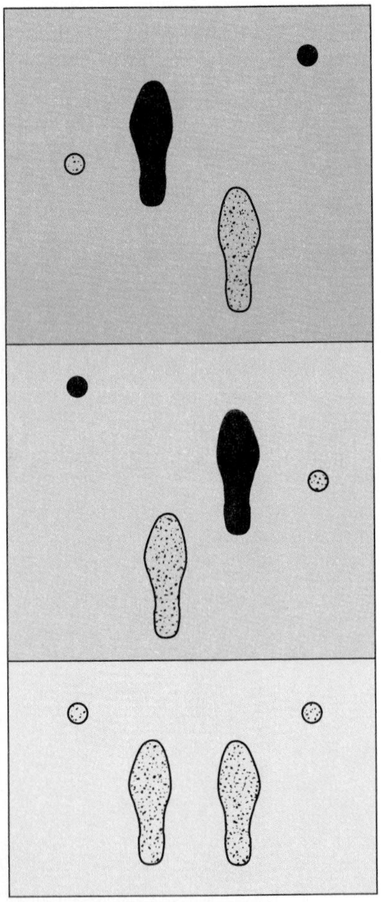

FIGURE 22-17 Two-point gait, with weight borne partially on each foot and each crutch advancing with opposing leg. Solid areas indicate leg and crutch tips bearing weight.

Three-point alternating or *three-point gait* requires the client to bear all of the weight on one foot. In a three-point gait, weight is borne on both crutches and then on the uninvolved leg, and the sequence is repeated (Figure 22-16). The affected leg does not touch the ground during the early phase of the three-point gait. Gradually the client progresses to touchdown and full weight bearing on the affected leg.

The *two-point gait* requires at least partial weight bearing on each foot (Figure 22-17). The client moves a crutch at the same time as the opposing leg, so the crutch movements are similar to arm motion during normal walking.

The *swing-through* or *swing-through gait* is frequently used by paraplegics who wear weight-supporting braces on their legs. With weight placed on the supported legs, the client places the crutches one stride in front and then swings to or through the crutches while they support the client's weight.

Crutch walking on stairs. When ascending stairs on crutches, the client usually uses a modified three-point gait (Figure 22-18). The client stands at the bottom of the stairs and transfers body weight to the crutches. The unaffected leg is advanced between the crutches to the stairs. The client then shifts weight from the crutches to the unaffected leg. Finally, the client aligns both crutches on the stairs. This sequence is repeated until the client reaches the top of the stairs.

To descend the stairs (Figure 22-19), a three-phase sequence is also used. The client transfers body weight to the unaffected leg. The crutches are placed on the stair, and the client begins to transfer body weight to the crutches, moving the affected leg forward. Finally, the unaffected leg is moved to the stairs with the crutches. Again, the client repeats the sequence until reaching the bottom of the stairs.

Because in most cases clients will need to use crutches for some time, they should be adequately taught to use crutches on stairs before discharge. This instruction applies to all crutch-dependent clients, not only those who have stairs in their homes.

Sitting in a chair with crutches. As with crutch walking and crutch walking up and down stairs, the procedure for sitting in a chair involves phases and requires the client to transfer weight (Figure 22-20). First, the client gets positioned at the center front of the chair with the posterior aspect of the legs touching the chair. Then the client holds both crutches in the hand opposite the affected leg. If both legs are affected, as with a paraplegic who wears weight-supporting braces, the crutches are held in the hand on the client's stronger side. With both crutches in one hand, the client supports body weight on the unaffected leg and crutches. While still holding the crutches, the client grasps the arm of the chair with the remaining hand and lowers the body into the chair. To stand, the procedure is reversed, and the client, when fully erect, should assume the tripod position before beginning to walk.

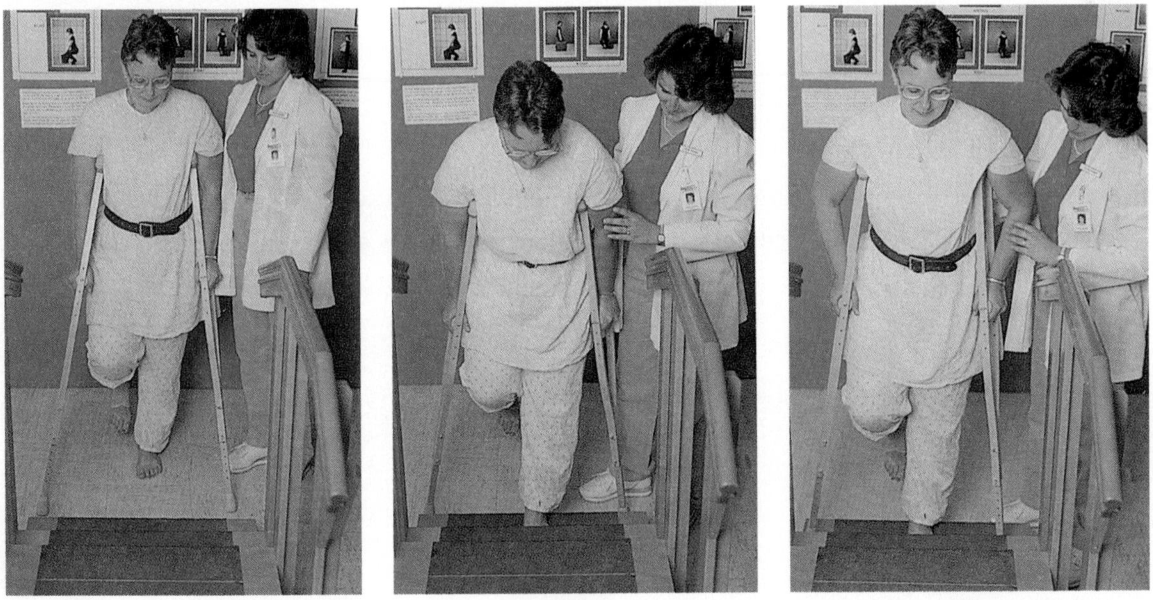

A B C

FIGURE 22-18 Ascending stairs. **A,** Weight is placed on crutches. **B,** Weight is transferred from crutches to unaffected leg on stairs. **C,** Crutches are aligned with unaffected leg on stairs.

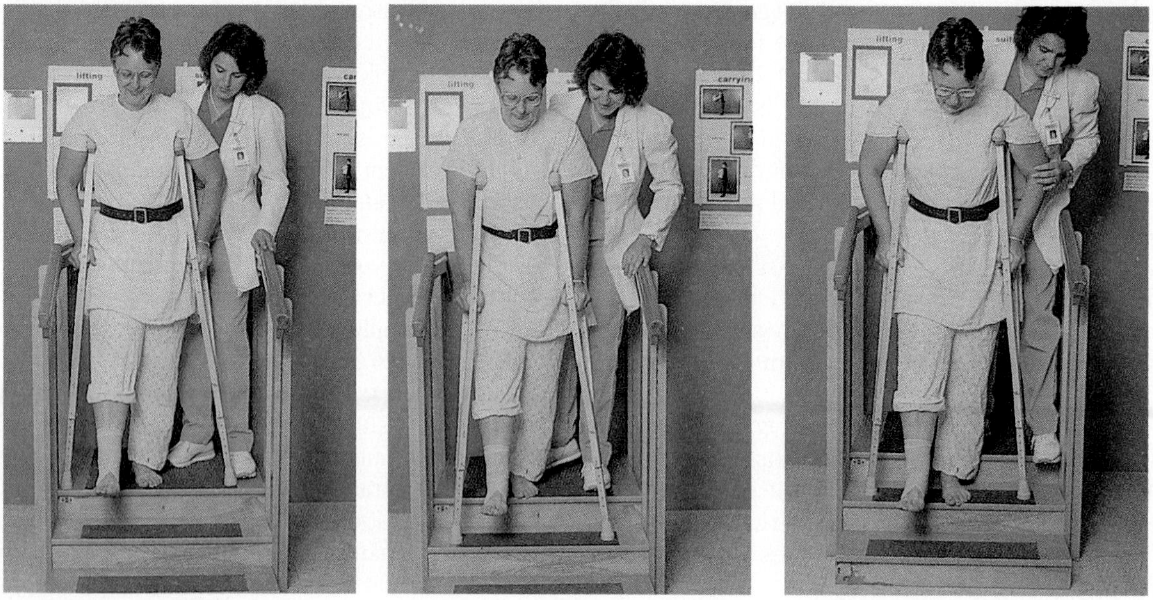

A B C

FIGURE 22-19 Descending stairs. **A,** Body weight on unaffected leg. **B,** Body weight transferred to crutches. **C,** Unaffected leg aligned on stairs with crutches.

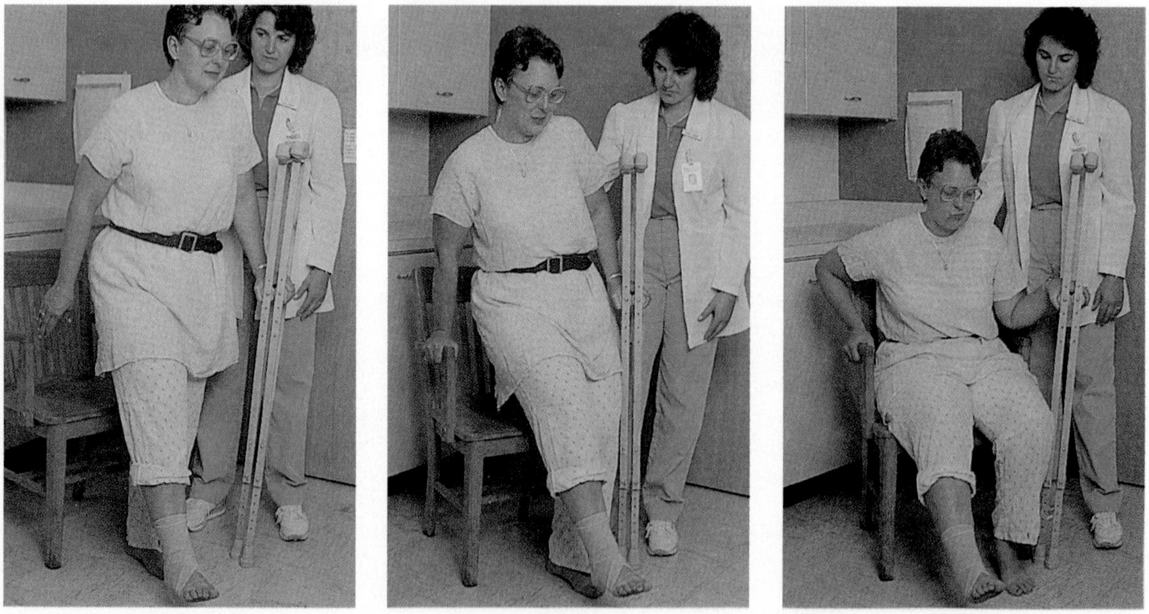

A B C

FIGURE 22-20 Sitting in a chair. **A,** Both crutches are held by one hand. Client transfers weight to crutches and unaffected leg. **B,** Client grasps arm of chair with free hand and begins to lower herself into chair. **C,** Client completely lowers herself into chair.

Evaluation

Evaluation of nursing care for clients with improper body alignment or impaired mobility is based on objective outcome criteria established for each nursing goal.

Goal: Client remains free of musculoskeletal disorders.

Outcome
Proper body alignment is maintained
Evaluative measures
Observe the client for proper body position while client is lying down, sitting, or standing
Observe the client in a lying-down, sitting, or standing position for signs of fatigue or discomfort

Outcome
Contractures are prevented
Evaluative measure
Inspect the musculoskeletal system for joint contractures

Outcome
All joints are movable
Evaluative measures
Palpate appropriate joints during range of motion activities
Measure range of joint motion

Goal: Client performs independent locomotion activities or assistive devices, as appropriate.

Outcome
Client ambulates twice daily
Evaluative measure
Observe ambulation

Outcome
Transfers to and from chair
Evaluative measure
Observe transfer to and from chair

Goal: Client increases activity tolerance.

Outcome
Verbalizes less fatigue
Evaluative measure
Ask client to rate fatigue on a scale of 1-10

Outcome
Increases participation in self-care activities
Evaluative measures
Ask client about the number of activities involved in
Following activity, observe client and obtain vital signs

Goal: Client remains free of bodily injury.

Outcome
Identifies factors that increase the potential for injury.
Evaluative measures
Inspect skin for pressure points
Inspect skin for impaired skin integrity
Inspect musculoskeletal system for joint contractures
Palpate integument for tenderness and inadequate muscle tone

SUMMARY

The nurse incorporates knowledge of the physiology of movement and the principles of body mechanics to transfer and position clients safely and to assist clients to use walkers and crutches safely. Using the nursing process, the nurse develops a nursing care plan for clients with potential or actual alterations in body alignment.

Correct body mechanics protects the nurse and client from injuries to the musculoskeletal system. For example, by using the principles of body mechanics, the nurse can transfer a client from bed to chair without self-injury or injury to the client.

CRITICAL THINKING ACTIVITIES

1. Mr. Kauffman, 69, is being released from the hospital today. He is going home with his daughter who will be caring for him. He will be confined to bed. List and discuss the guidelines you will give to Mr. Kauffman's daughter concerning body mechanics.
2. Identify the appropriate placement of equipment, positioning of the client, and movement of the nurse in the following situations:
   a. You are helping a client walk to the bathroom, when the client states he or she feels faint and starts to fall to the floor.
   b. You are moving a heavy client from a stretcher to the bed.
   c. You are giving an intramuscular injection into the left dorsogluteal muscle of a client in bed.
3. Your assigned client has a trapeze, trochanter rolls, a footboard, and side rails. Explain the rationale for each of these devices in maintaining proper body alignment.
4. Before your client with a full-leg cast can go home, he or she must be taught to ambulate with crutches and a three-point gait. Develop a teaching plan for your client.

KEY CONCEPTS

The term **body mechanics** describes the coordinated efforts of the musculoskeletal and nervous systems as the person moves, lifts, bends, assumes a standing, sitting, or lying position, and completes activities of daily living.

Coordinated body movement requires the integrated functioning of the skeletal system, skeletal muscles, and nervous system.

Muscles primarily associated with movement are located near the skeletal region, where movement results from leverage, which is characteristic of the movement of the upper extremities.

Muscles primarily associated with posture are located in the lower extremities, trunk, neck, and back.

Coordination and regulation of different muscle groups depend on muscle tone and the activity of antagonistic, synergistic, and antigravity muscles.

Balance is assisted through nervous system control by the cerebellum and inner ear.

Body alignment is the positioning of joints, tendons, ligaments, and muscles in various body positions.

Body balance is achieved when there is a wide base of support, the center of gravity falls within the base of support, and a vertical line falls from the center through the base of support.

Developmental stages influence body alignment and mobility.

Pathological conditions that affect body alignment and mobility include postural abnormalities, altered bone formation, altered joint mobility, impaired muscle development, damage to the central nervous system, and direct trauma to the musculoskeletal system.

Assessment of a client's mobility enables the nurse to determine the client's coordination, balance, and ability to complete activities of daily living and makes it possible to evaluate or plan an exercise program.

Range of joint motion is the maximal movement possible at a joint in one of the three planes of the body: sagittal, frontal, and transverse.

Assessing gait allows the nurse to draw some conclusions about the client's balance, posture, and ability to walk without assistance.

When lifting or transferring a client, the nurse considers the four basic principles of lifting: position of weight, height of object, body position, and maximal weight.

Clients with impaired body alignment require nursing interventions to maintain them in the supported Fowler's, supine, prone, side-lying, and Sims' positions.

Transfer techniques require the nurse to use correct body mechanics to move the client in bed, from bed to chair, and from bed to stretcher.

Mechanical devices to promote walking include canes and walkers, which require specific nursing interventions.

References

Carnevali DL, Patrick: *Nursing management for the elderly,* ed 3, Philadelphia, 1993, JB Lippincott.

Carpenito LJ: *Nursing diagnosis: application to clinical practice,* ed 5, Philadelphia, 1993, Lippincott.

Gordon M: Assessing activity tolerance, *Am J Nurs* 76:72, 1976.

Gröer MW and Shekleton ME: *Basic pathophysiology: a conceptual approach,* ed 3, St. Louis, 1989, Mosby.

Holm K: Immobility and bone loss in the aging adult, *Crit Care Nurs Q* 12(1):46, 1989.

Holm K, Walker J: Osteoporosis: treatment and prevention update, *Geriatric Nurs* 11(3), 140-142, 1990.

Jensen RC: Disabling back injuries among nursing personnel: research needs and justification, *Res Nurs Health* 10(1):29, 1987.

Lehmkuhl LD, et al.: Multidimensional treatment of joint contractures in patients with severe brain injury, *J Head Trauma Rehabil* 5(4):23, 1990.

Marchette L: Back injury: a preventable occupational hazard, *Orthop Nurse* 4(6):25, 1985.

McAbee RR: Nurses and back injuries: a literature review, *AAOHN J* 36(5):211, 1988.

McCance KL and Huether SE: *Pathophysiology: the biologic basis for disease in adults and children,* St. Louis, 1990, Mosby.

McConnell E: Placing your patient in the lateral position, *Nursing* 20(7):65, 1990.

Owen BD, Garg A: Back stress isn't part of the job, *AJN* 93(2):48-51, 1993.

Owen BD, Garg A: Reducing risks for back pain in nursing personnel, *AAOHN J* 39(1):24, 1991.

Owen BD: How to avoid that aching back, *Am J Nurs* 80:984, 1980.

Sine RD, et al.: *Basic rehabilitation techniques: a self-instructional guide,* ed 2, Rockville, Md., 1981, Aspen Publishers.

Stamps JL: "Back" to basics, *Emer Med Service* 18(2):38, 1989.

Bibliography

Aaronson L, Carlon-Wolf W, Schoener S: Pressures that fall on rising, *Geriatric Nurs* 12(12):67, 1990.

Eustace C: Back up and wait, *RN* 54(6):49-51, 1991.

Heeschen S: Getting a handle on patient mobility, *Geriatric Nurs* 10(3): 146-147, 1989.

Hogstel MO: *Clinical manual of gerontological nursing,* St. Louis, 1992, Mosby.

Lane PL, LeBlanc R: Crutch walking, *Orthopedic Nurs* 9(5):31, 1990.

Milde F: Impaired physical mobility, *J Gerontol Nurs* 14(3):20-24, 1988.

Mobily P, Kelly L: Iatrogenesis in the elderly: factors of immobility, *J Gerontol Nurs* 17(9):5-11, 1991.

Rogers-Seidl FF: *Geriatric nursing care plans,* St. Louis, 1992, Mosby.

23 Immobility

OBJECTIVES

Mastery of content in this chapter will enable the student to:

- Define the key terms listed.
- Describe mobility and immobility.
- Discuss the benefits and hazards of bed rest.
- Identify changes in metabolic rate associated with immobility.
- Describe physical changes associated with immobility.
- Describe musculoskeletal changes associated with immobility.
- Discuss factors that contribute to pressure ulcer formation.
- Describe psychosocial and developmental effects of immobilization.
- Complete a nursing assessment of an immobilized client.
- Develop a nursing care plan for an immobilized client.
- List appropriate nursing interventions for an immobilized client.
- State evaluation criteria for the immobilized client.

KEY TERMS

anthropometric
bed rest
bone resorption
chest physiotherapy
debridement
disuse osteoporosis
eschar
immobility
ischemia
isometric
joint contracture
mobility
negative nitrogen balance
orthostatic hypotension
pressure ulcer
renal calculi
sloughing
thrombosis
thrombus
Valsalva maneuver

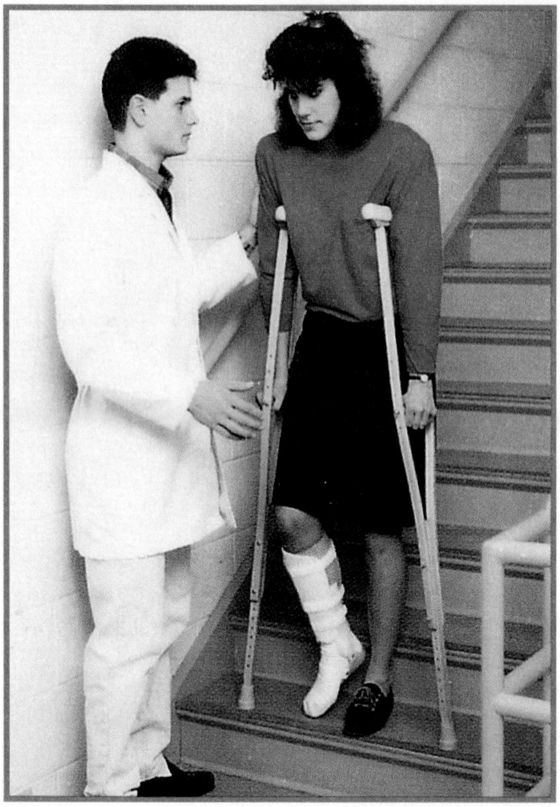

Mobility serves many purposes including expressing emotion, self-defense, attaining basic needs, completing activities of daily living, and performing recreational activities. In addition, mobility assists in maintaining the body's normal physiological activities. To maintain normal physical mobility, the nervous, muscular, and skeletal systems of the body must be intact and functioning (see Chapter 22).

When a body part or the entire body is immobilized for a time, secondary disabilities may develop in one or more body systems (Rubin, 1988b; Reddy, 1986; Holm, 1989). Factors that contribute to the amount of disability include the degree of immobility, the length of immobilization, and the severity of the illness.

Changes in the client's mobility may result from many types of health problems. Clients with certain illnesses or injuries become immobilized but return to mobility with rehabilitation. Other clients may experience a sudden or gradual shift from mobility to long-term or permanent immobility. Some clients are immobilized for therapeutic reasons; their ambulation may be restricted or they may be placed on bed rest.

MOBILITY AND IMMOBILITY

Mobility is a person's ability to move about freely. It is often essential to the client's perception of health (Oullett, 1992; Rubin, 1988a; Tompkins, 1980). Hogue (1985) views mobility as a result of the interaction between the physical and psychosocial aspects of the client and the resources in the environment. The aspects of the individual include motor skills, biological and psychological health, and sensory-perceptual capacity. The resources in the environment may include medical treatment, social support, physical barriers, and institutional policy and staffing patterns, if the client is in an institution. Complete, unrestricted mobility requires voluntary motor and complete sensory control of all body regions. It also requires an environment that enables movement. Nurses in most health care settings see clients at any point on the mobility-immobility continuum.

Clients with complete mobility may achieve needs and goals independently or with minimal guidance from the nurse. Often clients who are freely mobile require little help with self-care but may need the nurse's teaching and counseling skills to learn more about exercise or how to balance activity and rest.

Clients who are partially mobile usually have a motor or sensory impairment in a region of the body or a therapeutic restriction (e.g., a casted extremity). A partial loss of mobility may be temporary (e.g., the result of a fracture) or permanent (e.g., the result of paralysis). In some cases the restriction of mobility benefits the client's recovery, as with a casted extremity.

The hazards associated with partial mobility depend on the degree and duration of immobilization (Oullet, 1992; Rubin, 1988b) and the client's previous condition. The resulting hazards are usually temporary and resolve shortly after complete mobility is restored. Generally, clients who are relatively healthy before immobilization are more likely to have complete mobility restored.

The client with complete mobility restrictions is continually at risk for the hazards of immobilization. In a classic study, Deitrick et al. (1948) found that even young healthy men put on bed rest had physiological problems. Nursing care and education are directed toward minimizing these hazards because it is generally easier to prevent the complications than to treat or cure them (Reddy, 1986).

Immobility may be the result of either physical inactivity or physical restriction of movement. Physical inactivity such as bed rest causes a reduction in body movement. Physical inactivity may occur as a response to severe pain or as a result of sensory changes reducing the physical stimulus to move. It may also be a result of cognitive-emotional changes such as depression, or as a result of a treatment such as prescribed bed rest. Physical restriction or limitation of movement, such as by cast, traction, or restraints, results in an imposed reduction of movement. Both inactivity and restricted movement may cause changes in body position and posture that result in a loss of the body's ability to adapt to such changes. The degree of the client's immobility depends on the interaction of the conditions present (Gröer and Shekleton, 1989).

BED REST

Bed rest is an intervention in which the client is restricted to bed for therapeutic reasons. Bed rest has different meanings among nurses, physicians, and other health care professionals. The general objectives of bed rest include the following:

1. Reducing physical activity and the oxygen needs of the body
2. Allowing ill or debilitated clients to rest and regain strength
3. Preventing further injury to traumatized structures (e.g., spinal and vertebral injury)

Bed rest has physiological and psychological benefits only if the client finds it restful and if the client can freely move and change positions. Clients resistant to bed rest may actually expend more energy in fighting it than they would if allowed to move from bed to chair (Greenleaf, 1984).

Clients with a wide variety of conditions are placed on bed rest. The box below lists conditions often requiring bed rest. The list is not all inclusive and does not apply to all clients with these conditions. The duration of bed rest depends on the illness or injury and the client's prior state of health.

CONDITIONS REQUIRING BED REST

CARDIOVASCULAR CONDITIONS

Acute myocardial infarction
Congestive heart failure
Cardiomyopathies
Inflammation of myocardial tissues

NEUROLOGICAL CONDITIONS

Head injuries
Spinal cord trauma
Degenerative neurological conditions
Inflammatory diseases of the nervous system (e.g., Guillain-Barré syndrome)
Bleeding aneurysms

MUSCULOSKELETAL CONDITIONS

Multiple fractures of the lower extremities
Surgical reattachment of a traumatically amputated extremity

PULMONARY CONDITIONS

End-stage chronic lung diseases

OTHER CONDITIONS

Terminal phases of cancer
Clients awaiting major organ transplants
Morbid obesity

IMMOBILITY

Immobility occurs when a client is unable to independently move or change positions. The effects of immobility are systemic and functional. No body system is immune to the effects of immobility. Research has shown that healthy people exposed to periods of immobility or prolonged bed rest suffer physiological and psychological effects (Deitrick et al., 1948; Greenleaf, 1984; Ouullet, 1992).

These effects can be gradual or immediate. The greater the extent and the longer the duration of immobility, the more pronounced the consequences. The box on p. 560 lists the effects of immobilization in all dimensions.

Physiological Effects

Each body system is at risk for impairments resulting from immobility. The severity of the impairment depends on the client's age, overall health, and the degree of immobility. Frail older adult clients with chronic illnesses develop pronounced effects of immobility more quickly than younger clients (Reddy, 1986; Harper and Lyles, 1988). For an older adult client who has had a stroke, immobility-related problems can occur within a few days (Coletta and Murphy, 1992).

Metabolic Changes

Immobility disrupts normal metabolic functioning, including problems with the metabolic rate and the metabolism of carbohydrates, fats, and proteins. It can also cause fluid and electrolyte imbalances, problems with bone metabolism, and gastrointestinal disturbances.

Metabolic Rate. Decreased mobility results in a decrease in the basal metabolic rate (BMR). The client's BMR falls in response to the decreased energy requirement of body cells, which is directly related to cellular oxygen demands (Greenleaf, 1984; Gröer and Shekleton, 1989). However, fever or wound healing may increase the BMR because these conditions increase cellular oxygen requirements (McCance and Heuther, 1994).

EFFECTS OF IMMOBILITY IN ALL DIMENSIONS

PHYSIOLOGICAL EFFECTS

Metabolic system

Decreased basal metabolic rate (BMR)
Altered carbohydrate, fat, and protein metabolism
Fluid and electrolyte imbalances
Increased bone resorption
Gastrointestinal disturbances

Respiratory system

Decreased hemoglobin levels
Reduced lung expansion
Respiratory muscle weakness
Stasis of secretions

Cardiovascular system

Orthostatic hypotension
Increased cardiac workload
Thrombus formation

Musculoskeletal system

Loss of endurance
Decreased muscle mass
Atrophy
Decreased stability
Joint contractures
Disuse osteoporosis

Integument

Pressure ulcer formation

Urinary system

Renal calculi
Decreased urinary output
Urinary stasis
Urinary tract infection

PSYCHOSOCIAL EFFECTS

Depression
Behavioral changes
Altered sleep-wake cycles
Decreased coping abilities
Increased isolation
Sensory deprivation

DEVELOPMENTAL EFFECTS

Decreased progression through developmental tasks
Increased dependence

Data from Rubin M: The physiology of bedrest, *Am J Nurs* 88:53, 1988b; and Greenleaf SE: Physiological responses to prolonged bedrest and fluid immersion in humans, *J Appl Physiol* 57(3):619, 1984.

Metabolism of Carbohydrates, Fats, and Proteins. As bed rest continues, pancreatic activity decreases, as does the body's ability to tolerate glucose. Insulin production is not enough to lower serum glucose levels. These effects can be seen in as little as 3 days but can reverse 7 days after resuming activity (Rubin, 1988b).

As proteins are metabolized, nitrogen is produced as an end product. Nitrogen balance provides a reliable indicator of protein use by the body. A **negative nitrogen balance** exists when the excretion of nitrogen from the breakdown of protein exceeds intake (Gröer and Shekleton, 1989). During periods of immobility, urinary excretion of nitrogen rises, increasing the risk of a negative nitrogen balance. The urinary excretion of nitrogen increases about day 5 or 6 of immobilization (Gröer and Shekleton, 1989).

Decreased mobility results in changes in fat stores. The percentage of body fat increases because of the loss of lean body mass (Greenleaf, 1984).

Fluid and Electrolyte Imbalances. Because the client is in a recumbent position, major shifts in blood volume occur. An immediate diuretic response occurs during the first day of bed rest, and the client loses an additional average of 600 ml per day (Greenleaf, 1984). Urinary excretion of calcium, chloride, and sodium also increases (Greenleaf, 1984).

Bone Metabolism. The classic research on healthy, immobilized young men by Deitrick et al. (1948) demonstrated an increased excretion of calcium in the urine during bed rest. Later research showed the probable source of this calcium is bone resorption. Normally the kidneys are able to excrete excess calcium. However, if the kidneys are unable to respond appropriately, hypercalcemia results (Holm, 1989). Because of the hypercalcemia, an increase in fecal and renal excretion of calcium also occurs.

Gastrointestinal Changes. Although impairments in gastrointestinal functioning vary in clients, the symptoms are related to decreased motility. Constipation is common. Diarrhea, when it occurs, is frequently the result of a fecal impaction (Figure 23-1). The nurse must be aware this is not normal diarrhea but rather liquid stool passing around the area of impaction. Left untreated, this impaction can result in a mechanical bowel obstruction that may partially or completely occlude the intestinal lumen, blocking normal propulsion of liquid

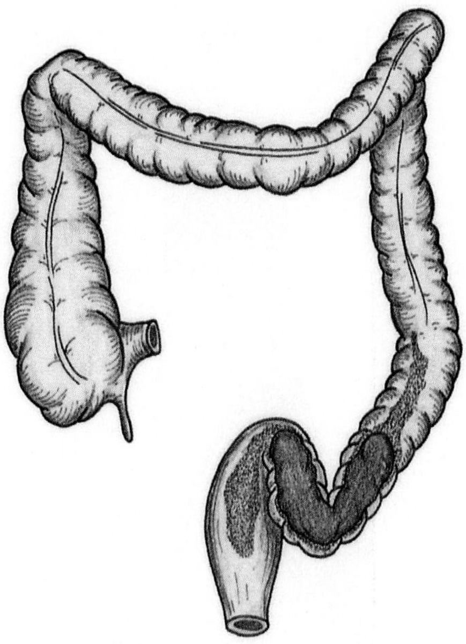

FIGURE 23-1 Fecal impaction with liquid stool passing around impaction.

and gas. The resulting fluid stasis in the intestine produces distention and increases intraluminal pressure. Finally, intestinal function becomes depressed, dehydration occurs, and absorption ceases. Thus fluid and electrolyte disturbances worsen.

Respiratory Changes

When a client assumes a recumbent position, the lungs shift position a full 90 degrees. Shifts in lung position and body fluids, along with the pressure of the abdominal contents pushing against the diaphragm, cause a change in lung volume (Rubin, 1988b). Respiratory problems occurring with immobility are caused by decreased hemoglobin, decreased lung expansion, generalized muscle weakness, and stasis of secretions.

Because of the diuretic response to bed rest, hypovolemia may result, causing transient elevations in hematocrit values on or about the eighth day of immobilization. Red blood cell mass and hemoglobin levels decline (Greenleaf, 1984). Hemoglobin transports oxygenated blood to the tissues, and when the oxygen carrying capacity is reduced, there is a reduction in oxygen delivery to the tissues. Initially the body tries to adapt by increasing the heart rate, but this is a short-term adaptive response and ultimately increases cardiac workload.

Immobilization decreases lung expansion. Changes in the client's position alter the distribution of ventilation and blood flow through the lung. As a result, the dependent lung is less effectively oxygenated. The exception to this principle occurs when the client has underlying lung disease. In addition, research has documented that all lung volumes are reduced during immobilization (Beckett et al., 1986; Convertino, et al., 1986; Sahn, 1991).

Limited physical activity and metabolic changes result in weakened and decreased respiratory muscles. Thus the work of breathing increases (Tyler, 1984), causing a proportional decline in the client's ability to cough productively. Ultimately the distribution of mucus in the bronchi increases, particularly when the client is in the supine, prone, or lateral positions (Figure 23-2). Mucus accumulates in the dependent regions of the

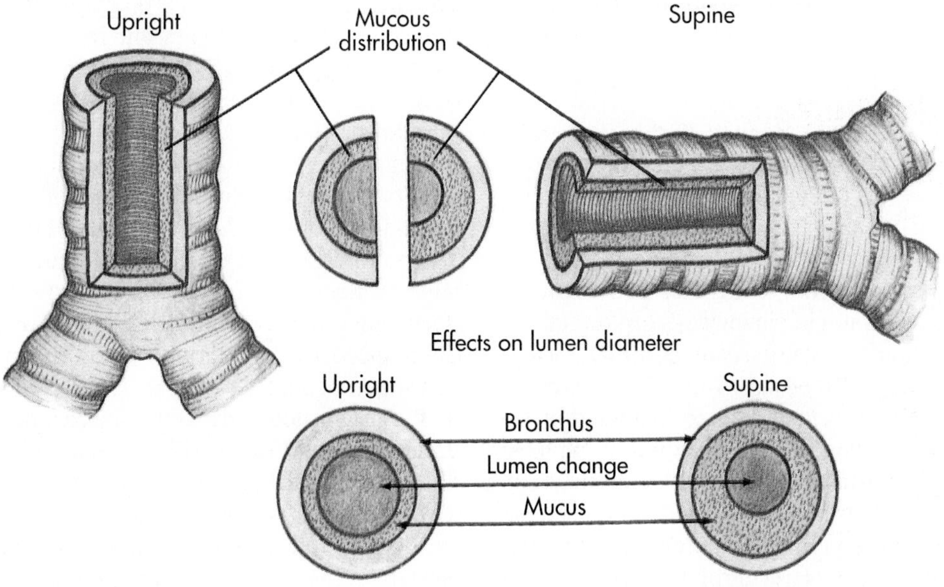

FIGURE 23-2 Effect of recumbency and gravity on distribution of respiratory tract mucus of bronchiolar lumen.

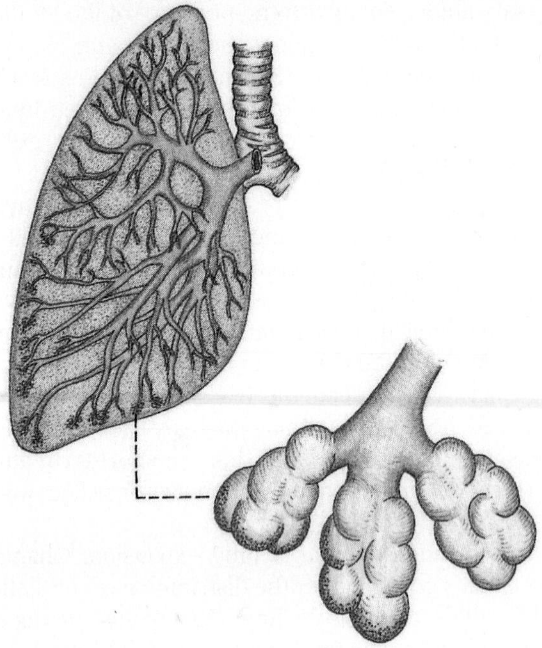

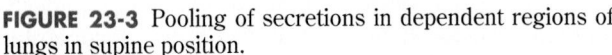

FIGURE 23-3 Pooling of secretions in dependent regions of lungs in supine position.

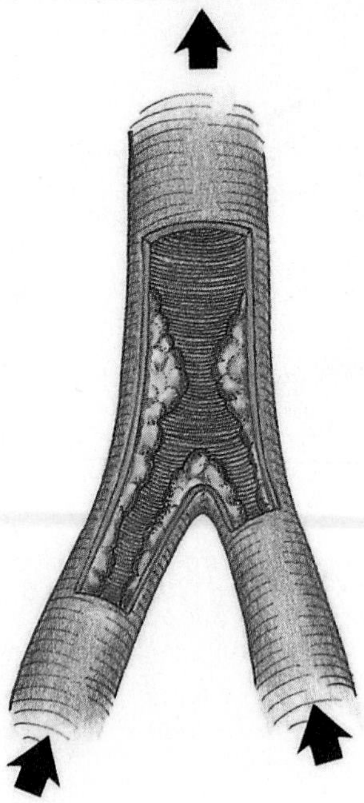

FIGURE 23-4 Thrombus formation in vessel.

bronchial tube, and because mucus is an excellent medium for bacterial growth, **hypostatic bronchopneumonia** may result.

With decreased lung expansion and weakened respiratory muscles, secretions stagnate or pool in the dependent lung regions (Figure 23-3). In addition, cilia become unable to move the secretions from the respiratory tract. Thus the potential increases for pneumonia and **atelectasis** (Mobily and Kelley, 1991). Atelectasis is a collapse of the alveoli that prevents the normal exchange of oxygen and carbon dioxide.

Cardiovascular Changes

The cardiovascular system is also affected by immobilization. The three major changes are orthostatic hypotension, increased cardiac workload, and thrombus formation.

Orthostatic hypotension occurs in the client on bed rest, but it also occurs in clients with prolonged immobility in the sitting position (Greenleaf, 1984). Orthostatic hypotension is a drop of 15 mm Hg or more in blood pressure when the client rises from a lying or sitting position to a standing position. In the immobilized client, there is decreased circulating fluid volume, pooling of blood in the lower extremities, and decreased autonomic response. These result in decreased venous return, central venous pressure, stroke volume, and a drop in systolic blood pressure when the client stands (McCance and Huether, 1994; Mobily and Kelley, 1991; Winslow, 1985).

Increased cardiac workload is demonstrated by rate changes. Prolonged bed rest increases the resting heart rate 4 to 15 beats per minute. When the immobilized client is asked to do physical activity such as with range of motion (ROM) exercises or activities of daily living, this increased rate is more pronounced (Winslow, 1985). As the workload of the heart increases, so does its oxygen consumption. The heart therefore works harder and less efficiently during prolonged rest. As immobilization increases, cardiac output falls, further decreasing cardiac efficiency and increasing the workload. In an earlier classic study, Coe (1954) noted that cardiac workload is increased almost 20% when the client is lying down.

Immobile clients are at risk for thrombus formation. A **thrombus** is an accumulation of platelets, fibrin, clotting factors, and cellular elements of the blood attached to the interior wall of a vein or artery, sometimes occluding the lumen of the vessel (Figure 23-4). Thrombi form for many reasons. Because of hypovolemia, the hematocrit level is increased, and the circulating blood is more viscous (Greenleaf, 1984). After 8 days of bed rest, more procoagulants are found, and thromboplastin time shortens (Rubin, 1988b). In addition, the weight of the legs on the bed compresses the blood vessels of the calves, causing stasis and injury to vessel linings (Gröer and Shekleton, 1989). Another problem in the venous system is the loss of the pumping action of the skeletal muscles. Normally, muscles aid venous return by squeezing blood through the legs back to the heart.

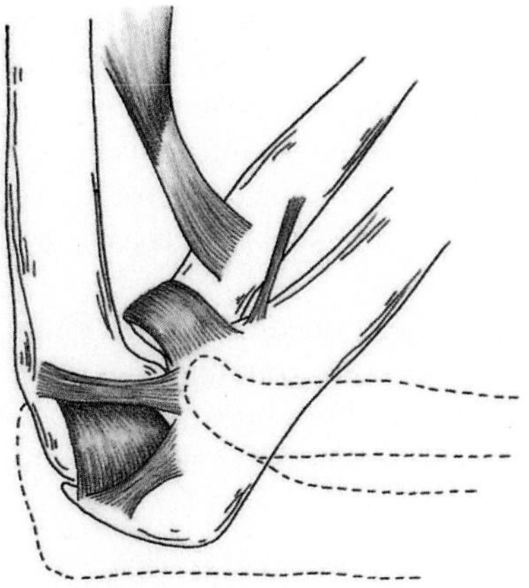

FIGURE 23-5 Flexion contracture of elbow resulting in permanent flexion of joint. Normally, elbow is able to extend to 90-degree angle *(dotted line)* and to 180-degree angle *(not shown)*.

However, this mechanism is reduced when the client is on bed rest or has a cast on a leg.

Venous thrombi put the client at risk for **pulmonary emboli,** a life-threatening complication. Pulmonary emboli are clots that have moved in the venous system and block a portion of the pulmonary artery system and thus disrupt blood flow to the lungs. Immobilized surgical and older adult clients are at high risk for developing pulmonary emboli.

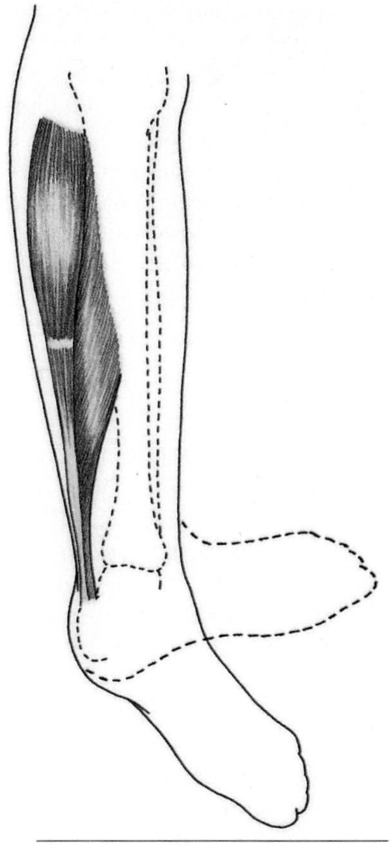

FIGURE 23-6 Footdrop. Ankle is fixed in plantar flexion.

Musculoskeletal Changes

The effects of immobility on the musculoskeletal system can include permanent impairment of mobility. Restricted mobility affects the client's muscles by loss of strength and endurance, decreased muscle mass, and decreased stability.

Muscle strength is lost when muscles are inactive. The rate of loss will vary with the degree of immobility but may be as high as 5% per day (Muller, 1970). These effects can be devastating to clients who are marginally functioning at home in the tasks of daily living. Hoenig and Rubenstein (1991) note that a 10% loss in function in some older adult clients may mean the loss of independence in their activities of daily living.

Reduced endurance results from changes in muscle strength and altered cardiovascular functioning. Because of the increased cardiac workload, muscle endurance is decreased due to the reduced ability of the cardiopulmonary system to meet the oxygen needs of the tissue (Winslow, 1985). In addition, because of the metabolic changes, the client loses lean body mass, which is composed partially of muscle. Therefore the reduced muscle mass is unable to sustain activity without fatigue.

Muscle mass decreases from metabolic causes and disuse. As immobility continues and the muscles are not exercised, muscle mass continues to decrease. Muscle atrophy resulting from immobility can be observed and measured. The muscle atrophies, and the size of the muscle decreases (Booth, 1982). The extensor muscles in the legs appear to be the most affected, lending support to the theory that the normal stresses of gravity are important in maintaining function, development, and therefore mobility (Gröer and Shekleton, 1989).

Decreased stability is the result of loss of endurance, decreased muscle mass, and joint abnormalities. Therefore clients are unable to move steadily, and their risk for falling increases.

Immobilization causes two skeletal changes. A **joint contracture** is an abnormal and usually permanent condition of a joint, characterized by flexion and fixation and caused by disuse, atrophy, and shortening of muscle fibers. When a contracture occurs, the joint cannot maintain its full range of joint motion. Contracture usually leaves the joint in a nonfunctional position (Figure 23-5). Footdrop contracture (Figure 23-6) results in the foot being permanently fixed in plantar flexion. Ambulation is difficult with the foot in this position.

The second skeletal change is **disuse osteoporosis,** the result of impaired calcium metabolism. Because immobilization results in bone resorption, bone tissue is less dense, osteoporosis results (Holm, 1989), and the client is at risk for pathological fractures. The link between disuse osteoporosis and immobility is twofold. Immobilization and non–weight-bearing activities increase the rate of bone resorption. **Bone resorption** also causes calcium to be released in the blood. If the kidneys cannot fully excrete this increased calcium, hypercalcemia results.

Integument Changes

The effect of immobility on the skin is compounded by impaired metabolism, the loss of lean body mass, and negative nitrogen balance (Greenleaf, 1984; Gröer and Shekleton, 1989). Any break in the skin's integrity is difficult to heal in the immobilized client. Older adult clients and clients with paralysis have a greater risk for developing pressure ulcers (AHCPR, 1992; Reddy, 1986).

A **pressure ulcer,** or decubitus ulcer, is an inflammation in the skin as a result of prolonged ischemia in tissues (see Chapter 24). Usually the ulcer forms over a bony prominence (Figure 23-7, *A* and *B*). Ischemia develops when the pressure on the skin is greater than the pressure inside the small peripheral blood vessels supplying blood to the skin (Knight, 1988).

Normally, tissue metabolism depends on the body's receipt of oxygen and nutrients from the blood supply and the elimination of metabolic wastes. Any factor that interferes with this process affects cellular metabolism and, as a result, the function or life of the cell. Pressure affects cellular metabolism by decreasing or obliterating tissue circulation.

When a client lies in bed or sits in a chair, the weight of the body is on bony prominences. The longer the pressure is applied, the longer the period of ischemia and therefore the greater the risk of skin breakdown (see Chapter 24).

Urinary Elimination Changes

Urinary elimination is altered by immobility. Urine flows out of the renal pelvis and into the ureter and bladder because of gravitational forces when the client is upright. When the client is recumbent, the kidneys and ureters move toward a more level plane, and urine formed by the kidney must enter the bladder against gravity. Because the peristaltic contractions of the ureters are insufficient to overcome gravity, the renal pelvis may fill before urine enters the ureters (Figure 23-8). This condition, called *urinary stasis,* increases the client's risk of urinary tract infection and renal calculi.

Renal calculi are calcium stones that lodge in the renal pelvis and pass through the ureters (Figure 23-9).

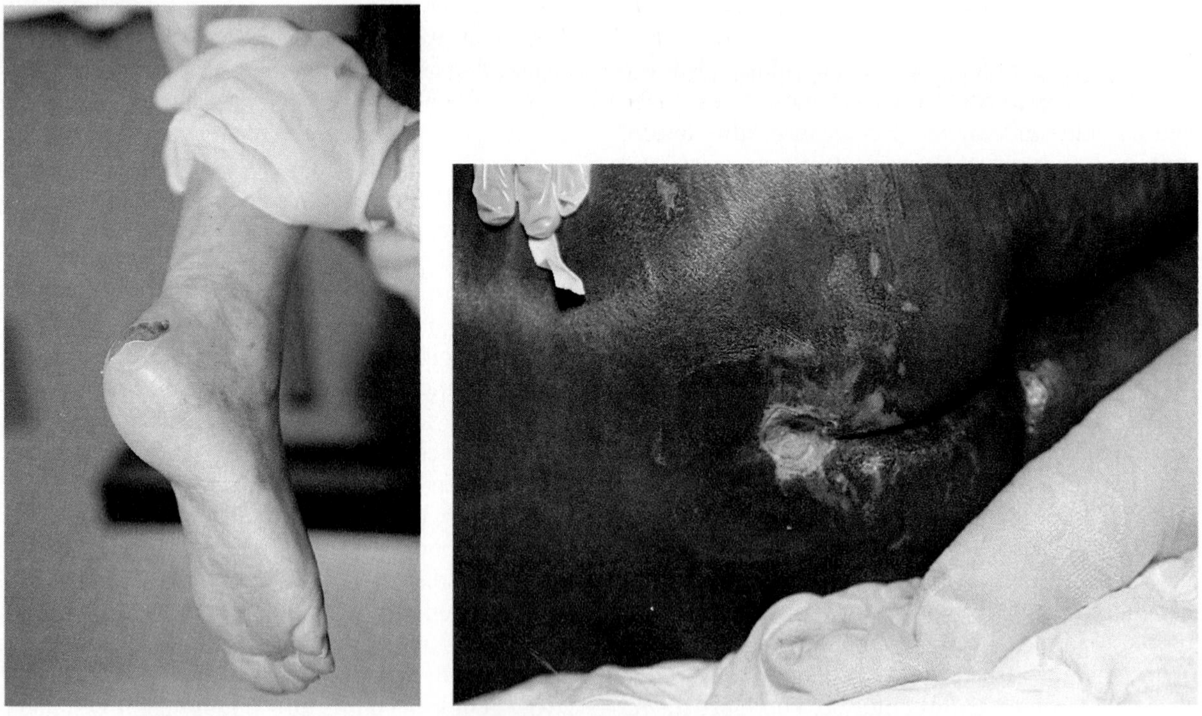

FIGURE 23-7 **A,** Formation of pressure sore on heel. **B,** Pressure ulcer with tissue necrosis on coccyx.

Immobilized clients are at risk for calcium stones because of altered bone metabolism and the resulting hypercalcemia.

During the initial period of immobility, urine volume is increased secondary to fluid shifts and a natural diuresis (Deitrick et al., 1948; Greenleaf, 1984). As immobility continues, fluid intake diminishes, and other causes such as fever increase the risk of dehydration. Because of these factors, urinary output declines on or about day 5 or 6. The urine then produced is usually highly concentrated.

This concentrated urine increases the risk for calculi formation and infection. Poor perineal care after bowel movements, particularly in women, increases the risk of urinary tract contamination by *Escherichia coli*. Another cause of urinary tract infections is indwelling urinary catheters, which provide pathways for pathogens to ascend into the urinary tract.

Immobility also increases the risk of incontinence. Barriers such as side rails, distant bathrooms, and lack of staff to help with toileting make incontinence a problem particularly for the older adult client. Burgio, Jones, and Engel (1988) found that clients who were incontinent had significantly more immobility than clients who were continent.

Psychosocial Effects

Immobilization may lead to emotional, intellectual, sensory, and sociocultural responses. However, the older adult may be more susceptible to these changes. As a result, the nurse may observe them earlier. The most common emotional changes are depression, behavioral changes, and impaired coping.

The immobilized client can become depressed because of changes in role, self-concept, and other factors. Depression is an affective disorder characterized by exaggerated feelings of sadness, melancholy, dejection, worthlessness, emptiness, and hopelessness out of proportion to reality. Depression can result from worrying about present and future levels of health, finances, and family needs. Because immobilization removes the client from a daily routine, he or she has more time to worry about disability. Worrying can quickly increase the client's depression, causing withdrawal. Assessing behavioral changes throughout restricted mobility helps the nurse to identify changes in self-concept, recognize early signs of depression, and develop nursing interventions.

Behavioral changes resulting from immobilization vary widely, depending on the client. Common behavioral changes include hostility, belligerence, giddiness, withdrawal, confusion, and anxiety. Early in the nursing process the nurse should interview the client's family and friends about normal behavioral patterns to gain baseline data. If unexpected behaviors are observed later, the nurse can intervene to reduce the effects of immobilization on the client's behavioral patterns.

The immobilized client requires constant nursing care. Because of physiological hazards, the client cannot be allowed to sleep for 8 hours without a change of position or other nursing care. Disruption of normal sleeping patterns can further cause behavioral changes. Nursing interventions should be used to ensure the client receives sufficient sleep (see Chapter 27). The client who is on bed rest and is able to change position during sleep does not require continuous physical nursing care directed at reducing the hazards of immobility. Unless other treatment activities are required during the night, the care plan for the physiologically stable client on bed rest can provide for uninterrupted sleep.

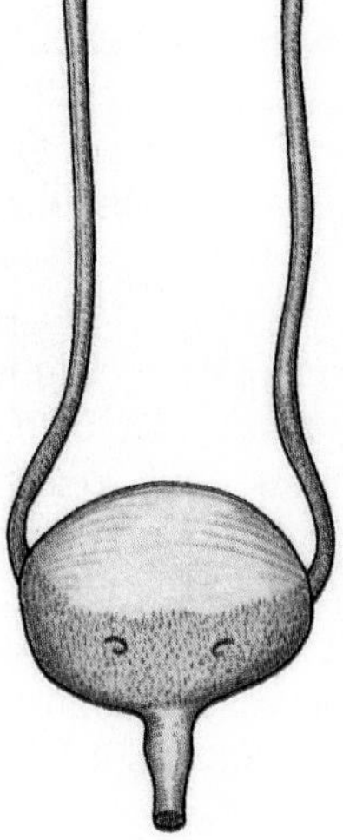

FIGURE 23-8 Stasis of urine.

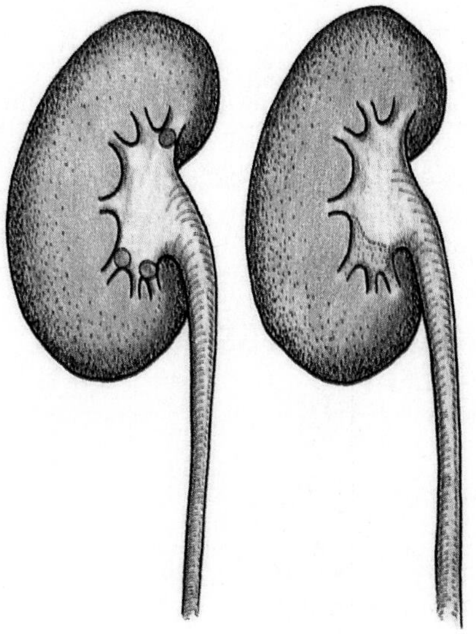

FIGURE 23-9 Renal calculi in renal pelvis.

Long-term immobility or bed rest can affect usual coping patterns. Such a client may withdraw and become passive. The passive client allows nurses to provide care and is not interested in increasing independence or involvement in care. Early in the care of an immobilized client the nurse should assess the client's normal coping mechanisms. The nurse then designs a nursing care plan that will allow the client to continue to use these coping abilities or will help him or her develop new ones.

Developmental Effects

More developmental changes tend to be associated with immobility in the very young and in the older adult. The immobilized young or middle-age adult may experience few, if any, developmental changes. However, there are exceptions to this guideline, and clients must be fully assessed for developmental implications. One exception might be a mother who has complications at childbirth and as a result cannot interact with the newborn as expected. When the infant, toddler, or preschooler is immobilized, it is usually because of trauma or the need to correct a congenital skeletal abnormality. Prolonged immobilization can delay the child's motor skill and intellectual development. Nurses caring for immobilized children should plan activities that provide physical and psychosocial stimuli. Other activities focus on the specific effects of immobilization.

Immobilization of older adult clients increases their physical dependence on others and accelerates functional losses in physiological systems. Immobilization of an older adult client usually results from a degenerative disease, neurological trauma, or a chronic illness. For some clients, immobilization occurs gradually and progressively, whereas for others—especially those who have had a stroke—immobilization is sudden. When providing nursing care for an older adult client, the nurse should develop a care plan that encourages the client to perform as many self-care activities as possible, thereby maintaining the highest level of mobility. Mobily and Kelley (1991) point out that nurses may inadvertently contribute to a client's immobility by providing unnecessary help with activities such as bathing and transferring.

NURSING PROCESS AND IMMOBILITY

Assessment

The assessment includes the client's present mobility and the potential effects of immobility.

Mobility. Assessment of the client's mobility focuses on range of joint motion, muscle strength, activity tolerance, gait, and posture. Chapter 22 describes the normal ROM for all joints in the body. Observation during activities of daily living enables the nurse to estimate the client's fatigability, muscle strength, and ROM. These assessment data assist the nurse in developing a care plan.

Finally, observing posture and gait helps the nurse to determine the type of assistance the client may require to change positions or transfer from bed to chair. This information helps the nurse to assess the client's overall level of mobility and coordination.

Risks and Indicators of Immobility. The nurse assesses immobilized clients for physiological changes resulting from immobility. A head-to-toe physical assessment (see Chapter 16) allows the nurse to assess the physical function. It also includes a review of psychosocial and developmental dimensions.

PHYSIOLOGICAL CONDITION. The nurse assesses body systems most likely to be affected by immobility.

METABOLIC SYSTEM. When assessing the client's metabolic functioning, the nurse uses anthropometric measurements to evaluate muscle atrophy. Intake and output records and laboratory data evaluate fluid and electrolyte status. Assessment of wound healing, evaluation of nutrients, food intake, and elimination patterns determine altered gastrointestinal functioning.

Anthropometric measurements include height, weight, mid-upper arm circumference, and triceps skinfold measurements. Ideally, this assessment should be done early in the period of immobilization and should be repeated at 3-week intervals. Assessment of height and weight are discussed in Chapter 16. A decrease in mid-upper arm circumference, measured in centimeters, or triceps skinfold, measured in millimeters, indicates a decline in muscle mass. This decline, with decreased serum protein levels and decreased white cell count, can indicate the client is breaking down more protein than he or she is building up. As a result, the client may be at risk for severe negative nitrogen imbalance. Measurements of the mid-upper arm circumference and triceps skinfold provide baseline information about the amount of subcutaneous fat, which may be lost during immobilization.

Intake and output measurements determine whether a fluid imbalance exists. Dehydration and edema can increase the speed of skin breakdown in an immobilized client. Laboratory tests, specifically measurement of serum electrolytes and calcium, can also indicate an electrolyte imbalance.

If an immobilized client has a wound, the speed of healing indicates how well nutrients are delivered to the tissues for use (see Chapter 35). The normal progression of wound healing indicates the metabolic needs of the injured tissues are being met.

Anorexia occurs commonly in immobilized clients. The nurse should assess food intake. Nutritional imbalances can be avoided if the nurse learns the client's dietary patterns and food preferences early in the immobilization.

Respiratory system. A respiratory assessment should be performed every 2 hours for acutely ill clients with restricted activity patterns. The nurse should inspect chest wall movements during the full inspiratory-expiratory cycle. The nurse should auscultate the entire lung region to identify regions of diminished breath sounds, crackles, or wheezes. Auscultation should focus on the dependent lung field, because pulmonary secretions tend to move to these lower regions. If a client has an atelectatic area, breath sounds may be asymmetrical. A complete respiratory assessment identifies the presence of secretions and can be used to determine nursing interventions necessary to maintain optimal respiratory function.

Cardiovascular system. The cardiovascular assessment of the immobilized client includes monitoring blood pressure, evaluating apical and peripheral pulses, and observing the venous system. Because of the risk for orthostatic hypotension, blood pressure should be measured, particularly when changing from lying to a sitting or standing position. In this way the client's ability to tolerate postural changes can be assessed.

The nurse also needs to assess the apical and peripheral pulses. Recumbency increases the cardiac workload and results in an increased pulse rate. In some clients, particularly the older adult, the heart may not be able to tolerate the increased workload, and a form of cardiac failure may develop. Monitoring the client's peripheral pulses allows the nurse to evaluate the heart's ability to pump the blood throughout the body. The absence of a peripheral pulse, particularly one that was previously present, should be documented and reported immediately.

Edema may indicate the heart's inability to handle the increased workload. Because fluid moves to dependent body regions, assessment of the immobilized client should include the sacrum, legs, and feet. If the heart is unable to tolerate the increased cardiac workload, the peripheral body regions such as the hands, feet, nose, and earlobes will be colder than the central body regions.

Finally, the nurse assesses the venous system because deep vein **thrombosis** is a hazard of restricted mobility. A dislodged thrombus, called an *embolus,* may travel through the circulatory system to the lungs and impair that organ's circulation. Emboli to the lungs (pulmonary emboli) pose a threat to the client's life.

To assess for a deep vein thrombosis, the nurse should remove the client's elastic stockings once every 8 hours and observe the calves for redness, warmth, and tenderness. The nurse should ask the client about calf pain. The nurse may also ask the client to dorsiflex the foot and assess for the presence of calf pain. Calf pain on dorsiflexion (positive Homan's sign) may indicate deep vein thrombosis. In addition, calf circumference should be measured daily in clients at high risk for developing thrombi. To do this, the nurse marks a point on each of the client's calves 10 cm from the midpatella. The circumference is measured each day using the mark as a reference point for placing the tape measure. One-sided increases in calf diameter can be an early indication of thrombosis. Because deep vein thrombosis can also occur in the thigh, thigh circumference measurements should be taken daily.

Musculoskeletal system. The major musculoskeletal abnormalities identified during assessment include decreased muscle strength, loss of muscle tone and mass, and contractures. Anthropometric measurements provide clues to muscle mass loss. Muscle strength and tone may be measured during ROM assessment. Disuse osteoporosis cannot be identified by physical assessment. However, postmenopausal women and clients with increased serum and urine calcium levels are at greater risk for bone demineralization. Clients who have joint pain (such as in the hip) or who complain of back pain may have an unrecognized fracture caused by disuse osteoporosis.

Integument. The nurse must continually assess the skin for signs of pressure ulcer formation. The neurologically impaired client, the chronically ill client in long-term care, the client with diminished mental status (Gosnell, 1987), and the orthopedic client are at high risk for developing pressure ulcers.

The nurse should look for specific factors such as sensory loss and anemia (Chapter 24) when assessing clients at risk for pressure ulcer formation. When assessing the client's skin, the nurse should view all pressure points to determine whether they are adequately protected and the skin is not exposed to body fluids.

Last, the nurse assesses the client's nutritional status and observes for signs of infection that increase the risk for pressure ulcers (Bergstrom et al., 1987).

Elimination system. The client's elimination status should be evaluated on each shift, and the total intake and output should be evaluated every 24 hours. The nurse should determine that the client is receiving the correct amount and type of fluids orally or parenterally (see Chapters 32 and 33).

Inadequate fluid and electrolyte balances or intake and output can increase the risk for renal impairment, ranging from recurrent infections to kidney failure. These conditions decrease the client's overall level of mobility and increase the duration and cost of care.

Assessment of elimination status should also include the frequency and consistency of bowel movements. The client's usual urine and bowel elimination patterns should be assessed to maintain consistency. Accurate assessment enables the nurse to intervene before fecal impaction occurs and may also prevent urine incontinence.

Psychosocial condition. Changes in psychosocial status usually occur slowly and are often overlooked by health care personnel. The nurse should observe for changes in emotional status (e.g., depression). The nurse also observes for behavioral changes (e.g., the cooperative client who becomes argumentative or the modest client who begins to expose himself or herself repeatedly). The nurse should try to determine the reasons for such behavioral alterations to identify specific nursing therapies.

Changes in the client's sleep-wake cycle such as difficulty falling asleep or frequent awakenings must be identified and corrected (see Chapter 27). Many sleep disruptions can be prevented or minimized. Finally, the nurse should observe for changes in the use of normal coping mechanisms to adapt to immobilization. Decreasing coping ability may cause the client to become disoriented, confused, or depressed, or to experience other behavioral changes. Clients may report sensory alterations such as seeing shapes and dots or seeing people and animals or hearing the wind or mechanical noises (Rubin, 1988b). The client may find these sensations disturbing and may be reluctant to mention them to the nurse. The nurse may need to watch and listen to the client closely to note these changes. The client may only refer to the sensations casually (e.g., "It sure sounded like a dog was in here last night"). Allowing clients to discuss sensory alterations will help to reassure them they are not losing touch with reality.

Development. Assessment of the immobilized client should include developmental considerations to ensure that all needs are identified. With a young child the nurse determines whether the child is able to meet developmental tasks and is progressing normally. Development may regress or be slowed because of immobilization. By identifying a child's overall developmental needs, the nurse can design nursing therapies to maintain normal development. When developmental delays are temporary, the nurse may also need to assure the parents.

Developmental assessment is as important with the older adult client as with the young child. The nursing assessment enables the nurse to determine the older adult client's ability to meet needs independently and to adapt to developmental changes. A decline in developmental functioning prompts investigation to determine the reasons the change occurred and the interventions necessary to restore the client to an optimal level of function (see Chapter 20).

NURSING DIAGNOSES FOR IMMOBILITY

- Impaired physical mobility
- Altered patterns of urinary elimination
- Ineffective airway clearance
- Ineffective breathing pattern
- Impaired gas exchange
- Actual or high risk for impaired skin integrity
- High risk for altered peripheral tissue perfusion
- High risk for infection
- Total incontinence
- High risk for fluid volume deficit
- Ineffective individual coping
- Social isolation
- Sleep pattern disturbance

Nursing Diagnosis

An immobilized client may have one or more nursing diagnoses related to the condition (see box below, left). Assessment reveals clusters of data that indicate whether a problem or potential problem exists. Assessment also identifies pertinent defining characteristics that support the diagnostic label and probable cause of the diagnosis. Locating the probable cause of the diagnosis (based on assessment data) is important to planning client-centered goals and subsequent nursing interventions that will best help the client.

Impaired physical mobility related to bed rest would require slightly different interventions than impaired physical mobility related to pain in the left shoulder. The first diagnosis would require interventions aimed at keeping the client as mobile as possible and encouraging the client to do self-care and ROM in bed. The second diagnosis would require the nurse to assist the client with comfort measures so the client would then be willing and more able to move. In both situations the nurse would explain the importance of activity to healthy body functioning.

Many alterations in physiological, sociocultural, and developmental functioning are related to immobility. Often, these problems are interrelated, and it is imperative that nursing care focus on all dimensions. Often the focus of immobility is on the easily visible physical problems such as skin impairment, but the psychosocial and developmental aspects of immobility should not be overlooked.

Immobilization of a family member changes the family's functioning. The family's response to this change may lead to problems, stress, and anxieties.

Nursing diagnoses for health needs in developmental areas reflect changes from the client's normal activities. Immobility can lead to a developmental crisis if the client is unable to resolve problems and continue to mature.

Planning

Clients at risk for hazards of immobility require nursing care plans directed at meeting their actual and potential needs (see nursing care plan). In addition, the nurse must develop client-centered goals aimed at preventing or reducing the hazards of immobility. Care planning is individualized to the client, taking into consideration the client's most immediate needs. The immediacy of any problem is determined by the effect the problem has on the client's mental and physical health. Actual breathing problems, for example, generally take precedence over recreational activity deficits when the nurse is setting priorities. The respiratory problem may cause life-threatening complications, whereas the leisure activity is not generally as serious.

Other client factors to be considered when setting priorities include everyday activities, family, and developmental stage. The nurse may need the help of another health team member such as a physical or occupational therapist when considering mobility needs. These factors are important for clients in institutional and in home settings. Discharge planning is begun when a client enters the health care system. Anticipating the client's discharge from an institution, a referral may be necessary to help the client remain mobile or regain mobility at home.

The care plan is developed with the client and significant others based on one or more client-centered goals. Goals, like diagnoses, must be prioritized and are formed based on the nursing assessment. General goals and expected outcomes that may serve as guidelines for developing care plans for clients with immobility problems include the following:

Goal: Client regains proper or optimal body alignment.

Outcomes

Maintains correct body alignment while sitting, standing, and lying

Maintains ROM in all joints

SAMPLE NURSING CARE PLAN
Immobility

ASSESSMENT

Clinical scenario: Mrs. Huebner, a 70-year-old client hospitalized with multiple fractures of the ribs and pelvis after a motor vehicle accident, is *immobilized in full traction.* Bilateral pedal pulses are strong at this time. Client can flex and extend both knees and move both feet while in traction. *Calves measure 35 cm in diameter on the right and 36 cm on the left.*

NURSING DIAGNOSIS

High risk for altered peripheral tissue perfusion related to decreased mobility.

PLANNING

Goal	Expected outcomes
Client will remain free of thrombus formation during hospitalization.	Diameters of both calves will remain within 1 cm of baseline measure. Calves will remain free of erythema. Peripheral pedal pulses will be palpable.

IMPLEMENTATION

Steps	Rationale
1. Administer low-dose heparin as ordered.	Administration of low-dose heparin has shown reductions in risk of vein thrombosis (Clagett and Reisch, 1988).
2. Apply elastic stockings and remove each shift for hygiene.	Application increases venous tone, improving venous return, and reduces venous stasis (Winslow, 1985).
3. Have client perform range of motion exercise to lower legs and feet hourly while awake.	Exercise promotes venous return and prevents venous stasis.

EVALUATION

Measure calves daily; report any increases in dimensions.
Inspect client's calves for erythema.
Palpate peripheral pulses in lower extremities.

Defining characteristics are shown in italic type.

Goal: Injuries to the client's skin and musculoskeletal system are reduced or prevented.

Outcomes

No reddened areas over bony prominences
Skin remains intact
Maintains ROM in all joints
Maintains muscle tone

Goal: Client maintains a patent airway.

Outcomes

Client coughs productively
Client's lungs are free of adventitious sounds

Goal: Client achieves optimal lung expansion by 6/12.

Outcomes

Chest wall excursion is symmetrical and full
Respirations remain under 24 at rest
Client inspires prescribe amount as measured by incentive spirometry by 6/10
Normal breath sounds heard throughout all lobes

Goal: Client increases activity tolerance by 6/15.

Outcomes

Client identifies factors that reduce activity tolerance (6/12)
Client resumes prehospital activities on discharge (6/14)
Client maintains baseline vital signs following activity
Client paces activity so as not to become fatigued

Goal: Client achieves optimal elimination patterns by 6/12.

Outcomes

Client maintains usual bowel routine while hospitalized
Client drinks at least 2000 cc of fluid a day
Client maintains urine output of at least 50 cc an hour

Goal: Client maintains normal sleep-wake patterns (6/12).

Outcomes

Client sleeps uninterrupted (6/10)
Client demonstrates one relaxation method before retiring (6/12)
Client states is not fatigued after night's rest

Goal: Client socializes with family.

Outcomes

Client participates in leisure activities
Client participates in organized activities

Goal: Client performs self-care activities.

Outcomes

Uses assistive devices for feeding
Uses assisitive devices for self-toileting
Participates in self-care by washing upper body

Goal: Client achieves physical and mental stimulation.

Outcomes

Participates in activities of daily care
Remains alert and oriented to surroundings

Implementation

Nursing interventions for the completely or partially immobilized client focus on preventing the hazards of immobility.

Metabolic System. The dietary needs of the immobilized client are based on many factors. These factors include infection, need for wound healing, food intolerances, functioning of the alimentary system, and daily caloric needs.

A dietary plan of carbohydrates, proteins, and fats is designed to meet the client's needs. Carbohydrates are needed to meet energy requirements. Proteins are necessary for tissue repair. Fats prevent further breakdown of nutritional stores. The specific caloric and diet prescription is determined from the nutritional assessment in conjunction with a qualified clinical dietitian (see Chapter 35).

If the client is unable to eat, nutrition including fluids must be provided enterally or parenterally. If the gastrointestinal system is able to ingest, digest, and absorb nutrients, the enteral (tube) method of feeding is best. If the client's gastric system does not function, the parenteral route of nutrition is selected (see Chapter 35).

Respiratory System. Nursing interventions for the respiratory system are aimed at promoting expansion of the chest and lungs, preventing stasis of pulmonary secretions, and maintaining a patent airway.

PROMOTING EXPANSION OF THE CHEST AND LUNGS. The nurse can counteract reduced chest expansion with several interventions. A healthy adult resting in bed will change position once every 11 to 12 minutes. Changing the client's position allows the dependent lung to expand. This maintains the elastic recoil property of the lungs and clears the dependent lung of pulmonary secretions. The minimum suggested timing for turning is every 2 hours, but that may not be enough. The nurse must judge the client's particular situation to determine the frequency of position changes. The most effective position in bed for lung expansion is high Fowler's, but the client in this position tends to slide down in bed, which then decreases lung expansion.

The nurse should encourage the client to deep breathe and cough every 1 to 2 hours while awake. Alert clients can be taught to deep breathe or yawn every hour. This action expands all lobes of the lungs and prevents atelectasis. Coughing reduces the stasis of pulmonary secretions. Some immobile clients, particularly after surgery, should use an incentive spirometer to aid in deep breathing (see Chapter 34).

Postoperative pain medications can depress the respiratory center so the rate of respiration or expansion of the lungs is decreased. The client may be drowsy as a result of the medication. Therefore, the nurse should actively reinforce coughing and deep breathing exercises and encourage early ambulation.

If abdominal binders or rib supports are required, they should be removed every 2 hours to allow the client to breathe deeply. Binders must be assessed for correct positioning and adjusted as necessary to prevent interference with respirations. Often clients will wear the binder only when ambulating. Specific physician instructions for the use of binders will vary.

Preventing stasis of pulmonary secretions. Stagnant secretions accumulating in the bronchi and lungs of the immobilized or bedridden client may lead to the growth of bacteria and the subsequent development of pneumonia. The stagnation of secretions can be reduced by changing the client's position every 2 hours. This change rotates the dependent lung, mobilizing the secretions.

The immobile client should take in a minimum of 2000 cc a day to help keep mucociliary clearance normal. In clients free from infection and with adequate hydration, pulmonary secretions will appear thin, watery, and clear. The client can easily remove the secretions with coughing. Without adequate hydration the secretions are thick and tenacious and difficult to remove (see Chapter 34). Encouraging fluids also benefits in helping with bowel and urine elimination and aids in maintaining circulation and skin integrity (see box at right).

Perhaps the best method for preventing pulmonary secretions is **chest physiotherapy,** which is the use of positioning techniques to drain secretions from specific segments of the bronchi and lungs into the trachea, from which the client expels the secretions by coughing. Respiratory assessment findings identify areas of the lungs requiring chest physiotherapy. Clients are then placed in appropriate positions to promote drainage. The nurse uses pillows and slant boards to position clients properly, and uses cupping, clapping, and vibrating techniques to dislodge and mobilize secretions. Chest physiotherapy is a precise procedure requiring specific nursing skills (see Chapter 34).

Maintaining a patent airway. Immobilized clients and those on bed rest are generally weakened. If the weakness progresses, the cough reflex gradually becomes inefficient. If the client is too weak or unable to cough up secretions, the nurse must maintain a patent airway by using suctioning techniques. The stasis of secretions in the lungs may be life threatening for an immobilized client because hypostatic bronchopneumonia can easily develop. Dislodging and mobilizing the stagnant secretions reduces the risk of pneumonia. Assessment findings indicating this condition include productive cough with greenish-yellow sputum, fever, and pain on breathing.

The nurse can implement the following therapies to maintain the patent airway. The nurse asks the client to deep breathe and cough every 1 to 2 hours while awake. In addition, the nurse uses nasotracheal or orotracheal suction to remove secretions in the upper airways of a weakened client unable to cough productively. This procedure must be performed aseptically. The nurse places a suction catheter in the nose or through the mouth and applies suction to remove secretions that have accumulated in the upper airways (see Chapter 34).

Finally, the nurse maintains a patent airway by suctioning secretions from an artificial airway such as an endotracheal or tracheal tube. Through suctioning, pulmonary secretions are removed from the upper and lower airways (see Chapter 34).

GERONTOLOGIC NURSING PRACTICES FOR THE CLIENT WHO NEEDS TO BE ENCOURAGED TO TAKE FLUIDS

- The older adult client may have diminished thirst because of age-related factors. Therefore offer fluids on a regular schedule.
- Because older adults sometimes mistakenly try to control urine incontinence and frequency by limiting fluid intake, the nurse should explain the importance of fluids to the body's functioning.
- Some older adults may never have acquired the taste for ice water, so it is important to assess what temperature the client prefers to have water kept.
- Because older adults may have reduced appetite (from illness and associated with the aging process), do not expect them to take in large amounts of fluids at meal time.
- Because arm mobility and dexterity may be decreased, make sure fluids are within reach and are in containers that are easily handled and opened.

Cardiovascular System. Nursing therapies are designed to minimize or prevent orthostatic hypotension, increased cardiac workload, and thrombus formation.

Reducing orthostatic hypotension. After bed rest, clients usually have an increased pulse rate, a decrease in pulse pressure, and an increase in fainting in response to a tilting or an erect posture (Winslow, 1985). Interventions should be directed toward reducing or eliminating the effects of orthostatic hypotension. The nurse attempts to get the client out of bed as soon as the physical condition allows, even if the move is only to a chair. This activity maintains muscle tone and increases venous return. **Isometric** exercises used during bed rest do not have any beneficial effect on orthostatic hypotension but may improve activity tolerance (Winslow, 1985).

When getting the client from a supine position into a chair, the nurse moves the client gradually. When performing this procedure, the nurse documents orthostatic changes. The nurse first obtains baseline blood pressure and pulse with the client in the supine position. The nurse then raises the client to a high Fowler's position and measures blood pressure and pulse again to detect decreases in blood pressure or elevations in pulse. The nurse remains with the client in the high Fowler's position for a few moments to allow the body to adapt. The nurse continually monitors the client for dizziness or lightheadedness and whether spots are seen. Then the nurse has the client sit at the side of the bed with the feet on the floor. If there is no dizziness, the nurse assists the client to a chair. When getting an immobile client up for the first time the nurse should usually gets the assistance of at least one other person. This is a precautionary step. The client would still be expected to do as much of the transfer the condition allows.

Encouraging clients to sit or stand minimizes the orthostatic effect of bed rest. These interventions counteract the fluid shift and redistribute venous volume (Winslow, 1985).

REDUCING CARDIAC WORKLOAD. The nurse uses interventions to reduce cardiac workload, which is increased by immobility. The nurse discourages the client from using the **Valsalva maneuver.** When using this maneuver, the client holds the breath and strains, increasing intrathoracic pressure, which decreases venous return and cardiac output. When the strain is released, venous return and cardiac output immediately increase and systolic blood pressure and pulse pressure rise. These pressure changes produce a reflex bradycardia. The Valsalva maneuver may be associated with sudden cardiac death in clients with heart disease (Metzger and Therrien, 1990).

Movements such as getting on and off a bedpan and moving up in bed increase the use of the Valsalva maneuver. The nurse teaches the client to breathe out while moving or being lifted up in bed to avoid straining. Supine and sitting exercises also increase endurance and reduce the loss of muscle mass and strength (Winslow, 1985; Greenleaf, 1984).

PREVENTING THROMBUS FORMATION. Many interventions reduce the risk of thrombus formation in the immobilized client. Leg exercises, encouraging fluids, position changes, and teaching should begin when the client becomes immobile. Preoperative clients should be given this information before surgery (see Chapter 34). Other interventions such as medications and intermittent pneumatic compression stockings require a physician's order.

Positioning techniques help reduce pressure to the skin. Proper positioning used with other therapies (e.g., heparin and elastic stockings) help reduce thrombus formation. When positioning clients, the nurse uses caution to prevent pressure on the posterior knee and deep veins in the lower extremities. Client teaching should include avoiding crossing the legs, not sitting for prolonged periods of time, not wearing tight clothing that constricts the legs or waist, not putting pillows under the knees, and avoiding massaging of the legs.

Range of joint motion exercises are designed to reduce the risk of contractures but can also prevent

INCORPORATING ACTIVE RANGE OF JOINT MOTION EXERCISES INTO ACTIVITIES OF DAILY LIVING

Nodding head "yes" exercises *neck* (flexion)
Shaking head "no" exercises *neck* (rotation)
Moving right ear to right shoulder exercises *neck* (lateral flexion)
Moving left ear to left shoulder exercises *neck* (lateral flexion)
Reaching to turn on overhead light exercises *shoulder* (extension)
Reaching to bedside stand for book exercises *shoulder* (extension)
Scratching back exercises *shoulder* (hyperextension)
Rotating shoulders toward chest exercises *shoulder* (abduction)
Rotating shoulders toward back exercises *shoulder* (adduction)
Eating, bathing, shaving, and grooming exercise *elbow* (flexion and extension)
All activities requiring fine motor coordination, such as writing and eating, exercise *fingers* and *thumb* (flexion, extension, abduction, adduction, and opposition)
Walking exercises *hip* (flexion, extension, and hyperextension)
Moving to side-lying position exercises *hip* (flexion, extension, and abduction)
Moving from side-lying position exercises *hip* (extension and adduction)
Rolling feet inward exercises *hip* (internal rotation)
Rolling feet outward exercises *hip* (external rotation)
Walking exercises *knee* (flexion and extension)
Moving to and from a side-lying position exercises *knee* (flexion and extension)
Walking exercises *ankle* (dorsiflexion and plantar flexion)
Moving toe toward head of bed exercises *ankle* (dorsiflexion)
Moving toe toward foot of bed exercises *ankle* (plantar flexion)
Walking exercises *toes* (extension and hyperextension)
Wiggling toes exercises *toes* (abduction and adduction)

thrombi (see Chapter 22). These exercises can be incorporated into activities of daily living (see box on p. 572). Activity causes contraction of the skeletal muscles, which in turn exerts pressure on the veins to promote venous return, thereby reducing venous stasis. Specific exercises that help prevent thrombophlebitis are ankle pumps, foot circles, hip rotation, and knee flexion. Ankle pumps, sometimes called calf pumps, include alternating plantar flexion and dorsiflexion. Foot circles require the client to rotate the ankle. This can be done by instructing the client to make the letters of the alphabet with the feet. Inward and outward rotation of the hip can be done while the client is supine or sitting. Knee flexion involves alternately extending and flexing the knee. In the high-risk patient, these exercises should be done hourly while awake.

When deep vein thrombosis is suspected, it should be reported immediately. The leg should be elevated, with no pressure on the area of the leg with the suspected thrombus. The family, client, and all health care personnel should be instructed not to massage the area because the thrombus may be dislodged.

Therapeutic elastic stockings with graded compressions reduce the risk of thrombus formation (Clagett and Reisch, 1988). Elastic stockings aid in maintaining pressure on the muscles of the lower extremities and are believed to promote venous return. The stockings must be applied properly (Procedure 23-1) and removed and reapplied at least once a shift. In addition, the stockings should always be clean and dry, and it may be necessary for the client to have two pairs. Clients often come to the hospital with stockings they have worn for years. These must be assessed for fit and to see if the client is wearing them properly. Clients may roll them at the knee, subsequently constricting venous return. An important teaching point is that clients should be told not to roll stockings.

Intermittent pneumatic compression (IPC) provides rhythmic, external extremity compression through inflatable "stockings." These stockings, also referred to as pulsating antiembolic stockings (PAS), are effective in reducing deep vein thrombosis in general surgical high-risk clients with malignant disease and clients with orthopedic or neurological conditions (Clagett and Reisch, 1988).

Immobilized clients are frequently placed on low-dose heparin therapy to minimize the risk of venous thromboembolism. This therapy requires a physician's order. The medication is usually administered every 8 hours. The usual route of administration is subcutaneous injection, although some clients may receive it through a heparin lock (e.g., Hep-Lock) catheter (Clagett and Reisch, 1988). Heparin is an anticoagulant and thus suppresses clot formation. Because of the action of this medication, the nurse must continually assess the client for signs of bleeding (e.g., increased bruising, guaiac-positive stools, and bleeding gums). These risks exist, although most clients do not experience side effects.

Musculoskeletal System. The immobilized client must receive some exercise to prevent excessive muscle wasting and atrophy and joint contractures. The amount of activity required to prevent physical disuse syndromes is only about 2 hours in a 24-hour period, but it must be scheduled so the client does not remain inactive for more than 1 hour at a time. However, the best method to prevent complications from impaired mobility is to encourage ambulation. Whenever possible, the nurse should encourage clients to participate in an activity program.

If the client is unable to move any part or all of the body, the nurse must perform passive range of joint motion exercises for all immobilized joints at least 3 or 4 times a day. If one extremity is paralyzed, the client can be taught to put that joint independently through its range of motion.

Some orthopedic and neurological conditions require more frequent passive ROM exercises to restore the injured joint or extremity to maximal function. Clients with such conditions may use automatic equipment for passive range of joint motion exercises. The equipment extends an extremity to a prescribed angle for a prescribed period. This method is beneficial when the client must gradually increase the degree and duration of extension to achieve optimal functioning of the affected area.

Clients on bed rest should have active range of joint motion exercises incorporated into the daily schedule (see Chapter 22). The client can perform these exercises during activities of daily living. The box on p. 572 describes the joint movements that occur with various daily activities.

Passive and active range of joint motion exercises maintain the functioning of the musculoskeletal system. The nurse should also plan interventions for the gradual return of mobility in clients who will be able to resume pre-illness activity patterns.

The best nursing intervention is establishing an individualized progressive exercise program. A progressive exercise program gradually increases the client's physical activity to reverse the deconditioning associated with bed rest (Winslow and Weber, 1980; Norman and Gibbs, 1991). Progressive exercise programs are used for clients with musculoskeletal, neurological, cardiopulmonary, renal, and other chronic diseases. General teaching guidelines for clients with limited mobility are given in the box on p. 575.

Integument. The major risk to the skin from restricted mobility is the formation of pressure ulcers (see Chapter 24). Nursing interventions therefore focus on

procedure 23-1

APPLYING ELASTIC STOCKINGS

Steps	Rationale
1. Identify need for elastic stockings, including immobility, lower extremity edema, and varicose veins.	These conditions increase the risk of thrombus formation.
2. Prepare equipment: a. Tape measure b. Stockings in proper size c. Talcum powder	Stockings must be measured according to directions of specific manufacturer. Measure calf circumference from foot to knee. For thigh-high stockings, measure calf circumference, thigh circumference, and length from foot to thigh.
3. Explain procedure to client.	Relieves anxiety and increases cooperation.
4. Wash hands.	Reduces transmission of microorganisms.
5. Elevate bed to comfortable position.	Promotes good body mechanics for nurse.
6. Place client in supine position.	Eases application.
7. After legs have been cleansed, apply small amount of talcum powder to each leg and foot.	Reduces friction and allows for easier application of stockings.
8. Turn elastic stocking partially inside out by placing one hand into sock, holding client's toe, and pulling (see illustration).	Allows easier application of stockings.
9. Place client's toe into foot of stocking, making sure that sock is smooth (see illustration).	Wrinkles in sock can impede circulation to leg and foot.
10. Slide remaining portion of sock over foot, being sure that toes are covered (see illustration).	If toes remain uncovered, they will become constricted by the elastic, and circulation can be reduced.
11. Slide sock over calf until sock is completely extended. Be sure sock is smooth and no ridges are present (see illustration).	Ridges impede venous return and can counteract purpose of stockings.

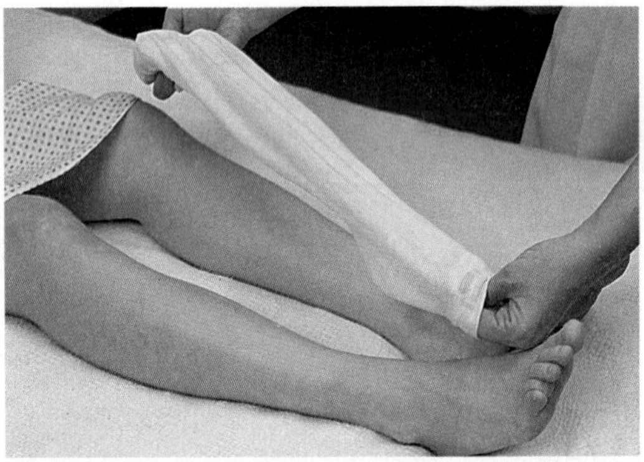

Step 8

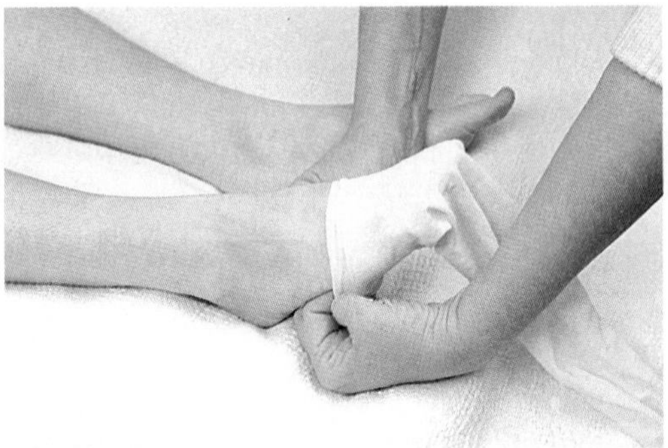

Step 9

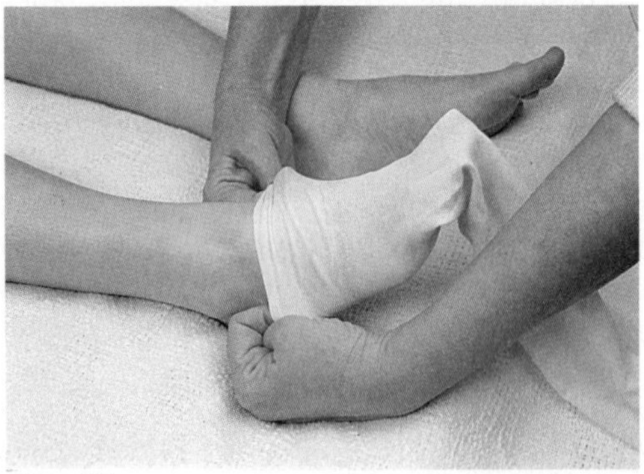

Step 10

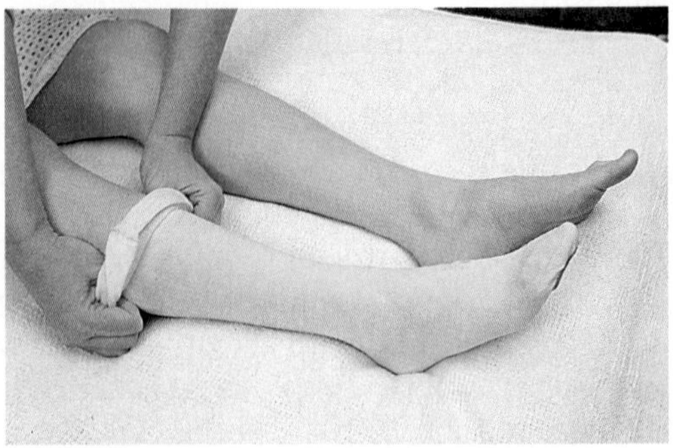

Step 11

Steps	Rationale
12. Instruct client not to roll socks partially down.	Rolling sock partially down will have constricting effect and impede venous return.
13. Help client to comfortable position.	Maintains body alignment and promotes comfort.
14. Wash hands.	Reduces transmission of microorganisms.
15. After 1 hour:	
a. Observe stockings for wrinkles in binding.	Leads to increased pressure to skin and impairs circulation.
b. Assess capillary refill in toes and palpate pulses in feet.	Ensures that circulatory status in lower extremities has not been compromised.
16. Remove stockings at least once a shift.	Provides for assessment of skin and circulatory status.
17. Record date and time of stocking application and condition of skin before application, circulatory status of lower extremities, and stocking length and size in nurses' notes.	Documents condition of lower extremities and performance of procedure.

preventing or treating these ulcers. Early identification of high-risk clients and their risk factors aids the nurse in preventing pressure ulcers. Interventions aimed at prevention are positioning, skin care, and the use of therapeutic devices such as pressure relief devices. The immobilized client's position should be changed according to the client's activity level, perceptual ability, and daily routines (Bergstrom et al., 1987). While turning every 1 to 2 hours is recommended for preventing ulcers, it may also be necessary to use pressure relief devices. The time a client sits uninterrupted in a chair should be limited to 1 hour or less, but this time interval is individualized. The client should be repositioned frequently because uninterrupted pressure will cause skin breakdown. The nurse should teach clients who are able to shift their weight every fifteen minutes. Chair-bound clients should have a pressure reducing device for the chair (AHCPR, 1992).

CLIENT TEACHING FOR LIMITED MOBILITY

Explain the need for position changes at regular intervals based on client needs.
Demonstrate passive and active range of joint motion exercises.
Describe the risk factors for pressure sores.
Describe early warning signs of immobility (e.g., continued erythema over a bony prominence) so interventions can be developed to prevent worsening of the condition.
Discuss activities to reduce the psychosocial problems of immobilization.
Encourage the client's participation in care and decision making.

Elimination System. Nursing interventions for maintaining optimal urinary functioning are directed toward keeping the client well hydrated without causing bladder distention and the reflux of urine into the ureters and, in some instances, the renal pelvis.

Adequate hydration helps to prevent renal calculi and urinary tract infections. The client should void large amounts of dilute urine. If the client is also incontinent, the nurse modifies the care plan so the increased urinary output does not cause skin breakdown.

To prevent bladder distention, the nurse assesses the frequency and amount of urinary output. A client who continually dribbles urine and whose bladder is distended has overflow incontinence. If the immobilized client does not have voluntary control of bladder elimination, bladder retraining may be necessary. If the client experiences bladder distention, the nurse may be required to insert a straight catheter or an indwelling Foley catheter (see Chapter 32).

The nurse must also record the frequency and consistency of bowel movements. A diet rich in fruits and vegetables can help to facilitate normal peristalsis. If a client is unable to maintain normal bowel patterns, the nurse may initiate a bowel training program and the physician may order stool softeners, cathartics, or enemas (see Chapter 33).

Psychosocial Problems. Assessment can identify the effects of prolonged immobilization on the client's psychosocial dimension. Clients with a tendency toward depression or mood swings are at greater risk for developing these changes during bed rest or immobilization.

The nurse should anticipate changes in psychosocial status to intervene with preventive measures. The nurse can provide routine and informal socialization for the client. Nursing activities are planned to give the client opportunities to interact with the staff. If possible, the client should be placed in a room with other mobile clients. If the client must remain in a private room, staff members are asked to visit with the client periodically throughout the client's waking hours.

The nurse also provides stimuli to maintain the client's orientation and to entertain the client. Bedside chats at appropriate moments orient the client to the schedule of nursing activities, meals, and visiting hours. Books from the hospital library help to occupy the client. If the client's condition permits, he or she can participate in craft activities.

Clients should be encouraged to wear their glasses or artificial teeth and to shave or apply makeup. These are normal activities through which people maintain body image.

In addition, the client should be encouraged to perform as much self-care as possible. Hygiene and grooming articles should be kept within easy reach so the client can attend to personal needs.

Nursing care between 10 PM and 7 AM should be scheduled to minimize sleep interruptions. The balance between rest and the physiological effects of bed rest must be weighed. Assessments may be kept to a minimum in a stable client who is able to turn in bed unassisted. More seriously ill clients may need medications, assessments, and skin care during the night. Nursing care should be coordinated to prevent as many interruptions as possible.

Finally, the nurse should observe the client for failure to cope with restricted mobility. If the nursing care plan is not improving the client's coping patterns, outside assistance may be required. Recommendations of consultants should be incorporated into the care plan.

Developmental Changes. Ideally, immobilized clients continue normal development. However, this goal is unrealistic for the very young or very old. Nursing interventions can help. Nursing care should stimulate the client mentally, as well as physically, particularly with a young child. Play activities can be incorporated into the nursing care plan. Puzzles, for example, can help to develop fine motor skills, and reading can help the child to learn and develop cognitively. An immobilized child should be placed in a room with children of the same age who are not immobilized, unless a contagious disease is present. Nursing activities can be designed to require the participation of the child. The nurse must recognize extreme changes from the child's normal behavioral patterns. If these behavioral changes continue, the nurse should consult a clinical nurse specialist, counselor, or other health care professional whose specialty is treating children.

Immobilization or restricted mobility of an older adult may require complex care and innovative approaches from the nurse. It is not uncommon for older adult clients to have one or more chronic illnesses. Because of deconditioning associated with age and chronic illness, older adults are at high risk for the hazards of immobility. After a chronically ill older adult has been immobilized, he or she may be unable to regain previous functional abilities.

Inactive older adults are at risk for cognitive changes and depression as a result of immobilization, chronic illnesses, and medications. Therefore the nurse should focus on activities to promote cognitive awareness of the client's surroundings. A calendar and a clock with a large dial should be in the client's room at all times. The calendar should be marked so the client can immediately identify the day and date (see Chapter 38). If the client has pictures and cards in the room, they should be inquired about. Explanations should be given before starting care.

Nursing care should be planned to allow the older adult client to perform as many activities of daily living as possible. The nurse should always remember the older adult client is extremely susceptible to all hazards of immobility. A nursing care plan for an older adult client with limited mobility should be designed to prevent or minimize these hazards, rather than to allow problems to develop and then treat them. The frail older adult client may need his or her position changed every hour instead of every 2 hours and may need more frequent range of joint motion exercises. Not only are the older adults more susceptible to the hazards of immobility, but the consequences of immobility appear more quickly and become severe more rapidly.

Health Promotion. Although many diseases and physical problems can cause or contribute to immobility, it is important to remember that structured exercise programs for immobile clients can enhance their feelings of well-being, as well as their endurance, strength, and health. The advantages of exercise can be seen with coronary clients, who are traditionally bedridden when first admitted to the hospital. Cardiac rehabilitation is standard in most settings for clients who have had myocardial infarctions. Diabetic clients have also been shown to benefit from exercise. Insulin needs may change considerably for diabetics who exercise.

Disuse may account for as much as 50% of functional decline in the older adult population (Webster, 1988). Therefore the older client need not accept muscle deterioration as inevitable and the nurse must be alert to preventing further disuse while the client is ill.

Nurses can contribute to promoting health for many types of clients by encouraging or starting managed ex-

GUIDELINES FOR ASSISTING CLIENTS TO EXERCISE

Teach clients breathing skills to help reduce anxiety and to fully oxygenate tissues.
Always know client's limitations.
Do not force a muscle or a joint during exercise.
Let each client move at own pace.
Keep a record of the client's progess and provide feedback as client exercises.
Posture, body alignment, and good body mechanics should be maintained during exercise.
Monitor vital signs before, during, and after exercise.
Stop exercise if client has pain, shortness of breath, or a change in vital signs.
Clients should wear shoes and comfortable clothing.

ercise programs. Even hospitalized clients can be encouraged to do stretching, ROM, and light walking within the limits of their condition. Postsurgical ambulation might be more enticing if others also participated. A lounge area can be used for ROM exercises where music and company may make the task more interesting to both client and nurse. Distances walked should be measured in feet and yards instead of "walked to the nurses' station and back to room × 1". Guidelines for exercise for the hospitalized client are outlined in the box above.

Evaluation

All nursing interventions for reducing the risks of immobility are evaluated by comparing the client's actual response to the expected outcomes for each goal. If expected outcomes are not achieved, the nurse will need to revise the care plan. The success in meeting each outcome is based on the nurse's use of evaluative measures. Examples of goals, outcomes, and corresponding evaluative measures include:

Goal: Client regains proper or optimal body alignment.

Outcomes

Maintains correct body alignment while sitting, standing, and lying
Maintains ROM in all joints

Evaluative measures

Observing client for improved body alignment while client is lying down, sitting, or standing
Inspecting musculoskeletal system for joint contractures

Goal: Injuries to the client's skin and musculoskeletal system are reduced or prevented.

Outcomes

No reddened areas over bony prominences
Skin ramains intact
Maintains ROM in all joints
Maintains muscle tone

Evaluative measures

Inspecting skin for breakdown at pressure points
Measure range of joint motion
Palpating skin for tenderness and adequate muscle tone

Goal: Client maintains a patent airway.

Outcomes

Patient coughs productively
Client's lungs are free of adventitious sounds

Evaluative measures

Observing client for symmetrical lung expansion
Observing client for productive cough
Inspecting and palpating for retractions and abnormal chest wall motion

Goal: Client achieves optimal lung expansion.

Outcomes

Chest wall excursion is symmetrical and full
Respirations remain under 24 at rest
Client inspires prescribed amount as measured by incentive spirometry
Normal breath sounds heard throughout all lobes

Evaluative measures

Inspecting and palpating for symmetrical lung expansion
Observing client for decreased dyspneic and tachypneic respirations
Observing client for increased lung expansion as demonstrated by incentive spirometry
Auscultating for normal breath sounds in all lung fields

Goal: Client increases activity tolerance.

Outcomes

Client identifies factors that reduce activity tolerance
Client resumes prehospital activities on discharge
Client maintains baseline vital signs
Client paces activity to avoid fatigue

Evaluative measures

Observing client for decreased fatigability
Observing for increased requests for self-care and recreational activities
Palpating pulse after exercise for return to resting level within 10 minutes

Goal: Client achieves optimal elimination patterns.

Outcomes

Client maintains usual bowel routine while hospitalized
Client drinks at least 2000 cc of fluid a day
Client maintains urine output of at least 50 cc an hour

Evaluative measures

Observing client for frequency of elimination patterns consistent with normal schedule

Observing intake and output for adequate fluid balance
Inspecting feces for impaction or constipation
Inspecting urine for foul odor, concentration, and increased sediment
Palpating abdomen for gas and intestinal distention

Goal: Client maintains normal sleep-wake patterns.

Outcomes

Client sleeps uninterrupted
Client demonstrates one relaxation method before retiring
Client is not fatigued after night's rest

Evaluative measures

Observing client for irritability, disorientation, daytime drowsiness
Observing client's nighttime nursing schedule for minimum of 6 hours of uninterrupted sleep
Observing client for reduction in episodes of awakening from sleep
Observing client for ability to fall asleep within 20 to 30 minutes
Observing client for return to sleep within minutes of awakening

Goal: Client achieves socialization.

Outcomes

Client participates in leisure activities
Client participates in organized activities

Evaluative measures

Observing staff for increased social visits to client
Observing client for assertiveness in interaction with staff, friends, and family

Goal: Client achieves completion of self-care activities.

Outcomes

Uses assistive devices for feeding
Uses assistive devices for self-toileting
Participates in self-care by washing upper body

Evaluative measures

Observing client for increased activity tolerance
Observing client for increased ability and willingness to feed, bathe, dress, and complete activities of daily living

Goal: Promoting physical and mental stimulation.

Outcomes

Participates in activities of daily care
Remains alert and oriented to surroundings

Evaluative measures

Observing client for prolonged daytime sleeping
Observing client for increased levels of orientation
Observing client for increased interaction with environment

SUMMARY

Immobilization can adversely affect the client in all dimensions. Although in some cases immobilization is necessary to promote wound healing, proper skeletal alignment, or rest after an illness, it involves many hazards and risks. Nursing care seeks to prevent adverse effects and to minimize them when they occur. Using the nursing process, the nurse assesses physiological, psychosocial, and developmental health needs. The nurse also diagnoses actual or potential problems related to immobilization, and plans and delivers nursing care to meet the client's needs and prevent or resolve problems.

KEY CONCEPTS

Normal physical mobility depends on intact and functioning nervous and musculoskeletal systems.
The risk of disabilities related to immobilization depends on the extent and duration of the immobilization.
Immobility may result from illness or trauma or may be prescribed for therapeutic reasons; in any case it presents hazards in the physiological, psychological, and developmental dimensions.
Pressure ulcers are one of the most common physiological hazards of immobility, but the nurse can take actions to prevent or treat them.
Effects of immobility include depression, behavioral changes, changes in the sleep-wake cycle, decreased coping abilities, and developmental effects.
The nurse uses the nursing process to provide care for clients experiencing or at risk for the adverse effects of immobility.
Assessment focuses on range of joint motion, musculoskeletal status, and complete physical examination for potential adverse effects in all body systems, as well as psychosocial and developmental effects.
After identifying nursing diagnoses, the nurse plans and implements interventions to prevent or minimize the hazards and complications of immobilization.
The use of therapeutic beds and mattresses for preventing or treating pressure ulcers does not eliminate the need for meticulous nursing care.
Maintaining cleanliness of the sore and skin surfaces is of prime importance in treating pressure ulcers.
The primary evaluation criterion for nursing care in the developmental dimension for immobilized clients is the prevention of any measurable decline in functioning or delay in development.

CRITICAL THINKING ACTIVITIES

1. You are caring for an 80-year-old female client with a fractured hip who has been healthy and independent until this hospitalization. What are your priorities for reducing the risk of complications from immobility?
2. You are assigned to care for a 35-year-old male with cancer. He is emaciated and has a stage II pressure ulcer on one heel and a stage III ulcer on his coccyx. What therapeutic bed would be best for him and why?
3. Your client is back from the recovery room after abdominal surgery. She is awake and alert and asking for something for pain. Her respirations are diminished in the lower bases. What other evaluations of her respiratory system must you make?
4. The client you are caring for is on complete bed rest and has a history of thrombophlebitis. You ask the client during your assessment if she is doing her leg exercises. She replies, "No, I don't need to. I have these fancy stockings." She raises her legs and shows you her elastic stockings. What do you reply and why?
5. Mrs. Williams is a client you are supposed to get up for the first time after her abdominal surgery. She has an IV and a Foley catheter. Before surgery she was active and in good health. What assessments must you make before you move her to a chair? How many people will you need to help move her?

References

AHCPR: *Pressure ulcers in adults: prediction and prevention,* Rockville, Md., 1992, U.S. Department of Health and Human Services.

Beckett WS, et al.: Effect of prolonged bedrest on lung volume in normal individuals, *J Appl Physiol* 61(3):919, 1986.

Bergstrom N, Braden BJ, et al.: The Braden scale for predicting pressure sore risk, *Nurs Res* 36:205, 1987.

Booth FW: Effect of limb immobilization on skeletal muscle, *J Appl Physiol* 52:1113, 1982.

Burgio L, Jones LT, and Engel BT: Studying incontinence in an urban nursing home, *J Gerontol Nurs* 15:40-45, 1988.

Clagett GP and Reisch JS: Prevention of venous thromboembolism in general surgical patients, *Ann Surg* 208(2):227, 1988.

Coe WS: Cardiac work and the chair treatment of acute coronary thrombosis, *Ann Intern Med* 40:42, 1954.

Coletta EM and Murphy JB: The complications of immobility in the elderly stroke patient, *JABFP* 5(4):389-397, 1992.

Deitrick JE, et al.: Effects of immobilization upon various metabolic and physiologic functions of normal men, *Am J Med* 4:3, 1948.

Gosnell DJ: Assessment and evaluation of pressure sores, *Nurs Clin North Am* 22(2):399, 1987.

Greenleaf JE: Physiological responses to prolonged bedrest and fluid immersion in humans, *J Appl Physiol* 57(3):619, 1984.

Gröer MW and Shekleton ME: *Basic pathophysiology: a conceptual approach,* ed 3, St. Louis, 1989, Mosby.

Harper CM and Lyles YM: Physiology and complications of bed rest, *J Amer Geriatrics Soc* 36:1047-1054, 1988.

Heath GW, Hagberg JM, et al.: A physiological comparison of young and older endurance athletes, *J Appl Physiol* 51:634-640, 1981.

Hoenig HM and Rubenstein LZ: Hospital associated deconditioning and dysfunction, *J Amer Geriatrics Soc* 39(2):220-222, 1991.

Hogue CC: Mobility. In Schneider EL, Wendland CJ, et al., editors: *The teaching nursing home,* New York, 1985, Raven Press.

Holm K: Immobility and bone loss in the aging adult, *Crit Care Nurs Q* 12(1):46, 1989.

Knight AL: Medical management of pressure sores, *J Fam Pract* 27(1):95, 1988.

McCance KL and Huether SE: *Pathophysiology: the biologic basis for disease in adults and children,* ed 2, St. Louis, 1994, Mosby.

Metzger BL and Therrien B: Effect of position on cardiovascular response during the Valsalva maneuver, *Nurs Res* 39(4):198-202, 1990.

Mobily PR and Kelley LS: Iatrogenesis in the elderly, *J Gerontol Nurs* 17(9):5-10, 1991.

Muller EA: Influence of training and of inactivity on muscle strength, *Arch Phys Med Rehabil* 51:449, 1970.

Norman GM and Gibbs JA: Why walk when you can ride? *J Gerontol Nurs* 17(8):28-35, 1991.

Oullet LL and Rush KL: A synthesis of selected literature on mobility: a basis for studying impaired mobility, *Nurs Diag* 9(2):72-80, 1992.

Rubin M: How bedrest changes perception, *Am J Nurs* 88:53, 1988a.

Rubin M: The physiology of bedrest, *Am J Nurs* 88:50, 1988b.

Sahn S: Continuous lateral rotational therapy and nosocomial infections, *Crit Care* 99(5):1263-1267, 1991.

Tompkins ES: Effect of restricted mobility and dominance on perceived duration, *Nurs Res* 31:333, 1980.

Tyler ML: The respiratory effects of body positioning and immobilization, *Respir Care* 29:472, 1984.

Webster JA: Key to healthy aging, *Gerontol Nurs* 14:8-15, 1988.

Winslow EH: Cardiovascular consequences of bedrest, *Heart Lung* 14(3):236, 1985.

Winslow EH and Weber TM: Progressive exercises to combat hazards of bedrest, *Am J Nurs* 80:440, 1980.

Bibliography

Fernsebner B: Sleep deprivation in patients, *AORN J* 37:35, 1983.

Feustel DE: Pressure sore prevention: age, there is the rub, *Nurs 82* 12:78, 1982.

Goldberg WG and Fitzpatrick JJ: Movement with the aged, *Nurs Res* 29:339, 1980.

Moore SR: Walking for health: a nurse managed activity, *J Gerontol Nurs* 15(7):26-28, 1989.

Pender NJ: *Health promotion in nursing practice,* ed 2, Norwalk, Conn., 1987, Appleton-Lange.

Pires M and Muller A: Detection and management of early tissue pressure indicators: a pictorial essay, *Progressions* 3(3):3, 1991.

Sullivan M: Atrophy and exercise, *J Gerontol Nurs* 13(7):26-31, 1987.

Weinstein LB: Aquatic activity benefits aging, *J Gerontol Nurs* 12(2):6-11, 1986.

24 Skin Integrity

OBJECTIVES

Mastery of content in this chapter will enable the student to:

- Define the key terms listed.
- Describe the economic consequences of pressure ulcers.
- Describe the role of AHCPR and NPUAP multidisciplinary expert panels in pressure ulcer prevention and treatment.
- Describe four risk factors for pressure ulcer development.
- Discuss 10 contributing factors to pressure ulcer formation.
- Discuss the pathogenesis of pressure ulcers.
- List the four classifications of pressure ulcers.
- Complete an assessment for a client with impaired skin integrity.
- List nursing diagnoses associated with impaired skin integrity.
- Develop a nursing care plan for a client with impaired skin integrity.
- List appropriate nursing interventions for a client with impaired skin integrity.
- State evaluation criteria for a client with impaired skin integrity.

KEY TERMS

abnormal reactive hyperemia
activity
AHCPR
anemia
blanching
cachexia
debridement
edema
eschar
friction
induration
maceration
mobility
normal reactive hyperemia
NPUAP
pressure ulcer
shearing force
sloughing
tissue ischemia

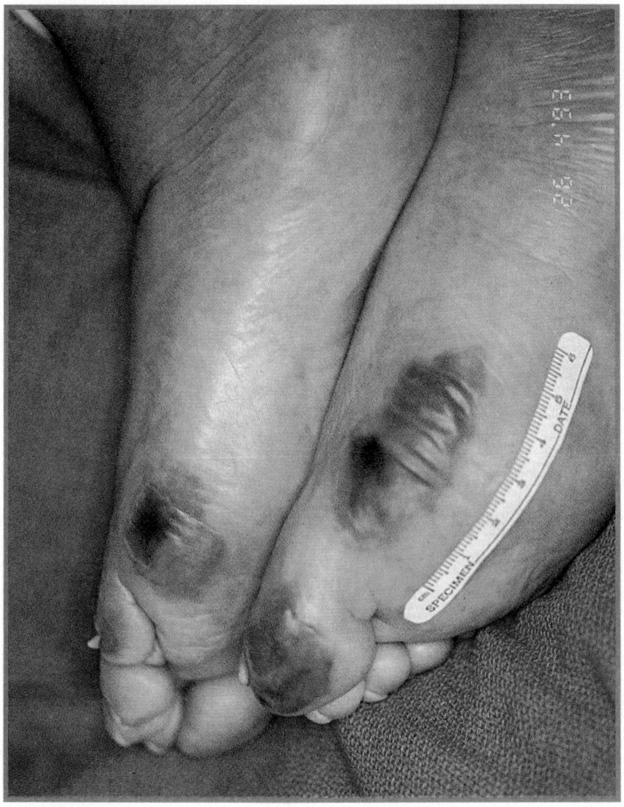

A major aspect of nursing care is the maintenance of skin integrity. Impaired skin integrity can occur from prolonged pressure, irritation of the skin, or immobility, leading to the development of pressure ulcers. A **pressure ulcer** is a localized area of tissue necrosis (death) that tends to develop when soft tissue is compressed between a bony prominence and an external surface for a prolonged period (National Pressure Ulcer Advisory Panel [NPUAP], 1989).

ECONOMIC CONSEQUENCES OF PRESSURE ULCERS

Pressure ulcers have been and continue to be a problem in acute and chronic care settings. The frequency of pressure ulcers ranges from 3% to 14% (NPUAP, 1989). Occurrence among clients admitted to nursing homes is between 2% and 25% (Ferrell, 1993). Furthermore, another study indicated that 58% of clients with pressure ulcers were adults over the age of 65 (Meehan, 1990).

When a pressure ulcer occurs, the length of stay in a hospital and the overall cost of health care increase. The actual cost of treatment is difficult to approximate; estimates for the increased cost of treatment of pressure ulcers are $4000 to $40,000 (Ferrell, 1993). Although treatment of pressure ulcers is more costly than prevention, the preventive measures themselves are expensive (Ferrell, 1993; Kemp, 1993). Thus the use of extra equipment such as special beds and mattresses and increased nursing time needed to administer these measures should be used on those clients identified as high pressure ulcer risk (Gosnell, et al., 1992; Maklebust, 1987).

Prediction and Prevention of Pressure Ulcers

Prediction. Prevention and treatment of pressure ulcers are major nursing priorities. In 1992 the Agency for Health Care Policy Research (AHCPR) developed guidelines for care of adult clients at risk for pressure ulcers. Predictive instruments for pressure ulcer development can identify those clients at highest risk for pressure ulcers. Clients with little risk for pressure ulcer development are spared the unnecessary expense of preventive treatments and the risk of complications (Stotts, 1988). Identifying clients at risk helps to reduce health care costs (Gosnell, et al., 1992; Norton,

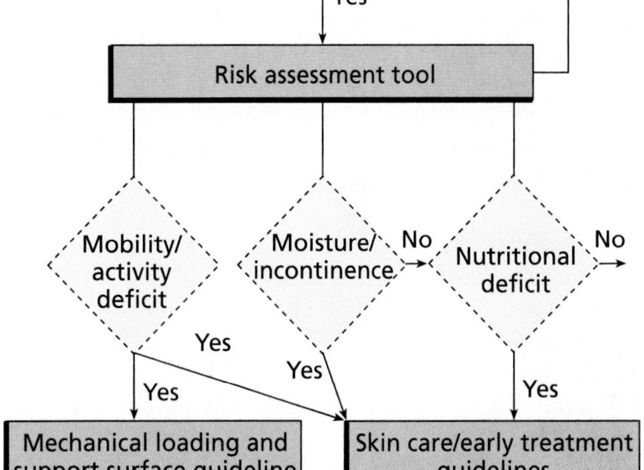

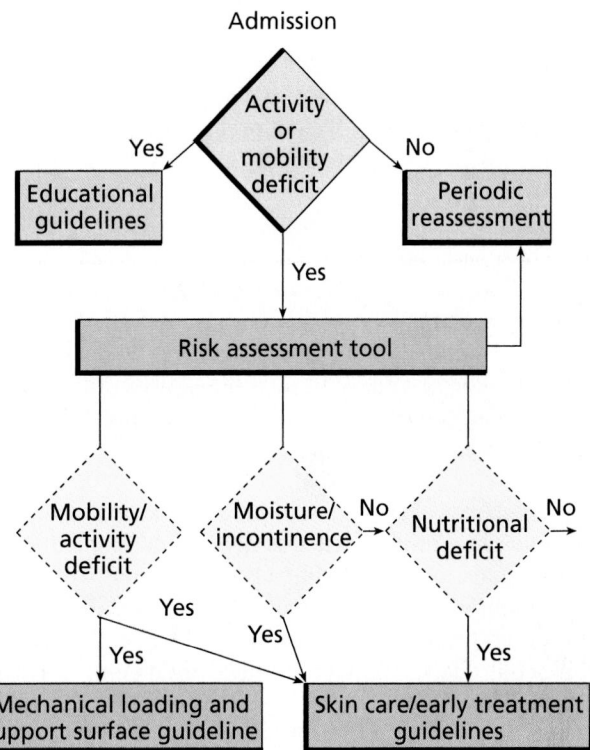

FIGURE 24-1 Pressure ulcer prediction and prevention algorithm. (Agency for Health Care Policy and Research (AHCPR): *Pressure ulcers in adults: prediction and prevention,* US Department of Health and Human Services, Public Health Service, Rockville, Md., 1992, Pub Nos. 92-0047, p. 31.)

table 24-1

NORTON RISK ASSESSMENT SCALE

		Physical condition	Mental condition	Activity	Mobility	Incontinent	
		Good 4 Fair 3 Poor 2 Very Bad 1	Alert 4 Apathetic 3 Confused 2 Stupor 1	Ambulant 4 Walk/help 3 Chairbound 2 Bad 1	Full 4 Sl. limited 3 V. limited 2 Immobile 1	Not 4 Occasional 3 Usually/Urine 2 Doubly 1	TOTAL SCORE
Name	Date						

From Centre for Policy on Ageing, London, England.

McLaren, Exton-Smith, 1962). The Norton Scale (Table 24-1) is designed to score five risk factors—physical condition, mental condition, activity, mobility, and continence. The range is 5 to 20, with a lower score indicating a higher risk for pressure ulcer development. This tool also offers descriptive information regarding potential risk factors (Bryant, 1992).

A second tool is the Braden Scale. The Braden Scale is composed of six subscales: sensory perception, moisture, activity, mobility, nutrition, and friction and shear (Table 24-2). A hospitalized adult with a score of 16 or below is considered at risk. In older clients, a score of 17 or 18 may be a more efficient prediction of risk (Bryant, et al., 1992). This instrument is highly reliable in the identification of clients at greatest risk for pressure ulcers (Bergstrom, et al., 1987a, 1987b).

These are only two examples of risk assessment tools. The Gosnell and Knoll instruments are also effective in pressure ulcer prediction. The overall objective of predictive instruments is to effectively and efficiently identify those clients with the greatest risk for pressure ulcer development. From this, risk identification and plan of care is devised (Figure 24-1).

Prevention. Prevention of pressure ulcers is a priority in caring for clients and is not limited to clients with restrictions in mobility. Impaired skin integrity is not a problem in healthy, immobilized individuals but is a serious and potentially devastating problem in the ill or debilitated client (AHCPR, 1992; Shekleton, Litwack, 1991).

PRESSURE ULCERS

Pressure ulcer, pressure sore, decubitus ulcer, and *bedsore* are terms used to describe impaired skin integrity (Figure 24-2). *Pressure ulcer* is the most current term and is consistent with the NPUAP and the AHCPR's Pressure Ulcer Guidelines Panel (Maklebust, 1991a, 1991b; Green, Katz, 1991; Hastings, 1991; AHCPR, 1992). An ill client experiencing decreased mobility, impaired neurological functioning, decreased sensory perception, or decreased circulation is at risk for pressure ulcer development.

Tissues receive oxygen and nutrients and eliminate metabolic wastes via the blood. Any factor that interferes with this affects cellular metabolism and the function or life of the cell. Pressure affects cellular metabolism by decreasing or obliterating tissue circulation, resulting in tissue ischemia.

Tissue ischemia is the localized absence of blood or a major reduction of blood flow resulting from mechan-

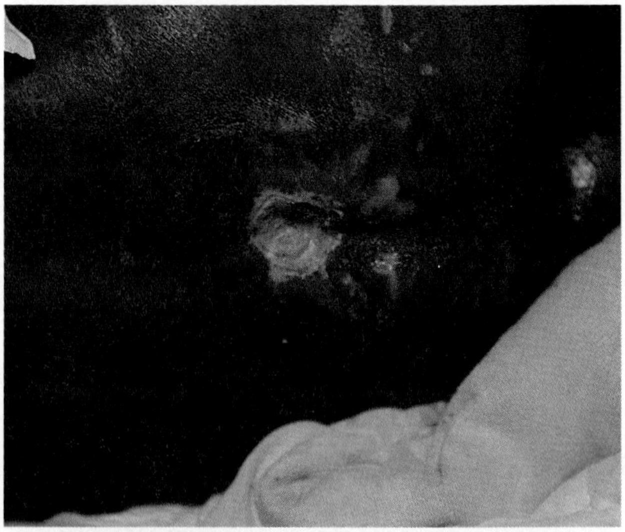

FIGURE 24-2 Pressure ulcer with tissue necrosis.

table 24-2

BRADEN SCALE FOR PREDICTING PRESSURE SORE RISK

	1 Point	2 Points	3 Points	4 Points
SENSORY PERCEPTION				
Ability to respond meaningfully to pressure-related discomfort	**Completely limited:** Unresponsive (does not moan, flinch, or grasp) to painful stimuli because of diminished level of consciousness or sedation. **or** Limited ability to feel pain over most of body surface.	**Very limited:** Responds only to painful stimuli. Cannot communicate discomfort except by moaning or restlessness. **or** Has a sensory impairment that limits the ability to feel pain or discomfort over half of body.	**Slightly limited:** Responds to verbal commands but cannot always communicate discomfort or need to be turned. **or** Has some sensory impairment, which limits its ability to feel pain or discomfort in 1 or 2 extremities.	**No impairment:** Responds to verbal commands. Has no sensory deficit that would limit ability to feel or voice pain or discomfort.
MOISTURE				
Degree to which skin is exposed to moisture	**Constantly moist:** Skin is kept moist almost constantly by perspiration, urine, etc. Dampness is detected every time patient is moved or turned.	**Very moist:** Skin is often, but not always, moist. Linen must be changed at least once a shift.	**Occasionally moist:** Skin is occasionally moist, requiring an extra linen change approximately once a day.	**Rarely moist:** Skin is usually dry; linen requires changing only at routine intervals.
ACTIVITY				
Degree of physical activity	**Bedfast:** Confined to bed.	**Chairfast:** Ability to walk severely limited or nonexistent. Cannot bear own weight and/or must be assisted into chair or wheelchair.	**Walks occasionally:** Walks occasionally during day, but for very short distances, with or without assistance. Spends majority of each shift in bed or chair.	**Walks frequently:** Walks outside the room at least twice a day and inside room at least once every 2 hours during waking hours.
MOBILITY				
Ability to change and control body position	**Completely immobile:** Does not make even slight changes in body or extremity position without assistance.	**Very limited:** Makes occasional slight changes in body or extremity position but unable to make frequent or significant changes independently.	**Slightly limited:** Makes frequent though slight changes in body or extremity position independently.	**No limitations:** Makes major and frequent changes in position without assistance.

Instructions: Score client in each of the six subscales. Maximum score is 23, indicating little or no risk. A score of ≤ 16 indicates "at risk"; ≤ 9 indicates high risk.

Continued.

table 24-2—cont'd

BRADEN SCALE FOR PREDICTING PRESSURE SORE RISK

	1 Point	2 Points	3 Points	4 Points
NUTRITION				
Usual food intake pattern	**Very poor:** Never eats a complete meal. Rarely eats more than one third of any food offered. Eats 2 servings or less of protein (meat or dairy products) per day. Takes fluids poorly. Does not take a liquid dietary supplement. **or** Is NPO and/or maintained on clear liquids or IVs for more than 5 days.	**Probably inadequate:** Rarely eats a complete meal and generally eats only about half of any food offered. Protein intake includes only 3 servings of meat or dairy products per day. Occasionally will take a dietary supplement. **or** Receives less than optimal amount of liquid diet or tube feeding.	**Adequate:** Eats over half of most meals. Eats a total of 4 servings of protein (meat, dairy products) each day. Occasionally will refuse a meal, but will usually take a supplement if offered. **or** Is on a tube-feeding or TPN regimen that probably meets most of nutritional needs.	Excellent: Eats most of every meal. Never refuses a meal. Usually eats a total of 4 or more servings of meat and dairy products. Occasionally eats between meals. Does not require supplements.
FRICTION AND SHEAR	**Problem:** Requires moderate to maximal assistance in moving. Complete lifting without sliding against sheets is impossible. Frequently slides down in bed or chair, requiring frequent repositioning with maximal assistance. Spasticity, contractions, or agitation leads to almost constant friction.	**Potential problem:** Moves feebly or requires minimal assistance. During a move skin probably slides to some extent against sheets, chair, restraints, or other devices. Maintains relatively good position in chair or bed most of the time but occasionally slides down.	**No apparent problem:** Moves in bed and in chair independently and has sufficient muscle strength to sit up completely during move. Maintains good position in bed or chair at all times.	

Copyright 1988. Used with permission of Barbara Braden, Ph.D., R.N., Professor, Creighton University School of Nursing, Omaha, Nebraska.
Instructions: Score client in each of the six subscales. Maximum score is 23, indicating little or no risk. A score of ≤ 16 indicates "at risk"; ≤ 9 indicates high risk.

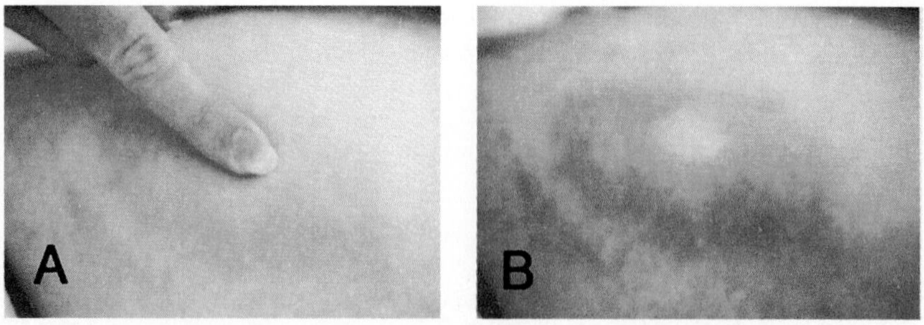

FIGURE 24-3 A, Reactive hyperemia. **B,** Blanches with fingertip pressure. (From Pires M, Muller A: *Progressions* 3(3):3, 1991.)

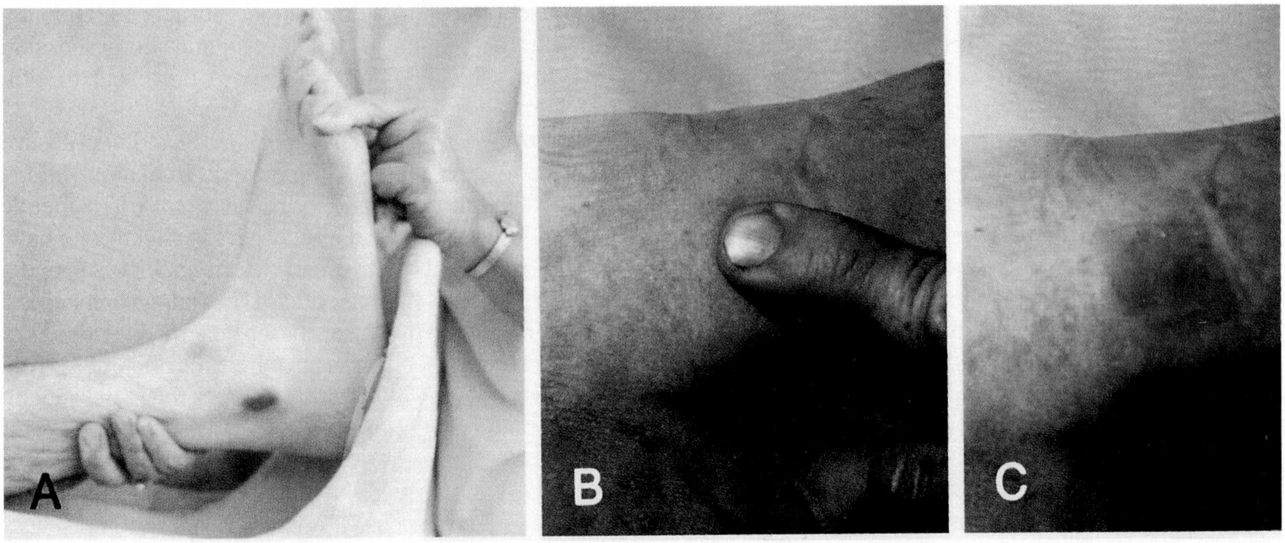

FIGURE 24-4 **A,** Abnormal reactive hyperemia. **B** and **C,** In abnormal reactive hyperemia the area is much darker than the surrounding skin and does not blanch with fingertip pressure. (From Pires M, Muller A: *Progressions* 3(3):3, 1991.)

ical obstruction (Pires, Muller, 1991). The reduction in blood flow causes blanching. **Blanching** is seen when the normal red tones of the skin are absent. Tissue damage occurs when the capillary closing pressure exceeds the normal range of 16 to 32 mm Hg (Kosiak, 1959; Maklebust, 1987).

After a period of ischemia the skin can undergo one of two hyperemic changes. **Normal reactive hyperemia** (redness) is the visible effect of localized vasodilation, the body's normal response to lack of blood flow to the underlying tissue (Figure 24-3, *A*). The area blanches with fingertip pressure (Figure 24-3, *B*). When a client is lying or sitting, the weight of the body is heavily placed on bony prominences. When the pressure is removed, there is a period of reactive hyperemia, or a sudden increase in blood flow to the region. Reactive hyperemia, which lasts less than 1 hour, is a compensatory response and is effective only if the pressure on the skin is removed before necrosis or damage occurs. **Abnormal reactive hyperemia** is an excessive vasodilation and induration in response to pressure. The skin appears bright pink to red. The **induration** is an area of localized edema under the skin. Abnormal reactive hyperemia (Figure 24-4) can last more than 1 hour up to 2 weeks after the removal of pressure (Pires, Muller, 1991).

Contributing Factors to Pressure Ulcer Formation

Impaired skin integrity resulting in pressure ulcers is primarily the result of prolonged pressure. However, additional factors can further increase the client's risk for pressure ulcer development. These include shearing force, moisture, poor nutrition, anemia, infection, fever, impaired peripheral circulation, obesity, cachexia, and age.

Shearing force is the pressure exerted against the skin when a client is moved or repositioned in bed by being pulled or being allowed to slide down in bed (Figure 24-5). When a shearing force is present, the skin and subcutaneous layers adhere to the surface of the bed, and the layers of muscle and even the bones slide in the direction of body movement. The underlying tissue capillaries are compressed and severed by the pressure (Knight, 1988; Bennett, Lee, 1988). As a result, minute layers of bleeding and necrosis occur deep within the tissue layers. Subcutaneous fat is more vulnerable to the effects of shearing and the resultant pressure from the underlying bony structure. Eventually a tract opens to the skin to allow drainage from the necrotic area.

Friction is an injury to the skin that has the appearance of an abrasion. Friction results from two surfaces

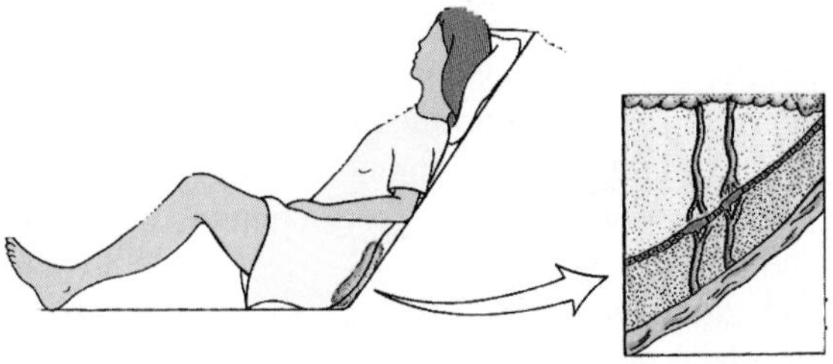

FIGURE 24-5 Diagrammatic sketch of shearing force exerted against sacral area.

rubbing against one another. The body surfaces most at risk to friction are the elbows and heels because abrasion of these surfaces occur when they are rubbed against the sheets during repositioning. Injury from friction is shallow without necrosis and is limited to the epidermis (Bryant, 1992).

Moisture on the skin increases the risk of ulcer formation. Moisture reduces the skin's resistance to other physical factors such as pressure or shearing force. Moisture can originate from wound drainage, perspiration, condensation from humidified oxygen-delivery systems, vomitus, and incontinence. The susceptibility to pressure ulcer formation increases with the duration of the exposure to moisture.

Poor nutrition increases the risk of pressure ulcer formation. Clients with poor nutrition experience muscle atrophy and decreases in subcutaneous tissue (see Chapter 31). Because of these changes, less tissue is present to serve as padding between the skin and underlying bone (Breslow, et al., 1993). Therefore the effects of pressure are increased on remaining tissue. The client can have protein deficiency and negative nitrogen balance and have an inadequate intake of vitamin C (Shekleton, Litwack, 1991). Poor nutritional status may be overlooked if the client has a weight equal to or above the ideal body weight (IBW).

Poor nutrition alters fluid and electrolyte balance. In clients with severe protein loss, hypoalbuminemia (serum albumin below 3.0 g/100 ml) leads to a shift of fluid from the extracellular fluid volume to the tissues, resulting in edema (Breslow, et al., 1993; Steinberg, 1990). **Edema** increases the affected tissue's risk for pressure ulcers. The blood supply to the edematous tissue is decreased, and waste products remain because of the changing pressures in the capillary circulation and capillary bed (Shekleton, Litwack, 1991). **Anemia** increases risk for pressure ulcer formation because decreased levels of hemoglobin reduce the oxygen-carrying capacity of the blood and the amount of oxygen available to tissues.

Optimal nutritional status can lower clients' risks for pressure ulcers. Adequate nutritional support is difficult to achieve by calorie ranges alone. A client's nutritional status depends on the client's sex, age, weight, underlying illnesses, and presence and severity of wounds. However, general guidelines assist in determining adequate nutrition. A healthy adult client requires 0.8 g protein/kilogram every 24 hours; however, in the presence of a wound this requirement must increase (Bryant, 1992). Continuous assessment of physical and laboratory data can alert the nurse to changes in nutritional status.

Infection results from the presence of pathogens in the body. A client with an infection usually has a fever. Infection and *fever* increase the metabolic needs of the body, making an already hypoxic tissue more susceptible to ischemic injury (Shekleton, Litwack, 1991). In addition, fever results in diaphoresis and increased skin moisture, which further predispose the client to skin breakdown.

Impaired peripheral circulation is related to pressure ulcer development. With decreased circulation the tissue becomes hypoxic and more susceptible to ischemic damage. Impaired circulation occurs in clients who have peripheral vascular diseases, who are in shock, spend a prolonged period of time on hard operating room tables, or who are receiving vasopressor-type medications.

Obesity can speed pressure ulcer development. Adipose tissue in small quantities protects the skin by cushioning bony prominences against pressure. However, adipose tissue is poorly vascularized, and the adipose and underlying tissues are more susceptible to ischemic damage. When excessive adipose is present, the client is more susceptible to pressure ulcers.

Cachexia is generalized ill health and malnutrition, marked by weakness and emaciation. It is usually associated with severe diseases such as cancer and end-stage cardiopulmonary or renal diseases. This condition increases the client's risk for pressure ulcers. Basically the cachexic client has lost the adipose tissue necessary to protect bony prominences from pressure.

Pressure ulcer development occurs more frequently in clients over 65 years of age. Studies by Stotts (1988), Kane, et al. (1994), and Gosnell, et al. (1992) note a greater incidence of ulcer development in this population.

This section lists those factors contributing to the risk of pressure ulcers. However, when these factors occur in combination over prolonged periods, the risk increases.

Pathogenesis of Pressure Ulcers

A pressure ulcer occurs as a result of an intensity-time-pressure relationship (Stotts, 1988). If this pressure is greater than 32 mm Hg and remains unrelieved to the point of hypoxia, the vessels collapse and thrombose (develop a clot) (Bergstrom, 1992). The greater the intensity and duration of the pressure, the greater the incidence of ulcer formation. The skin and subcutaneous tissue can tolerate some pressure. However, externally applied pressure greater than the pressure in the capillary bed decreases or obliterates blood flow to adjacent tissues. These tissues become hypoxic, and ischemic injury results. Second, duration influences the detrimental effects of pressure. Low intensity pressures over a long period of time can be just as damaging to the tissue as high intensity pressure over short periods of time (Bryant, 1992). If the pressure is relieved before the critical point, circulation to the affected tissues is restored through the physiological mechanism of reactive hyperemia. The coccyx-sacral areas, heels, and elbows are the most susceptible (Gosnell, et al., 1992; Maklebust, 1987). Last, tissue tolerance to pressure determines ulcer development. Tissue tolerance is influenced by the ability of the skin and underlying structures to work together to offset the load (pressure) from the surface of the tissues to the underlying skeleton (Bryant, 1992). The effect of pressure can be increased by unequal distribution of body weight.

The compensatory response of the tissues to ischemia, reactive hyperemia, permits ischemic tissue to be flooded with blood when pressure is removed. Increased blood flow increases delivery of oxygen and nu-

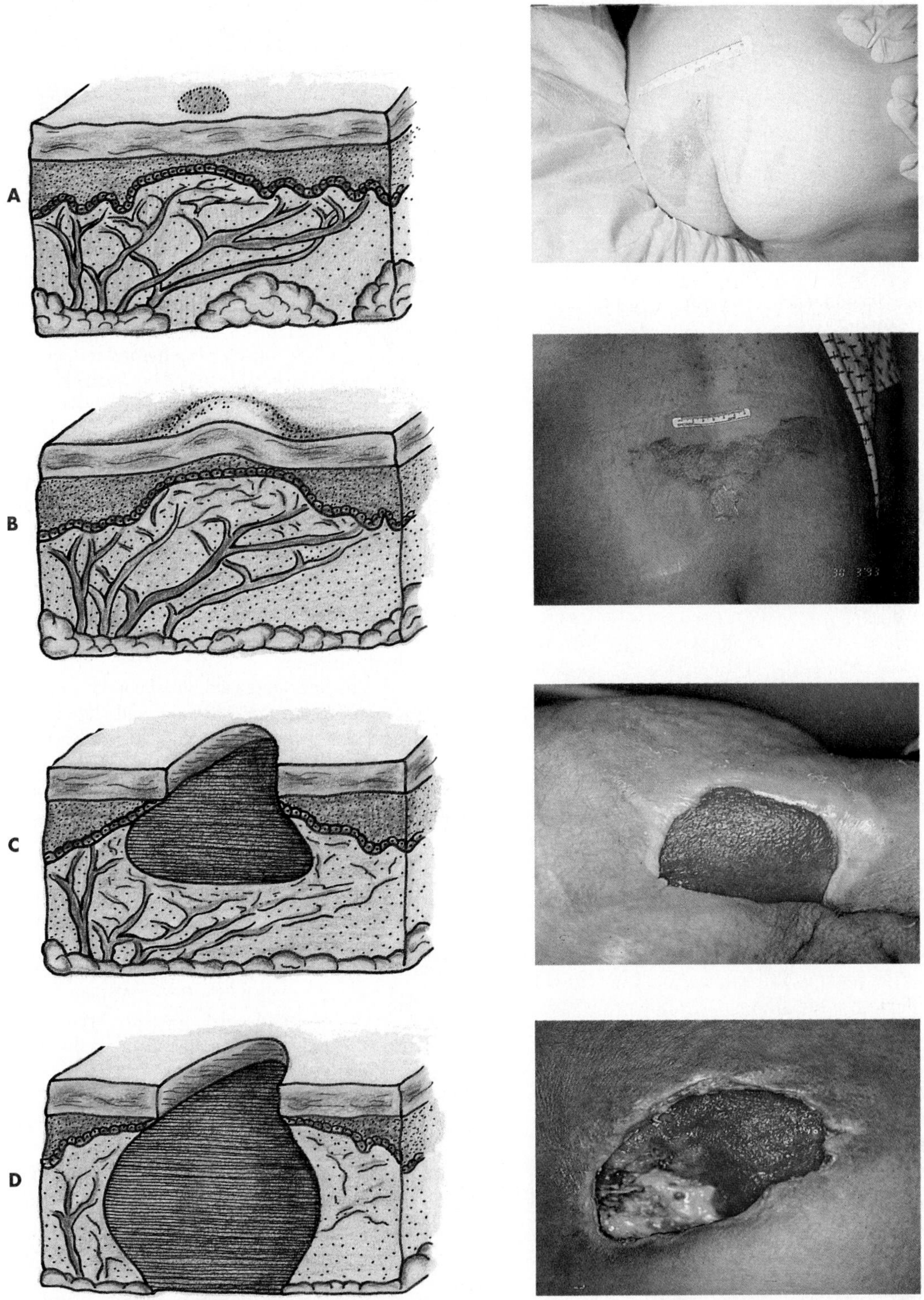

FIGURE 24-6 **A,** Stage I pressure ulcer. **B,** Stage II pressure ulcer. **C,** Stage III pressure ulcer. **D,** Stage IV pressure ulcer. (Photos from Laurel Wiersema, RN, MSN, Clinical Nurse Specialist, Barnes Hospital, St. Louis, MO.)

procedure 24-1

ASSESSMENT FOR RISK OF PRESSURE ULCER DEVELOPMENT

Steps	Rationale
1. Identify client's risk for pressure ulcer formation:	Determines need to administer preventive care and use topical agents for existing ulcers.
a. Paralysis or immobilization caused by restrictive devices	Client is unable to turn or reposition independently.
b. Sensory loss	Client feels no discomfort from pressure.
c. Circulatory disorders	Reduce perfusion of skin's tissue layers.
d. Decreased level of consciousness, sedation, or anesthesia	Client is unable to perceive pressure to turn or reposition independently.
e. Shearing force	Causes skin and underlying subcutaneous layers to adhere to surface of bed. Trauma occurs to underlying tissues.
f. Moisture: incontinence, perspiration, wound drainage, or vomitus	Reduces skin's resistance to pressure from shearing force.
g. Malnutrition	Can lead to weight loss, muscle atrophy, and reduced tissue mass. Less tissue is available to pad between skin and underlying bone. Poor protein, vitamin, and caloric intake limit wound-healing capabilities.
h. Anemia	Decreased hemoglobin level reduces oxygen-carrying capacity of blood and amount of oxygen available to tissues.
i. Infection	Causes increase in metabolic demands of tissues. Accompanying diaphoresis leaves skin moist.
j. Obesity	Poorly vascularized excess adipose tissue is more susceptible to pressure. Body weight against bony prominences places underlying skin at risk for breakdown.
k. Cachexia	Causes loss of adipose tissue that protects bony prominences from pressure.
l. Hydration: edema or dehydration	Edematous tissue has decreased blood supply and thereby is less tolerant of pressure, friction, and shearing force. Dehydrated skin is less elastic, and skin turgor is poor.
m. Older adulthood	Skin is less elastic and drier; tissue mass is reduced.
n. Existing pressure ulcers	Limits surfaces available for position changes, placing available tissues at increased risk.
2. Assess condition of skin over regions of pressure. Look for the following characteristics:	
a. Normal or abnormal reactive hyperemia	May indicate that tissue was under pressure. Normal reactive hyperemia is normal physiological response to hypoxemia. In dark-skinned persons, skin that was under pressure will appear darker than surrounding skin and may even take on purplish hue (Pires, Muller, 1991). Normal reactive hyperemia over pressure area lasts less than 1 hr. Affected area blanches at fingertip pressure (Pires, Muller, 1991). Abnormal reactive hyperemia lasts longer than 1 hr. Surrounding tissue does not blanch (Pires, Muller, 1991).
b. Blanching	Blanching is normal, expected response.
c. Induration	Localized edema beneath the skin surface, induration commonly occurs with abnormal reactive hyperemia (Pires, Muller, 1991).
d. Pallor and mottling	Persistent hypoxia in tissues that were under pressure is abnormal physiological response.
e. Absence of superficial skin layers	Represents early pressure ulcer formation.
f. Scabs, blisters, or pimples	Early signs of skin damage, but damage to underlying tissue may be more progressive (Pires, Muller, 1991).

Steps	Rationale
3. Assess client for areas of potential pressure:	Clients at high risk have multiple sites of pressure necrosis.
a. Nares	Pressure can occur from nasogastric tube or nasal O_2 cannula.
b. Tongue, lips	Oral airway and endotracheal tube are high-risk locations.
c. Intravenous sites (especially long-term access sites)	Stress occurs at catheter exit sites.
d. Drainage tubes	There is stress against tissue at exit site.
e. Foley catheter	There is pressure against labia, especially with edema.
4. Observe client for preferred positions when in bed or chair.	Weight of body will be placed on bony prominences. Contractures (flexion and fixation of joint) may result in pressure exerted in unexpected places. Phenomenon is best assessed through observation.
5. Observe client's mobility and ability to initiate and assist with position changes.	Potential for friction and shear increases when client is completely dependent for position changes.
6. Obtain risk score: a. Norton Scale (see Table 24-1) b. Braden Scale (see Table 24-2)	Risk score depends on instrument used and predicts client's need for preventive care (AHCPR, 1992).
7. Monitor length of time any area of redness persists:	Redness usually persists for half of time hypoxia occurred. For example, redness lasts 15 min, so hypoxia lasted approximately 30 min.
a. Determine appropriate turning interval, which should be (turning interval − hypoxia time = suggested interval)	For example, turning interval is 2 hr, hypoxia time is 30 min. 2 hr − 30 min = 1 ½ hr suggested turning interval.
b. Use pressure-relief device, if indicated	Short turning intervals (e.g., 1-2 hr) may not be realistic. Therefore use of device is recommended.
8. Obtain nutritional assessment data, including serum albumin level, total protein level, hemoglobin level, and IBW percentage (see Chapter 31).	Poor nutritional status decreases skin's and underlying tissue's tolerance to pressure, friction, and shearing force (Hanan, Scheele, 1991).
9. Assess client's and family's understanding of risks for pressure ulcers.	Provides opportunity to begin prevention education.
10. Document assessment findings.	Provides baseline data for skin integrity and risk of pressure ulcer development.

trients to tissue. The metabolic debt resulting from pressure can then be met. Healthy equilibrium is restored, and necrosis of the compressed tissue is avoided (Kosiak, 1959; Maklebust, 1991a, 1991b; Pires, Muller, 1991). Reactive hyperemia is effective only if pressure is removed before damage occurs.

Stages of Pressure Ulcers. Pressure ulcers may occur initially in the superficial layers of the skin. In 1992 the Agency for Health Care Policy and Research's Pressure Ulcer Guideline Panel revised the classification of pressure ulcers (AHCPR, 1992).

I. Nonblanchable erythema of the intact skin, the heralding lesion of skin ulceration, occurs (Figure 24-6, *A*).

II. Partial-thickness skin loss involves epidermis and/or dermis. Ulcer is superficial and presents clinically as an abrasion, blister, or shallow crater (Figure 24-6, *B*).

III. Full-thickness skin loss involves damage or necrosis of subcutaneous tissue that may extend down to but not through the underlying fascia. Ulcer presents clinically as a deep crater with or without undermining of adjacent tissue (Figure 24-6, *C*).

IV. Full-thickness skin loss occurs with extensive destruction, tissue necrosis, or damage to muscle, bone, or supporting structures (Figure 24-6, *D*).

NURSING PROCESS AND PRESSURE ULCERS

Assessment

Baseline and continual assessment data provide critical information about the client's skin integrity and the increased risk for pressure ulcer development. Assessment for pressure ulcers (Procedure 24-1) is not limited to the skin. Pressure ulcers have multiple etiological factors.

Predictive Measures. A benefit of the predictive instruments is to increase the nurses' early detection of clients at greatest risk for ulcer development. Once these clients are identified, appropriate interventions are instituted to maintain skin integrity.

It is best to use predictive instruments to assess risks for impaired skin integrity in those clients who are immobilized, malnourished, incontinent, or paralyzed. Prompt identification of such clients enables nurses to individualize costly resources to appropriate clients, and reduce their risk.

Skin. Assessment for tissue pressure indicators includes visual and tactile inspection of the skin (Pires, Muller, 1991). Baseline assessment is performed to determine the client's normal skin characteristics and any actual or potential areas of breakdown. The neurologically impaired client, the chronically ill client in long-term care, the client with diminished mental status

GERONTOLOGIC NURSING PRACTICES FOR THE CLIENT WITH IMPAIRED SKIN INTEGRITY

- Older adult's skin is less tolerant to pressure, friction, and shear because of decreased elasticity due to normal aging.*
- The older adult has decreased number of sweat glands, leaving the skin dry and less tolerant to shear and friction.
- Impaired skin integrity is a high risk to older adults; it is among the five most common nursing diagnoses for older adult clients in long-term care facilities.†
- Dermis of the older adult's skin is thinner due to the normal absence of subcutaneous fat, therefore making the older adult more susceptible to skin breakdown.*
- After the age of 50 epidermal cell renewal reduces by one third, and as a result wound healing is approximately 50% slower than a 35-year-old adult.*
- In the presence of chronic coronary or peripheral vascular diseases circulation to the extremities is reduced.

*From Ebersole P, Hess P: *Toward healthy aging: human needs and nursing response,* ed 3, St. Louis, 1990, Mosby.
†From Goodridge DM: Pressure ulcer risk assessment tools: what's new for gerontological nurses, *J Gerontol Nurs* 19(1):23, 1993.

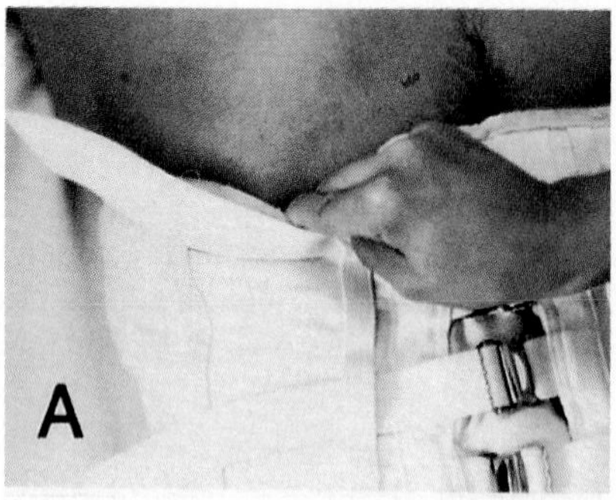

FIGURE 24-7 Benign devices such as this corset may result in scabbing or blistering, resulting from external pressure. (From Pires M, Muller A: *Progressions* 3(3):3, 1991.)

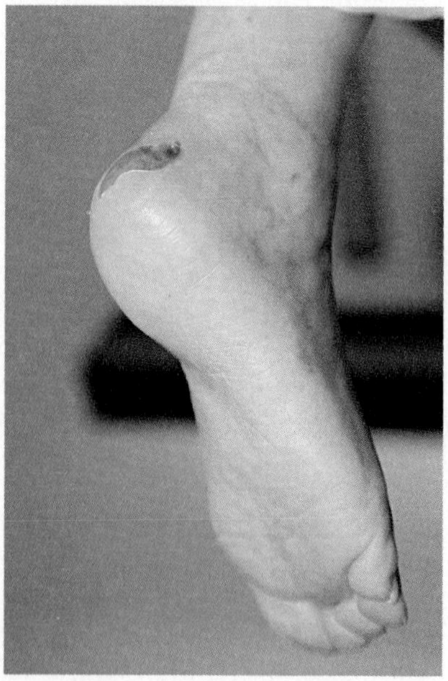

FIGURE 24-8 Formation of pressure ulcer on heel resulting from external pressure from mattress of bed.

(Gosnell, 1987), and the orthopedic client have increased potential for developing pressure ulcers. The skin of an older adult client is more fragile and has an increased risk for skin breakdown (see gerontologic nursing practice guidelines box on p. 590). The nurse pays particular attention to areas exposed to casts, traction, or splints. The frequency of systematic pressure assessment should occur at least once a day on those clients at greater risk for pressure ulcer development (AHCPR, 1992). Assessment also depends on the schedule of appliance application and the skin's response to the external pressure (Figures 24-7 and 24-8).

When hyperemia is noted, the nurse documents its location, size, and color and reassesses the area after 1 hour. If the nurse suspects abnormal reactive hyperemia, outlining the affected area with a marker makes reassessment easier. Another early warning sign of pressure damage is a blister or pimple over the weight-bearing area with possible hyperemia. Pires and Muller (1991) report that a frequently overlooked sign of early pressure is a scabbing over of the weight-bearing areas in the absence of trauma (Figure 24-9). All of these signs are very early indicators of impaired skin integrity, but damage to the underlying tissue may be more progressive. The nurse palpates the tissues adjacent to the observed area to acquire further data about induration and the damage to the skin and underlying tissues.

The nurse assesses for blanching with return to normal skin tones. The nurse also notes changes in color, temperature, and hardness of the surrounding skin and tissues (Pires, Muller, 1991).

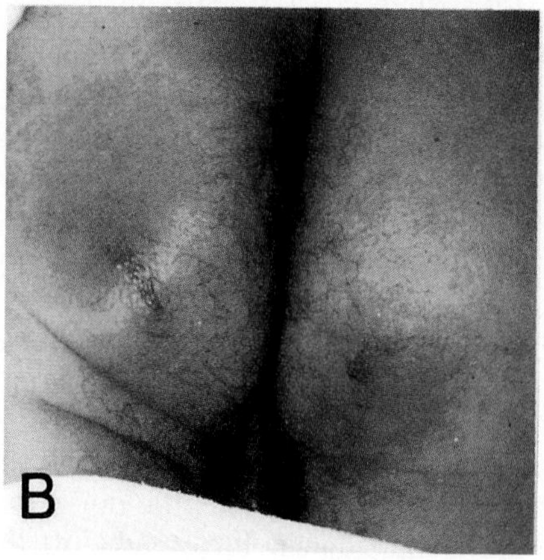

FIGURE 24-9 Scabbing over bony prominences is a sign of excessive pressure. (From Pires M, Muller M: *Progressions* 3(3):3, 1991.)

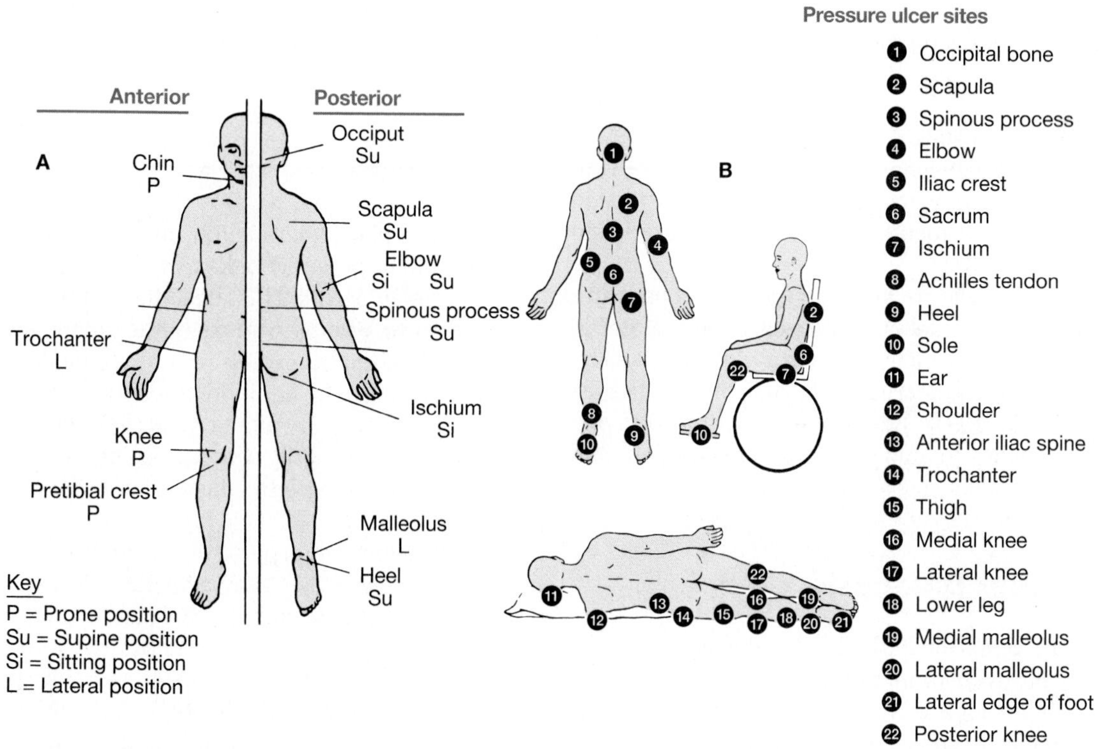

FIGURE 24-10 **A,** Bony prominence most frequently underlying pressure ulcer. **B,** Pressure ulcer sites. (From Trelease CC: *Ostomy/Wound Manage* 20:46, 1988.)

The nurse includes visual and tactile inspection over the body areas most frequently at risk for pressure ulcer development (Figure 24-10). When a client lays in bed or sits in a chair, body weight is heavily placed on certain bony prominences. Body surfaces subjected to the greatest weight or pressure are at greatest risk for decubitus ulcer formation.

Mobility. Assessment includes documenting level of mobility and the potential effects of impaired mobility on skin integrity. Assessment of mobility should also include obtaining data regarding the quality of muscle tone and strength. For example, the nurse determines whether the client can lift the weight off the ischial tuberosities and can roll the body to a side-lying position. The client may have adequate range of motion (ROM) to independently move into a more protective position. Finally the nurse notes the client's activity tolerance (see Chapter 23).

Mobility must be assessed as part of baseline data. If the client has some degree of independence in mobility the nurse reinforces the frequency of position changes and measures to relieve pressure.

Nutritional Status. An assessment of the client's nutritional status should be an integral part of the initial assessment data for clients at risk for impaired skin integrity (see Chapter 31). Albumin is a frequently measured variable used to evaluate the client's protein status. A client with a serum albumin level below 3.0 g/100 ml or body weight equal to more than 10% of ideal are at greater risk for pressure ulcers. Although serum albumin levels are slow to reflect changes in visceral proteins, they are the best predictors of malnutrition in all age-groups (Breslow, 1993; Hanan, Scheele, 1991). Other laboratory data such as white blood cells, serum transferrin, hemoglobin, and hematocrit are essential to the nutritional assessment of clients with impaired skin integrity (Chapter 31).

Total protein levels are also correlated with pressure ulcer development. Total protein levels below 5.4 g/100 ml decrease colloid osmotic pressure, which leads to interstitial edema and decreased oxygen to the tissues (Hanan, Scheele, 1991). Edema decreases the skin and underlying tissue's tolerance to pressure, friction, and shearing force.

Nursing Diagnosis

A client with actual or high risk for impaired skin integrity may have one or more nursing diagnoses related to the condition (see box above). Assessment reveals clusters of data that indicate whether an actual or a risk for impaired skin integrity exists. Assessment also identifies pertinent defining characteristics that support the diagnostic label and probable cause of the diagnosis. Identification of the probable cause is important to planning client-centered goals and subsequent nursing interventions.

NURSING DIAGNOSES FOR SKIN INTEGRITY

High risk for infection
Impaired physical mobility
Impaired skin integrity
High risk for impaired skin integrity
Sensory/perceptual alterations (kinesthetic, tactile)
Tissue perfusion: altered (peripheral)

Clients with the nursing diagnosis *high risk for impaired skin integrity* are in a state in which their skin is at risk of being adversely altered. The defining characteristics that support the diagnostic label are the presence of thermal, chemical, mechanical, or secretory irritants to the skin, as well as those clients whose mobility, circulation, sensation, or perception are altered (Kim, et al., 1993).

A client may have one or more problems related to impaired skin integrity, such as impaired mobility, diaphoresis, wound drainage, or incontinence. Many alterations in physiological functioning are related to skin breakdown, and impaired functioning in one system may affect another. For example, urinary stasis in the kidney can quickly lead to kidney infection, which produces fever and diaphoresis. The resulting increased skin moisture may then increase the potential for skin breakdown.

Planning

The nurse plans therapeutic interventions for clients with actual or potential risks to skin integrity (see nursing care plan on p. 593). These therapies are designed according to severity of risks to the client, and the plan is individualized according to developmental stage and level of health. In addition, the nurse must develop client-centered goals aimed at preventing or reducing impaired skin integrity. Care planning is individualized to the client, taking into consideration the client's most immediate needs.

Other client factors to be considered when setting priorities include everyday activities, family, and developmental stage. The nurse may need the help of another health team member, such as a physical or occupational therapist, when considering mobility needs. These factors are important for clients in institutional and in home settings. Discharge planning is begun when a client enters the health care system. Anticipating the client's discharge from an institution, a referral to a

SAMPLE NURSING CARE PLAN
Impaired Skin Integrity

ASSESSMENT

Clinical scenario: Mrs. Kless is a 66-year-old diabetic who is presently hospitalized for a cerebrovascular accident with left-sided hemiplegia. She is able to sit in a chair, but the *sacral area reddens easily;* there is *a 1 cm blister over her left ischial region.*

NURSING DIAGNOSIS

Impaired skin integrity related to reduced sensation and mobility.

PLANNING

Goals	Expected outcomes
Client's injury to the skin and underlying tissue will be reduced by 7/2.	Wound size will decrease (6/30). Skin will remain intact in unaffected areas (6/26). Normal reactive hyperemia will be observed in unaffected areas (6/26).

IMPLEMENTATION

Steps	Rationale
1. Instruct and assist client to shift body weight every 15 minutes when sitting.	Redistribution of body weight every 15 minutes when sitting relieves the downward pressure on the ischial tuberosities (Pires, Muller, 1991).
2. Reposition client every 90 minutes.	Repositioning removes pressure and allows normal hyperemic response (Maklebust, 1991a). This client's initial assessment noted excessive hyperemia after 2 hours in a single position. Therefore a more frequent positioning schedule is needed.
3. Obtain oscillating air mattress for client's bed.	Clients with pressure ulcer development are at greater risk for new ulcers; this mattress eliminates shear and friction.
4. Apply hydrocolloid dressing to wound.	Dressings protect underlying skin and remove any drainage from surface of wound (Maklebust, 1991b).

EVALUATION

Observe skin over bony prominences when client's position changes.
Palpate skin and underlying tissue over bony prominences with each position change.
Observe wound for drainage.
Measure wound diameter.
Observe and time reactive hyperemic response in affected and unaffected areas.

Defining characteristics are shown in italic type.

skilled nursing care facility or home health agency may be necessary to help the client remain or regain mobility at home.

The care plan is developed with the client and significant others based on one or more client-centered goals. Goals, like diagnoses, must be prioritized and are formed based on the nursing assessment. General goals and expected outcomes that may serve as guidelines for developing care plans for clients with impaired skin integrity include the following:

Goal: Identifying at-risk clients needing prevention and the specific factors placing them at risk (AHCPR, 1992).

Outcomes

Client has no areas of broken skin

Client's skin is free from excessive friction, moisture, shear force, and pressure

Goal: Client maintains and improves tissue tolerance to pressure in order to prevent injury (AHCPR, 1992).

Outcomes

Circulation to client's integument is maintained

Client's skin is free of abnormal reactive hyperemia
Client or family demonstrates proper skin care measures

Goal: Client avoids the adverse effects of external mechanical forces: pressure, friction, and shearing force (AHCPR, 1992, 1994).

Outcomes

Client's skin is intact
Client's skin lesion is clean and healing
Client's skin is free of abnormal reactive hyperemia

Goal: Client improves nutritional intake.

Outcomes

Client's nutritional lab values are at or are returning to normal limits
Client's weight returns toward ideal body weight
Client does not have any increased pitting edema

Implementation

When the client is immobile, the major risk to the skin is the formation of pressure ulcers. Nursing interventions focus on prevention or treatment of pressure ulcers.

Health Promotion and Prevention of Pressure Ulcers. Once risk factors are identified, the nurse then reduces environmental factors that accelerate pressure ulcer formation, such as high room temperature (causing diaphoresis), moisture, or wrinkled bed linen.

Early identification of high-risk clients and their risk factors aids the nurse in preventing pressure ulcers. Prevention minimizes the impact that risk factors or contributing factors may have on pressure ulcer development. Table 24-3 outlines some nursing interventions for the prevention of pressure ulcers. Three major areas of nursing interventions for prevention of pressure sores are hygiene and topical skin care, use of the 30-degree lateral position (Figure 24-11), and the use of therapeutic beds and mattresses.

table 24-3

A QUICK GUIDE TO PREVENTION

Risk factor	Nursing interventions
Immobility	Establish individualized turning schedule. Reduce shear and friction. Provide pressure-relief surface.
Inactivity	Provide assistive devices to increase activity.
Incontinence	Assess need for incontinence management. Clean and dry skin after soiling.
Malnutrition	Provide adequate nutritional and fluid intake. Consult dietitian for nutritional evaluation.
Diminished sensation, decreased mental status	Assess client's and family's ability to provide care. Educate care giver regarding pressure ulcer prevention.
Impaired skin integrity	Avoid pressure. Do not use donut-shaped cushions. Lubricate skin. Do not massage red areas. Do not use heat lamps.

Modified from Maklebust J, Sieggreen M: *Pressure ulcers: guidelines for prevention and nursing management,* West Dundee, Ill., 1991, S-N Publications.

HYGIENE AND TOPICAL SKIN CARE. The nurse must keep the client's skin clean and dry. In this initial line of defense for preventing skin breakdown, the client's skin must be continually assessed by nurses. In addition, the types of products available for skin care are numerous, and their uses need to be matched to the specific needs of the client (Maklebust, 1991a, 1991b).

When the skin is cleaned, soaps are avoided. Soaps and alcohol-based lotions cause drying and leave an alkaline residue. The alkaline residue discourages the growth of normal skin bacteria, thus promoting an overgrowth of opportunistic bacteria, which can then enter an open wound (Barnes, 1987).

After the skin is cleansed and completely dried, protective moisturizer should be applied to keep the epidermis well lubricated but not oversaturated. Cornstarch is a dry lubricant and helps to reduce friction (Maklebust, 1991b). A & D, Unicare, and Pericare are bland, water-repellent ointments that protect the skin from moisture (AHCPR, 1992). In addition, these ointments are easily cleansed from the skin (Barnes, 1987). When the nurse uses any water-repellent ointment, the nurse must completely clean the area on a routine basis. Ointment, when left in place too long, can be a medium for bacteria and can cause further skin problems such as maceration and infection.

When the client's skin is exposed to body fluids such as urine, bowel, or wound drainage, the area should be cleansed, and a skin barrier containing petrolatum (e.g., Vaseline) or zinc oxide is applied. These barriers protect the skin from excessive moisture and toxins from urine or stool (Maklebust, 1991b).

When clients are incontinent, absorptive underpads such as adult diapers or incontinence briefs can be used. Those products drain moisture away from the client's skin (AHCPR, 1992). The proper absorptive garments have a quilted lining and contain a polymer filling. The newer products also lubricate the skin as well as protect

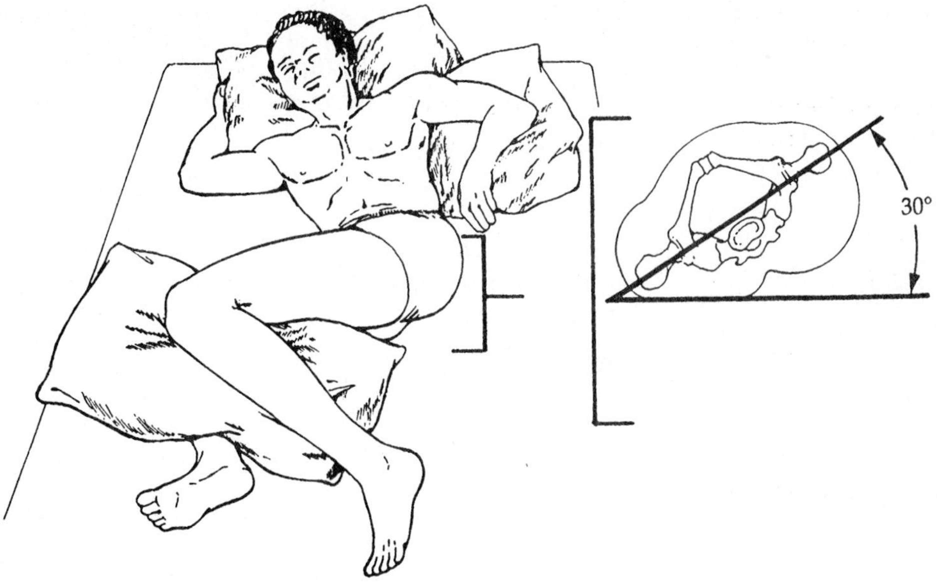

FIGURE 24-11 Thirty-degree lateral position to avoid pressure points. (From Bryant RA, et al.: Pressure ulcer. In Bryant RA, editor: *Acute and chronic wounds: nursing management,* St. Louis, 1992, Mosby.)

from moisture. These absorptive underpads (Senecare and Silopad [Silipos Silicone Technology, N.Y.]) are placed in direct contact with the skin. As the client moves, the skin is lubricated and friction is reduced and excess moisture is absorbed into the pad (Marchand, Lidowski, 1993). When providing skin care to the incontinent client, the health care team must also assess and treat the causes of incontinency (see Chapter 32).

POSITIONING. Positioning interventions are designed to reduce pressure and shearing force to the skin. The immobilized client's position should be changed according to activity level, perceptual ability, and daily routines (Pajk, et al., 1986; Bergstrom, et al., 1987a and 1987b). Therefore a standard turning interval of $1\frac{1}{2}$ to 2 hours may not prevent pressure sore development in some clients. The Wound Ostomy, Incontinence Nurses (WOCN) Association and AHCPR recommend reducing shear by keeping the client's head of bed below the 30-degree angle, using assistive devices when turning or transferring clients, using the bed gatch or foot board, and the 30-degree lateral position (Marchand, Lidowski, 1993; Bryant, 1992).

When the client can sit in a chair, the time should be limited to 2 hours or less. Again, the exact time interval is individualized (see Procedure 24-1). However, the nurse should not allow the client to sit for a period longer than the recommended time interval that was calculated during assessment. Thus if the timing interval is every $1\frac{1}{2}$ hours, the client should remain in a sitting position less than $1\frac{1}{2}$ hours. In the sitting position, the pressure on the ischial tuberosities is greater than when in the supine position (Pajk, et al., 1986). In addition, a high-risk client sitting in a chair should be taught or assisted to shift weight every 15 minutes. Shifting weight provides short-term relief on the ischial tuberosities. A client should also sit on gel or an air cushion to redistribute weight so that it is not all on the ischium. Rigid and donut-shaped cushions are contraindicated because they reduce blood supply to the area, resulting in wider areas of ischemia (Maklebust, 1991a).

After the client is repositioned, the nurse reassesses the skin and observes for normal reactive hyperemia and blanching. The reddened areas should *never* be massaged. This change in practice is a result of nursing research (Maklebust, 1991a; AHCPR, 1992; Bryant, 1992). Massaging the reddened areas increases breaks in the capillaries in the underlying tissues and increases the risk of pressure ulcer formation.

THERAPEUTIC BEDS AND MATTRESSES. A variety of special beds and mattresses have been designed to reduce the hazards of immobility to the skin and musculoskeletal system. However, none eliminates the need for meticulous nursing care. No single device eliminates the effects of pressure on the skin.

When selecting specialty beds, the nurse must thoroughly assess clients' needs. A flow diagram (Figure 24-12) assists the nurse in clinical decision making. In addition, Table 24-4 lists the specific device and pertinent nurse alerts for using the equipment safely. Clients and families need to be taught the reason for and proper use of the beds or mattresses (see box on p. 598). When used correctly, these mattresses and specialty beds assist in reducing pressure ulcers in high-risk clients (see box on p. 598).

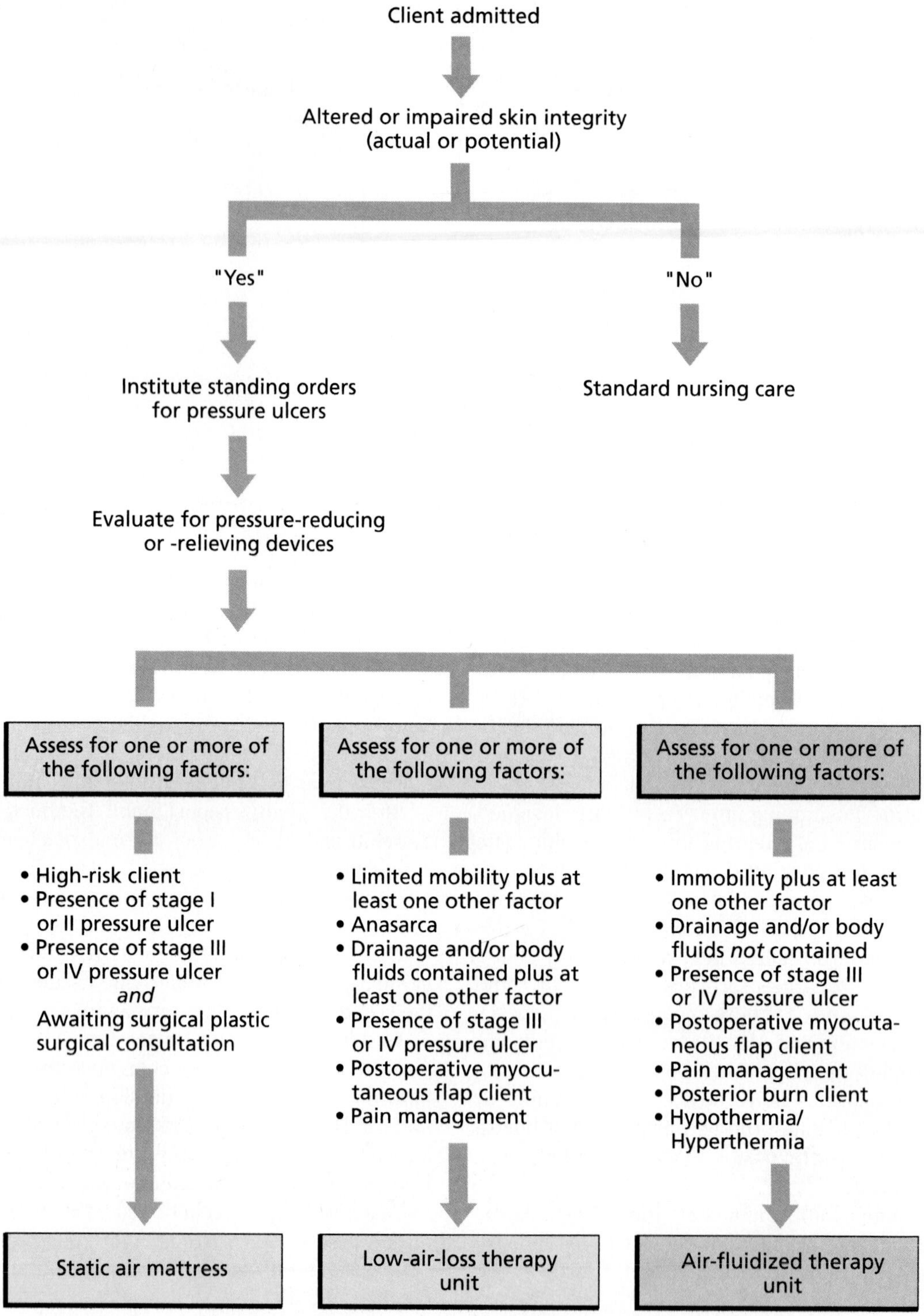

FIGURE 24-12 Flow diagram for ordering specialty beds. (From Thomas C: *Ostomy/Wound Manage* 23:51, 1989.)

table 24-4
SURFACE TYPES BY PURPOSE AND ADVANTAGES

Type	Examples	Purpose	Advantages	Disadvantages	Notes
Foam overlay	Geomatt Biogard	Pressure reduction, comfort	Low cost, ease of use, many sizes	Hot, traps moisture, life is limited, loses pressure reduction with use	Usually one-client use; washing removes flame-retardant chemicals; ease of use at home
Foam replacement	MaxiFloat DeCube Comfortex	Pressure reduction, comfort	Reduced bed height, reduces nursing time, multiple client use	High initial cost, difficult to evaluate when effectiveness is lost	Some have removable sections (cubes); may be rented or purchased
Fluid overlay	Lotus	Pressure reduction, comfort	Easily cleaned, multiple client use, readily available	Heavy, leaks with puncture, cannot raise head of bed	May be rented or purchased; baffled systems control motion
Air overlay	Sofcare Roho KoalaKare	Pressure relief	Ease of setup, single- or multiple-use products available	Lack of comfort, damaged by sharp objects, requires monitoring for inflation	May be rented or purchased; adapts to multiple settings
Low air loss	KinAir Flexicair Mediscus	Pressure relief	Ease of use, seat deflates for transfer, company offers support staff	Portable blowers are noisy, surface may be slippery, noisy	Generally rented; home unit is available
Air fluidized	Clinitron Fluidair Skytron	Pressure relief	Reduced friction and shear, facilitates control of high drainage, company offers support staff	Coughing may be less effective, heavy, circulating air may dehydrate, transfers are difficult	Available for home, but may be too heavy
Kinetic	Rotokinetic treatment table	Movement, skeletal stability	Mobilize secretions, skeletal stability, supports traction, company offers support staff	Must be kept in rotation or no pressure reduction, shearing if client position is not correct	Must be in rotation 21 hours/day, now available as low air loss version
Bariatric	Burke	Management of morbidly obese, staff safety	Facilitates client independence, converts to a chair	Width is standard so surface may not accommodate turning	Requires addition of special mattress and overlay for pressure relief

table 24-5
EXAMPLES OF TOPICAL CLEANSING SOLUTIONS

Name	Type	Comments
Acetic acid	Antimicrobial	Effective against *Pseudomonas aeruginosa.* Changes color of exudate. Thus can provide false assurance for elimination of infection.
Safclens	Detergent	Non-ionic surfactant.
Biolex	Detergent	Surfactant for wound cleansing.
Cara-Klenz	Detergent	Wound cleanser.
Sodium hypochlorite (Dakins)	Antimicrobial	Effective for odor control. Protect intact skin with zinc oxide. Discontinue use when necrotic tissue is gone.

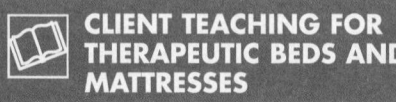

CLIENT TEACHING FOR THERAPEUTIC BEDS AND MATTRESSES

- Explain the reasons for the client's reduced mobility.
- Teach basic preventive care measures to reduce the hazards to the client's skin.
- Demonstrate how to optimize the client's safety by reducing risk of falls, using proper body mechanics, and using the equipment correctly.
- Teach client how to maintain optimal independence and mobility.
- Teach client that fluid intake must increase, and determine which type and amount of fluids are appropriate.

DEVICES USED TO PREVENT OR TREAT PRESSURE ULCERS

DEVICES TO SUPPORT PRESSURE AREAS

Flotation pads are pliable pads with a consistency like body fat, which disperse pressure over a larger area.

Pillows and bridging techniques lift the pressure site off the mattress and separate two points of pressure.

DEVICES TO AID IN TURNING A CLIENT

A Guttman bed rotates the client from prone to supine positions and from side to side.

Kinetic therapy continuously rotates the client 270 degrees every 3 minutes.

DEVICES TO MINIMIZE OR EQUALIZE PRESSURE

Alternating air mattresses made of polyvinyl air cells are attached to a pump that inflates and deflates them every 3-7 seconds, alternating pressure points.

Water mattresses disperse and evenly distribute the client's body weight.

High and low air loss beds allow deformation of bed surface to the body contours, thereby reducing tissue pressure below capillary closure. These beds also eliminate shear and friction and reduce moisture (Bryant, 1992).

Treating Pressure Ulcers

Skin. In addition to removing all pressure from the affected area and keeping pressure from the area, cleanliness of the ulcer area and all skin surfaces is essential (Procedure 24-2). Maintaining cleanliness may be extremely difficult with incontinent, feverish, or confused clients.

Moisture in and around an area of skin breakdown can cause further ulceration and infection. Many products are available for the care of pressure ulcers (Tables 24-5 and 24-6). Before instituting treatment measures, the nurse must thoroughly assess the client's pressure ulcer and determine the correct dressing based on the stage of ulcer development.

The nurse cleans the affected area to (1) remove bacterial and surface contaminants, and (2) protect the healing area. Clean proliferating wounds and infected necrotic wounds require different cleansing agents (Bryant, 1992). Therefore the nurse must select appropriate solutions (Procedure 24-2). Caution is needed because antiseptics can damage tissues unprotected by the dermis and may inactivate some drugs. The ulcer should be rinsed with normal saline to minimize the effect of antiseptic (Fowler, 1982).

An ulcer that has necrotic tissue or eschar or shows signs of sloughing must be debrided. **Eschar** is a thick, leathery devitalized necrotic tissue. **Sloughing** is the shedding of loose, stringy necrotic tissue as the result of skin ulceration. **Debridement** is the removal of devitalized tissue so that healthy tissue can regenerate.

For reddened areas or areas of broken skin integrity, skin care products that lubricate and protect, stimulate circulation, and promote wound healing are recommended. When the ulcer is pink with granulation tissue throughout, a dressing is indicated to promote healing. A clean, moist environment promotes migration of epithelial cells across the ulcer surface.

Nutritional status. Maintaining adequate protein intake and hemoglobin levels is important in treatment of pressure ulcers (see Chapter 31).

Protein status. Clients with a potential for or decreased serum albumin levels or poor protein intake need a nutritional evaluation to ensure proper caloric intake (Breslow, et al., 1993; Maklebust, 1991a). Increased protein intake, 2 to 4 times above the daily recommended requirement, helps rebuild epidermal tissue. Increased caloric and protein intakes help promote healing of pressure ulcers (Breslow, et al., 1993; Bodnar, Myron, 1992). Increased intake of vitamin C promotes protein synthesis and tissue repair (Shekleton, Litwack, 1991).

Hemoglobin. A low hemoglobin level decreases delivery of oxygen to the tissues and leads to further ischemia. When possible, hemoglobin should be maintained at 12 g/100 ml.

Evaluation

Nursing interventions for reducing and treating pressure ulcers are evaluated by determining the client's response to nursing therapies and by determining whether each goal was achieved. To evaluate outcomes

table 24-6

TREATMENT OPTIONS BY ULCER STAGE

Ulcer stage	Ulcer status	Dressing*	Comments	Expected change	Adjuvant
1	Intact	None Film, adherent Hydrocolloid	Allows visual assessment. Protects from shear. May not allow visual assessment.	Resolves slowly without epidermal loss over 7 to 14 days.	Turning schedule. Support hydration. Nutritional support. Silicone-based lotion to decrease shear. Pressure relief mattress or chair cushion.
2	Clean	Composite Hydrocolloid Hydrogel sheet	Viasorb, film plus telfa. Exudry. Limits shear. Change every 7 days if occlusive seal. Absorbent, requires secondary dressing of gauze or adherent film.	Heals through reepithelialization and epithelial budding.	See previous stage. Manage incontinence.
3	Clean	Hydrocolloid Hydrogel Exudate absorbers calcium alginate wound pastes Gauze, fluffy Growth factors	See Stage 2. Apply ¼-inch thick, cover with gauze or hydrocolloid. Change when strike through is noted on secondary dressing. Cover with gauze or hydrocolloid. Use with normal saline. Use with gauze.	Heals through granulation and reepithelialization. (NOTE: does not become a stage 2 ulcer as it heals.)	See previous stages. Electrical stimulation. Evaluate pressure relief needs.
	Eschar	Adherent film Hydrocolloid Gauze plus ordered solution None	Will facilitate softening of eschar. Will facilitate softening of eschar. Absorb drainage. Rarely, if eschar is dry and intact, no dressing is used, allowing eschar to act as physiologic cover.	Eschar will lift at the edges as healing progresses. Cross-hatching central area of eschar with a small blade will facilitate release from center.	See previous stages. Surgical consult for debridement. Surgical consult for closure.
4	Clean	Hydrogel Hydrocolloid plus hydrocolloid paste/beads Calcium alginate Gauze Growth factors	See Stage 3 Clean. See Stage 3 Clean; critical to treat areas of undermining.	Heals through granulation and reepithelialization. Because of contraction, surface may close more rapidly than base, leaving wound cavity.	See stages 1, 2, and 3 Clean
	Eschar	See Stage 3 Eschar	See Stage 3 Clean. Pack deeply undermined ulcers. Use with gauze.	See Stage 3 Eschar.	See Stage 3 Eschar.

NOTE: As with *all* occlusive dressings, wound should *not* be clinically infected.

and responses to care, the nurse measures the effectiveness of interventions. The optimal outcomes are to prevent injury to the skin and tissues, reduce injury to the skin and underlying tissues, and restore skin integrity.

The nurse also evaluates specific interventions designed to promote skin integrity and to teach the client and family to reduce future threats to skin integrity. The AHCPR (1992b) panel produced a *Patient's guide for pressure ulcers* that is short with clear illustrations

procedure 24-2

TREATING PRESSURE ULCERS

Steps	Rationale
1. Wash hands.	Reduces transmission of blood-borne pathogens. Gloves should be worn when handling items soiled by body fluids (CDC, 1988).
2. Close door or bedside curtains.	Maintains privacy.
3. Position client comfortably with area of pressure ulcer and surrounding skin easily accessible.	Area should be accessible for cleansing of ulcer and surrounding skin.
4. Assemble supplies at bedside. Open sterile packages and topical solution containers.	Sterile supplies should be ready for easy application so that nurse can use them without contaminating them.
a. Wash basin, warm water, washcloth, and towel	Used to bathe surrounding skin.
b. Cleansing agent (see Table 24-5)	
c. Prescribed topical agent:	
(1) Enzymes: collagenase, fibrinolysin, deoxyribonuclease, or sutilains	Proteolytic enzymes debride dead tissue to clean ulcer. Cleans wounds, especially with anaerobic bacteria. Decreases oxygen supply to devitalized tissues.
(2) Dextranomer beads: Debrisan	Cleans wounds with heavy exudate. Absorb fluid, protein, fibrin, fibrinogen, and all products of tissue breakdown and bacterial infection.
d. Sterile dressing (Table 24-6):	
■ Gauze type: 4 × 4 pads, fluffs.	Applied over ulcers treated with enzymes, oxidizing agents, and dextranomer beads.
■ Transparent dressings	Applied over superficial ulcers and skin subjected to shear.
■ Hydrocolloid type	Maintains moist environment to facilitate wound healing.
■ Hydrogel type	Maintains moist environment to facilitate wound healing. May be used to apply topical agents.
■ Calcium alginate type	Highly absorbent of wound exudate in heavily draining wounds.
■ Exudate absorbers	Highly absorbent of wound exudate.
■ Foam types	Protective and will prevent wound dehydration; also absorb small to moderate amounts of drainage.
e. Hypoallergenic tape or adhesive dressing sheet (Hypofix).	Used to secure nonadherent dressing. Prevents skin irritation and tearing.
5. Wash hands and apply clean gloves. Close room door or bedside curtains.	Reduces transmission of microorganisms and prevents accidental exposure to body fluids.
6. Position client to allow dressing removal.	Area should be accessible for dressing change. Proper disposal of old dressing promotes proper handling of contaminated waste.
7. Assess pressure ulcer and surrounding skin to determine ulcer stage (Table 24-6).	
a. Note color, moisture, and appearance of skin around ulcer and of ulcer itself.	Skin condition may indicate progressive tissue damage. Retained moisture causes maceration.
b. Measure two maximum perpendicular diameters.	Provides an objective measure of wound size. May influence size and type of dressing selected. Surface area = length × width
c. Measure depth of pressure ulcer using sterile cotton-tipped applicator or other device that will allow measurement of wound depth.	Depth measure is important for determining wound volume. While surface area adequately represents tissue loss in stage 1 and 2 ulcers, volume more adequately represents tissue loss in deeper stage 3 and 4 wounds. Volume = 2(L × D) + 2(W × D) + (L + D)

Steps	**Rationale**
d. Measure depth (d) of undermining skin by lateral tissue necrosis. Use a cotton-tipped applicator and gently probe under skin edges.	Undermining represents the loss of the underlying tissues (subcutaneous and muscle) to a greater extent than the skin (see illustration). Undermining may indicate progressive tissue necrosis.
8. Wash skin around ulcer gently with warm water and rinse area thoroughly with water.	Reduces number of resident bacteria. Soap can be irritating to skin.
9. Gently dry skin thoroughly by patting lightly with towel.	Retained moisture causes maceration of skin layers.
10. Change to sterile gloves.	Aseptic technique must be maintained during cleansing, measuring, and application of dressings. Refer to institutional policy regarding use of clean or sterile gloves.
11. Cleanse ulcer thoroughly with normal saline or cleansing agent: a. Use irrigating syringe for deep ulcers. b. Cleansing in the shower may be done with a hand-held shower head. c. Whirlpool treatments may be used to assist with wound cleansing and debridement.	Removes wound debris. Previously applied enzymes may require soaking for removal.
12. Apply topical agents, as prescribed:	Topical agents should be changed as wound heals or worsens:
a. Enzymes: ■ Keeping gloves sterile, place small amount of enzyme ointment in palm of hand.	Thick layer of ointment is not necessary. Thin layer absorbs and acts more effectively. Excess medication can irritate surrounding skin. Apply only to necrotic areas.
■ Soften medication by rubbing briskly in palm of hand.	Makes ointment easier to apply.

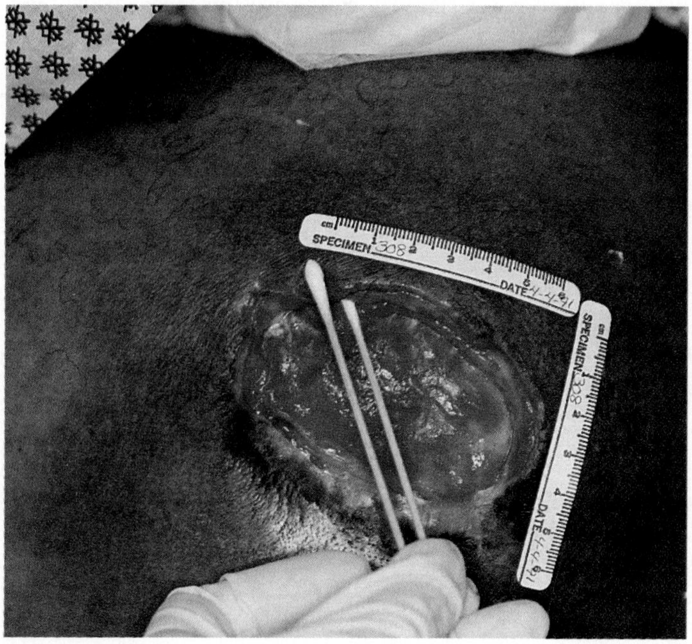

Step 7d

Continued.

procedure 24-2—cont'd

TREATING PRESSURE ULCERS

Steps	Rationale
■ Apply thin, even layer of ointment over necrotic areas of ulcer. Do not apply enzyme to surrounding skin.	Proper distribution of ointment ensures effective action. Enzyme can cause burning, paresthesia, and dermatitis to surrounding skin.
■ Moisten gauze dressing in saline and apply directly over ulcer.	Protects wound. Moist ulcer surface reduces time needed for healing. Skin cells normally live in moist environment.
■ Cover moistened gauze with single dry gauze and tape securely in place.	Prevents bacteria from entering moist dressing.
b. Antiseptics:	
■ Infected ulcers only: apply antiseptic ointment to dominant gloved hand and spread ointment in and around ulcer.	Antiseptic ointment causes minimal tissue irritation. All surfaces of wound must be covered to effectively control bacterial growth.
■ Apply sterile gauze pad over ulcer and tape securely in place.	Protects ulcer and prevents removal of ointment during turning or repositioning.
c. Dextranomer beads:	
■ Hold container of beads approximately 1 inch (2.5 cm) above ulcer site and lightly sprinkle 5 mm layer over wound.	A single layer of insoluble powder is needed to absorb wound exudate.
■ Apply gauze dressing over ulcer.	Holds beads in place and protects wound.
d. Hydrocolloid beads or paste:	
■ Fill ulcer defect to approximately half of the total depth with hydrocolloid beads or paste.	Hydrocolloid beads or paste assist in absorbing wound drainage. Highly draining wounds are best treated with hydrocolloid beads or granules.
■ Cover with hydrocolloid dressing, extend dressing 1 to 1½ inches beyond edges of wound.	Maintains wound humidity. May be left in place up to 7 days. Are not effective on dry eschar (Bryant, 1992).
e. Hydrogel agents:	
■ Cover surface of ulcer with Hydrogel using applicator or gloved hand.	Provides maintenance of wound humidity while absorbing excess drainage. May be used as carrier for topical agents.
■ Apply dry fluffy gauze or hydrocolloid or transparent dressing over gel to completely cover ulcer.	Holds Hydrogel against wound surface; absorbent.
f. Calcium alginates:	
■ Pack wound with alginate using applicator or gloved hand.	Provides maintenance of wound humidity while absorbing excess drainage.
■ Apply dry gauze, foam, or hydrocolloid over alginate.	Holds alginate against wound surface.
13. Reposition client comfortably off pressure ulcer.	Avoids accidental removal of dressings.
14. Remove gloves and dispose of soiled supplies. Wash hands.	Reduces transmission of microorganisms.
15. Report changes in ulcer's appearance to nurse in charge or physician.	Changes in ulcer's appearance indicate changes in prescribed topical agents and dressings. Condition may indicate need for additional therapy.
16. Record appearance of ulcer in nurse's notes. Describe type of topical agent used, dressing applied, and response.	Documents status of ulcer and specific treatment. Response documents evaluation of treatment.

(Ayello, 1993). The nurse also evaluates the client's and family's need for additional support services (e.g., home health care, physical therapy, and counseling) and initiates the referral process. Examples of goals, outcomes, and corresponding evaluative measures include:

Goal: Identifying at-risk clients needing prevention and the specific factors placing them at risk.

Outcomes

Client has no areas of broken skin

Clients skin is free from excessive friction, moisture, shear force, and pressure

Evaluative measures

Inspect the skin for breakdown

Observe for the presence of excessive friction, shear force, and pressure

Palpate the skin for moisture

Goal: Client maintains and improves tissue tolerance to pressure in order to prevent injury.

Outcome

Circulation to client's integument is maintained

Evaluative measure

Palpate the client's skin for temperature and adequate pulses.

Outcome

Client's skin is free of abnormal reactive hyperemia

Evaluative measure

Observe client's skin for hyperemic response following relief of pressure

Outcome

Client or family demonstrates proper skin care measures

Evaluative measure

Observe client or family providing skin care

Goal: Client avoids the adverse effects of external mechanical forces: pressure, friction, and shearing force.

Outcomes

Client's skin is intact

Client's skin lesion is clean and healing

Evaluative measure

Observe and palpate client's skin

Goal: Client improves nutritional intake.

Outcome

Client's nutritional lab values are within or are returning to normal limits

Evaluative measure

Monitor nutritional lab values

Outcome

Client's weight returns toward ideal body weight

Evaluative measure

Weigh client daily

Outcome

Client does not have any or increased dependent edema

Evaluative measure

Observe and palpate dependent body regions

SUMMARY

Pressure ulcers adversely affect the client in all health care settings. Although in some cases immobilization is necessary to promote wound healing, proper skeletal alignment, or rest after an illness, it involves risks. Nursing care prevents the adverse effects of reduced mobility on skin integrity. Using the nursing process, the nurse assesses the risk for pressure ulcers, diagnoses actual or potential problems related to impaired skin integrity, and plans and delivers nursing care to meet the client's needs. Because of the cost, increased nursing time, and prolonged hospital stay to treat pressure ulcers, nursing care aims first to prevent pressure ulcers and then to minimize the effects of pressure ulcers after they develop.

CRITICAL THINKING ACTIVITIES

1. Your client's mobility is severely restricted, and he is receiving a medication that causes peripheral vasoconstriction. What interventions are essential in reducing pressure ulcer formation?
2. You have just admitted a client from a nursing home to your division. On initial assessment, you assess a stage II pressure ulcer. How do you determine the type of care and dressing to use with this particular pressure ulcer?
3. You are assigned to care for an older adult with two stage III pressure ulcers. One of your interventions is to place this client on a therapeutic bed. What information do you need to obtain to order the proper therapeutic bed?

KEY CONCEPTS

Pressure ulcers remain a potential problem in acute and chronic care settings.

Pressure ulcers increase length of stay in hospitals and extended care settings, as well as the overall cost of nursing care needed to manage the wound.

The Agency for Health and Policy Research developed clinical guidelines for future research directions and for the prevention and treatment of pressure ulcers.

Prediction for development of pressure ulcers must focus on clients having the greatest risk for developing impaired skin integrity.

Alterations in mobility, sensory perception, exposure to moisture, level of consciousness, and nutrition, the use of casts, and the presence of severe infection or other debilitating diseases increase the risk for pressure ulcer development.

External pressure, shearing force, moisture, impaired peripheral circulation, edema, and obesity are also contributing factors to the development of pressure ulcers.

When the external pressure against the skin is greater than the pressure in the capillary bed, blood flow decreases to the adjacent tissues.

Decreased circulation to the tissues results in tissue hypoxia; if untreated, tissue necrosis results.

There are four classifications of pressure ulcers.

Meticulous assessment of the skin and underlying tissue and identification of risk factors are important in decreasing the opportunity for pressure ulcer development.

In addition to assessing the reactive hyperemia, the nurse must also palpate adjacent tissue for signs of induration.

Preventive skin care is aimed at controlling external pressure on bony prominences and keeping the skin clean, well lubricated and hydrated, and free of excess moisture.

Plastic-lined pads protect the bed, not the client's skin, because they do not remove moisture away from the client's skin.

Proper positioning should reduce the effects of pressure and guard against the shearing force.

Therapeutic beds and mattresses reduce the effects of pressure; however, selection is based on assessment data to identify the best bed for individual needs.

Cleansing and topical agents used to treat pressure ulcers vary according to the stage of the pressure ulcer. Assessment of the ulcer enables the nurse to select proper skin care agents.

Nutritional interventions are directed at improving wound healing through increasing protein and hemoglobin levels.

The risk of impaired skin integrity related to immobilization depends on the extent and duration of immobilization.

References

Agency for Health Care Policy and Research (AHCPR): *Pressure ulcers in adults: prediction and prevention,* US Department of Health and Human Services, Public Health Service, Rockville, Md., 1992, Pub Nos. 92-0047, 92-0050.

Agency for Health Care Policy and Research (AHCPR): *Preventing pressure ulcers: a patient's guide,* US Department of Health and Human Services, Public Health Service, Rockville, Md., 1992, Pub No. 92-0048.

Ayello EA: A critique of AHCPR's "Preventing pressure ulcers—a patient's guide" as a written instruction tool, *Decubitus* 6:44, 1993

Barnes SH: Patient/family education for the patient with a pressure necrosis, *Nurs Clin North Am* 22:463, 1987.

Bennett L, Lee BY: Vertical shear existence in animal pressure threshold experiments, *Decubitus* 1(1):18, 1988.

Bergstrom N: A research agenda for pressure ulcer prevention, *Decubitus* 5(5):22, 1992.

Bergstrom N, Demuth PJ, Braden, B: A clinical trial of the Braden Scale for predicting pressure sore risk, *Nurs Clin North Am* 22(2):417, 1987a.

Bergstrom N, et al.: The Braden Scale for predicting pressure sore risk, *Nur Res* 36:205, 1987b.

Bodnar B, Myron P: Portrait of practice: reducing the prevalence of pressure ulcers, *Decubitus* 5(2):49, 1992.

Breslow RA, et al.: The importance of dietary protein in healing pressure ulcers, *J Am Geria Soc* 41:357, 1993.

Bryant RA, et al.: Pressure ulcer. In Bryant RA, editor: *Acute and chronic wounds: nursing management,* St. Louis, 1992, Mosby.

Ebersole P, Hess P: *Toward healthy aging: human needs and nursing response,* ed 4, St. Louis 1994, Mosby.

Ferrell BA, et al.: A randomized trial of low-air-loss beds for treatment of pressure ulcers, *JAMA* 269(4):494, 1993.

Goodridge DM: Pressure ulcer risk assessment tools: what's new for gerontological nurses, *J Gerontol Nurs* 19(1):23, 1993.

Gosnell DJ: Assessment and evaluation of pressure sores, *Nurs Clin North Am* 22(2):399, 1987.

Gosnell DJ, et al.: Pressure ulcer incidence and severity in a community hospital, *Decubitus* 5(5):56, 1992.

Green E, Katz J: Practice guidelines for management of pressure ulcers, *Decubitus* 4(1):36, 1991.

Hanan K, Scheele L: Albumin vs. weight as a predictor of nutritional status and pressure ulcer development, *Ostomy/Wound Manage* 33:22-27, 1991.

Hastings KE: Legal aspects of the AHCPR pressure ulcer guidelines, *Decubitus* 4(2):36, 1991.

Hoff J: Effecting a change in nursing practice: pressure ulcer prevention, *J Nurs Qual Assur* 3(4):56, 1989.

Kane RL, et al.: *Essentials of clinical geriatrics,* ed 3, New York, 1994, McGraw-Hill.

Kemp MG, et al.: The role of support surfaces and patient attributes in preventing pressure ulcers in elderly patients, *Res Nurs Health* 16:89, 1993.

Kim MJ, McFarland GK, McLane AM: *Pocket guide to nursing diagnoses,* ed 5, St. Louis, 1993, Mosby.

Knight AL: Medical management of pressure sores, *J Fam Prac* 27(1):95, 1988.

Kosiak M: Etiology and pathology of ischemic ulcers, *Arch Phys Med Rehabil* 40:62, 1959.

Maklebust J: Impact of AHCPR pressure ulcer guidelines on nursing practice, *Decubitus* 4(2):46, 1991a.

Maklebust J: Pressure ulcer update, *RN* 41(12):56, 1991b.

Maklebust J: Pressure ulcers: etiology and intervention, *Nurs Clin North Am* 22(2):359, 1987.

Marchand AC, Lidowski H: Reassessment of the use of genuine sheepskin for pressure ulcer prevention and treatment, *Decubitus* 6(1): 44, 1993.

Meehan M: Multi-site pressure ulcer prevalence survey, *Decubitus* 3(4):14, 1990.

National Pressure Ulcer Advisory Panel (NPUAP): Pressure ulcers incidence, economics, risk assessment, Consensus Development Conference Statement, *Decubitus* 2(2):24, 1989.

Norton D, et al.: An investigation of geriatric nursing problems in a hospital, London, 1962, National Corporation for the Care of Old People.

Pajk M, et al.: Investigating the problem of pressure sores, *J Gerontol Nurs* 12(7):11, 1986.

Pires M, Muller A: Detection and management of early tissue pressure indicators: a pictorial essay, *Progressions* 3(3):3, 1991.

Shekleton ME, Litwack K: *Critical care nursing of the surgical patient,* Philadelphia, 1991, Saunders.

Steinberg J: Prevalence of decubitus ulcers: issues of concern, *Decubitus* 2(2):50, 1990.

Stotts NA: Predicting pressure ulcer development in surgical patients, *Heart Lung* 17(6):641, 1988.

Thomas C: Specialty beds: decision-making made easy, *Ostomy/Wound Manage* 23:51, 1989.

Trelease CC: Developing standards for wound care, *Ostomy/Wound Manage* 20:46, 1988.

Bibliography

Barnes S, Rutland BS: Air-fluidized therapy as a cost-effective treatment for a "worst case" pressure necrosis, *J Enterostom Ther* 13(1):27, 1986.

Berecek KH: Etiology of decubitus ulcers, *Nurs Clin North Am* 10:157, 1975.

Fournier L, et al.: A research-based risk assessment tool as the cornerstone of a pressure ulcer prevention program, *J Enterstom Ther* 19:155, 1992.

Gosnell DJ: An assessment tool to identify pressure sores, *Nurs Res* 22(1):55 1973.

Hedrick-Thompson JK: A review of pressure reduction device studies, *J Vas Nurs* 10(4):3, 1992.

Norton D, et al.: Pressure sores. In Horsley JA, editor: *Preventing decubitus ulcers: CURN project,* New York, 1981, Grune & Stratton.

Rubin M: How bedrest changes perception, *Am J Nurs* 88:55, 1988.

Rubin M: The physiology of bedrest, *Am J Nurs* 88:50, 1988.

Sideranko S, et al.: Effects of position and mattress overlay on sacral and heel pressures in a clinical population, *Res Nurs Health* 15:245, 1992.

Thompson-Bishop JY, Mottola CM: Tissue interface pressure and estimated subcutaneous pressures of 11 different pressure reducing support surfaces, *Decubitus* 5(2):42, 1992.

25

Infection Control

OBJECTIVES

Mastery of content in this chapter will enable the student to:

- Define the key terms listed.
- Identify the body's normal defenses against infection.
- Discuss the events in the inflammatory response.
- Describe the signs of a localized and systemic infection.
- Describe characteristics of each link of the infection chain.
- Assess clients at risk for acquiring an infection.
- Explain conditions that precipitate the onset of nosocomial infections.
- Describe precautions taken for Body Substance Isolation precautions.
- Explain universal blood and body fluid precautions.
- Identify principles of surgical asepsis.
- Describe nursing interventions designed to break each link in the infection chain.
- Correctly perform isolation barrier techniques.
- Perform proper procedures for handwashing.
- Properly apply a surgical mask and gloves.

KEY TERMS

aerosolization
antibodies
antigen
asepsis
Body Substance Isolation
carriers
Centers for Disease Control and Prevention (CDC)
colonized
communicable disease
contaminated
disinfection
endogenous infection
exogenous infection
exudate
iatrogenic infection
immunity
inflammation
isolation
leukocytosis
lymphocyte
macrophages
medical asepsis
microorganisms
necrotic
nosocomial infection
pathogens
sterilization
surgical asepsis
Universal Precautions
virulence

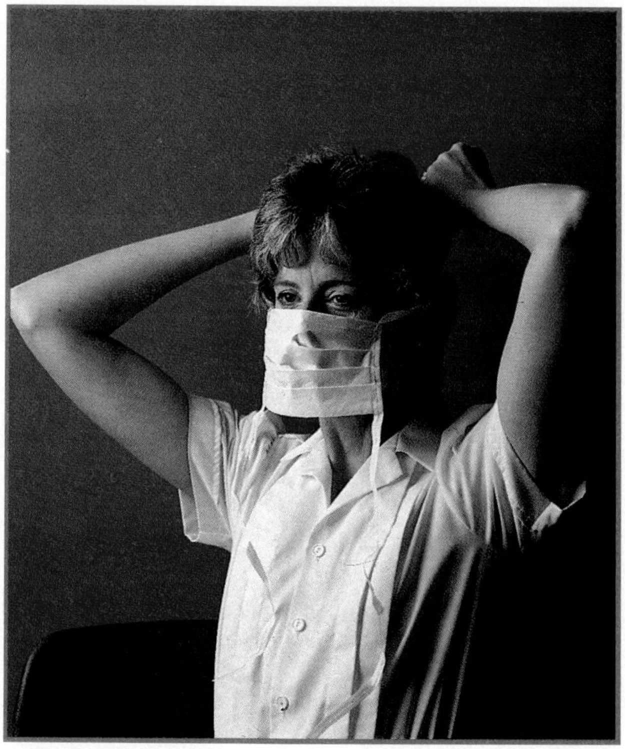

Infection control is one of the most important functions a nurse can perform. The nurse becomes the client's advocate by understanding the infectious process and practicing infection control principles. In addition, the nurse can ensure personal safety by using common sense with all clients.

Clients entering a variety of health care settings are at risk for infections related to numerous diagnostic and invasive procedures. Furthermore, many clients have a lower resistance to **microorganisms** and develop disease or infection after increased exposure. The nurse helps to protect clients from infections by controlling and/or eliminating sources. Clients and families must be able to recognize sources of infections and be able to initiate protective measures. The nurse should instruct them about the nature of infections, the mode of transmission, the reasons for susceptibility, and the measure of control.

With the introduction of new infections such as human immunodeficiency virus (HIV) and the recurrence of old infections such as tuberculosis, the nurse must practice infection control and barrier protection. This chapter will emphasize techniques for personal safety.

NATURE OF INFECTION

An infection is the invasion of the body by **pathogens** or microorganisms capable of producing disease. If the microorganisms fail to injure cells or tissues, infection is asymptomatic. Disease results if the pathogens multiply and alter normal tissue function. If the infectious disease can be transmitted directly from one person to another, it is a **communicable** or contagious **disease.**

Chain of Infection

The presence of a pathogen does not mean that an infection will begin. Development of an infection occurs in a cyclical process that depends on the following elements: the infectious agent or pathogen, reservoir for pathogen growth, portal of exit from the reservoir, means of transmission or vehicle, portal of entry to host, and susceptible host (Figure 25-1). Infection develops if this chain stays intact. The nurse's efforts to control infection are directed at breaking this chain.

Infectious Agent. Pathogenic organisms include bacteria, viruses, fungi, protozoa, and rickettsiae (Table 25-1). Pathogens on the skin are categorized as resident (normally present and stable in number) or transient (picked up when a person contacts another object). Resident pathogens are mostly found in superficial skin layers, but about 10% to 20% inhabit deep epidermal layers (Garner and Favero, 1985). They are not easily removed by handwashing unless considerable friction is used. Transient organisms attach loosely to the skin in dirt and grease or under fingernails and can be removed easily with thorough handwashing. The development of

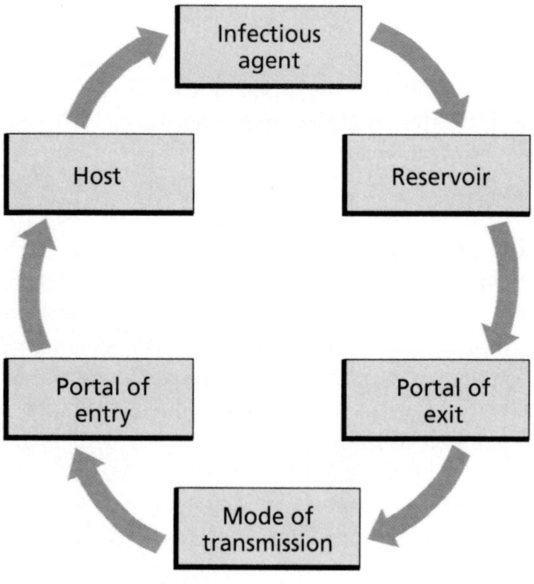

FIGURE 25-1 Chain of infection.

table 25-1

COMMON PATHOGENS AND SOME INFECTIONS OR DISEASES THEY PRODUCE

Organism	Primary reservoir	Infection or disease
BACTERIA		
Staphylococcus aureus	Skin, hair, anterior nares	Wound infection, pneumonia, food poisoning, cellulitis
Streptococcus (beta-hemolytic group A)	Oropharynx, skin, perianal area	"Strep throat," rheumatic fever, scarlet fever, impetigo
Streptococcus (beta-hemolytic group B)	Adult genitalia	Urinary tract infection, wound infection, endometritis, neonatal sepsis
Escherichia coli	Colon	Enteritis
Neisseria gonorrhoeae	Genitourinary tract, rectum, mouth, eye	Gonorrhea, pelvic inflammatory disease, infectious arthritis, conjunctivitis
VIRUSES		
Herpes simplex 1	Lesions of mouth, skin, blood, excretions	Cold sores, aseptic meningitis, sexually transmitted disease
Hepatitis A	Feces	Hepatitis A
Hepatitis B	Feces, blood, body fluids and excretions	Hepatitis B
Hepatitis C	Blood	Hepatitis C
Human immunodeficiency (HIV)	Blood, semen, and vaginal secretions	Acquired immunodeficiency syndrome (AIDS)
FUNGI		
Candida albicans	Mouth, skin, colon, genital tract	Thrush, dermatitis
Aspergillus	Dust, decaying vegetation	Aspergillosis
PROTOZOA		
Plasmodium falciparum	Mosquito	Malaria
RICKETTSIAE		
Rickettsia rickettsii	Wood tick	Rocky Mountain spotted fever

an infectious disease depends on the number of organisms, **virulence** or ability to produce disease, the ability to enter and survive in the host, and susceptibility of the host.

Reservoir. Microorganisms have many sources or reservoirs for growth. One of the most common is the human body. Organisms live on the skin and within body cavities, fluids, and discharges. An organism does not always cause illness. **Carriers** are persons or animals who show no symptoms of illness but who have pathogens on or in their bodies that can be transferred to others. Animals, plants, insects, food, water, and milk can also be reservoirs for infectious organisms. All organisms require food and a proper environment for growth. A dark, warm, moist habitat as in the oral cavity or under a dressing is ideal. The amount and degree of food, oxygen, water, temperature, pH, and light required for growth varies from organism to organism.

Portal of Exit. After microorganisms find a site in which to grow and multiply, they must find a portal or exit if they are to enter another host and cause disease. Microorganisms can exit through a variety of sites such as skin and mucous membranes, respiratory tract, gastrointestinal tract, reproductive tract, and blood.

Mode of Transmission. There are many vehicles for the transmission of microorganisms from the reservoir to the host. Table 25-2 summarizes common modes of transmission. Certain infectious diseases tend to be transmitted more commonly by specific modes. However, the same microorganism may be transmitted by more than one route. For example, herpes zoster may

table 25-2
MODE OF TRANSMISSION

Route and mode	Examples of organisms (diseases)
CONTACT	
Direct (direct physical contact between an infected source and a susceptible host): sexual contact with an infected person, direct client care	Hepatitis A, scabies, HIV, syphilis
Indirect (personal contact of susceptible host with contaminated inanimate object): needles, instruments and dressings	Hepatitis B virus, *Enterococcus, Pseudomonas,* HIV, and *Staphylococcus*
Droplet contact (infectious agent coming in contact with conjunctivae, nose, or mouth of susceptible host; droplets travel only up to 3 feet and therefore contact is not airborne): coughing and sneezing	Measles, streptococcal pharyngitis, influenza
AIR	
Droplet nuclei (residue of evaporated droplets remain suspended in air): coughing, sneezing, and talking	Tuberculosis, staphylococcus
Dust (contains infectious agent)	*Aspergillus* (aspergillosis)
VEHICLE	
Contaminated items	
Liquids	
Water	*Vibrio cholerae* (cholera)
Drugs and solutions	*Pseudomonas*
Blood	Hepatitis B virus and HIV
Food (improperly handled or stored items and fresh fruits and vegetables)	*Salmonella, Staphylococcus, Enterobacter,* and *Klebsiella*
VECTORS	
Insects	
Mosquitoes	*Plasmodium* (malaria)
Fleas, ticks, and lice	*Rickettsia typhi* and *R. prowazekii* (typhus)
Animals (cows and pigs)	*Brucella* (brucellosis)

be spread by the airborne route in droplet nuclei and also by direct contact with vesicle fluid.

Portal of Entry. Organisms can enter the body through the same routes they use for exiting. For example, obstruction to the flow of urine from a urinary catheter allows for organisms to travel up the urethra. Factors that reduce the body's defenses enhance the chances that pathogens will enter.

Susceptible Host. Susceptibility to an infectious agent depends on the individual's degree of resistance to pathogens. Although everyone is constantly in contact with large numbers of organisms, an infection does not develop until an individual becomes susceptible to the strength and numbers of those microorganisms. A person's natural defenses against infection and certain risk factors (see assessment section) affect susceptibility.

In addition, a host is no longer considered susceptible if it has acquired **immunity** from either a natural or artificially induced event. Natural acquired immunity results from having a certain disease, such as measles, and usually lasts a lifetime. Artificial immunity can be either active or passive. Active artificial immunity follows receipt of a vaccine such as the polio vaccine. The duration of active artificial immunity is variable and depends on the disease. For example, a booster vaccine is needed to maintain protection from diphtheria.

Another type of short-term artificial immunity results from use of immune serum globulin (i.e., serum that contains antibodies such as IgG for protection from hepatitis A.) A small amount of passive antibiotics is also transplacentally transferred. Passive immunity is usually of a short duration, several months at most.

Course of Infection

By understanding the infection chain, the nurse can assist in the prevention of infections. The nurse assesses

COURSE OF INFECTION

INCUBATION PERIOD

There is an interval between entrance of pathogen into the body and appearance of first symptoms (e.g., chickenpox 2 to 3 weeks, common cold 1 to 2 days, influenza 1 to 3 days, and mumps 18 days).

PRODROMAL STAGE OF ILLNESS

There is an interval from the onset of nonspecific signs and symptoms (malaise, low-grade fever, and fatigue) to more specific symptoms; during this time, microorganisms grow and multiply, and a client is more capable of spreading disease to others.

FULL STAGE OF ILLNESS

Client manifests signs and symptoms specific to type of infection (e.g., common cold manifested by sore throat, sinus congestion, rhinitis, and mumps manifested by earache, high fever, parotid and salivary gland swelling).

CONVALESCENCE

Acute symptoms of infection disappear; length of recovery depends on severity of infection and client's general state of health; recovery may take several days to months.

the risk for infection and takes appropriate actions to prevent its spread. Infections follow a progressive course (see the box above). The severity depends on the extent of the infection, the pathogenicity of the causative microorganisms, and the host's susceptibility.

If infection is localized, such as in a wound, antibiotic therapy and proper wound care may control the infection's spread and minimize the illness. The client will experience only localized symptoms such as pain, tenderness, and swelling at the wound site. An infection that affects the entire body instead of just a single organ or part is systemic and can be fatal.

DEFENSES AGAINST INFECTION

The body has normal defenses against infection. Normal flora, body system defenses, and inflammation are nonspecific defenses that protect against microorganisms, regardless of prior exposure. The immune system is composed of separate cells and molecules, some of which fight specific pathogens.

Normal Flora

The body normally contains large numbers of microorganisms that reside on the surface and deep layers of the skin, in the saliva and oral mucosa, and in the intestinal walls. Normal flora do not cause disease but instead help to maintain health. For example, the skin's flora inhibits multiplication of organisms landing on the skin. The number of flora maintains a sensitive balance with other microorganisms to prevent infection. Any factor that disrupts this balance places a person at serious risk for infection. For example, the use of broad-spectrum antibiotics for the treatment of infection can lead to a suprainfection. Antibiotics can eliminate or change normal bacterial flora. Microorganisms resistant to the antibiotic can then cause serious infection (Clark et al., 1990).

Body System Defenses

The skin, respiratory tract, and gastrointestinal tract are easily accessible to microorganisms, but they also have unique defenses against infection, physiologically suited to their structure and function (Table 25-3). Any conditions that impair an organ's specialized defenses increase susceptibility to infection.

Inflammation

The body's cellular response to injury or infection is **inflammation**. Inflammation is a protective vascular reaction that delivers fluid, blood products, and nutrients to interstitial tissues in an area of injury. The process neutralizes and eliminates pathogens or **necrotic** tissues and establishes a means of repairing body cells and tissues. Signs of inflammation include swelling, redness, heat, pain or tenderness, and loss of function in the affected body part. When inflammation becomes systemic, other signs and symptoms develop; these include fever, **leukocytosis** (increased number of white blood cells), malaise, anorexia, nausea, vomiting, and lymph node enlargement.

The inflammatory response may be triggered by many physical agents (e.g., temperature extremes and radiation), chemical agents (e.g., gastric acid or poisons), and microorganisms. Inflammation involves a series of well-coordinated events, including vascular and cellular responses, formation of inflammatory **exudate,** and tissue repair (Table 25-4).

Immune Response

When a foreign material **(antigen)** enters the body, a series of responses change the body's biological makeup

table 25-3

NORMAL BODY SYSTEM DEFENSE MECHANISMS AGAINST INFECTION

Defense mechanisms	Action	Factors that may alter defense
SKIN		
Intact multilayered surface, body's first line of defense against infection	Provides mechanical barrier to microorganisms	Cuts, abrasions, puncture wounds, areas of maceration
Shedding of outer layer of skin cells	Removes organisms that adhere to skin's outer layers	Failure to bathe regularly
Sebum	Contains fatty acid that kills some bacteria	Excessive bathing
MOUTH		
Intact multilayered mucosa	Provides mechanical barrier to microorganisms	Lacerations, trauma, extracted teeth
Saliva	Washes away particles containing microorganisms Contains microbial inhibitors (e.g., lysozyme)	Poor oral hygiene, dehydration
RESPIRATORY TRACT		
Cilia lining upper airways, coated by sticky mucous blanket	Traps inhaled microbes and sweeps them outward in mucus to be expectorated or swallowed	Smoking, high concentration of oxygen and carbon dioxide, decreased humidity, cold air
Macrophages	Engulfs and destroys microorganisms that reach lung's alveoli	Smoking
URINARY TRACT		
Flushing action of urine flow	Washes away microorganisms on lining of bladder and urethra	Obstruction to normal flow by urinary catheter placement, obstruction from growth or tumor, or delayed micturition
Intact multilayered epithelium	Provides barrier to microorganisms	Introduction of urinary catheter, continual movement of catheter in urethra
GASTROINTESTINAL TRACT		
Acidity of gastric secretions	Chemically destroys microorganisms incapable of surviving low pH	Administration of antacids
Rapid peristalsis in small intestine	Prevents retention of bacterial contents	Delayed motility from impaction of fecal contents in large bowel or mechanical obstruction by masses
VAGINA		
At puberty, normal flora causing vaginal secretions to achieve low pH	Acidic secretions inhibiting growth of many microorganisms	Antibiotics and birth control pills disrupting normal flora

so that reactions to future antigens are different from the first. In an immune response, the antigen is neutralized, destroyed, or eliminated.

There are two types of immunity: cell mediated and humoral. In cell-mediated immunity, T cells, a form of **lymphocyte,** bind with antigens. The T cell becomes sensitized and releases lymphokines, which attract **macrophages** and cause them to destroy antigens. In humoral immunity, B-lymphocytes cause synthesis of the **antibodies** that destroy antigens. After a B cell binds with an antigen, it causes formation of plasma cells and memory B cells. Plasma cells synthesize and secrete antibodies for greater immunity. Memory B cells prepare the body against future invasion.

table 25-4
INFLAMMATION

Physiological response	Signs and symptoms
VASCULAR AND CELLULAR RESPONSE	
Arterioles supplying infected or injured area dilate, delivering blood and leucocytes.	Redness Warmth
Tissue necrosis causes release of histamine, bradykinin, prostaglandin, and serotonin, which increase blood vessel permeability.	Edema
Fluid, protein, and cells enter interstitial spaces to cause swelling.	Pain
White blood cells (WBCs) enter tissues and phagocytose microorganisms. More WBCs are released into bloodstream.	WBC count normally 5,000 to 10,000/mm^3, 15,000 to 20,000/mm^3 common with inflammation
Phagocytic release of pyrogens from bacteria occurs.	Fever
INFLAMMATORY EXUDATE	
Fluid, dead cells, and WBCs form exudate at inflammatory site that later clears lymphatic drainage.	Serous or sanguineous exudate
TISSUE REPAIR	
Damaged cells are replaced with healthy new cells. Cells mature to take on structural characteristics and appearance of injured cells.	Tissue defects heal and close

RISKS FOR NOSOCOMIAL INFECTION

Multiple illnesses
Numerous invasive procedures (diagnostic and surgical)
Conditions monitored and treated using multiple invasive devices such as IV lines and urinary catheters
Use of broad-spectrum antibiotics that can cause resistant microorganisms to colonize in clients
Health care personnel who use poor aseptic or handwashing techniques
Multiple health care personnel caring for a client
Extended length of hospitalization

ASEPSIS AND NOSOCOMIAL INFECTION

Clients in health care settings, especially those in tertiary or extended care facilities, may be at a higher risk for infection (see box above) than those clients seen in the home setting. A **nosocomial** infection is defined as an infection that was not present or incubating upon admission and may or may not result from the delivery of health care (Garner, et al., 1988). Some nosocomial infections result when, because of the clients' lower immune system, they become infected with their own organisms. Unfortunately, most nosocomial infections are transmitted by the health care worker because of poor handwashing. For example, a wound infection may occur as a result of improper handwashing before a dressing change. **Iatrogenic** is a type of nosocomial infection resulting from a diagnostic or therapeutic procedure; an example could be a urinary tract infection that develops after a catheter insertion. The incidence of nosocomial infection may be lowered if nurses consciously practice handwashing and aseptic techniques.

Nosocomial infections may be exogenous or endogenous. An **exogenous infection** arises from microorganisms outside the individual, which do not exist as normal flora, such as *Salmonella, Clostridium tetani,* and *Aspergillus.* **Endogenous infections** can occur when part of the client's flora becomes altered and an overgrowth results (e.g., infections caused by enterococci, yeasts, and streptococci). When sufficient numbers of microorganisms normally found in one body cavity or lining are transferred to another body site, an endogenous infection develops. For example, transmission of enterococci, normally found in fecal material, from the hands to the skin is a cause of wound infections. The number of microorganisms needed to cause a nosocomial infection depends on the virulence of the organisms, the host's susceptibility, and the body site affected. Major sites for nosocomial infection include the urinary tract, surgical or trauma wounds, the respiratory tract, and the bloodstream (see the box on p. 613).

The nurse's efforts to minimize the onset and spread of infection are based on the principles of aseptic technique. Aseptic technique is the effort to keep the client as free from microorganisms as possible. The term **asepsis** means the absence of disease-producing microorganisms. The two types of aseptic technique that the nurse practices are medical asepsis and surgical asepsis.

Medical asepsis, or clean technique, includes procedures used to reduce the number of microorganisms and prevent their spread. Changing a client's bed linen daily, handwashing, and using clean medication cups

CAUSES AND SITES FOR NOSOCOMIAL INFECTIONS

SURGICAL WOUND INFECTION

Improper skin preparation before surgery
Colonization of health care worker
Improper handwashing
Use of contaminated instruments or solutions
Improper aseptic techniques during dressing change

PRIMARY BLOODSTREAM INFECTION/SEPSIS

Improper skin prep before insertion of IV catheter
Improper handwashing
Failure to change IV site at appropriate interval
Improper care of IV site
Contaminated IV equipment or solutions

PNEUMONIA

Improper handwashing
Improper aseptic techniques during suctioning
Contaminated equipment or tubing
Displacement of NG tube

URINARY TRACT INFECTION

Improper handwashing techniques
Insertion of urinary catheter
Open or disconnected drainage system
Improper specimen collection technique
Obstruction of drainage
Reflex of urine into bladder
Contaminated catheter or equipment

BONE AND JOINT INFECTION

Improper handwashing
Improper aseptic techniques during pin care or dressing care
Contaminated equipment

CARDIOVASCULAR SYSTEM INFECTION

Improper handwashing
Improper aseptic techniques during dressing change or following cardiac surgery
Contaminated equipment or dressings

CENTRAL NERVOUS SYSTEM INFECTION

Improper handwashing
Improper aseptic techniques during dressing changes or during monitoring of intercranial monitoring device
Contaminated equipment

EYE, EAR, NOSE, THROAT, AND MOUTH INFECTION

Improper handwashing
Contaminated equipment or dressings

GASTROINTESTINAL SYSTEM INFECTION

Improper handwashing
Contaminated food, water, or equipment

REPRODUCTIVE INFECTION

Improper handwashing
Contaminated equipment

SKIN AND SOFT TISSUE

Improper handwashing
Improper skin care

Modified from Garner JS, et al.: CDC definitions for nosocomial infections, *Am J Infec Control* 6(3):128, 1988.

are examples of medical asepsis. Principles of medical asepsis are commonly followed in the home, such as in the case of washing hands before preparing food.

Surgical asepsis, or sterile technique, includes procedures used to eliminate any microorganisms from an area. The process of sterilization destroys all microorganisms and their spores. This technique is practiced by operating room nurses when sterile instruments and supplies are used during a surgical procedure.

After an object becomes unsterile or unclean, it is **contaminated.** In medical asepsis an area or object is considered contaminated if it contains or is suspected of containing pathogens. For example, a used bedpan and a wet piece of gauze are contaminated. In surgical asepsis an area or object is considered contaminated if touched by any object that is not sterile. For example, a tear in a surgical glove exposes the outside of the glove to the skin surface, thus contaminating it.

The nurse is responsible for providing the client with a safe environment. The effectiveness of aseptic practices depends on the nurse's conscientiousness and consistency in using effective aseptic techniques. It is easy to forget key procedural steps or to take shortcuts that break aseptic procedures when hurried. However, the nurse's failure to be meticulous places the client at risk for an infection that can seriously impair his or her recovery.

The nurse should also assume responsibility for monitoring other health care team members who enter the client's environment. The nurse is the primary person at the client's bedside and is in a prime position to remind or educate others regarding the client's isolation status

ASSESSMENT OF CLIENT SUSCEPTIBILITY

FACTORS AFFECTING SUSCEPTIBILITY

Age

Infants have immature immune systems.

Children acquire more immunity but are susceptible to infectious diseases such as mumps and measles.

Young and middle-age adults have refined body system defenses and immunity.

Older adults' immune responses decline, and the structure and function of major organs change.

Nutritional status

A reduction in protein, carbohydrates, and fats as a result of illness, poor diet, or debilitation makes a client more susceptible to infection and impairs wound healing.

Conditions such as burns or trauma that increase protein requirements place an individual at greater risk.

Stress

Increased stress elevates cortisone levels, causing decreased resistance to infection.

Continuous stress exhausts energy stores.

Disease process

Diseases of the immune system such as AIDS or lymphoma weaken defenses against infection.

Chronic diseases like diabetes cause general debilitation and nutritional impairment.

Diseases that alter body system defenses increase the risk of infection.

Diagnostic and therapeutic procedures

Intravenous therapy, chemotherapy, and exploratory surgery increase risk of infection.

Heredity

Certain hereditary conditions impair the response to infection.

Medical therapy

Certain drugs and therapies compromise immunity to infection.

Inadequate defenses

Primary and secondary defenses may be altered (e.g., broken skin or mucosa, traumatized tissue, decreased ciliary action, suppressed inflammatory response, and low WBC count).

CLINICAL APPEARANCE

Localized infection

Redness, swelling, pain or tenderness, and restricted movement of a body part occur. There may be drainage from open lesions or wounds.

Systemic infections

Fever, fatigue, malaise, lymph node enlargement, loss of appetite, nausea, and vomiting may be found.

Laboratory data

Specific laboratory tests, including WBC count, iron level, cultures, erythrocyte sedimentation rate, and differential count, add to the data base for assessing infection.

Immunization status

Nonimmunized individuals are at risk for disease.

and to reinforce proper technique when procedures are performed.

NURSING PROCESS

Assessment

The nurse assesses the client's susceptibility, defenses, and knowledge of infection (see box above). A review of the disease history with the client and family may reveal a recent exposure to a communicable disease. By evaluating signs and symptoms, the client's clinical condition may indicate the onset or extension of an infection. The assessment would also include risk factors, previously discussed, for infections.

Laboratory data should be assessed as soon as available (Table 25-5). Laboratory values such as increased WBCs and/or positive blood culture may indicate infection. Sometimes these results may indicate the need for the use of barrier precautions or isolation. The nurse can consult with the Infection Control Department or refer to the facility's policy for assistance.

The early recognition of infection assists the nurse in making the correct nursing diagnosis and establishing a treatment plan. In addition, the nurse can alert the physician to the need for further investigation of the client's condition, facilitating initiation of prompt therapy.

The nurse must also assess ways in which an infection affects client and family needs. Clients with chronic or serious infection such as tuberculosis or AIDS may experience psychological and social problems from self-imposed isolation or rejection by friends and family. Clients or their families may not be able to afford the cost of medical care. Families, especially those in home care settings, may not be able to offer the physical or emotional support necessary to facilitate adjustment to disease. In such a situation the nurse should begin discharge planning. The nurse should also be able to assess the client's ability to adjust to the dis-

table 25-5

LABORATORY TESTS TO SCREEN FOR INFECTION

Laboratory value	Normal (adult) values	Indications
WBC count	5000-10,000/mm	Increased in acute infection, decreased in certain viral infections or in reduced immunity
Erythrocyte sedimentation rate	Up to 15 mm/hr for men and 20 mm/hr for women	Elevated in presence of inflammation
Iron level	60-90 g/dl	Decreased in chronic infection
Cultures of urine and blood	Normally sterile, without microorganism growth	Presence of greater than 100,000 colonies of microorganisms (clean catch urine specimen)
Cultures of wound, sputum, and throat	Possible normal flora	Presence of infectious microorganism growth
Differential count (percentage of each type of WBC)		
Neutrophils	55%-70%	Increased in acute suppurative infection, decreased in overwhelming bacterial infection (older adult)
Lymphocytes	20%-40%	Increased in chronic bacterial and viral infection, decreased in sepsis
Monocytes	2%-8%	Increased in protozoal, rickettsial, and tuberculosis infections
Eosinophils	1%-4%	Increased in parasitic infection
Basophils	0.5%-1%	Normal during infection

ease and the need for resources to manage health problems.

Nursing Diagnosis

Following assessment, the nurse clusters data that show a pattern of findings indicating an actual infection or risk for infection. Objective data might include an elevated temperature, open draining wound, or inflammation of an intravenous catheter site. Subjective findings might include client complaint of chills, malaise, or tenderness over a wound. The nurse's assessment also includes a review of laboratory data for findings such as an elevated WBC count. Other sources of data include a review of nursing documentation. For example, the record shows the date of insertion for the intravenous catheter currently in place.

Clusters of defining characteristics lead to the selection of a nursing diagnosis. The related factors, revealed in the assessment, ensure individualization of the diagnosis. For example, the nurse may diagnose "high risk for infection related to intravenous catheter placement" in a client with a decreased WBC count, multiple intravenous catheters, and inflammation around a catheter site. The related factor, intravenous catheter placement, will direct the nurse to change the catheter regularly and take measures to minimize microorganism transfer through the intravenous system. If the nursing diagnosis happened to be "high risk for infection related to malnutrition," the nurse's choice of interventions would include use of nutritional support. An accurate related factor ensures a more appropriate care plan.

Infection or its associated treatment may be the related factor for a number of nursing diagnoses (see box below). In the case of social isolation, the related factor will be the isolation precautions used for the client. Nursing interventions would then be directed at minimizing the effect isolation has on the client's ability to socialize.

Planning

The client's care plan is based on each nursing diagnosis and related factor. The use of aseptic technique is incorporated into appropriate interventions. Nursing interventions are selected in collaboration with the client,

NURSING DIAGNOSES FOR CLIENTS SUSCEPTIBLE TO OR AFFECTED BY INFECTION

High risk for infection
Altered nutrition: less than body requirements
Actual impaired skin integrity
Altered oral mucous membrane
Body-image disturbance
Social isolation
Impaired tissue integrity

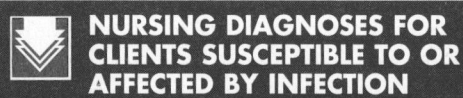

family, and other health care team members. The nurse, for example, may choose to involve the infection control nurse, dietitian, or enterostomal therapist in the client's care. As the nurse plans for discharge from an acute care setting, it will be important to determine the extent to which the family will be involved in caring for the client at home. The family may require instruction regarding infection control practices. If a client is to receive extended care in the home, the nurse must plan for the availability of resources such as dressing materials and solutions.

When the client has a known infection or the nurse has diagnosed a high risk for infection, the common goals and outcomes of care may include the following:

Goal: Control transmission of infectious organisms.

Outcomes

Client does not experience onset of nosocomial infection

Infection does not spread to other body parts

Goal: Control or decrease progression of infection.

Outcomes

Client's wound drainage decreases in 3 days

Inflammation over an involved site decreases in 5 days

Goal: Client's resistance to infection is maintained or increased.

Outcomes

Client achieves daily 2600 calorie intake

Client's WBC count remains in normal limits

Goal: Client uses self-care practices to control infection by the day of discharge.

Outcomes

Client demonstrates correct handwashing techniques by third hospital day

Client describes signs and symptoms of local wound infection by fourth hospital day

Once goals and outcomes are developed, the nurse sets priorities. For example, a client suffering from a debilitating illness develops an open draining wound and has been unable to tolerate solid foods. The priority the nurse should set in this situation is to promote wound healing before planning support of self-care activities in the home. As the client's condition changes, the priority of interventions will also change.

Implementation

Nurse's Role in Infection Control

The nurse prevents the onset and spread of infection and promotes measures for treatment of infection. To prevent an infection from developing or spreading, the nurse minimizes the numbers and kinds of organisms transmitted to potential infection sites. Eliminating reservoirs of infection, controlling portals of exit and entry, and avoiding actions that transmit microorganisms prevent bacteria from finding a site to grow. Disinfection and sterilization of supplies and good handwashing are examples of aseptic methods used to control the spread of microorganisms. A final preventive measure is strengthening a potential host's defenses against infection. Nutritional support, rest, maintenance of physiological protective mechanisms, and immunization protect a client from invasion by pathogens.

When a client develops an infection, the nurse continues preventive care so that health care personnel and other clients do not acquire the infection. Good handwashing continues to be a major step in minimizing exposure of staff and clients to infection. Clients with communicable diseases and infections that are easily transmissible to others require special precautions. Isolation precautions involve control of a client's environment by forming barriers against bacterial spread. Interventions for the older adult require recognition of risk factors that are caused by the aging process (see box below).

Treatment of an infectious process includes identification and elimination of the organism and support of the client's defenses. The nurse collects specimens of body fluids or drainage from infected body sites for cultures. When the disease process or causative organism has been identified, the physician prescribes the antiinfective or antibiotic drug most effective for the situation.

GERONTOLOGIC NURSING PRACTICE FOR INFECTION CONTROL INTERVENTIONS

The older adult experiences an alteration in oral mucosa integrity. The nurse should promote careful oral hygiene and regular dental care.

The older adult experiences a decrease in the production of digestive acid. The nurse teaches the older client to carefully wash hands before food preparation, to adequately cook foods, and to refrigerate unused portions promptly.

The dermal and epidermal skin layers of the older adult become thinner, and elasticity is decreased. The nurse turns the bedridden client frequently and carefully observes the skin for breakdown.

The older adult experiences urethral stricture, neurogenic bladder, and in older men, prostatic enlargement. In the older client with an indwelling Foley catheter, the nurse assesses for adequate drainage and maintains cleanliness of the urethra at the insertion site.

Older adults experience a decrease in rib cage movement during inspiration. Caring for older adults postoperatively, the nurse elevates the head of the bed (if indicated) and encourages the client to cough and breath deeply and to get out of bed as soon as possible.

The nurse administers antibiotics carefully, watching for allergic reactions, assessing the progress of the client's infection, and administering the drugs by the proper methods.

Systemic infections require measures to prevent the complications of fever (see Chapter 15). Maintaining intake of fluids prevents dehydration resulting from diaphoresis. Increased metabolism requires an adequate nutritional intake. Rest preserves energy for the healing process.

Localized infections often require measures to facilitate removal of infectious organisms. Wet-to-dry dressings (see Chapter 37) are used to remove infected drainage from wound sites. Application of heat compresses promotes blood flow to an infected site and thus the delivery of blood components needed to fight an infection. Drainage tubes may be inserted to remove infected drainage from body cavities. The nurse uses medical and surgical aseptic techniques to manage wounds and ensures the correct handling of infected drainage or body fluids.

During any infection, the nurse supports the client's body defense mechanisms. For example, if a client is known to have infectious diarrhea, the nurse must maintain skin integrity to prevent breakdown and entrance of microorganisms. Routine hygiene measures such as cleansing the oral cavity and bathing further protect the skin and mucous membranes from organism spread.

A client with an infection may have many needs. By monitoring the infection's course carefully, the nurse can choose the most appropriate measures to maintain or restore the client's health.

Medical Asepsis

The nurse follows certain principles and procedures when preventing infection and controlling its spread. Basic medical aseptic techniques break the infection

SAMPLE CARE PLAN
High Risk for Infection

ASSESSMENT

Clinical scenario: Mr. Russel is a 35-year-old client diagnosed with *chronic myelocytic leukemia.* A *WBC count* shows an *abnormal elevation* of 100,000/mm^3 with *immature neutrophils.* Mr. Russel has fatigue, *a small ulceration of the oral mucosa, enlarged cervical and axillary lymph nodes,* and a *20-pound weight loss* over the last month.

NURSING DIAGNOSIS

High risk for infection related to inadequate immune defenses

PLANNING

Goals	Expected Outcomes
Infection of oral mucosa will not develop during hospitalization.	Oral mucosa will remain free of additional ulcerations. Existing ulceration will heal within 1 week. Client will experience no further weight loss during hospitalization.

IMPLEMENTATION

Steps	Rationale
1. Offer foods high in protein, vitamins A and C, zinc, and copper.	Physiological processes of wound healing depend on availability of protein, vitamins, and trace minerals.
2. Use thorough handwashing with antimicrobial soap before administering mouth care.	In care settings where clients are at high risk of infection, antimicrobial soaps are more effective in reducing microorganisms on hands (Larson, 1989).
3. Provide mouth care routinely after all meals, using solution of ½ to 1 tsp. of salt or baking soda to 1 pint of water.	Solution effectively removes mucus (Greifze, et al., 1990). Soft toothbrush minimizes bleeding gums. Systematic oral care may be more effective than a particular oral care regimen (Kenny, 1990).
4. Apply liquid topical antibiotics as ordered.	Promotes healing of ulcer.

EVALUATIVE MEASURES

Inspect condition of mucosa before and after mouth care.
Weigh client daily in morning.

chain. The nurse uses precautions for all clients, even when an infection has not been diagnosed. Aggressive preventive measures can be highly effective in reducing nosocomial infections.

Control or Elimination of Infectious Agents. With the increased use of disposable equipment, nurses may become less aware of disinfection and sterilization procedures. The proper cleaning, disinfection, and sterilization of contaminated objects significantly reduce and often eliminate microorganisms. In large health care centers, a central supply department does most of the disinfection and sterilization of reusable supplies, which in most cases involve surgical aseptic technique. However, at times, nurses use medical aseptic techniques in preparing items. Many of these principles also apply in the home.

CLEANING. **Cleaning** is the process of removing foreign materials (e.g., organic material such as blood or inorganic material such as soil) from objects. Generally, this is accomplished by the use of water, a detergent, and proper mechanical scrubbing action. Cleaning must occur before disinfection and sterilization procedures (Rutala, 1989). When cleaning objects soiled by blood or body fluids, the nurse should first don personal protection equipment (PPE) such as gloves, goggles, and mask to protect from splash. Items may be cleaned using a soft-bristle brush, water, and detergent. In addition, the nurse should check the health care facility's policy before cleaning. Wearing PPE, the nurse may follow these steps for the cleaning of an object:

1. Rinse or soak the contaminated object with cold water to remove organic materials. Care should be taken not to rinse under running water as splashing and aerosolization may occur. Hot water coagulates the protein in organic material, making it sticky and difficult to remove.
2. After rinsing or soaking, wash the object with a detergent and warm water. Detergents lower the surface tension of water and emulsify dirt or remaining material. Rinse the object thoroughly to remove the emulsified dirt.
3. Use a soft brush to remove dirt or material in grooves or seams. Stiff-bristle brushes can damage delicate objects such as surgical instruments.
4. Rinse the object in copious amounts of water. Some objects such as surgical instruments should have distilled water as the final rinse.
5. Dry the object and prepare it for disinfection or sterilization.
6. Cleaning equipment should be disposed of according to the health care facility's policy.

DISINFECTION AND STERILIZATION. Physical and chemical processes are used for disinfection and sterilization. Both processes disrupt the internal functioning of microorganisms by destroying cell proteins. **Disinfection** is a process that eliminates almost all pathogenic organisms on objects, with the exception of bacterial spores, whereas **sterilization** is a process that eliminates or destroys all forms of microbial life (Rutala, 1989). The level of disinfection and sterilization required depends on the type and usage of the contaminated item. The items used for client care are divided into three categories (see box above). It is important for the nurse to be familiar with the health care agency's policies and procedures for the cleansing, disinfecting or sterilization, handling, and delivery of client care items. Workers specially trained in disinfection and sterilization procedures perform most of these procedures. The nurse does have the responsibility of checking for package integrity and/or out dates before using an object designated as sterile. Any object not meeting the aforementioned criteria should be disposed of or sent to the sterilization processing department. Table 25-6 lists examples of methods of disinfection and sterilization.

CATEGORIES FOR STERILIZATION, DISINFECTION, AND CLEANING

CRITICAL ITEMS—STERILIZATION

Items that enter sterile tissue or vascular system present a high risk of infection if the items are contaminated with any microorganisms and spores. Items must be sterile. Some of these items follow:

- Surgical instruments
- Cardiac catheters
- Urinary catheters
- Needles
- Implants

SEMICRITICAL ITEMS—DISINFECTION

Items that come in contact with skin that is not intact or mucous membranes also present risks. These objects must be free of all microorganisms (except bacterial spores). Some of these items follow:

- Respiratory therapy equipment
- Endotracheal tubes
- Gastrointestinal endoscopes
- Reusable mercury thermometers

NONCRITICAL ITEMS—CLEANING

Items that come in contact with intact skin but not mucous membranes must be clean. Some of these items follow:

- Bedpans
- Blood pressure cuffs
- Crutches
- Linens
- Food utensils

table 25-6

EXAMPLES OF PROCESSES FOR DISINFECTION AND STERILIZATION

Characteristics	Examples of use
MOIST HEAT	
Moist heat includes steam (moist heat under pressure) or free steam. When exposed to high pressure, water vapor can attain a temperature above boiling point to kill all pathogens and spores. Free steam is used to sterilize objects that would otherwise be destroyed at higher temperature of autoclave.	Steam autoclave sterilizes surgical instruments, parenteral solutions, and surgical dressings.
RADIATION	
Ionizing radiation penetrates deeply into objects for effective sterilization and disinfection.	Radiation sterilizes drugs, foods, and other heat-sensitive items.
CHEMICALS	
Effective disinfectants when used appropriately. Selection depends on the item to be disinfected and its use, correct concentration and temperature of chemical, and correct exposure time of the item.	Chemicals are used for disinfection of instruments and equipment such as respiratory therapy equipment.
ETHYLENE OXIDE GAS	
This gas destroys spores and microorganisms by altering cells' metabolic processes. Fumes are released within an autoclave-like chamber. Ethylene oxide gas is toxic to humans and proper aeration after sterilization is essential.	This gas sterilizes rubber, paper, and plastic items. (Check manufacturer's recommendations.)
BOILING WATER	
Boiling is least expensive for use in home. Bacterial spores and some viruses resist boiling. It is not used in hospitals.	The items (e.g., glass baby bottles) should be boiled for at least 15 minutes.
DRY HEAT	
Sterilizing process occurs when heat is absorbed by the exterior surface of an article and then passes inward to the next layer. Death of the microorganism is accomplished by the coagulation of protein of the cells.	Dry heat is used for sterilization of glassware, powders or oils, and instruments that could corrode easily.

Control or Elimination of Reservoirs. To control or eliminate infection in reservoir sites the nurse eliminates sources of body fluids, drainage, or solutions that might harbor microorganisms. The nurse also carefully discards articles that become contaminated with infectious material (see box on p. 620).

Control of Portals of Exit. To control organisms exiting through the respiratory tract, the nurse avoids talking, sneezing, or coughing directly over a surgical wound or sterile dressing field. The nurse covers the mouth or nose when sneezing or coughing. The nurse also teaches clients to protect others when they sneeze or cough and gives clients disposable wipes or tissues to control spread of microorgansims.

A nurse who has a mild cold and continues to work with clients should wear a mask, especially when changing a dressing or performing a sterile procedure. The nurse should refrain from working with clients who are highly susceptible to infection.

Another way of controlling the exit of microorganisms is the careful handling of exudate such as urine, feces, and wound drainage. The nurse should wear disposable gloves if there is a chance of contact with any exudate. Soiled items are appropriately bagged and discarded.

Control of Transmission. Effective control of infection requires a nurse to know the modes of transmission and ways to control them. In the hospital, home, or ex-

INFECTION CONTROL TO REDUCE RESERVOIRS OF INFECTION

Bathing. Use soap and water to remove drainage, dried secretions, excess perspiration, or sediment from disinfectants.
Dressing changes. Change dressings that become wet and soiled (see Chapter 37).
Contaminated articles. Place tissues, soiled dressings, or soiled linen in moisture-resistant bags for proper disposal.
Contaminated needles. Place syringes and hypodermic needles and intravenous needles in moisture-resistant, puncture-proof containers. (Do not recap needles or attempt to break them.)
Bedside unit. Keep table surfaces clean and dry.
Bottled solutions. Do not leave bottles open for long periods. Keep solutions tightly capped.
Surgical wounds. Keep drainage tubes and collection bags patent to prevent accumulation of serous fluid under the skin's surface.
Drainage bottles and bags. Empty and rinse suction bottles according to agency policy. Empty all drainage systems on each shift unless otherwise ordered by a physician.

tended care facility, a client should have a personal set of care items. Sharing thermometers, bedpans, urinals, bath basins, and eating utensils can easily lead to transmission of infection. Electronic thermometers significantly reduce the transmission of infection. Glass thermometers, even when individually used, require special care. Because the client's mucus can become a source for microorganism growth, the thermometer is washed in soap and water and dried after each use.

Because certain microorganisms travel easily through the air, linens or bedclothes should not be shaken. Dusting with a treated or dampened cloth prevents dust particles from entering the air.

To prevent transmission of microorganisms through indirect contact, soiled items and equipment must not touch the nurse's clothing. A common error is to carry dirty linen in the arms against the uniform. Special linen bags should be used, or soiled linen should be carried with the hands held out from the body.

Anything that touches the floor is contaminated. If the nurse accidentally drops a piece of equipment, it should be discarded. Clean or soiled linen should never be put on the floor.

HANDWASHING. The most important and most basic technique in preventing and controlling transmission of pathogens is handwashing. Handwashing is a vigorous, brief rubbing together of all surfaces of lathered hands, followed by rinsing under a stream of water (Garner and Favero, 1985).

The need for handwashing depends on the type, intensity, duration, and sequence of activity. For example, if a nurse simply touches an object that is not visibly soiled, handwashing is not required. In contrast, contact with any client, especially one with wound drainage, requires thorough handwashing. It is recommended that nurses wash their hands in the following situations:

1. Before and after contact with each client, especially those susceptible to infection (e.g., newborn infants or immunosuppressed clients)
2. After touching organic material
3. Before performing invasive procedures such as injections, catheterization, and suctioning
4. Before and after handling dressings or touching open wounds
5. After handling contaminated equipment

The ideal duration of handwashing is not known. The **Centers for Disease Control and Prevention (CDC)** note that washing times of at least 10 to 15 seconds (Garner and Favero, 1985) remove most transient microorganisms from the skin. In addition, antimicrobial soaps must be in contact with the skin at least 10 seconds to have a desired effect (Larson, 1989b). Washing the hands more often also improves the effectiveness of antiseptic soaps (Larson, 1989a). Agency policies often recommend that staff wash hands for as long as 1 to 2 minutes after working in high-risk areas. Routine handwashing may be performed with bar, liquid, or granule soap, or soap-impregnated tissue.

Use of antimicrobial-containing soaps is encouraged when nurses work in special care units, perform invasive procedures, or care for clients with known multiple resistant bacteria (Larson, 1989a). Larson et al. (1987) also found that using 3 to 5 ml of antiseptic soap can significantly reduce bacteria on the hands. In the same study, bacterial counts were the same after using 1, 3, or 5 ml of plain soap. Procedure 25-1 lists the steps for handwashing.

Handwashing must be performed without risk to the care giver. Excessive washing may crack the skin and alter its pH. Products that are less harsh to the skin are now available. At one time, hand lotion was felt to harbor microorganisms. Studies now show that hand lotion may reduce shedding of viable microorganisms from the skin (Hall et al., 1986). Larson (1989b) recommends using hand lotion dispersed from small containers and avoiding application right after washing or right before giving direct care.

Nurses often omit handwashing when gloves are worn. However, gloves do not provide complete protection as they may have tiny holes. Microorganisms can multiply on hands inside gloves. Handwashing is also required after removing gloves (CDC, 1988).

Nurses must instruct clients and visitors about

procedure 25-1

HANDWASHING

Steps	Rationale
1. Use sink with warm running water, soap or disinfectant, and paper towels.	Running water facilitates removal of organisms. Paper towels are easy to discard.
2. Push wristwatch and long uniform sleeves above wrists. Remove jewelry, except plain band, from fingers and arms.	Provides complete access to fingers, hands, and wrists. Jewelry may harbor microorganisms.
3. Keep fingernails short filed, and free of nail polish or artificial fingernails.	Dirt and secretions that lodge under fingernails contain microorganisms. Long fingernails can scratch skin.
4. Inspect surface of hands and fingers for breaks or cuts in skin and cuticles. Report such lesions when caring for highly susceptible clients.	Open cuts or wounds can harbor high concentrations of microorganisms. Such lesions may serve as portals of exit, increasing client's exposure to infection, or as portals of entry, increasing nurse's risk of acquiring infection.
5. Stand in front of sink, keeping hands and uniform away from sink surface. (If hands touch sink during handwashing, repeat.) Use sink where it is comfortable to reach faucet.	Inside of sink is contaminated area. Reaching over sink increases risk of touching edge, which is contaminated.
6. Turn on water by pressing knee or foot pedals or turning hand-operated faucet (see illustration).	
7. Avoid splashing water against uniform.	Microorganisms travel and grow in moisture.
8. Regulate flow of water so that temperature is warm.	Warm water is more comfortable. Hot water opens pores of the skin, causing irritation.

Step 6

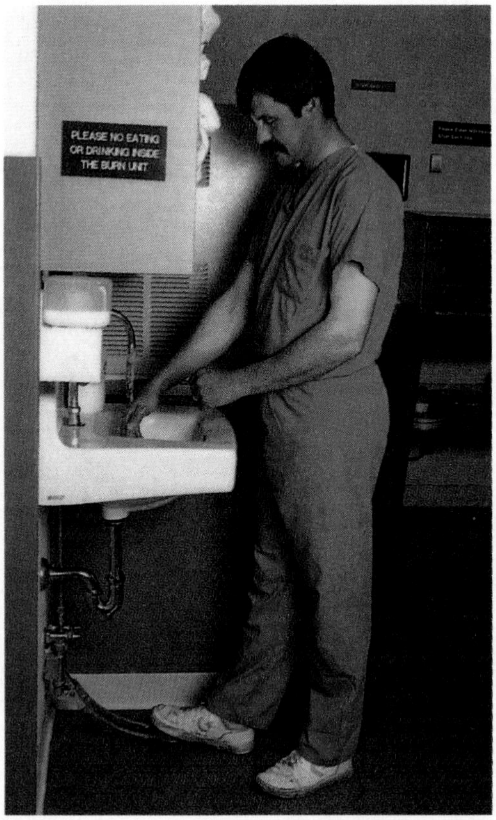

Continued.

procedure 25-1—cont'd

HANDWASHING

Steps	Rationale
9. Wet hands and lower arms thoroughly under running water. Keep hands and forearms lower than elbows during washing.	Hands are the most contaminated parts to be washed. Water flows from least to most contaminated area, rinsing microorganisms into sink.
10. Apply 1 ml of regular or 3 ml of antiseptic liquid soap to hands, lathering thoroughly (Larson, 1988). If bar soap is used, hold it throughout lathering. Soap granules and leaflet preparations may be used.	Bar soap should be rinsed before returning it to soap dish. Soap dish that allows water to drain keeps soap firm. Jellylike soap permits growth of microorganisms.
11. Wash hands using plenty of lather and friction for at least 10 to 15 seconds. Interlace fingers and rub palms and back of hands with circular motion at least 5 times each (see illustration).	Soap cleanses by emulsifying fat and oil and lowering surface tension. Friction and rubbing mechanically loosen and remove dirt and transient bacteria. Interlacing fingers and thumbs ensures that all surfaces are cleansed.
12. If areas underlying fingernails are soiled, clean them with fingernails of other hand and additional soap or clean orangewood stick. Do not tear or cut skin under or around nail.	Mechanical removal of dirt and sediment under nails reduces microorganisms on hands.
13. Rinse hands and wrists thoroughly, keeping hands down and elbows up (see illustration).	Rinsing mechanically washes away dirt and microorganisms.
14. Repeat steps 10 through 12 but extend period of washing to 1 to 3 minutes.	Greater the likelihood of hands being contaminated, greater the need for thorough handwashing.
15. Dry hands thoroughly from fingers to wrists and forearms.	Drying from cleanest (fingertips) to least clean (forearms) area avoids contamination. Drying hands prevents chapping and roughened skin.
16. Discard paper towel in proper receptacle.	Prevents transfer of microorganisms.
17. Turn off water with foot and knee pedals. To turn off hand faucet, use clean, dry paper towel.	Wet towel and hands allow transfer of pathogens by capillary action.

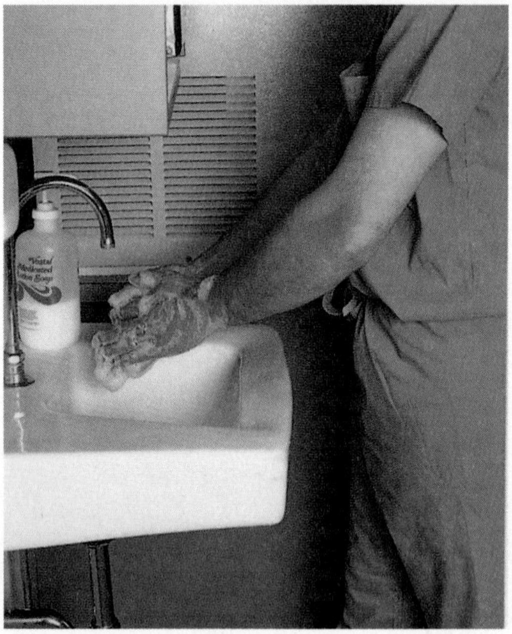

Step 11

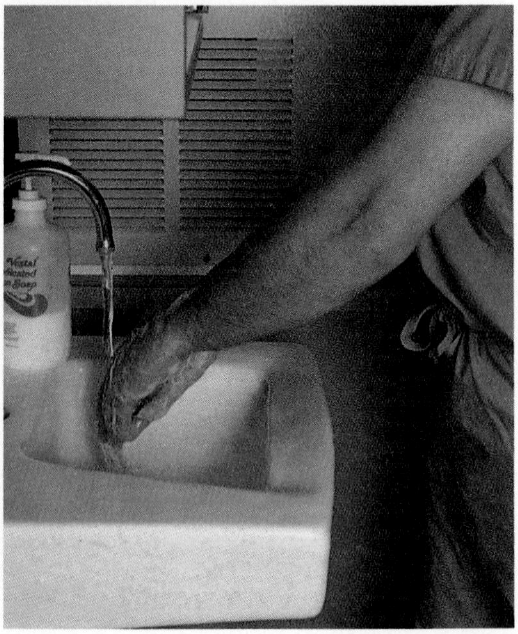

Step 13

proper techniques and times for handwashing, especially if the client's health care is to continue at home. Visitors are encouraged to wash their hands before eating or handling food, after coming in contact with infected clients, and after handling contaminated equipment or organic material.

Isolation and barrier protection. Clients often have infection and/or communicable disease that can be transmitted to other clients, family members, or health care workers without the use of proper barrier protection. In addition, special precautions and/or barrier protection may be required to protect clients with lower immunity. Barriers such as gloves or masks may prevent the transmission of infections; isolation and/or private rooms may keep pathogens in a confined area. For example, since TB is transmitted by the inhalation of infectious droplet nuclei, health care workers wear either masks or respirators to prevent the transmission of infections, and the client is placed in a special ventilated isolation room to keep the TB organism contained (CDC, 1993). Care givers should follow practices to prevent transmission of infected organisms.

In health care settings the nurse may see a variety of types of isolation precautions being utilized. Two of these types, **Body Substance Isolation** and **Universal Precautions,** stress the importance of barrier protection from blood or body fluid, even in a client with an undiagnosed disease. For this reason, a nurse must always use precaution when there is a potential for being exposed to an infectious agent. These isolation precautions are generally used with a combination of one or more types of isolation.

Lynch and Jackson (1988) described a system, Body Substance Isolation (see box at right), which is based on the premise that many organisms can be found in body substance regardless of whether a culture has confirmed the infection and a diagnosis has been made. They stressed that body substances such as feces, urine, gastric content, mucus, and wound drainage always contain organisms and that an isolation system that uses certain precaution for all clients is more likely to prevent the transmission of infection than a system initiated only after a diagnosis is made. Many hospitals today are implementing such a system (Lynch, et al., 1990).

A major concern about the risk of exposure to HIV and hepatitis B exists among health care providers. In 1987 the CDC recommended that blood and body fluid precautions be consistently used for all clients regardless of their blood-borne infection status. In other words, health care workers should consider all clients to be potentially infected with HIV, hepatitis B virus, or other blood-borne pathogens. These Universal Precautions are intended to prevent parenteral, mucous membrane, and nonintact skin exposures of health care providers to blood-borne pathogens. In 1988 the CDC

BODY SUBSTANCE ISOLATION

An isolation system that uses generic infection control practices for all clients.

Health care personnel use protective barriers when contacting any body fluid, mucous membranes, or nonintact skin.

Personnel change gloves between clients and between activities with the same client when gloves become excessively soiled.

Personnel wash hands for at least 10 seconds when the hands are soiled, before each new client contact, and after gloves are removed. (Wearing gloves does *not* eliminate the need to wash hands.)

Additional barriers such as gowns or plastic aprons, masks, goggles or glasses, hair covers, and shoe covers are used as needed to keep moist body substances off clothing, skin, and mucous membranes of the wearer. For example, the nurse wears masks and goggles when performing a procedure in which the face can be sprayed with mucus, blood, or any body fluid.

All sharp instruments and needles are discarded uncapped in a rigid, puncture-proof container located at the point of use such as client room or treatment area.

Laboratory specimens from all clients are handled as if they were infectious.

Handling and reprocessing practices are uniform for all articles and equipment used on all clients. For example, soiled reusable articles are transported in plastic bags or rigid containers.

Soiled linen is bagged securely before transport.

Private rooms are used for clients with communicable diseases transmitted via the air or clients who soil their environment uncontrollably with body substances. A large red sign reading *Stop* (see Figure 25-2) is placed at the door of this client's room; it also instructs all persons, "Check with the nurse before entering." For certain diseases (e.g., meningococcal meningitis), masks are worn when personnel or family enter the client's room. Roommates who are immune to the client's disease or who are currently infected with the same disease may share rooms (institutional policy may vary on this issue).

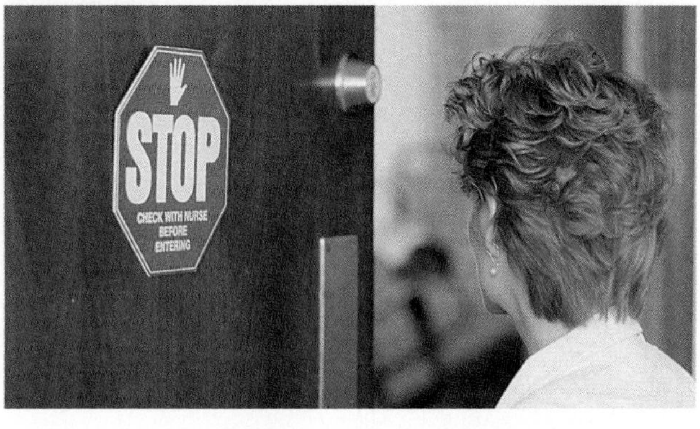

FIGURE 25-2 A visible stop sign is placed on the door of a client under special isolation precautions.

clarified that Universal Precautions apply to blood, cerebrospinal fluid, synovial fluid, pleural fluid, peritoneal fluid, pericardial fluid, amniotic fluid, semen and vaginal secretions, and to any other body fluid such as feces, nasal secretions, sputum, urine, and vomitus containing visible blood. Further, the CDC emphasized that blood is the most important source of HIV, hepatitis B, and other blood-borne pathogens. Use of Universal Precautions is now the minimum standard of health care practice as mandated by the Occupational Safety and Health Act of 1991 (Federal Register, 1991) (see box on p. 625).

Because of the resurgence of tuberculosis (TB), another type of isolation gaining increased importance is AFB or respiratory isolation (some facilities use these terms interchangeably). The CDC (1993) has produced guidelines for the prevention of transmission of TB in the health care worker and stresses the importance of isolation for known or suspected TB clients in specially vented negative pressure rooms. In addition, a room should have at least six air exchanges and the door closed to maintain control of direction of air flow. A special high filtration particulate respirator should be used when entering an AFB isolation room or when caring for a cough-producing client. The disposable respirator looks like a cup-shaped surgical mask. Types of masks may be dictated by the state or local OSHA; however they must be able to fit health care workers with different facial sizes and characteristics. When worn correctly, the particulate respirators and masks (Figure 25-3, *A* and *B*) have a tighter face seal than routine surgical masks.

The CDC (1983) published specific guidelines for the isolation of clients in controlled settings. Although not all these system categories may be seen in today's health care facilities, nurses should be aware of these and the general premise for each type. One is the disease-specific system; a sign is placed on the client's door designating types of barriers required. Unfortunately, all too often, the actual disease (e.g., hepatitis, tuberculosis) is also stated on the door sign and/or front of the chart, thus breaching client confidentiality. The other system is designated as category-specific isolation. Diseases requiring similar isolation precautions are determined by the manner in which organisms are transmitted. The category Universal Precautions was formerly called Blood and Body Fluid Precautions. A sign is placed outside the client door to alert health care workers to use proper barrier protection (Table 25-7 lists CDC categories).

Regardless of the type of isolation or barrier protection utilized, the nurse must follow certain basic principles:

1. The hands should be washed thoroughly before entering and leaving the room of a client.

A
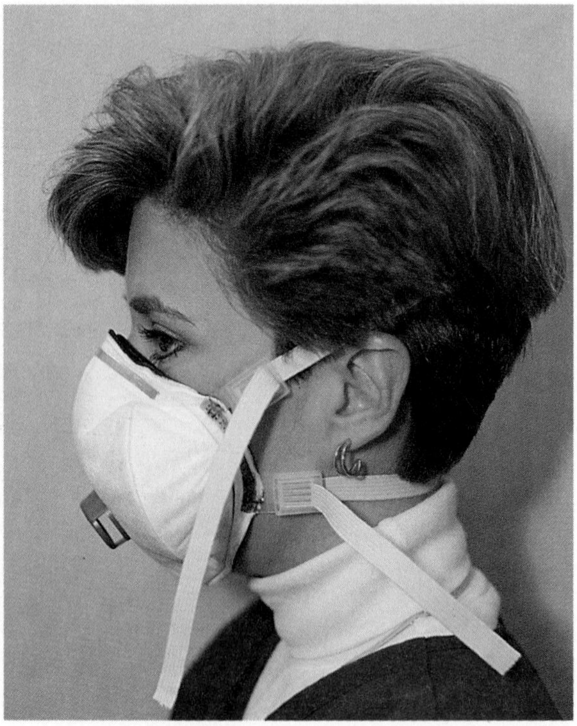

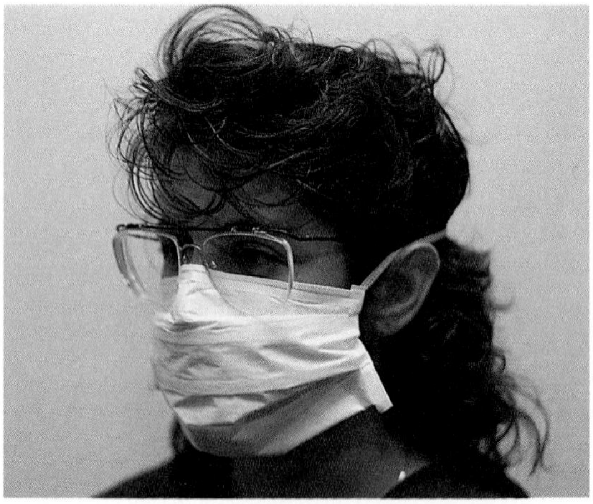
B

FIGURE 25-3 A, Disposable HEPA air-purifying respirator. **B,** 0.1-micron filtration surgical facemask.

UNIVERSAL PRECAUTIONS

Occupational exposure means reasonably anticipated skin, eye, mucous membrane, or parenteral contact with blood or other potentially infectious materials that may result from the performance of an employee's duties. In this definition parenteral refers to piercing mucous membranes or the skin barrier through such events as needlesticks, human bites, cuts, and abrasions.

Other potentially infectious materials means:

1. The following human body fluids: semen, vaginal secretions, cerebrospinal fluid, synovial fluid, pleural fluid, pericardial fluid, peritoneal fluid, amniotic fluid, saliva in dental procedures, any body fluid that is visibly contaminated with blood, and all body fluids in situations in which it is difficult or impossible to differentiate between body fluids
2. Any unfixed tissue or organ (other than intact skin) from a human (living or dead)
3. HIV-containing cell or tissue cultures, organ cultures, and HIV- or HBV-containing culture medium or other solutions

Health care personnel at risk for exposure to potentially infectious materials shall use **personal protective equipment** such as, but not limited to, gloves, gowns, laboratory coats, face shields or masks, and eye protection and mouthpieces, resuscitation bags, pocket masks, or other ventilation devices. Personal protective equipment will be considered "appropriate" only if it does not permit blood or other potentially infectious materials to pass through to the employee's work clothes, street clothes, undergarments, skin, eyes, mouth, or other mucous membranes. Masks, eye protection (such as goggles or glasses with solid side shields), and face shields shall be worn whenever there is risk of splashes, spray, spatter, or droplets of blood or other infectious materials being generated.

Employers shall ensure that appropriate personal protective equipment in the appropriate sizes is readily accessible at the worksite.

Hands and other skin surfaces shall be washed immediately and thoroughly if contaminated with blood or other fluids and after removal of gloves or other personal protective equipment. Personnel wash hands for at least 10 seconds when the hands are soiled, before each new client contact, and after gloves are removed. (Wearing gloves does not eliminate the need to wash hands.)

Contaminated needles and other contaminated sharps shall not be bent, recapped, or removed except as noted later. Shearing or breaking of contaminated needles is prohibited. Contaminated needles and other sharps shall not be recapped or removed unless the employer can demonstrate that no alternative is feasible or that such action is required by a specific medical procedure. Such recapping or needle removal must be done through the use of a mechanical device or a one-handed technique.

Immediately or as soon as possible after use, contaminated reusable sharps shall be placed in appropriate containers until properly reprocessed. These containers shall be puncture resistant, labeled or color-coded, and leakproof on the sides and bottom.

Eating, drinking, smoking, applying cosmetics or lip balm, and handling contact lenses are prohibited in work areas where there is reasonable likelihood of occupational exposure.

Food and drink shall not be kept in refrigerators, freezers, shelves, cabinets, or on countertops or benchtops where blood or other potentially infectious materials are present.

All procedures involving blood or other potentially infectious materials shall be performed in such a manner as to minimize splashing, spraying, spattering, and generation of droplets of these substances.

Specimens of blood or other potentially infectious materials shall be placed in a container that prevents leakage during collection, handling, processing, storage, transport, or shipping.

Regulated waste means liquid or semi-liquid blood or other potentially infectious materials—contaminated items that would release blood or other potentially infectious materials in a liquid or semi-liquid state if compressed. Items that are caked with dried blood or infectious materials are included. Contaminated sharps are considered regulated waste.

Regulated waste shall be placed in containers that are closable, constructed to contain all contents and prevent leakage of fluids during handling, storage, or transporting. The containers shall be color-coded for ease of identification and closed before removal to prevent spillage or protrusion of contents. If the outside of a container is contaminated, it shall be placed in a second container and closed before removal.

An employer shall make available the hepatitis B vaccine and vaccination series to all employees who have occupational exposure, and postexposure evaluation and follow-up to all employees who have had an exposure incident. This service shall be made available at no cost to the employee.

From OSHA: Bloodborne pathogens: rules and regulations, *Fed Register* 58:64175-64182, 1991.

table 25-7

ISOLATION CATEGORIES

Type of isolation (specific category)	Purpose	Examples of disease or condition	Room
Strict	Prevents transmission of highly contagious or virulent infections spread by air and contact	Chickenpox; diphtheria	Private room with door closed
Contact	Prevents transmission of highly transmissible infections spread by close or direct contact, which do not warrant strict precautions	Acute respiratory infections in infants and young children; impetigo; herpes simplex; infections by multiple resistant bacteria	Private room; clients infected with same organism may share room
Respiratory	Prevents transmission of infectious diseases over short distances by air droplets	Measles; meningitis; mumps; pneumonia; *Haemophilus* influenza (in children)	Private room; clients infected with same organism may share room
Acid-fast bacillus isolation (AFB)	Is special category for clients with pulmonary tuberculosis who have positive results on sputum or chest x-ray examination indicating active disease	Pulmonary or laryngeal tuberculosis	Private room with special ventilation (air from adjacent rooms and corridors must flow into, not out of, isolation room). Exhaust air must not be recirculated; door closed
Enteric precautions	Prevents infections transmitted by direct or indirect contact with feces	Cholera; diarrhea of an infectious cause; hepatitis A; gastroenteritis caused by highly infectious organism	Private room if client's hygiene is poor (does not wash hands, shares contaminated items); clients with same organism may share room
Drainage/secretion precautions	Prevents infections transmitted by direct or indirect contact with purulent material or drainage from infected body site	Abscess; burn infection; infected wound; minor infections not included in contact isolation	Private room not indicated
Universal precautions*	Prevents transmission of blood-borne pathogens by direct or indirect contact; must be practiced with *all clients* as a minimum standard	Acquired immune deficiency syndrome (AIDS); hepatitis B; syphilis	Private room indicated if client's hygiene is poor
Neutropenic precautions	Protects uninfected client with lowered immunity and resistance from acquiring infectious organisms	Leukemia; lymphoma; aplastic anemia	Private room with door closed

*Formerly blood and body fluid precautions.

Gown	Gloves	Mask	Precautions
Required of all persons entering room	Required of all persons entering room	Required of all persons entering room	Discard or bag and label articles contaminated with infective materials. Send reusable articles for disinfection and sterilization.
Indicated if soiling or contact likely	Indicated for persons touching infective material	Indicated for persons coming close to client	Discard or bag and label articles contaminated with infective material. Send reusable items for disinfection and sterilization.
Not indicated	Not indicated	Indicated for persons who come close to client	Discard or bag and label articles contaminated with infective material. Send reusable items for disinfection and sterilization. Bathroom should not be shared with clients.
Indicated only if needed to prevent gross contamination of clothing	Not indicated	Well-fitting, high-filtration mask. *Ordinary surgical masks offer little protection* (ATS, 1992)	Articles are rarely involved in transmission of tuberculosis. Articles should be thoroughly cleansed, disinfected, or discarded.
Indicated if soiling is likely	Indicated when touching infective material	Not indicated	Discard or bag and label articles contaminated with infective material. Send reusable items for disinfection and sterilization. Bathroom should not be shared with clients.
Indicated if soiling or contact with infective material likely	Indicated for touching infective material	Not indicated	Discard or bag and label articles contaminated with infective material. Send for disinfection or sterilization.
Indicated during procedures likely to generate splashes of blood or body fluids	Indicated for touching blood or body fluids containing visible blood, mucous membranes or nonintact skin of all clients; indicated for touching soiled items	Indicated during procedures likely to generate droplets of blood	Discard or bag and label articles contaminated with blood or body fluids. Disinfect and sterilize articles. Avoid needle stick injuries. Dispose of used needles in properly labeled, puncture-resistant container. Clean blood spills promptly with 5.25% solution of sodium hypochloride diluted 1:10 with water.
Required of all persons entering room	Required of all persons entering room	Indicated for persons coming in contact with client	For open wound or burns, use sterile gloves.

2. All contaminated supplies and equipment should be disposed of in a manner that prevents spread of microorganisms to other persons.
3. Knowledge of a known disease process and the means of infection transmission should be applied when using protective barriers.
4. All persons who might be exposed during transport of a client outside the isolation room must be protected.

Psychological implications of isolation. Implementing isolation precautions creates a forced solitude that could deprive the client of normal social relationships. This situation can be psychologically harmful, especially for children.

As a result of the infectious process, the client's body image may be altered. He or she may feel unclean, rejected, lonely, or guilty. The aseptic practices the nurse follows add to these feelings. Isolation in a private room limits sensory contact. The nurse acts to minimize the client's feelings of psychological and physical isolation.

Before isolation measures are instituted, the client and family must understand the nature of the client's condition, the purposes of the precautions, and ways to carry out specific precautions. If the client and family can participate in maintaining isolation precautions, the chances of reducing the spread of infection and lowering the client's risk of complications are great. The client and family are taught the proper way to wash hands and don gowns, masks, or gloves. Each procedure should be demonstrated, and the client and family should be given an opportunity for practice. The nurse also explains the way infectious organisms can be transmitted so that the client understands the difference between contaminated and clean objects. Unless family members know that their clothing becomes contaminated by contact with infected secretions, efforts at controlling infection are wasted.

The nurse also improves the client's sensory stimulation during isolation. Reading materials, a radio or television set, a clock, and hobby materials should be available. The room environment should be clean and pleasant looking. The room drapes or shades should be opened and excess supplies or equipment removed. The nurse must take the opportunity to listen to the client's concerns or interests; if the nurse rushes through care or shows a lack of interest in the client's needs, the client will feel rejected and even more isolated. Mealtime is a good opportunity for conversation. Providing comfort measures such as repositioning or a back massage increases physical stimulation. The nurse encourages the client to walk and sit up in a chair when possible.

The nurse explains the client's risk of depression or loneliness to family members. Visitors should be encouraged to avoid expressions or actions that convey revulsion or disgust. The nurse advises family members on ways to provide meaningful stimulation.

Environment. When BSI or Universal Precautions are in place, all clients are treated as though they are potentially infected. In the past a private room was recommended for reducing the possibility of transmission of infection by separating susceptible clients from those who might have an infection. The room also served as a reminder for personnel to wash their hands and use medical asepsis. Today, private rooms are only used for infection control when a client soils the environment, uses poor hygiene, or fits into a special CDC isolation category (check agency policy). When a private room is recommended, the nurse posts a card on the client's room door, listing the precautions for the isolation category. The card is a handy reference for health care personnel and visitors and alerts all who enter the room of any special precautions.

The protective environment should contain handwashing, bathing, and toilet facilities. Soap and antiseptic solutions are also available. Personnel and visitors wash their hands before coming to the client's bedside and again before leaving the room. If toilet facilities are unavailable, there are special procedures for handling portable commodes, bedpans, or urinals (check agency policy). Isolation supplies can be stored in an anteroom between the room and hallway or in a special isolation cart in the hallway. The nurse keeps ample supplies of gowns, masks, and gloves in the storage area.

Each isolation room contains a special impervious bag for soiled or contaminated linen, as well as a trash container with plastic liners. These receptacles prevent transmission of microorganisms by preventing seepage to and soiling of the outside surface. A disposable, impervious container should be available in the room to discard used needles, sharps, and syringes.

The nurse avoids taking any article or piece of equipment into a client's room that is to be reused outside the isolation area. If such an article becomes contaminated with infected material, it must be discarded or disinfected and sterilized.

Gowns. The primary reason for gowning is to protect health care personnel from contacting infectious organisms in blood and body fluids. Gowns used for barrier protection are made of a fluid-resistant material and changed immediately if damaged or heavily contaminated. If visitors are likely to contact infectious waste, they should learn to wear gowns routinely while in client rooms.

Isolation gowns usually open at the back and have ties or snaps at the neck and waist to keep the gown closed and secure. A gown should be long enough to cover all outer garments. Long sleeves with tight-fitting cuffs provide added protection. No special technique is required for donning a gown as long as it is fastened securely. Occasionally, a nurse reuses an isolation gown for the same client. If a gown is to be reused, it must not be visibly soiled.

Masks. A mask protects a nurse from inhaling mi-

procedure 25-2

DONNING A SURGICAL MASK

Steps	Rationale
1. Find top edge of mask (usually has thin metal strip along edge).	Pliable metal fits snugly against bridge of nose.
2. Hold mask by top two strings or loops. Tie two top ties at top of back of head, with ties above ears (see illustration). (Alternative: slip loops over each ear.)	Provides tight fit. Ties over ears may cause irritation.
3. Tie two lower ties snugly around neck with mask well under chin (see illustration).	Prevents escape of microorganisms through sides of mask as nurse talks or breathes.
4. Gently pinch upper metal band around bridge of nose.	Prevents microorganisms from escaping around nose.

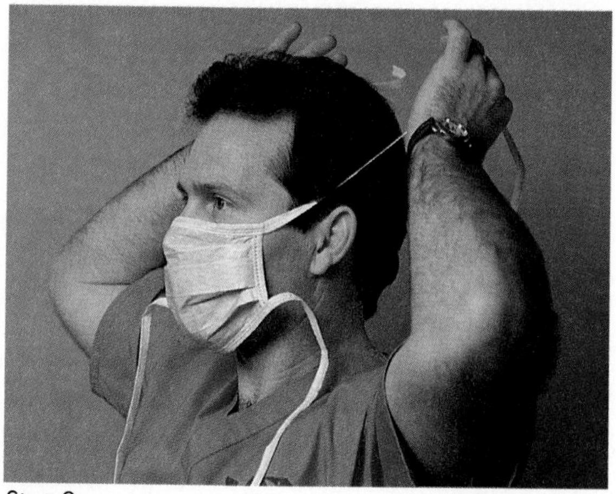
Step 2

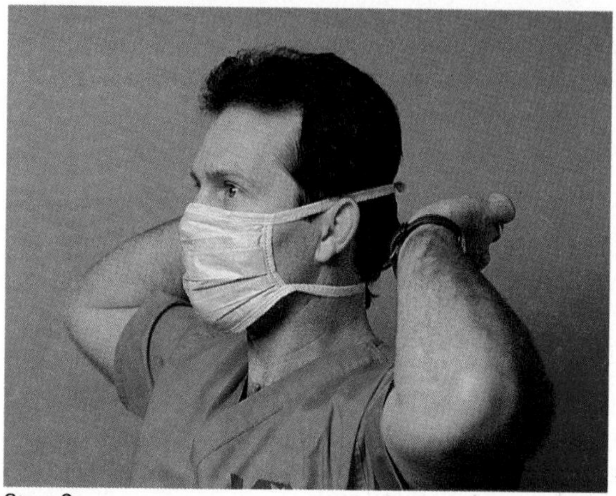
Step 3

croorganisms from a client's respiratory tract and prevents the transmission of pathogens from the nurse's respiratory tract. The mask protects a wearer from inhaling large-particle aerosols that travel short distances (3 feet) and small-particle droplet nuclei that remain suspended in the air and travel longer distances. At times a client who is susceptible to infection wears a mask to prevent inhalation of pathogens. Clients receiving respiratory precautions who are transported outside their rooms should wear masks during transit to protect other clients and personnel.

According to the CDC, masks may prevent the transmission of infections by direct contact with mucous membranes (Williams, 1983). A mask discourages the wearer from touching the eyes, nose, or mouth.

A properly applied mask fits snugly over the mouth and nose so that pathogens and body fluids cannot enter or escape through the sides (Procedure 25-2). If a person wears glasses, the top edge of the mask fits below the glasses so they will not cloud over as the person exhales. Talking should be kept to a minimum while wearing a mask. A mask that has become moist is ineffective and should be discarded. A mask should never be reused. Clients and family members should be warned that a mask can cause a sensation of smothering. If family members become uncomfortable, they should leave the room and discard the mask. It should be noted that special high filtration masks may be required when a client is in AFB isolation (consult agency policy). Before removing a mask, a person should remove gloves (if worn) and wash the hands.

Gloves. Gloves prevent transmission of pathogens by direct and indirect contact by the nurse. The CDC (Williams, 1983) cites the following reasons for wearing gloves:

1. Reduces the possibility of personnel coming in contact with infectious organisms that infect clients
2. Reduces likelihood that personnel will transmit their own endogenous flora to clients
3. Reduces possibility that personnel will become transiently colonized with microorganisms that

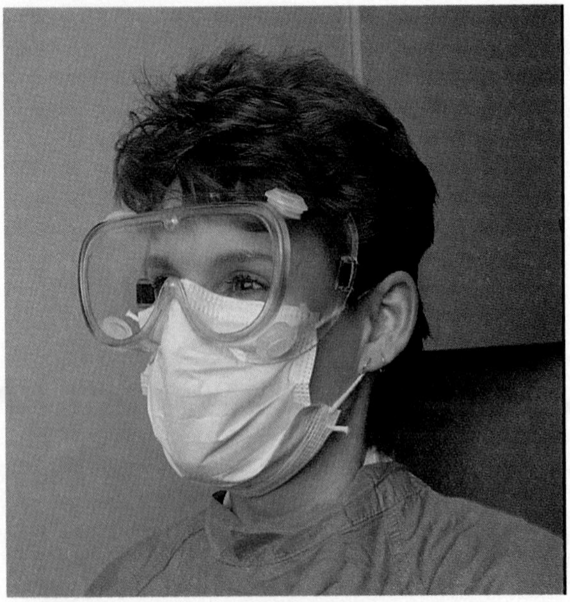

FIGURE 25-4 Nurse wearing protective goggles and mask.

can be transmitted to other clients (transient colonization can usually be prevented with handwashing)

Nurses apply gloves when there is a risk of exposure to potentially infectious material. In addition, gloves are recommended when the nurse has scratches or breaks in the skin; when performing venipuncture, finger, or heel sticks; and when the nurse is inexperienced (Dickerson, 1989). In most cases disposable, single-use gloves are worn. Gloves may be worn alone or in combination with other personal protective equipment. Before applying gloves, the nurse dons a mask and eyewear (if required), washes and dries the hands, and applies a gown. Disposable gloves are easily applied and designed to fit either hand. The glove's thin rubber can tear easily. The glove cuffs should be pulled up over the wrists or cuffs of a gown.

After contacting infectious material, the nurse changes gloves and washes hands if care is not completed. If the nurse's actions do not involve more client contact, reapplying gloves is unnecessary.

Family members often believe they can touch any object after they have applied gloves. The nurse should explain that gloves can also become contaminated after touching infectious material or contaminated objects (Larson, 1989a). A person should always wash hands immediately after removing gloves.

Eye protection and face shields. Properly fitted eye protection (glasses or goggles) (Figure 25-4) or chin-length face shields should be worn to protect the nurse during procedures in which the eyes or face could be splattered by blood or other infectious material. OSHA requires health care organizations to enforce policy that directs employees to protect their eyes, nose, or mouth during procedures in which splattering could occur. In many instances, care givers purchase their own eyewear with prescription lenses. Regular glasses are insufficient. Glasses must have side shields to prevent material from entering the eye between the glasses and face. Nurses working in high risk areas such as operating rooms, emergency, labor and delivery, or trauma units should be especially careful to protect themselves from exposure.

Delivery of care in an isolation room. With the development of Body Substance Isolation and Universal Precautions, all clients are potentially in some type of isolation room. The nurse should be aware of how diseases are transmitted and the barriers necessary to prevent transmission. For example, a nurse would not need to wear a gown or gloves when giving an oral medication, but may need these barriers when changing a dressing on a draining wound. But in the same manner, gloves may be appropriate when assisting a client with an oral medication if the client has visible draining oral herpes simplex. Care should be taken not to expose an article brought into a client's room to an infectious material. If an article such as a blood pressure cuff becomes contaminated with blood or any infectious material, it should be bagged according to the facility's policy and sent for decontamination. A contaminated article should not be used on or brought into the room of another client. The most protective procedure that can be practiced for the client or the health care worker is handwashing.

Specimen collection. A client with a suspected or actual infectious disease may undergo many laboratory studies. Body fluids and materials suspected of containing infectious organisms are collected for culture and sensitivity tests. The specimen is placed in a special medium that promotes the growth of organisms. A laboratory technologist then identifies the type of microorganisms growing in the culture. Additional sensitivity test results indicate the antibiotics to which the organisms are resistant or sensitive so that the proper medications will be used in the client's treatment.

The nurse obtains all culture specimens with sterile equipment. Collecting fresh material from the site of infection, as in the case of wound drainage, ensures that the specimen will not be contaminated by neighboring microbes. All specimen containers should be sealed tightly to prevent spillage and contamination of the outside of the container. The box on p. 631 describes the techniques for collecting specimens from the client. In each case, a clean container remains outside the client's room or on a clean paper towel in the client's bathroom. After the specimens are transferred to containers, the nurse labels each specimen properly with the client's name, the type of specimen, and the type of isolation.

SPECIMEN COLLECTION TECHNIQUES*

WOUND SPECIMEN

Use cotton-tipped swab or syringe to collect as much drainage as possible. Have clean test tube or culturette tube on clean paper towel. After swabbing center of wound site, grasp collection tube by holding it with paper towel. Carefully insert swab without touching outside of tube. After securing tube's top, transfer tube into bag for transport and then wash hands.

BLOOD SPECIMEN

Use syringe and culture media bottles to collect 10 ml of blood per culture bottle. Perform venipuncture at two different sites to decrease likelihood of both specimens being contaminated with skin flora. Place blood culture bottles on bedside table or other surface, swab off bottletops with alcohol. Inject appropriate amount of blood into each bottle. Remove gloves and transfer specimen into clean bag for transport.

STOOL SPECIMEN

Use clean cup with seal top (not necessary to be sterile) and tongue blade to collect small amount of stool, approximately the size of a walnut. Place cup on clean paper towel in client's bathroom. Using tongue blade, collect needed amount of feces from client's bedpan. Transfer feces to cup without touching cup's outside surface. Dispose of tongue blade, wash hands, and place seal on cup. Transfer specimen into clean bag for transport.

URINE SPECIMEN

Use syringe and sterile cup to collect 1 to 5 ml of urine. Place cup or tube on clean towel in client's bathroom. Use syringe to collect specimen if client has a Foley catheter. Have client follow procedure to obtain a clean voided specimen (see Chapter 32) if not catheterized. Transfer urine into sterile container by injecting urine from syringe or pouring it from used container. Wash hands and secure top of container. Transfer specimen into clean bag for transport.

From Pagana KD, Pagana TJ: *Diagnostic testing and nursing implications,* ed 3, St. Louis, 1989, Mosby.
*Agency policies may differ on type of containers and amount of specimen material required.

Nurses place the specimen containers in labeled impervious bags before transporting them to the laboratory.

Bagging articles. The nurse uses special bagging procedures for removing contaminated items from the client's environment. Bagging articles prevents accidental exposure of personnel to contaminated articles and prevents contamination of the surrounding environment.

The CDC recommends that a single bag is adequate for discarding or wrapping items if the bag is impervious and sturdy and if the article can be placed in the bag without contaminating the outside of the bag (Williams, 1983). The nurse typically discards reusable equipment such as stethoscopes, forceps, or suction bottles in single bags. The CDC recommends double bagging if it is impossible to prevent contamination of the bag's outer surface. When linen bags become filled, the CDC suggests the following guidelines (Weinstein et al., 1989) for handling isolation linen:

1. Soiled linen should be placed in a laundry bag in the client's room.
2. The bag should be labeled or it should be a specific color designated for such linen so that it is easily recognized.
3. Linen requires less handling if the bag is soluble in hot water. However, such a bag may need to be double bagged because it punctures or tears easily.

Double bagging is often still required in many hospitals. However, studies have shown that this procedure is not necessary to control for infection (Maki, et al., 1986; Weinstein et al., 1989). Use of one standard-sized linen bag that is not overfilled and that is tied securely and is intact is adequate to prevent infection transmission. The same rule applies to trash bags.

If double bagging is followed in an agency, the procedure requires the nurse in the client's room to place all soiled linen into a bag and close it tightly. The nurse then places the first bag into a second bag held by a "clean nurse" or into a self-supporting hamper outside the client's room. The outer bag is specially labeled or colored. The "clean nurse" outside the room secures the outer bag and sends it to the laundry. The nurse should consult agency policy for the proper procedure.

Removing protective clothing. The nurse removes gloves, mask, eyewear, and gown before leaving the isolation room. The order of removal depends on the protective equipment worn by the nurse at the time. In the example in which all four protective items are worn, the nurse first removes the gloves because they are more likely to be contaminated. If the nurse unties a gown with gloves still on, there is a chance of contaminating hair or a portion of the uniform. When gloves are pulled off, the cuff should be grasped with the other gloved hand and pulled off, turning the glove inside out (Figure 25-5, *A*). With the ungloved hand the nurse tucks the fin-

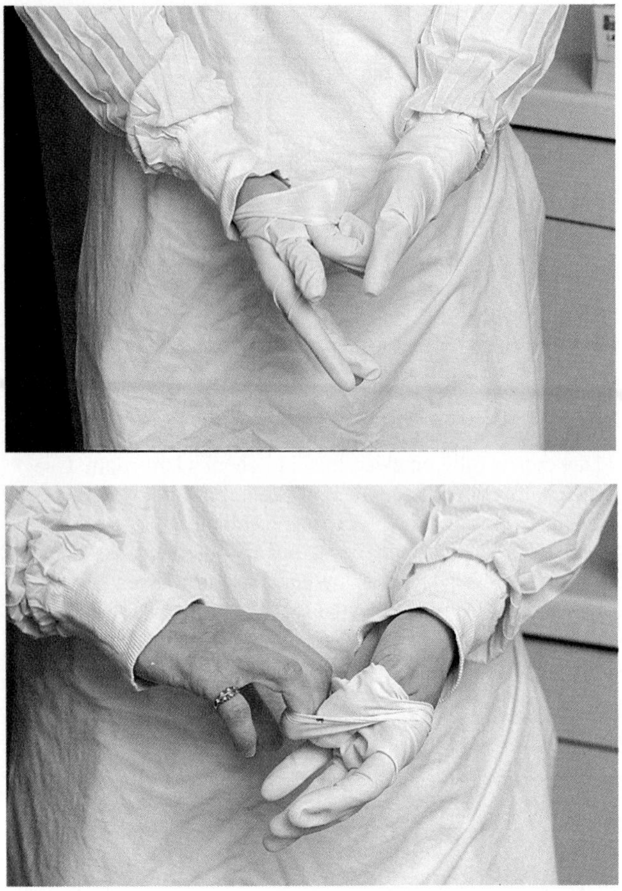

A

B

FIGURE 25-5 Removing disposable gloves. **A,** Nurse places gloved finger inside cuff to pull first glove off hand. **B,** Second glove is removed as nurse slides finger inside glove cuff and pulls.

gers inside the cuff of the remaining glove and pulls it off, turning the glove inside out (Figure 25-5, *B*). The gloves are discarded in a plastic-lined receptacle.

Masks are disposable and made of a specially prepared paper or cotton fiber. The nurse unties the top string first, then the bottom, and pulls the mask away from the face while holding the strings. The outside surface of the mask should not be touched. The nurse simply discards the mask in a plastic-lined receptacle.

To remove a gown, the nurse first unties the waist and neck ties. The nurse allows the gown to fall gently from the shoulders. Care should be taken to remove the hands from the sleeves without touching the outside of the gown (Figure 25-6). The sleeves should not be allowed to turn inside out. The gown is held at the shoulder seams and folded in half with the outside surfaces touching to reduce contact with the soiled gown. The gown is then discarded in the soiled receptacle.

The last step is to remove eyewear. Goggles and glasses are reusable. The nurse refers to agency policy for cleaning procedures. Once eyewear is removed, the nurse completes a thorough handwashing.

TRANSPORTING CLIENTS. Clients infected with virulent organisms should leave their rooms only for essential purposes such as diagnostic procedures or surgery. Before transferring the client to a wheelchair or stretcher, the nurse gives the client the appropriate barrier protection. For example, a client who is infected by an organism transmitted by the respiratory tract must wear a mask. Personnel transporting the client should practice the appropriate precautions while in the client's room.

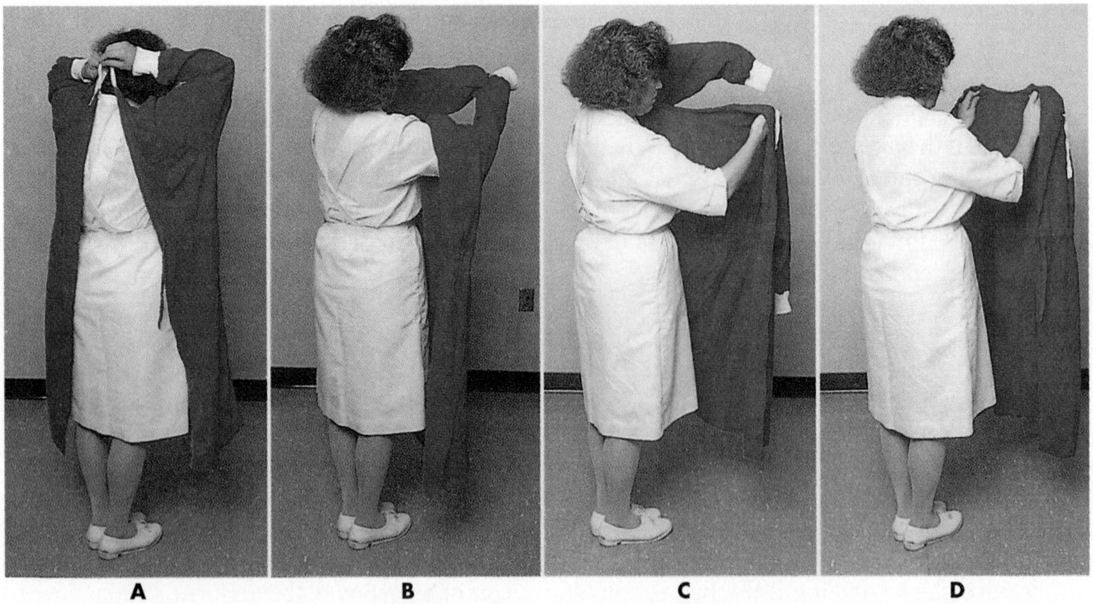

A B C D

FIGURE 25-6 Removing isolation gown. **A,** Nurse loosens neck ties. **B,** Hands are carefully removed from sleeves. **C,** Sleeves are not allowed to be turned inside out. **D,** Gown is folded with outside surfaces touching.

Personnel in diagnostic areas or the operating room should be notified that the client is on isolation. The nurse records the type of isolation on the client's chart and explains ways to avoid transmitting infection during transport.

Control of Portals of Entry. Many measures that control the exit of microorganisms also control the entrance of pathogens. The nurse makes sure that the microorganisms do not enter sterile environments. The box below lists examples of nursing interventions.

Protection of the Susceptible Host. A client's resistance to infection improves as the nurse protects normal body defenses against infection. The nurse also intervenes to maintain the body's normal reparative processes (see box below, right).

Role of the Infection Control Department. Most hospitals employ health professionals who are specially trained in the area of infection control. Roles and responsibilities of the infection control department include the following:

1. Providing staff education on infection control
2. Reviewing infection control policies and procedures
3. Gathering statistics regarding the epidemiology of nosocomial infections
4. Investigation of outbreaks oi infection
5. Providing input regarding selection of patient-care products
6. Research related to infection control activities
7. Liaison and consultant to pertinent hospital committees
8. Liaison with regulatory agencies

An effective infection control program can reduce the risk of infection in both clients and the health care team as well as reduce the cost of health care.

Health Promotion in Hospital Personnel and Clients

Hospital workers are exposed occasionally to infectious microorganisms. An employee who becomes ill can expose susceptible clients to any of a number of infectious

INFECTION CONTROL OF PORTALS OF ENTRY

INTACT SKIN AND MUCOSA

Keep skin clean and well lubricated.
Avoid positioning clients on tubes or objects that might cause breaks in skin.
Use dry, wrinkle-free linen.
Offer frequent oral hygiene (see Chapter 30).
Provide frequent position changes for clients with impaired mobility.

URINARY TRACT

Teach women to clean rectum and perineum by wiping from area of least contamination (urinary meatus) toward area of most contamination (rectum).
Do not allow urine in drainage bags and tubes to flow back into the bladder. Never raise a drainage system above the level of the bladder.
Keep points of connection between catheter or drain and tubing closed.

INVASIVE TUBES AND LINES

When obtaining specimens from drainage tubes or inserting needles into intravenous lines, disinfect tubes and ports by wiping them liberally with a disinfectant solution before entering the system.

WOUND CARE

Keep draining wounds covered so that drainage is contained.
Clean outward from a wound site using a clean swab for each application.

INFECTION CONTROL: PROTECTING THE SUSCEPTIBLE HOST

PROTECTING NORMAL DEFENSE MECHANISMS

Regular bathing removes transient microorganisms from the skin's surface. Lubrication helps to keep the skin hydrated and intact.
Regular oral hygiene removes proteins in the saliva that attract microorganisms. Flossing removes tartar and plaque that can cause infection.
Maintenance of an adequate fluid intake promotes normal urine formation and a resultant outflow of urine to flush the bladder and urethral lining of microorganisms.
For physically dependent or immobilized clients, encourage routine coughing and deep breathing to keep lower airways clear of mucus.
For physically dependent or immobilized clients, provide frequent position changes to decrease the risk of skin breakdown at bony prominences.
Encourage proper immunization of children or adult clients who become exposed to certain infectious microorganisms (e.g., influenza, measles).

MAINTAINING REPARATIVE PROCESSES

Promote intake of a well-balanced diet containing essential proteins, vitamins, carbohydrates, and fats. Use measures to increase client's appetite (see Chapter 31).
Promote a client's comfort and sleep so that energy stores are replaced daily (see Chapters 28 and 27).
Assist client in learning techniques to reduce stress.

diseases. For these reasons the following are elements of a personnel health service that will assist in infection control.

1. Placement evaluation. A health assessment evaluates an employee's risk for acquiring or transmitting an infectious disease in the workplace. An immunization history, history of previous infectious disease, and a physical examination determine whether an employee is a carrier of a disease (e.g., tuberculosis) or has any condition (e.g., immunodeficiency) that increases susceptibility to infection.
2. Personnel health and safety education. A hospital's health service should plan educational programs to orient personnel to the policies and procedures for infection control. Employee health or infection control departments can coordinate such an effort. Written policies and guidelines should be provided for all levels of personnel.
3. Immunization programs. An immunization program safeguards personnel and protects clients from becoming infected by personnel. It is especially important to immunize employees who work in high-risk areas. Nurses working in obstetric clinics should be immunized against rubella to protect pregnant clients. According to the Occupational Safety and Health Act (OSHA) of 1991, all health care workers who are occupationally exposed to blood should be offered immunization to hepatitis B.
4. Work restrictions and control of job-related illnesses. When an employee is exposed to an infectious disease, the employee health service must determine whether the employee can continue working. The hospital has the responsibility of preventing the spread of infection to clients and employees.
5. Protocols for management of job-related exposures to infectious diseases. Hospitals also have the responsibility of providing prompt follow-up for job-related exposures to such diseases as AIDS, hepatitis, and tuberculosis (CDC, 1987).
6. Health counseling. Hospital personnel should know about infection risks. Personnel with certain clinical conditions require health counseling. Female employees who are pregnant or who might become pregnant should know about risks to the fetus from work assignments and measures to reduce these risks.

Client Education. Clients and families must often learn to use infection control practices at home. Aseptic technique becomes almost second nature to the nurse practicing it daily. However, the client is less aware of the factors that promote the spread of infection or of the ways to prevent its transmission. The home does not always lend itself to the practice of aseptic technique. A nurse must often help a client to improvise with the resources available to maintain hygienic techniques. For example, a client may use a laundered washcloth instead of expensive sterile gauze to wash around his or her open wound.

After clients are at home, they determine their own compliance with infection control practices. The nurse educates clients about the nature of infection and the techniques to use in preventing or controlling its spread (see teaching box above). Family members must also become involved in the teaching plan. Teaching efforts involve a commonsense approach to controlling and preventing infection.

CLIENT TEACHING FOR INFECTION CONTROL

Teach client basic handwashing practices (when and how).
Instruct client about hygiene practices that reduce organism growth and spread.
Provide a simple explanation of clean versus contaminated items.
Discuss the client's susceptibility to infection.
Explain that family members are at risk for acquiring infections.
Teach the application of aseptic principles to self-care activities such as wound care and medication administration.
Instruct client about proper methods for food handling and storage.
Discuss preventive health care (e.g., diet and immunizations).

Surgical Asepsis

Surgical asepsis requires more stringent precautions than medical asepsis. The nurse working with a sterile field or with sterile equipment must understand that the slightest break in technique results in contamination. Surgical asepsis requires the absence of all microorganisms, including spores, from an object. The nurse also practices surgical asepsis to keep microorganisms away from an area (e.g., when filling a syringe or changing a dressing on a wound).

Although surgical asepsis is commonly practiced in the operating room, labor and delivery area, and major diagnostic areas, the nurse may also use surgical aseptic techniques at the client's bedside (e.g., when inserting intravenous catheters). Surgical asepsis is indicated during procedures that require intentional perforation of the client's skin (e.g., surgical incision), when the skin's integrity is broken related to trauma or burns, and during procedures that involve insertion of catheters or surgical instruments into sterile body cavities.

Assessment. Because surgical asepsis requires exact techniques, the nurse must have the client's cooperation. Therefore the nurse must assess the client's understanding of sterile procedure and identify whether special precautions are necessary to prevent contamination during procedures.

CLIENT KNOWLEDGE. The nurse determines whether a client has undergone a sterile procedure in the past. If not, the nurse explains how the procedure will be performed and what the client can do to avoid contaminating sterile objects:

1. Avoiding sudden movements of body parts covered by sterile drapes
2. Refraining from touching sterile supplies, drapes, or the nurse's sterile gloves and gown
3. Avoiding coughing, sneezing, or talking over a sterile area

PRECAUTIONS. Certain sterile procedures may last a long time. The nurse assesses the client's needs and anticipates factors that may disrupt a procedure. If a client is in pain, the nurse tries to administer analgesics no more than 30 minutes before a sterile procedure begins. The nurse allows the client to care for elimination needs. Clients must often assume relatively uncomfortable positions during sterile procedures; the nurse helps the client to assume the most comfortable position possible. Finally, the client's condition may result in actions or events that contaminate a sterile field (e.g., the client with a respiratory infection who transmits organisms by coughing or breathing). The nurse anticipates such a problem (e.g., offering a mask to the client).

Principles of Surgical Asepsis. When beginning a surgically aseptic procedure, the nurse follows certain principles to ensure maintenance of asepsis. Failure to follow each principle conscientiously endangers clients, placing them at risk for an infection. The following principles are important:

1. A sterile object remains sterile only when touched by another sterile object. This principle guides the nurse in placement of sterile objects and how to handle them.
   a. Sterile touching sterile remains sterile; for example, sterile gloves are worn to handle objects on a sterile field.
   b. Sterile touching clean becomes contaminated; for example, if the tip of a syringe touches the surface of a clean disposable glove, the object is contaminated.
   c. Sterile touching contaminated becomes contaminated; for example, when the nurse touches a sterile object with an ungloved hand, the object is contaminated.
   d. Sterile touching questionable is contaminated; for example, when a tear or break in the covering of a sterile object is found, it is discarded regardless of whether the object appears untouched.
2. Only sterile objects may be placed on a sterile field. All items are properly sterilized before use. Sterile objects are kept in clean and dry storage areas for only a prescribed time; thereafter they are considered unsterile. The package or container holding a sterile object must be intact and dry. A package that is torn, punctured, wet, or open is unsterile.
3. A sterile object or field out of the range of vision or an object held below a person's waist is contaminated. Nurses never turn their backs on a sterile tray or leave it unattended. Any object held below waist level is considered contaminated because it cannot be viewed at all times. Sterile objects should be kept either on or out over the sterile field.
4. A sterile object or field becomes contaminated by prolonged exposure to the air. The nurse avoids activities that may create air currents, such as excessive movements or rearranging linen after a sterile object or field becomes exposed. When sterile packages are opened, the nurse minimizes the number of people walking into the area. Microorganisms also travel by droplet through the air. No one should talk, laugh, sneeze, or cough over a sterile field or when gathering and using sterile equipment. When opening a tray and adding sterile equipment, the nurse should wear a mask. Microorganisms traveling through the air can fall on sterile items or fields if the nurse reaches over the work area.
5. A sterile object or field becomes contaminated by capillary action when a sterile surface comes in contact with a wet contaminated surface. Moisture seeps through a sterile package's protective covering, allowing microorganisms to travel to the sterile object. When stored sterile packages become wet, the nurse discards the objects immediately or sends the equipment for resterilization. Spilling solution over a sterile drape contaminates the field unless the drape cannot be penetrated by moisture.
6. Fluid flows in the direction of gravity. A sterile object becomes contaminated if gravity causes a contaminated liquid to flow over the object's surface. To avoid contamination during a surgical hand scrub, the surgical nurse holds the hands above the elbows. This allows water to flow downward without contaminating the nurse's hands and fingers. The principle of water flow by gravity is also the reason for drying from fingers to elbows with the hands held up, after the scrub.

7. The edges of a sterile field or container are contaminated. A 2.5 cm (1-inch) border around a sterile towel or drape is considered contaminated. The edges of sterile containers become exposed to air after they are open and are thus contaminated. After a sterile needle is removed from its protective cap or after forceps are removed from a container, the objects must not touch the container's edge. The lip of an opened bottle of solution also becomes contaminated after it is exposed to air. When pouring a sterile liquid, the nurse first pours a small amount of solution and discards it. The solution washes away any microorganisms on the bottle lip. The nurse then pours a second time to fill a container with the desired amount of solution.

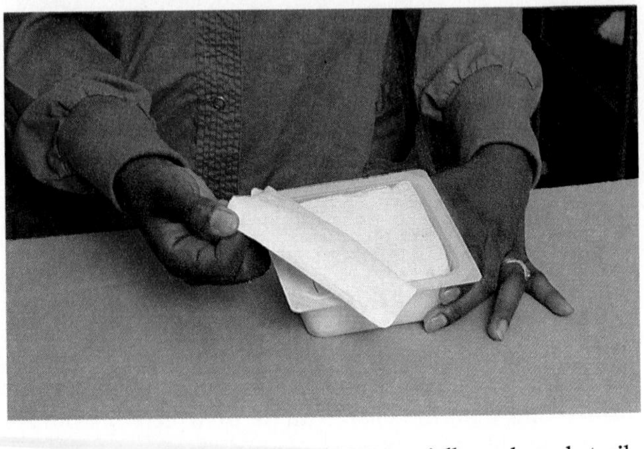

FIGURE 25-7 When opening a commercially packaged sterile item, the nurse tears the wrapper away from the body.

Performing Sterile Procedures. All the equipment that will be needed should be assembled before a procedure. The nurse should anticipate equipment required so that equipment is not left unattended. A few extra supplies should be available in case objects accidentally become contaminated. Before the sterile procedure, each step should be explained so that the client can cooperate fully. Another nurse should be in attendance during the procedure in case assistance in acquiring supplies is needed. If an object becomes contaminated during the procedure, the nurse should not hesitate to discard it.

DONNING AND REMOVING CAPS AND MASKS. For sterile procedures on a general nursing division, the nurse may wear a surgical mask without a cap. For sterile surgical procedures, the nurse first applies a clean paper or cloth cap that covers all the hair and then the surgical mask. A mask must fit snugly around the face and nose to prevent contamination by droplet nuclei. After a mask is worn for several hours, the area over the mouth and nose often becomes moist. Moisture promotes the spread of microorganisms. When operating room nurses' masks become wet, nurses must change them with the aid of the circulating room nurse or by stepping out of the room at an appropriate time. Before permanently removing a mask and cap, the nurse removes sterile gloves to prevent contamination of the hair, neck, and facial area. After untying the mask, the nurse holds it by the ties and discards it with the cap; then the nurse washes hands thoroughly.

OPENING STERILE PACKAGES. Sterile items such as syringes, gauze dressings, or irrigation trays are packaged in paper or plastic containers impervious to microorganisms as long as they are dry and intact. Plastics are pliable and resistant to tearing. Some agencies wrap reusable sterile items in a double thickness of linen. Sterile items are kept in clean, enclosed storage cabinets and never in the same room as dirty equipment.

Sterile supplies have dated labels or chemical tapes that indicate the date when the sterilization period expires. The tapes change color during the sterilization process. Failure of the tapes to change color means the item is not sterile. A sterile supply or piece of equipment should never be used after the expiration date. The item is discarded or returned to the institution's supply area for resterilization.

Before opening a sterile item, the nurse washes the hands thoroughly. The nurse assembles the supplies in the work area such as bedside table or countertop. The work area should be above waist level. Sterile supplies should not be opened in a confined space where a dirty object might fall on or strike them.

OPENING A STERILE ITEM ON A FLAT SURFACE. Sterile packaged items can be opened without contaminating the contents. Commercially packaged items are usually designed so that the nurse only has to tear away or separate the paper or plastic cover. The item is held in one hand while the wrapper is pulled away with the other (Figure 25-7). Care is then taken to keep the inner contents sterile before use. When opening items wrapped in linen or paper, the nurse follows the following steps:

1. Place item flat in center of work surface.
2. Remove any tape or seal indicating sterilization date.
3. Grasp the outer surface of the tip of the outermost flap.
4. Open the outer flap away from the body, keeping the arm outstretched and away from the sterile field (Figure 25-8, *A*).
5. Grasp the outside surface of the first side flap.
6. Open the side flap, allowing it to lie flat on the work surface. Keep the arm to the side and not over the sterile surface (Figure 25-8, *B*). Do not allow flaps to spring back over the sterile contents.
7. Grasp the outside surface of the second side flap, again keeping the arm to the side (Figure 25-8, *C*).
8. Grasp the outside surface of the last flap.

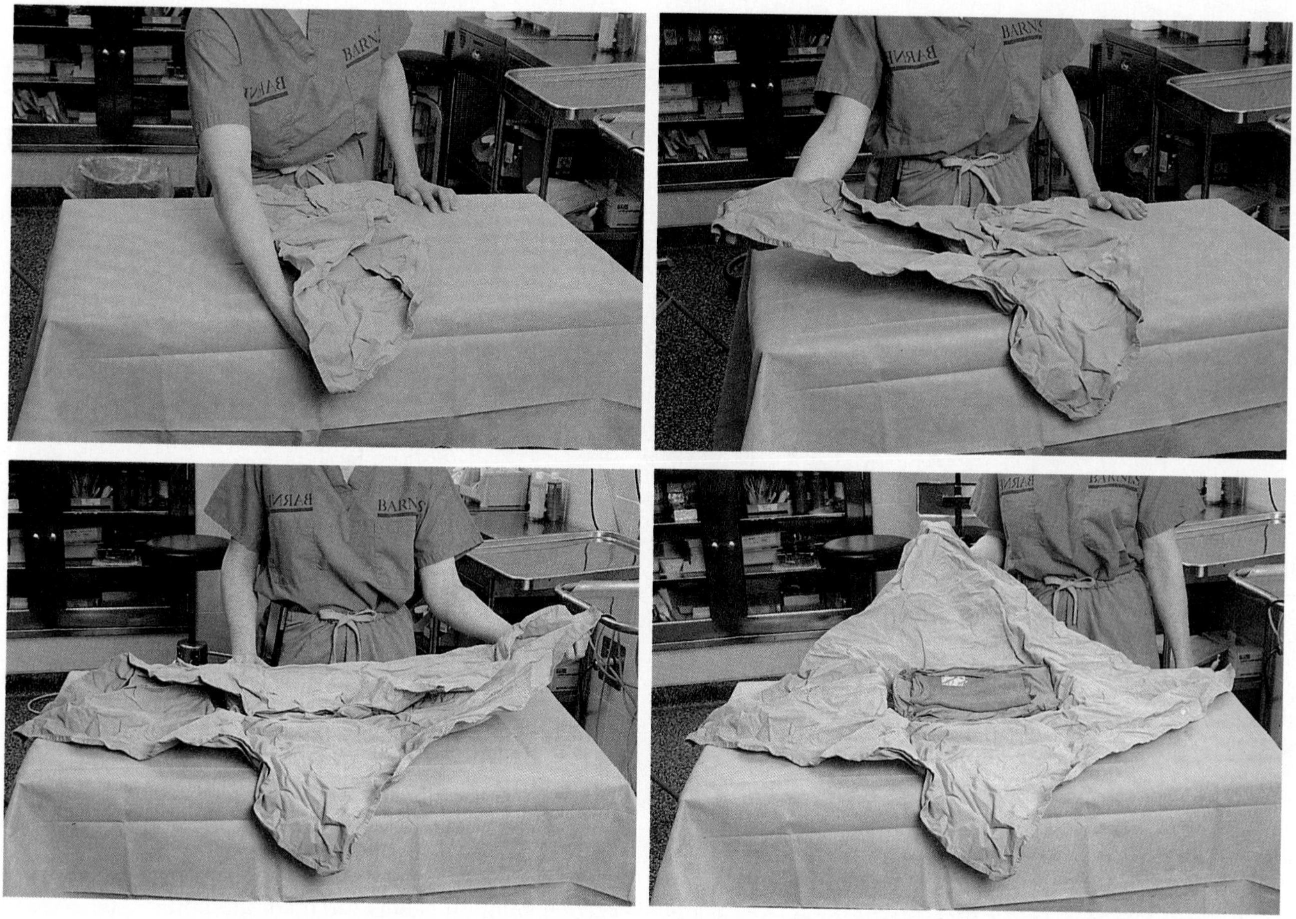

FIGURE 25-8 Opening sterile packaged items on a flat surface. **A,** Nurse opens the top flap away from the body. **B,** The nurse's arm is kept out, away from the sterile field while opening a side flap. **C,** The second side flap is opened. **D,** The back flap is opened.

9. Stand away from the sterile package and pull the flap back, allowing it to fall flat on the surface (Figure 25-8, *D*).
10. Use the inner surface of the linen package (except for the 1-inch border around the edges) as a field to add additional items because it is sterile. Grasp the 1-inch border to move the field over the work surface.

To close a package, the nurse reverses the order of the steps used to unwrap an item. The nurse does not touch the inside contents or reach over the field. This practice may be used in an operating room.

Preparing a sterile field. To perform sterile procedures, the nurse needs a sterile work area for handling and placing sterile items. A sterile field is an area free of microorganisms and prepared to receive sterile items. A field may be created by using the inner surface of a sterile wrapper laid flat or by preparing a sterile drape. Drapes are available in cloth, paper, and plastic. The ideal drape is waterproof.

When preparing a sterile field, the nurse may use gloved or ungloved hands. Gloved hands make the procedure easier because the nurse can touch the entire drape. If gloves are not worn, the nurse may touch only a 1-inch border along the drape's edge. The most important principle to follow in preparing a field is to avoid contamination—by not reaching over a drape, not allowing the drape to touch the uniform, and not allowing the drape's sterile surface to touch the client. The nurse prepares a sterile field by using the following steps:

1. Wash hands thoroughly.
2. Place pack containing sterile drape on work surface and open as described under "opening sterile items on a flat surface."
3. With fingertips of one hand, pick up the folded top edge of the sterile drape.
4. Gently lift the drape up from its outer cover and let it unfold by itself without touching any object. Discard the outer cover with the other hand.
5. With the other hand, grasp an adjacent corner of the drape and hold it straight up and away from the body (Figure 25-9, *A*).

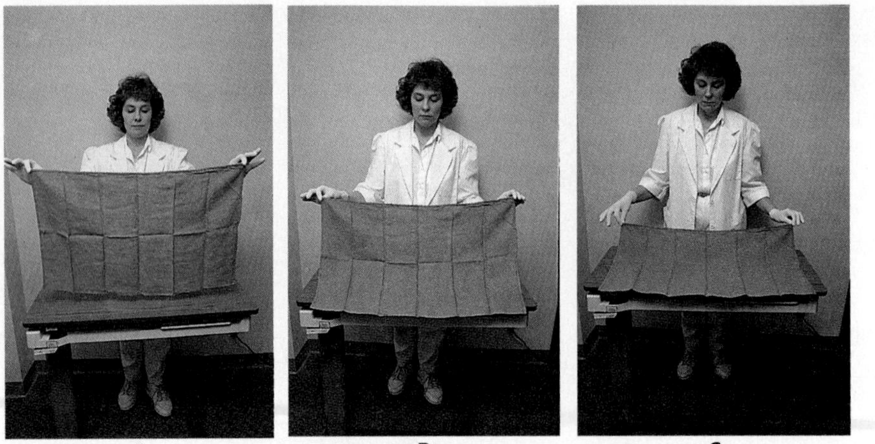

FIGURE 25-9 Creating a sterile field. **A,** Holding drape out, above work surface. **B,** Nurse lays bottom half over work surface. **C,** Top half of drape is placed over work surface.

6. Holding the drape, first position and lay the bottom half over the intended work surface (Figure 25-9, *B*).
7. Allow the top half of the drape to be placed over the work surface last (Figure 25-9, *C*).
8. Grasp the 1-inch border around the edge to position as needed.

ADDING STERILE SUPPLIES TO A STERILE FIELD. Occasionally the nurse will add sterile supplies to a sterile field. For example, after opening a gauze pack wrapped in linen, the nurse may add sterile instruments to the field. To add supplies the nurse opens the item to be transferred by grasping its outside wrapper in the nondominant hand. After the wrapper is peeled over on the nondominant hand, the item is still sterile and the nurse can safely drop the item onto the sterile field. If the wrapper is long and could fall on the sterile field, the nurse takes the dominant hand and carefully holds the wrapper around the wrist of the nondominant hand.

When transferring sterile items, the nurse must carefully place objects onto the sterile field. An object that comes in contact with the edge of the sterile field must be discarded.

POURING STERILE SOLUTIONS. The nurse must often pour sterile solutions into sterile containers. A bottle containing a sterile solution is sterile on the inside and contaminated on the outside, including the bottle's neck. The inside of the bottle cap is also sterile. After a cap or lid is opened, it is held in the hand or placed sterile side (inside) up on a clean surface. This means that the inside of the lid can be seen as it rests on the table surface. A bottle cap or lid should never rest sterile side down on a sterile surface because the outer edge of the cap is unsterile and would contaminate the surface. Likewise, placing a sterile cap down on an unsterile surface may increase the chances of the inside of the cap becoming contaminated.

The bottle should be held with its label in the palm of the hand to prevent the solution from wetting and fading the label. Before pouring the solution into the container, the nurse pours a small amount (1 to 2 ml) into a disposable cup or plastic-lined waste receptacle. The discarded solution cleans the lip of the bottle. The edge of the bottle is kept away from the edge or inside of the receiving container. The nurse pours the solution slowly to avoid splashing the drape or field. The bottle should also be kept low to reduce splashing during pouring. The bottle should be held outside the edge of the sterile field.

SURGICAL HANDWASHING. During surgical handwashing, the nurse scrubs from the fingertips to elbows with a brush and antimicrobial surgical hand scrub preparation before each operation or sterile procedure (Procedure 25-3). Regular handwashing is satisfactory before routine sterile procedures on a general nursing division. Surgical handwashing or scrubbing should take at least 5 minutes before the first procedure of the day (Garner, 1985). The AORN (1992) recommends a 5- to 10-minute surgical scrub before each surgical procedure. For maximum elimination of bacteria, the nurse removes all jewelry and keeps fingernails short, clean, and free of polish.

DONNING STERILE GLOVES. After the nurse scrubs the hands, sterile gloves act as an additional barrier to bacterial transfer. However, bacteria multiply rapidly under gloves and can contaminate a wound or sterile object through a puncture. Use of antiseptic detergents retards bacterial growth under gloves.

There are two gloving methods: open and closed. Nurses commonly use the open method in the clinical

procedure 25-3

SURGICAL HANDWASHING

Steps	Rationale
1. Use deep sink with foot pedals or knee controls for dispensing soap and controlling water temperature and flow.	Minimizes risk of hands and lower arms touching dirty surface.
2. Use appropriate antimicrobial agent.	Reduces number of microorganisms on hands.
3. Have two hand brushes and an orange stick or disposable nail file available.	Brushes enhance mechanical friction during handwashing. Orange stick facilitates cleansing under fingernails.
4. Remove all jewelry.	Jewelry harbors microorganisms.
5. Apply face mask, making certain to cover nose and mouth snugly. Apply eyeglasses or goggles.	Prevents escape of microorganisms into air, which can contaminate hands. Protects eyes from possible splash.
6. Adjust water flow to lukewarm temperature.	Removes protective oils from skin and increases skin's sensitivity to soap.
7. Wet hands and forearms liberally, keeping hands above level of elbows. NOTE: Nurse's scrub dress or uniform must be kept dry.	Water runs by gravity from fingertips to elbows. Hands become the cleanest part of upper extremity. Keeping hands elevated allows water to flow from least to most contaminated area.
8. Dispense liberal amount of soap (2 to 5 ml) into hands and lather hands and arms to 5 cm (2 in) above elbows.	Washing wide area reduces risk of contaminating overlying gown that nurse later applies.
9. Clean nails with orange stick or file under running water (see illustration).	Removes dirt and organic material that harbor large numbers of microorganisms.
10. Rinse hands and arms thoroughly.	Removes transient bacteria from fingers, hands, and forearms.
11. Lather hands and arms, keeping hands above level of elbows. Scrub each hand with brush for 45 sec. Then using same brush, scrub each arm to 5 cm (2 in) above elbow, dividing arm into thirds: scrub each lower forearm 15 sec, each upper forearm 15 sec, and 5 cm above each elbow 15 sec (see illustration).	Loosens resident bacteria that adhere to skin.
12. Discard brush and rinse hands and arms thoroughly.	After touching skin, brush is contaminated. Rinsing removes resident bacteria.
13. Using second brush, scrub each hand for 30 sec. Then use same brush to scrub each arm up to elbow by dividing arm in half: scrub each lower forearm 15 sec and each upper forearm 15 sec.	Ensures thorough cleansing of hands and forearms. Number of resident microorganisms remaining on skin will be minimal.

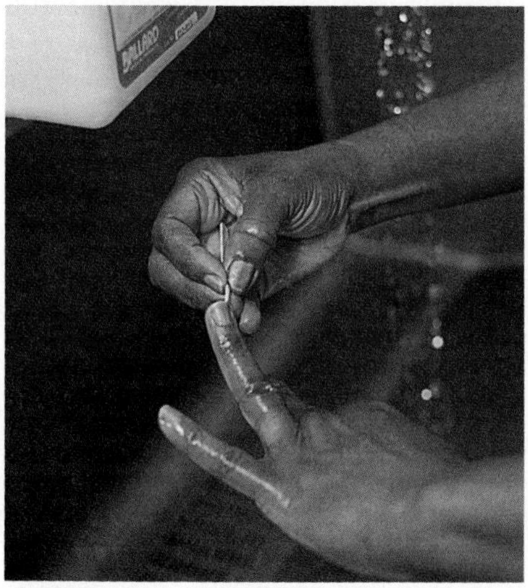

Step 9

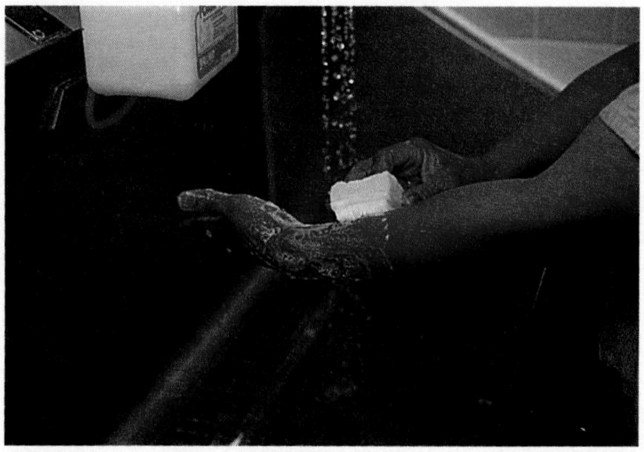

Step 11

Continued.

procedure 25-3—cont'd

SURGICAL HANDWASHING

Steps	Rationale
14. Discard brush and rinse hands and arms thoroughly (see illustration). Turn off water with knee or foot pedal.	
15. Move into sterile work area, keeping hands above elbow. Use sterile towel to dry one hand thoroughly, moving from fingers to elbow. Dry in rotating motion. NOTE: Nurses wishing to apply sterile gloves for use in regular clinical area need not use brushes or dry hands with sterile towels. Thorough lathering and friction performed twice according to procedure ensures clean hands. In this situation, nurse may use clean paper towels for drying.	Dry from cleanest to least clean area. Drying prevents chapping and facilitates donning of gloves.
16. Repeat drying method for other hand, using different area of towel or new sterile towel.	

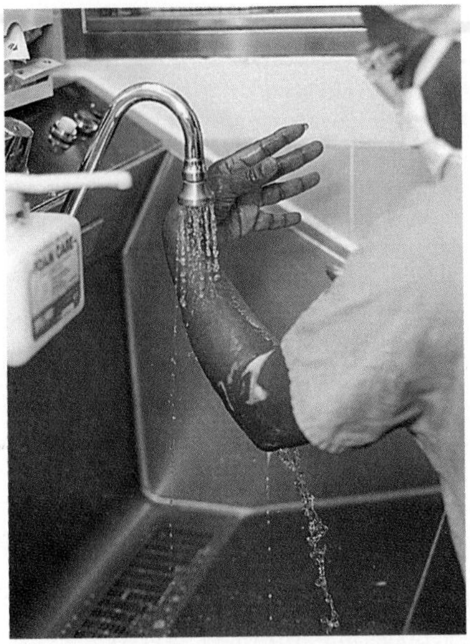

Step 14

Steps	Rationale
17. Keep hands higher than elbows and away from body.	Prevents accidental contamination.
18. Proceed into operating room, labor and delivery area, or treatment room.	

area before changing dressings, inserting catheters, or suctioning a client's airway. Both methods are acceptable in operating rooms, but closed gloving is more frequently used for initial gloving and the open method for changing a contaminated glove during an operative procedure. Procedure 25-4 reviews steps for open gloving. The proper glove size should be chosen. The glove should not stretch so tightly that it can easily tear; yet it should be tight enough that objects can be picked up easily.

After a sterile procedure the nurse disposes of gloves in the following manner to minimize hand contamination.

1. The outside of one cuff is grasped with the other gloved hand (taking care not to touch the wrist).
2. The glove is peeled off, turned inside out, and discarded in the proper receptacle.
3. The fingers of the bare hand tuck inside the remaining glove's cuff. (The outside of the glove is not touched.)
4. The glove is peeled off, turned inside out, and discarded in the proper receptacle.

STERILE GOWNING. The nurse wears a sterile gown in the operating and delivery room so that sterile objects can be easily handled with less risk of contamination. The sterile gown acts as a barrier to microorganisms. The nurse dons a gown after applying a mask, goggles, and cap and after surgical handwashing. The nurse can pick up only the inside surface of the gown at the collar. The gown is held straight up at arm's length away from the body. The nurse holds the gown by the inside open shoulder seams while placing each hand through the armholes. The hands are kept inside the cuffs so that gloves can later be applied (closed method). Only a certain portion of the gown—the area from the anterior waist to but not including the collar and the anterior sur-

procedure 25-4

OPEN GLOVING

Steps	Rationale
1. Perform thorough handwashing.	Reduces transmission of infection.
2. Remove outer package wrapper by carefully peeling apart sides.	Prevents inner glove package from accidentally opening and touching contaminated objects.
3. Grasp inner package and lay it on clean, flat surface just above waist level. Open package, keeping gloves on wrapper's inside surface.	Sterile object held below waist is contaminated. Inner surface of glove package is sterile.
4. If gloves are not prepowdered, take packet of powder and apply lightly to hands over sink or wastebasket.	Powder allows gloves to slip on easily. (Some physicians do not use powder for fear of promoting growth of microorganisms.)
5. Identify right and left glove. Each glove has cuff approximately 5 cm (2 in) wide. Glove dominant hand first.	Proper identification of gloves prevents contamination by improper fit. Gloving of dominant hand first improves nurse's dexterity.
6. With thumb and first two fingers of nondominant hand, grasp edge of cuff of the glove for the dominant hand. Touch only glove's inside surface (see illustration).	Inner edge of cuff will lie against skin and thus is not considered sterile.
7. Carefully pull glove over dominant hand, leaving cuff and being sure cuff does not roll up wrist. Be sure thumb and fingers are in proper spaces (see illustration).	If glove's outer surface touches hand or wrist, it is contaminated.
8. With gloved dominant hand, slip fingers underneath second glove's cuff (see illustration).	Cuff protects gloved fingers. Sterile touching sterile prevents glove contamination.

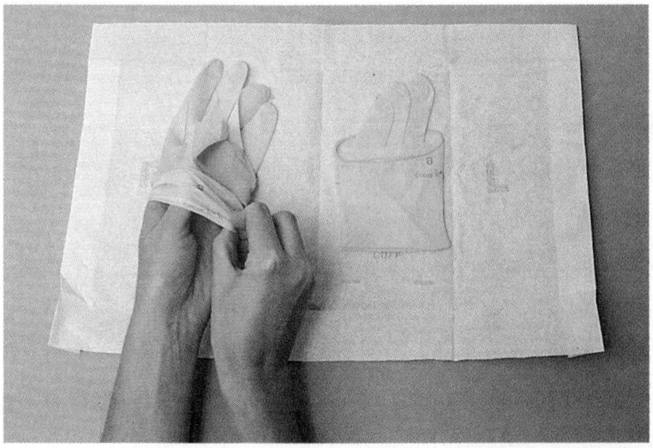

Step 6

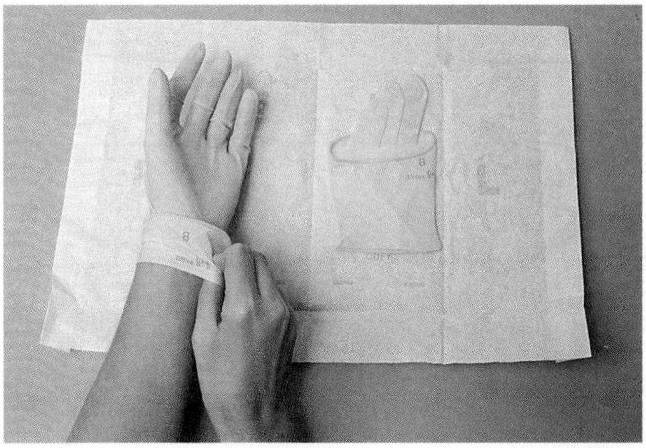

Step 7

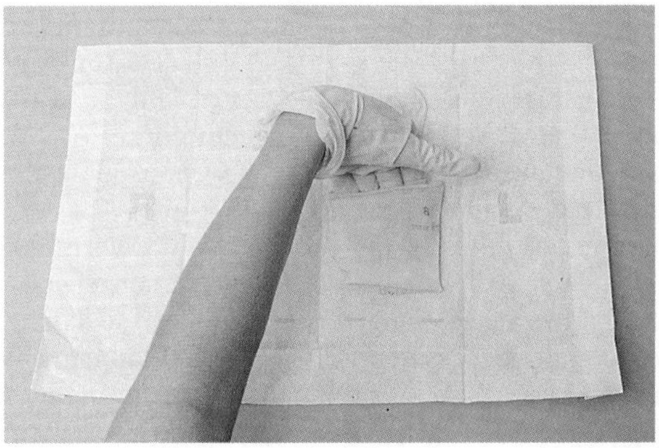

Step 8

procedure 25-4—cont'd

OPEN GLOVING

Steps	Rationale
9. Carefully pull second glove over nondominant hand. Do not allow fingers and thumb of gloved dominant hand to touch any part of exposed nondominant hand. Keep thumb of dominant hand abducted (see illustration).	Contact of gloved hand with exposed hand results in contamination.
10. After second glove is on, interlock hands (see illustration). Cuffs usually fall down after application. Be sure to touch only sterile sides.	Ensures smooth fit over fingers.

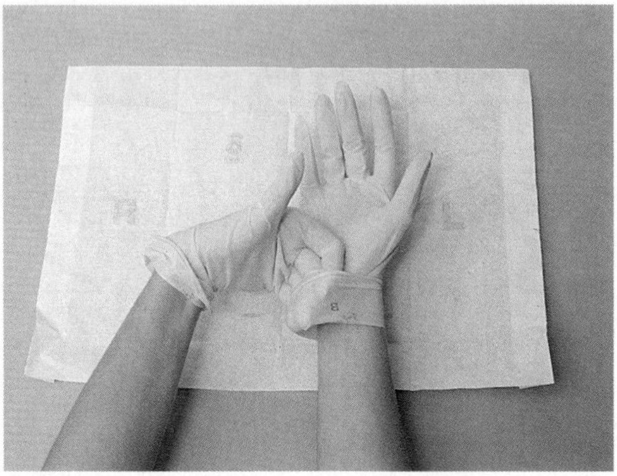

Step 9

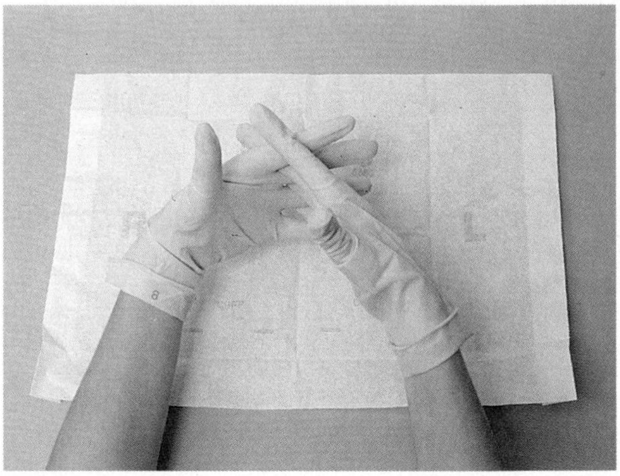

Step 10

face of the sleeves—is considered sterile. A circulating nurse in the operating room ties the back of the nurse's gown to prevent contamination.

Evaluative Measures

As the nurse delivers care to the client, it is important to evaluate the result of interventions so that the nurse can either continue, revise nursing care therapies, or determine that a problem has been resolved. Evaluation of nursing care is based on the goals and outcomes established during the planning phase of the nursing process. Because a client's condition can change at any time, evaluation is ongoing. The nurse must use assessment skills to determine the client's progress over time.

The nurse will use evaluative measures for each of the established expected outcomes. The information gathered determines the status of each client goal.

Goal: Control transmission of infectious organisms.

Outcome

Client does not experience onset of nosocomial infection

Evaluative measures

Nurse assesses client's temperature; observes any wound sites for redness, swelling, tenderness, or discharge; inspects character of any body fluids such as urine or sputum

Outcome

Client's infection does not spread to other body part

Evaluative measure

Nurse inspects other wound sites for early signs of infection, such as increased drainage, change in color of drainage, or redness

Goal: Control or decrease the progression of infection.

Outcome

Client's wound drainage decreases in 3 days

Evaluative measure
Nurse inspects amount of drainage on a dressing or measures the amount of drainage collected in a drainage device
Outcome
Inflammation over the involved site decreases in 5 days
Evaluative measure
Size of inflamed area is inspected over consecutive intervals. Nurse palpates involved site to note reduction in tenderness

Goal: Client's resistance to infection is maintained or increased.
Outcome
Client achieves daily 2600-calorie intake
Evaluative measure
Nurse conducts a calorie count in collaboration with dietitian
Outcome
Client's WBC count remains in normal limits
Evaluative measure
Nurse checks laboratory report for WBC count

Goal: Client uses self-care practices to control infection by day of discharge.
Outcome
Client demonstrates correct handwashing techniques by third hospital day
Evaluative measure
Nurse observes client perform handwashing in home setting
Outcome
Client describes signs and symptoms of local wound infection by fourth hospital day
Evaluative measure
Nurse asks client to describe signs and symptoms of local wound infection during a dressing change

SUMMARY

In every aspect of practice, the nurse encounters situations that present a risk of an infection developing or being transmitted. Knowledge of the body's normal defenses against infection helps the nurse to recognize clients most at risk for acquiring infections. The nature of the infection chain is a useful concept in identifying nursing interventions for infection control.

Nurses use two types of infection-control practices, medical and surgical asepsis, to prevent infection transmission. Each calls for a conscientious and knowledgeable application of infection control principles. Failure to follow these principles seriously hampers a client's recovery or maintenance of good health.

KEY CONCEPTS

- Normal body flora resist infection by releasing antibacterial substances and inhibiting multiplication of pathogenic microorganisms.
- Immunity to infection is measured by the capacity to produce antibodies in response to exposure to an antigen.
- An infection can develop as long as the six elements comprising the infection chain are uninterrupted.
- A microorganism's virulence depends on its ability to resist attack by the body's normal defenses.
- Microorganisms are transmitted by direct and indirect contact, by airborne spread, and by vectors and contaminated vehicles.
- Increasing age, poor nutrition, stress, inherited conditions, chronic disease, and treatments or conditions that compromise the immune response increase susceptibility to infection.
- Masks in combination with eye protection devices such as goggles or glasses with solid side shields shall be worn whenever splashes or spray of blood or potentially infectious material may be generated.
- Invasive procedures, medical therapies, long hospitalization, and contact with health care personnel increase a hospitalized client's risk for acquiring a nosocomial infection.
- Surgical asepsis requires more stringent techniques than medical asepsis and is directed toward eliminating microorganisms.
- The CDC recommends that health care workers consider all clients as potentially infected with HIV and other blood-borne pathogens and to reduce risk of exposure to blood and body fluids.
- Body substance isolation involves taking precautions before waiting for a client to be diagnosed with an infection.
- Following aseptic principles is the key to a nurse's success in preventing clients from acquiring infections.
- A client receiving isolation precautions is subject to sensory deprivation because of the restricted environment.
- Lack of handwashing is the main cause of nosocomial infections.
- An infection control health professional monitors the incidence of infections within an institution and provides educational and consultative services to maintain aseptic practices.
- If the skin is broken or if the nurse performs an invasive procedure into a body cavity normally free of microorganisms, surgical aseptic practices are enforced.
- A sterile object becomes contaminated by direct contact with a clean or contaminated object, by exposure to airborne microorganisms, and by contact with a wet medium containing microorganisms.

CRITICAL THINKING ACTIVITIES

1. Identify the six elements of the chain of infection. Identify those elements of the chain that are broken when the nurse does not wash hands between contact with clients.
2. Explain the elements of the CDC Universal Precautions and the elements of Body Substance Isolation. How do these isolation systems differ?
3. Each year health care facilities spend millions of dollars for isolation barrier protection (e.g., gloves, gowns, goggles, masks). For this reason, nurses must carefully choose the right personal protective equipment (PPE) in clinical situations without creating additional costs for their facility. In the following client care situations, select the appropriate PPE and give rationale: (a) starting an IV catheter; (b) B/P checks on a client with Hepatitis B; (c) changing the bed linen for an incontinent client; (d) entering the room of a client with meningococcal meningitis; (e) entering the room of a client with *Mycobacterium avium;* (f) emptying a suction bottle containing bloody fluid; and (g) bathing a baby born to a mother who is HIV positive.
4. The nurse has admitted Mr. Cobbs to a general medical unit with a diagnosis of tuberculosis. The physician has not ordered isolation precautions. Should the client be on isolation? If so, what kind?
5. Mr. Stamm is an 86-year-old client whose diagnosis includes vomiting and diarrhea presumed secondary to a food-borne illness. Develop a discharge teaching plan.

References

American Health Consultants: *Hosp Infect Control* 21(8):107, 1994.

American Thoracic Society: Control of tuberculosis in the United States, *American Rev of Resp Disease,* vol 146, 1992.

Association of Operating Room Nurses, Inc.: *AORN standards and recommended practices,* Denver, 1992.

Benenson AS: *Control of communicable disease in man,* ed 15, Washington, D.C., 1990, American Public Health Association.

Bennett SV, Brackman PS: *Hospital infection,* ed 3, Boston, 1992, Little, Brown, & Co.

Centers for Disease Control: Guidelines for isolation precautions in hospitals. In *Guidelines for the prevention and control of nosocomial infections,* Atlanta, 1983, CDC.

Centers for Disease Control: Recommendations for prevention of HIV transmission in health care settings, *MMWR* 36:55, 1987.

Centers for Disease Control: Update: Universal Precautions for prevention of transmission of human immunodeficiency virus, hepatitis B virus, and other blood borne pathogens in health-care settings, *MMWR* 37:377, 1988.

Centers for Disease Control: Guidelines for preventing the transmission of tuberculosis in health care settings, with special focus on HIV-related issues, *MMWR* 39(RR-17), 1990.

Centers for Disease Control: Surveillance, prevention, and control of nosocomial infections, *MMWR* 41:783, 1992.

Centers for Disease Control: Draft guidelines for preventing the transmission of tuberculosis in healthcare facilities, *DHHS,* Oct. 12, 1993.

Clark JB, et al.: *Pharmacological basis of nursing practice,* St. Louis, 1986, Mosby.

Department of Labor: Joint advisory notice: Department of Labor/Department of Health and Human Services, *HBV/HIV 52:* Oct. 30, 1987.

Dickerson M: Protecting yourself from AIDS: infection control measures, *Crit Care Nurs* 9(10):26, 1989.

Ebersole P, Hess P: *Toward healthy aging,* ed 3, St. Louis, 1989, Mosby.

Garner JS: *Guidelines for prevention of surgical wound infections,* Atlanta, 1985, Hospital Infections Program, CDC, PHS, and U.S. Department of Health and Human Services.

Garner JS, Favero MS: *Guidelines for handwashing and hospital environmental control,* Atlanta, 1985, Hospital Infections Program, CDC, PH, and U.S. Department of Health and Human Services.

Garner JS, Simmons BP: CDC guidelines for isolation precautions in hospitals, *Infect Control* 4(4):249, 1983.

Garner JS, Simmons BP: CDC guidelines for the prevention and control of nosocomial infections: guidelines for isolation precautions in hospitals, *Am J Infect Control* 12:103, 1984.

Greifze S, Radjeski D, and Winnick B: Oral care is part of cancer care, *RN* 53:43,1990.

Gurevich I: Infection Control: applying theory to clinical practice. In Block SS, editor: Disinfection, sterilization, and preservation, Philadelphia, 1991, Lea & Febiger.

Hall GS, et al.: The dispersal of bacteria and skin scales from the body after showering and after application of a skin lotion, *J Hyg (Lond)* 97:289, 1986.

Kenny SA: Effect of 2 oral care protocols on the incidence of stomatitis in hematology patients, *Cancer Nurs* 13:345, 1990.

Krumholz HM, Cummings S, and York M: Blood culture phlebotomy: switching needles does not prevent contamination, *Ann Intern Med* 113(4):290, 1990.

Larson E: Guidelines for use of topical and microbial agents, *Am J Infect Control* 16: 253-266, 1988.

Larson E: Handwashing: it's essential even when you use gloves, *Am J Nurs* 89:934, 1989a.

Larson EL: Effects of handwashing agent, handwashing frequency, and clinical area on hand flora, *Am J Infect Control* 12:76, 1984.

Larson EL, et al.: Physiological and microbiologic changes in skin related to frequent handwashing, *Infect Control* 7:59, 1986.

Larson EL, et al.: Quantity of soap as a variable in handwashing, *Infect Control* 8:371, 1987.

Larson E, et al.: Influence of two handwashing frequencies on reduction in colonizing flora with three handwashing products used by health care personnel, *Am J Infect Control* 17:83, 1989b.

Leisure MK, Moore DM, et al.: Changing the needle when inoculating blood cultures, a no-benefit and high-risk procedure, *JAMA* 264(16):2111, 1990.

Lynch P and Jackson MM: Isolation practices: how much is too much or not enough? *Asepsis* 10(3):12, 1988.

Lynch P, et al.: Implementing and evaluating a system of generic infection precautions: body substance isolation, *Am J Infect Control* 18(1):1, 1990.

Maki DG, et al.: Double-bagging of items from isolation rooms is unnecessary as an infection control measure: a comparative study of surface contamination with single and double-bagging, *Infect Control* 7(11):535, 1986.

Occupational Safety and Health Administration: Blood born pathogens rules and regulations, *Federal Register* 58:64175-64182, 1991.

Pagana KD, Pagana TJ: *Diagnostic testing and nursing implications,* ed 3, St. Louis, 1989, Mosby.

Pugliese G and Lampinen T: Prevention of human immunodeficiency virus infection: our responsibilities as health care professionals, *Am J Infect Control* 17(1):1, 1989.

Rutala WA: Draft guideline for selection and use of disinfectants, *Am J Infect Control* 17(1):24A, 1989.

Simmons BP: Guidelines for prevention of surgical wound infections, *Am J Infect Control* 11(4):133, 1983.

Smith PW, editor: *Infection control in long-term care facilities,* New York, 1984, John Wiley & Sons.

Thibodeau GA: *Anatomy and physiology,* ed 12, St. Louis, 1987, Mosby.

Weinstein SA, et al.: Bacterial surface contamination of patient's linen: isolation precautions versus standard care, *Am J Infect Control* 17(5):264, 1989.

Williams WW: CDC guidelines for infection control in hospital personnel, *Infect Control* 4(4):325, 1983.

Bibliography

Centers for Disease Control: Guidelines for preventing the transmission of tuberculosis in health-care settings, with special focus on HIV-related issues, *MMWR* 39:1, 1990.

Centers for Disease Control: Recommendations for HIV testing services for inpatients and outpatients in acute-care hospital settings, *MMWR* 42:157, 1993.

Conly JM, et al.: Handwashing practices in an intensive care unit: the effects of an educational program and its relationship to infection rates, *Am J Infect Control* 17(6):330, 1989.

Crow S: Asepsis: an indispensable part of the patient's care plan, *Crit Care Nurs Q* 11(4):11, 1989.

Favero MS and Bond WW: Chemical disinfection of medical and surgical materials. In Block SS editor: *Disinfection, sterilization and preservation,* Philadelphia, 1991, Lea & Febiger.

Hoffmann KK, Weber DJ, et al.: Transparent polyurethane film as an intravenous catheter dressing. A meta analysis of the infection risks, *JAMA* 267(15):2072, 1992.

Jackson MM: Infection prevention and control (review), *Crit Care Nurs Clin North Am* 4(3):401, 1992.

Landry SL, et al.: Hospital stay and mortality attributed to nosocomial enterococcal bacteremia: a controlled study, *Am J Infect Control* 17(6):323, 1989.

Maki DG, Botticelli DB, and LeRoy M: Prospective study of replacing IV administration sets at 48 hour versus 72 hour intervals, *JAMA* 258(13):1777, 1987.

Maki DG, Ringer M: Evaluation of dressing regimens for prevention of infection with peripheral intravenous catheters, *JAMA* 258(17), 1987.

McCrary E and Martone WJ: Preventing HIV exposure among patients and staff, *AIDS Patient Care* 1:32, 1987.

Shorein J, et al.: MRSA: Pandora's box for hospitals. Methicillin-resistant *Staphylococcus, Am J Nurs* 92(2):48, 1992.

26

Administering Medications

OBJECTIVES

Mastery of content in this chapter will enable the student to:

- Define the key terms listed.
- Discuss the nurse's legal responsibilities in drug prescription and administration.
- Describe the physiological mechanisms of drug action, including absorption, distribution, metabolism, and excretion of medications.
- Differentiate among toxic, idiosyncratic, allergic, and side effects of drugs.
- Discuss developmental factors that influence drug pharmacokinetics.
- Discuss factors that influence drug actions.
- Discuss methods of educating a client about prescribed medications.
- Describe the roles of the pharmacist, physician, and nurse in drug administration.
- Describe factors to consider when choosing routes of drug administration.
- Correctly calculate a prescribed drug dosage.
- Discuss factors to include in assessing a client's needs for and response to drug therapy.
- List the "five rights" of drug administration.
- Correctly prepare and administer subcutaneous, intramuscular, intradermal injections, and intravenous medications; oral and topical skin preparations; eye, ear, and nose drops; vaginal instillations; rectal suppositories; and inhalants.

KEY TERMS

absorption
anaphylactic reaction
apothecary system
bioavailability
biotransformation
buccal
concentration
detoxify
drug abuse
drug allergy
drug interaction
idiosyncratic reaction
infusion
inhalation
injection
instillation
intradermal (ID)
intramuscular (IM)
intravenous (IV)
irrigation
metered dose inhaler (MDI)
metric system
narcotics
nurse practice acts
ophthalmic
parenteral administration
pharmacokinetics
prescriptions
serum half-life
side effects
solution
subcutaneous (SQ)
sublingual
synergistic effect
therapeutic effect
toxic effect
Z-track injection

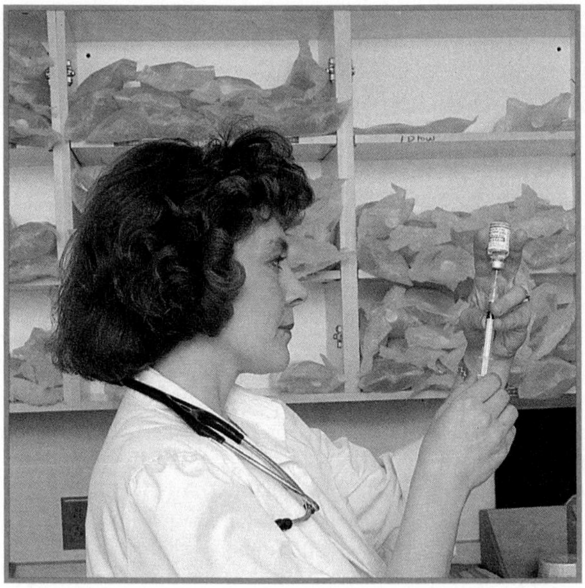

The safe and accurate administration of medications is one of the nurse's most important responsibilities. Drugs are a primary therapy for clients with health alterations, but any drug can cause harmful effects. The nurse is responsible for understanding a drug's expected and unexpected effects, administering the drug correctly, monitoring the response, and helping the client self-administer drugs correctly.

In addition to knowing about a specific drug's action, the nurse must also understand the client's previous and current health problems to determine whether a particular medication is safe to give. The nurse's judgment is critical for proper drug administration.

DRUG NOMENCLATURE AND FORMS

A drug or medication is a substance used in the diagnosis, treatment, cure, relief, or prevention of disease. Physicians and dentists prescribe the majority of medications in the United States and Canada. However, in many states within the United States, nurse practitioners may prescribe medications under a collaborative agreement with a physician. Physician's assistants and nurses in expanded roles may prescribe under written protocols or standing orders.

Names

A drug may have as many as three different names. A drug's chemical name provides an exact description of the drug's composition and molecular structure. An example of a chemical name is acetylsalicylic acid, which is commonly known as aspirin. The generic or nonproprietary name is given, with USAN (United States Adopted Name Council) approval, by the manufacturer who first develops the drug. Aspirin is an example of a generic name. The generic name becomes the official name that is listed in official publications such as the *United States Pharmacopeia (USP)*. The trade name, brand name, or proprietary name is the name under which a manufacturer markets a drug. The trade name has the symbol ® at the upper right of the name, indicating that the manufacturer has copyrighted the drug's name (e.g., Bufferin, Ecotrin, and Anacin).

Manufacturers have chosen names that are easy to pronounce, spell, and remember so that laypersons will recognize trade names. Many companies may produce the same drug, so similarities in trade names can be confusing. Hospital and clinic pharmacies attempt to consistently dispense medications with the same trade names so nurses can become familiar with them. However, the nurse finds drugs under a variety of different nomenclatures or names and must be careful to obtain the exact name and spelling for a particular drug.

Classification

Nurses learn to categorize medications with similar characteristics by their class. Drug classification indicates the effect of the drug on a body system, the symptoms the drug relieves, or the drug's desired effect. Each class contains drugs prescribed for similar types of health problems. The physical and chemical composition of drugs within a class are not necessarily the same. A drug may also be part of more than one class. For example, aspirin is an analgesic, an antipyretic, and an antiinflammatory drug.

It is important to learn the general characteristics of medications in each class. Each class has certain nursing implications for proper administration and monitoring. Nursing implications for all drugs within a class provide guidelines for safe and effective client care.

Drug Forms

Drugs are available in a variety of forms or preparations. The form of the drug determines its route of administration. The composition of a drug is designed to enhance its absorption and metabolism. Many drugs are made in several forms such as tablets, capsules, elixirs, and suppositories. When administering a medication,

table 26-1

FORMS OF MEDICATIONS

Form	Description
Aerosol	Powder, liquid, or foam deposited in a fine layer on the skin or mucous membranes
Caplet	Solid dosage form for oral use; shaped like capsule and coated for ease of swallowing
Capsule	Solid dosage form for oral use; medication in powder, liquid, or oil form and encased by gelatin shell; capsule colored to aid in product identification
Elixir	Clear fluid containing water and/or alcohol; designed for oral use; usually has sweetener added
Enteric-coated tablet	Tablet for oral use coated with materials that do not dissolve in stomach; coatings dissolve in intestine where medication is absorbed
Extended/sustained release	Drugs usually in tablet or capsule form that allow for effect over a longer period of time
Extract	Concentrated drug form made by removing active portion of drug from its other components (e.g., fluid extract is drug made into solution from vegetable source)
Glycerite	Solution of drug combined with glycerin for external use; contains at least 50% glycerin
Liniment	Preparation usually containing alcohol, oil, or soapy emollient that is applied to skin
Lotion	Drug in liquid suspension applied externally to protect skin
Ointment	Semisolid, externally applied preparation, usually containing one or more drugs
Paste	Semisolid preparation, thicker and stiffer than ointment; absorbed through skin more slowly than ointment
Powder/granule	Finely ground loose or molded drugs, given with or without liquids
Solution	Liquid preparation that may be used orally, parenterally, or externally; can also be instilled into body organ or cavity (e.g., bladder irrigations); contains water with one or more dissolved compounds; must be sterile for parenteral use or when instilled into body cavity
Suppository	Solid dosage form mixed with gelatin and shaped in the form of pellet for insertion into a body cavity (rectum or vagina); melts when it reaches body temperature, releasing the drug for absorption
Suspension	Finely divided drug particles dispersed in liquid medium; when suspension left standing, particles settle to bottom of container; commonly is oral medication and is not given parenterally
Syrup	Medication dissolved in concentrated sugar solution; may contain flavoring to make drug more palatable
Tablet	Powdered dosage form compressed into hard disks or cylinders; in addition to primary drug, contains binders (adhesive to allow powder to stick together), disintegrators (to promote tablet dissolution), lubricants (for ease of manufacturing), and fillers (for convenient tablet size)
Tincture	Alcohol or water-alcohol drug solution
Transdermal disk or patch	Medication contained within semipermeable membrane disk or patch; allows medications to be absorbed through skin slowly over a longer period (24 hours)
Troche (lozenge)	Flat, round dose form containing drug, flavoring, sugar, and mucilage; dissolved in mouth to release drug

the nurse must be certain to use the proper form (Table 26-1).

DRUG LEGISLATION AND STANDARDS

Drug Standards

In 1906 the U.S. government set standards for drug quality and purity as a result of the Pure Food and Drug Act. Official publications—the *United States Pharmacopeia (USP)* and the *National Formulary*—set standards for drug strength, quality, purity, packaging, safety, labeling, and dose form. In Canada the *British Pharmacopoeia (BP)* sets similar standards. Physicians, nurses, and pharmacists depend on such standards to ensure that clients receive pure drugs in safe and effective doses. Accepted standards must be met in five areas:

1. **Purity.** Standards control type and concentration of extraneous substances allowed in drug products.
2. **Potency.** The concentration of active drug in the preparation affects strength or potency.

3. **Bioavailability.** The ability of a drug to be released from its dosage form and dissolved, absorbed, and transported by the body to its site of action.
4. **Efficacy.** Detailed laboratory studies determine a drug's effectiveness.
5. **Safety.** All drugs should be continually evaluated to determine their side effects.

Legislation and Control

The Pure Food and Drug Act of 1906 focused on the purity of food but also set official standards for drugs. Manufacturers were required to label drugs accurately and to ensure that the strength and purity of drugs conformed to their claims. Since that time, federal law has extended and refined controls on drug sales and distribution, drug testing, naming and labeling, and the regulation of controlled substances (e.g., the Controlled Substances Act, 1970).

State drug laws must conform with federal legislation. States can also have additional controls. Local governmental bodies also regulate the use of alcohol and tobacco.

Health care institutions establish individual policies that must meet federal, state, and local regulations. The size of an institution, the types of services it provides, and the types of professional personnel it employs influence policies. Institutional policies are often more restrictive than governmental controls. An institution is concerned primarily with preventing health problems resulting from drug use. For example, a common institutional policy is the automatic discontinuation of antibiotic therapy after a set number of days. Although a physician may reorder the antibiotic, this policy helps to control unnecessarily prolonged drug therapy.

Federal, state, and local legislation governs nursing practice including the administration of medications. State **nurse practice acts** define and set limits on the scope of a nurse's professional functions and responsibilities. Institutions and agencies may interpret specific actions allowed under the acts, but they cannot modify, expand, or restrict the act's intent. The nurse practice acts protect the public from unskilled, undereducated, and unlicensed nurses.

Nurses must know the regulations affecting drug use in their practice area. When moving from one state to another, a nurse may discover significant differences in laws governing drugs. For example, laws concerning who may prescribe medications and administer drugs intravenously vary. In the past, only physicians prescribed medications. Today, several states have recognized the expanding role of the nurse and have revised nurse practice acts to include prescription of medications. In most cases, this privilege is limited to certified nurse practitioners, nurse specialists, nurse midwives, or nurse anesthetists.

Administering medications directly into a vein is a responsibility most nurses now assume. Because the intravenous injection of medications may cause serious adverse effects, nurses who perform this function must be qualified through proper training, education, and experience.

The nurse is responsible for following legal provisions when administering controlled substances or narcotics (drugs that affect the mind and behavior), which are carefully controlled through federal and state guidelines. Violations of the Controlled Substances Act are punishable by fines, imprisonment, and loss of nurse licensure. Hospitals and other health care institutions have policies for the proper storage and distribution of narcotics (see box at left).

GUIDELINES FOR SAFE ADMINISTRATION AND CONTROL OF CONTROLLED SUBSTANCES AND NARCOTICS

Store all controlled substances and narcotics in a locked, secure cabinet or container.

Nurses in charge carry sets of keys for the controlled substances and narcotics cabinet.

During an institution's change-of-shift, the nurse going off duty counts all controlled substances and narcotics with the nurse coming on duty. Both nurses sign the record to indicate that the count is correct.

Discrepancies in counts are reported immediately.

A special inventory record is used each time a controlled substance or narcotic is dispensed (Some agencies have computerized narcotic dispensing with automatic record printouts).

The record is used to document the client's name, the date, time of drug administration, name of drug, dosage, and signature of nurse dispensing the drug.

The form provides an accurate, ongoing count of medications used and remaining.

If only one part of a premeasured dose of a controlled substance or narcotic is given, a second nurse witnesses disposal of the unused portion and documents such on the record form.

Nontherapeutic Drug Use

Despite legislative controls, some people use drugs for reasons other than their prescribed purpose. The indiscriminate use of drugs poses serious health problems for users, families, and the community. In the past, the misuse or abuse of medications was related to use for therapeutic qualities such as the relief of pain or reduction in anxiety. Today, factors such as peer pressure, curiosity, and the pursuit of pleasure are motivators for drug use. Problems with nontherapeutic drug use involve heroin, cocaine, other "hard" drugs, alcohol, and over-the-counter drugs. It takes only a few minutes of watching television, with its frequent advertisements for pain relievers, decongestants, and antacids, to realize that our society is drug conscious. The box below lists terms associated with the nontherapeutic use of drugs.

The nurse is ethically and legally responsible to understand the problems of persons using drugs improperly. When caring for clients with suspected drug problems, nurses must be aware of their own values and attitudes about drug-using clients. The nurse cannot develop a therapeutic relationship with clients if personal values interfere with acceptance or understanding of their needs. Knowledge of the physical, psychological, and social changes resulting from drug abuse allows the nurse to identify clients with drug problems.

A problem involving the misuse of drugs by health professionals also exists. Stress in the workplace, personal problems, and the strong desire to perform well are some factors that may cause nurses to rely on drugs. Nurses must recognize and understand the problems of colleagues involved in **drug abuse.**

TERMS ASSOCIATED WITH THE NONTHERAPEUTIC USE OF DRUGS

ABUSE

A maladaptive pattern of substance use indicated by at least one of the following in a 12-month period:
- Recurrent substance use resulting in a failure to fulfill major role obligations at work, school, or home (e.g., repeated absences or poor work performance).
- Recurrent substance use in situations in which it is physically hazardous (e.g., driving an automobile or operating a machine when impaired by substance use).
- Recurrent substance-related legal problems (e.g., arrests for substance-related disorderly conduct).
- Continued substance use despite having persistent or recurrent social or interpersonal problems caused or exacerbated by the effects of the substance (e.g., arguments with spouse about consequences of intoxication, physical fights).

DEPENDENCE

At least three of the following in a 12-month period:
- Substance often taken in larger amounts or over a longer period than the person intended
- Persistent desire or one or more unsuccessful efforts to cut down or control substance use
- A great deal of time spent in activities necessary to get the substance, taking the substance, or recovering from its effects
- Frequent intoxication or withdrawal symptoms when expected to fulfill major role obligations at work, school, or home
- Important social, occupational, or recreational activities given up or reduced because of substance use
- Continued substance use despite knowledge of having a persistent or recurrent social, psychological, or physical problem caused or exacerbated by the use of the substance
- Marked tolerance, need for markedly increased amounts of the substance to achieve intoxication or desired effect, or markedly diminished effect with continued use of the same amount

Modified from American Psychiatric Association: *Diagnostic and statistical manual of mental disorders (DSM-IV)*, rev 4, Washington, DC, 1994, The Association.

NATURE OF DRUG ACTIONS

Medications produce therapeutically useful effects. A drug does not create a function in a tissue or organ but rather alters physiological functions. Drugs may protect cells from the influence of other chemical agents, promote cell function, or accelerate or slow cell processes. A drug may also replace a substance that is missing in the body (e.g., insulin or estrogen).

Mechanisms of Action

Drugs produce their actions by altering body fluids, altering cell membranes, or interacting with receptor sites. The drug, aluminum hydroxide gel, exerts its effect by altering the chemical properties of a body fluid. Specifically, the stomach's acid contents become neutralized. Drugs such as general anesthetic gases interact with cell membranes. After properties of the cells become altered, the drug exerts its effects. The most common mechanism of drug action is the binding of drugs to a cell's receptor sites. The drug and receptor bind together much like a lock-and-key fit. When receptors and drugs lock together, the therapeutic effects occur. Receptors localize drug effects. Each tissue or cell in the body possesses a unique group of receptors. For example, receptors in the myocardial cells respond to digitalis preparations.

Pharmacokinetics

Pharmacokinetics is the study of how drugs enter the body, reach their site of action, are metabolized, and exit the body. The nurse uses knowledge of pharmacokinetics when timing drug administration, selecting the route of administration, judging the client's risk for alterations in drug action, and observing the client's response.

Absorption. **Absorption** is the passage of drug molecules into the blood. Most drugs, except those applied topically for local effects, must enter the systemic circulation to exert therapeutic effect. Factors influencing drug absorption include route of administration, ability of the drug to dissolve, and conditions at the site of absorption.

The nurse administers drugs by several routes. Each route has a different influence on drug absorption, depending on the physical structure of the tissues. Skin absorption is slow. The mucous membranes and respiratory airways allow quick drug absorption. Orally administered drugs have a slow absorption rate because they must pass through the gastrointestinal tract. Intravenous (IV) injection produces more rapid absorption, with direct access to the systemic circulation. Drugs that are inhaled may produce immediate effects by acting directly on the "target" site and being rapidly absorbed across the pulmonary capillary network.

The ability of an oral medication to dissolve depends largely on its form or preparation. Solutions and suspensions already in a liquid state are absorbed more readily than tablets or capsules. Acidic drugs pass through the gastric mucosa rapidly. Drugs that are basic are not absorbed before reaching the small intestine.

Conditions at the site of absorption influence how easily medications enter the systemic circulation. When skin is abraded, topical drugs are absorbed easily. This may create serious reactions when the topical substance is absorbed through the skin layers. The absorption of parenterally administered medications depends on the blood supply of the tissues. Because muscles have a richer blood supply than subcutaneous tissues, a drug given intramuscularly is absorbed more quickly than one injected subcutaneously. In some instances a delayed subcutaneous absorption is preferable to produce long-lasting drug effects. If a client's tissue perfusion is poor, as in the case of circulatory shock, the intravenous route is best. Intravenous administration provides the most rapid and dependable absorption.

Oral medications are absorbed more easily when administered between meals. When the stomach is filled with food, the contents are emptied slowly into the duodenum, thus slowing drug absorption. Certain foods and antacids cause drugs to bind into complexes that cannot pass through the gastrointestinal tract lining. For example, milk interferes with the absorption of iron and tetracycline.

Some drugs are destroyed by the increased acidity of gastric contents and protein digestion during a meal. Enteric coatings on certain tablets resist dissolution in gastric juices and prevent certain medications from being digested in the upper gastrointestinal tract. The coating also protects the stomach lining from irritation by the medication. Enteric-coated medication should never be crushed or dissolved for administration.

The nurse often has little choice concerning the route by which to administer a medication. However, the nurse may request a drug be given by a different route or in another form, based on client assessment. Knowledge of factors that alter or impair drug absorption helps the nurse to administer drugs correctly. Nurses should be aware that food, milk, antacids, and other medications may alter absorption and should schedule medications appropriately. There are examples of medications given ½-hour before, ½-hour after, and with meals. Some clients take many medications, making a medication schedule difficult to achieve and follow. Before administering a drug by injection, the nurse assesses for local factors that may impair drug absorption.

Distribution. After a drug is absorbed, it is distributed within the body to tissues and organs and ultimately to its specific site of action. The rate and extent of distribution depend on the physical and chemical properties of drugs and the physiology of the person taking the drug.

Body size. There is a direct relationship between the amount of drug administered and the amount of body tissue in which it is distributed. Most medications are distributed to body fat or body water (Simonson, 1984). An increase in the percentage of body fat may cause a longer duration of drug action because of slower distribution throughout the body. In obese clients a lower concentration accumulates in the body tissues that are the targets for drug action. The less a client weighs, the greater the concentration of a drug in tissues and the more powerful the effects. The older adult experiences a reduction in tissue mass and height and often require lower drug doses than younger clients.

Circulation. Drugs pass more easily from interstitial to intravascular spaces than between body compartments. Blood vessels are permeable to most dissolved substances unless drug particles are large or bound to serum proteins. The concentration of a drug at a specific site depends on the number of blood vessels in tissues, the degree of local vasodilation or vasoconstriction, and the rate of blood flow to a tissue site. For example, a warm compress applied to an intramuscular (IM) injection site results in vasodilation, increasing drug distribution.

Biologic membranes may serve as barriers to the passage of drugs. The *blood-brain* barrier allows only fat-soluble drugs to pass into the brain and cerebral spinal fluid. Central nervous system infections require treatment with antibiotics injected directly into the subarachnoid space in the spinal cord. Older clients may experience adverse effects (e.g., confusion) as a result of the change in the permeability of the blood-brain barrier, with easier passage of fat-soluble drugs. The placental membrane is a nonselective barrier to drugs. Fat and non–fat soluble agents may cross the placenta and produce fetal deformities, respiratory depression and, with narcotic abuse, withdrawal symptoms. Women need to be aware of the possible hazards associated with drug use during pregnancy.

PROTEIN BINDING. The degree to which drugs bind to serum proteins such as albumin affects drug distribution. Most medications bind to this protein to some extent. When drugs bind to albumin, they cannot exert any pharmacological activity. The unbound or "free" drug is the active form of the drug. Older adults have a decrease in albumin in the bloodstream, probably caused by change in liver function. The same is true for clients with liver disease or malnutrition. Because of the potential for more drug being unbound, the older adult may be at risk for an increase in drug activity or toxicity, or both.

METABOLISM. After a drug reaches its site of action, it becomes metabolized into an inactive form that is more easily excreted. Biotransformation occurs under the influence of enzymes that **detoxify,** degrade (break down), and remove biologically active chemicals. Most biotransformation occurs within the liver, although the lungs, kidneys, blood, and intestines also metabolize drugs.

The liver is especially important because its specialized structure oxidizes and transforms many toxic substances. The liver degrades many harmful chemicals before they become distributed to the tissues. If a decrease in liver function occurs, such as with aging or liver disease, a drug may be eliminated more slowly, resulting in an accumulation of the drug.

If the organs that metabolize drugs are altered, clients are at risk for drug toxicity. For example, a small sedative dose of a barbiturate may cause a client with liver disease to lapse into a hepatic coma.

EXCRETION. After drugs are metabolized, they exit the body through the kidneys, liver, bowel, lungs, and exocrine glands. The chemical makeup of a drug determines the organ of excretion. Gaseous and volatile compounds such as nitrous oxide and alcohol exit through the lungs. Deep breathing and coughing (see Chapter 36) help the postoperative client to eliminate anesthetic gases more rapidly.

The exocrine glands excrete lipid-soluble drugs. When medications exit through sweat glands, the skin may become irritated. The nurse assists the client in good hygiene practices (see Chapter 30) to promote cleanliness and skin integrity. If a drug exits through the mammary glands, there is a risk that a nursing infant will ingest the chemicals. Mothers should check on the safety of any drug used while breastfeeding.

The gastrointestinal tract is another route for drug excretion. Many drugs enter the hepatic circulation to be broken down by the liver and excreted into the bile. After chemicals enter the intestines through the biliary tract, they may be reabsorbed by the intestines. Factors that increase peristalsis (e.g., laxatives and enemas) accelerate drug excretion through the feces, whereas factors that slow peristalsis (e.g., inactivity and improper diet) may prolong a drug's effects.

The kidneys are the main organs for drug excretion. Some drugs escape extensive metabolism and exit unchanged in the urine. Other drugs must undergo biotransformation in the liver before being excreted by the kidney. If renal function declines, a client is at risk for **drug toxicity.** If the kidney cannot adequately excrete a drug, it may be necessary to reduce the dose. Maintenance of an adequate fluid intake (50 ml/kg/day) promotes proper elimination of drugs for the average adult.

Types of Drug Action

Therapeutic Effects. The therapeutic effect is the expected or predictable physiological response a drug causes. Each drug has a desired therapeutic effect for which it is prescribed. For example, nitroglycerine is used to reduce the cardiac workload and increase myocardial oxygen supply. Drug actions are also influenced by other individual and environmental factors (see box on p. 654). Clients may therefore respond differently to the same drug (Table 26-2).

Side Effects. Predictably a drug will cause other, secondary effects. Side effects may be harmless or injurious. If the side effects are serious enough to negate the beneficial effects of a drug's therapeutic action, the physician may discontinue the drug. Clients often stop taking medications because of side effects.

Toxic Effects. Toxic effects develop after intake of high doses of medication, when a drug accumulates in the blood because of impaired metabolism or excretion, or with unexpected sensitivity to a drug. Excess amounts of a drug within the body may have lethal effects, depending on the drug's action. For example, toxic levels of morphine may cause severe respiratory depression and death. Antidotes are available to treat specific types of drug toxicity. For example, Narcan is used to reverse the effects of opioid toxicity.

Idiosyncratic Reactions. Medications may cause unpredictable effects such as an idiosyncratic reaction in which a client overreacts or underreacts to a drug or has a reaction different from normal. For example, a child receiving an antihistamine (Benadryl) may become extremely agitated or excited instead of drowsy. It is impossible to assess clients for idiosyncratic responses.

Allergic Reactions. Allergic reactions are another unpredictable response to a drug; they make up 5% to 10% of all drug reactions. A client can become sensitized immunologically to the initial dose of a medication. With

table 26-2

INFLUENCE OF DRUG ACTIONS ON OLDER ADULTS

Physiological change	Drug action/client response	Nursing interventions
GASTROINTESTINAL TRACT		
Oral cavity		
Loss of elasticity in oral mucosa, which becomes dry and easily abraded	Difficulty swallowing tablets or capsules Sensitivity to drugs that cause dryness of mouth Susceptibility to gum disease and dental caries	Rinse oral cavity frequently with tepid clear water. Floss daily; brush teeth, gums, and tongue gently. Use substitute saliva.
Esophagus		
Delayed esophageal clearance because of weakened contractions and failure of lower esophageal sphincter to relax	Difficulty swallowing large tablets or capsules Tissue erosion caused by drugs such as aspirin and uncoated potassium chloride	Position client upright. Administer full glass of permitted liquid with drug. Crush tablets and mix with food (if gastric pH does not affect absorption).
Stomach		
Decrease in gastric acidity and peristalsis	Potentiation of irritating effects of highly acidic drugs (e.g., aspirin) Alteration of solubility of certain drugs	Have client drink full glass of water and take medication with nonfat snack to reduce gastric distress.
Large intestine		
Reduced colon muscle tone Loss of defecation reflex Decreased intestinal blood flow	Slowing of drug excretion Overuse and abuse of laxatives by client Drug absorption delayed	Provide normal fluid intake. Instruct client to eat bulk-forming foods and avoid use of constipating drugs.
SKIN AND VASCULATURE		
Reduced subcutaneous skin fold thickness in extremities (less body fat) Reduced elasticity in skin and vasculature	Fragile blood vessels Client prone to bleeding after injection	Avoid using veins in hand for IV injections. Apply pressure to injection sites after drug administration. Observe injection sites for bleeding.
LIVER		
Reduced liver size Decline in hepatic blood flow	Longer biotransformation time Longer-than-normal duration of drug action Greater risk for drug sensitivity and toxicity	Monitor for signs of liver impairment (jaundice, pruritus, or dark urine). Question dosages for clients with known liver disease.
KIDNEY		
Reduced glomerular filtration Decreased tubular function and renal blood flow	Risk of drug accumulation and toxicity	Prevent urinary retention (keep catheters free flowing; observe frequency of urination). Monitor for signs of renal impairment (reduced output, difficulty urinating). Question dosages for clients with renal disease.

FACTORS INFLUENCING DRUG ACTIONS

GENETIC DIFFERENCES

A person's genetic makeup can influence drug metabolism. Members of a family may share a sensitivity to a medication.

PHYSIOLOGICAL VARIABLES

Variables such as sex, age, body weight, nutritional status, and disease states all affect drug actions.

Hormonal differences between men and women affect drug metabolism.

Children require lower drug doses than adults. The changes accompanying aging alter the influence of drugs (Table 26-2).

There is a direct relationship between the amount of medication administered and the amount of body tissue in which it is distributed. Proper drug metabolism relies on good nutrition.

Diseases that impair the function of organs responsible for normal pharmacokinetics also impair drug action.

ENVIRONMENTAL CONDITIONS

Stress and the exposure to heat and cold affect drug actions. Clients receiving vasodilators, for example, require lower drug dosages in warm weather.

The setting in which a drug is administered can influence a client's reaction. If a person is alone or isolated, more pain medication may be needed than if he or she is in a room with other clients.

PSYCHOLOGICAL FACTORS

A client's attitude, reaction to the meaning of a drug, and the nurse's behavior affect drug actions. If a client understands and accepts the need for a drug and if it is administered with a supportive behavior, the drug's effect is enhanced.

DIET

Drug and nutrient interactions can alter a drug's action or the effect of a nutrient. For example, mineral oil decreases the absorption of fat-soluble vitamins.

repeated administration the client develops an allergic response to the drug, its chemical preservatives, or a metabolite. The drug or chemical acts as an antigen, triggering the release of the body's antibodies. A client's **drug allergy** may be mild or severe. Allergic symptoms vary, depending on the individual and the drug.

Among the different classes of drugs, antibiotics cause a high incidence of allergic reactions. Common, mild allergy symptoms are summarized in Table 26-3. Severe or anaphylactic reactions are characterized by sudden constriction of bronchiolar muscles, edema of the pharynx and larynx, and severe wheezing and shortness of breath. Antihistamines, epinephrine, and bronchodilators may be used to treat anaphylactic reactions.

The client may also become severely hypotensive, necessitating emergency resuscitation measures. A client with a known history of an allergy to a medication should avoid reexposure and wear an identification bracelet or medal, which alerts nurses and physicians to the allergy if the client is unconscious when receiving medical care.

table 26-3

MILD ALLERGIC REACTIONS

Symptom	Description
Urticaria (hives)	Raised, irregularly shaped skin eruptions with varying sizes and shapes Eruptions: reddened margins and pale centers
Rash	Small raised vesicles that are usually reddened and often distributed over a person's entire body
Pruritus	Itching of skin accompanying most rashes
Rhinitis	Inflammation of mucous membranes lining the nose, causing swelling and clear watery discharge

Drug Interactions

When one drug modifies the action of another drug, a **drug interaction** occurs. Drug interactions are common in individuals taking several medications. A drug may potentiate or diminish the action of other drugs, and may alter the way in which another drug is absorbed, metabolized, or eliminated from the body. When two drugs act synergistically, the effect of the two drugs combined is greater than the effect of the drugs when given separately. Alcohol is a central nervous system depressant that has a **synergistic effect** on antihistamines, antidepressants, barbiturates, and narcotic analgesics.

A drug interaction is not always undesirable. Often a physician orders combination drug therapy to create a drug interaction for the client's therapeutic benefit. For example, a client with moderate hypertension typically receives several drugs such as diuretics and vasodilators that act together to control blood pressure.

Drug Dose Responses

When a medication is prescribed, the goal is a constant blood level within a safe therapeutic range. Repeated doses are required to achieve a constant therapeutic concentration of a medication because a portion of a drug is always being excreted. When absorption ceases, only metabolism, excretion, and distribution continue. The highest serum concentration (peak concentration) of the drug usually occurs just before the last of the drug is absorbed (Clark, et al., 1993). After peaking, the serum drug concentration falls progressively. With intravenous infusions, the peak concentration occurs quickly, but the serum level also begins to fall immediately.

All drugs have a **serum half-life,** which is the time it takes for excretion processes to lower the serum drug concentration by half. To maintain a therapeutic plateau, the client must receive regular fixed doses. After an initial medication dose the client receives each successive dose when the previous dose reaches its half-life (Figure 26-1). In this way an almost constant therapeutic drug concentration is maintained.

The client and nurse must follow regular dosage schedules and adhere to prescribed doses and dosage intervals. Knowledge of the time intervals of drug action also helps the nurse to anticipate a drug's effect:

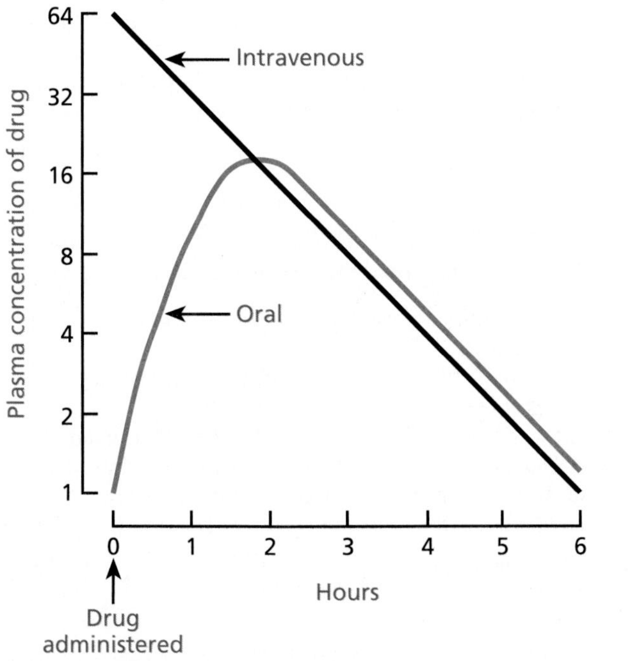

FIGURE 26-1 Curve showing therapeutic blood levels. (From Clark J, Queener S, and Karb V: *Pharmacological basis of nursing practice,* ed 4, St. Louis, 1993, Mosby.)

1. Onset of drug action. Period of time it takes after a drug is administered for it to produce a response.
2. Peak action. Time it takes for a drug to reach its highest effective concentration.
3. Duration of action. Length of time during which the drug is present in a concentration great enough to produce a response.
4. Plateau. Blood serum concentration of a drug reached and maintained after repeated fixed doses.

An effective way to achieve a constant therapeutic drug level is continuous IV infusions, which eliminate the fluctuating effects of intermittent doses.

ROUTES OF ADMINISTRATION

The route prescribed for administering a drug depends on the drug's properties and desired effect and on the client's physical and mental condition (Table 26-4). A nurse collaborates with the physician in determining the best route for a client's medication, as in the following hypothetical situation:

The client, Mr. Huels, has progressively worsened physically. His temperature is 39.2° C. He complains of nausea and is unable to tolerate oral fluids. The nurse checks Mr. Huels' order, which reads, "Aspirin 600 mg orally for temperature above 38.5° C." On the basis of the assessment, the nurse believes that Mr. Huels will not be able to tolerate an oral dose of aspirin. By consulting the physician, the nurse acquires an order for a rectal suppository instead.

Oral Routes

Oral Administration. The oral route is the easiest and the most commonly used. Medications are given by mouth and swallowed with fluid. Oral medications have a slower onset of action and a more prolonged effect than parenteral medications. Clients generally prefer the oral route.

Sublingual Administration. Some drugs are designed to be readily absorbed after being placed under the tongue to dissolve. A drug given sublingually should not be swallowed or the desired effect will not be achieved. Nitroglycerin is commonly given sublingually. A drink should not be taken by the client until the drug is completely dissolved.

Buccal Administration. Administration of a drug by the buccal route involves placing the solid medication in the mouth and against the mucous membranes of the cheek until the drug dissolves. Clients should be taught to alternate cheeks with each subsequent dose to avoid mucosal irritation. Clients are also warned not to chew

table 26-4

FACTORS INFLUENCING CHOICE OF ADMINISTRATION ROUTES

Advantages	Disadvantages or contraindications
ORAL, SUBLINGUAL, AND BUCCAL ROUTES	
Routes are convenient and comfortable for client. Routes are economical. Medications may produce local or systemic effects. Routes rarely cause anxiety for client.	Oral route is avoided when client has alterations in gastrointestinal function (e.g., nausea, vomiting), reduced motility (after general anesthesia or bowel inflammation), and surgical resection of portion of gastrointestinal tract. Some drugs are destroyed by gastric secretions. Oral administration is contraindicated in clients unable to swallow (e.g., clients with neuromuscular disorders, esophageal strictures, mouth lesions). Oral medications cannot be given when client has gastric suction and are contraindicated in clients before some tests or surgery. Unconscious or confused client is unable or unwilling to swallow or hold medication under tongue. Oral medications may irritate lining of gastrointestinal tract, discolor teeth, or have unpleasant taste.
SQ, IM, IV, INTRADERMAL ROUTES	
Routes provide means of administration when oral drugs are contraindicated. More rapid absorption occurs than with topical or oral routes. IV infusion provides drug delivery when long-term therapy is required. If peripheral perfusion is poor, IV route is preferred over injections.	There is risk of introducing infection and drugs are expensive. Clients must experience repeated needlesticks. The SQ, IM, and intradermal routes may be avoided in clients with bleeding tendencies. There is risk of tissue damage with SQ injections. IM and IV routes are dangerous because of rapid absorption. These routes cause considerable anxiety in many clients, especially children.
SKIN	
Topical	
Topical skin applications primarily provide local effect. Route is painless. Limited side effects occur.	Extensive applications may be bulky and cause difficulty in maneuvering. Clients with skin abrasions are at risk for rapid drug absorption and systemic effects.
Transdermal	
Transdermal applications provide prolonged systemic effects, with limited side effects.	Application leaves oily or pasty substance on skin and may soil clothing.
MUCOUS MEMBRANES	
Therapeutic effects are provided by local application to involved sites. Aqueous solutions are readily absorbed and capable of causing systemic effects. Mucous membranes provide route of administration when oral drugs are contraindicated.	Mucous membranes are highly sensitive to some drug concentrations. Insertion of rectal and vaginal medication often causes embarrassment. Client with ruptured eardrum cannot receive irrigations. Rectal suppositories are contraindicated if client has had rectal surgery or if active rectal bleeding is present.
INHALATION	
Inhalation provides rapid relief for local respiratory problems. Route provides easy access for introduction of general anesthetic gases.	Some local agents can cause serious systemic effects.

or swallow the drug or to take any liquids with it. A buccal medication acts locally on the mucosa or systemically as it is swallowed in a person's saliva.

Parenteral Routes

Parenteral administration involves injecting a drug into body tissues. The four major sites of injection are:

1. **Subcutaneous:** Injection into tissues just below the dermis of the skin
2. **Intramuscular (IM):** Injection into a muscle
3. **Intravenous (IV):** Injection into a vein
4. **Intradermal:** Injection into the dermis just under the epidermis

A physician may use additional routes for parenteral injections, including the intrathecal or intraspinal, intracardiac, intrapleural, intraarterial, intraosseous, and intraarticular routes.

Strict sterile technique must be used when preparing medications for parenteral injection. Contamination of medication solutions, syringe needles, or the syringe itself can lead to infection (see Chapter 25).

Skin and Mucous Membrane Route

Drugs applied to the skin and mucous membranes generally have local effects. Medications are applied to the skin by painting or spreading them over an area, applying moist dressings, soaking body parts in a solution, or giving medicated baths. Systemic effects can occur if a client's skin is thin, if the drug concentration is high, or if contact with the skin is prolonged.

Some medications (e.g., nitroglycerin, scopolamine, and estrogens) have systemic effects because they are applied topically by a transdermal disk or patch. The disk secures the medicated ointment to the skin. These topical applications may be applied for as little as 8 hours or as long as 7 days.

Mucous membranes differ in their sensitivity to medications. The cornea of the eye and nasal mucous membranes are very sensitive. The client may complain of a burning sensation when the nurse administers eye or nose drops. Medications are generally less irritating to vaginal or rectal mucosa. The nurse uses several methods for applying medications to mucous membranes:

1. Direct application of liquid or ointment (e.g., eye drops, gargling, swabbing the throat)
2. Insertion of drug into a body cavity (e.g., placing a suppository in rectum or vagina or inserting medicated packing into vagina)
3. Instillation of fluid into body cavity (e.g., ear drops, nose drops, or bladder and rectal instillation [fluid is retained])
4. Irrigation of body cavity (e.g., flushing eye, ear, vagina, bladder, or rectum with medicated fluid [fluid is not retained])
5. Spraying (e.g., instillation into nose and throat)

Inhalation Route

The deeper passages of the respiratory tract provide a large surface area for drug absorption. The vascular alveolar-capillary network readily absorbs gases and mists introduced through the airways. Medications introduced into the lung's airways must not interfere with normal gas exchange such as constricting bronchioles.

Inhaled medications may have local effects. Drugs such as oxygen and general anesthetics create general systemic effects. Some medications given by inhalation are designed to produce local effects but have potentially dangerous systemic side effects. Cocaine, when sniffed or snorted, produces vasoconstriction and hypertension—physical dangers associated with the abuse of this drug. Administration of local-acting medications with hand-operated **inhalers** must be carefully taught to the client by the nurse.

SYSTEMS OF DRUG MEASUREMENT

The proper administration of a medication depends on the nurse's ability to compute drug doses accurately and measure medications correctly. A careless mistake in placing a decimal point or adding a zero to a dose can lead to a fatal error. The nurse is responsible for checking the dose before giving a drug and teaching clients about prescribed doses.

The metric, apothecary, and household systems of measurement are used in drug therapy. Most nations, including Canada, use the metric system as their standard of measurement. Although the U.S. Congress has not officially adopted the metric system, most health professionals in the United States use it and the apothecary system. Prescriptions to be self-administered are often written in household measures for clients.

Metric System

As a decimal system, the **metric system** is the most logically organized. Metric units can easily be converted and computed through simple multiplication and division. Each basic unit of measurement is organized into units of 10. Multiplying or dividing by 10 forms secondary units. In multiplication, the decimal point moves to the right; in division, the decimal moves to the left. For example:

$$\mathbf{10.0\ mg \times 10 = 100.\ mg}$$

$$\mathbf{10.0\ mg \div 10 = 1.0\ mg}$$

The basic units of measurement in the metric system are the meter (length), the liter (volume), and the gram (weight). For drug calculations the nurse uses only the volume and weight units. In the metric system, small or large letters are used to designate basic units:

Gram = g or Gm

Liter = l or L

Small letters are abbreviations for other units:

Milligram = mg

Milliliter = ml

A system of Latin prefixes designates subdivision of the basic units: *deci-* (1/10 or 0.1), *centi-* (1/100 or 0.01), and *milli-* (1/1000 or 0.001). Greek prefixes designate multiples of the basic units: *deka-* (10), *hecto-* (100), and *kilo-* (1000). When writing drug doses in metric units, physicians and nurses use fractions or multiples of a unit. Fractions are always in decimal form:

500 mg or 0.5 g, *not* ½ g

10 ml or 0.01 L, *not* 1/100 L

When fractions are used, a zero is always placed in front of the decimal to prevent error.

Apothecary System

The **apothecary system** is an older system of measurement familiar to most people in the United States and Canada. The basic unit of weight is a grain. Units of weight derived from the grain are the dram, ounce, and pound. The apothecary unit for volume or fluid measurement is the minim. The minim is the approximate amount of water that weighs a grain. The fluidram, fluid ounce, pint, quart, and gallon are measures derived from the minim. In the apothecary system, small letters or symbols are used for measurement units:

Grain = gr

Ounce = oz or ℥

Fluid ounce = f℥

Minim = m

Dram = ʒ

Lower-case Roman numerals designate the amounts of the apothecary units. The Roman numeral follows the unit of measure:

3 grains = gr iii

Physicians often use fractions and symbols with apothecary units:

2½ fluid ounces = f℥ iiss

½ fluid ounce = f℥ ½ or f℥ ss

Household Measurements

Household units of measure are familiar to most people. The disadvantage with household measures is their inaccuracy. Household utensils such as teaspoons and cups often vary in size. Scales to measure pints or quarts are often not well calibrated. Household measures include drops, teaspoons, tablespoons, and cups for volume and pints and quarts for weight. Although pints and quarts are considered household measures, they are also used in the apothecary system.

The advantage of household measurements is their convenience and familiarity. When the accuracy of a drug dose is not critical, it is safe to use household measures. For example, many over-the-counter drugs can safely be measured by this method. Table 26-5 gives common equivalents from each measurement unit.

Solutions

The nurse uses solutions of various concentrations for injections, irrigations, and infusions. A **solution** is a

table 26-5

EQUIVALENTS OF MEASUREMENT

Metric (volume)	Apothecary	Household
1 ml	15 minims (m) or 16 minims	15 drops (gtt)
4-5 ml	1 fluidram (fʒ)	1 teaspoon (tsp)
15 ml	4 fluidrams (fʒ)	1 tablespoon (tbsp)
30 ml	1 fluid ounce (f℥)	2 tablespoons (tbsp)
240 ml	8 fluid ounces (f℥)	1 cup (c)
480 ml (approximately 500 ml)	1 pint (pt)	1 pint (pt)
960 ml (approximately 1 L)	1 quart (qt)	1 quart (qt)
3840 ml (approximately 4000 ml)	1 gallon (gal)	1 gallon (gal)

given mass of solid substance dissolved in a known volume of fluid or a given volume of liquid dissolved in a known volume of another fluid. When a solid is dissolved in a fluid, the **concentration** is in units of mass per units of volume (e.g., g/ml, g/L, mg/ml). A concentration of a solution may also be expressed as a percentage. A 10% solution, for example, is 10 g of solid dissolved in 100 ml of solution. A proportion also expresses concentrations. A $\frac{1}{1000}$ solution represents a solution containing 1 g of solid in 1000 ml of liquid or 1 ml of liquid mixed with 1000 ml of another liquid.

CONVERTING MEASUREMENT UNITS

A pharmacist does not always dispense a medication in the unit of measure in which it is ordered. Drug companies package and bottle certain standard equivalents. For example, the physician may order 250 mg of a medication that is available only in grams. The nurse is responsible for converting available units of volume and weight to the desired doses. Therefore the nurse should be aware of approximate equivalents in all major measurement systems.

Drug administration is not the only function in which nurses use volume and weight conversions (see box below). Conversions are used in a variety of nursing activities.

Conversions Within One System

Converting measurements within one system is relatively easy. In the metric system the nurse simply divides or multiplies. To change milligrams to grams, the nurse divides by 1000, moving the decimal 3 points to the left.

1000 mg = 1 g

350 mg = 0.35 g

To convert liters to milliliters, the nurse multiplies by 1000 or moves the decimal 3 points to the right.

1 L = 1000 ml

0.25 L = 250 ml

To convert units of measurement within the apothecary or household system, the nurse must consult an equivalent table. For example, when converting fluid ounces to quarts the nurse must first know that 32 ounces is the equivalent of 1 quart. To convert 8 ounces to a quart measurement, for example, the nurse divides 8 by 32 to get the equivalent, $\frac{1}{4}$ or 0.25 quart.

Conversion Between Systems

The nurse must frequently determine the proper dose of a medication by converting weights or volumes from one system of measurement to another. Commonly, apothecary and metric units must be converted to equivalent household measures for use at home. When the time comes to make actual drug calculations, it is necessary to work with units in the same measurement system. Tables of equivalent measurements are available in all health care institutions. The pharmacist is also a good resource.

Before making a conversion, the nurse compares the measurement system available with that ordered. For example, a physician orders morphine gr $\frac{1}{6}$ IM. The medication is available in milligrams. To convert grains to milligrams, the nurse must know the equivalents:

1 mg = $\frac{1}{60}$ **gr**

or

60 mg = 1 gr

Therefore, by converting gr $\frac{1}{6}$ to milligrams, the nurse will have the measurements needed to make the eventual dose calculation. The nurse divides by 6:

60 mg ÷ 6 = $\frac{1}{6}$ **gr**

10 mg = $\frac{1}{6}$ **gr**

After calculating that the physician's order for morphine gr $\frac{1}{6}$ is the same as 10 mg morphine, the nurse can accurately prepare the medication based on the available dosage.

Dosage Calculations

The nurse can use a simple formula in many different types of dosage calculations. The following formula can be applied when preparing solid or liquid forms:

$$\frac{\text{Dose ordered}}{\text{Dose on hand}} \times \text{Amount on hand} = \text{Amount to administer}$$

The *dose ordered* is the amount of pure drug the physician prescribes. The *dose on hand* is the weight or volume of drug available in units supplied by the phar-

COMMON REASONS FOR DRUG CONVERSIONS

- Converting fluid ounces to milliliters for measurement of intake and output
- Converting body weight from pounds to kilograms and vice versa
- Converting volume equivalents to calculate IV flow rates, prepare wound irrigation solutions, enemas, or bladder irrigations

macy; it may be expressed on the drug label as the contents of a tablet or capsule or as the amount of drug dissolved per unit volume of liquid. The *amount on hand* is the basic unit or quantity of the drug that contains the dose on hand. For solid drugs the amount on hand may be one capsule; the amount of liquid on hand may be a milliliter or liter depending on the container. The *amount to administer* is the actual amount of available medication the nurse will administer. The amount to administer is always expressed in the same unit as the amount on hand.

The following example illustrates how to apply the formula. The physician orders the client to receive Demerol 50 mg IM. Thus the dose ordered is 50 mg. The drug is available only in ampules containing 100 mg per milliliter. Thus the dose on hand is 100 mg in an amount on hand of 1 ml. The formula is applied as follows:

$$\frac{\textbf{50 mg}}{\textbf{100 mg}} \times \textbf{1 ml} = \textbf{Volume of milliliter to administer}$$

To simplify the $^{50}/_{100}$ fraction, divide numerator and denominator by 50:

$$\frac{\textbf{1}}{\textbf{2}} \times \textbf{1 ml} = \textbf{½ ml to administer}$$

Syringes are calibrated only in decimals. After converting the fraction ½ to 0.5, the nurse can more accurately draw up the correct dose.

Another example demonstrates how the formula applies with solid dose forms. The physician orders 0.125 mg PO* of digoxin. The drug is available in tablets containing 0.25 mg.

$$\frac{\textbf{0.125 mg}}{\textbf{0.250 mg}} \times \textbf{1 tablet} = \textbf{Tablets to administer}$$

The fraction $^{0.125}/_{0.250}$ equals ½ or 0.5. Therefore,

$$\textbf{0.5} \times \textbf{1 tablet} = \textbf{0.5 or ½ tablet to be administered}$$

Many tablets come with scores or indentations across the center of the tablet. A scored tablet is easy to break in half for divided doses. In some institutions pharmacists are responsible for scoring tablets. The potential for giving an incorrect dosage is high when the nurse estimates amounts by breaking unscored tablets.

Often, liquid drugs come prepared in volumes greater than 1 ml. The formula still applies. For example, the order is, "Erythromycin suspension 250 mg po." The pharmacy delivers 100 ml bottles with the labels stating, "5 ml contains 125 mg of erythromycin."

$$\frac{\textbf{250 mg}}{\textbf{125 mg}} \times \textbf{5 ml} = \textbf{Volume to administer}$$

The fraction $^{250}/_{125}$ equals 2. Therefore,

$$\textbf{2} \times \textbf{5 ml} = \textbf{10 ml to administer}$$

Here the nurse ignores the total volume available and instead uses the values noted on the label. If the nurse calculated the dose on the basis of 100 ml available, the following error would occur:

$$\frac{\textbf{250 mg}}{\textbf{125 mg}} \times \textbf{100 ml} = \textbf{200 ml to administer}$$

On the basis of this calculation the client would receive 20 times the desired dose. The nurse should always double-check calculations or confer with another professional if an answer seems unreasonable.

Pediatric Dosages

Calculating children's drug dosages requires caution. Children are unable to metabolize many drugs as readily as adults. The child's body size also requires smaller dosages. In most cases, physicians calculate the safe dose for a child before ordering the medication. However, nurses should be aware of the formulas used to calculate pediatric dosages and recheck all dosages before administration. Most drug references list the normal ranges for pediatric dosages.

Body Surface Area. The most accurate method of calculating pediatric dosages is based on a child's body surface area. Body surface area is estimated on the basis of the child's weight. Standard nomograms or charts list a child's body surface area by weight and approximate age (Figure 26-2). The formula is a ratio of the child's body surface area compared with the body surface area of an average adult (1.7 square meters, or 1.7 m^2).

$$\textbf{Child's dose} = \frac{\textbf{Surface area of child}}{\textbf{1.7 m}^2} \times \textbf{Normal adult dose}$$

For example, what dose of ampicillin does a child weighing 12 kg require if the normal single adult dose for ampicillin is 250 mg? A nomogram shows that a child weighing 12 kg has a surface area of 0.54 m^2.

$$\textbf{Child's dose} = \frac{\textbf{0.54 m}^2}{\textbf{1.7 m}^2} \times \textbf{250 mg}$$

The m^2 units are constant and can be ignored.

$$\textbf{Child's dose} = \frac{\textbf{0.54}}{\textbf{1.7}} \times \textbf{250 mg}$$

$$\frac{\textbf{0.54}}{\textbf{1.7}} = \textbf{0.3}$$

$$\textbf{Child's dose} = \textbf{0.3} \times \textbf{250 mg} = \textbf{75 mg}$$

*PO is the abbreviation for the Latin phrase *per orum,* by mouth.

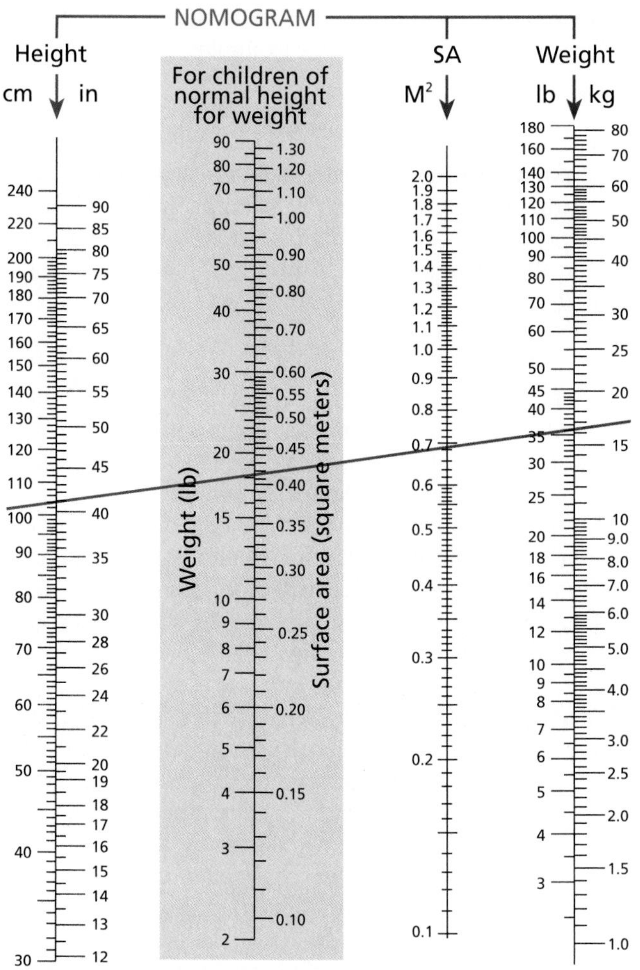

FIGURE 26-2 West nomogram for estimation of surface areas in children. Straight line is drawn between height and weight. Point where the line crosses surface area column is estimated body surface area. (From Behrman RE and Vaughan VC, editors: *Nelson textbook of pediatrics,* ed 14, Philadelphia, 1992, WB Saunders; modified from data of Boyd E by West CD.)

Body Weight. Another method of calculating pediatric dosages is by using the child's body weight in kilograms. In this method the drug is prescribed in amounts per kilogram of body weight. The child's weight must be converted from pounds to kilograms. For example, what dosage range of acetaminophen is required for a child weighing 44 lbs.? To determine the weight in kilograms, 44 lbs. must be divided by 2.2 kg/lb.

$$\frac{44 \text{ lbs.}}{2.2 \text{ kg/lb}} = 20 \text{ kg}$$

The safe dosage range for acetaminophen is 10-15mg/kg q4h. The kilogram weight is then multiplied by the range values.

$$20 \text{ kg} \times 10 \text{ mg/kg} = 200 \text{ mg}$$

$$20 \text{ kg} \times 15 \text{ mg/kg} = 300 \text{ mg}$$

In this case the safe range for administration of the acetaminophen is 200-300 mg q4h. Although not as precise as the body surface area calculation, this method is used quite frequently.

ADMINISTERING MEDICATIONS

The nurse does not have sole responsibility for drug administration. The physician and pharmacist also help to ensure the right medication gets to the right client. However, the nurse administering medications is accountable for knowing what medications are prescribed, their therapeutic and nontherapeutic effects, and the client's needs and abilities.

Physician's Role

The physician prescribes the client's drugs (unless a state's nurse practice act allows nurse practitioners or other advance practice nurses to prescribe under collaborative agreements). The physician writes an order on a form in the client's medical record, in a physician's order book, on a legal prescription pad, or through a computer terminal. In some situations such as an emergency, a physician may also order a medication by telephone or by giving the nurse a verbal order.

The nurse enters and signs all telephone and verbal orders, writes the name of the physician ordering the drug, and later has the physician countersign the order. Most institutions require a physician's signature within 24 hours after the order is made.

Institutional policies vary regarding the personnel who can take verbal or telephone orders. In many institutions, nursing students cannot take medication orders. *No medication is to be given without an order.* If the technology is available, a physician may Fax orders to the unit.

Common abbreviations are used when writing orders. The abbreviations indicate dosage frequencies or times, routes of administration, and special information for giving the drug (see box on p. 662).

Types of Orders. The four common types of medication orders are based on the frequency of drug administration.

STANDING ORDERS. A standing order is carried out until the physician cancels it by another order or until a prescribed number of days elapse. A standing order may indicate a final date or number of treatments or dosages. Many institutions have policies for automatically discontinuing standing orders. The following are

ESSENTIAL COMPONENTS OF DRUG ORDERS

CLIENT'S FULL NAME

This information distinguishes the client from other persons with the same last name.

DATE AND TIME ORDER IS WRITTEN

The day, month, year, and time are included. Designating the time an order is written helps to clarify when certain orders are to automatically stop. If an incident involving a drug error occurs, it will be easier to document what happened when this information is available.

DRUG NAME

The physician usually orders a generic or trade-name drug. Correct spelling is essential in differentiating names with similar spelling.

DOSAGE

The amount and strength of the drug are included.

ROUTE OF ADMINISTRATION

The physician uses common abbreviations for drug routes. Accuracy is important because certain drugs are given by more than one route.

TIME AND FREQUENCY OF ADMINISTRATION

The nurse needs to know when to start drug therapy and how often the drug will be administered.

SIGNATURE OF PHYSICIAN OR NURSE PRACTITIONER

The signature makes the order a legal request.

examples of standing orders:

Tetracycline 500 mg PO q6h*
Decadron 10 mg qd × 5 days

PRN ORDERS. The physician may order a drug when a client requires it. This is a prn order. The nurse uses discretion in determining the client's need. Often the physician sets maximum intervals for the time of administration. The nurse may decide to lengthen the interval if the client does not need the drug.

Examples of prn orders:

Morphine gr ¼ IM q3-4h prn for incisional pain
Maalox 30 ml po prn for gastric discomfort

SINGLE (ONE-TIME) ORDERS. A physician will often order a drug to be given only once at a specified time. This is common for preoperative drugs or drugs given before diagnostic examinations. For example:

Atropine 0.4 mg IM on call to OR
Valium 10 mg po at 0900

STAT ORDERS. A stat order signifies that a single dose of a medication is to be given immediately and only once. Stat orders are often written for emergencies when the client's condition changes suddenly. For example:

Give Apresoline 10 mg IM stat

Some conditions change the status of a client's medication orders. For example, surgery automatically cancels all of a client's preoperative medications (see Chapter 36). Because the client's condition changes after surgery, the physician must write new orders. When a client is transferred to another health care agency or a different medical service within a hospital or is discharged, the physician should review the medications and write new orders as indicated.

Prescriptions. The physician writes **prescriptions** for clients who are to take drugs outside the hospital. The prescription includes more detailed information than a regular order because the client must understand how to take the drug and when to refill the prescription if necessary. The parts of a prescription include:

1. Superscription. The client's name, address, age, and date are given for identification purposes. The symbol R_x ("take thou") is at the top of the form.
2. Inscription. This is the drug name, strength, and dose.
3. Subscription. Directions regarding the number of tablets or amount to be dispensed are given to the pharmacist.
4. Signature. The physician signs the prescription. If the drug is a controlled substance, the physician includes his or her registration number and address.
5. Personal data. Information to be written on the label (e.g., directions to the client, and directions for refilling the prescription, and whether the drug name should be included on the label) is included.

Pharmacist's Role

The pharmacist prepares and distributes prescribed drugs. The pharmacist is responsible for filling prescriptions accurately and for being sure that prescriptions are valid. If there is any question that a prescription is forged or that the prescribing physician is unlicensed, the pharmacist should not fill the prescription. The pharmacist calls the physician if an ordered dosage seems outside of the safe therapeutic range.

The pharmacist in a health care agency rarely has to

**q*, every; *h*, hour; *qd*, every day.

mix compounds or solutions, except in the case of IV additive solutions. Most drug companies deliver drugs in a form ready for use. Dispensing the correct drug, in the proper dosage and amount, with an accurate label is the pharmacist's main task. The pharmacist can also provide information about drug side effects, toxicity, interactions, and incompatibilities.

Distribution Systems

Systems for storing and distributing drugs vary. Pharmacists provide the drugs, but nurses distribute drugs to clients. Institutions providing nursing care have a special area for stocking and dispensing drugs. Special drug rooms, portable locked carts, computerized drug cabinets, and individual storage units next to clients' rooms are some of the facilities used. Nurses must make sure that storage areas are locked when unattended.

Stock Supply. With a stock system, drugs are available in quantity in larger, multidose containers. This system is time-consuming and costly because a nurse must dispense each drug separately for a client.

Individual Client Supply. A separate supply of drugs for each client can be kept in specially labeled drawers or storage bins. Generally the pharmacist dispenses only the amount of a drug a client will use for a limited period of time. Nurses distribute a client's drugs only from the client's supply. This system reduces the time it takes to dispense drugs.

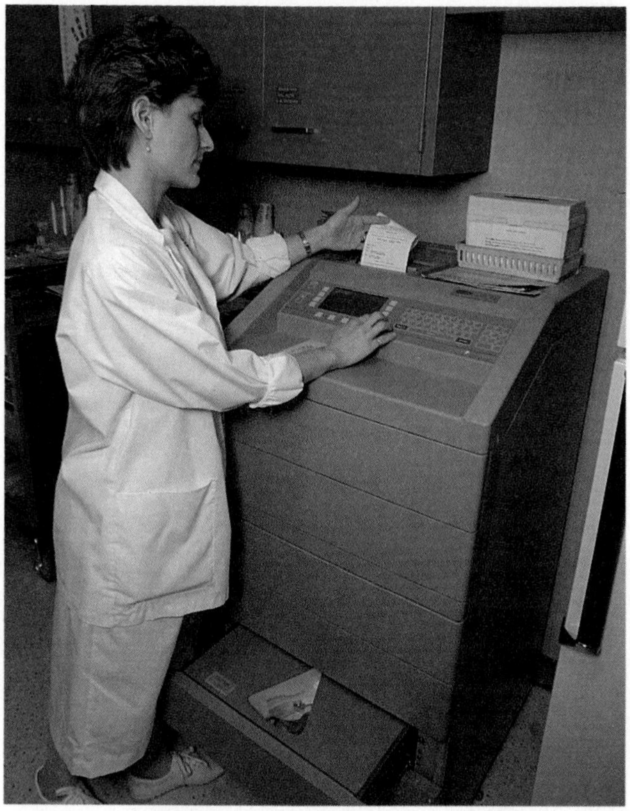

FIGURE 26-3 Computer-controlled dispensing system.

Unit Dose. The unit-dose system uses portable carts containing a drawer with a 24-hour supply of medications for each client. The unit-dose is the ordered dose of medication the client receives at one time. Each tablet or capsule is wrapped in a foil or paper container. At a designated time each day the pharmacist refills the drawers in the cart with a fresh supply. The cart also contains limited amounts of prn and stock drugs for special situations. The unit-dose system is designed to reduce the number of medication errors and saves steps in dispensing drugs.

Computer-Controlled Dispensing Systems. Computer-controlled dispensing systems are used successfully throughout the country (Figure 26-3). They are especially useful for the delivery and control of narcotics. Each nurse has a security code allowing access to the system. Then the client's identification number is entered. In these systems the nurse is then allowed to select the desired drug, dosage, and route. The system delivers the drug to the nurse, records it, and charges it to the client.

Nurses may also scan bar codes (Figure 26-4) to identify the client, drug (name, dosage, route), and nurse administering the drug (Abdoo, 1992). This information is then automatically recorded on a computerized data base.

Nurse's Role

The nurse's role extends beyond simply giving drugs to a client. The nurse assesses the client's ability to self-administer drugs, determines whether a client should receive a drug at a given time, administers drugs correctly, and monitors the effects of prescribed drugs.

FIGURE 26-4 UPC bar code symbol.

Client and family education about proper drug administration and monitoring is an integral part of the nurse's role. The nurse uses the nursing process to integrate drug therapy into care.

NURSING PROCESS

Assessment

To determine the need for and potential response to drug therapy, the nurse assesses many factors.

MEDICAL HISTORY. A medical history provides indications or contraindications for drug therapy. Disease or illness may place clients at risk for adverse drug effects. Long-term health problems such as diabetes or arthritis, which require medicinal therapies, suggest to the nurse the type of drugs a client is taking. A client's surgical history may indicate use of medications.

HISTORY OF ALLERGIES. If the client has a history of allergies to medication, the nurse informs other members of the health care team. Food allergies should also be carefully documented because many drugs have ingredients also found in food sources. One example is shellfish. If clients are allergic to shellfish, the client may be sensitive to any product containing iodine. In a hospital, clients wear identification bands listing medications to which they are allergic. All allergies should be noted on the nurse's admission notes, medication records, and physician's history.

DRUG DATA. The nurse assesses information about each drug, including action, purpose, normal dosages, routes, side effects, and nursing implications for administration and monitoring. Common questions to ask are: Is the smallest possible dose ordered (a question pertinent to older adults)? Can a certain drug interact with other drugs being used? Are there special instructions for administering the drug? Often, several resources must be consulted to gather needed information. Pharmacology textbooks, nursing journals, the *Physicians' Desk Reference (PDR)*, drug package inserts, and the pharmacist are valuable resources. The nurse is responsible for knowing as much as possible about each drug given. Many nursing students prepare or purchase cards containing drug data to use as a quick resource.

DIET HISTORY. A diet history reveals normal eating patterns and food preferences. The nurse can then plan the dosage schedule more effectively and advise the client in avoiding foods that may interact with medications.

CLIENT'S PERCEPTUAL OR COORDINATION PROBLEMS. For a client with perceptual or coordination limitations, self-administration may be difficult. The nurse must assess the client's ability to prepare doses and take medications correctly. If the client is unable to self-administer drugs, the nurse may need to assess whether family or friends will be available to assist.

CLIENT'S CURRENT CONDITION. The ongoing physical or mental status of a client may affect whether a drug is given or how it is administered. The nurse should assess a client carefully before giving any drug. For example, the nurse checks blood pressure before giving an antihypertensive. A client who is nauseated may be unable to swallow a tablet. Assessment findings also serve as a baseline in evaluating the effects of drug therapy.

CLIENT'S ATTITUDE ABOUT DRUG USE. The client's attitude about drugs may reveal the level of drug dependence. Clients often do not express feelings about drugs, particularly if dependence is a problem. To assess attitudes, the nurse observes the client's behavior for evidence of drug dependence.

CLIENT'S KNOWLEDGE AND UNDERSTANDING OF DRUG THERAPY. The client's knowledge and understanding of drug therapy influence the willingness or ability to follow a drug regimen. Unless a client understands a drug's purpose, the importance of regular dosage schedules and proper administration methods, and the possible side effects, compliance is unlikely. When assessing knowledge of a drug, the nurse asks: What is it for? How is it taken? When is it taken? What side effects have there been? Has the client ever stopped taking doses? Is there anything else the client does not understand and would like to know about the drug? When the client has a history of poor compliance, the nurse should also review resources available for purchase of medications.

CLIENT'S LEARNING NEEDS. By assessing the client's level of knowledge about a medication, the nurse determines the need for instruction. It may be necessary for the nurse to explain the action and purpose of the drug, expected side effects, correct administration techniques, and ways to help the client to remember the drug regimen. If a client has been placed on a newly prescribed drug, instruction may need to be more involved.

Nursing Diagnosis

Assessment provides data about the client's condition, ability to self-administer drugs, and drug use patterns,

NURSING DIAGNOSES FOR DRUG THERAPY

- Knowledge deficit regarding drug therapy
- Noncompliance regarding drug regimen
- Impaired physical mobility
- Sensory/perceptual alterations: visual
- Anxiety
- Impaired swallowing

which can be used to determine actual or potential problems with drug therapy (see box on p. 664). Certain data are defining characteristics, which when clustered together reveal nursing diagnoses. For example, a client's admission of missing a dosage, evidence that a medication has not reversed symptoms, and evidence that the client has not progressed indicates noncompliance regarding a drug regimen. Once the diagnosis is selected, the nurse identifies the related factor. The related factors of inadequate resources versus lack of knowledge require different interventions. If the client's noncompliance is related to inadequate finances, the nurse will collaborate with family members, social workers, or community agencies to help a client receive necessary medications. If the related factor is lack of knowledge, the nurse will implement an extensive teaching plan and follow-up.

There are diagnoses such as impaired physical mobility and sensory alteration that can place a client at risk during drug therapy. In these cases the nurse must ensure safe methods for drug administration. Again, education of the client or significant others will be important.

Planning

The nurse organizes care activities to ensure the safe administration of drugs. Undue haste can cause errors. The nurse can also plan to use time during drug administration to teach clients about their medications. It is important to collaborate with the client's family or friends when instruction is given. Family members will often reinforce the importance of drug regimens in the home setting. When clients are hospitalized, it is important for the nurse to not postpone instruction until the

SAMPLE NURSING CARE PLAN
Knowledge Deficit

ASSESSMENT

Clinical scenario: Mr. Grimes is an 18-year-old *newly diagnosed* diabetic. The physician has *prescribed insulin therapy* for the client. The client is alert, responsive to all questions, and able to read printed literature on diabetes. Mr. Grimes has *asked the nurse for information on insulin administration.*

NURSING DIAGNOSIS

Knowledge deficit regarding self administration of insulin related to inexperience

PLANNING

Goal	Expected outcomes
Client will self-administer insulin correctly within 3 days.	Client will prepare insulin correctly in syringe within 2 days. Client will prepare proper dose within 2 days. Client will administer injection safely into subcutaneous site within 3 days.

IMPLEMENTATION

Steps	Rationale
1. Provide client with syringe and let him handle parts.	Client becomes familiar with working parts of syringe.
2. Explain and demonstrate aseptic technique for preparing dosage from vial.	Provides learner with clear mental image of how skill is performed; demonstration is method most suited for teaching a psychomotor skill (Redman, 1988).
3. Discuss importance of proper dose.	Insulin can create serious side effects if improper dose is administered.
4. Explain and demonstrate method for administering subcutaneous injection (have client stand behind nurse).	Demonstration provides image of injection technique; over-the-shoulder view provides clear image of how to do action (Redman, 1988).

EVALUATIVE MEASURES

Have client perform return demonstration of preparing dose in a syringe.
Ask client to describe ordered insulin dosage and implications of receiving incorrect dosage.
Have client perform return demonstration of administering self- injection.

Defining characteristics are shown in italic type.

day of discharge. In order for the client to understand medications and self-administration guidelines, there must be time for questions and discussion. Early planning is critical.

Whether a client attempts self-administration or the nurse assumes responsibility for administering medications (see care plan on p. 665), the following goals and expected outcomes must be met:

Goal: Client and family understand drug therapy.

Outcomes

- Client and family describe information about drug, dosage, schedule, purpose, and adverse effects
- Client and family identify situations that require medical intervention
- Client and family demonstrate appropriate administration technique (e.g., placement of transdermal patch)

Goal: Client gains therapeutic effect of the prescribed medications without discomfort or complications.

Outcomes

- Client demonstrates physiological and psychological responses consistent with desired therapeutic effect of medication
- Client states positive responses to prescribed medications

Goal: Client has no complications related to the route of administration.

Outcomes

- Client swallows oral medications without difficulty
- Client does not have localized or systemic reactions to parenteral administration

Goal: Client safely self-administers medications.

Outcomes

- Client follows prescribed treatment regimen
- Client performs techniques correctly
- Client identifies available resources for obtaining necessary medication

Implementation

CORRECT TRANSCRIPTION AND COMMUNICATION OF ORDERS. The nurse or a designated unit secretary writes the physician's complete order on the appropriate medication forms (Figure 26-5). The transcribed order includes the client's name, room, and bed number, drug name, dosage, frequency, and route of administration. Each time a drug dosage is prepared the nurse refers to the medication form. With the unit-dose system, only one transcription is necessary, limiting the opportunity for errors. When transcribing orders, the nurse

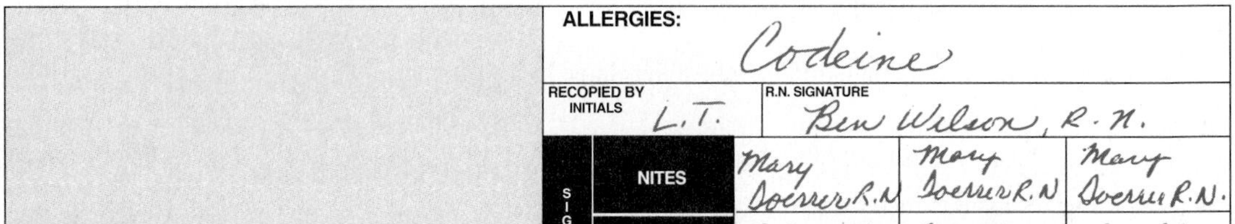

BARNES HOSPITAL PATIENT ROUTINE MEDICATION RECORD

ALLERGIES: Codeine

RECOPIED BY INITIALS: L.T. R.N. SIGNATURE: Ben Wilson, R.N.

SIGNATURES			
NITES	Mary Doerrer R.N.	Mary Doerrer R.N.	Mary Doerrer R.N.
DAYS	Pat Little R.N.	Pat Little R.N.	Pat Little R.N.
EVES	Donna C Gail R.N.	Donna C Gail R.N.	

ORDER DATE / EXP DATE	INIT	ROUTINE MEDICATION Name of drug, strength and frequency	RTE	SCHEDULE	SHIFT	DATE 2/6/94	DATE 2/7/94	DATE 2/8/94
2/6	PL	Lanoxin 0.25 mg q.d.	PO		NITES			
				10	DAYS	0950 PL	1000 PL	1010 PL
					EVES			
2/7	DG	Lasix 40 mg b.i.d.	PO		NITES			
				10	DAYS			1010 PL
				16	EVES		1545 DG	
2/7	DG	Ancef Gm i q6°	IVPB	06	NITES			06 MD
				12	DAYS		1215 PL	1200 PL
				18-24	EVES		18 DG 2345 DG	
2/8	PL	Nitro Paste 1 inch q8°	Top	06	NITES			
				14	DAYS			1410 PL
				22	EVES			
2/8		Neosporin Ophthalmic Oint. OD	Top		NITES			
				10	DAYS			1010 PL
				22	EVES			

FIGURE 26-5 Example of medication record. (Courtesy Barnes Hospital, St Louis.)

should be sure that names, dosages, and symbols are legible. The nurse rewrites any smudged or illegible transcriptions.

In some institutions a computer printout lists all currently ordered medications with dosage information. Orders are entered directly into the computer, preventing the need for transcription of orders. The same printout may be used to record medications given.

A registered nurse checks all transcribed orders against the original order for accuracy and thoroughness. If an order seems incorrect or inappropriate, the nurse consults the physician. The nurse who gives the wrong medication or an incorrect dose is legally responsible for the error.

ACCURATE DOSAGE CALCULATION AND MEASUREMENT. When measuring liquid drugs, the nurse uses standard measuring containers. The procedure for drug measurement is systematic to lessen the chance of error. The nurse calculates each dose when preparing the drug, pays close attention to the process of calculation, and avoids interference from other nursing activities.

CORRECT ADMINISTRATION. For safe administration, the nurse uses aseptic technique and proper procedures when handling and giving medications. Promoting client comfort (e.g., positioning) increases efficiency. Certain drugs require the nurse to perform assessments (e.g., assessing heart rate before giving antidysrhythmic medications).

RECORDING DRUG ADMINISTRATION. After administering a drug, the nurse records it immediately on the appropriate record form (see Figure 26-5). *The nurse never charts a drug before administering it.* Recording immediately after administration prevents errors.

The recording of a drug includes the name of the drug, dosage, route, and exact time of administration. Often the drug forms are prepared and the nurse need only record the time. Agency policies may also require that the nurse record the location of an injection.

If a client refuses a drug or is undergoing tests or procedures that result in a missed dose, the nurse explains the reason the drug was not given in the nurse's notes. Some agencies require the nurse to circle the prescribed administration time on the drug record when a dose is missed.

Health Promotion and Maintenance

The nurse, in promoting or maintaining the client's health, identifies factors that may improve or diminish well-being. Health beliefs, personal motivations, socioeconomic factors, and habits (e.g., smoking) can influence the client's compliance with the medication regimen.

Teaching the client and family about the prescribed medications can promote adherence to the regimen and foster independence. Integrating the client's health beliefs and cultural practices into the treatment plan can assist the nurse in establishing a schedule or routine with the client. The nurse may make referrals to community resources if the client is unable to afford, or get out to obtain, necessary medications.

The nurse, as a care giver and client advocate, is also responsible for knowing about the medications and determining if they may adversely affect the client, especially if there are multiple prescriptions.

CLIENT AND FAMILY TEACHING. Unless a client is properly informed about drugs, he or she may take the drugs incorrectly or not at all. The nurse provides information about the purpose of medications and their actions and effects. Many health care institutions offer easy-to-read leaflets on specific types of drugs. A client must know how to take a drug properly and the effects if he or she fails to do so. For example, after receiving a prescription for an antibiotic, a client must understand the importance of taking the full prescription. Failure to do this can lead to a worsening of the condition, as well as the development of bacteria resistant to the drug.

Nurses teach proper self-administration of drugs to clients who depend on daily injections. The client learns to prepare and administer an injection correctly using aseptic technique. Family members or friends should be taught to give injections in case the client becomes ill or physically unable to handle a syringe. Nurses can provide specially designed equipment such as syringes with enlarged calibrated scales for easier reading or braille-labeled medication vials for clients with visual alterations.

Clients must be aware of the symptoms of drug side effects or toxicity. For example, clients taking anticoagulants learn to notify the physician immediately when signs of bleeding or bruising develop. Family members should be informed of drug side effects such as changes in behavior because they are often the first persons to recognize such effects. Clients are better able to cope with problems caused by drugs if they understand how and when to act. All clients should learn the basic guidelines for drug safety. These guidelines ensure the proper use and storage of drugs in the home (see box on p. 668).

MAINTAINING CLIENTS' RIGHTS. In accordance with the Patient's Bill of Rights (see Chapter 6) and because of the potential risks related to drug administration, a client has the right to:

1. Be informed of drug name, purpose, action, and potential undesired effects
2. Refuse a medication regardless of the consequences
3. Have qualified nurses or physicians assess a drug history, including allergies
4. Be properly advised of the experimental nature of drug therapy and to give written consent for its use

CLIENT TEACHING FOR DRUG SAFETY

Instruct the client to:
- Keep each drug in its original labeled container.
- Protect drugs from exposure to heat and light, as required.
- Check that labels are legible.
- Discard outdated medications.
- Always finish a prescribed drug unless otherwise instructed and never save a drug for future illnesses.
- Dispose of drugs in a sink or toilet and never place drugs in the trash within reach of children.
- Never give a family member a drug prescribed for another.
- Refrigerate drugs that require it.
- Read labels carefully and follow all instructions.
- Notify physician or practitioner of side effects.

5. Receive labeled medications safely without discomfort in accordance with the "five rights" of drug administration (see section on medication delivery)
6. Receive appropriate supportive therapy in relation to drug therapy
7. Not receive unnecessary medications

The nurse must be aware of these rights and handle all inquiries by clients and families courteously and professionally. A nurse should not become defensive if a client refuses drug therapy. The nurse must have the necessary knowledge and skill to satisfy the responsibilities of safe and effective drug administration.

Evaluative Measures

The nurse monitors a client's response to medications on an ongoing basis. This requires that the nurse know the therapeutic action and common side effects of each medication. A change in a client's condition can be physiologically related to health status or may result from medications or both. The nurse must be alert for reactions in a client taking several medications. The goal of safe and effective drug administration involves a careful evaluation of technique and the client's response to therapy and ability to assume responsibility for self-care.

To evaluate the effectiveness of nursing interventions when meeting established goals of care, the nurse uses evaluative measures to identify if client outcomes were met. The following are examples of goals, expected outcomes, and corresponding evaluative measures:

Goal: Client and family understand drug therapy.

Outcome

Client and family describe information about drug, dosage, schedule, purpose, and adverse effects

Evaluative measure

Have client write out medication schedule for a 24-hour period

Ask client to describe purpose, dosage, and adverse effects of each prescribed medication

Outcome

Client and family identify situations that require medical intervention

Evaluative measure

Have family describe what to do when a client has adverse effects from a medication

Outcome

Client and family demonstrate appropriate administration technique

Evaluative measure

Have client demonstrate filling of an insulin syringe and self-injection

Goal: Client gains therapeutic effect of prescribed medications without discomfort or complications.

Outcome

Client demonstrates physiological and psychological responses consistent with desired therapeutic effect of medication

Evaluative measure

Compare physical assessment findings before drug initiation (e.g., blood pressure, fever, pain) to same assessment findings after course of medication

Outcome

Client states positive response to prescribed medications

Evaluative measure

Ask client if symptom relief is noted

Goal: Client has no complications related to route of administration.

Outcome

Client swallows oral medications without difficulty

Evaluative measure

While administering oral medications, give a single tablet or capsule with full glass or water and observe client swallowing

Outcome

Client does not have localized or systemic reactions to parenteral administration

Evaluative measure

Observe injection site for evidence of bruises, inflammation, localized pain, or bleeding

Evaluative measure

Ask if client notes numbness or tingling at injection site

Goal: Client safely self-administers medications.

Outcome

Client follows prescribed treatment regimen

Evaluative measure

Have family keep log of client's compliance with therapy for 1 week

Outcome

Client performs techniques correctly

Evaluative measure

Observe client instill eye drops

Outcome

Client identifies available resources for obtaining necessary medication

Evaluative measure

Ask family to identify how to contact local pharmacy, community clinic, American Cancer Society for necessary medications

MEDICATION DELIVERY

Preparing and administering medications requires accuracy by the nurse, who must pay full attention to preparing medications and must not attempt to do other tasks simultaneously. The nurse uses five guidelines to ensure safe drug administration—the "five rights" of drug administration:

1. The *right* drug
2. The *right* dose
3. The *right* client
4. The *right* route
5. The *right* time

Right Drug

When drugs are first ordered, the nurse compares the medication recording form or computer orders with the physician's written orders. When administering drugs, the nurse compares the label of the drug container with the medication form. The nurse does this three times: (1) before removing the container from the drawer or shelf, (2) as the amount of drug ordered is removed from the container, and (3) before returning the container to storage. With unit-dose prepackaged drugs, the nurse checks the label with the medicine form a third time even though there is no permanent container. Unit-dose medications may be checked before opening at the client's bedside.

Nurses administer only the drugs they prepare. If an error occurs, the nurse who administers the drug is responsible for its effects. If a client questions the medication a nurse prepares, it is important not to ignore these concerns. An alert client will know whether a drug is different from those received before. In most cases the client's drug order has been changed; however, the client's questions might reveal an error. The nurse should withhold the drug until the preparation can be rechecked against the physician's orders.

Clients who self-administer drugs should keep them in their original labeled containers, separate from other drugs, to avoid confusion.

The nurse never prepares medications from unmarked containers or containers with illegible labels. If a client refuses a drug, the nurse should discard it rather than return it to the original container. Unit-dose packaged drugs can be saved if they are unopened.

Right Dose

The unit-dose system minimizes errors. When a drug must be prepared from a larger volume or strength than needed or when the physician orders a system of measurement different from what the pharmacist supplies, the chance of error increases. When performing drug calculations or conversions, the nurse should have another qualified nurse check the calculated doses.

After calculating dosages, the nurse prepares the drug using standard measurement devices. Graduated cups, syringes, and scaled droppers can be used to measure medications accurately. At home, clients should use kitchen measuring spoons rather than teaspoons and tablespoons, which vary in volume.

When it is necessary to break a scored tablet, the break should be even. A tablet may be cut in half by using a knife edge or by using a cutting device. Tablets that do not break evenly are discarded. The two halves are given in successive doses if the second half was repackaged and labeled.

Often a nurse prepares a tablet by crushing it so that it can be mixed in food. The crushing device should always be cleaned completely before the tablet is crushed. Remnants of previously crushed drugs may increase a drug's concentration or result in the client receiving a portion of an unprescribed drug. Crushed medications should be mixed with very small amounts of food or liquid. The client's favorite foods or liquids should not be used because a medication may alter their taste and decrease the client's desire for them.

Right Client

An important step in administering drugs safely is being sure the drug is given to the right client. It is difficult to remember every client's name and face. To identify a client correctly, the nurse checks the medicine card or form against the client's identification bracelet (Figure 26-6) and asks the client to state his or her name.

If an identification bracelet becomes smudged or illegible, or is missing, the nurse must acquire a new one for the client. When asking the client's name, the nurse should not merely speak the name and assume that the client's response indicates that he or she is the right per-

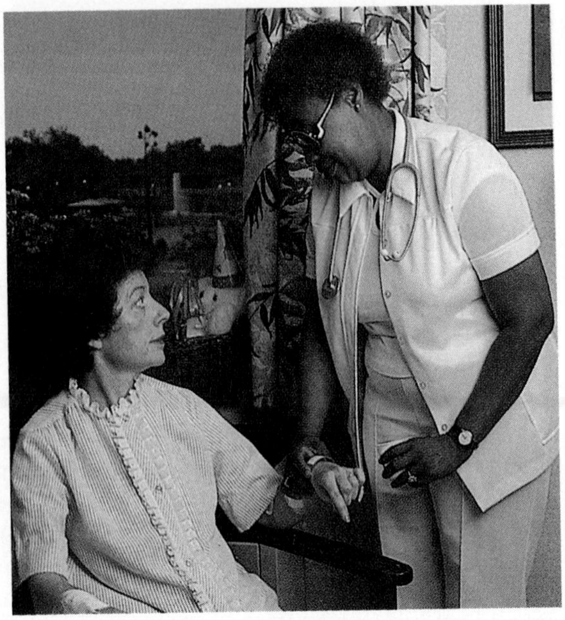

FIGURE 26-6 Before administering any medication, nurse checks client's identification bracelet to be sure right client receives drug.

son. Instead, the nurse asks the client to state his or her full name. To avoid making the client feel uneasy, the nurse simply states that the question is routine for giving a drug.

Clients who self-administer medications at home should be cautioned never to give a family member or friend one of their medications. A physician should be consulted before one person uses a prescription meant for another.

Right Route

If a physician's order does not designate a route of administration, the nurse consults the physician. Likewise, if the specified route is not the recommended route, the nurse should alert the physician immediately.

When the nurse administers injections, precautions are necessary to ensure that the drugs are given correctly. It is also important to prepare injections only from preparations designed for parenteral use. The injection of a liquid designed for oral use can produce local complications, such as a sterile abscess, or fatal systemic effects. Drug companies label parenteral drugs for "injectable use only."

Right Time

The nurse must know why a drug is ordered for certain times of the day and whether the time schedule can be altered. For example, two drugs are ordered, one q8h (every 8 hours) and the other t.i.d. (3 times a day). Both medications are to be given 3 times within a 24-hour period. The physician intends the q8h medication to be given around the clock to maintain therapeutic blood levels of the drug. In contrast, the t.i.d. medication is given during the waking hours. Each institution has a recommended time schedule for medications ordered at frequent intervals.

The physician often gives specific instructions about when to administer a medication. A preoperative medication to be given on call means that the nurse is to administer the drug when the operating room notifies the nursing division. A drug ordered pc (after meals) is to be given within half an hour after a meal when the client has a full stomach. A stat medication is to be given immediately.

Drugs that must act at certain times are given priority. For example, insulin should be given at a precise interval before a meal. All routinely ordered medications should be given within 30 minutes of the times ordered (30 minutes before or after the prescribed time).

Some drugs require the nurse's clinical judgment in determining the proper time for administration. A prn sleeping medication should be administered when the client is prepared for bed or at a time appropriate for maximum benefit. A nurse also uses judgment when administering prn analgesics. For example, the nurse may need to obtain a stat order from the physician if the client requires a drug before the prn interval has elapsed.

At home a client may have to take several medications throughout the day. The nurse helps to plan schedules based on preferred drug intervals and the client's daily schedule. For clients who have difficulty remembering when to take drugs, the nurse can make a chart that lists the times when each drug is to be taken or prepare a special container to hold each timed dose.

Avoiding Errors

Most medication errors occur when a nurse fails to follow routine procedures. Unfortunately, many medication errors are never identified (Table 26-6).

An error should be acknowledged immediately. After assessing the client's status, the nurse has the ethical and professional responsibility for reporting the error to the client's physician and the risk manager of the institution. Measures to counteract the effects of the error may be necessary. The nurse is also responsible for completing an incident report that describes the incident. The report is not an admission of guilt or the basis for punishment and is not a part of the client's legal medical record. The report provides an objective analysis of what went wrong and is a means of monitoring for the institution's risk management personnel. Without incident reports, nursing supervisory personnel have

table 26-6

WAYS TO PREVENT DRUG ADMINISTRATION ERRORS

Precaution	Rationale
Read drug labels carefully.	Many products come in similar containers, colors, and shapes.
Question administration of multiple tablets or vials for single dose.	Most doses are one or two tablets or capsules or one single-dose vial. Incorrect interpretation of order may result in excessively high dose.
Be aware of drugs with similar names.	Many drug names sound alike (e.g., digoxin and digitoxin, Keflex and Keflin, Orinase and Ornade).
Check decimal point.	Some drugs come in quantities that are multiples of one another (e.g., Coumadin in 2.5 and 25 mg tablets, Thorazine in 30 and 300 mg spansules).
Question abrupt and excessive increases in dosages.	Most dosages are made gradually so that physician can monitor therapeutic effect and response.
When a new or unfamiliar drug is ordered, consult resource.	If physician is also unfamiliar with drug, there is greater risk of inaccurate dosages being ordered.
Do not administer drug ordered by nickname or unofficial abbreviation.	Many physicians refer to commonly ordered medications by nicknames or unofficial abbreviations. If nurse or pharmacist is unfamiliar with name, wrong drug may be dispensed and administered.
Do not attempt to decipher illegible writing.	When in doubt, ask physician. Unless nurse questions order that is difficult to read, chance of misinterpretation is great.
Know clients with same last name. Also have clients state their full names. Check name bands carefully.	It is common to have two or more clients with same or similar last names. Special labels on Kardex or medication book can warn of potential problem.
Do not confuse equivalents.	When in hurry, it may be easy to misread equivalents (e.g., milligram instead of milliliter).

difficulty in identifying errors and solving recurrent problems.

Special Considerations for Age-Groups

A client's developmental level is a factor in the way nurses administer medications. Knowledge of a client's developmental needs helps the nurse to anticipate responses to drug therapy.

Infants and Children. Children vary in age, weight, surface area, and the ability to absorb, metabolize, and excrete medications. Children's drug dosages are lower than those of adults, so special caution is needed when preparing medications for them. Drugs are usually not prepared and packaged in standardized dose ranges for children. Preparing an ordered dosage from an available amount requires careful calculation.

A child's parents are valuable resources for learning the best way to give a child medications. Sometimes it is less traumatic for the child if a parent gives the drug and the nurse supervises.

All children require special psychological preparation before receiving medications. Supportive care is needed if a child is expected to cooperate. The nurse explains the procedure to a child, using short words and simple language appropriate to the child's level of comprehension. Long explanations may increase a child's anxiety, especially for painful procedures such as an injection. The nurse must approach a child with confidence and act as though the child is expected to cooperate (Whaley and Wong, 1991). If it is possible to involve the child, the nurse may have greater success giving a medication. For example, saying "It's time to take your tablet now. Do you want it with water or juice?" allows a child to make a choice. *Never* give the child the option of not taking a medication. After a drug is given, the nurse

TIPS FOR ADMINISTERING DRUGS TO CHILDREN

ORAL MEDICATIONS

Liquid forms are safer to swallow to avoid aspiration.

Offer juice, a soft drink, or frozen juice bar after a drug is swallowed.

Carbonated beverages poured over finely crushed ice reduce nausea.

When mixing drugs with palatable flavorings such as syrup or honey, use only a small amount. (The child may refuse to take all of a larger mixture. Avoid mixing the drug with food or liquids the child enjoys because the child may then refuse them.)

A plastic disposable syringe is the most accurate device for preparing liquid dosages. (Cups, teaspoons, and droppers are inaccurate.)

When administering liquid drugs, a spoon, plastic cup, or syringe (without needle) are useful.

INJECTIONS

Be very careful when selecting intramuscular injection sites. Infants and small children have underdeveloped muscles.

Children can be unpredictable and uncooperative. Have someone available to hold a child if needed.

Always awaken a sleeping child before giving an injection.

Distracting the child with conversation or a toy may reduce pain perception.

Give the injection quickly and do not fight with the child.

GERONTOLOGIC NURSING PRACTICE

- Position the client upright to reduce the chance of aspiration
- Allow time for assessment, explanation, and administration
- Provide ample fluid (as permitted) to assist the client in swallowing tablets or capsules
- Obtain liquid forms of medications if the client has difficulty swallowing
- Select an injection site that has sufficient tissue or muscle mass (e.g., ventrogluteal)
- Monitor intravenous (IV) infusions carefully to reduce the risk of fluid overload

praises the child and may even offer a simple reward such as a star or token. Depending on the route of administration, tips exist for effective drug administration for children (see box above).

Older Adults. Older adults also require special consideration during drug administration (see box, right). Age affects the absorption, distribution, metabolism, and excretion of drugs. In addition to physiological changes of aging, behavioral and economic factors influence an older person's use of drugs.

Noncompliance with drug therapy is the failure of clients to follow instructions regarding the use of medication, which is a problem more complicated than simply forgetting to take a medication. Noncompliance may involve failure to take a medication by choice, intentional reduction in drug dosage, failure to take a drug at the right time, increasing the frequency of dose, or prematurely discontinuing use of a drug. Older clients may also deny an illness and therefore choose not to take a medication.

Although noncompliance may occur in any age-group, it is a special problem for the older adult. An older person is more prone to suffer serious physical effects from a particular disease when medications are not taken. Simonson (1984) summarizes the following client-related factors that may relate to noncompliance with drug therapy in older adults:

1. Lack of understanding of drug therapy. Older clients can easily become confused when prescribed several medications.
2. Poor self-medication practices. Clients may consume more nonprescription drugs than needed. These drugs can interfere with the action of prescription drugs.
3. Lack of social supervision. Persons living alone are less likely to comply with prescribed drug therapy than those living with another person.
4. Feeling too ill or tired to take medication. These feelings may be complicated by an older person's difficulty with ambulating and adverse effects of certain drugs.
5. Sensory losses. Visual alterations make it difficult to read prescriptions. Hearing problems may alter the ability to understand oral instructions.
6. Keeping old prescriptions and self-dosing. These medications may be inappropriate or have little therapeutic effect.
7. Economic status. The high costs of certain medications are not affordable for many clients on a fixed income.

Compliance can be improved by offering clients simple, realistic plans for drug therapy. The least possible number of medications and regimens should be prescribed to complement daily habits (e.g., meals and bedtime). Eliopoulos (1992) makes the following recommendations for instructing and assisting the older adult with drug regimens:

1. Provide a detailed written and oral description to the client or care giver. Outline the drug's name,

GUIDELINES FOR GIVING DRUGS THROUGH A NASOGASTRIC TUBE, J-TUBE, G-TUBE, OR SMALL-BORE FEEDING TUBE

Determine the placement of the tube before administering any medications.
Administer medications in a liquid form (suspension, elixer, or solution) when possible to prevent tube obstruction.
Read medication labels carefully before crushing a tablet or opening a capsule.
Do *not* administer buccal, sublingual or enteric-coated tablets or sustained action medications through an enteral feeding tube.
Dissolve crushed tablets, powders, and soft gelatin capsules in warm water.
Irrigate the tube before and after each medication is given with 50 to 100 ml of water.
Avoid giving syrups or medications with a pH of less than 4.
Do not attempt to give whole or undissolved medications.

Modified from Petrosin BM, et al.: *Crit Care Nurs Q* 12:1, 1989.

schedule, route of administration, action, special precautions, incompatible foods or drugs, and adverse reactions.
2. Offer a color-coded schedule for persons who have visual deficits or are illiterate.
3. Be sure all medication labels are typed in large print.
4. Provide medicine containers with easy-to-remove caps for weak or arthritic hands.
5. Offer memory aids to remind clients of medication schedules (e.g., a partitioned plastic box containing prescribed doses for 1 week, labeled plastic baggies holding each timed dose, or a color-coded chart describing each drug and time to be taken).

ORAL ADMINISTRATION

The most desirable way to administer medications is by mouth (Procedure 26-1). For clients with nasogastric feeding tubes, liquid medications are preferred but some tablets can be crushed and capsules opened to mix in a solution for administration (see box above). Most tablets and capsules should be swallowed and administered with approximately 60 to 100 cc of fluid (as allowed).

When administering medications orally, the nurse must protect the client against possible aspiration. Positioning the client in a sitting or side-lying position will prevent liquid or solid medication from accumulating in the back of the throat. A client who swallows slowly should not be forced to take a large amount of liquid with each swallow. Such a client should take only one tablet or capsule at a time. If a client begins to cough while taking a medication, the nurse withholds the remaining portion of the drug until the client can breathe more easily. If the client has difficulty with swallowing tablets or capsules, other forms of the medication should be considered.

Some medications such as narcotic analgesics (e.g., Sublimaze) have been added to lollipops so they can be absorbed across the oral mucosa (Ashburn et al., 1989). The nurse should follow guidelines when administering oral medications (see box above).

ORAL ADMINISTRATION GUIDELINES

Always administer a drug with adequate fluid.
For clients with nasogastric feeding tubes, give a liquid form or crush tablets and mix with fluid.
Cola is effective in keeping tubes patent.
Never crush or break enteric-coated tablets.
Mix powdered drugs with liquids and administer immediately.
Administer effervescent powders and tablets immediately after dissolving in water or juice.
Never allow clients to chew or swallow lozenges.
Avoid giving fluids immediately after a client swallows a syrup. The syrup exerts local medicating effects on the oral mucosa.
Protect client against aspiration through positioning in sitting or side-lying position.
Protect client against aspiration by giving one tablet or capsule at a time.

PARENTERAL ADMINISTRATION

Administering an injection is an invasive procedure that must be performed using aseptic techniques (see box on p. 677). After a needle pierces the skin, there is risk of infection. Each type of injection requires certain skills to ensure that the drug reaches the proper location. The effects of a parenterally administered drug can develop rapidly, depending on the rate of drug absorption. The nurse closely observes the client's response.

Equipment

A variety of syringes and needles are available, each designed to deliver a certain volume of a drug to a specific

procedure 26-1

ADMINISTERING ORAL MEDICATIONS

Steps	Rationale
1. Assess for contraindications to client receiving oral medication: difficulty swallowing, nausea or vomiting, bowel inflammation or reduced peristalsis, recent gastrointestinal surgery, reduced or absent bowel sounds, gastric suction, decreased level of consciousness.	Factors may interfere with drug distribution, absorption or excretion, and client's ability to swallow.
2. Determine client's preferences and tolerances for fluids.	Offering fluids can increase fluid intake (unless contradicted by heart, lung, or renal diseases).
3. Prepare needed supplies and equipment:	
a. Medication record forms or printout	
b. Medication cart	
c. Disposable medication cups	
d. Glass of water, juice, or preferred liquid	
e. Drinking straw	
f. Pill crushing device	Crushes tablets for clients who have difficulty in swallowing.
g. Knife (optional)	Used to cut scored tablets.
h. Paper towels	
4. Check accuracy and completeness of each medication form or printout with physician's written medication order. Check client's name and drug name, dosage, route of administration, and time for administration. Report discrepancy in order to charge nurse or physician.	Physician's order is legal record of drugs client is to receive.
5. Prepare drug:	
a. Wash hands.	Reduces transfer of microorganisms.
b. Arrange medication cups in medicine room or move medication cart to position outside client's room.	Saves time and reduces error.
c. Unlock medicine drawer or cart (see illustration). (Narcotics are generally stored in double-locked box separate from medicine drawers or carts.)	Medications are safeguarded when locked in cabinet or cart.
d. Prepare medications for one client at a time. Keep medication forms for each client together.	Prevents preparation errors.
e. Select correct drug from stock supply or unit-dose drawer. Compare label of medication with medication form, or printout.	Reduces error.

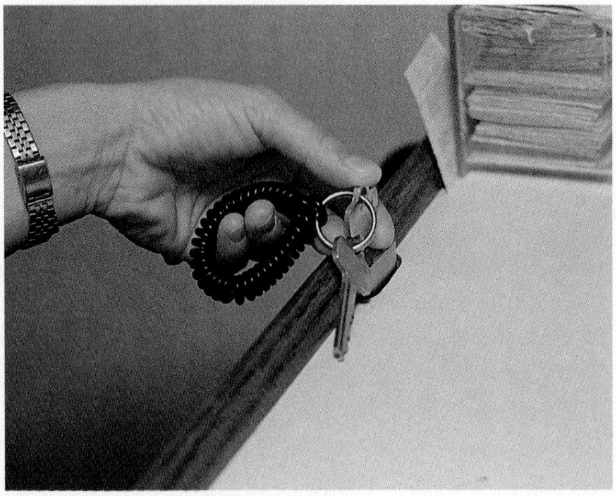

Step 5c

Steps	Rationale
f. Calculate correct drug dose. Take time. Double check calculation.	Calculation is more accurate when information from drug label is at hand.
g. To prepare tablet or capsules from bottle, pour required number into bottle cap and transfer to medication cup. Do not touch with fingers. Extra tablets or capsules may be returned to bottle.	Maintains cleanliness of drugs.
h. To prepare unit-dose tablets or capsules, place packaged tablet or capsule directly into medicine cup. (Do not remove wrapper.) (See illustration.)	Wrappers maintain cleanliness and identification of medications. Unopened medications may be returned to pharmacy if they are refused.
i. Place all tablets or capsules given at same time in one cup except for those requiring preadministration assessments (e.g, pulse rate or blood pressure).	Keeping medications requiring preadministration assessments separate makes it easier to withhold drugs as necessary.
j. If client has difficulty in swallowing, grind tablets in crushing device. Place tablet in device and crush. Continue to crush fragments until smooth powder remains. Alternative method is to place tablet between two medication cups and grind with blunt instrument. Again, continue to crush fragments until fine powder is achieved. Mix crushed tablet in small amount of soft food such as custard or applesauce. CAUTION: Do not crush enteric-coated or sustained-action medications.	Large tablets can be difficult to swallow. Ground tablet mixed with palatable soft food is usually easy to swallow. Verify that medication can be crushed before doing so; enteric-coated medications are not designed to be absorbed in stomach.
k. Prepare liquids:	
(1) Remove bottle cap from container, place cap upside down, and hold bottle with label against palm of hand while pouring.	Prevents contamination of inside of cap. Spilled liquid will not soil or fade label.
(2) Hold medication cup at eye level or place on counter and fill to desired level on scale (see illustration). (Scale should be even with fluid level at its surface or base of meniscus, not edges.)	Ensures accuracy of measurement.

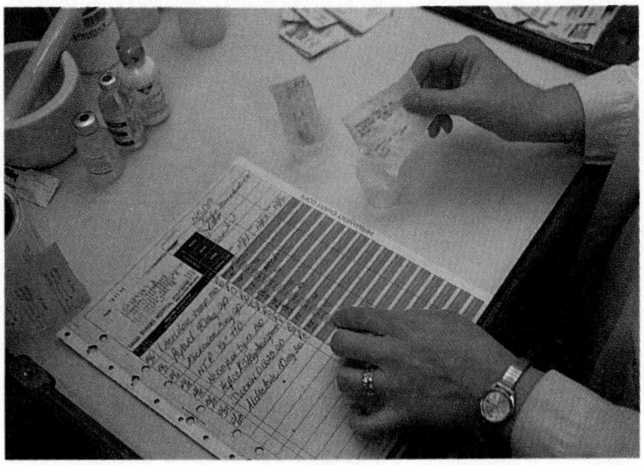
Step 5h

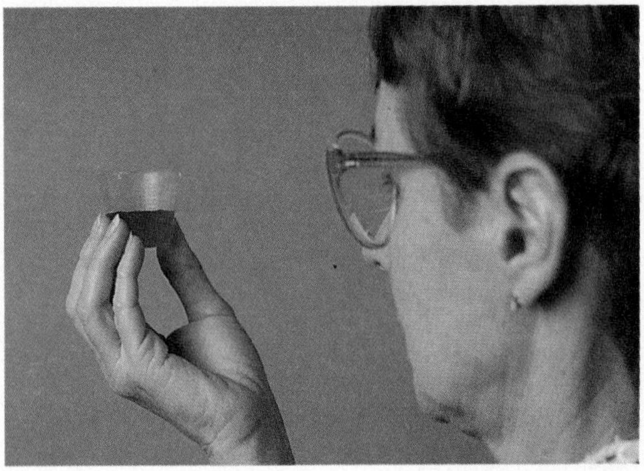
Step 5k

Continued.

procedure 26-1—cont'd

ADMINISTERING ORAL MEDICATIONS

Steps	Rationale
(3) Discard excess liquid in cup into sink. Wipe lip of bottle with paper towel.	Prevents contamination of bottle's contents and prevents bottle cap from sticking.
(4) Draw volumes of less than 10 ml in syringe (without needle). To prevent accidental injection during administration, never use needle to draw up oral medication.	Ensures accuracy of small volume.
l. When preparing narcotic, check narcotic record for previous drug count, compare with supply available, remove drug, and complete necessary information on narcotic form and sign.	Controlled substance laws require careful monitoring of dispensed narcotics.
m. Compare medication form or printout with prepared drug and container.	Reading label second time reduces error.
n. Return stock containers or unused unit-dose medications to shelf or drawer and read label again.	Third check of label reduces errors.
o. Place medications, forms, or printouts together on tray or cart.	Drugs are labeled at all times for identification.
p. Do not leave drugs unattended.	Nurse is responsible for safekeeping of drugs.
6. Administer medications:	
a. Take medications to client at correct time.	Medications are given within 30 minutes before or after prescribed time to ensure intended effect. Stat or single-order medications should be given at time ordered.
b. Identify client by comparing name on form or printout with name on client's identification bracelet. Ask client to state full name.	Identification bracelets are most reliable source of identification. Missing or faded bracelets are replaced to avoid errors.
c. Check label of unit-dose medications before opening.	Reduces error with unit-dose medications.
d. Perform necessary preadministration assessment for specific medications (e.g., blood pressure or pulse).	Assessment data determine whether specific medications should be given at that time.
e. Explain purpose of each medication and its action to client. Allow client to ask questions about drugs.	Client has right to be informed, and understanding of medication improves compliance with therapy.
f. Assist client to sitting or side-lying position.	Prevents aspiration during swallowing.
g. Administer drugs properly:	
(1) Ask if client wishes to hold solid medications in hand or cup before placing in mouth.	Client learns to know medications by seeing each drug.
(2) Offer full glass of water or juice with drugs to be swallowed.	Choice of fluid promotes comfort and can improve fluid intake.
(3) For sublingual administered drugs, have client place medication under tongue and allow it to dissolve completely. Caution client against swallowing.	Drug is absorbed through blood vessels of undersurface of tongue. If swallowed, drug is destroyed by gastric juices or rapidly detoxified by liver reducing therapeutic blood levels.
(4) Mix powdered medications with liquids at bedside and give to client to drink.	When prepared in advance, powdered drug forms may thicken and even harden, making swallowing difficult.
(5) Caution client against chewing or swallowing lozenges.	Drug acts through slow absorption through oral mucosa, not gastric mucosa.
(6) Give effervescent powders and tablets immediately after dissolving.	Effervescence helps improve unpleasant taste of drug.
h. If client is unable to hold medications, place medication cup to lips and gently introduce each drug into mouth, one at a time. Do no rush.	Prevents contamination of medications. Administering single tablet or capsule eases swallowing and prevents aspiration.

Steps	Rationale
i. If tablet or capsule falls to floor, discard it and repeat preparation.	Drug is contaminated when it touches floor.
j. Stay with client until each medication has been swallowed. If uncertain whether medication has been swallowed, ask client to open the mouth.	Nurse must ensure client receives ordered dosage. If left unattended, client may not take dose or may save drugs, causing risk to health.
k. For highly acidic medications (e.g., aspirin), offer nonfat snack (e.g., crackers).	Reduces gastric irritation.
l. Assist client in returning to comfortable position.	Maintains comfort.
m. Dispose of soiled supplies and wash hands.	Reduces transmission of microorganisms.
n. Return medication forms or printouts to appropriate file for next administration time.	Forms and printouts are used as reference for when next dose is due. Loss can lead to administration error.
o. Replenish stock such as cups and straws, return cart to medicine room, and clean work area.	Clean working space assists other staff in completing duties efficiently.
7. Record actual time that each drug was administered on medication record or computer. Include initials or signature (see Figure 26-5).	Prompt documentation prevents errors such as repeated doses. Signature establishes accountability for administration.
8. Return within 30 minutes to evaluate response to medications.	Used to assess drug's therapeutic benefit and detect onset of side effects or allergic reactions.

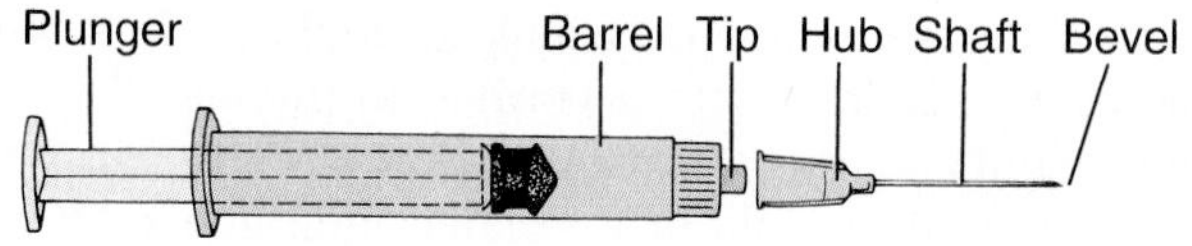

FIGURE 26-7 Parts of syringe and hypodermic needle.

PREVENTING INFECTION DURING AN INJECTION

To prevent contamination of solution, draw medication from an ampule quickly; do not allow ampule to stand open.

To prevent needle contamination, avoid letting needle touch contaminated surface (e.g., outer edges of ampule or vial, outer surface of needle cap, nurse's hands, countertop, or table surface).

To prevent syringe contamination, avoid touching length of plunger or inner part of barrel; keep tip of syringe covered with cap or needle.

To prepare skin, wash skin soiled with dirt, drainage, or feces with soap and water and dry. Use friction and a circular motion while cleaning with an antiseptic swab; swab from center of site and move outward in a 2-inch radius.

type of tissue. The nurse uses judgment when determining the syringe or needle that will be most effective.

Syringes. Syringes consist of a cylindrical barrel with a tip designed to fit the hub of a hypodermic needle and a close-fitting plunger (Figure 26-7). Most health care institutions use disposable, single-use plastic syringes, which are inexpensive and easy to manipulate.

The nurse fills a syringe by aspiration, pulling the plunger outward while the needle tip remains immersed in the prepared solution. The nurse may handle the outside of the syringe barrel and the handle of the plunger. To maintain sterility, the nurse avoids letting any unsterile object touch the tip or inside of the barrel, the shaft of the plunger, or the needle.

Syringes come in a number of sizes, from 0.5 to 60 ml (Figure 26-8). Larger syringes are used to prepare intravenous medications. A 1-ml syringe is appropriate for subcutaneous injections. A 3-ml syringe is usually adequate for intramuscular injections. Many hypodermic syringes come prepackaged with a needle attached. However, the nurse may change needle sizes. The hypodermic has two scales along the barrel; one is divided into minims and the other into tenths of a milliliter.

An insulin syringe holds 0.5 to 1 ml and is calibrated in units. Insulin syringes that hold 0.5 ml are known as low-dose syringes. Insulin syringes are U-100s, de-

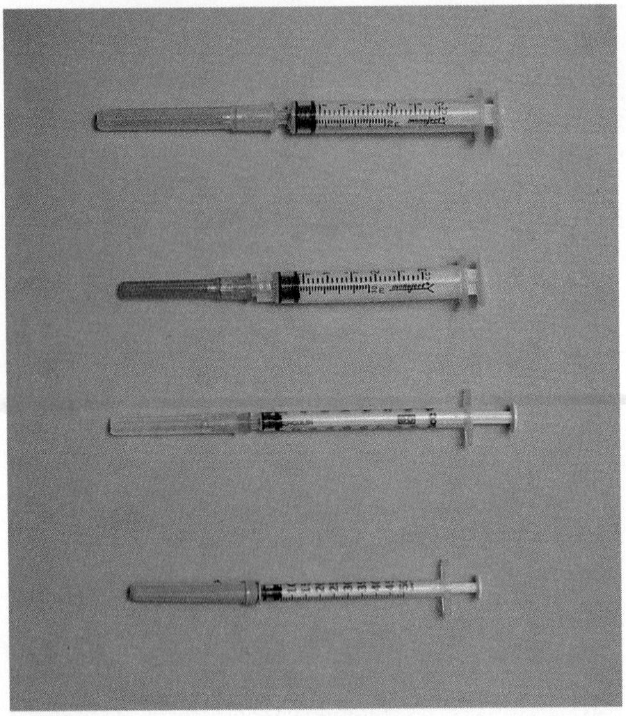

FIGURE 26-8 Types of syringes. *From top to bottom:* disposable 3-ml hypodermic syringe (intramuscular), 3-ml hypodermic syringe (subcutaneous), tuberculin syringe, and insulin syringe.

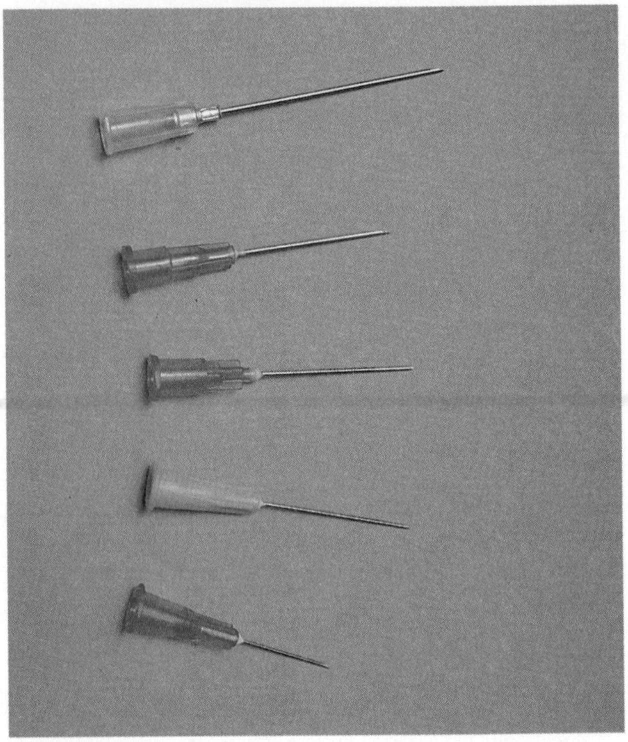

FIGURE 26-9 Hypodermic needles arranged in order of gauge. *Top to bottom:* 19-gauge, 20-gauge, 21-gauge, 23-gauge, and 25-gauge.

signed for use with U-100 strength insulin. Each milliliter of solution contains 100 units of insulin.

The tuberculin syringe has a long, thin barrel and may also come with a preattached needle. The syringe is calibrated in sixteenths of a minim and hundredths of a milliliter and has a capacity of 1 ml. The nurse uses a tuberculin syringe to prepare small amounts of potent drugs. A tuberculin syringe is also useful when preparing small precise doses for infants or young children. The nurse uses large syringes to administer certain intravenous drugs, add medications to intravenous solutions, and irrigate wounds or drainage tubes.

Needles. Needles come packaged in individual sheaths to allow flexibility in choosing the right needle for a client. Some needles are preattached to standard-sized syringes. Most needles are made of stainless steel and are disposable.

The needle has three parts: the hub, which fits onto the tip of a syringe; the shaft, which connects to the hub; and the bevel or slanted tip (see Figure 26-7). The nurse may handle the needle hub when securing a tight fit on the syringe. However, the shaft and bevel must remain sterile at all times.

Each needle has the following features: the slant of the bevel, the length of the shaft, and the needle gauge or diameter. Long bevels are sharper, which minimizes the discomfort caused by subcutaneous and intramuscular injections. Needles vary in length from 1/4 to 5 inches, although 1 1/2 inches is the most commonly used to give intramuscular injections to adults. The nurse chooses a needle length according to the client's size and weight and the type of tissue into which the drug is to be injected. A child or a slender adult generally requires a shorter needle. The nurse uses a longer needle (usually 1 to 1 1/2 inches) for intramuscular injections and a shorter needle (usually 3/8 to 5/8 inch) for subcutaneous injections.

The smaller the gauge, the larger the needle diameter (Figure 26-9). The selection of a gauge depends on the viscosity of the fluid to be injected or infused. An intramuscular injection usually requires a 19- to 23-gauge needle, depending on the viscosity of the medication. Subcutaneous injections require smaller-diameter needles such as a 25-gauge needle. A 26-gauge needle is used for an intradermal injection.

Disposable Injection Units. Disposable, single-dose, prefilled syringes are available for some medications. The nurse needs to check the dose and expel any unneeded portion of the drug.

The Tubex and Carpuject injection systems include reusable plastic or metal syringes that hold prefilled, disposable, sterile cartridge-needle units (Figure 26-10). The nurse slips the cartridge into the mechanism, secures it (per package directions), and checks for air bubbles. The nurse advances the plunger to obtain the

A

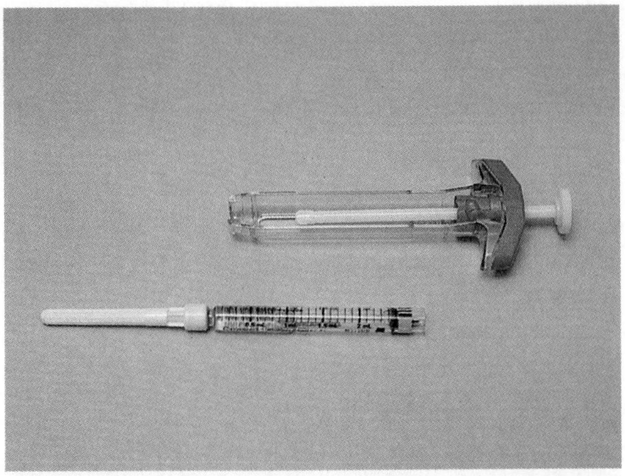

FIGURE 26-10 **A,** Carpuject syringe and prefilled sterile cartridge with needle. **B,** Assembling the Carpuject. **C,** Cartridge slides into syringe barrel, turns, and locks at needle end. Plunger then screws into cartridge end.

B

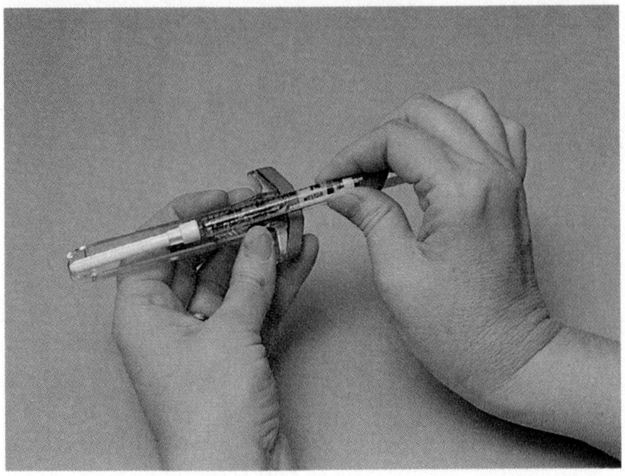

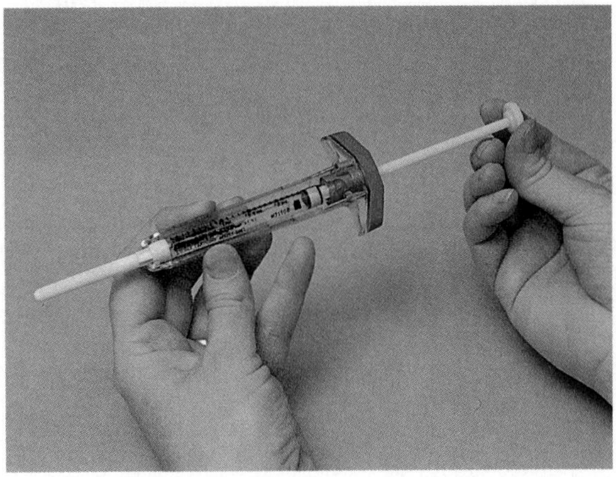

C

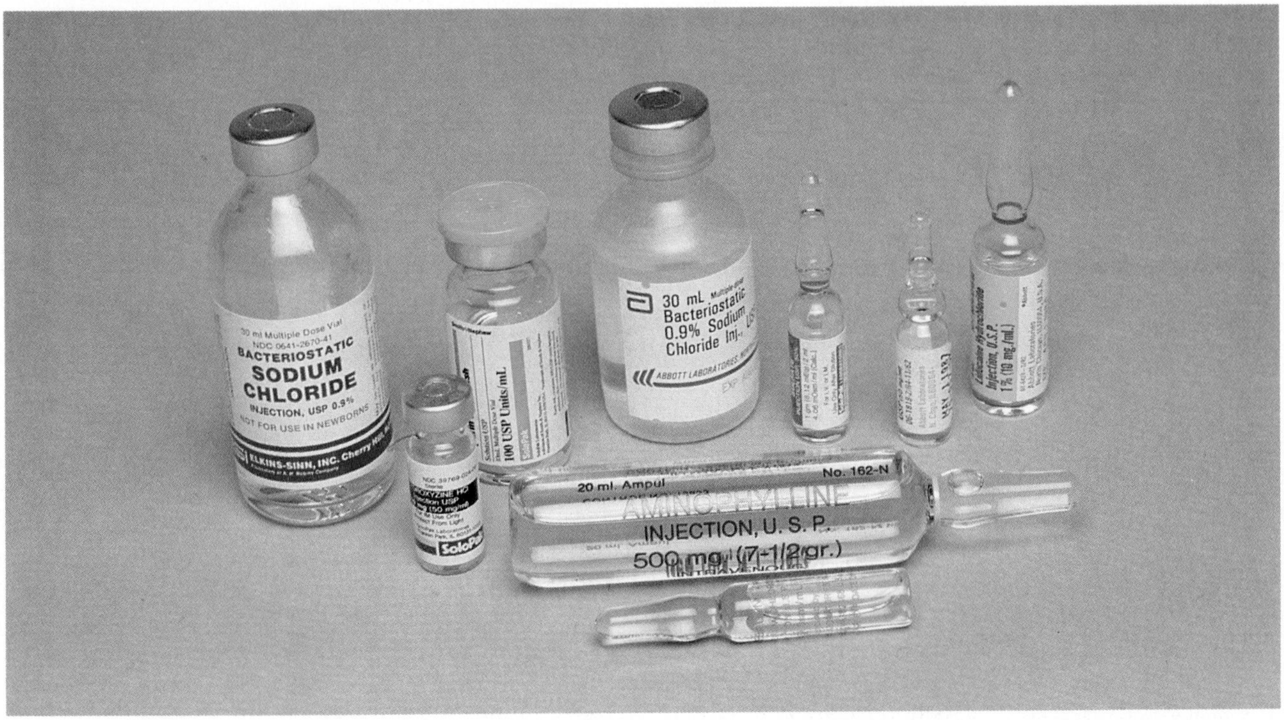

FIGURE 26-11 Variety of vials and ampules.

procedure 26-2

PREPARING INJECTIONS FROM AMPULES AND VIALS

Steps	Rationale
1. Wash hands.	Reduces transmission of infection.
2. Prepare needed equipment and supplies:	
a. Ampules:	
(1) Ampule containing medication	
(2) Syringe and needle	
(3) Small gauze pad or alcohol swab	
(4) Container for disposing of glass	
b. Vials:	
(1) Vial with medication	
(2) Syringe and needle	
(3) Alcohol swab	
(4) Diluent (e.g., normal saline or sterile water)	Used to dissolve drugs in dry form.
c. Medication forms or printouts	Verifies order.
3. Assemble supplies at work area.	Makes procedure orderly.
4. Check each medication form or computer printout against label on each ampule or vial.	Ensures that right drug and dosage are prepared.
5. Ampule preparation:	
a. Tap top of ampule lightly and quickly with finger until fluid leaves neck (see illustration).	Dislodges fluid that collects above neck. All solution moves into lower chamber.
b. Place small gauze pad or dry alcohol swab around neck of ampule.	Protects your fingers from trauma as glass tip is broken off.
c. Snap neck quickly and firmly away from hands (see illustration).	Prevents shattering glass toward or in your fingers or face.
d. Draw up medication quickly. Hold ampule upside down (see illustration) or set it on flat surface. Insert syringe needle into center of ampule opening. Do not allow needle tip or shaft to touch rim of ampule.	Broken rim of ampule is considered contaminated. As long as needle tip or shaft does not touch rim, solution does not dribble out.
e. Aspirate medication into syringe by gently pulling back on plunger (see illustration).	Withdrawal of plunger creates negative pressure within syringe barrel, which pulls fluid into syringe.
f. Keep needle tip below surface of liquid. Tip ampule to bring all fluid within reach of needle.	Prevents aspiration of air bubbles.

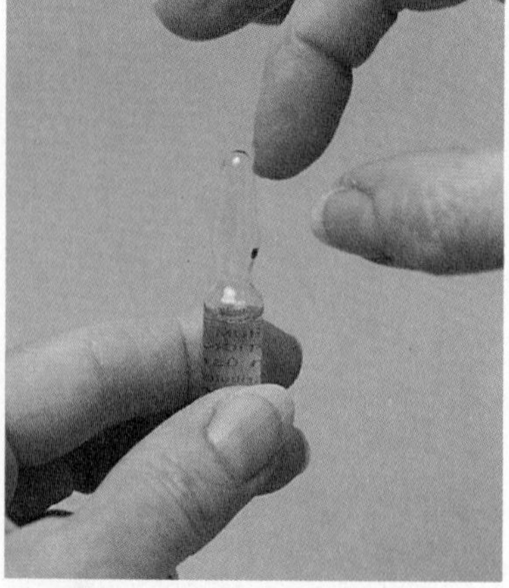
Step 5a

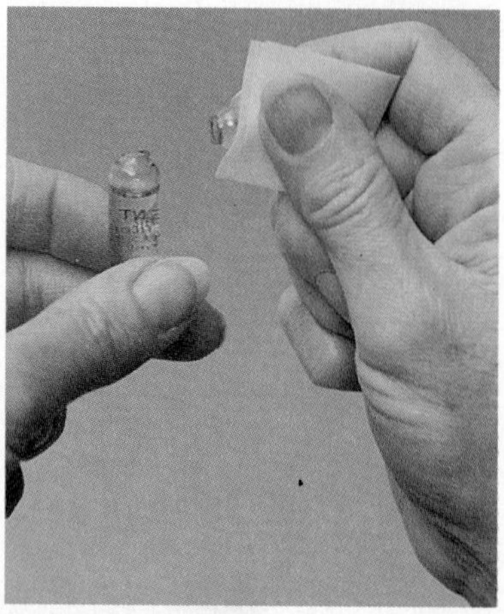
Step 5c

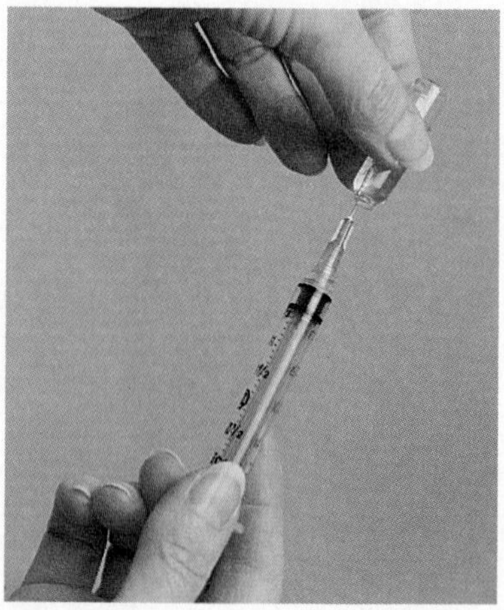
Step 5d

Steps	Rationale
g. If air bubbles are aspirated, do not expel air into ampule.	Air pressure may force fluid out of ampule, and medication will be lost.
h. To expel excess air bubbles, hold syringe with needle pointing up. Tap side of syringe to cause bubbles to rise toward needle. Draw back slightly on plunger, and push plunger upward to eject air. *Do not eject fluid.*	Withdrawing plunger too far will pull it from barrel. Holding syringe vertically allows fluid to settle in bottom of barrel. Pulling back on plunger allows fluid within needle to enter barrel so that fluid is not expelled. Air at top of barrel and within needle is then expelled.
i. If syringe contains excess fluid, use sink for disposal. Hold syringe vertically with needle tip up and slanted slightly toward sink. Slowly eject excess fluid into sink. Recheck fluid level in syringe by holding it vertically.	Medication is safely dispersed into sink. Position of needle allows medication to be expelled without flowing down needle shaft. Rechecking fluid level ensures proper dose.
j. Cover needle with sheath or cap. Change needle on syringe.	Prevents contamination of needle. Changing needle is required if you suspect that medication is on needle shaft. New needle prevents tracking medication through skin and SQ tissues.
k. Dispose of soiled supplies. Place broken ampule in special container for glass.	Controls transmission of infection. Proper disposal of glass prevents accidental injury to personnel.
6. Prepare injection from vial:	
a. Remove metal cap covering top of unused vial. Expose rubber seal.	Vial comes packaged with cap to prevent contamination of rubber seal.
b. Wipe off surface of rubber seal with alcohol swab, if vial had been previously opened.	Removes dust or grease but does not sterilize surface.
c. Take syringe and remove needle cap. Pull back on plunger to draw amount of air into syringe equivalent to volume of medication to be aspirated from vial (see illustration).	To prevent buildup of negative pressure in vial when aspirating medication, air must first be injected into vial.
d. Insert tip of needle, with bevel pointing up, through center of rubber seal (see illustration). Apply pressure to tip of needle during insertion.	Center of seal is thinner and easier to penetrate. Keeping bevel up and using firm pressure prevents cutting rubber core from seal
e. Inject air into vial, holding on to plunger.	Air must be injected to equalize pressure and assist in aspirating fluid. Plunger may be forced backward by air pressure within vial.

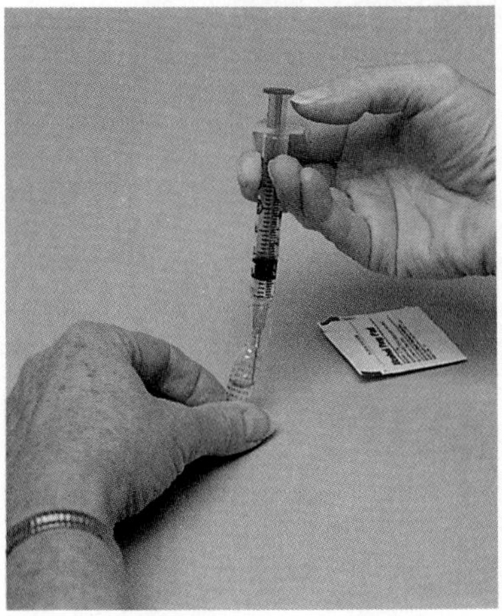
Step 5e

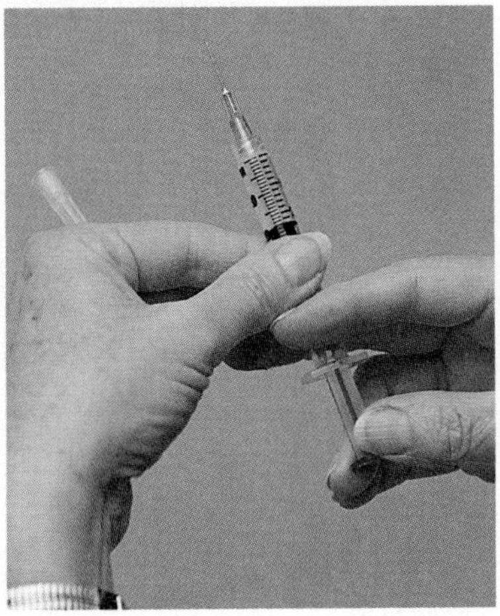
Step 6c

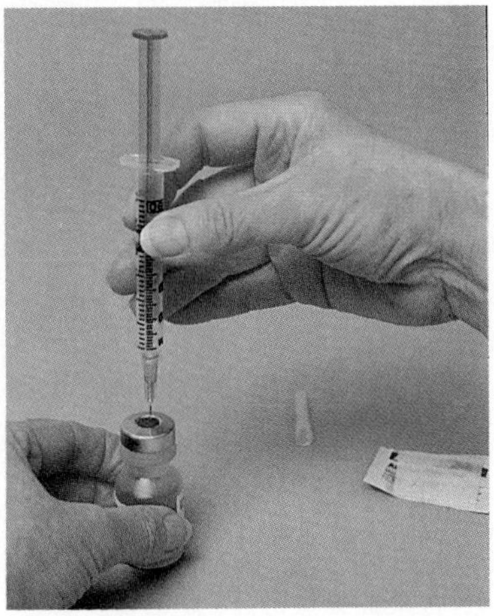
Step 6d

Continued.

procedure 26-2—cont'd

PREPARING INJECTIONS FROM AMPULES AND VIALS

Steps	Rationale
f. Invert vial while keeping firm hold on syringe and plunger. Hold vial between thumb and middle fingers of nondominant hand. Grasp end of syringe barrel and plunger with thumb and forefinger of dominant hand.	Inverting vial allows fluid to settle in lower half of container. Position of hands prevents movement of plunger and permits easy manipulation of syringe.
g. Keep tip of needle below fluid level.	Prevents aspiration of air.
h. Allow air pressure to fill syringe gradually with medication. Pull back slightly on plunger if necessary (see illustration).	Positive pressure within vial forces fluid into syringe.
i. Tap side of syringe barrel carefully to dislodge air bubbles. Eject air remaining at top of syringe into vial.	Forcefully striking barrel while needle is inserted in vial may bend needle. Accumulation of air displaces medication and causes errors.
j. After correct volume is obtained, remove needle from vial by pulling back on barrel of syringe.	Pulling plunger rather than barrel causes separation from barrel and loss of medication.
k. Remove remaining air from syringe by holding it and needle upright. Tap barrel to dislodge air bubbles (see illustration). Draw back slightly on plunger, and then push plunger upward to eject air. Do not eject fluid.	Holding syringe vertically allows fluid to settle in bottom of barrel. Pulling back on plunger allows fluid within needle to enter barrel so that fluid is not expelled. Air at top of barrel and within needle is then expelled.
l. Recap needle and change needle.	Inserting needle through rubber stopper may blunt bevel. New needle is sharper, and because no fluid is along shaft, it will not track medication through tissues.
m. For multidose vial, make label that includes date and time of mixing, concentration of drug per milliliter, and your initials.	Ensures that future doses will be prepared correctly. Certain drugs should be discarded after set number of days after mixing of vial.
n. Dispose of soiled supplies in proper containers.	
7. Clean work area. Wash hands.	Reduces transmission of microorganisms.
8. Check fluid level in syringe and compare with desired dose.	Ensures that accurate dose has been prepared.
9. Check medication form, etc. with label on ampule/vial.	Reduces errors.

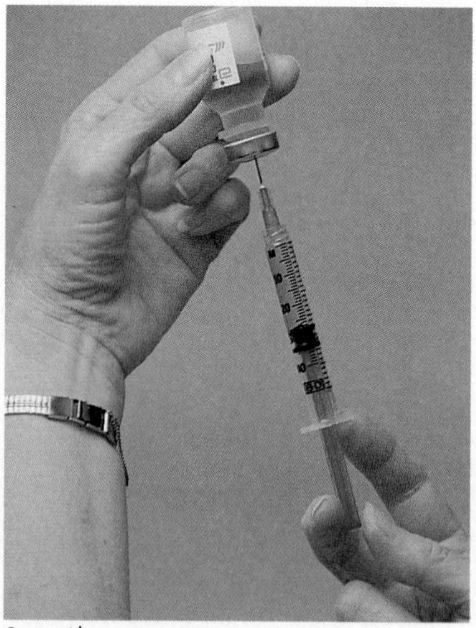

Step 6h

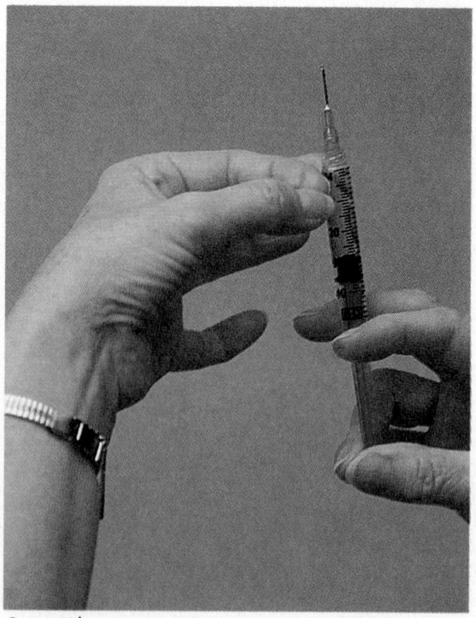

Step 6k

correct dosage and then to expel the medication, as in a regular syringe.

Needleless Devices. Approximately 800,000 accidental needle stick and sharps injuries occur annually in health care settings (Jagger, 1990). These injuries commonly occur when nurses forget and recap needles, mishandle intravenous lines and needles, or contact stray needles left at a client's bedside. The risk of exposure of health care workers to blood-borne pathogens has led to the development of "needleless devices" or special needle safety devices.

Special syringes are designed with a sheath or guard that covers the needle after it is withdrawn from the skin. The needle is immediately covered, eliminating the chance for a needle stick injury. The syringe and sheath are disposed of together in a receptacle. The CDC and OSHA have recommended use of "needleless" devices to reduce the risk to health care workers of needle sticks and sharps injuries (AJIC, 1993).

Intravenous catheters have been designed with blunt-edged cannulas, valves, or needle guards to minimize injuries during IV insertion or medication delivery. In addition, IV tubing with recessed and shielded needle connectors have been designed, further reducing needle sticks.

Preparing an Injection from an Ampule

Ampules contain single doses of medication in a liquid. Ampules are available in several sizes, from 1 ml to 10 ml or more (Figure 26-11). An ampule is made of glass with a constricted neck that must be snapped off to allow access to the medication. A colored ring around the neck indicates where the ampule is prescored to be broken easily. Aspiration of the drug into a syringe occurs easily (Procedure 26-2) and may be completed with a filter needle (if available).

Preparing an Injection from a Vial

A vial is a single-dose or multidose glass container with a rubber seal at the top (see Figure 26-11). A metal cap protects the seal until it is ready for use. Vials contain liquid or dry forms of medications. Drugs that are unstable in solution are packaged dry. The vial label specifies the solvent or diluent used to dissolve the drug and the amount of diluent needed to prepare a desired drug concentration. Normal saline and sterile distilled water are solutions commonly used to dissolve drugs.

Unlike the ampule, the vial is a closed system, and air must be injected into it to permit easy withdrawal of the solution. Failure to inject air when withdrawing creates a vacuum within the vial that makes withdrawal difficult (see Procedure 26-2).

To prepare a powdered drug, the nurse draws up the amount of diluent or solvent recommended on the vial's label. The nurse injects the diluent into the vial in the same manner as injecting air into the vial. Most powdered drugs dissolve easily, but it may be necessary to withdraw the needle to mix the contents thoroughly. Gently shaking or rolling the vial between the hands will dissolve the powdered drug. The needle is reinserted to draw up the dissolved medication. After mixing multidose vials the nurse makes a label that includes the date and time of mixing and the concentration of drug per milliliter. Multidose vials may require refrigeration after the contents are reconstituted.

Mixing Medications

If two drugs are compatible, it is possible to mix them in one injection. Most nursing units have charts that list common compatible drugs. If there is any uncertainty about drug compatibilities, consult a pharmacist.

Mixing Medications from Two Vials. The nurse follows these principles when mixing medications from two vials:

1. Do not contaminate one medication with another.
2. Ensure the final dosage is accurate.
3. Maintain aseptic technique.

Only one syringe is needed to mix medications from two vials (Figure 26-12). The nurse takes a syringe and aspirates the volume of air equivalent to the first drug's dose (vial A). The nurse injects the air into vial A, making sure the needle does not touch the solution. The nurse withdraws the needle, aspirates air equivalent to the second drug's dose (vial B), and then injects the volume of air into vial B. The nurse immediately withdraws the medication from vial B into the syringe. At this point the drug from vial A has not contaminated vial B. The nurse applies a new sterile needle to the syringe and inserts it into vial A, being careful not to push the plunger and expel the drug within the syringe into the vial. The nurse then withdraws the desired amount of drug from vial A into the syringe. If a vial has excess positive pressure, the plunger may move before the nurse is ready, causing an accidental withdrawal of too much of the drug. After withdrawing the necessary amount, the nurse withdraws the needle, applies a new needle, and sheathes the syringe.

Mixing Medications from One Vial and One Ampule. Mixing medications from a vial and an ampule is simple because it is not necessary to add air to withdraw medication from an ampule. The nurse prepares medication from the vial first and then, using the same syringe and needle, withdraws medication from the ampule. This technique prevents contamination of the solution in the vial and the needle.

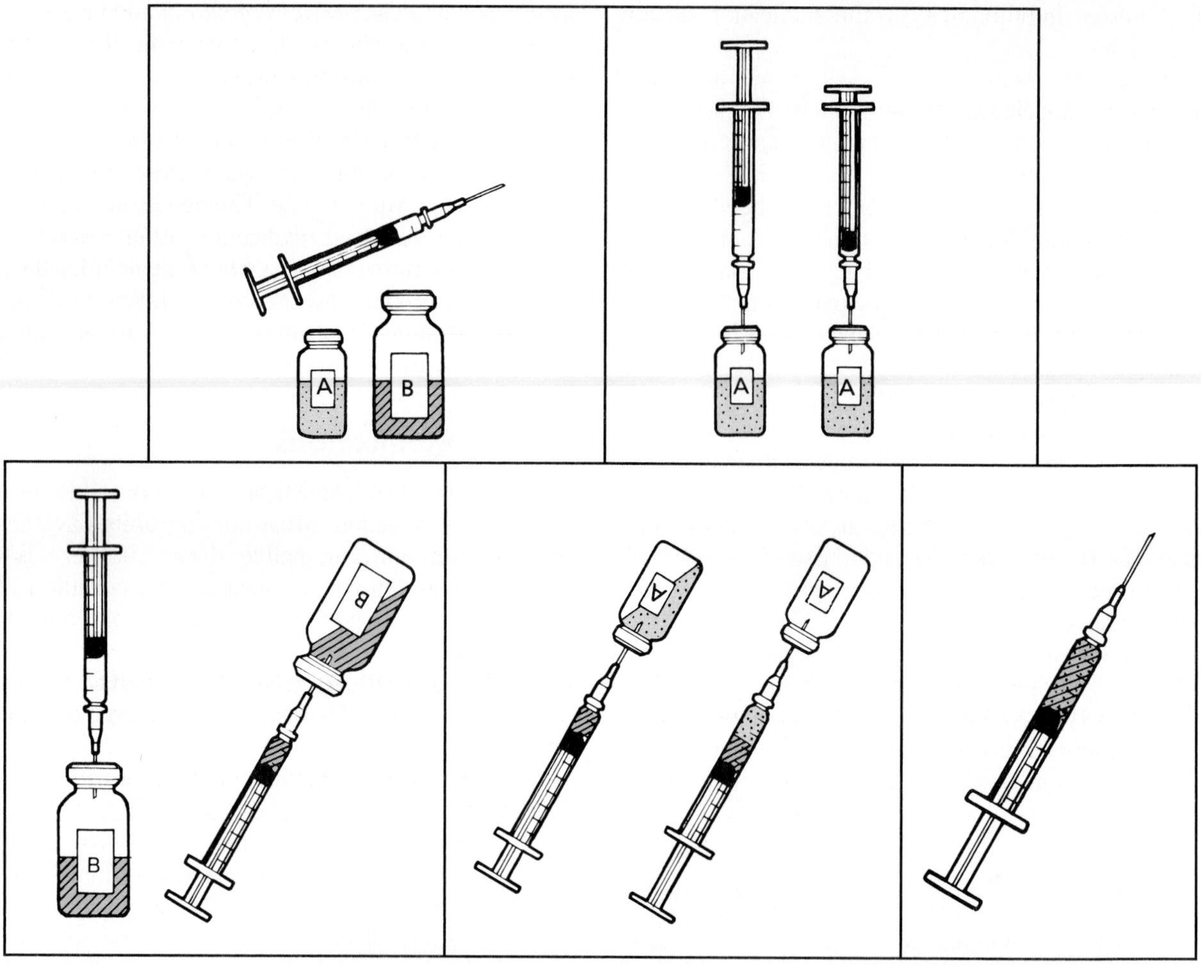

FIGURE 26-12 Steps in mixing single and multidose vials.

Insulin Preparation. Insulin is the hormone used to treat diabetes. It must be administered by injection because it is broken down and destroyed in the gastrointestinal tract. In the United States and Canada, the drug is available in 100 units per milliliter of solution. When preparing insulin, the correct syringe must be used; for example, a 100-unit scaled syringe is used to prepare 100-unit insulin.

Insulin is classified by rate of action, including rapid, intermediate, and long-acting. A client with diabetes may require more than one type of insulin. For example, by receiving a rapid-acting (Regular) and an intermediate-acting (NPH) insulin, a client receives more sustained control of blood sugar over 24 hours.

Regular unmodified insulin is a clear solution that acts rapidly and can be given either subcutaneously or intravenously. Other types of insulin are cloudy because of the addition of a protein, which slows absorption. These slower acting insulins can be given only subcutaneously.

Insulin is ordered by specific dosage at select times or by a sliding scale. A sliding scale dictates a certain dosage based on the client's blood sugar level. Only Regular insulin is used for sliding scales. Before mixing different types of insulin, each vial should be rotated at least 1 minute between both hands. This resuspends the modified insulin preparations and helps to warm the medication. The nurse should not shake insulin vials. Shaking causes bubbles to form, which take up space and alter the dosage. The following guidelines should be used for mixing two kinds of insulin in the same syringe:

1. Regular insulin can be mixed with any other type of insulin.
2. Insulin zinc suspensions (lente insulins) can be mixed with each other and with Regular insulin only.

To prepare insulin from two vials, the nurse or client follows these steps:

1. With an insulin syringe and needle, inject air, equal to the dose of insulin to be withdrawn, into the vial of modified insulin (cloudy vial). Do not touch the tip of needle to the solution.

2. Remove the syringe from the vial of modified insulin.
3. With the same syringe, inject air, equal to the dose of insulin to be withdrawn, into the vial of unmodified (Regular) insulin (clear vial). Then withdraw the correct dose.
4. Remove the syringe from the unmodified (Regular) insulin. Carefully remove air bubbles in the syringe to ensure correct dosage.
5. Return to the vial of modified insulin and withdraw the correct dose.
6. Administer mixture of insulins within 5 minutes of preparing it. Regular insulin binds with modified (NPH) insulin, thus reducing the action of the Regular insulin.

Always prepare the unmodified (Regular) insulin first. This prevents adding modified insulin to the unmodified (Regular) vial. If two modified forms are mixed, it makes no difference which vial is prepared first.

Administering Injections

Each injection route is unique in regard to the type of tissues into which the medication is injected. The characteristics of the tissues influence the rate of drug absorption and thus the onset of drug action. Before injecting a drug the nurse should know the volume of the drug to administer, the drug's characteristics, and the location of anatomical structures underlying injection sites (Procedure 26-3).

A nurse's inability to administer injections correctly can have negative consequences. Failure to select an injection site in relation to anatomical landmarks can result in nerve or bone damage during needle insertion. If the nurse fails to aspirate the syringe before injecting a drug, the drug may accidentally be injected directly into an artery or vein. Injecting too large a volume of medication for the site selected causes extreme pain and may result in local tissue damage.

Many clients, particularly children, fear injections. Clients with serious or chronic illness often are given several injections daily. The nurse may be able to minimize the client's discomfort in the following ways:

1. Using a sharp-beveled needle in the smallest suitable length and gauge
2. Positioning the client as comfortably as possible to reduce muscular tension
3. Selecting the proper injection site, using anatomical landmarks
4. Applying ice to the injection site to create local anesthesia before needle insertion
5. Diverting the client's attention from the injection through conversation
6. Inserting the needle quickly and smoothly to minimize tissue pulling
7. Holding the syringe steady while the needle remains in tissues
8. Injecting the medication slowly and steadily
9. Massaging the injected area gently for several seconds unless contraindicated

Subcutaneous Injections. Subcutaneous injections involve placing drugs into the loose connective tissue under the dermis (see Procedure 26-3). Because subcutaneous tissue is not as richly supplied with blood as the muscles, drug absorption is somewhat slower than with intramuscular injections. However, drugs are absorbed completely if the client's circulatory status is normal. Because subcutaneous tissue contains pain receptors, the client may experience some discomfort.

The best subcutaneous injection sites include the outer posterior aspect of the upper arms, the abdomen from below the costal margins to the iliac crests, and the anterior aspects of the thighs (Figure 26-13). The site most frequently recommended for heparin injections is the abdomen. Other sites include the scapular areas of the upper back and the upper ventral or dorsal gluteal areas. The injection site chosen should be free of skin lesions, bony prominences, and large underlying muscles or nerves. Clients with diabetes should practice intrasite rotation of insulin injections.

Use of the same part of the body for a sequence of injections provides more consistency in the absorption of

Text continued on p. 690.

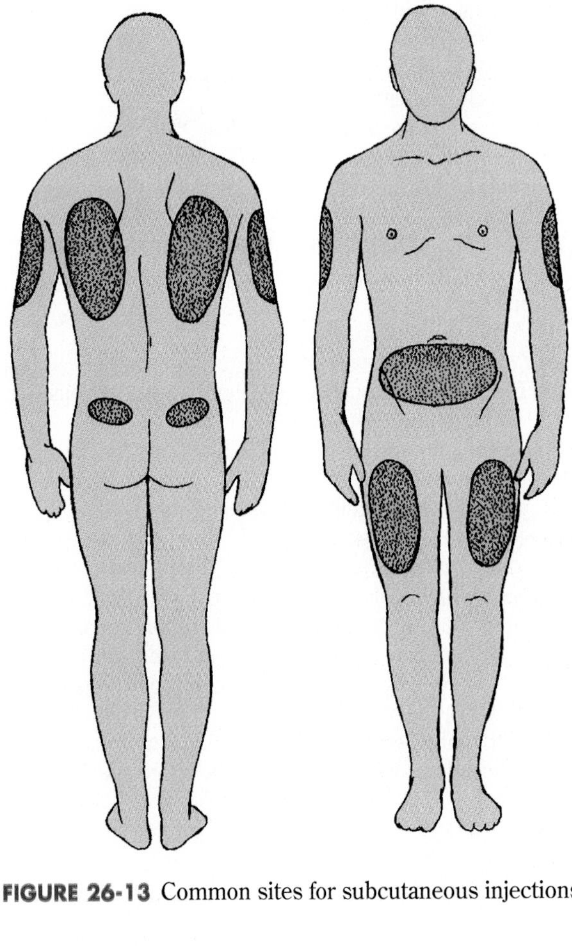

FIGURE 26-13 Common sites for subcutaneous injections.

procedure 26-3

ADMINISTERING INJECTIONS

Steps	Rationale
1. Assess indications for proper route for medication.	Ensures proper drug absorption and distribution through tissues to enhance drug action. Ensures proper route appropriate for client per physician orders.
2. Assess medical history and history of allergies.	Alerts nurse to any precautions to observe for during administration. History of allergies may cancel order for drug.
3. Observe verbal and nonverbal responses toward receiving injection.	Injections can be painful. Clients may have anxiety, which can increase pain.
4. Wash hands.	Reduces transmission of microorganisms.
5. Prepare needed equipment and supplies:	
a. Proper-size syringe:	Volume injected should be compatible with tissue type.
(1) SQ: 1 ml, 100 U insulin	
(2) IM: 2 to 5 ml for adult, 1 to 2 ml for child	
(3) ID: 1-ml tuberculin	
b. Proper-size needle:	Prevents client injury and ensures drug distribution.
(1) SQ: 25- to 27-gauge and 3/8 to 5/8 in in length	
(2) IM: 19- to 23-gauge and 1 to 1 1/2 in in length for adults, 25- to 27-gauge and 1/2 to 1 in in length for child and 5/8 in for newborn (Whaley, Wong, 1991)	
(3) ID: 26- to 27-gauge	
c. Antiseptic swab (Betadine or alcohol)	Used to cleanse skin.
d. Disposable gloves	
e. Medication ampule or vial	
f. Medication forms or printouts	Identifies medication dose ordered and client's name.
6. Check medication order.	Ensures accuracy.
7. Prepare correct medication dose from ampule or vial. (Procedure 26-2). Check carefully. Be sure all air is expelled. (For IM medications that are particularly irritating to tissues, draw 0.2 cc of air into syringe, being careful not to expel drug dose. See air-lock technique.	Ensures that medication is sterile. Preparation techniques differ for ampule and vial. Injection of a small volume of air clears the needle of medication and prevents tracking of the drug.
8. For IM injection, change needle if medication is irritating to SQ tissue.	Prevents tracking of irritating substance through tissues as needle passes into muscle.
9. Apply disposable gloves.	Injections could cause mild seepage of blood at injection site. Gloves reduce risk of exposure.
10. Identify client by checking identification armband and asking name.	Ensures that correct client is receiving prescribed medication.
11. Explain procedure to client and proceed in calm, confident manner.	Helps client anticipate actions. Calm approach minimizes anxiety.
12. Close room curtains or door.	Provides for privacy.
13. Keep sheet or gown draped over body parts not requiring exposure.	Proper selection of injection site may require exposure of body parts.
14. Select appropriate injection site. Inspect skin surface over sites for bruises, inflammation, or edema:	Injection sites should be free of abnormalities that may interfere with drug absorption. ID site should be clear so that results of skin test can be seen and interpreted correctly.
a. SQ: palpate sites for masses of tenderness.	
b. IM: note integrity and size of muscle and palpate for tenderness.	
c. ID: note lesions or discolorations of forearm.	
15. If injections are given frequently, rotate sites.	Site used repeatedly can become hardened from lipohypertrophy (increased growth in fatty tissue).

Steps	Rationale
16. Assist client to comfortable position:	
a. SQ: have client relax arm, leg, or abdomen, depending on site chosen.	Relaxation of site minimizes discomfort.
b. IM: have client lie flat, on side, or prone or have client sit, depending on site chosen.	Reduces strain on muscle and minimizes discomfort of injections.
c. ID: have client extend elbow and support it and forearm on flat surface.	Stabilizes site for easiest accessibility.
Talk with client about subject of interest.	Distraction reduces anxiety.
17. Relocate site using anatomical landmarks.	Accurate injection requires insertion in correct site to avoid injury to underlying tissues, blood vessels, nerves, or bone.
18. Cleanse site with antiseptic swab. Apply swab at center of site and rotate outward in circular direction for about 5 cm (2 in) (see illustration).	Mechanical action of swab removes secretions containing microorganisms.
19. Hold swab between third and fourth fingers of nondominant hand.	Swab remains readily accessible when needle is withdrawn.
20. Remove cap from needle by pulling it straight off.	Prevents contamination.
21. Hold syringe correctly between thumb and forefinger of dominant hand:	Quick, smooth injection requires proper manipulation of syringe parts.
a. SQ: hold as dart (see illustration)	
b. IM: hold as dart.	
c. ID: hold bevel of needle pointing up.	With bevel up, medication will more likely be deposited into the tissues below dermis.

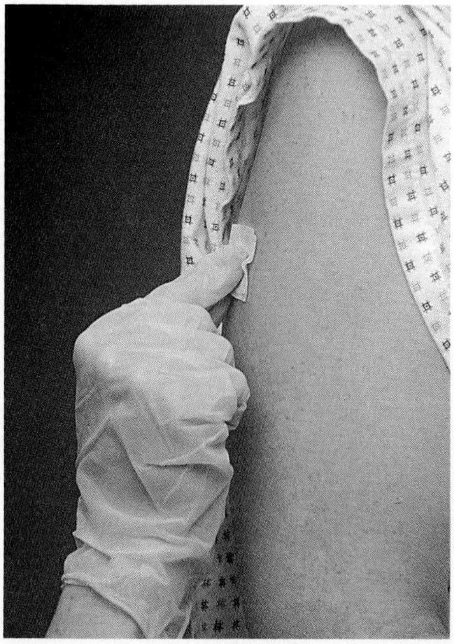

Step 18

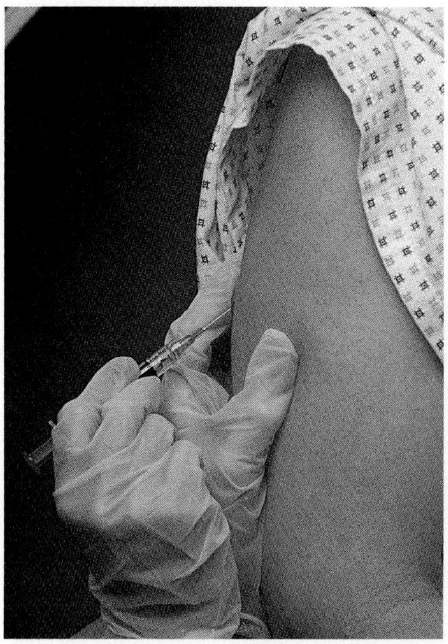

Step 21a

Continued.

procedure 26-3—cont'd

Steps	Rationale
22. Administer injection:	
a. SQ:	
(1) For average-size client, spread skin tightly across injection site or pinch skin with nondominant hand, depending on client assessment.	Needle penetrates tight skin easier than loose skin. Pinching skin elevates SQ tissue and may desensitize area.
(2) Inject needle quickly and firmly at 45- to 90-degree angle. (Then release skin, if pinched.)	Quick, firm insertion minimizes discomfort. (Injecting medication into compressed tissue irritates nerve fibers.)
(3) For obese client, pinch skin at site and inject needle below tissue fold.	Obese clients have fatty layer of tissue above SQ layer. Pinching skin elevates the SQ tissue for injection.
b. IM:	
(1) Position nondominant hand at proper anatomical landmarks and spread skin tightly. Inject needle quickly at 90-degree angle into muscle.	Speeds insertion and reduces discomfort.
(2) If client's muscle mass is small, grasp body of muscle between thumb and other fingers.	Ensures that medication reaches muscle mass.
(3) If medication is irritating, use Z-track method (see section on Z-track methods on p. 693).	Used to prevent tracking of drug through SQ tissue.
c. ID:	
(1) With nondominant hand, stretch skin over site with forefinger or thumb.	Needle pierces tight skin more easily.
(2) With needle almost against client's skin, insert it slowly at 5- to 15-degree angle until resistance is felt. Then advance needle through epidermis to approximately 3 mm (1/8 in) below surface. Needle tip can be seen through skin.	Ensures that needle tip is in dermis.

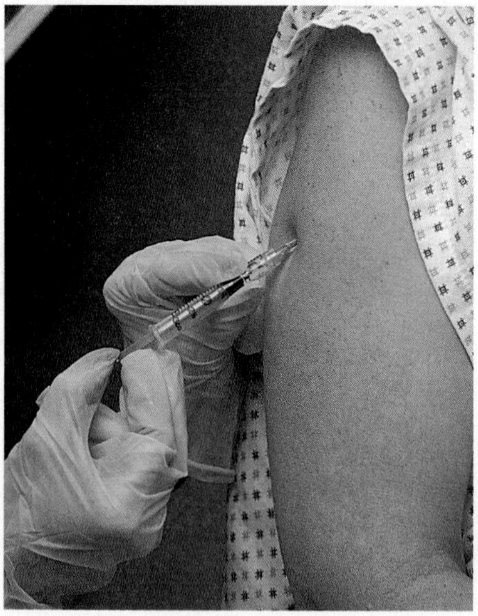

Step 23

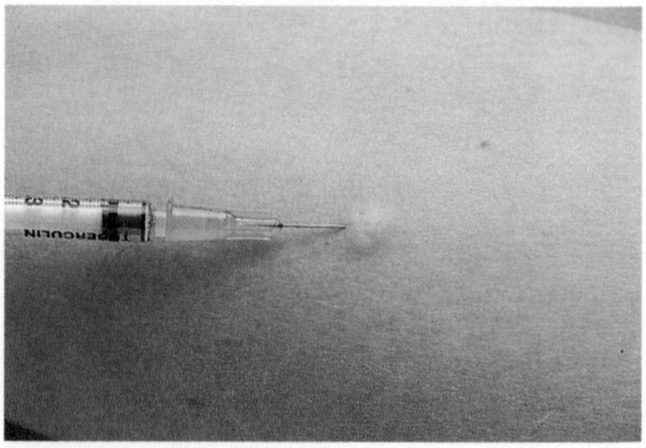

Step 25

Steps	Rationale
23. After needle enters site of SQ or IM injections *only,* grasp lower end of syringe barrel with nondominant hand. Move dominant hand to end of plunger. Avoid moving syringe while slowly pulling back on plunger to aspirate drug (see illustration). If blood appears in syringe, remove needle, discard medication and syringe and repeat procedure. (It is unnecessary to aspirate ID injection.) Do not aspirate when giving heparin by SQ route.	Properly performed injection requires smooth manipulation of syringe parts. Movement of syringe may displace needle and cause discomfort. Aspiration of blood into syringe indicates IV placement of needle. SQ and IM injections are not for IV use (dermis is relatively vascular). Aspiration of heparin injection may cause the needle to move, creating tissue damage and bleeding.
24. Inject medication slowly. (For ID injections, it is normal to feel resistance; if not, needle is too deep.)	Minimizes discomfort and trauma at site. (Dermal layer is tight and does not expand easily.)
25. During ID injection, note formation of small bleb on skin's surface (see illustration).	Indicates that medication is deposited into dermis.
26. Withdraw needle while applying alcohol swab gently above or over injection site.	Supports tissues around injection site to minimize discomfort during needle withdrawal.
27. For SQ or IM injections, massage skin lightly. Do not massage after SQ injection of heparin or insulin. OPTIONAL: Apply bandage. For ID injections, *do not massage site.*	Stimulates circulation and improves drug distribution. Massage of site after heparin injection may cause bleeding. Massage may increase absorption rate of insulin. Massage of ID site may disperse medication into underlying tissue layers and alter test results. (e.g., tuberculin test).
28. Assist client to comfortable position.	Gives client sense of well-being.
29. Discard an uncapped needle or needle enclosed in safety shield and attached syringe in appropriately labeled receptacle. When nurse is unable to leave client's bedside, a one-handed technique can be done to recap a needle (see p. 703).	CDC and OSHA mandate that needles not be re-capped for prevention of needle sticks and disease transmission.
30. Remove disposable gloves. Wash hands.	Reduces transmission of microorganisms.
31. For ID injection, draw circle around perimeter of injection site with skin pencil.	Site must be read at various intervals to determine test results. Pencil mark makes site easier to find.
32. For SQ and IM injections, chart medication dose, route, and site and time and date given in medication record. Correctly sign according to institutional policy.	Timely documentation prevents administration errors.
33. For ID injections, record area of injection, amount and type of testing substance, and date and time on medication record.	Timely documentation prevents administration errors and allows for follow-up assessment.
34. Return to room and ask if client feels acute pain, burning, numbness, or tingling at injection site. Observe for allergic reaction after ID injection.	Continued discomfort may indicate injury to underlying bones or nerves. Anaphylactic reaction may occur suddenly after ID injection because of drug's toxicity.
35. Return to evaluate response to medication in 10 to 30 min.	IM medications absorb quicker than SQ; undesired effects may also develop rapidly. Observations determine efficacy of drug action.

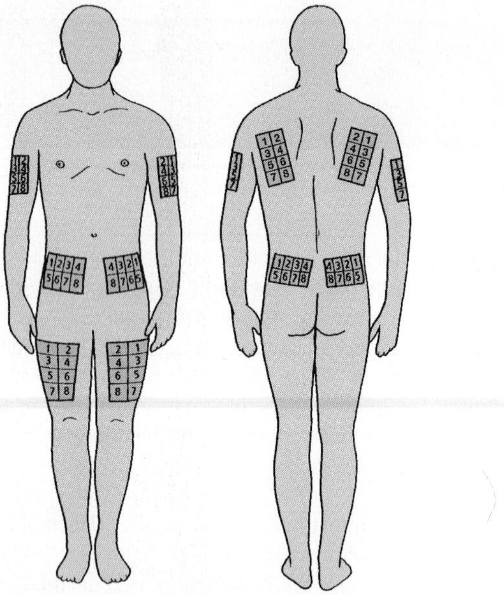

FIGURE 26-14 Subcutaneous injection sites for clients who rotate sites.

the insulin. For example, if the morning insulin is injected into the client's arm, then a subsequent injection should also be given in the arm. A box diagram (Figure 26-14) or clock pattern (e.g., 12 o'clock, 3 o'clock, etc.) may be used to plan for regular injections. With either method, the injections are to be given at least an inch away from the previous site. The client or nurse may mark the site used on a diagram (see Figure 26-14) or on the site itself with a small bandage. No injection site should be used again for at least 1 month.

Only small doses (0.5 to 1 ml) of water-soluble drugs should be given subcutaneously because the tissue is sensitive to irritating solutions and large volumes of drugs. Collection of drugs within the tissues can cause sterile abscesses, which appear as hardened, painful lumps under the skin.

A client's body weight indicates the depth of the subcutaneous layer. Therefore the nurse must choose the needle length and angle of insertion based on weight. Generally a 25-gauge ⅝-inch needle inserted at a 45-degree angle (Figure 26-15), or a ½-inch needle inserted at a 90-degree angle deposits drugs into the subcutaneous tissue of a normal-sized client. A child may require only a ½-inch needle. If the client is obese, the nurse often pinches the tissue and uses a needle long enough to insert through fatty tissue at the base of the skinfold. The preferred needle length is one-half the width of the skinfold. With this method the angle of insertion may be between 45 and 90 degrees. Thin clients may have insufficient tissue for subcutaneous injections. The upper abdomen is the best site for injection when a client has little peripheral tissue. It is important to rotate injection sites. Repeated use of the same site causes tissue sloughing and lesions that impair drug absorption.

Insulin syringes generally come with 26-29-gauge needles. To ensure the insulin reaches the subcutaneous tissue, the nurse follows this rule: if 2 inches of tissue can be grasped, the needle should be inserted at a 90-degree angle; if 1 inch of tissue can be grasped, the needle should be inserted at a 45-degree angle.

Clients with diabetes self-administer their insulin whenever possible. A new device, the insulin cartridge "pen" (Novalin) allows for clients to self-administer the injection when they cannot handle a syringe. With the "pen," clients dial up and inject the correct dosage easily.

Intramuscular Injections. The intramuscular route provides faster drug absorption than the subcutaneous

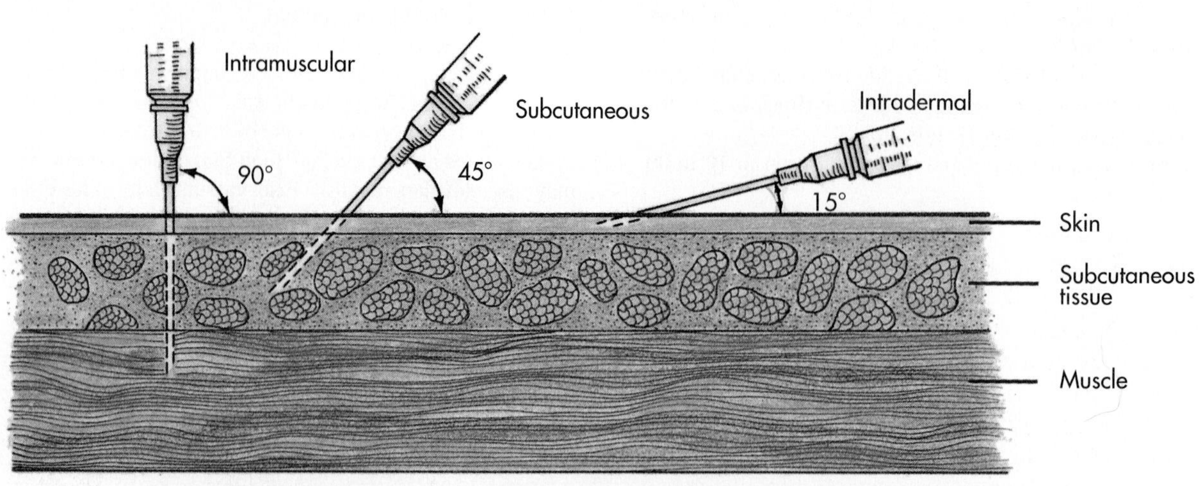

FIGURE 26-15 Comparison of angles of insertion for intramuscular (90 degrees), subcutaneous (45 degrees), and intradermal (15 degrees) injections.

because of muscle's greater vascularity. There is less danger of causing tissue damage when drugs enter deep muscle, but the risk of inadvertently injecting drugs directly into blood vessels exists. The nurse uses a longer and heavier-gauge needle to pass through subcutaneous tissue and penetrate deep muscle tissue (see Procedure 26-3). Weight and the amount of adipose tissue can influence needle size selection. For example, an obese client may require a needle 3 inches long, and a thin client may only require a 1/2- to 1-inch needle.

The angle of insertion for an intramuscular injection is 90 degrees (see Figure 26-15). Muscle is less sensitive to irritating and viscous drugs. A normal, well-developed client can tolerate 3 ml of medication into a larger muscle without severe muscle discomfort. A larger volume of medication is unlikely to be absorbed properly. Children, older adults, and thin clients can tolerate only 2 ml of an intramuscular injection. Whaley and Wong (1991) recommend giving no more than 1 ml to small children and older infants.

The nurse assesses the integrity of a muscle before giving an injection. The muscle should be free of tenderness. Repeated injections in the same muscle can cause severe discomfort. With the client relaxed, the nurse can palpate the muscle to rule out any hardened lesions. The nurse can minimize discomfort during an injection by helping the client assume a position that will help reduce muscle strain.

Sites. When selecting an intramuscular site, the nurse considers the following: Is the area free of infection or necrosis? Are there local areas of bruising or abrasions? What is the location of underlying bones, nerves, and major blood vessels? What volume of medication is to be administered? Each site has certain advantages and disadvantages (see box at right).

Vastus lateralis. The vastus lateralis muscle is a preferred injection site for adults, children, and infants. The muscle is located on the anterior lateral aspect of the thigh and extends in an adult from a handbreadth above the knee to a handbreath below the greater trochanter of the femur (Figure 26-16, *A* and *B*). The middle third of the muscle is the best site for injection. In width the site extends from the midline of the thigh's top to the midline of the thigh's outer side. See Figure 26-17 for children.

With young children or cachectic clients, it helps to grasp the body of the muscle during injection to be sure that the drug is deposited in muscle tissue. To help to relax the muscle, the nurse asks the client to lie flat with the knee slightly flexed or in a sitting position.

Ventrogluteal. The ventrogluteal muscle involves the gluteus medius and minimus. The nurse locates the muscle by placing the heel of the nondominant hand over the greater trochanter of the client's hip. The nurse points the thumb toward the client's groin and fingers toward the client's head, places the index finger over the

CHARACTERISTICS OF INTRAMUSCULAR SITES

VASTUS LATERALIS

Lacks major nerves and blood vessels
Rapid drug absorption

VENTROGLUTEAL

A deep site, situated away from major nerves and blood vessels
Less chance of contamination in incontinent clients or infants
Easily identified by any prominent bony landmark

DORSOGLUTEAL

Risk of striking underlying sciatic nerve, greater trochanter, or major blood vessels
Not used with children under 3 years of age
Never use when client is standing

DELTOID

Easily accessible but muscle not well developed in most clients
Used for small amounts of drugs
Not used in infants or children with underdeveloped muscles
Potential for injury to radial and ulnar nerves or brachial artery

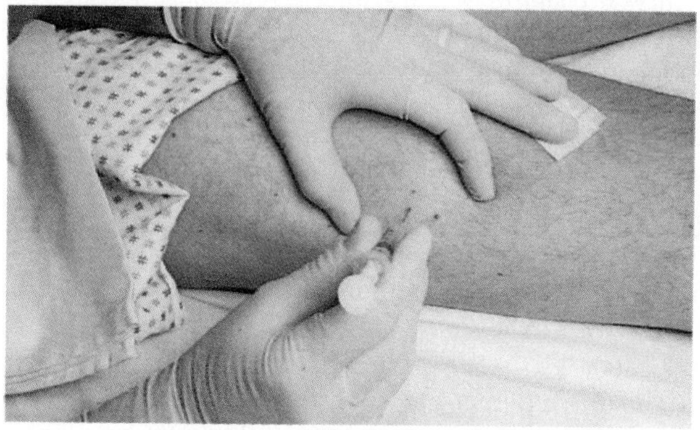

A

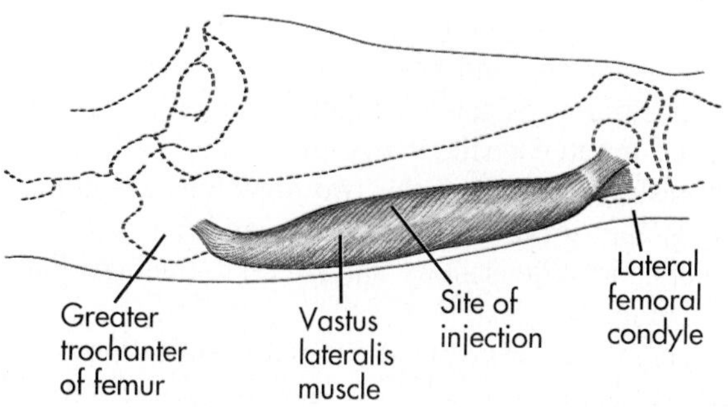

B

FIGURE 26-16 A, Injection site into vastus lateralis muscle. **B,** Anatomical view of site for intramuscular injection into vastus lateralis muscle.

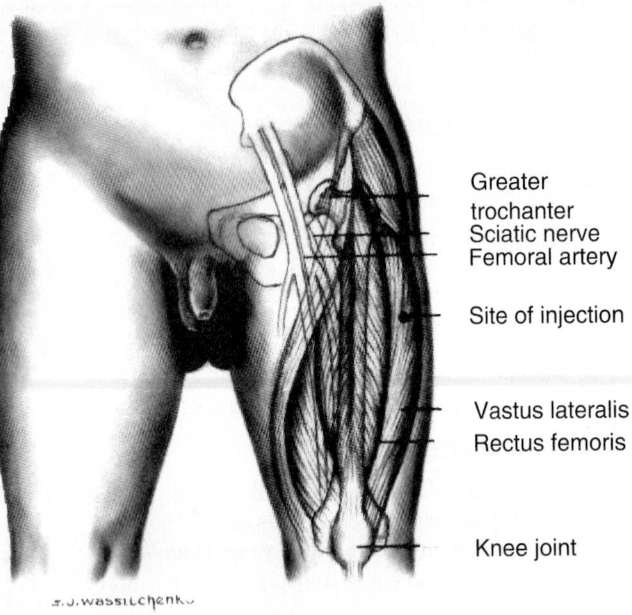

FIGURE 26-17 Acceptable IM site for children, the vastus lateralis muscle. (From Whaley LF, Wong DL: *Nursing care of infants and children,* ed 4, St. Louis, 1991, Mosby.

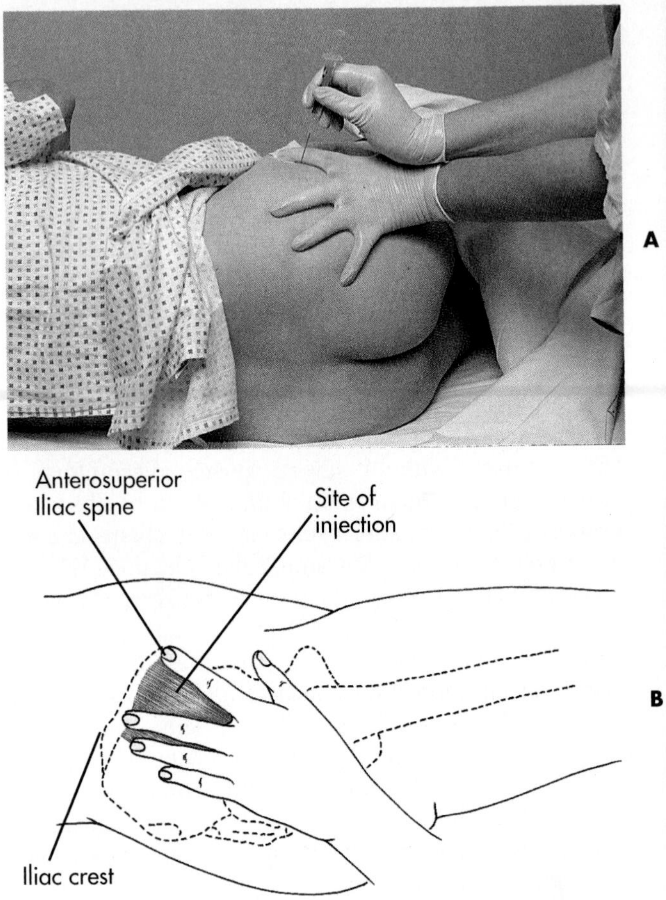

FIGURE 26-18 A, Injection site into ventrogluteal muscle avoids major nerves and blood vessels. **B,** Anatomical view of ventrogluteal muscle injection site.

anterior superior iliac spine, and extends the middle finger back along the iliac crest toward the buttock. The index finger, the middle finger, and the iliac crest form a V-shaped triangle, and the injection site is the center of the triangle (Figure 26-18, *A* and *B*). The client may lie on the side or back. Flexing of the knee and hip helps a person to relax.

Dorsogluteal. The dorsogluteal muscle has been a traditional site for intramuscular injections. However, accidental insertion of a needle into the sciatic nerve can cause permanent or partial paralysis of the involved leg. Major blood vessels and bone are also near the site. In clients with flabby, sagging tissues, this site is difficult to locate.

The dorsogluteal site is located in the upper outer aspect of the upper outer quadrant of the buttock, approximately 5 to 8 cm (2 to 3 inches) below the iliac crest. Clients may lie in the prone position with toes turned medially or in a side-lying position with the upper leg flexed at the hip and knee. To locate the dorsogluteal site, the nurse palpates the poster superior iliac spine and the greater trochanter of the femur. An imaginary line is drawn between the two anatomical landmarks. The sciatic nerve runs parallel to and below the line. The injection site is above and lateral to the line (Figure 26-19, *A* and *B*).

Nurses may use the dorsogluteal injection site in adults and children (at least 3 years of age) with well-developed gluteal muscles.

Deltoid. In some adults and most children the deltoid muscle is not well developed. The radial and ulnar nerves and brachial artery lie within the upper arm along the humerus. The nurse uses the deltoid site to administer small volumes of medication (usually no more than 2 ml) or when other injection sites are inaccessible because of dressings, casts, or other obstructions.

To locate the deltoid muscle the nurse has the client expose the upper arm and shoulder fully. A tight-fitting sleeve should not be rolled up. The nurse has the client relax the arm at the side and flex the elbow (Figure 26-20, *A*). The client may sit, stand, or lie down. The nurse palpates the lower edge of the acromion process, which forms the base of a triangle in line with the midpoint of the lateral aspect of the upper arm (Figure 26-20, *B*). The injection site is in the center of the triangle, about 2.5 to 5 cm (1 to 2 inches) below the acromion process. The nurse may also locate the site by placing four fingers across the deltoid muscle, with the top finger along the acromion process. The injection site is then 3 finger breadths below the acromion process.

Air lock technique. Intramuscular injections using the air lock technique are less irritating to subcutaneous tissues. When a small volume of air is injected behind a

A
B
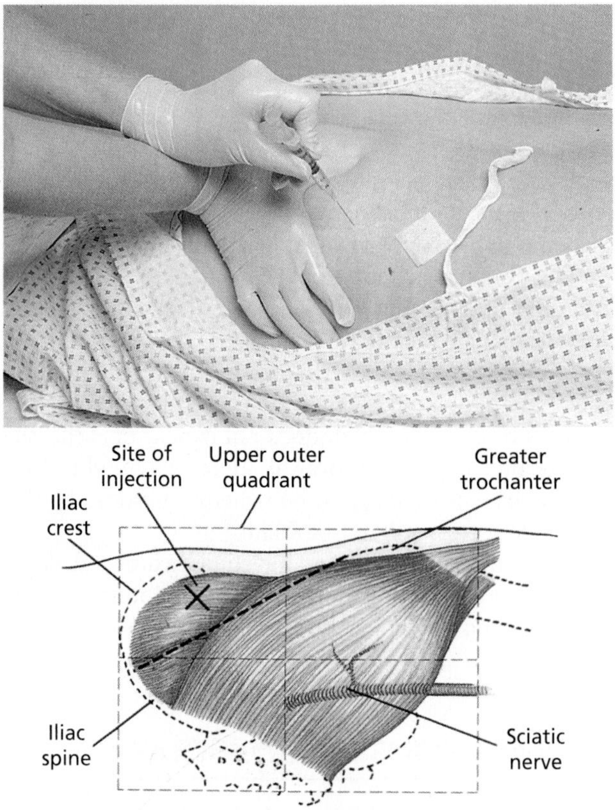

FIGURE 26-19 **A,** Site of injection into dorsogluteal muscle. **B,** Imaginary diagonal line extending from the posterosuperior iliac spine to the greater trochanter is the landmark for selecting the dorsogluteal injection site.

bolus of medication, the air clears the needle of medication, preventing tracking of the drug through subcutaneous tissues. This technique is recommended in the drug information insert of only a few medications. Examples include Inferon, Wyeth's vaccines prepared with aluminum adjuvant, diphtheria and tetanus toxoid, and the pertussis vaccine.

After preparing the proper dose, the nurse draws up 0.2 ml of air. The needle then must be injected downward at a 90-degree angle so that the air rises to the top of the drug toward the plunger. As the nurse injects the drug into the muscle, the air follows the medication, creating an air lock (Figure 26-21). If the nurse administers the drug with the needle at an angle less than 90 degrees, the air collects along the barrel of the syringe and enters the muscle too soon. Medication can then easily leak back into subcutaneous tissues.

Z-TRACK METHOD. The Z-track technique is recommended for administering intramuscular injections (especially drugs irritating to subcutaneous tissue). The technique reduces discomfort and tissue irritation by sealing the drug in muscle tissue (Keen, 1980; Taylor, 1992). However, it should not be used for clients with insufficient muscle mass, such as infants, children, or debilitated adults.

The nurse selects an intramuscular site, preferably in larger, deeper muscles such as the ventrogluteal muscle. It is important to apply a new needle to the syringe after preparing the drug so that no solution remains on the outside needle shaft. The nurse draws up 0.2 ml of

A
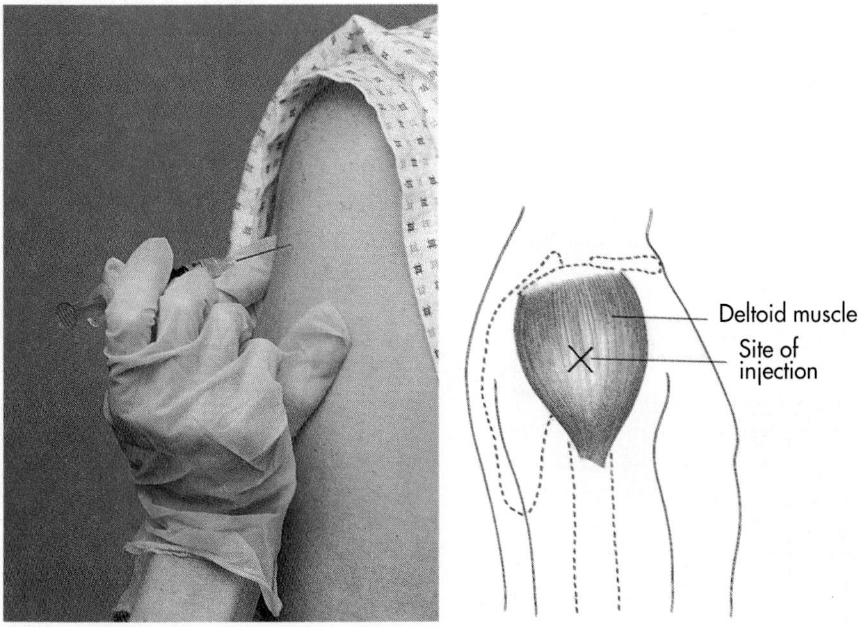

B

FIGURE 26-20 **A,** Site of intramuscular injection into deltoid muscle. **B,** Anatomical view of site of deltoid muscle injection below acromial process.

air to create an air lock. After preparing the site with an antiseptic swab, the nurse pulls the overlying skin and subcutaneous tissues approximately 2.5 to 3.5 cm (1 to $1^{1}/_{2}$ inches) laterally to the side. Holding the skin taut with the nondominant hand, the nurse injects the needle deep into the muscle. With practice the nurse learns to hold the syringe and aspirate with one hand. The nurse injects the drug and air slowly if there is no blood return on aspiration. The needle remains inserted for 10 seconds to allow the medication to disperse evenly. The nurse then releases the skin after withdrawing the needle. This leaves a zigzag path that seals the needle track where tissue planes slide across each other (Figure 26-22). The drug cannot escape from the muscle tissue.

Intradermal Injections. The nurse typically gives intradermal injections for skin testing (e.g., tuberculin screening and allergy tests). Because these drugs are potent, they are injected into the dermis, where blood supply is reduced and drug absorption occurs slowly. A client may have a severe anaphylactic reaction if the medications enter the circulation too rapidly.

Skin testing requires that the nurse be able to clearly see the injection sites for changes in color and tissue integrity. Intradermal sites should be lightly pigmented, free of lesions, and relatively hairless. The inner forearm and upper back are ideal locations.

The nurse uses a tuberculin or small hypodermic syringe for skin testing. The angle of insertion for an intradermal injection is 5 to 15 degrees (see Figure 26-15). As the nurse injects the drug, a small bleb resembling a mosquito bite should appear on the skin's surface (see Procedure 26-3). If a bleb does not appear or if the site bleeds after needle withdrawal, there is a good chance the medication entered subcutaneous tissues. In this case, test results will not be valid.

Data from an intradermal injection include a description of the precise location and time of administration. The injection site must be "read" within a prescribed time.

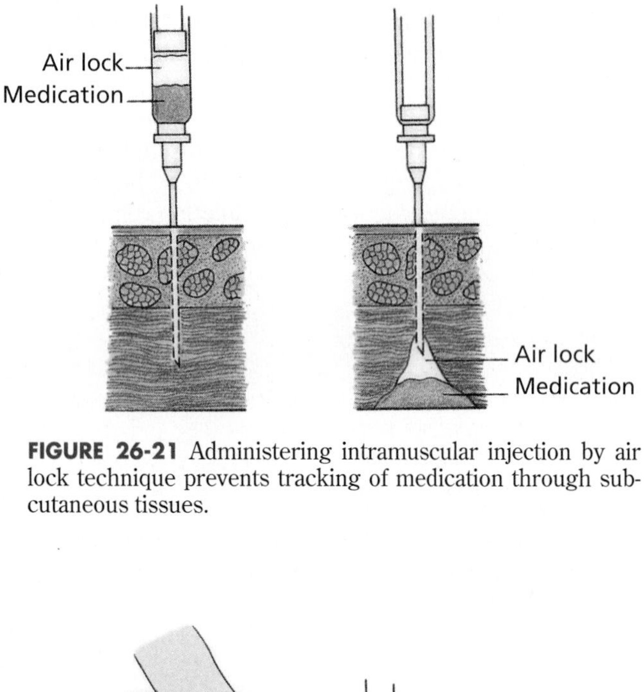

FIGURE 26-21 Administering intramuscular injection by air lock technique prevents tracking of medication through subcutaneous tissues.

INTRAVENOUS ADMINISTRATION

The nurse administers drugs intravenously by the following methods:

1. As mixtures within large volumes of IV fluids
2. By injection of a bolus or small volume of medication through an existing intravenous **infusion** line or intermittent venous access (heparin lock).
3. By "piggyback" infusion of a solution containing the prescribed drug and a small volume of IV fluid through an existing IV line.

In all three methods the client has either an existing IV infusion line or an IV access site such as an intermittent infusion (heparin lock). In most institutions, policies and procedures list persons who may give IV medications

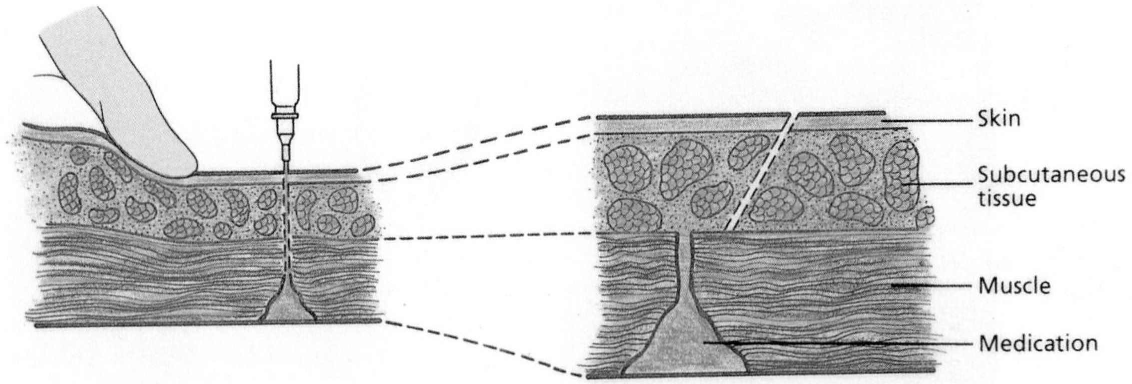

FIGURE 26-22 Z-track method of injection prevents deposit of medication into sensitive tissues.

HOW TO PLAY LOTTO GEORGIA

- Select 6 numbers per play by placing a heavy vertical mark in ea chosen number box. DO NOT use red ink. If you make a mistake, m the VOID box. DO NOT ERASE.
- If you would like the computer to randomly select your numbers, m the Quik Pik **(QP)** box at the bottom of each area that you wish to ha played.
- To play your numbers for more than one drawing at a time, mark appropriate box next to multi draw. This will play all your selection play panels "A" through "E" for that number of drawings. If you mak mistake mark the void box. Do not erase.
- **CASH OPTION** - If you match 6 of 6 numbers, all (or your portion if th are multiple winners) of the grand prize pool will be paid in 30 ann payments. If you prefer to receive all (or your portion if there are mult winners) of the **current cash value** of the grand prize pool, mark "Cash Option" box. This must be done **PRIOR** to submitting y playslip to the retailer.
- Review your playslip carefully before giving it to the retailer to purcha your valid ticket. A ticket may not be voided or canceled. **ALL SAL ARE FINAL**.
- You will receive a ticket from the On-Line Terminal which lists y chosen numbers and draw date(s). **You are responsible for check the draw date(s) and numbers before you leave the retaile ensure that they are the ones you selected.**

PRIZE CATEGORIES	**ODDS**
All 6 of 6 winning numbers	1 in 9,366,819
Any 5 of 6 winning numbers	1 in 39,028
Any 4 of 6 winning numbers	1 in 801
Any 3 of 6 winning numbers	1 in 47
Overall odds	1 in 45

All LOTTO Georgia prize payouts are calculated by a pari-mutuel form

HOW TO CLAIM YOUR PRIZE

- Sign the back of the ticket. Ticket is a bearer instrument until sign
- Present winning tickets of $599 or less to any On-Line Retailer validation and payment of prize. A winning ticket of greater than $5 may be claimed at any Georgia Lottery District Office claim cente mailed with a completed claim form to the Georgia Lottery, P.O. 56966, Atlanta, GA. 30343. Claim forms are available at all Geo Lottery retailer locations and district offices.
- Grand Prize Winners must claim at INFORUM Claims Center, Williams St., Atlanta, GA 30303.
- Winning tickets must be claimed within 180 days after the draw date the ticket.

LOTTO GEORGIA RULES

- All tickets, transactions and winners are subject to the rules rgia Lotter tion and applicable State L ssued is the only v

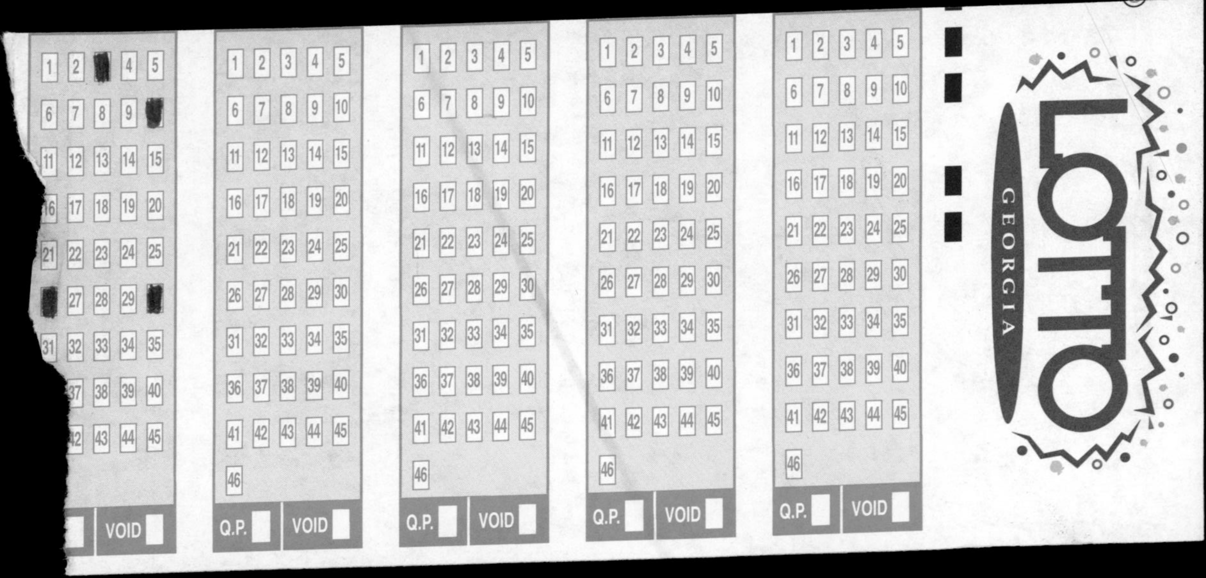

LOTTO
GEORGIA
Q.P.
VOID

and the situations in which they may be given. These policies are based on the drug, capability and availability of staff, and type of monitoring equipment available.

Chapter 35 describes the technique for performing venipuncture and establishing continuous IV fluid infusions. Medication administration is only one reason for supplying IV fluids. IV fluid therapy is used primarily for fluid replacement in clients unable to take oral fluids and as a means of supplying electrolytes and nutrients.

Despite the method of IV drug used, the nurse must observe clients closely for symptoms of adverse reactions. After a drug enters the bloodstream, it begins to act immediately, and there is no way to stop its action. Thus the nurse takes special care to avoid errors in dose calculation and preparation. The nurse should double-check the "five rights" of safe drug administration and know the desired action and side effects. If the drug has an antidote, it must be available during administration. When administering potent drugs, the nurse assesses vital signs before, during, and after infusion.

Administering drugs by the IV route has advantages. Often the nurse uses the IV route in emergencies when a fast-acting drug must be delivered quickly. The IV route is also best when it is necessary to establish constant therapeutic blood levels. Some medications are highly alkaline and irritating to muscle and subcutaneous tissue. These drugs cause less discomfort when given intravenously.

Large-Volume Infusions

Of the three methods of administering IV medications, mixing drugs in large volumes of fluids is the safest and easiest. Drugs are diluted in large volumes (500 ml or 1000 ml) of compatible IV fluids such as normal saline or lactated Ringer's solution. In most institutions the pharmacist adds drugs to the primary container of IV solution to ensure asepsis. Because the drug is not in a concentrated form, the risk of side effects or fatal reactions is minimal when infused over the prescribed time frame. Vitamins and potassium chloride are two types of drugs commonly added to IV fluids. However, there is a danger with continuous infusion; if the IV fluid is infused too rapidly, the client may suffer circulatory fluid overload (see Chapter 35 and Procedure 26-4).

Intravenous Bolus

An IV bolus involves introducing a concentrated dose of a drug directly into the systemic circulation (see box above). Because a bolus requires only a small amount of fluid to deliver the drug, it is an advantage when the amount of fluid the client can take is restricted. The IV bolus is the most dangerous method for administering drugs because there is no time to correct errors. In addition, a bolus may cause direct irritation to the lining of blood vessels. Before administering a bolus the nurse confirms placement of the IV line. This involves obtaining a blood return through the IV catheter or needle. The inability to obtain a blood return suggests that the needle or catheter is in the client's tissues or resting against the vein wall. A drug should never be given intravenously if the insertion site appears puffy or edematous or the IV fluid cannot flow at the proper rate. Accidental injection of a medication into the tissues around a vein can cause pain, sloughing of tissues, and abscesses, depending on the drug's composition.

GUIDELINES FOR GIVING MEDICATIONS BY IV BOLUS

- Check physician's order for type of medication to be administered, dosage, and route.
- Wash hands and apply gloves.
- Prepare ordered medication. Carefully read package directions for proper dilution of medication.
- Carefully check client's identification by looking at armband and asking name.
- Assess intravenous insertion site for signs of infiltration or phlebitis. If present, do not give medication; restart IV line or intermittent venous access (Chapter 35) in another site.
- Use small-gauge needles (21- or 25-gauge) to insert through IV tubing ports.
- Start IV push through intravenous lock:
  - Clean off injection port with antiseptic swab.
  - Aspirate for blood return.
  - Clear lock with 1 ml saline. (A central venous port may require 5 to 10 ml saline.)
  - Administer medication.
  - Clear lock with 1 ml saline.
  - Inject heparin 10 units/ml (may be omitted depending on institution's policy).
- Start IV push through existing line:
  - Select injection port closest to client.
  - Clean off injection port with antiseptic swab.
  - Occlude intravenous line by pinching tubing just above injection port.
  - Gently aspirate for blood return and inject medication.
- Administer medication over specified time recommended. (Check manufacturer's directions.) Use a watch to time administration.
- Dispose of gloves and wash hands.
- Observe client closely for adverse reactions as the drug is administered and for several minutes thereafter.
- Dispose of uncapped needles or needle enclosed in safety shield and attached syringes in proper container.
- Record drug, dosage, route, time administered, and length of time medication given on medication form. Note adverse reactions.

procedure 26-4

ADDING MEDICATIONS TO IV FLUID CONTAINERS

Steps	Rationale
1. Check physician's order for type of IV solution, medication, and dose.	Overall physical condition determines type of solution to use. Ensures safe and accurate drug administration.
2. When more than one medication is to be added to solution, assess for drug compatibility. Check the compatibility of the drug with the IV fluid.	Certain drugs are incompatible when mixed. May result in clouding or crystallization of fluids or cause drug interaction that is not visible.
3. Prepare equipment and supplies:	
a. Vial or ampule of prescribed medication	
b. Syringe of appropriate size (5 to 20 ml)	
c. Sterile needle (1 to 1½ in, 19- to 21-gauge) with special filters (optional)	Larger needle gauge ensures easy aspiration of drugs from vial or ampule. Filter prevents particles from entering syringe and thus avoids transfer to fluid container.
d. Correct diluent (e.g., sterile water or normal saline)	Certain IV medications are prepared in dry powder form. Solvent must be added for mixing.
e. Sterile IV fluid container (bag or bottle, 500 to 1000 ml in volume)	Solution bags are kept sterile by being stored in separate intact plastic bag. Bottles have plastic or metal seal over bottle cap.
f. Alcohol or antiseptic swab	
g. Label to attach to IV bag or bottle	Continuously infusing medication must be labeled properly for all nurses to observe.
4. Wash hands thoroughly.	Reduces transfer of microorganisms when handling sterile equipment.
5. Assemble supplies in medication room.	Ensures that procedure will be orderly with less likelihood of contaminating supplies.
6. Prepare prescribed medication from vial or ampule (Procedure 26-2). (If filter needle is used, replace it with regular needle before injecting medication into IV fluid container.)	Different techniques are used for each type of container.
7. Identify client by reading identification band and asking name.	Ensures that correct client receives ordered medication.
8. Prepare client by explaining that medication is to be given through existing IV line or one to be started. Explain that no discomfort should be felt during infusion. Encourage client to report symptoms of discomfort.	Allows client to understand procedure and minimizes anxiety. Most IV medications will not cause discomfort when diluted. However, potassium chloride can be irritating. Pain at insertion site may be early indication of infiltration.
9. Add medication to new container:	
a. Locate medication injection port on IV solution bag:	
(1) Remove plastic cover over port. Port has small rubber stopper at end. Do not select port for IV tubing insertion or air vent.	Medication injection port is self-sealing to prevent introduction of microorganisms after repeated use.
b. Locate injection site on IV solution bottle:	
(1) Remove metal or plastic cap and rubber disk. Place cap upside down on counter top.	Cap seals bottle to maintain sterility. Inside of cap may remain sterile for reuse.
(2) Locate medication injection site on bottle's rubber stopper. Site is usually marked by X, circle, or triangle.	Accidental injection of medication through main tubing port or air vent can alter pressure within bottle and cause fluid leaks through air vent.
c. Wipe off port or injection site with alcohol or antiseptic swab (see illustration).	Reduces risk of introducing microorganisms into bag during needle insertion.
d. Remove needle cap from syringe and insert needle of syringe through center of injection port or site, and inject medication (see illustration).	Injection of needle into sides of port may produce leak and lead to fluid contamination.

Steps	Rationale
e. Withdraw syringe from bag or bottle.	
f. Mix medication and IV solution by holding bag or bottle and turning it gently end to end.	Allows medication to be distributed evenly.
g. Complete medication label with name and dose of medication, date, time, and your initials. Stick it upside down on bottle or bag (see illustration).	Label can be easily read during infusion of solution. Informs nurses and physicians of contents of bag or bottle.
h. Spike bag or bottle with IV tubing and hang (see Chapter 35). Regulate infusion at ordered rate.	Prevents rapid infusion of fluid.
10. Add medication to existing container:	
a. Prepare vented IV bottle or plastic bag:	
(1) Check volume of solution remaining in bottle.	Proper volume is needed to dilute medication adequately.
(2) Verify dilution of medication desired (amount of medication per milliliter).	
(3) Close off IV infusion clamp.	Prevents medication from directly entering circulation as it is injected into bag or bottle.
(4) Wipe medication port with alcohol or antiseptic swab.	Mechanically removes microorganisms that could enter container during needle insertion.
(5) Lower bag or bottle from IV pole. Insert syringe needle through injection port and inject medication.	Injection port is self-sealing and prevents fluid leaks.

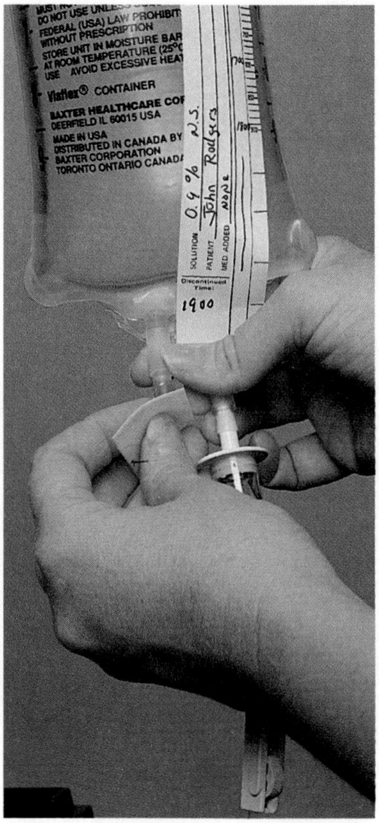

Step 9c

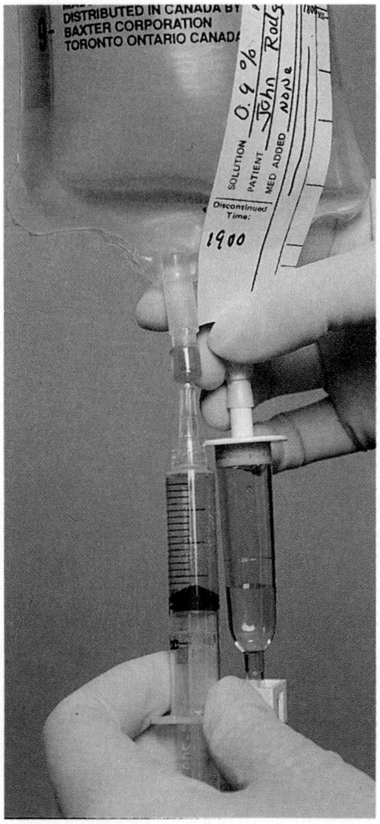

Step 9d

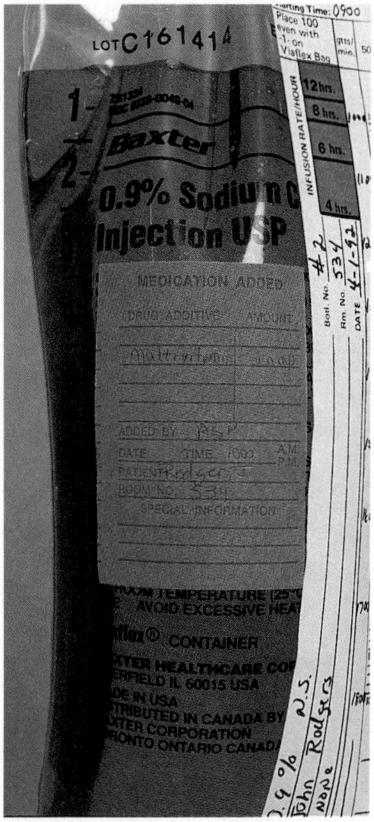

Step 9g

Continued.

procedure 26-4—cont'd

ADDING MEDICATIONS TO IV FLUID CONTAINERS

Steps	Rationale
(6) Gently mix bottle or bag.	Ensures that medication is evenly distributed.
(7) Rehang bag and regulate infusion to desired rate.	Prevents rapid infusion of fluid.
b. Complete medication label and stick it to bag or bottle.	Informs nurses and physicians of contents of bag or bottle.
11. Dispose of equipment and supplies; wash hands.	Reduces transmission of microorganisms.
12. Record solution and medication added to parenteral fluid on appropriate form.	Information used to monitor type of solutions client receives and fluid intake over 24 hours.
13. Report side effects (e.g., change in pulse rate, noisy respirations, or change in blood pressure) to nurse in charge or physician.	Reaction may require therapeutic intervention.

The rate of administration of an IV bolus medication is usually determined by the amount of drug that can be given each minute. The nurse should look up each medication to determine the recommended concentration and rate of administration. The purpose for which a drug is prescribed and any potential adverse effects related to the rate or route of administration must be considered when a nurse gives a drug IV push.

Volume-Controlled Infusions

Another way of administering IV medications is through small amounts (50 to 100 ml) of compatible IV fluids. The fluid is within a secondary fluid container separate from the primary fluid bag. The container connects directly to the primary IV line or to a separate tubing that inserts into the primary line. The two types of containers are volume control administration sets (e.g., Volutrol or Pediatrol) and piggyback sets. Using volume-controlled infusions has several advantages:

1. Reduces risk of rapid-dose infusion by IV push. Medications are diluted and infused over longer time intervals (e.g., 30 to 60 minutes)
2. Allows for administration of drugs (e.g., antibiotics) that are stable for a limited time in solution
3. Allows for control of IV fluid intake

Volume-control administration sets are small (100 to 150 ml) containers that attach just below the primary infusion bag or bottle (Procedure 26-5). The set is attached and filled in a manner similar to a regular IV infusion (see Chapter 35). However, the priming or filling of the set is different, depending on the type of filter (floating valve or membrane) within the set. Package directions should be followed during priming, or the set will not function properly.

Piggyback sets are small (50 or 100 ml) IV bags or bottles connected to short tubing lines that connect to the upper Y-port of a primary infusion line or an intermittent venous access. The piggyback tubing is a microdrip or macrodrip system. The sets are called piggyback because the small bag or bottle is set higher than the primary infusion bottle in some sets.

Intermittent Venous Access

An intermittent venous access **(heparin lock)** is an IV catheter with a small "well" or chamber covered by a rubber diaphragm (Figure 26-23). Special rubber-seal injection caps serve as wells and can be inserted into most IV catheters (see Chapter 35). Advantages to intermittent venous access include:

1. Cost savings resulting from the omission of continuous IV therapy

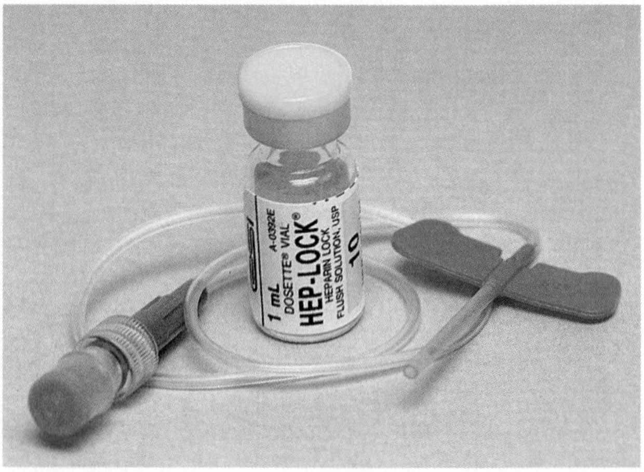

FIGURE 26-23 Intravenous lock with vial of flush solution.

procedure 26-5

ADMINISTERING IV MEDICATIONS BY PIGGYBACK OR VOLUME ADMINISTRATION SETS

Steps	Rationale
1. Check physician's order to determine type of medication dosage, route, and time.	Client's overall physical condition determines types of solution used. Ensures safe and accurate drug administration.
2. Assess patency of existing IV infusion line (see Chapter 35) by noting infusion rate of main IV line.	IV line must be patent and fluids must infuse easily for medication to reach venous circulation effectively.
3. Assess insertion site for signs of infiltration or phlebitis and blood return. (see Chapter 35).	Confirmation of placement of needle or catheter and integrity of surrounding tissues ensure that medication is administered safely.
4. Prepare following equipment and supplies: a. Piggyback set: (1) Medication prepared in a 50- to 100-ml, labeled infusion bag with IV line, microdrip or macrodrip infusion tubing set with "needleless" connector or 21- or 23-gauge needle. (2) Adhesive tape (optional) (3) Antiseptic swab	Used for piggyback administration. Most piggybacks are prepared by pharmacies. Medication is "piggybacked" or connected to main infusion line through injection port. "Needleless" connectors reduce the chance of needle sticks.
(4) Metal/plastic hook	Used to lower primary infusion bag below smaller infusion bag (only if tubing is shorter than primary tubing).
(5) Disposable gloves b. Volume-control administration set: (1) Volutrol, Pediatrol, or Burette	Graduated container connects to main IV solution.
(2) Infusion tubing	Connected to administration set used to inject medication into set.
(3) Syringe (5 to 20 ml) (4) Needle (1 to $1\frac{1}{2}$ in, 21- or 23-gauge) (5) Vial or ampule of ordered medication (6) Medication label	
5. Wash hands and apply gloves.	Reduces transmission of microorganisms. During handling of IV equipment, there is some risk of blood exposure.
6. Administer medications by piggyback set: a. Assemble supplies at bedside.	Drug preparation is usually not required. May assemble infusion tubing and bag of medication in medication or client's room.
b. Connect infusion tubing to medication bag (see Chapter 35). Allow solution to fill tubing by opening regulator flow clamp.	Infusion tube should be filled with solution and free of air bubbles to prevent air embolus.
c. Hand medication bag at or above level of main fluid bag. Hook may be used to lower main bag (see illustration).	Height of fluid bag affects rate of flow to client.

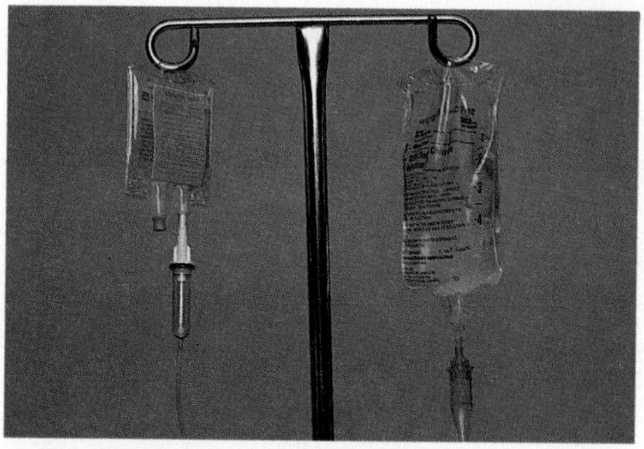

Step 6c

Continued.

procedure 26-5—cont'd

ADMINISTERING IV MEDICATIONS BY PIGGYBACK OR VOLUME ADMINISTRATION SETS

Steps	Rationale
d. Connect covered sterile needle to end of infusion tubing.	Cover keeps needle sterile before connecting it to main line.
e. Check client's identification by looking at armband and asking name.	Ensures that drug is administered to correct client.
f. Clean injection Y-port of main line with antiseptic swab.	Prevents introduction of microorganisms during connection.
g. **Needle:** Remove cover and insert needle of secondary piggyback line through injection port of main line. Secure with strip of adhesive tape if necessary. **Needleless Device:** Use needle-lock device to secure needle of secondary piggyback line through injection port of main line (see illustrations).	Establishes route for medication to enter main IV line. Needle-lock devices or tape prevents needle from slipping out of port, which could result in improper dose of medication. "Needleless" or sheathed connections reduce the risk of needlestick injury to health care workers.
h. Regulate flow rate appropriate or as ordered by physician. Pharmacist may recommend infusion rate.	Intermittent infusion of medication maintains therapeutic blood levels. For optimal effect, drug should infuse in prescribed time interval.
i. After medication has infused, check flow regulator on primary infusion. Piggyback set hung at level of primary bag has backcheck valve that automatically stops flow of primary infusion until medication infuses. Primary infusion should automatically begin to flow after piggyback is empty.	Valve prevents backup of medication into main infusion line. Checking flow rate ensures proper administration of fluids.
j. Regulate main infusion line to desired rate, if necessary.	Infusion of piggyback may interfere with main line infusion rate.

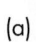

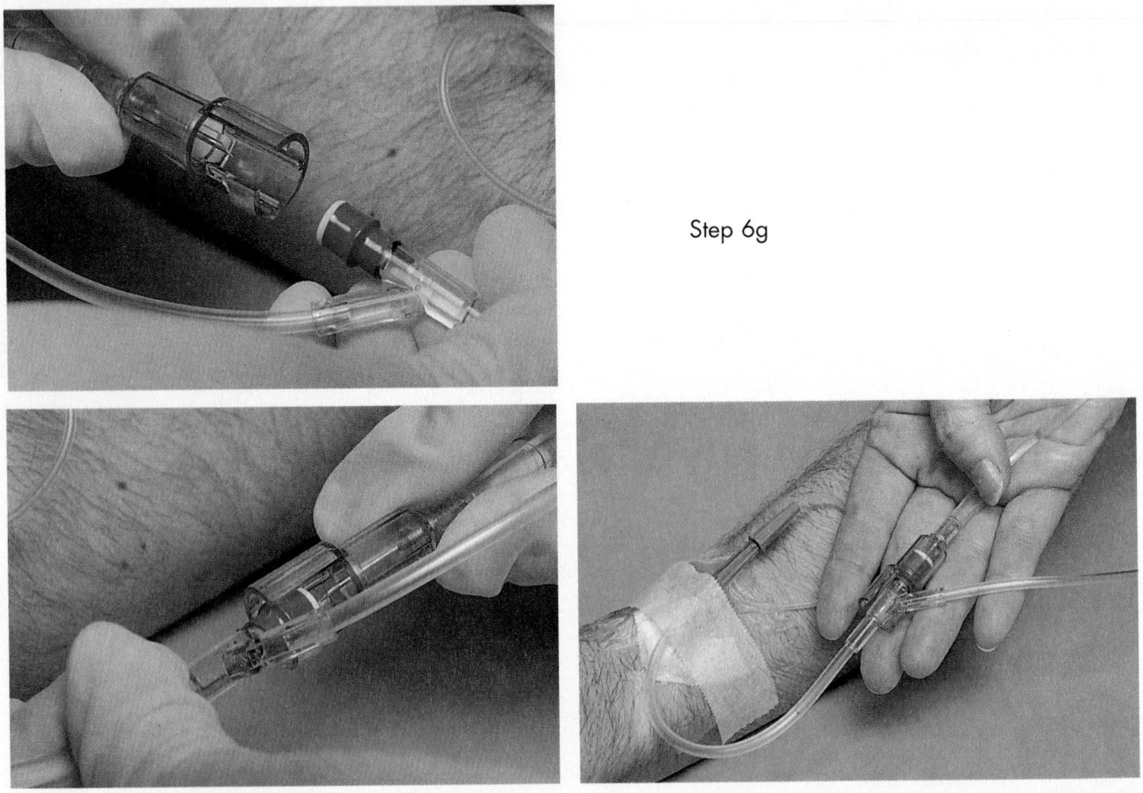

(a) (b) (c)

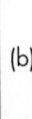

Step 6g

Steps	Rationale
k. Leave secondary bag, tubing, and inserted needle in place for future drug administration or discard in appropriate containers (check agency policy).	Establishment of secondary line produces route for microorganisms to enter main line. Repeated changes in tubing or needles increase risk of infection transmission.
7. Administer medication by volume-control administration set (e.g., Volutrol):	
a. Assemble supplies in medication room.	Controls risk of contaminating IV solution.
b. Prepare medication from vial or ampule (Procedure 26-2).	
c. Check client's identification by looking at armband and asking name.	Ensures drug administered to correct client.
d. Fill Volutrol with desired amount of fluid (50 to 100 ml) by opening clamp between Volutrol and main IV bag (see illustration).	Small volume of fluid dilutes medication and reduces risk of too-rapid infusion.
e. Close clamp and check to be sure clamp in air vent of Volutrol chamber is open.	Prevents additional leakage of fluid into Volutrol. Air vent allows fluid in Volutrol to exit at regulated rate.
f. Clean injection port on top of Volutrol with antiseptic swab.	Prevents introduction of microorganisms during needle insertion.
g. Remove needle cap and insert syringe needle through port, and then inject medication (see illustration). Gently rotate Volutrol between hands.	Rotating mixes medication with solution in Volutrol to ensure equal distribution.
h. Regulate IV infusion rate appropriate for medication. Follow physician or pharmacist's recommendations for infusion rates.	For optimal therapeutic effect, drug should infuse in prescribed time interval.
i. Label Volutrol with name of drug, dose, total volume including diluent, and time of administration.	Alerts nurses to drug being infused. Prevents other medications from being added to Volutrol.
j. Dispose of uncapped needle and syringe in proper container.	Prevents accidental needlesticks.
8. Remove and dispose of gloves. Wash hands.	Prevents transmission of microorganisms.
9. Observe client for signs of adverse reactions.	IV medications act rapidly.
10. During infusion, periodically check infusion rate and condition of IV site.	IV line must remain patent for proper drug administration. Development of infiltration necessitates discontinuing infusion.
11. Record drug, dose, route, and time administered on medication form (Figure 26-5). Record volume of fluid in medication bag or Volutrol on intake and output form (see Chapter 35).	Timely documentation prevents medication errors (e.g., repeated doses). Fluid balance is regulated and monitored on basis of total fluid intake.

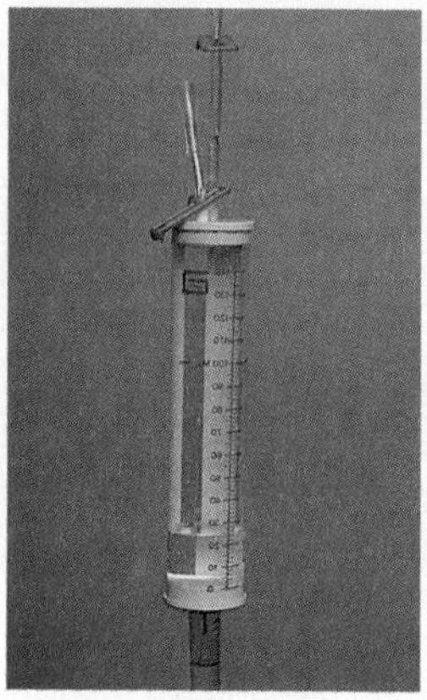

Step 7d(a)

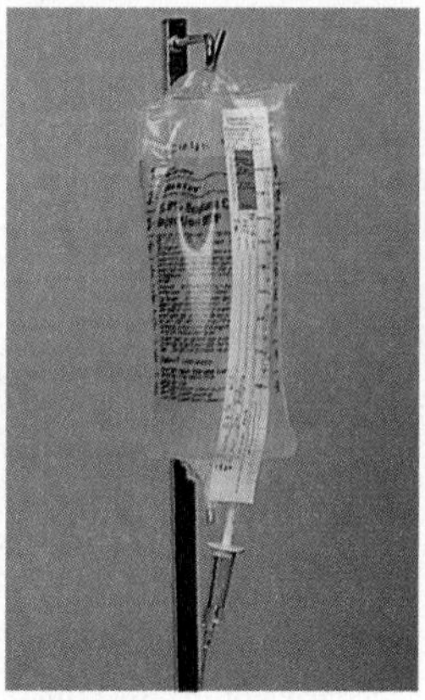

Step 7d(b)

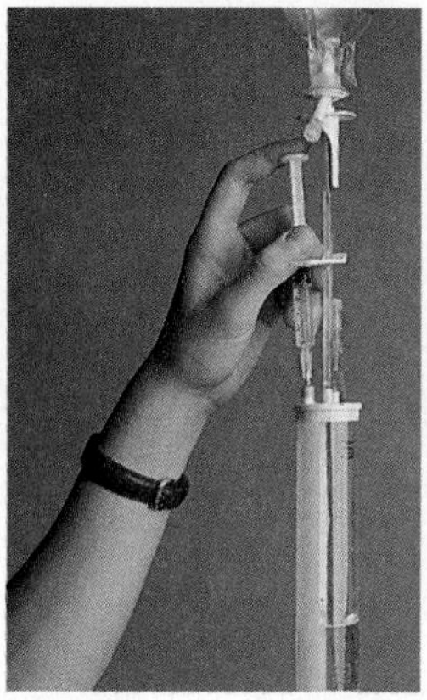

Step 7g

Continued.

2. Convenience to the nurse by eliminating constant monitoring of flow rates
3. Increased mobility, safety, and comfort for the client

After an IV bolus or piggyback medication has been administered through an intermittent venous access, the access must be flushed with a solution to keep it patent. Disagreement exists about the type of solution to use to keep the access free of clots. A heparin flush solution (1 ml = 100 units) or a saline flush may be used to keep the intermittent venous access patent. The nurse needs to be aware of different agency policies regarding this procedure.

Normally, checking for a blood return in an IV lock before bolus administration is unnecessary. However, if the needle site becomes puffy or the client complains of discomfort, the well must be aspirated for a blood return.

DISPOSAL OF EQUIPMENT

After administering injections, the nurse must properly dispose of used equipment (Figure 26-24). A stray needle can injure the client, nurse, housekeeper, or other health care personnel. A needle stick can be the source of hepatitis B or acquired immunodeficiency syndrome (AIDS).

The Occupational Safety and Health Administration (OSHA) mandates that *needles should not be capped before disposal.* Covering a needle may predispose the nurse to a needlestick injury and transmission of bloodborne pathogens. The nurse discards the needle and syringe intact into clearly marked, appropriate containers. Containers should be puncture- and leak-proof, closable, labeled, and color-coded. These containers should be placed as close as possible to the area of use. *Needles and plungers should not be broken.* A needle should never be forced into a full needle disposal receptacle. Used needles and syringes should not be placed in wastebaskets, in the nurse's pocket, or at the client's bedside.

A needle especially designed to prevent sticks is available. It is equipped with a plastic guard sheath that slips over the needle as it is withdrawn from the skin. The guard locks in place, preventing accidental needle sticks and eliminating the need to recap the needle. The guard and needle are disposed of as a single unit (Figure 26-25, *A* and *B*).

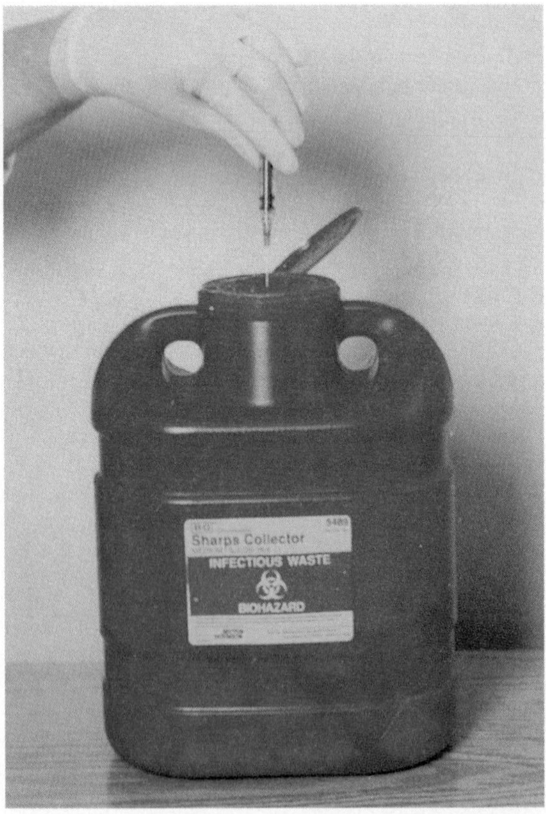

FIGURE 26-24 Special containers are available in nursing units for disposal of contaminated syringes.

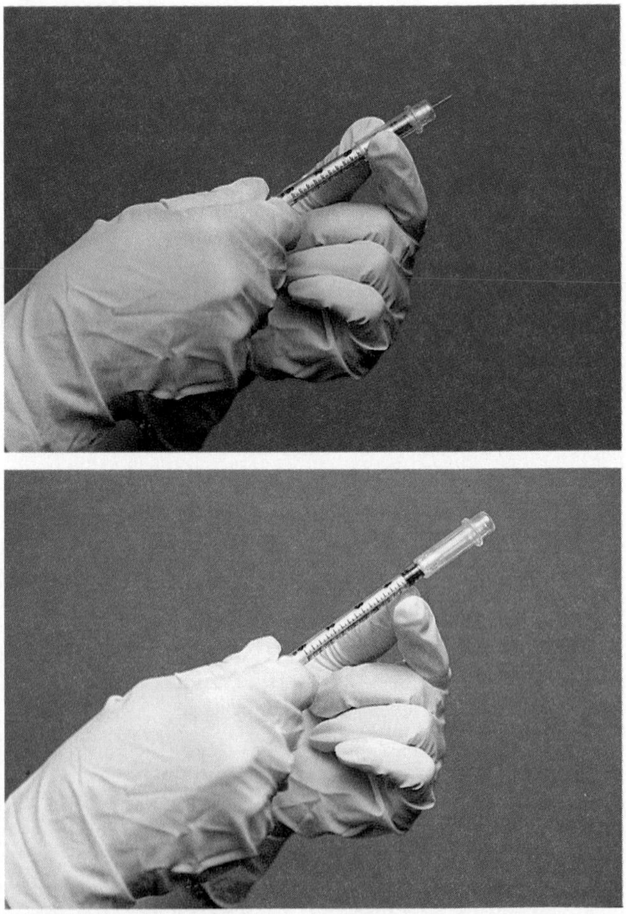

FIGURE 26-25 Needle with plastic guard to prevent needlesticks. **A,** Position of guard before injection. **B,** After injection, the guard locks in place, covering the needle.

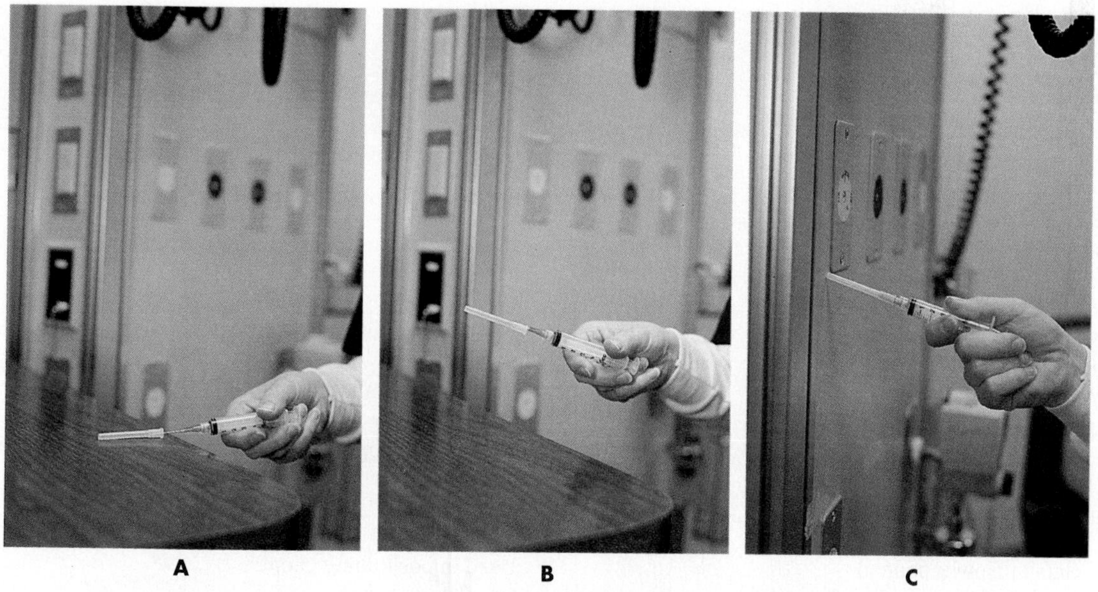

FIGURE 26-26 One-handed technique for recapping needle. **A,** Nurse uses one hand to slip needle into cap. **B,** Nurse scoops up cap to cover length of needle. **C,** Nurse presses cap against firm surface.

In special circumstances it may be necessary to recap a needle. If this procedure must be done, the nurse needs to be extremely cautious and follow a one-handed technique (Haiduven et al., 1992). It is expected that the nurse employs Universal Precautions when administering medications to clients and disposing of used equipment.

One-Handed Needle Recapping Technique

In administering injections it may be necessary, for client safety reasons, to recap a contaminated needle. For example, the nurse may be assisting with emergency measures at the bedside and cannot reach a disposable container. If a commercially made recapping device is not available, then the following procedure is recommended to reduce the risk of accidental needlesticks (Craft, 1990):

1. Position the needle cap on its side at the edge of a table or counter (Figure 26-26, *A*).
2. Hold the syringe with the dominant hand and scoop up the cap with the tip of the needle, being careful not to contaminate a sterile needle (Figure 26-26, *B*).
3. Press the syringe, needle, and cover against a flat, vertical surface (e.g., a wall or cabinet door) to get the cap firmly in place (Figure 26-26, *C*).

To reduce the temptation of using two hands, it is suggested that the nondominant hand be held behind the back during the recapping procedure. Craft (1990) also recommends that needlesticks may be prevented by the nurse carefully assessing the client and the environment and properly disposing of materials in puncture-proof containers as soon as possible.

OTHER ROUTES OF ADMINISTRATION

Topical Drug Applications

Skin Applications. Because many locally applied drugs such as lotions, pastes, and ointments can create systemic and local effects, the nurse should apply these drugs using gloves and applicators. Sterile technique is used if the client has an open wound.

Skin encrustations and dead tissues harbor microorganisms and block contact of medications with the tissues to be treated. Simply applying new medications over previously applied drugs does little to prevent infection or offer therapeutic benefit. Before applying medications, the nurse cleans the skin thoroughly by washing the area gently with soap and water, soaking an involved site, or locally debriding tissue.

When applying ointments or pastes, the nurse spreads the medication evenly over the involved surface and covers the area well without applying an overly thick layer. Opaque ointments prevent visualization of underlying skin. Physicians may order a gauze dressing to be applied over the medication to prevent soiling of

procedure 26-6

ADMINISTERING NASAL DROPS AND SPRAYS

Steps	Rationale
1. Review physician's medication order for client's name, drug name, concentration of solution, number of drops, and time of administration.	Ensures safe and correct administration of medication.
2. Refer to medical record to determine which sinus is affected.	Will affect positioning that client assumes during drug instillation.
3. Wash hands.	Reduces transmission of microorganisms.
4. Prepare equipment and supplies:	
a. Prepared medication with clean dropper	Dropper or applicator need not be sterile but should be clean.
b. Medication forms or printout	
c. Facial tissue	
d. Small pillow (optional)	Used in positioning client.
e. Washcloth (optional)	Used to clean nares.
5. Check client's identification by reading identification bracelet and asking name.	Ensures that correct client receives medication.
6. Inspect condition of nose and sinuses (see Chapter 16). Palpate sinuses for tenderness.	Findings provide baseline to monitor effect of medication. Discharge will interfere with drug absorption.
7. Explain procedure regarding positioning and sensations to expect, such as burning or stinging of mucosa or choking sensation as medication trickles into throat.	Helps reduce anxiety.
8. Arrange supplies and medications at bedside.	Ensures smooth, orderly procedure.
9. Instruct client to blow nose unless contraindicated (e.g., risk of increased intracranial pressure or nose bleeds).	Removes mucus and secretions that can block distribution of medication.
10. Administer nasal drops:	
a. Assist client to supine position.	Position provides access to nasal passages.
b. Position head properly:	Position allows medication to drain into affected sinus.
(1) Posterior pharynx—tilt client's head backward.	
(2) Ethmoid or sphenoid sinus—tilt head back over edge of bed or place pillow under shoulder and tilt head back (see illustration).	

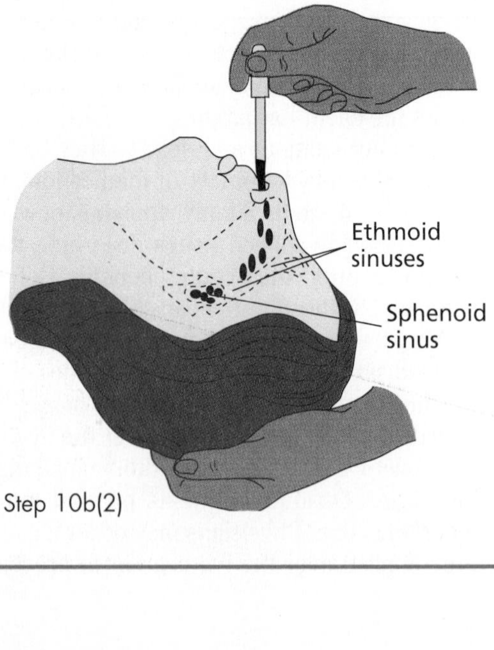

Step 10b(2)

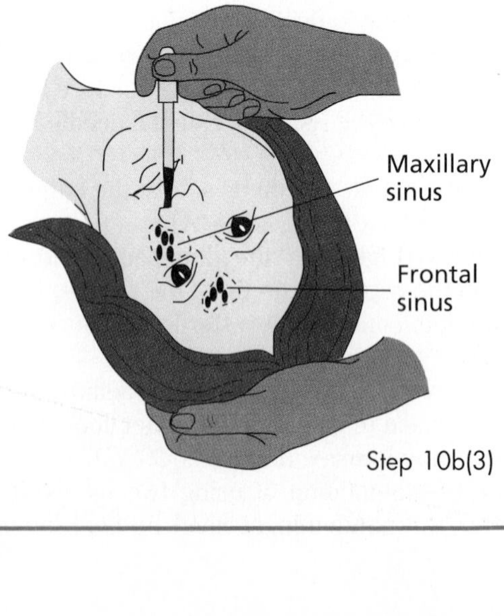

Step 10b(3)

Steps	Rationale
(3) Frontal and maxillary sinus—tilt head back over edge of bed or pillow with head turned toward side treated (see illustration).	
Support client's head with nondominant hand.	Prevents straining of neck muscles.
c. Instruct client to breathe through mouth.	Reduces chance of aspirating nasal drops into trachea and lungs.
d. Hold dropper 1 cm (½ in) above nares and instill prescribed number of drops toward midline of ethmoid bone.	Avoids contamination of dropper. Instilling toward ethmoid bone facilitates distribution of medication over nasal mucosa.
e. Have client remain in supine position 5 min.	Prevents premature loss of medication through nares.
f. Offer facial tissue to blot runny nose, but caution against blowing nose for several minutes.	Allows maximum amount of medication to be absorbed.
11. Administer nasal spray.	
a. Assist client to supine position.	Position provides access to nasal passages.
b. Position head properly:	
(1) Tilt client's head backward.	Position allows medication to reach nasal passages.
Support client's head with nondominant hand.	Prevents straining of neck muscles.
For children, keep head in upright position.	Prevents swallowing of spray.
c. Hold tip of container just inside nares.	Position provides best access for spray to reach nasal passages.
d. Instruct client to inhale as the spray enters the nasal passages.	Promotes maximum amount of medication to reach nasal passages.
12. Assist client to a comfortable position after drug has been absorbed.	Restores comfort.
13. Dispose of soiled supplies in proper container and wash hands.	Maintains neat, orderly environment. Reduces spread of microorganisms.
14. Record medication administration, including drug name, concentration, number of drops, nostril into which drug was instilled, and time of administration.	Timely documentation prevents drug errors (e.g., repeated doses).
15. Observe client for side effects 15 to 30 min after administration.	Drugs absorbed through mucosa can cause systemic reaction.

clothes and wiping away of the drug. Each type of medication, whether an ointment, lotion, powder, or other type, should be applied a specific way to ensure proper penetration and absorption. The nurse applies lotions and creams by smearing them lightly onto the skin's surface; rubbing may cause irritation. A liniment is applied by rubbing it gently but firmly into the skin. A powder is dusted lightly to cover the affected area with a thin layer. During any application the nurse should assess the skin thoroughly. To record administration, the area applied, name of medication, and condition of skin should be noted.

Nasal Instillations. Clients with nasal sinus alterations may receive drugs by spray, drops, or tampons (Procedure 26-6). The most commonly administered form of nasal **instillation** is decongestant spray or drops, used to relieve symptoms of sinus congestion and colds. Clients must be cautioned to avoid abuse of drugs because overuse can lead to a rebound effect in which the nasal congestion worsens. When excess decongestant solution is swallowed, serious systemic effects may also develop, especially in children. Saline drops are safer as a decongestant for children than nasal preparations that contain sympathomimetics (e.g., Afrin or Neo-Synephrine).

It is easier to have the client self-administer sprays, since the client can control the spray and inhale as it enters the nasal passages. For clients who use nasal sprays repeatedly, the nurse checks the nares for irritation. Nasal drops are effective in treating sinus infections. The nurse learns the proper way of positioning clients to

procedure 26-7

ADMINISTERING EYEDROPS AND OINTMENT

Steps	Rationale
1. Review physician's medication order, including client's name, drug name, concentration, number of drops (if a liquid), time, and eye (right or left) to receive medication.	Ensures correct administration of medication.
2. Wash hands.	Reduces transmission of microorganisms.
3. Prepare equipment and supplies:	
a. Medication bottle with sterile eye dropper or ointment tube	Ophthalmic drops come in plastic or glass bottles. Ointments are prepared in small tubes.
b. Medication form or printout	
c. Cotton ball or tissue	
d. Wash basin filled with warm water and wash cloth	
e. Eye patch and tape (optional)	
f. Disposable gloves	
4. Check client's identification by looking at identification bracelet and asking name.	Ensures that correct client receives medication.
5. If eye patch is present, remove it.	
6. Assess condition of external eye structures (see Chapter 16).	Provides baseline to later determine whether local response to medications occurs. Also indicates need to clean eye before drug application.
7. Explain procedure to client.	Client often becomes anxious about medication being instilled into eye because of potential for discomfort.
8. Arrange supplies at bedside and apply gloves.	Ensures smooth, orderly procedure. Gloves reduce exposure to infectious drainage.
9. Ask client to lie supine or sit back in chair with head slightly hyperextended.	Provides easy access to eye for medication instillation and minimizes drainage of medication through tear duct.
10. If crusts or drainage are present along eyelid margins or inner canthus, gently wash away. Soak crusts that are dried and difficult to remove by applying damp washcloth or cotton ball over eye for few minutes. Always wipe clean from inner to outer canthus.	Crusts and drainage harbor microorganisms. Soaking allows easy removal, thus preventing pressure from being applied directly over eye. Cleansing from inner to outer canthus avoids entrance of microorganisms into lacrimal duct.
11. Hold cotton ball or clean tissue in nondominant hand on client's checkbone just below lower eyelid.	Cotton or tissue absorbs medication that escapes eye.
12. With tissue or cotton resting below lower lid, gently press downward with thumb or forefinger against bony orbit.	Technique exposes lower conjunctival sac. Retraction against bony orbit prevents pressure and trauma to eyeball and prevents fingers from touching eye.
13. Ask client to look at ceiling.	Action retracts sensitive cornea up and away from conjunctival sac and reduces stimulation of blink reflex.
14. Instill eyedrops:	
a. With dominant hand resting on client's forehead, hold filled medication eye dropper approximately 1 to 2 cm (½ to ¾ in) above conjunctival sac (see illustration).	Helps prevent accidental contact of eyedropper with eye structures, thus reducing risk of injury to eye and transfer of infection to dropper. Ophthalmic medications are sterilized.
b. Drop prescribed number of drops into conjunctival sac.	Conjunctival sac normally holds 1 to 2 drops. Applying drops to sac provides even distribution across eye.
c. If client blinks or closes eye or if drops land on outer lid margins, repeat procedure.	Therapeutic effect is obtained only when drops enter conjunctival sac.
d. When administering drugs that cause systemic effects, cover finger with clean tissue and apply gentle pressure to client's nasolacrimal duct for 30 to 60 sec.	Prevents overflow of medication into nasal and pharyngeal passages. Prevents absorption into systemic circulation.
e. After instilling drops, ask client to close eye gently.	Helps distribute medication. Squinting or squeezing of eyelids forces medication from conjunctival sac.

Steps	Rationale
15. Instill eye ointment:	
a. Holding ointment applicator above lid margin, apply thin stream of ointment evenly along inside edge of lower eyelid on conjunctiva (see illustration).	Distributes medication evenly across eye and lid margin.
b. Ask client to look down and apply thin stream of ointment along upper lid margin on inner conjunctiva.	Distributes medication evenly across eye and lid margin without excess blinking.
c. Have client keep eyes closed for several seconds.	Further distributes medication without traumatizing eye.
16. If excess medication is on eyelid, gently wipe it from inner to outer canthus.	Promotes comfort and prevents trauma to eye.
17. If client has eye patch, apply clean one by placing it over affected eye so that entire eye is covered. Tape securely without applying pressure to eye.	Reduces chance of infection.
18. Dispose of soiled supplies in proper receptacle. Remove and dispose of gloves. Wash hands.	Maintains neat environment at bedside and reduces transmission of microorganisms.
19. Observe response to medication, noting signs and symptoms of potential systemic effects and condition of eye.	Evaluates reaction to medication.
20. Record drug, concentration, number of drops, time of administration, and eye (left, right, or both) that received medication.	Timely documentation prevents drug errors (e.g., repeated or missed doses).

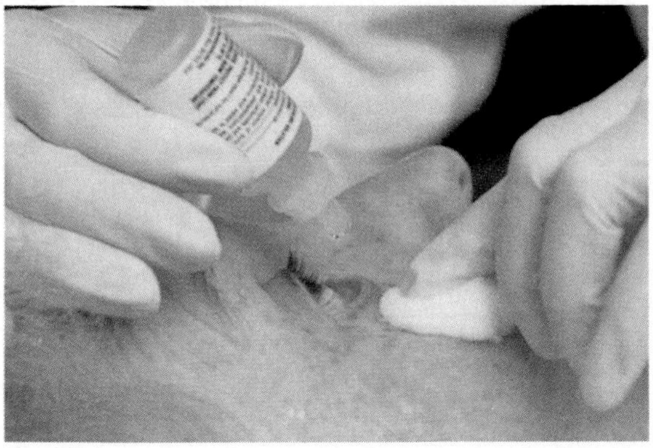

Step 14a

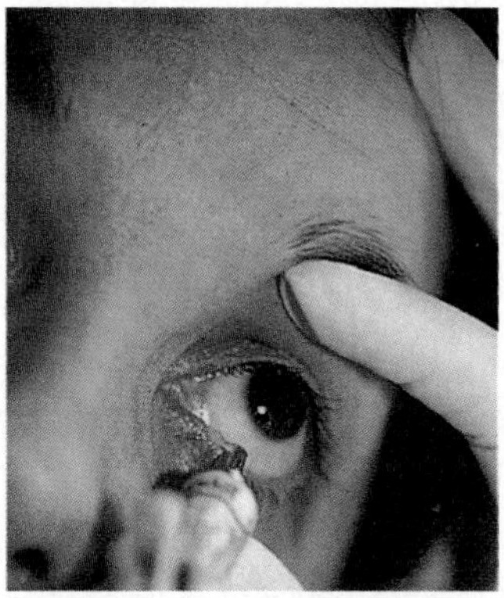

Step 15a

permit the medication to reach the affected sinus. Severe nosebleeds are usually treated with packing or nasal tampons, which are treated with epinephrine, to reduce blood flow. Usually a physician places nasal tampons.

Eye Instillations. A common medication used by clients is eye drops and ointments, including over-the-counter preparations such as artificial tears and vasoconstrictors (e.g., Visine and Murine) (Procedure 26-7). However, many clients receive prescribed ophthalmic drugs for eye conditions, such as glaucoma, and after cataract extraction. A large percentage of clients receiving eye medications are older adults. Age-related problems including poor vision, hand tremors, and difficulty grasping or manipulating containers affect the ease with which the older adult can self-administer eye medications. The nurse instructs clients and family members about the proper techniques for administering eye medications. The nurse may determine the client and family's ability to self-administer through a return demonstration of the procedure. Showing clients each step of

procedure 26-8

ADMINISTERING EARDROPS

Steps	Rationale
1. Review physician's medication order for client's name, drug name, concentration, time of administration, number of drops to instill, and ear (right or left) to receive medication.	Ensures safe and correct administration of medication.
2. Wash hands.	Reduces transmission of microorganisms.
3. Prepare equipment and supplies: a. Medication bottle and dropper b. Medication form or printout c. Cotton-tipped applicator d. Tissue e. Cotton ball (optional) f. Disposable gloves (optional)	c. Used to remove visible cerumen or drainage.
4. Identify client by reading identification bracelet and asking name.	Ensures that correct client receives medication.
5. Apply gloves if client has ear drainage.	Reduces exposure to microorganisms.
6. Assess condition of external ear structures and canal (see Chapter 16).	Provides baseline to determine whether local response to medication occurs, client's condition improves, or cleansing will be necessary before instillation.
7. Explain procedure to client.	Reduces anxiety.
8. Arrange supplies at bedside.	Ensures smooth procedure.
9. Have client assume side-lying position with ear to be treated facing up.	Provides easy access to ear for instillation of medication. Ear canal is in position to receive medication.
10. If cerumen or drainage occludes outermost portion of ear canal, wipe out gently with cotton-tipped applicator. Do *not* force wax inward to block or occlude canal.	Cerumen and drainage harbor microorganisms and can block distribution of medication into canal. Occlusion of canal interferes with normal sound conduction.
11. Straighten ear canal by pulling auricle down and back (children) or upward and outward (adult).	Straightening of ear canal provides direct access to deeper external ear structures.
12. Instill prescribed drops holding dropper 1 cm ($\frac{1}{2}$ in) above ear canal (see illustration).	Forcing drops into occluded canal can cause injury to eardrum.
13. Ask client to remain in side-lying position 2 to 3 min. Apply gentle massage of pressure to tragus of ear with finger (see illustration).	Allows complete distribution of medication. Pressure and massage move medication inward.
14. At times, physician orders placement of cotton ball into outermost part of canal. Do not press cotton into innermost part of canal.	Inserting cotton into outer canal prevents escape of medication when client sits or stands. Cotton should not block canal to impair hearing.
15. Remove cotton in 15 min.	Promotes drug distribution and absorption.
16. Dispose of soiled supplies and gloves and wash hands.	Keeps bedside neat. Reduces transmission of infection.
17. Assist client to comfortable position after drops are absorbed.	Restores comfort.
18. Evaluate condition of external ear between drug instillations.	Determines response to medication.
19. Record drug, concentration, number of drops, time administered, and ear into which drops were instilled on medication form.	Timely documentation prevents drug errors (e.g., repeated doses).
20. Record condition of ear canal in nurses' notes.	Documents client's status and response to therapy.

Step 12

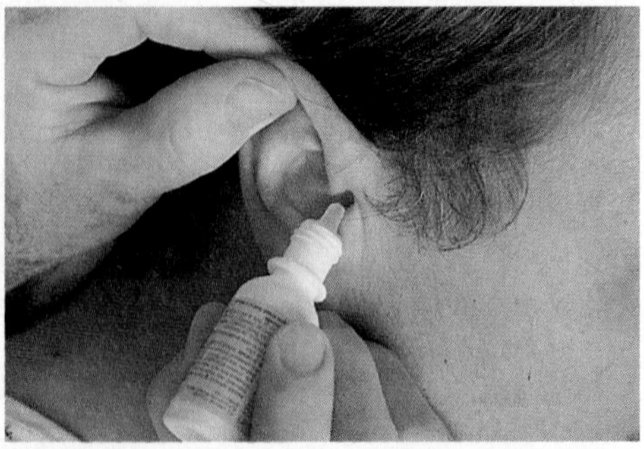

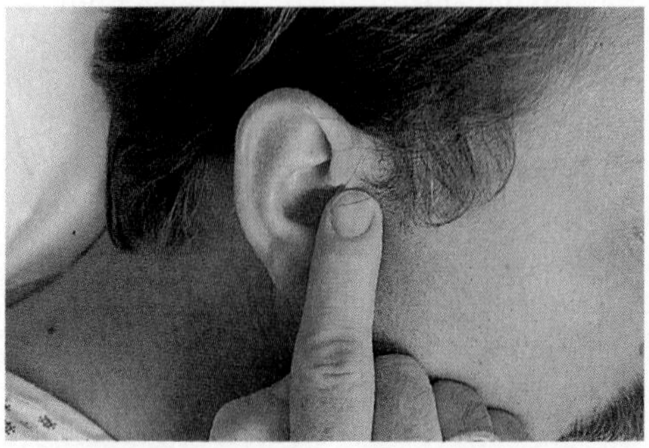

Step 13

the procedure for instilling eye drops can improve their compliance. The following principles can be followed when administering eye medications:

1. The cornea of the eye is richly supplied with pain fibers and thus very sensitive to anything applied to it. Avoid instilling any form of eye medication directly onto the cornea.
2. The risk of transmitting infection from one eye to the other is high. Avoid touching the eyelids or other eye structures with eye droppers or ointment tubes.
3. Use eye medication only for the client's affected eye.
4. Never allow a person to use another's eye medications.

Ear Instillations. Internal ear structures are very sensitive to temperature extremes. Failure to instill ear drops or irrigating fluid at room temperature may cause vertigo (severe dizziness) or nausea. Although the structures of the outer ear are not sterile, it is wise to use sterile drops and solutions in case the eardrum is ruptured. The entrance of nonsterile solutions into middle ear structures could result in infection. With ear drainage, the nurse should check with the physician to be sure the client does not have a ruptured eardrum. A nurse should never occlude the ear canal with the dropper or irrigating syringe. Forcing medication into an occluded ear canal creates pressure that may injure the eardrum.

External ear structures of children differ from those of adults. When instilling drops or irrigating solutions (Procedure 26-8), the nurse must straighten the ear canal. In infants and young children the nurse straightens the cartilaginous canal by grasping the auricle of the ear and pulling it gently down and backward. In adults the ear canal is longer and composed of underlying bone and is straightened by pulling the auricle upward and backward. Failure to straighten the canal properly may prevent medicinal solutions from reaching the deeper external ear structures.

Vaginal Instillations. Vaginal medications are available as suppositories, foam, jellies, or creams. Suppositories come individually packaged in foil wrappers. Storage in a refrigerator prevents the solid, oval-shaped suppositories from melting. After a suppository is inserted into the vaginal cavity, body temperature causes it to melt and be distributed and absorbed. Foam, jellies, and creams are administered with an inserter or applicator (Procedure 26-9). A suppository is given with a gloved hand in accordance with Universal Precautions. Clients often prefer administering their own vaginal medications and should be given privacy. After instillation of the drug, a client may wish to wear a perineal pad to collect drainage. Because vaginal medications are often given to treat infection, discharge may be foul-smelling. Aseptic technique should be followed, and the client should be offered frequent opportunities to maintain perineal hygiene (see Chapter 30).

Rectal Instillations. Rectal suppositories are thinner and more bullet-shaped than vaginal suppositories. The rounded end prevents anal trauma during insertion. Rectal suppositories contain medications that exert local effects such as promoting defecation or systemic effects such as reducing nausea. Rectal suppositories are stored in the refrigerator until administered.

During administration, the nurse must place the suppository past the internal anal sphincter and against the rectal mucosa (Procedure 26-10). Otherwise the suppository may be expelled before it can dissolve and be absorbed into the mucosa. With practice a nurse learns to recognize the sensation of the sphincter relaxing around the finger. The suppository should not be forced into a mass of fecal material. It may be necessary to clear the rectum with a small cleansing enema before a suppository can be inserted.

Inhalation

Drugs administered with hand-held inhalers are dispersed through an aerosol spray, mist, or powder that penetrates lung airways. The alveolar-capillary network absorbs medications rapidly. Metered dose inhalers (MDIs) are usually designed to produce local effects such as bronchodilation. However, some medications can create serious systemic side effects.

Clients who receive drugs by inhalation frequently suffer chronic respiratory disease such as chronic asthma, emphysema, or bronchitis. Drugs given by inhalation provide these clients with control of airway obstruction, and because these clients depend on medications for disease control, they must learn about them and ways to administer them safely.

A metered dose inhaler (Procedure 26-11) delivers a measured dose of drug with each push of a canister. Approximately 5 to 10 pounds of pressure must be used to activate the aerosol. However, hand strength diminishes with age and from chronic respiratory disease. A three-point or lateral hand position is effective in activating a canister. Some clients may require two hands or an adapted inhaler device.

Irrigations

Medications may be used to irrigate or wash out a body cavity and are delivered through a stream of solution. Irrigations most commonly use sterile water, saline, or antiseptic solutions on the eye, ear, throat, vagina, and urinary tract. If there is a break in the skin or mucosa, the nurse uses aseptic technique. When the cavity to be ir-

Text continued on p. 716.

procedure 26-9

ADMINISTERING VAGINAL MEDICATIONS

Steps	Rationale
1. Review physician's order including client's name, drug name, form (cream or suppository), route, dosage, and time of administration.	Ensures safe and correct administration of medication.
2. Wash hands.	Reduces transfer of microorganisms.
3. Prepare supplies:	
a. Suppository insertion:	
(1) Vaginal suppository	Stored in refrigerator to maintain solid shape.
(2) Clean, disposable gloves	
(3) Lubricating jelly	Eases insertion of suppository.
(4) Clean tissues	
(5) Perineal pad (optional)	
(6) Medication card, form, or printout	
b. Cream or foam instillation:	
(1) Vaginal cream or foam	Prepared in plastic tube or can.
(2) Plastic applicator	
(3) Clean, disposable gloves	
(4) Paper towel	
(5) Perineal pad (optional)	
(6) Medication form or printout	
4. Check client's identification by reading identification bracelet and asking name.	Ensures that correct client receives medication.
5. Inspect condition of external genitalia and vaginal canal (see Chapter 16).	Findings provide baseline to monitor effect of medication.
6. Assess client's ability to manipulate applicator or suppository and to position self to insert medication.	Mobility restriction indicates level of assistance required from nurse.
7. Explain procedure to client. Be specific if client plans to self-administer medication.	Promotes understanding. Will enable client to self-administer drug if physically able.
8. Arrange supplies at bedside.	Ensures smooth procedure.
9. Close room curtain or door.	Provides privacy.

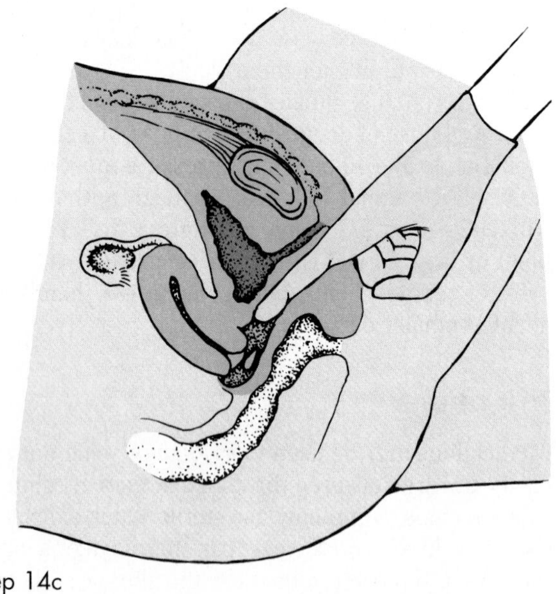

Step 14c

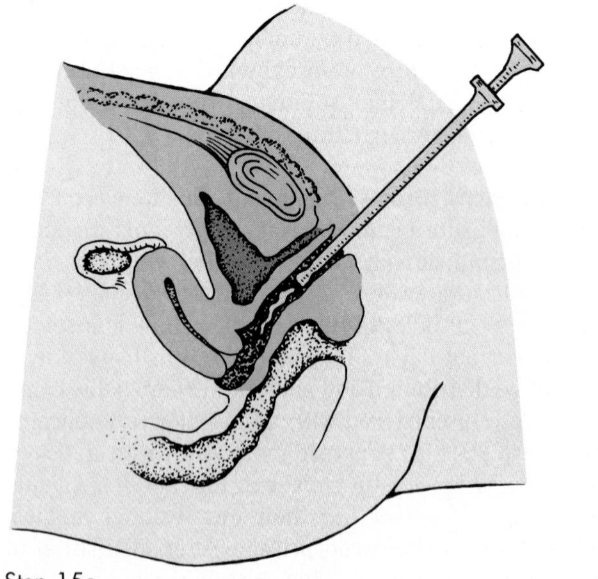

Step 15c

Steps	Rationale
10. Assist client to lie in dorsal recumbent position.	Provides easy access to and good exposure of vaginal canal. Also allows suppository to dissolve without escaping through orifice.
11. Keep abdomen and lower extremities draped.	Minimizes embarrassment.
12. Apply disposable gloves.	Prevents transmission of infection between you and client.
13. Be sure vaginal orifice is well-illuminated by room light or gooseneck lamp.	Proper insertion requires visualization of external genitalia.
14. Insert suppository with gloved hand:	
a. Remove suppository from foil wrapper and apply liberal amount of water-soluble lubricant to smooth or rounded end. Lubricate gloved index finger of dominant hand.	Lubrication reduces friction against mucosal surfaces during insertion.
b. With nondominant gloved hand, gently retract labial folds.	Exposes vaginal orifice.
c. Insert rounded end of suppository along posterior wall of vaginal canal entire length of finger (7.5-10 cm or 3-4 in) (see illustration).	Proper placement ensures equal distribution of medication along walls of vaginal cavity.
d. Withdraw finger and wipe away remaining lubricant from around orifice and labia.	Maintains comfort.
15. Apply cream or foam:	
a. Fill cream or foam applicator following package directions.	Dosage is prescribed by volume in applicator.
b. With nondominant gloved hand, gently retract labial folds.	Exposes vaginal orifice.
c. With dominant gloved hand, insert applicator approximately 5-7.5 cm (2-3 in). Push applicator plunger to deposit medication into vagina (see illustration).	Allows equal distribution of medication along vaginal walls.
d. Withdraw applicator and place on paper towel. Wipe off residual cream from labia or vaginal orifice.	Residual cream on applicator may contain microorganisms.
16. Instruct client to remain on back for at least 10 min.	Medication will be distributed and absorbed evenly throughout vaginal cavity and not be lost through orifice.
17. If applicator is used, wash with soap and warm water, rinse, and store for future use.	Vaginal cavity is not sterile. Soap and water assist in removal of bacteria and residual cream.
18. Remove gloves by pulling them inside out and discard in appropriate receptacle. Wash hands.	Reduces transfer of microorganisms.
19. Offer client perineal pad when she resumes ambulation.	Provides comfort.
20. Record drug name, dosage, route, and time of administration on medication record.	Timely recording prevents drug errors.
21. Inspect condition of vaginal canal and external genitalia between applications.	Evaluates whether vaginal medication effectively reduced irritation or inflammation of tissues.

procedure 26-10

ADMINISTERING RECTAL SUPPOSITORIES

Steps	Rationale
1. Review physician's order, including client's name, drug name, form, route, and time of administration.	Ensures safe and correct administration of medication.
2. Review medical record for rectal surgery or bleeding.	Conditions contraindicate use of suppository.
3. Wash hands.	Reduces transfer of microorganisms.
4. Prepare equipment and supplies: a. Rectal suppository b. Water-soluble lubricant c. Clean, disposable gloves d. Tissue e. Medication form or printout	
5. Apply disposable gloves.	Prevents contact with infected fecal material.
6. Check client's identification by reading identification bracelet and asking name.	Ensures that correct client receives medication.
7. Explain procedure. Be specific if client wishes to self-administer drug.	Promotes understanding and cooperation. Will enable client to self-administer drug if physically able.
8. Arrange supplies at bedside.	Ensures smooth procedure.
9. Close room curtain or door.	Maintains privacy and minimizes embarrassment.
10. Assist client in assuming Sims' position. Keep client draped with only anal area exposed.	Exposes anus and helps client relax external anal sphincter. Maintains privacy and facilitates relaxation.
11. Examine condition of anus externally and palpate rectal walls as needed (see Chapter 16). If gloves become soiled, dispose of them by turning them inside out and placing them in proper receptacle.	Determines presence of active rectal bleeding. Palpation determines whether rectum is filled with feces, which may interfere with suppository placement. Reduces transmission of infection.
12. Apply disposable gloves (if previous gloves were discarded).	Minimizes contact with fecal material and reduces transmission of microorganisms.
13. Remove suppository from wrapper and lubricate rounded end. Lubricate index finger of dominant hand with a water-soluble lubricant.	Lubrication reduces friction as suppository enters rectal canal.
14. Ask client to take slow deep breaths through mouth and relax anal sphincter.	Forcing suppository through constricted sphincter causes pain.
15. Retract buttocks with nondominant hand. Insert suppository gently through anus, past internal sphincter and against rectal wall, 10 cm (4 in) in adults, 5 cm (2 in) in children and infants.	Suppository must be placed against rectal mucosa for eventual absorption and therapeutic action.
16. Withdraw finger and wipe anal area with tissue.	Provides comfort.
17. Discard gloves by turning them inside out, and dispose of them in appropriate receptacle.	Reduces transfer of microorganisms.
18. Ask client to remain flat or on side for 5 min.	Prevents expulsion of suppository.
19. If suppository contains laxative or fecal softener, place call light within reach.	Provides client with sense of control over elimination. Allows client to obtain assistance to bedpan or toilet.
20. Wash hands.	Reduces risk of transfer of infection.
21. Return within 5 min to determine whether suppository was expelled.	Reinsertion may be necessary.
22. Record drug name, dosage, route, and time of administration on medication record.	Timely recording prevents errors.
23. Observe for effects of suppository (e.g., bowel movement, relief of nausea) 30 min after administration.	Evaluates effectiveness of medication and relief of client's symptoms.

procedure 26-11

USING METERED DOSE INHALERS

Steps	Rationale
1. Review physician's medication order, including client's name, drug name, dosage, number of inhalations, and time of administration.	Ensures safe and correct administration of medication.
2. Assess client's ability to hold and manipulate inhaler.	Impairment of grasp, muscle strength, or tremors of hands interferes with ability to depress inhaler canister.
3. Assess drug schedule and number of inhalations prescribed for each dose.	Influences explanations nurse provides for use of inhaler.
4. Have client prepare equipment and supplies:	
a. MDI with medication canister	
b. Facial tissues (optional)	
c. Wash basin or sink with warm water	Used to clean inhaler.
d. Paper towel	
5. Instruct client in comfortable environment by sitting in chair in hospital room or at kitchen table in home.	Client will be more likely to remain perceptive of explanation.
6. Allow client to manipulate inhaler and canister. Explain and demonstrate how canister fits into inhaler.	Client must be familiar with how to use equipment.
7. Explain *metered dose* and warn client about overuse of inhaler, including drug side effects.	Client must not arbitrarily decide to administer excessive inhalations because of risk of serious side effects. If given in recommended doses, side effects are uncommon.
8. Explain steps used to administer inhaled dose of medication. (Demonstrate steps when possible.)	Use of simple, step-by-step explanations allows client to ask questions at any point during procedure. Nurse demonstrates depression of canister without self-administering drug dose.
a. Remove cap and hold inhaler upright, grasping it with thumb and first two fingers.	
b. Shake inhaler.	Mixes medication evenly within solution so that aerosol drug concentration is even.
c. Tilt head back slightly and breathe out.	Maximizes airway exposure to medication from inhaler.
d. Position inhaler in one of following ways:	
(1) Open mouth with inhaler 0.5-1 cm (1-2 in) away from mouth (see illustration).	Avoids rapid influx of inhaled medication and subsequent airway irritation.
(2) OPTION: Attach spacer to mouthpiece of inhaler (see illustration).	Eliminates rapid influx of particles from inhaled drugs, which reduces irritant properties and tendency to cough. Also eliminates sores/lesions on the posterior pharynx caused by medication deposits and pressure of inhaled spray. Spacer is recommended for young children (National Heart, Lung, and Blood Institute, 1991).
(3) Place mouthpiece of inhaler or spacer in mouth (see illustration).	

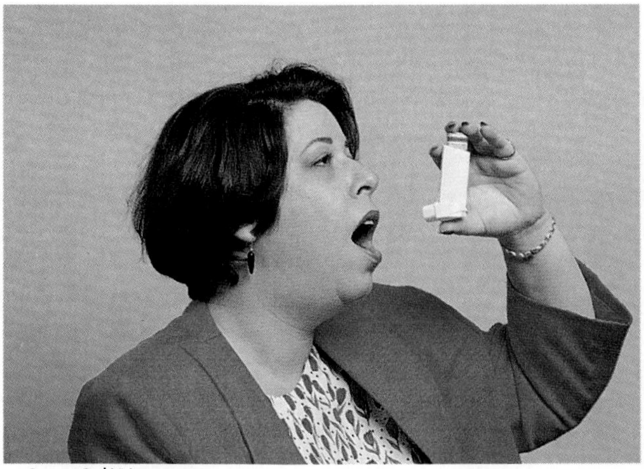

Step 8d(1)

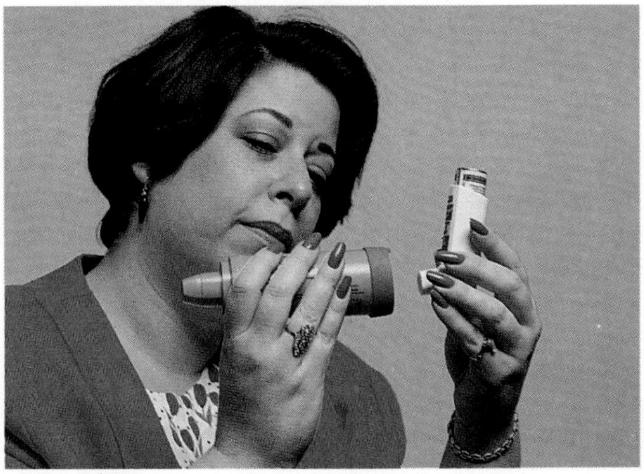

Step 8d(2)

procedure 26-11—cont'd

Steps	Rationale
e. Press down on inhaler to release medication (one puff) while inhaling slowly (see illustration).	Medication is distributed to airways during inhalation. Inhalation through mouth rather than nose draws medication more effectively into airways.
f. Breathe in slowly for 2 to 3 sec.	As client inhales, particles of medication are delivered to airway (National Heart, Lung, and Blood Institute, 1991).
g. Hold breath for approximately 10 sec.	Allows tiny drops of aerosol spray to reach deeper branches of airways.
h. Repeat puffs as ordered, waiting 1 min between puffs.	Allows maximal airway effect from first puff of medication. Therefore airways are more open for second delivery. Thus more particles are delivered directly to airways.
9. If two inhaled medications are prescribed, wait 5 to 10 min between inhalations or as ordered by physician.	Drugs must be inhaled sequentially. Usually bronchodilators are given first to maximize airway opening, followed by other inhaled medications such as steroids.
10. Explain that client may feel gagging sensation in throat caused by droplets of medication on pharynx or tongue.	Results when inhalant is sprayed and inhaled incorrectly.
11. Instruct client in removing medication canister and cleaning inhaler in warm water.	Accumulation of spray around mouthpiece can interfere with proper distribution during use. Accumulation at mouthpiece increases risk of microorganism accumulation and oral infections.
12. Ask if client has questions.	Allows clarification of misconceptions or misunderstanding.
13. Have client demonstrate use of inhaler and explain drug schedule.	Provides feedback for measuring learning. Improves likelihood of compliance with therapy (Redman, 1988).
14. Instruct client against repeating inhalations before next scheduled dose.	Drugs are prescribed at intervals during day to provide constant bronchodilation and minimize side effects.
15. Describe in nurses' notes content of skill taught and client's ability to perform skill.	Provides continuity to teaching plan so that other members of nursing staff will not teach same material.

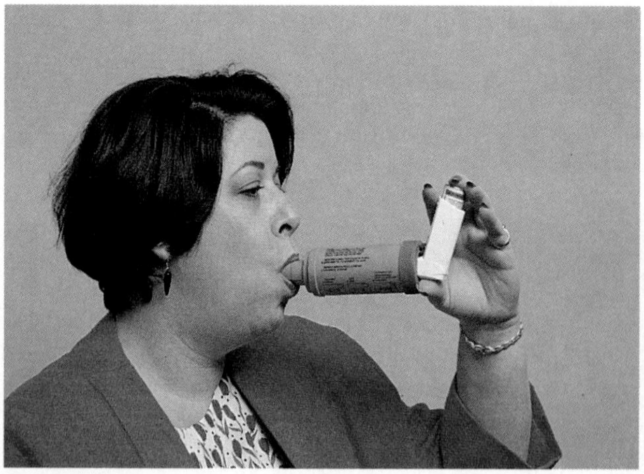

Step 8d(3)

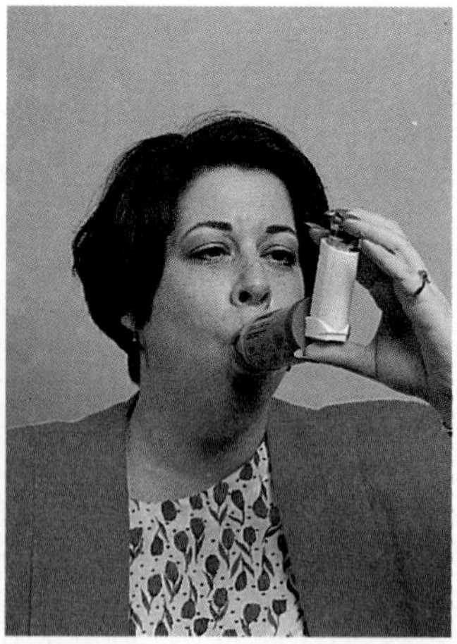

Step 8e

procedure 26-12

EAR IRRIGATIONS

Steps	Rationale
1. Review physician's order for client name, purpose of irrigation, type of irrigant ordered, and time of administration.	Ensures safe and correct administration of irrigation.
2. Check client's identification by reading identification bracelet and asking name.	Ensures that correct client receives irrigation.
3. Wash hands.	Reduces transfer of microorganisms.
4. Assess condition of external ear structures and canal for redness, swelling, and discharge (see Chapter 16).	Evidence of signs of infection serves as baseline data in determining effectiveness of irrigation.
5. Determine whether client is experiencing localized tenderness or discomfort.	Indicates inflammation of outer ear structures.
6. Prepare equipment and supplies:	
a. Container of sterile irrigating solution warmed to room temperature	Warmed solution minimizes chance of causing client to feel dizzy when solution comes in contact with tympanic membrane.
b. Disposable gloves.	
c. Irrigating syringe (rubber bulb or Asepto)	Used to introduce solution under low pressure.
d. Kidney-shaped basin	Used to collect irrigating solution.
e. Towel	
f. Applicator swab and cotton balls	Used to clean and dry ear canal.
7. Explain procedure. Warn that irrigation may cause sensation of dizziness, fullness, and warmth.	Prepares client to anticipate effects of irrigation and promotes cooperation.
8. Arrange supplies at bedside.	Ensures smooth procedure.
9. Close curtain or room door.	Maintains privacy.
10. Assist client to assume sitting or lying position with head tilted or turned toward affected ear. Place towel under client's head and shoulder and have client hold basin under affected ear. Wash hands and apply gloves.	Position minimizes leakage of fluids around neck and facial area for comfort. Solution will flow from ear canal to basin.
11. Gently clean auricle and ear canal with cotton applicator. Do *not* force drainage or cerumen into ear canal.	Prevents infected material from reentering ear canal.
12. Fill irrigating syringe with solution (approximately 50 ml).	Enough fluid is needed to provide steady irrigating stream.
13. Gently grasp auricle and straighten ear canal by pulling it down and back (children) or upward and outward (adult).	Allows fluid to flow length of canal.
14. Slowly instill irrigating solution by holding tip of syringe 1 cm (½ inch) above opening of ear canal. Allow fluid to drain out during instillation. Continue until canal is cleansed or all solution is used.	Slow instillation prevents buildup of pressure in ear canal and ensures contact of medication with all of canal surfaces.
15. Do *not* occlude canal with tip of syringe.	Buildup of fluid in canal under forced pressure could cause rupture of tympanic membrane.
16. Dry off outer ear canal with cotton ball. Leave cotton loosely in place for 5 to 10 min.	Maintains comfort. Absorbs excess moisture in ear canal.
17. If client was in a lying position, assist client to sitting position.	Maintains comfort.
18. Wash hands and dispose of gloves and supplies.	Reduces transmission of infection.
19. Record and report irrigation solution used, character of ear structures, appearance of fluid return or discharge, and client's response.	Documents response to therapy.

rigated is not sterile, as in the case with the ear canal (Procedure 26-12) or vagina, clean technique is acceptable. In health care settings, however, use sterile solutions. Irrigations can cleanse an area, instill a medication, or apply hot or cold to injured tissue. When performing irrigations, the nurse follows these principles:

1. Avoid further injury to tissue
2. Prevent transmission of infection
3. Maintain client's comfort

SUMMARY

The nurse is responsible for safely and effectively administering medications, which requires understanding of legal guidelines affecting drug prescription and administration. The nurse's care of clients also involves making decisions about the need for drug therapy. The nurse must have detailed knowledge about a drug and the client receiving it. A thorough assessment of the client's physical condition, medical history, allergies, diet, and medication history ensures that accurate judgments will be made about drug therapy.

Preparation of drugs requires accurate calculation and a methodical approach. Application of physiological, anatomical, and aseptic principles ensures safe administration of drugs. When monitoring a response to medications, the nurse uses physical assessment skills and knowledge of expected drug effects. The nurse also teaches clients and families to administer drugs safely and to follow schedules for drug therapy. If medications are given incorrectly, they can injure the client. A client's well-being depends on the nurse's application of all principles of drug administration.

KEY CONCEPTS

- Learning drug classifications improves understanding of nursing implications for administering drugs with similar characteristics.
- Nurse practice acts define and set limits on the scope of a nurse's professional functions and responsibilities in giving medications.
- Federal drug legislation regulates the production, distribution, prescription, and administration of drugs.
- All controlled substances are handled according to strict procedures that account for each drug.
- The nurse applies understanding of the physiology of drug action when timing administration, selecting routes, initiating actions to promote drug efficacy, and observing responses to drugs.
- The older adult's body undergoes structural and functional changes that alter drug actions and influence the manner in which nurses provide drug therapy.
- Children's drug doses are computed on the basis of body surface area or weight.
- Repeated doses of a drug are required to achieve constant therapeutic blood levels.
- Drugs given parenterally are absorbed more quickly than drugs administered by other routes.
- Each drug order should include the client's name, the order date, the drug name, dosage, route and time of administration, and the physician's signature.
- A medication history reveals allergies, drugs a client is taking, and client's compliance with therapy.
- The nursing process should be used when administering medication.
- A teaching plan for drug therapy should include guidelines for drug safety.
- The "five rights" of drug administration ensure accurate preparation and administration of drug doses.
- Nurses administer only medications they prepare.
- Prepared medications are never left unattended.
- The nurse never administers a drug without accurately identifying a client.
- Drugs should be charted immediately after administration.
- A nurse uses clinical judgment in determining the best time to administer prn medications.
- Clients with alterations in kidney or liver function are at risk for drug toxicity.
- The nurse reports a drug error immediately.
- When preparing medications, the nurse checks the drug container label against the medication card, form, or printout three times.
- Air locks prevent tracking of medication through subcutaneous tissues and localize the drug in muscle tissue.
- The Z-track method for intramuscular injections protects subcutaneous tissues from irritating parenteral fluids.
- When administering medications to children, the nurse should attempt to eliminate their fear or negative feelings associated with taking medications.
- Sensory changes in the older client may lead to errors in self-administration of drugs.
- Failure to select injection sites by anatomical landmarks may lead to tissue, bone, or nerve damage.
- The nurse rotates injection sites during repeated parenteral administrations.

CRITICAL THINKING ACTIVITIES

1. Your 84-year-old client is having visual difficulties. What specific interventions should you use to promote compliance and safety in administering medications?
2. When you and another nurse are checking the narcotics at the beginning of the shift, you notice the morphine count is incorrect. What actions should you take? What legal guidelines are involved?
3. In preparing to administer the client's medications, you notice there is no identification band. What are your next actions?
4. After administering all of a client's medications you are informed by another nurse that they were already given 30 minutes before but not charted. What actions are indicated? What actions could prevent future occurrences?
5. In preparing a medication, you discover the physician's order is illegible and you are unsure of the drug dosage. The primary nurse informs you he wrote it correctly on the medication record. What should you do?
6. How is your nursing approach modified when administering medications to infants and children?

References

Abdoo YM: Designing a patient care medication and recording system that uses bar code technology, *Computers in Nursing* 10(3):116, 1992.

American Psychiatric Association: *Diagnostic and statistical manual of mental disorders (DSM-IV),* rev 4, Washington, DC, 1994, The Association.

Ashburn MS, et al.: Oral transmucosal fentanyl citrate for the treatment of breakthrough cancer pain: a case report, *Anesthesiol* 71:615, 1989.

Clark JB, et al.: *Pharmacological basis of nursing practice,* ed 4, St. Louis, 1993, Mosby.

Craft K: Do you really know how to handle sharps?, *RN* 53(8):33, 1990.

Eliopoulos C: Geriatric pharmacology. In Eliopoulos C: *Gerontological nursing,* ed 3, Philadelphia, 1992, JB Lippincott.

Haiduven D, et al.: A five-year study of needlestick injuries: significant reduction associated with communication, education, and convenient placement of sharps containers, *Infect Control Hosp Epidem* 13(5):265, 1992.

Keen MF: Get on the right track with Z-track injections, *Nurs* 20(8):59, 1990.

National Heart, Lung, and Blood Institute: *Guidelines for the diagnosis and management of asthma,* National Asthma Education Program, Expert Panel Report, Pub No 91-3042, Bethesda, Md., 1991, The Institute.

Petrosin BM, et al.: Implications of selected problems with hasoenteral tube feedings, *Crit Care Nurs Q* 12:1, 1989.

Redman BK: *The process of patient education,* ed 6, St. Louis, 1988, Mosby.

Simonson W: *Medications and the elderly: a guide for promoting proper use,* Rockville, Md., 1984, Aspen Publishers.

Taylor HJ: Patients deserve painless injections. . . Z-track technique, *RN* 55(3):25, 1992.

Whaley LF and Wong DL: *Nursing care of infants and children,* ed 4, St. Louis, 1991, Mosby.

Bibliography

Albanese JA and Nutz PA: *Mosby's nursing drug cards,* St. Louis, 1993, Mosby.

Ali N: Promoting safe use of multiple medications by elderly persons, *Geriatric Nurs* 13(3):157, 1992.

Bernstein LH, et al.: Portable medicine pumps in primary care, *Patient Care* 27(3):91, 1993.

Cawley MM: Recent advances in chemotherapy: administration and nursing implications, *Nurs Clin North Am* 25(2):377, 1990.

Cohen MR: Even night drug cabinet can cause problems, *Nursing* 22(7):9, 1992.

Cohen MR: Help new nurses avoid making errors, *Nursing* 22(4):21, 1992.

Decker M: The OSHA blood-borne hazard standard, *Infect Control Hospital Epidem* 13(7):407, 1992.

Dick L: Warning: take only as directed, *RN* 52(10):83, 1989.

Dickerson RJ: 10 tips for easing the pain of intramuscular injections, *Nursing* 22(8):55, 1992.

Drass J: What you need to know about insulin injections, *Nursing* 22(8):55, 1992.

Faut-Callahan M: Update on drug interventions, *Nurs Clin North Am* 26(2):xi, 1991.

Ferris M: Proper med pass techniques ensure resident safety, *Provider* 18(3):46, 1992.

Gahart BL: *A handbook of intravenous medications,* ed 7, St. Louis, 1992, Mosby.

Glassman SK and Measel CP: A makeshift mini-bottle: accurate small fluid or oral medication administration to infants, Neonatal Network-*J Neonatal Nursing* 7(4), 1989.

Hahn K and Wietor G: Helpful tools for medication screenings, *Geriatric Nurs* 13(3):160, 1992.

Helliwell M and Taylor D: Solid oral dosage forms, *Professional Nurse* 8(5):313, 1993.

Irvine L and Vogt T: We put IV therapy down on paper, *RN* 56(1):34, 1993.

Kudzma E: Drug response: all bodies are not created equal, *Am J Nurs* 92(12):48, 1992.

McConnell EA: Applying nitroglycerin ointment correctly, *Nursing* 20(8):70, 1990.

McFarland GK and McFarlane E: *Nursing diagnosis and intervention,* ed 3, St. Louis, 1993, Mosby.

McKenry L and Salerno E: *Pharmacology in nursing,* ed 18, St. Louis, 1992, Mosby.

McMullen A, et al.: Heparinized saline or normal saline as a flush solution in intermittent intravenous lines in infants and children, *J Mat Child Nurs* 18(2):78, 1993.

Messner R and Gardner S: Start with the medicine cabinet, *RN* 56(1):51, 1993.

Newton M, et al.: Reviewing the "big three" injection routes, *Nursing* 22(2):34, 1992.

Pauca AL: Constant-rate drug infusions: two methods of preparation, *AANA Journal* 56(6):537, 1988.

Radcliff RK and Ogden SJ: *Calculations of drug dosages,* ed 4, St. Louis, 1991, Mosby.

Rudy D: A drop or a dropper: the risk of overdose, *J Ped Health Care* 6(1):40, 1992.

Rydberg S: Robo-Pill, *Computers in Nursing* 11(1):6, 1993.

Santo-Novak D and Edwards RM: Rx: take caution with drugs for elders, *Geriatric Nurs* 10(2):72, 1989.

Sharts-Engel NC: Inhaled steroids for children with asthma, *Am J Mat Child Nurs* 17(2):112, 1992.

Sherman JJ and Clinefelter K: Medication variances: a multi-hospital comparison, *Nurs Management* 20(5):56, 1989.

Skidmore-Roth L: *Mosby's 1993 nursing drug reference,* St. Louis, 1993, Mosby.

Todd B: Intravenous drug hazards: interactions, adsorption, and inadequate mixing, *Geriatric Nurs* 9(1):20, 1988.

Williams PJ: How do you keep medicines from clogging feeding tubes?, *Am J Nurs* 89(2):29, 1989.

Wink DM: Giving infants and children drugs: precision + caution = safety, *Am J Mat Child Nurs* 16(6):317, 1991.

Wolf ZR: Medication errors and nursing responsibility, *Holistic Nurs Pract* 4(1):8, 1989.

27 Sleep

OBJECTIVES

Mastery of content in this chapter will enable the student to:

- Define the key terms listed.
- Compare the characteristics of sleep and rest.
- Explain the effect of a 24-hour sleep-wake cycle on biological function.
- Discuss the mechanisms that regulate sleep.
- Describe the stages of a normal sleep cycle.
- Explain the functions of sleep.
- Compare the sleep requirements of different age-groups.
- Identify factors that normally promote and disrupt sleep.
- Discuss characteristics of common sleep disorders.
- Conduct a comprehensive sleep history
- Identify nursing diagnoses appropriate for clients with sleep alterations.
- Identify nursing interventions designed to promote a normal sleep cycle for clients of all ages.
- Describe ways to evaluate sleep therapies.

KEY TERMS

apnea
biological clock
bulbar synchronizing region (BSR)
central sleep apnea
circadian rhythm
insomnia
monoamine oxidase inhibitor
narcolepsy
nocturnal enuresis
nonREM sleep
obstructive sleep apnea
polysomnogram
rapid eye movement (REM) sleep
reticular activating system (RAS)
sleep
sleep deprivation
sleep disorder

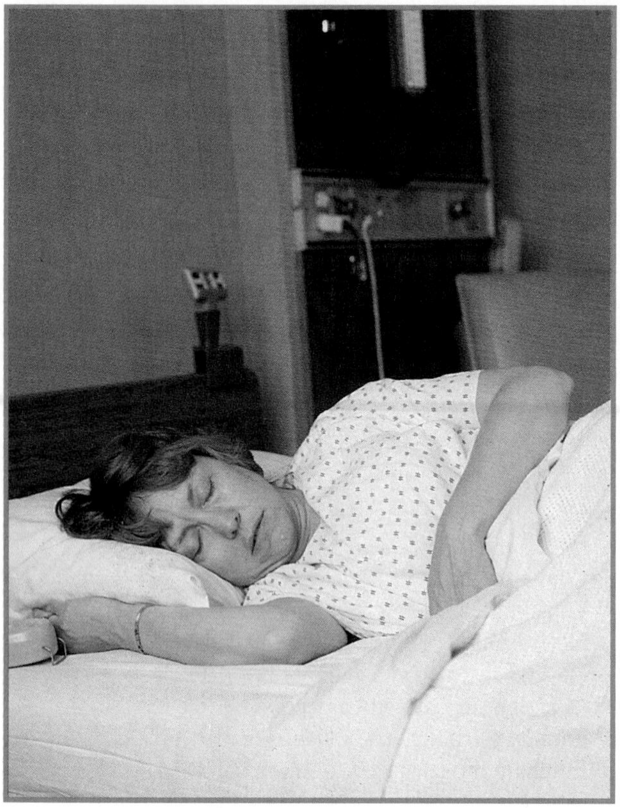

Sleep and rest are basic to the quality of life. Different people need different amounts and qualities of rest and sleep. Without rest and sleep, the ability to concentrate, make judgments, and participate in daily activities decreases while irritability increases. The nurse cares for clients who have preexisting sleep disturbances and clients who develop sleep problems as a result of health alterations.

A sleep disturbance may cause a client to seek health care or problems may go unnoticed for years. When a person becomes ill, increased rest and sleep are often required for normal recovery. However, the nature and implications of an illness may prevent the client from gaining adequate rest and sleep. Hospitalized clients must face the problem of inadequate rest and sleep as a result of the routines health care personnel follow. Unpredictable scheduling and the hectic-paced environment of a hospital make it difficult for clients to sleep.

To help a client gain needed rest and sleep, a nurse must understand the nature of sleep, the factors influencing it, and each client's unique sleep habits. Each client requires an individualized approach. A nurse's interventions can be effective for short- and long-term sleep disturbances.

SLEEP AND REST

A person at rest feels mentally relaxed, free from anxiety, and physically calm. Rest is a state of decreased mental and physical activity that leaves a person feeling refreshed, rejuvenated, and ready to resume the activities of the day. Each person has personal habits for gaining rest such as reading a book, practicing a relaxation exercise (Chapter 28), or taking a long walk. Physical inactivity such as bed rest does not always imply a state of rest because such a client may have emotional worries that prevent complete relaxation.

Sleep is a recurrent, altered state of consciousness that occurs for sustained periods, restoring a person's energy and well-being. Fordham (1988) defines sleep in two ways: first as a discrete state of reduced responsiveness to external stimuli, from which a person can be aroused; second as a continuous cyclical change in level of consciousness. These definitions help explain why people occasionally have problems with the state of sleep or with the scheduling of sleep, and sometimes with both (Hodgson, 1991).

The rest and sleep habits of clients entering a health care facility can easily be changed by illness or disruptions within the health care environment. Illness may have already caused a sleep disturbance. The nurse plays an important role in understanding the causes of sleep disturbances and helping clients to learn the value of rest and ways to promote it at home or in the health care environment. Conditions that promote proper rest include the following:

1. Physical comfort
   a. Eliminating sources of physical irritation
      Keeping sheets dry and smooth
      Providing frequent mouth care
   b. Controlling sources of pain
      Providing analgesics before pain becomes severe
   c. Providing warmth
      Controlling room temperature
      Offering extra blankets
   d. Maintaining hygiene
      Keeping the skin clean and dry
      Providing dry clothing
   e. Maintaining proper anatomical alignment or positioning
      Turning frequently
      Supporting painful extremities
   f. Removing environmental distractions
      Closing room doors
   g. Providing adequate ventilation
2. Freedom from worry
   a. Making decisions
      Asking a neighbor to pick up medications from a pharmacy
      Choosing not to attend a social event

b. Participating in personal health care
Following a daily exercise routine
c. Gaining an understanding of health problems and their implications
Attending a support group
d. Practicing restful activities regularly
Reading a book nightly
e. Knowing the environment is safe
Installing dead bolt locks and an outdoor lighting system for the home

3. Sufficient sleep
a. Obtaining average hours of sleep needed to avoid fatigue
Going to bed at a regular hour
b. Following good sleep hygiene habits
Avoiding intake of caffeine before bedtime

PHYSIOLOGY OF SLEEP

Sleep is a set of complex physiological processes resulting from the interaction of many different neurochemical systems within the brain and associated with changes in the peripheral nervous, endocrine, cardiovascular, respiratory, and muscular systems (Hoch and Reynolds, 1986; Closs, 1988; and Hodgson, 1991). Each sequence can be identified by specific behaviors, physiological responses, and patterns of brain activity. Sleep is a cyclical phenomenon.

Circadian Rhythms

Each person's life is a series of cyclical rhythms influencing and regulating physiological function and behavioral responses. The most familiar rhythm is the 24-hour, day-night cycle known as the diurnal or **circadian rhythm.** The fluctuation and predictability of body temperature, heart rate, hormone and electrolyte secretions, and mood depend on the circadian cycle. Another rhythm is the woman's menstrual cycle, an **infradian rhythm** (longer than 24 hours). Biological cycles lasting less than 24 hours are called **ultradian rhythms.**

Circadian rhythms, including daily sleep-wake cycles, are most affected by light and temperature; other stimuli such as social and occupational habits can also be influential. All people have **biological clocks** that synchronize their sleep cycle. People have different preferred sleep times and function best at different times of the day. Hospitals or extended-care facilities often fail to adapt care to an individual's preference for sleep. If a person's sleep-wake cycle is altered significantly, poor quality sleep results. Reversals of the sleep-wake cycle can signal serious illness.

The biological rhythm of sleep frequently becomes synchronized with other bodily functions such as body temperature. When a person's sleep-wake cycle changes (e.g., by rotating job shifts), numerous physiological functions may also change.

Sleep Regulation

A single cause for sleep has not been discovered. The control of sleep is not confined to one localized part of the brain (Hodgson, 1991). Instead many different neurochemical systems interact within the brain to regulate sleep. Areas of the brain believed to influence sleep control are the **reticular activating system (RAS)** located in the upper brainstem and the **bulbar synchronizing region (BSR)** in the pons and medial forebrain. These systems are believed to work together, alternately activating and suppressing the brain's higher centers to control sleep.

The RAS is believed to contain special cells that maintain alertness and wakefulness. The RAS receives visual sensory input and auditory, pain, and tactile stimuli. Activity from the cerebral cortex (e.g., emotions) also stimulates the RAS. Biddle and Oaster (1990) and Chuman (1983) suggest that wakefulness results from neurons in the RAS releasing neurotransmitters such as norepinephrine, dopamine, and GABA (gamma-aminobutyric acid). Biddle and Oaster (1990) write that sleep is a complex intertwining of the central nervous system, its neurotransmitters, and a person's behavior.

Sleep may be produced by the release of serotonin from specialized cells in the BSR. Whether a person stays awake or falls asleep depends on a balance of impulses received from the cerebral cortex (e.g., thoughts), peripheral sensory receptors (e.g., sound or light) and the limbic system (emotions) (Figure 27-1).

As a person begins to fall asleep and relax, stimuli to the RAS decline. If the room is generally dark and quiet, activation of the RAS further declines. At some point the BSR takes over, causing a person to fall asleep.

Stages of Sleep

Sleep involves two phases: nonrapid eye movement **(NREM)** and rapid eye movement **(REM)** sleep (see box on p. 722). During NREM a sleeper progresses through four stages during a typical sleep cycle. These stages do not occur once but cycle back and forth several times during the course of sleep (Hodgson, 1991). At the end of each NREM phase, REM sleep typically occurs. Various factors interfere with the sleep stages. The nurse learns to choose therapies that foster sleep or attempts to eliminate factors that can disrupt sleep.

Sleep Cycle. The normal adult sleep pattern begins with a presleep period during which the person is aware only of a gradually developing drowsiness. Presleep usually lasts 10 to 30 minutes, but if a person has trouble falling asleep, it may last more than 1 hour.

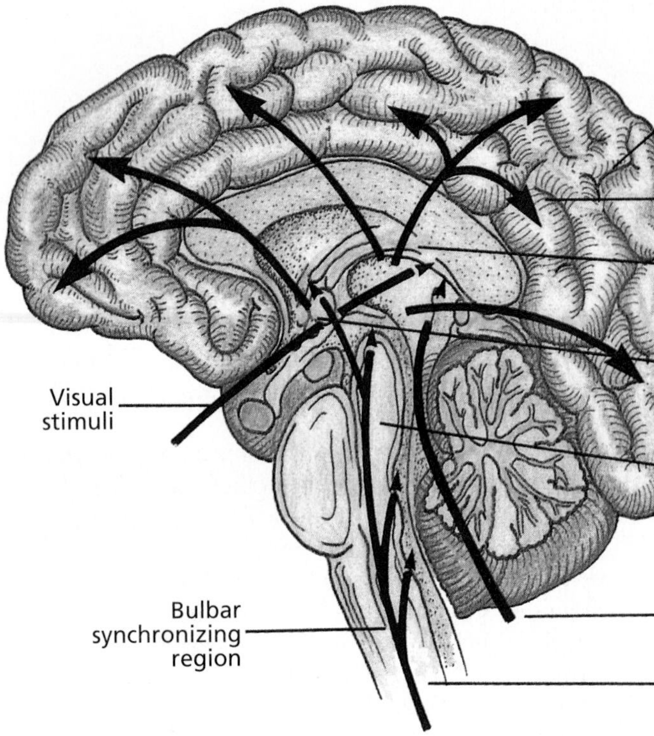

FIGURE 27-1 RAS and BSR control sensory input, intermittently activating and suppressing brain's higher centers to control sleep and wakefulness.

STAGES OF SLEEP

STAGE 1: NONREM

Lightest level of sleep
Lasts a few minutes
Decreased physiological activity beginning with a gradual fall in vital signs and metabolism
Person easily aroused by sensory stimuli such as noise
If person awakes, feels as though daydreaming has occurred
Reduction in autonomic activities (e.g., heart rate)

STAGE 2: NONREM

Period of sound sleep
Relaxation progresses
Arousal still easy
Lasts 10 to 20 minutes
Body functions still slowing

STAGE 3: NONREM

Initial stages of deep sleep
Sleeper difficult to arouse and rarely moves
Muscles completely relaxed
Vital signs decline but remain regular
Lasts 15 to 30 minutes
Hormonal response includes secretion of growth hormone

STAGE 4: NONREM

Deepest stage of sleep
Very difficult to arouse sleeper
If sleep loss has occurred, sleeper will spend most of night in this stage
Restores and rests the body
Vital signs significantly lower than during waking hours
Lasts approximately 15 to 30 minutes
Possible sleepwalking and enuresis
Hormonal response continues

REM SLEEP

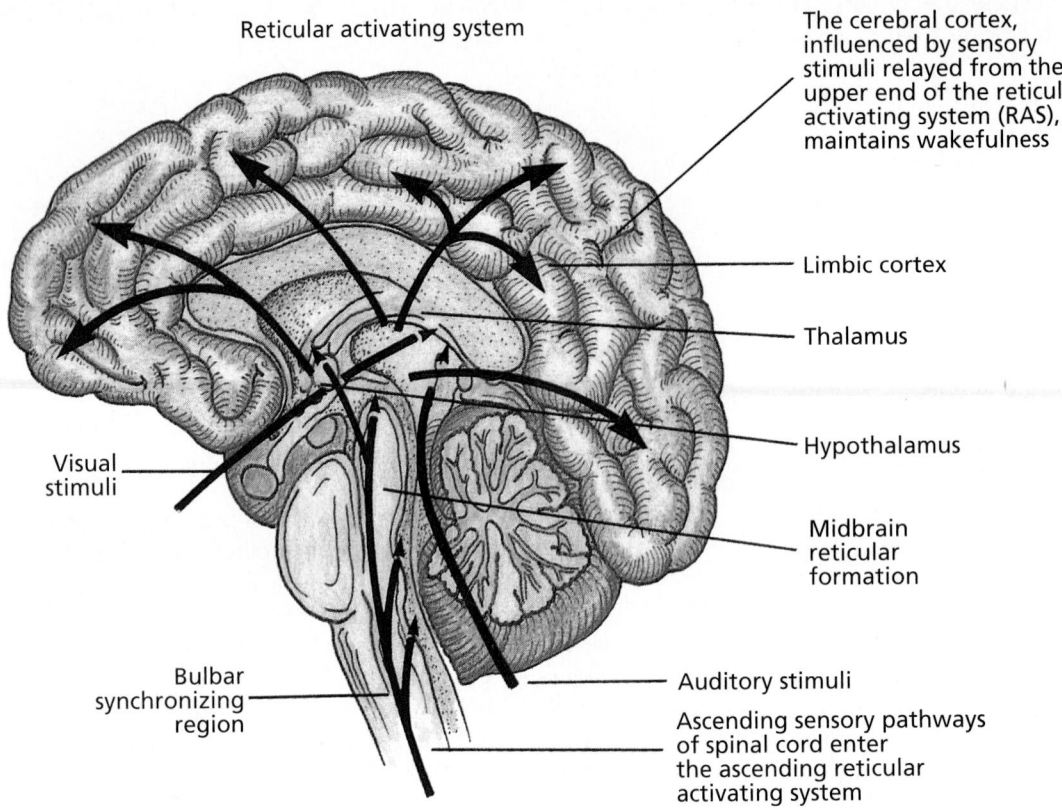

Stage of vivid, full-color dreaming (less vivid dreaming may occur in other stages)
First occurs approximately 90 minutes after sleep has begun, thereafter occurs at end of each NREM cycle
Typified by autonomic response of rapidly moving eyes, fluctuating heart and respiratory rates, and increased or fluctuating blood pressure
Loss of skeletal muscle tone
Responsible for mental restoration
Stage in which sleeper is most difficult to arouse
Duration increasing with each cycle and averaging 20 minutes

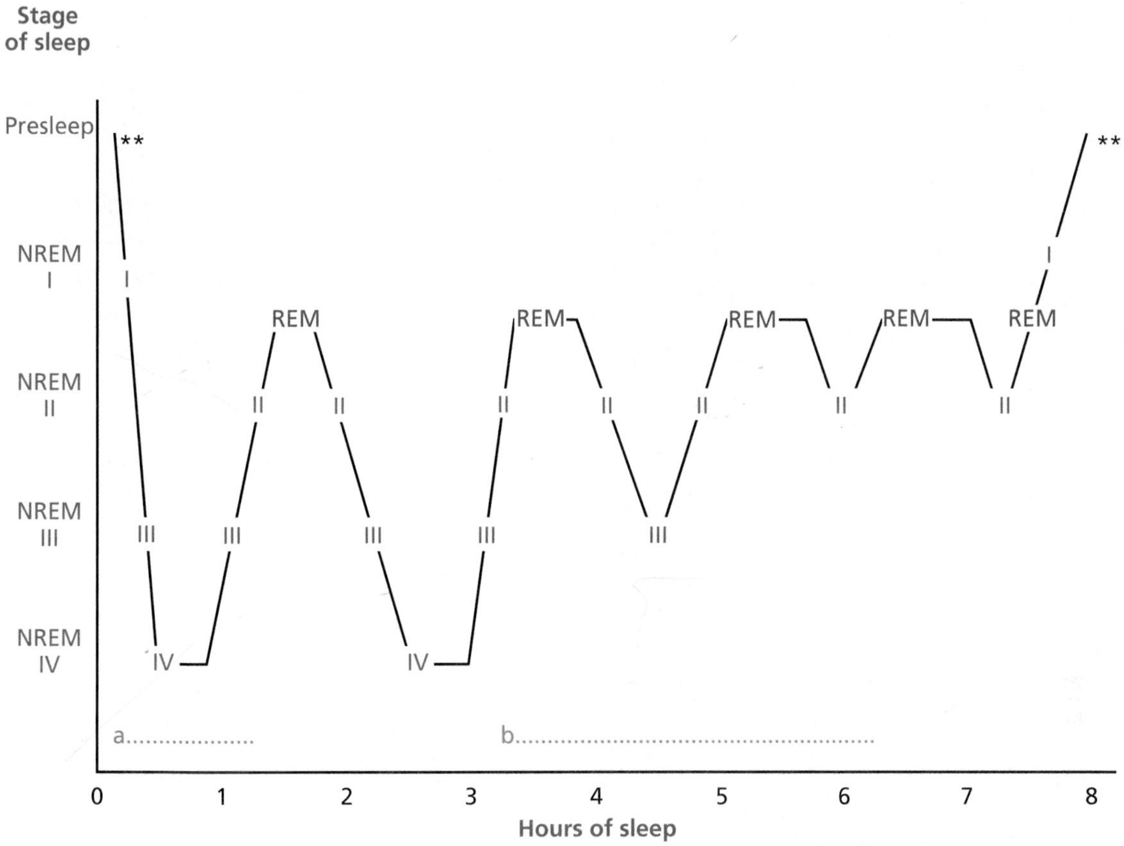

FIGURE 27-2 Normal adult sleep cycle and the stages of sleep. (Modified from Biddle C and Oaster TRF: *J Am Assoc Nurs Anesthet* 58(1):36, 1990.)

Following presleep, the first 90 minutes or so of human sleep is characterized by NREM, with a person moving progressively through four stages into a deep sleep (Biddle and Oaster, 1990). As a sleeper progresses through NREM sleep, the quality of sleep becomes increasingly deep. Light sleep is characteristic of stages 1 and 2, and a person is easily arousable. Stages 3 and 4 involve a deeper sleep. After reaching stage 4, the sleep pattern reverses back from stage 4 to 3 to 2, ending with a period of REM sleep (Figure 27-2). During REM the sleeper is very difficult to arouse.

With each full sleep cycle, stages 3 and 4 shorten, and the period of REM lengthens. REM sleep may last 30 to 60 minutes during the last sleep cycle. If a person awakens from sleep during any stage, sleep begins again at stage 1. Consistent interruption in the sleep cycle can ultimately lead to sleep deprivation.

Not all people progress consistently through the sleep stages. The amount of time spent in each stage also varies. The number of sleep cycles depends on the total amount of time a person sleeps.

FUNCTIONS OF SLEEP

Researchers have proposed sleep to be restorative, protective, instinctive, and serving to readjust or conserve biological systems (Hodgson, 1991; and Chuman, 1983). During NREM sleep a person's biological functions slow. For example, a healthy adult's heart rate averaging 70 to 80 beats per minute drops during sleep to around 60 to 70 beats per minute or less, thereby decreasing the heart's workload. In normal sleep, systemic blood pressure declines an average 5 to 10 percent in stages 3 and 4 NREM sleep (Parish and Shepard, 1990).

Much discussion centers around the theory that sleep serves to repair and renew epithelial and specialized cells such as brain tissue. Children experience more stage 4 NREM sleep, during which the production of growth hormone for bone growth and protein synthesis is triggered. Energy is conserved during NREM sleep by the absence of muscular contraction and a lowered basal metabolic rate. Some human tissue (e.g., the epidermis) has an increase in cell division within usual sleep periods. The question is, are most of these physiological responses caused by sleep or do they occur at a time of day coincident with sleep?

Hodgson (1991) notes that evidence for the function of sleep has been obtained from studying the effects of lack of sleep (sleep deprivation). People who experience sleep deprivation have been shown to undergo behavioral changes. When tested in skills requiring speed and prolonged concentration, sleep deprived persons have difficulty maintaining focused attention. Undemanding, tedious, uninteresting, and simple tasks are the first to become impaired. These effects on mental functioning suggest that sleep is necessary for brain restitution.

Horne (1983) is a researcher who suggests that not all human sleep is essential. She asked volunteers to take 1 to 2 hours less sleep per day for at least 8 to 12 months. The subjects of the study did not experience day-time sleepiness or any other consequences. Horne suggests that interrupted or disturbed sleep is the major cause of daytime sleepiness, and not simply less sleep. Therefore 5 to 6 hours of sound sleep is better than 8 hours of disturbed sleep.

REM sleep appears to be a critical cycle of brain activity important for learning, memory, and behavioral adaptation. Deprivation of REM sleep can affect mood and basic drives. Gribbin (1990) suggests that REM sleep is more important than non-REM sleep for a person's well-being. Experiments have shown that a minimum ration of fantasy dreams is needed each day. Sleep and dreaming enable a person to solve problems, gain new insights, clarify emotions, and prepare the mind for events of the next day. REM sleep comprises only one quarter of total adult sleep. As long as one's normal quota of REM sleep is achieved, the total length of the sleep period is unimportant. This may explain why some people require less overall sleep than others (Hodgson, 1991).

Dreams

Dreams occur during NREM and REM sleep. The dreams of REM sleep are more vivid and elaborate. REM dreams progress in content during the night from dreams about current events to emotional dreams of childhood or the past. Personality can also influence the quality of dreams; for example, a depressed person often dreams of helplessness.

Most people dream about immediate concerns such as an argument with a spouse. Sometimes a person is unaware of fears represented in bizarre dreams. Psychologists attempt to analyze the symbolic nature and occurrence of dreams as a basis for psychotherapy. Sigmund Freud believed that dreams were a product of unconscious wishes that released psychological tensions. Jung suggested that dreaming is a kind of processing that is ongoing but surfaces in sleep (Hartmann, 1984). Another theory suggests that dreams serve to erase fantasies or nonsensical memories. Dreaming may be the brain's way of sorting and filing our recent experiences (Biddle and Oaster, 1990).

Most dreams are forgotten because during REM sleep consolidation of short-term memory is impaired. To remember a dream, a person must consciously think about it on awakening. People who recall dreams vividly usually awake just after a period of REM sleep.

Normal Sleep Requirements and Patterns

Sleep duration and quality vary among age-groups (see box on p. 725). One person may function well with 4 hours of sleep, whereas another requires 10 hours. Figure 27-3 shows the change in the distribution of sleep stages during life.

FACTORS AFFECTING SLEEP

Sleep is not always easy to attain. Factors that promote sleep in one person may hinder sleep in another. Physiological and psychological factors may alter the quality and quantity of sleep (see box on p. 726).

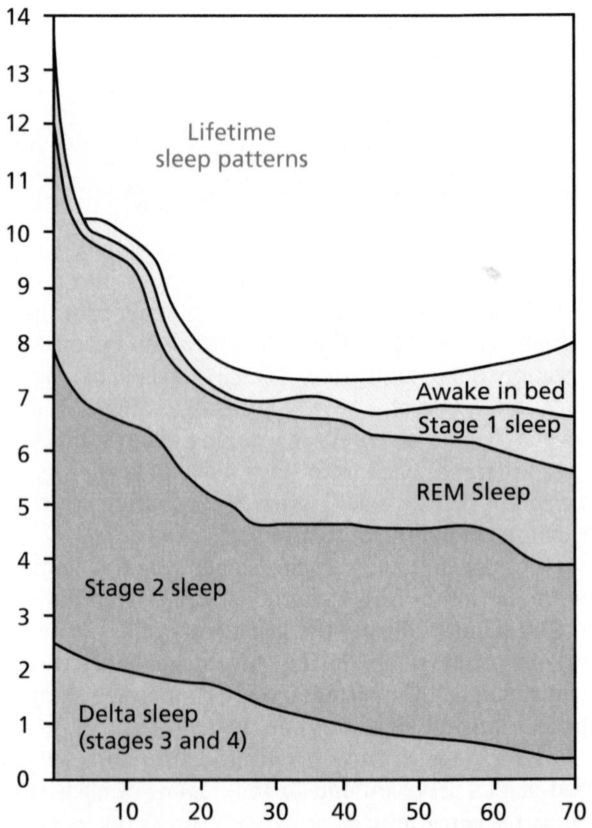

FIGURE 27-3 Distribution of sleep stages over life span. (From Berman TM, Nino-Murcia G, Roehrs T: *Patient Care* 24:85, 1990.)

SLEEP REQUIREMENTS OF DIFFERENT AGE-GROUPS

NEONATES*

Average 16 hours of sleep daily with a range of 10 to 23 hours.

Infants born of unmedicated mothers enter the world in a state of wakefulness with eyes wide open and sucking is vigorous.

Hunger, pain, and cold often cause crying.

During first week, neonate sleeps almost constantly to recover from birth with almost 50% of sleep being REM sleep.

The newborn experiences five distinct states of sleep: regular sleep, irregular sleep, drowsiness, alert inactivity, and waking and crying.

INFANTS*

Active infants sleep less than quiet infants.

Develop nighttime pattern of sleep by 3 to 4 months of age.

Infant may take several naps daily but usually sleeps an average of 8 to 10 hours during the night.

Breast-fed infants usually sleep less, with frequent waking, than a bottle-fed infant.

An infant between 1 month and 1 year of age sleeps an average of 14 hours daily with REM sleep predominating.

TODDLERS*

By age 2, children usually sleep through the night and take daily naps.

Total sleep averages 12 hours daily.

Daily naps are common but cease at 3 years.

PRESCHOOLERS

Child averages 12 hours of sleep nightly and rarely takes naps.

Preschooler has difficulty relaxing or quieting down after an active day.

A preschooler has problems with bedtime fears, waking during the night, or nightmares.

Bedtime rituals help parents to get active preschoolers to bed.

SCHOOL-AGE CHILDREN

Amount of sleep required varies by state of activity and level of health.

Naps are usually not required.

Older children may resist sleeping because of an unawareness of fatigue or a need to be independent.

90-minute adult sleep cycle is in place.

Child will be tired the following day if allowed to stay up later than usual.

ADOLESCENTS

Adolescent averages 8 to 9 hours of sleep nightly.

Because of staying up late, an adolescent often sleeps late in the mornings.

Rapid physical growth and an active life-style can cause fatigue.

YOUNG ADULTS

Adult requires rest and sleep but busy life-style may interrupt sleep pattern.

Young adults average 6 to 8½ hours of sleep nightly.

Stress often leads to use of medications, but their long-term use disrupts sleep patterns and causes other health problems.

MIDDLE ADULTS

Total time spent sleeping at night begins to decline with the amount of stage 4 NREM sleep falling.

Sleep disturbances are common and generally caused by anxiety, depression, or certain physical ailments.

Women with menopausal symptoms may experience insomnia.

OLDER ADULTS

The total amount of sleep does not change as age increases, but this is due to an increase in time asleep during daily naps.

The need for increased rest occurs earlier than the need for increased sleep.

Duration of nighttime sleep declines with shortening of REM sleep and a decrease in stage 3 and 4 NREM sleep.†

Older adults awaken more during the night and often take more time to fall asleep.‡

Changes in the CNS, sensory impairment, and chronic illnesses influence an older adult's sleep pattern.

*Data from Whaley, LF, Wong, DL: *Nursing care of infants and children,* ed 4, St. Louis, 1991, Mosby.

†Kales A, Kales J: Sleep disorders; recent findings in the diagnosis and treatment of disturbed sleep, *N Engl J Med* 290:487, 1974.

‡Ross MS, et al.: When sleep won't come: helping our elderly clients, *Can Nurs* 82:14, 1986.

SLEEP DISORDERS

Sleep disorders are conditions that repeatedly disrupt a person's pattern of sleep. They are common among clients. Research shows that most adults in the United States have significant sleep debts from cumulative sleep losses (Berman, et al., 1990). The best way to diagnose sleep disorders is by a nighttime **polysomnogram,** which uses electrodes to measure a sleeping client's electrical brain waves (EEG), extraocular eye movements (EOG), and chin and facial muscle movements (EMG).

FACTORS AFFECTING SLEEP

PHYSICAL ILLNESS

Pain or physical discomfort result in difficulty falling or staying asleep.

Chronic pain may have a circadian rhythm of increasing intensity at night, thus disrupting sleep (Glyn et al., 1976).

Illness may force clients to sleep in positions to which they are unaccustomed.

Respiratory diseases interfere with the rhythm of breathing or influence the position a person must assume to breath easily. Both factors can disturb sleep.

Clients with heart disease are often afraid to go to sleep at night.

Hypertension causes early morning awakening and fatigue.

Nocturia and "restless leg syndrome" disrupt sleep, causing clients to awaken during the night and often result in difficulty resuming sleep.

Conditions that increase intracranial pressure or alter central nervous system physiology alter sleep patterns and can cause excessive day-time sleeping.

ANXIETY AND DEPRESSION

As anxiety and depression increase, so does lack of sleep and, as sleep decreases, anxiety and depression increase (Hodgson, 1991).

The bereaved often experience sleep problems related to fear of intruders, loneliness, and the dreams or nightmares that occur involving the lost loved one.

DRUGS AND SUBSTANCES

Various drugs and substances affect the pattern and quality of sleep (see box on p. 727).

Older adults often take several drugs, the combined effects of which disrupt sleep.

L-Tryptophan, a protein found in foods such as milk, cheese, and meats, may help induce sleep.

LIFE-STYLE

Daily routines such as working rotating shifts influence sleep patterns. Only after several weeks of working a night shift does a person's biological clock adjust.

Performing unaccustomed heavy work, late-night social activities, and changing evening mealtimes are activities that can disrupt sleep.

SLEEP PATTERNS

Sleep patterns include starting time and duration of sleep.

The most significant cause of daytime sleepiness is inadequate or abnormal sleep at night (Berman et al., 1990).

Everyone has an increased sleep tendency from 2 AM to 7AM and to a lesser degree from 2 AM to 5 PM (Mitler et al., 1988). When sleep patterns are disrupted, the natural tendency to be sleeping at select times increases.

Sleep patterns influence succeeding attempts to fall asleep because of changes in circadian rhythm. Sleeping 1 hour later results in falling asleep 1 hour later the next night.

Chronic lack of sleep can alter the ability to perform daily functions such as driving.

STRESS

Stress resulting from personal problems or situational crises causes tension and may cause a person to try too hard to fall asleep, to awaken frequently, or to oversleep.

Stress causes release of corticosteroids and adrenalin, which leads to catabolism and sleeplessness.

Clients with advanced cancer or chronic illness often are afraid to sleep in case they might die.

Older clients experience losses such as retirement or death of a loved one. Thus older adults can suffer delays in falling asleep, earlier REM sleep, frequent awakening, increased total bed time, and feelings of sleeping poorly (Colling, 1983).

ENVIRONMENT

Environmental factors influence the ability to fall and remain asleep. Significant factors include ventilation, lighting, type of bed, sound level, and the presence or absence of a bed partner.

In hospitals, unfamiliar noises and higher noise levels such as that created by wall suction, opening packages, ringing alarms, and flushing toilets can cause sleep deprivation.

Intensive care units are sources for high noise levels.

EXERCISE AND FATIGUE

Exercise and fatigue in moderation usually facilitate restful sleep, but excess fatigue from exhausting or stressful work can make falling asleep difficult.

Exercise 2 hours before bedtime allows the body to cool down and promotes relaxation.

NUTRITION

Weight gain causes longer sleep periods with fewer interruptions and later awakening.

Weight loss can cause reduction in total sleep along with broken sleep and earlier awakening.

DRUGS AND THEIR EFFECTS ON SLEEP

HYPNOTICS

Interfere with reaching deeper sleep stages
Provide only temporary (1 week) increase in quantity of sleep
Eventually cause "hangover" during day: excess drowsiness, confusion, decreased energy
May worsen sleep apnea in older adults

DIURETICS

Cause nocturia

ANTIDEPRESSANTS AND STIMULANTS

Suppress REM sleep

ALCOHOL

Speeds onset of sleep
Disrupts REM sleep
Awakens person during the night and causes difficulty in returning to sleep

CAFFEINE

Prevents person from falling asleep
May cause person to awaken during night

DIGOXIN

Causes nightmares

BETA BLOCKERS

Cause nightmares
Cause insomnia
Cause awakening from sleep

VALIUM

Decreases stages 2, 4, and REM sleep
Decreases awakenings

NARCOTICS (MORPHINE/DEMEROL)

Suppress REM sleep
If discontinued quickly, can increase risk of cardiac dysrythmias because of "rebound REM" periods
Cause increased awakenings and drowsiness

Insomnia

Insomnia is a symptom wherein a person has chronic difficulty falling asleep (initial insomnia), difficulty remaining asleep (intermittent insomnia), or inability to resume sleep after awakening (terminal insomnia). The client with insomnia complains of insufficient quantity and quality of sleep but usually sleeps more than he or she realizes. Insomnia can cause daytime sleepiness, fatigue, depression, and anxiety, and it may signal an underlying physical or psychological disorder.

Insomnia may be temporary as a result of situational crises (e.g., jet lag or illness) or may continue for years. It can develop at any age. Insomnia may recur, but between episodes the client is able to sleep well. A temporary case of insomnia, however, can lead to a chronic problem.

Insomnia is most commonly associated with poor sleep habits. If the condition continues, the fear of not being able to sleep can cause wakefulness. Because there are many causes of insomnia, management involves several approaches. First, it is important to treat underlying emotional or medical problems. Treatment is usually symptomatic, including improved sleep hygiene measures, biofeedback, and relaxation techniques. In drug dependence insomnia the client is unable to fall asleep because of excessive use of hypnotics. A gradual withdrawal of the drug should help.

Sleep Apnea

Sleep apnea is the cessation of breathing for a time during sleep. Apnea is the cessation of airflow through the nose and mouth for at least 10 seconds, resulting in a reduction in oxygen level of a person's blood. A serious decline in arterial oxygen levels can create risks for cardiac dysrhythmias, right heart failure, angina, stroke, and hypertension. The most frequent time of naturally occurring death is between 4AM and 6AM, and some researchers believe sleep apneas are a cause (Berman, et al., 1990). There are three types: central, obstructive, and mixed.

The most common form, **obstructive sleep apnea,** occurs when muscles or structures of the oral cavity or throat relax during sleep. The upper airway becomes blocked and nasal airflow stops. The person still tries to breathe because chest and abdominal movement continue. During apnea, each successive diaphragmatic movement becomes stronger until the obstruction is relieved. Structural abnormalities such as a deviated septum or enlarged tonsils can result in obstructive apnea. However, most clients with sleep apnea have anatomically normal airways (Berman, et al., 1990).

Central apnea involves defects in the brain's respiratory center. The impulse to breathe temporarily fails, and nasal airflow and chest wall movement cease. The condition is seen in clients with brain stem injury, muscular dystrophy, and encephalitis. No treatment exists for central sleep apnea. **Mixed sleep apnea** involves a combination of decreased ventilatory drive and upper airway obstruction.

A person with sleep apnea typically snores. Obstruction of the upper airway may last as long as 30 to 60 seconds. The client rarely awakens. The client is also deprived of deep sleep periods. Complaints of daytime sleepiness, sleep attacks, fatigue, morning headaches, and decreased sex drive are common. Treatment includes therapy for underlying cardiac or respiratory complications and emotional problems. Sleep hygiene and weight-loss therapy can also help. One of the most effective therapies is use of a nasal continuous positive airway pressure (CPAP) device at night. CPAP requires a client to wear a mask over the nose. Room air is delivered through the mask at a high pressure, which keeps the airway open. In cases of severe obstructive apnea, surgical removal of portions of the pharynx and palate may be attempted.

Narcolepsy

Narcolepsy is a chronic, incurable dysfunction of REM sleep processes and of mechanisms regulating sleeping and waking states (Bergstrom and Keller, 1992). During the day a person experiences excessive sleepiness. A person may suddenly feel an overwhelming wave of sleepiness and fall asleep, even in unusual situations such as while having a conversation. REM sleep can occur within 15 minutes of falling asleep. These attacks may occur 2 to 6 times a day and last for more than 30 minutes. **Cataplexy** is a symptom of narcolepsy involving a brief sudden loss of muscle control occurring during intense emotions such as anger, sadness, or laughter. This symptom may result in a client falling or collapsing. A client with narcolepsy may also have hallucinations just when falling asleep. The client may not know the difference between a dream and reality. Sleep paralysis, or the feeling of being unable to move or talk just before waking or falling asleep, is another symptom. Studies show a genetic link for narcolepsy (Kales, et al., 1987).

The greatest problem with narcolepsy is falling asleep at inappropriate times. Attacks are most likely to occur in sedentary, unstimulating situations, such as watching television or driving (Bergstrom and Keller, 1992). Persons suffering narcolepsy often have driving accidents. Unless a client and family understand the disorder, a sleep attack can easily be mistaken for laziness, lack of interest in activities, or drunkenness. A client with narcolepsy frequently experiences psychosocial consequences that may affect interpersonal relations, vocation and educational endeavors, and marital and family relationships.

Combination drug therapy may help to control the symptoms of narcolepsy. Sleep attacks are treated with central nervous system stimulants such as Ritalin (methylphenidate) and Cylert (pemoline), which increase alertness and wakefulness and diminish the sense of fatigue. Brief daytime naps no longer than 20 minutes help reduce narcoleptic attacks. Factors that increase a narcoleptic's drowsiness (e.g., liquor or exhausting activities) should be avoided.

Sleep Deprivation

Although not a true sleep disorder, **sleep deprivation** is a problem for many clients. It involves a decrease in the amount, quality, and consistency of sleep. When sleep becomes interrupted or fragmented, changes in the normal sequence of sleep stages occur, and cycles cannot be completed (Fisher, 1984). Over time, cumulative sleep deprivation occurs in persons who receive "usual" hours of sleep. Thus a person with insomnia may develop sleep deprivation. Sleep deprivation is a common problem for those who care for loved ones with advanced disease at home. A care giver can experience serious sleep deprivation, as a result of circadian rhythms being disrupted over the long term (Hodgson, 1991).

A client's response to sleep deprivation is highly variable. Clients may experience physiological symptoms such as hand tremors, decreased reflexes, slowed response time, reduced word memory, and decreased reasoning and judgment. Other physiological effects include fall in body temperature, slight changes in cardiovascular and respiratory function, slight hormonal changes, and changes in control of eye movements and musculature (Canavan, 1986; Horne, 1983). Psychological symptoms include mood swings, disorientation, irritability, decreased motivation, fatigue, sleepiness, hyperactivity, and agitation. The severity of symptoms is often related to the duration of sleep deprivation. Causes may include illness, sleep disorders, emotional stress, aging, medications, environmental disturbances, and changes in sleep patterns. The most effective treatment for sleep deprivation is to eliminate or correct factors that disrupt the sleep pattern.

Other Sleep Disorders

Sleep problems common in children include **somnambulism** (sleep walking), night terrors, nightmares, **nocturnal enuresis** (bedwetting), and **bruxism** (tooth grinding). When adults have these problems, it may indicate more serious disorders. Specific treatment for these disorders varies. However, in all cases, it is important to support clients and maintain their safety. For example, sleepwalkers are unaware of surroundings and are slow to react. Thus the risk of falls is great. A nurse should not startle sleepwalkers but instead gently awaken them and lead them to bed.

NURSING PROCESS AND SLEEP

Assessment

To promote a normal, restful sleep for clients, the nurse assesses their sleep histories (see box on p. 729), including factors that normally influence sleep. If sleep is

COMPONENTS OF A SLEEP HISTORY

Description of client's sleeping problem, including symptoms
Normal sleep pattern during health
Current sleep pattern
Medical history
Present medications
Current life events
Emotional and mental status
Bedtime rituals and environment
Sleep-wake log
Wake-time behavior

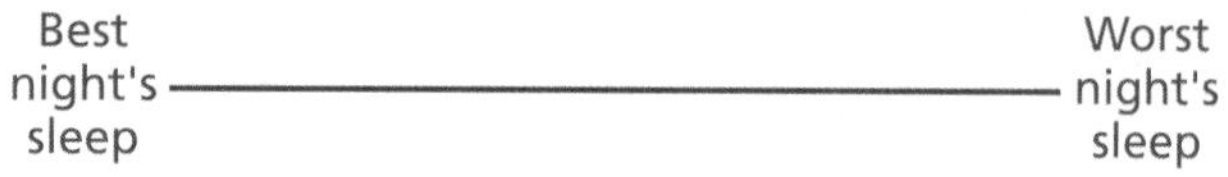

FIGURE 27-4 Visual analog scale to assess sleep quality.

adequate the nursing history can be brief. Sleep is subjective. Only the client can report if it is restful. If the client is satisfied with the amount of sleep received, it may be considered normal (Closs, 1988). If a client admits to or the nurse suspects a sleep problem, a more detailed history is needed.

During the history the nurse notes the client's behaviors. Lethargy, apathy, lack of concentration, and failure to remain alert during questioning are relevant observations that may indicate inadequate sleep.

Sleep Assessment Tools. Most people can give a reasonably accurate estimate of their normal and current sleep patterns, particularly if any changes have occurred. One of the most effective subjective methods for assessing sleep quality is a visual analog scale (Closs, 1988). The nurse draws a straight horizontal line about 100 mm (4 inches) long (Figure 27-4). Opposing statements such as "best night's sleep" and "worst night's sleep" are at each end of the line. The middle represents an average night's sleep. Clients are asked to place marks on the horizontal line at points corresponding to their perceptions of the previous night's sleep. The distance of the mark along the line can be measured in millimeters and offers a numerical value for sleep satisfaction. The scale can be reused to show change over time.

The choice of sleep therapies for a client will depend on an assessment of factors and conditions that normally promote sleep or cause a sleep problem. For example, if a client reads before falling asleep, it will make sense to offer reading material at bedtime. Assessment also reveals the characteristics of any sleep problem and the client's usual sleep habits. Clapin-French (1986) recommends using a sleep history, particularly in caring for older clients. In a study of 102 older adults residing in a long-term care facility, Clapin-French discovered that 71% received some type of sleep medication regularly. Significant shifts in sleep patterns occurred after admission for those on medication. However, only 54% had sleep histories gathered by nurses. Clients may receive inappropriate sleep therapy without accurate assessments. This is just one example of why a sleep assessment is critical to understanding a client's health care needs.

Figure 27-5 is one example of a sleep questionnaire used to assess a hospitalized client's sleep patterns. The tool focuses on the nature of a sleep problem and the review of factors that potentially contribute to the problem. In many institutions sleep and comfort are combined as a single category in assessment tools.

Sources for Sleep Assessment. The client is the best resource for a sleep assessment. The client can report the extent to which a sleep problem represents a change from normal. Parents are often the best source of information about children's sleep problems.

Description of Sleeping Problems. When a client reports a sleep problem or shows behaviors suggesting a problem, the nursing history must be detailed. Open-ended questions help a client to describe a problem more fully. A general description of a problem followed by more focused questions usually reveal specific characteristics used in planning care. To begin, the nurse needs to understand the type of sleep disturbance and the nature of the problem. The following questions will ensure a complete assessment:

1. **Nature of the problem**—Tell me what type of problem you have sleeping. Tell me why you think your sleep is inadequate.
2. **Signs and symptoms**—Describe for me how easy it is to fall asleep. Tell me about the times when you awaken during the night. Tell me what your wife has said about your snoring. Are you tired or irritable during the day? Do you fall asleep at inopportune times? Describe how often you take naps during the day.
3. **Onset and duration**—Tell me about the time when you first noticed a problem with sleeping. How long has the problem lasted?
4. **Severity**—Describe how long it usually takes to fall asleep. How often during the week do you have trouble falling asleep? Tell me how many hours of sleep you got this week; compare that to normal.
5. **Predisposing factors**—Tell me what you do just before going to bed. Have you recently had problems at work or at home?

THE SLEEP QUESTIONNAIRE

At home, what do you do at bedtime to help you sleep?____________________

Some of the statements may *appear* to be the same, but each is different and should be rated as such.*

A. I think I have difficulty with sleep
   a. in the hospital
   b. at home
B. I sleep more at home than in the hospital.
C. When I awaken in the hospital, I feel fatigued and groggy.
D. It takes me longer than 30 minutes to fall asleep in the hospital.
E. Since I've been in the hospital, I awaken frequently at night.
F. In the hospital, if I wake up in the middle of the night it takes me longer then 30 minutes to fall back to sleep.
G. It bothers me that I now go to bed at a different time than I would like.
H. It bothers me that I get up at a different time each morning.
I. Hospital staff awaken me while I'm sleeping.
J. I am awakened at night for treatments.
K. During the day, there is little time for rest.
L. At night I am awakened by noises.
M. At night I am awakened by light.
N. The mattress in the hospital bothers my sleep.
O. The pillow in the hospital bothers my sleep.
P. Having a roommate in the hospital affects my sleep.
Q. I sleep in a very warm room.
R. I have pain at night.
S. The medicines I take keep me awake.
T. My illness keeps me awake at night.

1. I drink coffee, tea, cola, or cocoa during the day.
2. I drink coffee, tea, cola, or coca around sleeping time.
3. I exercise during the day.
4. I exercise around sleeping time.
5. I smoke during the day.
6. I smoke around sleeping time.
7. I have unpleasant conversation during the day.
8. I have unpleasant conversation around sleeping time.
9. I have negative thoughts during the day.
10. I have negative thoughts around sleeping time.
11. I think about what happened during the day and at sleeping time plan for tomorrow.
12. I read during the day.
13. I read around sleeping time.
14. I eat around sleeping time.
15. I watch TV during the day.
16. I watch TV around sleeping time.
17. I have pleasant conversation during the day.
18. I have pleasant conversation around sleeping time.
19. I have positive thoughts during the day.
20. I have positive thoughts around sleeping time.
21. I drink alcohol around sleeping time.

*Response choices were: *Never, Rarely, Sometimes, Often, Very Often.*

FIGURE 27-5 Sleep questionnaire can be used to assess sleep patterns. (From McNeil BJ, et al.: Sleep questionnaire, *Am J Nurs* 86(1):261, 1986. Reproduced with permission from *Am J Nurs* Company.)

6. **Effect on client**—Tell me how the loss of sleep has affected you? Ask a spouse, friend, or parent: What changes in behavior have you noticed since your spouse developed a sleep problem?

Normal Sleep Pattern. The nurse must gain an understanding of a client's normal sleep pattern compared with the current reported sleep pattern. To determine a client's sleep pattern, the nurse asks the following questions:

1. What time do you usually go to sleep?
2. How quickly do you fall asleep?
3. What is the average number of hours you sleep during the night?
4. How many times do you awaken at night?
5. When do you typically awaken in the morning?
6. Do you rise once you awaken or do you stay in bed?

Findings from the assessment are compared with the norm for the client's age. The nurse begins to assess for identifiable patterns such as insomnia. It is important to recognize that hospitalized clients usually need or want more sleep as a result of illness, or they may require less sleep because they are less active. These changes can disrupt sleep patterns and lead to more serious problems.

Medical History. The nurse determines if the client has any preexisting health problems that might affect sleep. Psychiatric illness is significant. For example, a manic depressive client sleeps more when depressed than when manic. Chronic diseases (such as thyroid disease) and painful disorders (such as arthritis) interfere with sleep. The nurse also assesses the client's medication history, including over-the-counter and prescribed drugs. If a client takes sleeping medications the nurse determines the dosage. The nurse also assesses daily caffeine intake.

If the client has recently had surgery the nurse expects to assess a sleep disturbance. The effect on sleep depends on the severity of the surgery (Kavey and Anderson, 1986). Clients often awaken frequently during the first night after surgery and receive little deep or REM sleep. Depending on the type of surgery, it may take several days for a normal sleep cycle to return.

Current Life Events. The nurse learns if the client is experiencing any stressful events in life. Change in job or marital status, financial difficulties, loss of a loved one, and the uncertainty of a medical diagnosis are examples of changes sufficient to disrupt sleep. The client should be asked whether any such stressor precipitated the sleep alteration.

Emotional and Mental Status. If a client is anxious, excitable, or angry, mental preoccupations can seriously disrupt sleep. It is common for a person who is emotionally upset to lay awake for hours at a time. A client's emotional stress may be related to changes in current life events. Often clients with psychiatric disorders require mild sedation to achieve sleep. The nurse assesses the effectiveness of the medication and its effect on daytime function.

Bedtime Rituals. The nurse asks the client about bedtime rituals such as reading, eating, or exercise. It is important to determine habits that are beneficial compared with those that disturb sleep. Hospitalization often interferes with rituals. Illness may prevent the client from eating, drinking, or exercising normally. Ultimately the nurse will want to introduce rituals into the client's health care routine.

The nurse should pay special attention to a child's bedtime rituals. The parents can report if it is necessary, for example, to read to the child or engage in quiet play.

Bedtime Environment. The nurse asks the client to describe normal bedroom conditions such as light, sound, temperature, and type of bed. Is the bedroom usually dark? Does any type of noise prevent the client from falling asleep? After determining the answers to such questions, the nurse can try to reproduce an environment conducive to sleep in the health care facility or help the client to make changes in the home. The nurse should pay special attention to a child's sleeping environment. Many children fear the dark or are unable to fall asleep without the presence of a parent.

Sleep-Wake Log. If the cause of a sleep problem is unclear, a client and bed partner can keep a sleep-wake log for 2 weeks. The nurse should not rely only on the client's casual description of the problem. Descriptions of the worst sleeping nights may distort the real problem. A sleep-wake log is completed every morning to provide information on day-to-day variations in sleep-wake patterns over long periods. Entries into the log include physical activities, mealtimes, alcohol and caffeine intake, time and length of naps, evening and bedtime rituals, the time the client tries to fall alseep, nighttime awakenings, and the time of morning awakening. The log is helpful, but sometimes its completion can distract clients. It is not a technique for acutely ill clients who have short hospital stays.

Wake Time Behavior. A client's behaviors can reveal the nature of certain sleep disorders. Some clients are unaware of their sleep problems. The nurse observes for behaviors such as irritability, disorientation (similar to a drunken state), and slurred speech. A friend or spouse may be aware of changes in behavior such as impaired memory or slowed judgment. If sleep deprivation exists, psychotic behavior such as delusions and paranoia may develop.

Clients with chronic sleep disorders usually have mild symptoms of sleep deprivation. More acute sleep deprivation can occur with clients hospitalized in intensive care units. Constant environmental stimuli within an ICU, such as strange noises from equipment, ever-present lights, and care activities, prevent a client from gaining needed rest and sleep. Sleep deprivation is a stressor that can consume a client's energy needed for recovery (Richards and Bairnsfather, 1988). As a result of the acute change in sleep pattern a client may display behaviors such as confusion, irritability, and aggressiveness.

Nursing Diagnosis

The nurse gathers findings from the assessment and validates the accuracy with the client or significant other. Once the data base is complete, the nurse clusters data that begin to form a recognizable pattern describing the client's sleep problem. This pattern includes the defining characteristics for a nursing diagnosis. The nursing diagnosis of *sleep pattern disturbance* has defining characteristics of verbal complaint of falling asleep, awakening earlier or later than desired, interrupted sleep, and complaints of not feeling rested (Kim, et al., 1993). The client may also have exhibited behavioral changes (such as disorientation or lethargy). Accurate selection of the nursing diagnosis is essential; otherwise nursing care can be misdirected (see box below). For example, if the nurse selects *fatigue* instead of *sleep pattern disturbance,* the choice of nursing therapies will not necessarily improve the real problem, disturbed sleep.

Assessment should also identify the probable cause of the sleep disturbance such as a noisy environment or stress involving loss of job. These causes are the related factors that direct the nurse's interventions. For example, if a client has insomnia as a result of a noisy environment, the nurse will offer basic recommendations for promoting sleep such as controlling the noise of hospital equipment and reducing interruptions. In contrast, if the insomnia is due to emotional stress, the nurse's actions will involve introduction of coping strategies. If the related factors are incorrectly defined, the client may not benefit from nursing care.

Sleep problems may affect clients in other ways and be the related factor for nursing diagnoses. For example, a nurse may find that a client with sleep apnea has problems with a spouse who is frustrated over the client's snoring. In addition, the spouse is worried about the client's state of health. The nursing diagnosis of *ineffective family coping related to spouse's sleep disturbance* indicates that the nurse must support the client and spouse so that they can understand sleep apnea and obtain necessary medical care.

NURSING DIAGNOSES FOR SLEEP DISTURBANCES

Sleep pattern disturbance (difficulty falling asleep)
Sleep pattern disturbance (frequent awakenings)
High risk for injury
Ineffective breathing pattern
Knowledge deficit regarding sleep hygiene measures
Altered thought processes
Ineffective family coping
Relocation stress syndrome
Fatigue

Planning

After identifying each nursing diagnosis, the nurse develops a plan of care (see the nursing care plan on p. 733). An individualized plan can be developed only after understanding the client's normal sleep pattern, the client's current sleep pattern, the factors disrupting the client's sleep, and the effect sleep disturbance has on other health problems. Together the nurse and client develop interventions for promoting rest and sleep. The client's bed partner will often have useful suggestions for the plan of care. The nurse conveys caring by offering the client choices in establishing an optimal sleep environment.

It is important for the nurse to recognize that controls can be set in a health care setting to create a pleasing, comfortable environment for sleep. In a hospital the nurse schedules treatments or routines to minimize interruptions and provide time periods for rest and sleep. All staff members should know the plan of care so that they can work together to reduce awakenings. The success of sleep therapy depends on an approach that fits the client's life-style and the nature of any sleep disorder.

There may be a need for consultations to assist in developing a plan of care. If the client is experiencing emotional problems, a social worker or pastoral care representative can be helpful. If sleep is disrupted by pain or discomfort, a nurse specialist might be able to provide specific pain relief therapies or referral to a pain clinic by the physician may be in order.

When developing a plan of care, the nurse's selection of time frames for goals and outcomes may be long term, since sleep disturbances may not disappear quickly. Short-term goals may be directed more toward establishing routine sleep patterns, whereas long-term goals will be directed to improving the general state of

SAMPLE NURSING CARE PLAN
Sleep Pattern Disturbance

ASSESSMENT

Clinical scenario: Mr. Raines, a 76-year-old client hospitalized with deep vein thrombosis of the left leg, reports pain in the left thigh during movement. An IV line is inserted into Mr. Raines' left arm, adding to his discomfort. He reports that it is *difficult to fall asleep* as a result of his pain. He has been *awakened during the last two nights* because of noises in the hallway and visits by nurses to his room. *Normally* he *goes to sleep at 10 PM* but has been *unable to fall asleep until midnight.* He *feels fatigued,* and the nurses report he is *restless.* He *tries to nap* during the day *without success.*

NURSING DIAGNOSIS

Sleep pattern disturbance (difficulty falling asleep) related to environmental irritants and sleep habit disruptions.

PLANNING

Goals	Expected outcomes
Client will obtain sense of restfulness after sleep within 72 hours. Client will establish healthy sleep pattern.	Client will report increased satisfaction with amount of sleep within 48 hours. Client will fall asleep within 30 minutes of going to bed. Client will have no more than one period of awakening during sleep each night. Client reports 4 to 5 hours of uninterrupted sleep nightly (Hodgson, 1991).

IMPLEMENTATION

Steps	Rationale
1. Offer analgesic (Tylenol 650 mg as ordered) for leg pain 1 hour before bedtime (9 PM).	Peak action of analgesic will occur as client goes to sleep. Tylenol (acetaminophen) has peak effects between 1 and 3 hours (McKenry and Salerno, 1989).
2. Provide client with glass of milk 30 minutes before bedtime (9:30 PM).	Milk contains L-tryptophan, natural amino acid that induces sleep (Ross, et al., 1986).
3. Check patency and status of IV and vital signs before bedtime.	Checking prevents unnecessary interruptions after client falls asleep.
4. Control sources of environmental noise inside and outside of client's room by closing room door, delaying flushing of toilet, avoiding conversation outside of room.	Routine hospital activities create noises of significantly high decibels. With doors closed, sound levels fall 6 to 18 decibels (Hilton, 1987). Noises in the hospital are new and strange and will likely awaken clients (Webster and Thompson, 1986).

EVALUATION

Ask client to report overall satisfaction with sleep using visual analog scale.
Ask client to report number of awakenings and duration of sleep.
Observe client's nonverbal expressions and behaviors once awake.

Defining characteristics are shown in italic type.

restfulness. Setting time frames will be influenced by the duration of the sleep disturbance.

When the client has a known sleep disturbance, the goals and outcomes of care may include the following:

1. **Goal:** Client acquires an adequate amount of sleep within 1 month.

   Outcomes

   Client reports satisfaction with amount of sleep

   Client displays behaviors reflecting attentiveness and alertness.

2. **Goal:** Client establishes a regular healthy sleep pattern within 2 weeks.

   Outcomes

   Client falls asleep within 30 minutes of going to bed

   Client reports no episodes of awakening during the night

Client sleeps preferred number of hours each night

3. **Goal:** Client follows sleep hygiene practices nightly.

   Outcomes

   Client uses relaxation therapies nightly

   Client eats foods containing L-tryptophan before bedtime

   Client participates in regular exercise at least 2 hours before bedtime.

4. **Goal:** Client identifies factors that promote or disrupt sleep by next home visit.

   Outcomes

   Client describes environmental factors that disrupt sleep

   Client discusses the effect caffeine-containing beverages have on sleep

   Client explains influence physical illness has on sleep

Implementation

In an acute care setting, sleep is sometimes given less importance than therapies or procedures. However, unless clients obtain necessary rest and sleep, their physical conditions can deteriorate. In the home the ability to acquire sleep depends largely on the client's willingness and ability to use sleep therapies. The selection of appropriate sleep therapies will lessen interruption of the sleep cycle and foster a more normal, restful environment for the client. The nurse's creativity is important in helping clients to integrate sleep therapies into daily routines.

Health Promotion

Nearly 4 out of every 10 Americans do not regularly receive a good night's sleep (Berman, et al., 1990). Most persons are aware of the value of physical fitness and a balanced diet. But in the busy world of today, many individuals ignore the importance of adequate sleep. Research has shown that persons receiving inadequate sleep are in more accidents and show poor performance in their work (Berman et al., 1990). To develop good sleep habits at home, clients and their bed partners should learn ways to promote sleep and to avoid conditions that interfere with sleep (see box above). Parents can also learn good sleep habits to enforce with their children. Improved sleep habits will be reflected in how a person feels during work and play.

Clients benefit most from instructions that can easily be applied in their daily lives. Information about good sleep hygiene, the practices that promote a sound, uninterrupted sleep cycle, should apply to the client's personal routines. For example, a suggestion to exercise regularly, a few hours before bedtime, should be given to clients who return home in enough time to do so. In contrast, suggestions for controlling noise may do little for the client who lives near a busy airport. The nurse must know the client's routines and preferences for sleep therapies to be effective. Suggestions for relaxing bedtime activities should include activities the client enjoys.

> **CLIENT TEACHING FOR PROMOTING GOOD SLEEP HABITS**
>
> Exercise daily (walking, light jogging, swimming, and bicycling are beneficial).
>
> Decide on a regular bedtime and arising time and observe it daily.
>
> Avoid lengthy sleeping on weekends and holidays.
>
> Limit naps to no more than 20 minutes (adults under 65).
>
> Install carpets, window shades, and heavy draperies to soundproof and darken the bedroom.
>
> A warm hot bath before bedtime can be relaxing.
>
> If unable to sleep after a half hour or so, get out of bed, stay quiet, and relax in another room.

Environmental Controls

All clients require a sleeping environment with a comfortable room temperature and ventilation, minimal noise, a comfortable bed, and proper lighting. Infants sleep best in room temperatures of 18° to 21° C (65° to 69.8° F) at night. Cribs should not be near open windows or drafts. The infant is covered with a light, warm blanket. Wrapping an infant snugly in a blanket tends to promote sleep. Children and adults vary more in regards to comfortable room temperature. Some prefer to sleep without covers. Older adults often require extra blankets or covers. Many older adults sleep wearing socks.

It helps to eliminate distracting noises so the bedroom is as quiet as possible. Noise and other environmental factors can cause chronic fatigue. In a hospital the nurse can control noise in several ways (see box on p. 735). Nurses should also make equipment manufacturers aware of the need for quiet in future product designs. At home, it may require the cooperation of people living with the client to reduce noise (e.g., turning down TV or radio volume, closing doors of rooms where people are gathered, and lowering voices).

A bed and mattress should provide support and comfortable firmness. Bed boards can be placed under mattresses to add support. The position of the bed in the room may make a difference for some clients.

Infants' beds must be safe. To reduce the chance of

CONTROL OF NOISE IN THE HOSPITAL

Close doors to a client's room.
Reduce volume of nearby telephone and paging equipment.
Wear rubber-soled shoes.
Turn off bedside equipment not in use, such as oxygen or suction equipment.
Avoid abrupt loud noise such as moving furniture.
Keep necessary conversations at low levels, particularly at night.
Conduct discussions or nursing reports in a private, separate area away from client rooms.
Turn off the television or radio unless client prefers soft music.

suffocation, pillows or the ends of loose blankets should not be placed in cribs. Loose-fitting plastic mattress covers should not be used because infants might pull them over their faces.

For clients prone to confusion or falls, the nurse should check the client often during the night. The raising of siderails is a precaution nurses routinely use. However, the confused client can become more restless and disoriented when awakening with a side rail up. In this situation, a client may be safer with the side rails down. Many beds are equipped with an alarm that goes off when a client at risk for falling gets out of bed. A call light should also be placed within the client's reach so the client may request help.

Clients vary in the amount of light they prefer at night. Infants sleep best in softly lit rooms. Light should not shine directly on their eyes. Older adult clients may sleep best with dimmed lights that reduce the chance of confusion and prevent falls en route to the bathroom. If street lights shine through windows or if clients sleep during the day, heavy shades, drapes, or slatted blinds are helpful. Nurses should close curtains between clients in semiprivate rooms. Lights on a hospital nursing unit can be dimmed at night.

Promoting Comfort

People fall asleep only after feeling comfortable and relaxed. Even minor irritants may cause wakefulness.

Newborns and infants should be put to bed in dry diapers and soft cotton nightclothes. Children and adults need loose-fitting nightwear and dry, unwrinkled bed linens. The nurse should remove any moist, wrinkled sheets or equipment that a client may lie on.

A client's sense of comfort is also improved by personal hygiene at bedtime, such as dental and denture care, a warm bath or shower, and an opportunity for the bed-restricted client to wash the face and hands. At home, a client whose sleep is disturbed by the bed partner may need to temporarily sleep in another room.

When a sleep disorder results from a painful illness, the nurse should encourage the administration of analgesics at least ½ hour before bedtime. Application of dry or moist heat to a painful area (see Chapter 37) may help to reduce inflammation or muscle tension and promote relaxation. Proper positioning also can be useful in eliminating stress on painful body parts, whereas a gentle backrub can ease muscle tension and aches. Measures designed to alleviate the client's pain can promote restful sleep (see Chapter 28).

Establishing Periods of Rest and Sleep

In a hospital or extended-care setting it is hard to give clients the time needed for rest and sleep. However, the nurse schedules care activities to avoid awakening clients for nonessential tasks. The nurse can help by scheduling assessments, treatments, procedures, and routines for times when clients are awake. For example, if a client has been physically stable, the nurse may decide to avoid checking vital signs. Unless maintaining a drug's therapeutic blood level is essential, drugs should be given during waking hours. When a client's condition demands more frequent monitoring, the nurse can combine activities (such as dressing changes, specimen collection, and IV assessment) to allow for extended rest periods. If the nurse plans to check the client or the room equipment, it helps to make sure the path to the bed is uncluttered so that tables and chairs will not be bumped. It may also be necessary to limit the number of visitors. Although important to a client's well-being, visitors may stay much too long and prevent a client from gaining needed rest.

In an intensive care environment the nurse uses monitors to check a client's condition. To make sure monitors are valid, the nurse checks blood pressure using both cuff and monitor readings to acquire a baseline. The nurse can then track trends without awakening a client for vital sign assessment (Littrell and Schumann, 1989).

In the home, it may help to encourage clients to stay physically active during the day so they are more likely to sleep at night. Increasing daytime activity lessens problems with falling asleep. It is common for older adults to nap during the day. Hayter (1985) suggests that older clients take afternoon naps for physical restoration. Hoch and Reynolds (1986) recommend taking naps the same time each day to maintain a consistent schedule.

Controlling Physiological Disturbances

The nurse can help clients control the symptoms of physical illness that disrupt sleep. For example, a client with respiratory problems should sleep with two pillows in a semisitting position in bed or sleep in a recliner chair to ease breathing. A client with a hiatal hernia also needs special care. After meals the client may have a burning sensation as a result of gastric reflux. To prevent sleep problems, the client should eat a small meal several hours before bedtime and sleep in a semisitting position.

Clients will not sleep if they are in pain or suffer from other recurrent symptoms. Symptom-relieving medications such as analgesics and antiemetics should be given so the drug's peak action takes effect at bedtime. Analgesia can be provided during the night with use of controlled-release morphine (Hodgson, 1991). Often a client's pain worsens at night because of fear, anxiety, and lack of distraction. The nurse can spend time offering information to alleviate the client's fears before bedtime.

Stress Reduction

Emotional stress interferes with sleep. The inability to sleep can make clients irritable and tense. Forcing sleep may lead to insomnia and bedtime may become associated with the inability to relax. A client who has difficulty falling asleep may find it helpful to get up and pursue a relaxing activity rather than stay in bed and think about sleep. Relaxation exercises can be useful in extending a person's sleep period. Slow, deep breathing for 1 or 2 minutes induces calm. Rhythmic contraction and relaxation of muscles reduces tension and prepares the body for rest. Guided imagery, praying, and yoga may also promote sleep.

In health care settings nurses should take time to sit and talk with clients unable to sleep. This helps in determining factors keeping clients awake. Explaining procedures or answering questions may give clients needed peace of mind. If a sedative is indicated, the nurse confers with the physician to be sure the lowest dosage is used initially. Older adults can be vulnerable to the side effects of sedatives, hypnotics, or analgesics because the drugs are metabolized slowly (see box above).

For clients with chronic sleep problems such as sleep apnea and narcolepsy, it is important for nurses to assist clients and families in developing appropriate coping strategies. Uncomfortable social situations such as negative labeling of clients with narcolepsy may affect work or school success (Bergstrom and Keller, 1992). The nurse can suggest ways for clients to improve study habits, facilitate employment choices, and achieve productivity. These may include stimulating environments, job choices in areas where there is less monotony, and employer or teacher education about the disorder (Bergstrom and Keller, 1992). The nurse must also help clients find ways to retain their family relationships. The symptoms and treatment of sleep disorders may disrupt the family unit. Marital counseling and child care referrals can prove helpful. There are also social support groups such as the American Narcolepsy Association that can provide invaluable aid to clients and families.

Children often have bedtime fears, awaken during the night, or have nightmares. After nightmares, parents should enter children's rooms immediately and talk to them briefly about fears to calm them down. Children are comforted but left in their own beds. Their fears should not be used as excuses to delay bedtime.

GERONTOLOGIC CONSIDERATIONS FOR SLEEP THERAPY: ADMINISTRATION OF SEDATIVES

Older adults are susceptible to the side effects of antianxiety and sedative agents because of changes in metabolism.

Administer short-acting benzodiazepines only: oxazepam, lorazepam, temazepam, alprazolam, and triazolam (McKenry and Salerno, 1992). Try these after other therapies fail.

Initial sedative or hypnotic doses should be small, and increments are added gradually based on client response.

Excessive doses of sedatives may cause incontinence, confusion, and impaired mobility in normal, healthy, older clients.

Antihistamines may be used for sedation, but the client should be aware of tolerance with long-term use (Ebersole and Hess, 1990).

Powerful tranquilizers such as butyrophenone (Haldol) have the highest incidence of **extrapyramidal** side effects such as involuntary movement, abnormal posture, and changes in muscle tone. The drugs can also create amnesia and confusion in older adults.

Nutritional Therapy

Some clients enjoy bedtime snacks, whereas others cannot sleep after eating. A perfect light snack includes a dairy product such as warm cocoa that contains L-tryptophan and a small serving of fruit or crackers. A full meal before bedtime can often cause gastrointestinal upset and interfere with the ability to fall asleep. Generally, clients should avoid spicy foods just before bedtime.

Clients with sleep apnea may benefit from a weight loss diet. The condition is more common in obese clients. The mechanism by which weight reduction improves the syndrome is unknown (Feinsilver, 1992). It is known that small degrees of weight loss improve a client's oxygenation and reduce daytime somnolence.

The ingestion of alcohol or stimulants such as caffeine before bedtime can affect the client's sleep cycle.

Caffeine impairs the ability to fall asleep and can cause cardiac dysrhythmias. Alcohol interrupts sleep cycles and reduces the amount of deep sleep. Caffeine drinks and alcohol act as diuretics and may cause a client to awaken in the night to void.

Infants require special measures to minimize nighttime awakenings for feeding. Many children need middle-of-the-night bottle or breast-feeding. Whaley and Wong (1991) recommend offering the last feeding as late as possible. Eventually it may help to gradually reduce the amount of formula or duration of breastfeeding. Infants should not be given bottles in bed.

Promoting Bedtime Rituals

Bedtime rituals relax clients in preparation for sleep. Newborns and infants sleep through so much of the day that a specific ritual is hardly necessary. However, quieting activities such as holding them snugly in blankets, singing or talking softly, and gentle rocking, will help infants fall asleep. Whaley and Wong (1991) recommend placing a child in a crib or cradle while awake. When infants fall asleep in their parents' arms and are then transferred to their crib, they will awaken in unfamiliar surroundings.

A bedtime ritual such as the same hour of bedtime or a quiet activity used consistently helps young children avoid attempts to delay sleeping. Toddlers and preschoolers may be too excited and full of energy to sleep. Parents should ignore attention-seeking behaviors and instead reinforce patterns of preparing for bedtime. Reading stories or sitting on the nurse's lap while listening to music, are routines that can be associated with preparing for bed. Quiet activities such as coloring and reading work well for school-agers. A child should never be put to bed as punishment.

Adults should learn to follow normal bedtime routines as closely as possible. Physical exercise at least 2 hours before bedtime can promote sleep. Reading, watching television, or listening to music may also help. A client should not try to finish office work or resolve family problems before bedtime. It is usually best to associate the bedroom only with sleep. Working toward a consistent time for sleep and voiding before retiring helps most clients gain a healthy sleep pattern and strengthens the rhythm of the sleep-wake cycle.

In a hospital or health care facility, part of the bedtime ritual is assuring clients of their safety and wellbeing. A client should know that a nurse is available at all times. A call light should be placed within reach so the client may obtain assistance when needed.

Administering Sleep Medications

Sleep medications can help a client if used short term. However, their long-term use can disrupt sleep and lead to more serious problems. Benzodiazepines, including flurazepam (Dalmane), temazepam (Restoril), triazolam (Halcion) and alprazolam (Xanax) are relatively safe. They do not cause general CNS depression like other **sedatives** or **hypnotics** do. The benzodiazepines create muscle relaxation, antianxiety, and hypnotic effects. The antianxiety effects usually occur at safe, nontoxic doses. The benzodiazepines are generally not available to children under 12 to 18 years of age, depending on the specific drug.

Pregnant clients should avoid benzodiazepines because of their association with the risk of congenital problems. Nursing mothers should not take the drugs because they are excreted in breast milk. Older adults should use caution in taking benzodiazepines.

One group of clients particularly at risk when taking sedatives are those with sleep apnea. These clients suffer serious sleep deprivation and may try anything for a night's sleep. Sedatives and hypnotics can decrease ventilatory drive and worsen the apnea.

Clients benefit from knowing the risks of nonprescription sleeping medications, especially the long-term effects of sleep disruption. Behavioral therapy can often cure sleep problems more safely. Regular use of any sleep medication can lead to tolerance, withdrawal, and eventual rebound insomnia. Routine medical monitoring of any sleeping medication is important.

A client who takes sleep medications should know about risks and possible side effects. Nurses should caution clients against taking benzodiazepines with alcoholic beverages, opioid analgesics, or monoamine oxidase inhibitors (MAO) and tricyclic antidepressants to avoid CNS depression. Clients should learn to not take more than the prescribed dose if a drug seems less effective.

Evaluation

Each client has a different need for sleep and rest. For this reason evaluation of therapies designed to promote a client's sleep and rest must be individualized. As in the case of assessment, the client is the best source for evaluating whether the quality of sleep has improved or if other health care problems are eliminated through the improvement in sleep.

The nurse must determine if the established plan of care is effective. Is the client meeting the expected outcomes established for the goals of care? If goals are being met, then the nursing diagnosis is resolved. If goals are unmet, the nurse may need to revise nursing therapies or reconsider if the correct nursing diagnosis was chosen.

During evaluation the nurse must remain aware of priorities. The client's physical condition might change, necessitating therapies that may interfere with sleep. In this case the nurse adjusts the plan accordingly to provide opportunity for the client to rest.

The nurse may evaluate the client's response to interventions shortly after a therapy has been tried (e.g., observing if a client falls asleep after reducing noise and darkening a room). Other evaluative measures may be used after a client awakens from sleep (e.g., asking a client to describe the number of awakenings during the night). It may take several weeks before the nurse is able to determine if a client's sleep pattern has permanently improved. The client and bed partner can usually provide accurate evaluative information.

The nurse will use evaluative measures for each of the expected outcomes. The information gathered determines the status of each client goal.

Goal: Client acquires an adequate amount of sleep within 1 month.

Outcome
Client reports satisfaction with amount of sleep.

Evaluative measure
Nurse asks client to rate satisfaction with sleep on a visual analog scale using a range of 1 to 10. The nurse compares the score with previous measurements.

Outcome
Client displays behaviors reflecting attentiveness and alertness.

Evaluative measure
Nurse observes client behavior during repeated visits to clinic or after several days of hospitalization.

Goal: Client establishes a regular healthy sleep pattern within 2 weeks.

Outcome
Client falls asleep within 30 minutes of going to bed.

Evaluative measure
Nurse has bed partner report when client was observed to fall asleep. Another option: nurse checks on client 30 minutes after client goes to bed.

Outcome
Client reports no episodes of awakening during the night.

Evaluative measure
Nurse asks client the next morning to report on any occurrences of awakening.

Outcome
Client sleeps preferred number of hours each night.

Evaluative measure
Nurse asks client to report the next morning on total hours of sleep during the night.

Goal: Client follows sleep hygiene practices nightly.

Outcome
Client uses relaxation therapies nightly.

Evaluative measure
Nurse asks client to demonstrate relaxation therapies and then asks client to report on frequency exercises are performed at home.

Outcome
Client eats foods containing L-tryptophan before bedtime.

Evaluative measure
Nurse has spouse report on type of snack client regularly has at bedtime.

Outcome
Client participates in regular exercise at least 2 hours before bedtime.

Evaluative measure
Nurse asks client or spouse to report on when exercise is routinely performed.

Goal: Client identifies factors that promote or disrupt sleep by next home visit.

Outcome
Client describes environmental factors that disrupt sleep.

Evaluative measure
Have client explain factors in the home setting that disrupt sleep.
Have client explain factors in the home setting that promote sleep.

Outcome
Client discusses the effect caffeine-containing beverages have on sleep.

Evaluative measure
Nurse asks client to explain which of the following contain caffeine: cocoa, cola, milk, or tea.
The nurse asks the client to explain how ingestion of cocoa, cola, and tea affect sleep.

Outcome
Client explains influence physical illness has on sleep.

Evaluative measure
Nurse asks client to describe how thyroid disease affects sleep.

SUMMARY

Each day a person needs sleep to protect and restore body functions. Normally the sleep-wake cycle follows a 24-hour rhythm coordinated with other physiological functions such as body temperature. Sleep is a rhythm within a rhythm. After falling asleep, a person passes through a series of stages that help the body to rest and recover.

All age-groups have different sleep requirements and sleep habits. A person's age affects the type of sleep therapies used by the nurse. The nurse's care may differ in the home compared with a health care setting.

Many factors can promote or disrupt sleep. The nurse must thoroughly assess a client's sleep history to plan an individualized and effective approach to sleep therapy. To help a client achieve a normal sleep pattern, the nurse should use therapies that foster relaxation and sleep and eliminate factors that disrupt sleep.

KEY CONCEPTS

- Sleep is an altered state of consciousness that occurs for sustained periods, restoring a person's energy and well-being.
- The 24-hour sleep-wake cycle is a circadian rhythm influencing physiological function and behavior.
- The control and regulation of sleep depend on a balance of central nervous system regulators.
- During a night's sleep, a person passes through four to six sleep cycles, each of which has five stages.
- No specific number of hours of sleep is needed by each person to rest.
- During sleep, many physiological functions slow down, the body conserves energy, and brain activity promotes memory and learning.
- Sleep may be disrupted by disease processes, long-term use of sleeping pills, hectic life-style, emotional and psychological stress, and alcohol ingestion.
- An environment conducive to sleep is a darkened room with reduced noise, a comfortable bed, and good ventilation.
- The most common type of sleep disorder is insomnia, which is characterized by the inability to fall or remain asleep during the night.
- Assessment of a client's sleep history involves an analysis of the normal sleep pattern, nature of the sleep disturbance, and identification of factors impairing sleep.
- A bedtime ritual of relaxing activities prepares a person physically and mentally for sleep.
- One of the most important nursing interventions for promoting sleep is establishing periods for sleep and rest.

CRITICAL THINKING ACTIVITIES

1. You are the nurse working in the outpatient medical clinic for a small community hospital. A patient who has recently been diagnosed with cancer is in for testing and is accompanied by his wife. The patient has had a great deal of pain lately. The wife's appearance is listless. She has difficulty following the conversation with her husband. What areas of assessment would you include for this family? What is the potential sleep problem they may be experiencing?
2. Take a tour of a general nursing division. After doing so, answer the following question: Consider a client newly admitted to this nursing division. What factors on the division have you identified that may serve as barriers to this client's ability to receive adequate sleep?
3. Ms. Sims is a 32-year-old account executive with a major corporation. She has been moving up the corporate ladder for a number of years. She travels frequently, sometimes to Europe. She freely admits that her sleep schedule is erratic due to frequent, late evening meetings. She has trouble falling asleep at night because she is so "wound up." She knows that she needs to be getting more sleep. "I just don't feel that well in the morning. It takes me awhile to get energized." Ms. Sims drinks at least 10 cups of coffee daily. What factors in Ms. Sims' history suggest a sleep disturbance problem may exist? What additional factors would you like to assess about her? Develop a plan of care based on your findings.
4. Explain the difference in the choice of nursing therapies for treatment of insomnia in a young adult compared with an older adult.

References

Bergstrom DL and Keller C: Narcolepsy: pathogenesis and nursing care, *J Neurosci Nurs* 24(3):153, 1992.

Berman TM, et al.: Sleep disorders: take them seriously, *Patient Care* 24:85, 1990.

Biddle C, and Oaster TRF: The nature of sleep, *J Am Assoc Nurs Anesth* 58(1):36, 1990.

Canavan T: The functions of sleep, *Nurs* 3(9):321-324, 1986.

Chuman MA: The neurological basis of sleep, *Heart Lung* 12:177, 1983.

Clapin-French E: Sleep patterns of aged persons in long-term care facilities, *J Adv Nurs* 11:57, 1986.

Closs SJ: Assessment of sleep in hospital patients: a review of methods, *J Adv Nurs* 13:501, 1988.

Colling J: Sleep disturbances in aging: a theoretical and empiric analysis, *ANS* 6:36, 1983.

Ebersole P and Hess P: *Toward healthy aging: human needs and nursing response,* ed 3, St. Louis, 1990, Mosby.

Feinsilver SH: Recognizing and treating the sleep apnea syndromes, *Emergency Med* 24:83, 1992.

Fisher ME: ICU syndrome, *Crit Care Nurse* 4:39, 1984.

Fordham M. In *patient problems: a research base for nursing care,* 1988, Wilson-Barnett J and Bateup L, eds: London, 1988, Scutari Press.

Glyn CJ, et al.: The diurnal variation in perception of pain, *Proc Royal* Soc Med 69:369, 1976.
Gribbin M: All in a night's sleep, *New Scientist* 7(36):1-4, 1990.
Hartmann E: *The nightmare: the psychology and biology of terrifying dreams,* New York, 1984, Basic Books.
Hayter J: Sleep behavior of older persons, *Nurs Res* 32:242, 1983.
Hayter J: To nap or not to nap? *Geriatr Nurs* 6:104, 1985.
Hilton, A: The hospital racket: how noisy is your unit? *Am J Nurs* 87:59, 1987.
Hoch C and Reynolds C III: Sleep disturbances and what to do about them, *Geriatr Nurs* 7:24, 1986.
Hodgson LA: Why do we need sleep? Relating theory to nursing practice, *J Adv Nurs* 16:1503-1510, 1991.
Horne JA: Sleep and tissue repair, *Psychiatry Practice,* 2(18):9-12, 1983.
Kales A and Kales J: Sleep disorders: recent findings in the diagnosis and treatment of disturbed sleep, *N Engl J Med* 290:487, 1974.
Kales A, et al.: Sleep disorders: sleep apnea and narcolepsy, *Ann Intern Med* 106:434, 1987.
Kavey NB, Anderson D: Why every patient needs a good night's sleep, *RN* 49:16, 1986.
Kim MJ, et al.: *Pocket guide to nursing diagnoses,* ed 5, St. Louis, 1993, Mosby.
Littrell K and Schumann L: Sleep in the CCU, the impossible dream? *Nurs* 89, 7:32u-32y, Nov., 1989.
McKenry LM, Salerno E: *Mosby's pharmacology in nursing,* St. Louis, 1989, Mosby.
McNeil BJ, et al.: Sleep questionnaire, *Am J Nurs* 86(1):261, 1986.
Mitler MM, et al.: Catastrophies, sleep and public policy: consensus report, *Sleep* 11:100, 1988.
Parish JM, Shepard JW: Cardiovascular effects of sleep disorders, *Chest* 97 (5):1220-1226, 1990.
Richards KC and Bairnsfather L: A description of night sleep patterns in the critical care unit, *Heart Lung* 17(1):35-41, 1988.
Ross MS, et al.: When sleep won't come: helping our elderly clients, *Can Nurse* 82:14, 1986.
Webster RA and Thompson DR: Sleep in hospital, *J Adv Nurs* 11:447, 1986.
Whaley LF and Wong DL: *Nursing care of infants and children,* ed 4, St. Louis, 1991, Mosby.

Bibliography

Ali NJ, et al.: The acute effects of continuous positive airway pressure and oxygen administration on blood pressure during obstructive sleep apnea, *Chest* 101(6):1526, 1992.
Barndt-Maglio B: Sleep pattern disturbance: the pediatric ICU, *DCCN* 5(6):342, 1986.
Potempa K, et al.: Chronic fatigue, *Image* 18:165, 1986.
Turpin G: Psychophysiology of sleep, *Nurs* 3(9):313, 1986.
Weaver TE and Millman RP: Broken sleep, *Am J Nurs* 86:146, 1986.

28 Comfort

OBJECTIVES

Mastery of content in this chapter will enable the student to:

- Define the key terms listed.
- Discuss common misconceptions about pain.
- Describe the physiology of pain.
- Identify components of the pain experience.
- Discuss the three phases of behavioral responses to pain.
- Explain how the gate control theory relates to selecting nursing therapies for pain relief.
- Assess a client experiencing pain.
- Develop appropriate nursing diagnoses for a client in pain.
- Describe guidelines for selecting and individualizing pain therapies.
- Describe applications for use of nonpharmacological pain therapies.
- Discuss nursing implications for administering analgesics.
- Describe interventions for the relief of acute pain following operative or medical procedures.
- Describe the sequence of activities related to pain management in cancer clients.
- Successfully evaluate a client's response to pain therapies.

KEY TERMS

analgesics
anesthesia
cutaneous stimulation
endorphins
epidural infusion
exacerbations
guided imagery
intractable pain
local anesthesia
narcotic
neurotransmitters
nociceptors
pain
patient-controlled analgesia (PCA)
perception
placebo
prostaglandins
reaction
reception
relaxation
remissions
synapse
threshold
tolerance
transcutaneous electrical nerve stimulation (TENS)

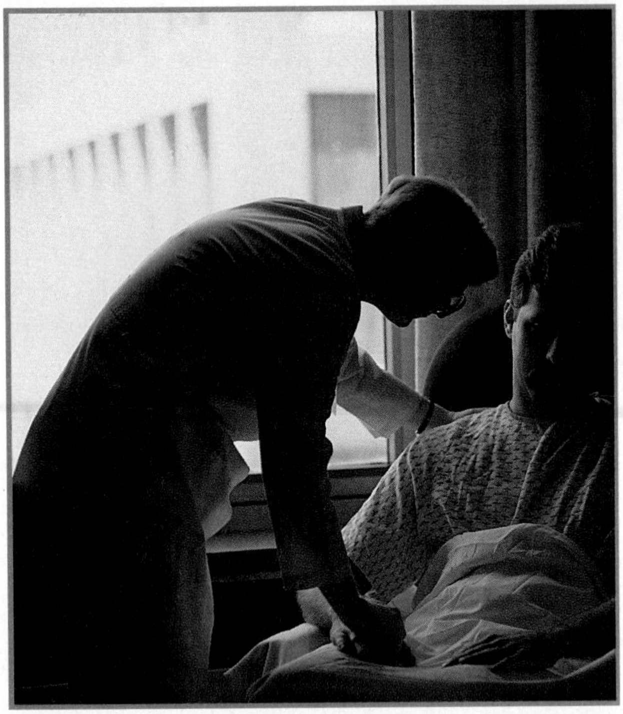

Every person has experienced some type or degree of **pain.** It is the most common reason to seek health care. Persons in pain feel distress or suffering and seek relief. The nurse can use many interventions to bring relief or restore comfort. However, the nurse cannot see or feel the client's pain. Pain is subjective; no two persons experience pain in the same way, and no two painful events create identical responses or feelings. The International Association for the Study of Pain (IASP, 1979) defined pain as "an unpleasant, subjective sensory and emotional experience associated with actual or potential tissue damage, or described in terms of such damage." Pain can be a major factor inhibiting the ability and willingness to recover from illness.

Nurses care for clients in many settings and situations in which interventions are provided to promote comfort. Since the experience of pain is dynamic, the nurse must understand the pain experience. The nurse, client, family, and members of the health care team must collaborate to find the most effective approach to pain control. Nurses are ethically responsible to manage pain and relieve suffering. Effective pain management not only reduces physical discomfort but also promotes earlier mobilization, shortened hospital stays and reduced health care costs.

COMFORT

Comfort is a concept central to the art of nursing. Donahue (1989) summarized "through comfort and comfort measures . . . nurses provide strength, hope, solace, support, encouragement, and assistance." A variety of nursing theorists refer to comfort as a basic client need for which nursing care is delivered.

The concept of comfort is as subjective as that of pain. Each individual brings physiological, social, spiritual, psychological, and environmental characteristics that influence how comfort is interpreted and experienced. Yolcaba (1991) has attempted to define comfort in a manner consistent with clients' subjective experiences. She defines comfort as the state of having met basic human needs for ease (contentment that promotes routine performance), relief (need being met), and transcendence (state in which one rises above problems or pain).

A holistic view of comfort helps to identify four contexts:

Physical—Pertaining to bodily sensations

Social—Pertaining to interpersonal, family, and societal relationships

Psychospiritual—Pertaining to internal awareness of self, including esteem, sexuality, and meaning in life

Environmental—Pertaining to the external background of human experience; light, noise, temperature, color, and natural elements

An appreciation of the context of comfort gives a nurse a larger range of choices when selecting pain therapies. Pain management is more than administering analgesics. The nurse must first understand how the pain experience affects a client's comfort level and then use therapies that meet the unique needs of clients.

NATURE OF PAIN

Pain is more than a single sensation caused by a specific stimulus. It is subjective and highly individualized. The person experiencing pain is the only authority on it. According to McCaffery and Beebe (1989), "Pain is whatever the experiencing person says it is, existing whenever he says it does." Pain cannot be objectively measured in pounds or inches. Often the only way a nurse can assess pain is by relying on the client's words and behavior. To help a client gain relief, the nurse must believe the pain exists.

Pain is a protective physiological mechanism, resulting from a harmful stimulus. A client with a sprained ankle avoids bearing full weight on the foot to prevent further injury. Pain can also be a warning of tissue damage, which should be the nurse's first consideration when assessing pain (Clancy and McVicar, 1992). Clients unable to feel sensations, such as after spinal cord injury, are unaware of pain-inducing injuries.

Pain is a leading cause of disability. As the population ages, more people have chronic disease, in which pain is a common symptom. Medical advances have resulted in diagnostic and therapeutic measures that are often uncomfortable. Nurses care daily for clients in pain. One of the earliest fears of any client with a diagnosed illness is the concern over possible pain.

Health care personnel often hold prejudices against clients in pain. Unless clients have objective signs of pain, a nurse may not believe they are uncomfortable. Nurses' attitudes about pain are due in part to the traditional medical model of illness that suggests that physical problems result from physical causes. Thus pain is viewed as a physical response to an organic dysfunction. When no obvious source of pain can be found, nurses may stereotype clients as complainers or difficult clients.

The extent to which nurses make assumptions about clients in pain seriously limits the ability to offer pain relief. Too often, nurses allow misconceptions about pain (see box below) to affect their willingness to intervene. Many nurses even avoid acknowledging a client's pain because of their own fear and denial.

To help a client gain comfort, the nurse must view the experience through the client's eyes. Acknowledging personal prejudices or misconceptions helps the nurse to address the client's problem more professionally. Often a nurse who has personally experienced pain is better able to provide support. Holm et al. (1989) found that assessment of a client's pain is significantly influenced by the intensity of a nurse's personal pain experience. They found that nurses who have had intense pain are generally more sympathetic to a client in pain. The nurse who is an active, knowledgeable observer of a client in pain makes a more objective assessment and applies skills and techniques that will give relief.

COMMON BIASES AND MISCONCEPTIONS ABOUT PAIN

Drug abusers and alcoholics overreact to discomforts.
Clients with minor illnesses have less pain than those with severe physical alterations.
Administering analgesics regularly leads to clients' tolerance and drug dependence.
The amount of tissue damage in an injury accurately indicates pain intensity.
Health care personnel are the best authorities on the nature of pain.
Psychogenic pain is not real.
Illness and its associated suffering are an inevitable part of aging.
Severe pain can be controlled only by narcotics.

PHYSIOLOGY OF PAIN

Pain is a complex mixture of physical, emotional, and behavioral reactions. To understand the pain experience, it helps to describe its three physiological components of reception, perception, and reaction. A client in pain cannot discriminate among the components. An understanding of each component helps the nurse recognize factors that cause pain, symptoms that accompany pain, and the rationale and actions of therapies.

Reception

Any cellular damage caused by thermal, mechanical, chemical, or electrical stimuli (Table 28-1) results in the release of pain-producing substances. Exposure to hot or cold, pressure, friction, and chemical stimuli release substances such as histamine, bradykinin, and potassium, which combine with receptor sites on nociceptors (receptors that respond to harmful stimuli) to initiate the neural transmission associated with pain (Clancy and McVicar, 1992).

Not all tissues contain receptors that transmit pain signals. The brain and alveoli of the lung are insensitive to pain. When the combination with pain receptors reaches **threshold** (minimum level of stimulus intensity required to evoke a nervous impulse), then activation of pain neurons occurs. Because of the variation in body shapes and sizes, the distribution of pain receptors in parts of the body varies. This explains anatomical subjectivity to pain (Clancy and McVicar, 1992). In addition, individuals have different production capacities of pain-producing substances, which are controlled by the person's genes.

Nerve impulses resulting from the painful stimulus travel along afferent peripheral nerve fibers. Two types of peripheral nerve fibers conduct painful stimuli: the fast, myelinated A-delta fibers and the small, slow unmyelinated C fibers. The A fibers send sharp, localized, and distinct sensations. The small C fibers relay impulses that are poorly localized, visceral, and persistent (Puntillo, 1988). For example, after stepping on a nail, a person initially feels a sharp localized pain, which is the result of A fiber transmission. Within a few seconds the pain becomes more diffuse and widespread until the whole foot aches because of C fiber innervation.

A-delta and C fibers transmit impulses from peripheral projections to the end of the fiber in the dorsal horn of the spinal cord. Within the dorsal horn, an excitatory **neurotransmitter,** substance P, is released. This causes a **synaptic** transmission from the afferent (sensory) peripheral nerve to spinothalamic tract nerves

table 28-1

EXAMPLES OF PHYSICAL SOURCES OF PAIN

Type of stimulus	Source	Pathophysiological process
Mechanical	Alteration in body fluids	Edema distending body tissues
	Duct distention	Overstretching of duct's narrow lumen (e.g., passage of kidney stone through ureter)
	Space-occupying lesion (tumor)	Irritation of peripheral nerves by growth of lesion within confined space
	Pressure	Decreases or obliterates tissue circulation, causing tissue ischemia
Chemical	Perforated visceral organ	Chemical irritation by secretions on sensitive nerve endings (e.g., ruptured appendix, duodenal ulcer)
Thermal	Burn (heat or extreme cold)	Inflammation or loss of superficial layers of epidermis, causing increased sensitivity of nerve endings
Electrical	Burn	Skin layers burned with muscle and subcutaneous tissue injury, causing injury to nerve endings

(Paice, 1991). This allows the pain impulse to be transmitted further within the central nervous system. Pain stimuli travel through nerve fibers in the spinothalamic tracts that cross to the opposite side of the spinal cord. Pain impulses then travel up the spinal cord. Figure 28-1 shows the normal pain reception pathway. After the pain impulse ascends the spinal cord, information is sent quickly to higher centers in the brain, including the reticular formation, limbic system, thalamus, and sensory cortex.

A protective reflex response also occurs with pain reception (Figure 28-2). A fibers send sensory impulses to the spinal cord, where they synapse with spinal motor neurons. The motor impulses travel via a reflex arc along efferent nerve fibers back to a peripheral muscle near the stimulation site. Muscle contraction leads to a protective withdrawal from the source of pain. When superficial fibers in the skin are stimulated, a person moves away from the pain source. If internal tissue such as muscle becomes stimulated, tightening and guarding of muscles occur.

Pain reception requires an intact peripheral nervous system and spinal cord. Common factors that disrupt pain reception include trauma, drugs, tumor growth, and metabolic disorders.

Neuroregulators. **Neuroregulators,** or substances that affect the sending of nerve stimuli, are divided into neurotransmitters and neuromodulators (see box at left). Neurotransmitters such as substance P send electrical impulses across the synaptic cleft between two nerve fibers. They either excite or inhibit nerve transmission. Neuromodulators such as endorphins modify neuron activity without directly transferring a nerve signal through a synapse. They are believed to act indirectly by increasing and decreasing the effects of neu-

NEUROREGULATORS OF PAIN

NEUROTRANSMITTERS

Substance P

Found in the dorsal horn (excitatory peptide)
Needed to transmit pain impulses from the periphery to higher brain centers
Causes vasodilation and edema

Serotonin

Released from the brain stem and dorsal horn (inhibitory)

Prostaglandins

Generated from the breakdown of phospholipids in cell membranes
Believed to increase sensitivity to pain

NEUROMODULATORS

Endorphins

Body's natural supply of morphine-like substances
Activated by stress and pain
Located within the brain, spinal cord, and gastrointestinal tract
Cause analgesia when they attach to opiate receptors in brain

Bradykinin

Released from plasma that leaks from surrounding blood vessels at tissue injury site
Binds to receptors on peripheral nerves, increasing pain stimuli
Binds to cells that cause the chain reaction producing prostaglandins

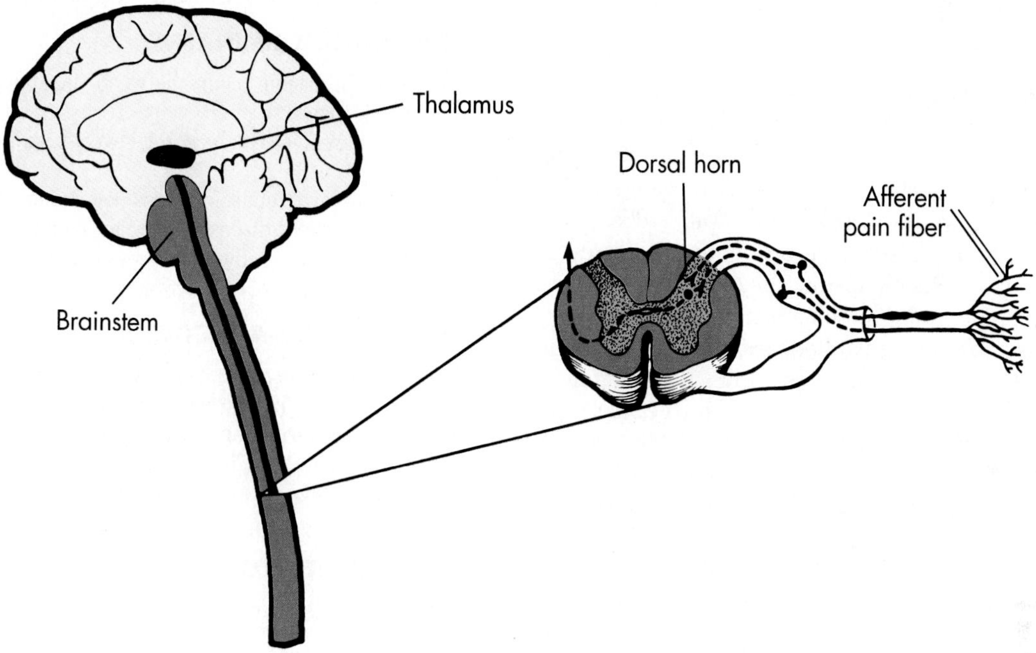

FIGURE 28-1 Pain reception pathway.

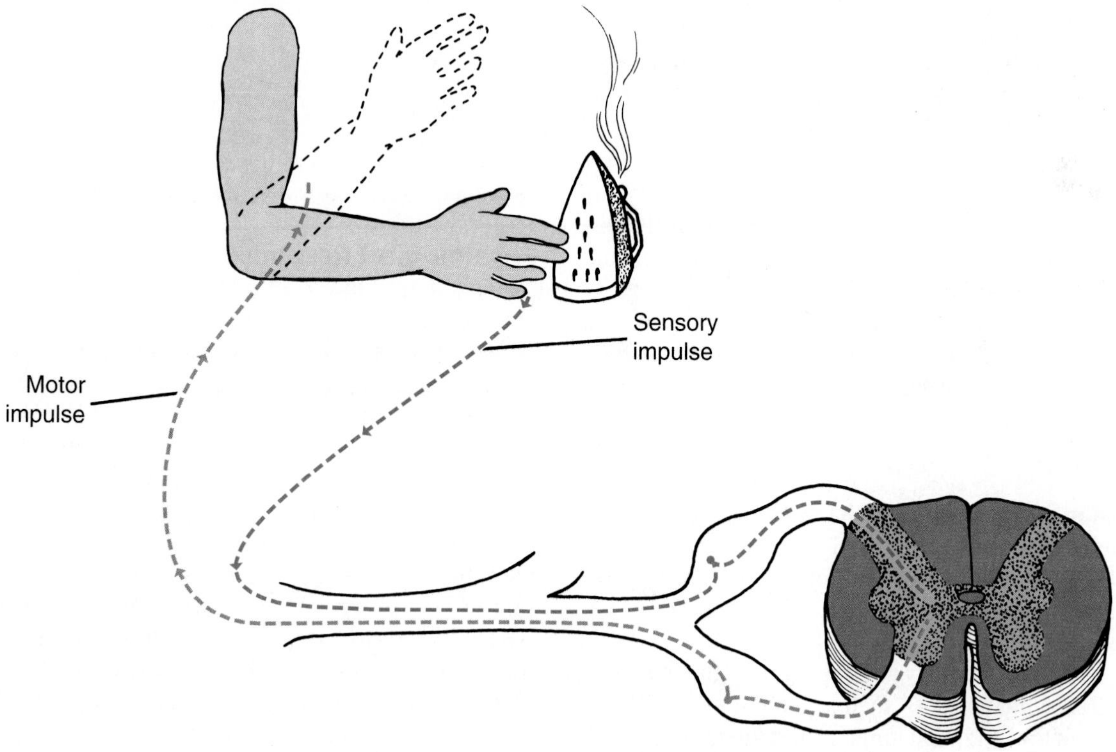

FIGURE 28-2 Protective reflex to pain stimulus.

rotransmitters (Whipple, 1987). Pain perception is influenced by the balance of neurotransmitters and the descending pain control fibers originating from the cerebral cortex.

Gate Control Theory of Pain. Researchers know there is no specific pain center in the nervous system (Fordham, 1986). The gate control theory gives the nurse a conceptual basis for pain-relief measures. The gate control theory of Melzack and Wall (1965) suggests that pain impulses can be regulated or even blocked by gating mechanisms along the central nervous system. The gating mechanism occurs within the spinal cord's substantia gelatinosa (SG) cells, present in the dorsal horn, as well as sites within the thalamus, reticular formation, and limbic system (Clancy and McVicar 1992; Melzack and Wall, 1988). The theory suggests that pain impulses pass through when the gate is open and not while it is closed. Closing of the gate is the basis for pain relief therapies.

A balance of activity from sensory neurons and descending control fibers from the brain regulate the gating process. The A-delta and C neurons release substance P to transmit impulses through the gating mechanisms. In addition there are mechanoreceptor, thicker, faster A-beta neurons that release inhibiting neurotransmitters. If dominant input is from A-beta fibers, the gating mechanisms will close. It is believed this influence can be seen when a nurse delivers a gentle backrub. The massage stimulates mechanoreceptors. If dominant input is from A-delta and C fibers, the gates likely open and the client perceives pain. Even if pain impulses flow to the brain, there may be higher cortical centers in the brain to modify pain perception. Descending neural pathways release endogenous opiates such as endorphins and dynorphin, the body's own natural pain killers. These neuromodulators close gating mechanisms by inhibiting substance P's release. Distraction, counseling, and placebo techniques are ways to release endorphins. Researchers do not know how some people can activate their endorphins.

Perception

Perception is the point at which a person is aware of pain. Meinhart and McCaffery (1983) describe three interactional systems of pain perception as sensory-discriminative, motivational-affective, and cognitive-evaluative (see box above).

The gate-control theory suggests gating mechanisms can be altered by thoughts, feelings, and memories. The cerebral cortex and thalamus can influence whether pain impulses reach a person's consciousness. Individuals also produce different amounts of pain-producing substances such as prostaglandins and substance P (Clancy and McVicar, 1992).

INTERACTIONAL SYSTEMS OF PAIN PERCEPTION

SENSORY-DISCRIMINATIVE

Nerve transmission occurs between the thalamus and sensory cortex.
A person perceives the location, severity, and character of pain.
Factors that lower consciousness (e.g., analgesics, anesthetics, cerebral disease) decrease pain perception.
Factors that increase the awareness of stimuli (e.g., anxiety, sleep deprivation) increase pain perception.

MOTIVATIONAL-AFFECTIVE

Interaction between the reticular formation and limbic system results in pain perception.
The reticular formation creates a defensive response, causing a person to interrupt or avoid pain stimuli.
The limbic system controls emotional response and coping with pain.

COGNITIVE-EVALUATIVE

Higher cortical centers in the brain influence perception.
Culture, experience with pain, and emotions influence a person's evaluation of the pain experience.
Helps a person to interpret the intensity and quality of pain so that action can be taken.

Reaction

The **reaction** to pain is the physiological and behavioral responses that occur after pain is perceived.

Physiological Responses. As pain impulses ascend the spinal cord toward the brain stem and thalamus, the autonomic nervous system is stimulated as part of the stress response. Pain of low to moderate intensity and superficial pain elicit the flight-or-fight reaction of the general adaptation syndrome (see Chapter 4). Stimulation of the sympathetic branch of the autonomic nervous system results in the physiological responses summarized in Table 28-2. If pain is unrelenting, severe, or deep, typically involving visceral organs, the parasympathetic nervous system goes into action. Sustained physiological responses to pain could cause serious harm. Except in cases of severe traumatic pain, which may place a client into shock, most clients adapt, with physical signs returning to normal. Thus a client in pain will not always have physical signs.

Behavioral Responses. The phases of a pain experience are anticipation, sensation, and aftermath (Meinhart and McCaffery, 1983). Anticipation occurs

table 28-2
PHYSIOLOGICAL REACTIONS TO PAIN

Response	Cause or effect
SYMPATHETIC STIMULATION*	
Dilation of bronchial tubes and increased respiratory rate	Provides greater oxygen intake
Increased heart rate	Provides greater oxygen transport
Peripheral vasoconstriction (pallor, elevation in blood pressure)	Elevates blood pressure with shift of blood supply from periphery and viscera to skeletal muscles and brain
Increased blood glucose level	Provides additional energy
Diaphoresis	Controls body temperature during stress
Increased muscle tension	Prepares muscles for action
Dilation of pupils	Afford better vision
Decreased gastrointestinal motility	Frees energy for more immediate activity
PARASYMPATHETIC STIMULATION†	
Pallor	Causes blood supply to shift away from periphery
Muscle tension	Results from fatigue
Decreased heart rate and blood pressure	Results from vagal stimulation
Rapid, irregular breathing	Causes body defenses to fail under prolonged stress of pain
Nausea and vomiting	Causes return of gastrointestinal function
Weakness or exhaustion	Results from expenditure of physical energy

*Pain of low to moderate intensity and superficial pain.
†Severe or deep pain.

before pain is perceived. A person knows pain will occur. Therefore anticipation allows a person to learn about pain and its relief through instruction and support. Nurses are important in helping clients during the anticipatory phase. An example involves the nurse explaining the stinging sensation of a needle stick. Proper explanation helps clients control their anxiety. In cases in which clients are too fearful, anticipation of pain can heighten pain perception.

Sensation of pain occurs when pain is felt. People react to pain in different ways. A person's **tolerance** to pain is the point at which there is an unwillingness to accept pain of greater severity or duration. Tolerance depends on attitudes, motivation, and values.

Pain threatens physical and psychological well-being. However, pain may not be expressed if the client believes such expression would inconvenience others or signal loss of self-control. The client with high pain tolerance is able to endure severe pain without assistance. Often a nurse must encourage such a client to accept pain-relieving measures. In contrast, a client with low tolerance may seek relief before pain occurs. The client's ability to tolerate pain influences the nurse's perceptions of the degree of discomfort. The nurse is often more than willing to attend to the client whose pain tolerance is high. Yet it is unfair to discount or ignore the needs of a client unable to tolerate even minor pain.

Typical body movements and facial expressions that indicate pain include clenching the teeth, holding the painful part, bent posture, and grimaces. A client may cry or moan, be restless, or make frequent requests of the nurse. The nurse soon learns to recognize patterns of behavior that reflect pain. However, lack of pain expression does not mean the client is not having pain. Unless a client openly reacts to pain, it is difficult to assess the nature and extent of the discomfort. The nurse helps the client communicate the pain response more effectively. Knowledge of the disease or illness helps the nurse to anticipate the character of a client's pain. For example, a ruptured lumbar intravertebral disk causes severe low back pain and a burning pain that radiates or extends down the leg.

The aftermath phase occurs when pain is reduced or stopped. Even though the source of pain is controlled, a client may still require the nurse's attention. Pain is a crisis. During the aftermath, clients may have physical symptoms such as chills, nausea, vomiting, anger, or depression. If a client has pain again and again, aftermath responses in themselves can become serious health problems.

ACUTE AND CHRONIC PAIN

Minor discomforts such as the ache of overexercised muscles or the burning discomfort of eye strain rarely cause a person to seek health care. The pain nurses most often observe in clients includes acute, chronic malignant, and chronic nonmalignant pain (National Institutes of Health, 1986). Acute pain follows acute injury, disease, or types of surgery and has a rapid onset, varies in intensity (mild to severe), and lasts briefly. Acute pain warns people of impending injury or disease. It eventually resolves with or without treatment after a damaged area heals.

Clients in acute pain are frightened, anxious, and expect relief quickly. The time sequence of acute pain usually results in a willingness by health team members to treat acute pain aggressively. However, conflict between nurse and client may arise if the nurse does not provide quick relief. Acute pain is self-limiting, and the client therefore knows an end is in sight.

Acute pain seriously threatens a client's recovery by hampering the client's ability to become active and involved in self-care. Rehabilitation may be delayed and hospitalization prolonged if acute pain is not controlled. There cannot be physical or psychological progress as long as pain continues because the client focuses on pain relief. Efforts at teaching or motivation toward self-care will often be useless. After acute pain is relieved, the client can direct full attention toward recovery.

Chronic pain is prolonged, varies in intensity, and usually lasts more than 6 months (McCaffery, 1986). Chronic pain caused by uncontrolled cancer or its treatment, or other progressive disorders is called **intractable pain** (malignant pain). It can last until death.

Chronic nonmalignant pain such as low-back pain results from nonprogressive or healed tissue injury. However, the pain is ongoing and often does not respond to treatment. Frequently the cause is unknown. In chronic pain, endorphins often cease to function.

Health care workers are usually less willing to treat chronic pain as aggressively as acute pain. However, the AHCPR reports that up to 90% of the 8 million Americans who have cancer can have their pain managed with relatively simple means (Jacox, Carr, and Payne, 1994). Too often these clients are undertreated. If the cause of pain is unclear, care givers may question the severity of a client's discomfort. For cancer sufferers, clients may be unwilling to take pain medications and family members may be unwilling to give needed narcotics for fear of causing side effects such as lethargy and drug dependence.

Clients with chronic pain often have periods of **remissions** (partial or complete disappearance of symptoms) and **exacerbations** (increases in severity). This unpredictability frustrates the client, often leading to depression. Chronic pain is a major cause of psychological and physical disability, leading to problems such as job loss, inability to perform simple daily activities, sexual dysfunction, and social isolation.

The client with chronic pain often does not show overt symptoms and does not adapt to the pain but seems to suffer more with time because of physical and mental exhaustion. Symptoms of chronic pain include fatigue, insomnia, anorexia, weight loss, depression, hopelessness, and anger.

The life of a client with chronic pain can be tragic. The desperate search for pain relief may make the client susceptible to quackery, alcohol abuse, and undesirable side effects from mixing medications obtained from various sources. Fortunately, pain clinics throughout the United States and Canada can help clients find more acceptable methods of pain control. Exercise, biofeedback, cognitive distraction, and other methods taught in pain clinics may relieve chronic pain when pharmacological remedies do not.

Caring for the client with chronic pain is an unusual challenge. The nurse should not become frustrated or offer any false hope for a cure. The nurse must minimize or reduce the client's perception of pain.

FACTORS INFLUENCING PAIN

Numerous factors influence the pain experience (Figure 28-3). The nurse considers all factors affecting the client in pain to accurately assess the client's pain and to select appropriate pain therapies.

Age

Developmental differences influence how children and older adults react to pain. Children's behavioral responses to pain change with age. Young children have trouble understanding pain and the procedures that nurses administer that may cause pain. Young children without full vocabularies also have difficulty verbally describing and expressing pain to parents or care givers. Children's temperaments affect how they cope with pain. Broome, et al. (1990) found that children who are passive and cooperative may rate pain as more intense than children who use active coping such as resisting or attacking. Children often describe procedures (e.g., intravenous catheters, lumbar punctures, and dressing changes) as the most distressing aspect of disease or hospitalization. Aggressive efforts to reduce pain are necessary (AHCPR, 1992).

Studies have shown that children are grossly undermedicated for pain. When comparing children with adults having the same medical diagnoses, children received fewer medication doses (Eland and Anderson, 1977; Beyer et al., 1983). In addition, analgesic doses are often too small or given too infrequently to be effective. The nurse assesses pain in children using the same criteria used with adults. The nurse must understand the responses of children in each age-group. For example, the nurse observes children who cannot yet speak for

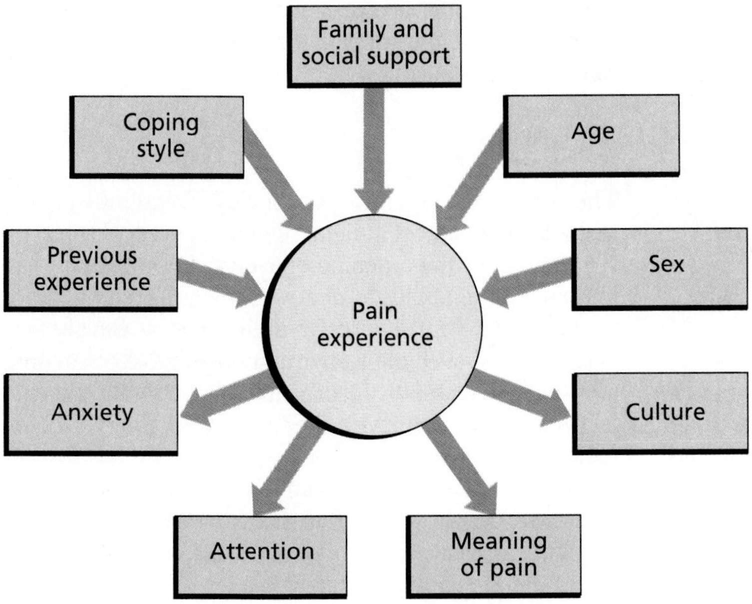

FIGURE 28-3 Factors that influence the pain experience. (From Gil K: *Anesthes Report* 2(2):246, 1990.)

behavioral changes such as irritability, loss of appetite, unusual quietness, disturbed sleep patterns, restlessness, and rigid posturing (Whaley and Wong, 1991). A child's response to medication may also indicate pain. If a behavior such as crying changes after a child receives an analgesic, it was probably caused by pain.

A nurse must use simple but appropriate communication techniques to help children understand and describe pain. The nurse will measure the child's pain using self-report and behavioral observation tools.

Pain is not a natural part of aging. However, older adults often suffer acute and chronic painful disease, have multiple diseases, and take many medications. Older adults can suffer serious loss of functional status as a result of pain. Mobility, self-care activities, socialization, and activity tolerance can all be reduced. A client with cognitive impairment may have trouble recalling pain experiences and providing detailed explanations.

The ability of older adults to interpret pain can be complicated by multiple diseases and vague symptoms affecting similar parts of the body. When older clients have more than one source of pain, a nurse must gather detailed assessments. Different diseases can cause similar symptoms. Herr and Mobily (1991) note that older adults may not report pain because they may believe pain is a part of aging, fear the unknown, fear death, use inadequate terms to describe pain, or believe showing pain is unacceptable.

Sex

Generally, men and women do not differ significantly in pain responses (Gil, 1990). However, cultural influences on gender may produce different expressions of pain (e.g., making it acceptable for a little boy to be brave and not cry, whereas a little girl in the same situation may cry). Burns, et al. (1989) found that male and female clients differed in their degree of pain tolerance after abdominal surgery.

Culture

Culture influences how people learn to react to and express pain. Understanding cultural background, socioeconomic status, and personal characteristics helps the nurse more accurately assess pain and its meaning for clients. Miller and Shuter (1982) found that European Americans expressed pain more often than African Americans. Several studies have shown that more educated and affluent clients respond quicker to symptoms and seek medical care for conditions that persons in lower social classes ignore. Clancy and McVicar (1992) suggest that cultural socialization determines one's psychological behavior. This in turn may affect the physiological output of endogenous opiates and thus pain perception. The nurse should be concerned with managing a type of pain rather than different treatment approaches for a client's portrayal of pain. For example, an acute muscle sprain can be effectively managed with cold application. The nurse must administer therapies known to be effective, while respecting how the client responds to the nurse's interventions.

Meaning of Pain

The meaning a client associates with pain affects the pain experience. Clients perceive pain differently if it suggests a threat, loss, punishment, or challenge. Frequently, a client will report unbearable pain before a hospital admission. After admission, some clients report that the pain lessens or even disappears, without the source of pain having been treated. Clancy and McVicar suggest that the fear of a serious diagnosis may cause an increase in release of endogenous opiates. The degree and quality of pain perceived by a client are related to the meaning of pain.

Attention

The degree to which a client focuses on pain can influence pain perception. Increased attention has been associated with increased pain, whereas distraction has been associated with decreased pain (Gil, 1990). Nurses apply this concept in pain-relief therapies such as relaxation and guided imagery. By focusing a client's attention and concentration on other stimuli, the nurse places pain on the periphery of awareness. Usually, increased tolerance for pain lasts only during the time of distraction.

Anxiety

There is a relationship between pain and anxiety. Elevated anxiety levels cause an increase in pain perception (Seers, 1987). In addition, pain may also cause anxiety. Autonomic arousal patterns are similar in pain and anxiety (Gil, 1990). Emotionally healthy persons are usually able to tolerate moderate or even severe pain better than those less stable emotionally. Endorphins may cause differences in pain tolerance because anxiety over pain may release endorphins.

Fatigue

Fatigue heightens pain perception. This intensifies pain and decreases coping abilities. Pain is often experienced less after restful sleep than at the end of a tiring day.

Previous Experience

Just because a client has had a previous pain experience does not necessarily mean the client will accept pain more easily in the future. Frequent episodes of pain without relief or bouts of severe pain may produce anxiety or fear. In contrast, experiences with the same type of pain that has successfully been relieved makes it easier for the client to interpret the pain sensation. As a result, the client is better prepared to take steps to relieve the pain.

A client who has had no experience with pain may have an impaired ability to cope with it. For example, a postoperative client, unprepared for surgical incisional pain, may be reluctant to ambulate or increase activity. The nurse should prepare such a client with a clear explanation of the type of pain that will be experienced and methods to reduce it.

Coping Style

The experience of pain can be lonely. Frequently clients feel a loss of control in being unable to control their environments or the outcome of events. Coping style thus influences the ability to deal with pain. Clients with internal loci of control perceive themselves as having personal control over their environments and the outcome of events (Gil, 1990). In contrast, clients with external loci of control perceive other factors in their environments, such as nurses, as being responsible for the outcome of events. Those with an internal loci of control report less severe pain than those with external loci (Schultheis et al, 1987). This concept is applied in the use of patient-controlled analgesia (PCA).

Pain can strip persons of their dignity. Geach (1987) acknowledges the active role many clients play in dealing with pain. This view casts more respect than that of seeing clients as "passive sufferers." Seeing clients "doing pain work" underlines the collegial relationship necessary for health care providers to offer comfort measures. To assist a client in "pain work," the nurse must know the client's strengths and failings that influence the work. Similarly the nurse should work with clients in a way that the memories of the experience are positive.

Family and Social Support

A client often depends on the support of spouse, family, or friends when coping with pain. Although pain still exists, the presence of a loved one can minimize loneliness and fear. Clients of different sociocultural groups have different expectations of people to whom they complain about pain. Clients in pain often depend on family members for support, assistance, or protection. Absent family or friends can often make the pain experience more stressful. The presence of parents is especially important for children in pain.

NURSING PROCESS AND PAIN

Nurses need to approach pain management systematically to understand a client's pain and to provide appropriate therapy. The reporting of pain is a social transaction between nurse and client (AHCPR, 1992). Successful assessment depends in part on establishing a positive relationship between health care provider, clients, and families. Clients must then become active participants in their care. Pain management extends beyond pain relief, encompassing the client's quality of life and ability to work productively, to enjoy recreation, and to function normally in the family and society (Jacox, Carr, and Payne, 1994).

Assessment

Accurate and factual pain assessment is necessary for judging clients' progress and response, arriving at proper nursing diagnoses, and selecting appropriate therapies. Pain assessment is one of the most common and one of the most difficult activities a nurse performs. The nurse assesses the pain experience from the client's perspective. Nurses cannot allow personal biases to prejudice pain assessment. It is important to carefully interpret pain cues and remember that psychological and physical components of pain influence the reaction to it.

The Agency for Health Care Policy and Research (AHCPR) has established specific guidelines for assessing clients who are to have surgery or other procedures. The focus is planning successful pain management therapies before pain is experienced. Because it involves a collaborative approach, the AHCPR pain treatment flow chart (Figure 28-4) provides a useful conceptual approach to acute pain control in general. Clients must understand that informed reporting of pain is valuable and necessary if the health care team is to manage pain in an individualized and effective way.

Nurses must be sensitive to a client's level of discomfort. If pain is acutely severe, it is unlikely the client can provide a detailed description. During an episode of acute pain, the nurse primarily assesses how the client feels, determining physiological responses to pain and the location, severity, and quality of pain. A more thorough pain assessment takes time and should be done when the client becomes more alert and attentive. Sofaer (1983) suggests that nurses should reduce a client's anxiety before trying to quantify the client's perception of pain. Physical reassurance may have analgesic qualities.

For clients with chronic pain, assessment may best be focused on affective and evaluative aspects of the pain experience and on its history and context (NIH, 1986). For clients with chronic nonmalignant pain, assessment should include level of function because it may be impossible to achieve complete pain relief. The AHCPR recommends that families of cancer clients learn how to assess pain so as to promote continuity of effective pain management (Jacox, Carr, and Payne, 1994). The nurse should be aware of possible errors in pain assessment (Harrison, 1991). Bias (overestimating or underestimating level of pain), vague or unclear assessment questions, and use of unreliable or invalid pain assessment tools will not provide accurate data. The nurse should recognize clients who do not provide complete, pertinent, or accurate pain information.

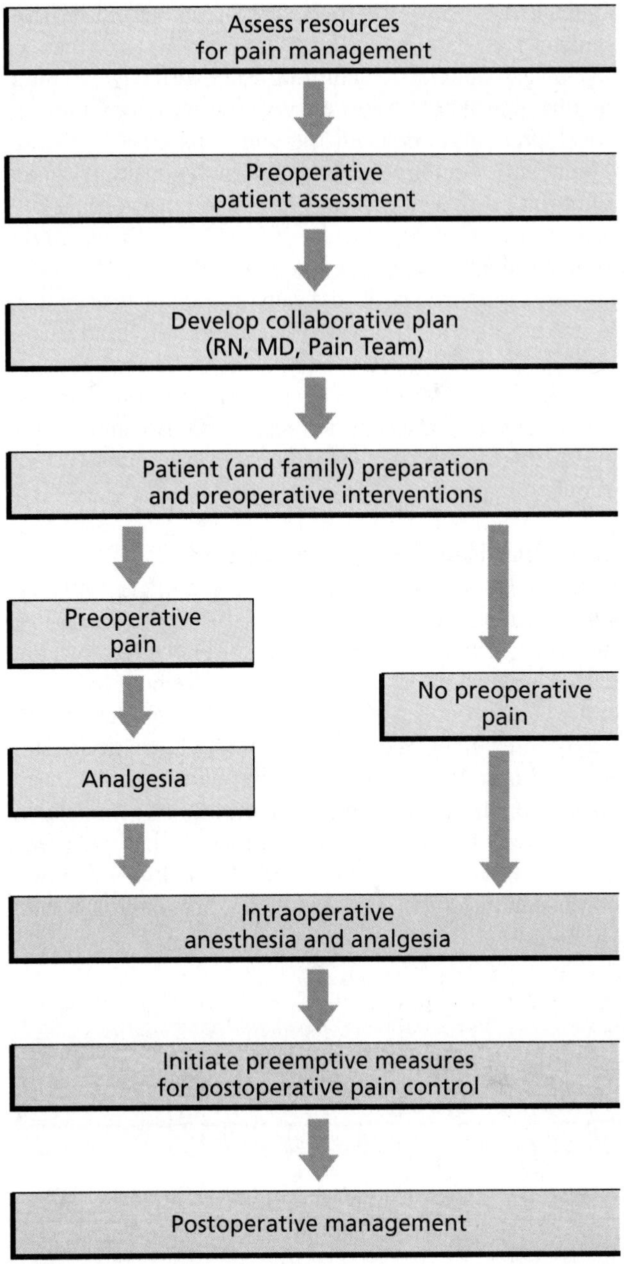

FIGURE 28-4 Pain treatment flow chart: preoperative and intraoperative phases. (Acute pain management guideline panel: *Acute pain management: operative or medical procedures and trauma. Clinical practice guideline,* AHCPR Publication No. 92-0032. Rockville, Md.: Agency for Health Care Policy and Research, Public Health Service, U.S. Department of Health and Human Services, Feb. 1992.)

Client's Expression of Pain. Clients often fail to report or discuss pain. To complicate assessment, nurses frequently believe that clients will report pain if they have it. A nurse should ask about pain regularly. A client must trust a nurse and perceive the nurse's willingness to help before discussing pain openly. The nurse should learn verbal or nonverbal ways that the client communicates discomfort. Grimacing, splinting a body part, and unusual posturing are examples of nonverbal expressions of pain.

Clients unable to communicate effectively often require special attention during assessment. Children, developmentally delayed persons, psychotic clients, clients with dementia and non-English speaking clients all require different approaches. Children's verbal statements are most important (Whaley and Wong, 1991). Young children may not know what the word "pain" means, and therefore assessment may require the nurse to use words such as "owie," "boo-boo," or "hurt." Cognitively impaired clients require simple assessment approaches involving close observation of behavior. If a client speaks a different language, a family member or interpreter may be needed. Clients in pain often confide in only one person.

Classification of the Pain Experience. It can help to know the phase of pain clients are undergoing because it influences not only clients' symptoms but also the types of therapies most likely to relieve pain. Clients in the anticipatory phase such as those scheduled for diagnostic procedures or surgery may be anxious or fearful, or they may ask questions about upcoming pain. Studies have shown that providing clients with physiological coping (positioning, deep breathing), sensory information (description of discomforts to be expected), and procedural information leads to clients with fewer complications, reporting less pain, and using less analgesia (Fortin and Kirouac, 1976; Van Aernam and Lindeman, 1971; AHCPR, 1992).

Clients in the sensation phase generally show signs of discomfort. Clients who are sensing pain, especially severe pain, want relief fast. After the pain has been relieved, the nurse must assess carefully for physical and psychological effects.

The nurse assesses if the client's pain is acute or chronic. If the pain is acute in nature, a detailed assessment of pain characteristics is needed. With chronic pain the nurse determines if it is intermittent, persistent, or limited. After the phase or type of pain is assessed, findings direct the nurse to assess further to determine specific interventions.

Characteristics of Pain. Characteristics of pain can be detailed only by the client. Client self-report to assess pain characteristics is the single most reliable indicator of the existence and intensity of pain and any related discomfort (NIH, 1987).

ONSET AND DURATION. The nurse asks questions to determine the onset, duration, and time sequence of pain. When did the pain begin? How long has it lasted? Does it occur at the same time each day? How often does it recur?

It may be easier to diagnose the nature of pain by identifying time factors. The onset of sudden and severe pain is easier to assess than gradual, mild discomfort. Knowing the time cycle of a client's pain helps the nurse to intervene before the pain occurs or worsens (Table 28-3).

LOCATION. To assess pain location, the nurse asks the client to point to all areas of discomfort. To localize the pain more specifically, the client traces the area

table 28-3

IMPLICATIONS OF PAIN ASSESSMENT FOR NURSING INTERVENTIONS

Assessment criteria	Nursing interventions
Onset and duration	Administer analgesics before pain becomes severe so that peak action occurs when pain is most acute (e.g., during dressing change or exercise therapy).
Location	Position client off affected area. Apply local treatments (e.g., elastic bandage and splinting) directly over painful site.
Severity	Change or revise interventions, depending on success of one intervention.
Precipitating or aggravating factors	Avoid activities that cause or aggravate pain. Teach client or family to avoid same activities.
Relief measures	Use measures that client uses to relieve pain, as long as they are safe and appropriate.

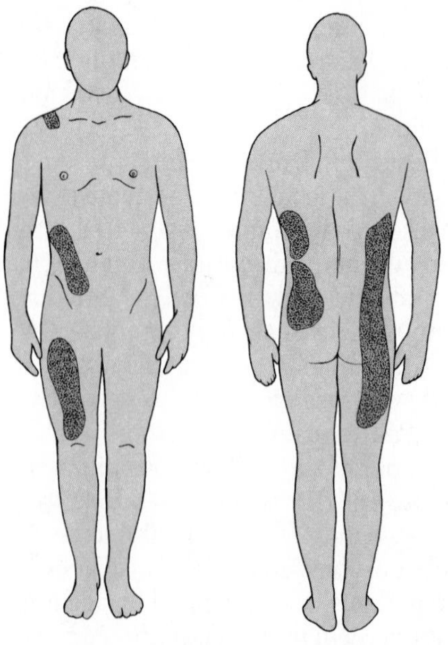

FIGURE 28-5 Diagrammatic figures to locate a client's pain.

from the most severe point outward. This is difficult to do if pain is diffuse, involves several sites, or involves large parts of the body. A drawing showing the location of pain can be used as a baseline if the pain changes (Figure 28-5). The nurse uses anatomical landmarks and descriptive terminology to record pain location (e.g., "Pain is in the right upper abdominal quadrant"). Pain classified by location may be superficial or cutaneous, deep or visceral, localized or diffuse, or referred or radiating (Table 28-4).

Severity. The most subjective characteristic of pain may be its severity or intensity. Clients are often asked to describe pain as mild, moderate, or severe. However, the meaning of these terms differs for the nurse and client.

Descriptive scales measure pain severity objectively (Figure 28-6). A verbal descriptor scale (VDS) consists of a line with three- to five-word descriptors equally spaced along the line. The descriptors are ranked from "No pain" to "Unbearable pain." The nurse shows the client the scale and asks the client to determine the current intensity of pain. In addition, the nurse asks how much does the pain hurt at its worst and how much does

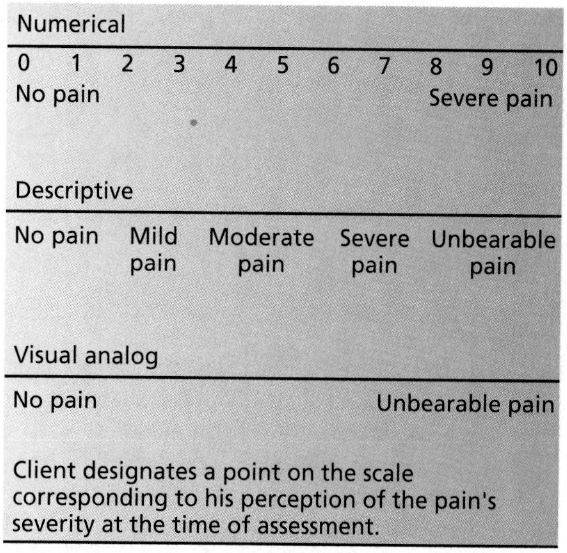

Numerical
0 1 2 3 4 5 6 7 8 9 10
No pain
Severe pain
Descriptive
No pain
Mild pain
Moderate pain
Severe pain
Unbearable pain
Visual analog
No pain
Unbearable pain
Client designates a point on the scale corresponding to his perception of the pain's severity at the time of assessment.

FIGURE 28-6 Sample pain scales. **A,** Numerical. **B,** Descriptive. **C,** Visual analog.

table 28-4

CLASSIFICATION OF PAIN BY LOCATION

Definition	Characteristics	Examples
SUPERFICIAL OR CUTANEOUS		
Pain resulting from stimulation of skin	Pain is of short duration and is localized. It usually is sharp sensation.	Needle stick; small cut or laceration
DEEP VISCERAL		
Pain resulting from stimulation of internal organs	Pain is diffuse and may radiate in several directions. Duration varies but it usually lasts longer than superficial pain. Pain may be sharp, dull, or unique to organ involved.	Crushing sensation (e.g., angina pectoris); burning sensation (e.g., gastric ulcer)
REFERRED		
Common phenomenon in visceral pain because many organs themselves have no pain receptors; entrance of sensory neurons from affected organ into same spinal cord segment as neurons from areas where pain is felt; perception of pain in unaffected areas	Pain is felt in part of body separate from source of pain and may assume any characteristic.	Myocardial infarction, which may cause referred pain to jaw, left arm, and left shoulder; kidney stones, which may refer pain to groin
RADIATING		
Sensation of pain extending from initial site of injury to another body part	Pain feels as though it travels down or along body part. It may be intermittent or constant.	Low-back pain from ruptured intravertebral disk accompanied by pain radiating down leg from sciatic nerve irritation

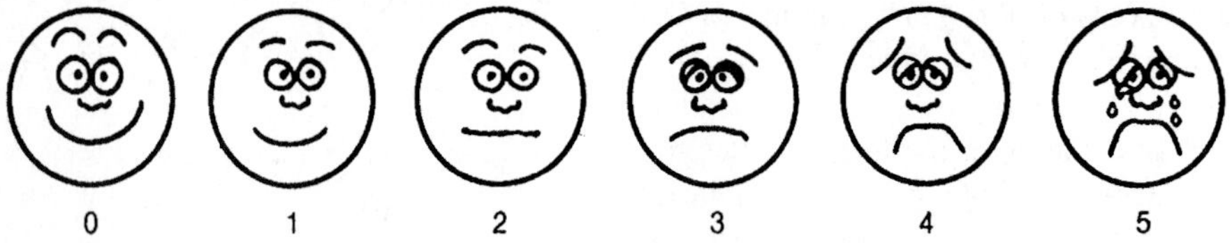

FIGURE 28-7 Faces Scale. (From Whaley L and Wong D: *Nursing care of infants and children,* ed 4, St. Louis, 1991, Mosby.)

it hurt at its best. The VDS enables a client to choose a category for describing pain. Numerical rating scales (NRS) may be used instead of word descriptors. In this case clients rate pain on a scale of 1 to 10. The scales work best when assessing pain intensity before and after therapeutic interventions. When scales are used to rate pain, a 10 cm baseline is recommended (AHCPR, 1992).

A visual analog scale (VAS) consists of a straight line without labeled subdivisions. The straight line shows a continuum of intensity and has labeled endpoints. A client indicates pain by marking the appropriate point on the VAS. This scale gives the client total freedom to identify pain severity. The visual analog scale may be a more sensitive measure of pain severity because clients mark at any point on the continuum rather than having to choose one word or number (McGuire, 1984).

Wong and Baker (1988) developed a Faces Scale to assess pain in children (Figure 28-7). The scale consists of six cartoon faces ranging from very happy, smiling face for "no pain" to increasingly less happy faces to a final sad, tearful face for "worst pain." Children as young as 3 years of age can use the scale. Researchers are beginning to test the Faces Scale with older adults. The advantage is that clients do not have to interpret the meaning of numbers or adjectives. The faces more clearly and quickly depict the concept of pain or discomfort.

A pain scale should be designed so it is easy to use and not time consuming for clients. If a client can easily read and understand a scale, the description of pain should be more accurate. Descriptive scales are useful not only in assessing the severity of pain but also in evaluating changes in a client's condition. The nurse does not use pain scales to compare one client with another.

Quality. Another subjective characteristic of pain is quality. When assessing the quality of pain, the nurse should not provide descriptive words for the client. Assessment is more accurate if a client can describe the sensation in his or her own words after open-ended questions. For example, the nurse might say, "Tell me what your pain feels like." The only time the nurse offers to list descriptive terms is when the client cannot describe pain. The qualities of pricking, burning, and aching are useful to describe pain initially (McCaffery and Beebe, 1989). Later the client may choose more descriptive terms. Copp (1990) reported on characteristics of pain named by clients; these included mean, hateful, detestable, sneaky, intense, dark, sharp, loud, clawing, and wicked.

There is some consistency in the way clients describe certain types of pain. The pain of a myocardial infarction is often described as *crushing or viselike,* whereas the pain of a surgical incision is often described as *sharp and stabbing.* When the descriptions fit the pattern forming in the nurse's assessment, a clearer analysis can be made of the nature and type of pain.

Pain pattern. Many factors affect the character of pain. It helps to assess specific events or conditions that precipitate or aggravate pain. The nurse asks the client to describe activities that elicit pain, such as physical activity, coffee or alcohol ingestion, urination, swallowing, or emotional stress. The nurse may ask the client to demonstrate actions that elicit painful responses such as coughing or turning in a certain manner. After identifying specific factors, it is easier to plan interventions to avoid worsening the pain.

Some clients experience suffering, the response to pain, even before the pain begins (Copp, 1990). These clients anticipate pain and its consequences. The fear of having pain may create warning symptoms of restlessness, uneasiness, irritability, and physical symptoms such as diarrhea, vomiting, and muscle aches. Knowledge of these factors may help the nurse plan preventive therapies.

Relief measures. The nurse should know if a client has an effective way for relieving pain such as changing position, using ritualistic behavior (pacing, rocking, rubbing), eating, or applying heat or cold to the painful site. The client's methods often work for the nurse, too. Clients gain comfort from knowing the nurse is willing to try their relief measures. Copp (1990) discovered that clients develop methods to reduce the intensity of oncoming pain. They used a range of muscular activities, verbal methods (prayer and cursing), and concentration exercises. In the home, the nurse must be sure relief measures are used safely. Assessment of relieving factors should also include identifying practitioners (e.g., internist, chiropractor, acupuncturist, faith healer) whose services the client has sought. Clients with chronic pain are more likely to try alternative health care methods.

Concomitant symptoms. Concomitant symptoms are those that often occur with pain, including nausea, headache, dizziness, urge to urinate, constipation, and restlessness. Certain types of pain have predictable symptoms. For example, severe rectal pain often causes constipation. These symptoms can be as much a problem to a client as the pain itself.

Effects of Pain on the Client. Pain is a stressful event that can alter life-style and psychological well-being. By recognizing the effects of pain on a client, the nurse can identify the nature and existence of the pain.

Physical signs and symptoms. The physiological response to pain can reveal the existence and nature of pain and the potential threat to the client's welfare. When a client has pain, the nurse should assess vital signs, conduct a focused physical examination, and observe for autonomic nervous system involvement (see Table 28-2). In the case of cancer clients, a neurologic examination is especially important (Jacox, Carr, and Payne, 1994). Physiological signs can reveal pain in a client who tries not to complain or admit pain. There is no predictable level or extent of change in a client's condition that indicates pain.

At the onset of acute pain, the heart and respiratory rates and blood pressure increase. The nurse compares vital sign values with baseline measurements recorded before onset. A change in vital signs is significant, but the nurse should take into account all signs and symptoms before determining that pain is the cause. The nurse should not confuse signs and symptoms of pain with other pathological changes. The nurse performs a physical and neurologic assessment based on the client's pain history. The painful area should be examined to see if palpation or manipulation of the site increases pain (Jacox, Carr, and Payne, 1994). During a general overview (Chapter 16), the nurse observes for cues indicating pain (e.g., posturing, restricting limb movement, or guiding a painful area).

If pain is unrelieved, the nurse looks for signs of physical exhaustion. Decreasing vital sign values indicate parasympathetic nerve response. The client becomes less responsive to stimuli within the environment. The nurse should measure vital signs more often if the client's condition deteriorates.

Behavioral effects. When clients have pain, the nurse assesses verbalization, vocal response, facial and body movements, and social interaction (see box above). A verbal report of pain is a vital part of assessment. The nurse must be willing to listen and understand. Many clients cannot verbalize discomfort because of an inability to communicate. In these cases the nurse must be alert for behaviors that indicate pain. Marzinski (1991) studied clients with Alzheimer's disease in an attempt to identify pain behaviors in older adults who could not verbalize symptoms. Staff reported that clients who normally moaned and rocked became quiet and withdrawn when in pain. In addition, clients who were outgoing cried easily and withdrew. Nurses must watch for subtle indicators of pain in nonalert older adults.

Subtle facial expressions or body movements often reveal more about the character of pain than vocalizations. In addition, some nonverbal expressions characterize sources of pain. The client with chest pain, for example, often grabs or holds the chest. Nonverbal expressions of pain may support or contradict other information about pain.

The nature of pain causes a client to attend to the discomfort and fight it or give in and withdraw. The extent to which a client interacts with the environment can provide a clue for the nurse about the intensity or nature of pain. Severe pain can seriously hamper a client's life-style.

Influence on activities of daily living. Clients who live with daily pain are less able to participate in routine activities. Assessment reveals the extent of the disability

BEHAVIORAL INDICATORS OF EFFECTS OF PAIN

VOCALIZATIONS

Moaning
Crying
Screaming
Gasping

FACIAL EXPRESSIONS

Grimace
Clenched teeth
Wrinkled forehead
Tightly closed or opened eyes or mouth
Lip biting

BODY MOVEMENT

Restlessness
Immobilization
Muscle tension
Increased hand and finger movements
Pacing activities
Rhythmic or rubbing motions

SOCIAL INTERACTION

Avoidance of conversation or social contacts
Focus only on activities for pain relief
Reduced attention span

ASSESSING THE INFLUENCE OF PAIN ON ACTIVITIES OF DAILY LIVING

SLEEP

Does the client have difficulty in falling asleep?
Does pain awaken the client at night?
Are sleeping pills or other aids needed?

HYGIENE

Does pain hinder the client's ability to use eating utensils or bathe, dress, or perform other hygiene measures independently?
Are family members or friends available or needed to assist?

SEXUAL FUNCTION

Do physical conditions such as arthritis or back pain prevent the client from assuming usual positions during intercourse?
Does pain or fatigue reduce the client's desire for sex?
Are clients fearful that pain will increase as a result of intercourse?

WORK ACTIVITIES

Is physical activity required in the job, and is activity now limited by pain?
If pain is related to emotional stress, does the job involve tension-filled decision making?
Must the client stop activities momentarily to relieve pain?

SOCIAL ACTIVITIES

Does the client regularly socialize?
To what extent has pain disrupted activities?

NURSING DIAGNOSES FOR PAIN

Anxiety
Pain
Chronic pain
Hopelessness
Ineffective individual coping
Impaired physical mobility
High risk for injury
Self-care deficit; bathing/hygiene
Self-care deficit; dressing/grooming
Self-care deficit; feeding
Sexual dysfunction
Sleep pattern disturbance

and the adjustments that will be necessary for participation in self-care (see box above).

Neurological Status. A client's neurological function can easily influence the pain experience. Any factor that interrupts or influences normal pain reception or perception affects the client's awareness and response to pain. Some therapies also influence pain perception and response. For example, analgesics, sedatives, and anesthetics depress the central nervous system. The nurse should assess the neurological status of a client at risk for being insensitive to pain in order to provide preventive care.

Nursing Diagnosis

Accurate nursing diagnoses for clients in pain result from thorough data collection and analysis (see box above, right). A nurse must not diagnose pain simply if it is presumed that a client will be uncomfortable. Too often a nurse may choose the diagnosis of *pain* simply because a client is about to have a painful procedure or a specific disease implies pain.

An accurate diagnosis is made after reviewing clusters of defining characteristics. In the example of *pain* the nurse may assess the client's withdrawal from communication, rigid posturing, moaning, and the client's verbalization of discomfort. In contrast, the diagnosis of *anxiety* may be made by observing a client's facial tension and appearance, poor eye contact, restlessness, and verbalization of feeling scared. The two diagnoses have similar defining characteristics, but the nurse sorts out patterns to reveal pain versus anxiety.

The related factor for the diagnostic statement focuses on the specific nature of the client's problem. Pain related to physical trauma versus pain related to natural childbirth processes require very different nursing interventions. Successful identification of related factors ensures that nursing therapies will be directed toward relieving the client's discomfort.

The nurse may make diagnoses other than pain. The extent to which pain affects a client's life-style and general state of health determines whether other nursing diagnoses are relevant. Sleep pattern disturbance or altered physical mobility are examples of problems that may exist as a result of pain.

Planning

The nurse develops an individualized plan of care for each nursing diagnosis identified (see nursing care plan on p. 757). The nurse and client set realistic expectations for pain relief and the degree of pain relief to expect. In the home, the nurse probably uses some of the client's remedies, as long as they are safe. The client

SAMPLE NURSING CARE PLAN
Pain

ASSESSMENT

Clinical scenario: Ms. Dennis reports having had chronic back pain for more than a year. It was first noted by a pulling sensation in her lower back after a new exercise routine. She now *reports* a *dull, localized pain (rating 6 on a scale of 1 to 10)* in the lumbosacral area. Previous x-rays suggest a mild herniation of a lumbar disk. She *cannot, without discomfort, bend at the waist while standing, dressing, or performing other self-care activities.* She also reports *difficulty sleeping* and a *hesitancy to participate in social events.* She responds to questions alertly but *grimaces while turning* during the physical examination.

NURSING DIAGNOSIS

Chronic pain related to compression of spinal nerves.

PLANNING

Goals	Expected outcomes
Client will achieve a sense of pain relief within 1 month.	Client will report pain at 3 on a scale of 0 to 10 following relaxation therapy. Client will exhibit less grimacing during turning and movement within 2 weeks.
Client will perform self-care measures with less discomfort on self-report within 14 days.	Client will demonstrate less restriction in postural movement during self-care. Client will initiate return to social activities within a month.

IMPLEMENTATION

Steps	Rationale
1. Have client take analgesics or muscle relaxants approximately 30 minutes before client begins self-care activities. During instruction, tell client that drug will relax muscles and reduce pain.	Medication will exert peak effect when client begins activities. An added placebo effect is brought into play when client's attention is focused on action and purpose of analgesic. Then medication is taken with assurance that it will work (McCaffery, 1982; Clancy and McVicar, 1992).
2. Instruct family member on technique for performing slow stroke back massage before client's self-care routines.	Cutaneous stimulation may activate mechanoreceptor A-beta fibers, thus inhibiting transmission of pain by releasing inhibitory neurotransmitters (Clancy and McVicar, 1992).
3. Apply warm, moist heat externally to lower back.	Heat promotes muscle relaxation and reduces pain from spasm or stiffness.
4. Instruct client on method for performing relaxation exercise, to be used when back tightness or stiffening increases.	Distraction is believed to reduce pain perception by modifying the gating process through release of endogenous opiates (e.g., endorphins, which inhibit substance P release) (Melzack and Wall, 1988).

EVALUATION

Observe client's freedom of movement and facial expressions for signs of discomfort.
Ask if client experiences discomfort during self-care activities.
Observe client perform dressing and/or bathing as appropriate, noting range of motion.
Ask client to rate pain on a scale of 1 to 10 and compare with baseline assessment. Use after nursing therapies are administered.

Defining characteristics are shown in italic type.

should understand that complete pain relief cannot be guaranteed, but it will be attempted.

Essential elements for planning pain relief include development of a therapeutic relationship with the client and education regarding pain. The client in pain is highly vulnerable and needs someone to trust. If the nurse cannot establish a therapeutic relationship, any resultant mistrust can heighten the client's awareness of pain and cause an inappropriate reaction to it. The nurse can best help by seeing the client as a total person, listening carefully to concerns, attending promptly to his or her needs, and respecting any response to pain. In a successful nurse-client relationship, the nurse recognizes that the client knows more about his or her own pain and its relief.

The client who understands pain will be better prepared to cope with discomfort. Such understanding reduces anxiety and enhances self-control by allowing the client to focus on pain management. A client can better prepare for an impending painful experience, such as postoperative pain or a diagnostic test, after being properly informed. During the anticipatory phase of the pain experience, the nurse plans to teach clients about procedures and their associated discomfort. This can improve pain tolerance. However, for some clients, early warning can be a problem. Highly anxious or fearful clients often become irrational and are unable to learn. If clients seem unlikely to benefit from advanced preparation, it is best to explain invasive procedures a short time before they occur.

When developing the care plan, the nurse selects priorities based on the client's level of pain and its effect on the client's condition. For acute severe pain, it is important to provide quick relief. Analgesics can be very effective. After a client gains some relief from pain, the nurse plans other therapies such as relaxation or the application of heat to enhance the effect of analgesics.

A comprehensive plan includes a variety of resources for pain control such as family and friends. The family may need to administer care in the home. In an acute-care setting the family must understand the nature and extent of the client's pain and the choice of therapies. Family members or friends who show a disinterest or prejudice toward pain can slow recovery. Additional resources available include nurse specialists, physical therapists, and occupational therapists. An oncology nurse specialist knows therapies for chronic, malignant pain. Physical therapists can plan exercises that strengthen muscle groups and lessen pain. Occupational therapists may devise splints to support painful body parts.

When developing a plan of care, the nurse establishes goals and expected outcomes so that progress toward the goals can be evaluated over time. Client-centered goals of care and outcomes might include:

Goal: Client obtains a sense of well-being and comfort within 3 days.

Outcomes

- Client expresses a reduction in pain as measured on a visual analog scale following pain therapies within 24 hours
- Client demonstrates nonverbally (e.g., facial expression, posture, tone of voice) relief from pain within 48 hours

Goal: Client regains ability to perform self-care independently within 48 hours.

Outcome

- Client bathes and grooms self without hesitancy or restriction in movement within 24 hours

Goal: Client maintains existing physical and psychosocial function.

Outcomes

- Client ambulates independently without restriction in range of motion 3 days postoperatively
- Client participates in social functions with friends within 1 week

Goal: Client understands the pain experience.

Outcomes

- Client describes the sensations to anticipate during a diagnostic procedure
- Client uses options for pain relief following surgery

Implementation

The nature of pain and the extent to which it affects an individual's physical and psychosocial well-being determine the choice of pain relief therapies. Copp (1990) challenges nurses to allow clients to teach them about the nature of suffering so that nurses may help clients cope. Pain therapy requires an individualized approach, perhaps more so than any other client problem. The nurse and client must be partners in using pain control measures. Nurses administer and monitor therapies ordered by physicians for pain relief and independently use pain-relief measures that complement those prescribed by a physician. Client remedies are often most successful, especially when the client has already had experience with pain. Generally, the least invasive or safest therapy should be tried first. If there is doubt about a nursing therapy, the nurse should consult a physician.

Guidelines for Individualizing Pain Therapy. When providing pain-relief measures, the nurse chooses therapies suited to the client's unique pain experience. McCaffery (1979) suggests guidelines for individualizing pain therapy (see box on p. 759).

GUIDELINES FOR INDIVIDUALIZING PAIN THERAPY

Use different types of pain relief measures.

This produces an additive effect in reducing pain and allows for changes in the character of pain.

Provide pain relief measures before pain becomes severe.

It is easier to prevent severe pain than to relieve it after it exists.

Use measures the client believes are effective.

The client's beliefs may make pain therapy successful, so include those remedies as long as they are not harmful.

A client may have ideas about measures to use and times to use them.

Consider the client's ability or willingness to participate in pain-relief measures.

Suggest measures that require little physical effort for clients unable to actively assist with pain therapy because of fatigue or altered levels of consciousness. Do not force participation.

Choose pain relief measures on the basis of client behavior that reflects the severity of pain.

Never administer a potent analgesic for mild pain. Only the client can determine the potency of an effective therapy.

If a therapy is ineffective at first, encourage the client to try it again before abandoning it.

Client anxiety or doubt may prevent therapy from relieving pain, or the measure may require adjustment or practice to become effective.

Keep an open mind about ways to relieve pain.

Rejecting nonconventional therapies leads to mistrust. Be sure all therapies are safe.

Keep trying.

When efforts at pain relief fail, do not abandon the client but reassess the situation and consider alternative therapies.

Protect the client.

Pain therapy should not cause more distress than the pain itself; the nurse wants to relieve pain without disabling the client mentally, emotionally, or physically.

Educate the client about pain.

The nurse should explain the cause of pain, times when analgesics can be given, and alternative therapies.

Caring in Promoting Pain Relief. Regardless of the type of therapies used, the nurse's ability to show caring toward a client can maximize pain control. Clancy and McVicar (1992) suggest that reducing client anxiety or using a confident approach during nursing care may be ways to enhance the effects of naturally occurring opiates in the body. Clients are able to perceive a nurse's caring approach. This reinforces the trust that builds as a nurse forms a relationship with a client. Caring involves a sense of dedication to an individual, but it involves more than having concern for another person; it involves integrating behaviors into everyday nursing practice.

Pain can be minimized through caring behaviors such as gentle handling and touch. Burnside (1988) suggests that two types of touching—*task-oriented* and *affective*—can be effective with clients. Task-oriented touching occurs when a nurse takes a client's blood pressure or helps the client walk. Affective is less routine and intended to show concern, such as giving a client a hug. Often one can combine task-oriented and affective touching (e.g., placing a hand on the client's shoulder while administering a tablet). Simply sitting and holding a client's hand, allowing a client to move at his or her own speed, speaking in a soft tone of voice, and staying with a client for a time after a procedure are all caring behaviors. The nurse's use of nonverbal expressions to reinforce words of encouragement and support also convey caring. When a nurse can successfully convey compassion, maintain the client's dignity, and consistently strive to minimize discomfort or suffering, pain-relieving measures will be more successful.

Promoting Wellness. Pain can seriously disable and immobilize a person, which can impair the ability to perform self-care activities. Pain also causes social isolation, depression, and changes in self-concept. Change in function can mean a significant loss to a client. The nurse helps clients and families learn to discuss their feelings about the loss so as to find ways to cope with pain and the life-style it imposes.

The nurse minimizes the effects of immobilization from pain by using good positioning techniques (see Chapter 22). Painful body parts can be further protected by using elastic bandages, braces, splints, or pillows for support. These devices can be used in the home as well as in any health care facility. If crutches or other assistive devices are needed, the nurse ensures that they are used safely and properly.

The nurse may refer clients who have difficulty eating, bathing, grooming, and dressing to an occupational therapist. Some agencies may require a physician's order to ultimately initiate occupational therapy. Devices designed to maintain function, even when finger movement or grasp is impaired, can help. The therapist can attach eating utensils, a comb, or a toothbrush to extension devices that have enlarged handles or splints for easy use. Clothing fasteners made of Velcro tape allow clients to remove or apply clothing by themselves.

Measures that promote a sense of well-being in a client with pain include warm baths, thorough personal hygiene measures, and a schedule for adequate rest. The nurse should plan rest periods before exhaustive procedures or visits by friends. Clients with chronic pain should rest before social activities in the home.

A client with pain may avoid sexual activity. The need for sexual warmth is not negated by pain. Clients can learn to express themselves sexually by assuming alternative positions during intercourse and learning more about ways to make their partner feel sexually stimulated. Nurses should caution clients that some pain medications can decrease libido and potency.

Nonpharmacologic Pain Relief Measures. One of the most basic nursing responsibilities is protecting the client from harm. There are a number of nonpharmacologic therapies that lessen the reception and perception of pain. Similarly, these therapies can be used in combination with pharmacologic measures. The AHCPR guidelines for acute pain management (1992) cite nonpharmacologic interventions to be appropriate for clients who:

- Find such interventions appealing
- Express anxiety or fear
- May benefit from avoiding or reducing drug therapy
- Are likely to experience and need to cope with a prolonged interval of postoperative pain
- Have incomplete pain relief after use of pharmacologic therapies

In the case of cancer patients, the nurse's responsibility is to evaluate the effects of nonpharmacologic measures to ensure pain relief occurs so that clients are not excluded from use of pharmacologic therapies as needed.

Reducing pain reception. One simple way to promote comfort is by removing or preventing painful stimuli (see box below, left). This is especially important for clients who are immobilized or unable to sense discomfort. Pain can also be prevented by anticipating painful activities (e.g., ambulation or turning). Before performing a procedure the nurse considers the client's condition, aspects of the procedure that are painful, and ways to avoid causing pain. It takes only simple consideration of the client's comfort and a little extra time to avoid pain-producing situations.

Cutaneous stimulation. Cutaneous stimulation is the stimulation of the skin to relieve pain. A massage (see box below), warm bath, ice bag, and transcutaneous electrical nerve stimulation (TENS) are simple ways to reduce pain perception. The specific way in which cutaneous stimulation works is unclear. One suggestion is that it releases endorphins. The gate-control theory suggests that cutaneous stimulation activates

CONTROLLING PAINFUL STIMULI IN THE CLIENT'S ENVIRONMENT

Tighten and smooth wrinkled bed linen.
Position client off tubing or other equipment.
Loosen constricting bandages (unless applied as pressure dressing).
Change wet dressings or bed linen.
Position client correctly.
Check temperature of hot or cold applications, including bath water.
Lift client up in bed; do not pull.
Position client correctly on bed pan.
Avoid exposing skin or mucous membranes to irritants (e.g., diarrheal stool or wound drainage).
Prevent urinary retention by keeping Foley catheters patent and free flowing.
Prevent constipation with fluids, diet, and exercise.

TECHNIQUES FOR MASSAGE AND BACKRUB

Massage one or more body parts.
Help client to assume comfortable lying or sitting position.
Massage each body part at least 10 minutes:
Hands. Make contact first with one hand and then the other. Using both hands, slowly open the client's palm, gliding the fingers over the palmar surface. While supporting the hand, use both thumbs to apply friction to the palm and use them in a circular motion to stretch the palm outward. Massage each finger outward and then separately, using a corkscrew-like motion from base of finger to the tip. With thumb and finger, knead each small muscle in the client's fingers. Glide hands smoothly from fingertips to wrists. Repeat for other hand.
Arms. Use a gliding stroke to massage from the client's wrist to forearm. With thumb and forefinger of both hands, knead muscles from forearm to shoulder. Continue kneading biceps, deltoid, and triceps muscles. Finish with gliding strokes from the wrist to the shoulder.
Neck. Support the neck at the hairline with one hand and massage up it with a gliding stroke. Knead muscles on one side. Switch hands to support neck and knead other side. Stretch the neck slightly, with one hand at the top and the other at the bottom.

larger, faster transmitting A-beta sensory nerve fibers. This decreases pain transmission through small-diameter A-delta and C fibers. Synaptic gates close to the transmission of pain impulses. Meek (1993) suggests that touch and massage are sensory integration techniques that influence autonomic nervous system activity. When a person perceives touch to be relaxing, the relaxation response is elicited.

An advantage to cutaneous stimulation is that the measures can be used in the home, giving clients and families some control over pain symptoms and treatment. The proper use of cutaneous stimulation can reduce pain perception and help to reduce muscle tension that might otherwise increase pain. When slow stroke back massage has been used with terminally ill clients, there has been a decrease in systolic and diastolic blood pressure, suggesting relaxation (Meek, 1993). When using cutaneous stimulation methods, the nurse eliminates sources of environmental noise, helps the client to assume a comfortable position, and explains the purpose of the therapy. Cutaneous stimulation should not be used directly on sensitive skin areas (e.g., burns, bruises, skin rashes, inflammation, and underlying bone fractures).

Cold and heat applications (Chapter 37) relieve pain and promote healing. The selection of heat versus cold therapies varies with clients' conditions. For example, moist heat relieves the early morning stiffness of arthritis, but cold applications reduce the acute pain and inflamed joints of the disease (Ceccio, 1990). When using any form of heat or cold application, the nurse instructs the client to avoid injury to the skin. Especially at risk are clients with spinal cord or other neurological injury, older adults, and confused clients.

Ice massage is one therapy particularly effective. It involves use of a large ice cube or a small paper cup filled with water and frozen. A nurse or the client can apply the ice with firm pressure to the skin, followed by a slow, steady, circular massage over the area. Cold may be applied near the pain site, on the opposite side of the body corresponding to the pain site, or on a site between the brain and pain site (McCaffery, 1986). It takes 5 to 10 minutes to apply cold. Application near the actual site of pain tends to work best. A client feels cold, burning and aching sensations, and numbness. When numbness occurs, the ice should be removed. Cold is particularly effective for tooth and mouth pain and before invasive needle punctures.

Another form of cutaneous stimulation sometimes called counterstimulation is **transcutaneous electrical nerve stimulation (TENS),** involving stimulation of the skin with a mild electrical current passed through external electrodes. It requires a physician's order. The TENS unit (Figure 28-8) consists of a battery-powered transmitter, lead wires, and electrodes. The electrodes are placed directly over or near the site of pain. Hair or skin preparations should be removed before attaching the electrodes. When a client feels pain, the transmitter is turned on and a buzzing or tingling sensation is created. The tingling sensation can be applied until pain relief is achieved. TENS is useful in managing postoperative pain and in reducing pain caused by postoperative procedures (e.g., removing drains) (Hargreaves and Lander, 1989). It is easy to use and is contraindicated for only a few clients.

DISTRACTION. With meaningful sensory stimuli, a client can ignore or become unaware of pain. Pleasurable stimuli cause the release of endorphins. Distraction directs a client's attention to something else and thus can reduce the awareness of pain and even increase tolerance. Distraction may work best for short, intense pain lasting a few minutes such as during an invasive procedure or while waiting for an analgesic to work.

Useful forms of distraction include singing, listening to music, describing photos out loud, telling jokes, and playing games. Music can be used in many clinical situations. Soothing music is played in some operative recovery areas. Whipple (1987) found that soothing music and stimulating music can significantly elevate pain thresholds (see box on p. 762). Musical selections should match a client's mood and taste (Bailey, 1985).

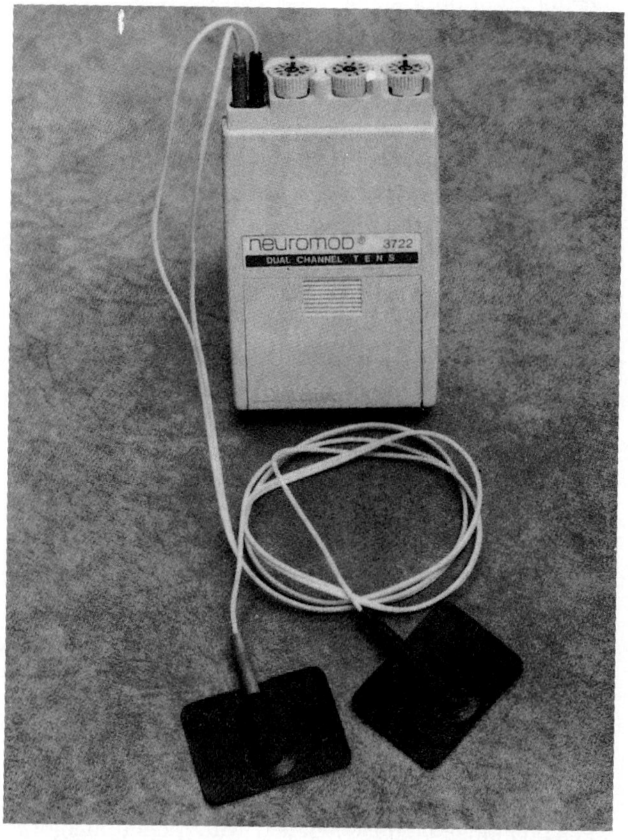

FIGURE 28-8 Transcutaneous electrical nerve stimulation (TENS) unit.

USING MUSIC TO CONTROL PAIN

Use earphones to avoid annoying others and help client to concentrate on music.
If pain is acute, increase volume of music. As pain decreases, reduce the volume.
Have client concentrate on the music and emphasize rhythm by tapping fingers or patting the thigh.
Encourage clients to use music, particularly when it is enjoyed in the home.

Earphones with audio cassettes avoid annoying other clients or staff and help the client to concentrate on the music. If pain becomes acute, it helps to increase the volume of the music. The client can concentrate better by rhythmically tapping fingers or patting the thigh to the beat.

Relaxation. The ability to relax physically promotes mental relaxation. Relaxation techniques provide clients with self-control when pain occurs, reversing the physical and emotional stress of pain. Clients who use relaxation techniques successfully go through physiological and behavioral changes (e.g., decreased pulse and blood pressure, decreased muscle tension, heightened concentration on a single idea, and decreased oxygen consumption). Relaxation strategies include simple relaxation, imagery, hypnosis, biofeedback, and music-assisted relaxation. Relaxation and imagery techniques can be simple and have been successful in reducing self-reported pain and analgesic use (Wells, 1982). The techniques require periodic reinforcement through encouragement and coaching (AHCPR, 1992). Supportive family and friends or the use of audiotapes can sustain client skills.

Relaxation is mental and physical freedom from tension or stress. For effective relaxation the client needs to participate and cooperate. Relaxation techniques are taught only when the client is not in acute discomfort and thus is able to concentrate. The nurse explains the technique in detail and notes that considerable practice is needed for consistent pain control. The nurse describes common sensations that the client may experience (e.g., a decrease in temperature, a feeling of heaviness, or numbness of a body part). The client uses these sensations as feedback. Acting as a coach, the nurse guides the client slowly through the steps of the exercise. The environment should be free of noises or other irritating stimuli. The client should sit in a comfortable chair in good alignment or lie in bed. A light sheet or blanket keeps the client warm and comfortable. Relaxation may be done alone or with guided imagery.

In **guided imagery,** the client creates an image in the mind, concentrates on that image, and gradually becomes less aware of pain. The nurse coaches the client in forming the image and concentrating on the sensory experience. Initially the nurse asks the client to think of a pleasant scene or experience that promotes using all senses. The client describes the image and the nurse records it so that it can be used later. The nurse uses only specific information given by the client and makes no changes in the image. The following is an example of a portion of guided imagery exercise:

Imagine yourself lying on a cool bed of grass with the sounds of rushing water from a nearby stream. It's a warm, balmy day. You turn to see a patch of blue wildflowers in bloom and can smell their fragrance.

The nurse sits close enough to the client to be heard but is not intrusive. A calm, soft voice helps the client to focus more completely on the suggested image. While relaxing, the client focuses on the image, and it becomes unnecessary for the nurse to speak continuously. If the client shows signs of agitation, restlessness, or discomfort, the nurse should stop the exercise and begin later when the client is more at ease.

Progressive relaxation exercises involve a combination of controlled breathing exercises and a series of contractions and relaxations of muscle groups. The client begins by breathing slowly and diaphragmatically, allowing the abdomen to rise slowly and the chest to expand fully. When the client establishes a regular breathing pattern, the nurse coaches the client to locate any area of muscular tension, think about how it feels, tense the muscles fully, and then completely relax them. This creates the sensation of removing all discomfort and stress. Gradually the client can relax the muscles without first tensing them. After the client achieves full relaxation, pain perception is lowered, and anxiety toward the pain experience becomes minimal. The following is an example of how a nurse coaches a client:

Let's begin by finding as comfortable a position as possible. Arms at your sides. . . . legs uncrossed. . . . Move until you feel at ease. . . . Take a deep breath. Feel your stomach and chest slowly rise. . . . Relax. . . . Now breathe out slowly . . . slowly . . . and relax. Breathe in slowly again . . . and let it out. Your body is beginning to relax. . . . Think relax. . . . Feel the parts of your body. . . . Notice any tension in your muscles. . . . Continue to breathe slowly . . . and relax. Concentrate on any tension in your hands. . . . Notice how it feels. . . . Now make a fist. A tight fist! As you begin to exhale, relax your fist. . . . Good! Notice how your hand feels. . . . Think relax. . . . Your hand may feel warm or cool . . . heavy or light. . . . Just relax more . . . and more. Now focus on your forearms. . . . Notice any tension. . . . Relax your arms. . . . Feel your body relaxing. . . . Let the feelings of relaxation spread from your fingers and hands through the muscles of your arms.

If the client becomes agitated or uncomfortable, the nurse stops the exercise. If the client reports having difficulty relaxing only part of the body, the nurse slows the progression of the exercise and concentrates on the tensed body part. The client may stop the exercise at any time. With practice, the client can learn to perform relaxation exercises independently.

Relaxation techniques are particularly effective for chronic pain, labor pains, and relief of procedure-related pain. The techniques are less effective for episodes of acute or severe pain.

ANTICIPATORY GUIDANCE. Modifying anxiety directly associated with pain relieves pain and adds to the effects of other pain-relief measures. Moderate anxiety can help when a client anticipates pain. Clients can learn what is to be expected during a painful event. Knowledge about pain helps a client control anxiety and gain a level of relief. The AHCPR (1992) reports that giving clients detailed descriptions of all medical procedures, expected postoperative discomfort, and instruction aimed at decreasing treatment- and mobility-related pain can decrease self-reported pain, analgesic use, and postoperative length of stay. Clients should receive sufficient procedural and sensory information (e.g., prick of a needle during blood draw or burning during urinary catheter insertion) to satisfy their interest and enable them to assess, evaluate, and communicate pain.

BIOFEEDBACK. Biofeedback is a behavioral therapy that involves providing information about physiological responses (such as blood pressure or tension) and ways to exercise voluntary control over those responses. Special training and equipment are necessary. For example, in the treatment of chronic headaches a client wears temporal electrodes, which measure skin tension in microvolts. A polygraph machine visibly records the tension level for the client to see. The client learns to relax, using feedback from the polygraph; as relaxation increases, tension declines. The therapy takes several weeks to learn.

HYPNOSIS. Hypnosis can help alter pain perception through the influence of positive suggestion. Some people can induce self-hypnosis while others cannot. Formal hypnosis requires the service of a hypnotist. Self-hypnosis is similar to daydreaming. The intense concentration reduces apprehension and stress as a person concentrates on only one thought.

Pharmacological Pain Therapy

Several pharmacological agents provide pain management. All require a physician's order. The nurse's judgment in the use of medications with or without other pain therapies ensures the best pain relief possible.

Acute Pain Management. Nurses care for clients who undergo surgery, medical procedures, and who are victims of trauma. The approach to therapy ranges from no set strategy to a comprehensive team approach. The AHCPR (1992) has established a pain treatment flow chart (Figure 28-9) for the aggressive treatment of postoperative pain. The guidelines can also be applicable to patients recovering from painful medical procedures and trauma. The systematic approach ensures quick response on the part of care givers to client discomfort.

Analgesics. Analgesics are the most common method of pain relief. Although analgesics can effectively relieve pain, nurses and physicians tend to undertreat clients because of incorrect drug information, concerns about addiction, anxiety over errors in judgment while using narcotic analgesics, and administration of less medication than was ordered. Nurses must understand the drugs available for pain relief and their pharmacological effects.

The three types of analgesics are nonnarcotic and nonsteroidal anti-inflammatory drugs (NSAIDs), opioids, and adjuvants or coanalgesics (Table 28-5). NSAIDs are effective in treating mild to moderate pain. They act by inhibiting the synthesis of prostaglandins (McKenry and Salerno, 1993) and by inhibiting the cellular responses during inflammation. Most NSAIDs act on peripheral nerve receptors to diminish transmission and reception of pain stimuli. One exception, acetaminophen, acts on central nervous system prostaglandins. Opioid or narcotic analgesics are generally used for severe pain. They act on the central nervous system to produce a combination of depressing and stimulating effects. Adjuvants such as sedatives, antianxiety agents, and muscle relaxants enhance pain control or relieve other symptoms associated with pain such as depression and nausea. They may be given alone or with analgesics.

Narcotic analgesics such as morphine and meperidine (Demerol) act on higher centers of the brain and spinal cord by binding with opiate receptors to modify perception of and reaction to pain. Morphine is a derivative of opium. It raises the pain threshold (reducing pain perception), reduces anxiety and fear (components of the reaction to pain), and induces sleep. Morphine and other narcotic analgesics can depress vital nervous system functions such as respirations. Clients may also have side effects such as nausea, vomiting, constipation, and altered mental processes. Characteristics of an ideal analgesic include:

1. Rapid onset
2. Prolonged effectiveness
3. Effectiveness in all age-groups
4. Oral and parenteral use
5. Lack of severe side effects
6. Nonaddicting nature
7. Inexpensive

The proper use of analgesics requires careful assessment, application of pharmacological principles (see Chapter 26), and common sense (see box on p. 766). Re-

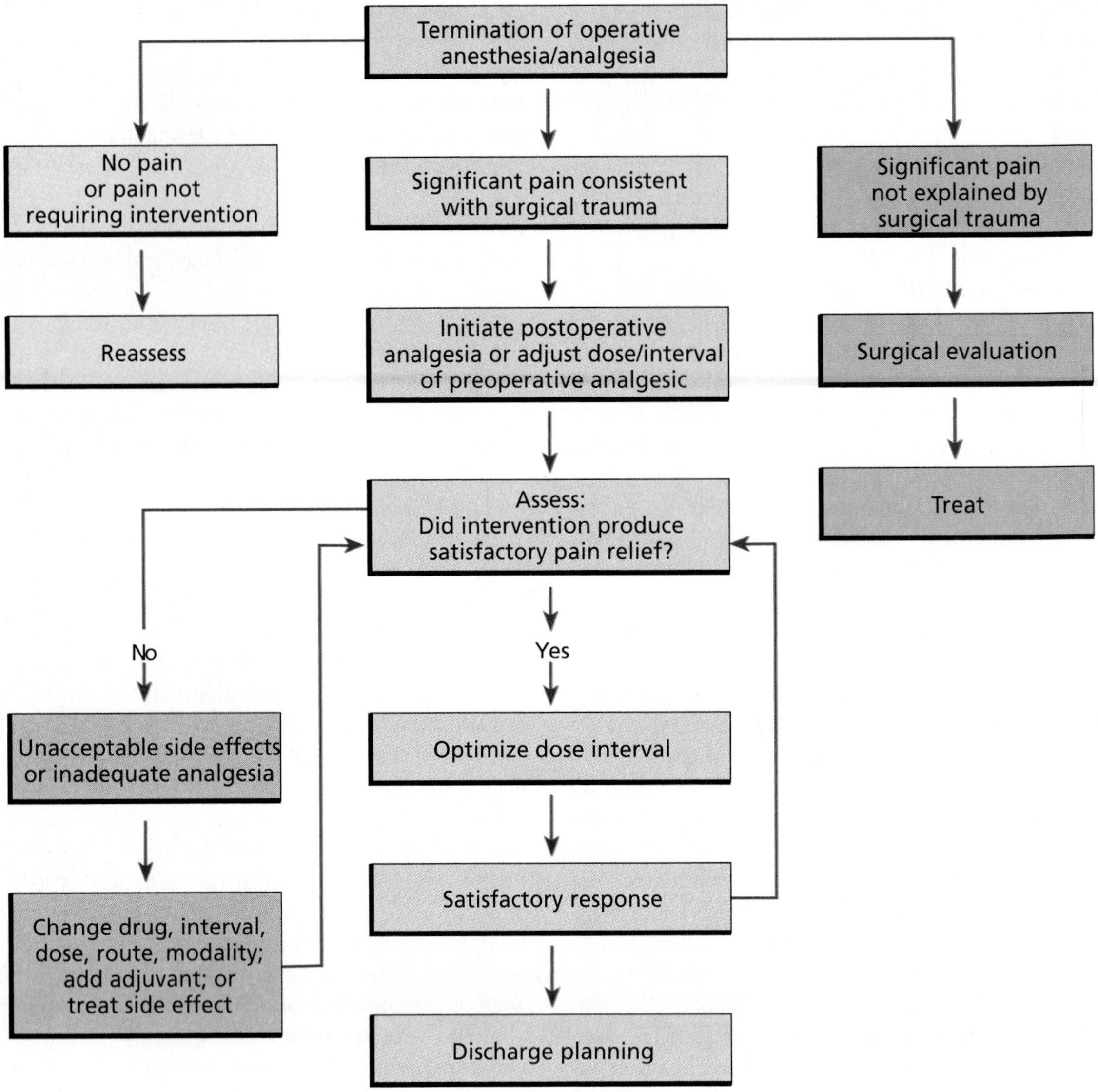

FIGURE 28-9 Pain treatment flow chart: postoperative phase. (From Acute pain management guideline panel. Acute pain management: Operative or medical procedures and trauma, *Clinical practice guideline.* AHCPR Pub No 92-0032. Rockville, Md. AHCPR, Public Health Service, USDHHS, Feb. 1992.)

sponses to analgesics are highly individualized. An NSAID may be as effective as a potent narcotic for some clients, or an orally administered analgesic may bring the same relief as an injectable form. Nurses must remain familiar with comparative doses of different analgesics. In addition, nurses on succeeding shifts must know the route of administration most effective for a client so that controlled, sustained pain relief is achieved.

Children require careful calculation of drug doses. Equianalgesic charts that convert recommended adult doses to children's doses are available. These charts consider age and body size. Older adults also require special considerations (see box on p. 766).

Patient-Controlled Analgesia. Clients benefit from having control over pain therapy. When clients depend on nurses for analgesia, an erratic cycle of alternating pain and analgesia often occurs. The client feels pain and asks for a drug, but the nurse may be unable to give it promptly. Within 1 hour analgesia finally occurs, but pain relief may last only 1/2 hour and the client may be sedated as long as 1 hour. Then the client feels pain again, and the cycle starts over.

Patient controlled analgesia (PCA) is a safe

table 28-5
ANALGESIC INDICATIONS

Drug category	Indications
NON-NARCOTIC ANALGESICS	
• Acetaminophen (Tylenol, Datril) • Acetylsalicylic acid (aspirin) • Choline magnesium trisalicylate (Trilisate)	Postoperative pain Rheumatic and nonrheumatic inflammation Fever Dysmenorrhea Vascular headaches
NSAIDS	
• Ibuprofen (Motrin, Nuprin) • Naproxen (Naprosyn) • Naproxen sodium (Anaprox) • Indomethacin (Indocin) • Tolmetin (Tolectin) • Piroxicam (Feldene)	
NARCOTIC ANALGESICS	
• Meperidine (Demerol) • Methylmorphine (Codeine) • Morphine sulfate (Morphine) • Fentanyl (Sublimaze) • Butorphanol (Stadol) • Hydromorphone HCl (Dilaudid)	Postoperative pain Severe traumatic pain Cancer pain (except for Meperidine) Myocardial infarction
ADJUVANTS	
• Amitriptyline (Elavil) • Hydroxyzine (Vistaril) • Caffeine • Chlorpromazine (Thorazine) • Diazepam (Valium)	Anxiety Depression Nausea Vomiting

method for postoperative, traumatic, labor and delivery, and cancer pain management that most clients prefer to intermittent injections. It is a drug delivery system that allows clients to administer pain medications when they want them. Systemic PCA usually involves IV drug administration, but it can also be given subcutaneously. PCAs are portable infusion pumps containing a chamber for a syringe (Figure 28-10, *A*) or specifically designed devices like the wristwatch (Figure 28-10, *B*) that deliver a small preset dose of medication (usually morphine). To receive a dose, the client pushes a button attached to the PCA device. The system is designed to deliver no more than a specified number of doses either every hour or 4 hours (depending on pump) to avoid overdoses. For example, a typical PCA prescription relies on a series of "loading" doses: for example, 3 to 5 mg of morphine, repeated every 5 minutes until initial postoperative pain diminishes. A low-dose basal infusion (0.5 to 1 mg/hr) at night allows uninterrupted sleep. On-demand doses typically add 1 mg of morphine every 6 minutes, with a total hourly limit of 10 mg (AHCPR, 1992). Most pumps have locked safety systems to prevent tampering. Even though a dose can be released only over a select number of minutes, a small bell alarms each time the client pushes the button. The bell acts as a placebo. The client believes a dose is delivered with each ring.

Benefits of PCA include clients having control over pain, pain relief not depending on nurse availability, clients tending to take less medication, and small doses of narcotics delivered at short intervals stabilizing serum drug concentrations for sustained pain relief. Client preparation and teaching is critical to the safe and effective use of PCA (see teaching box on p. 766). Clients must be able to understand the use of the equipment and be physically able to locate and press the button to deliver the dose.

Nurses must check the intravenous line and PCA device regularly to ensure proper functioning. Certain pumps keep track of accumulative dosage and print out

NURSING PRINCIPLES FOR ADMINISTERING ANALGESICS

Know the client's previous response to analgesics.

Determine if relief was obtained.
Ask if a nonnarcotic was as effective as a narcotic.
Identify previous doses and routes of administration to avoid undertreatment.
Determine if the client has allergies.

Select proper medications when more than one is ordered.

Use NSAIDs or milder narcotics for mild-to-moderate pain.
The concurrent use of opioids and NSAIDs often provides more effective analgesia than either drug class alone.
Use of NSAIDs can help reduce opioid side effects.
Morphine and hydromorphone are the narcotics of choice for long-term management of severe pain.
Know that injectable medications act quicker and can relieve severe pain within 1 hour and that oral medication may take as long as 2 hours to relieve pain.
For chronic pain, give an oral drug for longer, more sustained relief.

Know the accurate dosage.

Remember that doses at the upper end of normal are generally needed for severe pain.
Dosage typically requires adjustment over time.
Adjust doses, as appropriate, for children and older adults.
Know the comparative potencies of analgesics (refer to drug manual or pharmacy) in oral and injectable form (e.g., Demerol 100 mg equals approximately 13 mg morphine intramuscularly).

Select the right time and interval for administration.

Administer analgesics as soon as pain occurs and before it increases in severity.
Do not give analgesics only on "as-needed" schedules. An around-the-clock administration schedule is usually best, especially for cancer clients (Jacox, Carr, Payne, 1994).
Give analgesics before pain-producing procedures or activities.
Know the average duration of action for a drug and the time of administration so that the peak effect occurs when pain is most intense.
Choose the right route.
Oral route is preferred.
Intramuscular administration should be avoided because this route can be painful and absorption is not reliable (Jacox, Carr, and Payne, 1994).

GERONTOLOGIC CONSIDERATIONS FOR PAIN CONTROL

In older adults there is fear that pain will result in crippling and forced dependency.
Older adults are at high risk for pain inducing situations.
Several pain-producing conditions may coexist.
The potential for lowered pain tolerance exists with diminished adaptive capacity.
Changes in peripheral vascular function, skin, and transmission of pain impulses place the older adult at risk for being unable to sense pain (Ebersole and Hess, 1990).
When administering analgesics, nurses should confer with physicians regarding proper dosing. Clients may be susceptible to side effects of narcotics because of changes in serum proteins, liver and renal function, and a reduction in cardiac output.
The risk for gastric and renal toxicity from NSAIDs is increased among older adults.
Older adults are more sensitive to the analgesic effects of opioid drugs as they experience a higher peak and longer duration of pain relief.

CLIENT TEACHING AND PREPARATION FOR PCA

Teach the use of PCA before surgery so that clients can understand how to use it after awakening from anesthesia. (Confused and unresponsive clients, clients with history of narcotic abuse, neurological disease, impaired renal or pulmonary function, and those unable to press the delivery button are not candidates for PCA.)
Instruct clients on the purpose of PCA, operating instructions, expected pain relief, precautions, and potential side effects (IVNS, 1990), emphasizing that the client controls medication delivery.
Explain that the pump prevents risks of overdose.
Tell family members or friends that they should not operate the PCA device for the client.
Have the client demonstrate use of the PCA delivery button.

A

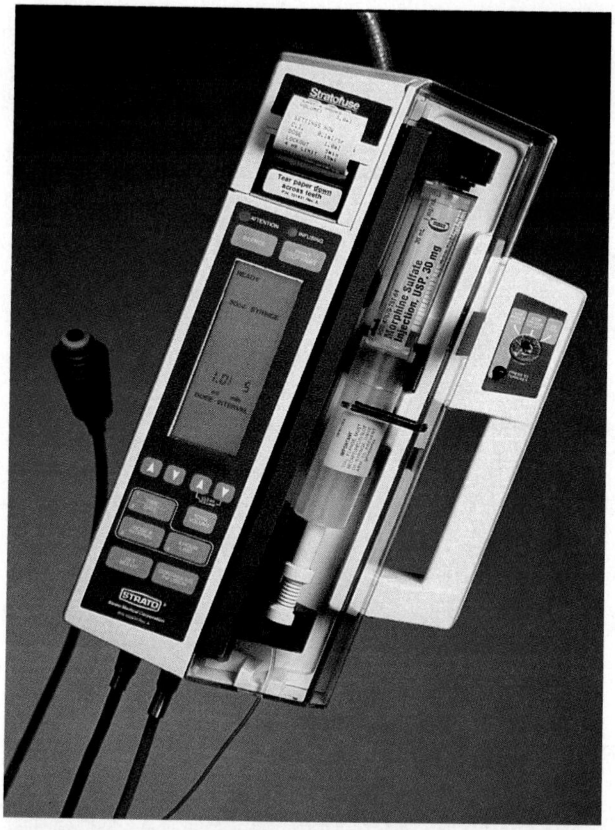

B

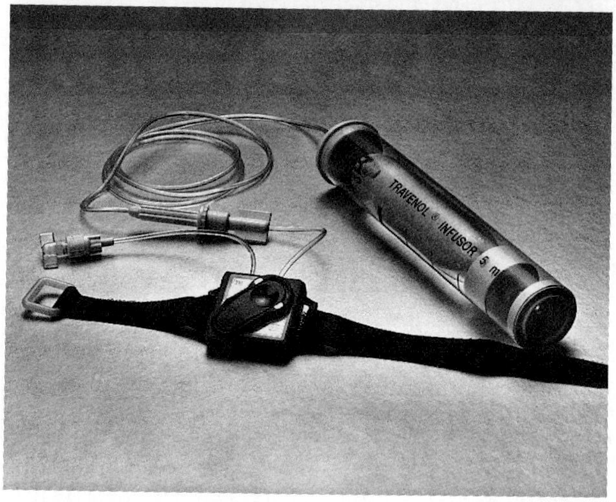

FIGURE 28-10 Patient-controlled analgesia devices. **A,** Computerized pump. **B,** Wristwatch device. (Courtesy Baxter Healthcare Corporation.)

the information on demand. Drug doses must be carefully documented, and any narcotics that are wasted or unused must be recorded (see Chapter 26).

Placebos. A **placebo** is a dose form that contains no pharmacologically active ingredient but may relieve pain. Commonly used placebos are normal saline, sterile water, and sugar. The pharmacy prepares placebos in forms (e.g., tablets) that make them look like medications. A doctor's order is required. Considerable argument exists over the way placebos work. Some researchers believe that they increase endorphin levels. Others believe that the placebo creates a psychological sense of pain relief, lowering pain perception. No matter the mode of action, when the placebo is administered correctly, the client is convinced that it will provide pain relief. The client's belief that a placebo is a true form of therapy may be the necessary factor in relieving pain. A nurse can also use a "placebo effect" when administering analgesics by telling clients that the drug will act to reduce pain. Belief that a medication will work and trust in the nurse increases the likelihood of pain relief. The nurse administers the placebo as though it were an actual pain medication, assesses the pain carefully, and evaluates the placebo's effects.

The use of placebos raises certain ethical questions. Is it appropriate to lie to a client even though a placebo proves effective? If a client learns that a placebo has been given, trust in the nurse may become threatened. The nurse must be a client advocate and determine whether use of a placebo is appropriate. Continuous use of narcotic agents, for example, is not beneficial to the client if placebos instead provide pain relief.

Local Anesthetics. **Local anesthesia** is the loss of sensation to a localized body part. Physicians use local anesthesia while suturing a wound, moving a painful body part, delivering an infant, and performing some surgery. Local anesthetics have fewer risks than general anesthetics, which cause loss of consciousness and depress vital functions. Local anesthetics can be given topically on skin and mucous membranes or injected to anesthetize a body part. The drugs produce temporary losses of sensation by inhibiting nerve conduction; they also block motor and autonomic functions when administered as nerve blocks (Table 28-6). Typically a client loses sensation in small sensory nerves before losing motor function; conversely, motor activity returns before sensation.

Local anesthetics can cause side effects, depending on their absorption. Itching, burning of the skin, or a localized rash are common with topical application. Application to vascular mucous membranes may cause systemic effects such as a change in heart rate. Injection increases the risk of systemic effects.

Table 28-6 summarizes the types of local anesthesia by injection. Each produces a different level of anesthesia as a result of the amount of drug used and the location of the spinal nerve affected.

The nurse provides emotional support to clients receiving local anesthesia by explaining insertion sites and warning clients that they will temporarily lose sensory function. Autonomic function (bowel and bladder control) may also be temporarily lost. To reassure the

table 28-6

LOCAL ANESTHESIA TECHNIQUES

Type	Area of injection	Area anesthetized	Indications for use
Infiltration	Under skin or mucous membranes	Small peripheral nerves in area treated	Small skin incisions, insertion of sutures to close cuts or wounds, minor dental repairs
Peripheral nerve block	In areas surrounding large peripheral nerve at point above bifurcation of nerve	Wider area than with infiltration, numbing entire body part (e.g., hand, or foot)	Major dental repairs, manipulation or reduction of extremity fractures, minor hand and foot surgery
Epidural or peridural nerve block	In lumbosacral region of spinal cord, around major nerve roots exiting base of spinal cord at site outside dura mater	Lower trunk and extremities	Delivery of newborn, major surgery to lower trunk and extremities (e.g., hemorrhoidectomy, vascular repair), cancer pain in lower trunk
Spinal nerve block	Around major nerve root within subarachnoid space of spinal cord	Lower trunk and extremities	Major surgery to lower trunk and extremities, clients at risk with general anesthesia

client, the nurse explains application of the anesthetic and the sensations experienced. Injection can be painful unless the physician numbs the injection site. The nurse prepares clients for such discomfort. Before a client receives an anesthetic, the nurse checks for allergies. To monitor systemic effects, the nurse assesses blood pressure and pulse. Spinal anesthesia may also cause respiratory changes.

After administration of a local anesthetic the nurse protects the client from injury until full sensory and motor function return. Pain is a protective mechanism. Until a local anesthetic is absorbed and metabolized the client must be careful in using an anesthetized body part. Clients can easily injure themselves without knowing it.

Epidural analgesia. Epidural analgesia is a form of local anesthesia and an effective therapy for the treatment of acute postoperative pain and chronic pain, especially that associated with cancer (McNair, 1990). It permits control or reduction of severe pain without the sedative effects of narcotics. Epidural analgesia can be short or long term, depending on the client's condition and life expectancy. Short-term therapy is used for pain after intrathoracic, abdominal, and orthopedic surgery. Long-term therapy is used for intractable pain in the lower part of the body, particularly when bilateral (DuPen and Williams, 1992). McNair (1990) lists several advantages of epidural analgesia including:

- Production of excellent analgesia
- Occurrence of minimal sedation
- Action of long duration
- Facilitation of early ambulation
- Avoidance of repeated injections
- No significant effect on sensation
- Little effect on blood pressure or heart rate

Epidural analgesia is administered into the spinal epidural space usually while the client is in the operating room or in a postanesthesia care unit. A physician inserts the catheter into the level of the vertebral interspace nearest to the area requiring analgesia or at the L_4 to L_5 space depending on physician preference (Figure 28-11). Once the catheter is advanced into the epidural space (Figure 28-12) and the needle removed, the remainder of the catheter is secured with occlusive dressing and taped up the back of the client (McNair, 1990). If the catheter is only temporary, it is connected to tubing positioned along the spine and over the client's shoulder. The end of the catheter can then be placed on

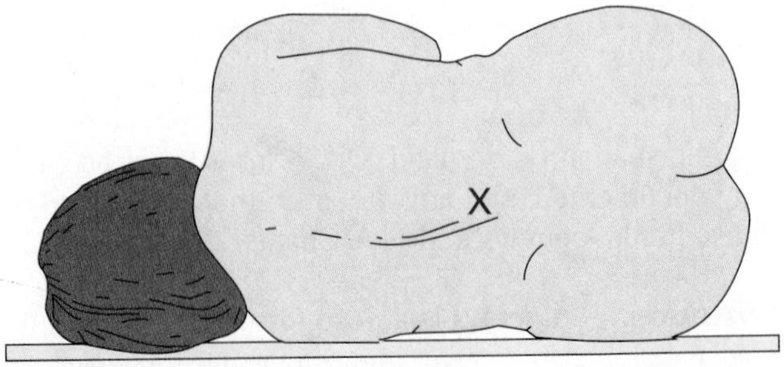

FIGURE 28-11 Positioning of client for epidural catheter insertion.

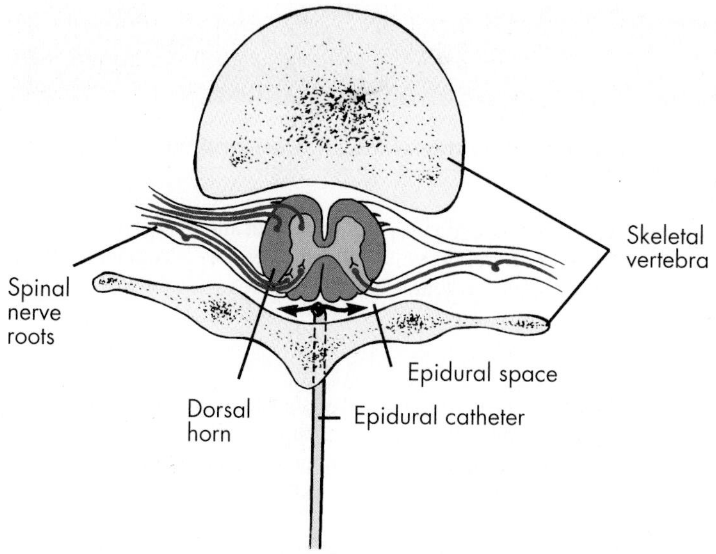

FIGURE 28-12 Anatomic drawing of epidural space.

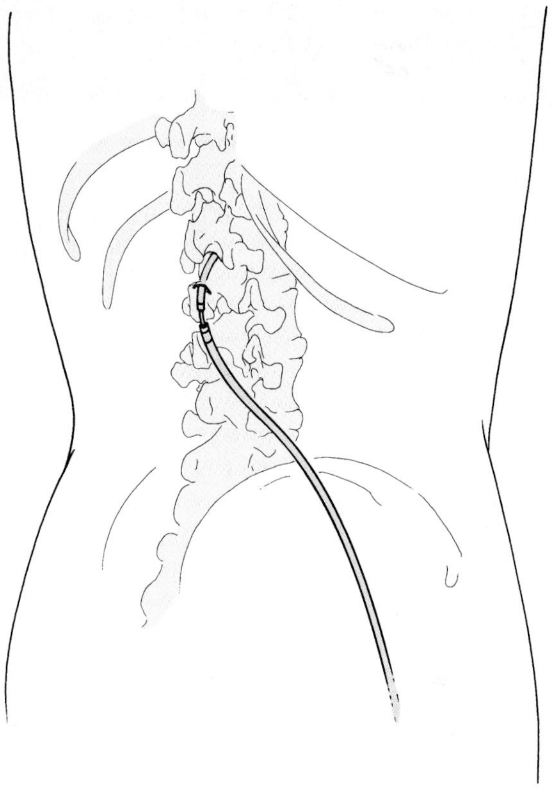

FIGURE 28-13 Epidural catheter.

table 28-7

NURSING CARE OF CLIENTS WITH EPIDURAL INFUSIONS

Goal	Actions
Prevent catheter displacement	Secure catheter carefully to outside skin.
Maintain catheter function	Observe external dressing or tape around catheter insertion site for dampness or discharge. (Leak of cerebrospinal fluid may develop.) Use of transparent, adhesive dressing aids inspection. Inspect catheter for breaks.
Prevent infection	Use strict aseptic technique when caring for catheter. Do not routinely change dressing over site. Change tubing every 24 hours.
Monitor for respiratory depression	Monitor vital signs, especially respirations, routinely per policy. Pulse oximetry and apnea monitors may be used.
Prevent undesirable complications	Assess for pruritis (itching) and nausea and vomiting. Administer antiemetics as ordered.
Maintain urinary and bowel function	Monitor intake and output. Assess for bladder and bowel distention. Assess for discomfort, frequency and urgency.

the client's chest for the nurse's access (Lonsway, 1988). Permanent catheters may be tunneled through the skin and exit at the client's side (Figure 28-13).

The catheter is connected to a continuous epidural infusion pump, a port or reservoir, or is capped off for bolus injections. To reduce the risk of accidental epidural injection of drugs intended for intravenous use, it helps to place a brightly colored intermittent injection cap on the catheter tubing. Labeling the catheter "epidural catheter" also helps. Continuous infusions must be administered through electronic infusion devices for proper control (IVNS, 1990). Because of the catheter location, strict surgical aseptic technique is needed to prevent a serious and potentially fatal infection. Physicians are notified immediately of any signs or symptoms of infection or pain at the insertion site.

Narcotics used commonly for epidural analgesia include preservative-free morphine sulfate, fentanyl, methadone, and meperidine. Morphine has a long-lasting effect but also causes more side effects (Sabbe and Yaksh, 1990). The medications act like the neurotransmitter enkephalin, an endorphin, blocking transmission of pain stimuli in the spinal cord (McNair, 1990).

Nursing implications for managing epidural analgesia are numerous (Table 28-7). Monitoring for drug effects differs, depending on if infusions are intermittent or continuous. Complications of epidural narcotic use include respiratory depression (rare), nausea and vomit-

table 28-8

NEUROSURGICAL PROCEDURES FOR PAIN RELIEF

Procedure	Indications	Nursing implications/special considerations
NEURECTOMY		
Surgical excision of a peripheral nerve	Pain well localized in a single peripheral nerve (e.g., trigeminal neuralgia)	Assess for paresthesias (reduced sensation) of area supplied by peripheral nerve. Protect affected area from exposure to pressure or temperature extremes
RHIZOTOMY		
Surgical destruction of (dorsal) posterior nerve roots as they enter spinal cord	Useful for well-defined nerve root involvement (e.g., pain in upper trunk)	See above Assess for loss of temperature sensation of affected area. Client may have surgical incision (laminectomy) or percutaneous wound. The percutaneous approach is less risky.
SYMPATHECTOMY		
Interruption of sympathetic afferent nerve fibers either through chemical block or by resection	Causalgia, phantom limb pain	Explain to client that pain may persist.
CORDOTOMY		
Resection of pain pathways in spinothalamic tract of spinal cord	Unilateral for pain of extremity or pelvis; bilateral for midline pain	Assess for bowel and bladder dysfunction, loss of motor function, loss of temperature and pain sensation. Clients with bilateral approach may suffer respiratory complications because of high resection.

ing, urinary retention, constipation, and pruritis. When clients are started on epidural analgesia, monitoring occurs as often as every 15 minutes, including assessment of respiratory rate, respiratory effort, and skin color. Pulse oximetry may be used. If a client remains stable, monitoring can move to every hour. Clients should be informed about the potential for respiratory depression and instructed to notify a nurse if breathing difficulty develops. If respiratory depression develops, the infusion is turned off immediately.

Surgical Measures for Pain Relief. When a client's pain persists despite medical treatment and it is clear that the pain is physical and not psychological, surgical therapies may give relief (Table 28-8). These therapies involve resection of either peripheral nerve roots or pain pathways in the spinothalamic tract. When nurses care for these clients, it is important to be aware of the area of resection so as to assess for paresthesias, change in temperature sensation, and loss of motor function. When performed correctly, these procedures can relieve persistent pain without causing serious neurological deficits.

Clients With Intractable Pain. Intractable pain cannot be permanently relieved. It can become so debilitating that clients will try anything to gain relief. Cleeland (1984) reports that one in three people with metastatic cancer reports pain that interferes with the quality of life. Recently the AHCPR released clinical practice guidelines for the management of cancer pain (Jacox, Carr, and Payne, 1994). The guidelines are designed to treat cancer pain in a more comprehensive and aggressive manner. Similiarly, they provide clients and families more options for pain relief. Figure 28-14 is a flowchart depicting cancer pain management from assessment to various treatment measures. The best choice of treatment often changes as the client's condition and the characteristics of pain change. Nonpharmacologic as well as pharmacologic therapies can be beneficial.

Administering analgesics to treat cancer-related pain requires applying principles different from those used to treat acute pain. The World Health Organization (1990) recommends a three-step approach to managing cancer pain (Figure 28-15). Therapy begins with NSAIDs and/or adjuvants and then progresses to strong opioids if pain persists. When a client with cancer first has pain, it is best to begin with a higher dosage than will be needed for relief. The physician can slowly decrease the dosage to the amount needed, thus giving the client immediate relief. Side effects of analgesia are aggressively treated so analgesia can be continued.

Studies show that drug dependence is low among

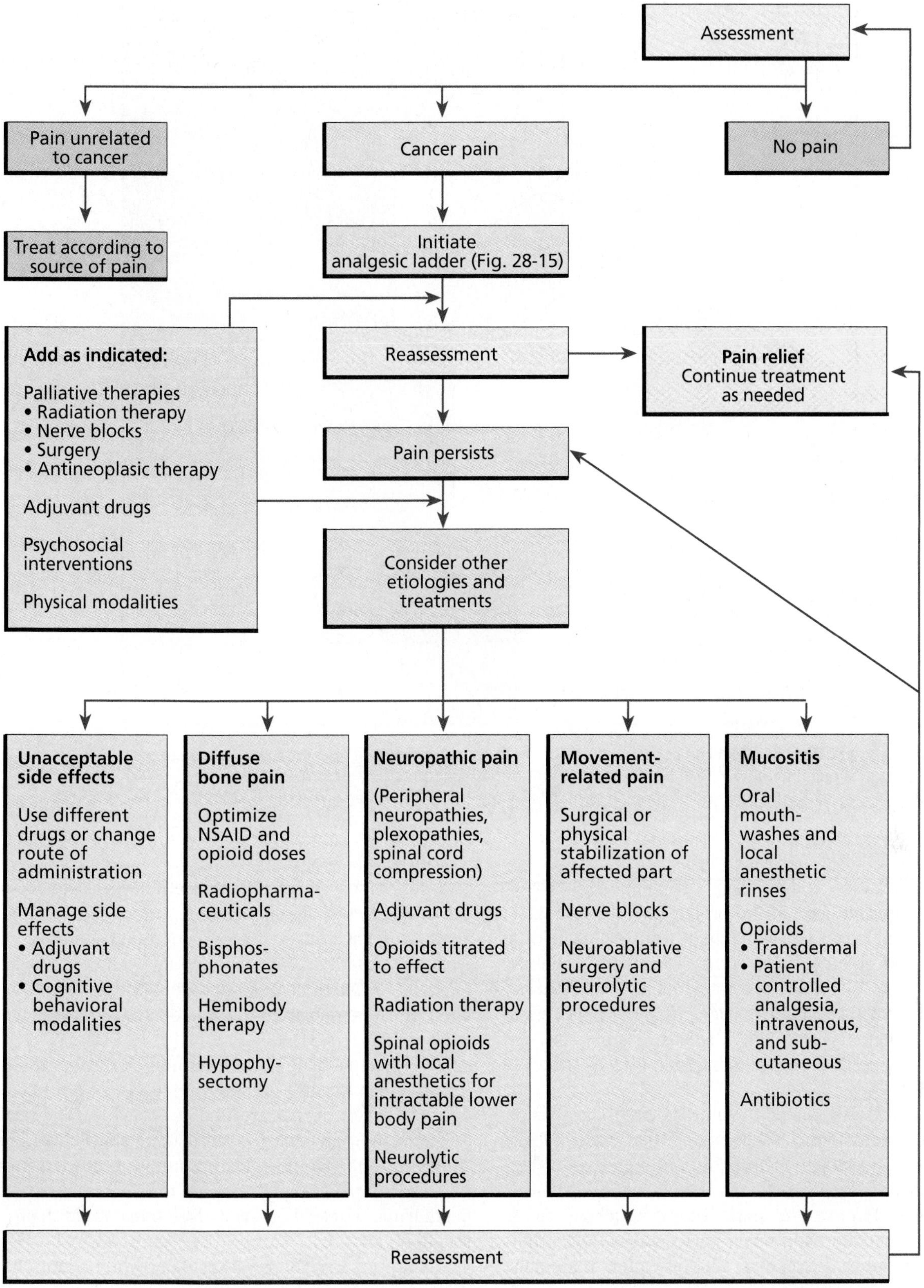

FIGURE 28-14 Flowchart: continuing pain management in patients with cancer. (From Jacox A, Carr DB, Payne R, et al.: Management of cancer pain. Clinical practice guideline No. 9. AHCPR Pub. No. 94-0592, Rockville, Md., Agency for Health Care Policy and Research, U.S. Department of Health and Human Services, Public Health Service, March, 1994.)

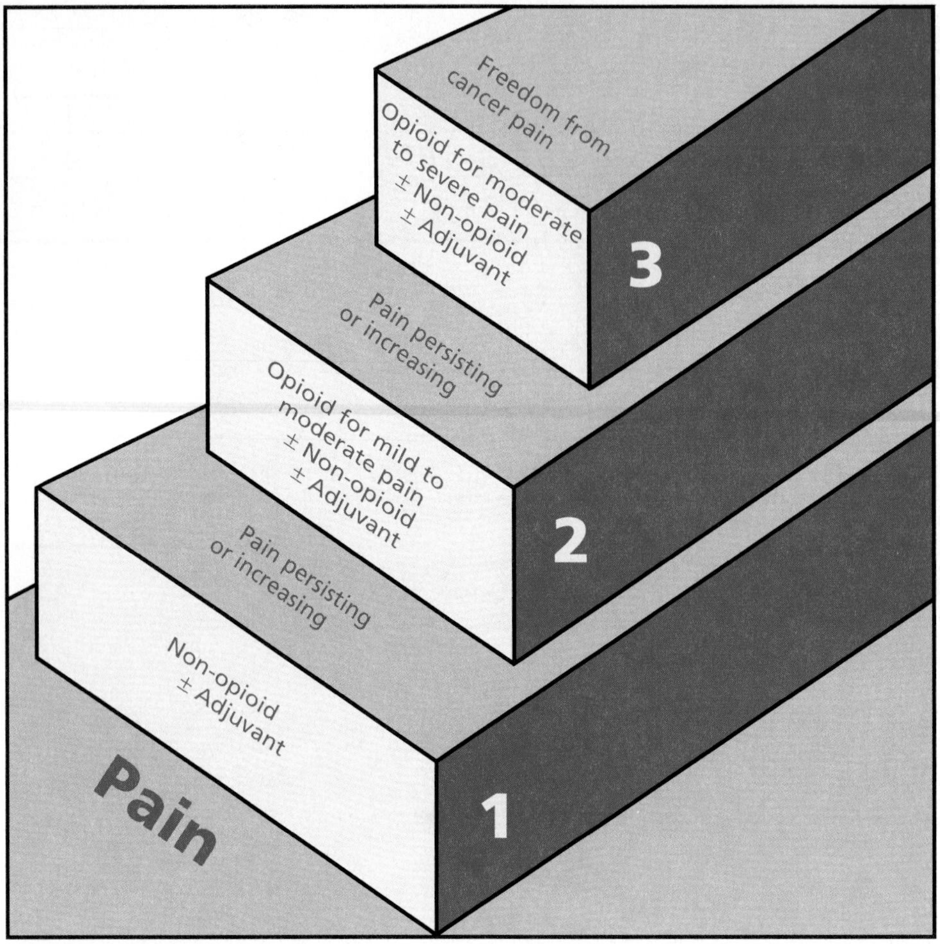

FIGURE 28-15 WHO's analgesic ladder is a three-step approach to using drugs in cancer pain management. +/−, adjuvant, with or without adjuvant medications. (From World Health Organization: *Cancer pain relief and palliative care: report of a WHO expert committee,* WHO Tech Rep Series No 804, Geneva, 1990, The Organization.)

clients with cancer-related pain. Giving the right drug and the required dose at the proper interval alleviates the fear of pain, protects the client from drug-seeking behavior, and reduces dependence. Terminally ill clients with prolonged pain develop a tolerance to analgesics. They thus require higher dosages to attain pain relief. Higher dosages are not lethal because clients also develop tolerance to life-threatening side effects (McCaffery, 1986).

For clients with cancer, the aim of drug therapy is to anticipate and minimize pain rather than cure it. It is therefore necessary to give required dosages regularly. Prescribing analgesics on an as-needed basis for cancer clients is ineffective and causes more suffering. Analgesics are needed even when pain, nausea, and other symptoms subside. Regular administration maintains blood levels for ongoing pain control.

Various medications and routes of administration can provide some relief for chronic pain sufferers. Epidural analgesia has been highly effective. Intrathecal infusion (administration of opioids via catheters placed within the brain's ventricles) is becoming more common. New analgesics have fewer side effects. Long-acting or controlled-release morphine sulfate has been very successful. Two of these medications are MS Contin and Roxanol SR with a duration of action of 8 to 12 hours (McKenry and Salerno, 1992).

Transdermal drug systems administer drugs such as fentanyl over predetermined rates up to 24 hours. This is useful when clients are unable to take drugs orally. Self-adhesive patches release the drug slowly over time, achieving effective analgesia. Caution is needed in administering transdermal patches to clients who are hyperthermic. Hyperthermia causes more rapid drug absorption.

Analgesics may be given rectally when clients have nausea and vomiting or are fasting before or after surgery (Jacox, Carr, and Payne, 1994). The route is contraindicated if clients have diarrhea or if cancerous lesions involve the anus or rectum. Morphine, hy-

CLIENT TEACHING FOR AMUBULATORY INFUSION PUMPS

Tell client and family to observe for side effects:
Drowsiness, drop in blood pressure, dizziness or fainting, nausea, vomiting, slower and shallow respirations, constipation, mood changes, euphoria, inability to empty bladder fully, dry mouth, weakness, agitation, tremors, and strange dreams.
Instruct family on how to administer naloxone (Narcan) intramuscularly to reverse respiratory depression.
Teach client to keep the central venous catheter patent, maintain the minimum pump flow rate, and irrigate the catheter routinely with heparin flush.
Tell client how to prevent air from entering central venous catheter and clamp catheter when infusion has stopped.
Explain ways to prevent infection at catheter site and keep site clean with soap and water.
Have client follow a preventive bowel routine using stool softeners, laxatives, dietary fiber, hydration, and routine exercise.

dromorphone and oxymorphone are available as suppositories.

Another measure to treat severe intractable cancer pain is morphine given by continuous intravenous drip or intermittently by a PCA pump. Continuous infusions provide improved, uniform pain control because lower dosages are used. Thus there are fewer side effects. The total daily dosage may be less than with regular intramuscular injections. Candidates for continuous infusions include clients with severe pain for which oral or injectable narcotics provide minimal relief, clients with severe nausea and vomiting, clients with clotting disorders who bruise from injections, clients with delirium, confusion, or other mental status changes, and clients unable to swallow oral medications.

Continuous-drip morphine is given in acute care settings and the home. Morphine mixed in intravenous solution is delivered by an infusion control pump to ensure safe and accurate administration. Each agency has guidelines for morphine dose and infusion rates. The drug can cause numerous side effects (see teaching box above) that require the nurse's ongoing assessment. Adjuvant drugs such as antiemetics, corticosteroids, anticonvulsants, neuroleptics, biphosphonates, and calcitonin (bone pain), or antidepressants may be needed to enhance pain control and prevent side effects (Murphy, 1990; Paice, 1991; Jacox, Carr, and Payne, 1994).

When a client is first placed on continuous-drip morphine, it is essential that an intravenous access is patent and the intravenous site is without complications (see Chapter 35). To prevent overdose and central nervous system depression, the nurse records baseline blood pressure and respiratory rates before the infusion begins. After the infusion starts, the nurse monitors vital signs as often as every 15 to 30 minutes for the first few hours until the client gains relief at a constant dosage. If blood pressure or respirations decrease, the infusion rate is reduced according to the physician's order or agency policy.

If the client shows signs of severe respiratory depression, the physician will order the infusion discontinued. The narcotic antagonist naloxone (Narcan) should be available to reverse respiratory depression.

In the home, clients may use ambulatory infusion pumps. The pumps are lightweight, compact (about the size of a transistor radio), and allow free movement. The pump is battery powered and worn in a pouch attached to a belt or harness. The bag of medication and intravenous fluid fits inside the pump. A dose of morphine, delivered continuously over 24 hours, is usually slowly infused into a central venous catheter either by way of a peripherally inserted central catheter (PICC) or a more traditional subclavian placed catheter. Both catheters can be left in place for an extended period of time. The pumps differ from PCA devices, which deliver only small, preset doses of medication. The client and family learn to manage the pump, observe for drug side effects, and maintain function of the central venous catheter (see teaching box at left). Because the client is initially managed on morphine in the hospital before going home, the risk of side effects is not as great unless the client or family member increases dosages. A home health nurse makes routine visits to be sure the client manages the pump correctly.

Hospice and Pain Clinics

Hospices are programs to care for the terminally ill (see Chapter 21). Hospice is Latin for a place to rest. Hospices are often affiliated with hospitals. The programs help terminally ill clients to continue to live at home in comfort and privacy with the help of a health care team. Pain control is a priority. Clients receive the proper dosage and forms of analgesics to provide pain relief. Families learn to monitor the client's symptoms and become primary care givers.

Pain clinics have evolved to provide pain management for a variety of clients. A comprehensive pain center can treat clients in the hospital or in outpatient clinics. Nurses, physicians, physical therapists, and dietitians collaborate to find the most effective pain relief therapies. Diverse therapies, as well as research into new treatments, are among the center's services.

There are also syndrome-oriented and modality-oriented pain centers. A syndrome-oriented center cares for clients with specific types of pain such as back pain or arthritis. Modality-oriented centers offer only specific types of treatment such as biofeedback, acupuncture, or TENS.

Evaluation

The client is the best resource for evaluating the effectiveness of pain relief measures. Having pain can be a lonely and frightening experience. Unless a nurse communicates closely with clients, attending responsively to their needs, pain control is less likely to be achieved. Continuous evaluation allows the nurse to determine whether new or revised therapies are required and if new nursing diagnoses have developed.

To evaluate the effectiveness of nursing interventions in meeting the goals of care, the nurse identifies actual outcomes using evaluative measures. Comparisons are made with baseline pain assessments to determine if the severity and other characteristics of pain have changed. Similarly the nurse evaluates if the client's response to pain (e.g., ability to socialize or perform self-care) has changed. Outcomes are compared with expected outcomes to determine the client's health status. The following are examples of goals and corresponding outcomes and evaluative measures:

Goal: Client obtains a sense of well-being and comfort within 3 days.

Outcome

Client expresses a reduction in pain as measured on a visual analog scale

Evaluative measure

Offer client visual analog scale to rate pain severity and compare with client's previous rating score

Outcome

Client demonstrates nonverbally relief from pain within 48 hours

Evaluative measure

Observe client's facial expression, body movements, and posturing, noting if there is more spontaneous freedom of movement

Goal: Client regains ability to perform self-care independently within 48 hours.

Outcome

Client bathes and grooms self without hesitancy or restriction in movement within 24 hours

Evaluative measure

Ask client to report ease of performing self-care in the home environment.

Observe client perform grooming activities

Goal: Client maintains existing physical and psychosocial function.

Outcome

Client ambulates independently without restriction in range of motion

Evaluative measure

Observe client ambulate down hallway and during ascent and descent of stairs

Outcome

Client participates in social functions with friends within 1 week

Evaluative measure

Ask family or friends to report on frequency client participates socially

Goal: Client understands the pain experience.

Outcome

Client describes sensations to anticipate during a diagnostic procedure

Evaluative measure

Have client describe the anticipated sensation following discussion of the procedure

Outcome

Client uses options for pain relief following surgery

Evaluative measure

Observe client using relaxation or positioning techniques

SUMMARY

The experience of pain is different for each person. The meaning pain conveys, the threat to comfort, and the implications of serious illness make the experience highly subjective but very real. Pain is a problem faced by clients in every health care setting. The nurse is most effective in providing comfort by understanding the nature of pain and the client's perceptions, eliminating personal prejudices about pain, and working closely with the client to find the best relief measures.

CRITICAL THINKING ACTIVITIES

1. Mrs. Wiegand is a 76-year-old woman, married, and coming to the outpatient clinic with complaints, in her words, of severe burning pain in her hands and wrists. She has been diagnosed with arthritis for more than 1 year. What type of questions might you ask of Mrs. Wiegand to assess how this pain has affected her life-style?
2. Mr. Jasper and Mr. Stern are clients experiencing back pain. Mr. Jasper's pain resulted following a fall from a ladder 48 hours ago. Mr. Stern's pain has been bothering him for more than 8 months with no known cause. As the nurse caring for both clients, how might you anticipate differences in assessment and treatment?

3. Consider the example of Mr. Stern above. What might influence your approach to assessment if Mr. Stern were 39 versus 80 years of age?
4. Ms. Rogers is receiving morphine by way of a PCA device following abdominal surgery for a hysterectomy. During your assessment, you note Ms. Rogers to be more drowsy and her respirations have decreased from 16 a minute to 10. What actions should you take?
5. Mr. Lake is a 45-year-old man who experienced a traumatic injury to his left arm following an industrial accident 24 hours ago. His arm is in a very bulky dressing, and pain is aggravated when he lies on his left side. He has an intravenous line with a continuous infusion of IV fluids in his right arm. What nonpharmacologic pain relief measures might be helpful for Mr. Lake?

KEY CONCEPTS

Pain, a protective mechanism that warns a person of tissue injury, is largely a subjective experience.

Misconceptions about pain can lead to undertreatment.

Knowledge of the three components of the pain experience—reception, perception, and reaction—provides the nurse with guidelines for determining relief measures.

An interaction of psychological and cognitive factors affects pain perception.

The pain experience is influenced by a client's age, sex, anxiety, culture, experience, and the meaning of pain.

A client's pain tolerance influences the nurse's perceptions of the seriousness of the discomfort.

The difference between acute and chronic pain involves the duration of discomfort, physical signs and symptoms, and the client's perceptions regarding relief.

Pain scales are used to objectively evaluate the severity of pain and the effectiveness of pain therapies.

Building trust with a client enhances a nurse's success in accurately assessing pain and providing needed interventions.

The client's family and friends can be a key resource in pain assessment.

An assessment of a client in pain may lead to a nursing diagnosis of *pain* or diagnoses related to the physical and behavioral problems resulting from pain.

The nurse individualizes pain therapy by collaborating closely with the client, using assessment findings, trying a variety of therapies, and maintaining the client's well-being.

The AHCPR's clinical practice guideline for acute pain management emphasizes a collaborative, interdisciplinary approach to pain control that uses pharmacologic and nonpharmacologic therapies.

Eliminating sources of painful stimuli is a basic nursing measure for promoting comfort.

Nonpharmacologic cutaneous therapies are effective in altering client perception of pain, promoting muscle relaxation, and giving the client control over pain experienced.

Using a regular schedule for analgesic administration is more effective than an as-needed schedule.

A patient-controlled analgesic device gives clients pain control with the low risk of overdose.

The nurse's primary role in caring for a client who receives local anesthesia is protecting the client from injury.

The aim of therapy for cancer clients is to anticipate and prevent pain rather than treat it.

The most serious side effect of morphine infusions is respiratory depression, which can be reversed with intravenous Narcan.

Evaluation of pain therapy requires consideration of the changing character of pain, response to therapy, and the client's perceptions of a therapy's effectiveness.

References

AHCPR, Acute pain management guideline panel: acute pain management in infants, children and adolescents: operative or medical procedures and trauma. *Clinical practice guideline,* AHCPR Pub No 92-0032. Rockville, Md.: Agency for Health Care Policy and Research, PHS, USDHHS, Feb., 1992.

Bailey LM: Music's soothing charms, *Am J Nurs* 85:1280, 1985.

Beyer J, et al.: Patterns of postoperative analgesic use with adults and children following cardiac surgery, *Pain* 17:71-81, 1983.

Broome M, et al.: Children's medical fears, coping behaviors and pain perceptions during a lumbar puncture, *Oncol Nurs Forum* 17(3): 361-367, 1990.

Burns JW, et al.: The influence of patient characteristics on the requirements for postoperative analgesia, *Anaesthesia* 44:2, 1989.

Burnside I: *Nursing and the aged,* ed 3, St. Louis, 1988, Mosby.

Ceccio CM: Heat vs cold as treatment for arthritic pain, *RN* 53:83, 1990.

Clancy J, McVicar A: Subjectivity of pain, *Brit J Nurs* 1(1):8-11, 1992.

Cleeland CS: The impact of pain on the patient with cancer, *Cancer* 54(suppl):2635, 1984.

Copp LA: The spectrum of suffering, *Am J Nurs* 90:35-39, Aug. 1990.

Donahue P: *Nursing: the finest art,* St. Louis, 1989, Mosby.

DuPen SL, Williams AR: Management of patients receiving combined epidural morphine and bupivaccine for the treatment of cancer pain, *J Pain Symptom Manage* 7(2):125-127, 1992.

Ebersole P, Hess P: Toward healthy aging, ed 3, St. Louis, 1990, Mosby.

Eland JM and Anderson JE: The experience of pain in children. In Jacox, A, editor, *Pain: a source book for nurses and other health professionals,* Boston, 1977, Little, Brown & Co.

Fordham M: *Neurophysiological pain,* London, 1986, Bailliere Tindall.

Fortin F and Kirouac S: A randomized controlled trial of preoperative patient education, *Int J Nurs Stud* 13:11-24, 1976.

Geach B: Pain and coping, *J Nurs Sch Image* 19(1):12-15, 1987.

Gil K: Psychologic aspects of acute pain, *Anesthesiol Report* 2(2):246, 1990.

Hargreaves A, Lander J: Use of transcutaneous electrical nerve stimulation for postoperative pain, *Nurs Res* 38(3):159, 1989.

Harrison A: Assessing patients' pain: identifying reasons for error, *J Adv Nurs* 16:1018, 1991.

Herr KA, Mobily PR: Complexities of pain assessment in the elderly, *J Gerontol Nurs* 17(4):12, 1991.

Holm K, et al.: Effect of personal pain experience on pain assessment, *J Nurs Sch Image* 21(2):72, 1989.

International Association for the Study of Pain, Subcommittee on Taxonomy: Pain terms: a list with definitions and notes on usage, *Pain* 6:249, 1979.

Intravenous Nurses Society: Intravenous nursing standards of practice, *JIV Nurs,* S70-S71, suppl. 1990.

Jacox A, Carr DB, Payne R, et al.: Management of cancer pain. Clinical Practice Guideline No. 9. AHCPR Pub. No. 94-0592, Rockville, Md., Agency for Health Care Policy and Research, U.S. Dept. HHS, PHS, March, 1994.

Lonsway RA: Care of the patient with an epidural catheter: an infection control challenge, *JIV Nurs* 11(1):52, 1988.

Marzinski LR: The tragedy of dementia: clinically assessing pain in the confused, nonverbal elderly, *J Gerontol Nurs* 17(6):25-28, 1991.

McCaffery M: *Nursing management of the patient with pain,* ed 2, Philadelphia, 1979, Lippincott.

McCaffery M: *Pain: assessment and intervention in nursing practice, course syllabus,* St. Louis 1986, Barnes Hospital.

McCaffery M: Would you administer placebos for pain? These facts can help you decide, *Nurs 82* 12:22, 1982.

McCaffery M, Beebe A: *Pain: clinical manual for nursing practice,* St. Louis, 1989, Mosby.

McGuire DB: The measurement of clinical pain, *Nurs Res* 33(3):152, 1984.

McKenry LM, Salerno E: *Pharmacology in nursing,* ed 18, St. Louis, 1992, Mosby.

McNair ND: Epidural narcotics for postoperative pain: nursing implications, *J Neurosci Nurs* 22(5):275-279, 1990.

Meek SS: Effects of slow stroke back massage on relaxation in hospice clients, *J Nurs Sch Image* 25(1): 17-21, 1993.

Meinhart NT, McCaffery M: *Pain: a nursing approach to assessment and analysis,* Norwalk, Conn., 1983, Appleton-Century-Crofts.

Melzack R and Wall PD: *The challenge of pain,* Harmondsworth, 1988, Penguin.

Melzack R and Wall PD: Pain mechanisms: a new theory, *Science* 150:971, 1965.

Miller KF, Shuter R: An exploratory study of pain expression styles among blacks and whites, *Int J Intercult Rel* 6:281, 1982.

Murphy D: Home pain management, *JIN* 13(6):355-359, 1990.

National institutes of health consensus develop panel: New gains against pain, *Emerg Med* Nov. 1986, p. 143.

Paice JA: Unraveling the mystery of pain, *Oncol Nurs Forum* 18(5):843, 1991.

Puntillo KA: The phenomenon of pain and critical care nursing, *Heart Lung* 17:262-273, 1988.

Sabbe MB and Yaksh TL: Pharmacology of spinal opioids, *J Pain Symptom Manag* 5(3):191-203, 1990.

Seers K: Perceptions of pain, *Nurs Times* 83:37-39, 1987.

Sofaer B: Pain relief—the core of nursing practice, *Nurs Times* 79:38-42, 1983.

Schultheis K, et al.: Preparation for stressful medical procedures and person x treatment interactions, *Clin Psych Rev* 7:329, 1987.

Taylor AG, et al.: Duration of pain, condition, and physical pathology as determinants of nurses' assessment of patients in pain, *Nurs Res* 33:4, 1984.

Van Aernam B, Lindeman C: Nursing intervention with the presurgical patient: the effects of structured and unstructured preoperative teaching, *Nurs Res* 20:319-332, 1971.

Whaley L, Wong D: *Nursing care of infants and children,* ed 4, St. Louis, 1991, Mosby.

Whipple B: Methods of pain control: a review of research and literature, *J Nurs Sch Image* 19(3):142, 1987.

Wong D and Baker C: Pain in children: comparison of assessment scales, *Pediat Nurs* 14(1):9-17, 1988.

World Health Organization: Cancer pain relief and palliative care, Report of a WHO expert committee [World Health Organization Technical Report Series, 804] Geneva, Switzerland. WHO:1990, pp. 1-75.

Yolcaba KY: A taxonomic structure for the concept comfort, *J Nurs Sch Image* 23(4):237-240, 1991.

Bibliography

American Pain Society: Principles of analgesic use in the treatment of acute pain and chronic cancer pain: A concise guide to medical practice, ed 2, Skokie, Ill., 1989, American Pain Society.

Baquie ML: What matters most in chronic pain management, *RN* 52:46, 1989.

Berde CB: Pediatric analgesic trials. In Max MB, Portenoy RK, and Laska EM, editors: *Advances in pain research and therapy: the design of analgesic clinical trials* (vol 18) New York, 1991, Raven Press.

Bodnar B and Galligan A: An effective PCA documentation tool, *Nurs Manag* 23(10):48-50, 1992.

Brady B: Using the right touch, *Nurs 91* 21:46-47, 1991.

Broome ME, et al.: Pain interventions with children: a meta-analysis of research, *Nurs Res* 38(3):154, 1989.

Chapman CR and Syrjala KL: Measurement of pain. In Bonica JJ, editor: *The management of pain,* ed 2, vol 1, Philadelphia, 1990, Lea and Febiger.

Cook JD: Music as an intervention in the oncology setting, *Cancer Nurs* 9:23, 1986.

Craig KD: Social modelling influences in pain. In Sternbach RA, editor: *The psychology of pain,* ed 2, New York, 1986, Raven Press.

Egbert AM, et al.: Randomized trial of postoperative patient controlled analgesia vs intramuscular narcotics in frail elderly men, *Arch Int Med* 150:1897-1903, 1990.

Ferrel BA: Pain management in elderly people, *J Am Geriat Soc* 39:64-73, 1991.

Hurley RJ and Johnson MD: Spinal opioids in the management of obstetric pain, *J Pain Symptom Manag* 5(3):146-151, 1990.

Jones NH: Creative analgesic dosing in the elderly, *Am J Nurs* 89:1285, 1989.

Keller E, Bzdek VM: Effects of therapeutic touch on tension headache pain, *Nurs Res* 35:101, 1986.

Krieger D: Therapeutic touch: the imprimatur of nursing, *Am J Nurs* 75:784, 1975.

Lonsway RA: Care of the patient with an epidural catheter: an infection control challenge, *J Intraven Nurs* 11(1):52, 1988.

Martinelli AM: Pain and ethnicity: how people of different cultures experience pain, *AORN J* 46(2):273, 1987.

Melzack R: The McGill pain questionnaire: major properties and scoring methods, *Pain* 1:277, 1975.

Rahr V: Giving intrathecal drugs, *Am J Nurs* 86:829, 1986.

Ready LB: Spinal opioids in the management of acute and postoperative pain, *J Pain Symptom Manag* 5(3):138-144, 1990.

Shade P: Patient-controlled analgesia: can client education improve outcomes? *J Adv Nurs* 17:408-413, 1992.

Shapiro C: Pain in the neonate: assessment and intervention, *Neonatal Network* 8(1):7-21, 1989.

Tesler MD, et al.: Children's words for p
Key aspects of comfort: management
New York, 1989, Springer.

Whaley L and Wong D: *Nursing care of inf*
Louis, 1991, Mosby.

Williams DJ: Pushbutton pain relief puts
85:1458, 1985.

Witte M: Pain control, *J Gerontol Nurs* 15(3):32,

Funk SG, et al., editors:
fatigue, and nausea,
ildren, ed 4, St.
n control,

Safety

OBJECTIVES

Mastery of content in this chapter will enable the student to:

- Define the key terms listed.
- Describe how unmet basic physiological needs of oxygen, fluids, nutrition, and temperature can threaten safety.
- Discuss methods to reduce physical hazards and the transmission of pathogens and parasites.
- Discuss the specific risks to safety as they pertain to developmental age.
- Identify factors to assess when a client is placed in restraints.
- Describe four categories of safety risks in a health care agency.
- State nursing diagnoses associated with risks to safety.
- Develop a nursing care plan for clients whose safety is threatened.
- Describe nursing interventions specific to the client's age for reducing risk of falls, fires, poisonings, and electrical hazards.
- Describe methods to evaluate interventions designed to maintain or promote safety.

KEY TERMS

air pollution
carbon monoxide
carcinogen
decibels
Food and Drug Administration (FDA)
food poisoning
noise pollution
parasite
pathogen
poison
poison control center
pollutant
relative humidity
water pollution

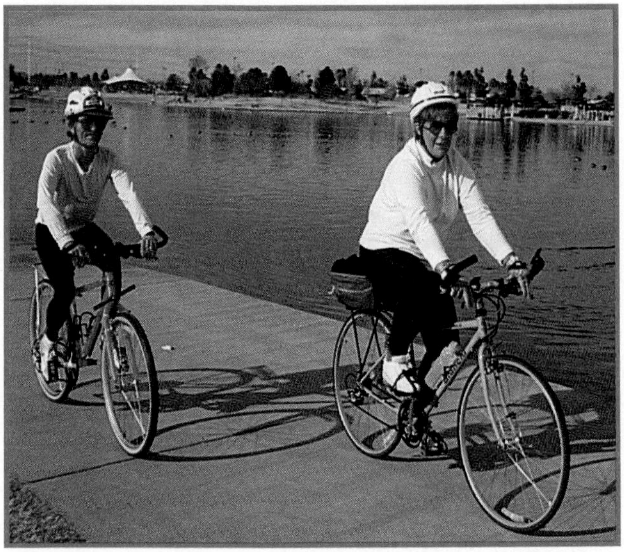

Nursing care directed toward health maintenance and illness prevention includes promotion of the client's safety in the community or health care environment. Protection and safety are basic, lifelong needs. The nurse can increase the client's safety by including interventions for a safe environment in the care plan and with every nursing procedure.

Defined broadly, an environment is all of the many factors, physical and psychosocial, that influence or affect the life and survival of the client. A safe environment in a health care agency is comfortable, maintains the client's privacy, and reduces to a minimum the risks of injury, infection, and untoward effects from treatments or medications. A safe environment in the home, workplace or school, and neighborhood reduces the risk of accidents and illnesses and the subsequent need for health care service.

NURSING PROCESS FOR CLIENTS WITH SAFETY NEEDS

Assessment

Nurses provide care to clients and families in their homes or communities, as with community health nursing, or within an institutional setting, such as a hospital or extended care facility. Ill, disabled, illiterate, poor, or older adult clients often require the nurse's help in achieving a safe environment. To do this the nurse needs to understand factors contributing to a safe environment in the home or health care agency and then thoroughly assess the environment for threats to safety.

Environment

A safe environment is one in which basic needs are achievable, physical hazards are reduced, exposure to carcinogens is reduced, transmission of pathogens and parasites is reduced, sanitation is regulated, and pollution is controlled.

Basic Needs. Meeting basic human needs includes achieving safety and security needs. Frequently the basic physiological needs—including oxygen, degree of humidity, nutrition, and optimal temperature—influence safety.

The nurse must know about environmental hazards that threaten the client by decreasing the amount of available oxygen. One such hazard is **carbon monoxide,** a colorless, odorless, poisonous gas produced by the combustion of carbon or organic fuels. This gas binds strongly with hemoglobin, preventing the formation of oxyhemoglobin and thus reducing the supply of oxygen delivered to the tissues (see Chapter 34). Carbon monoxide is most commonly introduced into the client's environment by an improperly functioning furnace or by automobile exhaust fumes.

Another environmental variable that may affect the client's health and safety is **relative humidity,** the amount of water vapor in the air compared with the maximum amount of water vapor the air could contain at the same temperature. The skin's moisture evaporates more quickly as the relative humidity decreases. Most people are comfortable when the humidity is between 60% and 70%. People at risk from high environmental temperatures, such as older adults or very young, should avoid extremely hot, humid environments. Modern air conditioners and forced air furnaces enable people to control the temperature of the home and work environments but also remove humidity.

Other environmental threats to safety arise in connection with nutritional needs. Unrefrigerated perishable foods or food products with expired dates for use may contain harmful organisms. Unwashed fresh vegetables and fruits can harbor insecticides, dirt, and pathogens. Improper home canning may cause botulism poisoning. Lack of water supply or garbage collection leads to unsanitary conditions that also threaten safety.

Temperature extremes, which frequently occur during the winter and summer, affect comfort, productivity, and safety. Exposure to severe cold for prolonged periods causes frostbite and hypothermia, a lowering of the core body temperature to 35° C (95° F) or below (see Chapter 15). The risk of hypothermia is increased by advanced age, chronic or acute illness, and alcohol consumption. Exposure to extreme heat can change the body's electrolyte balance and raise the core body temperature, resulting in heat stroke or heat exhaustion. Chronically ill, older adults, young clients, and clients without financial resources are at greater risk for injury from extreme heat.

Physical Hazards. Physical hazards in an environment may threaten a client's safety and result in physical or psychological injury. Possible hazards to be assessed include inadequate lighting, clutter, and lack of security measures.

Inadequate lighting can cause eyestrain as the client carries out daily activities and can increase the risk of injury from falls. The risk of crime is also higher in poorly lit areas. The nurse should evaluate the adequacy of illumination in areas the client moves and works, particularly outside walkways, steps, garages, doorways, and in interior halls and staircases.

The client's home should be assessed for clutter because injuries frequently result from inadvertent contact with objects on stairs, floors, bedside tables, closet shelves, refrigerator tops, and bookshelves. The risk of injury from clutter is greatest for older adults, clients with impaired vision, and clients who require adaptive aids, crutches, and walkers for ambulation. Clients with impaired mobility are at great risk for falls. The nurse should assess the condition of stairways, bathrooms, and hard-to-get-to areas to be sure safety devices are in place. For example, handrails around toilets or railings along stairways can help.

People need to take precautions to secure their homes from intruders, who constitute a threat to physical and mental safety. When observing the home for security measures, the nurse should assess the presence and quality of locks on doors and windows and the adequacy of exterior lighting.

table 29-1

KNOWN CARCINOGENIC RISKS AND CANCERS

Carcinogen	Cancer
Asbestos	Lung
Smoking	Lung
High dietary fat intake	Colorectal Breast
Pesticides	Lung Lymphatic Leukemias
Vinyl chloride	Leukemias
Saccharin	Bladder
Exposure to cytotoxic drugs	Multiple
Anesthetic gas wastes	Multiple

Carcinogens. There is a high correlation between life-style habits and occupational exposures to cancers. Health care workers are frequently exposed to biological and chemical hazards in the course of their jobs (Jacobsen, 1987). These agents or risks are called *carcinogens.* A **carcinogen** is a substance or agent that causes the development or increases the risk of cancer.

Consumer groups and health care professionals work with legislators to enact laws to protect the public against known carcinogens. In addition, right-to-know laws require employers to teach employees about toxic agents used in the workplace, ways workers can be harmed, and specific safety measures to use to avoid toxic exposures.

When doing health assessments, nurses must first be aware of carcinogens and their cancer risk factors (Table 29-1). Nurses must also assess for past and present occupational or life-style exposures.

Pathogens and Parasites. Pathogens and parasites pose a threat to client safety. A **pathogen** is any microorganism capable of producing an illness (see Chapter 25). A **parasite** is an organism living in or on another organism and obtaining nourishment from it. Pathogens and parasites can be found in water, food, people, insects, and animals. Factors to be assessed include food sanitation, insect and rodent control, and human waste disposal.

Improperly processed or contaminated food can cause illness and death by transmitting pathogens and parasites. **Food poisoning** is the toxic process resulting from ingesting a food contaminated by toxic substances or by bacteria containing toxins. The **Food and Drug Administration (FDA)** is a federal agency responsible for enforcing federal regulations regarding the manufacture and distribution of food, drugs, and cosmetics to protect consumers against the sale of impure or dangerous substances. The FDA guidelines require commercial food processors to comply with sanitation and preparation standards that decrease the risk of contamination.

Insects and rodents are carriers of pathogens. The *Anopheles* mosquito is a carrier of malaria, and the rat or mouse can transmit rat-bite fever. Uncontrolled mosquito and rodent populations increase the risk of these diseases.

Sanitation. The transmission of pathogens and parasites is also controlled by adequate disposal of human waste through proper construction and repair of sewers and drains. Without a satisfactory sewer and waste system, the population is at risk for illnesses such as typhoid fever and hepatitis.

Health care agencies are also faced with problems concerning the processing of biohazardous wastes. Needles, surgical dressings, and syringes must be disposed of in such a manner that neither the general population nor employees are at risk for exposure. In addition, some disposable items, including some respiratory, orthopedic, and hemodynamic equipment, are reused. The reprocessing of disposable equipment must meet JCAHO and CDC guidelines (Radany, et al., 1987).

Pollution. A healthy environment is free of air, water, or noise pollution. A **pollutant** is a harmful, chemical, or waste material discharged into the water or atmosphere. **Air pollution** is the contamination of the environmental atmosphere with pollutants. In urban regions, industrial wastes and vehicle exhausts commonly contribute to air pollution. Cigarette smoke is the primary indoor air pollutant. Prolonged exposure to air pollution increases the risk for pulmonary disease.

Water pollution is the contamination of lakes, rivers, and streams, usually by industrial pollutants. Properly functioning water treatment facilities filter harmful contaminants from the water, but flooding may damage a treatment station, requiring boiling of drinking water. Before the introduction of water purification standards, many communities had epidemics of cholera, dysentery, and typhoid fever, all caused by water-borne pathogens.

Noise pollution occurs when the noise level in an environment becomes uncomfortable to its inhabitants. Noise levels are measured in units of sound intensity called **decibels.** Noise level tolerances vary among individuals and are influenced by health status. Noise often prevents clients from receiving adequate rest or sleep. A high noise level over time can produce hearing loss, and even a lower level of noise may produce a syndrome called *sensory overload* (see Chapter 38).

RISKS TO CLIENT SAFETY

Risks at Developmental Stages

Threats to safety within the community are influenced by developmental stage, life-style habits, mobility status, sensory impairments, and safety awareness. In the United States and Canada, accidents are the leading cause of death in people between 1 and 44 years of age (National Center for Health Statistics, 1993).

Infant, Toddler, and Preschooler. Home accidents kill, disfigure, and permanently disable thousands of children each year, with children less than 5 years of age being at greatest risk for death. Accidents involving children are largely preventable, but parents frequently need to be shown the specific dangers by nurses and other health care professionals. As the infant grows, accident potential increases. The newborn's accident potential is influenced by people or external agents, but growth and the acquisition of new motor skills place the active toddler and preschooler at risk for injuries (Table 29-2). Accident prevention thus requires health education for parents and removal of dangers where possible.

School-Age Child. When children enter school, their environment expands to include the school and the means of transportation to and from school. Children should be taught to cross the street safely and to refrain from talking to or accepting rides or gifts from strangers. School-age children involved in team and contact sports should be taught to play safely and to use protective safety equipment.

Adolescent. As children enter adolescence, they begin to develop a sense of identity and personal values, which may conflict with parental values. In addition, the adolescent begins to separate emotionally from the family, and the peer group begins to have a stronger influence.

The struggle toward identity may cause the teenager to experience shyness, fear, and anxiety, with resulting dysfunction at home, at school, or within the peer group. Psychoactive substances such as drugs and alcohol may make the world more bearable for the troubled teenager. Unfortunately, substances used for this purpose put the adolescent at a high risk for continued alcohol or drug abuse (Robinson and Greene, 1988). The use of alcohol and drugs also increases the risk for motor vehicle accidents, which are a leading cause of death and injury in adolescents (American Academy of Pediatrics, 1992).

Long-term habitual use of drugs or alcohol results in subtle but recognizable physiological and behavioral changes. The nurse should be aware, however, that medical and emotional problems can produce similar behavioral changes. Moodiness and confusion are typical adolescent behavior patterns (Acee and Smith, 1987). When assessing the adolescent for possible substance abuse, the nurse must look for environmental and psychosocial clues. Environmental clues include drug-oriented magazines, beer and liquor bottles, drug paraphernalia, blood spots on clothing, or the continual wearing of long-sleeved shirts in hot weather and dark glasses indoors. Psychosocial clues include failing grades, change in dress, increased absenteeism from school, increased aggressiveness, changes in interpersonal relationships, isolation, erratic behavior, avoidance of eye contact, bragging about drug abuse, and increased time spent in the bathroom.

Adult. The threats to an adult client's safety are frequently related to life-style habits. The client who excessively uses alcohol or drugs, for example, is at greater risk for motor vehicle accidents. The long-term smoker has a greater risk of cardiovascular or pulmonary disease. The adult experiencing a high level of stress is at greater risk for accidents, as well as certain

table 29-2

EXPECTED MOTOR DEVELOPMENT CHANGES THAT INCREASE THE RISK OF INJURY IN INFANTS AND TODDLERS

Age	Motor development	Hazard
1 month	Can hold head midline and parallel to body Unable to hold head erect	If not supported, infant's head flops forward or backward.
2 months	Has grasp reflex: grasps and holds object for few moments or longer	Infant is able to grasp electrical cords and other dangerous items on floor.
3 months	May begin to roll from back to abdomen Bears weight on forearms	There is increased risk of falling off bed, changing table, and counter.
4 months	Has increased grasping ability and explores new objects with mouth	Child is able to pick up small objects, which usually go immediately into mouth.
	Can roll from abdomen and from side to side and move in rocking motion	There is increased risk of falling from surfaces.
5 months	Has increased ability of locomotion through rocking, rolling, and twisting	Infant is able to purposefully move self toward objects that may be dangerous.
	Can grasp bottle but should not be left unattended	There is risk of choking on contents; drinking from bottle in supine position can increase risk of ear infections and dental caries in baby and permanent teeth.
	Can grasp small objects	There is increased risk of choking on small objects.
6 months	Creeps by propelling self on abdomen and steering with arms and legs	Child is able to move to potential dangers, such as electrical outlets and household cleaners.
7 months	May be crawling Able to sit alone for short periods	Infant is able to rapidly move from one spot to another.
8 months	May be able to pull self to standing position Able to sit unsupported	Child can easily fall unless helped back to sitting or lying position.
9 months	Begins to crawl up stairs Can stand and move by using furniture for support (walking may occur any time after 8 months)	Infant can lose balance and fall down stairs, can lose balance with wobbly furniture, and can bruise self on sharp corners of tables and bookcases.
10 months	Climbs up and tries to climb down from chairs Can change from prone to sitting position	Child may fall from chair and unable to judge distances or his or her own limits.
11 months	Interested in feeding self	Unless foods are cut into small pieces, child may choke.
12 months	May climb out of crib (although rare at this age)	There is increased risk of falling out of crib or playpen.
	Takes covers off plastic screw-top containers	Infant is able to open and possibly taste harmful substances.
15 months	Walks with help; cannot walk around corners or stop suddenly without losing balance	Child loses sense of balance and easily falls.
18 months	Runs clumsily and falls often	Toddler may injure head from severe falls.
	Moves and climbs on furniture	Child may pull furniture over on self or fall off furniture.
24 months	Can turn doorknobs	Toddler can independently open closed door and may ingest harmful products stored in cabinet, closet, or bathroom.

Modified from Whaley LF and Wong DL: *Nursing care of infants and children,* ed 4, St. Louis, 1993, Mosby; and Potter PA and Perry AG: *Fundamentals of nursing: concepts, process, and practice,* ed 3, St. Louis, 1993, Mosby.

stress-related illnesses such as headaches, gastrointestinal disorders, and infections (see Chapter 4).

Older Adult. Accidental injury from falls, driving accidents, and thermal injuries account for many hospitalizations of older adults, most of whom are unable to return to their previous level of independence (Ebersole and Hess, 1994). Falls are the leading cause of death by injury among the older adult population (Lowenstein and Hunt, 1990). Approximately 60% of falls by people 65

table 29-3

CAUSES OF FALLS IN OLDER ADULTS

Normal aging process	Pathological process
NEUROLOGICAL/SENSORY CHANGES	
Vision changes: presbyopia (farsightedness) or reduction in light that reaches retina	Vision changes: glaucoma or cataracts
Auditory impairment: decreased acuity	Auditory impairment: vertigo
Central processing: decreased proprioceptive reflexes	Central processing: senile epilepsy, cerebrovascular accident, or neurosyphilis
MUSCULOSKELETAL CHANGES	
Fibrotic changes in joints, muscles, tendons, and ligaments Loss of muscle size, strength, and speed of contraction	Gait abnormalities: shuffling; waddling; slow, short, deliberate steps; or muscle rigidity Arthritis Osteoporosis
CARDIOVASCULAR CHANGES	
Impaired regulation of cerebral blood flow Decreased baroreceptor sensitivity Progressive decrease of cerebral blood flow	Orthostatic hypotension Postprandial hypotension Carotid sinus hypersensitivity—excessive cardiac slowing or hypotension Supraventricular and ventricular dysrhythmias—sudden reduction in cardiac output or systemic blood pressure Drop attacks
GENITOURINARY/ENDOCRINE CHANGES	
Low estrogen in postmenopausal women	Stress incontinence in postmenopausal women

From McFarland GK and McFarlane EA: *Nursing diagnosis and intervention:* planning for patient care, ed 2, St. Louis, 1993, Mosby.

years of age or older occur at home (Tideiksaar, 1989). Older adults are more likely to fall because of physiological changes or acute or chronic diseases that result in weakness (Table 29-3). In addition, changes in mental status related to multiple medications or emotional responses that can accompany a loss can increase the risk of falls (Spellbring, Gannon, et al., 1988; Berryman, Gaskin, et al., 1989).

Other Risk Factors

Life-style. Life-style can increase safety risks. At greater risk of injury are people who drive or operate machinery while under the influence of chemical substances, who work at jobs that are inherently more dangerous, and who are risk-takers or daredevils. In addition, people experiencing great stress or anxiety are more accident prone because they often are too preoccupied with stressors to notice the source of potential accidents, such as a cluttered stair or a stop sign.

Mobility. A client with impaired mobility has many kinds of safety risks. Immobilization can predispose a client to other physiological and emotional hazards, which in turn can further restrict mobility and independence (see Chapter 23). A client with impaired mobility is at risk for injury when entering motor vehicles and buildings not equipped for the handicapped. Physically challenged clients are also at greater risk for automobile and other kinds of accidents.

Sensory Impairments. Clients with visual, hearing, or communication impairments are at greater risk for injury in the community. Such clients may not be able to perceive a potential danger or express needs for assistance.

Safety Awareness. Some clients are unaware of safety precautions, such as keeping medicine, poisonous plants, or other poisons away from children or reading the expiration date on food products. A complete nursing assessment should help the nurse to identify the client's level of knowledge regarding home safety so that deficiencies can be corrected with an individualized care plan.

Allergic Reactions. The majority of insect bites and stings are not serious, but the danger of death resulting from insect allergy always exists. Immediate emergency medical treatment is required for an allergic reaction (Missouri Poison Control System, 1987). A complete assessment should include allergies to insects and medications.

Risks in the Health Care Agency

The basic types of risks to safety within the health care environment are falls, client-inherent accidents, procedure-related accidents, and equipment-related accidents. The nurse learns to recognize factors associated with these risks and to take steps to prevent or minimize accidents.

An accident necessitates the filing of an incident report, a confidential document that completely describes any client accident occurring on the premises of a health care agency. The incident report is for internal use and is filed with the agency's insurance, risk management, and quality assurance office. In the event of a lawsuit, the incident report is available to the hospital attorneys (see Chapter 6). Incident reports are also collected by risk managers who monitor trends and frequencies of incidents in the workplace. Repeated occurrences will lead managers to take preventive actions.

In addition to completing the incident report, the nurse must document the accident in the client's medical record and describe its effects on the client's health status. The nurse does not write "incident report completed" in the medical record because the incident report is for internal use only.

Falls. Falls account for 29% to 89% of all incidents reported in hospitals (Raz and Baretich, 1987). A study conducted by Whedon and Shedd (1989) attempted to review the literature for accurate high-risk assessment profiles in predicting client falls. In the research it was noted that the most comprehensive data were incident

RISK FOR FALLS ASSESSMENT TOOLS

TOOL 1: RISK ASSESSMENT TOOL FOR FALLS

Directions: Place a check mark in front of elements that apply to your client. The decision of whether a client is at risk for falls is based on your nursing judgment. Guideline: A client who has a checkmark in front of an element with an asterisk (*) or four or more of the other elements would be identified as at risk for falls.

General data

__ Age over 60
__ History of falls before admission*
__ Postoperative/admitted for operation
__ Smoker

Physical condition

__ Dizziness/imbalance
__ Unsteady gait
__ Diseases/other problems affecting weight-bearing joints
__ Weakness
__ Paresis
__ Seizure disorder
__ Impairment of vision
__ Impairment of hearing
__ Diarrhea
__ Urinary frequency

Mental status

__ Confusion/disorientation*
__ Impaired memory or judgment
__ Inability to understand or follow directions

Medications

__ Diuretics or diuretic effects
__ Hypotensive or CNS suppressants (e.g. narcotic, sedative, psychotropic, hypnotic, tranquilizer, antihypertensive, antidepressant)
__ Medication that increases GI motility (e.g., laxative, enema)

Ambulatory devices used

__ Cane
__ Crutches
__ Walker
__ Wheelchair
__ Geriatric (Geri) chair
__ Braces

TOOL 2: REASSESSMENT IS SAFE "KARE" (RISK) TOOL

Directions: Place a check in front of any element that applies to your client. A client who has a check mark in front of any of the first four elements would be identified as at risk for falls. In addition, when a high-risk client has a check mark in front of the element "Use of a wheelchair," the client is considered to be at greater risk for falls.

__ Unsteady gait/dizziness/imbalance
__ Impaired memory or judgment
__ Weakness
__ History of falls
__ Use of a wheelchair

From Brians LK, et al.: *Rehabil Nurs* 16(2):67, 1991.

reports but not all falls were reported. Although authors try to define characteristics for potential falls, it must be remembered that studies gather data after the fall has occurred. Brians et al. (1991) have developed a risk assessment tool for early recognition of potential falls (see box on p. 784). Such tools might enable the nurse to assess potential risks before accidents and injuries result.

Client-Inherent Accidents. Client-inherent accidents are accidents other than falls in which the client is the primary factor. Examples are self-inflicted cuts, injuries, and burns; ingestion or injection of foreign substances; self-mutilation or setting fires; and pinching fingers in drawers or doors.

The nurse must file a complete and accurate incident report for client-inherent injuries. A thorough report describing the client's physical and behavioral status, as well as the incident, is necessary for studying risk factors within the agency that require preventive action and for protecting the institution and health care professionals from lawsuits (see Chapter 6).

Procedure-Related Accidents. Procedure-related accidents occur during therapy. They include medication and fluid administration errors, improper application of external devices, and improper performance of procedures, such as dressing changes.

The nurse can prevent many procedure-related accidents. For example, correct administration of medications, using the "five rights" described in Chapter 26, helps to prevent errors. In addition, proper administration of intravenous fluids prevents fluid overload or deficit (see Chapter 35). Also, injury from the introduction of pathogens is reduced when surgical asepsis is used for sterile dressing changes (see Chapter 36) or invasive procedures such as insertion of a Foley catheter (see Chapter 32). The nurse can protect clients, self, and other health care workers by practicing universal precautions and body substance isolation procedures (see Chapter 25). Finally, correct use of body mechanics and transfer techniques reduces the risk of injuries from transfer procedures (see Chapter 22).

Equipment-Related Accidents. Equipment-related accidents result from the malfunction, disrepair, or misuse of equipment or from an electrical hazard. To avoid injury, personnel should not operate monitoring or therapy equipment without instruction.

A checklist should be used to assess potential electrical hazards to reduce the risk of electrical fires, electrocution, or injury from improperly wired equipment (see box below, left).

Nursing Diagnosis

The nurse's assessment reveals sets of data in the form of defining characteristics that reveal a pertinent nursing diagnosis. Defining characteristics such as impaired vision, presence of household chemicals, and poorly lighted staircases are clustered to support a specific nursing diagnosis. They include signs and symptoms, laboratory and diagnostic data, or risk factors that make an individual more vulnerable to injury. The nursing diagnosis identifies risks to a client's safety and thus the predisposition to injury (see box below).

The nursing diagnosis should include specific causative factors so that nursing care measures can be individualized. For example, the nursing diagnosis "high risk for injury" could be related to altered mobility or it could be related to sensory alteration (visual). Correct identification of the causative factor (such as altered mobility) would lead to selecting such nursing interventions as teaching and performing range-of-motion exercises or proper use of safety devices such as side rails, canes, or crutches. Visual impairment as the related factor would lead to selecting different interventions such as keeping the area well lighted, orienting the client to the surroundings, or keeping eyeglasses clean, handy, and well protected.

CHECKLIST FOR ELECTRICAL HAZARDS

Ungrounded equipment
Frayed cords
Circuits overloaded by too many appliances in one area
Improperly functioning equipment
Use of extension cords
Tangled or cluttered cords
Use of electrical appliances near sink, bathtub, shower, or damp areas
Electrical cords or appliances within range of young children
Noninsulated wiring in basement or crawl-space

NURSING DIAGNOSES FOR SAFETY RISKS

- High risk for injury
- High risk for poisoning
- High risk for suffocation
- High risk for trauma
- Altered thought processes
- Impaired home maintenance management
- Knowledge deficit
- High risk for altered body temperature
- Impaired physical mobility
- Sensory/perceptual alterations

Planning

Clients with actual or potential risks to safety require a nursing care plan directed at meeting their safety needs. The planning phase may identify nursing interventions to prevent threats to safety and to meet safety needs. Planning and goal setting need to be done in collaboration with the client, family, and other members of the health care team. Consideration must be given to the client's developmental stage, physical and psychosocial status, and economic and environmental resources. The total plan should address all aspects of client needs and utilize resources of the health care team and the community when appropriate (see nursing care plan below).

When the plan has been developed, priority goals should be identified. Priorities are based on those that are most important in terms of risks to safety and health promotion. The plan is based on one or more of the following client-centered goals and expected outcomes for these goals.

Goal: Client's environment is adapted to motor, sensory, and cognitive developmental needs.

Outcome

Modifiable hazards in the home reduced by 100% by 2 weeks

Goal: Client learns potential threats to personal safety within 1 month.

Outcomes

Client will list hazards within the home by 1 week

SAMPLE NURSING CARE PLAN
Potential Threat to Safety

ASSESSMENT

Clinical scenario: Cathy and Mike Morrow are *adolescent parents of an active 2-year-old* boy, Tommy. Tommy has just been admitted to the *emergency room for ingesting dishwasher powder, which was located under the kitchen sink in the family's apartment.* Both parents are visibly upset because their child is ill and because *they did not know about the harmful effects of dishwasher powder.*

NURSING DIAGNOSIS

Knowledge deficit regarding information about household poisons related to unfamiliarity with child care safety

PLANNING

Goal	Expected outcomes
Parents will understand potential threats to child's safety within 1 week.	Parents will correctly identify hazards in home and community. Parents will reduce modifiable hazards in the home by 100%.

IMPLEMENTATION

Steps	Rationale
1. Conduct home assessment with parents and make a list of threats to child's safety.	Accurate home assessment more readily identifies threats to safety than does information provided by nursing history alone (Whaley and Wong, 1993).
2. Stress importance of safeproofing the home and give parents specific instructions for preventing burns, poisoning, drowning, falls, aspiration, and suffocation.	Advance guidance is important in preventing potential injuries (Pridham, 1993).
3. Instruct parents about local poison control center. 4. Provides parents with poison control center's phone number.	Poison control centers should be contacted first when home poisonings occur. Syrup of ipecac is given *after* instruction from health care professional (Woolf, et al., 1987).

EVALUATIVE MEASURES

Observe environment for potential threats to safety.

Obtain feedback from parents about actions to take if an accidental poisoning occurs in the future.

Defining characteristics are shown in italic type.

Home will be free of hazards in 1 month
Client will correctly use medication, equipment, or treatments in 2 weeks

Goal: Client's potential for injury will be reduced.

Outcomes

Side effects or adverse effects of medications will be absent
Skin and tissues will be intact. Musculoskeletal system will be free of injury
Electrical grounding and functioning of equipment will be correct

Goal: Client's risk of accidental poisoning will be reduced.

Outcomes

Client will correctly administer medications
Safe sanitation practices are followed
Medications, household cleaners, poisonous plants, and other poisonous substances are properly stored and marked and kept out of reach of children.
Syrup of ipecac will be in the home, and client can describe its correct use
Phone number of poison control center will be accessible

Implementation

Nursing interventions are directed toward maintaining the client's safety in the home and in health care agencies. Nursing measures for providing a safe environment include health promotion, developmental considerations, and environmental protection.

Health Promotion

The emphasis in health care today is on health promotion. Wellness (which is synonymous with health promotion) depends on safety. Edelman and Mandle (1994) describe passive and active strategies aimed at health promotion. Passive strategies are implemented through government legislation (e.g., sanitation and clean water laws). Active strategies are those in which the individual is actively involved through changes in life-style and participating in wellness programs.

The nurse participates by supporting legislation and acting as a positive role model. Because environmental and community values have the greatest impact on health promotion, community nurses can assess and recommend safety measures in the home, school, neighborhood, and workplace. Some specific health promotion strategies for safety are teaching adolescents about proper nutrition and the dangers of alcohol and drugs, instructing clients about safety measures in the workplace, and advising older adults about smoking and its relationship to fires in the home and potential cancer risks. Nurses can also promote healthy life-styles by teaching stress avoidance and by participating in community programs aimed at reducing stress, stop smoking clinics, CPR training, and baby-sitting safety courses. Other measures include promotion of safety awareness such as safeproofing the home, planning and practicing home fire drills, and the appropriate use of safety belts and helmets for automobiles and cycles.

Social and cultural issues frequently influence safety measures affecting health promotion (Foss, 1987). Nurses can thus promote health indirectly by assisting clients to build value systems that include safety measures and decision making.

Developmental Considerations

Infant, Toddler, and Preschooler. Growing, curious children depend on adults to protect them from injury. Nurses can frequently educate young parents or guardians about reducing risks of injuries for children. Nurses working in prenatal clinics and in community health programs can teach parents to promote safety in their homes. The pediatric nurse can also teach the child about safety. Other nursing interventions that should be incorporated into the care plan for safety of a child are listed in Table 29-4 and illustrated in Figure 29-1.

School-Age Child. School-age children increasingly explore their environment. They have friends outside their immediate neighborhood; they may walk to school, and they become more active in school, church, and community activities. All of these activities help the child to develop social skills and independence, but they also increase the risk of injury. Some nursing interventions help to guide the parent to provide for the safety of the school-age child (Table 29-5).

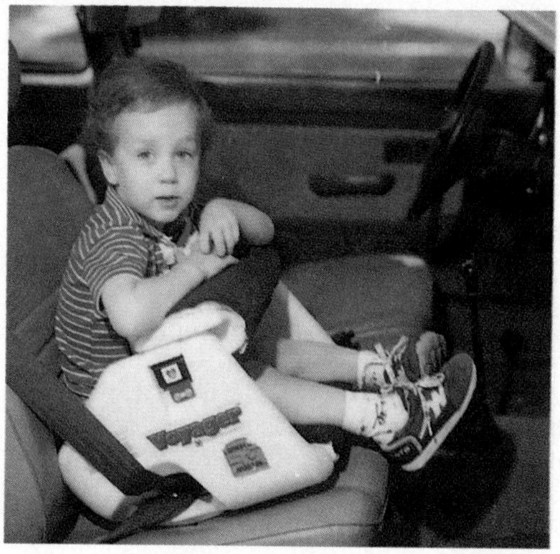

FIGURE 29-1 Toddler car seat.

table 29-4

NURSING INTERVENTIONS TO PROMOTE SAFETY OF INFANTS, TODDLERS, AND PRESCHOOLERS

Intervention	Rationale
Use large soft toys without plastic eyes, nose, or mouth.	Small parts can be dislodged by baby, and accidental aspiration can occur.
If playpen with mesh sides is used, do not leave one side down.	Baby's head can become wedged between playpen pad and lowered mesh side, and asphyxiation can occur.
Never leave sides of crib down or turn away from baby on changing table.	Child can suddenly roll and fall from crib or changing table.
Hold baby at feeding time; do not prop bottle.	This increases bonding with parent and reduces risk of choking.
If formula is used, be sure to read instructions. Most formulas must be diluted with water.	Using undiluted formula can cause fluid and electrolyte imbalances in newborn.
Discontinue use of infant seat at 3 months or earlier if infant is very mobile.	At 3 months, active infants may be able to propel themselves out of seat and fall.
Baby-proof house for small objects, sharp objects, and toxic and poisonous substances.	Babies explore their world with their hands and mouths, and small objects can result in choking. Toxic and poisonous substances require prompt action (see later section on poison).
Cover electrical outlets with protective covers.	Electrical wall outlets are at babies' eye level and stimulate their curiosity. Crawling baby will frequently attempt to play with electrical wall plates regardless of number of toys available.
Use guardrails at top and bottom of stairs and at doorway of rooms considered off-limits to crawling or walking toddler.	This prevents child from falling down stairs or being exposed to rooms with unguarded dangers.
Never leave baby unattended in infant seat, walker, stroller, or high chair.	Active child can easily slide out of these devices and fall.
Never leave baby or child unattended in bath or wading pool.	Accidental drowning may occur.
Never attach pacifier to child with string around neck.	String may become easily tangled and strangulation can result.
Restrain child in back seat of automobile. Children under 4 should be in approved car seat (Figure 29-1). Older children should be restrained with seat belt.	In case of sudden stop or accident, unrestrained child is bounced against hard, sharp surfaces of vehicle's interior, and injuries result.
Remove plastic bags, such as those for storing fruit or dry cleaning, from home.	If child places these over head, air supply decreases, and child suffocates.
Install strong, dead-bolt locks on doors well beyond toddler's reach, even when child is standing on chair.	This prevents child from leaving home without parent's knowledge, reducing danger of child getting lost, freezing to death, or being abducted.
Use words "no" and "don't" to convey that object or action increases child's risk of injury, such as playing with matches.	Improperly using these words renders them meaningless to child.
Teach child to swim at early age but always provide supervision.	Child will be able to enjoy water safely. Child who knows how to swim can still get in difficulty in water and needs supervision.
Teach child how to cross street and walk in parking lots.	This provides child with self-protection against dangers from automobiles.
Teach child not to talk to or accept anything from stranger and to notify parents or responsible adult if approached by stranger.	This reduces risk of injury or abduction by stranger. Reporting stranger's presence helps law enforcement personnel to investigate and remove threat.
Do not allow child to run with sucker or popsicle in mouth.	Child may fall, and stick from sucker or popsicle can cause puncture or a foreign body in child's airway.
Teach child not to eat anything found on street or in grass.	Substance may be poisonous and can cause severe illness.
Use back burners on stoves and turn pot handles toward wall.	This reduces risk of child pulling down pot of hot liquid and being burned.
Remove doors from unused refrigerators and freezers, and instruct child not to hide in these items.	Door may latch and on older models cannot be released from inside; as result, asphyxiation can occur.

table 29-5

NURSING INTERVENTIONS TO PROMOTE SAFETY OF SCHOOL-AGERS*

Intervention	Rationale
Teach child safe use of equipment for play and work.	Child needs to learn the difference between play and work equipment and that improper use can result in injury.
Teach child how to ride a bicycle safely and responsibilities that go with bicycling.	If bicycling is prohibited on sidewalks, child must learn to obey traffic signals and ride with traffic patterns.
Teach child to wear protective helmets and knee and elbow pads when roller skating or skate boarding.	Protective devices reduce risk of serious injury in falls.
Never allow child to operate appliances while alone.	If electrical mishap occurred, no one would be available to help child.
If parent chooses to have firearms in house, teach parent to keep them unloaded, locked up, and out of reach.	This prevents injury from accidental discharge or improper use.

*In addition to interventions in Table 29-4 that are appropriate for school-age child.

CLIENT TEACHING FOR ACCIDENT PREVENTION FOR ADOLESCENTS

Enroll teenagers in a driver's education course and make practice drives with them in good and bad weather. Teach them to handle a motor vehicle in a skid.
Teach them to wear seat belts while driving or as passengers.
Instruct them not to drive after using a psychoactive substance or enter an automobile when the driver has been using such substances.
Form a contract with teenagers: if they drink at a party, they will call home for a ride with no questions asked.
Help them to develop safe eating, sleeping, and relaxation habits.
Inform them of the dangers of psychoactive substances.
Recognize changes in adolescents' behavior and mood.
Listen to them.
Do not try to be a buddy; remain a parent.

Adolescent. When children approach adolescence, much of their time is spent away from home and with their peer group. During adolescence young persons learn to drive. Risks to the adolescent's safety therefore involve many factors outside the home. Adults serve as role models for adolescents and can help adolescents to minimize risks to their safety through example and education. The box above, right, lists measures by which nurses and parents can help the adolescent to prevent accidents.

Adult. Risks to young and middle adults frequently result from life-style factors such as child rearing, high stress states, inadequate nutrition, and abuse of drugs or alcohol. Adults need to be taught their safety is in fact threatened, and as a result, their life-style needs to be modified. Chapters 2 and 4 detail appropriate nursing interventions.

Older Adult. Most injuries to older adults involve falls, auto accidents, and burns (Lowenstein and Hunt, 1990). Advancing age and the concurrent physiological changes in vision, hearing, mobility, reflexes, circulation, and the ability to make quick judgments all predispose older adults to falls (see Chapter 20). Kilpeck, et al. (1991) reported mental status change and mobility deficit as the most frequent risk factor for falls. Certain disease states, such as arthritis or cerebrovascular accidents common to older adults, increase chances of injury. In addition, the effects of many medications such as sedatives, diuretics, and laxatives given to older adults make falls more likely (Berryman, 1989). Nursing interventions designed to compensate for the physiological changes of aging are listed in Table 29-6 and in the box on gerontological nursing practice on p. 791.

Automobile accidents are more likely to occur with older adults because of changes in visual acuity and depth perception, hearing acuity, and nervous system response. Interventions directed toward preventing automobile accidents are designed to compensate for these changes (see box on p. 791).

Pedestrian accidents can also be reduced by persuading older adults to take five precautions: (1) wear reflectorized garments when walking at night, (2) stand on the sidewalk, not in the street, when waiting to cross a street, (3) always cross at corners, not in the middle of the block, particularly if the street is a major one, (4) when possible, cross with the traffic light, not against it, and (5) look left, right, and left again before entering the street or crosswalk.

Burns and scalds are also more apt to occur with older adults who are at greater risk for several reasons. They may forget and leave hot water running or become confused when turning the dials on a stove. Impaired visual acuity and sense of smell increases the danger that they may not detect smoke or gas fumes (Cooper,

table 29-6

MEASURES TO PREVENT FALLS BY OLDER ADULTS

Measure	Rationale
STAIRS	
Install treads with uniform depth of 9 inches (22.5 cm) and 9-inch risers (vertical face of steps).	If stairs are of uniform size, older adult does not have to continually adjust vision.
Install uniform-textured or plain-colored surfaces on each tread, and mark edge of tread with contrasting color.	Uniform textures or color help to decrease vertigo. Marking edge of tread provides obvious visual clue to end of stair.
Ensure proper lighting of each tread. Block sun or lightbulb glare with translucent shades or screen, or use lower-wattage bulbs.	Older adults' vision is unable to adjust quickly to changes in lighting.
Ensure adequate head room so that users do not have to duck to negotiate stairs.	Sudden changes in head position may result in dizziness.
Remove protruding objects from staircase walls.	Decreased peripheral vision may prevent client from seeing object.
Maintain outdoor walkways and stairs in good condition and free of holes, cracks, and splinters.	Decreased visual acuity can prevent client from seeing any structural defect.
HANDRAILS	
Install smooth but slip-resistant handrail at least 2 inches (5 cm) from wall.	Two-inch distance allows client to grasp handrail firmly for support.
Secure handrail firmly so that user's weight is supported, especially at bottom and top of stairway.	Older adult has greatest risk of falling at top and bottom of stairs because center of gravity is being shifted and balance is unstable.
Install grab rails in bathroom near toilet and tub.	This enables client to have support while rising from sitting to standing position.
FLOOR COVERINGS	
Ensure clients wear properly fitting shoes or slippers with nonskid surface.	Reduces chances of slipping.
Secure all carpeting, mats, and tile; place nonskid backing under small rugs.	Sudden slip may cause dizziness and inability to regain balance.
ORIENTATION	
Place disoriented clients in rooms near nurses' station.	Provides for more frequent observation on the part of nursing staff.
Maintain close supervision of confused clients.	Confused client often attempts to wander out of bed or room.

1983). Nursing measures developed for preventing burns are designed to minimize the risk from impaired vision and hearing (see box on p. 792).

The nurse should also provide information regarding neighborhood resources to the older adult (Ebersole and Hess, 1990). Older adults frequently relocate to new neighborhoods and must get acquainted with new resources such as modes of transportation and church schedules. In addition, the food resources of some older adults (e.g., Meals on Wheels) make the difference in their ability to maintain an independent life-style. Although retired from their jobs, older adults have a wealth of past experiences to aid volunteer organizations. In addition some retirees may enjoy reentering the work force in a new capacity. Information about assistance resources, such as daily "hello" programs, emergency services, and elder abuse hot lines are often helpful. Nurses able to provide this information to older adults assist them in maintaining an independent life-style.

Environmental Considerations

Nursing interventions directed at eliminating environmental threats include general preventive measures such as meeting basic needs, reducing physical hazards, reducing pathogen and parasite transmission, and controlling pollution effects. They also include specific measures to reduce the risk of accidental injuries from falls, fires, poisoning, and electrical hazards.

GERONTOLOGIC NURSING PRACTICE

Gerontological nursing practices for the client at risk for injury might include:

- Older adult clients frequently have visual impairments that increase their risk for accidents. The nurse will teach clients to keep living areas well-lighted and clutter-free, to keep eyeglasses in good condition, and to avoid night driving.
- Older adults have musculoskeletal changes that make movement difficult and increase the risk of falling. The nurse will teach clients to use assistive devices in proper working order (canes, rails in tub and bathroom, elevated seats).
- Older adults have sensory impairments that increase their risks for burns. The nurse will advise clients to avoid smoking in bed, to lower thermostats on water heaters, to avoid overloading electrical outlets, and to install and maintain smoke detectors in the home.
- Older adults have slowed reaction time from impaired cerebral blood flow. The nurse will teach clients safety tips for avoiding automobile accidents.
- Older adults frequently have some impairment of memory that increases their risk for accidental poisoning. The nurse will teach clients about the proper handling and storage of food and safe methods of scheduling and taking medications.
- Older adults have physiological changes that result in slower metabolism of drugs. The nurse teaches clients about drug interactions and signs and symptoms of drug toxicity to report to their health care provider.

CLIENT TEACHING FOR PREVENTION OF AUTOMOBILE ACCIDENTS IN OLDER ADULT CLIENTS

Tell client to see his or her physician if a hearing problem is suspected.

Instruct client to leave car windows partially open in order to hear warning signals.

Instruct client to set the air conditioner or heater and the radio low so that their noise does not mask outside sounds.

Tell client to place mirrors on both sides of the car, and use them and a wide rear-view mirror when changing lanes or passing other vehicles.

Instruct client to stop frequently to stretch muscles and rest eyes.

Advise client to schedule regular eye examinations to check for vision changes or health problems that may affect vision.

Tell client to follow the physician's recommendations, if any, about limiting when and where to drive.

Tell client to allow time to adjust to new lenses, especially bifocals or trifocals, before driving.

Instruct client to wear good quality sunglasses to reduce glare and wear them only during the day.

Tell client to keep windshield and all windows clean inside and out, replace worn wiper blades, and keep headlights, tail lights, and turn signals clean to maintain maximum lighting.

Instruct client about medication's long- and short-term effects on driving ability.

Tell client not to smoke while driving at night because smoking impairs vision.

Instruct client not to drive after drinking alcohol.

Encourage client to enroll in a driver training course through the state motor vehicle department.

Instruct client to take circuitous routes to avoid freeways.

Modified from Cooper S: Accidents and older adults. Copyright 1981, *American Journal of Nursing Company.* Reprinted with permission from *Geriatric Nursing*, July/August, vol 2.

General Preventive Measures. Nursing interventions can contribute to a safer environment by helping the client to meet the basic physiological needs of oxygen, humidity, nutrition, and temperature. To ensure that oxygen availability is not threatened, the client's furnace should be periodically inspected for proper functioning. To achieve a comfortable level of humidity in the home, the client might attach a humidifier to the furnace or, in the case of upper respiratory tract infection, use a room humidifier while the client sleeps. The nurse can teach basic techniques for food handling and preparation so that nutritional needs are met safely. Education regarding frostbite, hypothermia, heatstroke, and heat exhaustion can help clients to avoid conditions caused by temperature extremes.

Adequate lighting and security measures in and around the home, including the use of night lights, exterior lighting, and locks on doors and windows, enable the client to reduce the risk of injury from falls or crime. The nurse should also encourage removing clutter from halls, stairs, traffic areas, and furniture such as bedside tables to further reduce the risk of falls.

Nurses use effective and efficient methods to control pathogen transmission. These include techniques of medical asepsis, removing or destroying disease-causing organisms or infected material, and surgical asepsis, protection against infection by the use of sterile techniques. Pathogen transmission from person to person can be reduced or prevented by immunization, the process by which resistance to an infectious disease is acquired through the administration of an antigen and

CLIENT TEACHING FOR PREVENTION OF BURNS IN OLDER ADULT CLIENTS

- Instruct client not to smoke in bed or when sleepy.
- Tell client not to wear loose-fitting clothing (bathrobes, nightgowns, or pajamas) when cooking.
- Encourage client to learn to use a microwave oven.
- Tell client to set thermostats for water heater or faucets so that water does not become too hot.
- Encourage client to install a portable hand fire extinguisher and smoke detectors in the kitchen.
- Advise client to keep access to outside doors unobstructed.
- Advise client to identify emergency exits in public buildings.
- Tell client that before entering a boarding or foster home, check to see that it has smoke detectors, a sprinkler system, and fire extinguishers.
- Instruct client to wear clothing that is nonflammable or treated with a permanent flame-retardant finish. Fabrics of animal hair, wool, or silk are less flammable.
- Advise client to use several electrical outlets to avoid overloading.

Modified from Cooper S: Accidents and older adults. Copyright 1981, *American Journal of Nursing Company.* Reprinted with permission from *Geriatric Nursing,* July/August, vol 2.

CLIENT TEACHING TO REDUCE THE RISK OF FALLS

- Instruct family to place bedside tables and over-bed tables close to the client.
- Encourage the client to rise from the bed or chair slowly to prevent dizziness resulting from postural hypotension.
- Tell the family to remove clutter from bedside tables, hallways, bathrooms, and grooming areas.
- Encourage the family to mount grab bars around toilets and showers; instruct the client how to use them (Figure 29-2).
- Advise that rugs and carpets be securely attached to floors and stairs.
- Advise that bath mats and nonskid strips be attached to bathtubs and the floors of shower stalls.
- Advise that electrical cords be secured against baseboards so that the client cannot easily trip over them.
- Ensure that the call bell is within easy reach of the hospitalized client, who should be shown the location of emergency call bells in bathrooms. (Nurses must respond to call lights quickly, especially for clients needing assistance to the bathroom.)
- See that wheelchairs remain locked when transporting a client from bed to wheelchair or back to bed.
- Instruct care givers to check that side rails are up and safety straps secured around the client who is on a stretcher (Figure 29-3).

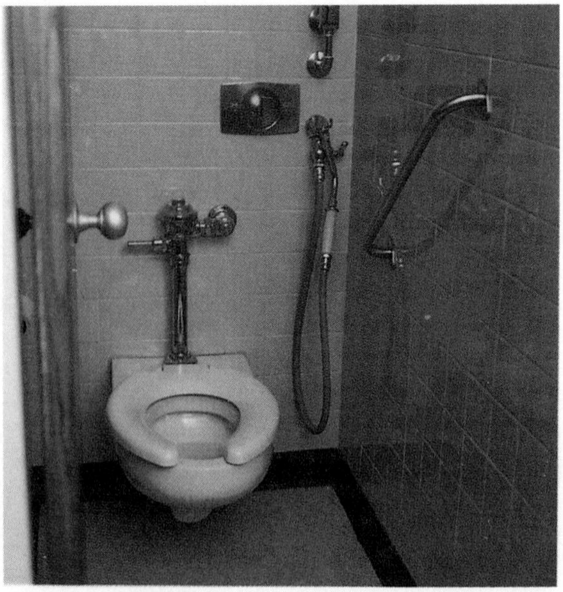

FIGURE 29-2 Safety bars beside toilets.

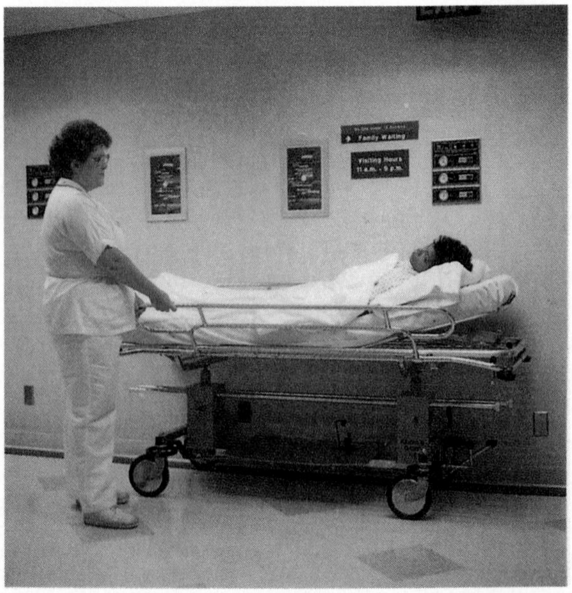

FIGURE 29-3 Raising side rails to "up" position on stretcher.

the body's consequent production of an antibody. In the home, awareness of safe methods of food handling helps to reduce the risk of pathogen and parasite transmission through contaminated food.

The nurse should provide information about any potential threat from air, water, and noise pollution in the client's environment so the client can eliminate the pollutant where possible and otherwise limit exposure.

Specific Safety Concerns. The nurse should take measures to help the client to avoid falls, fires, poisons, and electrical hazards.

FALLS. Modifications in the client's home or health care environment can easily reduce the risk of falls. A heavy or debilitated client in a bed or wheelchair or on a toilet should be properly secured or supported. Excess furniture and equipment should be removed, and a weakened client should wear rubber-soled shoes or slippers for walking or transferring. Clients should be instructed to inspect canes, walkers, and crutches to be sure the rubber tip is intact.

With clients in the home or hospital, certain safeguards can be implemented or taught to the family to minimize the risk of falls (see box on p. 792 and Figures 29-2 and 29-3). In addition, confused and disoriented clients or clients who repeatedly try to remove medical devices (e.g., O_2 equipment, IVs, dressings) may require the use of restraints and side rails to keep them from falling out of bed.

RESTRAINTS. A physical restraint is a device used to immobilize a client or extremity. In addition to physical restraints, drugs may also be prescribed to calm clients and restrain their level of activity (Fletcher, 1990). Because of the risks of restraints, current legislation is moving toward reducing the use of restraints in nursing homes and extended care facilities (Blakeslee, et al., 1991). In addition, regulatory agencies such as JCAHO are enforcing standards for the safe use of restraints in inpatient settings. The impetus is for health care organizations to move to a more "restraint free" environment. Nurses should use alternatives such as more frequent observation, involvement of family during visitation, fre-

table 29-7

GUIDELINES FOR THE USE OF RESTRAINTS

Guidelines	Rationale
A physical restraint should be selected to reduce client's movement only as much as necessary.	Overrestraining client so that activities are unduly restricted can exacerbate hazards of immobility and increase client restlessness.
If restraint is necessary, nurse should carefully explain type of restraint and reasons for its use.	Restraint can increase confusion or hostility in the client and family. Explanation of restraint can reduce or even prevent some of these negative perceptions.
Restraint should not exacerbate client's health problem.	Restraints that are too tight can impair circulation to distal extremities.
Restraint should not interfere with treatment.	Restraints placed over intravenous sites can impede flow of fluid into circulation. Restraints attached to fractured or dislocated extremities can impair healing.
Bony prominences should be padded before applying restraint.	Padding reduces risk of injury to skin from pressure.
Restraints should be changed when they become soiled or damp.	Soiled or damp restraints increase risk of skin breakdown.
Restraints should be secured away from a client's reach. A care giver should be able to quickly release the device.	When client is able to undo restraints, purpose of the restraint is negated. Quick release ties ensure that client can be released quickly to avoid injury.
Restraint applied to client in bed should be attached to bed frame (see step 9 illustration in Procedure 29-1), not side rails.	Release of side rails while restraint remains attached can result in injury to client's musculoskeletal system.
Restraints should be removed a minimum of every 2 hours (see agency policy). Client should not be left unattended when restraints are removed.	Removal provides opportunity to assess skin integrity, circulation, respiratory function (in the case of a rest restraint), and client's behavior. Skin care is provided as needed. Previously restrained client who is left unattended can cause self-injury or can injure others.
Frequent (up to every 1 hour) circulation checks should be performed when extremity restraints are used (see agency policy).	Checks reduce risk of vascular extremity injury from poor distal circulation caused by tightening of restraint.

procedure 29-1

APPLYING RESTRAINTS

Steps	Rationale
1. Identify clients whose behavior places them at risk for injury: confused or disoriented clients; clients who are combative; clients awakening from sedation.	Restraints are used to reduce risk of client falling out of bed, chair, or wheelchair; prevent interruption of therapy such as traction, intravenous infusions, or nasogastric tube feedings; prevent confused or combative client from injuring self by removing Foley catheters, surgical drains, or life support equipment; and reduce risk of injury to others by client.
2. Check physician's order for time restraint is to be applied, rationale for restraint, and assess type of restraint to be used.	Physician's order protects nurse from liability.
3. Explain carefully to client and family reasons restraint is necessary, type of restraint selected, and anticipated duration of restraint.	Restraints can increase confusion or combativeness in client. In addition, family may express anger about restraint. Explanation and reinforcement can reduce or even prevent some of these negative perceptions.
4. Prepare equipment: a. Proper restraint	Nurse is able to complete restraining procedure without having to leave client partially restrained.

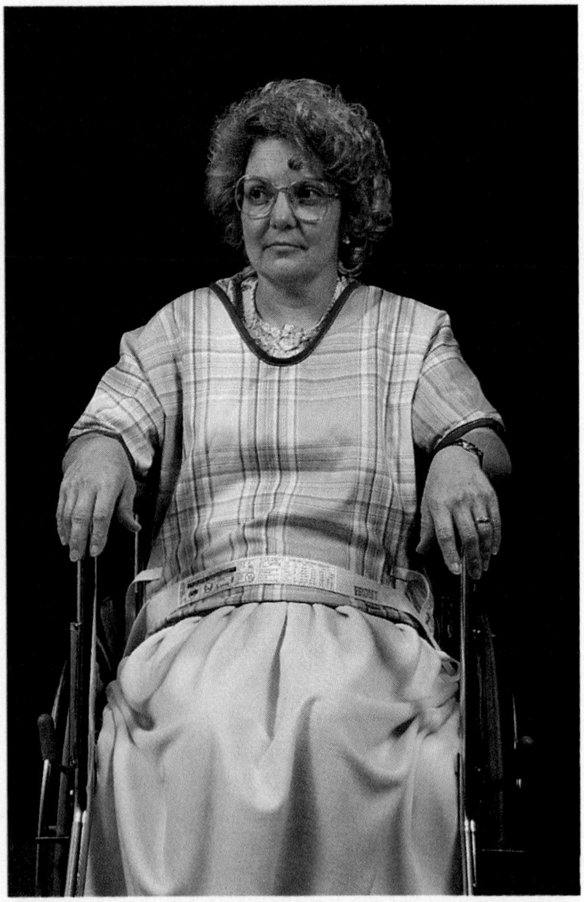

Step 7a

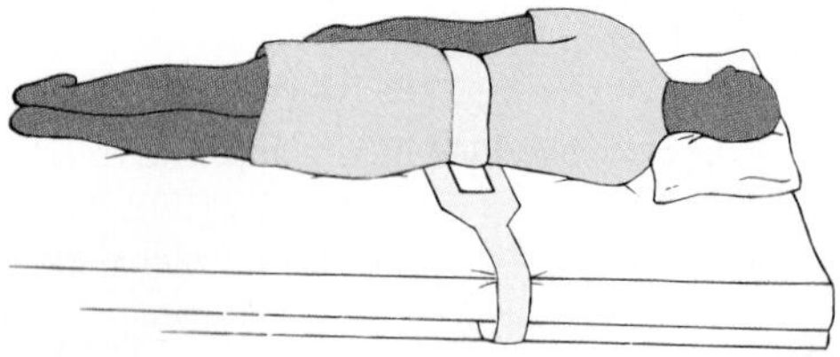

Step 7b

Steps	Rationale
b. Padding to protect bony prominences	Padding protects circulation to distal portion of extremity if wrist or ankle restraints are selected.
5. Wash hands.	Reduces transmission of microorganisms.
6. Pad bony prominences before applying restraint.	Padding decreases injury to underlying skin.
7. Apply selected restraint:	
a. Jacket restraint: vestlike garment that crosses or closes in back of client (see manufacturer's directions) (see illustration).	Restrains client while lying or reclining in bed or sitting in chair or wheelchair. Are useful in home care settings but should not be used unless other methods have failed.
b. Belt restraint: Device that secures client on stretcher (see illustration). Avoid placing belt too tightly across client's chest or abdomen.	Restrains center of gravity and prevents client from rolling off or sitting up while on stretcher.
c. Extremity restraints (ankle or wrist): Designed to immobilize one or all extremities. Commercially available limb restraints are composed of sheepskin and foam pad that comes in contact with skin. Restraints are designed so that client can pull against it without device tightening against extremity.	Maintains immobilization of extremity to protect client from injury from fall or accidental removal of therapeutic device such as an intravenous tube or Foley catheter.
d. Mitten restraint: thumbless mitten devices (see illustration) to restrain hands.	Prevents clients from dislodging invasive equipment, removing dressings, or scratching.
e. Elbow restraint: Piece of fabric with slots in which tongue blades are placed so that elbow joint remains rigid (see illustration).	Used with infants and children to prevent elbow flexion.

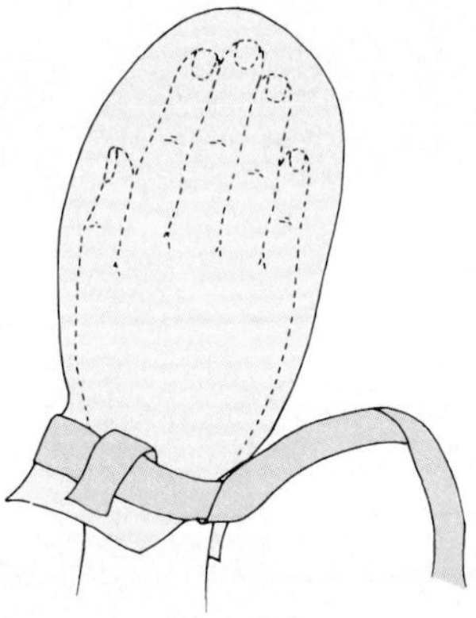

Step 7d

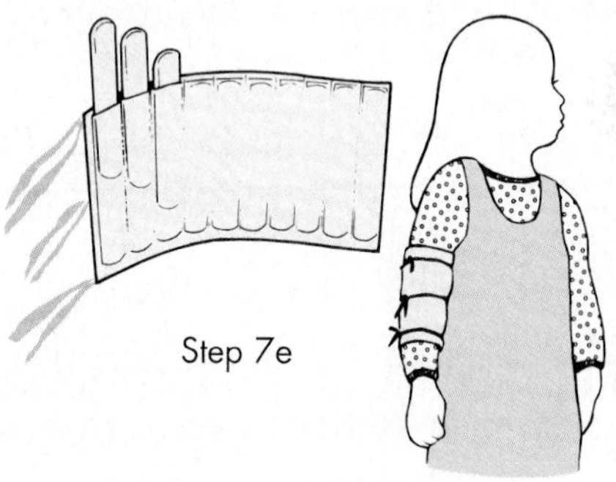

Step 7e

Steps	Rationale
f. Mummy restraint: Blanket or sheet is opened on bed or crib with one corner folded toward center. Child is placed on blanket with shoulders at fold with feet toward opposite corner. With child's right arm straight down against the body, right side of blanket is pulled firmly across right shoulder and chest and secured beneath left side of body. Left arm is placed straight against side, and left side of blanket is brought across shoulder and chest and locked beneath child's body on right side. Lower corner is folded and brought over body and tucked or fastened securely with safety pins (Whaley and Wong, 1993).	Maintains short-term restraint of small child or infant for examination or treatment involving head and neck. Effectively controls movement of torso and extremities.

Continued.

procedure 29-1—cont'd

APPLYING RESTRAINTS

Steps	Rationale
8. Secure ties of jacket or extremity restraints by wrapping them around stable parts of the bed, bed frame, or chair (legs or under frame of wheelchair) (see illustrations).	When client is able to undo restrains, purpose of restraint is negated.
9. **Do not tie the end of a restraint in a knot. Use a quick release tie for all restraints** (see illustration).	A client can become improperly positioned in a restraint—requiring immediate release.
10. Wash hands.	Reduces transmission of microorganisms.
11. Completely remove restraints briefly at least every 2 hr and document in nurse's notes. Client should not be left unattended. Observe color of extremity and palpate pulses below extremity. Have client move extremity.	Provides opportunity to assess circulation, ROM, and respiration, and to provide skin care. Timely assessment enables nurse to routinely observe musculoskeletal system and prevent complications from restraint device.
12. Observe for correct application of restraint and condition of restrained extremity or body part every 1 hour.	Incorrect application of restraints can result in injury to client.
13. Attempt a trial release when client's behavior begins to improve.	A trial release is a period when the nurse reassesses client to determine if continued use of restraint is needed.
14. Record in nurse's notes nursing assessment before and after restraints were used, focusing on client's safety, level of orientation, type of restraint selected, response to restraint.	Documents that client's physical safety was at risk and that specific restraint was warranted.

(a)

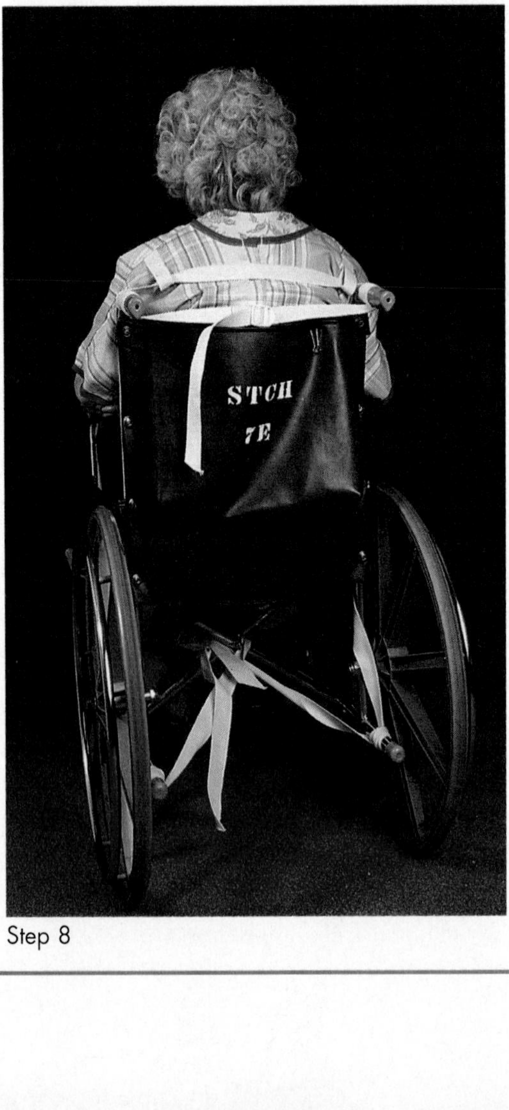

Step 8

(b)

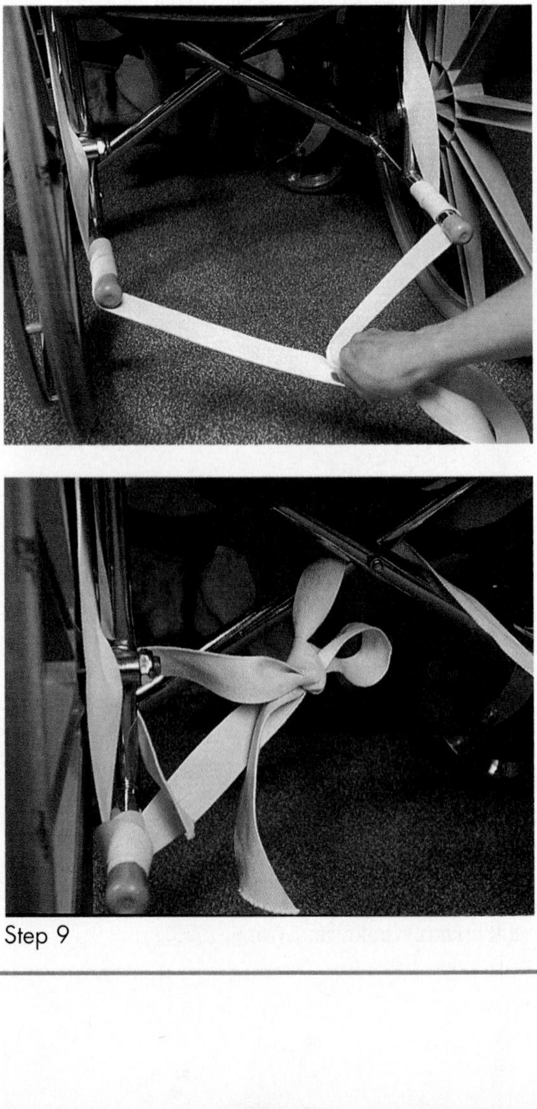

Step 9

quent reorientation, and introducing familiar stimuli within the environment to reduce behaviors that often lend to restraint use. The use of restraints involves a psychological adjustment for the client and family, and the nurse should assist them in adapting to this change when it is necessary (Table 29-7). Nursing homes must now obtain informed consents from family members before using restraints. As with other procedures, the nurse must follow specific guidelines when using physical restraints (Procedure 29-1). The overall objectives for restraints follow:

1. Reducing the risk of client injury from falls
2. Preventing interruption of therapy such as traction, intravenous infusions, nasogastric tube feeding, or Foley catheter
3. Preventing the confused or combative client from removing life support equipment
4. Reducing the risk of injury to others by the client

In keeping with current trends toward health promotion, improved assessment techniques and modifications of the environment are being offered as alternatives to restraints (Brower, 1991; Radar, 1991; Strumph and Evans, 1991). Often the decision to restrain causes a conflict between the need to provide client protection and the client's belief about the nurse's professional behavior (Strumph and Evans, 1988; Scherer, et al., 1991).

For legal purposes the nurse must be familiar with agency policy and procedures for appropriate use and monitoring of restraints. Institutions require a physician's order that is time limited and designates the patient behavior for which restraints are to be used. When making an independent judgment to apply restraints, the nurse should document the assessment of the client's activity and behavior, the conclusions about the client's status, the nursing action, and the fact that the action was explained to the client and family. In addition, the nurse should note the type of restraint selected and where it was applied.

Side rails. Chapter 22 discusses side rails as a device for increasing the client's mobility and stability in bed or when moving from bed to chair. Side rails also help to prevent the unconscious client from falling out of bed. However, the use of side rails alone for a disoriented client may cause only more confusion and further injury. Frequently a confused client or one determined to get out of bed because of pain, toileting needs, or anxiety attempts to climb over the side rail or climbs out at the foot of the bed. Either attempt usually results in a fall. Nursing interventions to reduce a client's confusion should first focus on the cause of the confusion. Frequently, nurses mistake confusion for a client's attempt to explore his or her environment or to self-toilet. If all efforts to reduce confusion or restlessness fail, restraints may become necessary.

Fires. A fire is always possible at the home and hospital. Accidental home fires typically result from smoking in bed, careless extinguishing of cigarette butts in trash cans, grease fires, or electrical fires resulting from faulty wiring or appliances. Institutional fires typically result from a client smoking in bed or from an electrical or anesthetic-related fire.

FIRE PREVENTION GUIDELINES

Know the telephone number for reporting a fire, and be sure the number is attached to all telephones.
Know the agency's or unit's fire drill or fire evacuation routine.
Post accurate, easy-to-follow routes for the location of fire exits.
Know the location of fire extinguishers, how to use them, and which type of extinguisher to use for specific fires (Table 29-8).
Report a fire before attempting to extinguish it, regardless of its size.
Keep hallways free of unnecessary equipment or furniture.
Keep fire hoses clear at all times.
Periodically check the efficiency of fire extinguishers.
Post signs on the outside of elevators warning people to take the stairs in the event of a fire.

The interventions described here are directed toward fires occurring in health care agencies, but the same principles apply for fires in the home. It is important to have a plan of action in the event of fire (see box above).

If a fire occurs in a health care agency, the nurse protects clients from injury and attempts to contain the fire. When observing a fire, the nurse should immediately report its exact location and may then attempt to extinguish it if there is no immediate threat to clients.

When hospital or institutional fires occur, all personnel are mobilized to evacuate clients. Clients who are close to the fire, regardless of its size, are at risk of injury and should be moved to another area. If a client requires oxygen but not life support, the nurse discontinues the oxygen, which is combustible and can fuel an existing fire. If the client is on life support, the nurse may need to maintain the client's respiratory status manually with an Ambu bag (see Chapter 34) until the client is moved away from the fire. Ambulatory clients can be directed to walk by themselves to a safe area and in some cases may be able to assist in moving clients in wheelchairs. Bedridden clients are generally moved from the scene by a stretcher, their bed, or a wheelchair. If none of these methods is appropriate, the clients must be carried from the area. If a client must be carried, the nurse should be careful not to overextend physical limits for lifting because injury to the nurse can result in further injury to the client. If fire department personnel are on the scene, they can help to evacuate the clients.

table 29-8

FIRE EXTINGUISHERS AND THEIR USES

Class of fire	Use	Precautions
CARBON DIOXIDE (CO_2)		
Grease Electrical	Direct CO_2 into flame, thus cutting off fire's oxygen supply.	
SODA AND ACID (WATER EXTINGUISHER)		
Paper and rubbish Wood	Turn canister upside down, thereby mixing soda and acid. CO_2 is then produced, releasing water extinguisher under pressure. To stop flow, turn canister right side up.	Ineffective against grease and electrical fires because it causes grease to spatter, thereby spreading fire, and because water conducts electricity
DRY CHEMICAL		
Rubbish Electrical	Pull pin or press level on extinguisher, blanketing fire with foam and thus cutting off fire's oxygen supply.	Ineffective against grease because it causes grease to spatter and thus spreads fire
WATER PUMP		
Rubbish Wood	Pump handle while pointing nozzle toward fire.	Ineffective against grease and electrical fires because grease can spatter, spreading fire, and because water conducts electricity
ANTIFREEZE OR WATER		
Rubbish Wood Grease Anesthetics	Pull pin and handle of extinguisher, and direct extinguisher toward fire.	Ineffective against electrical fires because water conducts electricity

After a fire has been reported and clients are out of danger, nurses and other personnel must take measures to contain or put out the fire, such as closing doors and windows, turning off oxygen and electrical equipment, and using a fire extinguisher. The three basic types of fires for which extinguishers are used are paper and rubbish (type A), grease and anesthetic gas (type B), and electrical (type C). The appropriate extinguisher must be used for each type (Table 29-8).

Of course the best intervention is to prevent fires. Nursing measures aimed at primary prevention are complying with the agency's smoking policies and keeping combustible materials away from heat sources (Collins, 1988). Some agencies have fire doors that are held open by magnets and close automatically when a fire alarm sounds. It is important to keep equipment away from these doors.

POISONING. A **poison** is any substance that impairs health or destroys life when ingested, inhaled, or absorbed by the body. Specific antidotes or treatments are available for only some types of poisons. The capacity of body tissue to recover from poison determines the reversibility of the effect. Poisons can impair the respiratory, circulatory, central nervous, hepatic, gastrointestinal, and renal systems of the body. Accidental poisonings are a greater risk for the toddler, preschooler, and young school-age child. The nurse can help parents to reduce the risk of accidental poisoning by teaching them to keep hazardous substances out of the reach of children. With adolescents and young or middle-age adults, poisonings are often caused by insect or snake bites. Drug and other substance poisonings in these age-groups are commonly related to suicide attempts or drug experimentation. Older adults are also at risk for poisoning because diminished eyesight may cause an accidental ingestion of a toxic substance. The impaired memory of some older adult clients may result in an accidental overdose of prescribed medications.

In the home the two major sources of poisons are plants (see box on p. 799) and household cleaners (see box on p. 800). Experts recommend that when poisoning is suspected, the nurse or family member call a **poison control center.** The center provides information regarding all aspects of intoxication, treatment, and re-

POISONOUS PLANTS

These plants contain a wide variety of poisons, and symptoms may vary from a mild stomach ache, skin rash, and swelling of the mouth and throat to involvement of the heart, kidneys, or other organs. The poison control center can give more specific information on these plants or others that may be poisonous and are not on this list. Many plants do not cause toxicity unless ingested in very large amounts.

Acorn (oak)
Akee fruit
Anemone
Angel trumpet tree
Apricot (kernels, leaves)
Arrowhead
Autumn crocus
Avocado (leaves)
Azalea
Baneberry
Belladonna
Betel nut palm
Bird of paradise
Bittersweet
Black locust
Bleeding heart
Buckeye
Buttercup
Caladium
Calla lily
Castor bean
Century plant
Cheries (pits)
Chinaberry
Choke cherry
Christmas rose
Climbing nightshade
Cowbane
Daffodil
Daphne
Deadly nightshade
Delphinium
Desert potato
Devil's ivy
Dieffenbachia
Dumbcane
Dutchman's breeches
Elderberry
Elephant ear
English ivy
Euonymus
Fava bean
Flags (iris)
Four o'clock
Foxglove
Goldenchain
Holly berries
Horsetail reed
Hyacinth
Hydrangea
Indian turnip
Inkberry
Iris
Jack-in-the-pulpit
Janpanese yew
Jasmine
Jequirty bean
Jerusalem cherry
Jimson weed seeds
Jonquil
Lantana
Larkspur
Lingustrum
Lily of the valley
Lobelia
Locoweed
Lucky nut
Marsh marigold
Mayapple
Mistletoe berries
Monkshood
Moonseed
Morining glory
Mother-in-law plant
Mountain laurel
Mulberries (green,)
Narcissus
Nightshade
Oleander
Peach (seeds)
Pencil tree
Peony
Periwinkle
Peyote
Philodendron
Pigeonberry
Poinsettia
Poison hemlock
Poison ivy
Pokeweed/pokeberries
Potato (all green parts)
Primrose
Privet
Ranunculus
Phododendron
Rhubarb leaves
Rosary pea
Snow drop
Sorrel
Star of Bethelem
Swiss cheese plant
Thornapple
Threadleaf
Tobacco
Tomato (all green parts)
Tulip bulb
Virginia creeper
Water hemlock
Wisteria
Yellow jessamine
Yew berries

From Missouri Poison System: *Poisonous plants,* St. Louis, 1987, Cardinal Glennon Memorial Hospital for Children.

ferrals. The nurse should teach parents that calling such a center for information before attempting home remedies can save their child's life.

Procedure 29-2 lists accepted interventions for accidental poisonings the nurse may teach to a parent or guardian. In addition, the parent may be instructed to give milk to neutralize an acid substance or lemon juice or vinegar to neutralize an alkaline substance.

ELECTRICAL HAZARDS. Much of the equipment used in health care settings is electrical and must be well maintained in a safe condition to prevent electrical hazards. Improperly grounded or malfunctioning electrical equipment increases the risk of electrical injury and fire. The use of a prevention checklist when assessing the client's environment can reduce injuries from electrical sources in the health care agency and home (see box on p. 801).

procedure 29-2

INTERVENING IN ACCIDENTAL POISONING

Steps	Rationale
1. Identify the type and amount of substance ingested.	Will help to determine correct type and amount of antidote needed for victim.
2. Call poison control center before attempting intervention.	Centers have information needed to treat poisoned client or to offer referral to treatment centers.
3. If instructed to induce vomiting: a. Infants up to 12 months: ipecac administered only under direction of a physician b. Children (1 to 12 years): 1 tablespoon (15 ml) of ipecac c. Adults: 2 tablespoons (30 ml) of ipecac	Households should keep syrup of ipecac in easily accessible place. Ipecac causes vomiting and emptying of stomach, rather than gagging or retching. Experts recommend these doses and do not advise inducing vomiting with substances other than ipecac (Aronow, et al., 1985). Vomiting should be induced only under physician's instruction and is not induced with ingestion of gasoline or other caustic poisons.
4. Give oral fluids to assist vomiting: a. Children (1 to 12 years): 5 to 15 ml/kg, up to 8 oz of water b. Adults: 16 oz of water	Assists in emptying of stomach and further avoids gagging and retching.
5. If requested to do so, save vomitus and deliver to poison control center.	Laboratory analysis can determine further treatment.
6. Place victim with head turned to side.	Reduces the risk of aspiration.
7. Vomiting is never induced for the following substances: lye, household cleaners, grease or petroleum products, and furniture polish.	Vomiting can increase area of internal burns (in case of lye) and risk of aspiration.
8. Vomiting is never induced in an unconscious victim.	Vomiting increases risk of aspiration.
9. If instructed by poison control center to take person to emergency room, call ambulance.	Ambulance personnel will be able to provide emergency measures if needed. In addition, parent or guardian may be too upset to drive safely.

COMMON POISONOUS HOUSEHOLD CHEMICALS

Alcoholic beverages
Ammonia
Antifreeze
Ant syrup or paste
Automotive products
Bathroom bowl cleaner
Bleach
Boric acid
Campho-Phenique
Charcoal lighter
Cleaning fluid
Clinitest tablets
Cologne
Copper and brass cleaners
Corn and wart remover
Detergents
Dishwasher detergents
Disinfectants
Drain cleaners
Epoxy glue kit
Furniture polish
Garden sprays
Gasoline
Gun cleaners
Hair dyes
Insecticides
Iodine
Iron medications
Kerosene
Lighter fluid
Model cement
Muriatic acid
Mushrooms
Nail polish
Nail polish remover
Oven cleaner
Paint
Paint remover
Paint thinner
Perfume
Permanent wave solutions
Pesticides
Pine oil
Plants
Prescription and nonprescription medicines
Rat poisons
Rubbing alcohol
Shaving lotion
Silver polish
Snail bait
Spot removers
Strychnine
Sulfuric acid
Super glue
Turpentine
Veterinary products
Weed killers
Window wash solvent

From Missouri Poison Center Network: Poisonous household chemicals, St. Louis, 1987, Cardinal Glennon Memorial Hospital for Children.

PREVENTION OF ELECTRICAL HAZARDS

Use only grounded equipment.
Check electrical equipment for frayed cords or visible signs of damage before use.
Avoid overloading outlets.
If extension cords must be used, make sure they are taped to the ground with electrical tape to prevent others from tripping over the cord and pulling out the plug.
Never pull a plug using the cord. Pull a plug by gripping it firmly and pulling it straight out of the wall socket.
Send equipment that has been dropped to the biomedical department before use.
Report shocks experienced while using equipment.
Believe a client who reports a tingling sensation or shocks from equipment, and have the equipment evaluated for stray current. If possible, unplug equipment until evaluation takes place.
If you do not understand how to operate a piece of equipment, ask for assistance.

Modified from Cooper KC: *Focus* 10:17, 1983.

Evaluative Measures

Nursing interventions for reducing threats to safety are evaluated by comparing the client's response to the expected outcomes for each goal of care. When expected outcomes are not met, interventions must be revised. The nurse applies evaluative measures to determine a client's progress toward outcomes and goals. Examples of goals, outcomes, and corresponding evaluative measures include:

Goal: Client's environment is adapted to motor, sensory, and cognitive developmental needs.
Outcome
Modifiable hazards in the home reduced by 100% by 2 weeks
Evaluative measures
Observe environment for elimination of threats to safety
Reassess motor, sensory, and cognitive status for appropriate environmental modifications

Goal: Client learns potential threats to personal safety within 1 month.
Outcome
Client will list hazards within the home by 1 week
Evaluative measure
Observe client identifying potential hazards
Outcome
Home will be free of hazards within 1 month
Evaluative measure
Observe home environment for removal of hazards
Outcome
Client will correctly use medication, equipment, or treatments within 2 weeks
Evaluative measure
Observe client for safe use of home appliances, medications, oxygen equipment, and power lawn mowers

Goal: Client's potential for injury will be reduced.
Outcomes
Skin and tissues will be intact
Musculoskeletal system will be free of injury
Evaluative measure
Inspect skin and musculoskeletal system for impairment in tissue integrity
Outcome
Electrical grounding and functioning of equipment will be correct
Evaluative measure
Observe equipment for correct electrical grounding and functioning

Goal: Client's risk of accidental poisoning will be reduced.
Outcome
Client will correctly administer medications
Evaluative measure
Observe client self-administer medications
Outcomes
Safe sanitation practices are followed
Medications, household cleaners, poisonous plants, and other poisonous substances are properly stored and marked and kept out of reach of children
Evaluative measure
Observe environment for potential poisonings from chemicals, plants, cleaning substances, or unsafe sanitation
Outcome
Syrup of Ipecac will be in the home, and client can describe its correct use
Evaluative measure
Observe for Syrup of Ipecac in home, and ask client to state its proper use
Outcome
Phone number of poison control center will be accessible

Evaluative measure

Observe for posted poison control phone number

SUMMARY

A safe environment is essential for maintaining and restoring a client's health. Nurses working in a structured health care setting or in a community-based agency are the client's first line of defense against falls, environmental hazards, medication errors, poisoning, and other injuries.

The client's risk for injury increases with declining health status, mobility, and reduced functioning of special senses. In addition, clients at opposite ends of the life span, the very young and the very old, have greater risks to safety.

The nursing process is used to reduce the risk of injury through specific nursing interventions and client education. The nurse promotes a safe environment by removing threats to safety and by teaching clients and families about hazards in their homes.

KEY CONCEPTS

A safe environment in a health care agency is comfortable, maintains the client's privacy, and reduces the risks of injury, infection, and untoward effects of treatment or medications.

A safe health care environment reduces the length of treatment or hospitalization, the frequency of treatment-related accidents, the potential for lawsuits, the number of work-related injuries to personnel, and the overall cost of health service.

Safety in the home reduces the risk of accidents, illnesses, and the need for health care services.

In the community, a safe environment is one in which basic needs are achievable, physical hazards are reduced, transmission of pathogens and parasites is reduced, pollution is controlled, and sanitation is maintained.

The transmission of pathogens and parasites is reduced through medical and surgical asepsis, immunization, food sanitation, insect and rodent control, and disposal of human wastes.

Every developmental stage involves specific safety risks the nurse should assess.

Children under 5 years of age are at greatest risk for home accidents that may result in severe injury and death.

The school-age child is at risk for injury at home, at school, and traveling to and from school.

Adolescents are at risk from injury due to the effects of drug and alcohol abuse.

Threats to an adult's safety are frequently associated with life-style habits.

Risks of injury for older adults are directly related to the physiological changes of the aging process.

Risks to client safety within a health care agency include falls and client-inherent, procedure-related, and equipment-related accidents.

Nursing interventions for promoting safety are individualized for developmental state, life-style, and the environment.

Nursing interventions are developed to modify environment for protection from falls, fires, poisonings, and electrical hazards.

The nursing care plan to promote safety is continually evaluated to identify new or continued risks to the client.

Physical restraints should be used only as a last resort when client behavior places them at risk for injury.

CRITICAL THINKING ACTIVITIES

1. During a home care visit for a client you notice several loose throw rugs, a filled ash tray next to the bed, and food out on the counter. What interventions are appropriate?
2. Mr. Jones is a disoriented older adult who likes to wander the halls in the long-term care facility where you are assigned. Restraining him adds to his disorientation and causes him to become agitated. Describe alternative nursing measures that could be used to ensure his safety.
3. You are assigned to a pediatric clinic and notice that when Mrs. Lopez arrives she and her three children are all sitting in the front seat and none are using seatbelts. Her 3-month-old infant is being held by her 5-year-old and her 2-year-old is sitting in the middle. How would you approach her about the hazards of this practice? What interventions are appropriate?

4. During your clinical rotation you admit an older adult, blind client to the nursing unit. The client is mobile but unaccustomed to the surroundings. What measures would you take to ensure the client's safety?
5. The fire alarm sounds in the medical center where you are working, indicating there is a fire on your unit. You are giving a bath to a client with limited mobility. Describe the sequence of actions you would take to best provide for the safety of your clients and personnel.

References

Acee AM and Smith D: Crack, *Am J Nurs* 87:614, 1987.
American Academy of Pediatrics: Teen auto safety update, *Safe Ride News* 11(1):7, 1992.
Aronow R, et al.: Comments from AAPCC to U.S. Food and Drug Administration on poison treatment drug products, *Vet Hum Toxicol* 28:343, 1985.
Berryman E, Gaskin D, et al.: Point by point-predicting elder's falls, *Geriatric Nurs* 10(4):199-201, 1989.
Blakeslee J, Goldman B, et al.: Making the transition to restraint free care, *J Gerontol Nurs* 17(2):4-8, 1991.
Brians L, Alexander K, et al.: The development of the RISK tool for fall prevention, *Rehabi Nurs* 16(2):67-69, 1991.
Brower HT: The alternatives to restraints, *J Gerontol Nurs* 17(2):18-21, 1991.
Collins H: Who'd survive a fire on your unit, *RN* 51(7):32-36, 1988.
Cooper KL: Electrical safety: the electrically sensitive ICU patient, *Focus* 10:17, 1983.
Cooper S: Common concern—accidents and older adults, *Geriatric Nurs* 2:287, 1981.
Ebersole P and Hess P: *Toward healthy aging: human needs and nursing response,* ed 3, St. Louis, 1994, Mosby.
Edelman CL and Mandle CL: *Health promotion throughout the life span,* ed 2, St. Louis, 1990, Mosby.
Fletcher K: Restraints should be a last resort, *RN* 53(1):56-58, 1990.
Foss R: Sociocultural perspective on child occupant protection, *Pediatics* 80(6):886, 1987.
Jacobsen E: New hospital hazards—how to protect yourself, *Am J Nurs* 90(2):36-41, 1990.
Kilpack, et al.: Using research based interventions to decrease patient falls, *Appl Nsg Res* 4(2):50-51, 1991.
Lowenstein SR and Hunt D: Injury prevention in primary care (editorial), *Ann Intern Med* 113(4):261, 1990.
McFarland GK and McFarlane EA, *Nursing diagnosis: planning for patient care,* ed 2, St. Louis, 1993, Mosby.
Missouri Poison Control System: *Poisonous and nonpoisonous plants,* St. Louis, 1987, Cardinal Glennon Hospital for Children.
National Center for Health Statistics: *Health United States 1987,* DHHS publication no (PHS) 88-122, Washington DC, Public Health Service, US Government Printing Office.
Potter P and Perry A: *Fundamentals of nursing: concepts, process, and practice,* ed 3, St. Louis, 1993, Mosby.
Pridham K: Anticipatory guidance of parents of new infants—potential contribution of the internal working model construct, *Image* 25(1):49-56, 1993.
Radany MH, Perry S, and McCullum D: Is it safe to reuse disposables? *Am J Nurs* 87(1):35, 1987.
Radar J: Modifying the environment to decrease use of restraints, *J Gerontol Nurs* 17(2):9-13, 1991.
Raz T and Baretich MF: Factors affecting the incidence of patient falls in hospitals, *Med Care* 25(3):185, 1987.
Robinson D and Green J: The adolescent alcohol and drug problem—a practical approach, *Ped Nurs* 14(4):305, 1988.
Scherer Y, Janelli L, et al.: The nursing dilemma of restraints, *J Gerontol Nurs* 17(2):14-17, 1991.
Spellbring MS, Gannon ME, et al.: Improving safety for hospitalized elderly, *J Gerontol Nurs* 14(2):31-37, 1988.
Strumph NE and Evans LK: Physical restraints of the hospitalized elderly—perceptions of patients and nurses, *Nurs Res* 37:132, 1988.
Strumph NE and Evans L: The ethical problems of prolonged physical restraints, *J Gerontol Nurs* 17(2):27-30, 1991.
Tideiksaar R: Home safe home, practical tips for fall-proofing, *Geriatric Nurs* 10(6):280-284, 1989.
Whaley L and Wong D: *Essentials of pediatric nursing,* ed 4, St. Louis, 1993, Mosby.
Whedon M and Shedd P: Prediction and prevention of patient falls, *Image* 21(21):108-114, 1989.
Woolf A, et al.: Prevention of childhood poisoning—efficiency of an educational program carried out in an emergency clinic, *Pediatrics* 80(3):359, 1987.

Bibliography

Cutchins CH: Blueprint for restraint free care, *American Journal of Nursing* 91:36, 1991.
Easterling M: Which of your clients is heading for a fall? *RN* 53(1):56-58, 1990.
Gordon M: *Manual of Nursing Diagnosis,* ed 6, St. Louis, MO, 1993, Mosby-Year Book, Inc.
Haley B, Nagy M, and Roberts S: Care versus control—the key to unlocking physical restraints, *Chart* 88(4):5, 1991.
Houston K and Lach H: Restraints— How do you score? *Geriatric Nursing* 11(5):231-232, 1990.
Jaffe E: Working with troubled teens, *RN* 54(2):58-62, 1991.
Johnson D: Make your own chairbound alternatives, *Geriatric Nursing* 12(1):18-19, 1991.
Levy G and Hickey J: Fighting the battle against drugs, *RN* 54(4):44-46, 1991.
Meyer C: New evidence in the case against restraints, *American Journal of Nursing* 92(5):14, 1992.
Morgan KJ: Motor vehicle-related fatalities—Implications for home health care, *Home Health Care Nurse* 9(3):18-22, 1991.
Stillwell E: Nurses education related to the use of restraints, *Journal of Gerontological Nursing* 17(2):23-25, 1991.
Wright B, Aizenstein S, Vogler G, Paine M, and Miller C: Frequent fallers, *Journal of Gerontological Nursing* 16(4):15-18, 1990.

30

Assisting Clients With Hygiene

OBJECTIVES

Mastery of content in this chapter will enable the student to:

- Define the key terms listed.
- Identify common skin problems and related interventions.
- Describe factors that influence personal hygiene practices.
- Discuss conditions that may put a client at risk for impaired skin integrity.
- Describe the types of bathing techniques used for various physical conditions and for clients of various age-groups.
- Develop a care plan based on client preferences and hygiene practices.
- Perform a complete bed bath and back rub.
- Discuss factors that influence the condition of the nails and feet.
- Explain the importance of foot care for the diabetic client.
- Describe the methods used for cleaning and cutting the nails.
- Discuss conditions that may put a client at risk for impaired oral mucous membranes.
- Discuss measures used to provide special oral hygiene.
- Assist with or provide oral hygiene.
- List common hair and scalp problems and their related interventions.
- Offer hygiene to meet the needs of clients requiring eye, ear, and nose care.
- Describe how hygienic care for the older adult client may differ from the younger client.
- Make an occupied, unoccupied, and surgical hospital bed.

KEY TERMS

acne
afternoon care
AM care
apocrine glands
cerumen
complete bed bath
dental caries
dermis
eccrine glands
epidermis
hirsutism
morning care
oral hygiene
partial bed bath
perineal care
PM care
sebum
stratum corneum
subcutaneous layer
tepid sponging

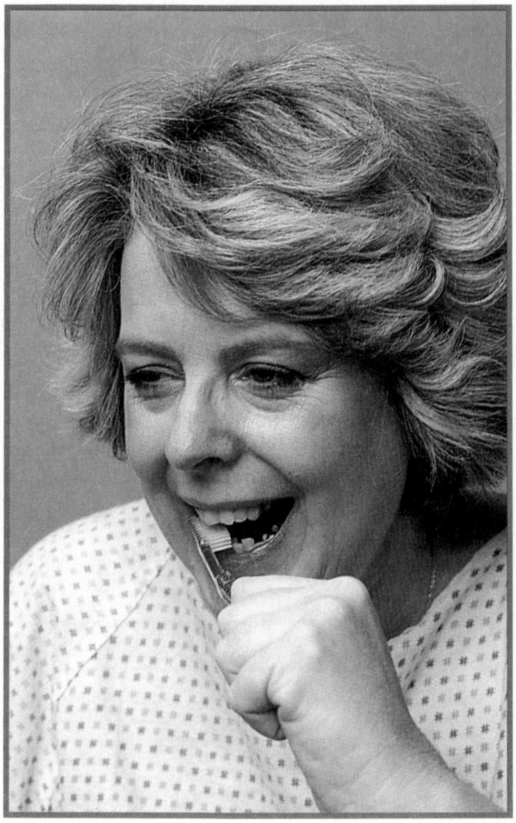

Good physical hygiene is necessary for comfort, safety, and well-being. Whereas well people are usually capable of meeting their own hygiene needs, ill people may require assistance. Several factors influence hygiene practice (see box on p. 806). The nurse determines a client's ability to perform self-care and provides hygiene care according to the client's needs and preferred practices.

Hygiene care is never routine. During the bath the nurse assesses physical conditions such as skin turgor and condition, areas of potential breakdown, and tissue perfusion. Because hygiene care often requires intimate contact with the client, the nurse uses communication skills to promote the therapeutic relationship and to learn about a client's emotional needs.

During hygiene care the nurse can also assess readiness to learn and teach health promotion practices. The nurse must also consider clients' specific physical limitations, beliefs, values, and habits. Individual hygiene preferences do not significantly affect health and can usually be included in the plan of care. The nurse preserves as much of the client's independence as possible, ensures privacy, and fosters physical well-being.

TYPES OF HYGIENE CARE

The nurse carries out many hygiene measures each day. These are commonly performed at specified times (see box on p. 806). However, these times may change because of factors affecting how the nurse organizes and schedules care. These include the client's preferences and habits, other scheduled activities or procedures, the nurse's other assignments, and the nurse-client staffing ratio.

CARE OF THE SKIN

The skin is an active organ. It protects, secretes, excretes, regulates temperature, and is a sense organ (Table 30-1). The three primary layers of the skin are epidermis, dermis, and subcutaneous tissue.

The **epidermis** has several thin layers of cells in different stages of maturation. It shields underlying tissue against water loss and mechanical and chemical injury. It also prevents entry of disease-producing microorganisms. The innermost layer generates new cells that move slowly toward the skin's surface or top layer (the **stratum corneum**), where they replace the dead cells continuously shed from the outer surface. The epidermis also contains melanocytes. These are special cells that produce the melanin or dark pigment of the skin. Bacteria commonly reside on the skin's outer surface.

The **dermis** is a thicker skin layer that contains nerve fibers, blood vessels, sweat glands, sebaceous glands, and hair follicles. Sebaceous glands secrete **sebum,** an oily, odorous fluid, into the hair follicles and lubricate the skin and hair. **Eccrine glands** are found throughout the skin but are more abundant in the forehead, palms, and soles. The sweat excreted cools the body by evaporation. **Apocrine glands** are in the axillary and genital areas. Sweat from these glands causes body odor. In the ears, ceruminous glands secrete **cerumen** into the external ear canal. Cerumen traps foreign material entering the ear.

The oral mucosa does not have sebaceous or sweat glands, hair follicles, or ceruminous glands. Instead, salivary glands secrete saliva through ducts at the base of the mouth. Saliva helps to clean and moisten the external mucosa. The skin is generally tough and pliable, but mucous membranes are more sensitive and need to be cleaned carefully.

The **subcutaneous layer** contains blood vessels, nerves, lymph, and loose, connective tissue filled with fat cells. The fatty tissue insulates the body. Subcutaneous tissue cushions the skin, enabling it to withstand stresses and pressure without injury.

The skin and mucosa exchange oxygen, nutrients, and fluids with underlying blood vessels. They also make new cells and eliminate dead cells. They require

FACTORS INFLUENCING HYGIENE PRACTICE

BODY IMAGE

The way clients look and feel about themselves indicates the importance of hygienic practices. The nurse must not convey feelings of disapproval if the client's hygiene is poor. When body image changes from surgery or illness, the nurse takes extra care to provide hygiene.

ECONOMIC STATUS

Hygienic practices are influenced by the economic resources available to clients. The nurse determines whether clients can afford hygiene supplies.

KNOWLEDGE

Clients' knowledge about the importance of proper hygiene influences motivation and practice. Often, learning about the illness or condition encourages clients to improve hygiene.

SOCIOCULTURAL VARIABLES

The client's cultural beliefs, age, personal values, and familial practices influence hygiene care. Clients from diverse cultural backgrounds follow different self-care practices.

PERSONAL PREFERENCES

Each client has individual desires and preferences concerning hygiene. The nurse incorporates the client's schedule and care practices into the plan.

PHYSICAL CONDITION

Certain illnesses, surgical procedures, and devices, such as casts or traction, may exhaust, incapacitate, or decrease the dexterity of clients. The nurse may need to assist with or perform total hygiene care.

adequate nutrition, hydration, and circulation to resist injury and disease. The skin often reflects a change in physical condition by alterations in color, thickness, texture, turgor, temperature, and hydration (see Chapter 16).

NURSING PROCESS

Assessment

Nursing assessment is an ongoing process. The nurse does not assess all body regions before a bath or hair shampooing. However, the nurse must determine whether the client can tolerate hygiene procedures, which can often be exhausting.

Most assessment occurs as the nurse cares for the client's hygienic needs. For example, during oral care, the condition of the teeth and mucosa can be observed. Hygiene care allows the nurse to assess for a variety of health care problems and thus helps to set health care priorities.

Physical Assessment of Skin. While assisting a client with personal hygiene, the nurse assesses all external body surfaces. Using inspection and palpation (see Chapter 16), the nurse looks for alterations, determines the need for hygiene, and notes skin changes in response to therapies.

HYGIENE CARE SCHEDULE

EARLY MORNING CARE

Nursing personnel on the night shift provide basic hygiene to clients getting ready for breakfast, scheduled tests, or early morning surgery. "AM care" includes offering a bedpan or urinal if the client is not ambulatory, washing the client's hands and face, and assisting with oral care.

MORNING OR AFTER-BREAKFAST CARE

In care performed after breakfast, the nurse assists by offering a bedpan or urinal to clients confined to bed; providing a bath or shower; providing oral, foot, nail, and hair care; giving a backrub; changing the client's gown or pajamas; changing the bed linens; and straightening the client's bedside unit and room. This is often referred to as "complete AM care."

AFTERNOON CARE

Hospitalized clients often undergo many exhausting diagnostic tests or procedures in the morning. In rehabilitation centers, clients may participate in physical therapy during the morning. Afternoon hygiene care includes washing the hands and face, assisting with oral care, offering a bedpan or urinal, and straightening bed linen.

EVENING OR HOUR-BEFORE-SLEEP CARE

Before bedtime the nurse offers personal hygiene care that helps a client relax to promote sleep. "PM care" may include changing soiled bed linens, gowns, or pajamas; assisting the client in washing the face and hands; providing oral hygiene; giving a back massage; and offering the bedpan or urinal to nonambulatory clients.

table 30-1

FUNCTION OF THE SKIN AND IMPLICATIONS FOR CARE

Function/description	Implications for care
PROTECTION	
Epidermis is relatively impermeable layer that prevents entrance of microorganisms. Although microorganisms reside on skin surface and in hair follicles, relative dryness of surface inhibits bacterial growth. *Sebum* removes bacteria from hair follicles. Acidic pH of skin further slows bacterial growth.	Weakening of epidermis occurs by scraping or stripping its surface as by use of dry razors, tape removal, or improper turning or positioning techniques. Excessive dryness causes cracks and breaks in skin and mucosa that allow bacteria to enter. Emollients soften and prevent moisture loss, soaking improves moisture retention, and hydration of mucosa prevents dryness. However, constant exposure to moisture causes maceration or softening, which interrupts dermal integrity and promotes ulcers and bacterial growth. Bed linen and clothing should be kept dry. Misuse of soap, detergents, cosmetics, deodorant, and depilatories can cause chemical irritation. Alkaline soaps neutralize protective acid condition of skin. Cleansing removes excess oil, sweat, dead skin cells, and dirt that can promote bacterial growth.
SENSATION	
Skin contains sensory organs for touch, pain, heat, cold, and pressure.	Friction should be minimized to avoid loss of stratum corneum, which can result in pressure sores. Smoothing linen removes sources of mechanical irritation. The nurse should remove rings to prevent injuring client's skin. Bath water should not be too hot or cold.
TEMPERATURE REGULATION	
Body temperature is controlled by radiation, evaporation, conduction, and convection.	Factors that interfere with heat loss can alter temperature control. Wet bed linen or gowns interfere with convection and conduction. Excess blankets or bed coverings can interfere with heat loss through radiation and conduction. Coverings can conserve heat.
EXCRETION AND SECRETION	
Sweat promotes heat loss by evaporation. Sebum lubricates skin and hair.	Perspiration and oil can harbor microorganism growth. Bathing removes excess body secretions, although excessive bathing can cause dry skin.

The nurse observes the skin's color, texture, thickness, turgor, temperature, and hydration. The box below describes normal skin characteristics. The nurse gives special attention to the characteristics most influenced by hygiene measures. Is the skin dry from too much bathing? Are there calluses of the feet that may benefit from soaking?

NORMAL SKIN CHARACTERISTICS

Skin is intact and has no abrasions.
Skin feels warm when palpated.
Localized changes in texture can be palpated across skin's surface.
There is good turgor (elastic and firm), with skin generally smooth and soft.
Skin color varies from body part to body part.

Certain conditions place clients at risk for impaired skin integrity (see Chapter 24). Nurses must be particularly alert when assessing clients with reduced sensation, vascular insufficiency, and immobility. The development of pressure sores is a common complication that extends hospital stays (Hill, 1992) (see box on p. 808).

While inspecting the skin, the nurse notes the presence and condition of lesions (see Chapter 16). Certain common skin problems affect hygiene (Table 30-2). Special care is also given to assess less obvious surfaces, such as under the female client's breasts or around perineal tissues. The nurse who observes skin problems should explain proper skin care to the client. The nurse may also educate the client about avoiding irritants, which can worsen the skin condition.

Developmental Changes. Age influences the normal condition of the skin and the type of hygiene required. The neonate's skin is relatively immature and

RISKS FOR IMPAIRED SKIN INTEGRITY

The nurse should consider the following conditions when assessing the risk for impaired skin integrity:

IMMOBILIZATION

Skin breakdown can result from immobilization.

Dependent body parts are exposed to pressure from underlying surfaces (e.g., mattress or wrinkled linen).

Client needs to be turned frequently to ensure proper circulation and comfort.

Pressure is the primary cause of pressure ulcers.

REDUCED SENSATION

Skin irritation can occur when the client cannot sense skin injuries.

Clients with paralysis, impaired circulation, or local nerve damage may not sense excessive heat, cold, pressure, or friction.

The client's skin needs increased protection, and the nurse minimizes the risk of injury.

VASCULAR INSUFFICIENCY

Impaired blood supply to tissues can cause tissue ischemia, skin breakdown, and a high risk for infection.

BROKEN SKIN

Any break in skin integrity may lead to infection or a pressure ulcer.

NUTRITIONAL AND HYDRATION ALTERATIONS

Limited caloric and protein intake impair tissue synthesis.

Poor digestion and excessive protein metabolism or loss cause nutritional imbalances.

Nutritional and hydration imbalances and impaired tissue synthesis result in thinner and less elastic skin and a loss of subcutaneous tissue. This can result in impaired or delayed tissue healing.

Hospitalized clients who are NPO over several days are at risk for nutritional problems unless adequate support is given.

MOISTURE

Moisture on the skin's surface provides a medium for bacterial growth and can cause local irritation, soften cells, and macerate the skin.

Areas under the woman's breasts, in the perineal area, or under the arms require special attention.

EXTERNAL DEVICES

Casts, bandages, and restraints can exert pressure on underlying surfaces, causing irritation and skin breakdown.

thin. The epidermis and dermis are loosely bound together. The nurse must handle the neonate carefully during bathing to avoid friction, which can result in bruising. A break in skin can easily cause infection.

The toddler's skin layers are more tightly bound together and thus have a greater resistance to infection and skin irritation. However, because the child is more active and does not have regular hygienic habits, care givers must be attentive.

During adolescence, growth and maturation of the skin are increased. In girls, estrogen secretion causes the skin to become soft, smooth, and thicker in texture with increased vascularity. In boys, male hormones produce an increased thickness of the skin with some darkening in color. Sebaceous glands become more active, resulting in **acne.** Eccrine and apocrine sweat glands become fully functional during puberty. More frequent bathing and use of antiperspirants become necessary to reduce body odors. Increased growth and distribution of body hair have a characteristic pattern the nurse can assess. Some girls and women have increased androgen levels causing **hirsutism,** or growth of facial hair.

The condition of an adult's skin depends on hygiene practices and exposure to environmental irritants. Normally the skin is elastic, well hydrated, firm, and smooth. With age the skin loses its resiliency and moisture, and sebaceous and sweat glands become less active. This encourages dry, cracked skin. Daily bathing, inadequate fluid and nutrition, and the use of some soap products may cause the skin of an older adult client to become too dry (see gerontologic nursing practice box on p. 810). The epithelium thins and elastic collagen fibers shrink, making the skin fragile and subject to bruising and breaking. The nurse uses caution when turning and repositioning an older adult client.

Assessment of Self-Care Ability. When a client becomes unable to bathe or perform personal skin care, the nurse provides assistance. To determine whether a client requires a bed bath instead of a tub bath or shower, the nurse should assess balance, activity tolerance, and muscle strength and coordination. The degree of assistance needed by a client during bathing may also depend on vision, the ability to sit without support, hand grasp, and range of motion (ROM) of extremities. If cognitive function is impaired, the nurse's help will probably be needed.

table 30-2

COMMON SKIN PROBLEMS

Characteristics	Implications	Interventions
DRY SKIN		
Flaky, rough texture on exposed areas such as hands, arms, legs, or face	Skin may become infected if epidermal layer is allowed to crack.	Bathe less frequently. Rinse body of all soap well because residue left on skin can cause irritation and breakdown. Add moisture to room air through use of humidifier. Increase fluid intake when skin is dry. Use moisturizing lotion to aid in healing process. Lotion forms protective barrier and helps to maintain fluid within skin. Use creams to clean skin that is dry or allergic to soaps and detergents.
ACNE		
Inflammatory, papulopustular skin eruption, usually involving bacterial breakdown of sebum; appears on face, neck, shoulders, and back	Infected material within pustule can spread if area is squeezed or picked. Permanent scarring can result.	Wash hair and skin thoroughly each day with hot water and soap to remove oil. Cosmetics should be used sparingly because oily cosmetics or creams accumulate in pores and tend to make condition worse. Dietary restrictions may be necessary. Foods found to aggravate condition should be removed from diet. Exposure to ultraviolet rays, either from sunshine or heat lamp, may help to control acne. Caution should be used to prevent burning of skin. Use prescribed topical antibiotics for severe forms of acne.
HIRSUTISM		
Excessive growth of body and facial hair, especially in women	Hirsutism may cause negative body image by giving woman a male appearance.	Depilatories (can cause infection, rashes, or dermatitis); shaving (safest method); electrolysis (permanently removes hair by destroying hair follicles); tweezing (temporary); bleaching of hair (temporary) may be used to remove unwanted hair.
SKIN RASHES		
Skin eruption that may result from overexposure to sun or moisture or from allergic reaction; may be flat or raised, localized or systemic, pruritic or nonpruritic	If skin is continually scratched, inflammation and infection may occur. Rashes can also cause discomfort.	Wash area thoroughly and apply antiseptic spray or lotion to prevent further itching and aid healing. Warm or cold soaks may relieve inflammation.
CONTACT DERMATITIS		
Inflammation of skin characterized by abrupt onset with erythema, pruritus, pain, and scaly oozing lesions; seen on face, neck, hands, forearms, and genitalia	Dermatitis is often difficult to eliminate because client is usually in continual contact with substance causing reaction. Substance may be hard to identify.	Condition usually disappears when exposure to causative agents (e.g., cleansers and soaps) is avoided.
ABRASION		
Scraping or rubbing away of epidermis; may result in localized bleeding and later weeping of serous fluid	Infection occurs easily because of loss of protective skin layer.	Nurses should be careful not to scratch clients with jewelry or fingernails. Wash abrasions with mild soap and water. Dressing or bandage could increase risk of infection because of retained moisture.

GERONTOLOGIC NURSING PRACTICE

- Older clients produce less sebum and perspire less and thus generally need to bathe less frequently. However, personal preference must always be considered.
- Older client's skin is often more fragile; avoid hot water and use only a mild cleansing agent. Some authorities suggest the use of bath oils; use with caution because this increases the danger of falling in a slippery tub.
- The majority of older clients have some degree of itching and skin sensitivity (Fenske et al., 1992); hydrocortisone cream, superfatted soaps, and petrolatum can offer relief.
- Dryness and redness is a common problem as skin ages, which worsens in cold, dry air; humidity should be kept above 40% (PPPUA, 1993).
- Elder abuse affects between 1 to 2 million persons a year (Anetzberger, 1993); unexplained bruises and skin trauma should not be ignored.

Nursing Diagnosis

An assessment reveals the condition of the skin and the client's need for and ability to maintain personal hygiene. The nurse reviews all data gathered (e.g., the client's risk for physical immobilization, presence of secretions, or altered circulation and sensation). Clustering defining characteristics reveals the diagnosis of impaired skin integrity. Accurate selection of a diagnosis ensures the client's needs are met (see box above, right).

A nursing diagnosis is accurate only if the appropriate related factors are selected. The diagnosis influences the nursing therapies chosen. For the diagnosis "impaired skin integrity related to pressure" the nurse must use therapies designed to reduce pressure to the skin. Frequent turning or repositioning, using a proper support surface, and removing underlying tubing are good measures. In contrast, the diagnosis "impaired skin integrity related to exposure to body excretions" requires a nurse to choose different therapies. Frequent skin cleansing, controlling sources of wound drainage or incontinence, and timely bed linen changes would be good measures to control the irritation of excretions. Selecting an incorrect related factor for a diagnosis can result in inappropriate and ineffective nursing care.

Whether a client has an actual alteration in skin integrity or is at high risk determines the focus of the nursing intervention. Preventive nursing measures are used when clients are at risk for skin breakdown. More aggressive therapies such as wound care for pressure ulcers (Chapter 24) become necessary when there is skin impairment. If the client has skin breakdown, the nurse must provide care to promote healing the injured skin surfaces and to prevent infection. The nurse also eliminates factors that may lead to further tissue injury.

NURSING DIAGNOSES FOR SKIN INTEGRITY AND THE NEED FOR THOROUGH SKIN CARE

Impaired skin integrity
High risk for impaired skin integrity
Altered peripheral tissue perfusion
Bathing/hygiene self-care deficit
Impaired tissue integrity

Planning

The plan for providing skin care should focus on the types or methods of care and on the many care measures the nurse can perform as a client bathes (see nursing care plan on p. 811). The nurse can teach, provide emotional support, and assist with ROM exercises.

Considering a client's hygiene preferences before planning is important. The type of hygiene the client desires or requires will determine the supplies and equipment the nurse must prepare.

The condition of a seriously ill, older adult, or inactive client must be considered so that bathing is adequate and not exhausting. The nurse must establish priorities based on the client's activity tolerance.

The nurse should also schedule hygiene care around tests and procedures. The plan is based on one or more of these goals:

Goal: Client maintains skin integrity and control of body odors.

Outcomes

Client's skin will be smooth, supple, clean, and free of odors following bathing

Client's skin will be free of localized redness or hyperemia at time of discharge

Goal: Client maintains or improves joint ROM.

Outcomes

Client demonstrates baseline ROM during bathing

Joints are stable and move freely during passive exercise

Goal: Client achieves relaxation and comfort.

Outcome

Client expresses sense of comfort and cleanliness following bathing

SAMPLE NURSING CARE PLAN
Skin Care

ASSESSMENT

Clinical scenario: Mr. Heinz is a 48-year-old man *immobilized for trauma to the spinal cord.* He has periods of *diaphoresis.* He has had *liquid diarrhea for the last 48 hours.* The *skin on Mr. Heinz' back, sacral regions, and buttocks is dry and intact, with 2 cm area of redness around the sacrum.*

NURSING DIAGNOSIS

High risk for impaired skin integrity related to immobilization and secretions.

PLANNING

Goal	Expected outcomes
Skin will remain intact during hospitalization.	Skin will remain free of pressure. Skin will have reduced or absent secretions. Skin will be dry, warm, and smooth.

IMPLEMENTATION

Steps	Rationale
1. Provide perineal care after each diarrheal episode.	Minimizing skin exposure to moisture decreases irritation and susceptibility to injury (PPPUA, 1993).
2. Change linen after diaphoresis or diarrheal episode.	Changing linen keeps skin free of moisture, which promotes bacterial growth (NPUAP, 1989).
3. Apply lotion to areas that can easily become dried and chapped.	Lotion reduces drying and chapping of skin. Dry, chapped skin impairs skin integrity and is port of entry for bacteria.
4. Monitor length of time any area of redness persists. Determine turning interval. Turning interval − hypoxia time = suggest interval (e.g., 2 hours − 30 min = 1½ hr).	Repositioning reduces pressure and allows for normal hyperemic response (Maklebust, 1991).
5. Place oscillating air mattress on client's bed.	Static air mattress is best support surface for client at high risk for pressure ulcer (Thomas, 1989).
6. Do **not** massage reddened area.	Massage increases breaks in capillaries in underlying tissues (Maklebust, 1991; USDHHS, 1992).

Goal: Client participates in hygiene.
Outcomes
- Client begins hygiene measures independently 2 days before discharge
- Client makes decisions regarding hygiene schedule by day of discharge

Goal: Client completes hygiene without fatigue.
Outcome
- Client denies feeling of fatigue after bathing

Implementation

Bathing a Client. Bathing may be done for cleanliness or for a specific therapy, depending on the type of bath (see box on p. 812). A physician's order is necessary for therapeutic baths (see box on p. 812).

The extent of the bath and the methods used for bathing depend on the client's physical abilities, health problems, and the degree of hygiene required. A **complete bed bath** is for clients who are dependent and require total hygiene care (see Procedure 30-1).

A **partial bed bath** involves bathing only body parts that would cause discomfort or odor if left unbathed. Aging or dependent clients in need of only partial hygiene or self-sufficient bedridden clients unable to reach all body parts receive partial bed baths.

The tub bath or shower can be used to give a more thorough bath than a bed bath (see Procedure 30-1). Washing and rinsing all body parts are easier. Safety is of primary concern because the surface of a tub or shower stall is slippery. Clients vary in how much help they will need.

Tepid sponging is used when a client's temperature is high. It can be soothing but also uncomfortable, depending on the client's skin temperature. Tepid water is

PURPOSES OF BATHING

CLEANSING THE SKIN

Cleansing removes perspiration, some bacteria, sebum, and dead skin cells, which minimizes skin irritation and reduces the chance of infection.

STIMULATION OF CIRCULATION

Good circulation is promoted through the use of warm water and gentle stroking of the extremities.

IMPROVED SELF-IMAGE

Bathing promotes relaxation and a feeling of being refreshed and comfortable.

REDUCTION OF BODY ODORS

Excessive secretion of sweat from apocrine glands located in the axillae and pubic areas causes unpleasant body odors. Bathing and use of antiperspirants minimize odors.

PROMOTION OF RANGE OF MOTION (ROM)

Movement of the extremities during bathing maintains joint function.

TYPES OF THERAPEUTIC BATHS

HOT WATER TUB BATH

Immersion in hot water helps to relieve muscle soreness and spasm. However, there is a danger of burns. Water temperature should be 45° to 46° C (113° to 115° F).

WARM WATER TUB BATH

Bathing in warm water relieves muscle tension. Water temperature should be 43° C (109° F).

COOL WATER BATH

Bathing in cool water can relieve tension or lower body temperature. Precautions must be taken to avoid chilling. Water temperature should be tepid (37° C [98.6° F]) rather than cold. This type of bath is especially effective in reducing the body temperature of a small child with fever.

SOAK

Local application of water or medicated solution can remove dead tissue or soften crusted secretions. Aseptic technique is necessary when cleaning open or abraded areas of the skin. Soaks are also useful in reducing pain and swelling of inflamed or irritated skin surfaces.

SITZ BATH

A sitz bath cleanses and reduces inflammation of the perineal and anal areas of a client who has had rectal surgery, given birth, or who has local rectal irritation from hemorrhoids or fissures. Water temperature depends on the client's condition but is usually 43° to 45° C (109° to 113° F). Cold sitz baths are more effective in relieving perineal pain in the postpartum period.*

*Data from Ramler D and Roberts J: A comparison of cold and warm sitz baths for relief of postpartum perineal pain, *JOGNN* 15:471, 1986.

used to avoid the chilling effect of cold water and to promote slow cooling, which avoids temperature fluctuations (Procedure 30-2).

Despite the type of bath the client receives, the nurse should follow the following guidelines:

1. Provide privacy. Close the door or pull room curtains around the bathing area. While bathing the client, expose only the areas being bathed.
2. Maintain safety. Keep side rails up while away from the client's bedside. (This is particularly important for dependent or unconscious clients.) Place the call light in the client's reach if leaving the room temporarily.
3. Maintain warmth. The room should be kept warm because the client is partially uncovered and may easily be chilled. Control drafts and keep windows closed.
4. Promote the client's independence as much as possible during bathing activities. Offer assistance as needed.

Perineal Care. Perineal care is usually part of the complete bed bath (see Procedure 30-3). Clients most in need of perineal care are at greatest risk for acquiring an infection (e.g., clients who have indwelling urinary catheters or who are recovering from rectal or genital surgery or childbirth). A client able to perform self-care should be allowed to do so. Many nurses are embarrassed about providing perineal care, particularly to clients of the opposite sex. This should not cause the

Text continued on p. 819.

procedure 30-1

BATHING A CLIENT

Steps	Rationale
1. Assess client's preferences for bathing practices: frequency, time of day preferred, type of hygiene products used.	Promotes participation in care and sense of comfort.
2. Review orders for precautions concerning movement or positioning.	Prevents accidental injury during bathing.
3. Explain procedure and ask client for suggestions or ways to prepare supplies. If partial bath is to be performed, ask how much of bath client wishes to complete.	Promotes cooperation and participation.
4. If shower or tub bath is to be done, schedule use of facilities if private bath unavailable.	Prevents unnecessary waiting that can cause fatigue.
5. Adjust room temperature and ventilation, and close room doors and windows. Close curtains around bed.	Warm room, free of drafts, prevents rapid loss of body heat during bathing. Ensures privacy.
6. Prepare necessary equipment and supplies:	
a. Two bath towels b. Two washcloths	Separate towel and washcloth are used for face and body to enhance feeling of cleanliness.
c. Washbasin (for complete or partial bed bath)	
d. Soap and soap dish	
e. Bath blanket (for complete or partial bed bath)	Bath blanket maintains warmth during procedure.
f. Clean gown or pajamas	
g. Hygienic aids, such as skin lotion, deodorant, or powder	
h. Bedpan or urinal and toilet paper	For client to use before bath.
i. Linen hamper or laundry bag	
j. Disposable gloves	Prevents contact with potentially infected body secretions.
k. Bed linen (optional)	
COMPLETE OR PARTIAL BED BATH	
1. Offer client bedpan or urinal. Provide towel and washcloth.	Client feels more comfortable after voiding. Prevents interruption.
2. Wash hands. OPTION: Apply gloves if drainage on skin.	Reduces transmission of microorganisms.
3. Lower side rail and assist client in assuming comfortable position maintaining body alignment.	Aids nurse's access to client. Maintains client comfort throughout procedure.
4. Bring client toward side closest to nurse. Place hospital bed in high position.	Minimizes strain on back muscles.
5. Loosen top covers at foot of bed. Place bath blanket over top sheet. Fold and remove top sheet from under blanket. If possible, have client hold bath blanket while the nurse withdraws sheet.	Removal of top linens prevents their becoming soiled or moist during bath. Blanket provides warmth and privacy.
6. If top sheet is to be reused, fold it for replacement later. If not, dispose in laundry bag, taking care not to allow linen to contact uniform.	Proper disposal prevents transmission of microorganisms.
7. Remove client's gown or pajamas while maintaining privacy. If extremity is injured or has reduced mobility, begin removal from unaffected side. If client has IV tube, remove gown from arm without IV first, then lower IV container and slide gown covering affected arm over tubing and container. Rehang IV container and check flow rate (see illustrations).	Provides full exposure of body parts. Undressing unaffected side first allows easier manipulation of gown over body part with reduced range of movement.

Continued.

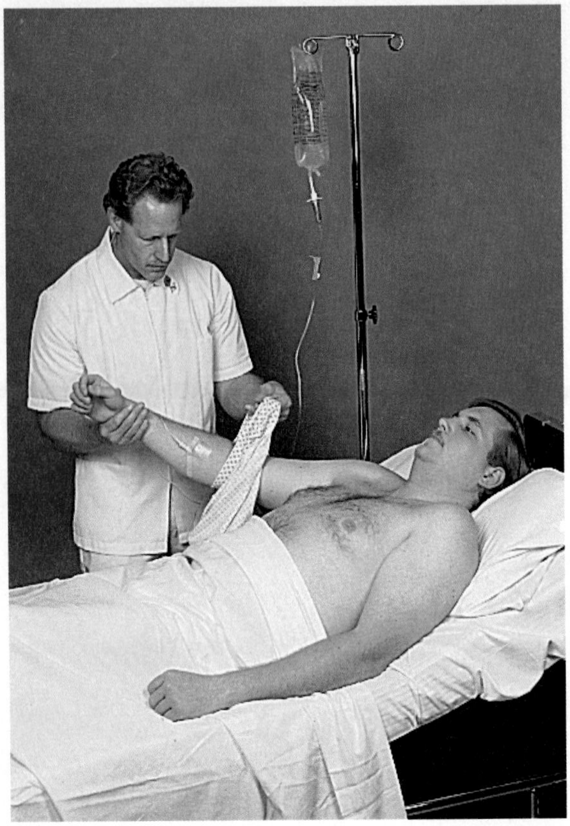

Step 7(a)

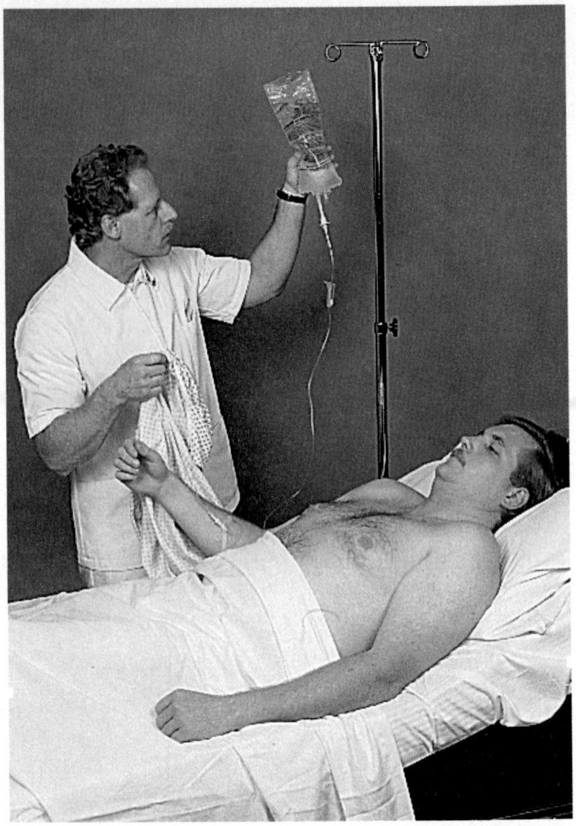

Step 7(b)

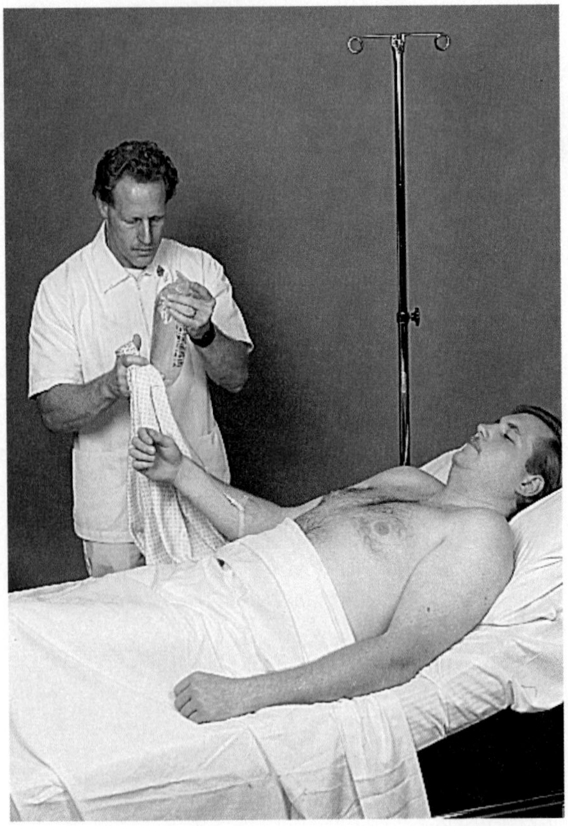

Step 7(c)

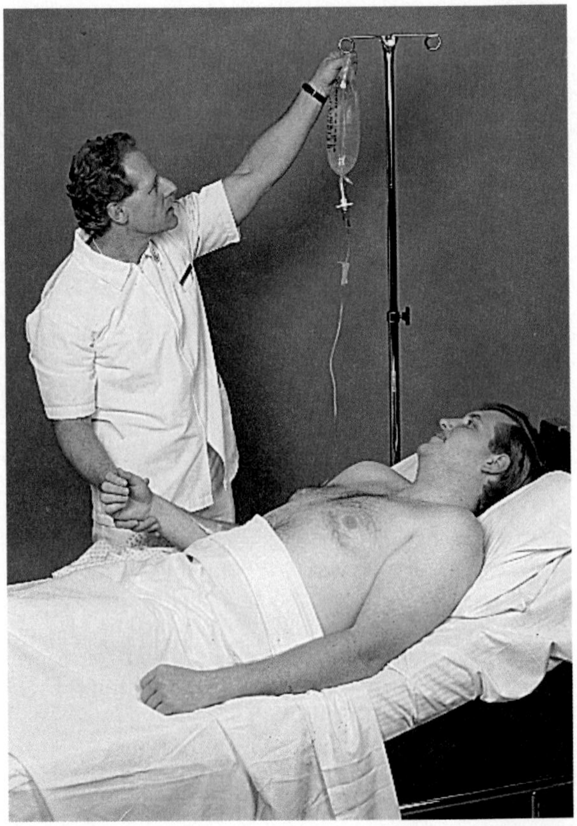

Step 7(d)

procedure 30-1—cont'd

Steps	Rationale
8. Pull side rail up. Fill washbasin two-thirds full, with warm water. Have client place fingers in water to test temperature tolerance. OPTION: Place plastic container of bath lotion in bath water.	Raising side rail maintains safety. Warm water promotes comfort and prevents unnecessary chilling. Testing temperature prevents accidental burning of skin. Keeps lotion warm for application.
9. Lower side rail. Remove pillow if allowed and raise head of bed 30 to 45 degrees. Place bath towel under client's head.	Makes it easier to wash client's ears and neck. Prevents soiling of bed linen.
10. Place bath towel over client's chest.	Prevents soiling of bath blanket.
11. Fold washcloth around fingers of the hand to form mitt (see illustrations). Immerse mitt in water and wring thoroughly.	Mitt retains water and heat better than loosely held washcloth, keeps cold edges from brushing against client, and prevents splashing.
12. Wash client's eyes with plain warm water. Use different section of mitt for each eye. Move mitt from inner to outer canthus (see illustration). Soak crustations on eyelid for 2 to 3 minutes with damp cloth before attempting removal. Dry eye thoroughly but gently.	Soap irritates eyes. Use of separate sections of mitt reduces infection transmission. Bathing eye from inner to outer canthus prevents secretions from entering nasolacrimal duct. Pressure can cause internal injury.
13. Ask client about preference for using soap on face. Wash, rinse, and dry forehead, cheeks, nose, neck, and ears. (Men may wish to shave at this point or after bath.)	Soap tends to dry face more quickly because it is exposed to air more than other body parts.

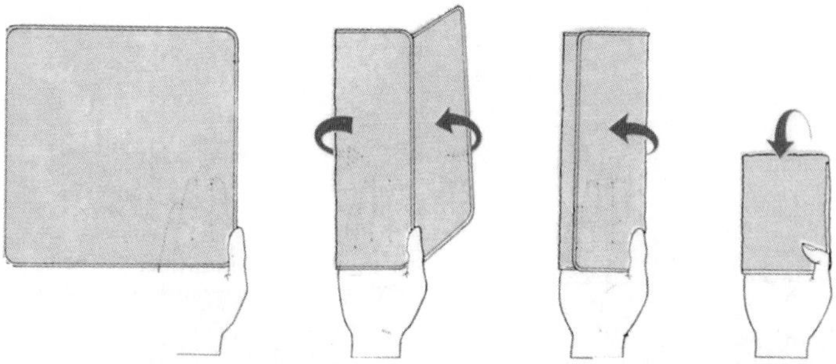

Step 11

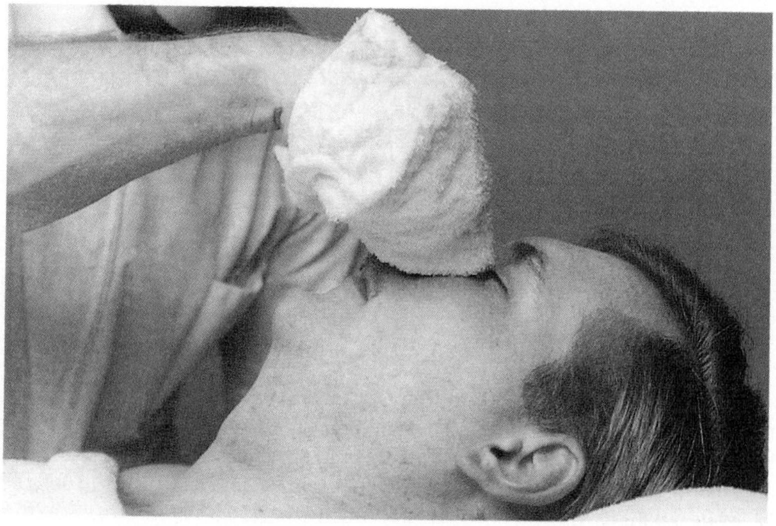

Step 12

Continued.

procedure 30-1—cont'd

Steps	Rationale
14. Remove bath blanket from client's arm closest to nurse. Place bath towel lengthwise under arm.	Prevents soiling of bed linen.
15. Bathe arm with soap and water using long, firm strokes from distal to proximal areas (fingers to axilla). Raise and support arm above head (if possible) while thoroughly washing axilla.	Soap lowers surface tension and facilitates removal of debris and bacteria when friction is applied during washing. Long, firm strokes stimulate circulation. Movement of arm exposes axilla and exercises joint's normal range of motion.
16. Rinse and dry arm and axilla thoroughly. If client uses deodorant or talcum powder, apply it.	Excess moisture causes skin maceration or softening. Deodorant controls body odor.
17. Fold bath towel in half and lay it on bed beside client. Place basin on towel. Immerse client's hand in water. Allow hand to soak for 3 to 5 min before washing it and fingernails (Procedure 30-5). Remove basin and dry hand.	Soaking softens cuticles and calluses and loosens debris beneath nails and enhances feeling of cleanliness. Thorough drying removes moisture from between fingers.
18. Raise side rail and go to other side of bed. Lower side rail and repeat Steps 14 to 17 for other arm.	
19. Check temperature of bath water and change water if necessary. (Do not leave side rail down if there is risk of fall.)	Use of warm water maintains comfort.
20. Cover client's chest with bath towel and fold bath blanket down to umbilicus.	Prevents unnecessary exposure of body parts.
21. With one hand, lift edge of towel away from chest. With mitted hand, bathe chest using long, firm strokes. Take special care to wash skinfolds under female client's breasts. It may be necessary to lift breast upward. Keep client's chest covered between wash and rinse periods. Dry well.	Towel maintains warmth and privacy. Secretions and dirt collect easily in areas of tight skinfolds.
22. Place bath towel lengthwise over chest and abdomen. (Two towels may be needed.) Fold blanket down to just above pubic region.	Prevents chilling and exposure of body parts.
23. With one hand, lift bath towel. With mitted hand, bathe abdomen, giving special attention to bathing umbilicus and abdominal folds. Stroke from side to side. Keep abdomen covered between washing and rinsing. Dry well.	Moisture and sediment that collect in skinfolds predispose client to skin maceration and irritation.
24. Apply clean gown or pajama top. If one extremity is injured or immobilized, always dress affected side first. (This step may be omitted until completion of bath; gown should not become soiled during remainder of bath.)	Maintains warmth and comfort. Dressing affected side first allows easier manipulation of gown over body part with reduced range of motion.
25. Cover chest and abdomen with top of bath blanket. Expose far leg by folding blanket over toward midline. Be sure perineum is draped.	Prevents unnecessary exposure.
26. Bend client's leg at knee by positioning nurse's arm under leg. While grasping client's heel, elevate leg from mattress slightly and slide bath towel lengthwise under leg.	Towel prevents soiling of bed linen. Support of joint and extremity during lifting prevents strain on musculoskeletal structures.
27. Ask client to hold foot still. Place bath basin on towel on bed and secure its position next to foot to be washed.	Sudden movement by client could cause spilling of water. (This step is omitted if client unable to hold leg in basin.)
28. With one hand supporting lower leg, raise it and slide basin under lifted foot. Make sure foot is firmly placed on bottom of basin. Allow foot to soak while washing leg (see illustration).	Proper positioning of foot prevents pressure from being applied from edge of basin against calf. Soaking softens calluses and rough skin. (NOTE: If client is unable to hold leg, do not immerse; simply wash with washcloth.)

Steps	Rationale
29. Unless contraindicated, use long, firm strokes in washing from ankle to knee and from knee to thigh. Dry well.	Promotes venous return.
30. Cleanse foot, making sure to bathe between toes. Clean and clip nails as needed (Procedure 30-5). Dry well. If skin is dry, apply lotion.	Secretions and moisture may be present between toes. Lotion helps to retain moisture and soften skin.
31. Raise side rail and move to other side of bed. Lower side rail and repeat Steps 25 to 30 for other leg and foot.	
32. Cover client with bath blanket, raise side rail for safety, and change bathwater.	Drop in water temperature during bathing can cause chilling. Clean water reduces microorganism transmission.
33. Lower side rail. Assist client in assuming prone or side-lying position (as applicable). Place towel lengthwise along client's side.	Exposes back and buttocks for bathing.
34. Keep client draped by sliding bath blanket over shoulders and thighs.	Maintains warmth and prevents unnecessary exposure.
35. Apply disposable gloves (if not done in step 2).	Prevents contact with microorganisms in body secretions.
36. Wash, rinse, and dry back from neck to buttocks using long, firm strokes (see illustration). Pay special attention to folds of buttocks and anus. (Give backrub. [Procedure 30-4]).	Skinfolds near buttocks and anus may contain fecal secretions that harbor microorganisms.
37. Change bathwater and washcloth.	Prevents transfer of microorganisms from anal area to genitalia.
38. Assist client in assuming side-lying or supine position. Cover chest and upper extremities with towel and lower extremities with bath blanket. Expose only genitalia. (If client can help, covering entire body with bath blanket may be preferable.) Wash, rinse, and dry perineum (Procedure 30-3). Give special attention to skinfolds.	Maintains privacy. Clients capable of performing partial bath usually prefer to wash their own genitalia. Skinfolds are site for accumulation of secetions or moisture.

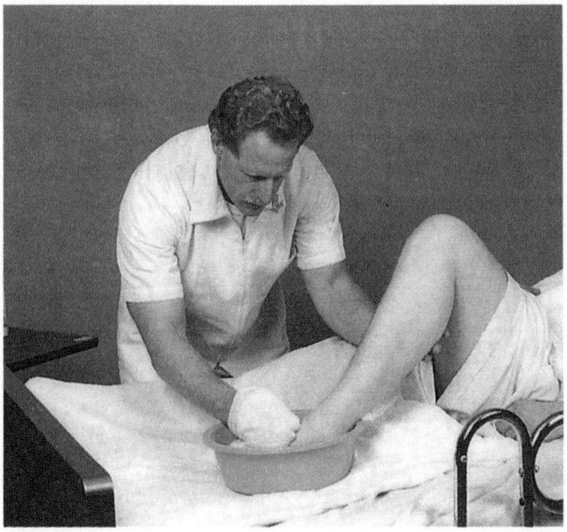

Step 28

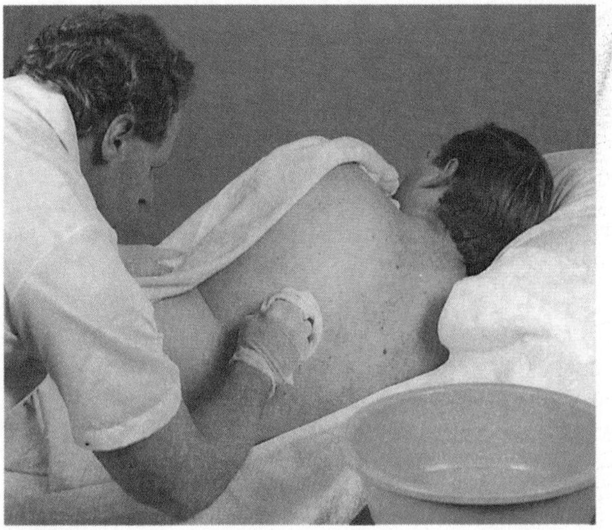

Step 36

Continued.

procedure 30-1—cont'd

Steps	Rationale
39. Dispose of gloves in receptacle.	Prevents transmission of microorganisms.
40. Apply additional body lotion or cream as desired.	Prevents dry, chapped skin.
41. Assist client in dressing.	
42. Comb client's hair. Women may want to apply makeup.	Maintains body image.
43. Make bed (Procedures 30-11 and 30-12).	Provides clean surrounding environment.
44. Remove soiled linen and place in dirty linen bag. Clean and replace bathing equipment. Replace call light and personal possessions and raise side rails as needed. Leave room as clean and comfortable as possible.	Prevents transmission of infection. Promotes client comfort. Promotes client safety.
45. Wash hands.	Reduces transmission of microorganisms.
TUB BATH OR SHOWER	
1. Check tub or shower for cleanliness. Use cleaning techniques according to agency policy. Place rubber mat on tub or shower bottom. Place disposable bathmat or towel on floor in front of tub or shower.	Cleaning prevents transmission of infection. Mats prevent slipping and falling.
2. Collect all hygiene aids, toiletry items, and linen requested by client. Place within easy reach of tub or shower.	Prevents possible falls when client reaches for equipment.
3. Assist client to bathroom if necessary. Have client wear robe and slippers en route to bathroom.	Prevents accidental falls. Prevents chilling.
4. Demonstrate how to use call signal for assistance when in hospital or extended care facility.	Bathrooms are equipped with signaling devices in case client feels faint or weak or needs immediate assistance. Clients prefer privacy during bath if safety is not jeopardized.
5. Place "occupied" sign on bathroom door when in hospital or extended care facility.	Maintains privacy.
6. Fill bathtub halfway with warm water. Ask client to test water, and adjust water temperature if it is too warm or too cold. Explain which faucet controls hot water. If client is taking shower, turn shower on and adjust water temperature before client enters stall.	Prevents accidental burns. Older adults and clients with neurological alterations (for example, spinal cord injuries) are at high risk for burns due to reduced sensation.
7. Instruct client to use safety bars when getting in and out of tub or shower.	Prevents slipping and falls.
8. Caution client against use of bath oil in tub water.	Oil causes tub surfaces to become slippery, predisposing client to accidental falls.
9. Instruct client not to remain in tub longer than 20 min. Check on client every 5 min.	Prolonged exposure to warm water may cause vasodilation and pooling of blood, leading to lightheadedness or dizziness.
10. Return to bathroom when client signals, and knock before entering.	Provides privacy.
11. For client who is unsteady, drain tub of water before client attempts to get out of it. Place bath towel over client's shoulders.	Prevents accidental falls. Client may become chilled as water drains.
12. Assist client in getting out of tub as needed and assist with drying.	Moisture may cause excessive softening of skin and promote spread of infection.
13. Assist client as needed in donning clean gown or pajamas, slippers, and robe. (In home, client may don regular clothing.)	Maintains warmth to prevent chilling.
14. Assist client to room and help to assume comfortable position in bed or chair.	Maintains relaxation gained from bathing.

Steps	Rationale
15. Clean tub or shower according to agency policy. Remove soiled linen and place in dirty linen bag. Discard disposable equipment in proper receptacle. Place "unoccupied" sign on bathroom door. Return supplies to storage area.	Prevents transmission of infection through soiled linen and moisture.
16. Wash hands.	Reduces transfer of microorganisms.
17. Observe client's behavior and ask if fatigue or discomfort is felt.	
18. Note areas on skin that were previously soiled, reddened, or showed early signs of breakdown.	Determines client's tolerance to bathing activities.
19. Record type of bath and client's tolerance of bathing. Also note condition of skin and significant findings such as reddened areas or joint or muscle pain. Record level of assistance required by client.	Techniques used during bathing should leave skin clean and clear.
	Maintains accuracy of client record. Condition of skin documents response to therapy such as turning and positioning.

Illustrations from Sorrentino SA: *Mosby's textbook for nursing assistants,* ed 3, St. Louis, 1994, Mosby.

nurse to overlook the client's hygiene needs. A professional, dignified attitude can reduce embarrassment and put the client and the nurse at ease.

If a client performs self-care, various problems such as vaginal or urethral discharge, skin irritation, and unpleasant odors may go unnoticed. The nurse must be alert for complaints of burning during urination, localized soreness or excoriation, or perineal pain. The nurse also inspects bed linen for signs of discharge.

Backrub. A backrub usually follows the bath. It promotes relaxation, relieves muscular tension, stimulates skin circulation, and is generally well tolerated by even critically ill clients (Tyler, et al., 1990). During the backrub the nurse can assess skin condition.

An effective backrub takes 3 to 5 minutes. The nurse should first ask whether the client would like a backrub because some clients dislike physical contact. The nurse should also consult the client's record for contraindications (Procedure 30-4).

Bathing an Infant. An infant can be bathed in much the same way as an adult, either by a sponge bath or in a small tub. However, there are special precautions. Because an infant's temperature control mechanisms are still immature, prolonged exposure of body parts may cause rapid cooling. When giving a bath, the nurse keeps the infant covered as much as possible, and the nurse should work quickly. Bathing a newborn by immersion causes less heat loss and less crying. The infant's thin, sensitive skin requires gentle handling and avoiding substances that might irritate the skin. Care of the umbilical cord is a special consideration for the newborn. The neonate must have sponge baths until the cord falls off and the skin heals. Immersing the umbilicus in a tub of water before the skin heals can cause a serious infection. The nurse gives special care to infants who have been circumcised. A small amount of bleeding normally occurs from the penis. The physician applies a sterile gauze dressing with petrolatum jelly around the circumcised area. The nurse instructs the parents to periodically clean the penis with moistened cotton balls until the dressing can be removed permanently (Whaley and Wong, 1991).

In hospitals where there is rooming-in of the infant and mother, the infant's bath is a good time to involve the parents in the child's care. The parents can examine the infant's body parts and learn about normal skin variations.

Since mothers return home quickly after delivery, the nurse may provide instruction on baby care in the home. The mother learns bathing techniques while using facilities in the bathroom or kitchen.

SPONGE BATH. A sponge bath is given to newborns until the umbilicus heals. Washing a newborn immediately after birth is unnecessary except to cleanse

procedure 30-2

TEPID SPONGING

Steps	Rationale
1. Assess body temperature and pulse.	Provides baseline for evaluating response to therapy. Sudden circulatory changes may alter pulse.
2. Explain purpose of tepid sponging is to cool body slowly. Briefly describe steps.	Procedure can be uncomfortable because of cool applications. Anxiety can increase body temperature.
3. Prepare necessary equipment and supplies:	
a. Bath basin	
b. Tepid water (37° C or 98.6° F)	Tepid water prevents sudden heat loss and chilling.
c. Bath thermometer	
d. Washcloths	
e. Waterproof pad	
f. Bath blanket	
g. Thermometer	
h. Disposable gloves (optional)	
4. Close room door or curtain.	Ensures privacy.
5. Wash hands. OPTION: Don gloves if drainage on skin.	Reduces transfer of microorganisms.
6. Place waterproof pads under client and remove gown.	Prevent soiling of bed linen. Provides access to all skin surfaces.
7. Keep bath blanket over body parts not being sponged. Close windows and door to prevent drafts.	Prevents chilling.
8. Check water temperature.	Prevents chilling.
9. Immerse washcloths in water and apply wet cloths under each axilla and over groin. If using tub, immerse client for 20 to 30 min.	Axilla and groin contain large superficial blood vessels. Application of washcloths promotes cooler temperature of body's core by conduction. Immersion provides more effective heat loss.
10. Gently sponge an extremity for 5 min. Note response. Opposite extremity may be covered by cool washcloth. In tub, gently squeeze water over back and chest.	Prevents sudden temperature fall and minimizes risk of developing chills.
11. Dry extremity and reassess pulse and body temperature. Observe response.	Response is monitored to prevent sudden temperature change.
12. Continue sponging other extremities, back, and buttocks for 3 to 5 min each. Reassess temperature and pulse every 15 min.	Prevents sudden temperature fall and minimizes risk of developing chills.
13. Change water and reapply sponges to axilla and groin as needed.	Water temperature rises as result of exposure to warm body surface.
14. When body temperature falls to slightly above normal, discontinue.	Prevents temperature drift to subnormal level. Follow institutional guidelines.
15. Dry extremities and body parts thoroughly. Cover client with light bath blanket or sheet.	Prevents chilling. Excessively heavy covering may increase body temperature.
16. Dispose of equipment and change bed linen if soiled. Wash hands.	Controls transmission of infection.
17. Measure body temperature and pulse.	Temperature indicates response to therapy. Dysrhythmias may be complication of therapy.
18. Record time procedure was started and terminated, vital sign changes, and response.	Communicates care provided in accurate and timely fashion.

procedure 30-3

PERINEAL CARE

Steps	Rationale
1. Identify clients at risk for developing infection of genitalia, urinary, or reproductive tract (e.g., indwelling catheter, fecal incontinence, or surgical incision).	Secretions that accumulate on surface of skin around genitalia act as reservoir for infection. Traumatized tissues provide route for introduction of infectious organisms.
2. Explain procedure and its purpose to client.	Helps to minimize anxiety during procedure that is often embarrassing to nurse and client.
3. Prepare necessary equipment and supplies:	Used when administering bed bath.
a. Washbasin	
b. Soap dish with soap	
c. Two or three washcloths	
d. Bath towel	
e. Bath blanket	
f. Waterproof pad or bedpan	Prevents soiling of bed linen.
g. Toilet tissue	
h. Disposable gloves	Prevents contact with microorganisms in body secretions.
Additional supplies when pericare is given during times other than a bath:	
a. Cotton balls or swabs	Used for cleansing menstruating women or around indwelling catheters.
b. Solution bottle or container filled with warm water or prescribed rinsing solution	
c. Waterproof bag	For disposal of cotton balls.
4. Assemble supplies at bedside.	Ensures orderly procedure.
5. Wash hands.	Reduces transmission of microorganisms.
6. Pull curtain around bed or close room door.	Maintains privacy.
7. Raise bed to comfortable working position.	Facilitates good body mechanics.
8. Lower side rail and assist client in assuming dorsal recumbent (female) or supine (male) position.	Provides easy access to genitalia.
9. Apply disposable gloves.	Decreases contact with body secretions.
10. Position waterproof pad under buttocks or place bedpan under client.	Prevents bed linen from becoming wet.
11. Fold top bed linen toward foot of bed and raise client's gown above genital area.	Exposes perineal area for easy accessibility.
12. Drape client by placing bath blanket with one corner between legs, one corner pointing toward each side of bed, and one corner over chest. For female, tuck side corners around legs and under hips (see illustrations).	Prevents unnecessary exposure of body part and maintains warmth and comfort.
13. Raise side rail. Fill washbasin with warm water.	Prevents accidental falls. Proper water temperature prevents burns to perineum.

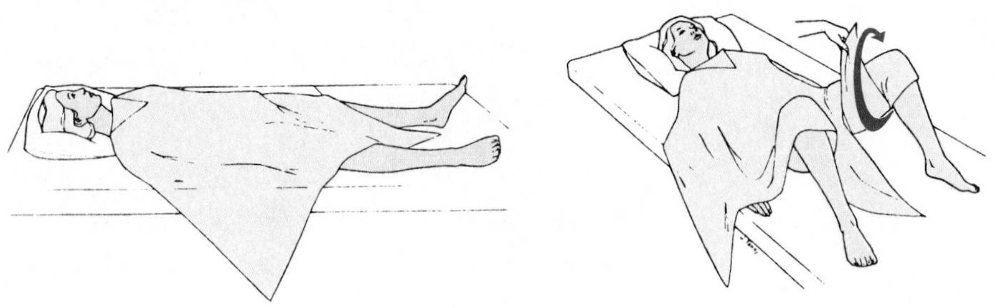

Step 12

Continued.

procedure 30-3—cont'd

Steps	Rationale
14. Place washbasin and toilet tissue on overbed table. Place washcloths in basin.	Equipment placed within nurse's reach prevents accidental spills.
15. Provide female genital care:	
a. Lower side rail and help client flex knees and spread legs.	Provides full exposure of female genitalia.
b. Fold lower corner of bath blanket between legs back onto abdomen.	Keeping client draped until procedure begins minimizes anxiety.
c. Wash and dry upper thighs.	Buildup of perineal secretions can soil surrounding skin surfaces.
d. Wash labia majora. Then use nondominant hand to gently retract labia from thigh; with dominant hand, wash carefully in skinfolds. Wipe in direction from perineum to rectum. Repeat on opposite side using separate section of washcloth. Rinse and dry area thoroughly.	Skinfolds may contain body secretions that harbor microorganisms. Wiping from perineum to rectum reduces chance of transmitting fecal organisms to urinary meatus.
e. Separate labia with nondominant hand to expose urethral meatus and vaginal orifice. With dominant hand, wash downward from pubic area toward rectum in one smooth stroke (see illustration). Use separate section of cloth for each stroke. Cleanse thoroughly around labia minora, clitoris, and vaginal orifice.	Reduces transfer of microorganisms to urinary meatus. (For menstruating women or clients with indwelling urinary catheters, cleanse with cotton balls.)
f. If client is on bedpan, pour warm water over perineal area.	Removes soap and microorganisms more effectively than wiping.
g. Dry perineal area thoroughly.	Retained moisture harbors microorganisms.
h. Fold lower corner of bath blanket back between legs and over perineum. Ask client to lower legs and assume side-lying position for anal care.	Side-lying position provides access to anal area for cleansing.
16. Provide male genital care:	
a. Lower side rail.	Provides access to client.
b. Lower top corner of bath blanket below perineum. Gently raise penis and place bath towel underneath.	Towel prevents moisture from collecting in inguinal area.
c. Gently grasp shaft of penis. If client is uncircumcised, retract foreskin. If client has an erection, defer procedure until later.	Gentle handling reduces chance of client having an erection. Secretions capable of harboring microorganisms collect underneath foreskin.

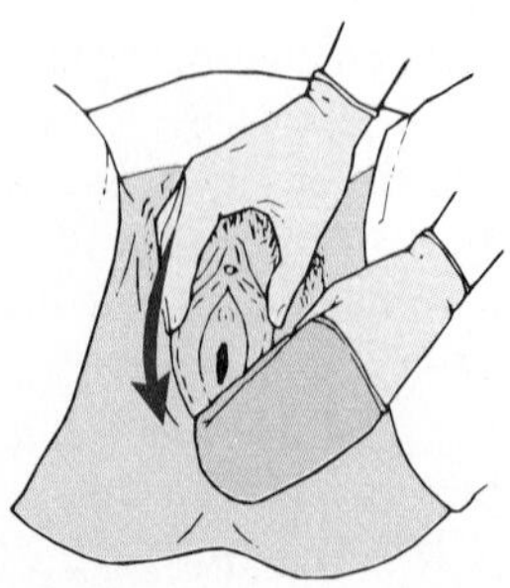

Step 15e

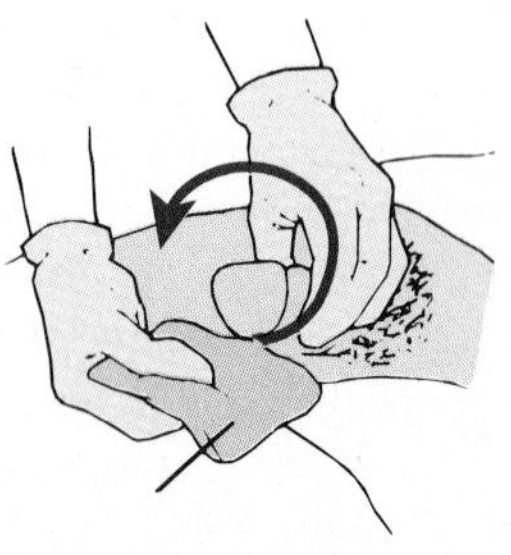

Step 16d

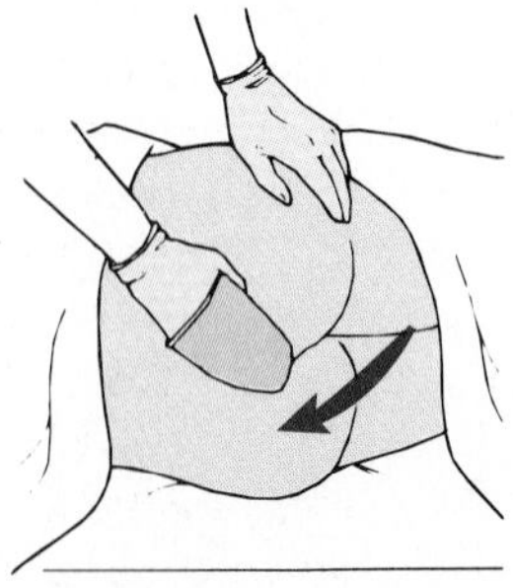

Step 17a

Steps	Rationale
d. Wash tip of penis at urethral meatus first. Using circular motion, cleanse from meatus outward and then down the shaft. Discard washcloth and repeat with clean cloth until penis is clean. Rinse and dry gently (see illustration).	Direction of cleansing moves from area of least contamination to area of most contamination, preventing microorganisms from entering urethra.
e. Return foreskin to natural position.	Tightening of foreskin around shaft of penis can cause local edema and discomfort.
f. Wash shaft of penis with gentle but firm downward strokes. Pay special attention to underlying surface.	Vigorous massage of penis can lead to erection, which can cause embarrassment for client and nurse. Underlying surface may have greater accumulation of secretions.
g. Rinse and dry penis thoroughly. Instruct client to spread his legs apart slightly.	Abduction of legs provides easier access to scrotal tissues.
h. Gently cleanse scrotum. Lift it carefully and wash underlying skinfolds. Rinse and dry.	Pressure on scrotal tissues can be very painful. Secretions collect between skinfolds.
i. Fold bath blanket back over perineum and assit client in turning to side-lying position.	Draping promotes comfort and minimizes anxiety. Side-lying position provides access to anal area.
17. Clean anal area:	
a. Clean anal area by first wiping off fecal material with toilet tissue. Wash by wiping from vagina toward anus with one stroke. Discard washcloth. Repeat with clean cloth until skin is clear of fecal material (see illustration).	Fecal material contains microorganisms that can cause vaginal or urinary tract infection.
b. Rinse area well and dry with bath towel.	Rinsing removes soap and microorganisms.
c. Remove disposable gloves and dispose in proper receptacle.	Moisture and body secretions on gloves can harbor microorganisms.
d. Assist client in assuming comfortable position and cover with sheet.	Client comfort minimizes emotional stress.
e. Remove bath blanket and dispose of all soiled bed linen. Return unused equipment to storage area.	Reduces transmission of infection.
f. Raise side rail and lower bed to proper height. Return room to condition before procedure.	Prevents client from accidentally falling. Clean environment enhances comfort.
g. Wash hands.	Reduces transmission of infection.
18. Inspect surface of external genitalia and surrounding skin after cleansing.	Thick secretions may cover underlying skin lesions or areas of breakdown. Evaluation can determine need for additional therapy.
19. Record procedure and abnormal findings (e.g., discharge or condition of genitalia).	Ensures accurate and timely documentation of care.

blood from the face and head. The vernix caseosa, a grayish white, cheeselike substance covering the infant's skin, can temporarily provide insulation and prevent infection. The vernix caseosa dries and disappears within 24 to 48 hours.

Supplies for the bath include a shirt, a diaper (disposable or plain cloth), safety pins, a soft washcloth, cotton balls, a towel, and facial tissue. Plain water is best for the bath to minimize irritation. Oils and powders should not be used. Optional supplies include alcohol for cleansing the umbilical cord, petrolatum jelly to prevent diaper rash, and lotion to provide pleasurable tactile stimulation for the infant during skin massage.

The nurse prepares a basin with water so it feels comfortably warm when tested on the inside surface of the forearm. To prevent cooling, the nurse washes portions of the head and face, with the other body parts covered. The nurse cleans the infant's eyes and ears with clean, moistened cotton balls or a washcloth. The eyes are gently wiped from the inner to the outer canthus, making sure each stroke is done with a clean surface. While washing the face the nurse inspects the nares for

Steps	Rationale
1. Identify factors or conditions such as age, rib or vertebral fractures, burns, or open wounds that contraindicate backrub.	Massage of sensitive tissues might lead to ischemia or tissue injury. Because of age-related skin changes, massage is not recommended in routine skin care for older adults (Rousseau, 1988).
2. For clients with history of hypertension or dysrhythmias, assess pulse and blood pressure.	Massage may cause autonomic nervous system stimulation that induces changes in heart rate and blood pressure. Research has not shown consistent relationships between human touch and the cardiac response of those being touched (Weiss, 1986).
3. Explain procedure and desired position to client.	Helps to promote relaxation.
4. Prepare necessary equipment and supplies: a. Bath blanket b. Bath towel c. Skin application (lotion, alcohol, or powder)	Lotion lubricates skin and prevents friction during massage. Alcohol cools skin but has drying effect. Powder reduces friction during massage.
5. Adjust bed to high, comfortable position.	Ensures proper body mechanics and prevents strain on nurse's back muscles.
6. Adjust light, temperature, and sound within room.	Promotes relaxation.
7. Lower side rail and help client to assume prone or side-lying (Sims') position with back toward nurse. Close curtain around bed.	Position makes it easier to apply necessary pressure to back muscles. Privacy promotes relaxation.
8. Expose back, shoulders, upper arms, and buttocks. Cover rest of body with bath blanket. Lay towel along back.	Prevents unnecessary exposure of body parts. Prevents excess lotion from touching linens.
9. Wash hands in warm water. Warm lotion in hands or by placing container under warm water. Place small amount of lotion in hands.	Cold causes muscle tension.
10. Explain that lotion will feel cool and wet.	Reduces startle response.
11. Apply hands first to sacral area and then down to buttocks (see illustration) massaging in circular motion. Stroke upward from buttocks to shoulders. Massage over scapulas with smooth, firm stroke. Continue in one smooth stroke to upper arms and laterally along sides of back down to iliac crests. Do not allow hands to leave skin. Continue massage pattern for 3 min.	Gentle, firm pressure applied to all muscle groups promotes relaxation. Continuous contact with skin's surface is soothing and stimulates circulation to tissues.

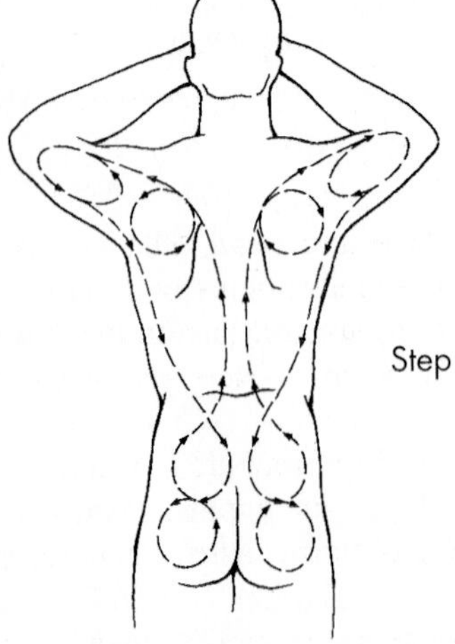

Step 11

Steps	Rationale
12. Knead skin by grasping tissue between thumb and fingers. Knead upward along one side of spine from buttocks to shoulders and around nape of neck. Knead or stroke downward toward sacrum. Repeat along other side of back.	Kneading increases circulation to muscles. Continuous motion is soothing and relieves muscle tension.
13. End massage with long stroking movements and tell client massage is ending.	Long stroking is most soothing of massage movements.
14. If lying on side, ask client to turn to opposite side, and massage other hip.	
15. Wipe excess lubricant from back with bath towel. Retie gown or assist with pajamas. Help client to comfortable position. Open curtain and raise side rails as needed.	Excess lotion can be an irritant. Comfortable position enhances backrub's effects.
16. Dispose of soiled towel and wash hands.	Promotes infection control.
17. Ask client about comfort or note any areas of muscle pain or tension.	Degree of relief depends on length of massage, ability to relax, and degree of discomfort before.
18. Reassess pulse and blood pressure.	Gentle back massage may increase heart rate and systolic blood pressure.
19. Record response to massage and condition of skin.	Accurate documentation describes response to therapy.

crusted secretions. Cotton-tipped swabs should not be used to clean the nares or ears. Sudden movement by the infant could cause a damaged eardrum or nasal passage. A rolled wisp of dampened cotton or the twisted end of the washcloth works best. The infant's scalp can be cleaned by wiping secretions off with a washcloth. However, if shampooing is necessary, the nurse secures the baby's head with one hand and holds it over the bath basin. A mild soap is best for shampooing. The nurse rinses the scalp by pouring water from a small cup over the infant's head. Thorough drying prevents heat loss.

The nurse undresses the infant to continue the bath. Because of the infant's sensitive skin, little rubbing should be done when cleansing. However, the nurse gives special attention to the folds in the neck, umbilicus, axillae, and creases at joints. After bathing the trunk, the nurse applies a clean shirt.

The nurse bathes the infant's buttocks and genitalia last. For a girl it is important to retract the labia fully to remove the vernix caseosa. If the vernix caseosa is thick and adherent, the nurse may choose to remove it gradually during successive diaper changes to avoid unnecessary irritation. The vulva is cleaned from front to back to avoid spreading microorganisms from the anus to the urethra.

In male infants the nurse washes carefully around the penis and scrotum. Noncircumcised infants should not initially have the foreskin retracted. Later, after the foreskin loosens, the nurse should teach the parents to retract the foreskin, cleanse the area, and return the foreskin to its position. No special care is required around a circumcised penis.

Any fecal material can be removed with facial tissue, using a mild soap. A thin layer of petrolatum jelly helps to retain skin moisture and prevent diaper rash.

After the bath the nurse applies a clean diaper, which should fit snugly around the thighs and abdomen to prevent leakage. If the child is circumcised, the diaper should fit loosely to avoid friction. The diaper should always be below the umbilical site until it is completely healed. The nurse fastens the diaper with the back overlapping the front to permit full hip flexion.

TUB BATH. Infants can be given a tub bath after the umbilicus has healed. Supplies are the same as for a sponge bath. The face, neck, ears, eyes, and scalp are washed before the infant is undressed and put in the tub. The nurse lowers the infant slowly into the tub to avoid startling. The head and back must always be held firmly with one hand. A child is never left unattended. Body creases are easier to clean and rinse in a tub bath. After the bath the nurse wraps the infant completely in a towel and gently pats the child dry, paying special attention to body creases.

CLIENT TEACHING FOR SKIN HYGIENE

- Stress importance of hygiene care (bath, skin care, oral hygiene)
- Inspect skin for changes (redness, rashes, changes in moles)
- Protect against falls in the tub or shower
- Stress importance of consistent use of sunscreen with a protection factor of at least 15 and to avoid unneccessary sun exposure

Health Promotion/Restoration Activities

Nurses can instruct clients to follow a few general rules to promote skin health and restore optimal function (see box above). Clients should bathe daily unless contraindicated, preferably in the morning. They should use lotions to moisturize dry skin and bathe in a warm environment, avoiding cold drafts. Drinking at least eight glasses of water daily helps to maintain hydration. Clients should report any changes in skin color and texture. The client should handle the skin gently, avoiding excessive rubbing. Finally, clients should be encouraged to eat nutritious foods rich in vitamins and minerals.

Evaluative Measures

During and after bathing and skin care, the nurse evaluates the success of interventions. The process is dynamic, because the client's condition may change. The nurse must always be prepared to revise the care plan based on the evaluation. For example, if a client's skin continues to be reddened over the sacrum, more frequent turning may be necessary. Systematic evaluation requires the nurse to determine if expected outcomes have been met. Examples of goals, outcomes, and corresponding evaluative measures include:

Goal: Client maintains skin integrity and control of body odor.

Outcome

Client's skin will be smooth, supple, clean, and free of odor following bathing

Evaluative measures

Inspect skin's texture, turgor, and cleanliness

Note presence of body odor

Outcome

Client's skin will be free of localized redness or hyperemia at time of discharge

Evaluative measure

Inspect potential pressure sites for redness or hyperemia

Goal: Client maintains or improves joint ROM.

Outcome

Client demonstrates baseline ROM during bathing

Evaluative measure

Observe client's joint movements while bathing

Outcome

Joints are stable and move freely during passive exercise

Evaluative measures

Palpate joints while performing passive exercise during bathing

Goal: Client achieves relaxation and comfort.

Outcome

Client expresses sense of comfort and cleanliness following bathing

Evaluative measure

Ask client to describe level of comfort or fatigue following bathing

Goal: Client participates in hygiene.

Outcome

Client begins hygiene measures independently 2 days before discharge

Evaluative measure

Observe client beginning and assisting with bathing activities

Outcome

Client makes decisions regarding hygiene schedule by day of discharge

Evaluative measure

Observe whether client makes choices about proper self-care measures

Goal: Client completes hygiene without fatigue.

Outcome

Client denies feeling of fatigue after bathing

Evaluative measures

Question client about level of exertion or fatigue while bathing

Observe client's willingness to continue self-care during bathing

Observe client for shortness of breath or increased breathing rate

CARE OF THE FEET AND NAILS

The feet and nails often require special attention to prevent infection, odor, and injury. Problems result from abuse or poor care.

The feet are important to physical and emotional health. Foot pain can often change a walking gait, causing strain on different muscle groups. Discomfort while standing or walking can lead to physical and emotional stress.

The nails are epithelial tissues that grow from the root of the nail bed, located in the skin at the nail groove. A normal healthy nail is transparent, smooth, and convex, with a pink nail bed and translucent white

table 30-3

COMMON FOOT AND NAIL PROBLEMS

Condition	Characteristics	Implications	Interventions
Callus	Thickened portion of epidermis, consisting of mass of horny, keratotic cells; usually flat, painless, and on undersurface of foot or on palm; caused by local friction or pressure	Condition may cause discomfort when wearing tight-fitting shoes.	Advise client to wear gloves when using tools or objects that may create friction on palmar surfaces. Encourage client to wear comfortable shoes. Soak callus in warm water and Epsom salts to soften cell layers. Use pumice stone to remove callus after it softens. Applications of creams or lotions can reduce reformation.
Corns	Keratosis caused by friction and pressure from shoes; seen mainly on toes and over bony prominence; usually cone shaped, round, and raised	Conical shape compresses underlying dermis, making it thin and tender. Pain is aggravated when tight-fitting shoes are worn. Tissue can become attached to bone if allowed to grow. Client may suffer alteration in gait because of pain.	Surgical removal may be necessary, depending on severity of pain and size of corn. Avoid use of oval corn pads, which increase pressure on toes and reduce circulation.
Plantar warts	Fungating lesion that appears on sole of foot; caused by papilloma virus	Warts may be contagious. They are painful and make walking difficult.	Treatment ordered by physician may include applications of salicylic acid, electrodesiccation (burning with an electrical spark), or freezing with solid carbon dioxide.
Athlete's foot (tinea pedis)	Fungal infection of foot; scaliness and cracking of skin between toes and on soles of feet; small blisters containing fluid may appear; apparently induced by wearing constricting footwear (e.g., sneakers)	Athlete's foot can spread to other body parts, especially the hands. It is contagious and frequently recurs.	Feet should be well ventilated. Drying feet well after bathing and applying powder help to prevent infection. Wearing of clean socks or stockings reduces incidence. Physician may order application of griseofulvin, miconazole, or tolnaftate.
Ingrown nails	Toenail or fingernail growing inward into soft tissue around nail; often results from improper nail trimming	Ingrown nails can cause localized pain when pressure is applied.	Treatment is frequently hot soaks in antiseptic solution and removal of portion of nail that has grown into skin. Instruct client on proper nail trimming techniques.
Ram's horn nails	Unusually long curved nails	Attempt by nurse to cut nails may result in damage to nail bed with risk of infection.	Refer client to a podiatrist.
Paronychia	Inflammation of tissue surrounding nail after hangnail or other injury; occurs in people who frequently have their hands in water; common in diabetic clients	Area can become infected.	Treatment is hot compresses or soaks and local application of antibiotic ointments. Paronychia can be prevented by careful manicuring
Foot odors	Result of excess perspiration promoting microorganism growth	Condition may cause discomfort as a result of excess perspiration.	Frequent washing, use of foot deodorants and powders, and wearing clean footwear prevent or reduce this problem.

ASSESSMENT OF NAILS AND FEET

DEVELOPMENTAL CHANGES

Consider special needs of older adult clients unable to maintain hygiene because of poor vision, hand tremors, or obesity.

Common problems with aging include skin fissures, dry feet, thickened nails, and fungal infections.

Assess home remedies used by older adults with chronic feet problems. Such remedies may cause burns or ulcerations.

FOOTWEAR

Assess types of footwear used. Shoes should be snug but not tight, with support to the arch.

Assess for ill-fitting shoes, socks, garters, and knee-high nylons.

Assess cleanliness of footwear.

PHYSICAL CHANGES

Inspect all skin surfaces, particularly areas between toes.

Assess gait, differentiating between alterations caused by skin and musculoskeletal problems.

Assess circulation to the feet. Check pedal pulses, skin color and temperature, pain, and sensation.

Inspect condition of nails. Inflammatory lesions of the nail bed cause formation of thickened, horny nails, which can separate from the nail bed.

KNOWLEDGE OF FOOT AND NAIL CARE PRACTICES

Does the client know how to cut nails?

Does the client use over-the-counter products?

Does the client see a podiatrist regularly?

tip. Disease can cause changes in the shape, thickness, and curvature of the nail (see Chapter 16).

NURSING PROCESS

Assessment

The nurse assesses clients for nail and foot problems by reviewing developmental factors contributing to alterations, determining the client's type of footwear, and assessing hygiene care practices (see box above). The nurse inspects the condition of the nails and looks for lesions, dryness, inflammation, or cracking (Table 30-3).

Nursing Diagnosis

After a thorough assessment, the nurse gathers and clusters all defining characteristics of specific foot and nail problems. These may include the presence or absence of discomfort or pain, swelling, lesion formation, changes in mobility, or altered circulation. The nurse selects the appropriate nursing diagnosis based on these factors (see box below, left).

NURSING DIAGNOSES FOR FOOT AND NAIL PROBLEMS

- Pain
- Bathing/hygiene self-care deficit
- Impaired skin integrity
- High risk for impaired skin integrity
- High risk for infection
- Knowledge deficit regarding foot/nail care
- Impaired physical mobility

The determining factors help the nurse to plan care for the client. For the diagnosis "impaired skin integrity related to improper nail-cutting practices" the nurse designs interventions to evaluate the client's nail-cutting technique and foot care practices. In contrast, "impaired skin integrity related to friction of shoes" requires the nurse to take a different approach. The nurse should assess the type, size, and quality of shoes worn, observe the client while walking, and make recommendations to reduce any source of friction. Effective nursing care and appropriate nursing interventions result from selecting the correct related factors for a nursing diagnosis.

Planning

The nurse may provide foot and nail care during the bed bath or at another time according to the client's preference. Many home health nurses visit clients at home to provide foot and nail care. Some foot and nail care problems are too complex for nursing intervention and require consulting a podiatrist. The nurse's care plan is based on the following goals:

Goal: Client achieves comfort while walking.

Outcomes

Client uses normal gait

Client reports increased comfort when wearing shoes

procedure 30-5

NAIL AND FOOT CARE

Steps	Rationale
1. Identify conditions that put clients at risk for foot or nail problems including:	
a. Older adult clients	Changes in sensory and motor function with aging impair self-care practices. Physiological changes of aging alter condition of feet and nails.
b. Clients with diabetes	Vascular changes associated with diabetes reduce blood flow to peripheral tissues.
c. Clients with heart failure or renal disease	Conditions that can cause tissue edema and reduced blood flow to tissues.
d. Clients who have had cerebrovascular accident or stroke	Residual paralysis or reduced sensation can cause abnormal walking patterns resulting in friction and pressure on feet.
2. Explain procedure, including that proper soaking requires several minutes.	Client must be willing to place fingers and feet in basin for 10 to 20 min. Client may become anxious or fatigued.
3. Prepare necessary equipment and supplies: a. Washbasin b. Emesis basin c. Washcloth d. Bath or face towel e. Nail clippers f. Orange stick g. Emery board h. Body lotion i. Disposable bath mat j. Paper towels k. Disposable gloves (optional)	
4. Obtain physician's order for cutting nails if agency policy requires it.	Client's skin may be accidentally cut. Certain clients are more at risk for infection, depending on medical condition.
5. Wash hands. Arrange equipment on overbed table.	Reduces transmission of infection. Prevents delays.
6. Pull curtain around bed or close room door (if desired).	Maintaining privacy reduces anxiety.
7. Assist client to bedside chair if possible. Place disposable bath mat on floor under client's feet. Place call light within client's reach.	Sitting in chair makes it easier to immerse feet in basin. Bath mat protects feet from exposure to soil or debris. Call light maintains safety.
8. Fill washbasin with warm water. Test temperature of water.	Warm water softens nails and thickened epidermal cells, reduces inflammation of skin, and promotes local circulation. Proper water temperature prevents burns.
9. Place basin on bath mat and help client to place feet in basin.	Clients with muscular weakness or tremors may have difficulty positioning feet.
10. Adjust overbed table to low position and place it over client's lap.	Prevent accidental spills.
11. Fill emesis basin with warm water and place it on paper towels on overbed table.	Warm water softens nails and thickened epidermal cells.
12. Instruct client to place fingers in emesis basin and place arms in comfortable position.	Prolonged positioning can cause discomfort unless normal anatomical alignment is maintained.
13. Allow feet and fingernails to soak for 10 to 20 min. Rewarm water in 10 min.	Softening of corns, calluses, and cuticles ensures easy removal of dead cells and easy manipulation of cuticle.
14. Clean gently under fingernails with orange stick while fingers are immersed. Then remove emesis basin and dry fingers thoroughly.	Orange stick removes debris under nails that harbors microorganisms. Thorough drying impedes fungal growth and prevents maceration of tissues.
15. With nail clippers, clip fingernails straight across and even with tops of fingers (see illustration). Shape nails with emery board.	Cutting straight across prevents splitting of nail margins and formation of sharp nail spikes that can irritate lateral nail margins. Filing prevents cutting nail too close to nail bed.
16. Push cuticle back gently with orange stick.	Reduces incidence of inflamed cuticles.
17. Move overbed table away from client.	Provides easier access to feet.

Continued.

procedure 30-5—cont'd

Steps	Rationale
18. Put on disposable gloves; scrub callused areas of feet with washcloth.	Prevent transmission of fungal infection. Removes dead skin layers.
19. Clean gently under nails with orange stick. Remove feet from basin and dry thoroughly.	Reduces chances of infection.
20. Clean and trim toenails using procedures in Steps 14 and 16.	
21. Apply lotion to feet and hands; assist client back to bed and into comfortable position.	Lubricates dry skin by helping to retain moisture.
22. Remove disposable gloves and dispose in receptacle. Clean and return equipment and supplies to proper place. Dispose of soiled linen in hamper. Wash hands.	Prevents transmission of infection.
23. Inspect nails and surrounding skin after soaking and nail trimming.	Evaluates condition of skin. Allows nurse to note rough nail edges.
24. Record procedure and observations. Report breaks in skin.	Documents procedure and response. Abnormalities may pose risk of infection.

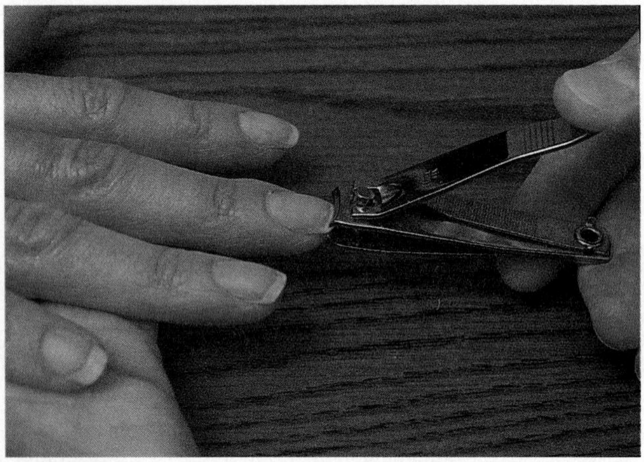

Step 15(a)

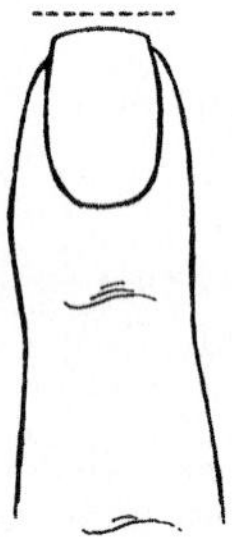

Step 15(b)

Goal: Client maintains skin integrity and clean, trimmed nails.

Outcome

Client's toes and nails exhibit no redness or swelling

Goal: Client reduces risk for further tissue injury.

Outcomes

Client identifies signs and symptoms of impending tissue injury

Client identifies proper type of footwear

Client explains factors that may cause tissue injury

Goal: Client demonstrates proper foot and nail care practices.

Outcomes

Client correctly trims nails and cleans feet

Client explains footcare regimen

Implementation

Foot and nail care involves soaking to soften cuticles and layers of horny cells, thorough cleansing, drying, and proper nail trimming. The nurse may provide the care in bed for an immobilized client or have the client sit in a chair (Procedure 30-5). The nurse must take time during the procedure to teach the client proper techniques for cleaning and nail trimming. Measures to prevent infection and promote good circulation should be stressed.

A client with diabetes or peripheral vascular disease is at risk for foot and nail problems because of impaired circulation. Although ongoing good foot care can help prevent toe amputation, studies have shown that many clients have not learned proper care (Christensen, et al., 1991). The nurse instructs clients on the following precautions during foot and nail care:

1. Wash the feet daily using lukewarm water. Thoroughly pat the feet dry, and dry well between the toes.
2. Do not cut corns or calluses or use commercial removers. Consult a physician or podiatrist.
3. If the feet perspire, apply a bland foot powder.
4. If dryness is noted along the feet or between the toes, apply lanolin, baby oil, or even corn oil and rub gently into the skin.
5. File the toenails straight across and square; do not use scissors or clippers. Consult a podiatrist as needed.
6. Do not use over-the-counter preparations to treat athlete's foot or ingrown toenails. Consult a physician or podiatrist.
7. Teach the client to avoid wearing elastic stockings, knee-high hose, or constricting garters. Do not cross the legs. Both impair circulation to the lower extremities.
8. Inspect the feet daily, including tops and soles of the feet, heels, and the area between the toes. Use a mirror to inspect all surfaces.
9. Wear clean socks or stockings daily. Socks should be dry and free of holes or darns that might cause pressure.
10. Do not walk barefoot.
11. Wear shoes that fit properly. Soles of shoes should be flexible and should not slip. Lamb's wool can be used between toes that rub or overlap. Shoes should be sturdy, closed in, and not restrictive.
12. Exercise regularly to improve circulation to the lower extremities. Walk slowly, elevate, rotate, flex, and extend the feet at the ankle. Dangle the feet over the side of the bed 1 minute, then extend both legs and hold them parallel to the bed while lying supine for 1 minute, and finally rest 1 minute (Jordan and Nickerson, 1982).
13. Avoid applying hot-water bottles or heating pads to the feet. Use warm soaks or extra coverings instead.
14. Minor cuts should be washed immediately and dried thoroughly. Only mild antiseptics (e.g., Neosporin ointment) should be applied to the skin. Avoid iodine or mercurochrome. Contact a physician to treat cuts or lacerations.

Health Promotion/Restoration Activities

For proper foot and nail care, clients should be instructed to protect the feet from injury, keep the feet clean and dry, and wear footwear that fits properly. The nurse can also help the client learn the proper way to inspect the feet for lesions, dryness, or signs of infection. Any of these conditions should be reported to the nurse. Finally, to maintain and promote foot and nail health, clients should visit a podiatrist when necessary.

Evaluative Measures

A client's response to nail and foot care is best evaluated over several days. Existing medical problems may take time to improve. Evaluation based on expected outcomes requires the nurse to determine the success of the interventions. Based on evaluative findings, the nurse must be prepared to revise the care plan. For example, if the client continues to have discomfort while walking, a different style of footwear may be needed. The nurse also instructs the client about ways to evaluate nail and foot care practices to prevent further problems. Goals, expected outcomes, and evaluative measures for client's receiving foot care include:

Goal: Client achieves comfort while walking.

Outcome

Client uses normal gait

Evaluative measure

Observe client walking

Outcome

Client reports increased comfort when wearing shoes

Evaluative measure

Ask client about pain occurring while walking or wearing shoes

Goal: Client maintains skin integrity and clean, trimmed nails.

Outcome

Client's toes and nails exhibit no redness or swelling

Evaluative measure

Observe skin and nail edges for cracks, abrasions, or lesions

Evaluative measure

Palpate nail edges for rough areas

Goal: Client reduces the risk for further tissue injury.

Outcome

Client identifies signs and symptoms of impending tissue injury

Evaluative measure

Ask client about sensations of pain on or around the nail beds

Outcome

Client explains factors that may cause tissue injury

table 30-4

PHYSIOLOGICAL DEVELOPMENT OF THE MOUTH

Developmental level	Changes
Infant	Deciduous teeth begin to erupt at about 5 months of age.
	Solid food can be taken at 5 to 6 months, with chewing beginning by 6 to 8 months.
18 months to 6 years	Twenty deciduous teeth are present.
	By age 2, child can begin to brush teeth and learn hygiene practices from parents.
	Dental caries may become a problem if dental hygiene is neglected.
6 to 12 years	Deciduous "baby teeth" begin to fall out and are replaced by permanent teeth. All permanent teeth are present by age 12 except second and third molars.
	Definite food preferences become apparent.
	Dental caries and irregularity in spacing of teeth are significant health poblems.
12 to 18 years	All permanent teeth are present.
	Dental hygiene practices improve because of increased awareness of body image.
18 to 40 years	Third molars appear.
	Good oral hygiene and nutrition practices are needed to avoid problems in later years.
Pregnancy	Changes in female sex hormones may exaggerate the reaction to irritants in dental plaque, causing gingivitis and increased risk of severe periodontal disease.*
40 to 65 years	Periodontal disease is common and increases risk for tooth loss.
	Many people over age 55 have lost some or all of their teeth because of poor oral care.
65 years and over	Aging teeth become brittle, drier, and darker in color.
	Teeth become uneven, jagged, and fractured after years of crushing and grinding.
	Gums lose vascularity and tissue elasticity, causing dentures to fit poorly.
	Eating habits often change, and malnutrition may be problem.

*Data from Deliefde B: The dental care of pregnant women, *NZ Dent J* 80:41, 1984.

Evaluative measure

Have client list three factors that can injure tissues surrounding nails

Goal: Client demonstrates proper foot and nail care practices.

Outcome

Client correctly trims nails and cleans feet

Evaluative measure

Observe client performing nail and foot care

Outcome

Client explains foot care regimen

Evaluative measure

Ask client to describe techniques for cutting nails and cleaning feet

ORAL HYGIENE

The major part of a tooth is the dentin, an ivory substance harder than bone. Dentin surrounds a tooth's pulp cavity. A layer of enamel covers the upper portion of each tooth at the crown. The periodontal membrane, just below the gum margins, surrounds the tooth root and holds it firmly in place. Healthy teeth are white, smooth, shiny, and properly aligned. Table 30-4 summarizes the physiological development of the mouth.

Oral hygiene helps to maintain the healthy state of the mouth, teeth, gums, and lips. Brushing cleans the teeth of food particles, plaque, and bacteria. It also massages the gums and relieves discomfort resulting from unpleasant odors and tastes. Complete oral hygiene enhances well-being and stimulates the appetite. The nurse's responsibilities in oral hygiene are maintenance and prevention. The nurse can help clients to maintain good oral hygiene by teaching correct techniques or by performing hygiene for weakened or disabled clients.

NURSING PROCESS

Assessment

A thorough assessment for problems related to oral hygiene should be included in every client's care (see box on p. 833). During the assessment the nurse can inform the client about good oral hygiene habits. The nurse may also refer the client to a specialist if common oral problems are found (see box on p. 833). Early identification of poor oral hygiene practices and common oral problems can reduce the risk of gum disease and **dental caries** or cavities.

ASSESSMENT OF ORAL HYGIENE

PHYSICAL CHANGES

Inspect all areas of the oral cavity (Chapter 16).
Check for dental caries, broken or jagged teeth, missing teeth, and halitosis among clients with poor hygiene practices.
Wear gloves and wash hands before and after the examination.

DEVELOPMENTAL CHANGES

Assess client's developmental level (Table 30-4) for normal changes in teeth, gums, and mucosa.
Evaluate socioeconomic and economic factors influencing hygiene habits.

HYGIENE PREFERENCES

Identify errors and deficiencies.
Ask clients about habits and preferences (e.g., frequency of brushing and flossing, dental products used, denture care, and visits to dentist).
Have client demonstrate practices.

RISK FACTORS FOR ORAL HYGIENE PROBLEMS

Assess for physical disability or emotional factors that may prevent clients from performing self-care.
Identify conditions that can cause alterations in oral cavity tissues (e.g., dehydration, mouth breathing, oxygen administration, chemotherapeutic drugs, radiation therapy, or oral surgery).
Be aware of the forms of treatment that can injure oral mucosal surfaces (e.g., endotracheal tubes, oral airways, or suction catheters).

COMMON ORAL PROBLEMS

DENTAL CARIES (CAVITIES)

Caries are most common among young people.
Buildup of plaque causes acid destruction of tooth enamel. Initially appears as chalky, white discoloration of the tooth.
Prevention involves reducing intake of carbohydrates, brushing within 30 minutes after eating sweets, using fluoridated water, brushing after each meal and before bedtime, and flossing daily.

PERIODONTAL DISEASE (PYORRHEA)

Periodontal disease is most common after age 35.
It involves destruction of gingiva (gums) and other supporting structures with bleeding gums, inflammation, and receding gum lines.
Prevention involves regular flossing and brushing.

OTHER PROBLEMS

Stomatitis (inflammation of the mouth)
Glossitis (inflammation of the tongue)
Gingivitis (inflammation of the gums)
Halitosis (bad breath)
Cheilosis (cracked lips)
Oral malignancy (mouth lumps or ulcers)

Nursing Diagnosis

The nurse's assessment can reveal if the client is at risk for or has an actual alteration in oral integrity. These findings may also indicate the client's need for assistance with oral hygienic care. The nurse clusters all defining characteristics to select appropriate nursing diagnoses for the client's problems. Examples of nursing diagnoses related to oral hygiene are shown in the box at right.

The nurse should carefully select a nursing diagnosis appropriate for the related factors displayed by the client. Selection influences the choice of nursing interventions. For example, for the diagnosis "altered oral mucous membranes related to trauma" the nurse must design therapies to prevent further mucosal injury. Special rinses, suctioning, and nutritional support may be ordered. In contrast, "altered mucous membranes related to ineffective oral hygiene" requires the nurse to take a different approach. Observing the client brushing and flossing, teaching good oral care practices, and helping the client to select the proper oral care equipment can assist the client to improve oral hygiene.

NURSING DIAGNOSES FOR ORAL HYGIENE PROBLEMS

Altered oral mucous membrane
Pain
Altered nutrition: less than body requirements
Bathing/hygiene self-care deficit
Body-image disturbance
Knowledge deficit regarding oral hygiene
High risk for infection

Planning

Developing a care plan for maintaining oral hygiene involves considering the client's personal preferences and physical and emotional status. The nurse must establish a good relationship with the client to assist with oral hygiene. Some clients are sensitive about the condition of their mouths and are reluctant to let someone else care for them. In many cases, clients are also unaware they are at risk for serious dental and periodontal disease and thus need instruction.

The nurse's care plan is based on the following goals:

Goal: Client maintains an intact, well-hydrated oral mucosa free of odor.

Outcomes

Client's oral mucosa will be moist, pink, and odor free

Client consumes at least 3 liters of liquids daily

Goal: Client's oral mucosa is free of infection and dental caries.

Outcomes

Client chews food without discomfort

Client's mucous membranes have no localized redness or swelling

Client's teeth will have no plaque, tartar, or caries

Goal: Client maintains or improves comfort level.

Outcomes

Client verbalizes sense of comfort following oral care

Client denies mouth pain

Goal: Client assumes oral hygiene care daily.

Outcomes

Client explains oral hygiene practices

Client demonstrates correct oral hygiene techniques

Implementation

Administration of Oral Hygiene

Good oral hygiene involves cleanliness, comfort, and the moisturizing of mouth structures. Proper care will prevent oral disease. Unfortunately, clients in hospitals or long-term care facilities often do not receive the aggressive care they need. Oral care must be provided on a regular basis (see box above).

Brushing, flossing, and irrigation are necessary for proper cleansing. Clients also benefit from a proper diet, which excludes foods promoting plaque formation and tooth decay. The diet should include foods that promote healthy periodontal structures.

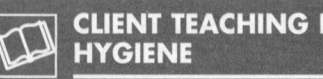

Diet. To prevent tooth decay, clients may have to change eating habits (e.g., reducing intake of carbohydrates, especially sweet snacks between meals). Sweet or starchy food adheres to tooth surfaces. After eating sweets, a client should brush within 30 minutes to reduce the action of plaque. Eating acidic foods (e.g., apples and fibrous vegetables) also reduces plaque. The acidic quality of fruits eliminates bacteria that forms on teeth. A well-balanced diet ensures the integrity of oral tissues.

CLIENT TEACHING FOR ORAL HYGIENE

Brush with an even, rounded brushing surface with soft nylon bristles.
Hard nylon toothbrushes can cause gum injury.
Select a toothpaste that contains fluoride.
Brush a minimum of four times a day.
Thoroughly rinse after brushing.
Stress importance of a proper diet.

Brushing. Thorough tooth brushing at least 4 times a day (after meals and at bedtime) is basic to an effective oral hygiene program. A toothbrush should have a straight handle and brush small enough to reach all areas of the mouth. Older adult clients with reduced dexterity and grip may require an enlarged handle with an easier grip.

All tooth surfaces should be brushed thoroughly. Commercially made foam rubber toothbrushes are useful for clients with sensitive gums. Electric toothbrushes can be used, but the nurse must check for electrical hazards. Lemon-glycerin sponges should be avoided since they dry mucous membranes and erode teeth enamel (Pettigrew, 1989). Moi-Stin is a salivary supplement that improves moisture and texture of the tongue and mucosa (Poland, 1987).

When teaching clients about mouth care, the nurse should recommend they do not share toothbrushes with family members or drink directly from a bottle of mouthwash. Cross-contamination occurs easily. The amount of assistance needed by the client when brushing the teeth may vary (Procedure 30-6).

Unconscious clients need special attention. While providing hygiene to an unconscious client, the nurse must protect the client from choking and aspirating. The safest technique is to have two nurses provide the care. One does the actual cleaning, and the other removes secretions with suction equipment. While cleansing the oral cavity, the nurse should never use fingers to hold the mouth open. A human bite is highly contaminated. It may be necessary to perform mouth care at least every 2 hours. The nurse explains the steps of mouth care and the sensations the client will feel. The nurse also tells the client when the procedure is completed (Procedure 30-7).

Flossing. Dental flossing is necessary to remove plaque and tartar between teeth. Flossing involves in-

procedure 30-6

BRUSHING AND FLOSSING TEETH OF A DEPENDENT CLIENT

Steps	Rationale
1. Determine client's ability to grasp and manipulate toothbrush.	Older adult clients or those with changes in level of consciousness or musculoskeletal or nervous system alterations may be unable to hold toothbrush with firm grip or manipulate brush. Nurse can determine level of assistance required.
2. Explain procedure and discuss preferences regarding use of hygienic acids.	Some clients feel uncomfortable about having nurse care for basic needs. Client involvement minimizes anxiety.
3. Prepare necessary equipment and supplies:	
a. Toothbrush with straight handle and small, soft, rounded bristles	Soft, rounded bristles stimulate gums without causing bleeding.
b. Toothpaste or dentifrice	
c. Dental floss	
d. Water glass with cool water	
e. Mouthwash (optional)	Serves to provide aftertaste.
f. Straw	
g. Emesis basin	
h. Face towel and paper towels	
i. Disposable gloves	Prevents contact with oral secretions.
4. Wash hands.	Reduces transmission of microorganisms.
5. Place paper towels on overbed table and arrange other equipment within easy reach.	Towels collect moisture and spills from emesis basin.
6. Pull curtain or close room door (optional if client is only brushing teeth).	Provides for privacy. When brushing is part of bathing and total hygiene, privacy is essential.
7. Raise bed to comfortable working position. Raise head of bed (if allowed) and lower side rail. Move client or help client to move toward nurse. Side-lying position can be used.	Raising bed and positioning client prevent nurse from experiencing muscle strain. Semi-Fowler's position helps to prevent client from choking or aspirating.
8. Place towel over client's chest.	Prevents soiling of gown and bed linen.
9. Position overbed table within easy reach and adjust height as needed.	Easy accessibility of supplies ensures smooth, safe procedure.
10. Don gloves.	Prevents contact with microorganisms in saliva.
11. Apply toothpaste to brush, holding brush over emesis basin. Pour small amount of water over toothpaste.	Moisture aids in distribution of toothpaste over tooth surfaces.
12. Hold toothbrush bristles at 45-degree angle to gum line (see illustrations). Be sure tips of bristles rest against and penetrate under gum line. Brush inner and outer surfaces of upper and lower teeth by brushing from gum to crown of each tooth. Use short, vibrating strokes and brush each tooth separately. Clean biting surfaces of teeth by holding top of bristles parallel with teeth and brushing gently back and forth. Brush sides by moving bristles back and forth.	Angle allows for brush to reach all tooth surfaces and to clean under gum line where plaque and tartar accumulate. Back-and-forth motion dislodges food particles caught between teeth and along chewing surfaces.

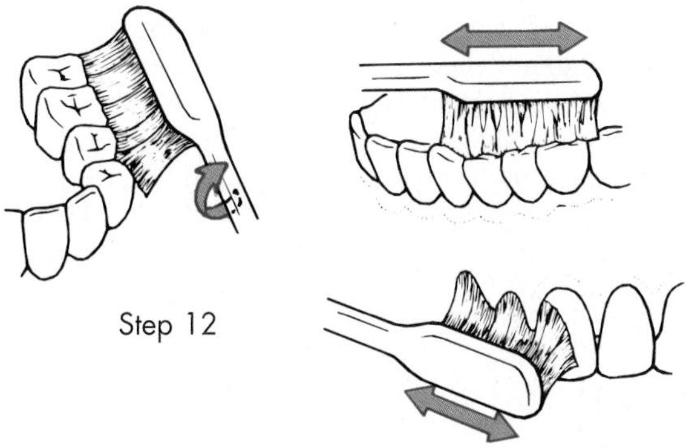

Step 12

Continued.

procedure 30-6—cont'd

Steps	Rationale
13. Hold brush at 45-degree angle and lightly brush over surface and sides of tongue. Avoid initiating gag reflex.	Microorganisms collect and grow on tongue's surface. Gagging is uncomfortable and may cause aspiration of toothpaste.
14. Allow client to rinse mouth thoroughly by taking several sips of water, swishing it across all tooth surfaces, and spitting it into emesis basin.	Removes food particles.
15. Allow client to gargle or rinse mouth with mouthwash.	Leaves pleasant taste in mouth.
16. Remove curved basin and assist in wiping mouth.	Promotes comfort.
17. Prepare for flossing by having client wash hands, if client is to floss independently.	Reduces transmission of microorganisms.
18. Prepare two pieces of dental floss approximately 25 cm (10 in) in length. Opinion differs over use of waxed versus unwaxed floss. Waxed floss frays less easily. Food particles adhere to unwaxed floss.	Adequate length needed to grasp floss firmly and insert over surfaces of teeth.
19. Wrap ends of floss around third finger of each hand. Using thumb and index finger, stretch floss and insert between two upper teeth. Move floss up and down in seesaw motion between teeth from under the gum lines up to top of each tooth's crown. Be sure to clean outer surface of back molar. Make figure "C" around edge of tooth being flossed. Work systematically along each set of teeth.	Proper insertion and movement along tooth surfaces removes plaque and tartar.

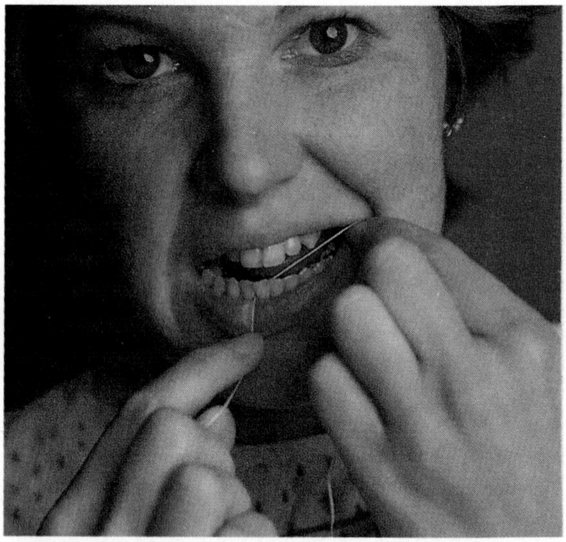

Step 20

Steps	Rationale
20. Take clean piece of floss and wrap around third finger of each hand. Using two index fingers, stretch floss and insert between two lower teeth (see illustration).	Frayed floss becomes caught between teeth and can be torn off, leading to gum inflammation and infection. Position of hands helps to reach lower tooth surfaces.
21. Move floss up and down, between gum lines and crown of lower teeth, one at a time.	Removes plaque and tartar.
22. Allow client to rinse mouth thoroughly with tepid water and spit into emesis basin. Assist in wiping mouth.	Removes plaque and tartar from oral cavity.
23. Assist client to comfortable position, remove bedside table, raise side rail, and lower bed to original position.	Provides comfort and safety.
24. Wipe off overbed table, discard soiled linen and paper towels in appropriate containers, remove and discard soiled gloves, and return equipment to proper place.	
25. Wash hands.	Prevents transmission of microorganisms.
26. Inspect condition of oral cavity.	Determines effectiveness of brushing and rinsing.
27. Record procedure and note condition of oral cavity in nurse's notes. Report bleeding or lesions.	Documents response to hygiene measures and status of oral cavity. Bleeding may indicate serious systemic problem. Oral lesions may be cancerous.

procedure 30-7

PERFORMING MOUTH CARE FOR AN UNCONSCIOUS OR DEBILITATED CLIENT

Steps	Rationale
1. Assess for gag reflex.	Reveals risk for aspiration.
2. Position client in Sims' or side-lying position with head turned well toward dependent side (see illustration).	Allows secretions to drain from mouth instead of collecting in back of pharynx. Prevents aspiration.
3. Explain procedure.	Unconscious client may retain ability to hear.
4. Prepare necessary equipment and supplies:	
a. Antiinfective solution (e.g., hydrogen peroxide diluted in equal parts of water)	Loosens crustations and acts as antiinfective.
b. Sponge toothbrush or tongue blade wrapped in single layer of gauze; small toothbrush	Brush cleans teeth most effectively. Sponge or swab stimulates and cleans gums and mucosa.
c. Padded tongue blade	Keeps mouth open and teeth separated during procedure without traumatizing oral structures.
d. Face towel	
e. Emesis basin	
f. Paper towels	
g. Water glass with cool water	
h. Petrolatum jelly	Lubricates lips.
i. Portable suction machine (optional) with rubber catheter	Removes retained oral secretions while oral cavity is cleansed.
j. Disposable gloves	Oral cavity contains many highly infectious microorganisms.
5. Wash hands and apply disposable gloves.	Reduces transfer of microorganisms.
6. Place paper towels on overbed table and arrange equipment. Turn on suction machine and connect tubing to suction catheter.	Prevents soiling of tabletop. Ensures smooth, safe procedure.
7. Pull curtain around bed or close room door.	Provides privacy.
8. Raise bed to highest horizontal level; lower side rail.	Prevents injury to nurse and client.
9. Bring client close to side of bed and near nurse; be sure head is turned toward mattress.	Proper positioning of head prevents aspiration.
10. Place towel under face and emesis basin under chin.	Prevents soiling of bed linen.
11. Carefully retract upper and lower teeth with padded tongue blade by inserting blade quickly but gently between back molars. Insert when client is relaxed, if possible.	Prevents client from biting down on nurse's fingers and provides access to oral cavity.

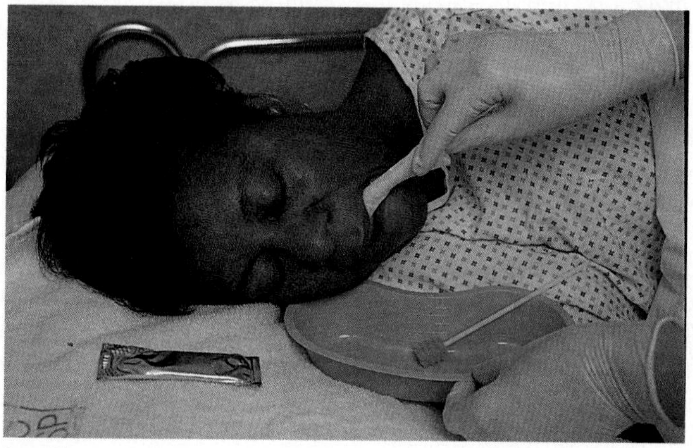

Step 2

Continued.

procedure 30-7—cont'd

Steps	Rationale
12. Clean mouth using brush or tongue blade moistened with peroxide and water (half and half). Have second nurse suction as secretions accumulate during cleansing. Clean chewing and inner tooth surfaces first. Clean outer tooth surfaces. Swab roof of mouth and inside cheeks. Gently swab or brush tongue but avoid stimulating gag reflex (if present). Moisten clean swab or toothette with water to rinse. Repeat rinse several times. Suction remaining secretions.	Brushing action removes food particles between teeth and along chewing surfaces. Swabbing helps to remove secretions and crustations from mucosa and moistens mucosa. Suction removes secretions and fluid that can collect in posterior pharynx. Repeated rinsing removes peroxide that can be irritating to mucosa.
13. Apply thin layer of petrolatum jelly to lips.	Lubricates lips to prevent drying and cracking.
14. Explain that procedure is completed.	Provides meaningful stimulation.
15. Remove gloves and dispose in proper receptacle.	Prevents transmission of microorganisms.
16. Reposition client comfortably, raise side rail, and return bed to original position.	Maintains comfort and safety.
17. Clean equipment and return to its proper place. Place soiled linen in proper receptacle.	Prevents spread of infection.
18. Wash hands.	Reduces transmission of microorganisms.
19. Inspect oral cavity. (Additional pair of gloves may be needed if nurse is to contact saliva.)	Determines efficiency of cleansing. After thick secretions are removed, underlying inflammation or lesions may be revealed.
20. Record procedure, including pertinent observation (e.g., bleeding gums, dry mucosa, ulcerations, or crusts on tongue) and report unusual findings to nurse in charge or physician.	Documents response to therapy. Bleeding may indicate more serious systemic problems. Lesions can be cancerous.

serting waxed or unwaxed dental floss between all tooth surfaces, one at a time. The seesaw motion used to pull floss between teeth removes plaque and tartar from tooth enamel. If toothpaste is applied to the teeth before flossing, fluoride can come in direct contact with tooth surfaces, aiding in cavity prevention. Flossing once a day is sufficient. Because it is important to clean all teeth surfaces thoroughly, the nurse should not rush to complete flossing. Placing a mirror in front of the client will help the nurse to demonstrate the proper methods for holding the floss and cleaning between the teeth.

Fluoride Use. Even though fluoride has not been proven to eliminate tooth decay, it is known to prevent dental caries (Whaley and Wong, 1991). People who do not have fluoridated water available can obtain fluoride in the form of mouthwash, toothpaste, or supplements. Fluoride supplements can be given to children beginning at 2 weeks of age. The family dentist should be consulted concerning the amount of fluoride to be given. Excessive fluoridation can result in discolored tooth enamel.

Denture Care. Dentures should be cleansed as often as natural teeth to prevent gingival irritation and infection (Procedure 30-8). Clients can be particular about the type of dentifrice or soaking solution they use. The nurse should always store dentures in an enclosed, labeled cup during soaking or when the dentures are not being worn.

Health Promotion/Restoration Activities

To encourage health promotion and restoration, the nurse should instruct clients to brush their teeth after each meal and before bedtime and to floss once daily. Clients should also reduce their intake of carbohydrates, especially sweet snacks. Acidic fruits in the client's diet can reduce plaque formation. All clients should visit a dentist regularly every 6 months for check-ups.

procedure 30-8

CLEANING DENTURES

Steps	Rationale
1. Ask client if dentures are loose and if there is tenderness or irritation of gum or mucous membrane. After dentures are removed, nurse should inspect oral cavity and denture surfaces.	Ill-fitting dentures rub against gums and mucous membranes. Area of irritation may require special care.
2. Explain procedure to client and assure that individual preferences will be used (when appropriate).	Promotes understanding and cooperation.
3. Prepare necessary equipment and supplies:	
a. Soft-bristled toothbrush	Used to brush gums and tongue.
b. Denture toothbrush	
c. Emesis basin or sink	
d. Denture dentifrice or toothpaste	
e. Water glasses (for warm and cool water)	
f. Single 4 × 4 gauze	Used to remove dentures.
g. Washcloth	
h. Plastic denture cup	
i. Disposable gloves	Prevents contact with microorganisms in saliva.
4. Wash hands.	Reduces transmission of microorganisms.
5. Arrange supplies on bedside table or near sink.	Ensures smooth, organized procedure.
6. Pour emesis basin half full with tepid water or place washcloth in sink and run water until it is approximately 1 in deep.	Water aids in distribution of dentifrice over denture surfaces. Cloth protects dentures against breakage. Hot water can cause warping or softening of dentures.
7. Don disposable gloves.	Reduces transmission of infection.
8. Ask client to remove dentures and place them in emesis basin. If client is unable to remove dentures, grasp upper plate at front with thumb and index finger wrapped in gauze. Use steady downward pull. Gently lift lower denture from jaw and rotate one side downward to remove from mouth. Place dentures in emesis basin.	Gauze prevents accidental slipping while handling dentures. Rotating denture at angle reduces pulling of lips during removal.
9. Apply dentifrice to denture and brush surfaces of dentures (see illustrations). Hold dentures close to water. Hold brush horizontally and use back-and-forth motion to cleanse biting surfaces. Hold brush horizontally and use short strokes from top of denture to biting surfaces of teeth to clean outer tooth surface. Hold brush vertically and use short strokes to clean inner tooth surfaces. Hold brush horizontally and use back-and-forth motion to clean undersurface of dentures.	Cleansing prevents food and bacteria from collecting on denture surfaces and prevents odor and stain buildup. Holding dentures close to water reduces chance of breakage because water will break fall if dentures slip.

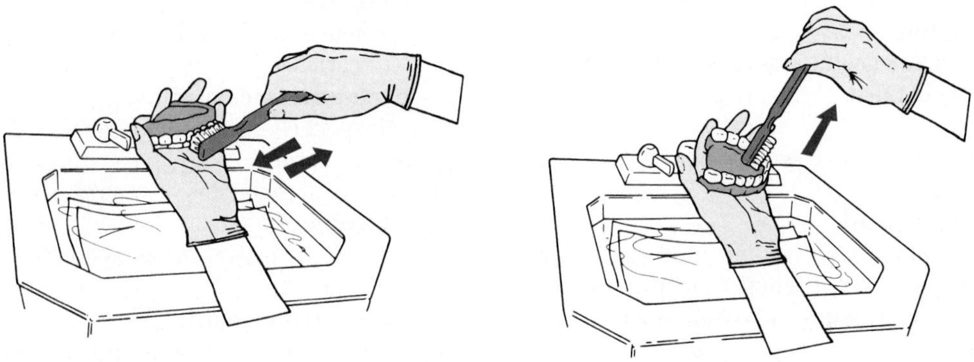

Step 9

Continued.

procedure 30-8—cont'd

Steps	Rationale
10. Rinse dentures thoroughly in tepid water.	Warm water dilutes and rinses dentifrice more effectively than cool water.
11. Return dentures to client or store in tepid water in denture cup.	Protects dentures from breakage. Tepid water keeps dentures well moistened to make insertion easier; plastic dentures become brittle and warp if not kept moist.
12. Empty emesis basin and add fresh cool water. Apply toothpaste to soft toothbrush and gently brush client's gums, palate, and tongue.	Helps to stimulate circulation to gums and removes residual film of debris on gums and mucosa.
13. Have client rinse mouth thoroughly.	Removes all food particles and secretions.
14. Reinsert dentures if client desires or allow client to do so. Begin by gently inserting moistened upper denture. Have client use finger to press denture firmly in place, then insert moistened lower denture.	Bulkier upper denture is easier to insert first when client has upper and lower plates. Moistening lubricates denture for easier insertion. Applying gentle pressure to upper denture seals it against palate.
15. Dispose of gloves in proper receptacle. Clean and store supplies. Wash hands.	Controls spread of infection.
16. Ask client if dentures feel comfortable.	Removes sources of irritation.
17. Record procedure on flow sheet or nurses' notes.	Maintains accuracy of client's record.

Evaluation

The expected outcomes of oral hygiene may not be seen for several days. Repeated cleansing is often needed to remove thick encrustations on the tongue and to restore the mucosa's normal hydration. The nurse evaluates the success of interventions to maintain mucosa integrity or to prevent further injury to the oral mucosa. The care plan is designed to be changed when the client's condition changes. If interventions are not successful, the nurse may have to initiate more aggressive actions. For instance, it will take weeks of rigorous hygiene to reduce the incidence of dental caries. The following goals, outcomes, and corresponding evaluative measures apply to clients requring oral hygiene.

Goal: Client maintains an intact, well-hydrated oral mucosa free of odor.

Outcome

Client's oral mucosa will be moist, pink, and odor free

Evaluative measure

Inspect client's lips and oral mucosa (tongue, gums, and floor of mouth) for ulcers or dryness. Note presence of broken teeth

Outcome

Client consumes at least 3 liters of liquids daily

Evaluative measure

Measure client's intake for 24 hours over 7 days

Goal: Client's oral mucosa is free of infection and dental caries.

Outcome

Client chews food without discomfort

Evaluative measure

Ask client about dental or localized areas of pain

Outcome

Client's mucosa membranes have no localized redness or swelling

Evaluative measure

Inspect oral mucosa for ulcers, swelling, or redness. Note presence of odor

Outcome

Client's teeth will have no plaque, tartar, or caries

Evaluative measure

Inspect client's teeth for increased plaque, tartar, or caries

Goal: Client maintains or improves comfort level.

Outcome

Client verbalizes sense of comfort following oral care

Evaluative measure

Ask client after brushing to describe level of comfort or signs of discomfort

Outcome
Client denies mouth pain
Evaluative measure
Observe client's nonverbal behavior for signs of discomfort

Goal: Client assumes oral hygiene care daily.
Outcome
Client describes oral hygiene practices
Evaluative measure
Ask client to explain oral hygiene practices
Outcome
Client demonstrates correct oral hygiene techniques
Evaluative measure
Observe client brushing and flossing teeth

HAIR CARE

A person's appearance and feeling of well-being often depend on the way the hair looks and feels. Illness or disability may prevent a client from maintaining daily hair care. An immobilized client's hair soon becomes tangled. Dressings may leave sticky blood or antiseptic solutions on the hair. Proper hair care is important to the client's body image. Brushing, combing, and shampooing are basic hygiene measures for all clients. Clients should be permitted to shave when their condition allows.

Hair growth, distribution, and pattern can indicate general health status (see Chapter 16). Hormonal changes, emotional and physical stress, aging, infection, and certain diseases can affect hair characteristics. The hair shaft is an inert structure. Changes in its color or condition result from hormonal activity and nutrient supply to the follicle. Table 30-5 describes common hair and scalp problems and nursing interventions.

ASSESSMENT OF HAIR CARE

PHYSICAL CHANGES

Assess condition of hair and scalp (Chapter 16). Consider age-appropriate changes.
Consider racial or ethnic differences
Determine reasons for change in distribution or loss of hair.
Check oiliness and texture of hair.
Inspect scalp for lesions, inflammation, infection, or parasites.

SELF-CARE ABILITY

Assess client's ability to grasp comb or brush.
Determine client's ability to physically care for hair.
Does client become easily fatigued?

HAIR-CARE PRACTICES

Assess client's preferences in hair styling.
Identify client's preferences for hair care and shaving products.
Assess adequacy of client's hygiene practices.
Determine client's perceptions of own appearance.
Assess client's socioeconomic background.

NURSING PROCESS

Assessment

Before performing hair care, the nurse must assess the condition of the hair and scalp (see box below, left). Findings will reveal the frequency and extent of care needed. A client's self-care ability can be altered by conditions such as arthritis, fatigue, and the presence of physical encumberences (e.g., cast or IV). The nurse assesses the client's physical ability to perform hair care. It is also essential to consider a client's personal hair care practices so every effort can be made to maintain the client's preferred appearance.

Nursing Diagnosis

Assessment of the hair and scalp indicates the client's need for and ability to maintain personal grooming. Conditions of the hair and scalp may reveal findings such as coarse or silky hair, or the presence or absence of secretions, lacerations, or infestations. The nurse reviews and clusters all defining characteristics to select appropriate nursing diagnoses (see box below). The diagnoses may focus primarily on grooming and comfort.

NURSING DIAGNOSES FOR HAIR AND SCALP CARE

Dressing/grooming self-care deficit
Impaired skin integrity
Pain
Body-image disturbance
High risk for infection

table 30-5
HAIR AND SCALP PROBLEMS

Problem	Characteristics	Implications	Interventions
Dandruff	Scaling of scalp accompanied by itching; in severe cases, dandruff on eyebrows	Dandruff causes embarrassment. If dandruff enters eyes, conjunctivitis may develop.	Shampoo regularly with medicated shampoo. In severe cases physician's advice may be needed.
Ticks	Small gray-brown parasites that burrow into skin and suck blood	Ticks transmit several diseases to people. Most common are Rocky Mountain spotted fever, tularemia, and Lyme disease.	Do not pull ticks from skin because sucking apparatus remains and may become infected. Placing drop of oil or ether on tick or covering it with petrolatum jelly eases removal. Oil suffocates tick.
Hair loss (alopecia)	Occurs in all races, mostly in women; balding patches seen in periphery of hairline; hair becomes brittle and broken; causes are use of hair curlers, picks, tight braiding, and hot comb.	Patches of uneven hair growth and loss alter client's appearance.	Stop hair-care practices that damage hair.
Pediculosis (lice)	Tiny, grayish white parasite insects that infest mammals		
Pediculosis capitis (head lice)	Found on scalp attached to hair strands; eggs look like oval particles, similar to dandruff; bites or pustules may be observed behind ears and at hairline	Head lice are difficult to remove and may spread to furniture and other people if not treated.	Shampoo with Kwell shampoo and repeat 12 to 24 hours later. Change bed linens.
Pediculosis corporis (body lice)	Tend to cling to clothing so may not be easily seen; suck blood and lay eggs on clothing and furniture	Client itches constantly. Scratches seen on skin may become infected. Hemorrhagic spots may appear on skin where lice suck blood.	Client should bathe or shower thoroughly. After skin is dried, Kwell lotion should be applied. After 12 to 24 hours another bath or shower should be taken. Bag infested clothing or linen until laundered.
Pediculosis pubis (crab lice)	Found in pubic hair; are grayish white with red legs	Lice may spread through bed linen, clothing, or furniture or between persons via sexual contact.	Shave hair off affected area. Cleanse as for body lice. If lice were sexually transmitted, partner must be notified.

However, when abnormalities of the scalp are identified, nursing diagnoses focus on scalp integrity.

Selecting appropriate related factors influences the nurse's care plan. For the diagnosis "impaired skin integrity related to parasite infestation" the nurse must design actions to remove the infestation. Shampooing and showering with special products, isolating all linens, and client teaching are good measures. The diagnosis "impaired skin integrity related to scalp laceration" will require measures to promote healing. Maintaining an intact suture line, preventing infection, and removing secretions may be necessary. Nursing interventions are designed to meet actual alterations or alterations a client may be at risk of developing.

Planning

Good hair-care practices must be performed routinely to meet the client's hygiene needs. The nurse should remember the client is aware of appearance at all times. Therefore an effective plan allows the client to initiate and participate in hygiene measures. Goals for clients in need of hair and scalp care include the following:

Goal: Client's hair and scalp will be clean and healthy.

Outcomes

Client's hair and scalp will be free of excess oil, secretions, and matting

Client verbalizes that hair feels clean

Goal: Client achieves a sense of comfort and self-esteem.

Outcomes

Client expresses positive feelings about appearance

Client requests hair to be groomed in a specific way

Goal: Client will participate in hair care practices.

Outcomes

Client grooms hair with assistance

Client shampoos hair independently

Implementation

Brushing and Combing. Frequent brushing helps to keep hair clean and distributes oil evenly along hair shafts. Combing prevents hair from tangling. The client should be encouraged to maintain routine hair care. However, clients with limited mobility and poor coordination and those who are confused or seriously weakened by illness require help. Clients in a hospital or extended care facility appreciate the opportunity to have their hair brushed and combed before being seen by others.

Long hair can easily become matted after a client is confined to bed, even for a short period. When lacerations or incisions involve the scalp, blood and topical medications can also cause tangling. Frequent brushing and combing keeps long hair neatly groomed. Braiding can help to avoid repeated tangles. The nurse asks permission before braiding a client's hair.

To brush hair the nurse parts the hair into two sections and separates each into two more sections. It is easier to brush smaller sections of hair. Brushing from the scalp towards the hair ends minimizes pulling. Moistening the hair with water or alcohol frees tangles for easier combing. The nurse never cuts a client's hair without written consent.

Shampooing. Frequency of shampooing depends on a client's daily routines. The nurse should remind hospitalized clients that staying in bed, excess perspiration, or treatments that leave blood or solutions in the hair may require more frequent shampooing. For clients at home the nurse's greatest challenge may be to find ways the client can shampoo the hair without injury.

If the client is able to take a shower or bath, the hair can usually be shampooed without difficulty. A shower chair may be used for the ambulatory client who becomes tired or faint. Handheld shower nozzles allow clients to wash the hair during a tub bath or shower. Clients allowed to sit in a chair can usually be shampooed in front of a sink. If the client is forced to sit at the bedside, the hair can be shampooed as the client leans forward over a washbasin.

If a client is unable to sit but can be moved, the nurse may transfer the client to a stretcher for transportation to a sink or shower equipped with a handheld nozzle. The nurse places a towel or small pillow under the client's head and neck, allowing the head to hang slightly over the stretcher's edge. Caution is needed with clients with neck injuries because hyperextension of the neck could cause further injury.

If the client is unable to sit in a chair or be transferred to a stretcher, shampooing must be done with the client in bed. Many institutions require a physician's order for the procedure (Procedure 30-9).

The hair of African Americans has a natural tendency to be dry. Normally, daily shampooing is unnecessary. The nurse asks the client how often shampooing is preferred. Similarly, clients' hair becomes drier and more brittle with advancing age. Frequently, older adults will shampoo only once a week.

Shaving. Shaving facial hair can be done after the bath or shampoo. Women may prefer to shave their legs or axillae while bathing. When assisting a client, the nurse should take care to avoid cutting the client with razor blades. Clients prone to bleeding (e.g., those receiving anticoagulants or high doses of aspirin) should use an electric razor. Before using an electric razor, the nurse should check for electrical hazards.

When a razor blade is used for shaving, the skin must be softened to prevent pulling, scraping, or cuts. For example, placing a warm washcloth over the male client's face for a few seconds, followed by application of shaving cream or a lathering of mild soap, softens the skin. If the client is unable to shave, the nurse may perform the shave. To avoid causing discomfort or razor cuts, the nurse gently pulls the skin taut and uses short, firm razor strokes in the direction the hair grows. Short downward strokes work best to remove hair over the upper lip. A client usually can explain to the nurse the best way to move the razor across the skin.

procedure 30-9

SHAMPOOING HAIR IN BED

Steps	Rationale
1. Determine if any risks exist that might contraindicate shampooing or positioning.	Some medical conditions (e.g., cervical neck injuries, open incisions, or tracheostomy) may place client at risk of injury because of positioning, exposure to moisture, or manipulation of scalp.
2. Review physician's orders to determine if medicated shampoo is ordered.	For conditions such as lice or dandruff, special shampoos may be ordered.
3. Explain procedure to client.	Client may be anxious about positioning or risk of water entering eyes.
4. Prepare necessary equipment and supplies:	
a. Two bath towels	
b. Face towel or washcloth	
c. Shampoo (hair conditioner and cream rinse optional)	Conditioner reduces tangles.
d. Water pitcher	Used to pour water over hair.
e. Plastic shampoo trough	Diverts water to basin to prevent soiling bed linen.
f. Washbasin	
g. Bath blanket	
h. Waterproof pad	
i. Clean comb and brush	
j. Hair dryer	
k. Bottle of hydrogen perioxide (optional)	Cleans hair matted with blood.
l. Disposable gloves (optional)	
5. Wash hands. (Apply gloves if scalp lacerations or lesions are present.)	Reduces transmission of microorganisms.
6. Arrange equipment in convenient place and lower side rail.	Prevents interruptions.
7. Place waterproof pad under shoulders, neck, and head. Position client supine with head and shoulders at top edge of bed. Place plastic trough under head and washbasin at end of trough, being sure trough spout extends beyond edge of mattress.	Prevents soiling of bed linen.
8. Place rolled towel under neck and bath towel across shoulders.	Minimizes water draining down back of neck.
9. Brush and comb client's hair.	Removing tangles results in more thorough cleansing.
10. Obtain warm water. Clients usually prefer warm water to avoid chilling. Check temperature by placing small amount of water on inner aspect of nurse's forearm.	Prevents burns to face and scalp.
11. Ask client to hold face towel or washcloth over eyes.	Prevents shampoo or water from entering eyes.
12. With water pitcher, slowly pour water over hair until it is completely wet. Apply small amount of shampoo.	Water aids in distribution of shampoo suds over hair.
13. Work up lather with both hands. Start at hairline and work toward back of neck. Life head slightly with one hand to wash back of head. Shampoo sides of head. Massage scalp by applying pressure with fingertips.	Systematic progression over hair and scalp ensures thorough cleansing. Massage increases scalp circulation. Use of fingernails during massage can cause scratching of scalp.
14. Rinse hair with water. Make sure water drains into basin. Repeat rinsing until hair is free of soap. To speed drainage from trough, press down on its spout.	Retained soap leaves dull finish on hair. Dried soap may cause scalp irritation.
15. Repeat Steps 12 to 14.	Ensures thorough cleansing.
16. Apply conditioner or rinse if requested and rinse hair thoroughly.	Conditioner prevents excess drying. Cream rinse makes combing and brushing easier.

Steps	Rationale
17. Wrap head in bath towel. Dry face with cloth used to protect eyes. Dry moisture on neck or shoulders.	If client is ill, retained moisture may cause cooling and chills.
18. Dry client's hair and scalp. Use second towel if first becomes saturated.	
19. Comb hair to remove tangles and dry with dryer or remaining towel as quickly as possible.	Drying prevents chilling.
20. Assist client to comfortable position and complete styling of hair.	Promotes sense of well-being.
21. Return equipment to its proper place. Discard soiled linen in linen hamper. Wash hands.	Maintains cleanliness of environment and controls transmission of infection.
22. Ask client how the hair feels.	Client will experience sense of cleanliness after shampooing.
23. Inspect condition of hair.	Shampooing should leave hair in clean condition.
24. Record procedure and any pertinent findings related to condition of hair or scalp.	Documents response to therapy and condition of hair or scalp in case further treatment is necessary.

Mustache and Beard Care. Clients with mustaches or beards require daily grooming. Keeping these areas clean is important, because food particles and mucus can easily collect in the hair. If the client is unable to carry out self-care, the nurse should do so at the client's request. The nurse never shaves off a mustache or beard without the client's consent.

Health Promotion/Restoration Activities

To best promote and restore hair and scalp health, clients should be instructed to keep hair clean, combed, and brushed regularly. Clients may also need to know how to check for and remove parasites. The nurse should tell clients they need to notify the primary health care provider of changes in the texture and distribution of hair.

Evaluative Measures

Evaluative measures for care of a client's hair are dynamic and change as the client's condition changes. As the care plan is being developed, the nurse must always be prepared to make necessary changes. For example, if the client becomes unable to provide care because of immobility, the nurse initiates and maintains good hair grooming techniques until the client or family is able to do so. Evaluative measures include:

Goal: Client's hair and scalp will be clean and healthy.

Outcome
Client's hair and scalp will be free of excess oil, secretions, and matting
Evaluative measure
Inspect client's hair and scalp for excess oil and matting
Outcome
Client verbalizes hair feels clean
Evaluative measure
Ask client whether hair feels clean

Goal: Client achieves a sense of comfort and self-esteem.

Outcome
Client expresses positive feelings about appearance
Evaluative measure
Observe client's behavior regarding appearance, noting posture, reference to own appearance, willingness to be seen by others
Outcome
Client requests hair to be groomed in a specific way
Evaluative measure
Ask client about preferences in hair style

Goal: Client will participate in hair care practices.

Outcomes
Client grooms hair with assistance
Client shampoos hair independently
Evaluative measure
Observe client grooming hair. Check during home visits if shampooing done regularly

CARE OF THE EYES, EARS, AND NOSE

Special attention is given to cleansing the eyes, ears, and nose during the client's bath. Care focuses on preventing infection and maintaining normal organ function.

Eyes

Normally no special care is required for the eyes because they are continually cleansed by tears and the eyelids and lashes prevent entrance of foreign particles. Unconscious clients are at risk for eye injury because of reduced lacrimation and blink reflex. Excessive drainage frequently collects along eyelid margins. Special attention is also needed for clients who have had eye surgery or who have conjunctivitis or external eye irritation resulting from increased discharge or drainage.

Ears

Hygiene of the ears affects hearing acuity only when wax or foreign substances collect in the external ear canal and interfere with sound conduction. The nurse should assess for any behavioral cues that might indicate a hearing impairment (see Chapter 38). When caring for a client with a hearing aid, the nurse must use communication techniques that promote hearing the spoken word.

Nose

The nose provides for the sense of smell but also controls the temperature and humidity of inhaled air and prevents foreign particles from entering the respiratory system. Crusted secretions within the nares can impair sensation and breathing. Irritation of nasal mucosa can cause swelling, leading to obstruction. Hygiene care of the nose is typically simple, but clients with nasogastric, enteral feeding, or endotracheal tubes that enter the nose may require special attention.

NURSING PROCESS

Assessment

Physical Assessment. The nurse carefully inspects all external eye structures (see Chapter 16). Normally the conjunctivae are clear and not inflamed. The eyelid margins are in close approximation with the eyeball, and the lashes are turned outward. The lid margins are normally without inflammation, drainage, or lesions. Flaking skin around the eyebrows may indicate dandruff.

Assessment of the external ear structures includes inspecting the auricle, external ear canal, and tympanic membrane (see Chapter 16). When performing hygiene, the nurse is most concerned with presence of accumulated cerumen or drainage in the ear canal, local inflammation, or pain.

The nurse inspects the nares for signs of inflammation, discharge, lesions, edema, and deformity (see Chapter 16). The nasal mucosa is normally pink, clear, and without discharge. For clients with any form of tubing exiting the nose, the nurse should check for tissue sloughing, localized tenderness, inflammation, and even bleeding.

Use of Sensory Aids. For clients who wear eyeglasses, contact lenses, artificial eyes, or hearing aids, the nurse assesses the client's knowledge and methods used to care for the aids, as well as any problems caused by them (see box above). The nurse's findings may indicate a need for client education.

Self-Care Ability. The nurse assesses a client's physical ability to perform eye, ear, and nose care, as well as care of any sensory aids. Clients who are unable to grasp small objects, have limited upper extremity mobility, have reduced vision, or are seriously fatigued require assistance.

ASSESSING CLIENT'S USE OF SENSORY AIDS

- Eyeglasses
  - Purpose for wearing
  - Cleansing method
- Contact lenses
  - Type of lens worn
  - Frequency and duration of time lenses are worn
  - Cleansing and storage techniques (including type of solutions used)
  - Use of eyedrops or ointments
- Artificial eye
  - Method for insertion and removal
  - Cleansing method
- Hearing aid
  - Type of aid worn
  - Cleansing method
  - Client's ability to change battery and adjust aid volume

Nursing Diagnosis

The nurse's assessment may reveal an actual alteration in the function of sensory organs, a problem in the cli-

NURSING DIAGNOSES FOR EYE, EAR, OR NOSE PROBLEMS

Bathing/hygiene self-care deficit
Knowledge deficit regarding personal hygiene
Pain
High risk for infection
Sensory/perceptual alterations (visual, auditory, or olfactory)

ent's ability to perform personal hygiene, or a deficit in the client's understanding of how to perform hygiene. Clustering defining characteristics such as physical limitation, visual impairment, or irritation of the eyes, ears, or nares help the nurse to form accurate nursing diagnoses (see box above).

Each nursing diagnosis requires a series of nursing interventions to meet the client's needs. The interventions are selected based on diagnostic related factors and the goals established for the client's care. When the client is at risk for developing a problem, the care plan is designed to prevent its occurrence. The nurse also seeks to eliminate any problem that could cause serious injury to the ear, eye, or nose.

Planning

The client's personal preference and habits are considered when the nurse plans hygienic care. When bathing a client, the nurse uses extra care to avoid injury to the eyes, ears, or nose. These areas are sensitive to irritating or painful stimuli. Children and older adult clients are especially susceptible. In the home environment, family members or friends should be familiar with a client's hygiene routines. Sensory aids must be clean and functional for the client to interact within the environment. The goals of care for clients requiring eye, ear, or nose care include the following:

Goal: Client's eyes, ears, or nose will be free of infection.

Outcome

Client's eyes, ears, or nose have no redness, discharge, or pain

Goal: Client will have normal sensory organ function.

Outcomes

Client's vision, hearing, or smell will be intact

Client maintains orientation to person, place, and time

Goal: Client performs daily care for the eyes, ears, and nose.

Outcomes

Client explains methods of cleaning the eyes, ears, or nose

Client explains care of adaptive aids (hearing aids)

Client demonstrates care of adaptive aids

Client demonstrates appropriate methods for cleaning eyes, ears, or nose

Implementation

Basic Eye Care. Cleansing the eyes simply involves washing with a clean washcloth moistened in water. Soap may cause burning and irritation (see Procedure 30-1). Direct pressure should never be applied over the eyeball because it may cause serious injury.

The unconscious client may require more frequent eye care. Secretions may collect along the lid margins and inner canthus when the blink reflex is absent or when the eye does not totally close. It may be necessary to place an eye patch over the involved eye to prevent corneal drying and irritation. Lubricating eye drops may be given according to physician's orders.

Eyeglasses. Glasses are made of hardened glass or plastic that is impact resistant to prevent shattering. Nevertheless, because of the cost, the nurse should be careful when cleaning glasses and should protect them from breakage or other damage when they are not worn. Glasses should be put in a case and in a drawer of the bedside table when not in use.

Warm water is sufficient for cleaning glass lenses. A soft cloth is best for drying to prevent scratching the lens. Plastic lenses in particular are scratched easily, and special cleansing solutions and drying tissues are available.

Contact Lenses. A contact lens is a small, round, sometimes colored disk that fits over the cornea of the eye. Rigid lenses are relatively easy to clean and handle and are durable and optically precise. Soft lenses are more comfortable but are less durable because they are thin and pliable and tear easily. Although soft lenses and the newer rigid lenses are gas permeable, all lenses still restrict flow of oxygen to the eye's surface. Consequently, all lenses must be periodically removed to prevent eye infection and corneal abrasions and ulcers. Rigid and daily wear soft lenses should not be worn longer than 12 to 14 hours. Extended-wear soft lenses should not be left in place longer than 1 week (Egan, et al., 1988). Clients who cannot remove their own lenses require assistance. Care includes cleaning, proper application and removal, and storage (Procedure 30-10).

Text continued on p. 852.

procedure 30-10

TAKING CARE OF CONTACT LENSES

Steps	Rationale
1. Assess client's ability to manipulate and hold contact lens.	Determines level of assistance required in care.
2. After lenses are removed, inspect eye for signs of corneal irritation.	Signs of corneal irritation may require client to refrain from contact use.
3. Prepare equipment and supplies for removal of lenses:	
a. Contact lens storage container	Separate cups labeled *R* for right lens and *L* for left lens hold lenses and protect them from breakage.
b. Suction cup (optional)	Used to remove hard lenses from unconscious, debilitated, or confused clients.
c. Sterile saline solution	Used to moisten cornea before lens removal.
d. Bath towel	
4. Prepare equipment and supplies for cleansing and insertion:	
a. Lenses in storage container	
b. Thermal disinfecting kit (optional)	Heats up to 80° C (176° F) to sterilize soft lenses.
c. Surfactant cleaner	
d. Rinsing solution	
e. Sterile lens disinfectant and/or enzyme solution (see illustration)	Cleans lens surfaces and reduces number of microorganisms present.
f. Sterile wetting solution for hard lenses	Allows lens to glide easily over cornea during insertion.
g. Cotton ball or cotton-tipped applicator	Used to spread lens cleaner over surface of hard lens.
h. Bath towel	
i. Emesis basin	
j. Glass of warm tap water	
5. Discuss procedure with client.	Client can assist in planning by explaining technique he or she feels may aid in removal and insertion. Client may be anxious as nurse retracts lids and manipulates lenses.
6. Have client assume supine or sitting position in bed or chair.	Provides easy access while retracting eyelids and manipulating lens.
REMOVING SOFT LENSES	
1. Wash hands.	Prevents transmission of microorganisms.
2. Place towel just below client's face.	Catches lens if it accidentally falls from eye.
3. Add few drops of sterile saline to eye.	Lubricates eye to facilitate lens removal.

Step 4e

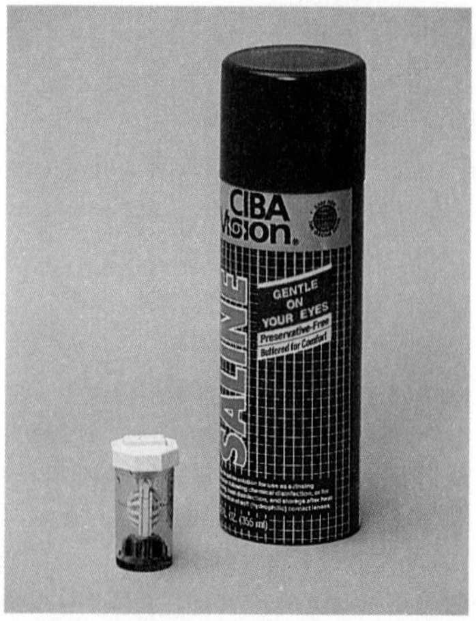

Steps	Rationale
4. Tell client to look straight ahead.	Eases tipping of lens during removal.
5. Using middle finger, retract lower eyelid.	Exposes lower edge of lens.
6. With pad of index finger of same hand, slide lens off cornea onto white of eye.	Prevents injury to cornea and damage to lens. Positions lens for easy grasping.
7. Pull upper eyelid down gently with thumb of other hand and compress lens slightly between thumb and index finger.	Causes soft lens to double up. Air enters underneath lens to release suction.
8. Gently pinch lens and lift out.	Protects lens from damage. Prevents lens edges from sticking together.
9. If lens sticks together, place it in palm and soak thoroughly with sterile saline. Gently roll lens with index finger in back-and-forth motion. If gentle rubbing does not separate lens edges, soak in sterile solution.	Assists in returning lens to normal shape.
10. Clean and rinse lens (see section on cleansing and disinfecting contact lenses). Place lens in proper storage case compartment: *R* for right lens and *L* for left. Be sure lens is centered.	Ensures proper lens will be reinserted into correct eye. Proper storage prevents cracking or tearing.
11. Repeat Steps 3 to 10 for other lens. Secure cover over storage case.	Proper storage prevents damage.
12. Dispose of towel; wash hands.	Reduces transmission of infection.
REMOVING RIGID LENSES	
1. Wash hands.	Prevents transmission of microorganisms.
2. Place towel just below face.	Catches lens if it accidently falls from eye.
3. Be sure lens is positioned directly over cornea. If it is not, have client close eyelids; place index and middle fingers of one hand behind lens. Gently but firmly massage lens back into place.	Allows for easy removal from eye.
4. Place index finger on outer corner of eye and draw skin gently back toward ear.	Tightens lids against eyeball.
5. Tell client to blink. Do not release pressure on lid until blink is completed.	Causes lens to dislodge and pop out. Lid margins must clear top and bottom of lens until blink.
6. If lens fails to pop out, gently retract eyelid beyond edges of lens. Press lower eyelid gently against lower edge of lens.	Causes upper edge of lens to tip forward.
7. Allow eyelids to close slightly and grasp lens as it rises from eye.	Causes lens to slide off easily.
8. Cup lens in hand.	Protects lens from breakage.
9. Cleanse and rinse lens (see section on cleansing and disinfecting contact lenses). Place lens in proper compartment: *R* for right and *L* for left. Center lens in storage case, convex side down.	Both lenses may not have the same prescription. Proper storage prevents cracking, tearing, or chipping.
10. Repeat Steps 3 to 9 for other lens. Secure cover over storage case.	Proper storage prevents damage.
11. Dispose of towel; wash hands.	Controls spread of infection and keeps client's environment neat.
CLEANSING AND DISINFECTING CONTACT LENSES	
1. Wash hands.	Reduces transmission of microorganisms.
2. Assemble supplies at bedside.	Provides easy access to supplies.
3. Place towel over work area.	Helps to prevent lens breakage.

Continued.

procedure 30-10—cont'd

Steps	Rationale
4. Open lens container carefully, taking care not to flip lens caps open suddenly.	Prevents lenses from being accidentally spilled or flipped out of case.
5. On removal of lens from eye, apply 1 to 2 drops of daily surfactant cleaner on lens in palm of hand (use cleanser recommended by lens manufacturer or eye care practitioner).	Removes tear components, including mucus, lipids, and proteins that collect on lens.
6. Rub lens gently but thoroughly on both sides for 20 to 30 sec. Use index finger (soft lenses) or little finger or cotton-tip applicator soaked with cleaner (hard lenses) to clean inside lens. Be careful not to contact or scratch lens with fingernail.	It is easier to manipulate and clean lenses using fingertips. Cleans all surfaces of microorganisms.
7. Holding lens over emesis basin, rinse thoroughly with rinsing solution recommended by manufacturer (soft lenses) or cold tap water (rigid lenses).	Prevents loss or breakage if lens are dropped.
8. Place lenses in storage case; fill with solution recommended by manufacturer or practitioner.	Disinfects lenses, removes residue, enhances wettability of lens, and prevents scratches from a dry case.

INSERTING RIGID LENSES

Steps	Rationale
1. Wash hands thoroughly with mild, noncosmetic soap. Rinse well; dry with clean, lint-free towel or paper towel.	Lint or film on hands from soaps containing perfumes, deodorants, or complexion creams can be transferred to lens and cause eye irritation.
2. Place towel over chest.	Catches dropped lens and avoids breakage.
3. Remove right lens from storage case; attempt to lift lens straight up.	Sliding lens out can cause scratches.
4. Rinse with cold tap water.	Hot water causes lens to warp.
5. Wet lens on both sides using prescribed wetting solution.	Lubricates lens so that it slides easily over and adheres to cornea.
6. Place right lens concave side up on tip of index finger of dominant hand.	Ensures easy insertion. Inner surface of lens should face up so that it is applied against cornea.
7. Instruct client to look straight ahead while retracting upper and lower eyelids; place lens gently over center of cornea.	Hard lens is rigid and can be placed as client looks straight ahead. Retraction of lids promotes easy insertion between lid margins.
8. Ask client to close eyes briefly and avoid blinking.	Helps to secure position of lens.
9. Be sure lens is centered properly by asking client if vision is blurred.	If lens slips to side of cornea or into conjunctival sac, vision will blur.
10. Repeat Steps 3 to 9 for left eye.	
11. Assist client to comfortable position.	
12. Discard soiled supplies. Discard solution in storage case; rinse case thoroughly and allow to air dry. Wash hands.	Use fresh solution daily. Prevents infection.

INSERTING SOFT LENSES

Steps	Rationale
1. Wash hands with mild, noncosmetic soap. Rinse well; dry with clean, lint-free or paper towel.	Lint or film left on hands from cosmetic or deodorant soaps can be transferred to lens and irritate the eye.
2. Place towel over chest.	Catches lens to avoid scratching or tearing.
3. Remove right lens from storage case and rinse with recommended solution (see illustration). Inspect lens for foreign materials, tears, or other damage.	Removes disinfectant solution. Prevents irritation or damage to eye.
4. Check to be sure lens is not inverted (inside out).	Soft lens is inverted if bowl has lip; it is in the correct position if curve is even from base to rim.

Steps	Rationale
5. Using middle or index finger of opposite hand, retract upper lid until iris is exposed.	Soft lenses do not adhere as easily as hard lenses. Separating lids as much as possible allows room for lens to contact cornea without touching lids or lashes.
6. Use middle finger or hand holding lens to pull down lower lid.	
7. Tell client to look straight ahead and "through" the lens and finger. Gently place lens directly on cornea. Release lens slowly, starting with lower lid (see illustration).	Ensures secure fit and comfort.
8. If lens is on sclera rather than cornea, tell client to slowly close eye and roll it toward lens.	Centers soft lens over cornea.
9. Tell client to blink.	Ensures that lens is centered, free of trapped air, and comfortable.

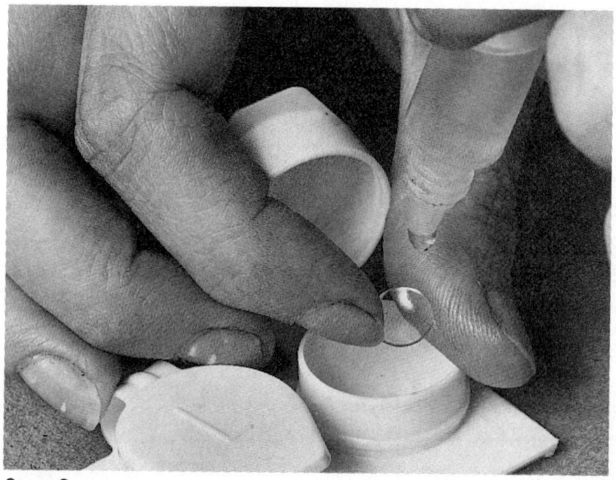

Step 3

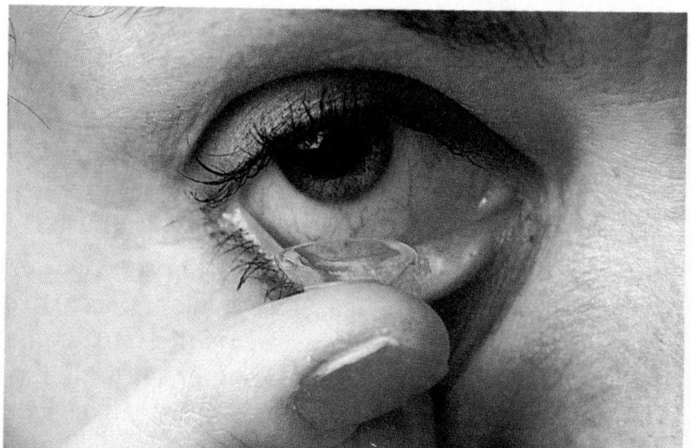

Step 7(a)

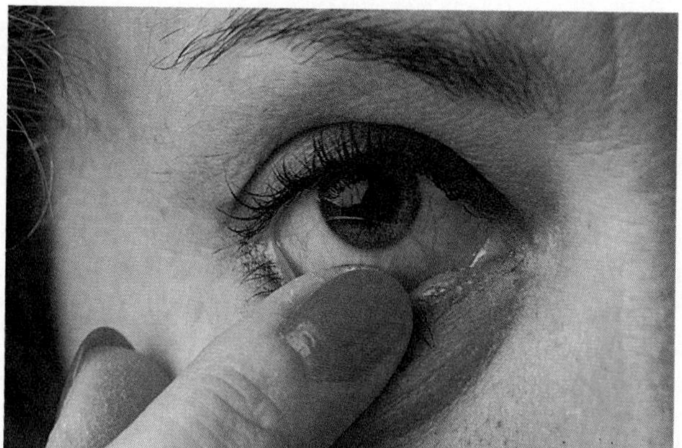

Step 7(b)

Continued.

procedure 30-10—cont'd

Steps	Rationale
10. Be sure lens is centered properly by asking client if vision is blurred.	If lens slips to side of cornea or into conjunctival sac, vision will blur.
11. If client's vision is blurred:	
a. Retract eyelids.	Repositions lens over center of cornea as client looks toward lens.
b. Locate position of lens.	
c. Ask client to look in direction opposite of lens; with index finger, apply pressure to lower eyelid margin and position lens over cornea.	
d. Have client look slowly toward lens.	
12. Repeat Steps 3 to 11 for other eye.	
13. Assist client to comfortable position.	
14. Discard soiled supplies. Discard solution in storage case; rinse case thoroughly and allow to air dry. Wash hands.	Prevents infection.

Artificial Eyes. Clients with artificial eyes have had an enucleation of an entire eyeball as a result of tumor growth, severe infection, or eye trauma. Some artificial eyes are permanently implanted. Others should be removed daily for cleansing. Clients with artificial eyes usually prefer to care for their own eyes rather than having a nurse assist them. If the client is unconscious, incapable of using the arms, or unable to move the head or neck, the nurse must assist with removing the eye.

To remove an artificial eye, the nurse retracts the lower eyelid and exerts slight pressure just below the eye. The nurse may also use a small, rubber-bulb syringe or medicine dropper bulb to create a suction. The suction created by placing the bulb tip directly over the eye and squeezing lifts the artificial eye from the socket.

The artificial eye is usually made of glass or plastic. Warm normal saline is effective for cleaning. The nurse should also clean the edges of the eye socket and surrounding tissues with saline or clean tap water. Any signs of infection should be reported immediately because bacteria can spread to the neighboring eye or underlying sinuses or brain tissue. To reinsert the eye, the nurse retracts the lower lid and gently slips the eye into the socket, fitting it neatly under the upper eyelid.

Cleaning the Ears. The nurse makes sure ear cleansing occurs as part of the complete bed bath (see Procedure 30-1). The clean end of a moistened washcloth, rotated gently into the ear canal, works best for cleaning. When cerumen is visible, gentle downward retraction at the entrance of the ear canal may cause the wax to loosen and slip out. The nurse instructs clients never to use sharp objects to cleanse the ears. Cotton-tipped applicators, which compact cerumen in the canal, should also be avoided.

Children and older adults commonly have impacted cerumen, which can be removed only by irrigation. The procedure first involves instilling 1 to 2 drops of mineral oil or other over-the-counter softeners (e.g., Debrox) in the impacted ear twice daily for 4 to 5 days (Watkins, 1984). Then the instillation of approximately 250 ml of warm water (37° C or 98.6° F) into the ear canal mechanically washes away loosened wax.

Hearing Aids. Chapter 38 discusses the need for and use of hearing aids. The nurse must remember to clean the earpieces daily with mild soap and water. Cleansing prevents the buildup of wax and other debris that could interfere with sound amplification. Batteries should be checked to maintain proper working order.

There are four basic types of hearing aids. One is the behind- the-ear hearing aid, shaped like a shrimp, which fits around and behind the ear. It is the most common hearing aid (Figure 30-1, *A*). Another is the in-the-ear hearing aid (Figure 30-1, *B*), which is a small device that fits in the external auditory ear. An eyeglass aid fits into the ear canal and attaches to a battery located on the arm of the eyeglass frame. Another device is the in-the-canal aid. It fits entirely in the ear canal.

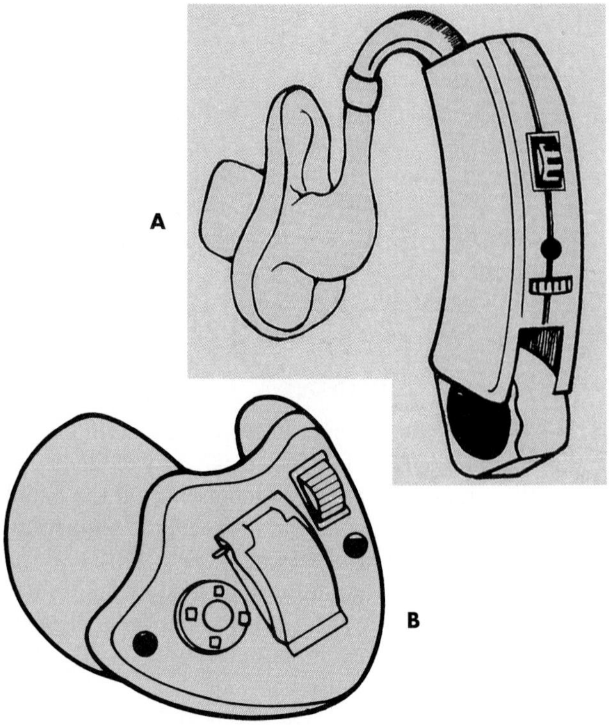

FIGURE 30-1 **A,** Behind-the-ear hearing aid. **B,** In-the-ear hearing aid.

Nose Care. The client can usually remove secretions from the nose by gently blowing into a soft tissue. The nurse cautions the client against harsh blowing that creates pressure capable of injuring the eardrum, nasal mucosa, and even sensitive eye structures. Bleeding from the nares is a key sign of harsh blowing.

If the client is unable to remove nasal secretions, the nurse assists by using a wet washcloth or a cotton-tipped applicator moistened in water or saline. The applicator should never be inserted beyond the length of the cotton tip. Excessive nasal secretions can also be removed by gentle suctioning.

When clients have tubes inserted through the nose, the nurse should change the tape anchoring the tube at least once a day. When tape becomes moist from nasal secretions, the skin and mucosa can easily become macerated. Friction causes tissue sloughing. The nurse should know how to tape tubing correctly to minimize tension or friction on the nares (see Chapter 34). When sloughing occurs, it may be necessary for the nurse to remove the tube and insert one through the other naris.

Health Promotion/Restoration Activities

To maintain optimal health, clients should be instructed in the proper methods of caring for the eyes, ears, and nose (see box upper, right). Clients with specific health concerns involving these structures should see the appropriate specialist regularly for check-ups and ongoing care. When active, clients should know the best ways of protecting these sensitive organs (e.g., eye protective devices). The older adult experiences a variety of changes in sensory function. The nurse adapts practice approaches to consider their special needs (see box above).

CLIENT TEACHING FOR EYE, EAR, AND NOSE CARE

- Encourage regular eye examinations.
- If an irritating substance enters the eye, rinse liberally with cool water for 5 to 10 minutes.
- Cleanse secretions from the lid margins without rubbing or applying pressure to the eye.
- Have client demonstrate care of any sensory adaptive aids.
- Caution against putting foreign objects in the ears and nose.
- Stress importance of daily hygiene care.

GERONTOLOGIC NURSING PRACTICE

- Although health promotion increases longevity and improves quality of life, older adults have been neglected (Pascucci, 1992); encourage appropriate protection and care of the senses.
- Maintaining and improving eyesight is an important aspect of an independent and satisfying life for older adults. The nurse:
  Encourages regular eye exams
  Discusses vision changes that occur naturally with aging
  Describes signs and symptoms of major eye diseases associated with aging
- 25% to 40% of people 65 years of age and older are hearing impaired (Ney, 1993); speak slowly and articulate carefully. However, do not shout and do not assume that *all* older clients have difficulty hearing.
- Ear wax tends to be drier in older people, impacts more easily, and takes longer to soften. Complaints of feeling of fullness, itching or ringing, and "blocked hearing" warrants regular assessment (Mahoney, 1993).

Evaluative Measures

Evaluation of eye, ear, and nose care must be based on the client's existing sensory function and the expected outcomes for the care plan's goals. Hygienic care alone will not improve sensory function beyond a client's baseline level. The evaluation process is ongoing. The nurse revises the care plan when the client's needs change. For example, if the client's hearing is altered because of a faulty hearing aid, the nurse may need to seek advice from other health care providers to correct the problem. Evaluative measures include:

Goal: Client's eyes, ears, or nose will be free of infection.

Outcome

Client's eyes, ears, or nose will have no redness, discharge, or pain

Evaluative measure

Inspect client's eyes, ears, or nose for redness, pain, or discharge

Goal: Client will have normal sensory organ function.

Outcome

Client's vision, hearing, or smell will be intact

Evaluative measures

Ask client about any perceived change in sight, hearing, or smell

Assess client's eyes, ears, and nose for objective changes in function (visual and hearing acuity, ability to identify aromas)

Outcome

Client maintains orientation to person, place, and time

Evaluative measure

Ask client to identify name, time of day, and place

Goal: Client performs daily care for the eyes, ears, and nose.

Outcome

Client explains methods of cleaning the eyes, ears, or nose

Evaluative measure

Ask client to describe methods of cleaning the eyes, ears, or nose

Outcome

Client explains care of adaptive aids

Evaluative measure

Ask client to describe the daily care of adaptive aids (contact lenses or hearing aids)

Outcome

Client demonstrates care of adaptive aids

Evaluative measure

Observe client clean adaptive aids

Outcome

Client demonstrates appropriate methods for cleaning eyes, ears, and nose

Evaluative measure

Observe client cleanse eye, ear, and nose during bathing

CLIENT'S ROOM ENVIRONMENT

Attempting to make a client's room as comfortable as the home is one of the nurse's priorities. The client's room should be comfortable, safe, and large enough to allow the client and visitors to move about freely. The nurse can control room temperature, ventilation, noise, and odors to create a more comfortable environment. Keeping the room neat and orderly also contributes to the client's sense of well-being.

Maintaining Comfort

The nature of what constitutes a comfortable environment depends on the client's age, severity of illness, and level of normal daily activity. Depending on the client's age and physical condition, the room temperature should be maintained between 20° and 23° C (68° and 74° F). Infants, older adults, and the acutely ill may need a warmer room. However, certain critically ill clients benefit from cooler room temperatures to lower the body's metabolic demands.

A good ventilation system keeps stale air and odors from lingering in the room. The nurse must protect the acutely ill, infants, and older adults from drafts by ensuring they are adequately dressed and covered with a lightweight blanket.

Good ventilation also reduces lingering odors caused by draining wounds, vomitus, bowel movements, and unemptied bedpans and urinals. Room deodorizers can help remove many unpleasant odors. Nurses should always empty and rinse bedpans or urinals promptly. Thorough hygiene measures are the best way to control body or breath odors. Most health care institutions also now prohibit smoking.

Ill clients seem to be more sensitive to common hospital noises. Until the client is familiar with hospital noises, the nurse should try to control the noise level. The nurse also explains the source of any unfamiliar noises.

Proper lighting is necessary for everyone's safety and comfort. A brightly lit room is usually stimulating, but a darkened room is best for rest and sleep. Room lighting can be adjusted by closing or opening drapes, regulating overbed and floor lights, and closing or opening room doors.

Room Equipment

A typical hospital room contains certain basic pieces of furniture: overbed table, bedside stand, chairs, lamp, and bed. The overbed table rolls on wheels and can be adjusted to various heights over the bed or a chair. Usually two storage areas are under the tabletop. The table provides ideal working space for the nurse performing

A

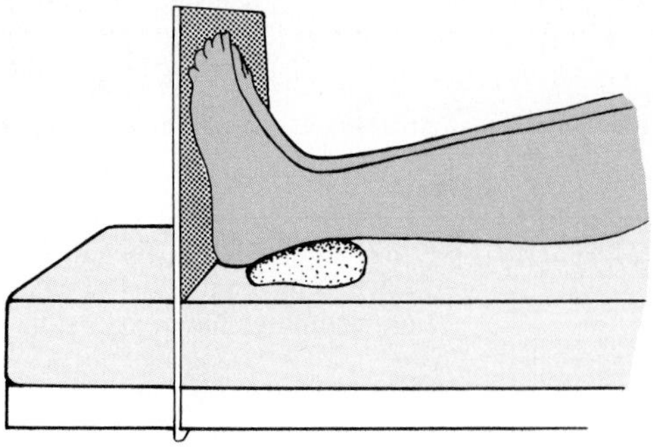

procedures. It also provides a surface to place meal trays, toiletry items, and objects frequently used by the client. The bedpan and urinal should not be placed on the bedside table. The bedside stand is used to store the client's personal possessions and hygiene equipment. The telephone, water pitcher, and drinking cup are commonly found on a bedside table.

Most hospital rooms contain an armless straight-backed chair and an upholstered lounge chair with arms. The lounge chair is used by the client and visitors and is usually placed at the foot of the bed or beside it. Straight-backed chairs are convenient when temporarily transferring the clients from the bed, such as during bedmaking.

Each room usually has an overbed light and a floor or table lamp. Movable lights that extend over the bed from the wall should be positioned for easy reach but moved aside when not in use. Gooseneck or special examination lights are portable standing lights used to provide extra light during bedside procedures.

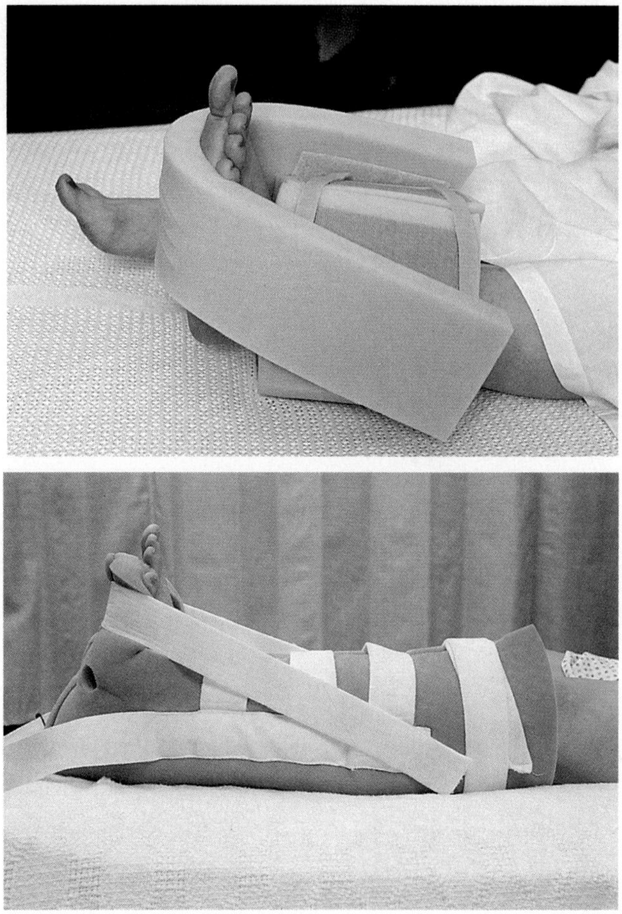

B

C

FIGURE 30-2 **A,** Footboard. **B,** Foot boots. **C,** Foot boot with lower leg extension.

SPECIAL ROOM EQUIPMENT

FOOTBOARD

A flat, plastic or wood panel placed at the foot of the bed above the mattress level helps keep the feet in the dorsiflexion position to prevent footdrop. A footboard also keeps bed covers up and off the feet. Works best for mobile clients who can push against board. Not as effective as foot boots.

FOOT BOOTS

Sheepskin- or foam-lined boots made of smooth plastic or foam support each foot in dorsiflexion. They are preferred over footboards because they allow clients to assume a variety of positions.

BED CRADLE

A bed cradle is a curved, semicircular device made of metal that can be placed over a portion of the client's body. The cradle keeps the top bed linens off of the feet, legs, or abdomen. Bed cradles come in many sizes.

SPECIAL MATTRESS

Many special mattresses are available to support specific pressure-prone areas of the body and provide client comfort (see Chapter 24). Flotation pads and alternating air mattresses disperse pressure from the client's body weight over a large area and thus reduce risk of pressure sores.

BED BOARD

A long wooden or Plexiglas board, the length of a regular bed mattress, is placed under a mattress to provide added support. Clients with back pain frequently use bed boards. The boards are rigid or hinged so that the foot or end of the bed can be elevated.

table 30-6

COMMON BED POSITIONS

Position	Description	Uses
Fowler's 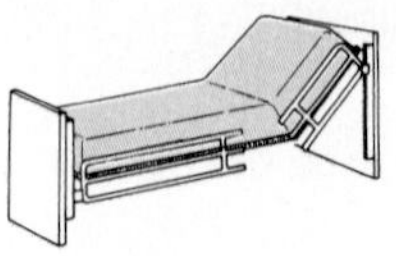	Head of bed raised to angle of 45 degrees or more; semisitting position.	Preferred while client eats; used during nasogastric tube insertion and nasotracheal suction; promotes lung expansion.
Semi-Fowler's 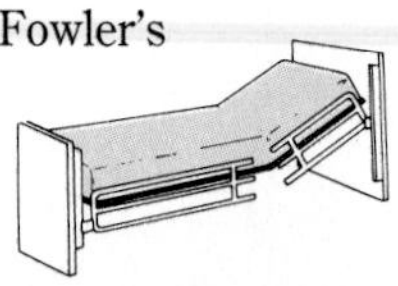	Head of bed raised approximately 30 degrees; incline less than Fowler's position.	Promotes lung expansion.
Trendelenburg 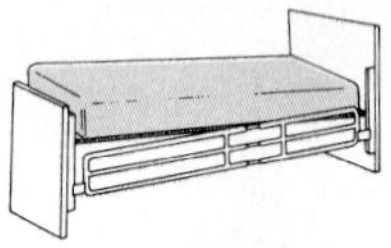	Entire bed tilted downward with head of bed down.	For postural drainage; facilitates venous return in clients with poor peripheral perfusion.
Reverse Trendelenburg 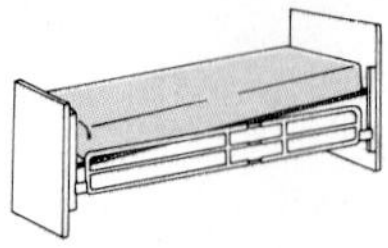	Entire bed frame tilted downward with foot of bed down.	Used infrequently; promotes gastric emptying and prevents esophageal reflux.
Flat 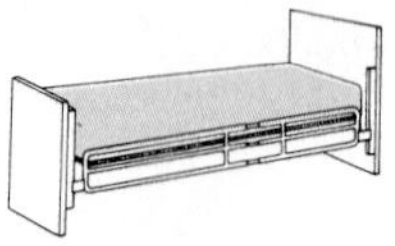	Entire bed frame horizontally parallel with floor.	For clients with vertebral injuries and in cervical traction; used by hypotensive clients; generally preferred by clients for sleeping.

Other equipment usually found in a client's room includes a call light, a television set or radio, a blood pressure gauge, oxygen and vacuum wall outlets, and personal care items. Special equipment designed for comfort or positioning clients includes footboards and foot boots (Figure 30-2, *A, B,* and *C*), special mattresses, bed boards, and bed cradles (see box on p. 855).

Beds. Seriously ill clients may remain in bed for a long time. Because a bed is the piece of equipment used most by a client, it should be designed for comfort, safety, and adaptability for changing positions.

The typical hospital bed has a firm mattress on a metal frame that can be raised and lowered horizontally (Table 30-6). The frame is divided into three sections so that the operator can raise and lower the head and foot of the bed, in addition to inclining the entire bed with the headboard up or down. Different bed positions are used to promote lung expansion, postural drainage, and other interventions (see Chapter 23).

The position of a bed is usually changed by electrical controls on the side or foot of the bed or in a bedside cable. Clients can thus raise or lower sections of the bed without expending much energy. Nurses should instruct clients on the proper use of controls and caution them against raising the bed to a position that might cause harm. A hospital bed is usually 65 to 70 cm (26 to 28 inches) above the floor at its lowest level. In the home, most beds are 50 to 55 cm (20 to 22 inches) high. The greater height of a hospital bed prevents undue musculoskeletal strain on the nurse and client.

Beds contain safety features such as locks on the wheels or casters (Figure 30-3). Wheels should be locked when the bed is stationary to prevent accidental movement. Side rails protect clients from accidental falls. The headboard can be removed from most beds.

Text continued on p. 866.

procedure 30-11

MAKING AN UNOCCUPIED BED

Steps	Rationale
1. Assess potential for client being incontinent or having excess drainage on bed linen.	Determines need for protective waterproof pads or bath blankets on bed.
2. Assess activity orders and physical mobility.	Determines level of activity allowed, including whether client should be out of bed.
3. If client is in bed, explain that you wish to change bed while he or she is sitting up. Ask if he or she feels able to sit in chair and assist as necessary.	Client should not feel inconvenienced by procedure. Client may feel anxious if uncomfortable or fatigued.
4. Prepare needed equipment and supplies:	
a. Linen bags b. Mattress pad (changed only when soiled) c. Bottom sheet (flat or fitted)	Collecting linen top to bottom in order of use makes it easier to make bed without delays.
d. Drawsheet	Used to help to lift or move client and to protect bottom sheet from soiling.
e. Top sheet (flat) f. Blanket g. Bedspread	
h. Waterproof pads or bath blankets (optional)	To lay under client at points where drainage is expected. Reduces soiling of bed linen.
i. Pillowcases	
j. Bedside chair or table	Used to place linen on in order of use.
k. Disposable gloves (optional)	Worn when removing soiled linen.
5. Wash hands.	Reduces transmission of microorganisms.
6. Assemble and arrange equipment on bedside chair or table. Remove unnecessary equipment, such as overbed table.	Provides for smooth procedure and ensures comfort. Placing linen on clean surface minimizes spread of infection.
7. Lower side rail on near side of bed and remove call light.	Provides easy access to bed.
8. Adjust bed height to comfortable working position.	Minimizes strain on nurse's back and muscles.
9. On near side, loosen linen, starting at top of bed. Move along sides and then down toward foot. Move to other side of bed, lower side rail, and loosen linen.	Makes linen easier to remove.
10. Remove bedspread and blanket separately by folding each into ball or folded square and discarding into linen bag if they are not to be reused. Do not allow uniform to come in contact with soiled linen (see illustration). Avoid fanning or shaking linen.	Reduces transmission of microorganisms.

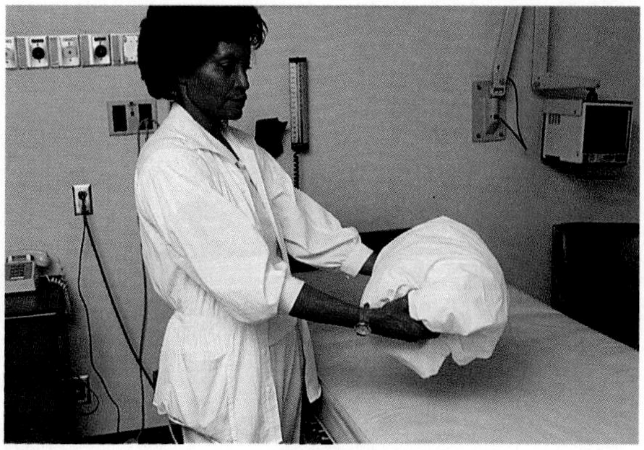

Step 10

Continued.

procedure 30-11—cont'd

Steps	Rationale
11. If spread or blanket is to be reused, fold as follows: fold each spread by grasping top edge with both hands, one hand at center, other hand at end. Fold top edge down, even with the bottom edge. Pick up spread at center and fold so that farthest side comes even with nearest side. Bring top and bottom edges together again. Place folded spread or blanket over back of chair.	Facilitates replacement and prevents wrinkling.
12. Remove soiled pillowcases by grasping closed end with one hand and slipping pillow out with other. Discard pillowcases in linen bag and place pillows on table.	Minimizes contact with soiled linen.
13. Fold each piece of remaining bed linen separately into ball or folded square and discard into linen bag.	Attempting to fold all soiled linen at once creates bulky bundle that is difficult to discard and may easily come in contact with uniform.
14. Slide mattress toward head of bed.	If mattress slides toward foot of bed when head of bed is raised, it is difficult to tuck in linen.
15. Wipe off moisture on mattress with washcloth moistened in antiseptic solution; dry thoroughly.	Reduces transmission of microorganisms.
16. Stand at side of bed where linen is placed. Spread mattress pad over mattress.	Time is saved by making half of bed first and then moving to opposite side.
17. Smooth out all wrinkles in pad.	Wrinkles or folds of linen are source of chronic irritation against client's skin.
18. Unfold bottom sheet lengthwise and place vertical center crease lengthwise along center of bed. Fold sheet's top layer toward opposite side of bed. Smooth bottom layer of sheet across mattress on near side; bring edge over side of mattress. Allow it to hang 25 cm (10 in) over mattress edge. Lower hem of bottom sheet should lie seam down, even with bottom edge of mattress (see illustration). Pull remaining top portion of sheet over top edge of mattress.	Method of unfolding linen saves nurse's time and energy. Making one side of bed at a time avoids excess movement. Proper placement of linen ensures adequate length will be available to cover opposite side of bed. Keeping seam edge down eliminates source of irritation to cliet's skin. If bottom edge of sheet is not tucked in, it can later be changed without removing top linen.
19. While standing at head of bed, miter top corner of bottom sheet:	Mitered corner is not loosened easily.
a. Face head of bed diagonally. Place hand away from head of bed under top corner of mattress near mattress edge and lift.	
b. With other hand, tuck top edge of bottom sheet smoothly under mattress so side edges of sheet above and below mattress would meet if brought together.	
c. Face side of bed and pick up top edge of sheet approximately 45 cm (18 in) down from top of mattress (see illustration).	
d. Lift sheet and lay on top of mattress to form neat, triangular fold, with lower base of triangle even with mattress side edge (see illustration).	
e. Tuck lower edge of sheet, hanging free below mattress, under mattress. Tuck with palms down without pulling triangular fold (see illustration).	

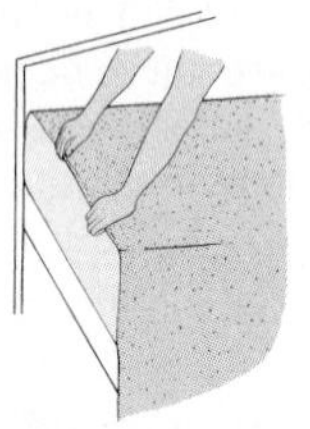

Step 18

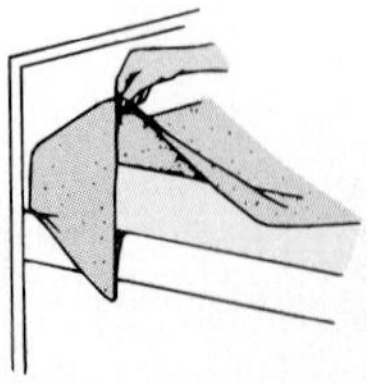

Step 19c

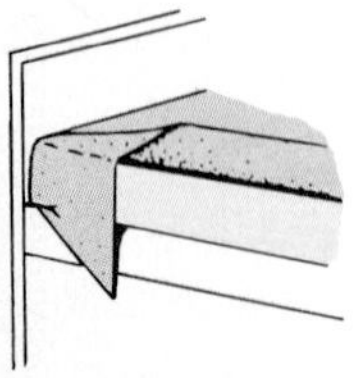

Step 19d

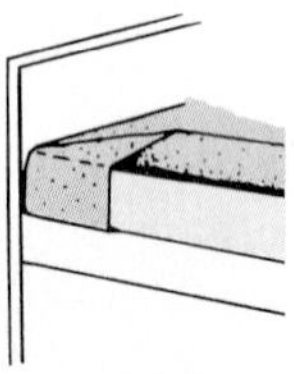

Step 19e

Steps	Rationale
f. Hold portion of sheet covering side edge of mattress in place with one hand. With other hand, pick up top of triangular linen fold and bring it down over side of mattress. Tuck this portion under mattress (see illustration).	
20. Tuck remaining portion of sheet under mattress. Keep linen smooth (see illustration).	Folds can irritate client's skin.
21. Open drawsheet so it unfolds in half. Lay center fold along middle of bed lengthwise. Fanfold top layer at center of bed. Smooth bottom layer of drawsheet over mattress.	Drawsheet is used to lift and reposition client. Placement under client's torso distributes most of body weight over sheet.
22. Tuck excess edge under mattress, keeping palms down.	Anchors sheet in place to prevent sliding and wrinkling.
23. Move to opposite side of bed.	One side of bed is completed before nurse moves to other side.
24. Spread fanfolded bottom sheet smoothly over edge of mattress from head to foot of bed.	Wrinkles can cause irritation.
25. Miter top corner of bottom sheet (Step 19). When tucking corner, be sure sheet is taut.	Taut sheet eliminates wrinkles and folds that can rub client's skin.
26. Facing side of bed, grasp remaining edge of bottom sheet, lean back, keeping back straight, and pull when tucking excess linen tightly under mattress. Proceed from head to foot of bed. (Avoid lifting mattress during tucking to ensure tight fit.)	Prevents injury to nurse.
27. Smooth folded drawsheet over bottom sheet. Grasp edge of drawsheet with palms down, lean back, and tuck sheet under mattress. Tuck first at middle, then at top, and then at bottom.	Tucking first at top or bottom may pull sheet sideways, causing poor fit. Loose bed sheets reduce friction and help to prevent pressure sores (Rousseau, 1988).
28. If needed, apply waterproof pad or bath blanket over drawsheet.	Pad collects body secretions and drainage, protecting linen from becoming soiled.
29. Move to side of bed when linen is located. Place top sheet over bed with vertical center fold lengthwise down middle of bed. Open sheet out from head to foot, being sure top edge of sheet is seam up and even with top edge of mattress. Spread excess sheet over bottom edge of mattress. (Do not fan top sheet over the bed.)	Placement ensures equal distribution of sheet over bed. Positioning sheet with seam up prevents irritation of client's skin. Fanning creates air currents that can spread microorganisms throughout room.
30. Make horizontal toe pleat: stand at foot of bed and fan fold in sheet 5 to 10 cm (2 to 4 in) across bed. Pull sheet up from bottom to make fold. Fold should be approximately 15 cm (6 in) from bottom edge of mattress.	Allows for free movement of client's feet and prevents friction against surface of toes.
31. Tuck in remaining portion of sheet on one side of foot of mattress (optional).	Anchors top sheet so that client can move freely.

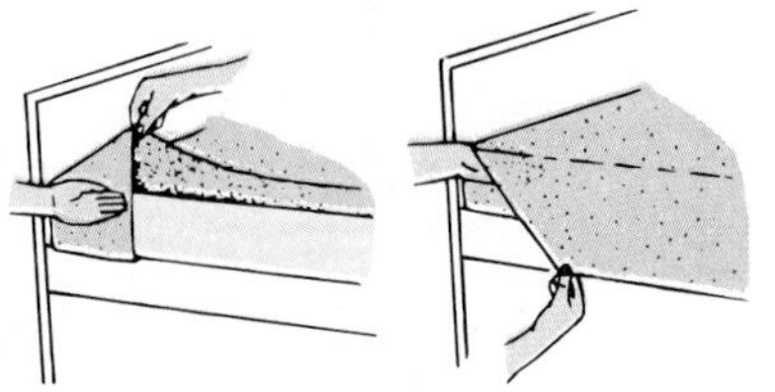
Step 19f

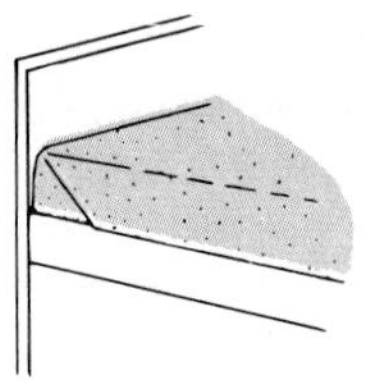
Step 20

Continued.

procedure 30-11—cont'd

Steps	Rationale
32. Place blanket on bed, unfolding it so that crease runs lengthwise along middle of bed. Top edge should be parallel with edge of top sheet and 15 to 20 cm (6 to 8 in) down from top mattress edge. Bottom edge should hang over mattress edge. Spread blanket evenly over bed.	Blanket provides adequate warmth. Cuff will be formed with sheet folded over top edge of blanket and spread.
33. Place spread over bed according to Step 32. Be sure top edge of spread extends about 2.5 cm (1 in) above blanket's edge. Then tuck top edge of spread over and under top edge of blanket.	Spread gives bed a neat appearance and provides extra warmth.
34. Make cuff by turning edge of top sheet down over top edge of blanket and spread.	Smooth cuff protects client's face from irritation.
35. Standing on one side at foot of bed, lift mattress corner slightly with one hand and with other hand tuck top sheet, blanket, and spread together under mattress. Be sure toe pleats of sheet are not pulled out so that linens are loose enough for client to move.	Pressure sores can develop on client's toes and heels if feet rub between tight-fitting bed sheets. Lifting mattress too high can loosen bottom linen.
36. Make modified mitered corner with top sheet, blanket, and spread: pick up side edge of top sheet, blanket, and spread approximately 45 cm (18 in) up from foot of mattress. Lift linens to form triangular fold and lay it on bed. Tuck loose edge hanging down under side of mattress. Pick up triangular fold and bring it down over mattress, holding linen in place along side of mattress. Do not tuck tip of triangle (see illustration).	Modified mitered corner secures top linen but keeps even edge of top sheet, blanket, and spread draped over mattress. 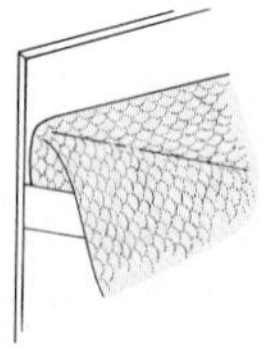 Step 36
37. Go to other side of bed: spread sheet, blanket, and spread out evenly. Fold top edge of spread over blanket and make cuff with top sheet (as in Step 34). Make modified mitered corner at foot of bed (as in Step 36).	Nurse saves time and energy by completing one side of bed at time.
38. Apply clean pillowcase. With one hand, grasp pillowcase at center of closed end. Gather case, turning it inside out over hand holding it. With same hand, pick up middle of one end of pillow. Pull pillowcase down over pillow with other hand. Be sure corners of case fit evenly over pillow.	This method makes it easy to slide case smoothly over pillow.
39. Position pillows at center of head of bed.	Maintains neat appearance.
40. Place call light within client's reach and return bed to comfortable height.	Provides for client's safety.
41. If client is to return to bed, fold back top covers to one side or fanfold them down to bottom third of bed.	Folding back covers makes it easy for client to return to bed.
42. Rearrange furniture and place any personal items within easy reach.	Neat environment promotes sense of well-being.
43. Discard dirty linen in linen hamper or chute. Wash hands.	Prevents transmission of microorganisms.
44. Evaluate client's tolerance to sitting up in chair. Compare heart rate to previous resting rate; ask if client feels weak, dizzy, or fatigued; assess blood pressure if client complains of dizziness or weakness.	Client's inability to tolerate exertion, even low levels of exercise, may be reflected in changes in vital signs or subjective report of symptoms.
45. Assist client in returning to bed.	

procedure 30-12

MAKING AN OCCUPIED BED

Steps	Rationale
1. Determine potential for client being incontinent or having excess drainage on bed linen.	Determines need for protective waterproof pads or extra bath blankets on bed.
2. Check chart for orders or specific precautions for movement and positioning.	Ensures safety and use of proper body mechanics for nurse and client.
3. Explain procedure to client, noting that client will be asked to turn on side to roll over linen.	Minimizes anxiety and promotes cooperation.
4. Prepare needed equipment and supplies:	
a. Linen bag	Collecting linen (top to bottom) in order of use makes it easier to make bed without delays.
b. Bath blanket	
c. Mattress pad (need only be changed when soiled)	
d. Bottom sheet (flat or fitted)	
e. Drawsheet	Used to help lift or move client at points where drainage is expected. Reduces soiling of bed linen.
f. Top sheet (flat)	
g. Blanket	
h. Bedspread	
i. Waterproof pads (optional)	Lay under client at points where drainage is expected. Reduces soiling of bed linen.
j. Pillowcases	
k. Bedside chair or table	
l. Disposable gloves (optional)	Worn when removing soiled linen.
5. Wash hands.	Minimizes spread of infection.
6. Assemble and arrange equipment on bedside chair or table. Remove unnecessary equipment.	Provides for smooth procedure and ensures comfort.
7. Draw room curtain around bed or close door.	Maintains privacy, thus promoting emotional and physical comfort.
8. Lower side rail on near side of bed. Remove call light.	Provides easy access to bed and linen.
9. Adjust bed height to comfortable working position.	Minimizes strain on nurse's back. It is easier to remove and apply linen evenly to bed in flat position.
10. Loosen top linen sheet at foot of bed.	Makes linen easier to remove.
11. Remove bedspread and blanket separately by folding them into squares and placing them in linen bag (if not to be reused). Do not allow linen to contact uniform. Do not fan or shake linen.	Reduces transmission of microorganisms.
12. If blanket and spread are to be reused, fold by bringing top and bottom edges together. Fold farthest side over onto nearer bottom edges. Place folded linen over back of chair.	Facilitates replacement and prevents wrinkling.
13. Cover client with bath blanket in following manner: unfold bath blanket over top sheet. Ask client to hold top edge of bath blanket. If client is unable to help, tuck top of bath blanket under shoulder. Grasp top sheet under bath blanket at client's shoulders and bring sheet down to foot of bed. Remove sheet and discard it in linen bag.	Bath blanket provides warmth and keeps body parts covered during linen removal.
14. With assistance from another nurse, slide mattress toward head of bed.	If mattress slides toward foot of bed when head of bed is raised, it is difficult to tuck linen and is uncomfortable for client.

Continued.

procedure 30-12—cont'd

Steps	Rationale
15. Position client on the side on far side of bed, facing away. Adjust pillow under head. Be sure side rail is up.	Provides space for placement of clean linen. Side rail ensures safety.
16. Loosen bottom linens, moving from head to foot of bed.	Prepares for removal of bottom linen simultaneously.
17. Fanfold bottom sheet and drawsheet toward client; first drawsheet, then bottom sheet. Tuck edges of linen just under buttocks, back, and shoulders. Do not fanfold mattress pad if it is to be reused.	Provides maximum work space for placing, clean linen. Later, when client turns to other side, soiled linen can be easily removed.
18. Wipe off moisture on mattress with towel and appropriate disinfectant.	Reduces transmission of microorganisms.
19. Apply clean linen to exposed half of bed:	
a. Place clean mattress pad on bed by folding it lengthwise with center crease in middle of bed. Fanfold top layer over mattress. (If pad is reused, simply smooth out wrinkles.)	Applying linen over bed in successive layers minimizes energy and time nurse uses in bedmaking.
b. Unfold bottom sheet lengthwise so center crease is situated lengthwise along center of bed. Fanfold sheet's top layer toward center of bed alongside client. Smooth bottom layer of sheet over mattress and bring edge over near side (see illustration). Allow sheet's edge to hang about 25 cm (10 in) over mattress edge. Lower hem of bottom sheet should lie seam down and even with bottom edge of mattress.	Proper positioning of linen on one side ensures that adequate linen will be available to cover opposite side of bed. Keeping seam edges down eliminates irritation to client's skin.
20. Miter bottom sheet at head of bed:	Mitered corner cannot be loosened easily, even if client moves about frequently in bed.
a. Face head of bed diagonally. Place hand away from head of bed under top corner of mattress, near mattress edge, and lift.	
b. With other hand, tuck top edge of bottom sheet smoothly under mattress so side edges of sheet above and below mattress would meet if brought together.	
c. Face side of bed and pick up top edge of sheet at approximately 45 cm (18 in) down from top of mattress.	

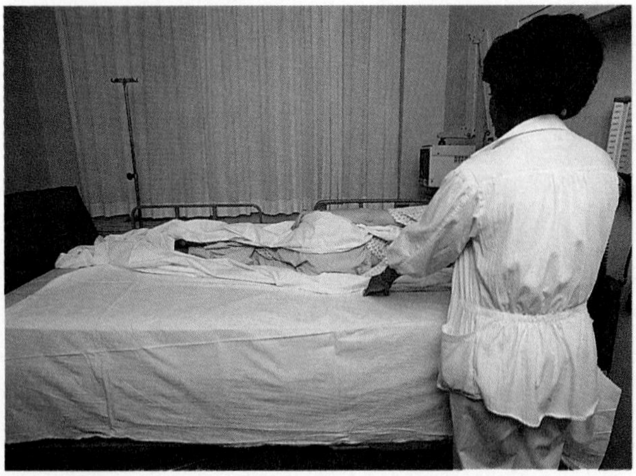

Step 19b

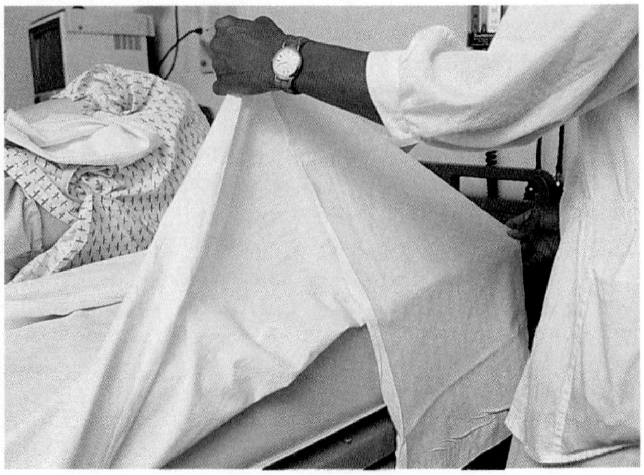

Step 20d

Steps	Rationale
d. Lift sheet and lay it on top of mattress to form neat triangular fold, with lower base of triangle even with mattress side edge (see illustration).	
e. Tuck lower edge of sheet, which is hanging free below mattress, under mattress. Tuck with palms down without pulling triangular fold.	
f. Hold portion of sheet covering side edge of mattress in place with one hand. With other hand, pick up top of triangular linen fold and bring it down over side of mattress. Tuck this portion of sheet under mattress.	
21. Tuck remaining portion of sheet under mattress, moving toward foot of bed. Keep linen smooth.	Folds of linen are source of irritation.
22. Open drawsheet so it unfolds in half. Lay center fold along middle of bed lengthwise and position sheet so it will be under buttocks and torso (see illustration). Fanfold top layer toward client with edge alongside back. Smooth bottom layer out over mattress and tuck excess edge under mattress (keep palms down).	Drawsheet is used to lift and reposition client. Placement under client's torso distributes most of body weight over sheet.
23. Place waterproof pad over drawsheet with center fold against client's side. Fanfold far half toward client.	Used to protect bed linen from soiling.
24. Raise side rail on working side and go to other side.	Maintains safety.
25. Lower side rail. Assist client to roll slowly onto other side, over folds of linen.	Exposes opposite side of bed for removal of soiled linen and placement of clean linen.
26. Loosen edges of soiled linen from underneath mattress.	Makes linen easier to remove.
27. Without allowing dirty linen to touch uniform, remove soiled linen by folding it into a bundle or square, with soiled side turned in. Discard it in linen bag.	Reduces transmission of microorganisms.
28. Spread clean, fanfolded linen smoothly over edge of mattress from head to foot of bed.	Smooth linen will not irritate client's skin.
29. Assist client in rolling back into supine position. Reposition pillow.	Client's comfort is maintained.

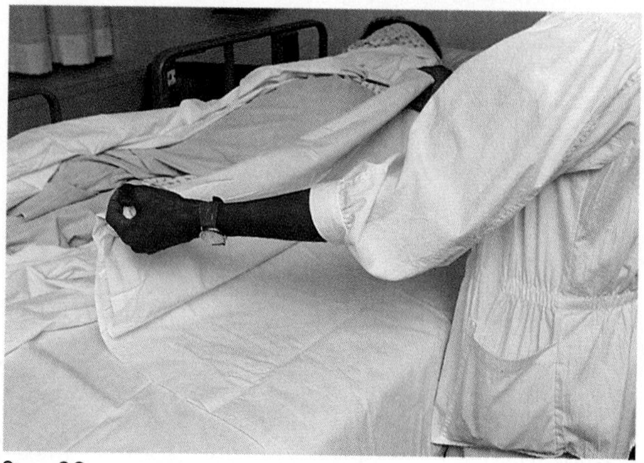

Step 22

Continued.

procedure 30-12—cont'd

Steps	Rationale
30. Miter top corner of bottom sheet (Step 20). When tucking corner be sure sheet is smooth and free of wrinkles.	Wrinkles and folds can cause mechanical irritation to skin.
31. Facing side of bed, grasp remaining edge of bottom sheet. Keep back straight and pull as excess linen is tucked under mattress (see illustration). Proceed from head to foot of bed. (Avoid lifting mattress during tucking to ensure fit.)	Proper use of body mechanics while tucking linen prevents injury to nurse.
32. Smooth fanfolded drawsheet over bottom sheet. Grasp edge of sheet with palms down, lean back, and tuck sheet under mattress. Tuck from middle to top and to bottom.	Tucking first at top or bottom may pull sheet sideways, causing poor fit.
33. Place top sheet over client with center fold lengthwise down middle of bed. Open sheet from head to foot and unfold it over client.	Sheet should be equally distributed over bed by correctly positioning center fold.
34. Without allowing dirty linen to touch uniform, ask client to hold clean top sheet, or tuck sheet around shoulders. Remove bath blanket and discard it into linen bag (see illustration).	Sheet prevents exposure of body parts. Having client hold sheet encourages participation in care.
35. Place blanket on bed, unfolding it so that crease runs lengthwise along middle of bed. Unfold blanket to cover client. Top edge should be parallel with edge of top sheet and 15 to 20 cm (6 to 8 in) down from top sheet's edge.	Blanket should be placed to cover client completely and provide adequate warmth.
36. Place spread over bed according to Step 31. Be sure top edge of spread extends about 2.5 cm (1 in) above blanket's edge. Tuck top edge of spread over and under top edge of blanket.	Spread gives bed neat appearance and provides extra wamth.
37. Make cuff by turning edge of top sheet down over top edge of blanket and spread.	Smooth cuff protects client's face from rubbing against blanket or spread.

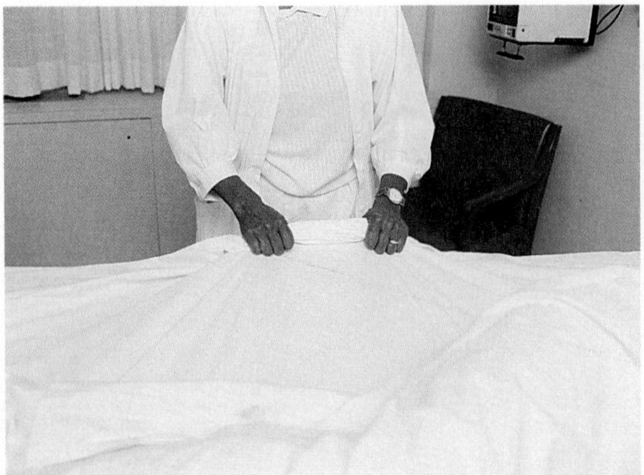
Step 31

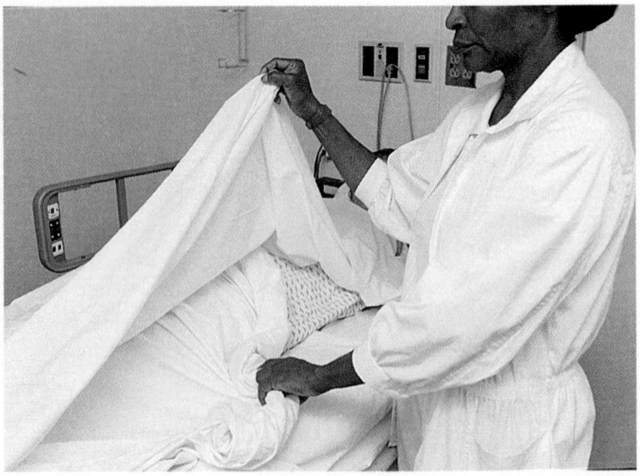
Step 34

Steps	Rationale
38. Standing on one side at foot of bed, lift mattress corner slightly with one hand and tuck top linens under mattress. Top sheet and blanket are tucked under together. Be sure linens are loose enough to allow for movement of client's feet. (Horizontal toe pleat may be made [Procedure 30-11, Step 30].)	Tucking all top linens together makes neat-appearing bed. Pressure sores can develop on client's toes and heels from feet rubbing between tight fitting bed sheets.
39. Make modified mitered corner with top sheet, blanket, and spread:	
a. Pick up side edge of top sheet, blanket, and spread approximately 45 cm (18 in) up from foot of mattress. Lift linens to form triangular fold and lay it on bed.	Modified mitered corner secures top linen but keeps an even edge of blanket and top sheet draped over mattress.
b. Tuck lower edge of sheet, which is hanging free below mattress, under mattress. Do not pull triangular fold.	
c. Pick up triangular fold and bring it down over mattress while holding linen in place along side of mattress. Do not tuck tip of triangle.	
40. Raise side rail. Make other side of bed; spread sheet, blanket, and bedspread out evenly; fold top edge of spread over blanket and make cuff with top sheet (Step 37); make modified corner at foot of bed (Step 39).	Side rail protects client from accidental falls.
41. Change pillowcase:	
a. Have client raise head. While supporting neck with one hand, remove pillow.	Prevents injury during flexion and extension of neck.
b. Remove soiled case by grasping pillow at open end with one hand and pulling case over pillow with other hand. Discard case in linen bag.	
c. Grasp clean pillowcase at center of closed end. Gather case, turning it inside out over hand holding it. With same hand pick up middle of one end of pillow. Pull pillowcase down over pillow with other hand.	Method makes it easy to slide pillowcase over pillow.
d. Be sure pillow corners fit evenly in corners of pillowcase.	Poorly fitting case constricts fluffing and expansion of pillow.
42. Support client's head under neck and place pillow under head.	Prevents hyperextension of neck muscles.
43. Place call light within client's reach; return bed to comfortable position.	Ensures safety and comfort.
44. Open room curtains. Rearrange furniture. Place personal items within easy reach on overbed table or bedside stand. Return bed to comfortable height.	Promotes sense of well-being.
45. Discard dirty linen in linen hamper or chute; wash hands.	Prevents transmission of microorganisms.

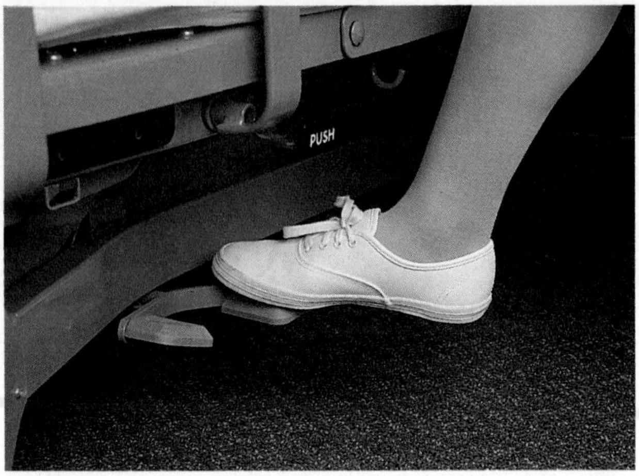

FIGURE 30-3 Lock on bed wheels.

This is important when the medical team must have easy access to the head during cardiopulmonary resuscitation (see Chapter 34).

Most beds have firm, water-repellent mattresses. Special rubber, water, and alternating air pressure mattresses can be placed on top of the mattress. These devices reduce pressure sores during prolonged immobilization (see Chapter 24). Special beds are also available for clients with severe mobility restrictions (see Chapter 23).

BEDMAKING. A client's bed should be kept as clean and comfortable as possible. This requires frequent inspections to be sure linen is clean, dry, and free of wrinkles.

The nurse usually makes a bed in the morning after the client's bath, as the client is bathing, or when the client is out of the room for tests or procedures. Throughout the day the nurse straightens linen that becomes loose or wrinkled. The bed linen should also be checked for food particles after meals and for wetness or soiling. Linen that becomes wet or soiled should be changed.

When changing the bed linen, the nurse follows basic principles of asepsis by keeping soiled linen away from the uniform. Soiled linen is placed in special linen bags before discarding it in the linen hamper. To avoid air currents, which can spread microorganisms, the nurse never fans linen. To avoid transmitting infection, the nurse should not place dirty linen on the floor. If clean linen touches the floor, it is immediately discarded.

During bedmaking the nurse must use proper body mechanics. The bed should always be raised to its highest position before changing linen so the nurse does not have to bend or stretch over the mattress. When making an occupied bed the nurse should also use principles of body mechanics (see Chapter 22).

The client's privacy, comfort, and safety are important when making a bed. Using side rails, keeping call lights within the client's reach, and maintaining the proper bed position help promote comfort and safety. After making a bed the nurse always returns it to the lowest horizontal position to prevent accidental falls.

When possible, the nurse should make the bed while it is unoccupied (Procedure 30-11). If the client is confined to bed, the nurse organizes bedmaking activities to conserve time and energy (Procedure 30-12). When making an unoccupied bed, the nurse follows the same basic principles as for bedmaking. The surgical, recovery, or postoperative bed is a modified version of the unoccupied bed. The top covers are folded to one side or fanfolded to the bottom third of the bed. After a client is discharged, all bed linen is sent to the laundry, the mattress and bed are cleaned by housekeeping personnel, and new bed linen is applied.

LINENS. Before bedmaking, it is important to collect not only bed linens but also the client's personal linens. Linens are pressed and folded to prevent the spread of microorganisms and to make bedmaking easier. Bed linens have a center crease that the nurse places in the center of the bed from the head to the foot. The linens unfold easily to the sides, with creases often fitting over the mattress edge. New linens are applied whenever there is soiling.

SUMMARY

Hygiene measures cover many basic physical needs clients are often unable to meet themselves. The nurse's responsibility includes assessing a client's physical condition, personal hygiene habits, and body image. The nurse should promote independence and participation in health care.

A nurse should be resourceful when delivering hygiene measures. There is time for therapeutic communication, client teaching, and emotional support. Likewise, when the client needs assistance, the nurse can conduct portions of a physical examination.

The nurse uses considerable judgment and planning to anticipate clients' hygiene needs. The nurse incorporates client preferences into hygiene care and ensures the client's comfort and safety.

CRITICAL THINKING ACTIVITIES

1. Mrs. Jones, a 70-year-old widow who lives alone, has been admitted to your unit. She is frail and unkempt. Her skin is extremely dry and cracked, with some reddened areas noted on the sacrum. Describe appropriate nursing intervention you would take in the situation. What other assessments are required in this situation?
2. Mrs. Lee, a 50-year-old newly diagnosed diabetic, has long toe nails and asks you to cut them. Describe the sequence of actions you would take and give a rationale for each.
3. Mrs. Sams gave birth to her first child 3 days ago. She complains of perineal discomfort. What type of therapeutic bath is appropriate for her? How would you ensure her safety?

KEY CONCEPTS

- The nurse provides clients' daily hygiene needs if they are unable to care for themselves adequately.
- Providing hygienic care gives the nurse the chance to assess external body surfaces and the client's emotional state.
- While providing daily hygiene needs, the nurse uses teaching and communication skills to develop a relationship with the client.
- The client's personal preferences must always be considered when the nurse plans daily hygiene care.
- The nurse must maintain privacy and comfort when providing the client's daily care.
- During assessment of the skin and oral mucosa, the nurse observes characteristics influenced by hygiene.
- Clients who are immobilized and poorly nourished and who have reduced sensation or peripheral circulation are at risk for altered skin integrity.
- Gloves should be worn by nurses during hygiene care when the risk of contacting body fluids is high.
- Clients with diabetes need nail and foot care.
- When administering oral care to unconscious clients, the nurse takes measures to prevent aspiration.
- Clients who wear contact lenses must learn proper self-care techniques to avoid corneal injury.
- Evaluation of hygiene care is based on the client's sense of comfort, relaxation, well-being, and understanding of hygiene techniques.

References

Anetzberger GJ, Lachs MS, et al.: Elder mistreatment: A call for help, *Patient Care* June:93, 1993.

Christensen MH, Funnell MM, et al.: How to care for the diabetic foot, *Am J Nurs* 91(3):50, 1991.

Egan D, et al.: Bethesda Eye Institute and St Louis University School of Medicine, Department of Ophthalmology: *Soft lens care and handling,* St. Louis, 1988, Bethesda Eye Institute.

Fenske N, Grayson L, and Newcomer V: Tips for treating aging skin, *Patient Care* March:61, 1992.

Hill L: The question of pressure sores, *Nurs Times* 88(12):76, 1992.

Jordan J, Nickerson D: Hygiene. In Guthrie D, Guthrie R, editors: *Nursing management of diabetes mellitus,* ed 2, St. Louis, 1982, Mosby.

Mahoney DF: Cerumen impaction: prevalence and detection in nursing homes, *J Gerontol Nurs* April:23, 1993.

Maklebust J: Pressure ulcer update, *RN* 41(12):56, 1991.

National Pressure Ulcer Advisory Panel (NPUAP), Pressure ulcer incidence, economics, risk assessment: Consensus Development Conference Statement, *Decubitus* 2(2):24, 1989.

Ney DF: Cerumen impaction, ear hygiene practices, and hearing acuity, *Geriatric Nurs* March/April:70, 1993.

Panel for the Prediction and Prevention for Pressure Ulcers in Adults (PPPUA): Assessing risk and preventing pressure ulcers, *Patient Care* April:36, 1993.

Pascucci MA: Measuring incentives to health promotion in older adults, *J Gerontol Nurs* March:16, 1992.

Pettigrew D: Investing in mouth care, *Geriatric Nurse* 10:22, 1989.

Poland JM: Comparing Moi-Stin to lemon glycerine swabs, *Am J Nurs* 87:422, 1987.

Ramler D, Roberts J: A comparison of cold and warm sitz baths for relief of postpartum perineal pain, *JOGGN* 15:471, 1986.

Rousseau P: Pressure sores in the aged: a preventable problem? *Contin Care* July 1988, p. 37.

Thomas C: *Ostomy and Wound Management* 23:51, 1989.

Tyler D, Winslow E, et al.: Effects of a 1-minute backrub on mixed venous oxygen saturation and heart rate, *Heart/Lung* 19(5):562, 1990.

United States Department of Health and Human Services: Prediction and Prevention, pub #92-0047, 92-0050, Rockville, Md., 1992, PHS, Agency for Health Care Policy and Research.

Weiss SJ: Psychophysiologic effects of care giver touch on incidence of cardiac dysrhythmias, *Heart Lung* 15(5):495, 1986.

Whaley LF and Wong DL: *Nursing care of infants and children,* ed 4, St. Louis, 1991, Mosby.

Bibliography

Brinkmann KL: Why can't your patient hear you? *RN* 54:46, 1991.

Ceccio C: Understanding therapeutic beds, *Orthop Nurs* 9(3):57, 1990.

Florey C: Skin assessment, *RN* June:22, 1992.

Futrell A, Forst S, et al.: Effects of occupied and unoccupied bedmaking on myocardial work in health subjects, *Heart/Lung* 20(2):161, 1991.

Kenny SA: Effect of two oral protocols on the incidence of stomatitis in hematology patients, *Cancer Nurs* 13(5/6):345, 1990.

McGovern M and Kuhn J: Skin assessment of the elderly client, *J Gerontol Nurs* 18(9):39, 1992.

Murray S and Thompson R: We've organized our approach to pressure sores, *RN* January:42, 1991.

Ruscin C, Cunningham G, and Blaylock A: Foot care protocol for the older client, *Geriatric Nurs* 14(4):210, 1993.

Spiller J: For whose sake—patient or nurse? Ritual practices in patient washing, *Prof Nurse* 7(7):431, 1992.

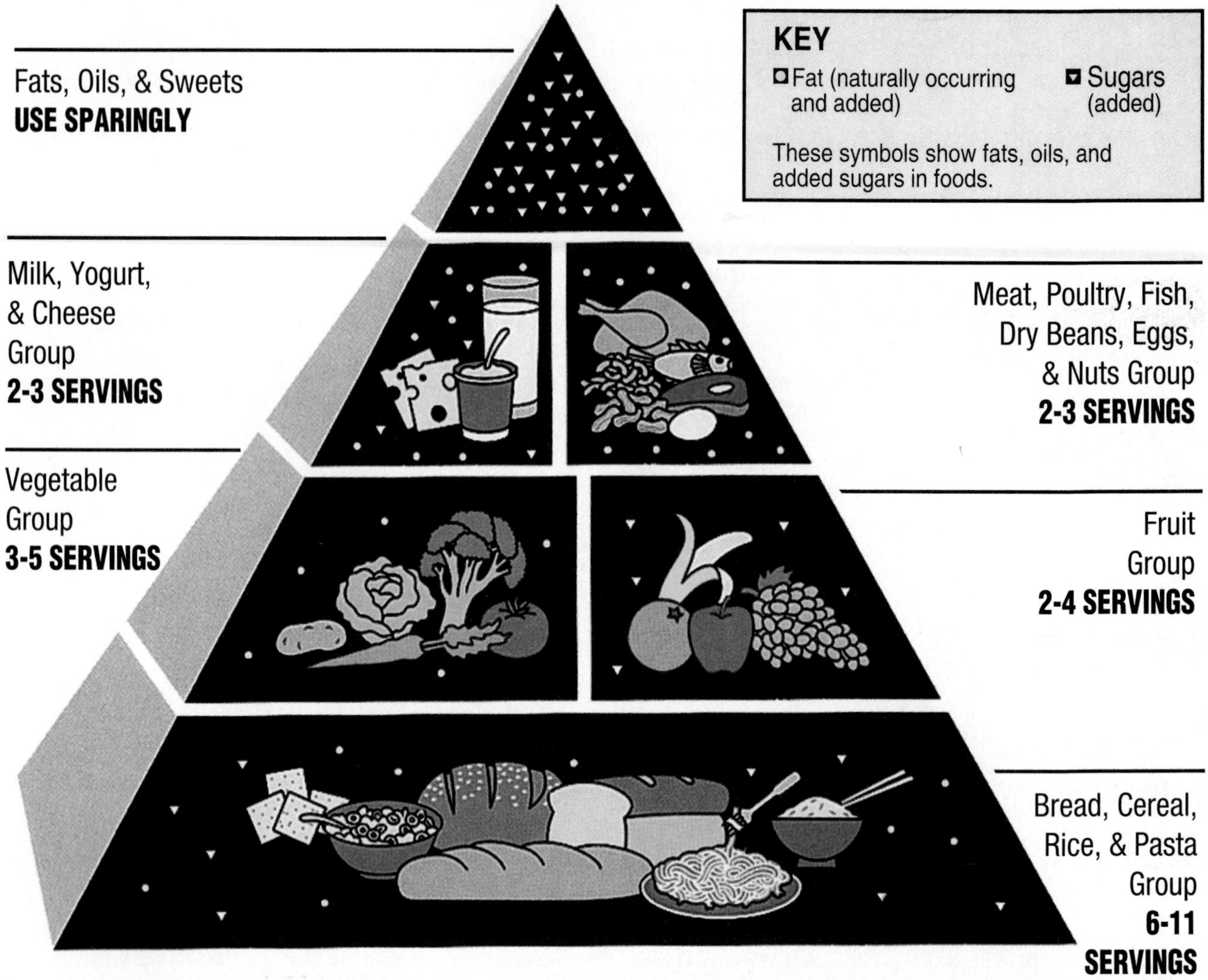
KEY
Fat (naturally occurring and added)
Sugars (added)
These symbols show fats, oils, and added sugars in foods.
Fats, Oils, & Sweets
USE SPARINGLY
Milk, Yogurt, & Cheese Group
2-3 SERVINGS
Meat, Poultry, Fish, Dry Beans, Eggs, & Nuts Group
2-3 SERVINGS
Vegetable Group
3-5 SERVINGS
Fruit Group
2-4 SERVINGS
Bread, Cereal, Rice, & Pasta Group
6-11 SERVINGS

unit six

BASIC PHYSIOLOGICAL NEEDS

31

Nutrition

OBJECTIVES

Mastery of content in this chapter will enable the student to:

- Define the key terms important in basic nutrition.
- List the six categories of nutrients and explain why each is necessary for nutrition.
- Explain the importance of a balance between energy intake and output.
- List the end products of carbohydrate, protein, and lipid metabolism.
- Explain the significance of saturated, unsaturated, and polyunsaturated lipids in nutrition.
- Describe the basic food groups (including the food pyramid) and their value in planning meals for good nutrition.
- Explain recommended daily allowances (RDAs).
- List USDA dietary guidelines and explain their importance in health promotion.
- Discuss the major areas of nutritional assessment.
- Identify three major nutritional problems and describe clients at risk for these problems.
- State goals of enteral nutrition.
- Describe the procedure for initiating and maintaining tube feedings.
- Describe methods to avoid the complications associated with tube feedings.
- State the goals of total parenteral nutrition.
- Describe the procedure for initiating and maintaining total parenteral nutrition.

KEY TERMS

anorexia nervosa
anthropometry
bulimia
carbohydrates
digestion
enzymes
gastrostomy feeding tube
hyperglycemia
hypoglycemia
jejunal feeding tube
lipid
malnutrition
metabolism
minerals
nitrogen balance
nutrients
obesity
proteins
recommended daily allowances (RDAs)
total parenteral nutrition (TPN)
vitamins

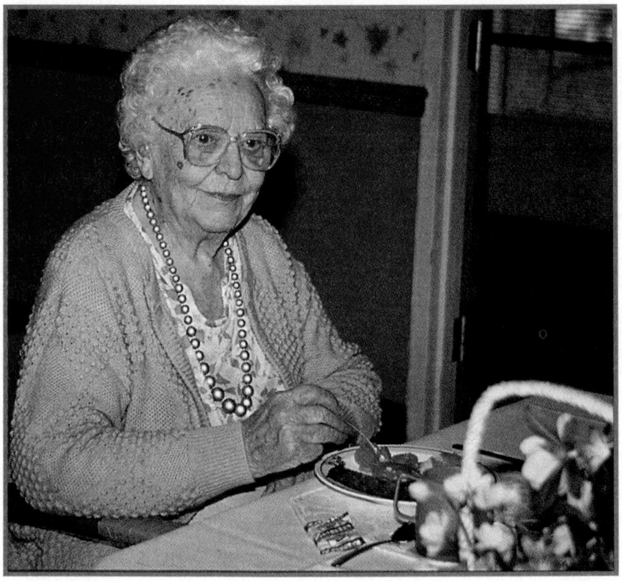

Nutrition is a basic component of all aspects of health. It is essential for normal growth, tissue maintenance and repair, and recovery from illness or surgery. An adequate supply of nutrients is needed for basic body cells to the special antibodies and cells of the immune system. Cardiovascular diseases, diabetes, cancer, and obesity are major diseases of our population that may be treated or prevented by optimal nutrition.

The nursing curriculum must incorporate scientific principles of the body's need for and use of nutrients. Today nursing students need a thorough understanding of all nutrients from the basic functions and how illnesses and their treatments affect nutrition. The focus needs to change from teaching diets to emphasizing healthy eating.

Research data are showing increasing evidence of the importance of nutrition in health maintenance and disease prevention. Today's nurse needs thorough knowledge of nutrition's role in reaching and maintaining health.

PRINCIPLES OF NUTRITION

The body requires food to provide energy for organ function, body movement, and daily activities, to maintain body temperature, and to provide raw materials for enzyme function, growth, replacement of body tissues, and repair.

Courtesy Michael S. Clement, MD, Mesa, Ariz.

Metabolism is the biochemical reactions within the body. It consists of anabolic reactions that build substances and body tissue and catabolic reactions that break down substances. Food is ingested, digested, and absorbed to produce energy needed for these reactions.

Energy requirements vary and are influenced by many factors. The energy requirement of an awake person at rest is called the basal metabolic rate (BMR). The BMR is the energy needed at the lowest level of cellular function. Age, body size and temperatures, activity, environmental temperature, growth, sex, nutritional and emotional states, and food intake affect individual energy requirements beyond the BMR.

Energy balance occurs when energy requirements are completely met by calorie intake in food and people maintain their activity level without weight change. When the number of calories ingested exceeds the energy needs, the person gains weight; when the number of calories ingested fails to meet energy requirements, weight loss occurs.

Nutrients are found in foods that are the elements necessary for body function. The six categories of nutrients are water, carbohydrates, proteins, lipids, vitamins, and minerals. Energy needs are met by the metabolism of carbohydrates, proteins, and lipids. Water is needed because nutrients must be in solution for absorption and transportation. Although vitamins and minerals do not provide energy, they are necessary in the chemical reactions that produce energy.

Water

Water is the most important nutrient because the function of cells depends on a fluid environment. A lean person's body contains more water than an obese person's body. Infants have the greatest percentage of total body weight as water; older adults have the least. The proportion of water in total body weight decreases with age. Infants and older adults are most vulnerable to water deprivation or water loss.

Fluid needs are met by the ingestion of liquids and solid foods such as fresh fruits and vegetables and by water produced when food is oxidized during digestion. In a healthy individual, the fluid intake from all sources equals the fluid output through elimination, respiration, and sweating. An ill person can have an increased need for fluids, as is the case with an increased body temperature or hypermetabolic state. In addition, an ill person can have a decreased need for fluid intake, as is the case in a client with cardiopulmonary or renal disease.

Thirst is a protective mechanism that alerts the oriented person to the need for fluids. Thirst is a less reliable guide for infants and confused clients. These clients are usually unable to communicate that they are thirsty.

Carbohydrates

Carbohydrates are composed of carbon, hydrogen, and oxygen and are obtained mainly from plant foods; the only important source of animal carbohydrate is the lactose in milk (milk sugar). People with limited financial resources tend to ingest more carbohydrates than those with more resources. Carbohydrates may contribute as much as 90% of the total caloric intake in parts of the world where grains are a major ingredient of every meal.

Carbohydrates are classified according to their sugar units or saccharides. A monosaccharide is a simple sugar that cannot be broken down into a more basic sugar unit (e.g., glucose [dextrose], galactose, and fructose).

A carbohydrate with two sugar units is a disaccharide (e.g., sucrose, lactose, and maltose). When two monosaccharides unite, they form a disaccharide and water. During digestion, the reverse occurs; a disaccharide takes up water and is split into two simple sugars.

Polysaccharides are composed of many sugar units, are insoluble in water, and are digested with varying degrees of completeness. Glycogen is a polysaccharide, synthesized from glucose and stored in the liver and muscles, and is the form in which the body stores carbohydrate.

Plants store carbohydrate as starch, which is made up of granules enclosed by cellulose walls. When starch is cooked, the granules swell and burst the cellulose wall. Raw starch foods are more difficult to digest than the same foods after cooking because the freeing of the granules from the cellulose permits greater contact with digestive enzymes and more complete digestion. The digestion of starch consists of several steps. Starch is first broken down into dextrose, then maltose, and finally glucose.

Some polysaccharides cannot be digested because humans do not have enzymes capable of breaking them down. Nevertheless, these polysaccharides have a role in human nutrition because they add fiber to the diet. Fiber is important in preventing and treating disease such as cancer and diabetes mellitus. An example of fiber is lignin, a woody substance added to breads.

The metabolism of 1 g of carbohydrate produces 4 calories (17 joules). Carbohydrate metabolism may produce three different results: catabolism into energy, carbon dioxide, and water; anabolism into glycogen for storage; and conversion into fat (adipose tissue) for storage. There are no specific required daily allowances for carbohydrates. Carbohydrates are the body's preferred energy source and are needed to metabolize lipids and spare protein for energy. To keep the body in acid-base balance, at least 50 to 100 g of carbohydrate are needed daily. Recent nutritional guidelines advocate an increase in the percentage of total daily calories provided by carbohydrates. This increase of 55% to 60% or more of total kilocalories should be derived from natural sugars and polysaccharides (Committee on Dietary Allowances, 1989; Pennington, 1989).

Proteins

Proteins are made of hydrogen, oxygen, carbon, and nitrogen; most proteins also contain sulfur and phosphorus. Because of their high molecular weight and tendency to form colloidal solutions, proteins do not readily pass through body membranes. Amino acids are the most important components of proteins; they are essential for synthesis of body tissue in growth, maintenance, and repair. Protein can also be used as a source of energy.

Protein foods tend to be expensive, and their contribution to total caloric intake is usually higher in affluent families and developed countries. Protein intake is of particular importance during periods of rapid growth and after disease and injury.

Proteins are classified as simple, conjugated, or derived. Simple proteins (e.g., albumin and globulin) are hydrolyzed into amino acids or their derivatives. The combination of a simple protein with a nonprotein substance produces a conjugated protein. Derived proteins are formed during the hydrolysis of protein (e.g., peptides and proteoses occur during stages in protein digestion).

Another method of classifying protein is based on its nutritional value, as complete or incomplete. A complete protein contains all essential amino acids in sufficient quantity to support growth and maintain nitrogen balance. Complete proteins are also referred to as *high-n-*

ESSENTIAL AND NONESSENTIAL AMINO ACIDS

ESSENTIAL	NONESSENTIAL
Histidine	Alanine
Isoleucine	Arginine
Leucine	Asparagine
Lysine	Aspartic acid
Methionine	Citrulline
Phenylalanine	Cysteine
Threonine	Cystine
Tryptophan	Glutamic acid
Valine	Glycine
	Hydroxyglutamic acid
	Hydroxyproline*
	Norleucine*
	Proline
	Serine
	Thyroxine*
	Tyrosine

*Whether these are true amino acids is questionable.

biological value proteins (e.g., meat, fish, poultry, milk, and eggs).

An incomplete protein does not contain all the essential amino acids or does not have them in sufficient quantity to support growth and maintain nitrogen balance (e.g., cereals, legumes, and vegetables). The combination of one incomplete protein with another incomplete protein in the same dish or meal may supply the essential amino acids to support growth and maintain nitrogen balance. Incomplete proteins that combine to act as complete proteins are called *complementary proteins* (e.g., grains and legumes). Amino acids are classified as essential or nonessential (see the box on p. 872).

Because the body cannot synthesize essential amino acids, they must be provided by the diet. Nonessential amino acids are not needed because the body manufactures them from the breakdown of other amino acids.

Protein is the body's only source of nitrogen, and 16% of protein is nitrogen. The body is in **nitrogen balance** when the intake and output of nitrogen are equal. When intake exceeds output, the body is in positive nitrogen balance (e.g., growth, normal pregnancy, and wound healing). Negative nitrogen balance occurs when the body loses more nitrogen than it takes in (e.g., infection, starvation, or injury). Increased nitrogen loss is the result of body tissue destruction.

Protein can be used to provide energy, but it must be spared to carry out its essential functions. A person must provide enough carbohydrate in the diet to meet the body's energy needs to spare protein for its role in nitrogen balance and tissue building.

Protein is metabolized to yield amino acids, nitrogen, and 4 kcal (17 joules) per gram. Amino acids are anabolized into tissues, hormones, and enzymes. Amino acids can also be converted to fat and stored as adipose tissue or catabolized into energy, carbon dioxide, and water.

The required daily allowance of protein ranges from 2.2 g/kg body weight for infants under 6 months to 56 g for males over 15 years. Pregnant women require an additional 30 g and lactating women an additional 20 g above the usual daily need of 44 to 46 g (Food and Nutrition Board, 1989).

Nutrition experts believe that the intake of protein in America is generally greater than required. Protein foods are expensive to buy and produce, and meats, whole milk, cheese, and eggs contain significant amounts of saturated fatty acids and cholesterol. Nutritional guidelines recommend reducing saturated fats and cholesterol in the diet along with increasing complex carbohydrates from fruits, vegetables, and whole grains (USDA, 1990).

Lipids

Lipid is a comprehensive term applied to compounds that are insoluble in water but soluble in organic solvents such as ethanol and acetone. Lipids include fats that are solid at room temperature and oils that are liquid at room temperature. Lipids are composed of carbon, hydrogen, and oxygen.

Lipids are simple, compound, or derived. Simple lipids (e.g., monoglycerides, diglycerides, and triglycerides) are esters of glycerol and fatty acids. Compound lipids are simple lipids combined with a nonlipid substance (e.g., carbohydrate in glycolipids). Derived lipids (e.g., cholesterol, steroid hormones, and fat-soluble vitamins) are produced during the breakdown of simple or compound lipids.

Approximately 98% of the lipids in foods and 90% of the lipids in the human body is in the form of triglycerides. High blood levels of triglycerides have been linked to cardiovascular diseases.

A saturated fatty acid contains as much hydrogen as it can hold. An unsaturated fatty acid can take up another hydrogen atom, and a polyunsaturated fatty acid can take up many more hydrogen atoms and become hydrogenated fat. Ingestion of saturated fatty acids appears to increase blood cholesterol levels. Ingestion of unsaturated fatty acids has a minimal effect on blood cholesterol. Polyunsaturated fatty acids appear to lower blood cholesterol levels.

Fatty acids are usually not purely saturated, unsaturated, or polyunsaturated. Most animal fats have high proportions of saturated fatty acids; most vegetable fats have higher amounts of unsaturated and polyunsaturated fatty acids (e.g., safflower oil is about 75% polyunsaturated, olive oil about 25%).

Linoleic acid is the only essential fatty acid. The body cannot synthesize it, so it depends on adequate dietary intake. Linoleic acid is polyunsaturated and is in safflower, soybean, corn, cottonseed, and peanut oils.

Fat is the body's form of stored energy. The glycerol portion of lipids can be converted to glucose by gluconeogenesis. All body cells except red blood cells and nerve cells can oxidize fatty acids for energy. After a period of starvation, even the central nervous system can adapt to amino acids and ketones as energy sources.

The metabolism of 1 g of lipid yields 9 kcal (38 joules), more than twice the energy provided by carbohydrates or proteins. Lipids account for 35% to 45% of the American diet; the percentage rises with affluence. Nutritional guidelines recommend a reduction of lipid intake to about 30% of the total caloric intake (American Heart Association, 1988).

Vitamins

Vitamins are organic substances present in small amounts in foods and are essential for normal metabolism. The body is unable to synthesize vitamins in the required amounts and depends on dietary intake. The National Research Council reviews new research and revises the recommended allowances for vitamins and other nutrients. Although contained in many foods, vita-

table 31-1

CHARACTERISTICS OF NUTRIENTS

Nutrient	Functions	Results of deficiency	Results of excess	Sources
WATER-SOLUBLE VITAMINS				
C (ascorbic acid)	Production of collagen, integrity of capillary walls, formation of red blood cells, metabolism of amino acids, reduction of iron salts, protection of other vitamins from oxidation	Scurvy, poor wound healing, bleeding gums, loose teeth, bruising	Kidney stones, scurvy on withdrawal, urinary tract infection	Citrus fruits, potatoes, cabbage, tomatoes, broccoli, strawberries, cantaloupe, green peppers
Vitamin B complex B_1 (thiamine)	Component of enzymes, carbohydrate oxidation	Beriberi (rare), polyneuritis, mental confusion, muscular weakness, ataxia, tachycardia, cardiac enlargement	Rapid pulse, headaches, weakness, irritability, insomnia	Pork, fish, eggs, poultry, dried beans, whole grains, wheat germ, oatmeal, bread, pasta
B_2 (riboflavin)	Metabolism of nutrients, essential for growth, oxidation and reduction of fat, carbohydrates, and proteins	Ariboflavinosis: cracks at mouth corners, scaly desquamation of skin around mouth, eye irritation, glossitis, photophobia	Ulcer, elevated blood glucose level, increased uric acid levels in blood	Milk, whole grains, green vegetables, liver
Niacin	Essential for protein use, glycolysis, fat synthesis, tissue repair	Pellagra: weakness, anorexia, lassitude, indigestion; severe pellagra: dermatitis, diarrhea, dementia	Ulcer, liver dysfunction, elevated blood glucose level, increased blood uric acid levels, diarrhea, nausea, flushing	Meats, dairy products, whole grains, cereals, tuna
B_6 (complex of pyridoxine, pyridoxal, pyridoxamine)	Metabolism of nutrients, synthesis of nonessential amino acids, conversion of tryptophan to niacin, proper function of blood and cells of central nervous system	Gastrointestinal upsets, irritability, weakness, nervousness, convulsions, anemia, skin lesions	Reverses antiparkinson effects of levodopa; megadoses: peripheral nerve damage, loss of sensation, numbness, awkward gait, depression	Whole grains, liver, fish, poultry, green beans, nuts, meats, potatoes
Folacin, folic acid	Metabolism of some amino acids, maturation of red blood cells	Macrocytic anemia	Diarrhea, insomnia, irritability; potentially harmful because body is able to store folacin	Liver, green leafy vegetables, meat, fish, poultry, whole grains
B_{12} (cobalamin)	Manufacture of enzymes essential to metabolism of nutrients, nucleic acid, and folic acid; proper function of cells of bone marrow, gastrointestinal tract, and nervous system	Absence of intrinsic factor in gastric juice preventing absorption of vitamin B_{12} and resulting in pernicious anemia, neurological disorders	None known	Milk, eggs, cheese, meat, fish, poultry, foods of animal origin (plant foods contain no vitamin B_{12})

Pantothenic acid	Metabolism of nutrients, synthesis of cholesterol and steroid hormones, activity of adrenal cortex	None known	Increased need for thiamine, occasional diarrhea, water retention	Meats, whole grain cereals, legumes
Biotin	Synthesis of fatty acids, use of glucose, metabolism of protein, use of vitamin B_{12} and folic acid	Produced by ingestion of large amounts of raw egg whites that contain protein substance, avidin, which binds biotin to itself	None known	Liver, kidneys, dark green vegetables, egg yolk, green beans
FAT-SOLUBLE VITAMINS				
A (retinol, retinal, and retinoic acid)	Growth and maintenance of epithelial tissue, maintenance of visual acuity in dim light	Night blindness, rough scaly skin, dry mucous membranes, decreased resistance to infection, faulty tooth and bone development	Nausea, vomiting, abdominal pain, and growth failure in children; weight loss in adults; megadoses: hair loss, bone swelling and tenderness, joint pain, hepatomegaly, splenomegaly, headache	Whole milk, whole milk products, eggs, green leafy vegetables, yellow fruits and vegetables
D (cholecalciferol, engosterol)	Absorption and use of calcium in bone and tooth development	Rickets and delayed dentition in children, osteomalacia in adults	Megadoses: loss of appetite, vomiting, diarrhea, fatigue, growth failure, drowsiness, kidney stones	Sunlight, fortified milk, fortified margarines, fish liver oils
E (tocopherol)	Protection of vitamins A and C and polyunsaturated fatty acids from oxidation, synthesis of heme	Increased hemolysis of red blood cells and macrocytic anemia in premature infants	Interference with the use of vitamins A and K, prolonged prothrombin time, intestinal irritability, fatigue, dizziness	Vegetable oils, green leafy vegetables, milk, eggs, meats, cereals
K	Essential to prothrombin formation and blood clotting	Hemorrhagic disease of the newborn, prolonged clotting time in adults	Hyperbilirubinemia in infants, vomiting in adults	Green leafy vegetables, synthesis in gastrointestinal tract
MACROMINERALS				
Calcium	Formation of teeth and bones, contraction of muscle fibers, transmission of nerve impulses, activation of enzymes, permeability of cell membranes, coagulation of blood, cardiac function	Tingling of fingers and around the mouth, muscle cramps, carpopedal spasm, tetany, convulsions, stunted growth, bone loss in adults, pathological fractures	Relaxed skeletal muscles, deep bone pain, kidney stones, cardiac irregularities	Milk, milk products, leafy green vegetables, fish

*Data from Grant JA and Kennedy-Caldwell C: *Nutritional support in nursing,* New York, 1988, Grune & Stratton; and Whitney EN, Cataldo CB, Rolfes SR: *Understanding normal and clinical nutrition,* St Paul, 1991, West.

†Data from Committee on Dietary Allowances, Food and Nutrition Board, National Academy of Sciences, National Research Council: *Estimated safe and adequate daily dietary intakes,* Washington, DC, 1989.

Continued.

table 31-1—cont'd

CHARACTERISTICS OF NUTRIENTS

Nutrient	Functions	Results of deficiency	Results of excess	Sources
Magnesium	Supports function of B vitamins; use of calcium, potassium, and protein; maintenance of electrical activity in nerves and muscles	Neuromuscular irritability, disorientation, confusion, leg cramps, hallucinations, tachycardia, convulsions, hypertension	Lethargy, respiratory dysfunction, coma, death	Whole grains, fish, nuts, legumes, green vegetables
Phosphorus	Formation of bone and teeth, activation of B vitamins, transfer of energy within cells, promotion of normal muscle and nerve activity, metabolism of carbohydrates, regulation of acid-base balance, transmission of hereditary traits	Hemolytic anemia, defective white blood cell function, delayed clotting, bone pain, pathological fractures	Erosion of jaw, calcium loss	Pork, beef, dried peas and beans, dairy products
MICROMINERALS				
Copper	Essential to hemoglobin formation, cofactor in synthesis of phospholipids, formation and activity of some enzymes, synthesis of prostaglandin	Abnormal blood cell development in infants, bone demineralization	Headache, dizziness, heartburn, weakness, nausea, vomiting, diarrhea, Wilson's disease	Liver, kidney, shellfish, nuts, raisins
Fluoride	Formation of teeth, prevention of dental caries	Poor dental health	Mottling, pitting, and discoloration of tooth enamel	Fluoridated water, seafood, toothpaste, mouthwash gels
Iodine	Basic component of thyroid hormones	Cretinism in infants, simple goiter in children and adults, depressed thyroid function	Toxic goiter	Iodized salt, seafood, food additives, dough oxidizers, dairy disinfectants, coloring agents
Iron	Essential to the formation of hemoglobin, synthesis of vitamins, purines, and antibodies	Anemia, fatigue, weakness, lethargy, lowered immunity	Hemosiderosis, acute iron poisoning from accidental ingestion in infants and children: cramps, abdominal pain, nausea, vomiting, black stools, cirrhosis	Liver, lean meats, whole grains, enriched breads and cereals, green vegetables
Zinc	Connective tissue integrity, involvement in immune response, formation of enzymes	Impaired wound healing, decreased sensations of taste and smell, delayed growth	Anemia, fever, nausea, vomiting, muscle pain, weakness, decreases calcium absorption	Oysters, liver, meats, poultry, legumes, nuts

mins are affected by processing, storage, and preparation. Vitamin content is usually highest in fresh foods used quickly after minimal exposure to heat, air, or water. Vitamins are classified as water soluble and fat soluble.

Water-Soluble Vitamins. Water-soluble vitamins are vitamin C and vitamin B complex, which consists of eight different vitamins. Water-soluble vitamins cannot be stored in the body and must be taken in daily. It was once assumed that, because water-soluble vitamins are not stored in the body, toxicity was not a problem with these vitamins. However, recent studies of people who took megadoses of vitamin C and vitamin B_6 indicate that toxicity can occur. Vitamins are used as catalysts in biochemical reactions. When there is enough of a vitamin to meet the catalyst demands, the rest of the vitamin supply acts as a free chemical and may be toxic to the body (Table 31-1).

Fat-Soluble Vitamins. Fat-soluble vitamins—A, D, E, and K—can be stored in the body, and therefore daily intake is not needed. However, with the exception of vitamin D, these vitamins should be provided by dietary intake. Toxicity to some fat-soluble vitamins, usually the result of megadoses of synthetic vitamins, has been recognized. Processing, storage, and preparation of foods have less effect on fat-soluble vitamin content, and many foods are fortified by the addition of vitamins A and D (see Table 31-1).

Minerals

Minerals are inorganic elements essential to the body because of their role as catalysts in biochemical reactions. Minerals are classified as macrominerals when the daily requirement is 100 mg or more and microminerals when less than 100 mg is needed daily. Because the required amount of microminerals is usually very small or a trace, they are also called trace elements (see Table 31-1). In addition to the microminerals in Table 31-1, arsenic, nickel, silicon, tin, vanadium, and possibly cadmium play unidentified roles in nutrition.

Digestion

The only nutrients the body can use in their ingested form are monosaccharides, water, vitamins, and some minerals. All other foods must be broken down into simpler forms for absorption.

Digestion consists of breaking down nutrients by chewing, mixing with fluid, and chemical reactions. Hormones control the flow of digestive juice. **Enzymes** are essential for digestion. They are protein-like substances that act as catalysts to speed up biochemical reactions. Most enzymes have one specific function, although some can enter into several closely related reactions. Enzyme activity is regulated by the pH of the intestinal contents; each enzyme functions best at a specific pH and is inactivated by major variations from that level. Secretions of the gastrointestinal tract have vastly different pH levels; saliva is relatively neutral, gastric juice is highly acidic, and small intestine secretions are alkaline.

The mechanical, chemical, and hormonal activities of digestion are interdependent. Enzyme activity depends on the mechanical breakdown of food to increase its surface area for chemical action. Hormones regulate the flow of digestive secretions needed for enzyme supply. Digestion may be slowed or speeded up by strong emotional states.

Digestion begins in the mouth, where food is mechanically broken down by chewing. The food is mixed with saliva, which contains ptyalin (salivary amylase), an enzyme that acts on cooked starch to begin its conversion to maltose. The longer food is chewed, the more starch digestion occurs in the mouth. Proteins and fats are broken down physically but remain unchanged chemically because there are no enzymes in the mouth. Chewing reduces food to a size suitable for swallowing, and saliva provides lubrication.

Swallowed food enters the esophagus and is moved along by peristaltic waves. At the upper opening of the stomach, the presence of food causes the sphincter to relax and allows the food to enter the stomach.

The stomach acts as a reservoir. Food remains in it for varying periods (i.e., an average of 3 hours but ranging from 1 to 7 hours) depending on type of meal, gastric motility, and psychological influences. In general, carbohydrate meals spend the least amount of time in the stomach, lipid meals the longest, and protein meals an intermediate period. Large food intake decreases gastric motility and increases the length of time food remains in the stomach.

The activity of ptyalin continues until hydrochloric acid decreases pH to inactivate it. The stomach mixes food with gastric secretions and further breaks down nutrients. The acidic environment favors the action of pepsin, an enzyme that splits proteins into proteoses and peptones. Lipase, an enzyme that functions best in alkaline media, acts on emulsified fats such as butter, egg yolk, milk, and cream at near-neutral pH levels. Lipase then splits emulsified fats into fatty acids and glycerol.

Food leaves the stomach at the pyloric sphincter as an acid, liquefied mass called *chyme.* Chyme flows into the duodenum and is quickly mixed with bile, intestinal juices, and pancreatic secretions. Bile emulsifies or breaks down fat to permit digestive enzyme action, and it holds fatty acids in solution. Intestinal secretions contain seven enzymes to digest fats, proteins, and carbohydrates. Pancreatic juice contains five enzymes for the digestion of starch, fats, and proteins.

Peristalsis continues in the small intestine, causing secretions to mix with chyme. The mixture becomes increasingly alkaline, inhibiting the action of the gastric enzymes and promoting the action of the duodenal secretions. The major portion of digestion occurs in the small intestine, producing glucose, fructose, and galactose from carbohydrates, amino acids from proteins, and fatty acids and glycerol from lipids.

Absorption

The small intestine is also the site of absorption of simple nutrients. It is lined with villi that project into the lumen and greatly increase the surface area available for absorption. Cholesterol, vitamins E and K, folic acid, riboflavin, and thiamine are absorbed in the upper duodenum; glucose, amino acids, and fats are absorbed in the lower duodenum and upper jejunum, and sucrose, lactose, and maltose are absorbed in the lower jejunum and ileum.

Intestinal contents move by peristaltic action into the large intestine. Water is the only nutrient absorbed from the large intestine. Other nutrients remaining in the intestinal contents when they reach the large intestine are excreted as waste products. When intestinal motility is increased, such as in diarrhea, the body loses nutrients that move through the small intestine too quickly for complete absorption.

Metabolism

Nutrients absorbed in the intestines, including water, are transported through the circulatory system to body tissues. Through metabolism, nutrients are converted into necessary substances for cell function. Carbohydrates, protein, and fat produce chemical energy and maintain a dynamic balance of tissue buildup and breakdown. The chemical energy produced by metabolism is converted to other types of energy by different tissues. Muscle contracture involves mechanical energy; the nervous system involves electrical energy, and the mechanisms of heat production involve thermal energy. These forms of energy all originate in metabolism.

The two basic types of metabolism are anabolism and catabolism. Anabolism is the production of more-complex chemical substances by synthesis of nutrients. Catabolism is the breakdown of body tissues into simpler substances. Although catabolism produces some energy, both processes require energy, which must be provided from food or stored sources.

Storage

The body's major form of stored energy is fat in the adipose tissue, which has an almost unlimited capacity. Glycogen is stored in small reserves in liver and muscle tissue, and protein is stored in muscle mass. When the body's energy requirements exceed the energy supplied, stored energy is used; unused energy is stored, principally in fat.

Fat-soluble vitamins are also stored in limited reserves and are released to meet the body's needs when not provided sufficiently by dietary intake. Water-soluble vitamins are not stored and therefore must be provided by daily intake.

Elimination

The intestinal contents move through the large intestine by peristalsis (see Chapter 33). As the material moves toward the rectum, water is absorbed into the mucosa. The longer the material stays in the large intestine, the more water is absorbed and the firmer the remaining solid material becomes. The end products of digestion include cellulose and similar fibrous substances the body is unable to digest. Sloughed cells from the intestinal walls, mucus, digestive secretions, water, and microorganisms are also eliminated.

FOUNDATIONS OF AN ADEQUATE DIET

Food Guide Pyramid

The basic four food groups were introduced in 1956 as one of the earliest recommendations by the USDA. It was suggested that selecting foods from a wide variety of milk, meat, bread and cereal products, and fruits and vegetables would ensure the required amounts of needed nutrients. The Food Guide Pyramid replaces the

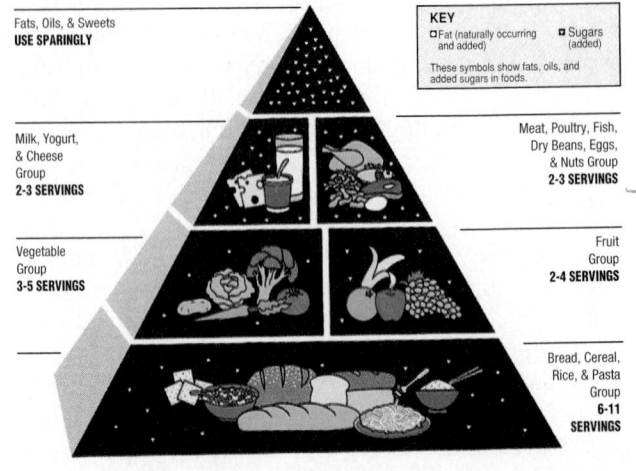

FIGURE 31-1 Food guide pyramid. (From US Department of Agriculture: *USDA's food guide pyramid,* USDA Human Nutrition Information Pub No 249, Washington, DC, 1992, US Government Printing Office.)

basic four food groups with five groups—milk, meat, fruit, vegetables, and grains (USDA, 1992).

The pyramid was designed as a guide for buying food and meal preparation (Figure 31-1). This basic plan provides for diets ranging from 1600 to 2800 kcal/day (USDA, 1992). Additional foods to round out meals and meet energy requirements can be selected from enriched cereals, complex carbohydrates, and additional grains.

Recommended Daily Allowances

The Committee on Dietary Allowances of the Food and Nutrition Board of the National Academy of Sciences has published a list of **recommended daily allowances (RDAs)** since 1943. The RDAs are the level of intake of essential nutrients considered, in the judgment of the committee and on the basis of scientific knowledge, to be adequate to meet the nutritional needs of healthy people (Table 31-2).

In 1990, Congress passed the Nutrition Labeling and Education Act (NLEA) to require mandatory nutrition labeling for most FDA-regulated foods. It also requires the Food and Drug Administration (FDA) to issue voluntary nutrition guidelines to food retailers for providing nutrition information on certain vegetables, fruits, and raw fish (Public Law 101-535, 1990). If retailers fail to comply substantially with the guidelines, the NLEA requires the FDA to issue mandatory requirements for these commodities.

A further proposal allows the use of health messages in the areas of fat and cancer, fat and heart disease, calcium and osteoporosis, and sodium and hypertension. In January 1991 the USDA announced that it would develop a mandatory nutrition labeling program for processed meat and poultry products and voluntary guidelines for fresh meat and poultry. The proposed nutrition label will clarify serving size, nutrient content, health claims, low-fat and low-cholesterol claims, and unclear terms such as *light* or *lite* to aid the consumer in understanding the actual nutritional content.

Other Dietary Guidelines

In 1980 the USDA and the USDHHS issued newer dietary guidelines. These guidelines consisted of seven categories and were revised in 1985 and in 1990 (see box at right).

In 1990 the USDHHS and Public Health Service (PHS), after a 4-year consensus process, published *Healthy People 2000, National Health Promotion and Disease Prevention Objectives.* The report defines national goals or objectives to be met in this decade to increase the proportion of Americans who live long, healthy lives.

All 21 nutrition-related goals for the year 2000 include baseline data. For example, one objective is to reduce the prevalence of overweight people to no more than 20% among people age 20 years and older, a decrease from the current baseline level of 26%. Other objectives are to reduce dietary fat intake to an average of 30% of total calories, down from the recent level of 36%, and to reduce saturated fat intake to less than 10%, down from the present 13%. Additional objectives include increasing intake of fruits, vegetables, and grain products and reducing sodium consumption.

1990 DIETARY GUIDELINES

Eat a variety of foods.
- Choose fruits and vegetables.
- Choose whole grain and enriched breads, cereals, and other grain products.
- Choose milk, cheese, yogurt, and other milk products.
- Choose meat, poultry, fish, eggs, and dry peas and beans.

Maintain healthy weight.

Choose a diet low in fat, saturated fat, and cholesterol.
- Choose lean meat, fish, and poultry.
- Use dry peas and beans as protein sources.
- Use low-fat milk and milk products.
- Use egg yolk and organ meats moderately.
- Limit consumption of butter, cream, heavily hydrogenated fats and oils, and food high in palm and coconut oil.
- Trim off excess fat on meats.
- Broil, bake, or boil rather than fry.

Choose a diet with plenty of vegetables, fruits, and grain products.
- Eat three or more servings of vegetables each day.
- Consume two or more servings of fruits daily.
- Eat six or more servings of grain products each day.

Use sugar in moderation
- Use less sugar and eat fewer high-sugar foods.
- Avoid between-meal sweets.
- Avoid foods whose labels contain sucrose, glucose, and lactose.
- Select foods canned without syrup or with light syrup.

Use salt in moderation.
- Learn to enjoy unsalted food.
- Cook with only a small amount of added salt.
- Add little or no salt at the table.
- Limit intake of salty foods.
- Read food labels.
- Use new, lower-sodium products.

If you drink alcohol, do so in moderation.

Data from USDA and USDHHS: *Nutrition and your health: dietary guidelines for Americans,* USDA/DHHS Home and Garden Bull No. 232, Washington, DC, 1990, US Government Printing office.

table 31-2

RECOMMENDED DIETARY ALLOWANCES*

Category	Age (yr) or condition	Weight† (kg)	Weight† (lb)	Height† (cm)	Height† (in)	kcal per day	Protein (g)	Fat-soluble vitamins: A (μg RE)‡	D (μg)§	E (mgαTE)‖	K (μg)
Infants	0.0-0.5	6	13	60	24	650	13	375	7.5	3	5
	0.5-1.0	9	20	71	28	850	14	375	10	4	10
Children	1-3	13	29	90	35	1300	16	400	10	6	15
	4-6	20	44	112	44	1800	24	500	10	7	20
	7-10	28	62	132	52	2000	28	700	10	7	30
Men	11-14	45	99	157	62	2500	45	1000	10	10	45
	15-18	66	145	176	69	3000	59	1000	10	10	65
	19-24	72	160	177	70	2900	58	1000	10	10	70
	25-50	79	174	176	70	2900	63	1000	5	10	80
	Over 51	77	170	173	68	2300	63	1000	5	10	80
Women	11-14	46	101	157	62	2200	46	800	10	8	45
	15-18	55	120	163	64	2200	44	800	10	8	55
	19-24	58	128	164	65	2200	46	800	10	8	60
	25-50	63	138	163	64	2200	50	800	5	8	65
	Over 51	65	143	160	63	1900	50	800	5	8	65
Pregnant						2500	60	800	10	10	65
Lactating:	1st 6 mo					3000	65	1300	10	12	65
	2nd 6 mo					3000	62	1200	10	11	65

From Food and Nutrition Board, *National Academy of Sciences—National Research Council: Recommended dietary allowances,* Washington DC, 1989, The Council.

*The allowances, expressed as average daily intakes over time, are intended to provide for individual variations among most normal persons as they live in the United States under usual environmental stresses. Diets should be based on a variety of common foods to provide other nutrients for which human requirements have been less well defined.

†Weights and heights of Reference Adults are actual medians for the U.S. population of the designated age.

‡Retinol equivalents. 1 RE = 1 μg retinol or 6 μg β-carotene. See text for calculations of vitamin A activity of diets as retinol equivalents.

§As cholecalciferol. 10 μg cholecalciferol = 400 U of vitamin D.

‖α-Tocopherol equivalents. 1 mg d-α-tocopherol = 1 α-TE.

¶1 NE niacin equivalent = 1 mg of niacin of 60 mg of dietary tryptophan.

The remaining challenge is to motivate consumers to put these dietary recommendations into practice. Health professionals can play a key role in promoting healthy dietary habits.

Alternative Food Patterns

Long before recommended allowances and guidelines were issued, many people followed special patterns of food intake based on religion, cultural background, ethics, health beliefs, personal preference, or concern for the efficient use of land to produce food. Such special diets are not necessarily more or less nutritional than diets based on the basic four food groups or other nutritional guidelines because good nutrition depends on a balanced intake of all required nutrients. A common dietary pattern is the vegetarian diet, which is the consumption of a diet consisting predominantly of plant foods. Vegetarians may be ovolactovegetarians, who avoid meat, fish, and poultry but eat eggs and milk, or lactovegetarians, who drink milk but avoid eggs. The pure vegetarian diet is not recommended for infants and young children unless it is carefully planned (Jacobs, Dwyer, 1988).

DEVELOPMENTAL VARIABLES IN NUTRITION

Infants

Infancy is marked by rapid growth and high energy requirements (Tasble 31-3). The average birth weight of an American baby is 3.2 to 3.4 kg (7 to 7½ lb). The infant usually doubles birth weight at 4 to 5 months and triples it at 1 year. An energy intake of approximately 108 kcal/kg of body weight is needed in the first half of in-

[redacted]

Water-soluble vitamins							Minerals						
C (mg)	Thiamin (mg)	Riboflavin (mg)	Niacin (mg NE)¶	B_6 (mg)	Folate (µg)	B_{12} (µg)	Calcium (mg)	Phosphorus (mg)	Magnesium (mg)	Iron (mg)	Zinc (mg)	Iodine (µg)	Selenium (µg) 35
30	0.3	0.4	5	0.3	25	0.3	400	300	40	6	5	40	10
35	0.4	0.5	6	0.6	35	0.5	400	500	60	10	5	50	15
40	0.7	0.8	9	1.0	50	0.7	400	800	80	10	10	70	20
45	0.9	1.1	12	1.1	75	1.0	800	800	120	10	10	90	20
45	1.0	1.2	13	1.4	100	1.4	800	800	170	10	10	120	20
50	1.3	1.5	17	1.7	150	2.0	1200	1200	270	12	15	150	40
60	1.5	1.8	20	2.0	200	2.0	1200	1200	400	12	15	150	50
60	1.5	1.7	29	2.0	200	2.0	1200	1200	350	10	15	150	70
60	1.5	1.7	19	2.0	200	2.0	800	800	350	10	15	150	70
60	1.2	1.4	15	2.0	200	2.0	800	800	350	10	15	150	70
50	1.1	1.3	15	1.4	150	2.0	800	1200	280	15	12	150	45
60	1.1	1.3	15	1.5	180	2.0	1000	1200	300	15	12	150	50
60	1.1	1.3	15	1.6	180	2.0	1000	1200	280	15	12	150	55
60	1.1	1.3	15	1.6	180	2.0	1000	800	280	15	12	150	55
60	1.0	1.3	13	1.6	180	2.0	1000	800	280	10	12	150	55
70	1.5	1.6	17	2.2	400	2.2	1500	1200	320	30	15	175	65
95	1.6	1.8	20	2.1	280	2.6	1200	1200	355	15	19	200	75
90	1.6	1.7	20	2.1	260	2.6	1200	1200	340	15	16	200	75

fancy and 98 kcal/kg in the second half (Food and Nutrition Board, 1989). A full-term newborn is able to digest and absorb simple carbohydrates, proteins, and a moderate amount of emulsified fat. Amylase, the starch-splitting enzyme, is not present until approximately 2½ or 3½ months. Infants need a high amount of fluid because a large portion of total body weight is water.

Breast-Fed Infants. Breast milk is the ideal food for infants. The current recommendation is that breast milk be the major source of nutrients for the first 4 to 6 months. Breast milk contains antibodies to protect against antigens in infant formulas and foods. As the infant grows, the gastrointestinal tract can fight against common bacteria and allergy-causing proteins.

Breast-feeding promotes bonding between mother and child (Figure 31-2). The lipid content of breast milk is better absorbed than that from other infant foods. Breast-feeding may prevent infant obesity and protect against hypercholesterolemia in later life. At the end of the nursing period, breast milk has a higher fat content. The high cholesterol level of breast milk is thought to foster the development of more efficient cholesterol metabolism.

Breast-fed infants need a source of vitamin C, fluoride, vitamin D, and iron. After 4 months, when the fetal store of iron is exhausted, the infant needs a dietary source of this nutrient.

Bottle-Fed Infants. Bottle-fed infants are usually given 5% to 10% glucose or sterile water 4 hours after birth. Infant formulas can also be fortified with vitamins and minerals to resemble human milk. Neither undiluted whole milk nor skim milk should be used as a basis for infant formulas. Whole milk has excess protein and requires dilution, and skim milk does not contain

table 31-3

HOW TO FEED YOUR BABY STEP-BY-STEP

Food group	Foods	Daily servings	Suggested serving size	Feeding tips
0-4 MO				
Milk	Breast milk or	8-12 or on demand		Nurse baby at least 5-10 min on each breast. Six wet diapers a day is good sign.
	Formula* 0-1 mo	6-8	2-5 oz	There is no need to force baby to finish bottle.
	1-2 mo	5-7	3-6 oz	Putting baby to bed with bottle could cause choking.
	2-3 mo	4-7	4-7 oz	
	3-4 mo	4-6	6-8 oz	Heating formula in microwave is not recommended.
4-6 MO				
Milk	Breast milk or formula*	4-6		May need to start baby cereal (iron-fortified).
		4-6	6-8 oz	Feed only one new cereal each week.
Grain	Baby cereal (iron-fortified)	2	1-2 tbsp	There is no need to add salt or sugar to cereal. Offer baby extra water. Use microwave with caution.
6-8 MO				
Milk	Breast milk or formula*	3-5		Add strained fruits and vegetables at first. Add mashed or finely chopped fruits and cooked vegetables later on.
	Baby cereal (iron-fortified)	3-5	6-8 oz	
Grain	Bread, bagel, or bun	2	2-4 tbsp	
	Crackers	Offer	1/2	Feed only one new fruit or vegetable each week.
			2 crackers	Take out of jar amount of food for one feeding. Refrigerate remaining food.
Fruit-vegetable	Fruit or vegetables	4	2-3 tbsp	
	Baby fruit juice	1	3 oz (from cup)	Try giving baby fruit juice in cup. Offer following foods only when baby has full set of teeth: apple chunks or slices, grapes, sausages, peanut butter, hard chunks of uncooked vegetables. Inform parents that these foods can cause choking.
8-12 MO				
Milk	Breast milk,	3-4		Ask your doctor if baby is ready for whole milk.
	Formula,* or whole milk	3-4	6-8 oz	
	Cheese		1/2 oz	
	Plain yogurt	Offer	1/2 cup	
	Cottage cheese		1/4 cup	
Grain	Baby cereal (iron-foritifed)	2	2-4 tbsp	
	Bread, bagel, or	2	1/2	Be patient. Babies make messes when they feed themselves.
	Crackers		2 crackers	
Fruit-vegetable	Fruit or vegetables	4	3-4 tbsp	Always test heated foods before serving them to baby.
	Baby fruit juice	1	3 oz (from cup)	
Meat	Chicken, beef, pork	2	3-4 tbsp	Add strained or finely chopped meats.
	Cooked, dried beans, or egg yolks			Feed only one new meat a week. Wait until baby's first birthday to feed egg whites. Some babies are sensitive to egg white. It is okay to give egg yolks.

From National Dairy Council: *Feeding guide for the first two years,* Rosemont, Ill, 1990, The Council.
Every baby is very special. Do not worry if your baby eats a little more or less than this guide suggests. In fact, this is perfectly normal. The suggested sizes are only guidelines to help you get started.
*If you are bottle feeding, most doctors recommend iron-fortified formula. Ask your doctor which formula is best for your baby.

table 31-3—cont'd

HOW TO FEED YOUR BABY STEP-BY-STEP

Food group	Foods	Daily servings	Suggested serving size	Feeding tips
12-24 MO				
Milk	Whole milk, yogurt	3	1/2 cup	Add whole milk now.
	Cheese		1/2 oz	Offer small portions and never force toddler to
	Cottage cheese		1/4 cup	eat.
Grain	Cereal, pasta, or rice	4	1/4 cup	"Food jags" are common now. Don't make big
	Bread, muffins, bagels,		1/2	deal out of them.
	rolls		2 crackers	Respect toddler's likes and dislikes. Offer re-
	Crackers			jected foods again.
Fruit-vegetable	All fruits and vegetables:	4		Make meals fun and interesting. Serve colorful
	Cooked, juice		1/4 cup	foods that are crunchy, smooth, or warm.
	Whole		1/2 medium	Feed toddler at least three snacks every day.
Meat	Fish, chicken, turkey, beef, pork	2	1 oz	
	Cook dried beans or peas		1/4 cup	
	Eggs		1	

linoleic acid and is too low in calories. Honey and corn syrup are potential sources of the botulism toxin and should not be used in the infant's diet. The toxin can be fatal in children under 1 year of age (Wardlaw, Insel, Seyler, 1992).

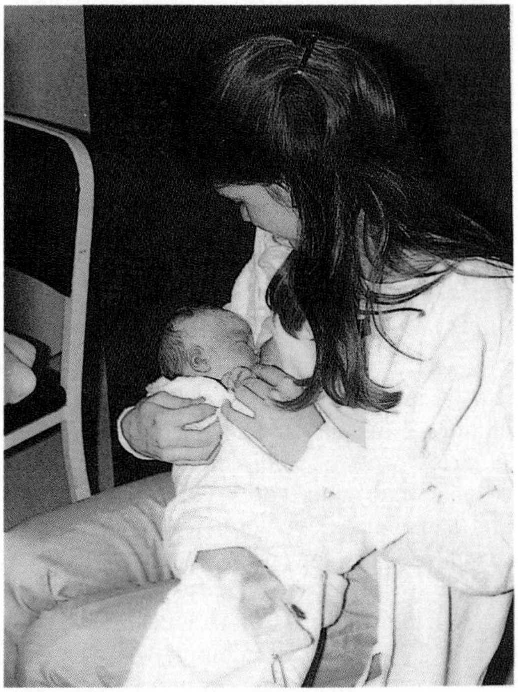

FIGURE 31-2 Bonding between mother and child. (From Dickason EJ, Silverman BL, Schult MO: Maternal-infant nursing care, ed 2, St. Louis, 1994, Mosby.)

Introduction to Solid Food. The ability to swallow voluntarily is not fully developed until 10 to 12 weeks of age. Before that time, swallowing must be stimulated by sucking. The amount of saliva needed to ease swallowing solid food is not secreted until about 3 months of age. Enzymes to digest complex carbohydrates (e.g., cereals) and taste sensation are not fully developed until 3 to 4 months of age.

Foods may be started gradually, beginning sometime between 4 and 6 months, depending on the infant's readiness. Indications of readiness can include the following:

1. Infant doubling the birth weight
2. Infant's ability to consume 8 oz of formula and to become hungry in less than 4 hours
3. Infant's ability to sit up
4. Infant's ability to consume 32 oz a day and want more
5. Six months of age

Toddlers and Preschoolers

The growth rate slows during the toddler period (1 to 3 years of age). The toddler needs fewer calories but an increased amount of protein in relation to body weight. Toddlers are more interested in their environment and increasing motor skills than in food.

The toddler needs a minimum of 16 ounces daily from the milk group to supply protein, calcium, riboflavin, and vitamins A and B_{12}. Fortified milk provides vitamin D and additional vitamin A. Whole milk should be used until the toddler reaches 2 years of age because of the linoleic acid in the milk fat. Half of the toddler's protein intake should consist of high-n-biological value proteins. Toddlers who consume more than 24 ounces of milk daily instead of other foods may develop a milk anemia. Lean red meats, as a part of the 1 to 3 ounces of meat group foods, are a good source of iron, as are whole grains, enriched cereals, and breads.

The toddler should receive four servings daily from the fruit and vegetable group. One serving should be a good source of vitamin C. Green leafy vegetables and deep yellow fruits and vegetables should be served frequently.

The toddler's four or more servings from the bread and cereal group should include whole grain or enriched breads, cereals, and pastas. Infant cereals may continue to be used because of their higher iron content. In addition to the food pyramid guidelines, the toddler should have 1 to 2 teaspoons of margarine or butter for vitamin A. The rate of growth slows after 12 to 14 months of age, but nutritional needs remain high. Good nutritional habits should be started early, with fruit desserts, custards, puddings, and ice cream emphasized instead of cake, pies, and cookies.

During the preschool years, children gain an average of 2 kg (4½ pounds) of body weight and 5 to 8 cm (2 to 3 inches) in height a year. At the end of the preschool period, the child's weight is double that at 1 year of age and height is 1½ times that at 1 year.

Daily protein needs are increased to 24 g, half of which should be high–biological value proteins. Calcium and iron remain important. Fruits and vegetables should be encouraged to provide vitamins A and C.

Preschoolers need 16 ounces of milk daily, 1 to 3 ounces from the meat group, four or more servings of fruits, vegetables (including a daily source of vitamin C and frequent servings of leafy green and deep yellow vegetables and fruits), four or more servings of whole grain or enriched foods, and 1 to 2 teaspoons of margarine or butter.

School-Age Children

School-age children, 6 to 12 years old, grow at a slower and more steady rate, with a gradual decline in energy requirements per unit of body weight. The school-age child gains 3 to 5 kg (6½ to 11 pounds) in weight and 6 cm (2½ inches) in height a year until puberty.

The appetites of school-age children are greater than those of younger children, and food intake is more varied. Recommended intake includes two to three servings from the milk group, 2 to 3 ounces of meat group foods, four to five servings of fruits and vegetables (with a daily source of vitamin C and a source of vitamin A every other day), six or more servings from whole grain and enriched breads and cereals, and 1 to 2 teaspoons of margarine or butter.

Despite better appetites and more varied food intake, the diets of school-age children should be carefully assessed for adequate protein and vitamin A and C.

The diets of American children exceed the recommended levels for dietary and saturated fats. Approximately 25 percent of children have blood cholesterol levels above acceptable levels (Gortmaker, et al., 1987, Expert Panel on Blood Cholesterol in Children and Adolescents, 1991).

Adolescents

During adolescence, physiological age is a better guide to nutritional needs than chronological age. Adolescence begins with the growth spurt of puberty at the end of childhood and ends with the completion of physical growth. Caloric needs are greatly increased to meet increased metabolic demands. Girls need approximately 2000 to 2500 kcal a day; boys need 2500 to 3000 kcal a day. Protein needs increase to a daily requirement of 45 to 59 g. Calcium is essential for the rapid bone growth of adolescence, and girls need a continuous source of iron to replace menstrual losses. Boys need increased iron for normal muscle development. Iodine supports increased thyroid activity, and B complex vitamins support the heightened metabolic activity.

Adolescents require three or more servings of dairy products; two or more meat/protein servings; four or more servings of fruit and vegetables (with a daily source of vitamin C and a source of vitamin A every other day); six to eleven servings of whole grain foods; and 1 to 2 tablespoons of margarine or butter.

Snacks provide approximately 25% of the teenager's total dietary intake (Whitney, Cataldo, Rolfes, 1991). The irregular eating pattern of skipping meals or eating meals and the wrong choice of snacks contribute to obesity and nutrient deficits. Snack food from the dairy and fruit-vegetable groups are good choices and contribute calcium, phosphorous, protein, zinc, vitamin A, vitamin C, and some of the B complex vitamins. Table 31-4 lists nutrients in some popular fast food restaurants.

The adolescent's diet is influenced by many factors other than nutritional needs, including concern about body image and appearance, desire for independence, and fad diets. Nutritional deficiencies may occur in adolescent girls as a result of dieting and using oral contraceptives. The nutrients that are involved are folic acid, vitamin B_6, vitamin C, thiamine, riboflavin, and iron. The adolescent boy's diet may be inadequate in iron and folic acid.

Pregnant teenage girls must meet their own nutritional needs, as well as the additional demands of pregnancy. Pregnancy occurring within 4 years after the menarche (which usually occurs at 10½ to 13 years in America) places mother and fetus at risk because of anatomical and physiological immaturity. The fetus has

table 31-4

REFERENCE GUIDE FOR POPULAR FAST FOODS

Item	Serving size	Calories*	Carbohydrates†	Protein†	Fat†	Sodium‡	Exchange*
ARBY'S							
Junior Roast Beef	3 oz	218	22	12	8	345	1½ starch, 1 ½ med. fat meat
Regular Roast Beef	5.2 oz	353	32	22	15	590	2 starch, 2 med. fat meat, 1 fat
Hot Ham 'n' Cheese sandwich	5.7 oz	353	33	26	13	1655	2 starch, 3 med. fat meat
Potato cakes	3 oz	201	22	2	14	425	1½ starch, 3 fat§
Roasted chicken Boneless breast	5 oz	254	2	43	7	930	6 lean meat
BURGER KING							
Hamburger	1	275	29	15	12	509	2 starch, 2 med. fat meat
Cheeseburger	1	317	30	17	15	651	2 starch, 2 med. fat meat, 1 fat
Whopper	1	628	46	27	36	880	3 starch, 3 med. fat meat, 4 fat§
Chicken specialty sandwich	1	688	56	26	40	1423	4 starch, 2 med. fat meat, 5 fat§
Chicken tenders	6 pc	204	10	20	10	636	1 starch, 2 med. fat meat
Onion rings	1 serving	274	28	4	16	665	2 starch, 3 fat
French fries	Regular	227	24	3	13	160	1½ starch, 2 fat
DAIRY QUEEN							
Single hamburger	1	360	33	21	16	630	2 starch, 2 med. fat meat, 1 fat
Hot dog	1	280	21	11	16	830	1½ starch, 1 med. fat meat, 2 fat
Fish fillet	1	430	45	20	18	674	3 starch, 2 med. fat meat, 1 fat
Chicken breast fillet	1	608	46	27	34	725	3 starch, 3 med. fat meat, 3 fat§
French fries	Regular	200	25	2	10	115	1½ starch, 2 fat
Onion rings	1 order	280	31	4	16	140	2 starch, 3 fat
Cone	Small	140	22	3	4	45	1½ starch, 1 fat
Chocolate sundae	Small	190	33	3	4	75	2 starch, 1 fat
Dilly Bar	1	210	21	3	13	50	1½ starch, 2 fat
DQ sandwich	1	140	24	3	4	40	1½ starch, 1 fat
DOMINO'S PIZZA							
Cheese pizza	12″ (2 slices)	340	52	18	6	660	3 starch, 1 med. fat meat, 1 vegetable
Pepperoni pizza	12″ (2 slices)	380	48	20	12	880	3 starch, 2 med. fat meat, 1 vegetable

From Franz M: *Fast food facts: nutritive and exchange values for fast food restaurants,* Minneapolis, 1984, International Diabetes Center.
*1 serving.
†In g.
‡In mg.
§Note high fat content.
Med., Medium; *NA,* not available.

Continued.

table 31-4—cont'd

REFERENCE GUIDE FOR POPULAR FAST FOODS

Item	Serving size	Calories*	Carbohydrates†	Protein†	Fat†	Sodium‡	Exchange*
KENTUCKY FRIED CHICKEN							
Original Recipe chicken center breast	1 (107 g)	257	8	26	14	532	1/2 starch, 3 med. fat meat
Extra Crispy chicken center breast	1 (120 g)	353	15	27	21	842	1 starch, 3 med. fat meat, 1 fat
Mashed potatoes	1 (80 g)	59	12	2	trace	228	1 starch
Corn-on-the-cob	1 (143 g)	176	32	5	3	21	2 starch
Cole slaw	1 (79 g)	103	12	1	6	171	2 vegetable or 1 starch, 1 fat
LONG JOHN SILVERS							
Fish & fries	3 pc fish	853	64	43	48	2025	4 starch, 4 med. fat meat, 5 fat§
Tender chicken plank dinner with fries, slaw	4 pc chicken	1037	82	41	59	2433	5 starch, 4 med. fat meat, 1 vegetable, 7 fat
Shrimp, fish, chicken dinner with fries, slaw, 2 hushpuppies	1 pc fish 2 shrimp 1 pc chicken	1022	87	34	60	2274	5 starch, 3 med. fat meat, 1 vegetable, 8 fat§
MCDONALD'S							
Hamburger	1 (100 g)	263	28	12	11	506	2 starch, 1 med. fat meat, 1 fat
Big Mac	1 (200 g)	570	39	25	35	979	2 1/2 starch, 3 med. fat meat, 4 fat§
Filet-O-Fish	1 (143 g)	435	36	15	26	799	2 1/2 starch, 1 med. fat meat, 4 fat§
Chicken McNuggets	1 (109 g)	323	15	19	20	512	1 starch, 2 med. fat meat, 2 fat
French fries	1 (68 g)	220	26	3	12	109	2 starch, 2 fat
Egg McMuffin	1 (138 g)	340	31	19	16	885	2 starch, 2 med. fat meat, 1 fat
PIZZA HUT							
Thin-n-Crispy pizza cheese	3 slices 1/2 10″ pizza	450	54	25	15	NA	3 1/2 starch, 2 med. fat meat, 1 fat
Thick-n-Chewy pizza Cheese	3 slices 1/2 10″ pizza	560	71	34	14	NA	5 starch, 3 med. fat meat
TACO BELL							
Bean burrito	1	343	48	11	12	272	3 starch, 2 fat
Burrito supreme	1	457	43	21	22	367	3 starch, 2 med. fat meat, 2 fat
Taco	1	186	14	15	8	79	1 starch, 2 lean meat
Tostada	1	179	25	9	6	101	1 1/2 starch, 1 med. fat meat

table 31-4—cont'd

Item	Serving size	Calories*	Carbohydrates†	Protein†	Fat†	Sodium‡	Exchange*
WENDY'S							
Single hamburger patty on white bun	1 (127 g)	350	26	24	16	360	2 starch, 3 med. fat meat
Plain baked potato	1 (250 g)	250	52	6	2	60	$3^{1}/_{2}$ starch
Sour cream & chives potato	1 (310 g)	460	53	6	24	230	$3^{1}/_{2}$ starch, 5 fat§
Chili (regular)	1 (236 g)	240	24	19	8	990	$1^{1}/_{2}$, 2 med. fat meat
Taco salad	1 (398 g)	430	43	22	19	1260	3 starch, 2 med. fat meat, 2 fat
Chicken breast fillet on bun	1 (87 g)	320	31	25	10	500	2 starch, 3 lean meat
Garden spot salad bar:							
Lettuce, iceberg, or romaine	3 cup (165 g)	20	3	Trace	Trace	20	1 vegetable
Cole slaw	$^{1}/_{4}$ cup	80	9	Trace	5	165	2 vegetable, 1 fat
Cottage cheese	$^{1}/_{2}$ cup	110	3	13	4	425	2 lean meat
American cheese	1 oz	90	trace	6	7	335	1 high fat meat
Sunflower seeds and raisins	1 oz	140	6	5	10	5	$^{1}/_{2}$ fruit, 1 high fat meat

an increased risk of low birth weight, malformation, and mortality.

The caloric intake of the pregnant adolescent should permit an 11 to 13 kg (24- to 31-pound) total weight gain, usually achieved by increasing the caloric intake by 300 kcal daily.

Most teenage girls do not want to gain weight. Counseling related to the nutritional needs of pregnancy may be very difficult, and suggestions are better than rigid directions. The diet of a pregnant adolescent is most apt to be deficient in calcium, iron, vitamin A, and vitamin C.

Young and Middle-Age Adults

The demands for most nutrients are reduced as the growth period ends. Mature adults need nutrients for energy, maintenance, and repair. Energy needs usually decline 2% to 8% per decade after age 20 (Hamel, 1989). Obesity may become a problem caused by decreased physical exercise, increased dining out, or the ability to afford more luxury foods.

Adult women who use oral contraceptives need extra folic acid, vitamin C, riboflavin, vitamin B_6, and vitamin B_{12}. Those who use intrauterine devices need additional vitamin C and iron to compensate for increased menstrual flow.

Young and middle-age adults are subject to the same recommendations for healthy eating: two or more servings of dairy foods, five or more servings of fruits and vegetables (with a daily source of vitamin C and three to four weekly servings of sources of vitamin A), six or more servings of whole grain foods, and 1 to 2 tablespoons of margarine or butter (see Figure 31-1).

Pregnancy. Poor nutrition during pregnancy can result in a low–birth-weight infant. If nutrient sources are not available from body stores and dietary intake, mother and fetus suffer. The nutritional status of the mother at the time of conception is important in terms of nutritional reserves and basic eating habits. Often, significant fetal growth and development occur before pregnancy is suspected.

The energy requirements of pregnancy are related to body weight and activity. Inadequate weight gain and excessive weight gain above 15 kg (35 lb) are not desirable. In the event of undesirable gains or losses, food intake should be evaluated.

Food intake in the first trimester should include balanced proportions of essential nutrients with emphasis on quality. Protein intake throughout pregnancy is increased to 60 g (Food and Nutrition Board, 1989). High-risk mothers are advised to double their normal protein intake.

Calcium intake should be increased to 1200 mg/day.

Calcium is needed for fetal tooth and bone development, muscle contraction, and blood clotting. Calcium intake is especially critical in the third trimester, when fetal bones mineralize.

Pregnant women need more iron than can be supplied by even the most ideal diet. Iron needs are increased to 30 mg/day, and a supplement is usually given. Iron is needed to correct preexisting deficiencies and to provide for increased maternal blood volume, for fetal storage, and for blood loss during delivery.

Iodine needs are increased to 30 μg (15% to 17%) because of increased activity of the thyroid gland. Vitamin A is needed for cell development, epithelial tissue maintenance, and tooth and bone development. Requirements are increased to 800 retinol equivalents (REs).

Pregnancy also increases requirements for B vitamins, which are needed for enzyme production necessitated by increased metabolic activity. Folic acid intake is particularly important for DNA synthesis and the growth of red blood cells. Inadequate intake may lead to megaloblastic anemia, a type of anemia seen in pregnancy.

Pregnant women should increase their fluid intake by drinking 6 to 8 glasses of water daily. They should avoid cigarette smoke, asparatame, saccharin, alcohol, excessive caffeine, and all drugs not specifically prescribed by the physician.

Lactation. The production of breast milk increases energy requirements. The lactating woman needs 500 kcal above her prepregnancy requirement.

Protein requirements are an additional 20 g above their usual need. The need for calcium remains the same as during pregnancy. There is an increased need for vitamin A, niacin, riboflavin, iodine, and zinc over pregnancy needs. The need for vitamins C, D, E, B_6, B_{12}, and thiamine and for the minerals calcium, phosphorus, and magnesium are the same for the pregnant and the lactating woman.

Increased calories should be provided by leafy green vegetables, citrus fruits, whole grains, milk, meats, and poultry to provide vitamins A and C, niacin, riboflavin, and zinc. Four servings from the dairy food group are needed. Fluid intake should total at least 3 quarts a day. The best fluid is water, and alcoholic or caffeinated beverages should be avoided. Drugs are excreted in breast milk and should be used only under a physician's supervision.

GERONTOLOGIC NURSING PRACTICES

- Obtain a complete medication history; medications have the potential to alter fluid, electrolyte, and nutritional status. In addition, multiple drug therapies have the potential to interact with one another; therefore potentiating or diminishing drug actions.*
- When the older adult is not interested in eating, foods with higher nutrient density (e.g., chicken or fish) should be recommended.*
- A decrease in taste sensitivity and decreased smell sensitivity can cause a decline in food intake. Offering foods that the client likes in an attractive and social environment can increase caloric intake.
- If constipation is a recurrent problem encourage client to eat regular meals and to include foods such as raw fruits and vegetables, whole grains, legumes, and water.†
- Exercise in older adults has the following nutritional benefits: retention of lean body mass, increased strength and flexibility, increased glucose clearance, retention of bone density, exposure to sunlight for vitamin D, and maintenance of normal appetite.†
- Encouraging the client to use auxiliary transportation services for dental and medical care as well as for social activities can prevent social isolation and subsequent poor nutritional intake.
- If the older adult must eat alone, encourage the client to maintain regular eating routines, participate in senior nutrition programs, watch TV, or listen to the radio while eating.†
- Have client buy meat in large quantities and request the butcher to repackage in smaller packages for freezing. This way the client receives the financial benefit of buying in bulk, and the store repackages the item for daily use.

*Mazy MA, Rauckhorst LH, Stoles SA: *Health assessment of the older individual,* ed 2, New York, 1993, Springer.
†Carnevali DL, Patrick M: *Nursing management for the elderly,* ed 3, Philadelphia, 1993, JB Lippincott.

Older Adults

Many factors determine the nutritional needs of the older adult (see box above). Physiological changes associated with aging affect nutritional status. The assumption that older adults have a reduced need for caloric requirements has been modified. The older adult who exercises needs increases in calorie, riboflavin, and vitamin B_6 intake (Roe, 1989). In addition, postmenopausal women have an increased need for calcium to reduce their risk for the development of osteoporosis (Hess, 1989; Roe, 1989; Kane, 1993).

Research has documented that the homebound and those living through long winters in northern climates are at risk for vitamin D deficiency. This deficiency is manifested as osteomalacia (Roe, 1989). Likewise, when exposed to high temperatures, older adults are at a greater risk for sodium depletion because of the loss of body fluids through sweating. Finally, because many older adults live alone, food shopping and preparation are more difficult. Living alone decreases the interest and pleasure of preparing and eating meals.

Taste acuity declines with age. The taste buds that recognize sweet and salt are the first to deteriorate, leaving bitter and sour as the dominant taste sensations. Zinc deficiency may cause diminished taste. Dentures also increase bitter and sour taste sensations. A normal decline in gastric secretions results in less efficient digestion.

The required amounts and types of food are the same as those for younger adults, although there may be some changes in the way foods are prepared or the types of foods selected. Diets of older adults are typically low in foods with protein, calcium, and high in breads, cakes, and cereals. Whole grain cereals and breads should be encouraged. Cream soups and meat-based vegetable soups are good for the older adult with chewing problems. The diet of the older adult should be low in fat and high in fiber and iron and should include good sources of calcium, vitamins B_{12} and B_6, and riboflavin.

NUTRITION AND THE NURSING PROCESS

Close daily contact with the hospitalized client enables nurses to make observations of physical status, food intake, and response to therapy. Nurses should inform the physician of observations that indicate nutritional problems and should incorporate approaches to solving the problem in care plans. They should investigate the reasons for reduced food intake and provide alternative types of food or methods of intake. An equally important nursing responsibility is awareness of indications that intravenous feedings can be replaced by oral feedings or that a nasogastric tube is no longer needed.

NURSING PROCESS

Assessment

Nutritional assessments should be a part of every nurse-client relationship. It is particularly important for clients

FACTORS INFLUENCING DIETARY PATTERNS

HEALTH STATUS

A good appetite is a sign of health.

Anorexia can be a symptom of disease, a side effect of drugs, or a response to an emotional crisis.

Nutritional support is an essential part of recovery from any medical treatment.

CULTURE AND RELIGION

Cultural and religious patterns and restrictions concerning food must be taken into account. The tendency to cling to these patterns increases during illness.

Special foods and diets should be given when appropriate.

SOCIOECONOMIC STATUS

Food expenses are not fixed, and spending varies according to the amount of available money.

Generally, but not always, people with higher incomes buy more proteins and fats and fewer carbohydrates, whereas poorer people do the opposite.

Whether someone is around to prepare food determines the amount of convenience foods used.

Advertising and lack of knowledge about contents of packaged foods also influence food buying.

PERSONAL PREFERENCE

Individual likes and dislikes are perhaps the strongest influence on diet.

Foods associated with pleasant memories tend to become favorite foods; those associated with unpleasant memories tend to be avoided.

PSYCHOLOGICAL FACTORS

Individual motivations to eat balanced meals and individual perceptions about diet are strong influences.

Food has strong symbolic value for many people (e.g., milk may symbolize helplessness; meat may symbolize strength).

ALCOHOL AND DRUGS

Alcohol and drug abuse contribute to nutritional deficiencies because money may be spent on alcohol instead of food, and alcohol may replace part of the diet and depress appetite.

Excess alcohol can affect gastrointestinal organs.

Drugs that depress appetite can lower intake of essential nutrients.

Drugs can deplete nutrient stores and lessen their absorption in the intestines.

MISINFORMATION AND FOOD FADS

Food myths can be the result of cultural background, peer pressure, and a desire to control one's own diet choices.

Food fads often involve erroneous beliefs that certain foods are especially healthful (e.g., yogurt is more nutritional than milk, oysters increase sexual potency, or honey is more healthy than sugar).

Nurses must be careful not to be condescending when teaching a client that foods may not have the qualities attributed to them.

at risk for nutritional problems related to hospitalization, life-style habits, and other factors (see box on p. 889).

Nutritional assessment goals (Forlaw, 1983) as outlined by the American Society of Parenteral and Enteral Nutrition (ASPEN) follow:

1. Identifying nutritional deficiencies that adversely affect health
2. Obtaining specific information to assist in planning and delivering nutritional care
3. Evaluating the efficacy of nutritional care and modifying the nutritional care plan as needed to obtain the desired result

The nutritional assessment consists of nursing history, observation, anthropometry, and laboratory data. In addition, the assessment is individualized to adequately assess each client to determine risks for nutritional alterations.

Nursing History. In addition to the general nursing history (see Chapter 7), the nurse can obtain a more specific diet history (see box below) to assess the client's actual or potential nutritional needs. The diet history focuses on habitual intake of food and liquids and information about preferences, allergies, and digestive problems.

A detailed record also can be kept of food intake over 3 days, including a weekend day. This record allows the nurse to calculate the client's nutritional intake and to compare it with the RDAs.

INFORMATION IN A DIET HISTORY

Name
Age
Present weight
Usual weight
Recent weight changes
Height
Number of meals and snacks a day
Person who prepares meals
Food preferences, allergies, and aversions
Foods that cause indigestion, diarrhea, or gas
Chewing or swallowing difficulties
Use of dentures
Usual bowel movements
Dietary problems
Use of medications
  Prescribed
  Over-the-counter
  Recreational
History of diseases, surgeries, or weight problems
Level of physical activity
Appetite changes
Type, time, and size of usual meals
Personal crises

The nurse also gathers information about the client's activity level to determine his or her energy need. The energy need is compared to food intake.

Observation. The nurse observes the client for signs of actual or potential nutritional needs. Inadequate nutrition affects all body systems; clues to malnutrition may be observed during physical assessment (see Chapter 16). When the general physical assessment is complete, the nurse can recheck pertinent areas to evaluate nutritional status. Clinical signs of nutritional status (Table 31-5) provide observation guidelines and are important noninvasive techniques.

Anthropometry. Anthropometry is a system of measurement of the size and makeup of the body at specific body sites. Anthropometric measurements that aid in identifying nutritional problems include weight, height, wrist circumference, mid-upper arm circumference, and triceps skinfold.

Unless contraindicated, height and weight measurements should be obtained during admission or entry into an outpatient care setting. A client should always be weighed at the same time each day, on the same scale, and with the same clothing or linen. Height and weight can be compared with the usual measurements and with standards for normal height-weight relationships.

Wrist circumference is used to estimate the client's body frame. A tape measure is used to measure the smallest portion of the wrist, distal to the styloid process. Normal values include 9 to 11 cm (small), 11 to 12 cm (medium), and 12 to 14 cm (large).

The mid-upper arm circumference (MAC) determines muscle wasting. The client should be sitting because measurements taken in the supine position may be less accurate. If the client is bedridden, the measurement can be obtained with the arm placed across the chest. The nondominant arm is relaxed, and the nurse measures the circumference at the midpoint of the arm, between the tip of the acromial process of the scapula and the olecranon process of the ulna. Measurement of the nondominant arm prevents false recordings secondary to increased muscle mass from activities of daily living or employment. The measurements in millimeters are then compared with percentiles of MAC by the client's age and gender.

Skinfold measurements are used to determine the fat content of subcutaneous tissue. The triceps skin fold (TSF) is the most common and easiest to measure. With the thumb and forefinger, the nurse pinches lengthwise a double fold of fat about 1 cm above the midpoint of the MAC. With the other hand, the nurse places the teeth of the calipers on either side of the fat fold. The nurse averages the measurements from three readings. The measurements in millimeters are then compared with percentiles of TSF thickness by the client's age and gen-

table 31-5
CLINICAL SIGNS OF NUTRITIONAL STATUS

Body area	Signs of good nutrition	Signs of poor nutrition
General appearance	Alert, responsive	Listless, apathetic, cachectic
Weight	Normal for height, age, body build	Overweight or underweight (special concern for underweight)
Posture	Erect, arms and legs straight	Sagging shoulders, sunken chest, humped back
Muscles	Well-developed, firm, good tone, some fat under skin	Flaccid, poor tone, underdeveloped, tender, "wasted" appearance, improper gait
Nervous control	Good attention span, not irritable or restless, normal reflexes, psychological stability	Inattentive, irritable, confused, burning and tingling of hands and feet (paresthesia), loss of position and vibratory sense, weakness and tenderness of muscles (may result in inability to walk), decrease or loss of ankle and knee reflexes
Gastrointestinal function	Good appetite and digestion, normal regular elimination, no palpable organs or masses	Anorexia, indigestion, constipation or diarrhea, liver or spleen enlargement
Cardiovascular function	Normal heart rate and rhythm, no murmurs, normal blood pressure for age	Rapid heart rate (above 100 beats per minute, tachycardia), enlarged heart, abnormal rhythm, elevated blood pressure
General vitality	Endurance, energetic, sleeps well, vigorous	Easily fatigued, no energy, falls asleep easily, looks tired, apathetic
Hair	Shiny, lustrous, firm, not easily plucked, healthy scalp	Stringy, dull, brittle, dry, thin, and sparse, depigmented, can be easily plucked
Skin (general)	Smooth, slightly moist, good color	Rough, dry, scaly, pale, pigmented, irritated, bruises, petechiae
Face and neck	Skin color uniform, smooth, pink, healthy appearance, not swollen	Greasy, discolored, scaly, swollen, skin dark over cheeks and under eyes, lumpiness or flakiness of skin around nose and mouth
Lips	Smooth, good color, moist, not chapped or swollen	Dry, scaly, swollen, redness and swelling (cheilosis), or angular lesions, fissures, or scars at corners of mouth, stomatitis
Mouth and oral membranes	Reddish pink mucous membranes in oral cavity	Swollen, boggy oral mucous membranes
Gums	Good pink color, healthy, red, no swelling or bleeding	Spongy, bleed easily, marginal redness, inflamed, gums receding
Tongue	Good pink color or deep reddish in appearance, not swollen or smooth, surface papillae present, no lesion	Swelling, scarlet and raw, magenta color, beefy (glossitis), hyperemic and hypertrophic papillae, atrophic papillae
Teeth	No cavities, no pain, bright, straight, no crowding, well-shaped jaw, clean, no discoloration	Unfilled caries, absent teeth, worn surfaces, mottled, malpositioned, fluorosis
Eyes	Bright, clear, shiny, no sores at corner of eyelids, membranes moist and healthy pink color, no prominent blood vessels or mount of tissue or sclera, no fatigue circles beneath	Eye membranes pale (pale conjunctivas), redness of membrane (conjunctival injection), dryness, signs of infection, Bitot's spots, redness and fissuring of eyelid corners (angular palpebritis), dryness of eye membrane (conjunctival xerosis), dull appearance of cornea (corneal xerosis), soft cornea (keratomalacia)
Neck (glands)	No enlargement	Thyroid enlarged
Nails	Firm, pink	Spoon shape (koilonychia), brittle, ridged
Legs and feet	No tenderness, weakness, or swelling; good color	Edema, tender calf, tingling, weakness
Skeleton	No malformations	Bowlegs, knock-knees, chest deformity at diaphragm, beaded ribs, prominent scapulas

From Worthington-Roberts BS and Williams SR: *Nutrition in pregnancy and lactation,* ed 4, St. Louis, 1990, Mosby.

der. Other anatomical areas for skinfold measurements include the biceps, scapula, and abdomen.

The mid-arm muscle circumference (MAMC) is an estimation of skeletal mass. It is calculated from the MAC and TSF anthropometric measures. The formula follows:

$$\text{MAMC} = \text{MAC} - (\text{TSF} \times 3.14)$$

Diagnostic Tests. Laboratory values useful in nutritional assessment include the complete blood count, serum albumin level, transferrin level, and urinary concentrations of sodium, potassium, urea nitrogen (BUN), and creatinine. A low red blood cell count and depressed hemoglobin value indicate anemia. The hemoglobin, hematocrit, and BUN values also reflect the state of hydration. Decreased serum levels of albumin and transferrin identify protein-calorie malnutrition (PCM). Reduced levels of albumin and transferrin in adults also indicate a visceral protein deficit.

Urine specimens collected every 24 or 48 hours help in assessing nutritional status. Urinary levels of sodium and potassium are useful indicators of renal function and response to intravenous electrolyte therapy. The BUN level is related to the use of exogenous protein and to nitrogen balance. Creatinine is used with height to indicate changes in lean tissue mass. Table 31-6 includes common laboratory tests to evaluate nutritional status.

Clients at Risk for Nutritional Problems. A client with a condition that interferes with the ability to ingest, digest, or absorb adequate nutrients should be considered at risk. Congenital anomalies and surgical revisions of the gastrointestinal tract interfere with normal function. Clients fed only by intravenous infusion of 5%-10% dextrose are at risk for nutritional deficiencies. Older adults, infants, or the malnourished are at greatest risk.

OBESITY. **Obesity** is a condition in which there is a

table 31-6

COMMON LABORATORY TESTS TO EVALUATE NUTRITIONAL STATUS

Test	Purpose	Abnormal findings
Serum albumin level (normal: 4-5.5 mg/100 ml)	Maintains serum protein levels Maintains fluid and electrolyte balance Determines prolonged protein wasting	Abnormal values may take up to 2 weeks before they are reflected in blood studies. Abnormalities in liver and kidney diseases, stress, dehydration, and infection may be reflected. Level of 3.5 mg/100 ml indicates protein depletion.
Transferrin level (normal: 170-250 mg/100 ml)	Is more specific indicator of protein-calorie malnutrition than albumin (blood protein binds with iron)	Abnormal values respond quickly to changes in protein intake. Decrease in liver disease and chronic renal failure are reflected.
Total lymphocyte count (normal: >1800)	Reflects depression of immune system caused by impaired nutritional intake	Lymphocyte count is depleted in all immunosuppressed clients and clients with protein deficiency.
Hemoglobin level (normal: 12-15 g/100 ml)	Measures oxygen and iron-carrying capacity of blood	Decrease may indicate some form of anemia, or level can be lowered with blood loss.
Blood urea nitrogen level (normal: 10-20 mg/100 ml)	Measures breakdown of dietary protein Measures urea production in liver and excretion in kidneys	Level is elevated with excessive protein intake. Level is depressed with low protein intake. Level is elevated in liver and renal disease. Level is falsely elevated in hypovolemic dehydration.
Creatinine excretion in 24-hour urine (normal: 0.6-1.3 mg/100 ml for men and 0.5-1.0 mg/100 ml for women)	Reflects total muscle mass Indirectly measures skeletal muscle mass depletion	Level is abnormally low in renal disease. Level is abnormally low in severe malnutrition and starvation.

20% increase above ideal body weight. Obesity cuts across all socioeconomic levels and is a health risk factor. Our culture stresses thinness, so excessive weight also causes psychological problems, inconvenience, and unhappiness.

To lose weight, a person must burn some of the body's store of fat. When insufficient calories are ingested to meet the daily energy needs, the body is forced to burn its reserve stores for energy. A person may lose weight by reducing food intake or increasing energy needs through increased activity. The best plan for weight loss combines reduced food intake with increased exercise and behavior modification. The best diet plan is to adopt a well-balanced diet for life.

Anorexia nervosa. **Anorexia nervosa** is a biopsychosocial disorder in which self-imposed starvation is used to establish identity and control, marked by denial of being underweight, hunger, and fatigue. It may be metabolic and familial. The desirability of a slender figure in today's society is considered a potent factor.

The client with anorexia nervosa is usually an adolescent girl. Extreme undernutrition leads to secondary endocrine disorders such as amenorrhea and delayed sexual development. The client may also go on food binges followed by self-induced vomiting or cathartic purges (binge-purge syndrome). The treatment of anorexia nervosa is a combination of psychotherapy, behavior modification, and dietary therapy. It is long term and should involve the whole family.

Bulimia. **Bulimia** or the binge-purge syndrome occurs in half of the clients with anorexia nervosa, but not all bulimic clients have anorexia nervosa. The syndrome seems to develop with an abnormal craving for food accompanied by the desire to remain slender. The client gorges on food to satisfy the craving and then induces vomiting to prevent digestion. The client may also use laxatives or enemas to increase gastric motility so that nutrients are not absorbed. The practice of secretly vomiting after eating usually starts with occasional binges and gradually becomes a daily activity and the preferred way of controlling weight. Frequent vomiting, laxative abuse, and overuse of enemas lead to electrolyte imbalances (hypokalemia being the most serious), esophageal lesions, dental caries, endocrine disturbances, and metabolic changes. Treatment includes dietary education, hospitalization, psychotherapy, drug therapy, group therapy, and behavioral modification.

Surgery. Surgery interferes with food intake. Preoperative preparation usually involves at least an 8-hour period of fasting. The resumption of food intake postoperatively varies with the client, surgical procedure, complications, and surgeon's protocol (see Chapter 36).

Unless the surgical procedure dictates an alternative feeding method, clients who have had surgery are usually given clear and then full liquid diets. The use of a straw may help increase a postoperative client's fluid intake, but in some cases such as dental surgery and cleft palate repairs straws are contraindicated. Soft foods are sometimes easier to swallow than liquids. Hot fluids, tart juices, and fiber should be avoided after throat and mouth surgery. Milk, yogurt, sherbet, ice cream, ginger ale, and diluted fruit juices are usually allowed.

When surgery is performed on the stomach and intestines, an alternative method of food intake is usually prescribed to allow the suture line to heal and edema to subside. Nasogastric suction may prevent gastric and intestinal secretions from irritating or stretching the resected areas. When oral intake is restricted, fluids are usually given intravenously. Gastric surgery may limit the amount of food that can be ingested at any time. Intestinal surgery may interfere with absorption of nutrients, depending on the length of intestine involved and the location.

The diversion of intestinal wastes through the creation of artificial openings in the abdomen (ileostomy or colostomy) affects fluid loss and electrolyte balance. Clients with ileostomies also lose some of the ability to absorb vitamin B_{12}. Clients with ileostomies and colostomies have dietary concerns related to the consistency of stool and control of odor. Foods that produce intestinal gas are usually limited or avoided.

Cancer and radiotherapy. Malignant cancer cells compete with normal cells for nutrients, increasing the metabolic needs of the client. Clients with cancer typically complain of anorexia and taste distortions. Optimal nutritional support and the correction of nutritional deficits can enable clients to benefit from therapies previously denied them and improves the quality of life.

Although radiotherapy destroys the rapidly dividing neoplastic cells, it also destroys normal cells. Clients in good nutritional states can tolerate larger doses of radiation. Radiotherapy usually causes anorexia, nausea, and vomiting. Irradiation of the head and neck can lead to taste and smell distortions, decreased salivation, and dysphagia. Irradiation of the abdomen and pelvis can result in malabsorption and diarrhea (Robuck and Fleetwood, 1992).

Cold foods are often preferred. Commercial preparations provide essential nutrients in a concentrated, palatable liquid form. Tube feedings or total parenteral nutrition can also be used for clients unable to eat.

Immobilization. Extended immobilization can result in deossification and osteoporosis of bones and in hypercalcemia. Hypercalcemia predisposes clients to kidney and bladder stones. Early ambulation is the best way to prevent immobilization problems. When ambulation is impossible, adequate quantities of high–biological value protein help to prevent skin breakdown and infections, and a high phosphorus intake in the early weeks of immobilization reduces blood calcium levels. Generous fluid intake also protects against kidney stones.

NURSING DIAGNOSES FOR CLIENTS WITH ALTERED NUTRITION

Aspiration, high-risk
Body image disturbance
Fluid volume deficit
Fluid volume deficit, high risk
Fluid balance excess
Nutrition, altered: less than body requirements
Nutrition, altered: more than body requirements
Nutrition, altered: high risk for more than body requirements
Oral mucous membrane, altered
Self-care deficit: feeding
Swallowing, impaired

Nursing Diagnosis

Following assessment, the nurse clusters relevant defining characteristics to determine whether actual or potential nutritional problems exist. The nursing diagnosis box above lists examples of the nursing diagnostic labels appropriate for clients with nutritional alterations. A deficit may occur when any nutrient is not ingested, is poorly digested, or is incompletely absorbed. A specific diagnosis indicates a nutritional deficiency. The nursing diagnosis may also involve a general nutritional deficiency or problems that place the client at risk for nutritional deficiencies.

The nursing diagnostic statement is based on supporting diagnostic characteristics in the assessment data base. In addition, the suspected cause or etiology of the diagnosis is stated. Identification of causes further individualizes the nursing diagnostic statement and subsequent plan of care.

Planning

Planning to maintain a proper nutritional status is better than having to correct deficits (see care plan on p. 31). The identification of clients at risk for nutritional problems should result in a care plan that will prevent or minimize nutritional problems. The client and family need to collaborate in the care plan. In addition, the dietitian and nutritional support clinical nurse specialists should be consulted to provide correct nutritional education and counseling, which are important for clients on regular diets to prevent disease and promote health. Clients on therapeutic diets who understand the rationale for the diets are more likely to comply.

In the health care setting and home, some clients with physiological conditions that cause more severe cases of malnutrition require total parenteral nutrition to meet fluid, electrolyte, and nutritional needs. Priority is given to those client-centered goals directed at restoring normal nutrition and fluid and electrolyte balance.

In total parenteral nutrition, a nutritionally adequate hypertonic solution consisting of glucose, amino acids, lipids, minerals, and vitamins is given through an indwelling peripheral or central intravenous catheter. The need for parenteral nutrition is determined by assessment.

Clients most likely to require TPN suffer from severe trauma, febrile states, cancer, or severe malnutrition. The care plan for clients receiving nutritional therapies should include one or more of the following goals and outcomes:

Goal: Client will return to within 10% of ideal body weight.

Outcomes

- Client gains 0.5 kg (1 lb) per week
- Client loses 0.5 kg (1 lb) per week
- Client selects appropriate foods to assist weight gain or loss

Goal: Client will maintain fluid and electrolyte balance within normal limits.

Outcomes

- Client does not have any assessments (e.g., edema, crackles, weight gain) associated with fluid volume excess
- Client does not have any assessments (e.g., poor skin turgor, sudden weight loss, tachycardia, decreased blood pressure) associated with fluid volume deficit
- Client's laboratory parameters show actual or steady return to normal values

Goal: The client will avoid any complications from therapies designed to assist clients to return to within 10% of ideal body weight.

Outcomes

- Client's blood glucose remains within normal limits
- Clients bowel elimination patterns remain normal
- Client verbalizes positive feelings about weight loss or gain

Goal: The client will state which foods to select for a properly balanced diet.

Outcomes

- Client states appropriate foods for balanced nutritional intake
- Client selects appropriate foods, as demonstrated by a twenty four hour diet diary

Implementation

Ill or debilitated clients usually have poor appetites despite the efforts of dietitians, nurses, families, friends,

SAMPLE NURSING CARE PLAN
Altered Nutrition

ASSESSMENT

Clinical scenario: Mrs. Adams is a 30-year-old mother of three with a *3-week history of diarrhea, 15-pound weight loss, and 1-week history of nausea and vomiting.* She was admitted last evening. Her electrolyte level showed *hypokalemia.* Her oral mucosa are *sore and inflamed.* Her orders include intravenous fluids and *NPO.*

NURSING DIAGNOSIS

Altered nutrition: less than body requirements related to the inability to retain nutrients

PLANNING

Goals	Expected outcomes
Client will return to within 10% of ideal body weight.	Client will gain 0.5 to 1 lb per week for 3 months. Client will be free of diarrhea. Serum electrolytes and other blood chemistry levels will indicate improving nutritional status.

IMPLEMENTATION

Steps	Rationale
1. Maintain client NPO for 24 hours.	Status prevents further loss of electrolytes and gastric irritation.
2. After 24 hours, initiate tube feedings gradually through small-bore feeding tube at half strength and progress as tolerated.	Initiation of gradual tube feedings permit client to adjust to nutrients. Full-strength formula can worsen symptoms of diarrhea (Grant, 1988).
3. Provide oral care as needed.	Promotes healing of inflamed mucosa to support oral intake later (Petrusino, 1989).

EVALUATION

Observe client's weight and compare with baseline.
Monitor intake and output.
Monitor serum electrolytes and blood chemistries.

Defining characteristics are shown in italic type.

and other support people. One of the primary responsibilities of nurses involved in the daily care of any client is the ongoing monitoring of overall nutritional status (Grant and Kennedy-Caldwell, 1988). Nurses can help by displaying interest in the client's intake, by understanding the influences that reduce appetite, and by being willing to do everything possible to improve intake.

One of the most disruptive influences on intake is diagnostic testing. Some blood and radiographic studies require the client to fast. Therefore the client's food is usually withheld until the client returns from the test or the testing is completed. Although microwave ovens make it possible for the client to have a hot meal after the test, he or she may be too fatigued to eat.

Stress also influences intake. Clients who are worried about their families, finances, employment, or illness may not be able to eat or eat enough to compensate for the effect of stress on metabolism.

Medications also affect intake and in some cases the utilization of nutrients. Medications can affect the sensations of taste or smell, and as a result, food is not appetizing. Medications can also cause nausea or vomiting; the client is anorexic due to the nausea, or the nutrients are lost. In addition, medications such as insulin and thyroid hormones can affect metabolism. Nurses keep these factors in mind when designing measures to promote nutrition.

Stimulating Appetite. A nurse can help to stimulate a client's appetite through environmental adaptations, consultation with a diet therapist, special diets and food preferences, and client and family counseling.

Providing a Comfortable Environment. Nurses should provide an environment conducive to eating. The client's room should be free of reminders of treatments and odors. Mouth care should be provided when necessary to remove unpleasant tastes. The client should be positioned comfortably so that the meal can be more enjoyable. If a client refuses a portion of the meal, every effort should be made to replace it with a suitable alternative.

Assisting Clients With Feeding. Nurses can improve client feeding by carefully protecting clients' dignity and actively involving them. Any material used to protect clothing should be referred to as a napkin, not a bib. The nurse should allow the client time to empty the mouth after every spoonful, attempting to match the speed of feeding to the client's readiness and asking frequently about the rate. The nurse should also allow clients to direct the order in which they wish to eat food items. Conversation about topics other than food should be used. Mealtime is a good time for nurses to instruct clients about the selection of appropriate foods and the importance of a balanced diet.

Disabled clients. Clients with disabilities that interfere with independent food intake should be allowed to do as much as possible for themselves. When necessary, the nurse should prepare the tray, cutting food into bite-sized pieces, buttering bread, and pouring liquids. Special eating utensils should be used. Some disabled clients may become tired from their efforts to feed themselves. The nurse should determine whether this client is still hungry and needs assistance (Figure 31-3). The results of self-feeding should be evaluated on the basis of food intake. Success should be recognized and commended. The nurse who finds a way to aid the disabled client to eat more independently should share this information by incorporating it into the care plan.

Providing Enteral Feedings. Enteral nutrition (EN) refers to nutrients given via the intestinal tract. This includes blended foods, modular formulas, and chemically defined elemental nutrients. The oral route is the preferred method of meeting nutritional needs if the client's gastrointestinal tract is functioning by providing safe, economical, nutritional support. For clients with eating difficulties, enteral nutrition may be supplied via nasogastric, jejunal, or gastrostomy tube (Robuck, Fleetwood, 1992). Problems with enteral feedings may be related to the following factors (Farley, 1988):

1. Negative attitudes by the client concerning tube feedings
2. Osmolality problems
3. Electrolyte imbalances
4. Gastrointestinal complications

Studies have demonstrated a beneficial effect in maintaining gastrointestinal function of enteral feedings over parenteral routes. Postoperative feeding by the enteral route can help reduce sepsis and enhance the immune response, and enteral nutrition is also preferable to TPN in protecting intestinal mucosal cells (Andressy, 1988; Randall, 1988).

Nutrient content in EN formulas varies in specific components, and the delivery is readily adjusted to meet the client's needs. EN products enriched with the amino acid glutamine benefit intestinal mucosal cells and their function (Alverdy, 1989).

Tube feedings. When the client cannot ingest, chew, or swallow food but can digest and absorb nutrients, a feeding tube is placed nasally into the stomach or small intestine or surgically into the stomach (gastrostomy) (Procedures 31-1 and 31-2).

Historically, large-bore tube placement has been verified by one of three techniques: withdrawing gastric contents from the tube, injecting air through the nasogastric tube while auscultating the stomach for a gurgling or bubbling sound, and asking the client to speak. These methods do not apply as readily to small-bore nasogastric tubes (Metheny et al., 1988).

The inability to satisfactorily measure gastric contents by gastric aspiration into a syringe interferes with the ability to measure gastric retention of the feeding. Thus it becomes even more important to assess the client for abdominal distention, nausea, and vomiting. Failure to note a markedly distended abdomen increases the client's risk of regurgitation and aspiration of gastric contents. The head of the client's bed needs to be elevated to prevent pulmonary aspiration.

Because of the difficulty in withdrawing fluid from small-bore feeding tubes, nurses frequently rely on the auscultatory method to confirm nasogastric tube placement. This method consists of insufflating 10 to 30 ml of air through the tube while auscultating the epigastrium or left upper quadrant for gurgling or bubbling. Yet, numerous sources in the literature report that "pseudoconfirmatory gurgling" can occur when the tube is elsewhere such as in the esophagus or lung (Miller, Tomlinson, and Sahn, 1985; Muthuswamy, Patel, and Rajendran, 1982). Metheny, Eisenberg, and McSweeney (1988) reported that nurses were unable to determine

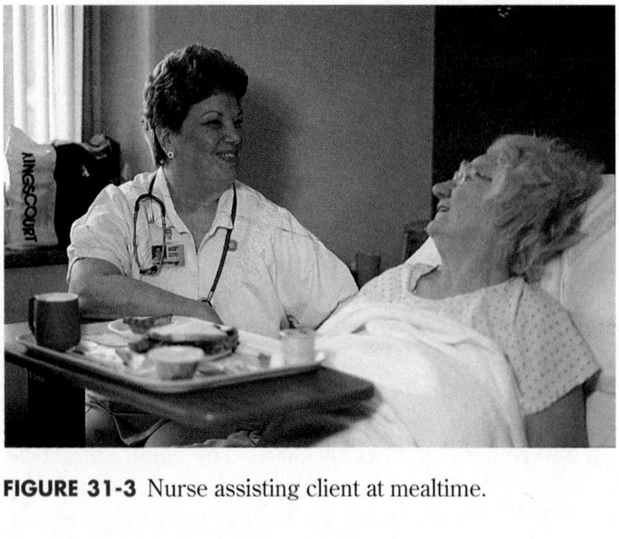

FIGURE 31-3 Nurse assisting client at mealtime.

procedure 31-1

INSERTING A SMALL-BORE NASOGASTRIC TUBE FOR ENTERAL FEEDINGS

Steps	Rationale
1. Assess client for enteral tube feeding and intubation: impaired swallowing, head or neck surgery, decreased level of consciousness, abdominal surgeries, facial trauma.	Identifying clients who need tube feedings before they become nutritionally depleted facilitates preparation of care plan and promotes client education.
2. Assess client for appropriate route of administration:	
a. Close each nostril alternatively and ask client to breathe.	Evaluates nares for patency. Nares may be obstructed. Assessment determines which naris to use.
b. Assess for gag reflex.	Identifies ability to swallow and reduces risk of aspiration.
c. Review client's medical history: nose bleeds, nasal surgery, deviated septum.	Nurse may need to seek physician's order to change route of nutritional support.
3. Review physician's order for type of tube and enteral feeding schedule.	Procedure and enteral feedings require physician's order.
4. Wash hands.	Reduces transfer of microorganisms.
5. Assemble equipment at bedside:	Organizes procedure and limits client discomfort.
a. Small-bore nasogastric tube (8-12 Fr)	
b. Large syringe: 30-ml Luer-Lok or tip	Larger syringe (greater than 30 ml) may rupture small-bore tube.
c. pH test strips	Used to measure gastric acidity.
d. Hypoallergenic tape and tincture of benzoin	Tincture of benzoin increases adhesion of tape to nose.
e. Glass of water and straw	Client drinks to activate swallowing reflex. Water also activates lubricant for small-bore tube (see Step 11d).
f. Emesis basin	Nasogastric intubation may activate gag reflex and cause vomiting.
g. Tongue blade	Essential for testing gag reflex.
h. Penlight or flashlight	Used to visualize posterior pharynx for tube placement.
i. Towel	
j. Clean gloves	
k. Facial tissues	
l. Guidewire or stylet	Used to place soft, flexible feeding tube (e.g., Dobbhoff and Keofeed).
m. Safety pin and rubber band	
6. Explain procedure to client.	Ensures cooperation.
7. Stand on right side of bed if right handed (or on left side if left handed) and assist client to high Fowler's position with pillows behind head and shoulders. Place comatose clients in semi-Fowler's position	Allows easier manipulation of tube. Promotes ability to swallow.
8. Place bath towel over chest. Keep facial tissues within client's reach.	Prevents soiling of gown. Insertion through nasal passages may cause tearing.
9. Instruct client to relax and breathe normally.	Tube passes more easily when client is relaxed and breathing normally.
10. Determine length of tube to be inserted and mark with tape:	Determines approximate depth of insertion.
a. Traditional method: measure distance from tip of nose to earlobe to xiphoid process to sternum (see illustration).	Length provides distance from nose to stomach in 98% of clients. For duodenal or jejunal tubes, additional 20-30 cm are required (Grant, Kennedy-Caldwell, 1988).
b. Hanson method: first mark 50 cm point on tube, and then do traditional measurement. Tube insertion should be to midway point between 50 cm (20 in) and traditional mark.	

Continued.

procedure 31-1—cont'd

Steps	Rationale
11. Prepare for intubation:	
a. Do not ice plastic tubes.	Tubes will become stiff and inflexible, causing trauma to mucous membranes.
b. Inject 10 ml of water from 30-ml Luer-Lok tip syringe into tube.	Aids in guidewire or stylet insertion.
c. Insert guidewire or stylet into tube, making certain that it is securely positioned against weighted tip and that both Luer-Lok connections are snugly fitted together.	Promotes smooth passage of tube into gastrointestinal tract. Improperly positioned stylet can induce serious trauma.
d. Dip weighted tip of tube into glass of water.	Activates lubricant to facilitate passage of tube.
e. Cut 10-cm (4-in) piece of tape. Split one end lengthwise 5 cm (2 in).	Ensures timely anchoring of tube after its placement is verified.
12. Apply clean gloves.	Protects nurse from transmission of infection.
13. Insert tube through nostril to back of throat (posterior nasopharynx). Client may gag. Direct tube back and down toward ear.	Natural contours facilitate passage of tube.
14. Flex head toward chest after tube has passed through nasopharynx. Allow client to relax.	Closes off glottis and reduces risk of tube entering trachea. Allows client to "catch breath" (Grant, Kennedy-Caldwell, 1988).
15. Encourage client to swallow by giving small sips of water or ice chips when possible. Advance tube as client swallows. Rotate tube 180 degrees while inserting while emphasizing need to mouth breathe and swallow.	Facilitates passage of tube past oropharynx. Decreases friction. Mouth breathing and swallowing facilitate passage of tube and alleviates fears.
16. Advance tube each time client swallows until desired length has been passed.	Reduces discomfort and trauma.
a. Do not force tube. When resistance is met or client starts to gag, cough, choke, or become cyanotic, stop advancing tube and pull tube back. Check for position of tube in back of throat with tongue blade.	Tube may be coiled or kinked or in oropharynx trachea.

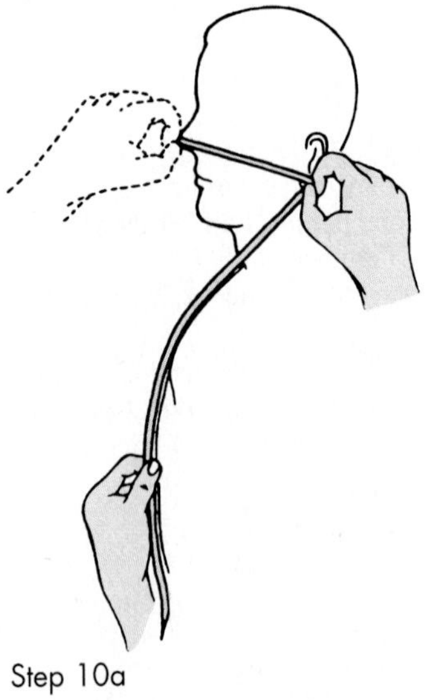

Step 10a

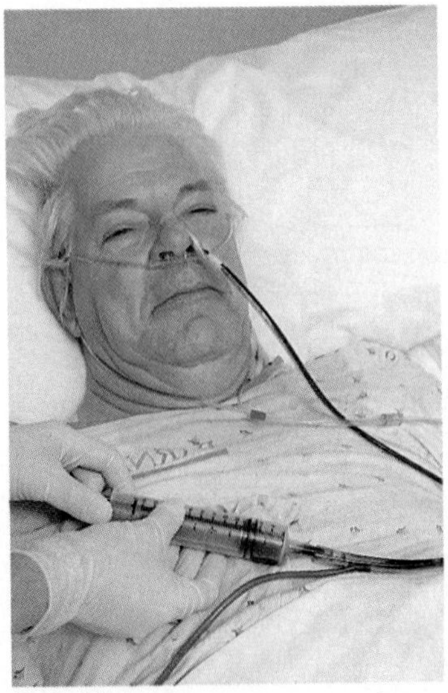

Step 17a

Steps	Rationale
17. Check placement of tube:	Ensures proper position before initiating feedings.
a. Aspirate gastric contents with Luer-Lok syringe. (Insufflation of air into tube followed by auscultation of sound is no longer considered reliable in determining tube placement) (see illustration).	Aspiration of contents provides measurement of pH of secretions and verification that tube is in gastrointestinal tract. (Sounds transmitted by insufflation may be transmitted from pleural space into upper abdomen, thus giving false impression of tube placement [Metheny, Spies, Eisenberg, 1988; Metheny, et al., 1989].)
b. Measure pH of aspirate with color-coded pH paper with range of whole numbers from 1-11 (see illustration).	Gastric aspirates have decidely acidic pH values; preferable value is 4 or less (Metheny, et al., 1989).
c. Obtain x-ray film of tube placement.	Determines correct tube placement. Physician's order is required.
18. Apply tincture of benzoin on tip of nose and tube. Allow to dry.	Helps tape adhere better.
19. Secure tube with tape and avoid pressure on naris.	Prevents trauma to nasal mucosa and permits mobility.
a. Take 10-cm (4-in) piece of tape that was split. Place intact end of tape over bridge of nose. Carefully wrap two ends around tube (see Step 32b, Procedure 36-3).	Secures tape to nose in manner that reduces pressure on nares.
b. Fasten end of tube to gown by looping rubber band around tube in slip knot. Pin rubber band to gown.	Reduces friction on nares in case client moves head. Pinning rubber band provides slack if client moves.
20. Position client on right side when possible until radiological confirmation of correct placement is verified.	Allows tube to pass into small intestine (duodenum or jejunum).
21. Leave stylet in place until correct position is ensured by x-ray study. Never attempt to reinsert partially or fully removed stylet while feeding tube is in place.	Guidewire or stylet may perforate gastrointestinal tract, especially esophagus or nearby tissue, and injure client.
22. Remain and talk with client.	Decreases anxiety.
23. Administer oral hygiene frequently (see Chapter 30). Cleanse tubing at nostril.	Promotes comfort and integrity of oral mucous membranes.
24. Remove gloves, dispose of equipment, and wash hands.	Reduces transmission of microorganisms.
25. Record type of tube placed, aspirate returned, and client tolerance.	Documents exact procedure.

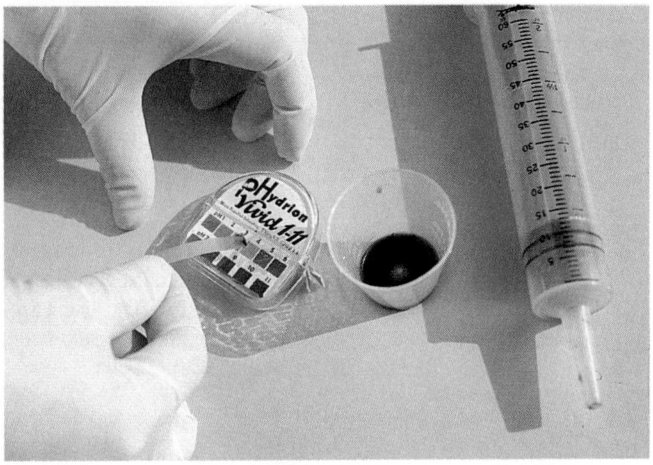

Step 17b

procedure 31-2

INITIATING ENTERAL TUBE FEEDINGS

Steps	Rationale
1. Assess client for enteral tube feedings: impaired swallowing, head or neck surgery, decreased level of consciousness.	Identify clients who need tube feedings before they become nutritionally depleted.
2. Verify physician's order.	Tube feedings must be ordered by physician. Order should include formula, route, amount, and frequency.
3. Place client in high-Fowler's position.	Reduces risk of pulmonary aspiration in case client vomits or regurgitates feeding.
4. Assemble following equipment:	Ensures prompt, efficient completion of feeding.
a. Disposable gavage bag and tubing	
b. Asepto syringe (60-ml size)	Formula can be administered via syringe for bolus feedings. Syringe can also be used to verify placement of large-bore feeding tubes.
c. Prescribed formula and amount	
d. Infusion pump designed for feeding tubes.	Pump is necessary to regulate continuous tube feedings.
e. Disposable gloves	Prevents transmission of microorganisms.
5. Wash hands. Apply gloves.	Prevents transmission of infection from gastric contents.
6. Determine placement of feeding tube (see Procedure 31-1, Step 17):	Verifies placement of tube in stomach. These measures have been proved effective and safe for large-bore tubes.
a. Aspirate gastric secretions and check gastric residual.	Indicates whether gastric emptying is delayed, which means that 150 ml or more remain in stomach. Small-bore tubes may collapse on aspiration (Petrosino, et al., 1989). Inability to satisfactorily measure gastric contents via aspiration interferes with ability to measure gastric retention.
b. Observe for abdominal distention.	Assessment for abdominal distention assists in recognizing delayed gastric emptying and reduces risk of regurgitation and pulmonary aspiration related to gastric distention (Petrosino, et al., 1989).
7. Auscultate for bowel sounds.	Indicates presence of peristalsis and ability of gastrointestinal tract to digest nutrients.
8. Administer tube feeding.	
a. *Bolus or intermittent feeding:*	
(1) Pinch proximal end of feeding tube.	Prevents air from entering client's stomach.
(2) Attach syringe to end of tube and elevate 18 in above client's head.	
(3) Fill syringe with formula. Allow syringe to empty gradually, refilling until prescribed amount has been delivered to client.	Gradual emptying reduces risk of diarrhea induced by bolus tube feedings.
(4) For gavage feeding, fill bag and tubing with prescribed amount of formula. Attach tubing to end of feeding tube and raise bag 18 in above client's head. Regulate flow gradually.	
b. *Continuous-drip method:*	
(1) Hang gavage bag to IV pole.	Method is designed to deliver prescribed rate of feeding that reduces risk of diarrhea. Clients who receive their feedings should have gastric residuals checked every 6 to 8 hours. Also decreases risk of feeding tube developing clogs that would occlude tube entirely (Petrosino, et al., 1989).
(2) Connect end of bag tubing to proximal end of feeding tube.	
(3) Connect infusion pump and set rate.	

Steps	Rationale
9. Administer additional water as ordered.	Ensures adequate hydration, which is supplement to tube-feeding formula (Haynes-Johnson, 1986).
10. Remove and dispose of gloves in proper receptacle. Wash hands.	Prevents transmission of microorganisms.
11. When tube feedings are not being administered, clamp proximal end of feeding tube.	Prevents air from entering the stomach between feedings.
12. Administer water via feeding tube as ordered with or between feedings.	Provides client with source of water to help maintain fluid and electrolyte balance.
13. Record amount and type of feeding in nurses' notes.	Documents administration of feeding.

gastric tube location by the auscultatory method. For example, the nurses reported hearing air when the tube was located in the esophagus, duodenum, jejunum, and stomach.

The ability to speak is generally hindered by the inadvertent respiratory placement of a firm, large-bore feeding tube. However, a number of clients report being able to speak when small-bore tubes accidentally enter the respiratory tract (Rombeau and Barot, 1981; McDanal, Wheeler, and Ebert, 1983). Thus this method is not a reliable means to test for accidental respiratory placement of small-bore pliable tubes.

Little has been written of how the nurse should check for placement of small-bore nasointestinal feeding tubes. Nurses in practice frequently report using the auscultatory method, even though its reliability has been questioned.

Another study by Metheny, Spies, and Eisenberg (1986) examines the incidence of nasoenteral feeding tube displacement. In this study, 92% of subjects were fed with small-bore tubes, and a sizable number of these tubes were found by radiological examination to be spontaneously displaced. That is, the distal tips of the tubes dislocated upwardly in the gastrointestinal tract while the proximal external portion remained taped in place. Displacement was associated with risk factors such as coughing, vomiting, suctioning, and decreased level of consciousness.

Bedside methods of testing placement of small-bore feeding tubes are frequently ineffective. The most reliable method is radiographic verification. This method is costly and has some risk from repeated exposure to x-ray equipment. Therefore new methods to test placement such as pH testing are being researched. In the meantime, the nurse must use meticulous assessment skills to find tube displacement.

In addition to the nasoenteral route, a gastrostomy or jejunostomy feeding tube is placed for EN. A **gastrostomy feeding tube** is a long, hollow, flexible tube inserted into the stomach through a surgical stoma inserted in the upper left abdominal quadrant.

Jejunal feedings, via jejunal feeding tube, are another method of EN. A **jejunal feeding tube** is a large-bore tube surgically inserted into the jejunum for the administration of liquified nutrition (Procedure 31-3).

The solutions used for tube feedings must be nutritionally adequate, tolerated by the client, and appropriate to the area of the gastrointestinal tract to which they are delivered. A wide variety of commercial products is available for tube feedings. They are easy to prepare and offer standard nutritional content. The commercial preparations differ in osmolarity, digestibility, caloric density (ranging from 1 to 2 kcal/ml), lactose content, viscosity, and lipid content.

Clients may be maintained indefinitely on tube feedings, which can provide all the essential nutrients except fiber. Although cramping and diarrhea are commonly associated with tube feedings, these symptoms usually subside when the flow rate or concentration of the solution is reduced or a formula containing fiber is used.

Providing Total Parenteral Nutrition. **Total parenteral nutrition (TPN)** is a complex form of therapy that provides daily nutritional requirements by the intravenous route. The success of this form of nutrition depends on the dietary prescription, management of the intravenous catheter, dressing care, and related complications (Grant and Kennedy-Caldwell, 1988).

Clients unable to ingest or digest enteral nutrition are candidates for TPN. It is contraindicated in clients whose gastrointestinal tracts are functional within 7 to 10 days after illness, surgery, or trauma; when clients

procedure 31-3

ADMINISTERING ENTERAL FEEDINGS VIA GASTROSTOMY OR JEJUNAL TUBE

Steps	Rationale
1. Assess client's need for enteral tube feedings: impaired swallowing, decreased level of consciousness, head or neck surgery, facial trauma, surgery of upper alimentary canal.	Identifies clients who need tube feedings before they become nutritionally depleted.
a. Auscultate for bowel sounds before feeding.	Indicates presence of peristalsis and ability of gastrointestinal tract to digest nutrients.
b. Observe for abdominal distention.	Assessment for abdominal distention assists in recognizing delayed gastric emptying and reduces risk of regurgitation and pulmonary aspiration related to gastric distention (Petrosino, et al., 1989).
c. While wearing gloves, assess gastrostomy or jejunostomy site for breakdown, irritation, drainage.	Infection, pressure from gastrostomy tube, or drainage of gastric secretions can cause skin breakdown.
2. Verify physician's order for formula, rate, route, and frequency.	Tube feedings must be ordered by physician.
3. Wash hands and apply clean gloves.	Reduces transmission of microorganisms.
4. Assemble equipment:	
a. Disposable gavage bag and tubing	Serves as container in which to place formula.
b. 60-ml catheter tip syringe	Formula can be administered via syringe for bolus feedings. Syringe is also used to check tube placement.
c. Stethoscope	Used to auscultate air entering stomach.
d. Formula	
e. Infusion pump (Use pump designed for tube feedings.)	Helps regulate flow of continuous feeding.
5. Prepare bag and tubing to administer formula:	
a. Connect tubing and bag.	Tubing must be free of contamination to prevent bacterial growth.
b. Fill bag and tubing with formula.	Prevents excess air from entering gastrointestinal tract.
6. Explain procedure to client.	Ensures cooperation and relaxation.
7. Place client in high-Fowler's position or elevate head of bed 30 degrees.	Helps prevent chance of aspiration.
8. Verify placement of tube:	
a. *Gastrostomy tube:*	
(1) Aspirate gastric secretions and check gastric residual.	Presence of gastric contents indicates that end of tube is in stomach. Gastric residual determines whether gastric emptying is delayed. Delayed emptying means that 100 ml or more remains in stomach from previous feeding.
(2) Auscultate over left upper quadrant with stethoscope and inject 10-20 ml of air into tube.	Air (i.e., whooshing or gurgling sound) can be heard entering stomach.
b. *Jejunostomy tube:*	
(1) Aspirate intestinal secretions and check for residual.	Presence of intestinal fluid indicates that end of tube is in jejunum. Large residual indicates slow small intestinal emptying.
9. Initiate feeding:	
a. *Gastrostomy tube:*	
(1) Bolus or intermittent feeding:	
• Pinch proximal end of gastrostomy tube.	Prevents air from entering stomach.
• Attach syringe to end of tube and elevate to 18 in above client's abdomen.	
• Fill syringe with formula. Allow syringe to empty gradually, refilling until prescribed amount has been delivered to client.	Gradual emptying of tube feeding by gravity from syringe or gavage bag reduces risk of diarrhea induced by bolus tube feedings.

Steps	Rationale
• If gavage bag is used, attach bag to end of feeding tube and raise bag 18 in above client's abdomen. Fill bag with prescribed amount of formula, and allow bag to empty gradually over 30 min.	
(2) Continuous drip method: • Hang gavage bag to IV pole. • Connect end of bag to proximal end of gastrostomy tube. • Connect infusion pump and set rate.	Method is designed to deliver prescribed hourly rate of feeding and reduce risk of diarrhea. Clients who receive continuous drip feedings should have residuals checked every 4 hr.
(3) When tube feedings are not being administered, clamp proximal end of gastrostomy tube.	Prevents air from entering stomach between feedings.
(4) Administer water via feeding tube as ordered with or between feedings.	Provides client with source of water to help maintain fluid and electrolyte balance.
(5) Rinse bag and tubing with warm water after all bolus feedings.	Clears old tube feedings and prevents bacterial growth.
(6) Advance tube feeding.	Tube feedings should be advanced gradually to prevent diarrhea and gastric intolerance of formula.
b. *Jejunal tube:*	
(1) Initiate continuous tube feeding (see Step 9a(2)).	Jejunal feedings are given continuously to ensure proper absorption.
(2) Advance tube feeding.	To provide maximum nutrition, formula needs to be increased to meet client's nutritional requirements.
10. Change exit site dressing as needed. Inspect exit site every shift. Skin around feeding tube should be cleansed daily with warm water and mild soap; small gauze dressing may be applied to exit site.	Leakage of intestinal drainage may cause irritation and excoriation.
11. Dispose of supplies and wash hands.	Reduces transmission of microorganisms.
12. Evaluate client's tolerance of tube feeding, and observe stoma site for skin integrity.	Tolerance of tube feeding is evaluated by checking amount of aspirate (residual) every 4 hr. Gastric and intestinal secretions can cause injury and necrosis at stoma site.
13. Record amount and type of feeding.	Documents amount and type of feeding administered to client.
14. Record client's response to tube feeding, patency of tube, and any untoward effects.	Documents client's reaction to therapy and identifies presence of adverse reactions (e.g., aspiration).
15. Report to oncoming nursing staff: type of feeding, status of gastrostomy or jejunostomy tube, client's tolerance, and adverse effects.	Provides new nursing personnel with status of gastric feeding. Allows new nursing staff to plan for next feeding.

are well nourished; and when minimal stress and trauma are present. It is also of limited value in clients who have untreatable diseases such as advanced metastatic malignancy. It should not be used when the risks outweigh the benefits (Grant and Kennedy-Caldwell, 1988).

TPN solutions are hyperosmolar (i.e., highly concentrated) and as a result are infused through central venous lines. The solution itself is tailored to the client's specific nutritional needs; however, a typical solution consists of approximately 25% dextrose and 3% to 4% protein, supplying close to 1000 calories per liter. Electrolyte needs vary with the client's general status.

Fat emulsions. Clients may also require nutritional supplements through fat emulsions. Fat emulsions provide supplemental calories to prevent essential fatty acid deficiencies. These nutrients can be administered through a separate peripheral line, through the central line by means of Y connector tubing (see Chapter 33), or as an additive to the TPN solution. The last option is based on research findings that fats (also called *lipids*) can be added to the TPN solutions without causing incompatibility problems or compromising the stability of the solutions (Atkins and Oakley, 1986). Fat emulsions should be administered under sterile asepsis into a patent intravenous line. The emulsion should not be used if it appears oily or appears to have separated.

The recommended initial infusion rate for fat emulsions is 1 ml per minute. Reactions to this emulsion can include dyspnea, cyanosis, allergy, nausea, vomiting, headache, chest pain, back pain, pressure over the eyes, or dizziness. If symptoms appear, the nurse should stop the infusion and notify the physician. If the client tolerates the fat emulsion, the rate can gradually be increased as ordered by the physician.

INITIATING TPN. TPN requires a large-gauge intravascular catheter threaded into a central vein such as the jugular or subclavian or a large peripheral vein. Nurses do not insert central catheters but assist in the procedure.

After placement of the catheter, the needle is removed and an intravenous infusion is connected to the hub of the catheter (see Chapter 35). The physician sutures the catheter in place and covers the site with a sterile dressing. A chest x-ray film is used to confirm the location of the catheter.

Before beginning an infusion, the nurse verifies the solution prepared by the pharmacy with the physician's order. The nurse connects the TPN infusion tubing to a filter and places the insertion spike in the solution. The tubing is filled with the solution and hung at the bedside. The nurse attaches the tubing to the infusion pump. Clients initially receive low doses of TPN solution, such as 1 or 2 liters per 24 hours, typically gradually increasing to 3 liters per 24 hours. A single prepared solution should be delivered over 24 hours; the rate is included in the physician's orders.

Too-rapid administration of this hypertonic infusion can result in osmotic diuresis, dehydration, and death. Infusion pumps help to regulate the flow. If an infusion falls behind schedule, the nurse should not increase the flow rate in an attempt to catch up because a hyperosmotic reaction could result (Metheny, 1991).

CARING FOR THE CLIENT RECEIVING TPN. Nursing care for the client receiving TPN is based on four major nursing goals: (1) preventing infection, (2) maintaining the TPN system, (3) preventing complications, and (4) promoting the client's well-being.

PREVENTING INFECTION. To prevent infection, the infusion tubing should be changed every 24 hours. It is best to change the tubing with the first new bottle administered each day. The procedure is the same as that for changing infusion tubing (see Chapter 35) except that an in-line filter is added to trap bacteria. A 0.22 μm filter blocks all bacteria including *Pseudomonas.*

According to the recommendations of the CDC the venipuncture dressing should be changed every 48 hours (CDC, 1987). Some experts have found that the less the dressing is manipulated, the lower the infection rate, and that if the dressing remains clean, dry, and intact, it does not need to be changed more frequently than every 48 to 72 hours (CDC, 1987).

Clients receiving TPN should have vital signs measured and their blood and urine checked for sugar every 4 to 6 hours. The nurse should be alert for changes and report any to the physician. An increased temperature may be an early sign of line infection and should be reported to the physician. In addition, glycosuria is an indicator of glucose intolerance.

Medications or blood should not be given through the TPN line because it increases the risk of bacterial contamination. Also medications may be chemically altered because of the reaction with the TPN formula. In a life-or-death situation, the TPN line may be the only intravenous line available and will need to be used for emergency treatment.

PREVENTING COMPLICATIONS. After the catheter is inserted, a chest x-ray film is used to document correct placement in the superior vena cava, proximal to the right atrium. The film can also show a pneumothorax (collapse of a lung), which may occur if the needle punctures the pleura during insertion. Pneumothorax assessment findings include chest pain, difficulty in breathing, and coughing; the rapidity of onset and the degree of symptoms depend on the severity of the pneumothorax.

A second complication is the development of an air embolus during insertion of the catheter or changing of the tubing. This can be prevented by having the client do the Valsalva maneuver (Chapter 15) and placing the client in the Trendelenburg position (Chapter 30).

Hyperglycemia is caused by a high concentration of dextrose in the TPN solution. Risk factors include increased secretion of adrenal hormones, increased age, and renal disease (Colley, 1987). Hyperglycemia, which can cause dehydration, nausea, headache, and weakness, can also occur when the rate of infusion is too rapid. The risk of hyperglycemia can be reduced by giving the solution at the prescribed rate. If the solution falls behind schedule, the nurse should not increase the rate unless ordered by the physician. Checking the urine for glucose and acetone every 4 to 6 hours can identify signs of glucose intolerance. Clients receiving TPN may be given insulin injections to increase the body's ability to metabolize the increased glucose. After the TPN has been discontinued, the insulin injections are discontinued.

Hypoglycemia can occur if the infusion rate is too slow or TPN is abruptly discontinued. The high glucose concentration of the TPN solution stimulates the client's pancreas to secrete more insulin. The client may also receive supplemental insulin injections. If the TPN infu-

table 31-7

INTERVENTIONS FOR PREVENTING METABOLIC COMPLICATIONS OF TPN

Intervention	Rationale
Weigh client daily.	Documents that the client is maintaining or gaining weight and has a proper fluid balance.
Record intake and output.	Provides data base for ongoing fluid balance assessment.
If client is allowed oral intake, maintain calorie count of foods eaten.	Provides data needed to calculate TPN caloric requirement.
Test urine or blood every 4 to 6 hours to measure glucose.	Determines whether client is excreting glucose in the urine and an insulin supplement may be needed.
Obtain blood samples for measurement of iron, transferrin, and white blood cells.	Evaluates cellular nutritional status.
Continually assess fluid and electrolyte status.	Provides for early detection of circulatory overload or dehydration.
Maintain infusion rate as ordered. Do not speed or slow infusion unless instructed by the physician or a severe complication occurs.	P vents hyperglycemia, osmotic diuresis, hypoglycemia, d fluid overload.

sion is too slow or abruptly discontinued, there is too little blood glucose and too much insulin, and hypoglycemia occurs. Symptoms include occipital headaches, cold clammy skin, dizziness, tachycardia, and tingling of the extremities (Colley, 1987). Hypoglycemia can be prevented by maintaining an accurate infusion rate and a gradual reduction of the TPN solution. Gradual reduction allows the pancreas time to adapt to the decreased glucose load. If the TPN solution must be discontinued abruptly, a solution of 10% dextrose in half-strength normal saline, with appropriate potassium chloride, should be given at the previous parenteral nutrition rate until the pancreatic insulin rate decreases in about 12 to 24 hours (Grant, Kennedy-Caldwell, 1988).

Fluid overload causes an increase in extracellular fluid volume. If severe, fluid overload can result in pulmonary edema and congestive heart failure. Signs and symptoms include shortness of breath, tachycardia, weak pulse, hypertension or hypotension, confusion, decreased urine output, or pitting edema. Fluid overload can be prevented by maintaining an accurate rate of infusion and monitoring the client's central venous pressure. If signs of fluid overload occur, the nurse slows the infusion rate, notifies the physician, and remains with the client, continually assessing the client's status. Chapter 35 more fully describes fluid overload.

The major metabolic complications of TPN can be prevented by continually implementing seven nursing interventions (Table 31-7). These interventions are designed for early identification and treatment of these complications.

Diet Therapy in Disease Management. The specific dietary intake pattern that results in good nutrition mus often be modified for clients with specific diseases. iet modifications are necessary to correspond with e body's ability to metabolize certain nutrients, to co ect nutritional deficiencies related to the disease, and eliminate harmful foods from the diet. In all cases, th nurse works with the physician and diet therapist w n planning and implementing modified diets.

GASTROINTESTIN DISEASES. The treatment of ulcerative colitis may inclu a liquid diet in the acute stage, a low-residue diet durin ecovery, and thereafter a bland diet high in protein, ca es, vitamins, and minerals and low in fat. Vitamins and n supplements are generally required because absorp is decreased.

The treatment of diarr may include a diet high in vitamins to counteract de ased absorption, low in residue, and high in calorie the client is emaciated. The treatment of acute enter enerally involves fasting followed by a liquid diet an ereafter a bland diet.

Acute gastritis is generally t ed by a liquid diet, with a gradual transition to a low- due diet and thereafter a bland diet. The treatment fo ronic gastritis involves eliminating food or liquids t cause inflammation and thereafter permitting on asily digested foods.

The treatment of diverticulitis withou rforation cludes a liquid diet or low-residue diet un e infect subsides, after which a high-fiber diet is ge lly gi The diet therapy for peptic ulcer considers lari meals and medications that blocks hydrochl c acid secretion. A regular diet is usually modified to ivid ual client needs. Alcohol, meat broths and ext cof fee, tea, cola, and any food that causes distress usually omitted.

CARDIOVASCULAR DISEASES. The general goals of dietary treatment of cardiovascular diseases include preventing stomach distention to avoid pressure against the heart, reducing the client's weight if needed, and lowering blood lipids to lessen the risk of atherosclerosis. The treatment of myocardial infarction includes a liquid diet for several days, progressing to a low-fat, low-sodium, high-carbohydrate soft diet during recovery. Dietary therapy for treatment and prevention generally includes maintaining a recommended weight and a diet low in saturated fats, with less than 30% of total calories from fat and 300 mg of cholesterol. The treatment of hypertension includes weight reduction to normal if the client is overweight and a diet low in sodium and moderately low in fats.

Consistent with the Dietary Guidelines for Ameri cans, the newly released National Cholesterol Educ tion Program (NCEP) Report of the Expert Panel on Blood Cholesterol Levels in Children and Adoles nts (Expert Panel, 1991) recommends that all health children over 2 years of age and adolescents consum a diet that provides the following:

1. Less than 10% of total calories from satu ted fatty acids
2. An average of no more than 30% of al calories from fat
3. Less than 300 mg/day dietary cho sterol

In addition to fat and cholesterol levels protein range of 10% to 20% and 50% to 60% carbohy ates is also recommended to lower cholesterol an ipid levels (NIH, 1991). Current research demonstr s that a 1% reduction in cholesterol level reduces th isk of heart disease by approximately 2% (Rifkind, 19

DIABETES. Adult-onset diabe (non–insulin-dependent diabetes mellitus [NIDI or type II DM) can usually be controlled by diet rapy. Juvenile-onset diabetes (insulin-dependent di tes mellitus [IDDM] or type I DM) requires insul nd dietary restrictions. In both cases the diet is in dualized according to the client's age, build, weig and activity level. Foods for dietary planning are cl ified in six exchange groups. Meals are planned ar l balanced numbers of food exchanges, and foods be exchanged within groups.

RENAL DISEASES e dietary treatment of acute glomerulonephrit epends on individual tolerances but may begin w a limited liquid diet for a few days, gradually retur to a normal diet limited in protein. The diet for nic glomerulonephritis is generally high in carb rates and fat and low in sodium, with protein amo equal to normal plus the amount lost in ine.

Dietar atment for renal stones depends on the ty of s s. For calcium phosphate stones the diet is low n m and high in acid ash. For uric acid stones the di ow in purines. For calcium oxalate stones the diet a s all foods high in calcium and oxalates.

Evaluation

The value of the nurse's activities in meeting the client's nutritional needs is measured by an ongoing evaluation. Care plans must be constantly updated to avoid ineffective actions and to support effective interventions. Adequate time should be allowed to test a nursing approach to a problem. Behavior change in a client is as valid an indcator of success as weight gain or laboratory results.

Nurses use the established expected outcomes to valuate the interventions.

Goal: Client will return to within 10% of ideal body weight.

Outcomes

Client gains 0.5 kg (1 lb) per week

Client loses 0.5 kg (1 lb) per week

Evaluative measure

Weigh the client

Outcome

Client selects appropriate foods to assist weight gain or loss

Evaluative measure

Ask client to identify high-fat, high-cholesterol foods

Goal: Client will maintain fluid and electrolyte balance within normal limits.

Outcome

Client does not have any assessments (e.g., edema, crackles, weight gain) associated with fluid volume excess

Evaluative measure

Palpate the skin for edema and skin breakdown

Weight the client to detect weight loss or gain

Monitor vital signs for tachycardia, dysrhythmias, hypertension, and dyspnea

Auscultate the lungs for crackles, third heart sound, and absent or diminished breath sounds

CLIENT TEACHING FOR ALTERED NUTRITION

Help client to assess and incorporate meal preferences and budgetary limitations into diet.

Teach client how to incorporate menu planning in weekly shopping lists.

Provide list of community resources that can enable him or her to adhere more readily to prescribed diets.

Teach creativity within the guidelines of prescribed diets (e.g., creative menu planning and seasonings).

Outcome
Client does not have any assessments (e.g., poor skin turgor, sudden weight loss, tachycardia, decreased blood pressure) associated with fluid volume deficit
Evaluative measure
Palpate for poor skin turgor, edema, weak pulses, and tachycardia
Inspect the oral cavity for dry, sticky mucous membranes, decreased saliva, and lognitudinal furrows on the tongue
Monitor vital signs for tachycardia, dysrhythmias, and hypotension
Outcome
Client's laboratory parameters show actual or steady return to normal values
Evaluative measure
Monitor laboratory values

Goal: Client will avoid any complications from therapies designed to assist clients to return to within 10% of ideal body weight.
Outcome
Client's blood glucose remains within normal limits
Evaluative measure
Monitor serum glucose
Outcome
Client's bowel elimination patterns remain normal
Evaluative measure
Monitor client's bowel elimination patterns
Outcome
Client verbalizes positive weight loss or gain
Evaluative measures
Ask client about appearance
Observe client's body image

Goal: The client will state which foods to select for a properly balanced diet.
Outcome
Client will select appropriate foods, as demonstrated by a 24-hour diet diary
Evaluative measure
Review client's 24-hour diet history

SUMMARY

Nurses must understand the functions of the basic nutrients and how they are metabolized to produce energy. This knowledge is essential for teaching clients about and answering questions related to diet. Nurses should also know about research findings and their impact on dietary recommendations. They should be familiar with alternative food patterns and know about the influence of age on diet. Nurses must be able to assess nutritional status. They must also recognize that many factors influence food intake. Nurses must be able to identify clients at risk for nutritional problems and be aware of common nutritional conditions. They should be aware of the importance of their interaction with others in the area of food intake, be familiar with common hospital diets, and be able to assist clients at mealtime.

KEY CONCEPTS

The nutrients needed by the body to carry out vital functions are water, carbohydrates, proteins, lipids, vitamins, and minerals.
Body weight is maintained when food intake equals energy output.
Carbohydrates are anabolized into glycogen and adipose tissue or catabolized into energy.
Proteins are anabolized into tissue, hormones, or enzymes or catabolized into energy.
Lipids may be anabolized into adipose tissue or catabolized into energy.
Proteins are essential for growth, maintenance, and repair.
Essential amino and fatty acids must be supplied by dietary intake because the body is unable to synthesize them from other ingested substances.
Digestion is the mechanical and chemical process by which food is broken down into its simplest form for absorption. Digestion and absorption occur mainly in the small intestine.
Recommended daily allowances (RDAs) were formulated for population groups, not individuals.
Guidelines for dietary change advocate reduced intake of fat, saturated fat, salt, refined sugar, and cholesterol and increased intake of complex carbohydrates and fiber.
Age affects the requirements for essential nutrients. Periods of rapid growth increase the need for protein, vitamins, and minerals.
Because improper nutrition can affect all body systems, nutritional assessment includes a review of the total physical assessment.
Proper feeding techniques can protect the dependent client from loss of dignity and self-esteem.
Tube feedings can be used for clients unable to ingest food but able to digest and absorb foods.
Total parenteral nutrition (TPN) supplies essential nutrients in appropriate amounts to support life through the introduction of a concentrated nutrient solution into a large central vein or the right atrium of the heart.
Evaluation of the outcomes of intervention for nutritional support is essential in revising, updating, or continuing nursing activities.

CRITICAL THINKING ACTIVITIES

1. With a partner, role play the following situation. The nurse assists the client in developing a weekly diet plan based on the food pyramid. The client is a vegetarian or must follow specific ethnic-cultural dietary guidelines. The nurse must help the client to incorporate personal preferences and restrictions into a healthy diet plan.
2. You are assigned to work in a well baby clinic. You are doing an assessment on 8-month-old John Henry. His weight is 12 pounds, by history his mother states that he "mostly drinks milk." What additional assessment data do you need to determine the presence of a nutritional deficit in this client?
3. You've received morning report on Mr. Karl. Nasogastric tube feedings have been ordered. The night nurse stated that his abdomen was distended, and the feeding was withheld. What assessments do you need to make about Mr. Karl's tolerance to the tube feeding, the placement of the tube, and the resumption of tube feedings?

References

Alverdy JC: The GI tract as an immunologic organ, *Contemp Surg* 35:5a, 1989.

American Heart Association: *Dietary treatment for hypercholesterolemia: handbook for counselors,* vol 70-2001, Dallas, 1988, The Association.

Andressy RM: Preserving the gut mucosal barrier and enhancing immune response, *Contemp Surg* 21:2A, 1988.

Atkins JM, Oakley CW: A nurse's guide to TPN, *RN* 6:20, 1986.

Carnevali DL, Patrick M: *Nursing management for the elderly,* ed 3, Philadelphia, 1993, JB Lippincott.

Centers for Disease Control: Recommendations for prevention of HIV transmission in health care settings, *MMWR 36* (suppl 25):35, 1987.

Colley R: Parental nutrition. In Metheney N, editor: *Fluid and electrolyte balance: nursing considerations,* ed 3, Philadelphia, 1987, JB Lippincott.

Committee on Dietary Allowances Food and Nurtrition Board, National Academy of Sciences-National Research Council: *Estimated safe and adequate daily dietary intakes,* Washington, DC, 1989, The Academy.

DeBruyner, LK, Rolfer SR: *Life style nutrition conception through adolescent,* Whitner, 1989, St. Paul, Minn., West.

Expert Panel on Blood Cholesterol Levels in Children and Adolescents: *Report of the expert panel on blood cholesterol levels in children and adolescents,* NIH Publication No. 91-2732, Bethesda, Md. 1991, US Department of Health and Human Services.

Farley JM: Current trends in enteral feeding, *Crit Care Nurse* 8:(4):23, 1988.

Food and Nutrition Board: *Recommended dietary allowances,* ed 10, Washington DC, 1989, Nations Academy of Sciences.

Forlaw B, Grant P: *Introduction to nutritional and physical assessment of the adult client for the nurse,* Aspen, Colo., 1983, American Society for Parental and Enteral Nutrition (ASPEN).

Franz M: *Fast food facts: nutritive and exchange values for fast food restaurants,* Minneapolis, 1984, International Diabetes Center.

Gortmaker SL, et al.: Increasing pediatric obesity in the United States., *Am J Dis Child* 141:535, 1987.

Grant JA, Kennedy-Caldwell C: *Nutritional support in nursing,* New York, 1988, Grune & Stratton.

Hamel R: Food fight, *American Demog* 11(3):37, 1989.

Haynes-Johnson V: Tube feeding complications: causes, prevention, and therapy, *Nutr Supp Serv* 6(3):17, 1986.

Hess LV: Nutritional care of the geriatric patient, *J Home Health Care Prac* 2(1):29, 1989.

Jacobs C, Dwyer JT: Vegetarian children: appropriate and inappropriate diets, *Am J Clin Nutr* 48:811, 1988.

Kane RL, Ouslander JG, and Abrass IB: *Essentials of clinical geriatrics,* ed 3, New York, 1993, McGraw-Hill.

Mazy MA, Rauckhorst LH, Stoles SA: *Health assessment of the older individual,* ed 2, New York, 1993, Springer.

McDanal J, Wheeler D, Ebert J: A complication of nasogastric intubation: pulmonary hemorrhage, *Anesthesiology* 59:356, 1983.

Metheny NM, Eisenberg P, McSweeney M: Effect of feeding tube properties and three irrigants on clogging rates, *Nurs Res* 37(1):165, 1988.

Metheny NM: *Fluid and electrolyte balance: nursing considerations,* ed 2, Philadelphia, 1991, JB Lippincott.

Metheny NM, Spies M, Eisenberg P: Frequency of nasoenteral tube displacement and associated risk factors, *Nurs Res Health* 9(3):241, 1986.

Metheny NM, Spies M, Eisenberg P: Measures to test placement of nasogastric and nasointestinal feeding tubes: a review, *Nurs Res* 37:324, 1988.

Miller K, Tomlinson J, Sahn S: Pleuropulmonary complications of enteral tube feeding, *Chest* 88:203, 1985.

Muthuswamy P, Patel K, Rajendran R: Isocal pneumonia with respiratory failure, *Chest* 81:390, 1982.

National Dairy Council: *Feeding guide for the first two years,* Rosemont, Ill, 1990, The Council.

Petrosino BM, et al.: Implications for selected problems with nasoenteral tube feedngs, *Crit Care Q* 12(3):1, 1989.

Public Law 101-535. *Nutrition Labeling And Education Act of 1990.* 103 STAT. 2353.21 USC 301, Nov. 8, 1990.

Randall HT: Meeting protein and energy requirements in the postoperative period, *Contemp Surg* 2a:4, 1988.

Rifkind BM: Cholesterol lowering and reduced risk of coronary heart disease, *Proc Cardio* 14:(suppl)3, 1988.

Robuck J, Fleetwood J: Nutrition support in the client with cancer, *Focus Crit Care Nurs* 19(2):129, 1992.

Roe DA: Nutritional needs of the elderly: issues, guidelines, and responsibilities, *Fam Community Health* 12(1):59, 1989.

Rombeau J, Barot L: Enteral nutritional therapy, *Surg Clin North Am* 61:605, 1981.

US Department of Agriculture: *USDA's food guide pyramid,* USDA Human Nutrition Information Service Pub No 249, Washington, DC, 1992, US Government Printing Office.

US Department of Agriculture and US Department of Health and Human Services: *Nutrition and your health: dietary guidelines for Americans,* USDA/DHHS Home and Garden Bull No 232, Washington, DC, 1990, US Government Printing Office.

Wardlaw GM, Insel PM, Seyler MF: *Contemporary nutrition: issues and insights,* St. Louis, 1992, Mosby.

Whitney EN, Catallo CB, Rolfes SR: *Understanding normal and clinical nutrition,* ed 3, St Paul, Minn., 1991, West.

Worthington-Roberts BS, Williams SR, Vermeersch JA: *Nutrition in pregnancy and lactation,* ed 4, St. Louis, 1989, Mosby.

Bibliography

Campbell SM: Enteral nutritional support of patients in alternative care settings: feeding tubes and formulas, *J Home Health Care Prac* 1(4):67, 1989.

Cerrato PL: Spotting the patient who looks healthy but isn't, *RN* 52(3):81, 1989.

Collingsworth R and Boyle K: Nutritional assessment of the elderly, *J Gerontol Nurs* 15(12):17, 1989.

Eisenberg P, Metheny N, and McSweeney M: Nasoenteral feeding-tube properties and the ability to withdraw fluid via syringe, *Appl Nurs Res* 2(4):168, 1989.

Elston-Hurdle B, et al.: In vivo and in vitro bacterial contamination of enterofeeding systems, *Crit Care Nurse* 9(10):85, 1990.

McPherson ML: Drugs and dietary interactions: guidelines for counseling the home health care patient, *J Home Health Care Prac* 1(4):27, 1989.

Metheney N: Measures to test placement of nasogastric and nasointestinal feeding tubes: a review, *Nurs Res* 37:324, 1988.

Metheny N, et al.: Effectiveness of pH measurements in predicting feeding tube placement, *Nurs Res* 38:280, 1989.

Paige CP: Enteral feeding: NCJ for early and continued feeding, *Contemp Surg* 32:2a, 1988.

Pennington JAT: The food and drug administration and the dietary guidelines, *Fam Community Health* 12(1):1, 1989.

Steinborn PA: Total parenteral nutrition: the transition from hospital to home, *J Home Health Care Prac* 1(4):39, 1989.

Suitor CW: Nutritional status during pregnancy and lactation: a new food and nutrition board study, *Fam Community Health* 12(1):53, 1989.

32 Urinary Elimination

OBJECTIVES

Mastery of content in this chapter will enable the student to:

- Define the key terms listed.
- Explain the function of each organ in the urinary system.
- Describe the process of urination.
- Identify factors that commonly influence urination.
- Compare and contrast common alterations in urination.
- Obtain a nursing history from a client with an alteration in urination.
- Describe physical assessment techniques used to assess urinary elimination.
- Describe characteristics of normal and abnormal urine.
- Describe nursing implications of common diagnostic tests of the urinary system.
- Discuss nursing measures to assist the client with urinary elimination.
- Describe nursing measures to control incontinence.
- Discuss nursing measures to reduce urinary tract infections.
- Apply or insert an external or indwelling catheter.
- Understand basic principles in urinary catheter selection.

KEY TERMS

bacteriuria
catheterization
dysuria
enuresis
glomerulus
hematuria
micturition
nephrons
proteinuria
residual urine
ureterostomy
urinary incontinence
urinary reflux
urinary retention

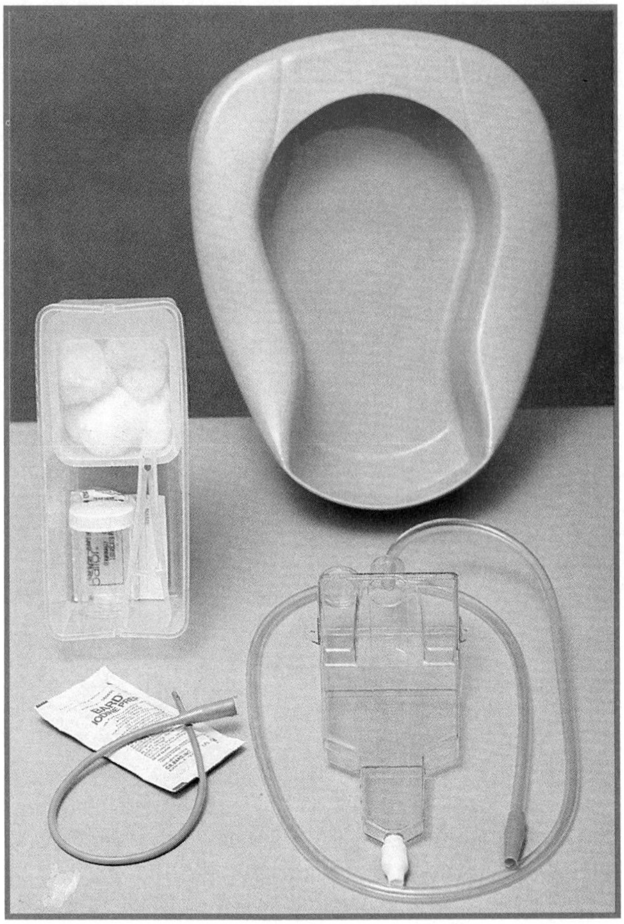

Normal elimination of urinary wastes is a function most people take for granted. When the urinary system fails to function properly, virtually all body systems can be affected. Clients with alterations in urinary elimination may also be affected by resulting body-image problems. The nurse provides understanding and sensitivity to the client's needs. With any client who has urinary elimination problems, the nurse must identify problems and acceptable solutions.

URINARY ELIMINATION

Urinary elimination depends on the function of the kidneys, ureters, bladder, and urethra. The kidneys remove wastes from the blood and urine. The ureters transport urine from the kidneys to the bladder. The bladder holds urine until the urge to urinate develops. The urine leaves the body through the urethra. All these organs must be intact and functional for the successful removal of urinary wastes (Figure 32-1).

Kidneys

The kidneys are reddish-brown, bean-shaped organs that lie on either side of the vertebral column behind the abdominal peritoneum and against the deep muscles of the back. The kidneys are level with the twelfth thoracic and third lumbar vertebrae. Normally the left kidney is 1.5 to 2 cm ($\frac{6}{10}$ to $\frac{8}{10}$ inch) higher than the right because of the anatomical position of the liver.

The kidneys contain functional units called **nephrons** that remove waste products from the blood and regulate water and electrolyte concentrations in body fluids (Figure 32-2). The kidneys can efficiently filter the blood of waste products in part because their blood flow is great, representing approximately 25% of the cardiac output. Blood reaches nephrons through the renal artery, which branches into smaller arteries, eventually becoming the afferent arterioles that directly supply the nephrons. A cluster of capillaries forms the **glomerulus,** which is the initial site of urine formation.

The glomerular capillaries filter water and glucose, amino acids, urea, uric acid, creatine, and major electrolytes. Normally, 180 liters of blood filter through the nephrons each day. Protein does not normally filter through the glomerulus. Therefore protein in the urine, **proteinuria,** is a sign of glomerular injury.

However, not all glomerular filtrate is excreted as urine. Approximately 99% is reabsorbed into the plasma. When the filtrate leaves the glomerulus, it passes through a system of tubules in which water and glucose, amino acids, uric acid, sodium, potassium, and bicarbonate ions are selectively reabsorbed into plasma. Hydrogen and potassium ions and ammonia are secreted into the tubules and become a part of the urine.

The normal range of urine production is 1 to 2 liters a day (McCance and Huether, 1994). Fluid intake and body temperature may affect urine production. Urine is usually 95% water and 5% solutes. These solutes include electrolytes and organic solutes (i.e., urea, uric acid, creatinine, and ammonia).

Ureters

Urine leaves the tubules and enters collecting ducts that transport it to the renal pelvis. A ureter is attached to each kidney pelvis and carries urinary wastes into the bladder. Ureters are long, tubular structures, 25 to 30 cm (10 to 12 inches) long and 1.25 cm ($\frac{1}{2}$ inch) in diameter in the adult. They extend behind the peritoneum to join at the floor of the bladder in the pelvic cavity. Urine draining from the ureters to the bladder is sterile.

Three layers of tissue form the wall of the ureter. The inner layer is a mucous membrane that lines the renal tubules and urinary bladder. The mucous lining is an excellent medium for the growth and spread of microorganisms. The middle layer consists of smooth muscle

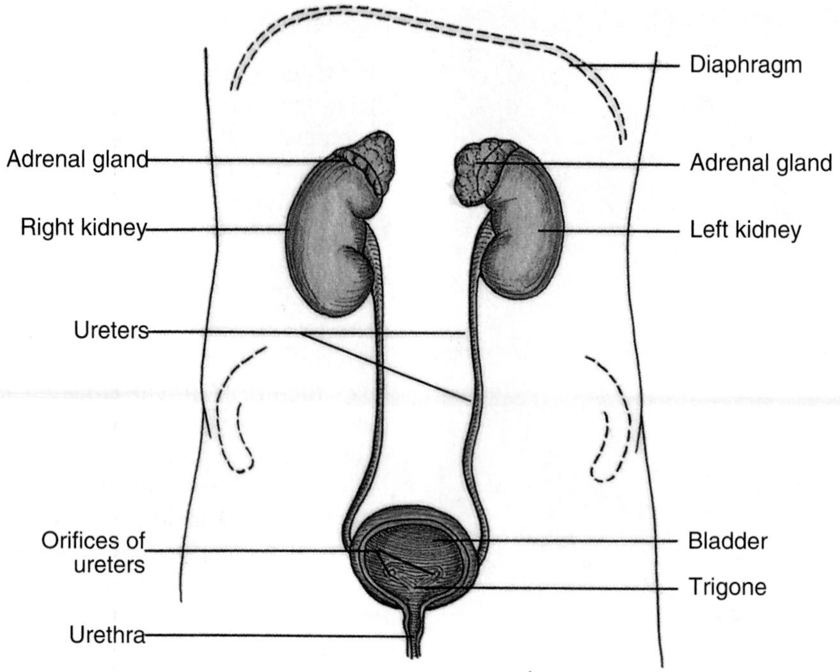

FIGURE 32-1 Organs of urinary system.

fibers; it helps to transport urine through the ureters by peristaltic waves. An outer layer of fibrous connective tissue supports the ureters.

Peristaltic waves cause the urine to enter the bladder in spurts rather than steadily. To prevent **urinary reflux,** a small, flaplike fold of mucous membrane acts as a valve and covers the juncture of the ureters and bladder. An obstruction within the ureters, such as a kidney stone (renal calculus), results in strong peristaltic waves that attempt to move the obstruction into the bladder. At the same time, a reflex response causes the renal arterioles to constrict to reduce urine production in the kidney on the affected side.

Bladder

The urinary bladder is a hollow, distensible, muscular organ that is a reservoir for urine. When empty, the bladder lies in the pelvic cavity behind the symphysis pubis. In the male, the bladder rests against the rectum posteriorly, and in the female it rests against the anterior wall of the uterus and vagina.

The bladder's shape changes as it fills with urine. Normally it holds approximately 600 ml of urine. When the bladder is full, its superior surface expands up into a dome and pushes above the symphysis pubis. A greatly distended bladder may reach the umbilicus. In a pregnant woman, the fetus pushes against the bladder, causing a feeling of fullness and reducing its capacity.

The trigone muscle is at the base of the bladder. An opening exists at each of the trigone's three angles: two for the ureters at its base and one for the urethra at its apex. The wall of the bladder has four layers: an inner mucous coat, a submucous coat of connective tissue, a muscular coat, and an outer serous coat. The muscular layer has bundles of muscle fibers that form the detrusor muscle. Parasympathetic nerve fibers supply this muscle during urination. The internal urethral sphincter, made of a ringlike band of muscle, is at the base of the bladder. The sphincter prevents the escape of urine and is under involuntary control.

Urethra

Urine travels from the bladder through the urethra and passes to the outside of the body through the urethral meatus. Mucous membrane lines the urethra, and urethral glands secrete mucus into the urethral canal. Thick layers of smooth muscle surround the urethra.

In women, the urethra is approximately 4 to 6.5 cm ($1\frac{1}{2}$ to $2\frac{1}{2}$ inches) long. The external urethral sphincter, located about halfway down the urethra, permits voluntary flow of urine. This short length in women and girls provides an easy access for microorganisms. In men, the urethra, which is also a passageway for cells and secretions from reproductive organs, is 20 cm (8 inches) long. It has three sections: the prostatic urethra, the membranous urethra, and the penile urethra.

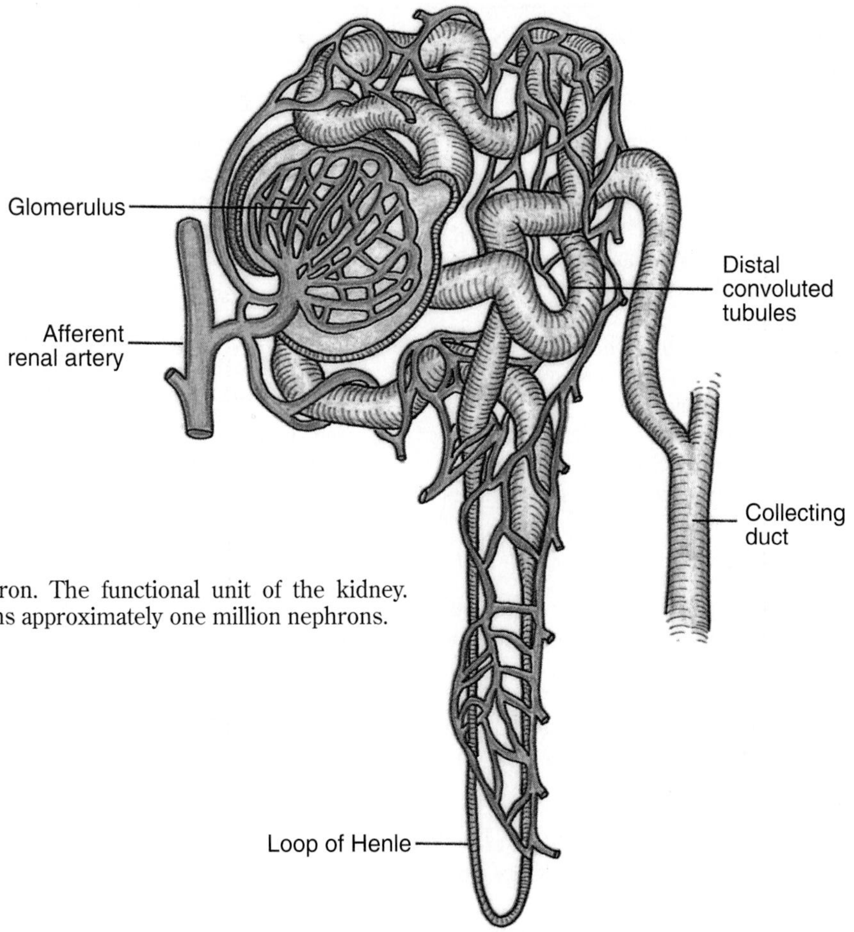

FIGURE 32-2 Nephron. The functional unit of the kidney. Every kidney contains approximately one million nephrons.

Act of Urination

Urination, **micturition,** and voiding are all terms for the process by which urine is expelled from the urinary bladder. The desire to urinate can be sensed when the bladder contains only a small amount of urine (150 to 200 ml in an adult and 50 to 100 ml in a child). As the volume of urine increases, the bladder wall stretches, sending sensory impulses for the sacral muscle to contract rhythmically. The internal urethral sphincter also relaxes so that urine may enter the urethra, although voiding does not yet occur. As the bladder contracts, nerve impulses travel to the midbrain and cerebral cortex. A person is thus conscious of the need to urinate. If the person chooses not to void, the external urinary sphincter remains contracted, and the micturition reflex is inhibited. However, when a person is ready to void, the external sphincter relaxes, the micturition reflex stimulates the detrusor muscle to contract, and urination occurs.

FACTORS INFLUENCING URINATION

Many factors influence urination (see box on p. 914). Normal urinary elimination can be affected by physiologic factors, psychosocial conditions, and diagnostic or treatment-induced factors. Knowledge of these factors enables the nurse to anticipate possible elimination problems.

COMMON URINARY ELIMINATION PROBLEMS

The most common urinary problems involve disturbances in micturition. These disturbances result from impaired bladder function, obstruction to urine outflow, or an inability to voluntarily control micturition. Some clients may have permanent or temporary changes in the normal pathway of urination. For example, the ureterostomy client has special problems because urine drains through an artificial opening (stoma) on the abdominal wall.

Urinary Retention

Urinary retention is an accumulation of urine in the bladder because the bladder is unable to empty. Urine collects in the bladder, stretching its walls and causing feelings of pressure, discomfort, tenderness over the

FACTORS INFLUENCING URINARY ELIMINATION

GROWTH AND DEVELOPMENT

Infants and young children cannot concentrate urine and reabsorb water effectively.

Children cannot control urination voluntarily until 18 to 24 months.

A child must be able to recognize the feeling of bladder fullness, to hold urine for 1 to 2 hours, and to communicate the sense of urgency to a parent.

With age, the ability to concentrate urine declines and the frequency of urination increases.

The process of aging may impair micturition.

Problems of mobility sometimes make it difficult for older adults to reach the toilet or bedside commode in time.

Chronic diseases, such as multiple sclerosis or stroke, alter urinary patterns.

SOCIOCULTURAL FACTORS

Cultural and gender norms vary on the privacy or publicness of urination. North Americans expect toilet facilities to be private, whereas some European cultures accept communal toilet facilities.

Social expectations (e.g., school recesses) influence the time of urination.

PSYCHOLOGICAL FACTORS

Anxiety and stress do not affect the characteristics of urine but may affect a sense of urgency and increase the frequency of urination.

Anxiety may prevent complete urination because tension makes it difficult to relax abdominal muscles.

PERSONAL HABITS

Privacy and adequate time to urinate are usually important to most people. Some people need distractions to relax.

MUSCLE TONE

Weak abdominal and pelvic floor muscles impair bladder contraction and control of the external sphincter.

Decreased muscle tone may be caused by immobility, childbirth, or trauma.

Muscle tone may also be lost with continuous drainage of urine through an indwelling catheter.

FLUID INTAKE

If fluids, electrolytes, and solutes are balanced, increased fluid intake increases urine production.

Alcohol stops the release of antidiuretic hormones, thus promoting urine production.

Fluids containing caffeine increase urinary output frequency.

Foods with high fluid content, such as fruits and vegetables, may increase urine production.

PATHOLOGICAL CONDITIONS

Diabetes mellitus and multiple sclerosis cause neuropathies that alter bladder function.

Rheumatoid arthritis, degenerative joint disease, and parkinsonism slow or hinder physical activity and interfere with urination.

Acute renal disease reduces urine volume; chronic renal disease initially increases volume of poorly concentrated urine.

Febrile conditions reduce the amount of urine but increase its concentration.

Spinal cord injuries interrupt voluntary bladder emptying.

SURGICAL PROCEDURES

The stress response to surgery reduces the amount of urine output to increase circulatory fluid volume.

Anesthetics and pain-killing drugs slow the filtration rate and reduce urine output.

Local trauma during surgery and lower abdominal and pelvic surgery may obstruct urine flow, so indwelling catheters may be needed.

MEDICATIONS

Diuretics prevent reabsorption of water and certain electrolytes, and urine output increases.

Some drugs also change the color of urine (e.g., amitriptyline turns it blue-green, and methyldopa turns it red; warfarin sodium turns it orange, and indomethacin turns it green).

DIAGNOSTIC EXAMINATIONS

Following intravenous pyelograms, monitor client for complications such as hypersensitivity reactions and acute renal failure.

Cystoscopy may cause localized edema of the urethral passageway and bladder sphincter spasm, resulting in urinary retention and the passing of red or pink urine.

symphysis pubis, restlessness, and diaphoresis. Key assessments include an absence of urine output over several hours and a distended bladder. The client under the influence of anesthesia or analgesia may perceive only pressure, but the alert client has worsening discomfort resulting in severe pain as the bladder distends beyond its normal capacity. In severe urinary retention, the bladder may hold as much as 2000 to 3000 ml of urine.

Eventually, retention with outflow may develop. Pressure in the bladder builds so that the external urethral sphincter is unable to hold back urine. The sphincter opens to allow a small volume of urine (25 to 60 ml) to

table 32-1

CAUSES OF URINARY ELIMINATION DISORDERS

Disorder	Causes
URINARY RETENTION	
Urine flow is obstructed; urine accumulates in bladder. Low fluid intake can lead to retention.	Prostate gland enlargement, fecal impaction, pregnancy in third trimester, urethral stricture or edema after childbirth, and urethral edema after surgery or diagnostic examination may obstruct urine flow. Spinal cord and peripheral nerve trauma and degeneration of peripheral nerves (e.g., diabetic neuropathy) alter sensory and motor innervation. Emotional anxiety and muscle tension may alter ability to relax sphincters.
LOWER URINARY TRACT INFECTION	
Microorganisms may be introduced resulting in bacterial spread, causing inflammation of bladder muscle.	Kinked or blocked urethral catheter and urinary retention can cause obstruction of urine flow. Poor perineal hygiene, frequent sexual intercourse, ingredients in bubble baths, improperly handled diagnostic instruments, improperly sterilized instruments, and contaminated urine receptacles can cause spread of bacteria.
URINARY INCONTINENCE	
Incontinence involves incompetent or weakened sphincter and loss of control of voiding.	Multiple childbirths, pelvic organ surgery, and removal of prostate gland can weaken sphincter. Mental confusion, sedatives or analgesics, spinal cord injury, bladder spasm, and bladder atrophy can cause loss of voiding control.

escape, after which the bladder pressure falls enough to allow the sphincter to close. The client voids small amounts of urine 2 or 3 times an hour with no relief of distention or discomfort. Bladder spasms may occur with voiding, further increasing discomfort.

Slow urine production can cause retention by filling the bladder gradually, thus preventing activation of the stretch receptors. After distending beyond a certain point, the bladder cannot contract. Retention can occur because of many other factors (Table 32-1).

Lower Urinary Tract Infections

Urinary tract infections account for 40% of hospital-acquired (nosocomial) infections in the United States (Burgener, 1987). It is important to identify these infections because bacteria in the urine, **bacteriuria,** may lead to the spread of organisms into the bloodstream and kidneys.

Microorganisms can enter the urinary tract through the urethral meatus or the bloodstream. However, the ascending route through the urethra is more common. Bacteria inhabit the vagina in women and the distal urethra and external genitalia in men and women. Organisms enter the urethral meatus easily and travel up the inner mucosal lining to the bladder. Women are more susceptible to urinary tract infection because of the proximity of the anus to the urethral meatus and because of a short urethra. In the male, the length of the urethra and the antibacterial substance in prostatic secretions reduce the risk of urinary tract infection.

In a healthy person with good bladder function, organisms are flushed out during voiding. However, bladder distention reduces blood flow to the mucosal and submucosal layer, and tissues become more susceptible to bacteria. **Residual urine** (urine that remains in the bladder after urination) is an ideal site for microorganism growth.

The causes of infection include invasive instrumentation of the urinary tract, contaminated hands of health personnel and the objects they use, poor perineal hygiene (especially women), frequent sexual intercourse, and some ingredients in bubble baths.

Clients with urinary tract infections have pain or burning during urination **(dysuria).** Fever, chills, nausea and vomiting, and malaise develop. An irritated bladder causes a frequent and urgent sensation of the need to void. Irritation to bladder and urethral mucosa results in blood-tinged urine **(hematuria).** The urine appears concentrated and cloudy because of bacteria. If infection spreads to the kidneys **(pyelonephritis),** fever, flank pain, tenderness, and chills are common symptoms.

Urinary Incontinence

Urinary incontinence is the loss of control over micturition. It may be temporary or permanent. The client cannot control the external urethral sphincter. Leakage may be continuous or intermittent. There are five types of incontinence (Newman and Smith, 1989) (Table 32-2).

Incontinence can develop in people of every age, although it is more common in adults. It has an impact on body image. Clothing becomes wet with urine, and the accompanying odor adds to embarrassment. Clients with this problem often avoid physical and social activities.

Older adults have special problems with incontinence because of physical limitations and the environment in which they live. An older person with restricted mobility has a greater chance of being incontinent because of the inability to reach toilet facilities in time. Low-set chairs and beds raised well above the floor may be obstacles for the older adult who must get up to reach a toilet. An older adult who has difficulty undoing buttons or manipulating zippers faces another obstacle. The older adult often lacks the energy to walk very far at one time, and if there is only one toilet in the home, the dis-

table 32-2

TYPES OF URINARY INCONTINENCE

Description	Causes	Symptoms
TOTAL		
Total uncontrollable and continuous loss of urine	Neuropathy of sensory nerves Trauma or disease of spinal nerves or urethral sphincter Fistula between bladder and vagina	Constant flow of urine at unpredictable times Nocturia Lack of awareness of bladder filling or incontinence
FUNCTIONAL		
Involuntary unpredictable passage of urine in client with intact urinary and nervous systems	Change in environment Sensory, cognitive, or mobility deficits	Strong urge to void with loss of urine before reaching appropriate receptacle
STRESS		
Increased intraabdominal pressure causing leakage of small amount of urine	Coughing, laughing, vomiting, or lifting with full bladder Obesity Full uterus pressing against bladder during third trimester of pregnacy Incompetent bladder outlet Weak pelvic musculature	Dribbling of urine with increased intraabdominal pressure Urinary urgency Frequency
URGE		
Involuntary passage of urine after strong sense of urgency to void	Decreased bladder capacity Irritation of bladder stretch receptors Alcohol or caffeine ingestion Increased fluid intake	Urinary urgency Abnormal frequency (more often than every 2 hours) Bladder contracture or spasm Nocturia Voiding in small (less than 100 ml) or in large (more than 550 ml) amounts
REFLEX		
Involuntary loss of urine occurring at somewhat predictable intervals when specific bladder volume is reached	Upper spinal cord injury or disease involving area above reflex arc, blocking cerebral awareness Lower spinal cord injury blocking impulses to reflex arc	Lack of awareness of bladder filling No urge to void Uninhibited bladder contraction or spasm at regular intervals

tance may be too far for the client with urge incontinence.

Continued episodes of incontinence can create skin breakdown. Acidic urine is irritating to the skin. The client who has frequent incontinence is especially at risk for pressure ulcers.

Enuresis

Enuresis is repeated involuntary urination in children who have reached the age when voluntary control is possible. This is usually around age 5 (Whaley and Wong, 1991; Gibson, 1989).

Episodes occur more commonly at night (nocturnal enuresis), usually during deep sleep. Enuresis may also occur during the day (diurnal enuresis) when the child who is engaged in play is unaware of a full bladder. Some children are enuretic during a temper tantrum or dispute with a sibling or playmate.

The child with primary enuresis has never had a long or symptom-free period. Secondary or acquired enuresis occurs after a dry period of at least 1 year.

Enuresis can be caused by many factors. Physiological causes have an organic basis such as urinary tract infections or obstructive uropathic conditions. There are also many psychological origins, including sex role conversion. Children who display neurotic, impulsive, or destructive behaviors often suffer from enuresis. In these children, enuresis can follow stressful events and may be only temporary. Some theorists believe that enuresis is hereditary or can be a dysfunction of the reticular activating system during deep sleep (Gibson, 1989).

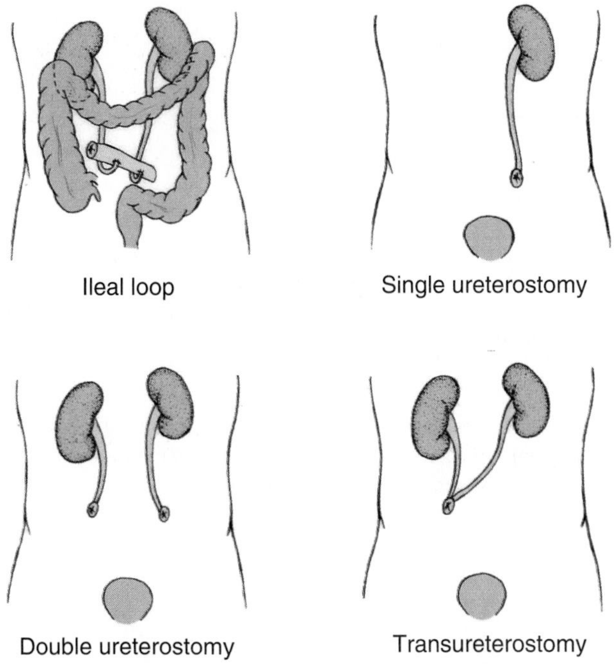

FIGURE 32-3 Types of ureterostomies.

Urinary Diversions

With surgery, it is possible to divert the drainage of urine from a diseased or dysfunctional bladder. A **ureterostomy** (urinary diversion) is any surgical procedure that creates stomas on the outer abdominal wall for urine drainage. Typically the client with a ureterostomy has had the bladder removed surgically because of a malignant growth, birth defects, or a spinal cord injury. A ureterostomy is the preferred treatment for chronic incontinence.

Figure 32-3 illustrates several types of ureterostomies. The ileal loop or conduit involves separating a loop of intestinal ileum with its blood supply intact. The surgeon implants the ureters into the ileum, which is an outlet for urine drainage. The ileum is not a reservoir. The remaining ileum is reconnected to the rest of the digestive tract. The disadvantage is that, if urine outflow becomes obstructed, the ileal conduit absorbs fluids and electrolytes and can cause metabolic alterations.

A ureterostomy involves bringing the end of one or both ureters to the abdominal surface. To avoid the need for two collecting devices, a transureterostomy connects the ureters and brings one out through the abdominal wall.

The client with a ureterostomy must wear a stomal pouch continuously because there is no sphincter control for regulation of urine flow. Because of continuous urinary drainage, the client must maintain skin integrity. Any obstruction within a ureterostomy may lead to serious fluid and electrolyte alterations.

A ureterostomy poses threats to body image. The client must wear an artificial device to collect urine and must learn to manage it. The client with a ureterostomy can wear normal clothing, engage in any physical activity, travel, and have sexual relations.

A client with a urinary diversion is referred to the enterostomal therapist (a nurse with specialized training in this area). This individual can serve as an invaluable resource to assist the client with matters pertaining to all aspects of care. The client should also be referred to the United Ostomy Association. This organization may be beneficial in providing information regarding support groups to enhance coping and adaptation to life-style and body-image changes.

NURSING PROCESS FOR ALTERATIONS IN URINARY ELIMINATION

Assessment

To identify a urinary elimination problem and gather data for a care plan, the nurse obtains a nursing history, performs a physical assessment, assesses the client's urine, and reviews information from diagnostic tests and examinations.

table 32-3

COMMON SYMPTOMS OF URINARY ALTERATIONS

Description	Causes or associated factors
URGENCY	
Feeling of the need to void immediately	Full bladder Inflammation or irritation to bladder mucosa from infection Incompetent urethral sphincter Psychological stress
DYSURIA	
Painful or difficult urination	Bladder inflammation Trauma or inflammation of urethra
FREQUENCY	
Voiding at frequent intervals	Increased fluid intake Bladder inflammation Increased pressure on bladder (e.g., pregnancy or psychological stress)
HESITANCY	
Difficulty in initiating urination	Prostate enlargement Anxiety Urethral edema
POLYURIA	
Voiding large amount of urine	Excess fluid intake Diabetes mellitus or insipidus Use of diuretics
OLIGURIA	
Diminished urinary output in relation to fluid intake	Dehydration Renal failure Urinary tract obstruction Increased secretion of antidiuretic hormone (ADH)
NOCTURIA	
Urination, particularly excessive, at night	Excess intake of fluids (especially coffee or alcohol before bedtime) Renal disease Cardiovascular disease
DRIBBLING	
Leakage of urine despite voluntary control of micturition	Urine retention from incomplete bladder emptying Stress incontinence
HEMATURIA	
Presence of blood in urine	Neoplasms of kidney, certain glomerular diseases, infections of kidneys or bladder, traumatic injury to urinary structure, calculi, blood dyscrasia
RETENTION	
Accumulation of urine in bladder, with inability of bladder to empty	Urethral obstruction, bladder inflammation, decreases sensory activity, neurogenic bladder, prostate enlargement after anesthesia, side effects of certain medications (e.g., anticholinergics, antispasmodics, antidepressants)
RESIDUAL URINE	
Volume of urine remaining in bladder after voiding (volumes of 100 mg or more)	Inflammation or irritation of bladder mucosa from infection, neurogenic bladder, prostatic enlargement, trauma or inflammation or urethra

Nursing History

The nursing history includes a review of the client's elimination patterns and symptoms of urinary alterations, as well as the following assessment of factors that may be affecting the ability to urinate normally:

1. Pattern of urination. Ask the client about daily voiding patterns, including frequency and times of day, normal volume at each voiding, and history of recent changes. Frequency varies among individuals. Most people void an average of 5 or more times a day. The client who voids frequently during the night may have renal or cardiovascular disease. Information about the pattern of urination is necessary to establish a baseline of comparison.
2. Symptoms of urinary alterations. Certain symptoms of alterations may occur in more than one type of urinary disorder. During assessment, the nurse asks the client about the symptoms listed in Table 32-3. The nurse also assesses whether the client is aware of conditions or factors that precipitate or aggravate symptoms.
3. Factors affecting urination. The nurse summarizes factors in the client's history that normally affect urination. These factors include the following:
   a. Medication history, including over-the-counter drugs.
   b. Environmental barriers in the home or health care setting. The client may need an elevated toilet seat, grab bars, or portable commode.
   c. Sensory restrictions (e.g., clients with visual problems who may have trouble reaching toilet facilities). If the client has difficulty with hand coordination, the nurse assesses the type of clothing and ease in using clothing fasteners.
   d. Past illness such as urinary tract infection or surgery increases the risk for recurrent problems. Chronic diseases (e.g., multiple sclerosis) that impair bladder function require the nurse to consider preventive care measures. Clients returning from surgery often have difficulty voiding the first few hours until the effects of anesthesia disappear.
   e. Presence of urinary diversion. If the client has a urinary diversion, the nurse assesses its location and function, condition of surrounding skin, and usual methods for management (type of appliance or pouch, type of skin barriers or applications, methods used to reduce skin irritation, frequency of appliance changes, and type of nighttime drainage system).
   f. Personal habits. If a client is hospitalized, the nurse assesses the extent to which personal habits are altered. Privacy is often difficult to accomplish in a health care setting, particularly if a client must use a bedpan.
   g. Presence of indwelling catheter. Clients recovering from major surgery and suffering critical illness or disability often have an indwelling catheter to aid urinary drainage and provide a measurement of urine output. A catheter places a client at risk for infection.
   h. Fluid intake. A client's physical condition affects the frequency with which the nurse monitors fluid intake (see Chapter 35). Regular intake and output measurements help to assess a client's overall fluid balance.

Physical Assessment

Skin and Mucosa. The nurse assesses the skin's hydration status by noting texture and turgor. The nurse also assesses skin integrity. Urinary incontinence, fluid imbalance, and electrolyte disturbances increase the risk for skin breakdown. Assessment of the oral mucosa also reveals whether hydration is adequate. To assess urinary function, the nurse examines the kidneys, bladder, and urethral meatus (see Chapter 16).

Kidneys. The only way to assess the position, shape, and size of the kidneys is by deep palpation of the abdomen. Much practice is needed to become adept at kidney palpation.

If the kidneys become infected or inflamed, flank pain typically develops. The nurse can assess for tenderness early in the disease by percussing the costovertebral angle (the angle formed by the spine and twelfth rib). Inflammation of the kidney results in pain on percussion.

Bladder. Normally the bladder rests below the symphysis pubis and cannot be examined by the nurse. When distended, the bladder rises above the symphysis pubis at the midline of the abdomen and just below the umbilicus. During physical assessment, the nurse may note a swelling or convex curvature of the lower abdomen. When distention is not visible, the nurse lightly palpates the lower abdomen. The bladder normally feels smooth and rounded. As the nurse applies light pressure to the bladder, the client may feel tenderness or even pain. Palpation also causes the urge to urinate.

Urethral Meatus. The female client assumes a dorsal recumbent position to provide full exposure of the genitalia. The nurse uses the gloved nondominant hand to retract the labial folds to see the urethral meatus. Normally the meatus is pink and appears as a small, slitlike opening below the clitoris and above the vaginal orifice. There is normally no discharge from the meatus. Drainage may indicate infection. The nurse notes the color and consistency of drainage. A clear, watery drainage is probably urine.

Women with vaginal infections are susceptible to urinary tract infections because vaginal discharge may travel easily to the urethral meatus. Older women may have vaginitis as a result of hormonal deficiencies. The nurse inspects the vaginal orifice carefully and describes any drainage. Infection is indicated by reddened, inflamed vaginal mucosa; discharge may be present.

The male's urethral meatus is normally a small opening at the tip of the penis. A hypospadias is a congenitally formed opening of the urethra on the undersurface of the penis. The nurse inspects the meatus for discharge and inflammation. It may be necessary to retract the foreskin in uncircumcised males to see the meatus.

Assessment of Urine

The assessment of urine involves measuring the client's fluid intake and urine output and observing the characteristics of the urine.

Intake and Output. The nurse assesses the client's average daily fluid intake. If a precise measurement of fluid intake is needed from the client who is at home, the nurse may ask the client to show a commonly used glass or cup on which the intake estimate is based.

In a health care setting, the nurse measures all fluid intake when the physician orders intake and output measurement (see Chapter 35). The nurse includes all sources of fluid intake.

Because it is often difficult for the client to estimate volumes of urine voided, the nurse must obtain measurements rather than depend on the client's estimate. A change in urine volume is a significant indicator of fluid imbalance or kidney disease. For example, in a catheterized postoperative client, hourly urinary output provides an indirect measure of circulating volume. If the urinary output falls below 30 ml an hour, the nurse must notify the physician and assess for other signs of shock.

While caring for the client, the nurse assesses volume by measuring (with plastic receptacles, bedpans or urinals, or a catheter bag) the urinary output with each voiding. Special urimeters attach to catheter drainage tubing and are a convenient means of measuring urine volume on a regular basis. A urimeter holds 100 to 200 ml of urine. After measuring urine from a urimeter, the nurse can drain the cylinder into the urinary drainage bag or into a receptacle for disposal.

Characteristics. The nurse inspects the client's urine for color, clarity, and odor.

COLOR. Normal urine ranges in color from a pale, straw color to amber, depending on its concentration. Urine is usually more concentrated in the morning. As the person drinks more fluids, it becomes less concentrated.

Bleeding from the kidneys or ureters usually causes urine to become dark red; bleeding from the bladder or urethra usually causes a bright red urine. Drugs can also change the urine's color. Beets, rhubarb, and blackberries may cause red urine. Special dyes used in intravenous diagnostic studies are eventually excreted by the kidneys and discolor the urine. Dark amber urine may be the result of high concentrations of bilirubin (urobilinogen) in clients with liver disease. The nurse reports any abnormal color to the physician.

CLARITY. Normal urine appears transparent at the time of voiding. Urine that stands several minutes in a container becomes cloudy. Freshly voided urine in clients with renal disease may appear cloudy because of protein concentration. Urine also appears thick and cloudy as a result of bacteria.

ODOR. Urine has a characteristic ammonia odor. The more concentrated the urine, the stronger the odor. As urine remains standing (e.g., in a collection device), more ammonia breakdown occurs, and the odor becomes stronger.

Testing

The nurse is frequently responsible for collecting urine specimens for laboratory testing. The type of test determines the method of collection. All specimens are labeled with the client's name, date, and time of collection. Table 32-4 lists routine urinary analysis and specific nursing interpretations for each.

Specimen Collection. The nurse collects several types of urine specimens for testing.

URINALYSIS SAMPLE. A simple urinalysis does not require a sterile urine specimen. The client may void into a clean urine cup, a urinal, or a bedpan. The client must void before defecating so that feces do not contaminate it. If a woman is menstruating, the nurse makes note of this on the specimen requisition in case red blood cells appear. The nurse transfers the urine to the proper container and sends it to the laboratory.

CLEAN-VOIDED OR MIDSTREAM SPECIMEN. To obtain a specimen relatively free of the microorganisms growing in the lower urethra, the nurse instructs the client on the method for obtaining a clean-voided specimen. Female and male clients wash the urethral meatus with soap or disinfectant. The woman should wipe from the meatus toward the rectum. The man cleans the meatus in a circular motion moving from the meatus up the glans penis. The nurse cautions the client against wiping repeatedly with the contaminated cloth.

The client receives a sterile urine cup. The nurse instructs the client to allow the first part of the urine stream to be discarded. The initial stream cleans or flushes the urethral orifice and meatus of resident bacteria. During the midstream or middle portion of voiding, the nurse or client collects the specimen. Immedi-

table 32-4

ROUTINE URINALYSIS VALUES

Measurement (normal value)	Interpretation
pH (4.6 to 8.0)	pH level helps to indicate acid-base balance. Urine that stands for several hours becomes alkaline from bacterial invasion. If pH is alkaline, selected antibiotics (e.g., neomycin and streptomycin) are more effective against urinary tract infections.
Protein (up to 8 mg/100 ml)	Protein is normally not present in urine. It is seen in renal disease because damage to glomerular membrane allows protein to enter urine. However, temporary presence of protein can occur after strenuous exercise, exposure to cold, or psychological stress.
Glucose (not normally present)	Diabetic clients have glucose in urine because of inability of tubules to reabsorb high serum glucose concentrations (over 180 mg/100 ml). Ingestion of high concentrations of glucose may cause some to appear in urine of healthy persons.
Ketones (not normally present)	With poor control of diabetes, clients experience breakdown of fatty acids. End product of fatty acid metabolism is ketones. Clients with dehydration, starvation, or excessive aspirin ingestion also have ketonuria.
Blood (up to two red blood cells)	Damage to glomerulus or tubules may cause blood cells to enter urine. Trauma or disease of lower urinary tract also causes hematuria.
Specific gravity (1.01 to 1.03)	Specific gravity tests measure concentration of particles in urine. High specific gravity reflects concentrated urine, and low specific gravity reflects diluted urine. Dehydration, reduced renal blood flow, and increase in ADH secretion elevate specific gravity. Overhydration and inadequate ADH secretion reduce it.

ately after obtaining the specimen the nurse places a sterile top securely over the container and sends it to the laboratory for testing. Urine specimens must reach the laboratory within 1 hour of collection or be refrigerated to 4° C. Urine that stands in a container at room temperature can grow bacteria.

STERILE SPECIMEN. Another method for collecting a sterile urine specimen for culture is by catheterizing a client (Procedure 32-1 on p. 933) or by obtaining the specimen from an indwelling catheter. Urine specimens should not be collected for culture from urine drainage bags unless it is the first urine drained into a new sterile bag. Bacteria grow rapidly in drainage bags and would give a false measurement of bacteria.

When catheterizing a client, the nurse collects the specimen as soon as urine flows from the catheter's end. After filling the sample container, the nurse withdraws the catheter or connects the indwelling catheter to a drainage tube.

If a client already has an indwelling catheter, the nurse uses a sterile syringe to withdraw urine. A 3 ml syringe with a 1-inch needle (21 to 25 gauge) is best to prevent creation of a hole in the catheter port. However, if blood is suspected in the urine, use of a large-bore needle prevents breakdown of red blood cells. It is safe to insert a needle directly into the end of a self-sealing rubber catheter. Silastic, plastic, or silicone catheters are not self-sealing. Some urine drainage tubes have special ports to withdraw specimens. First the nurse clamps the tubing just below the site chosen for specimen withdrawal, allowing fresh, sterile urine to collect in the tube. The nurse then wipes the catheter or port with a disinfectant swab. Insertion of the needle at a 30-degree angle ensures entrance into the catheter lumen. The nurse withdraws 3 ml for a culture (Figure 32-4). While aspirating urine the nurse must be careful not to raise the tubing, which would cause urine to return to the bladder.

After obtaining the specimen, the nurse transfers the urine into a sterile container using sterile aseptic technique. The laboratory requisition should indicate the way the specimen was collected.

TWENTY-FOUR–HOUR URINE SPECIMEN. Some tests of renal function and urine composition, such as measurements of levels of adrenocortical steroids and hormones and creatinine clearance tests, require a 24-hour collection of urine. The 24-hour collection period begins after the client urinates. The nurse indicates the starting time on the gallon container and on the laboratory requisition, and discards the first sample. The client then collects all urine voided in 24 hours. Any missed specimens make the results inaccurate, and the test must be restarted. The nurse should remind the client to void before defecating so that urine is not contaminated by feces. The 24-hour collection jar usually contains a preservative or requires refrigeration. The laboratory

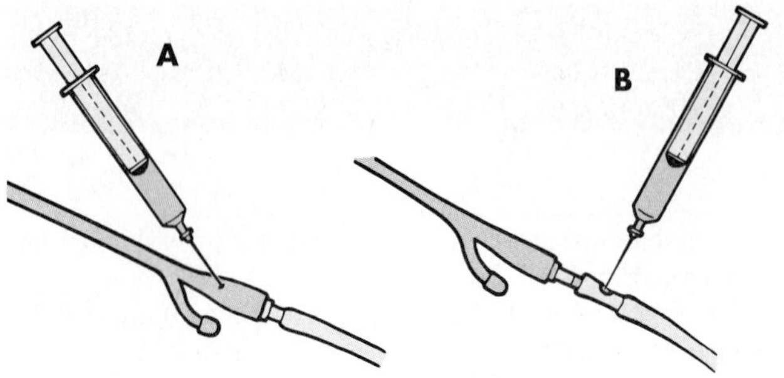

FIGURE 32-4 Urine specimen collection from an indwelling catheter. **A,** Aspiration of a urine specimen from a collection port in the drainage tubing of an indwelling catheter. **B,** Aspriation of a urine specimen from a collection port in the drainage tubing of an indwelling catheter. (Redrawn from McConnell EA: *Care of patients with urologic problems,* Philadelphia, 1983, Lippincott.)

should be consulted for instructions. The client should void the last specimen as close as possible to the end of the 24-hour period.

URINE COLLECTION IN CHILDREN. Specimen collection from infants and children is often difficult. Adolescents and school-age children can usually cooperate, although they may be embarrassed. Preschool children and toddlers have difficulty voiding on request. Offering a young child fluids 30 minutes before requesting a specimen may help. The nurse must use terms for urination that the child can understand. A young child may be reluctant to void in unfamiliar receptacles. A potty chair is usually more effective. The nurse must use special collection devices for infants or toddlers who are not toilet trained. Clear, plastic, single-use bags with self-adhering material can be attached over the child's urethral meatus.

The nurse prepares an infant by first washing the genitalia, perineum, and surrounding skin with soap and water or an antiseptic. Thorough drying is necessary because the bag's adhesive does not stick to a moist, powdered, or oily surface. The nurse attaches the bag from back to front, first to the perineum and then toward the symphysis pubis. In girls the perineum should be stretched tightly to ensure that the bag has a leak-proof fit. In boys the scrotum and penis fit inside the collection bag. A diaper is placed over the bag. The nurse checks the bag often and removes it as soon as urine is available. An active child can easily loosen the bag and cause a leak. For a clean-voided specimen, the nurse uses a sterile collection bag.

Common Urine Tests. Common urine tests include urinalysis, measurement of specific gravity, urine culture, and glucose and ketone levels.

URINALYSIS. The laboratory performs urinalysis on a routine or clean-voided specimen or on a specimen obtained from a catheter. Table 32-4 lists normal values. The urinalysis is a screening test for renal disease, metabolic disorders, lower urinary tract alterations, and fluid imbalances. For a quick screening, the nurse can perform certain portions of the urinalysis with special reagent strips. The nurse dips the strips into urine and watches for a color change, which indicates the presence of protein, blood, sugar, ketones, and other solutes. The nurse can also perform a specific gravity test on the patient care division.

GLUCOSE AND KETONES. An accurate measurement of glucose and ketones always requires a double-voided specimen. A Keto-Diastix or Multistix reagent strip easily detects glucose and ketone. The strips contain chemicals that change color when exposed to glucose and ketone. The nurse dips a stix in a urine specimen and pulls it out. After a select time period (10 to 15 seconds) the nurse compares the color of the stix with that of the color chart on the bottle. The color change indicates the glucose and ketone concentration.

SPECIFIC GRAVITY. To measure specific gravity, the nurse uses a urinometer and cylinder. The urinometer has a specific gravity scale at the top and a weighted mercury bulb at the bottom. The nurse pours a urine specimen into a clean, dry cylinder, and suspends the weighted urinometer into it. The concentration of dissolved substances in the urine determines the depth at which the urinometer will float. The point the level of urine reaches on the urinometer scale is the specific gravity measurement.

URINE CULTURE. A urine culture simply requires a sterile sample of urine. It takes approximately 72 hours before the laboratory can report significant findings of bacterial growth. If bacteria are present, an additional test for sensitivity determines the antibiotics that will be effective or ineffective.

Diagnostic Examinations

The urinary system is one of the few organ systems amenable to accurate diagnostic study by radiographic techniques. The two approaches for visualizing urinary structures, namely direct and indirect techniques, can be quite simplistic or very complex, requiring extensive nursing interventions. These procedures are further subdivided into invasive or noninvasive categories and will be briefly discussed under these headings in the following section. A discussion of the appropriate nursing responsibilities for each procedure is also provided.

Noninvasive Procedures

Abdominal Roentgenogram. Abdominal roentgenogram, also referred to as "plain film," "KUB," or "flat plate" of the abdomen, is commonly used to assess the gross structures of the urinary tract for abnormalities. It can be used to determine size, parity, shape, and location of the kidneys, ureters, and bladder structures. It is also useful in visualizing calculi or tumors in these organs. In addition, the ribs or other surrounding support structures can be assessed for fractures or abnormalities. This is of particular importance if the client has suffered some type of traumatic injury. The lack of positive findings on the roentgenogram does not rule out the possibility of abnormalities in the urinary tract. Additional diagnostic studies may be warranted.

The nursing implications for clients undergoing this procedure include explanation of the procedure and alleviation of client anxiety. No special bowel preparation is warranted unless the physician deems otherwise.

Intravenous Pyelogram. To view the entire urinary system, the physician orders the excretory urogram or intravenous pyelogram (IVP). This procedure provides visualization of the renal parenchyma and pelvis and outlines the ureters, bladder, and urethra (the latter two structures are better visualized by cystourethrogram). Although this procedure is noninvasive, it does require that the client receive an intravenous injection of a radiopaque dye. Normally, the injected medium takes only a few minutes to circulate and be excreted. Because the kidneys and ureters lie behind the intestines, it is necessary that the client receive a bowel preparation before the procedure. Procedures using barium should not be performed 2 to 3 days before an IVP because residual barium in the intestines will obscure the view (see Chapter 33).

During the IVP, x-ray studies are taken at specific intervals over a 30- to 60-minute period as the dye concentrates. The client may also be asked to void during the procedure to measure bladder emptying.

Diseases or disorders of the urinary tract that should be investigated by this means include renal artery occlusion, tumors, cysts or stones, vesicoureteral reflux, and traumatic injuries.

Nursing implications before the test include recognizing clients at risk for alterations in renal function as a result of the intravenous injection of the contrast material. Any client with preexisting renal insufficiency is at risk. Older adults in particular are prone to the nephrotoxic effects of these substances because of their propensity for volume depletion during bowel preparation. Appropriate nursing assessment of volume status and its maintenance before this procedure is of utmost importance (see Chapter 35).

Additional nursing implications are as follows:

1. Observe client sign informed consent.
2. Assess client for history of shellfish or iodine allergy, which predicts allergies to the IVP dye.
3. Administer cathartic on evening before test.
4. Ensure that client has only clear liquids after midnight.
5. Explain that facial flushing is normal during dye injection and that client may feel dizzy or warm.
6. Explain that an intravenous infusion for dye injection is started before the test.
7. Explain that the test involves x-ray studies taken at several intervals and that client will void near the end of the test.

Not all agencies employ nurses in the radiology department. If a nurse is not present, the physician or radiology technician assumes these responsibilities. Implications during the test include the following:

1. Assess intravenous site for signs of infiltration of dye into tissues (e.g., swelling, redness, and pain).
2. Observe for signs of allergic reaction to dye (e.g., respiratory distress or fall in blood pressure).
3. Remind client of normal sensations caused by dye injection.

Nursing implications after the test include the following:

1. Ensure that client receives normal diet afterward.
2. Encourage fluid intake to minimize dehydration caused by fasting and to avoid the potential nephrotoxic effects of the contrast material.
3. Observe client for itchiness, rash, or hives, which indicates delayed hypersensitivity to IVP dye.
4. Monitor intake and output.

Renal Scan. Radionuclide tests such as renal scans allow indirect visualization of urinary tract structures after an intravenous injection of radioactive isotopes. Selection of radiopharmaceutical agents depends on the physiological process to be investigated. The emissions from the radionuclides can be photographed by special cameras. The isotope can be detected without the need of bowel preparation. A very low dosage of radioisotope is used. Its half-life is short. Therefore no precautions against radioactive exposure are needed.

After a radionuclide is injected, it circulates through the kidney and is excreted. The renal scan measures radioactive concentrations while the client assumes a supine, prone, or sitting position. Except for the venipuncture, it is painless. The scanning procedure is completed in approximately 1 hour. Information pertaining to renal blood flow, anatomical structures, and their excretory function can be obtained from this procedure. The physician can diagnose abnormalities such as renal artery occlusion, urinary obstruction, and many other diseases of the kidney. This procedure is indicated for clients unable to receive IVP dyes. The nurse does not routinely give a sedative before the test unless the physician views the client as highly anxious. Nursing implications before the test include the following:

1. Observe client sign informed consent.
2. Explain that radioisotope is injected intravenously through an existing IV line or needle.
3. Explain that client will feel no discomfort but must lie still.

4. Explain there is no risk of radioactive exposure.

Nursing implications during the test include the following:

1. Assist the client in changing positions during the test. (Technician may do this.)
2. Explain that the machine measuring the isotope uptake is similar to a Geiger counter.

Computerized Axial Tomography

Computerized axial tomography (CT) is a computerized x-ray procedure that is used to obtain detailed images of structures within a selected plane of the body. Through a series of complex manipulations, the computer is able to "reconstruct" the cross-sectional image as a recognizable photograph on the television monitor. With this procedure, it is possible to visualize abnormal pathology such as tumors, obstructions, retroperitoneal masses, and lymph node enlargement. Although this procedure is noninvasive, in some examinations oral and/or intravenous contrast material is used to enhance the areas under study. If intravenous contrast is used, it may be necessary to administer a bowel prep, especially if additional organs in the abdominal cavity are to be examined. The nursing implications before, during, and after this test are the same as those listed under the IVP examination. However, the nurse explains that the client will be placed in a large machine, which may precipitate feelings of claustrophobia in susceptible individuals.

Renal Ultrasound

Ultrasonography is a valuable noninvasive diagnostic tool in the assessment of urinary disorders. It makes use of high frequency, inaudible sound waves that reflect off tissue. A conductive gel that functions as a transmitter for sound waves is applied to the skin. The client is usually prone during the procedure but can be positioned in a sitting position. The ultrasound is used to identify gross renal anatomy, structural abnormalities of the kidneys or lower urinary tract, and to assist with percutaneous biopsy. Such abnormalities as tumors or cysts in the kidney are easily identified with this procedure. This procedure is painless. No biological hazards have been identified with energy or sound wave emissions from this procedure.

Nursing implications before the procedure involve explanation of the test and possibly encouraging the client to ingest oral fluids to cause bladder distention. No specific post test client care is indicated.

Invasive Procedures

Invasive procedures include cystoscopy, biopsy, and arteriogram.

Cystoscopy. To view the interior of the bladder and urethra, the physician performs a cystoscopy. The cystoscope looks like a urinary catheter, although it is not as flexible. It is inserted through the urethra.

The procedure is painful during instrument insertion. Unless the client lies still, the bladder may be perforated. Local, spinal, or general anesthesia may be administered. Because the test requires insertion of a foreign object into a sterile cavity, the client receives large amounts of fluids (intravenously or orally) before and during the procedure to maintain a continuous urine flow and to flush out bacteria. Antibiotics may also be administered intravenously. During the test, urine and tissue specimens may be collected.

The physician usually performs the sterile cystoscopy in a hospital cystoscopy room. Special cystoscopy tables minimize the stress and fatigue that clients may experience from maintaining one position for a prolonged time. Nursing implications before the test include the following:

1. Observe client sign informed consent.
2. Perform a bowel preparation or enema or administer a cathartic on the evening before the test.
3. If local anesthetic will be used, encourage intake of oral fluids.
4. If general anesthetic is to be used, ensure that client takes nothing by mouth after midnight.
5. Explain that insertion of cystoscope is similar to insertion of urethral catheter.
6. Explain the importance of lying still during the test.
7. Explain that an intravenous line will be started to give fluids during the test.
8. Administer a sedative or analgesic per the physician's orders.

Nursing implications during the test include the following:

1. Assist client to assume a lithotomy position (see Chapter 16).
2. Prepare perineal area with antiseptic solution.
3. Explain (if client is awake) that insertion of cystoscope causes an urge to void.
4. Remind client to lie still.

Nursing implications after the test include the following:

1. Instruct the client to remain in bed as ordered.
2. Assess for signs of urinary retention and first voiding.
3. Observe characteristics of urine, noting bloody or cloudy urine.
4. Encourage increased fluid intake and monitor I & O.
5. Observe for fever, dysuria, or drop in blood pressure.
6. Administer medications to alleviate bladder spasms and/or lower back pain.

In addition to complete visual inspection of the bladder and urethra through the cystoscope, retrograde pyelography may also be performed. During this procedure, the physician passes a small catheter through the cystoscope into the bladder that allows catheterizing of the ureters and renal pelvis. Urine specimens are then collected separately from each ureter. Radiopaque dye can be instilled into the renal pelvis while serial x-rays are taken to examine the filling of the renal collecting system. Invasive examinations to visualize the bladder and urethra include retrograde cystograms, voiding cystourethrogram (VCUG), and cystourethrogram. All of these studies involve the instillation of a radiopaque fluid into the bladder via a catheter (urethral or suprapubic). Serial x-rays taken during these procedures will provide information regarding abnormalities in bladder mucosa, demonstrate vesicoureteral reflux, provide information regarding bladder function, as well as provide an assessment of the size and shape of the ureters.

Nursing implications for this procedure would be the same as those for the cystoscopy procedure.

Renal Biopsy. A renal biopsy is performed to determine the nature, extent, and prognosis of renal disease. This procedure involves obtaining a piece of renal cortical tissue for examination with sophisticated microscopic techniques. The procedure can be performed by either percutaneous (closed) or surgical (open) methods. The use of ultrasound examinations to localize the kidney has revolutionized the percutaneous approach. Tissue diagnosis allows differentiation between disease processes causing alterations in renal function.

Nursing implications before this procedure include:

1. Observe client sign informed consent.
2. Explain procedure and answers questions.
3. Obtain hematological studies for evaluation such as CBC, bleeding time, prothrombin time, platelet count, and type and crossmatch for possible blood transfusion.
4. Obtain urine specimens for routine analysis, culture, and sensitivity.
5. Instruct client in appropriate positioning and breathing techniques during the procedure.
6. Administer a sedative to relieve anxiety.

Nursing implications during the test include:

1. Nurse provides emotional support to the client.
2. Nurse coaches client regarding breathing and positioning techniques.
3. Nurse reminds client of normal sensations caused by the local administration of analgesics and the biopsy instrument.

Nursing implications after the test include:

1. Nurse observes color, amount, and character of urine, noting bloody urine.
2. Nurse monitors client's vital signs, noting changes consistent with hemorrhagic shock (see Chapter 36).
3. Nurse obtains post biopsy hematological studies (CBC).
4. Nurse encourages oral fluids.
5. Nurse instructs client to remain in bed for prescribed time period (usually 24 hours).
6. Nurse assesses biopsy site for signs of bleeding and/or client complaints of pain.
7. Nurse maintains pressure dressings on biopsy site.

Arteriogram (Angiogram). The renal angiogram is an invasive radiographical procedure with radiopaque contrast material that outlines the vascular supply to the kidneys. Most frequently, this procedure evaluates the arterial system; however, techniques to investigate the venous sytem (venogram) are available. The arteriogram is most often utilized to maintain the main renal artery and/or its segmental branches to detect narrowing or occlusion. In addition, this procedure is useful in the evaluation of mass lesions (e.g., neoplasms, cysts) to determine parity, collateral, or traumatic injury to blood vessels.

Venograms are most often performed to examine the excretory system and to allow for sampling of renal vein blood to assay various renal hormonal levels (e.g., renin, erythropoietin). The arteriogram is performed by placing a catheter into one of the femoral arteries and advancing it to the level of the renal arteries.

Pretest nursing implications are similar to those for the intravenous pyelogram procedure (IVP). In addition to those listed under the IVP procedure, nursing implications during the angiogram include:

1. Monitor client's vital signs.
2. Administer intravenous mannitol during the injection of contrast material to promote diuresis and excretion of the contrast. This is especially important in clients who may be prone to its nephrotoxic effects (e.g., older adults, individuals with renal insufficiency or a single kidney).

Nursing implications after the angiogram include:

1. Monitor client's vital signs hourly until stability is verified, then advance intervals to every 2 hours then 4 hours, respectively.
2. Ensure that client maintains bedrest for 8 to 12 hours. (If a venogram was performed, this time may be less.)
3. Check pulses and assess the circulation in the cannulated extremity.
4. Observe for bleeding, increased tenderness, or hematoma formation at the catheter insertion site for 24 hours.
5. Maintain a pressure dressing over the site for 24 hours.

6. Observe client for possible delayed reactions to the contrast material.
7. Monitor client's intake and output and report abnormalities in urine volume to the doctor.

Nursing Diagnosis

The nurse's thorough assessment of the client's urinary function may identify defining characteristics that support actual or potential elimination problems (see box below). Identification of the defining characteristics leads the nurse to select an appropriate diagnostic label. Specifying the appropriate related factors for each diagnosis allows the nurse to select individualized nursing interventions.

Associated problems require interventions that often have no direct effect on urinary elimination. Unless the nurse intervenes, however, these problems can continue. For example, when the client has a toileting self-care deficit related to limited lower extremity mobility, appropriate nursing interventions provide the client a means of easy access to toileting facilities. This may involve placing a bedpan or commode within close proximity or scheduling designated time intervals for a staff member to assist the client with toileting. However, if the nurse identifies the related factors in the aforementioned example to be loss of voluntary control of micturition, a different set of interventions would be appropriate. The nurse would then intervene by establishing outcome criteria to prevent incontinence. It is of utmost importance to identify the correct related factors for a given nursing diagnosis because this will affect the selection of the appropriate nursing interventions.

NURSING DIAGNOSES FOR URINARY ELIMINATION

Pain
Toileting self-care deficit
High risk for impaired skin integrity
Altered patterns of urinary elimination
Body-image disturbance
Functional incontinence
Knowledge deficit
High risk for infection
Reflex incontinence
Stress incontinence
Total incontinence
Urge incontinence
Urinary retention
High risk for altered health maintenance

Problems involved with urinary elimination alterations are often interrelated and complex. The nurse must also anticipate problems that may develop as a result of therapy.

Planning

The nurse plans therapeutic interventions for clients with urinary elimination problems, and preventive interventions may be required for clients with potential urinary problems (see nursing care plan on p. 927).

The client with actual or potential alterations in urinary elimination learns to recognize the signs of change and prevent serious problems. Alterations in urinary elimination pose a high risk to a client's overall state of health.

Planning should also include consideration of the client's home environment and normal elimination routines. Reinforcement of good health habits that are already followed improves the likelihood for compliance with the plan of care. In the hospital, planning care also includes preparations for discharge. The nurse determines any assistive devices that will be required and the client's educational needs. Teaching throughout the hospital stay is important. Theoretical concepts are continuously reinforced, and return demonstrations of psychomotor and self-care skills are performed by the client to ensure adherence to procedures and accuracy in their performance. Family members are also included in these teaching sessions. The need for home health services should be explored and appropriate referrals made. The nurse should enlist the assistance of other disciplines in this planning process (e.g., social services) to explore family financial resources or other influences that may affect the discharge process. The nurse's active and thoughtful role in planning these interventions will result in the client's progress toward improved urinary elimination.

The nurse and client work together to establish ways of maintaining client involvement in nursing care and to maintain normal elimination patterns when possible. Client-centered goals include the following:

Goal: Client understands normal urinary elimination.

Outcomes

Client will be able to state components of the lower urinary tract that assist to maintain continence

Client will understand that voluntary control over urination is influenced by the cerebral cortex

Client will be free of symptoms of urinary alterations

Goal: Client has normal micturition with complete bladder emptying within 1 month.

SAMPLE NURSING CARE PLAN
Urinary Retention

ASSESSMENT

Clinical scenario: Mrs. Kline, 2 days after giving birth, complains of a *frequent urge to void, dysuria, and dribbling.* The nursing assessment reveals a *distended bladder and small, frequent voidings.*

NURSING DIAGNOSIS

Urinary retention related to weakened detrusor muscle.

PLANNING

Goal	Expected outcomes
Client will achieve complete bladder emptying after voiding within 8 hours.	Bladder will not be distended after voiding. Client will deny feeling of bladder fullness after voiding. There will be less than 50 ml of residual urine.

IMPLEMENTATION

Steps	Rationale
1. Instruct client on use of pelvic floor (Kegel) exercises during nonvoiding times. Have client use exercise with each voiding.	Pelvic floor exercises assist in strengthening muscles when pelvic nerves are intact and functional (Touch, 1988).
2. Have client attempt voiding at regularly scheduled times.	Training bladder to empty regularly can reduce incidence of dribbling (Miller, 1990).
3. Have client use bladder compression (Credé method) during voiding.	Credé method helps to stimulate micturition and promotes bladder emptying.

EVALUATION

Palpate client bladder every 4 hours and after each voiding.
Ask client about sensation to void and bladder fullness.
Measure volume of each voiding; perform residual volume measurement with straight catheterization.

**Defining characteristics* are shown in italic type.

Outcomes

Client will ingest at least 2000 ml of fluids per day if not contraindicated

Client will empty the bladder using the procedural maneuvers taught within 1 week

The bladder will not be distended after voiding by second week

There will be less than 50 ml of residual urine

Client will experience gradual decrease in incontinent episodes within 1 month

Goal: Client understands how to prevent urinary tract infection.

Outcomes

Client will demonstrate appropriate hygiene measures to prevent infection.

Client will be free of symptoms of UTI.

Client will manage catheter care or urinary stoma appropriately.

Goal: Client's skin remains intact.

Outcomes

Skin around perineum, stoma, or condom catheter will be free of breakdown

Client will report an absence or decreased incidence of incontinence

Client will identify interventions to prevent incontinence

Goal: Client attains comfort.

Outcomes

Client's bladder will not become distended.

Client will report dryness that is personally satisfactory.

URINARY ELIMINATION HEALTH PROMOTION/RESTORATION ACTIVITIES

1. Maintain adequate hydration:
   A client with normal renal function who does not have heart disease or alterations requiring fluid restriction should drink 2000 to 2500 ml of fluid daily.
2. Promote micturition habits:
   Ensure client comfort and privacy.
   Allow sufficient time to void (at least 30 minutes).
   Integrating the client's habits into the care plan fosters a more normal voiding pattern.
   Offer the client use of toilet facilities if possible, avoiding bedpans.
   Ensure access to toilet facilities.
   Assist the client in the appropriate position for voiding (i.e., females—sitting, males—standing).
3. Encourage appropriate personal hygiene:
   Instruct female clients to cleanse the perineum and urethra from front to back after each voiding and bowel movement.
   Clients prone to UTIs should be encouraged to shower instead of bathe.
4. Promote complete bladder emptying:
   Clients who have difficulty starting or stopping the urine stream may benefit from exercises to strengthen pelvic muscles.
   Credé's method of manual bladder compression helps to stimulate urination and manually expels urine when bladder tone is reduced.
   Drug therapy alone or in conjunction with other therapies can be useful for treating problems of incontinence and retention.
5. Prevent infection:
   Ensure adequate fluid intake.
   Encourage good handwashing.
   Prevent breaks in closed catheter drainage systems.
   Follow tips for preventing infection in catheterized clients.
   Teach client how to keep urine acidic. Acid urine tends to inhibit growth of microorganisms. Meats, eggs, whole grain breads, cranberries, prunes increase urine acidity.
6. Maintain skin integrity:
   The skin is the first barrier of defense.
   The normal acidity of urine is irritating to the skin.
   Washing with mild soap and warm water is the best way to remove urine from the skin.
   After performing hygiene, dry clothing should be applied immediately on incontinent client.
   Clients with external urinary devices should receive assistance in selecting appliances that fit appropriately. They should also be taught preventive skin care measures.

Implementation

Clients should know basic mechanisms for urine production and voiding. The nurse focuses on client education, normal micturition, complete bladder emptying, prevention of infection, skin integrity, and comfort.

Health Promotion

Success of therapies aimed at optimizing normal urinary elimination depends in part on successful client education (see box below). The nurse instructs clients about their specific elimination problems. For example, a client who practices poor hygiene will benefit from learning about normal sterility of the urinary tract and ways to prevent bacterial invasion of the urinary tract. It may also be useful to discuss the basic mechanism for urine production and voiding for clients with elimination alterations. Knowledge of factors that promote normal urine production and voiding can also help. Health promotion skills should always be the initial focal point of teaching (see box at left).

The nurse can easily incorporate teaching during delivery of care. For example, if the nurse is attempting to increase the client's fluid intake, a good time to discuss benefits is while giving fluids with medications or meals. The nurse may be more successful in teaching about perineal hygiene during a bath or while giving catheter care. Much of the information the nurse offers is practical in nature. The nurse can easily include family members in informal discussions.

Promotion of Normal Micturition

Many nursing measures are designed to promote normal voiding in clients at risk for urination difficulties and

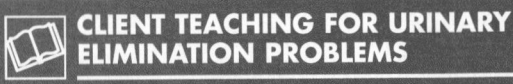

CLIENT TEACHING FOR URINARY ELIMINATION PROBLEMS

Instruct client or care giver about observations to make regarding urinary output.
Provide clients with pertinent signs and symptoms of infections.
Frequently remind ambulatory clients about intake and output measurements.
Reinforce correct perineal hygiene measures to reduce the risk of urinary tract infection.
Determine client's knowledge of medications and provide instruction on medications that affect urination, color of urine, and urine volume.
Instruct client and care giver regarding health promotion measures to prevent infection.

in clients with established urination problems. The nurse can independently initiate many measures.

Stimulating the Micturition Reflex. The client's ability to void depends on feeling the urge to urinate, on being able to control the urethral sphincter, and on being able to relax. The nurse can foster relaxation and stimulate the reflex to void by helping clients to assume the normal position for voiding.

Females are better able to void in a squatting position. This position promotes contraction of the pelvic and intraabdominal muscles that assist in sphincter control and bladder contraction. If the client cannot use a toilet, the nurse positions her on a bedpan or bedside commode.

The male client voids more easily in the standing position. At times it may be necessary for one or more nurses to assist the male client to stand. If the client cannot reach a toilet, he may stand at the bedside and void into a urinal (Figure 32-5).

Other measures to promote normal micturition include the use of sensory stimuli (e.g., turning running water on, putting a client's hand in a pan of warm water, or stroking the female client's inner thigh). Each tends to promote relaxation and the reflex to void.

Maintaining Elimination Habits. Many clients follow set routines of normal voiding. In a hospital or long-term care facility, the nurse's routines may conflict with those of the client. Integrating the client's habits into the care plan fosters a more normal voiding pattern.

The client usually requires time to void. The client should be given at least 30 minutes. The nurse must learn the times when a client normally voids and offer the opportunity to use a toilet at those times. The nurse must also respond in a timely manner to the client's urge to urinate. Delay in assisting the client to the bathroom may interfere with normal micturition. Research has shown that promptly assisting clients to toileting facilities reduces incontinence when the clients were able to perceive the urge to void (Kaltreider, et al., 1990). Older adults may also require other special interventions owing to the aging process (see box below).

Privacy is essential for normal voiding. If the client cannot reach the bathroom, the nurse makes sure the bedside area is private. In the home, the debilitated

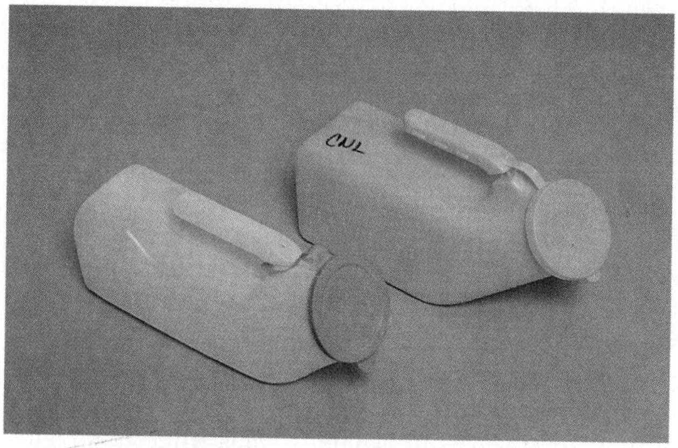

FIGURE 32-5 Types of male urinals.

GERONTOLOGIC NURSING PRACTICE

Kidney and urinary tract functions change with advancing age. There is a progressive decline in the glomerular filtration rate as well as changes in tubular function. As a result, the following gerontologic nursing practices for the client with altered patterns of urinary elimination might include:

- The older client may experience urinary incontinence problems as a result of mobility problems or neurological impairments. The nurse should be aware of these problems and arrange scheduled toileting and promote access to toileting facilities.
- The older client may be prone to physiological urinary retention as a result of diminished bladder muscle tone, capacity, and contractility (Wells, 1988; Kane, et al., 1993). This may increase their risk toward large post void residuals with a concomitant risk of frequent infections. Teaching sessions should include techniques to stimulate the voiding reflex, as well as provide for complete bladder emptying and prevention from infections.
- Older clients may also experience delayed sensations to void resulting in urgency. The nurse educates the client regarding any factor that interferes with the client's perceptions to void (Wells, 1988) (e.g., medications, emotional disturbances, or decreased fluid intake).
- Older adults experience the following physiological changes that make them more prone to incontinence. During teaching sessions, the nurse considers these normal physiological changes to plan appropriate interventions.
  1. Decreased renal blood flow secondary to decreased cardiac output.
  2. Decreased ability to concentrate urine secondary to decrease in nephron mass.
  3. Decreased tone of the pelvic floor muscles.
- Older adults in institutionalized settings (e.g., hospitals, nursing homes) are at the greatest risk for experiencing incontinence problems (Resnick and Yalla, 1985; Palmer, et al., 1991).
- Older adults may also experience sensory alterations such as diminished vision, which may delay attempts to locate toilet facilities (Kane, et al., 1993). During teaching sessions, the nurse orients clients to their environment with special emphasis on the location of toileting facilities, bedpans or urinals, and assistive devices (e.g., walkers, call light).

client may prefer using a bedside commode enclosed behind a partition or room divider. Some clients are embarrassed by the sound of voiding. Running water or flushing the toilet masks the sound effectively. Young children are often unable to void in the presence of persons other than parents.

If the client typically uses special measures to void (e.g., reading or listening to music), the nurse should encourage their continued use at home and, when possible, in the health care setting.

Maintaining Adequate Fluid Intake. A simple method of promoting normal micturition is maintenance of a good fluid intake. A client with normal renal function who does not have heart disease or alterations requiring fluid restriction should drink 2000 to 2500 ml of fluid daily. When fluid intake is increased, excreted urine flushes out solutes or particles that may collect in the urinary system. Because a client probably is not accustomed to drinking 2500 ml of water daily, the nurse should offer fluids the client prefers. At home, it may help to set a schedule for drinking fluids (e.g., with meals or medications). A simple trick is to encourage the client to drink a cup of water after voiding. Voiding becomes a natural cue to drinking fluids. A rigid schedule is not needed. To prevent nocturia, fluids should be avoided 2 hours before bedtime.

Promotion of Complete Bladder Emptying

Clients with urinary retention and incontinence are frequently unable to empty the bladder. Incontinence is a major nursing challenge. Choosing from a variety of treatment options, the client and nurse work together to design interventions that promote continence or control wetness (Table 32-5).

Strengthening Pelvic Floor Muscles. Clients who have difficulty starting and stopping the urine stream may benefit from exercises to strengthen pelvic muscles. The client may practice Kegel exercises anytime or anywhere (Table 32-6). The client first learns to feel the pelvic muscles. The client does this with each voiding.

Then while sitting or standing, the client tries to tighten the muscles around the anus without tensing leg, buttock, or abdominal muscles. This maneuver allows the client to identify the posterior muscles of the pelvic floor.

Sit-ups may also aid the bladder control by strengthening the abdominal muscles. Starting with a few at a time and gradually increasing the number of repetitions will improve pelvic muscle strength.

Manual Bladder Compression. By manually compressing the walls of the bladder, a person can improve bladder emptying. Credé's method helps to stimulate micturition and manually expels urine when bladder tone is reduced. The client places both hands flat on the abdomen below the umbilicus and above the symphysis pubis with the fingers pointed down toward the bladder's dome. The client compresses the hands downward against the bladder's walls while tightening the perineum, contracting the abdominal wall, and hold-

table 32-5

TREATMENT OPTIONS FOR INCONTINENCE

Primary treatment	Other treatments
ACUTE	
Management of acute illness.	Catheter.
Appropriate toileting schedule.	
Alteration of environment.	
Modification of drug regimen.	
Treatment of urinary tract infection.	Protective undergarments.
Treatment of atrophic urethritis and vaginitis.	
General supportive measures.	
URGE	
Anticholinergic drug therapy.	Biofeedback.
Treatment of associated urinary tract infection.	
Treatment of associated vaginitis.	Intravaginal electrical stimulation.
STRESS	
Conditioning (Kegel) exercises.	Estrogen. Alpha-adrenergic agonists.
Surgery.	Intravaginal electrical stimulation.
Bladder neck suspension.	Artificial sphincter.
OVERFLOW	
Surgery.	
Intermittent catheterization.	Indwelling catheter.
FUNCTIONAL	
Habit training.	Scheduled toileting. Protective undergarments. Environmental alterations. Supportive measures Indwelling and external catheters. Skin care.

From Orzeck S and Ouslander JG: Urinary incontinence: an overview of causes and treatment, *J Entero Ther* 14:24, 1987.

table 32-6
PELVIC FLOOR EXERCISES

Exercise steps	Rationale
EXERCISE I	
Instruct client to concentrate on pelvic muscles.	Assists client in feeling anterior muscles of pelvic floor.
Have client try to stop flow of urine during urination and then restart it. Practice with each voiding.	Teaches control technique.
EXERCISE II	
Have client assume sitting or standing position. Instruct client to tighten muscles around anus.	Assists client in feeling posterior muscles of pelvic floor.
EXERCISE III	
Have client tighten posterior muscles and then slowly contract anterior muscles while counting slowly to 4. Then have client relax muscles completely. Repeat exercise four times per hr while awake for 3 mo.	Improves pelvic muscle control, and aids relaxation of sphincters during voiding.
EXERCISE IV	
Instruct client to do sit-ups.	Strengthens abdominal muscles for bladder control.

ing the breath. When urine is in the bladder, Credé's compression causes the sensation of bladder fullness. The maneuver also promotes bladder emptying by relaxing the urethral sphincter.

Drug Therapy. Drug therapy alone or in conjunction with other therapies can be useful for treating problems of incontinence and retention. Commonly used drugs increase bladder emptying and decrease bladder hyperactivity (e.g., urge incontinence).

When urine is in the bladder, stress or urge incontinence may occur as a result of hyperactivity of the bladder muscle that suddenly increases pressure. Uncontrolled bladder contractions may be caused by local irritants such as stones or infection. Anticholinergic drugs (e.g., propantheline and methantheline) reduce incontinence caused by bladder irritation by relaxing the smooth muscle of the bladder. The anticholinergics can cause urinary retention by contracting the urinary sphincter and can cause cardiac dysrhythmias and should be used with caution in clients with heart disease.

When the bladder empties, the detrusor muscle contracts in response to stimulation. Incomplete bladder emptying results from impaired innervation or weakness of the detrusor muscle. As a result, the client experiences retention and overflow incontinence. Therapy with cholinergic drugs is aimed at increasing bladder contraction and improving emptying. Bethanechol (Urecholine) stimulates nerves to increase bladder wall contraction and relax the sphincter. It can be given subcutaneously or orally. The nurse should give the first dose 3 to 4 hours after the last voiding to be sure the bladder contains urine. To gain the peak effect of the drug, the nurse gives it shortly before micturition is attempted (15 to 30 minutes subcutaneously and 30 to 60 minutes orally). The effect of the drug can be augmented by using Credé's method or other measures for stimulating micturition.

Catheterization. Catheterization of the bladder involves introducing a rubber or plastic tube through the urethra and into the bladder. The catheter provides a continuous flow of urine in clients unable to control micturition or in clients with obstructions. Because bladder catheterization carries a high risk of urinary tract infection, the nurse first relies on other interventions to promote bladder emptying.

TYPES OF CATHETERIZATION. Intermittent and indwelling catheterization are the two forms of catheter insertion. With the intermittent technique, a straight, single-use catheter is introduced long enough to drain the bladder (5 to 10 minutes). When the bladder is empty, the nurse removes the catheter. Intermittent catheterization can be repeated as necessary. An indwelling or Foley catheter remains in place until a client is able to void completely and voluntarily. It may be necessary to change indwelling catheters periodically.

The straight, single-use catheter has a single lumen with a small opening approximately 1.3 cm (½ inch) from the tip. Urine drains from the tip, through the lumen, and to a receptacle. An indwelling Foley catheter has a small inflatable balloon that encircles the catheter just below the tip. When inflated, the balloon rests against the bladder outlet to anchor the catheter in place. The indwelling catheter also has as many as two or three separate lumens within the body of the catheter. One lumen drains urine through the catheter to a collecting tube. A second lumen carries sterile water to and from the balloon when it is inflated or deflated. A third (optional) lumen may be used to instill fluids or drugs into the bladder.

INDICATIONS FOR USE. Catheterization may be indicated for many reasons. When the need for catheterization is short term to minimize infection, the intermittent method is best. Indwelling catheterization is used for long-term bladder emptying. Intermittent catheterization is indicated in the following situations:

1. For immediate relief of acute bladder distention:
   a. Clients unable to void 8 to 12 hours after surgery.
   b. Clients with acute retention after trauma to the urethra.
   c. Clients unable to void as a result of the effects of sedatives or analgesics.
2. For long-term management of clients with incompetent bladders:
   a. Spinal cord injuries.
   b. Progressive neuromuscular degeneration.
3. To obtain a sterile urine specimen.
4. To assess for residual urine after voiding.

Intermittent catheterization with good aseptic technique has a lower risk of infection than indwelling catheterization. However, if a client's condition requires frequent intermittent catheterization, an indwelling catheter may be preferable. Indwelling catheterization is indicated in the following situations:

1. When there is an obstruction to urine outflow:
   a. Prostate enlargement.
   b. Urethral stricture.
2. For clients undergoing surgical repair of the urethra and surrounding structures (transurethral resection).
3. To prevent urethral obstruction from blood clots.
   a. Bladder tumors.
   b. Surgical repair of urethra.
4. To provide a means of accurately recording output in critically ill or comatose clients.
5. To prevent skin breakdown in comatose clients who are incontinent or severely disoriented.
6. To provide continuous or intermittent bladder irrigations.

CATHETER INSERTION. Urethral catheterization requires a physician's order. The nurse must use strict aseptic technique (see Chapter 25). Organizing equipment before the procedure prevents unnecessary interruptions. The steps for inserting an indwelling and a single-use straight catheter are the same. The difference lies in the procedure taken to inflate the indwelling catheter balloon and secure the catheter. The nurse can collect needed specimens while inserting an indwelling catheter. Procedure 32-1 lists steps for performing female and male urethral catheterization.

CLOSED DRAINAGE SYSTEMS. After inserting an indwelling catheter, it is necessary to maintain a closed urinary drainage system to minimize the risk of infection. Urinary drainage bags are plastic and can hold approximately 1000 to 1500 ml of urine. The bag should hang on the bed frame without touching the floor when the bed is in its lowest position. When the client ambulates, the nurse or client carries the bag below the level of the client's bladder. The nurse should never raise a drainage bag and tubing above the level of the client's bladder. Urine in the bag and tubing can become a medium for bacteria, and infection will probably develop if urine is returned to the bladder.

Most drainage bags contain an antireflux valve to prevent urine from reentering the drainage tubing and contaminating the bladder. A spigot at the base of the bag provides a means for the nurse to empty the bag. The spigot should always be clamped, except during emptying, and tucked into the protective pouch at the bag's side.

Some urinary drainage bags have special urimeters between the collection tubing and bag. The urimeter is a clear graduated cylinder that measures small volumes (100 to 200 ml) of urine. The urimeter is useful for clients requiring frequent urine output measurements. The nurse simply notes the volume of urine in the urimeter and opens the valve that allows urine from the urimeter to enter the drainage bag. When urine from the drainage bag is measured, it is best to use a separate graduated receptacle for accuracy.

To keep the drainage system patent the nurse checks for kinks or bends in the tubing, avoids positioning the client on drainage tubing, prevents tubing from becoming dependent, and observes for clots or sediment that may occlude the tubing.

ROUTINE CATHETER CARE. Special perineal hygiene is given to clients who have indwelling catheters (see Chapter 30). Secretions or encrustations that form at the insertion site are a source of infection and irritation. The nurse uses a sterile catheter care kit or individual supplies to wash the external genitalia and urethral meatus. The nurse may also use an antiseptic solution such as povidone-iodine to cleanse around the catheter. Sterile ointment is placed at the base of the catheter near the urethral meatus. The nurse replaces tape that becomes loose or soiled. Catheter care is performed twice daily and after bowel incontinence to help to minimize discomfort and infection.

REMOVAL OF INDWELLING CATHETER. When removing an indwelling catheter a nurse promotes normal bladder function and prevents trauma to the urethra. Loss of muscle tone in the bladder is a common problem after prolonged catheterization. Bladder reconditioning, which can reduce the loss of bladder tone, requires a physician's order and is begun at least 10 hours before catheter removal (Williamson, 1982; Orzeck and Ouslander, 1987). The nurse clamps the indwelling catheter to allow urine to accumulate. The volume of urine stretches the bladder's walls to stimulate muscle tone. The nurse unclamps the catheter 3 hours later and allows urine to drain for 5 minutes. The process is repeated two more times. After the conditioning procedure, the nurse removes the catheter. Clients who receive bladder conditioning can feel the urge to void sooner than clients who have no conditioning.

To remove a catheter, the nurse requires a clean, dis-

Text continued on p. 939.

procedure 32-1

INSERTING A STRAIGHT OR INDWELLING CATHETER

Steps	Rationale
1. Assess status of client	
a. When client last voided.	May indicate bladder fullness.
b. Level of awareness or developmental stage.	Reveals client's ability to cooperate during procedure.
c. Mobility and physical limitations (nurse can request additional nursing personnel to assist with procedure if necessary).	Affects way that nurse will position client and determines whether other personnel are needed to maintain client position.
d. Age.	Determines catheter size to use. No. 8-10 French gauge is generally used for children and 14-16 for women. No. 12 may be considered for young females. No. 16-18 is used for male clients unless larger size is ordered by physician.
e. Distended bladder.	Can indicate need to insert catheter if client is unable to void independently. Clients at risk for distention include postpartum women, postoperative clients, and men with prostatic hypertrophy.
f. Pathological condition that may impair passage of catheter (e.g., enlarged prostate gland).	Obstruction prevents passage of catheter through urethra into bladder.
g. Allergies.	Determines allergy to antiseptic, tape, or rubber.
h. Review physician's order for catheterization.	
2. Prepare equipment and supplies:	Ensures organized and efficient procedure.
a. Sterile gloves.*	Procedure is considered sterile.
b. Sterile drapes, one fenestrated.*	
c. Lubricant.*	Minimizes urethral trauma during insertion.
d. Antiseptic cleansing solution.*	
e. Cotton balls or gauze squares.	
f. Forceps.*	
g. Prefilled syringe with sterile water.*	Used to inflate balloon of indwelling catheter.
h. Catheters of correct size and type for procedure (intermittent or indwelling).*	An overly large catheter can cause trauma to urethral tissue. If catheter is too small, blood clots or urine sediment may obstruct urine outflow.
i. Flashlight or gooseneck lamp.	Helps in seeing urinary meatus of female client.
j. Bath blanket.	Promotes privacy by draping client.
k. Waterproof absorbent pad.	Positioning under client prevents soiling of bed linens.
l. Trash receptacle.	
m. Disposable gloves; basin with warm water, soap, face cloth, and towel.	Providing perineal care before introducing catheter helps to reduce risk of urinary tract infection. Provides opportunity to examine female's urethral meatus or to retract foreskin of uncircumcised male.
n. Sterile drainage tubing and collection bag (may be preattached to catheter), tape, safety pin, and elastic band.	If indwelling catheter will be inserted, tape, elastic band, and pin help to secure position of catheter, thus preventing trauma to external urethral sphincter.
o. Receptacle or basin (usually bottom of tray).	Provides area for urine to drain when straight or indwelling catheter is used.
p. Specimen container.*	Used to obtain sterile urine specimen to determine presence of bacteria.
3. Explain procedure. Also describe pressure sensation that will be felt during insertion.	Reduces anxiety and promotes cooperation.
4. Arrange for extra nursing personnel to assist, if appropriate.	May be necessary to assist with positioning dependent client. Promotes safety and use of correct body mechanics.
5. Wash hands.	Reduces anxiety and promotes cooperation.
6. Raise bed to appropriate working height.	Promotes use of proper body mechanics.

*These items may be contained on catheterization tray or may have to be added after sterile field is established. This may depend on whether disposable or nondisposable trays are used.

Continued.

procedure 32-1—cont'd

Steps	Rationale
7. Facing client, stand on left side of bed if right-handed (on right side if left-handed).	Successful catheter insertion requires nurse to assume comfortable position with all equipment easily accessible.
8. Raise siderail on opposite side of bed.	Promotes safety.
9. Close cubicle or room curtains.	Reduces embarrassment and aids in relaxation.
10. Place waterproof pad under client.	Prevents soiling of bed linen.
11. Position client:	
a. Female client:	
(1) Assist to dorsal recumbent position (supine with knee flexed). Ask client to relax thighs so they are externally rotated. (Legs may be supported with pillows.)	Provides good view of perineal structures.
(2) Position in side-lying (Sims') position, with upper leg flexed at knee and hip if unable to be supine (optional).	Alternate position if client cannot abduct leg at hip joint (e.g., arthritic joints). Also, position may be more comfortable. Support client with pillows, if necessary, to maintain position.
b. Male client, assist to assume supine position with thighs slightly abducted.	Supine position prevents tensing of abdominal and pelvic muscles.
12. Drape client:	Avoids unnecessary exposure of body parts and maintains comfort.
a. Female client, drape with bath blanket. Place blanket over client: one corner at neck, side corners over arms and sides, last over raised perineum. Raise gown above hips.	
b. Male client, drape upper trunk with bath blanket and cover lower extremities with bedsheets, exposing genitalia.	
13. Apply disposable gloves. Wash perineal area with soap and water as needed; dry.	Reduces presence of microorganisms near meatus.
14. Position lamp to illuminate perineal area. (When using flashlight, assistant holds it.)	Permits accurate identification and good view of urethral meatus.
15. Remove and dispose of gloves.	Prevents transmission of microorganisms.
16. Open catheterization kit and catheter (if packaged separately) according to directions, keeping bottom of container sterile.	Prevents transmission of microorganisms from table or work area to sterile supplies.
17. Put on sterile gloves.	Allows nurse to handle sterile supplies without contamination.
18. Organize supplies on sterile field; open inner sterile package of antiseptic solution in correct compartment containing sterile cotton balls; open packet containing lubricant; remove specimen container (lip should be loosely placed on top) and prefilled syringe from collection compartment of tray and set them aside on sterile field.	Maintains principles of surgical asepsis and organizes work area. All activities requiring nurse to use both hands are to be completed before cleaning meatus.
19. When inserting retention catheter, test catheter balloon by injecting fluid from prefilled syringe into balloon valve (see illustration). Balloon should inflate fully without leakage. Withdraw fluid and leave syringe on port of catheter.	Checks integrity of balloon. Balloon that leaks or inflates improperly is replaced.

Steps	Rationale
20. Apply sterile drape:	
a. Female client:	
(1) Allow top edge of drape to form cuff over both hands. Place drape on bed between thighs. Slip cuffed edge just under buttocks, taking care not to touch contaminated surface with gloves.	Outer surface of drape covering nurse's hands remains sterile until touched by buttocks. Sterile drape against sterile glove is sterile.
(2) Pick up fenestrated sterile drape and allow it to unfold without touching unsterile object. Apply drape over perineum, exposing labia and being sure not to touch contaminated surface.	Maintains sterility of work surface.
b. Male client: Apply drape over thighs just below penis. Pick up fenestrated sterile drape, allow it to unfold, and drape it over penis, with fenestrated slit resting over penis.	Maintains sterility of work surface.
21. Place sterile kit and its contents on sterile drape between thighs.	Provides easy access to supplies during catheter insertion.
22. Apply lubricant along sides of catheter tip:	Allows easy insertion of catheter tip through meatus.
a. Female client: 2.5 to 5 cm (1 to 2 in).	
b. Male client: 7.5 to 12.5 cm (3 to 5 in).	
23. Cleanse urethral meatus:	
a. Female client:	
(1) With nondominant hand, carefully retract labia to fully expose urethral meatus. Maintain position of nondominant hand throughout remainder of procedure.	Provides full visualization of meatus. Full retraction prevents contamination during cleansing. Closure of labia during cleansing requires that procedure be repeated because area has become contaminated.
(2) With dominant hand, pick up cotton ball with forceps and clean perineal area, wiping front to back from clitoris to anus. Use new, clean cotton ball for each wipe: near labial fold, along far labial fold, and directly over meatus.	Reduces number of microorganisms at urethral meatus. Use of single cotton ball for each wipe prevents transfer of microorganisms. Preparation moves from area of least contamination to that of most contamination. Dominant hand remains sterile.

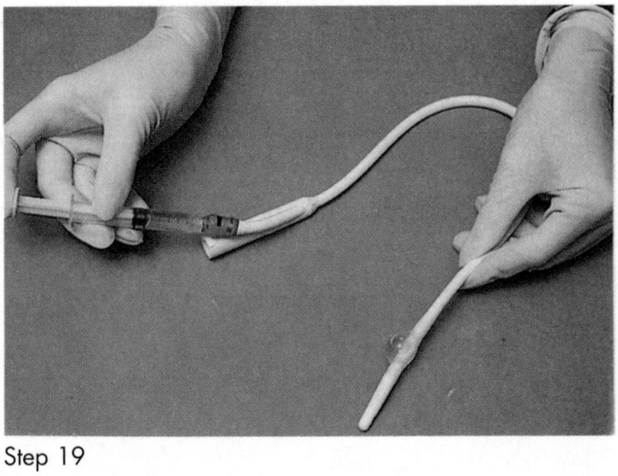

Step 19

Continued.

procedure 32-1—cont'd

Steps	Rationale
b. Male client:	
(1) If client is not circumcised, retract foreskin with nondominant hand. Grasp penis at shaft just below glans. Retract urethral meatus between thumb and forefinger. Maintain nondominant hand in this position throughout catheter insertion.	Minimizes chance of erection (if erection develops, discontinue procedure). Accidental release of foreskin or dropping of penis during cleansing requires process to be repeated because area has become contaminated.
(2) With dominant hand, pick up cotton ball with forceps and clean penis. Cleanse using cotton once around penis, starting at meatus and working toward base. Repeat this process 3 times, changing cotton ball each time.	Reduces number of microorganisms at meatus and moves from area of least to most contamination. Dominant hand remains sterile.
24. Pick up catheter with gloved, dominant hand approximately 5 cm (2 in) from catheter tip. Hold end of catheter loosely coiled in palm of dominant hand (optional: may grasp catheter with forceps). Place distal end of catheter in urine tray receptacle unless already attached to drainage bag.	Prevents soiling of bed linen and allows accurate measurement of urinary output.
25. Insert catheter:	
a. Female client *(see illustration)*, with nondominant hand continuing to retract labia:	

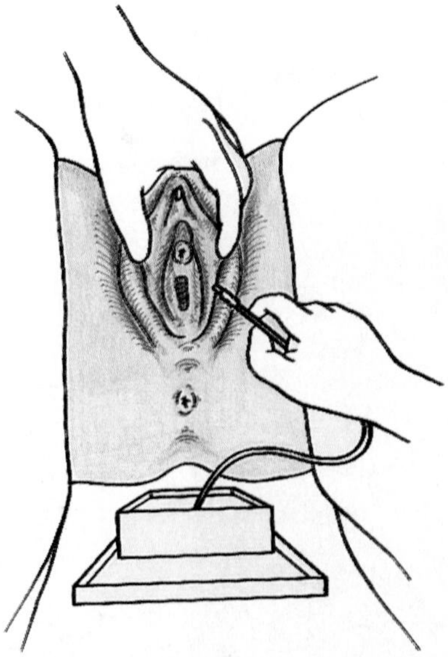

Step 25a

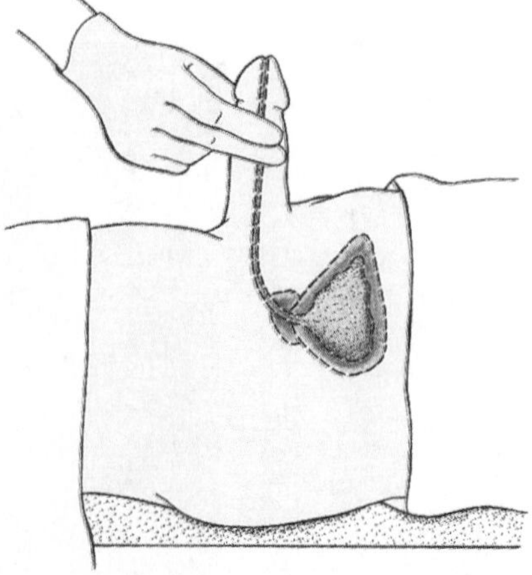

Step 25b

Steps	Rationale
(1) Ask client to take deep breath and slowly insert catheter through meatus. (If no urine appears, catheter may be in vagina. If catheter is in vagina, leave in place; obtain and insert another catheter and then remove first catheter.)	Aids in insertion of catheter. (Catheter in vagina is no longer sterile. Leaving first catheter in place helps to prevent inserting second catheter in vagina.)
(2) Advance catheter appoximately 5 to 7.5 cm (2 to 3 in) in adult, 2.5 cm (1 in) in child, or until urine flows out catheter's end. If inserting retention catheter, advance another 5 cm (2 in) after urine appears. Do not force catheter.	Female urethra is short. Appearance of urine indicates that catheter tip is in bladder or lower urethra. Further advancement ensures bladder placement. Balloon of retention catheter must be advanced into bladder. Forceful insertion may traumatize urethra.
(3) Release labia and hold catheter securely with nondominant hand.	Bladder or sphincter contraction may cause accidental expulsion of catheter.
b. Male client *(see illustration)*: lift penis to position perpendicular to body and apply light traction upward.	Straightens urethral canal to ease catheter insertion.
(1) Ask client to bear down as if to void and slowly insert catheter through meatus.	Relaxation of external sphincter aids in insertion of catheter.
(2) Advance catheter 17.5 to 22.5 cm (7 to 9 in) in adult and 5 to 7.5 cm (2 to 3 in) in young child, or until urine flows out catheter's end. If resistance is felt, withdraw catheter; do not force it through urethra. If inserting retention catheter, advance another 5 cm (2 in) after urine appears.	Adult male urethra is long. Appearance of urine indicates catheter tip is in bladder or urethra. Resistance may be caused by urethral strictures or enlarged prostate. Further advancement ensures proper placement. Ensures balloon is advanced into bladder.
26. Collect urine specimen as needed: Fill specimen cup or jar to desired level (20 to 30 ml) by holding end of catheter in dominant hand over cup (or collect specimen from sterile drainage bag). With dominant hand, pinch catheter to stop urine flow temporarily, then release catheter to allow remaining urine in bladder to drain into collection tray. Cover specimen cup and set it aside for labeling.	Allows sterile specimen to be obtained for culture analysis.
27. Allow bladder to empty fully, about 750 to 1000 ml (unless institution policy restricts maximum volume of urine to drain with each catheterization).	Retained urine may be reservoir for growth of microorganisms. Rapid emptying of large volume of urine may cause engorgement of pelvic blood vessels and alter blood pressure.
28. Remove straight single-use catheter. Withdraw slowly but smoothly until removed.	Minimizes discomfort.
29. Inflate balloon of indwelling catheter:	
a. While holding catheter with thumb and little finger of dominant hand at meatus, place end of catheter between first two fingers of nondominant hand.	Catheter should be anchored while syringe is manipulated.
b. With dominant hand, attach syringe to injection port at end of catheter. (In some sets, syringe is already connected).	Port connects to lumen leading to inflatable balloon.
c. Slowly inject total amount of solution. If client complains of sudden pain, aspirate back solution and advance catheter farther. Inject no more fluid than balloon size indicates.	Balloon within bladder is inflated. If balloon is malpositioned in urethra, pain will occur during inflation.
d. After inflating balloon fully, release catheter with nondominant hand and pull gently to feel resistance *(see illustration)*. Then move catheter slightly back into bladder. Disconnect syringe.	Anchors catheter tip in place above bladder outlet to prevent removal of catheter. Gentle pulling ensures proper placement and anchoring. Advancing catheter upward minimizes pressure on bladder neck.

Continued.

procedure 32-1—cont'd

Steps	Rationale
30. Attach end of catheter to collecting tube of drainage system, unless already connected to bag. Place drainage bag in a dependent position *(see illustration)*.	Establishes closed system for urine drainage. Dependent position of drainage bag promotes flow of urine away from bladder.
31. Tape catheter:	
a. Female client: tape catheter to inside of thigh with strip of nonallergenic tape. Allow for slack so that movement does not create tension on catheter.	Anchoring of catheter minimizes trauma to urethra and meatus during movement. Catheter positioned over the thigh prevents kinking. Nonallergenic tape prevents skin breakdown.

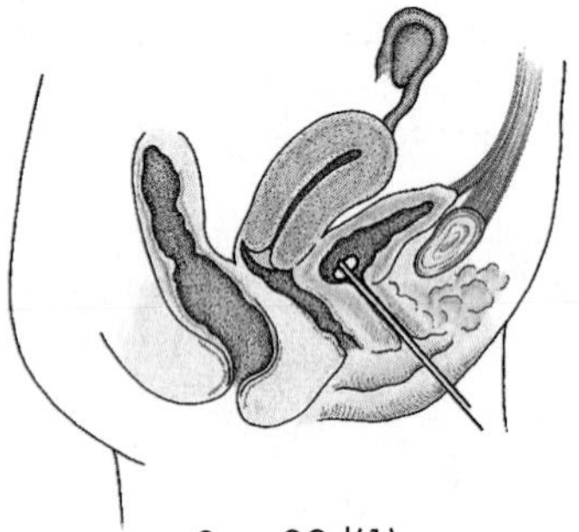

Step 29d(1)

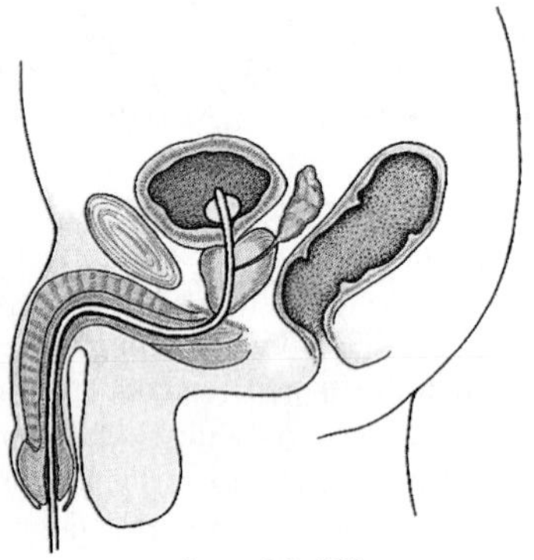

Step 29d(2)

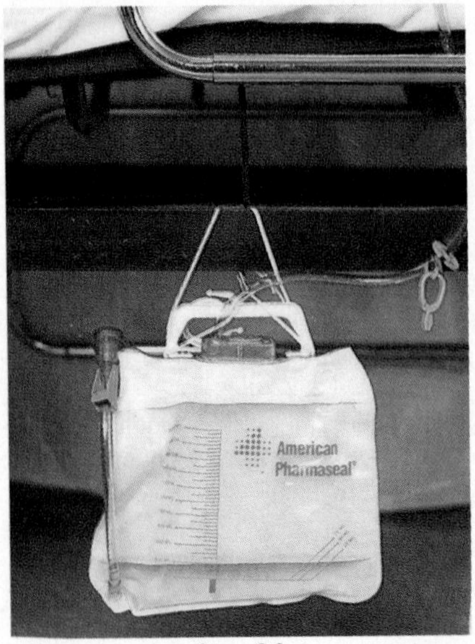

Step 30

Steps	Rationale
b. Male client: Tape catheter to top of thigh or lower abdomen (with penis directed toward abdomen). Allow for some slack in catheter so that movement does not create tension.	Anchoring catheter to lower abdomen is to reduce pressure on urethra at junction of penis and scrotum, thus reducing tissue necrosis in this area.
32. Be sure there are no obstructions or kinks in tubing. Place excess coil of tubing on bed and fasten it to bottom sheet with clip from drainage set or with rubber band and safety pin.	Allows free drainage of urine by gravity and prevents backflow of urine into bladder.
33. Remove gloves and dispose of equipment, drapes, and urine in proper receptacles.	Prevents transmission of infection.
34. Assist client to comfortable position, dispose of drapes and urine in proper receptacles.	Maintains comfort and security.
35. Instruct client on ways to lie in bed with catheter: side-lying facing drainage system with catheter and tubing draped over lower thigh and side-lying facing away from system, catheter and tubing extending between legs.	Urine should drain freely without obstruction. Placing catheter under extremities can result in obstruction from compression of tubing from client's weight. When client is on one side facing away from system, catheter should not be placed over upper thigh; this forces urine to drain uphill.
36. Caution client against pulling catheter.	Reduces trauma to urethral meatus.
37. Palpate bladder and ask whether client is uncomfortable.	Determines whether distention is relieved.
38. Wash hands.	Reduces spread of infection.
39. Observe character and amount of urine in drainage system.	Determines whether urine is flowing adequately.
40. Report and record: type and size of catheter inserted; amount of fluid used to inflate balloon; characteristics and amount of urine.	Communicates pertinent information to all members of health care team.

posable towel, a trash receptacle, clean gloves, and a sterile syringe the same size as the volume of solution within the catheter's inflated balloon. The end of each catheter contains a label that denotes the volume of solution (5 to 30 ml) within a balloon.

The nurse positions the client in the same position as during catheterization. Some institutions recommend collecting a sterile urine specimen at this time. After removing the tape, the nurse places the towel between the woman's or over the man's thighs. The nurse dons clean gloves and inserts the syringe into the injection port. Most ports are self-sealing and require that only the tip be inserted. To deflate the balloon, the nurse slowly withdraws all the solution. If a portion of the solution remains, the partially inflated balloon will traumatize the urethral canal as the catheter is removed. After deflation, the nurse explains that the client will feel a burning sensation as the catheter is withdrawn. The nurse then pulls the catheter out smoothly and slowly and disposes the catheter, tubing, and drainage bag in a proper receptacle.

The client normally experiences dysuria, especially if the catheter has been in place several days or weeks. The catheter causes inflammation of the urethral canal. Until the bladder regains full tone, the client may also have frequency of urination.

The nurse notes the time and the amount of the client's first void. If more than 8 hours elapse before the client voids, it may be necessary to catheterize the client again. If the volume of urine voided is small, residual urine may be in the bladder.

Alternatives to Catheterization. To avoid the risks associated with catheters inserted through the urethra, alternatives for urinary drainage exist. Suprapubic catheterization involves placing a catheter directly into the bladder through an abdominal incision to allow urine to drain into a collection bag. This method is use-

procedure 32-2

APPLYING A CONDOM CATHETER

Steps	Rationale
1. Assess status of client to determine need for condom catheter.	Client continuously incontinent of urine is at risk for skin breakdown.
2. Prepare equipment and supplies (see illustration):	
a. Rubber condom sheath (proper size).	
b. Strip of elastic tape and skin preparation.	
c. Urinary collection bag with drainage tubing or leg bag and straps.	Allows client to remain mobile.
d. Basin with warm water and soap.	
e. Towels and wash cloths.	
f. Disposable gloves.	Protects nurse's hands; reduces risk of infection.
g. Bath blanket.	
h. Hair clippers (optional).	
3. Explain procedure.	Reduces anxiety and promotes cooperation.
4. Close room door or bedside curtain.	Provides privacy and maintains self-esteem.
5. Assist client into supine position. Place bath blanket over upper torso. Fold sheets so that lower extremities are covered; only genitalia should be exposed.	Promotes comfort; draping prevents unnecessary exposure of body parts.
6. Wash hands and don gloves.	Reduces transmission of infection.
7. Assess condition of penis.	Provides baseline to compare changes in condition of skin after condom application.
8. Provide perineal care (see Chapter 30) and dry thoroughly. Clip hair at base of penis.	Removes irritating secretions. Rubber sheath rolls onto dry skin more easily. Hair adheres to condom, and pulls during removal.
9. Prepare urinary drainage collection bag and tubing or prepare leg bag for connection to condom, if necessary. Clamp off drainage exit ports. Secure collection bag to bed frame; bring drainage tubing through siderails onto bed.	Provides easy access to drainage equipment after condom is in place.
10. Apply skin preparation to penis and allow to dry.	Prepares penis for easy condom placement.
11. With nondominant hand, grasp penis along shaft. With dominant hand, hold condom sheath at tip of penis and smoothly roll sheath onto penis.	
12. Allow 2.5 to 5 cm (1 to 2 in) of space between tip of glans penis and end of condom catheter (see illustration).	Allows free passage of urine into collecting tubing when client passes urine. Prevents pressure on glans penis.

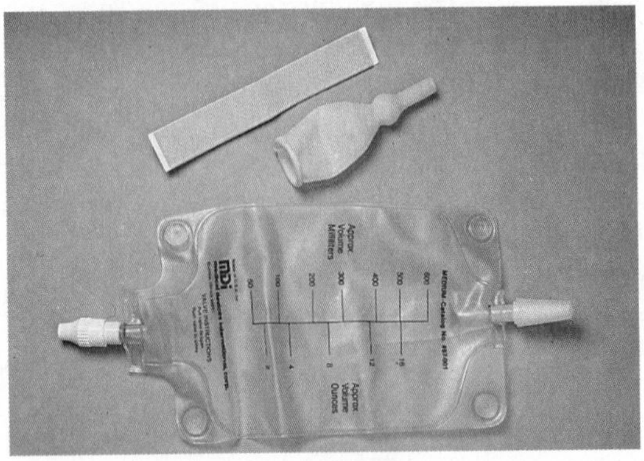

Step 2

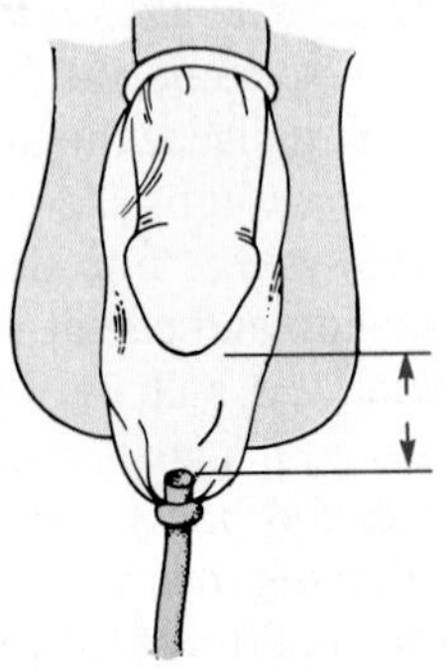

Step 12

Steps	Rationale
13. Encircle penile shaft with strip of elastic adhesive. Strip should touch only condom sheath. Apply snugly, but not tightly.	Condom must be secured so that it is snug and will stay on but not too tight to cause constriction of blood flow.
14. Connect drainage tubing to end of condom catheter. Be sure condom is not twisted.	Allows urine to be collected and measured. Keeps client dry. Twisted condom obstructs urine flow.
15. Place excess coiling of tubing on bed and secure to bottom sheet.	Prevents looping of tubing and promotes free drainage of urine.
16. Place client in safe, comfortable position.	Promotes comfort.
17. Remove gloves. Dispose of contaminated supplies and wash hands.	Prevents spread of infection.
18. Observe urinary drainage.	Determines whether normal voiding is occurring.
19. Regularly inspect skin on shaft for signs of breakdown or irritation.	Indicates whether condom or urine is causing irritation or whether adhesive is too restrictive.
20. Record and report: time of catheter application, condition of skin, and voiding pattern.	Provides data to determine change in elimination status.

ful in clients with chronic incontinence or loss of bladder control. Suprapubic catheterization reduces the risk of infection ascending along the urethra to the bladder. There is also less urethral irritation in the male. Bladder infection may still develop in the client with a suprapubic catheter. Spread of the infection to the kidneys may mean removing the catheter. The condom catheter is suitable for incontinent or comatose male clients who still have complete and spontaneous bladder emptying. The condom is a soft, pliable, rubber sheath that slips over the penis. A strip of special elastic tape fits around the top of the condom to secure it (Figure 32-6, *A*). Care must be taken not to tighten the band tightly, or the blood supply to the penis will be impaired. Standard adhesive tape should never be used to secure a condom catheter because it does not expand with change in penis size, and blood supply to the penis will be impaired.

The end of the condom fits into a plastic drainage tubing (Figure 32-6, *B*). A drainage bag can be attached to the side of the bed or strapped to the leg. The condom catheter poses little risk of infection. Infections, however, usually result from buildup of secretions around the urethra, trauma to the urethral meatus, or buildup of pressure in the outflow tubing. Procedure 32-2 reviews application of the condom catheter.

The nurse should change a condom catheter daily to check for skin irritation. The nurse cleans the urethral meatus and penis thoroughly with each catheter change. Twisting of the condom at the drainage tube attachment irritates the skin and obstructs urine outflow. The drainage tubing must be checked frequently for pa-

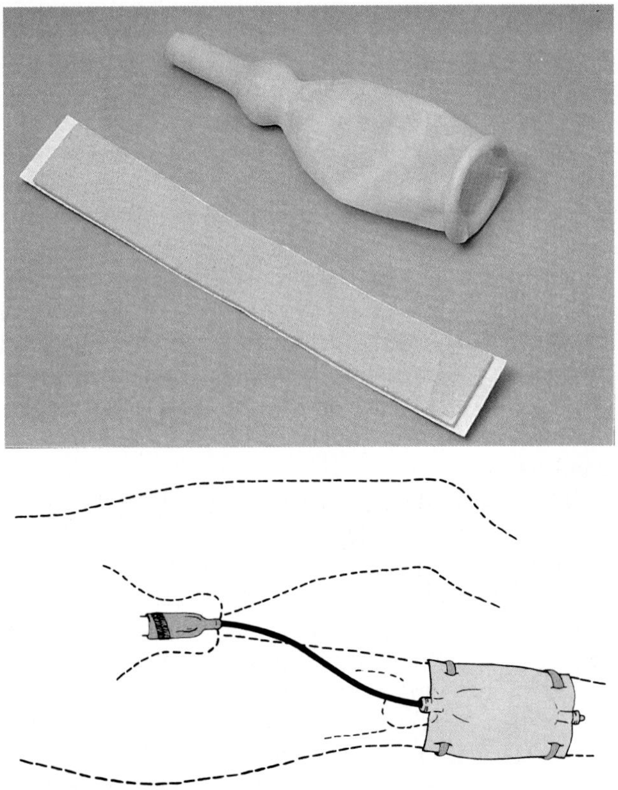

A

B

FIGURE 32-6 **A,** Condom catheter and elastic tape. **B,** Condom catheter with leg drainage bag.

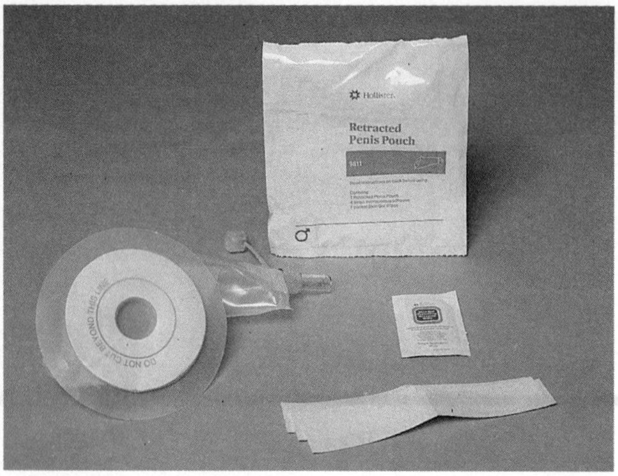

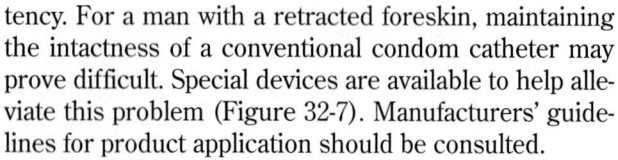

FIGURE 32-7 Retracted penis-pouch external urinary device.

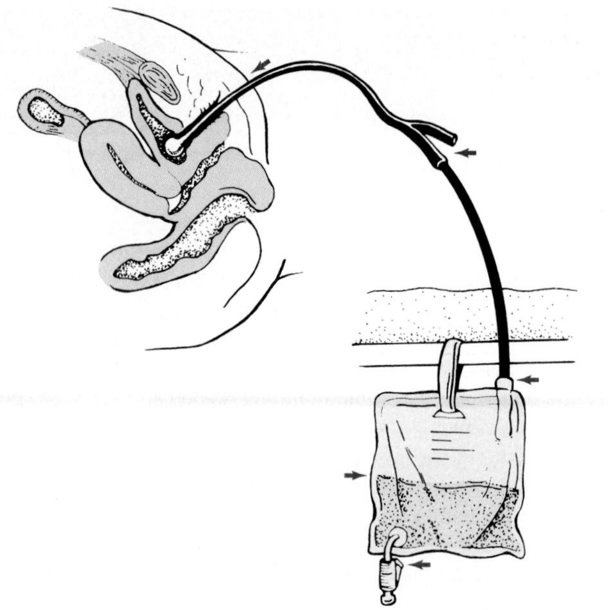

FIGURE 32-8 Potential sites for introduction of infectious organisms into urinary drainage system.

tency. For a man with a retracted foreskin, maintaining the intactness of a conventional condom catheter may prove difficult. Special devices are available to help alleviate this problem (Figure 32-7). Manufacturers' guidelines for product application should be consulted.

External incontinence devices for women are more difficult to design and fit (Pieper, et al., 1989). Women may also wear the newer absorbent pads and adult disposable undergarments. However, wearers of these disposable undergarments report skin irritation, odor, and increased infection rate. For the active, incontinent woman, these devices are options that can promote more independence.

Prevention of Infection

One of the most important considerations for a client with urinary alterations is the need to prevent infection. Good perineal hygiene involving cleansing the urethral meatus after each voiding is essential. A daily intake of 2000 to 2500 ml of fluids dilutes urine and promotes regular micturition, which flushes the urethra of microorganisms.

Infection can develop in a catheterized client in many ways. Maintaining a closed urinary drainage system is important in infection control. A break in the system can lead to introduction of microorganisms. Sites at risk are at the place of catheter insertion, drainage bag, spigot, tube junction, and junction of tube and bag (Figure 32-8). In addition, the nurse monitors the patency of the system to prevent pooling of urine. Urine in the drainage bag is an excellent medium for microorganism growth. Bacteria can travel up drainage tubing to grow in pools of urine. If this urine flows back into the bladder, an infection will probably develop. The box on p. 943 gives suggestions for ways to prevent infections in catheterized clients.

Handwashing. Good handwashing practices are basic to infection control. Handwashing is necessary before the nurse handles a catheter or the drainage system. When the nurse goes from a client with a catheter to one without, handwashing can prevent cross-contamination. The nurse also cautions clients against handling a catheter with unclean hands.

Acidifying Urine. Acid urine tends to inhibit growth of microorganisms. Meats, eggs, whole-grain breads, cranberries, prunes, and plums increase urine acidity. The foods metabolize into acid end products that eventually enter the urine. Cranberry juice increases urine acidity, whereas carbonated beverages and fruit juices such as orange or grapefruit juice produce an alkaline urine. High doses of ascorbic acid may lower the urine pH.

Maintenance of Skin Integrity

The normal acidity of urine is irritating to the skin. When urine becomes alkaline, encrustations or precipitate collects on the skin, fostering breakdown. Continuous exposure of the skin to urine leads to gradual maceration and excoriation. Washing with mild soap and warm water is the best way to remove urine from the skin. Body lotion keeps the skin moisturized and

TIPS FOR PREVENTING INFECTION IN CATHETERIZED CLIENTS

Follow good handwashing techniques.
Do not allow the spigot on the drainage bag to touch a contaminated surface.
Do not open the drainage system at connection points to obtain specimens or measure urine.
If the drainage tubing becomes disconnected, do not touch the ends of the catheter or tubing. Wipe the ends of the tube with antiseptic solution before reconnecting.
Each client should have a separate receptacle for measuring urine to prevent cross-contamination.
Prevent pooling of urine and reflux of urine into the bladder.
- Avoid raising the drainage bag above the level of the bladder.
- If it is necessary to raise the bag during transfer of the client to a bed or stretcher, clamp the tubing.
- Avoid allowing any dependent loops of tubing.
- Before client exercises or ambulates, drain all urine from tubing into bag.

Avoid prolonged clamping or kinking of the tubing (except during bladder conditioning).
Empty the drainage bag at least every 8 hours.
Remove the catheter as soon as possible after conferring with physician.
Tape the catheter to secure it in place, noting specific guidelines regarding the male client's taping procedure.
Perform routine perineal hygiene every shift and after defecation.

provides a barrier to the urine. Clients who wet their clothing should receive a clean set of clothes after each voiding.

When the skin becomes irritated or inflamed, the physician may prescribe a cream or spray containing steroids to reduce inflammation (e.g., Kenalog). If fungal growth develops, the antifungal drug nystatin (Mycostatin), available in cream or powder form, is effective.

The client with a ureterostomy has a special hygiene problem because urine drains from the ostomy site continuously. The drainage pouch or appliance frequently becomes moist and slips from the skin. Continual oozing of urine around the stoma causes skin breakdown. Skin barriers provide a layer of protection between the skin and ostomy pouch. When urine leaks, it frequently covers the outer skin barrier. An enterostomal therapist can help the client select an ostomy appliance that fits snugly against the skin's surface around the stoma.

Promotion of Comfort

Clients with urinary alterations can be uncomfortable as a result of the symptoms of urinary problems. Frequent or unpredictable voiding, dysuria, and painful distention are sources of discomfort.

The incontinent client gains comfort from having clean, dry clothing. When stress incontinence is the problem, a protective pad or sanitary belt offers protection against soiling. Wet clothing adheres to the skin and can cause rubbing and irritation.

Dysuria may be relieved by giving urinary analgesics that act on the urethral and bladder mucosa. Phenazopyridine helps to relieve dysuria, burning, and itching. It comes combined with sulfonamide antibiotics in preparations such as Azo Gantanol and Azo Gantrisin. The sulfonamide provides additional antibacterial action. Clients taking drugs with phenazopyridine should be aware that their urine may appear orange and their clothing is stained. They must drink large amounts of fluids to prevent toxicity from the sulfonamides and to maintain optimal flow through the urinary system.

If the client has local discomfort from an inflamed urethra, a warm sitz bath may provide pain relief. The warm water soothes inflamed tissues near the urethral meatus by improving blood supply. The client is often relaxed after a sitz bath, so voiding occurs easily.

The pain of distention cannot be relieved unless the client is able to empty the bladder. Methods for stimulating micturition may be the only sources of pain relief.

Evaluation

To evaluate the care plan the nurse uses the expected outcomes developed during planning to determine whether interventions were effective. This evaluation process is a dynamic one. The nurse uses this information to monitor the client's progress and direct future interventions. The optimal goal is the client's ability to urinate voluntarily without dysuria, urgency, or frequency. The client's urine should be an amber color, clear, without abnormal constituents, and within the normal range of pH and specific gravity.

The nurse can also evaluate specific interventions designed to promote normal urinary function and prevent complications of urinary alterations.

Goal: Client understands normal urinary elimination.

Outcomes

- Client will be able to state components of the lower urinary tract that assist to maintain continence.
- Client will understand that voluntary control over urination is influenced by the cerebral cortex.
- Client will be free of urinary alterations.

Evaluative measures

Ask the client to describe components of the urinary tract that influence continence.

Ask the client to describe what influences voluntary control over urination.

Ask the client to describe symptoms of urinary alterations.

Goal: Client has normal micturition with complete bladder emptying within 1 month.

Outcomes

Client will ingest at least 2000 ml fluids per day if not contraindicated.

Client will empty the bladder using the procedural maneuvers taught within 1 week.

The bladder will not be distended after voiding by second week.

There will be less than 50 ml of residual urine.

Client will experience gradual decrease in incontinent episodes within 1 month.

Evaluative measures

Measure urinary output equal to fluid intake.

Observe the client's ability to perform bladder compression or catheterization procedure.

Palpate the bladder after voiding.

Measure residual urine volume, as determined by straight catheterization.

Observe a reduced number of incontinent episodes.

Goal: Client understands how to prevent urinary tract infection.

Outcomes

Client will demonstrate appropriate hygiene measures to prevent infection.

Client will be free of symptoms of UTI.

Client will manage catheter care or urinary stoma appropriately.

Evaluative measures

Observe the urine for clarity. Obtain a urine culture showing negative bacterial growth.

Observe the handwashing techniques. Observe perineal cleansing techniques.

Assess client for dysuria, burning, itching at urethral meatus, urgency, or frequency.

Observe the client's stoma.

Goal: Client's skin remains intact.

Outcomes

Client will not demonstrate any areas of skin breakdown around perineum or stoma or condom.

Client will report an absence or decreased incidence of incontinence.

Client will identify interventions to prevent incontinence.

Evaluative measures

Inspect perineum for inflammation or excoriation.

Inspect skin around a ureterostomy stoma for dryness and inflammation.

Observe decreased need for clothing change.

Goal: Client attains comfort.

Outcomes

Client's bladder will not become distended.

Client will report dryness that is personally satisfactory.

Client will express confidence in utilizing the triggering mechanisms to initiate voiding.

Evaluative measures

Palpate bladder.

Observe the client's expression of a feeling of well-being.

Assess the client's ability to void without dysuria.

As nurses become more comfortable with the roles of client advocate and primary nurse, the delivery of quality care becomes a paramount goal. To this end, nurses are actively involved in developing methods to systematically evaluate the nursing process. Nursing research is being conducted to validate nursing interventions. Quality improvement is evolving as a tool to evaluate nursing care delivery. Its goal is to ensure the delivery of competent, state-of-the-art nursing care with positive outcomes for each client.

SUMMARY

The normal elimination of urinary wastes requires maintenance of urinary function. Each client has a different pattern of elimination. The nurse must assess this pattern and design nursing therapies to promote normal urinary elimination. When necessary, the nurse uses external devices such as a condom or an indwelling catheter to assist the client with urine elimination. The nurse must be understanding of, sensitive to, and supportive of the client's need for privacy and dignity.

CRITICAL THINKING ACTIVITIES

1. Mrs. Jaynes is 8 hours postpartum and has not voided. The physician has written an order for catheterization. What criteria do you use to determine if you will use a straight or indwelling catheter?
2. You have just removed an external condom catheter for routine hygiene care. What assessments are needed to determine the skin integrity of the client's penile skin and scrotum?

KEY CONCEPTS

Micturition or voiding is influenced by voluntary control from higher brain centers and involuntary control from the spinal cord.

Symptoms common to urinary disturbances include urgency, dysuria, polyuria, oliguria, and difficulty in starting the urinary stream.

When collected properly, a clean-voided urine specimen does not contain bacteria picked up from the urethral meatus.

A client can better understand the importance of perineal hygiene by knowing that the urinary tract is normally sterile.

Methods of promoting the micturition reflex assist clients in sensing the urge to urinate and controlling urethral sphincter relaxation.

An increased fluid intake results in urine formation that flushes particles and solutes from the urinary system.

Incontinence is classified as acute, urge, stress, overflow, and functional. Each type of incontinence has specific nursing interventions.

An indwelling urinary catheter remains in the bladder for an extended period, making the risk of infection greater than with intermittent catheterization.

Closed drainage systems deliver sterile solutions and medication to the bladder. Strict asepsis is necessary when caring for a client with a closed bladder drainage system.

Because urine drains almost continuously from a ureterostomy, there is risk of skin breakdown around a stoma site.

A primary function of the elimination process is fluid balance.

References

Burgener S: Justification of closed intermittent urinary catheter irrigation/installation: a review of current research and practice, *J Adv Nurs* 12:229, 1987.

Gibson LY: Bedwetting: a family's recurrent nightmare, *MCN* 14(4):270, 1989.

Kaltreider DL, et al.: Can reminders curb incontinence? *Geriatr Nurs* 11(1):17, 1990.

Kane RL, Ouslander JG, and Abrass IB: *Essentials of clinical geriatrics,* ed 3, New York, 1993, McGraw-Hill.

McCance KL and Huether SE: *Pathophysiology: the biologic basis for disease in adults and children,* ed 2, St. Louis, 1994, Mosby.

McConnell EA: *Care of patients with urologic problems,* Philadelphia, 1983, Lippincott.

Miller J: Assessing urinary incontinence, *J Gerontol Nurs* 16:15, 1990.

Orzeck S and Ouslander JG: Urinary incontinence: an overview of causes and treatment, *J Entero Ther* 14:24, 1987.

Palmer MH, et al.: Risk factors for urinary incontinence one year after nursing home admission, *Res Nurs Health* 14:405, 1991.

Piper B, et al.: Inventing urine incontinence devices for women, *Image* 21(4):205, 1989.

Resnick N and Yalla S: Diagnosing urinary incontinence in the elderly, *N Eng J Med* 5(13):800-805, 1985.

Touch DCH: Pelvic floor musculature exercises in treatment of anatomical urinary stress incontinence, *Phys Ther* 68(5):652, 1988.

Wells TJ: Research methods, outcomes, and issues, *J Gerontol Nurs* 14(1):11, 1988.

Whaley LF and Wong DL: *Nursing care of infants and children,* ed 4, St. Louis, 1991, Mosby.

Williamson ML: Reducing post-catheterization bladder dysfunction by reconditioning, *Nurs Res* 31:28, 1982.

Bibliography

Brogna L and Lakaszawski ML: The continent urostomy, *Am J Nurs* 96:160, 1986.

Carpenito LJ: *Nursing diagnosis application to clinical practice,* Philadelphia, 1992, Lippincott.

Greengold BA and Ouslander JG: Bladder retraining, *J Gerontol Nurs* 12:31, 1986.

Newman DK: The treatment of urinary incontinence in adults, *Nurs Pract* 14(6):21-32, 1989.

Newman DK and Smith DA: Incontinence: the problem patients won't talk about, *RN* 52:42, 1989.

Robb SS: Urinary incontinence verification in elderly men, *Nurs Res* 34:278, 1985.

Sampselle C, et al.: Pelvic muscle strength in childbearing women, *Nurs Res* 38(3):134, 1989.

Thomas B: Problem solving: urinary incontinence in the elderly, *J Gerontol Nurs* 6:553, 1980.

Tunink P: Alterations in urinary elimination, *J Gerontol Nurs* 14(R):25-30, 1988.

Wells T: Promoting urine control in older adults, *Geriatr Nurs* 1:236, 1980.

33 Bowel Elimination

OBJECTIVES

Mastery of content in this chapter will enable the student to:

- Define the key terms listed.
- Discuss the role of gastrointestinal organs in digestion and elimination.
- Describe four functions of the large intestine.
- Explain the physiology of normal defecation.
- List and discuss psychological and physiological factors that influence the elimination process.
- Describe common physiological alterations in elimination.
- Assess a client's elimination pattern.
- Perform a guaiac test for occult blood.
- List nursing diagnoses related to alterations in elimination.
- Describe nursing implications for common diagnostic examinations of the gastrointestinal tract.
- Administer an enema.
- List nursing measures aimed at promoting normal elimination and defecation.
- Discuss the relationship between the structure and function of a bowel diversion and nursing care required.

KEY TERMS

anorexia
bolus
cathartics
chyme
constipation
defecation
diarrhea
endoscope
enema
fecal impaction
fecal incontinence
feces
fissures
flatus
guaiac test
Harris flush
Haustral contractions
hemorrhoids
laxatives
masticate
melena
ostomy
peristalsis
prolapse
ptyalin
segmentation
smooth muscle
stoma
Valsalva maneuver

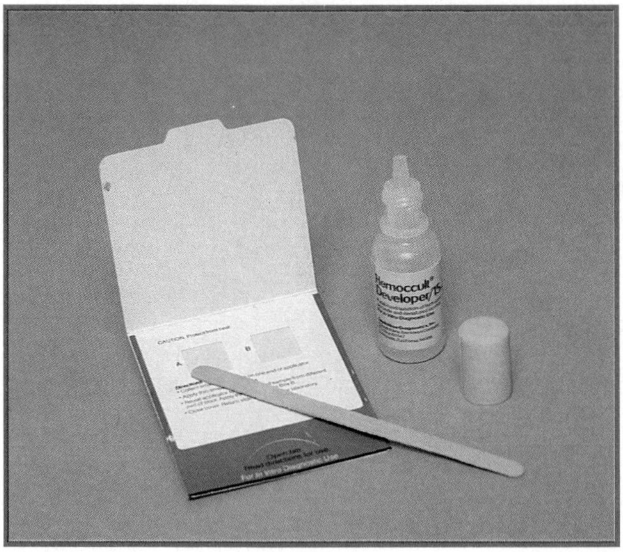

The regular elimination of bowel waste products is essential for normal body functioning. An alteration in normal bowel elimination can cause problems in other body systems and can be frustrating and embarrassing for a client. More importantly, recent evidence suggests that frequent high-volume defecation might reduce the possibility of colorectal cancer (Robinson and Weigley, 1989). Each client has a different pattern of defecation influenced by many factors. Diagnostic testing, illness, and surgical intervention can change an elimination pattern, creating the need for preventive and supportive nursing care. A client with elimination problems needs assistance, understanding, and sensitivity. Supportive nursing care respects the client's privacy and emotional needs. The nurse helps this client by promoting normal elimination for optimal health and well-being.

NORMAL DIGESTION AND ELIMINATION

The gastrointestinal (GI) tract is a series of hollow mucous membrane–lined muscular organs that have the primary purposes of absorbing fluid and nutrients and preparing food for absorption and use by the body's cells (Figure 33-1). The volume of fluid absorbed by the GI tract is high, making fluid balance one of its key functions. In addition to ingested fluids and foods, the GI tract also receives many secretions from organs such as the gallbladder and pancreas. A disorder that seriously impairs normal absorption or secretion of GI fluids causes fluid imbalance.

Mouth

The GI tract mechanically and chemically breaks down nutrients into suitable size and form. All digestive organs work together to ensure that the **bolus** (mass) of food reaches the area of nutrient absorption safely and effectively. Mechanical and chemical digestion begin in the mouth; teeth **masticate** (chew) food, breaking it down into a suitable size for swallowing. Salivary secretions contain enzymes such as **ptyalin** that initiate digestion of certain food elements. Saliva dilutes and softens the bolus of food in the mouth for easier swallowing.

Esophagus

As food enters the upper esophagus, it passes through the upper esophageal sphincter, a circular muscle that prevents air from entering the esophagus and food from **refluxing** (moving backward) into the throat. The bolus of food travels down the esophagus and is pushed along by slow peristaltic waves produced by alternating contractions of smooth muscle. As a portion of the esophagus contracts behind the food bolus, the circular muscle in front of the bolus relaxes. **Peristalsis** propels food toward the next wave and eventually throughout the length of the GI tract.

The bolus of food moves down the esophagus and reaches the lower esophageal sphincter in 15 seconds. The lower esophageal sphincter lies between the esophagus and the stomach, as a pressure difference exists at the lower end of the esophagus. The lower esophageal pressure is 10 to 40 mm Hg, whereas pressure within the stomach is 5 to 10 mm Hg. The pressure gradient normally prevents reflux of stomach contents back into the esophagus. Factors influencing lower sphincter pressure include antacids, which minimize reflux, and fatty foods and nicotine, which increase reflux.

Stomach

In the stomach, food is temporarily stored and mechanically and chemically broken down for digestion and absorption. The stomach secretes hydrochloric acid (HCl), mucus, the enzyme pepsin, and intrinsic factor. The concentration of HCl influences stomach acidity and the acid-base balance (see Chapter 35). For every HCl molecule secreted into the stomach, a bicarbonate (HCO_3^-) molecule enters the blood plasma. HCl helps to mix and break down food in the stomach. Mucus protects the stomach mucosa from acidity and enzyme activity. Pepsin digests proteins, although not much diges-

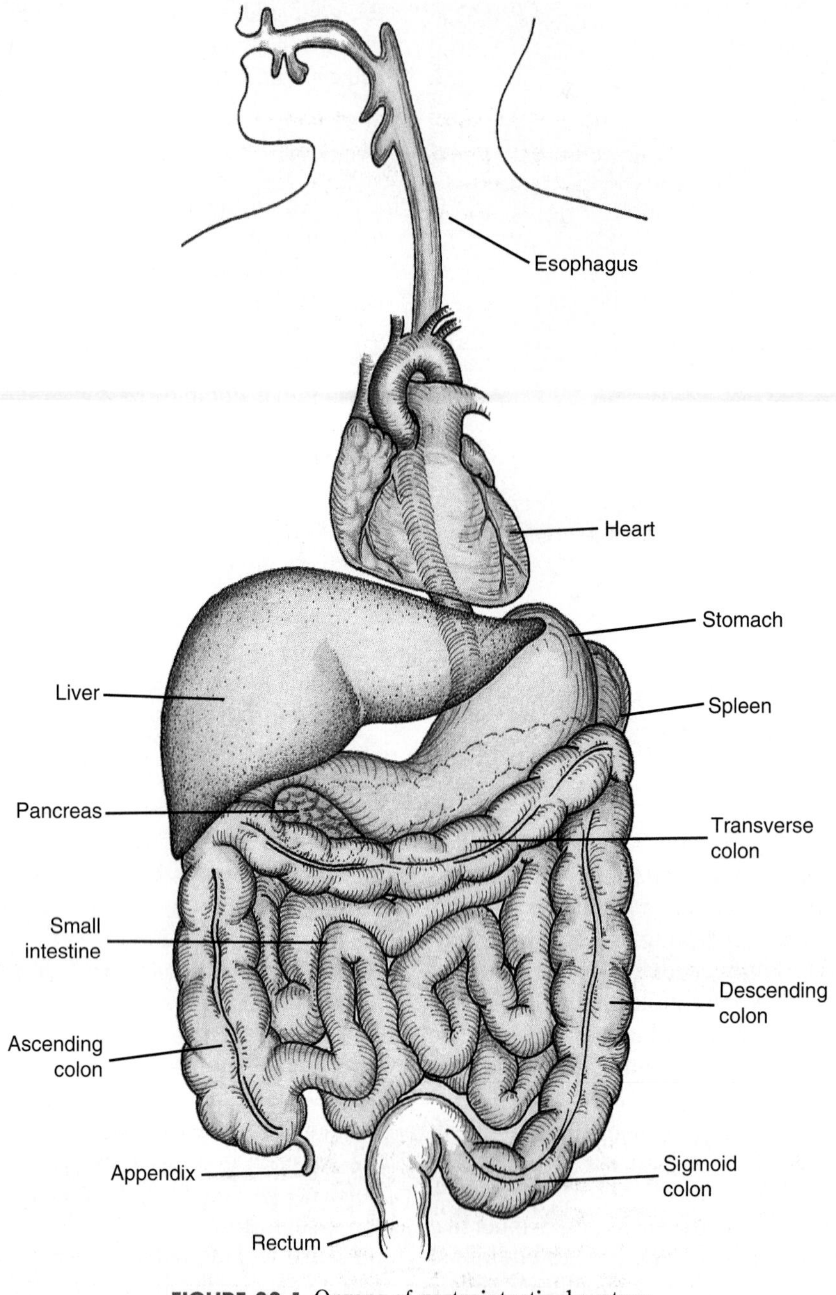

FIGURE 33-1 Organs of gastrointestinal system.

tion occurs in the stomach. Intrinsic factor is the essential component needed for vitamin B_{12} absorption in the intestine. Lack of it results in pernicious anemia.

Before food leaves the stomach, it is changed into a semifluid state, **chyme.** Chyme is more easily digested and absorbed than solid food. Clients who have portions of their stomach removed or who have rapid stomach emptying (as with gastritis) have serious digestive problems because food is not broken down into chyme. Food enters the small intestine before being adequately broken down to a semifluid form. Absorption is less efficient, and nutritional alterations can develop.

Small Intestine

During normal digestion, chyme leaves the stomach and enters the small intestine. The small intestine is a tube about 2.5 cm (1 inch) in diameter and 6 m (20 to 21 feet) long; it contains three divisions: duodenum, jejunum, and ileum. Chyme mixes with digestive enzymes (such as bile and amylase) while traveling through the small intestine. **Segmentation** (alternating contraction and relaxation of smooth muscle) churns the chyme, further breaking down food for digestion (Figure 33-2). As the chyme mixes, the forward peristaltic movement temporarily ceases in order to permit absorption. The

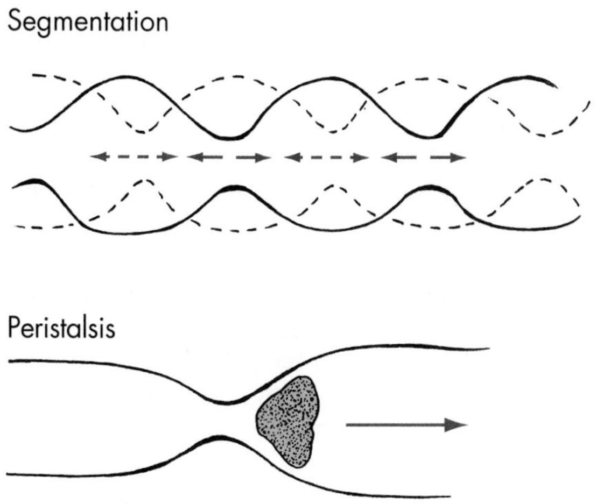

FIGURE 33-2 Segmental and peristaltic waves.

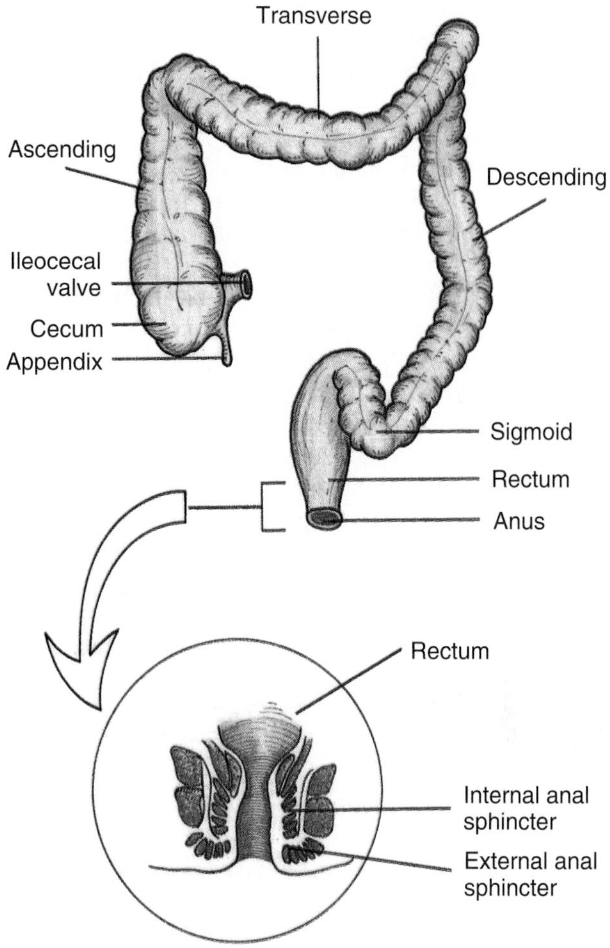

FIGURE 33-3 Divisions of large intestine.

chyme travels slowly through the small intestine to allow for absorption.

Most nutrients and electrolytes are absorbed in the small intestine. Enzymes from the pancreas and bile from the gallbladder are released into the duodenum. The intestine breaks down fats, proteins, and carbohydrates into basic elements (see Chapter 31). Nutrients are almost entirely absorbed by the duodenum and jejunum. The ileum absorbs certain vitamins, iron, and bile salts. If small intestine function is impaired, the digestive process is greatly altered. Conditions such as inflammation, surgical resection, or obstruction can disrupt peristalsis, reduce the area of absorption, or block the passage of chyme. Electrolyte and nutrient deficiencies then develop.

Large Intestine

Unabsorbed chyme enters the large intestine through the ileocecal valve, a circular muscle layer that prevents regurgitation (returning to the small intestine) of contents. The large intestine is the primary organ of bowel elimination. Its diameter is larger than that of the small intestine, but its length is shorter, 1.5 to 1.8 m (5 to 6 feet). Although watery chyme enters the colon, the volume of water lessens as the chyme moves along its length. Approximately 10 L of chyme passes through the large intestine daily, with 100 to 300 ml eventually expelled as feces.

The large intestine extends from the cecum to the anal canal (Figure 33-3). The colon is made of muscular tissue. The muscular quality of the colon allows it to accommodate and eliminate large quantities of waste.

The colon has four interrelated functions: absorption, protection, secretion, and elimination. A large volume of water and a significant amount of sodium and chloride are absorbed by the colon daily. As food passes through the large intestine, **haustral contractions** occur; these are similar to the segmental contractions of the small intestine but last longer—up to 5 minutes. The contractions produce large sacs in the colon's wall, providing a large surface area for absorption.

As much as 2.5 liters of water may be absorbed by the colon in 24 hours. On the average, 55 milliequivalents (mEq) of sodium and 23 mEq of chloride are absorbed daily. The amount of water absorbed from chyme depends on the speed at which the colonic contents move. The chyme is normally a soft, formed mass. If the speed of peristaltic contractions is abnormally fast (as in the case of colitis, irritable bowel syndrome, or intestinal virus), there is less time for the water to be absorbed, and the stool is watery. If peristaltic contractions slow, causing contents to remain in the colon too long, a hard mass of stool forms, resulting in constipation or impaction.

The colon protects itself by releasing mucus. The mucus lubricates the colon, preventing trauma. Lubrication is especially important near the distal end of the colon where contents become drier and harder.

The colon aids in electrolyte balance. Bicarbonate is

secreted in exchange for chloride. Approximately 4 to 9 mEq of potassium is released each day by the large intestine. Serious alterations in colon function can cause electrolyte imbalance.

Finally, the colon removes waste products and **flatus** (gas) that results from air swallowing and bacterial action on nonabsorbable carbohydrates. Fermentation of carbohydrates produces intestinal gas, which can stimulate peristalsis.

Slow peristaltic contractions move contents through the colon. Muscles of the colon are innervated by the autonomic nervous system. Parasympathetic stimuli increase peristalsis, and sympathetic stimuli decrease peristalsis. Intestinal contents are the main stimulus for contraction. Waste products and gas put pressure on the walls of the colon. The muscle layer stretches, stimulating the reflex that initiates contraction.

Mass peristaltic movements push undigested food toward the rectum. These movements are unlike the frequent peristaltic waves in the small intestine (usually heard on auscultation) in that they typically occur only 3 or 4 times daily. Large segments of the colon contract as a result of two reflex responses—gastrocolic and duodenocolic—that occur when the stomach or duodenum is filled with food. Filling initiates nerve impulses that stimulate the colon's muscular walls. Mass peristalsis is strongest during the hour after mealtime. Nursing measures designed to promote defecation should be timed with this natural reflex.

Rectum

Waste products that reach the sigmoid portion of the colon are called **feces.** The sigmoid stores feces until just before defecation. The rectum is the final division of the large intestine. Its length varies according to age.

Normally the rectum is empty of feces until defecation. It contains vertical and transverse folds of tissue that may help to temporarily hold fecal contents during defecation. Each vertical fold contains an artery and veins. If the veins become repeatedly distended from pressure during the straining of defecation, permanent dilations called *hemorrhoids* form. Hemorrhoids can make defecation painful.

Anus

Feces and flatus are eventually expelled from the rectum through the anal canal and anus. The anal canal is 2.5 to 4 cm (1 to 1.5 inches) long and opens into the perineum. The internal and external anal sphincters are located in the muscular walls of the anal canal. Contraction and relaxation of the sphincters, innervated by sympathetic and parasympathetic stimuli, aid in the control of defecation. The anal canal is richly supplied with sensory nerves that help to distinguish flatus from feces and thus help to control continence.

Defecation

When a fecal mass or gas moves into the rectum to distend its walls, the **defecation** reflex begins. The process involves involuntary and voluntary control. After the rectal walls are stretched, an awareness of the need to defecate is created. This spinal reflex produces parasympathetic relaxation of the smooth muscle of the internal anal sphincter, which allows feces to enter the anal canal. The striated muscle of the external anal sphincter voluntarily contracts as a person chooses whether to defecate. If the time for defecation is not right, voluntary constriction of the levator ani muscle closes the anus and defecation is delayed, only to return with the next distention of the rectum.

At the time of defecation, the external sphincter relaxes. Pressure can be exerted to expel feces through an increase in intraabdominal pressure or a Valsalva maneuver. A **Valsalva maneuver** is the voluntary contraction of abdominal muscles during forced expiration with a closed glottis (holding one's breath while straining). A Valsalva maneuver is contraindicated in persons with heart disease, glaucoma, or increased intracranial pressure. Relaxation of the levator ani muscle allows feces to be expelled. Defecation is aided by flexing the thigh muscles (which puts pressure on the abdomen) and sitting (which increases pressure down on the rectum). Normal defecation is painless, resulting in passage of soft, formed stool. The box on pp. 951-952 lists factors that influence elimination and defecation.

COMMON BOWEL ELIMINATION PROBLEMS

Bowel elimination problems result from physiological changes in the GI tract, surgical alteration of intestinal structures, or disorders that impair defecation.

Constipation

Constipation is a symptom, not a disease. It is a decrease in frequency of bowel movements, accompanied by prolonged or difficult passage of hard, dry stools. For many reasons, intestinal motility slows, causing prolonged exposure of the fecal mass to the intestinal walls. Most of the fecal water content is absorbed, leaving little to soften and lubricate the stool. Passage of a dry, hard stool can cause rectal pain.

There is no correct number of daily or weekly bowel movements. Each person has his or her own pattern. If a person has fewer than two bowel movements each week, there might be cause for concern, especially if this represents a change. Normal bowel function for 98% of the population varies from three movements daily to only three per week. Older adults often believe that cleaning out the colon is critical for maintaining good

FACTORS INFLUENCING BOWEL ELIMINATION

AGE

Infants have a small stomach capacity, less secretion of digestive enzymes, and more rapid intestinal peristalsis. The ability to control defecation does not occur until 2 to 3 years at toddlerhood.

Adolescents experience rapid growth of the large intestine and increased secretion of HCl.

The exercise and eating patterns and food selection of young and middle adults affect elimination patterns.

Older adults' teeth change as does the ability to chew food thoroughly. Partially chewed food cannot be digested because of a reduction in digestive enzymes. Peristalsis declines, and esophageal emptying slows. Absorption by the intestinal mucosa is impaired. They lose muscle tone in the perineal floor and anal sphincter, causing difficulty in controlling defecation (see gerontologic nursing practice box on p. 963). Hospitalized older adults are particularly susceptible to changes in bowel function (Ross, 1990).

DIET

Regular daily food intake promotes peristalsis.

High-fiber foods—raw fruits, cooked fruits, greens (cabbage and spinach), raw vegetables, and whole grains (cereals and breads)—promote peristalsis and defecation by creating bulk. High fiber foods have also been found to lower serum cholesterol (Davidson, et al., 1991; Van Horn, et al., 1991).

Low-fiber foods (pasta, lean meats, and milk) slow peristalsis.

Gas-producing foods (broccoli, cauliflower, onions, and dried beans) can stimulate peristalsis.

Persons with lactose intolerance lack the enzyme lactose, which is needed to digest the simple sugars in milk. This and other food intolerances can cause diarrhea and cramping.

POSITION DURING DEFECATION

Squatting allows a person to lean forward, exert intraabdominal pressure, and contract thigh muscles to normally defecate.

Older adults or those with arthritis may be unable to rise from a toilet seat.

Immobilized clients, required to use a bedpan while lying, cannot contract muscles to defecate.

PREGNANCY

As pregnancy advances and the fetus enlarges, pressure is exerted on the rectum. Constipation commonly occurs.

DIAGNOSTIC TESTS

Certain examinations involving visualization of gastrointestinal structures require the emptying of bowel contents.

The inability of a client to eat or drink and enema administration to cleanse the bowel before a test are factors that interfere with normal elimination.

Barium examinations require ingestion of barium, a mixture that can harden and cause serious constipation unless eliminated soon after a test. Cathartics or enemas are usually given after barium examinations.

FLUID INTAKE

An adult should drink a minimum of 6 to 8 glasses (1400 to 2000 ml) of fluid daily.

Hot beverages and fruit juices soften stool and increase peristalsis.

Fluid liquefies intestinal contents for easier passage.

Large quantities of milk may slow peristalsis and cause constipation.

ACTIVITY

Regular physical exercise promotes peristalsis.

Immobilization depresses colon motility.

The muscle tone of abdominal and pelvic muscles must be adequate to ease and control defecation.

PSYCHOLOGICAL FACTORS

Stress (anxiety or fear) initiates parasympathetic impulses, causing acceleration of digestion and peristalsis. Diarrhea and gaseous distention may result.

Emotional depression can decrease peristalsis and lead to constipation.

Stress placed on a child to become toilet trained can lead to chronic constipation.

PERSONAL HABITS

Personal habits (taking time to defecate, having privacy, and using one's own toilet facilities) promote normal elimination.

A busy work schedule can interrupt normal habits, causing constipation.

Hospitalized clients often share toilet facilities or use bedpans or bedside commodes. The resulting embarrassment causes them to ignore the urge to defecate.

PAIN

Hemorrhoids, rectal surgery, and abdominal surgery may cause discomfort during defecation. If a client suppresses defecation, constipation develops.

MEDICATIONS

Laxatives and cathartics soften stool and promote peristalsis. Chronic use of cathartics causes loss of intestinal muscle tone.

Antidiarrheal agents inhibit peristalsis.

Narcotic analgesics, opiates, and anticholinergic drugs depress peristalsis and can cause constipation.

Many antibiotics produce diarrhea.

Several medications may change the character of stool. Drugs that contain iron turn stool black. Antacids may cause a white discoloration. Blood in the stool may result from anticoagulants or aspirin.

Continued.

FACTORS INFLUENCING BOWEL ELIMINATION—cont'd

SURGERY AND ANESTHESIA

General anesthetics temporarily halt peristalsis (see Chapter 36).

Clients who receive local or regional anesthesia have fewer elimination problems because bowel activity is minimally affected.

Surgery involving bowel manipulation temporarily stops peristalsis (paralytic ileus) for 24 to 48 hours. Clients cannot eat or drink until peristalsis returns.

health and thus may use laxatives extensively (Ebersole and Hess, 1994).

Constipation often results from irregular bowel habits, such as ignoring the defecation reflex. Other contributing factors include an inadequate fluid intake, lack of exercise, immobilization, advanced pregnancy, and a low-fiber diet. In older adults, constipation commonly results from insufficient dietary bulk, inadequate fluid intake, laxative abuse, reduced muscle tone, postponement of defecation, lack of food intake or anorexia associated with depression, and organic illness (Ebersole and Hess, 1994).

A common cause of constipation is habitual laxative use. Individuals who rely on laxatives for regular bowel movements develop a physical dependence on them. Laxatives promote complete emptying of the colon, and a period of time is then necessary to refill the colon with bulk. However, the client may become anxious to have another bowel movement and take repeated doses of laxatives. The colon's normal reflexes eventually diminish; it loses its muscle tone and becomes responsive only to the stimulating effect of laxatives or enemas.

For many clients constipation is a significant hazard to health. Straining during defecation is a problem for the client who has had recent abdominal or rectal surgery. The effort to pass a stool can cause stress on the suture line, and sutures may rupture, reopening the wound.

Impaction

Fecal impaction results from unrelieved constipation. It is a collection of hardened feces, wedged in the rectum, that cannot be expelled. In cases of severe impaction, the mass may extend up into the sigmoid colon. Debilitated, confused, or unconscious clients are most at risk for impaction because they do not heed the defecation reflex. Frequent repetition of practices that produce constipation can also cause impaction, as can failure to pass barium contrast medium.

An obvious sign of impaction is the inability to pass a stool for several days, despite a repeated urge to defecate. The client with a history of constipation is most at risk. When a continuous oozing of diarrheal stool develops in such a client, impaction should be suspected. The liquid portion of feces located high in the colon seeps around the edges of the impacted mass. **Anorexia** (loss of appetite), abdominal distention and cramping, and rectal pain may occur. The nurse who suspects an impaction can gently perform a digital examination of the rectum and palpate the impacted mass. Some institutions require a physician's order for a nurse to perform a rectal examination because rectal stimulation may cause vagal slowing of the heart.

Diarrhea

Diarrhea is an increase in the number of stools and the passage of liquid unformed feces and is a symptom of disorders affecting digestion, absorption, and secretion in the GI tract. Intestinal contents pass through the small intestine and colon too quickly to allow fluid absorption. Irritation within the colon may result in an increased mucus secretion, and feces become watery. It is difficult to assess diarrhea in infants because of their wide variation in bowel habits. An infant who is bottle fed may have one firm stool every day or every other day, while a breast-fed baby may pass five to eight small, soft stools daily. The mother or nurse should note a sudden increase in the number of stools, a reduction in fecal consistency with an increase in fluid content, and a tendency for feces to be greenish.

The excess loss of fluid can result in serious fluid and electrolyte imbalance. Infants and the older adult are particularly susceptible (see Chapter 35). Diarrhea was once the chief cause of death in infancy. Because repeated passage of diarrheal stools also exposes the skin of the perineum and buttocks to irritating intestinal contents, meticulous skin care is needed to prevent skin breakdown.

Many conditions cause diarrhea (Table 33-1). The aim of treatment is first to remove all causative conditions (including eating and drinking) and then to slow peristalsis. Fluids may need to be given intravenously to maintain necessary hydration.

Incontinence

Fecal incontinence is the inability to control passage of feces and gas from the anus. Any condition that im-

table 33-1

CONDITIONS THAT CAUSE DIARRHEA

Condition	Physiological effects
Emotional stress (anxiety)	Increased intestinal motility
Intestinal infection (streptococcal or staphylococcal enteritis)	Inflammation of intestinal mucosa Increased mucus secretion in colon
Food allergies	Reduced digestion of food elements
Food intolerance (greasy foods, coffee, alcohol, or spicy foods)	Increased intestinal motility Increased mucus secretion in colon
Medications	
Iron	Irritation of intestinal mucosa
Antibiotics	Suprainfection, allowing overgrowth of normal flora Inflammation and irritation of mucosa
Laxatives	Increased intestinal motility
Colon disease (colitis, irritable bowel syndrome, or Crohn's disease)	Inflammation and ulceration of intestinal walls Reduced absorption of fluids Increased intestinal motility
Surgical alterations	
Gastrectomy	Loss of reservoir function of stomach Food dumping into duodenum too quickly for proper absorption
Colon resection	Reduced size of colon Reduced amount of absorptive surface

pairs function or control of the anal sphincter may cause fecal incontinence. Conditions that create frequent, loose, large-volume, watery stools also predispose to incontinence. Common physiological causes include spinal cord trauma, multiple sclerosis, cerebrovascular accidents, muscle flaccidity, and tumors or growths of the sphincter tissue. Schizophrenia, severe depression, and dementia may prevent the client from being aware of the need to defecate. Similarly, the use of sedatives can cause incontinence from depression of cerebral awareness and control over defecation (Ebersole and Hess, 1990).

Incontinence can harm body image. In many situations, the client is mentally alert but physically unable to avoid defecation. The embarrassment of soiling the clothes can lead to social isolation. The client must depend on the nurse for a very basic need. Clients with mental or sensory alterations are often unaware that they have passed a stool.

Like diarrhea, incontinence predisposes the client to skin breakdown. The nurse must check frequently to be sure that the client's anal and perineal regions are clean and dry.

Flatulence

As gas accumulates in the lumen of the intestines from swallowed air or decomposition of food in the colon, the bowel wall stretches and distends. It is a common cause of abdominal fullness, pain, and cramping. Normally intestinal gas escapes through the mouth (belching) or the anus (as flatus). However, if there is a reduction in intestinal motility resulting from opiates, general anesthetics, abdominal surgery, or immobilization, the client's flatulence may become severe enough to cause distention with shortness of breath. The accumulation of gas forces the diaphragm up and reduces lung expansion. This is especially problematic for a client with impaired respiration.

Hemorrhoids

Columns of mucosal tissue extend from the rectum down through the anal canal. These anal columns contain cross channels of anastomosing veins. When dilated, these veins are internal **hemorrhoids.** Veins that become varicosed at the lower end of the anal canal are external hemorrhoids. Increased venous pressure resulting from straining at defecation, pregnancy, congestive heart failure, and chronic liver disease can cause hemorrhoids. Internal hemorrhoids are characterized by the moist, red epithelium of the rectum. External hemorrhoids are protrusions of skin from the anal canal.

Hemorrhoids bleed easily when stretched. Passage of a hard stool commonly causes bleeding. The hemorrhoids become inflamed and tender, and clients may complain of itching and burning. Because pain worsens during defecation, the client may ignore the urge to defecate, resulting in constipation.

BOWEL DIVERSIONS

Certain diseases cause conditions that prevent normal passage of feces through the rectum. This creates the need for a temporary or permanent artificial opening **(stoma)** in the abdominal wall. Surgical openings are formed in the ileum (ileostomy) or colon (colostomy) (Figure 33-4). Ends of the intestines are then brought through the opening to create the stoma. The stoma is covered with a plastic pouch or bag to collect fecal material.

The location of the **ostomy** determines the consistency of stool. An ileostomy bypasses the entire large intestine. As a result, stools are frequent and liquid. The same is true for a colostomy of the ascending colon. A

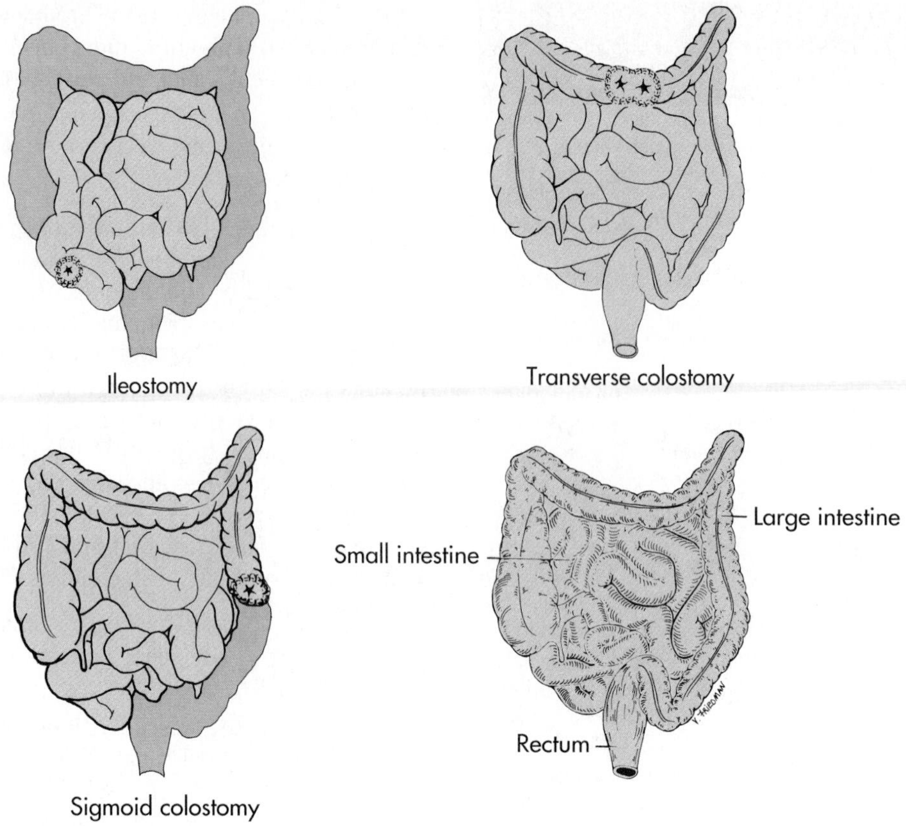

FIGURE 33-4 Types of colostomies.

colostomy of the transverse colon generally results in a more solid, formed stool. The sigmoid colostomy emits almost normal stool. The location of a colostomy is determined by the client's medical problem and the type of surgery required.

There are three types of colostomy construction: loop, end, and double-barrel. A loop colostomy involves pulling a loop of bowel onto the abdomen. Communication exists between the proximal and distal bowel. A plastic rod or catheter is temporarily placed underneath the bowel loop to keep it from slipping back. The loop ostomy is opened to create a proximal end that drains stool and a distal end that drains mucus. Eventually this temporary colostomy is closed. An end colostomy has one stoma formed from the proximal end of bowel with the distal end permanently removed. The double-barrel has two distinct stomas, a proximal functioning stoma and distal, nonfunctioning stoma. The bowel is severed.

A new option of bowel diversion, the ileoanal reservoir, preserves the integrity and function of the rectum (Dalton-Loehner, 1989). The surgery involves several stages: a colectomy (removal of colon), the dissection of rectal mucosa to leave only the muscle layers and sphincter intact, and creation of a J- or S-shaped pouch formed from the terminal end of the ileum. The ileum and anal canal are anastomosed. As the anastomosis heals, a client has a temporary ileostomy. Within 8 to 10 weeks after surgery, the ileostomy is closed, and a client regains defecation by being able to excrete ileal contents through the rectum.

Ostomies and ileoanal reservoirs create a management challenge. A bag or pouch into which frequent, liquid stools are emitted must always be worn on ileostomies. Regular defecation cannot be achieved because of continuous oozing of stool. The bag must be emptied, washed, and replaced throughout the day. However, some clients have been able to achieve continence through use of a new disposable colostomy plug, which allows the client to go for a period of time without a pouch (Cleague and Heald, 1990). Irrigation before plug application correlates positively with length of wear (Burcharth, Ballon, et al., 1986).

A colostomy in the descending or sigmoid colon is easier to manage. The client may wear a pouch at all times, even though bowel movements may occur only once or twice daily. Proper selection of foods and management of the ostomy through irrigations help to establish a regular elimination pattern so that eventually a pouch becomes unnecessary.

Skin care is important for clients with ostomies and ileoanal reservoirs. Liquid stool contains enzymes that can irritate and macerate skin. Diligent skin care by nurse and client is required.

An ostomy causes serious body image changes, particularly if it is permanent. Clients often perceive a stoma as a form of mutilation. Even though clothing conceals the ostomy, the client feels different. Many clients have difficulty in maintaining or initiating normal sexual relations. An important factor in the client's reaction is the character of fecal secretions and the ability to control them. Foul odors, spillage, or leakage of liquid stools and inability to regulate bowel movements give the client a loss of self-esteem.

NURSING PROCESS FOR THE CLIENT WITH BOWEL ELIMINATION PROBLEMS

Assessment

To assess bowel elimination patterns and to determine abnormalities, the nurse collects a nursing history, assesses the abdomen, inspects fecal characteristics, and reviews pertinent test results.

Nursing History

The nursing history reviews the client's normal bowel pattern and habits. The client's description of "normal" patterns may be different from factors and conditions that tend to promote normal elimination. Identifying normal and abnormal patterns and habits allows the nurse to determine the client's problems and anticipate possible problems. Much of the nursing history can be organized around the factors affecting elimination. The nurse then applies this knowledge through questions to determine the presence and extent of GI alterations. Family members can help if the client is unable to provide necessary information. A typical nursing history of a client's elimination status includes the following:

1. Determination of the usual elimination pattern. Frequency and time of day are included.
2. Identification of routines followed to promote normal elimination. Examples are drinking hot liquids, using a laxative, eating specific foods, or taking time to defecate during a certain part of the day.
3. Description of recent change in elimination pattern. This information is perhaps the most significant because elimination patterns vary, and the client can best detect change. Determine the time of the last bowel movement. If there were changes, ask the client to suggest a cause.
4. History of pain or discomfort. Ask the client whether there is a history of abdominal or anal pain. The location and nature of pain can help to locate the source of a problem (see Chapter 28).
5. Client's description of usual characteristics of stool. The nurse determines whether the stool is normally watery or formed, soft or hard, and the typical color. The client also describes a normal stool's shape. Ask whether there have been recent changes.
6. Diet history. Determine the client's dietary preferences for a day. The nurse measures servings of fruits, vegetables, cereals, and breads. Is mealtime regular or irregular, and are certain foods eaten infrequently?
7. Description of daily fluid intake. This includes the type and amount of fluid. The client may have to estimate the amount using common household measurements.
8. History of exercise. Ask the client to describe the type and amount of daily exercise. Simply asking the client whether the client exercises is not adequate because it leaves the judgment solely to the client.
9. Assessment of the use of artificial aids at home. The nurse assesses whether the client requires the use of enemas, laxatives, or special foods before having a bowel movement. If so, the nurse asks how often the client uses them.
10. History of surgery or illnesses affecting the GI tract. This information can often help to explain symptoms. In addition, it provides the nurse with an idea of the potential for maintaining or restoring a normal elimination pattern. It also helps to know whether there is a family history of cancer involving the GI tract.
11. Presence and status of artificial orifices. If the client has an ostomy, the nurse assesses the frequency of fecal drainage, character of feces, type of appliance used, and methods used to maintain the ostomy's function.
12. Medication history. Determine whether the client takes medications (such as laxatives, antacids, iron supplements, and analgesics) that might alter defecation or fecal characteristics.
13. Emotional state. Emotions can significantly alter the frequency of defecation. During assessment, observation of emotions, tone of voice, and mannerisms can reveal significant behaviors indicating stress.
14. Social history. If the client is not independent in bowel management, determine methods and degree of assistance required.

Physical Assessment

The nurse assesses the status of GI function to detect factors that may affect elimination and to gather data regarding the client's elimination problems (see Chapter 16).

Mouth. An assessment includes inspection of the teeth and gums. Poor dentition (arrangement of teeth) or poor-fitting dentures influence the ability to chew. The nurse also assesses the client's ability to swallow.

Abdomen. The nurse inspects all four abdominal quadrants for contour, shape, symmetry, and skin color. Inspection also includes noting masses, peristaltic waves, scars, venous patterns, stomas, or lesions. Normally, peristaltic waves are not visible. However, observable peristalsis might indicate intestinal obstruction.

Abdominal distention appears as an overall outward protuberance of the abdomen. Intestinal gas, large tumors, or fluid in the peritoneal cavity may cause distention. A distended abdomen feels tight and the skin appears taut, as if stretched. Daily measurement of the abdomen's girth using a tape measure reveals whether distention is increasing. Measurements should be taken over the same anatomical landmarks (e.g., umbilicus) to provide an accurate chronological measurement. If masses are present, they appear as localized bulges or protuberances.

The nurse auscultates the abdomen before palpation to avoid changing the frequency of bowel sounds. The diaphragm of the stethoscope is used to assess bowel sounds in each quadrant. While auscultating, the nurse notes the character and frequency of bowel sounds. The nurse assesses bowel sounds as normal or too loud, absent, hyperactive, or hypoactive. An increase in pitch or a "tinkling" sound may be heard with abdominal distention. Absent or hypoactive sounds occur with paralytic ileus after abdominal surgery. High-pitched and hyperactive bowel sounds occur with small intestine obstruction and inflammatory disorders.

The client should relax during palpation and percussion. Tense abdominal muscles interfere with palpation of underlying organs or masses. The nurse palpates with a light, gentle touch. Palpation of a tender or sensitive area causes a guarding or voluntary tightening of abdominal muscles. If the nurse locates an unusual mass, further assessment is done by the physician. The nurse should not apply deep palpation unless trained in the skill.

Percussion detects lesions, fluid, or gas within the abdomen. Familiarity with the five percussion notes also permits identification of underlying abdominal structures.

Rectum and Anus. Clients are easily embarrassed during rectal examination because of concern about cleanliness of the area or troubling symptoms. Fear can cause spasm of the anal sphincters and muscles of the buttocks, making the examination uncomfortable (Malasanos, et al., 1990). The nurse helps a client to relax through slow, deep breathing and proper draping and positioning.

The nurse inspects the area around the anus for skin color, skin tags, irritation, lesions, scars, inflammation, abscesses, fissures, hemorrhoids, or rectal prolapse. Having a client strain downward as though defecating reveals rectal **fissures, prolapse,** and internal hemorrhoids. The nurse describes findings by locating the position in relation to a clock.

The nurse uses gentle palpation for the remainder of the examination. After donning clean, disposable gloves, the nurse lubricates the index finger with a water-soluble lubricant. As the client strains downward, the pad of the index finger is gently placed against the anal opening; pressure is exerted until the external anal sphincter relaxes, and the finger is slowly inserted toward the client's umbilicus. The client is asked to tighten the sphincter around the finger to aid in assessing strength of the sphincter. The nurse next palpates the walls of the anal canal. The canal is short, 3 cm, equal to the distance from the fingertip to the first interphalangeal joint (Malasanos, et al., 1990). The mucosa should feel smooth.

The nurse can palpate 6 to 10 cm (2 to 4 inches) of the rectal canal with the examining finger. The nurse methodically palpates all sides of the rectal wall for abnormalities. The rectal mucosa is normally smooth and soft. Pushing the index finger forcefully against the rectal wall or extending the finger too far can cause discomfort. After completing the examination, the nurse cleans the anal area thoroughly, removes gloves, and thoroughly washes hands.

Fecal Characteristics

After examining the rectum, the nurse directly inspects feces on the glove for several characteristics (Table 33-2). If there is no feces on the glove, the nurse asks the client to describe a typical stool, noting recent changes. The client is probably the most knowledgeable about changes. The nurse should also determine whether the client passes an unusual amount of or little flatus.

Laboratory and Diagnostic Tests

Laboratory and diagnostic tests offer useful information concerning elimination problems. Laboratory analysis of fecal contents can detect tumors, hemorrhage, and infection. Diagnostic studies allow the physician to visualize all segments of the GI tract. Certain diagnostic tests such as endoscopy permit direct visualization of structures. Tests such as the barium enema or an upper gastrointestinal (UGI) series require ingestion of a contrast medium that outlines structures indirectly on x-ray examination.

Fecal Specimens. The nurse ensures that all specimens are accurately obtained, labeled properly in ap-

table 33-2

FECAL CHARACTERISTICS

Characteristic	Normal	Abnormal	Cause
Color	Infant: yellow Adult: brown	White or clay	Absence of bile
		Black or tarry	Iron ingestion or UGI bleeding
		Red	Lower GI bleeding and ingestion of beets
		Pale with fat	Malabsorption of fat
		Translucent mucous	Spastic constipation, colitis, and excessive straining
		Blood mucous	Neoplasm or inflammation
Odor	Pungent; affected by food type	Noxious change	Blood in feces or infection
Consistency	Soft, formed	Liquid	Diarrhea and reduced absorption
		Hard	Constipation
Frequency	Infant: 5 to 8 times daily (breast fed) or 1 daily or every other day (bottle fed) Adult: daily or 2 to 3 times a week	Infant more than 6 times daily or less than once every 1 to 2 days; adult more than 3 times a day or less than once a week	Hypomotility or hypermotility
Amount	150 g per day		
Shape	Resembles diameter of rectum	Narrow, pencil-shaped	Obstruction and rapid peristalsis
Constituents	Undigested food, dead bacteria, fat, bile pigment, cells lining intestinal mucosa, and water	Blood, pus, foreign bodies, mucus, and worms	Internal bleeding, infection, swallowed objects, irritation, and inflammation
		Excess fat	Malabsorption syndromes, enteritis and pancreatic disease, and surgical removal of section of intestine

propriate containers, and transported to the laboratory on time. Institutions provide special containers for fecal specimens. Certain tests require that the specimens be placed in chemical preservatives.

Medical aseptic technique should be used during the collection of any stool specimen (see Chapter 25). Bacteria can easily be acquired by a person who handles a specimen improperly. Gloving and handwashing are necessary for anyone who might come in contact with the specimen. The client is often capable of obtaining the specimen if properly instructed. Explain to the client that feces cannot be mixed with urine or water. For this reason the client defecates into a clean, dry bedpan or special container that is placed under the toilet seat.

Laboratory tests for occult (microscopic) blood in the stool and stool cultures require only a small sample. Minimum abrasions of the intestinal mucosa are thought to cause blood loss of 1 to 3 ml daily in feces (Malasanos, et al., 1990). Blood loss of over 50 ml appears as **melena.** To detect quantities less than 50 ml, laboratory analysis is needed. The nurse collects approximately an inch of formed stool or 15 to 30 ml of liquid diarrheal stool. To avoid contact with feces while transferring solid specimens to a container, the nurse applies gloves and uses a wooden tongue depressor. The nurse must pour the liquid specimens carefully into the proper container. Tests for measuring the output of fecal fat require the client to collect stools for 3 to 5 days. All fecal material must be saved throughout the test period.

After obtaining a specimen, the nurse tightly seals the container and completes laboratory requisition forms. The nurse then records all specimen collections in the client's medical record. The nurse avoids delays in sending specimens to the laboratory. Some tests require the stool to be warm. When stool specimens are allowed to stand at room temperature, bacteriological changes that alter test results can occur.

GUAIAC TEST. A common fecal laboratory test performed at the bedside is the **guaiac test,** which measures microscopic amounts of blood in the feces (Procedure 33-1). It is a useful diagnostic screening test for colon cancer (see box on p. 959). One positive result does not confirm GI bleeding. The test should be repeated at least 3 times while the client refrains from eating meat, poultry, fish, turnips, and horseradish, and using certain drugs such as steroids, iron, salicylates, etc.

MEASURING OCCULT BLOOD IN STOOL

Steps	Rationale
1. Assess client's medical history for bleeding or gastrointestinal disorder.	Routine screening can be instituted by nurse.
2. Assess type of medications client receives. Note drugs that can cause GI mucosal bleeding.	Anticoagulants increase risk of bleeding. Long-term use of steroids and acetylsalicylic acid (aspirin) can irritate mucosa.
3. Refer to physician's order for medication or dietary modifications or restrictions before test.	Rare meats and medications such as iron supplement and bismuth compounds cause stools to resemble melena.
4. Prepare equipment and supplies: a. Paper towel b. Hemoccult test supplies *(see illustration)*: (1) Cardboard Hemoccult slide (2) Wooden applicator (3) Hemoccult developing solution (4) Disposable gloves	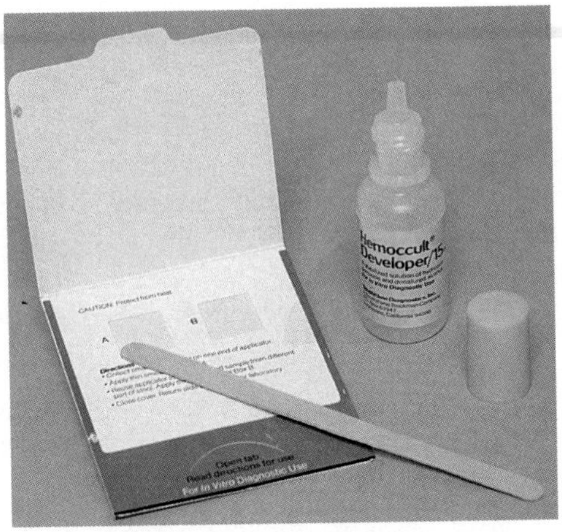
5. Explain purpose of test and ways client can assist.	Ensures cooperation and minimizes anxiety.
6. Be sure restrictions were followed.	Ensures accurate test results.
7. Wash hands.	Reduces transmission of infection.
8. Apply clean, disposable gloves.	Reduces transmission of microorganisms.
9. Obtain uncontaminated stool specimen.	Prevents incorrect test results.
10. Use tip of wooden applicator to obtain small portion of feces.	Small specimen is sufficient for measuring blood content in feces.
11. Perform Hemoccult slide test: a. Open flap of slide and apply thin smear of stool on paper in first box *(see illustration)*.	Guaiac paper inside box is sensitive to fecal blood content.
b. Obtain second fecal specimen from different portion of stool and apply thinly to slide's second box *(see illustration)*.	Findings of occult blood are more conclusive for GI bleeding when entire specimen is found to contain blood.
c. Close slide cover and turn slide over to reverse side *(see illustration)*. Open cardboard flap and apply 2 drops of Hemoccult developing solution on each box of guaiac paper *(see illustration)*.	Developing solution penetrates underlying fecal specimen. Blood is indicated by change in color of guaiac paper.
d. Read results of test after 30 to 60 sec *(see illustration)*. Note color changes.	Bluish discoloration indicates occult blood (guaiac positive). No change in color indicates negative results.
e. Dispose of test slide in proper receptacle.	Reduces transfer of microorganisms.
12. Wrap wooden applicator in paper towel, remove gloves, and dispose in proper receptacle.	Feces contain large numbers of microorganisms.
13. Wash hands.	Reduces spread of infection.
14. Record results of test in nurses' notes and note unusual fecal characteristics.	All test results should be documented promptly. Findings may indicate need for further diagnosis.

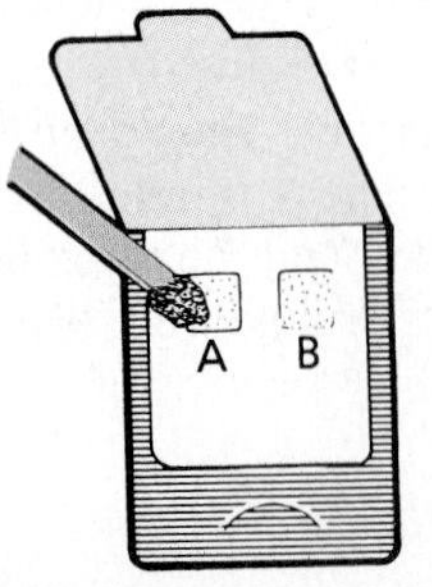

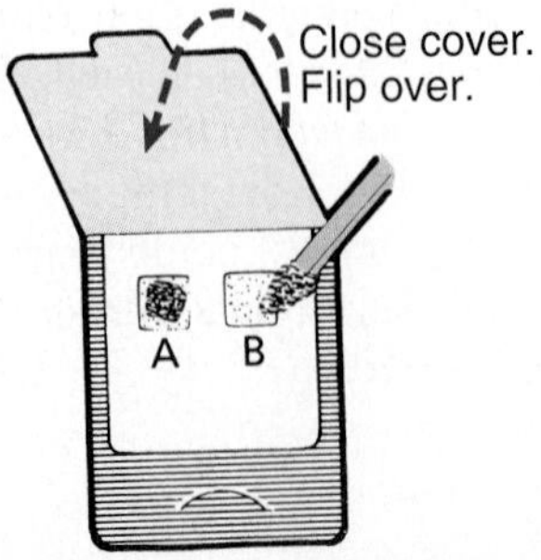

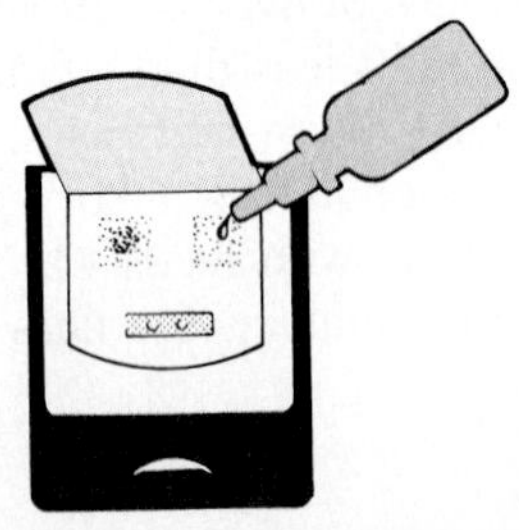

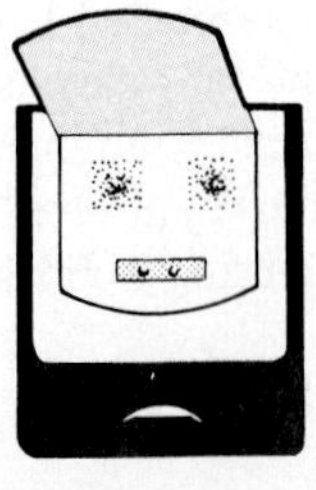

Step 11d

SCREENING FOR COLON CANCER

RISK FACTORS

Age: over 50
Family history: colon polyps
History of inflammatory bowel disease (colitis or Crohn's disease)
Living in urban area
Diet: high intake of fats and low fiber intake

WARNING SIGNS

Change in bowel habits
Rectal bleeding

SCREENING TESTS

Digital rectal examination every year after age 40
Guaiac test for occult blood every year after 50
Endoscopy every 3 to 5 years after age 50, after two annual negative examinations

Diagnostic Examinations

A client may have a diagnostic test as an outpatient or inpatient. Visualization of GI structures may be by a direct or an indirect approach.

DIRECT VISUALIZATION. Special instruments introduced through the mouth (upper GI viewing) or rectum (lower GI viewing) allow the physician to inspect the integrity of mucosa, blood vessels, and specific organ parts. A fiberoptic **endoscope** is an optical instrument with a lens viewer, a long flexible tube, and a light source at the end. It allows the physician to view structures at the tip of the tube and to insert special instruments for biopsy. The tube is flexible to minimize trauma and discomfort to the client.

Proctoscopes and sigmoidoscopes are rigid tube-shaped instruments with attached light sources. The proctoscope looks like a speculum with a light. These instruments are less flexible than fiberoptic scopes and more capable of causing the client discomfort.

UGI endoscopy or esophagogastroduodenoscopy allows visualization of the esophagus, stomach, and upper duodenum. The physician inspects for tumors, vascular changes, mucosal inflammation, ulcers, hernias, and obstructions. A gastroscope enables the physician to remove tissue specimens for biopsy, remove abnormal tissue growth (polyps), and coagulate sources of bleeding. Nursing implications before the test include the following:

1. Client signs informed consent after receiving explanation of purpose of test.
2. Client takes nothing by mouth after midnight or 6 to 12 hours before test.
3. Client removes dentures.
4. Nurse explains that a local anesthetic is sprayed on the mouth and throat, causing a bitter aftertaste and difficulty in swallowing.
5. Nurse explains that the client may feel fullness in the throat and a sense of gagging during the test.
6. Nurse explains that the client will be awake but unable to speak as the endoscope enters the esophagus.
7. Nurse gives a sedative and an anticholinergic.

Nursing implications during the test include the following:

1. Nurse describes steps of the test to the client.
2. Nurse positions the client in the left Sims' or left lateral position.
3. Nurse offers continuous emotional support.
4. Nurse measures baseline vital signs.
5. Nurse monitors any existing intravenous line.
6. Nurse places tissue specimens in a properly labeled container that is sealed tightly.
7. Nurse has emergency equipment available in case of respiratory complications.

Nursing implications after the test include the following:

1. Because the client's throat is anesthetized, nurse instructs the client to avoid eating or drinking until the gag reflex returns (2 to 4 hours).
2. Nurse explains that hoarseness and the sensation of a sore throat are normal for several days; cool fluids and gargling relieve soreness.
3. Nurse observes for fever, pain, difficulty in swallowing, difficulty in breathing, vomiting, and bloody or black stools (signs of perforation).
4. Nurse monitors vital signs according to agency policy.

Endoscopy allows visualization of the entire large intestine from the anal sphincter to ileocecal valve. The American Cancer Society (1993) recommends this examination every 3 to 5 years after the age of 50 (after two annual normal tests) to detect colorectal cancer. Nursing implications before the test include the following:

1. Nurse explains purpose and nature of test: a digital examination is followed by insertion of the endoscopy tube. Before insertion of the tube, an intravenous (IV) line is established and IV sedatives are administered as needed.
2. Client signs an informed consent.
3. Client receives an enema the night before and the morning of the test (check agency policy.)
4. Client may be allowed clear liquids.
5. Nurse explains that the client might feel minor discomfort and the urge to defecate as the tube is inserted.
6. During the test, the physician might use air to distend the bowel for better visualization; nurse explains that the client may feel "gas pains."

Nursing implications during the test include the following:

1. Nurse positions the client in a knee-chest position face down; Sims' position on the left side is acceptable.
2. Nurse drapes the client to avoid unnecessary exposure and minimize embarrassment.
3. Nurse keeps the client draped and observes for respiratory distress (especially in clients with lung disease who cannot tolerate a head-down position).
4. The nurse monitors O_2 saturation, BP, and pulse.
5. Nurse gives the physician long cotton swabs for removing mucus.
6. Nurse places tissue specimens in a properly labeled container that is tightly sealed.

Nursing implications after the test include the following:

1. Nurse observes for rectal bleeding, rectal or abdominal pain, and fever.
2. Nurse cautions the client to observe for any blood in stools and to report bleeding to a physician.
3. The nurse ensures that the client can stand and ambulate safely, and that a responsible person is available to provide transportation. The client is ready for discharge before all sedation has fully worn off.

INDIRECT VISUALIZATION. When direct visualization is impossible (as with deeper GI structures), the physician relies on indirect x-ray examination. The client ingests a radiopaque contrast medium, or the medium is given as an enema.

UGI is an x-ray study of an ingested contrast medium that allows the physician to visualize the lower esophagus, stomach, and duodenum. The physician notes ulcerations, strictures, motility problems, varices, hiatal hernias, inflammation, tumors, and anatomical malposition of the organs. The patency of the organs and the pyloric valve is also observed. Nursing implications before the test include the following:

1. Nurse explains the nature and purpose of the examination and that the test may take several hours and requires frequent position changes; nurse explains that discomfort is minimal except for lying on a hard examination table. A chalky-tasting barium preparation is given before the test.
2. Client signs an informed consent.
3. Client follows a low-residue diet 1 to 3 days before the test and takes nothing by mouth after midnight on the day of the test.

A nursing implication during the test follows:

1. The test is done in the radiology department; a technician explains the steps of the test.

Nursing implications after the test include the following:

1. Client may resume eating after the test if no further studies are ordered.
2. Client must expel the barium to avoid bowel impaction; nurse instructs the client to increase fluid intake (at least 2 liters after the test); the physician may order a mild laxative or enema; stools are lightly colored until the barium is expelled.

Small bowel follow-through (continuation of UGI) allows the physician to examine the small intestine. The flow of barium through the intestine may suggest motility problems. A barium enema allows indirect visualization of the colon to reveal location of tumors, polyps, and diverticula. The physician can also detect positional abnormalities. Nursing implications before the test include the following:

1. Nurse explains the nature and purpose of the test. Enemas or cathartics are given the evening or morning before the test to thoroughly cleanse the large intestine; cramping and the urge to defecate are normal sensations during the enema. Client will assume several positions while x-ray studies are taken.
2. Client signs informed consent.
3. Bowel preparation varies; client may receive any of the following the evening before the test:
   a. Clear liquids for lunch and supper
   b. One glass of water 8 to 10 hours before the test
   c. Stimulant cathartics
   d. An enema
4. On the day of the test, the client receives additional cathartic by suppository.
5. Nurse explains that a lengthy procedure may cause fatigue.
6. Nurse observes the results of all enemas and cathartics to ensure the bowel is empty before the test.

A nursing implication during the test includes the following:

1. Client expels barium after first set of x-ray films (30 minutes); a repeat film is taken to check for barium retention.

Nursing implications after the test include the following:

1. Client may resume eating after the test.
2. Nurse instructs the client to increase intake of oral fluids to promote barium evacuation and to counteract dehydrating effects of the cathartics.
3. Nurse instructs the client to observe stools for barium; physician may order a mild cathartic.

Nursing Diagnosis

Assessment of the client's bowel function reveals data that may indicate an actual or potential elimination problem or a problem resulting from elimination alterations (see box on p. 961). Associated problems such as body-image changes or skin breakdown may require interventions unrelated to controlling bowel function impairment. However, in some instances, the nurse must di-

NURSING DIAGNOSES FOR BOWEL ELIMINATION PROBLEMS

Constipation
Colonic constipation
Diarrhea
Bowel incontinence
Pain
Toileting self-care deficit
Impaired skin integrity
Body-image disturbance

rect as much attention to altered elimination as to the related problem, highlighting the importance of correctly identifying those related factors. For example, a client with constipation related to reduced activity would require increased ambulation, whereas a client with constipation related to inadequate fiber and fluid intake would require more hydration and bulk forming foods.

The nurse's ability to identify the correct diagnosis by clustering defining characteristics depends not only on the thoroughness of assessment but also on recognition of factors that affect elimination. The nurse should determine the risk and institute measures to ensure maintenance of normal bowel function. Heavy emphasis on promoting health and maintaining good habits already in place is vital.

Planning

After nursing diagnoses are defined, the nurse and client set goals and expected outcomes to direct interventions. The care plan should incorporate the client's elimination routines or habits as much as possible and reinforce those which promote health. However, if these habits caused the problem, the nurse helps the client to learn new ones. Defecation patterns vary among individuals. For this reason, the nurse and client work together to plan effective interventions (see nursing care plan on p. 962). Education is important so that clients can understand normal elimination patterns and the relatively easy ways to promote normal elimination. If clients are physically unable to follow elimination hygiene practices, the family should be included in the care plan. Dietitians and enterostomal therapists can be additional resources for the client. Goals of care for clients with elimination problems include the following:

Goal: Client attains regular defecation habits within 2 weeks.

Outcomes

- Client defecates on a predictable schedule by 1 week
- Client's stool is well formed within 3 days

Goal: Client understands normal elimination.

Outcomes

- Client verbalizes understanding of expected defecation pattern
- Client asks questions indicating appropriate understanding of normal elimination

Goal: Client maintains proper fluid and food intake within 1 week.

Outcomes

- Client increases intake of dietary fiber and whole grains
- Client increases fluid intake while maintaining appropriate urinary output within 3 days

Goal: Client achieves regular exercise program.

Outcomes

- Client maintains a diary demonstrating gradual, age-and-condition–appropriate increases in activities
- Client reports an improvement in defecation pattern as activity increases

Goal: Client's skin integrity is maintained.

Outcomes

- Existing skin breakdown resolves by 1 week
- Client expresses understanding of proper perineal hygiene to prevent skin breakdown

Implementation

The success of interventions depends on improving the client's and family members' understanding of bowel elimination. In the home, hospital, or long-term care facility, clients can be taught effective bowel habits.

Health Promotion Activities

Special emphasis should be on health habits already being practiced and acquiring new health promotion habits. The factors that normally promote bowel elimination—diet, exercise, and timing and privacy—become the nurse's interventions for helping clients to develop normal bowel habits.

Diet. The nurse's assessment will reveal a client's current diet pattern. Depending on the client's elimination problem, specific foods are recommended to ensure proper nutrient intake and normal defecation (see box on p. 963). There is increasing evidence that low fat intake and increases in dietary fiber and bulk forming foods reduce the client's risks of colorectal cancers, digestive diseases, and other cancers (American Cancer Society, 1993; Davidson, et al., 1991; Van Horn, et al., 1991). Assisting clients and their families in different food preparation practices, new menus, and healthy snacking can help to reduce the client's risks of disease.

SAMPLE NURSING CARE PLAN
Constipation

ASSESSMENT

Clinical scenario: Ms. Jefferies is a successful real estate agent who is in to see her physician for a routine checkup. Always on the go, she *rarely takes time to eat a balanced meal* and reportedly drinks about *3 to 4 glasses of fluids daily.* She admits, during the nurse's assessment, that she may *ignore the urge to defecate* if she is hurrying to meet a client. She resorts to *using over-the-counter laxatives* almost weekly. She reports having a bowel movement every 5 to 6 days, and the *stool* is *hard* and difficult to pass at times.

NURSING DIAGNOSIS

Constipation related to inadequate dietary and fluid intake.

PLANNING

Goals	Expected outcomes
Client will establish and maintain a normal defecation pattern within 1 month.	Client will pass soft, formed stools at least every 3 days. Diet will include high-fiber foods within 1 week. Client will drink a minimum of 5 to 6 glasses of fluids daily.

IMPLEMENTATION

Steps	Rationale
1. Suggest easy-to-prepare foods such as fresh fruits and vegetables and whole-grain breads to be included in daily diet.	High-fiber foods increase peristalsis and help propel intestinal contents through GI tract by increasing stool mass and fluid content (Brown, Everett, 1990).
2. Explain to client when gastrocolic reflex normally occurs and how she can time activities to plan for defecation.	Gastrocolic reflex normally occurs approximately 1 hour after breakfast, resulting in mass movement of colon contents (Goldfinger, 1991).
3. Recommend fluids client prefers: cranberry juice, water, grapefruit juice, and hot tea. Have client drink 8 full glasses daily.	Fluids keep fecal mass soft. Senna tea acts as mild laxative, causing increase in colon peristalsis (Ebersole and Hess, 1994).

EVALUATION

Observe character of stool specimen or have client describe it.

Ask client to keep diary of foods and liquids ingested for 1 week and review during a follow-up phone call.

Defining characteristics are shown in italic type.

Consideration must be given to whether a client can afford the foods recommended. In addition to solid foods, the nurse encourages the client to drink 2000 to 3000 ml of fluids daily, if not contraindicated by other medical conditions.

Exercise. An age-related exercise program also assists clients in maintaining healthy bowel patterns. Regular exercise, 3 to 5 times a week, promotes normal gastrointestinal motility. Walking, swimming, and cycling are excellent forms of exercise. A client immobilized by illness should ambulate as soon as possible. Clients restricted to bed may benefit from active range-of-motion exercises.

Timing and Privacy. One of the most important habits a nurse can teach a client regarding bowel habits is to take time for defecation. Ignoring the urge to defecate and not taking time to defecate completely are common causes of constipation. To establish regular bowel habits, a client must know when the urge to defecate normally occurs.

The nurse advises the client to begin establishing a routine during a time when defecation is most likely to occur, usually an hour after meals. If attempts are made to defecate during the time when mass colonic peristalsis occurs, the chances of success are great. If a client is restricted to bed or requires assistance in ambulating, the nurse should offer a bedpan or help the client to

GERONTOLOGIC NURSING PRACTICE

Changes in bowel function occurring with aging are similar to those changes in function that occur with reduced activity level. There are, however, certain nursing practices that can reduce the risk and occurrence of bowel elimination alterations in the older adult.

- Maintaining a proper diet, including appropriate intake of fluid and bulk, is important in reducing constipation. Fiber (4-6 g, which is equal to 3-4 tablespoons of bran per day) is recommended to reduce the risk of constipation (Kane, Ouslander, Abrass, 1994).
- Proper body position can facilitate bowel evacuation.
- Scheduling time periods for bowel elimination is important in assisting the older adult in maintaining normal elimination patterns.
- Educate older adults on the dangers of excessive laxative/cathartic use for bowel elimination. These medications may cause an atonic colon, thus contributing to chronic constipation (Kane, Ouslander, Abrass, 1994).
- Instruct clients that if their stool is soft and passes easily that it is not necessary to have a bowel movement daily. If clients should miss a daily movement, it does not mean that they are constipated and require a laxative.
- Instruct clients that travel changes in dietary intake can cause transient changes in bowel elimination patterns.

DIETARY RECOMMENDATIONS FOR ELIMINATION PROBLEMS

CONSTIPATION

Increase intake of high-fiber foods. Added fluids should accompany increase in fiber intake.

Vegetables (dried beans, brussels sprouts, corn, peas, and potatoes)

Fruits (apples with peels, raisins, and prunes)

Cereals (bran and whole wheat) and whole grain breads

For the older adult with poor dentition, offer chopped, not pureed, foods. Add extra chopped vegetables to soups.

Persons with difficulties in swallowing need mashed, not pureed, foods. Liquids such as fruit juices and hot tea are beneficial.

DIARRHEA

Avoid spicy or high-fiber foods.

Increase intake of low-fiber foods: chicken, fish, lean beef, pasta, and milk products.

If diarrhea causes serious fluid loss, replace with water, weak tea, gelatin, plain soda, and bouillon.

FLATULENCE

Avoid gas-producing foods: cauliflower, broccoli, brussels sprouts, onions, dried beans and lentils, and beer.

OSTOMIES

Remember that the location of an ostomy determines the type of diet needed for regular evacuation. Initially place clients on low-fiber diets to avoid irritation to mucosa and stomal obstruction.

Remind ostomy clients to eat slowly and chew food well when on low-fiber diets.

Avoid foods that may cause blockage: blackberries and raspberries, oranges, red apples with tough skins, bing cherries, large quantities of corn, Chinese bean sprouts in large amounts, stringy beef, popcorn, and hot dogs with heavy skins.

reach the bathroom. The nurse must be prompt in assisting before the urge disappears.

Many clients have established rituals for defecation. In a hospital or long-term care facility, the nurse should ensure that treatments do not interfere with the client's schedule. It is also important to provide privacy. When a client required to use a bedpan shares a room with another person, the nurse should pull the curtain around the client's area so that the client can relax, knowing that interruptions will not occur. The call light should always be placed within the client's reach. Bathroom doors should be closed, although the nurse may stand close by in case the client needs assistance.

Promotion of Normal Defecation

To help clients evacuate bowel contents normally and without discomfort, the nurse may use a number of interventions. These interventions stimulate the defecation reflex, affect the character of feces, or increase peristalsis.

Squatting Position. The nurse might need to assist clients who have difficulty in squatting because of muscular weakness and mobility problems. Regular toilets are too low for clients unable to lower themselves to a squatting position because of joint- or muscle-wasting diseases. Clients can purchase elevated toilet seats for the home. With such a seat, less effort is needed to sit or stand. In orthopedic and rehabilitation units in a health care center, toilet seats are elevated.

Positioning on Bedpan. A client restricted to bed must use a bedpan for defecation. Women use bedpans to pass urine and feces, whereas men use bedpans only for defecation. Sitting on a bedpan can be uncomfortable

procedure 33-2

ASSISTING A CLIENT ON AND OFF A BEDPAN

Steps	Rationale
1. Assess client's level of mobility and strength.	Determines degree of assistance required by nurse and safest positioning technique.
2. Plan to offer bedpan to coincide with duodenocolic or mass peristaltic reflex.	Reflex commonly occurs about 1 hour after meals.
3. Collect equipment:	
a. Bedpan	
b. Toilet tissue	
c. Disposable gloves	Used if there is chance nurse will contact fecal material.
d. Small, rolled towel	
e. Disposable cover for bedpan	
f. Talcum powder	
g. Handwashing supplies	
4. Wash, dry, and apply gloves.	
5. Assemble supplies at bedside and close curtains.	Organizes activities to increase efficiency. Provides privacy.
6. Explain procedure (especially if assistance is needed).	Ensures cooperation and participation.
7. If metal bedpan is used, run warm water over it.	Cold bedpan may cause client to tense muscles of abdomen and buttocks. Relaxation promotes defecation.
8. Raise bed to highest working level.	Minimizes strain on nurse's back and muscles while assisting client with bedpan.
9. Be sure client is positioned high in bed, with head elevated 30 degrees (unless contraindicated) with bedpan at side or foot of bed.	Prevents hyperextension of back and provides support to upper torso as client raises onto pan.
10. Fold back top linen to client's knees.	Provides for minimal exposure of client during bedpan placement.
11. Give client assistance if needed:	Allows client to effectively lift hips above level of pan with minimal energy. Supports client's back, with arm acting as lever in lifting.
a. Instruct client to bend knees and place weight on heels.	
b. Place hand, palm up, under client's sacrum, resting elbow on mattress.	
c. Have client lift hips while nurse slips bedpan into place with other hand (see illustration).	Uses minimal energy and prevents abrasion of pan against skin.
12. Aid immobile clients:	
a. Lower head of bed flat and have client roll onto one side.	Allows client to roll onto pan.
b. Apply powder lightly to lower back and buttocks.	Prevents skin from sticking to pan.
c. Place bedpan firmly against buttocks and push down into mattress with open rim toward client's feet.	Reduces size of pan over which client must roll.

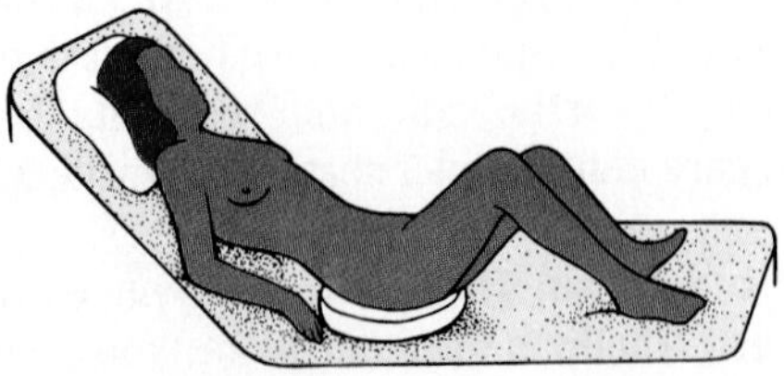

Step 11c

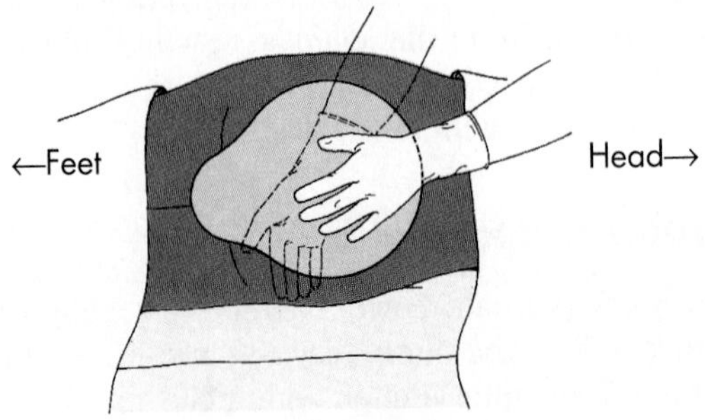

Step 12d

Steps	Rationale
d. Keeping hand against bedpan, place other around client's forehip. Ask client to roll onto pan, flat on bed (see illustration).	Client and pan roll as one unit, minimizing discomfort.
e. With client positioned comfortably, raise head of bed 30 degrees.	Allows client to strain more normally during defecation.
13. Place rolled towel under lumbar curve of client's back.	Offers added comfort, reducing strain on lumbar curve.
14. Place call light and toilet tissue within client's reach. Keep side rails up as appropriate.	Prevents falls.
15. Remove bedpan as client lifts hips up or as client carefully rolls off pan and to side. Hold pan firmly as client moves.	Prevents exposure to microorganisms in feces and accidental spillage of pan contents.
16. Assist client in wiping soiled anal area. Wipe from pubic area to anus. Replace top covers.	Promotes comfort and reduces transmission of microorganisms.
17. If specimen is required or intake and output are measured, do not dispose of tissue in bedpan. Place tissue in proper receptacle. Cover pan.	Tissue interferes with specimen analysis and output measurement.
18. Have client wash and dry hands.	Reduces transmission of microorganisms.
19. Empty bedpan contents and dispose of gloves and wash hands.	Reduces transmission of microorganisms.
20. Record intake and output, if ordered.	Diarrheal stool or urine is counted as output.

and awkward. The nurse should help to position the client comfortably.

Two types of bedpans are available. The regular bedpan, made of metal or hard plastic, has a curved smooth upper end and a sharp-edged lower end, and is about 5 cm (2 inches) deep. A fracture pan, designed for clients with body or leg casts or for whom semi-Fowler's position is contraindicated, has a shallow upper end about 1.3 cm (½ inch) deep. The upper end of either pan fits under the buttocks toward the sacrum, with the lower end just under the upper thighs. The pan should be high enough so that feces enter it. A metal bedpan should be warmed first.

The most important element for the nurse to consider in positioning the client is preventing muscle strain and discomfort. A client should never be placed on a bedpan and then left with the bed flat unless activity restrictions demand it. If the bed is flat, the client is forced to hyperextend the back to lift the hips onto the pan. It may sometimes be necessary to have the bed flat when placing the client on the bedpan. After the client is on it, the nurse raises the head of the bed 30 degrees. Raising the client to a 90-degree angle can make positioning difficult. In a sitting position, the client must rise straight up while using the strength of the arms as the nurse positions the pan. Most clients are too weak to accomplish this. Clients who have had abdominal surgery hesitate to exert strain on suture lines. Furthermore, the nurse risks injury in trying to lift the client onto the bedpan. Clients who have overhead trapeze frames can easily lift themselves by grasping the trapeze bar. Procedure 33-2 describes steps in assisting a client with a bedpan. A bedside commode can be a safe, effective alternative to a bedpan. Its use is less exhausting and allows the client to assume a more "normal or familiar" position for defecation.

Cathartics and Laxatives. A client is often unable to defecate normally because of pain, constipation, or impaction. **Cathartics** and **laxatives** have the short-term action of emptying the bowel. They are also used in bowel evacuation for clients undergoing GI tests and abdominal surgery. Although the terms *cathartic* and *laxative* are often used interchangeably, cathartics have a stronger effect on the intestines.

Cathartics and laxatives are available in oral, tablet, and powder suppository forms (see Chapter 26). The same medication can sometimes be classified as a cathartic or a laxative, depending on the amount used. Although the oral route is more commonly used, cathartics that come prepared as suppositories are more effective because of their stimulant effect on the rectal mucosa. Cathartic suppositories such as bisacodyl (Dulcolax) may act within 30 minutes. The nurse should give the suppository shortly before the client's usual time to defecate or immediately after a meal.

The nurse teaches clients about the potential harmful effects of repeated use of laxatives. The client should understand that laxatives and cathartics are not meant for long-term maintenance of bowel function.

Five types of cathartics are available. The classes are based on the method by which the agent promotes defecation.

Stimulant cathartics cause local irritation to the intestinal mucosa and inhibit reabsorption of water in the large intestine. Intestinal irritation increases intestinal motility. The rapid movement of feces causes retention of water in the stool. The drugs can cause formation of a soft to fluid stool in 6 to 8 hours. Clients tend to abuse stimulants more than other cathartics. Overuse leads to loss of intestinal tone. Commonly used stimulant cathartics include castor oil, cascara, phenolphthalein (Ex-Lax or Feen-A-Mint), and bisacodyl (Dulcolax). Nurses should warn mothers who breast feed that cascara is excreted in the milk. Phenolphthalein comes in a chewable gum or candy form and thus should be kept away from children because it can be toxic in large doses.

Saline or osmotic agents contain a salt preparation not absorbed by the intestines. The cathartic draws water into the fecal mass. This osmotic action increases the bulk of the intestinal contents and enhances lubrication. Rapid bowel evacuation may occur in 1 to 3 hours. Magnesium hydroxide (Milk of Magnesia) and sodium phosphate (Phospho-Soda) are saline cathartics. Clients with impaired kidney function should avoid using these drugs because of the toxic buildup of magnesium.

Wetting agents or stool softeners are detergents that lower the surface tension of feces, allowing penetration by water and fat. These drugs also inhibit absorption of water by the intestines. The fecal mass becomes large and soft. Commonly used wetting agents are dioctyl sodium sulfosuccinate (Colace) and dioctyl calcium sulfosuccinate (Surfak). A wetting agent is most effective when the goal is to prevent the client from straining during defecation. Several days can pass before effects of the drug are noted.

Bulk-forming cathartics consist of cellulose and polysaccharides that absorb water and increase solid intestinal bulk. The fecal bulk stretches the intestinal walls, stimulating peristalsis. Passage of stool will occur in 12 to 24 hours. Bulk laxatives are the least irritating and safest of all cathartics. When mixed with water, they can solidify if not swallowed quickly.

Clients should be encouraged to take bulk cathartics with plenty of fluids to prevent hardening of the drug and intestinal obstruction. Bulk-forming laxatives can also relieve a mild watery diarrhea by absorbing water to produce a soft-formed stool. Common bulk-forming cathartics are methylcellulose (Hydrolose) prune powder and psyllium hydrocolloid (Metamucil).

Lubricants soften the fecal mass, thus easing the strain of defecation. Clients with painful hemorrhoids particularly benefit from a lubricant. The only lubricant laxative available is mineral oil. Regular use of mineral oil interferes with absorption of the fat-soluble vitamins A, D, E, and K. The drug can also cause a dangerous form of pneumonia if aspirated.

Antidiarrheal Agents. For clients with diarrhea, the frequent passage of liquid stools becomes a problem. The most effective antidiarrheal agents are opiates such as codeine phosphate, paregoric, and diphenoxylate (Lomotil) and other drugs such as bismuth subsalicylate (Pepto-Bismol). Antidiarrheal agents decrease intestinal muscle tone to slow the passage of feces. Opiates inhibit peristaltic waves that move feces forward but also increase the segmental contractions that mix intestinal contents. As a result, more water is absorbed by intestinal walls. Antidiarrheal agents should be used with caution because opiates are habit forming.

Enemas. An **enema** is instillation of a preparation into the rectum and sigmoid colon. An enema is given primarily to promote defecation by stimulating peristalsis. The volume of fluid instilled breaks up the fecal mass, stretches the rectal wall, and initiates the defecation reflex. Enemas are also given as a vehicle for drugs that exert a local effect on rectal mucosa.

The most common use for an enema is temporary relief of constipation. Other indications include removing impacted feces; emptying the bowel before diagnostic tests, surgery, or childbirth; and beginning a program of bowel training.

Clients should be discouraged from relying on enemas to maintain bowel regularity. Enemas do not treat the cause of constipation. As with laxative abuse, frequent use destroys normal defecation reflexes.

Types. There are several types of enemas. Cleansing enemas promote complete evacuation of feces from the colon. They act by stimulating peristalsis through the infusion of a large volume of solution or through local irritation of the colon's mucosa. Suggested maximum volumes follow:

Infant	150 to 250 ml
Toddler	250 to 350 ml
School-age child	300 to 500 ml
Adolescent	500 to 750 ml
Adult	750 to 1000 ml

Cleansing enemas include tap water, normal saline, hypertonic saline, and soapsuds solution. Each solution exerts a different osmotic effect, causing the movement of fluids between the colon and interstitial spaces beyond the intestinal wall. Infants and children can tolerate only normal saline because they are at risk for fluid imbalance.

Tap water is hypotonic and exerts a lower osmotic pressure than fluid in interstitial spaces. After infusion into the colon, tap water escapes from the bowel lumen into interstitial spaces. The net movement of water is low; the infused volume stimulates defecation before large amounts of water leave the bowel. Tap water enemas should not be repeated because water toxicity or circulatory overload can develop if large amounts of water are absorbed.

Physiologically, normal saline is the safest solution to use because it exerts the same osmotic pressure as fluids in interstitial spaces around the bowel. The volume of infused saline stimulates peristalsis. Giving saline enemas does not create the danger of excess fluid absorption. If prepared saline is not available at home, 500 ml (1 pint) of tap water mixed with 1 teaspoon of table salt can be substituted.

Hypertonic solutions infused into the bowel exert osmotic pressure that pulls fluids out of interstitial spaces. The colon fills with fluid, and the resultant distention promotes defecation. Clients unable to tolerate large volumes of fluid benefit most from this type of enema.

Hypertonic enemas are contraindicated for dehydrated clients and young infants. A hypertonic solution of 120 to 180 ml (4 to 6 ounces) is usually effective. The Fleet's enema is most commonly used.

Soap solution may be added to tap water or saline to create the additional effect of intestinal irritation. Only pure castile soap is safe. Harsh soaps or detergents can cause serious bowel inflammation. The recommended ratio of soap to solution is 5 ml (1 teaspoon) of castile soap to 1000 ml of warm water or saline.

A physician may order a high or low cleansing enema. High enemas are given to cleanse the entire colon. Fluid is delivered at a high pressure by raising the enema container to a high level. During administration of a regular enema, the enema can or bag is held 30 to 45 cm (12 to 18 inches) above the client's hips. Thus with a high enema, the can is raised to 18 inches. The client is asked to turn from the left lateral to the dorsal recumbent, over to the right lateral position. The position change ensures that fluid reaches the large intestine. With a low enema, the nurse holds the enema bag 12 inches or less above the client's hips. A low enema cleans only the rectum and sigmoid colon.

Oil retention enemas lubricate the rectum and colon. The feces absorb the oil and become softer and easier to pass. To enhance action of the oil, the client retains the enema for several hours if possible.

Carminative enemas provide relief from gaseous distention. They improve the ability to pass flatus. An example of a carminative enema is MGW solution, which contains 30 ml of magnesium, 60 ml of glycerin, and 90 ml of water.

A return flow enema, or **Harris flush,** is a mild colonic irrigation that helps to expel flatus. The nurse first administers a small amount (100 to 200 ml) of mild enema solution into the rectum and colon. Then the nurse lowers the enema container to allow the solution to flow back through the rectal tube and into the container. Repeating this process several times aids in reducing flatus and promoting peristalsis.

Medicated enemas contain drugs. An example is polystyrene sodium sulfonate (Kayexalate), used to treat clients with dangerously high serum potassium levels. This drug contains a resin that exchanges sodium ions for potassium ions in the large intestine. Another medicated enema is neomycin solution, an antibiotic used to reduce bacteria in the colon before bowel surgery.

ADMINISTRATION. The nurse administers enemas in commercially packaged, disposable units or with reusable equipment prepared before use. Sterile technique is unnecessary because the colon contains bacteria. However, the nurse must wear gloves to prevent contact with microorganisms. Procedure 33-3 outlines the steps for enema administration.

The nurse should explain the procedure, including the position to assume, precautions to take to avoid discomfort, and the length of time necessary to retain the solution before defecation. If the client will receive the enema at home, the nurse explains the procedure to a family member.

The physician often orders "enemas till clear," which means that the enema is repeated until the client passes fluid that is clear and contains no fecal material. It may be necessary to give as many as three enemas, but the nurse should caution the client against using more than three. Excess enema use seriously depletes fluids and electrolytes. If the enema fails to return a clear solution after 3 times, the physician should be notified.

When an enema is given to a child, it helps to have a parent assist. The child should understand each step and be able to see the equipment for the procedure.

Giving an enema to a client unable to contract the external sphincter can cause difficulties. The nurse gives the enema with the client positioned on the bedpan. Giving the enema with the client sitting on the toilet is unsafe because the curved rectal tubing can abrade the rectal wall.

Digital Removal of Stool. For clients with an impaction, the fecal mass may be too large to be passed voluntarily. If enemas fail, the nurse must break up the fecal mass with the fingers and remove it in sections. The procedure can be very uncomfortable for the client. Excess rectal manipulation may cause irritation to the mucosa, bleeding, and stimulation of the vagus nerve, which can result in a reflex slowing of the heart rate. Because of the procedure's potential complications, in many institutions only physicians are allowed to remove

procedure 33-3

ADMINISTERING A CLEANSING ENEMA

Steps	Rationale
1. Assess status of client, last bowel movement, normal bowel patterns, presence of hemorrhoids, mobility, and external sphincter control.	Determines factors that indicate need for enema and influence method of administration.
2. Review physician's order for enema.	To determine number of enemas client will require; to determine type of enema to be given. Nurse must know this to organize equipment and prepare client.
3. Collect appropriate equipment:	Organizes activities, thereby increasing efficiency.
a. Disposable enema bag administration:	
(1) Disposable enema container with tubing and clamp	
(2) Appropriately sized rectal tube Adult: #22 to #30 French (Fr) Child: #12 to #18 Fr	Rectal tubing should be small enough to fit diameter of anus and large enough to prevent leakage of solution from around tube.
(3) Correct volume (average adult: 750 to 1000 ml) of warmed solution	Nurse must be aware of amount of fluid a client can safely tolerate. Hot water can burn intestinal mucosa; cold water can cause abdominal cramping and is difficult to retain.
(4) Additional additive such as soap or salt	Combined with solution, creates an osmotic effect to move fluids between colon and interstitial spaces.
(5) Lubricating jelly	Reduces friction and irritation to rectal mucosa.
(6) Waterproof pad	Prevents soiling bed linens.
(7) Bath blanket	Covers trunk and lower extremities and reduces exposure of body parts.
(8) Toilet tissue	
(9) Bedpan, plus commode chair or access to toilet	Depends on client's level of mobility.
(10) Disposable gloves	Protect nurse's hands and reduce spread of microorganisms.
(11) Washcloth, towel, and basin	Used to cleanse client after procedure, depending on level of mobility.
(12) Intravenous pole	Used to hang solution container.
b. Pepackaged enema:	
(1) Prepackaged disposable bottle with rectal tip	Contains solution and smooth tip for insertion.
(2) Disposable gloves	
(3) Lubricating jelly	
(4) Waterproof pad	
(5) Bath blanket	
(6) Toilet tissue	
(7) Bedpan or commode	
(8) Washcloth, towel, and basin	
4. Correctly identify client and explain procedure.	Reduces anxiety and promotes cooperation.
5. If using enema bag, assemble with appropriate solution and rectal tube.	
6. Wash, dry, and apply gloves.	Reduces transmission of infection.
7. Provide privacy by closing curtains around bed or closing door to room.	Reduces embarrassment.
8. Raise bed to appropriate working height and raise side rail on opposite side.	Promotes use of good body mechanics and client safety.

Steps	Rationale
9. Assist client into left side-lying (Sims') position with right knee flexed. Children may be placed in dorsal recumbent position. Position clients with poor sphincter control on bedpan in comfortable dorsal recumbent position.	Allows enema solution to flow downward by gravity along natural curve of sigmoid colon and rectum, thus improving retention of solution. (Clients with poor sphincter control cannot retain all enema solution.)
10. Place waterproof pad under hips and buttocks.	Prevents soiling linen.
11. Cover client with bath blanket, exposing only rectal area.	Provides warmth, reduces exposure of body parts, and allows client to feel more relaxed and comfortable.
12. Place bedpan or commode in easily accessible position. If client will be expelling contents in toilet, ensure that it is free.	Used in case client cannot retain enema solution.
13. Administer enema using prepackaged, disposable container:	
a. Remove plastic cap from rectal tip. Tip is already lubricated, but apply more jelly as needed.	Lubrication provides for smooth insertion of rectal tube without causing rectal irritation or trauma.
b. Gently separate buttocks and locate rectum. Instruct client to relax by breathing out slowly through mouth.	Breathing out promotes relaxation of external sphincter.
c. Insert tip of bottle gently into rectum. Advance tip: Adult: 7.5 to 10 cm (3 to 4 in) Child: 5 to 7.5 cm (2 to 3 in) Infant: 2.5 to 3.75 cm (1 to 1.5 in)	Prevents trauma to rectal mucosa.
d. Squeeze bottle until all solution has entered rectum and colon. (Most bottles contain about 250 ml).	Hypertonic solutions require only small volumes to stimulate defecation.
14. Administer enema using disposable enema bag:	
a. Add warmed solution to enema bag. (Warm tap water as it flows from faucet. Place saline container in basin of hot water before adding saline to enema bag.) Check temperature of solution by pouring small amount of solution over inner wrist. If a soap solution is ordered it is added *after* the solution.	Hot water can burn intestinal mucosa; cold water can cause abdominal cramping and is difficult to retain.
b. Raise container, release clamp, and allow solution to flow long enough to fill tubing.	Removes air from tubing.
c. Reclamp tubing.	Prevents further loss of solution.
d. Lubricate 7.5 to 10 cm (3 to 4 in) of tip of rectal tube with lubricating jelly.	Allows smooth insertion of rectal tube without risk of irritation or trauma to the mucosa.
e. Gently separate buttocks and locate anus. Instruct client to relax by breathing out slowly through mouth.	Breathing out promotes relaxation of external sphincter.
f. Insert tip of rectal tube slowly by pointing tip in direction of umbilicus. Length of insertion is: Adult: 7.5 to 10 cm (3 to 4 in) Child: 5 to 7.5 cm (2 to 3 in) Infant: 2.5 to 3.75 cm (1 to 1.5 in)	Prevents trauma to rectal mucosa from accidental lodging of tube against rectal wall. Insertion beyond proper limit can cause bowel perforation.
g. Hold tubing in rectum constantly until end of fluid instillation.	Bowel contraction can cause expulsion of rectal tube.
h. Open regulating clamp and allow solution to enter slowly with container at client's hip level.	Rapid infusion can stimulate evacuation of rectal tube.

Continued.

procedure 33-3—cont'd

Steps	Rationale
i. Raise height of enema container slowly to appropriate level above anus (see illustration): High enema: 45 cm (18 in) Low enema: 30 cm (12 in) Infant: 7.5 cm (3 in) Infusion time varies with volume of solution administered (e.g., 1 L in 10 min).	Allows for continuous, slow infusion of solution. Raising container too high causes rapid infusion and possible painful distention of colon. High pressure can cause rupture of the bowel in infants.

Step 14i

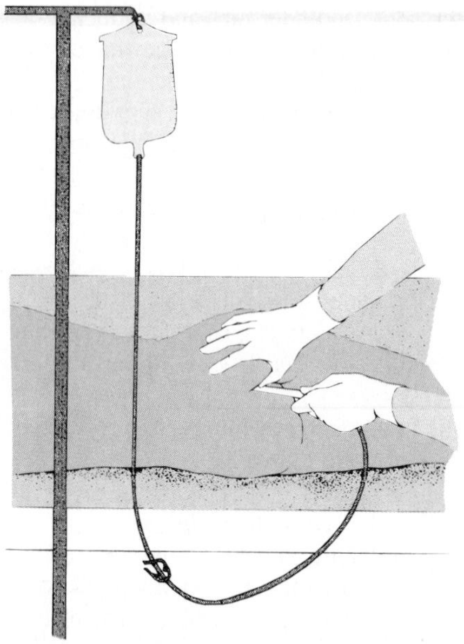

Steps	Rationale
j. Lower container or clamp tubing if client complains of cramping or if liquid escapes around rectal tube.	Temporary cessation of infusion prevents cramping, which may prevent client from retaining all fluid, altering effectiveness of enema.
k. Clamp tubing after all solution is infused.	Prevents entrance of air into rectum.
15. Place layers of toilet tissue around tube at anus and gently withdraw rectal tube.	Provides for comfort and cleanliness.
16. Explain to client that feeling of distention is normal. Ask client to retain solution for 5 to 10 min or as long as possible while lying quietly in bed. (For infant or young child, gently hold buttocks together for few minutes.)	Solution distends the bowel. Length of retention varies with type of enema and client's ability to contract anal sphincter. Longer retention promotes more effective stimulation of peristalsis and defecation.
17. Discard enema container and tubing in proper receptacle.	Controls transmission and growth of microorganisms.
18. Assist client to bathroom or help to position client on bedpan.	Normal squatting position promotes defecation.
19. Observe character of feces and solution. (Caution client against flushing toilet before inspection.)	When enemas are ordered "until clear," it is essential to observe contents of solution passed.
20. Assist client as needed to wash anal area with warm soap and water.	Fecal content can irritate skin. Hygiene promotes comfort.
21. Inspect character of stool and fluid passed.	Determines whether stool is evacuated or fluid is retained.
22. Remove gloves by pulling them inside out and discarding in proper receptacle.	Prevents transmission of microorganisms.
23. Wash hands.	Reduces transmission of infection.
24. Record pertinent information: a. Type and volume of enema given b. Color, amount, and consistency of fecal return	Communicates pertinent information to all members of health care team. Prompt recording improves documentation of treatment.

impactions digitally. If the nurse performs the procedure, a physician's order is necessary.

The steps for removing stool digitally include the following:

1. Explain the procedure and help the client to lie on the left side with knees flexed and back toward the nurse.
2. Drape the trunk and lower extremities with a bath blanket and place a waterproof pad under the buttocks. Keep a bedpan next to the client.
3. Apply disposable gloves, and lubricate the index finger of dominant hand with lubricating jelly.
4. Gently insert the index finger into the rectum and advance the finger slowly along the rectal wall toward the umbilicus.
5. Gently loosen the fecal mass by massaging around it. Work the finger into the hardened mass.
6. Work the feces downward toward the end of the rectum. Remove small pieces at a time and discard into bedpan.
7. Reassess the client's heart rate and look for signs of fatigue. Stop the procedure if the heart rate drops significantly or the rhythm changes.
8. Continue to remove feces, and allow the client to rest at intervals.
9. After completion, offer a washcloth and towel to wash and dry the buttocks and anal area. Assist as needed.
10. Remove bedpan and dispose of feces. Remove gloves by turning them inside out, then discard.
11. Assist client to toilet or clean bedpan if urge to defecate develops.
12. Wash hands. Record results of disimpaction by describing fecal characteristics.
13. Follow procedure with enemas or cathartics as ordered by physician.

Bowel Training. The client with incontinence cannot maintain bowel control. A bowel training program can help some clients, especially those who still have some neuromuscular control, to achieve normal defecation. The training program involves setting up a daily routine. By attempting to defecate at the same time each day and using measures that promote defecation, the client gains control of bowel reflexes. The program requires time, patience, and consistency. The physician determines the client's physical readiness and ability to benefit from bowel training. A successful program includes the following elements:

1. Explain the purpose of the program to the client, and involve him or her in the development of a plan to achieve bowel control.
2. Assess the client's normal elimination pattern, and record times of incontinence.
3. Choose a time in the client's pattern to initiate defecation-control measures.
4. Develop a plan for promoting normal elimination habits; include regular exercise, fiber and fluids in diet, and time to defecate.
5. Begin program with an empty bowel.
6. Begin daily training program. It usually takes 2 to 3 weeks before a regular pattern returns:
   a. Give stool softeners orally every day or a cathartic suppository at least 30 minutes before the selected defecation time.
   b. Offer a hot drink or fruit juice (or any fluid that normally stimulates peristalsis for the client) before the defecation time.
   c. Assist the client to the toilet at the designated time.
   d. Provide privacy and set a time limit for defecation (15 to 20 minutes).
   e. Instruct the client to lean forward at the hips while sitting on the toilet, to apply manual pressure with the hands over the abdomen, and to bear down but not strain to stimulate colon emptying.
   f. Do not criticize or convey frustration if the client cannot defecate.
   g. Encourage the client when measures are successful.

Care of Bowel Diversions

A client with a temporary or permanent bowel diversion has a unique health care problem. His or her elimination pattern differs from the pattern of clients with an intact

CLIENT TEACHING FOR STOMA CARE

Teach client to avoid use of alcohol to cleanse around a stoma. Alcohol dilates capillaries to cause bleeding of the stomal margin.

Instruct client to wash skin with mild soap and water or commercial preparations such as PeriWash. Pat or blot dry the skin thoroughly.

Tell client not to use cold cream on peristomal skin because it prevents pouches from adhering to skin.

Teach client to avoid use of peroxide around or on stoma because it irritates tissue.

If yeast infections develop, instruct client to wash thoroughly but gently, pat dry, apply medically prescribed Kenalog spray and Mycostatin topical powder to irritated skin.

Teach client to routinely inspect the appearance of the stoma and surrounding skin. (The stoma should be moist, shiny, and dark pink to red.) Bleeding around the stoma should be minimal. Tell client to report excess bleeding, abnormal color, or edema to the nurse or physician.

colon. This client wears a pouch or appliance to collect stool emitted from the stoma. Meticulous skin care is needed to prevent liquid stool from irritating skin around a stoma (see box on p. 971). Some clients irrigate their ostomies (similar to enema procedures) to establish regular bowel elimination routines. A client with an ostomy must also follow good health practices such as eating properly and exercising regularly. This client often faces psychological stress from changes in body image resulting from the stoma and body odors that sometimes accompany stool emissions. The nurse must involve this client early in self-care to promote independence and acceptance of the ostomy. The nurse's acceptance and understanding are essential to helping such a client achieve a more normal life-style. Many clients are reassured by the information and encouragement from ostomy support groups.

Pouching Ostomies. Ostomies require a pouch to collect fecal material. An effective pouching system protects the skin, contains feces, and is comfortable and inconspicuous. A person wearing a pouch should feel secure when participating in any activity.

Many pouching systems are available. To ensure that a pouch fits well and meets the client's needs, the nurse considers the type of ostomy, size and contour of the abdomen, condition of the skin around the stoma, physical activities of the client, client's personal preference, and cost of equipment. An enterostomal therapist (ET) is a specially trained nurse who can assist a client in selecting the correct system.

A pouching system consists of a pouch and skin barrier (Figure 33-5). Pouches come in disposable or reusable one- and two-piece systems. Skin barriers include wafers, pastes, powders, and a liquid film that is applied to the skin around the stoma. A good skin barrier protects the skin and prevents irritation from repeated pouch removal.

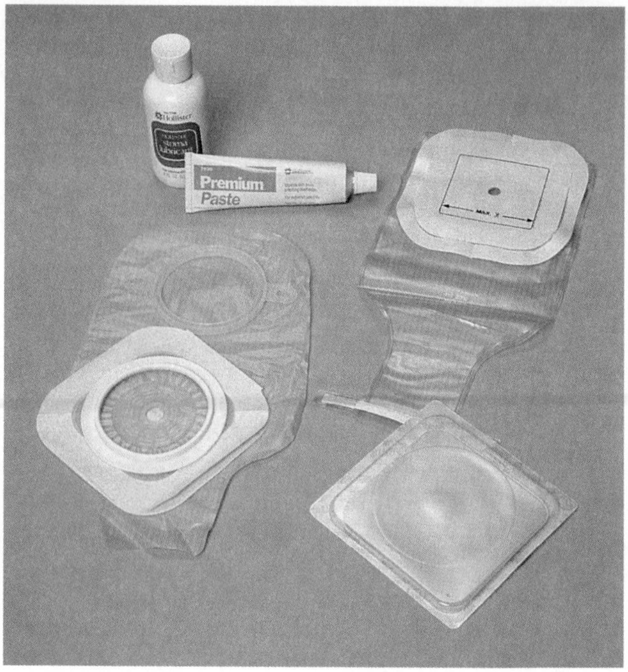

FIGURE 33-5 Ostomy pouches and skin barriers.

Before applying the pouch, the nurse removes the old pouch and thoroughly cleanses and dries the skin around the stoma. The nurse observes the condition of the skin and stoma. The client should participate in the procedure so that he or she can learn to recognize the normal appearance of the stoma, which is moist and red.

The pouch is changed when there is little drainage from the ostomy (e.g., before a meal or bedtime). After the skin is cleansed and thoroughly dried, the pouch and barrier are applied over the stoma. Care must be taken to not cut or constrict the stoma with the pouch system. The end of the pouch is clamped to collect drainage.

Ostomy Irrigation. To establish a pattern of regular defecation, clients with sigmoid colostomies may irrigate their colostomy daily or every other day. The irrigation procedure is identical to that of giving an enema; however, the shape of the stoma requires the use of a special cone-tipped irrigating tube (Figure 33-6). Care must be taken to avoid trauma to the stoma or bowel. Clients typically use warm tap water to cleanse the bowel. Emptying the bowel at a scheduled time prevents stomal discharges between irrigations. The client gains greater freedom without the need to wear a stomal pouch continuously.

Most clients prefer sitting on the toilet during irrigation. Because the stoma has no sphincter, the irrigating solution begins to drain when the cone is removed. The client wears a long plastic irrigating sheath or bag that extends from the stoma down into the toilet. The irrigating solution drains from the stoma into the toilet without soiling the skin. It may take up to an hour for feces and solution to be totally expelled. After the greatest portion has passed, the client may choose to close the bottom of the irrigating sheath and wear it as a bag until drainage stops. This allows the client to resume normal activity more quickly.

Promotion of Client Comfort

Many clients experience discomfort as a result of alterations in elimination. The client with hemorrhoids has pain when hemorrhoidal tissues are directly irritated. Flatulence can also create discomfort, particularly if abdominal distention develops.

The primary goal for the client with hemorrhoids is soft-formed stools. Proper diet, fluids, and regular exer-

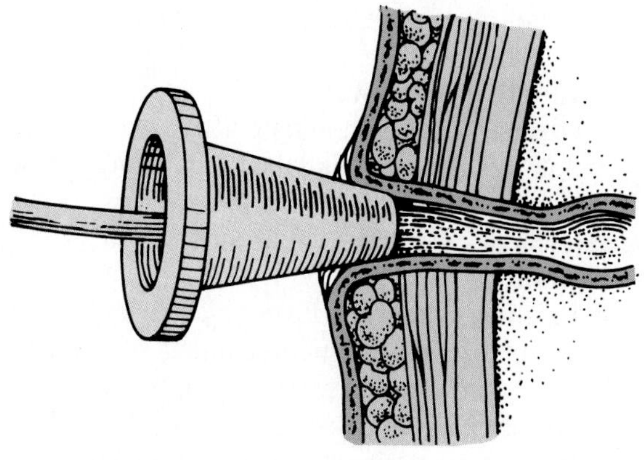

FIGURE 33-6 Irrigating cone and catheter used for ostomy irrigation.

cise improve the likelihood of soft stools. If the client becomes constipated, passage of hard stools will cause bleeding and irritation.

Local heat provides temporary relief to swollen hemorrhoids. A sitz bath is the most effective means of heat application.

Hemorrhoids often become so enlarged that they cover the rectum. To prevent trauma to tissues, the nurse must use caution when inserting rectal thermometers, suppositories, or rectal tubes. A generous amount of lubricating jelly reduces friction when an object is inserted past a hemorrhoid. Often the client is better able to insert an object safely into the rectum. The nurse should never attempt to force an object into the rectum without full view of the anus. When hemorrhoids cause chronic pain, surgical removal is the best treatment.

To relieve the discomfort of flatulence, the nurse should use measures that reduce flatus or promote its escape. Air swallowing increases flatus. The client can reduce the amount of air swallowed by not drinking carbonated beverages, not using straws for drinking, and not chewing gum or hard candies. When flatulence becomes severe as a result of reduced peristalsis, a nasogastric tube is often used.

When flatulence results in abdominal cramping, ambulation promotes the passage of flatus. Having the client walk down the hall may be enough to stimulate peristalsis and relieve gas.

When conservative measures fail, flatulence can be relieved by insertion of a rectal tube. The client assumes a side-lying position while the nurse inserts the tube in the same manner as for an enema (see Procedure 33-3). Because fluid is not instilled into the bowel, the nurse can advance the tube to reach areas where flatus has accumulated (15 cm or 6 inches in an adult and 5 to 10 cm or 2 to 4 inches in a child). If the client complains of pain with tube placement or resistance is met, the nurse should discontinue the procedure and notify the client's physician.

After inserting the tube, the nurse instructs the client to lie quietly in bed. To prevent the tube from being dislodged, the nurse tapes it to a buttock. A gauze dressing or waterproof pad placed around the open end of the rectal tube catches any liquid fecal material.

Continual use of rectal tubes can cause irritation and eventual excoriation of the anus and rectal mucosa. A rectal tube should not remain in place longer than 30 minutes. The physician will determine the frequency with which the tube can be inserted. If flatulence persists, the nurse notifies the physician.

Maintenance of Skin Integrity

The client with diarrhea or fecal incontinence is at risk for skin breakdown when fecal contents remain on the skin. The same problem exists for the client with a colostomy that drains liquid stool. Liquid stool is usually acidic and contains digestive enzymes. Irritation from repeated wiping with toilet tissue aggravates skin breakdown. Bathing the skin after soiling helps but may result in more breakdown unless the skin is thoroughly dried.

The nurse should instruct the client about cleansing the anal area with mild soap and water after each passage of stool. When caring for a debilitated, incontinent client who is unable to ask for assistance, the nurse should check frequently for defecation. The anal areas can be protected with petrolatum jelly, zinc oxide, or other ointment that holds moisture in the skin, preventing drying and cracking. Yeast infections can develop easily. Several powdered antifungal agents are effective against yeast. Baby powder or cornstarch should not be used because they have no medical properties and they frequently cake on the skin and become difficult to remove.

Evaluation

The effectiveness of nursing interventions is measured by the success of meeting the expected outcomes and goals of care. Optimally, the client can eliminate soft-formed stools regularly. The client gains information needed to establish a normal elimination pattern.

The nurse applies evaluation measures when determining a client's level of progress

Goal: Client attains regular defecation habits within 2 weeks.

Outcomes

Client defecates on a predictable schedule by 1 week

Client's stool is well formed within 3 days

Evaluative measures
Observe character of stools
Note the frequency of defection
Observe a recorded normal defection pattern over several days

Goal: Client understands normal elimination.

Outcomes
Client verbalizes understanding of expected defecation pattern
Client asks questions indicating appropriate understanding of normal elimination

Evaluative measures
Ask the client to describe factors affecting elimination
Ask the client to discuss factors in the history that place him or her at risk for elimination problems

Goal: Client maintains proper fluid and food intake within 1 week.

Outcomes
Client increases intake of dietary fiber and whole grains
Client increases fluid intake while maintaining appropriate urinary output within 3 days

Evaluative measures
Ask the client or family member to keep a diary of the client's food and fluid intake
Have the client develop a meal plan
Measure the client's fluid intake

Goal: Client achieves regular exercise program.

Outcomes
Client maintains a diary demonstrating gradual, age-and-condition–appropriate increases in activities
Client reports an improvement in defecation pattern as activity increases

Evaluative measures
Observe the client initiate active exercises daily
Ask the client to describe the benefits of regular exercise

Goal: Client's skin integrity is maintained.

Outcomes
Existing skin breakdown resolves by 1 week
Client expresses understanding of proper perineal hygiene to prevent skin breakdown

Evaluative measures
Inspect the perianal or peristomal skin
Ask the client to explain skin care measures

SUMMARY

Normal elimination of fecal wastes requires maintenance of gastrointestinal function. Each client has a different defecation pattern and presents risks for alterations in elimination. The nurse provides therapies to promote or minimize factors that affect peristalsis or the absorption and secretion of intestinal contents. Much of the nurse's care involves educating clients about daily activities or habits that affect defecation.

Clients depend on the nurse when the ability to control body functions is lost. The nurse's approach with clients who have elimination problems must be sensitive and understanding and will focus on restoring the client to a maximal level of self care.

KEY CONCEPTS

A primary function of the elimination process is fluid balance.
Mechanical breakdown of food elements, gastrointestinal motility, and selective absorption and secretion of substances by the large intestine influence the character of feces.
Mass peristalsis in the large intestine is strongest 1 hour after mealtime.
Food high in fiber content and an increased fluid intake keep feces soft.
Regular use of laxatives can lead to constipation.
Vagal stimulation, which slows the heart rate, may occur when straining while defecating, having a rectal temperature taken, and undergoing an enema.
The greatest danger from diarrhea is fluid and electrolyte imbalance.
The location of an ostomy influences the consistency of stool.
Assessment of an elimination pattern should focus on bowel habits, an analysis of factors that normally influence defecation, a review of recent changes in elimination, and a physical examination.
A guaiac test is recommended for clients who take anticoagulants, who have a bleeding disorder or gastrointestinal disorder causing bleeding, or who are at risk for colon cancer.
Indirect and direct visualization of the lower gastrointestinal tract requires cleansing of the bowel before the procedure.

The nurse should consider frequency of defecation, fecal characteristics, and effect of foods on gastrointestinal function when selecting a diet promoting normal elimination.

Proper positioning on a bedpan allows the client to assume a position similar to squatting without experiencing muscle strain.

Cathartics or laxatives should be administered shortly before the usual time of defecation.

Proper administration of an enema is the slow instillation of the proper volume of a warm solution.

Irrigation of an ostomy follows the same principles as an enema administration, except that a special irrigating tube is needed and the client cannot control passage of feces.

Dangers during digital removal of stool include traumatizing the rectal mucosa and promoting vagal stimulation.

Skin breakdown can occur after repeated exposure to liquid stool.

CRITICAL THINKING ACTIVITIES

1. A 25-year-old man with a history of good health is admitted to your unit following a motor vehicle accident. His injuries and treatments are such that he will be on bedrest for the next 2 weeks. What type of plan would you design to prevent him from becoming constipated during this period of immobility?
2. You are asked to provide an outpatient with material and instructions for three stool guaiac tests. Identify and explain four important points of information you would want to include in your instructions.
3. An elderly woman with a new, permanent colostomy is about to be discharged from your unit to her daugher's home. The skin around her stoma has no breakdown; both she and her daughter realize the importance of maintaining this skin integrity. How would you go about advising them?
4. This is your first day of caring for a bedridden, comatose, 87-year-old man. In reviewing his chart, you can find no entry of a bowel movement for the past 10 days. How would you proceed with your bowel assessment?
5. Dietary fiber is increasingly being recognized for its therapeutic effects. Identify and explain two of these.

References

American Cancer Society: *Cancer facts and figures—1993,* Atlanta, 1993, The Society.

Brown MK and Everett I: Gentler bowel fitness with fiber, *Geriatric Nurs* 11(1):26, 1990.

Burcharth F, Ballan A, et al.: The colostomy plug: a new disposable device for a continent colostomy, *Lancet* 2(8518):1062, 1986.

Cleague MB and Heald RJ: Achievement of stomal continence in one-third of colostomies by use of a disposable plug, *Surg Gynecol Obstet* 170(5):390, 1990.

Dalton-Loehner D and Connor PA: Beyond ileostomy: surgery for a normal life, *RN,* 12(7):29, 1989.

Davidson MH, et al.: The hypocholesterolemic effects of beta-glucan in oatmeal and oat bran: a dose-controlled study, *JAMA* 265(14): 1833-1839, 1991.

Ebersole P and Hess P: *Toward healthy aging: human needs and nursing response,* ed 4, St. Louis, 1994.

Goldfinger SE: Constipation: the hard facts. I. *Harvard Health Lett* 16(4):1, 1991.

Kane RL, Ouslander JG, Abrass IB: *Essentials of clinical geriatrics,* ed 3, New York, 1994, McGraw-Hill.

Malasanos L, et al.: *Health assessment,* ed 4, St. Louis, 1990, Mosby.

Robinson C and Weigley E: *Basic nutrition and diet therapy,* ed 6, New York, 1989, Macmillan.

Ross D: Constipation among hospitalized elders, *Orthop Nurs* 9(3):73, 1990.

Van Horn L, Moag-Stahlberg A, et al: Effects on serum lipids of adding instant oats to usual American diets, *Am J Pub Health* 81(2):183-188. 1991.

Bibliography

Beverly L and Travis I: Constipation: proposed natural laxative mixtures, *J Gerontol Nurs* 18(10):5-12, 1992.

Cameron JC: Constipation related to narcotic therapy: a protocol for nurses and patients, *Cancer Nurs* 15(5):372-377, 1992.

Carpenito LJ: *Nursing diagnosis: application to clinical practice,* ed 4, Philadelphia, 1992, JB Lippincott.

Castiglione G, Grazzini G and Ciatto S: Guaiac and immunochemical tests for fecal occult blood in colorectal cancer screening, *Brit J Cancer* 65(6):942-944, 1992.

Kovach T: Managing geriatric chronic constipation, *Home Healthcare Nurse* 10(5):57-58, 1992.

Lewis SM and Collier IC: *Medical-surgical nursing: assessment and management of clinical problems,* ed 3, St. Louis, 1992, Mosby.

McDonnell WM, Ryan JA, et al.: Effect of iron on the guaiac reaction, *Gastroenterology* 96(1):74-78, 1989.

Pieper B: A study of persons undergoing outpatient gastrointestinal radiography . . . upper gastrointestinal tract barium enema, *J Enterostomal Ther Nurs* 19(2):54-58, 1992.

Puet TA, Phen L and Hurst DL: Pulsated irrigation enhanced evacuation: new method for treating fecal impaction, *Arch Phys Med Rehabil* 72(11):935-936, 1991.

Stelling HP, Maimon HN, et al.: A comparative study of fecal occult blood tests for early detection of gastrointestinal pathology, *Arch Intern Med* 150(5):1001-1005, 1990.

Thibodeau GA and Patton K: *Anatomy and physiology,* ed 2, St. Louis, 1993, Mosby.

Whaley LF and Wong DL: *Nursing care of infants and children,* ed 4, St. Louis, 1991, Mosby.

Willis R: A nurse's invention teaches bowel control, *Austral Nurs J* 21(9):16-17, 1992.

Ziegler EE, et al.: Cow milk feeding in infancy: further observations on blood loss from the gastrointestinal tract, *J Pediatr* 116(1):11-18, 1990.

34 Oxygenation

OBJECTIVES

Mastery of content in this chapter will enable the student to:

- Define the key terms listed.
- Describe the gross structure and function of the cardiopulmonary system.
- Identify the processes in maintaining cardiac output, myocardial blood flow, and coronary artery circulation.
- Describe the electrical conduction system of the heart.
- Describe how cardiac output can be altered by preload, afterload, contractility, and heart rate.
- Identify the processes involved in ventilation, perfusion, and respiratory gas exchange.
- Describe neural and chemical regulation of respiration.
- Explain how level of health, age, life-style, and environment affect tissue oxygenation.
- Identify causes and effects of disturbances in conduction, altered cardiac output, impaired valvular function, myocardial ischemia, and impaired tissue perfusion.
- Identify causes and effects of hyperventilation, hypoventilation, and hypoxemia.
- Perform an assessment of the cardiopulmonary system.
- Develop nursing diagnoses for altered oxygenation.
- Describe nursing interventions to increase activity tolerance, maintain or promote lung expansion, promote mobilization of pulmonary secretions, maintain a patent airway, promote oxygenation, and restore cardiopulmonary function.
- Develop evaluation criteria for a care plan for the client with altered oxygenation.

KEY TERMS

afterload
airway resistance
angina pectoris
angiography
atelectasis
atrioventricular (AV) node
bronchoscopy
bundle of His
cardiac output
cardiopulmonary resuscitation (CPR)
chest percussion
chest tube
cyanosis
diaphragmatic breathing
diffusion
dyspnea
dysrhythmias
echocardiography
electrocardiogram (ECG)
electrophysiological (EP) study
exercise stress test
hematemesis
hemoptysis
hemothorax
Holter monitor
hyperventilation
hypoventilation
hypovolemia
hypoxia
incentive spirometry
myocardial infarction
myocardial ischemia
nasal cannula
nebulization
normal sinus rhythm (NSR)
orthopnea
oximetry
peak expiratory flow rate (PEFR)
pneumothorax
postural drainage
preload
productive cough
pulmonary function tests
Purkinje network
pursed-lip breathing
scintigraphy
sinoatrial (SA) node
stroke volume
thoracentesis
ventilation
wheezing

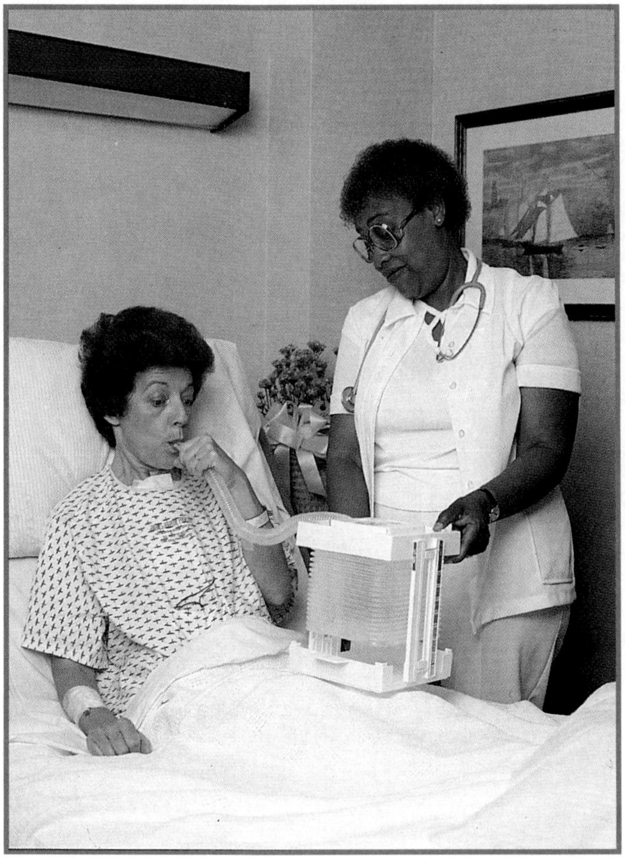

Oxygen is a basic human need and is required for life. The nurse often encounters clients who are unable to independently meet oxygen needs. To help clients meet their oxygen needs, the nurse must understand cardiac and respiratory physiology.

Cardiac physiology involves the delivery of oxygenated blood to the tissues and the delivery of deoxygenated blood to the pulmonary system. Once blood reaches the pulmonary circulation, the lungs oxygenate the blood. This oxygenated blood is returned to the left side of the heart and then delivered to the tissues.

Respiratory physiology involves oxygenation of the body through ventilation, perfusion, and transport of respiratory gases. Neural and chemical regulators control changes in respiratory rate and depth to meet tissue oxygen demands. Together, the cardiac and respiratory systems supply the body's oxygen demands.

CARDIOVASCULAR PHYSIOLOGY

The cardiac system delivers oxygen, nutrients, and other substances to the tissues and removes cellular waste products. These are achieved through the cardiac pump, the circulatory vascular system, and the integration of the respiratory, digestive, and renal systems (McCance, Huether, 1994).

Structure and Function

The heart pumps blood through the pulmonary circulation by way of the right ventricle and to the systemic circulation by way of the left ventricle. Both ventricles supply oxygen and nutrients to the tissues and remove wastes from the body. The circulatory system exchanges respiratory gases, nutrients, and waste products between the blood and the tissues.

Myocardial Pump. The pumping action of the heart maintains oxygen delivery. Diseases that decrease the pumping effectiveness of the heart lessen the volume of blood ejected from the ventricles. Conditions that affect circulating blood volume decrease the available blood for the heart to eject from the ventricles.

The chambers of the heart fill during diastole and empty during systole. A client's blood pressure reading helps determine the effectiveness of these diastolic and systolic events (see Chapter 15).

During ventricular filling, the myocardial fibers stretch. In a healthy heart, as the fibers stretch, the strength of the subsequent contraction also increases. This response is the Frank-Starling (Starling's) law of the heart.

In the diseased heart, the stretch of the myocardium is beyond physiological limits. The heart stretches or dilates, but the subsequent contraction results in insufficient ventricular ejection (volume). The heart loses its ability to pump the blood forward, and blood begins to "back-up" in the pulmonary (left heart failure) or systemic circulation (right heart failure).

Myocardial Blood Flow. The one-way flow of blood through the heart is ensured by the four heart valves (Figure 34-1). During ventricular diastole the atrioventricular (mitral and tricuspid) valves open and blood flows from the higher pressure atria into the relaxed ventricles. After ventricular filling, the systolic phase begins. As the systolic intraventricular pressure rises, the atrioventricular valves close. This prevents the back flow of blood into the atria, and ventricular contraction begins.

As the ventricles begin the systolic phase, ventricular pressure rises. This causes the semilunar (aortic and pulmonic) valves to open. As the ventricles eject blood past these open valves, the intraventricular pressure falls and the semilunar valves close. This prevents the back flow of blood into the ventricles.

Clients with valvular diseases may have back flow or regurgitation of blood through the incompetent valve. This regurgitation causes a murmur heard on ausculta-

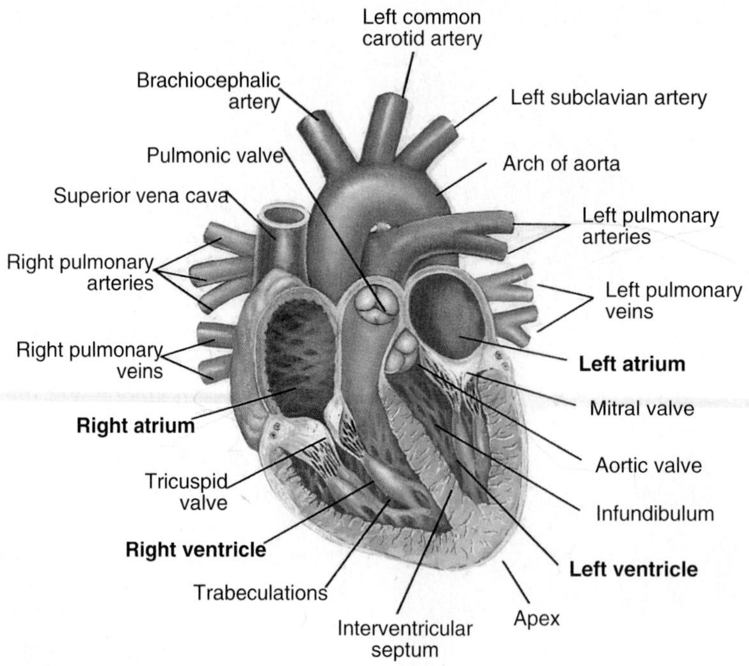

FIGURE 34-1 Structures that direct blood flow through the heart. Arrows indicate path of blood through chambers, valves, and major vessels. (Modified from Canobbio MM: *Cardiovascular disorders,* St. Louis, 1990, Mosby.)

tion over the specific auscultation areas for each valve (see Chapter 16).

Coronary Artery Circulation. The coronary circulation supplies oxygen and nutrients to and removes waste from the myocardium. These coronary arteries arise from the aorta just above and behind the aortic valve through openings called the *coronary ostia.* The most abundant blood supply feeds the left ventricular myocardium, which is more muscular and does most of the heart's work. The coronary arteries fill during ventricular diastole (McCance, Huether, 1990).

Systemic Circulation. The systemic arteries and veins deliver nutrients and oxygen to and remove waste from the tissues. Oxygenated blood flows from the left ventricle by way of the aorta and into large systemic arteries. These branch into smaller arteries and finally into arterioles. The arterioles branch further into the smallest vessels, the capillaries. At the capillary level, the exchange of respiratory gases, nutrients, and wastes occurs. The tissues are oxygenated, and nutrients are received. The waste products exit the capillary network by way of the venules that join to form veins. These veins form larger veins, which carry deoxygenated blood to the right heart to be returned to pulmonary circulation.

Regulation of Blood Flow. The amount of blood ejected from the left ventricle each minute is the **cardiac output.** The cardiac output changes according to the oxygen and metabolic needs of the body. For example, during exercise, pregnancy, and fever, the cardiac output increases. During sleep, the cardiac output decreases. Cardiac output is represented by the following formula:

$$\text{Cardiac output (CO)} = \text{Stroke volume (SV)} \times \text{Heart rate (HR)}$$

Stroke volume is the amount of blood ejected from the left ventricle with each contraction. It can be affected by the amount of blood in the left ventricle at the end of diastole (preload), the resistance to left ventricular ejection (afterload), and myocardial contractility.

Preload is essentially the end diastolic volume. As the ventricles fill, they stretch. According to the Frank-Starling law, the greater the stretch on the ventricle, the greater the contraction and the greater the stroke volume. In clinical situations, the preload and subsequent stroke volume can be manipulated by changing the amount of circulating blood volume. For example, in the client with hemorrhagic shock, fluid therapy and replacing blood volume increase volume. This increases the preload and subsequent cardiac output. If volume is not replaced, preload decreases, as does subsequent cardiac output. Ultimately the venous return to the right atrium decreases, which further decreases preload and cardiac output.

Afterload is the resistance to left ventricular ejection. For the left side of the heart, afterload is the work the

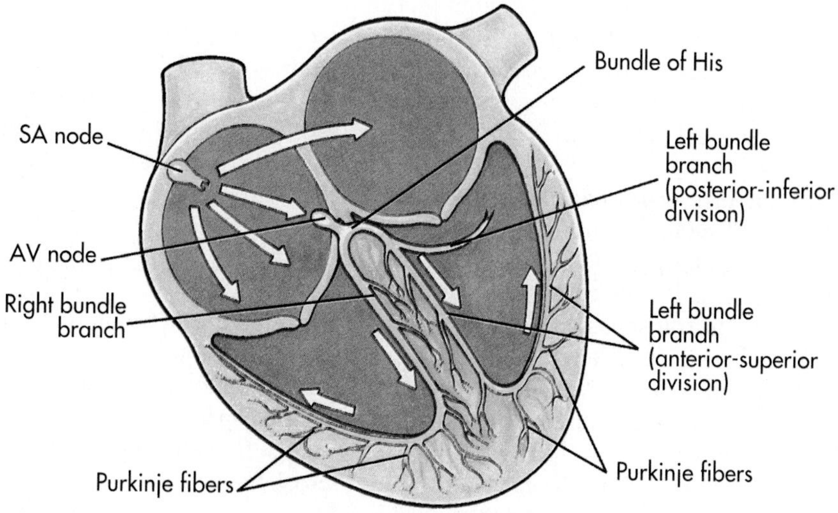

FIGURE 34-2 Electrical conduction system. (From Canobbio MM: *Cardiovascular disorders,* St. Louis, 1990, Mosby.)

heart must overcome to fully eject blood from the left ventricle. The diastolic aortic pressure measures afterload. In a client with an acute hypertensive crisis, the afterload and the cardiac workload increase. Afterload in this situation can be manipulated by decreasing systemic blood pressure.

Myocardial contractility also affects stroke volume and cardiac output. Poor contraction decreases the amount of blood ejected by the ventricles during each contraction. Myocardial contractility can be increased by drugs that increase the force of contraction, such as epinephrine.

Heart rate affects blood flow because of the interaction between rate and diastolic filling time. With a faster heart rate, particularly sustained rates greater than 160 beats/min, diastolic filling time decreases. As filling time decreases, stroke volume and cardiac output decrease.

Conduction System

The rhythmic relaxation and contraction of the atria and ventricles depend on continuous, organized transmission of electrical impulses. These impulses are generated and transmitted by the conduction system (Figure 34-2).

The heart's conduction system generates the necessary action potentials that conduct the impulses required to initiate the electrical mechanical chain of events. The autonomic nervous system influences the rate of impulse generation and the transmission speed through the conductive pathway and the strength of contractions. Sympathetic nerve fibers, which increase the impulse generation rate and the impulse transmission speed, supply the atria and ventricles. Parasympathetic fibers from the vagus nerve, which decrease this rate, also supply these parts along with the sinoatrial and atrioventricular nodes (McCance, Huether, 1994).

The conduction system originates with the **sinoatrial (SA) node.** This is "the pacemaker of the heart." The SA node is in the right atrium next to the entrance of the superior vena cava. Impulses are initiated at the SA node at an intrinsic rate of 60 to 100 beats/min.

The electrical impulses are then transmitted through the atria to the **atrioventricular (AV) node.** The AV node mediates impulses between the atria and the ventricles. It assists atrial emptying by delaying the impulse before transmitting it through the **bundle of His** and the ventricular **Purkinje network.**

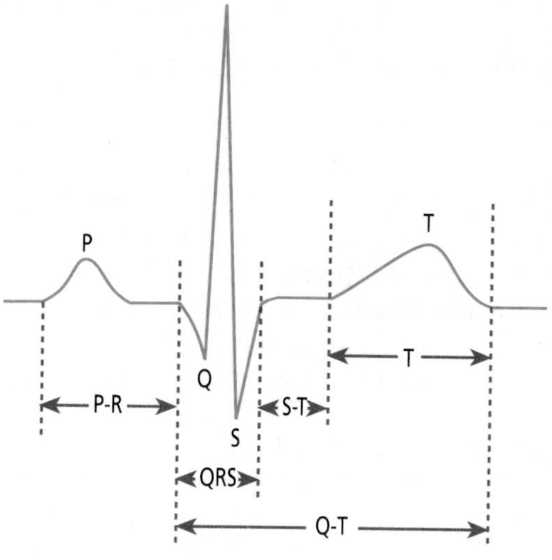

FIGURE 34-3 Normal ECG waveform. (From Canobbio MM: *Cardiovascular disorders,* St. Louis, 1990, Mosby.)

The electrical activity of the conduction system is reflected by an **electrocardiogram (ECG).** An ECG monitors the regularity and path of the electrical impulse through the conduction system. The normal sequence on the ECG is called *normal sinus rhythm (NSR)* (Figure 34-3).

NSR means the impulse originated in the SA node and followed the normal sequence through the conduction system. The P-wave on the ECG indicates that the atria have contracted. The PR interval provides information about the delay in transmission of the impulse through the AV node. The normal length for the PR interval is 0.12 to 0.20 seconds. An increase in the time indicates a block in the impulse transmission through the AV node. A decrease indicates the electrical impulse originated from a source other than the SA node. The QRS complex indicates the ventricles have contracted.

RESPIRATORY PHYSIOLOGY

Most cells in the body obtain much of their energy from chemical reactions involving oxygen. Cells must also eliminate carbon dioxide. The exchange of respiratory gases occurs between the environmental air and the blood. The three steps in oxygenation are ventilation, perfusion, and diffusion (McCance, Huether, 1994). The organs, nerves, and muscles of respiration must be intact for respiratory gas exchange. The central nervous system also must be able to regulate inspiration and expiration.

Structure and Function

Respiration can be altered by conditions or diseases that occur in the pulmonary system, resulting in structural and functional changes. The respiratory muscles, pleural space, lungs, and alveoli (Figure 34-4) are essential for ventilation, perfusion, and gas exchange (see box below).

Ventilation

Ventilation is the process by which gases are moved into and out of the lungs. Adequate ventilation requires coordination of the muscular and elastic properties of the lung and thorax and intact innervation. The major inspiratory muscle is the diaphragm, which is inner-

MAJOR ANATOMICAL STRUCTURES OF THE THORAX AND THEIR FUNCTIONS

INSPIRATORY MUSCLES

Diaphragm

Contraction causes the diaphragm to descend, creating a negative pleural pressure and increasing the vertical dimension of the lungs, which contributes to lung inflation. The increase in vertical dimension and the decrease in intrapulmonary pressure (negative with respect to atmospheric pressure) causes air to enter the lungs.

External Intercostal

Contraction elevates the anterior ends of the ribs, causing them to move upward and outward. This increases the anteroposterior dimension of the thorax.

Accessory Muscles

Accessory muscles include the scalene, sternocleidomastoid, and trapezius muscles. Contraction elevates the first two ribs and the sternum.

EXPIRATORY MUSCLES

Internal Intercostal

Contraction pulls ribs down and in, thereby decreasing the anteroposterior diameter of the thorax.

Abdominal Respiratory

Abdominal respiratory muscles contract to depress lower ribs, force the diaphragm up, and decrease the vertical dimension of the thoracic cavity.

PLEURAL SPACE

The pleural space is a potential space that is only a thin film of liquid lying between the outer layer of the lung (visceral pleura) and the inner layer of the chest cavity (parietal pleura). It permits a smooth, gliding movement of the lungs along the chest wall. Normally, air is not present in the pleural space.

LUNGS

Left (Two Lobes) and Right (Three Lobes)

The lungs transfer oxygen from the atmosphere into the alveoli and carbon dioxide from the alveoli to the lungs to be excreted as a waste product. They also filter toxic material from circulation and metabolize compounds such as angiotensin I, bradykinin, and prostaglandins.

Alveoli

Alveoli transfer oxygen and carbon dioxide to and from the blood through the alveolar membrane. These tiny air sacs expand during inspiration, greatly increasing the surface area over which exchange of gases occurs.

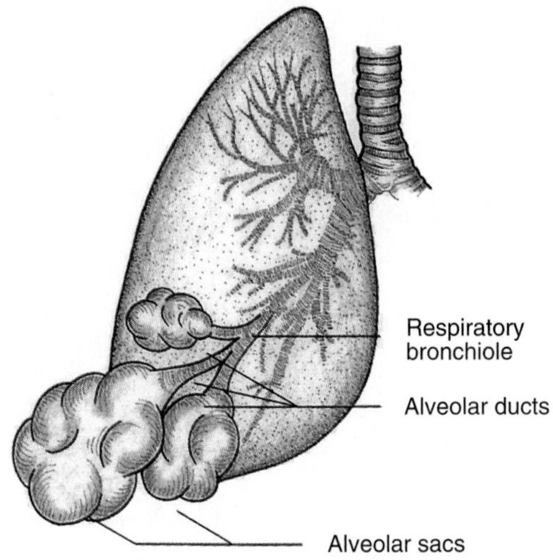

FIGURE 34-4 Alveoli at the terminal end of the lower airway. (From Gröer MW, Shekleton ME: *Basic pathophysiology: a holistic approach,* ed 3, St. Louis, 1989, Mosby.)

vated by the phrenic nerve. This nerve exits the spinal cord at the third, fourth, or fifth cervical vertebra. Spinal cord disruption at the fourth cervical level can sever the phrenic cervical nerve and impair the diaphragm's function.

Work of Breathing. Breathing is the effort required to expand and contract the lungs. It is determined by the degree of lung tissue compliance, airway resistance, active expiration, and accessory muscle use (Gröer, Shekleton, 1989).

Compliance is the ability of the lungs and thorax to distend (Dettenmeier, 1992). Compliance is decreased in diseases such as pulmonary edema and in congenital or structural abnormalities, such as kyphosis or fractured ribs.

Airway resistance is the pressure difference between the mouth and the alveoli in relation to the rate of flow of inspired gas. Airway resistance can be increased by an airway obstruction (such as a foreign body), small airway disease (such as asthma), and tracheal edema. When resistance is increased, the amount of air traveling through the anatomical airways is decreased.

Active expiration uses muscle to contract the lungs. Expiration is normally a passive process that depends on elastic recoil properties and requires little or no muscle work. Elastic recoil is produced by elastic fibers in lung tissue and by surface tension in the fluid film lining the alveoli (Dettenmeier, 1992).

Accessory muscles of respiration can increase lung volume during inspiration. Clients with chronic obstructive pulmonary disease, especially emphysema, frequently use these muscles to increase lung volume. During assessment the nurse may observe the client's clavicles being elevated during inspiration.

Decreased compliance, increased airway resistance, active expiration, or use of accessory muscles increases the work of breathing. This results in an increase in energy expenditure. To meet this expenditure, the body increases its metabolic rate. The need for oxygen and the need to eliminate carbon dioxide increase.

Volumes. Normal lung volumes are measured through pulmonary function testing. Some of these measurements are taken with a spirometer, which measures the volume of air entering or leaving the lungs. Lung volumes may vary with health states such as pregnancy, exercise, obesity, or obstructive and restrictive lung diseases. The amount of surfactant, degree of compliance, and strength of respiratory muscles can affect lung pressures and volumes.

Pressures. Gases are moved through the lungs by pressure changes (Figure 34-5). Intrapleural pressure is negative to (less than) atmospheric pressure, which is 760 mm Hg at sea level. For air to flow into the lungs, intrapleural pressure must become more negative. This sets up a pressure gradient between the atmosphere and alveoli, thus moving air into the lungs and alveoli.

Perfusion

The primary function of pulmonary circulation is to move blood to and from the alveolar-capillary membrane for gas exchange. Pulmonary circulation is also a reservoir for blood and filters blood to remove small thrombi before they reach the brain or other vital organs.

Pulmonary Circulation. Pulmonary circulation begins at the pulmonary artery, which receives mixed (poorly oxygenated) venous blood from the right ventricle. Blood flow through this system depends on the pumping ability of the right ventricle, which has an output of approximately 5 to 6 L/min. The flow continues through the pulmonary arterioles, capillaries, venules, and veins. Oxygen-rich blood returns to the left atrium.

Distribution. Pulmonary pressures are low when compared with the systemic circulatory system. The normal pulmonary systolic arterial pressure is between 20 and 30 mm Hg, the diastolic pressure is less than 12 mm Hg, and the mean pressure is less than 20 mm Hg (Daily, Schroeder, 1989). Because of low pressure and low resistance, the walls of the pulmonary vessels are thinner than those in the systemic circulation and contain less smooth muscle. The lung accepts the total cardiac output from the right ventricle and usually does not direct blood flow from one region to another.

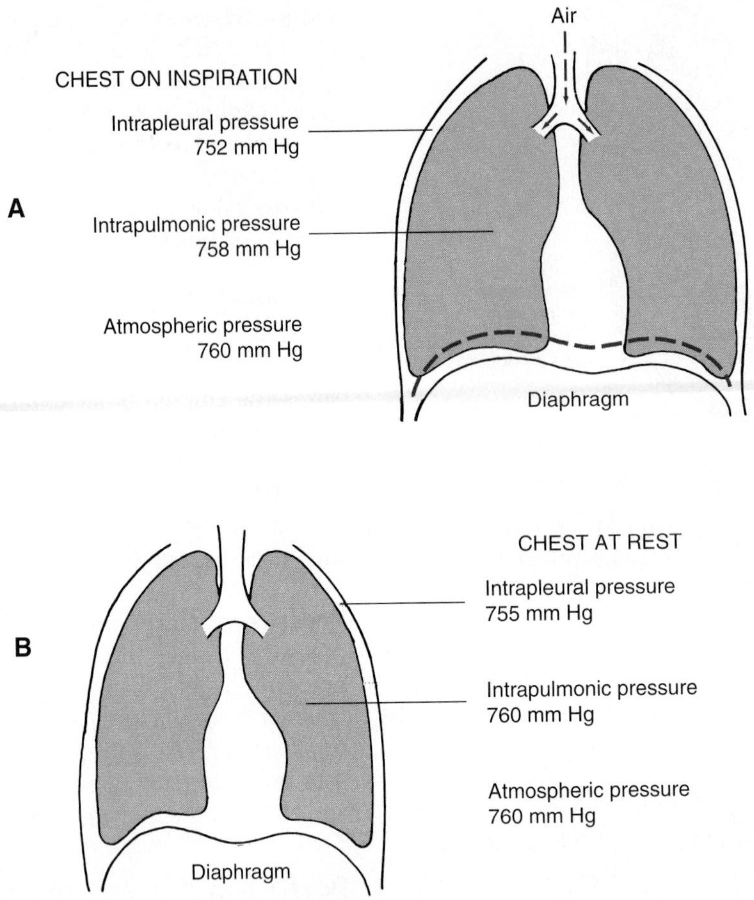

FIGURE 34-5 **A,** Contraction of the diaphragm to increase vertical dimensions of the lungs. **B,** Relaxation of the diaphragm, decreasing vertical dimensions of the lungs. (From Wade JF: *Comprehensive respiratory care,* ed 3, St. Louis, 1982, Mosby.)

Exchange of Respiratory Gases

Respiratory gases are exchanged in the alveoli of the lungs and the capillaries of the body tissues. Oxygen is transferred from the lungs to the blood, and carbon dioxide is transferred from the blood to the alveoli to be exhaled as waste. This transfer depends on diffusion.

Diffusion. **Diffusion** is the movement of molecules from an area of high concentration to an area of low concentration. Diffusion of respiratory gases occurs at the alveolar–capillary membrane. It can be affected by thickness of the membrane.

Increased thickness of the membrane (because of pulmonary edema) slows diffusion because gases take longer to transfer across the thickened space. Diffusion is slowed, and the delivery of oxygen to tissues is reduced. If the surface area of the membrane is reduced by disease or surgical removal of tissue, diffusion is also reduced.

Oxygen Transport. The oxygen transport system consists of the lungs and cardiovascular system. Delivery depends on the amount of oxygen entering the lungs (ventilation), blood flow to the lungs and tissues (perfusion), adequacy of diffusion, and capacity of the blood to carry oxygen. The capacity to carry oxygen is influenced by the amount of dissolved oxygen in the plasma, amount of hemoglobin, and tendency of hemoglobin to bind with oxygen (Ahrens, 1987, 1990).

Only 3% of the required oxygen is dissolved in the plasma. Most oxygen is transported by hemoglobin, which carries oxygen and carbon dioxide. The hemoglobin molecule combines with oxygen to form oxyhemoglobin. Oxyhemoglobin is easily reversible, allowing hemoglobin and oxygen to dissociate and oxygen to enter tissues.

Carbon Dioxide Transport. The transport of respiratory gases includes movement of carbon dioxide. Car-

NEURAL AND CHEMICAL REGULATION OF RESPIRATION

NEURAL REGULATION

Neural regulation maintains rhythm and depth of respiration, as well as the balance between inspiration and expiration.

Cerebral Cortex

Voluntary control of respiration delivers impulses to the respiratory motor neurons by way of the spinal cord. Voluntary control of respiration accommodates speaking, eating, and swimming.

Medulla Oblongata

Automatic control of respiration occurs continuously.

CHEMICAL REGULATION

Chemical regulation maintains appropriate rate and depth of respirations based on changes in the blood's carbon dioxide (CO_2), oxygen (O_2), and hydrogen ion (H^+) concentration.

Chemoreceptors

Chemoreceptors are located in the medulla, aortic body, and carotid body. Changes in chemical content of O_2, CO_2, and H^+ stimulate chemoreceptors, which in turn stimulate neural regulators to adjust the rate and depth of ventilation to maintain normal arterial blood gas levels. Chemical regulation can occur during physical exercise and in some illnesses. It is a short-term adaptive mechanism.

table 34-1

PHYSIOLOGICAL PROCESSES AFFECTING OXYGENATION

Process	Effect on oxygenation
Anemia	Decreases oxygen-carrying capacity of blood
Toxic inhalant (e.g., carbon monoxide)	Decreases oxygen-carrying capacity of blood; carbon monoxide displaces oxygen from hemoglobin and decreases capacity of blood to carry oxygen
Airway obstruction	Limits inspired oxygen delivered to alveoli
High altitudes	Decreases inspiratory oxygen concentration because atmospheric oxygen concentration is lower
Fever	Increases metabolic rate and tissue oxygen demand
Decreased chest wall motion (e.g., from musculoskeletal impairments)	Prevents lowering of diaphragm and reduces anteroposterior diameter of thorax on inspiration, thereby reducing volume of inspired air

bon dioxide diffuses into red blood cells and is rapidly hydrated into carbonic acid (H_2CO_3) because of carbonic anhydrase. The carbonic acid then dissociates into hydrogen (H^+) and bicarbonate (HCO_3^-) ions. The hydrogen ion is buffered by hemoglobin, and the HCO_3^- diffuses into the plasma (see Chapter 35). In addition, some of the carbon dioxide in red blood cells reacts with amino acid groups, forming carbamino compounds. This reaction can occur rapidly without an enzyme. Reduced hemoglobin (deoxyhemoglobin) can combine with carbon dioxide more easily and therefore venous blood transports most of the carbon dioxide.

Regulation of Respiration

Respiratory regulation supplies enough oxygen to meet the body's demands. It also promotes exhalation of carbon dioxide.

The two respiratory regulators are neural and chemical. Neural regulation includes the central nervous system control of respiratory rate, depth, and rhythm. Chemical regulation involves the influence of chemicals on the rate and depth of respiration (see box above).

FACTORS AFFECTING OXYGENATION

Adequacy of circulation, ventilation, perfusion, and transport of respiratory gases to the tissues are influenced by physiological, developmental, behavioral, and environmental factors.

Physiological Factors

Conditions that affect cardiopulmonary functioning also affect the body's ability to meet oxygen demands. Cardiac disorders include disturbances in conduction, impaired valvular function, myocardial hypoxia, cardiomyopathic conditions, and peripheral tissue hypoxia. Respiratory disorders include hyperventilation, hypoventilation, and hypoxia.

Other physiological processes also affect a client's oxygenation (Table 34-1). These include anemia, pregnancy, fever, and infection.

Decreased Oxygen-Carrying Capacity. Hemoglobin carries 97% of oxygen to tissues. Anything that lowers hemoglobin decreases the oxygen-carrying capacity of blood. Anemia and inhalation of toxic substances are two examples.

Anemia is characterized by low hemoglobin levels in the blood. Anemia reflects one or more of three basic processes: decreased hemoglobin production, increased red cell destruction, and blood loss. Clinical findings in clients with anemia include fatigue, decreased activity tolerance, increased breathlessness, pallor, and increased heart rate.

Carbon monoxide is the most common toxic inhalant decreasing the oxygen-carrying capacity of blood. A bond of the carbon monoxide molecule with the hemoglobin molecule is stronger than the bond between hemoglobin and oxygen. Because of the bond's strength, carbon monoxide is not easily dissociated from hemoglobin. This makes the hemoglobin unavailable for oxygen transport.

Decreased Inspired Oxygen Concentration. Decreased inspired oxygen concentration decreases the oxygen-carrying capacity of the blood. This can be caused by decreased environmental oxygen.

Hypovolemia. **Hypovolemia** is a reduced circulating blood volume resulting from fluid losses that occurs with conditions such as shock and severe dehydration. High fluid loss reduces the amount of fluid available for circulation. The body tries to adapt by increasing the heart rate and peripheral vasoconstriction to increase the volume of blood returned to the heart.

Increased Metabolic Rate. An increase in metabolic rate causes increased oxygen demand. If the body systems cannot meet this demand, the oxygenation level declines. An increased metabolic rate is a normal response of the body to pregnancy, wound healing, and exercise because the body is building tissue. Most people can meet the greater need for oxygen.

Fever increases metabolic demand, the tissues' need for oxygen, and carbon dioxide production. If the fever persists, the metabolic rate remains high and the body begins to break down protein stores. This results in muscle wasting, and the client has decreased muscle mass. Respiratory muscles are also wasted. The client may not be able to do the work of breathing and develops hypoxemia and hypercapnea.

During persistent fever, the body increases the rate and depth of respiration. This enables the body to rid itself of excess carbon dioxide by "blowing off" the carbon dioxide during expiration. It also increases the work of breathing. Clients, particularly those with pulmonary diseases, are thus at risk for hypoxemia and hypercapnea.

Conditions Affecting Chest Wall Movement. Any condition that reduces chest wall movement can decrease ventilation. If the diaphragm cannot fully descend with breathing, the volume of inspired air decreases and less oxygen is delivered.

PREGNANCY. As the fetus grows during pregnancy, the greater size of the uterus pushes abdominal contents up against the diaphragm. During the last trimester the woman's inspiratory capacity declines. She may be short of breath on exertion.

OBESITY. Obese clients often have a heavy lower thorax and abdomen. This reduces lung volumes, especially when the client is lying down. Some clients develop an obesity-hypoventilation syndrome. Oxygenation is decreased and carbon dioxide is retained, resulting in daytime sleepiness. The obese client is also at risk for pneumonia after an upper respiratory tract infection because the lungs cannot fully expand and secretions do not move out of the lower lobes.

MUSCULOSKELETAL ABNORMALITIES. Musculoskeletal impairments in the chest wall reduce oxygenation. They may result from abnormal structural configurations, trauma, muscle diseases, and central nervous system diseases.

ABNORMAL STRUCTURAL CONFIGURATIONS. Abnormal structural configurations include pectus excavatum (rib cage) and kyphosis (vertebral column). Pectus excavatum is a depression of the sternum that interferes with lung expansion. Kyphosis is caused by increased convexity of the thoracic spine. It produces a structural barrier to lung expansion. The angle of curvature can progress with time, resulting in severe hypoventilation and hypoxemia.

TRAUMA. Trauma to the chest wall may impede inspiration. A client with multiple rib fractures can develop a flail chest. The fractures cause instability in part of the chest wall and paradoxical breathing (the lung contracts on inspiration and bulges on expiration). This can result in hypoxia.

Chest wall or upper abdomen incisions may also decrease chest wall movement. The client may breathe shallowly to avoid pain.

MUSCLE DISEASES. Muscle diseases such as muscular dystrophy affect tissue oxygenation. If the client's ability to expand and contract the chest decreases, ventilation is impaired and atelectasis, hypercapnea, and hypoxemia can occur.

NERVOUS SYSTEM DISEASES. Nervous system diseases or conditions such as myasthenia gravis, Guillain-Barré syndrome, and poliomyelitis can affect respiratory functioning and result in hypoventilation. Myasthenia gravis interferes with normal impulse transmission from nerves to muscles. It involves the whole body, including respiratory muscles.

Guillain-Barré syndrome and poliomyelitis cause muscle inflammation and paralysis. Guillain-Barré syndrome usually results in an ascending paralysis. If paralysis ascends to the thoracic region, respiratory muscles become paralyzed. Poliomyelitis may lead to general or local paralysis.

CENTRAL NERVOUS SYSTEM ALTERATIONS. Alterations may impair respiration. When the medulla oblongata is affected, it alters the neural regulation of respiration and causes abnormal breathing. Spinal cord damage can affect respiration in two ways. If the phrenic nerve is damaged, the diaphragm may not descend, thus reducing inspiratory lung volumes and causing hypoxemia. Spinal cord trauma below the fifth cervical vertebra usually leaves the phrenic nerve intact but damages nerves that innervate the intercostal muscles. This prevents the chest from expanding in the anteroposterior diameter.

INFLUENCES OF CHRONIC DISEASE. Chronic diseases can decrease oxygenation levels either directly or indirectly. For example, cardiopulmonary diseases decrease oxygenation levels either by impaired ventilation in which there is inadequate oxygen in the alveoli or by a decrease in cardiac output in which there is a decline in the amount of oxygenated blood delivered to the tissues. Anemias decrease oxygen levels because of the reduced availability of the oxygen carrier, hemoglobin.

Developmental Factors

The developmental stage of the client and the normal aging process can affect tissue oxygenation.

Premature Infants. Premature infants are at risk for hyaline membrane disease, which is caused by a surfactant deficiency. The surfactant-synthesizing ability of the lungs develops late in pregnancy and may therefore be lacking in preterm infants (Gröer, Shekleton, 1989).

GERONTOLOGIC NURSING PRACTICE

The older adult has special risks and nursing interventions for altered respiratory status. Awareness of specific nursing practices can assist the nurse in providing individualized nursing care for the client.

- Older adults may have been exposed to tuberculosis (TB) as children. The disease can lie dormant with reactivation occurring in later life. The incidence of the disease increases with age and is probably due to the immunological changes of aging. Thus increased screening for exposure and active TB in this population is important (Burke, Walsh, 1992).
- Smoking cessation in the older adult is beneficial in the areas of pulmonary reconditioning and reduction in the incidence of respiratory tract infections.
- Older adult clients more frequently require home oxygen equipment. Assess their insurance status to determine their reimbursement status. Medicare guidelines restrict reimbursement for home oxygen use to clients with a documented oxygenation saturation under 85% or a PaO_2 under 55 mmHg (Kane, 1994; Burke, Walsh, 1992). Supplement insurance (e.g., Blue Cross) may have other reimbursement guidelines.
- Increase safety education. If home oxygen equipment is in use, determine the presence of environmental hazards.

Infants and Toddlers. Infants and toddlers are at risk for upper respiratory tract infections as a result of frequent exposure to other children. In addition, some infants develop nasal congestion while teething, which can cause bacterial growth and increases the risk for respiratory tract infection. Upper respiratory tract infections are usually not dangerous, and infants or toddlers recover with little difficulty. Common airway infections are epiglotittis, nasopharyngitis, pharyngitis influenza, and tonsillitis. Airway obstructions can occur with aspirated foreign objects.

School-Age Children and Adolescents. School-age children and adolescents are exposed to respiratory infections and respiratory risk factors such as smoking. A healthy child usually does not have adverse pulmonary effects from respiratory infections. A person who starts smoking in adolescence and continues to smoke into middle age, however, has an increased risk for cardiopulmonary disease (see Chapter 2).

Young and Middle-Age Adults. Young and middle-age adults are exposed to cardiopulmonary risk factors such as an unhealthy diet, lack of exercise, stress, and smoking. Reducing these factors may decrease the client's risk for cardiopulmonary diseases.

Older Adults. The cardiac and respiratory systems change throughout the aging process. The arterial system becomes clogged because of atherosclerotic plaques, and the systemic blood pressure may rise. The connective tissue and bronchial tree change as the lungs lose elasticity (Gröer, Shekleton, 1989). Ventilation and gas transfer decline with age. Some rib cage changes occur normally with aging. With these changes the lungs are unable to expand fully, lowering oxygenation levels (see box above).

Behavioral Factors

Behavior or life-style factors may directly or indirectly affect the body's ability to meet oxygen requirements.

Nutrition. Nutrition can affect cardiopulmonary function in several ways. Severe obesity can decrease lung expansion. Malnutrition may cause respiratory muscle wasting. Muscle weakness may also decrease the ability to cough productively. High-fat diets increase cholesterol and atherogenesis in the coronary arteries. Obese and malnourished clients are also at risk for anemia.

Exercise. Exercise increases the body's metabolic activity and thus oxygen demand. Respiratory rate and depth increase, enabling the person to inhale more oxygen and expire excess carbon dioxide. People who exercise regularly have a lower pulse rate and blood pressure, decreased cholesterol, increased blood flow, and greater oxygen extraction by working muscles. Fully conditioned people can increase oxygen consumption by 10% to 20% because of increased cardiac output.

Cigarette Smoking. Cigarette smoking is associated with heart disease, chronic obstructive lung disease, and lung cancer. It can also worsen peripheral vascular disease. The risk of lung cancer is 60 times greater for a person who smokes two packs of cigarettes a day than for someone who has never smoked. The mortality with lung cancer is high (greater than 70%), and it is frequently diagnosed only when it is advanced (Gröer, Shekleton, 1989).

Substance Abuse. Substance abuse can impair tissue oxygenation because of poor nutritional intake (which decreases hemoglobin production) and respiratory center depression (which decreases the amount of oxygen inhaled). In addition, injected subtances can cause pulmonary fibrosis and valvular heart diseases.

Anxiety. A continuous state of severe anxiety increases the body's metabolic rate and the oxygen demand. The body responds by an increased rate and depth of respiration. Most can adapt, but some, particularly those with chronic illnesses or acute life-threatening illnesses such as a myocardial infarction cannot tolerate the higher oxygen demands.

Environmental Factors

The environment can also influence oxygenation. The incidence of pulmonary disease is higher in smoggy, urban areas than in rural areas. Higher altitudes affect oxygen delivery because the concentration of atmospheric oxygen is less, and the client increases the respiratory rate to adapt. In addition, the client's workplace may increase the risk for pulmonary disease because of occupational pollutants such as asbestos, talcum powder, dust, and airborne fibers.

ALTERATIONS IN CARDIAC FUNCTIONING

Alterations in cardiac functioning are caused by illnesses and conditions that affect cardiac rhythm, strength of contraction, blood flow through the chambers, myocardial blood flow, and peripheral circulation.

Disturbances in Conduction

Some disturbances in conduction are called *dysrhythmias,* meaning a deviation from the normal sinus heart rhythm (Table 34-2). Dysrhythmias may be primary conditions or complications of other disorders. They are classified by cardiac response and site of impulse origin. Cardiac response can be tachycardiac (greater than 100 beats/min), bradycardic (less than 60 beats/min), premature (early beat), or blocked (delayed or absent beat).

Tachydysrhythmias and bradydysrhythmias can lower cardiac output and blood pressure. Tachydysrhythmias decrease diastolic filling time. Bradydysrhythmias decrease cardiac output because of lowered heart rate.

Abnormal impulses that originate above the ventricles are referred to as *supraventricular dysrhythmias.* The abnormality on the waveform is seen in the configuration and placement of the P-wave. Ventricular conduction usually remains normal with a normal QRS complex.

Junctional dysrhythmias are an abnormal site of impulse conduction at the A-V junction. The abnormality is identified by an abnormal P-wave, which can occur before, during, or after the QRS complexes. If the P-wave is visible, it is inverted. The QRS complex is usually normal.

Ventricular dysrhythmias are an abnormal site of impulse conduction within the ventricles. The abnormality on the waveform is seen in the configuration and placement of the QRS complex.

Altered Cardiac Output

Failure of the myocardial pump can decrease cardiac output and cause heart failure. It can result from primary coronary artery disease, cardiomyopathic conditions, valvular disorders, and pulmonary disease.

Left-sided heart failure is characterized by impaired functioning of the heart's left side and by elevated pressure and congestion in pulmonary veins and capillaries. If failure is significant, the amount of blood ejected from the left ventricle drops greatly and cardiac output falls. Falling cardiac output can cause tissue hypoxia. As the left ventricle continues to fail, blood begins to "back up" in the pulmonary circulation, causing congestion. This results in crackles, hypoxia, dyspnea, cough, and paroxysmal nocturnal dyspnea (Canobbio, 1990).

Right-sided heart failure is characterized by venous congestion in the systemic circulation. Right-sided heart failure more commonly results from pulmonary disease or as a sequelae to left-sided failure. The primary pathological factor in right-sided failure is elevated pulmonary vascular resistance (PVR). As the PVR rises, the right ventricle must generate more work, and the heart's oxygen demand increases. Continued failure reduces the amount of blood ejected from the right ventricle and blood begins to "back up" in the systemic circulation. Clinically, the client has weight gain, distended neck veins, abdominal organ distention, and dependent peripheral edema.

Impaired Valvular Function

Valvular heart disease is a cardiac valve disorder characterized by stenosis and obstructed blood flow or valvular degeneration and regurgitation of blood (Canobbio, 1990). When stenosis occurs in the semilunar valves (aortic and pulmonic valves), the adjacent ventricles must work harder to move the ventricular volume. Over time the stenosis can cause the ventricle to hypertrophy (enlarge). If left untreated, left- or right-sided heart failure can occur. If stenosis occurs in the atrioventicular valves (mitral and tricuspid valves), the atrial pressure rises. This causes the atria to hypertrophy.

When regurgitation occurs, blood flows back into an adjacent chamber. For example, in mitral regurgitation the mitral leaflets do not close completely. When the ventricle contracts, blood escapes back into the atria, causing a murmur. If left untreated atrial distention and dysrhythmias can occur.

Myocardial Ischemia

Myocardial ischemia results when the blood supply to the myocardium is insufficient to meet the oxygen demands. This ischemia commonly results in angina pectoris or myocardial infarction.

Angina pectoris is usually a transient imbalance between myocardial oxygen supply and demand, resulting in chest pain. Anginal chest pain can be aching, sharp, tingling, burning or feel like pressure. The pain may be on the left side or substernal and may radiate to the left or both arms, jaw, neck, and back. It may not radiate in some clients. The pain lasts from 3 to 15 minutes. Clients sometimes report that pain is brought on by exercise, anxiety, and stress. Anginal pain is relieved with rest and coronary vasodilators, such as nitroglycerine.

Myocardial infarction results from sudden decreases in coronary blood flow or an increase in myocardial oxygen demand. It occurs because of ischemia and necrosis of myocardial tissue and is not reversible (Canobbio, 1990).

Chest pain associated with myocardial infarction can be crushing, squeezing, or stabbing. The pain may be retrosternal and left precordial. If the pain radiates, it may move down the left arm and to the neck, jaws, teeth, epigastric area, and back and may be accompanied by sweating, nausea, and vomiting. It occurs at rest or exertion and lasts more than 30 minutes. It is unrelieved by rest, position change, or nitroglycerin use.

ALTERATIONS IN RESPIRATORY FUNCTIONING

Alterations in respiratory functioning are caused by illnesses and conditions that affect ventilation or oxygen transport.

Hyperventilation

Ventilation produces a normal arterial carbon dioxide tension ($Paco_2$) and indirectly maintains a normal arterial oxygen tension (Pao_2) (Dettenmeier, 1992). *Hyperventilation* and *hypoventilation* refer to alveolar ventilation and not to the client's respiratory rate.

Hyperventilation is ventilation in excess of that required to maintain normal carbon dioxide levels in body tissues. It can be induced by anxiety, infections, drugs, an acid-base imbalance, and hypoxia.

Many signs and symptoms of alveolar hyperventilation can be assessed (see box below). Hemoglobin does not release oxygen to tissues as readily, causing tissue hypoxia. As symptoms worsen, the client may become more agitated, which further increases the respiratory rate and can cause respiratory alkalosis.

Hypoventilation

Hypoventilation occurs when alveolar ventilation is inadequate to meet the body's oxygen demand or to remove enough carbon dioxide. As alveolar ventilation decreases, $Paco_2$ rises. Severe atelectasis can produce hypoventilation. **Atelectasis** is a collapse of the alveoli that prevents normal respiratory exchange of oxygen and carbon dioxide. In clients with chronic obstructive pulmonary disease, the inappropriate administration of oxygen can result in hypoventilation.

SIGNS AND SYMPTOMS OF ALVEOLAR HYPERVENTILATION

Tachycardia	Numbness (extremities, circumoral)
Shortness of breath	Tinnitus
Chest pain	Blurred vision
Dizziness	Disorientation
Lightheadedness	Tetany (carpopedal spasm)
Decreased concentration	
Paresthesia	

table 34-2

COMMON BASIC CARDIAC DYSRHYTHMIAS

Rhythm characteristics	Etiology	Clinical significance	Management
SINUS TACHYCARDIA			
Regular rhythm, rate 100-180 beats/min (higher in infants), normal P-wave, normal QRS complex	Rate increase may be normal response to exercise, emotion, or stressors such as pain, fever, pump failure, hyperthyroidism, and certain drugs (e.g., caffeine, nitrates, atropine, epinephrine, isoproterenol, nicotine)	May have hemodynamic consequence in client with damaged heart that is unable to sustain increased workloads (increased myocardial oxygen consumption) brought on by persistent increases in heart rate	Correct underlying factors, remove offending drugs

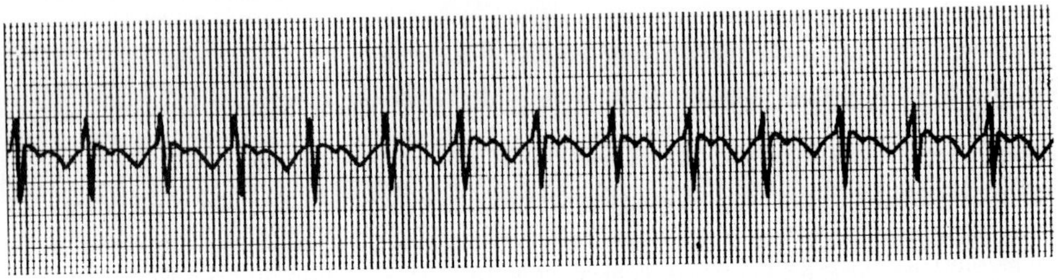

SINUS BRADYCARDIA			
Regular rhythm, rate less than 60 beats/min, normal P-wave, normal PR interval, normal QRS complex	Rate decrease may be normal response to sleep or in well-conditioned athlete; abnormal drops in rate may be caused by diminished blood flow to SA node, vagal stimulation, hypothyroidism, increased intracranial pressure, or pharmacological agents (e.g., digoxin, propranolol, quinidine, procainamide)	No clinical significance unless associated with signs of impaired cardiac output and symptoms of dizziness, syncope, chest pain	Correct underlying causes, administer atropine 0.5-1.0 mg IV, may need to implant transvenous pacemaker

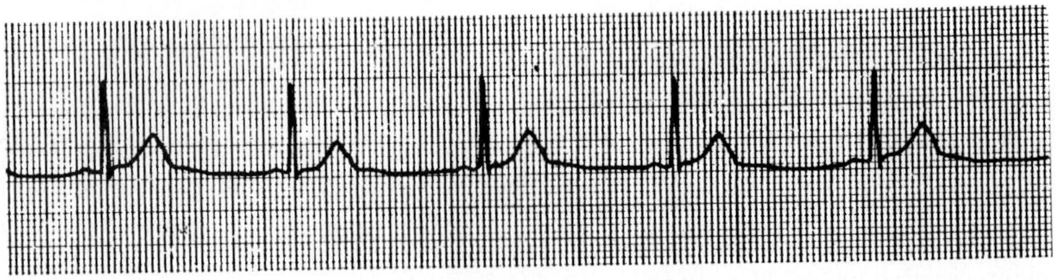

SINUS DYSRHYTHMIA			
Irregular rhythm; possibly phasic with respiration, slowing during inspiration and increasing with expiration; rate of 60-100 beats/min; normal P-wave; normal PR interval; normal QRS complex	Sinus rhythm with cyclic variation caused by vagal impulses that influence rhythm during respiration; occurs commonly in children, young adults, and older adults; usually disappears as heart rate increases	No clinical significance unless heart rate decreases and symptoms of dizziness occur with decreased rate	None indicated unless heart rate decreases and symptoms occur

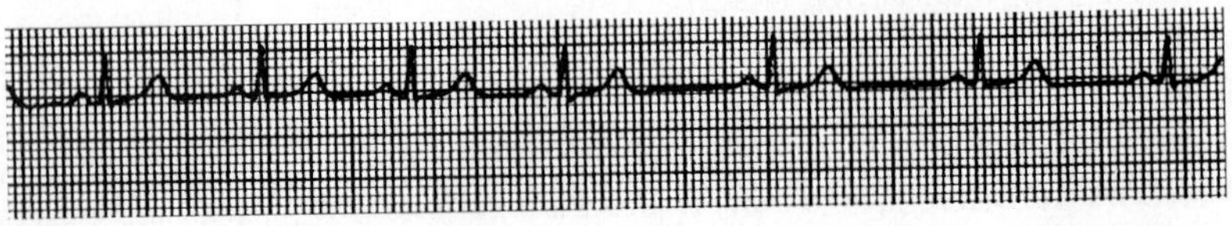

Modified from Canobbio MM: *Cardiovascular disorders,* St. Louis, 1990, Mosby.

Rhythm characteristics	Etiology	Clinical significance	Management
SUPRAVENTRICULAR TACHYCARDIA (SVT)			
Sudden, rapid onset of tachycardia with stimulus originating above AV node; regular rhythm; rate 150-250 beats/min; P-wave uniform, possibly buried in preceding T-wave; PR interval variable, often difficult to measure; normal QRS complex	May begin and end spontaneously or be precipitated by excitement, fatigue, or caffeine, smoking, or alcohol use	Usually no significant impairment; client complains of palpitations and shortness of breath; if persistent or occurring in client with preexisting organic heart disease, may cause decrease in cardiac output and/or blood pressure resulting in pump failure or shock	Perform vagal stimulation with carotid sinus massage. Physician may order drugs to decrease ventricular response with medication to block AV conduction: verapamil 5-10 mg IV push, propranolol slowly IV in 1 mg increments up to 4 mg [contraindicated in clients with heart failure], edrophonium, test dose 1 mg followed by 10 mg IV); perform cardioversion if resistant to preceding measures

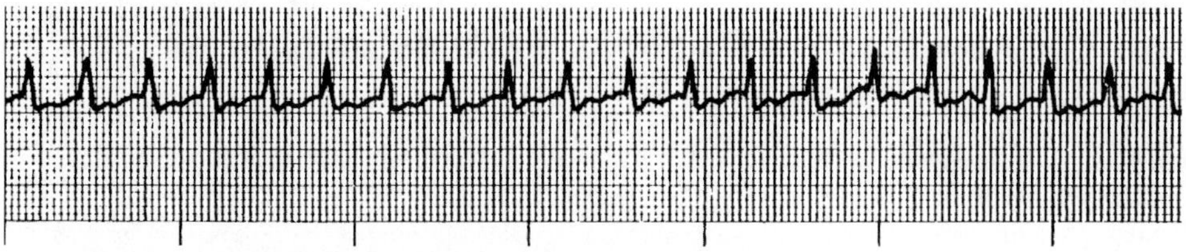

Rhythm characteristics	Etiology	Clinical significance	Management
PREMATURE VENTRICULAR CONTRACTIONS (PVCs)			
Irregular rhythm with ectopic beats followed by full compensatory pause; rate normal or increased depending on number of ectopic beats; P-wave absent in ectopic beat; PR interval absent; QRS complex widened and distorted; T-wave in opposition to R-wave	Caused by irritable focus within ventricle, commonly associated with myocardial infarction; other causes include hypoxia, hyopcalcemia, acidosis	PVCs occurring frequently (more than 6/min) or in pairs indicating increased ventricular irritability	Try to suppress PVCs; if PVCs frequent, administer IV bolus of lidocaine (50-100 mg) followed by continuous IV infusion; administer additional antiarrhythmic agents as needed

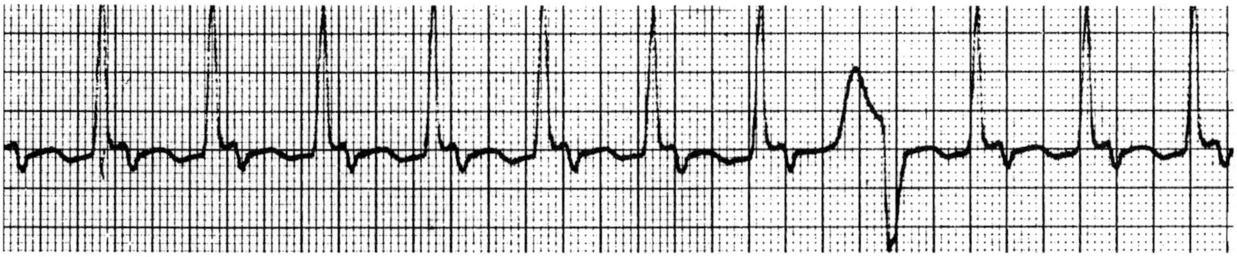

Rhythm characteristics	Etiology	Clinical significance	Management
VENTRICULAR TACHYCARDIA			
Rhythm slightly irregular, rate 100-200 beats/min, P-wave absent, PR interval absent, QRS complex wide and bizarre, >0.12 second	Caused by irritable ventricular foci firing repetitively, commonly caused by myocardial infarction	Often a forerunner of ventricular fibrillation; if condition persistent and rapid, causes decreased cardiac output because of decreased ventricular filling time	Most episodes terminate abruptly without treatment; administer lidocaine bolus 75-100 mg IV followed by continuous intravenous drip; perform cardioversion

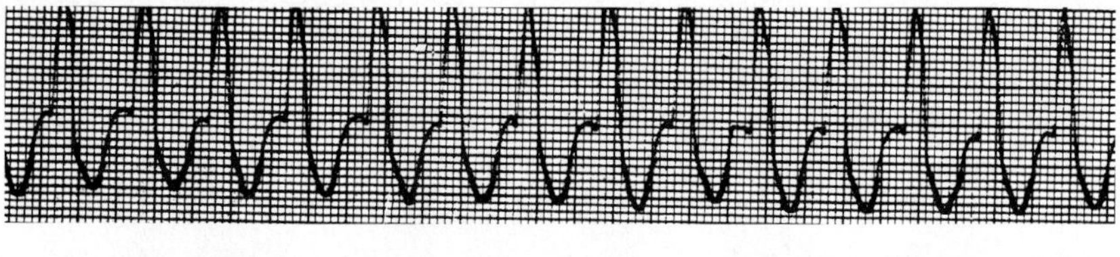

SIGNS AND SYMPTOMS OF ALVEOLAR HYPOVENTILATION

Dizziness	Cardiac dysrhythmias
Headache (may be occipital only on awakening)	Electrolyte imbalances
Lethargy	Convulsions
Disorientation	Coma
Decreased ability to follow instructions	Cardiac arrest

SIGNS AND SYMPTOMS OF HYPOXIA

Restlessness	Increased pulse rate
Apprehension, anxiety	Increased rate and depth of respiration
Decreased ability to concentrate	Elevated blood pressure
Decreased level of consciousness	Cardiac dysrhythmias
Increased fatigue	Pallor
Dizziness	Cyanosis
Behavioral changes	Clubbing
	Dyspnea

Many signs and symptoms of hypoventilation may be revealed through physical assessment (see box above). If untreated, convulsions, unconsciousness, and death can result. The goals of treatment are to treat the underlying cause while simultaneously restoring optimal ventilatory function, improving tissue oxygenation, and achieving acid-base balance (Gröer, Shekleton, 1989).

Hypoxia

Hypoxia is inadequate cellular oxygenation that results from deficient delivery or use of oxygen at the cellular level (Gröer, Shekleton, 1989). Hypoxia can be caused by a decreased hemoglobin level and lowered oxygen-carrying capacity of the blood, a diminished concentration of inspired oxygen such as may occur at high altitudes, the inability of the tissues to extract oxygen from the blood such as with cyanide poisoning, decreased diffusion of oxygen from the alveoli to the blood such as with pneumonia, poor tissue perfusion with oxygenated blood such as with shock, and impaired ventilation.

The clinical signs and symptoms of hypoxia are listed in the box above. The client with hypoxia is unable to lie down and appears fatigued and agitated. **Cyanosis,** a blue discoloration of the skin and mucous membranes caused by desaturated hemoglobin in capillaries, is a late sign of hypoxia. The nurse should observe other areas of the body besides the skin for signs of cyanosis, such as the conjunctivae, mouth, nail beds, and extremities. The presence or absence of cyanosis is not an absolute measure of oxygenation status. **Dyspnea,** shortness of breath or difficulty in breathing, is another clinical sign of hypoxia. It is the subjective sensation of difficult or uncomfortable breathing (Gift, 1990). Pathological dyspnea must be differentiated from physiological dyspnea, which is shortness of breath after exercise or excitement.

Hypoxia is a life-threatening condition. Untreated, it can produce fatal cardiac dysrhythmias. Hypoxia is managed by administering oxygen and by treating the underlying cause, such as shock or pneumonia.

NURSING PROCESS AND OXYGENATION

Assessment

The nursing assessment of a client's cardiopulmonary functioning should include data collected from a nursing history, physical examination, and diagnostic test results.

Nursing History. The nursing history should focus on the client's ability to meet oxygen needs. The nursing history for cardiac function includes information regarding pain, dyspnea, fatigue, peripheral circulation, cardiac risk factors, and past or current cardiac conditions. The nursing history for respiratory function includes cough, shortness of breath, wheezing, pain, environmental exposures, frequency of respiratory tract infections, pulmonary risk factors, past respiratory problems, smoking history, and medication use.

FATIGUE. Fatigue is a subjective sensation in which the client reports a loss of endurance. In the client with cardiopulmonary alterations fatigue is often an early sign of a worsening of the chronic underlying process. To provide an objective measure of fatigue, the client may be asked to describe changes in activity patterns or to rate the fatigue on a scale of 1 to 10, with 10 being the worst level of fatigue and 1 being no fatigue.

DYSPNEA. Dyspnea can occur with exaggerated respiratory effort, use of the accessory muscles during respiration, flaring of the nares, and a rapid increase in the rate and depth of respirations (Gröer, Shekleton, 1989). To provide an objective measure of dyspnea, the client may use a visual analog scale. The scale is a 100 mm vertical line with 0 equated with no dyspnea, and the 100 mm marker equated with extreme breathlessness. Its use to evaluate a client's dyspnea is valid and reliable (Gift et al., 1986; Gift, 1989).

The nursing history of dyspnea includes the circumstances under which it occurred and whether the client's perception of dyspnea affects the ability to lie flat. **Orthopnea** is the use of multiple pillows when lying down or having to sit to breathe. Orthopnea is usually described as two- or three-pillow orthopnea, depending on the conditions needed to overcome the dyspnea.

Cough. Cough is a sudden, audible expulsion of air from the lungs. The client breathes in, the glottis is partially closed, and the accessory muscles of expiration contract to expel the air forcibly. Coughing is a protective reflex to clear the trachea, bronchi, and lungs of irritants and secretions.

A **productive cough** is one that results in sputum. Sputum is material coughed up from the lungs that may be swallowed or expectorated through the mouth. It contains mucus, cellular debris, and microorganisms, and it may contain pus or blood. The nurse must collect data about the type and quantity of sputum (see box at right). The client should try to produce some sputum for inspection.

If **hemoptysis** (bloody sputum) is reported, the nurse determines if it is associated with coughing and bleeding from the upper respiratory tract and not from the gastrointestinal tract **(hematemesis).** It should be described according to amount, color, and duration and whether it is mixed with sputum. When a client reports bloody or blood-tinged sputum, diagnostic tests on sputum specimens or x-ray studies should be performed to determine the cause.

Coughing is classified as to the time when the client most frequently coughs. Clients with chronic sinusitis may cough only in the early morning or immediately after rising from sleep. This clears the airway of mucus resulting from sinus drainage. Clients with chronic bronchitis generally produce sputum all day, although greater amounts are produced after rising from a semirecumbent or flat position.

Wheezing. **Wheezing** is characterized by a high-pitched musical sound. It is caused by high-velocity air movement through a narrowed airway and may be associated with asthma and acute bronchitis. Clients can usually describe when they wheeze and whether wheezing is present during inspiration or expiration. The nurse should ask clients about any precipitating factors.

Pain. Chest pain must be thoroughly evaluated with regard to location, duration, radiation, and frequency. Cardiac pain does not occur with respiratory variations. It is most often on the left side of the chest and may radiate. Pericardial pain resulting from pericardial sac inflammation is usually nonradiating and may occur with inspiration.

Pleuritic chest pain is peripheral and may radiate to the scapular regions, worsens on inspiration, and lasts from minutes to hours. Pleuritic pain is often caused from an inflammation or infection in the pleural space. Clients often describe pleuritic pain as knifelike.

SPUTUM CHARACTERISTICS

COLOR

Clear, Green, White, Brown, Yellow, Red
Streaked with blood

CHANGES IN COLOR

Same color throughout the day
Clearing with coughing
Progressively darker

ODOR

None
Foul

QUALITY

Same as usual
Increased
Decreased

CONSISTENCY

Frothy
Watery
Tenacious, thick

PRESENCE OF BLOOD

Occasional
Early morning
Bright or dark red
Blood-tinged

Musculoskeletal pain may follow exercise, rib trauma, and prolonged coughing episodes. It is worsened on inspiration and may easily be confused with pleuritic chest pain.

Environmental or Geographical Exposures. Environmental exposure to many inhaled substances is closely linked with respiratory disease. The nurse should investigate exposures in the home and workplace to cigarette smoke (active or passive), radon, asbestos, coal, cotton fibers, fumes, or chemical inhalants. It is particularly important with clients who may have worked in places without regulations to protect workers from carcinogens. Exposure to other substances in certain geographical areas may result in diseases such as schistosomiasis and coccidioidomycosis (valley fever).

Respiratory Infections. A nursing history should contain information about the client's frequency and duration of respiratory tract infections, episodes of bronchitis or pneumonia, exposure to tuberculosis, and the results of tuberculin skin tests. Because the acquired immunodeficiency syndrome (AIDS) may initially be diagnosed after a *Pneumocystis carinii* infection is found, the nurse needs to assess the client for high-risk behaviors related to AIDS, including exposure to illicit intravenous drug use and multiple sexual contacts.

Risk Factors. The nurse assesses familial and environmental risk factors, including a family history of cancer, particularly lung cancer, or cardiovascular diseases, infectious diseases, particularly tuberculosis. The nurse should determine who in the client's household has been infected and the status of treatment.

Medications. The last component of the nursing history should be medications the client is using, including prescribed, over-the-counter, and illicit drugs and substances. Such medications may have adverse effects by

table 34-3

INSPECTION OF CARDIOPULMONARY STATUS

Abnormality	Cause
EYES	
Xanthelasma (yellow lipid lesions on eyelids)	Associated with hyperlipidemia
Corneal arcus (whitish opaque ring around junction of cornea and sclera)	Abnormal finding in young to middle-age adults associated with hyperlipidemia (normal finding in older adults with arcus senilius)
Pale conjunctivae	Associated with anemia
Cyanotic conjunctivae	Associated with hypoxemia
Petechiae on conjunctivae	Associated with fat embolus or bacterial endocarditis
SKIN	
Peripheral cyanosis	Vasoconstriction and diminished blood flow
Central cyanosis	Hypoxemia
Decreased skin turgor	Dehydration (normal finding in older adults as a result of decreased skin elasticity)
Dependent edema	Associated with right- and left-sided heart failure
Periorbital edema	Associated with kidney disease
FINGERTIPS AND NAIL BEDS	
Cyanosis	Decreased cardiac output or hypoxia
Splinter hemorrhages	Bacterial endocarditis
Clubbing	Chronic hypoxemia
MOUTH AND LIPS	
Cyanotic mucous membranes	Decreased oxygenation (hypoxia)
Pursed-lip breathing	Associated with chronic lung disease
NECK VEINS	
Distention	Associated with right-sided heart failure
NOSE	
Flaring nares	Air hunger, dyspnea
CHEST	
Retractions	Increased work of breathing, dyspnea
Asymmetry	Chest wall injury

From Dennison R: *Nurs 86* 16(4):34, 1986.

themselves or by interacting with other drugs. As with all medication, the nurse assesses clients' knowledge and ability to use the "five rights" of medication administration. Of particular importance is the assessment of clients' understanding of potential side effects.

When clients are prescribed drugs for which toxic levels can be monitored by blood analyses, the nurse must review these laboratory values. Toxic effects of these drugs can impair cardiopulmonary functioning. Illicit drugs, particularly inhaled or parenterally administered narcotics, are often diluted with talcum powder, which irritates lung tissues.

Physical Examination. The physical examination performed to assess level of tissue oxygenation includes evaluation of the entire cardiopulmonary system. Inspection, palpation, auscultation, and percussion techniques are used.

INSPECTION. Using inspection techniques, the nurse performs a head-to-toe observation of the client for skin and mucous membrane color, general appearance, level of consciousness, adequacy of systemic circulation, breathing patterns, and chest wall movement (Tables 34-3 to 34-5). Any abnormalities should be investigated during palpation, percussion, and auscultation.

table 34-4

ASSESSMENT OF BREATHING PATTERNS

Pattern	Causes
Eupnea—normal respiratory rate; adult range of 12-20 breaths/min; normal tidal volume of 5-7 ml/kg body weight*	
Tachypnea—increased respiratory rate above client's normal rate; shallow respirations	Exercise, pregnancy, fever, pulmonary diseases, anxiety, neurological conditions, bronchoconstriction
Bradypnea—decreased respiratory rate below client's normal rate	Drug overdose, central nervous system dysfunction, airway obstruction
Kussmaul respiration—abnormally deep, very rapid sighing type of respiration; increased tidal volume and rate	Diabetic ketoacidosis
Ataxic respirations—uncoordinated respiratory patterns; no coordinated rate or depth of respiration	Central nervous system disorders
Cheyne-Stokes respiration—breathing pattern characterized by alternating periods of apnea and deep rapid breathing; cycle beginning with slow, shallow breaths that gradually increase to abnormal depth and rate; respiration gradually subsiding as breathing slows and becomes shallow	Congestive heart failure, bronchopneumonia, drug overdose, sleep, central nervous system damage

*From Luce JM, Tyler ML, Pierson DJ: *Intensive respiratory care,* ed 2, Philadelphia, 1993, Saunders.

table 34-5

ASSESSMENT OF ABNORMAL CHEST WALL MOVEMENT

Abnormality	Cause
Retraction—visible sinking in soft tissues of chest between and around firmer tissue and cartilaginous and bony ribs; retractions having specific beginning point and worsening with need for increased inspiratory effort; possibly found at intercostal space, intraclavicular space, trachea, and substernally*	Any condition that causes increased inspiratory effort (e.g., airway obstruction, asthma, tracheobronchitis)
Paradoxical breathing—asynchronous breathing; chest contraction during inspiration and expansion during expiration	Flail chest
Increased anteroposterior diameter	Senile emphysema or chronic obstructive pulmonary disease

*Infants can experience sternal and substernal retractions with only slight inspiratory effort because of chest pliability.

PALPATION. Chest palpation documents the type and amount of thoracic excursion, elicits any areas of tenderness, and can identify tactile fremitus, thrills, and heaves. With palpation the nurse can locate the cardiac point of maximal impulse. Palpation also allows the nurse to feel for masses or lumps in the axilla and breast tissue. Palpation of the extremities provides data about the peripheral circulation.

PERCUSSION. With percussion, the nurse can detect abnormal fluid, air in the lungs, or diaphragmatic excursions.

AUSCULTATION. Auscultation enables the nurse to identify normal and abnormal heart and lung sounds. It should include assessment for normal S_1 and S_2 sounds, abnormal S_3 and S_4, and murmurs and rubs. The nurse identifies location, radiation, intensity, pitch, and quality of a murmur. Auscultation is also used to identify a bruit over the carotid arteries, abdominal aorta, and femoral arteries. Auscultation of lung sounds involves listening for air movement throughout all lung fields. It also evaluates the client's response to interventions for improving respiratory status.

Diagnostic Tests

TESTS TO DETERMINE ADEQUACY OF THE CARDIAC CONDUCTION SYSTEM. Tests used to determine the adequacy of the cardiac conduction system include electrocardiogram, Holter monitor, exercise stress test, and electrophysiological studies.

ELECTROCARDIOGRAM. The electrocardiogram (ECG) produces a graphic record of the heart's electrical activity. The ECG commonly detects abnormal impulse transmission and the electrical position of the heart (the axis).

HOLTER MONITOR. The **Holter monitor** is a portable device that records the heart's electrical activity and produces a continuous ECG over a specified period. It allows clients to continue with their normal activities while recording. This device enables clinicians to determine if activities such as walking and straining at stool are linked to abnormal electrical activity.

EXERCISE STRESS TEST. The **exercise stress test** evaluates the cardiac response to physical stress. Heart rate, electrical activity, and cardiac recovery time are reflected in the ECG tracing (Canobbio, 1990). Data about the client's blood pressure, chest pain, respiratory changes, and color are also monitored.

ELECTROPHYSIOLOGICAL STUDIES. An **electrophysiological (EP) study** measures electrical activity. An electrode catheter is inserted into the right atrium, usually via the femoral vein. Electrical stimulation is then delivered through the catheter. ECG monitors and computers record the heart's electrical response to the stimulus. It provides more specific information about difficult-to-treat dysrhythmias.

TESTS TO DETERMINE MYOCARDIAL CONTRACTION AND BLOOD FLOW. There are invasive and noninvasive tests used to determine myocardial contraction and blood flow.

ECHOCARDIOGRAPHY. **Echocardiography** evaluates the internal structures of the heart and heart wall and valve motion. Sonar (radar) technology is used to measure ultrasonic waves and translate them into formed images. The echocardiogram shows overall cardiac performance.

SCINTIGRAPHY. **Scintigraphy,** or radionuclide angiography, is an imaging technique that uses radioisotopes to evaluate cardiac structures, myocardial perfusion, and contractility (Canobbio, 1990).

CARDIAC CATHETERIZATION AND ANGIOGRAPHY. **Cardiac catheterization** and **angiography** is a procedure used to visualize cardiac chambers, valves, the great vessels, and coronary arteries. It also records pressures and volumes within the four chambers. A catheter is inserted into the heart via a percutaneous venous puncture. A contrast material is injected through the catheter, and fluoroscopic pictures are obtained of the vessels. Both right- and left-sided catheterizations can be performed.

TESTS TO MEASURE ADEQUACY OF VENTILATION AND OXYGENATION. Pulmonary function tests, peak expiratory flow rates, arterial blood gas tests, oximetry, and complete blood counts are used to assess ventilation and oxygenation.

PULMONARY FUNCTION TESTS. **Pulmonary function tests** determine ventilatory ability of the lungs. In combination with arterial blood gas tests and oximetry, a determination can be made of the lungs' efficiency in exchanging oxygen and carbon dioxide. Basic studies use a spirometer and recording device to measure volumes as the client breathes through a mouthpiece into a connecting tube. Measurements include tidal volume (TV), inspiratory reserve volume (IRV), residual volume (RV), and forced expiratory volume in 1 second (FEV_1).

Pulmonary function tests are usually performed in a pulmonary function laboratory. The nurse prepares the client by explaining the procedure. A nose clip prevents air from being inhaled or exhaled through the nose. The client breathes through a mouthpiece attached to a spirometer. The client is asked at certain times to inhale or exhale as much air as possible. The client must cooperate to ensure accurate results.

PEAK EXPIRATORY FLOW RATE. **Peak expiratory flow rate (PEFR)** is the point of highest flow during maximal expiration. It reflects changes in large airway sizes. The measure is similar to and correlates well with the FEV_1 (Walsh, 1992). The peak expiratory flow meter is a handheld instrument that allows clients with chronic asthma to follow the degree of airway openness.

ARTERIAL BLOOD GAS TESTS. Arterial blood gas tests are done together with pulmonary function tests to determine the hydrogen ion concentration, partial pressure of carbon dioxide and oxygen concentration, and oxyhemoglobin saturation. They provide information about diffusion of gas across the alveolar-capillary membrane and tissue oxygenation.

OXIMETRY. Continuous measurements of capillary oxygen saturation are available with cutaneous **oximetry** (Procedure 34-1). One of the most common is a finger oximeter. The nurse attaches a sensor to the client's finger, which noninvasively monitors capillary blood oxygen saturation. Continuous monitoring can assess sleep disorders, exercise tolerance, and transient decreases in oxygen saturation. However, clients with poor tissue perfusion such as with shock, hypothermia, and peripheral vascular diseases may not have reliable oximetry measures.

COMPLETE BLOOD COUNT. A complete blood count determines the number and type of red and white blood cells per mm^3 of venous blood. The nurse obtains a venous blood sample. Normal values for a complete blood count vary with age and gender. The complete blood count also measures the hemoglobin level. A deficiency in red blood cells (which contain hemoglobin) decreases the blood's oxygen-carrying capacity. When the

procedure 34-1

PULSE OXIMETRY

Steps	Rationale
1. Identify client who will benefit from pulse oximetry. a. Assess client's respiratory status: oxygen therapy, hemoglobin level. b. Review client's medical record for physician's order for pulse oximetry. c. Identify clients who may have oxygen desaturation with sleep, activity, suctioning.	Identifies hypoxemia before signs and symptoms develop. Allows nurse to monitor trends in client's level of oxygen. Enables nurse to use objective criteria to adjust nursing intervention to optimize oxygen saturation.
d. Clients receiving or who have received sedation.	Sedation can decrease respiratory rate and depth, which decreases oxygenation.
2. Obtain equipment and place at bedside (see illustration): a. Pulse oximeter b. Senser probe	Ensures error-free data regarding oxygen saturation.

Type of sensor	*Client's weight**
(1) Adhesive neonatal	Less than 3 kg (6.6 lb); more than 40 kg (88 lb)
(2) Adhesive infant	From 1 kg (2.2. lb) to 20 kg (44 lb)
(3) Adhesive pediatric	From 10 kg (22 lb) to 50 kg (110 lb)
(4) Adhesive adult	More than 30 kg (66 lb)
(5) Adhesive adult nasal	More than 50 kg (110 lb)
(6) Finger clip	More than 40 kg (88 lb)

c. Continuous printout (optional)

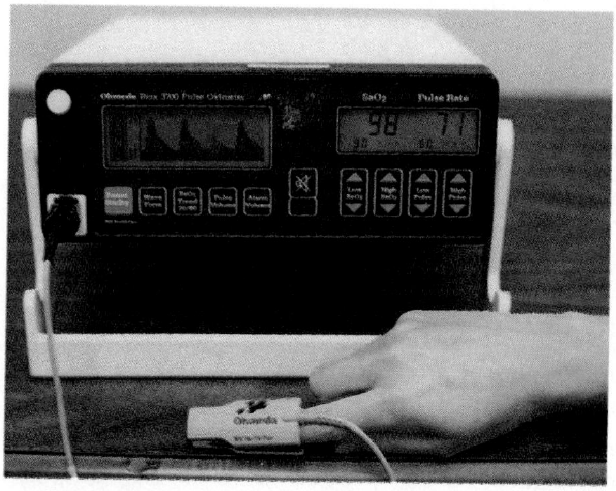

Step 2

Steps	Rationale
3. Explain purpose of procedure to client and family.	Ensures client and family understanding and increases compliance.
4. Wash hands.	Reduces transmission of microorganisms.
5. Select appropriate area on client to apply sensor based on peripheral circulation and extremity temperature.	
a. Determine adequacy of peripheral circulation by assessing capillary refill (toe and finger sites).	Peripheral vasoconstriction alters oxygen saturation.
b. Do not use adhesive adult nasal sensor if client has large-bore nasogastric tube or nasoendotracheal tube. c. Determine use of vasoactive drugs.	Prevents interference with oxygen saturation readings because of poor peripheral circulation and excessive equipment or dressings.
d. Align photoelectron and light-emitting diode.	Permits transmission of light. Alignment ensures accurate oxygen saturation readings.
6. Prepare selected site: a. Remove nail polish. b. Remove artificial nails. c. Remove earrings. d. Wash selected site, wipe with alcohol, and air dry.	Body oils, nail polish, and artificial nails interfere with transmission of light through nail, tissue, venous and arterial blood, and skin pigmentation (Sonnesso, 1991).
7. Attach sensor probe to finger, bridge of nose, earlobe, toe.	
8. Instruct client to breathe normally.	Prevents large fluctuations in minute ventilation and possible change in oxygen saturation.

*From Sonnesso G: *Nurs 91* 21(8):60, 1991.

Continued.

procedure 34-1—cont'd

Steps	Rationale
9. Attach oximeter sensor to pulse oximeter.	
a. Turn machine on.	
b. Listen for audible beep.	Senses with each pulse and indicates how well oximeter monitors pulse.
c. Observe waveform for bar of light.	Light or waveform fluctuates with each pulsation and reflects pulse strength. Poor light on small waveform usually indicates that signal is too weak to give accurate oxygen saturation reading.
10. Ensure that alarm limits for *both* high and low oxygen saturation and high and low pulse are set according to physician's order and *turned on.*	Manufacturers preset limits, and adjustments can be made according to client's underlying physical condition, therapy, and risks (Sonnesso, 1991). Provides an audible and visual signal that high or low limits have been exceeded.
11. Read saturation level as ordered and while performing nursing interventions.	Documents oxygen saturation levels at rest, with activity such as ambulation, during procedure such as suctioning, and with changes in physical condition.
12. Move a finger sensor every 4 hr and a spring-tension sensor every 2 hr.	Allows nurse to assess for and prevent impaired skin integrity caused by pressure from sensor.
13. Record in nurses' notes client's use of continuous pulse oximetry and record oxygen saturation.	Documents use of equipment for third-party payers, documents oxygen saturation.
14. Correlate oxygen saturation value with arterial blood gas measurements if available.	Documents reliability of oximeter.
15. Report oxygen saturation and respond to changes in therapy to oncoming shift.	Provides oncoming nurse with baseline information and response to therapy.

number of red blood cells is increased, the oxygen-carrying capacity of the blood is increased. However, abnormal elevations in red blood cells increase blood viscosity and the client's risk for thrombus formation.

TESTS TO VISUALIZE STRUCTURES OF THE RESPIRATORY SYSTEM. Chest x-ray examination, bronchoscopy, and lung scan are used to visualize the respiratory system.

CHEST X-RAY EXAMINATION. A chest x-ray examination consists of a radiograph of the thorax that allows the physician and nurse to observe the lung fields for fluid (as with pneumonia), masses (as with lung cancer), fractures (as with rib and clavicular fractures), lung expansion (as with pneumonothorax), and other abnormal processes (as with tuberculosis).

BRONCHOSCOPY. **Bronchoscopy** visualizes the trachea and bronchial tree. A narrow, flexible fiberoptic bronchoscope is used to obtain biopsy and fluid or sputum samples. It can also remove mucus plugs or foreign bodies lodged in the airways. The client fasts beforehand. The nurse also administers a sedative before the procedure. Atropine may also be administered to reduce oral secretions. The nurse observes the client after the procedure for signs and symptoms of respiratory distress or hypoxia. Assessment of the client's gag/swallow reflex is obtained before beginning oral fluids.

LUNG SCAN. The most common lung scan is the computed tomogram (CT) scan. CT scanning combines x-ray and computer technology. X-ray beams pass through a section or plane of the thorax from different angles. The computer calculates tissue absorption and displays a printout and scan picture of the tissues showing densities of various structures. A CT scan can identify abnormal masses by size and location but cannot identify tissue types, which requires a biopsy.

TESTS TO DETERMINE ABNORMAL CELLS OR INFECTION IN THE RESPIRATORY TRACT. Tests to determine abnormal cells or infection in the respiratory tract include throat cultures, sputum specimens, skin testing, and thoracentesis.

THROAT CULTURES. A throat culture sample is obtained by swabbing the oropharynx and tonsillar regions with a sterile swab. A culture and sensitivity test identifies microorganisms and the antibiotics to which they are most sensitive. When obtaining a throat culture, the nurse inserts the swab into the pharyngeal region and passes it along reddened areas and areas of exudate. An active gag reflex may make obtaining the specimen difficult. The client may be able to control gagging by sitting straight forward slightly.

Sputum specimens. Sputum specimens identify microorganisms and their drug sensitivities. This specimen is referred to as *sputum for culture and sensitivity* (C and S). A sputum specimen may also identify the tubercle bacillus (TB). This sputum specimen is called *sputum for acid-fast bacillus* (AFB). The AFB specimen is obtained 3 consecutive days in the early morning. Sputum specimens are also used to identify abnormal cells. This is called *sputum for cytology* and involves collecting three early morning sputum specimens. It identifies lung cancers by cell type. The nurse must ensure that the sputum specimens consist of mucus deep from the bronchus and not saliva. The nurse should record the color, consistency, amount, and odor of the sputum and document that the specimen was sent to a specific laboratory for analysis on a specific date and time.

Skin testing. Skin testing identifies exposure to bacterial, fungal, or viral pulmonary diseases. The antigen is injected intradermally (see Procedure 26-3). It should be properly injected, the injection site should be circled, and the client should be instructed not to wash off the circle. Positive results are based on the size of the induration, a palpable, elevated, hardened area around the injection site. It is caused by the antigen/antibody reaction. Indurations are measured in millimeters. Reddened flat areas are not positive reactions and should not be measured.

Thoracentesis. **Thoracentesis** is surgical perforation of the chest wall and pleural space with a needle to aspirate fluid for tests or to remove a biopsy specimen. It is performed with aseptic technique using a local anesthetic. The client usually sits upright with the anterior thorax supported by pillows or an over-the-bed table (Figure 34-6). Whether this procedure is painful depends on the client's pain tolerance. The nurse can reduce the client's anxiety by explaining the procedure and telling the client what to expect. The client must understand the importance of holding the breath and not coughing. Sudden movements of the thorax may result in the lung being punctured by the thoracentesis needle. The client should notify the physician before coughing or sneezing so the needle can be withdrawn. After the procedure the nurse monitors the client for signs of pneumothorax (Procedure 34-2).

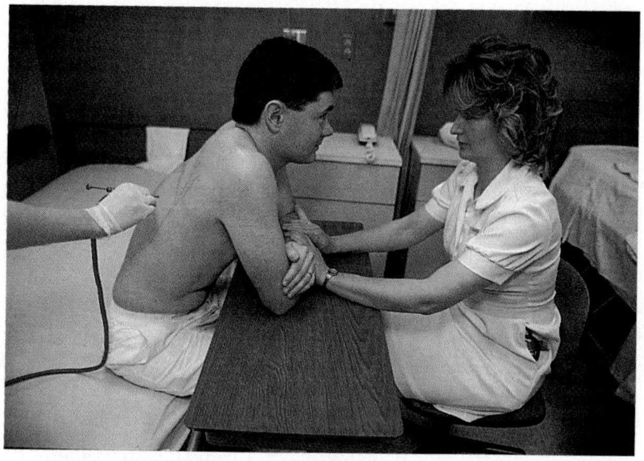

FIGURE 34-6 Position for thoracentesis. (From Wilson SF, Thompson JM: *Respiratory disorders,* St. Louis, 1990, Mosby.)

Nursing Diagnosis

Clients with an altered level of oxygenation can have nursing diagnoses that are primarily from a cardiovascular or pulmonary origin (see box below). After reviewing the subjective data, such as reports of increased fatigue, and objective findings, such as yellow sputum, the nurse clusters the data through critical thinking. Critical thinking distinguishes relevant from irrelevant data and determines patterns and relationships for accurate nursing diagnoses. Each nursing diagnosis should be based on specific defining characteristics and should include the related etiology. The diagnostic label is validated by the defining characteristics or signs and symptoms. Two nursing studies have validated nursing diagnoses resulting from pulmonary causes (McDonald, 1985; York, 1985). McDonald (1985) researched *ineffective airway clearance, ineffective breathing patterns,* and *impaired gas exchange.*

Planning

Clients with impaired oxygenation require a nursing care plan directed toward meeting the actual or potential oxygenation needs of the client (see p. 1000). The plan includes one or more of the following client-centered goals:

Goal: Client achieves improved activity tolerance.

Outcomes

Client reports less discomfort with exercise

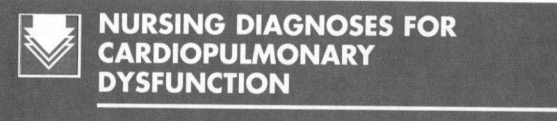

NURSING DIAGNOSES FOR CARDIOPULMONARY DYSFUNCTION

Ineffective airway clearance
Impaired gas exchange
Ineffective breathing pattern
Decreased cardiac output
High risk for infection
Activity intolerance

procedure 34-2

CARE OF THE CLIENT WITH CHEST TUBES

Steps	Rationale
1. Assess client for respiratory distress and chest pain, breath sounds over affected lung area, and stable vital signs.	Increase in respiratory distress and/or chest pain, decrease in breath sounds over the affected and nonaffected lungs, marked cyanosis, asymmetric chest movements, presence of subcutaneous emphysema around tube insertion site or neck, hypotension, tachycardia, and/or mediastinal shift are critical and indicate a severe change in client status, such as excessive blood loss or tension pneumothorax. Notify physician immediately.
2. Observe:	
a. Chest tube dressing	Ensures that dressing remains occlusive and notes any drainage.
b. Tubing for kinks, dependent loops, or clots	Maintains a patent, freely draining system, preventing fluid accumulation in chest cavity.
c. Chest drainage system, which should be upright and below level of tube insertion	System must be in this position to function properly.
d. Water seal for fluctuations with client's inspiration and expiration	Fluid should rise in water seal with inspiration and fall with expiration, indicating that system is functioning properly (Erickson, 1981a; Carroll, 1986).
e. Bubbling in water-seal bottle or chamber (see Table 34-6)	When system is initially connected to client, bubbles are expected in chamber from air that was present in system and in client's intrapleural space (Farley, 1988). After a short period, bubbling will stop. Fluid will continue to fluctuate in water seal on inspiration and expiration until lung is reexpanded or system becomes occluded.
f. Type and amount of fluid drainage: Nurse should note color and amount of drainage, client's vital signs, and skin color.	Sudden gush of drainage may be retained blood and not active bleeding. Increase in drainage can be result of client position change (Farley, 1988).
(1) Less than 50-200 ml/hr immediately postoperative in mediastinal chest tube (Johanson, et al., 1988); approximately 500 ml in first 24 hr; dark red drainage is expected early in postoperative period, turning serous with time.	Reexpansion of lungs forces drainage into tube. Coughing can also cause large gushes of drainage.
(2) Between 100-300 ml of fluid may drain in posterior chest tube during first 2 hr after insertion; rate will decrease after 2 hr, 500-1000 ml can be expected in first 24 hr; drainage will be grossly bloody during first several hours after surgery and then change to serous.	Excessive amounts and/or continued presence of frank, bloody drainage after first several hours of surgery should be reported to physician, along with client's vital signs and respiratory status.
g. Bubbling in the suction-control chamber (when suction is being used) (see Table 34-6)	Suction-control chamber has constant, gentle bubbling. Tubing to suction source should be free of obstruction, and suction source should be turned on to appropriate setting.
3. Provide two shodded hemostats for each chest tube. Shodded hemostats are usually attached to top of client's bed with adhesive tape or clamped to client's clothing during ambulation. Shodded hemostats have protective covering such as plastic over points. Covering prevents hemostat from penetrating chest tube.	Chest tubes are only clamped under specific circumstances: a. To assess air leak (see Table 34-6) b. To empty or change collection bottle or chamber (Farley, 1988); this procedure is performed only by physician or nurse who has received training in procedure c. To change disposable systems (Erickson, 1981b); have new system ready to be connected before clamping tube so that transfer can be rapid and drainage system reestablished d. To change a broken water-seal bottle in event that no sterile solution container is available

Steps	Rationale
	e. To assess if client is ready to have chest tube removed, which is done by physician's order (Farley, 1988); in this situation, nurse must monitor client for re-creation of pneumothorax (see Table 34-6)
4. Position the client:	Permits optimal drainage of fluid and/or air.
a. Semi-Fowler's to high Fowler's position to evacuate air (pneumothorax)	Air rises to highest point in chest. Pneumothorax tubes are usually placed on anterior aspect at midclavicular line, second or third intercostal space (Carroll, 1986).
b. High Fowler's position to drain fluid (hemothorax)	Permits optimal drainage of fluid. Posterior tubes are placed on midaxillary line, eighth or ninth intercostal space.
5. Maintain tube connection between chest and drainage tubes intact and taped.	Secures chest tube to drainage system and reduces risk of air leaks causing breaks in airtight system.
a. Water-seal vent must be without occlusion.	Permits displaced air to pass into atmosphere.
b. Suction-control chamber vent must be without occlusion when suction is used.	Provides safety factor of releasing excess negative pressure into atmosphere.
6. Coil excess tubing on mattress next to client. Secure with rubber band and safety pin or system's clamp.	Prevents excess tubing from hanging over edge of mattress in dependent loop. Drainage could collect in loop and occlude drainage system.
7. Adjust tubing to hang in straight line from top of mattress to drainage chamber. If chest tube is draining fluid, indicate time (e.g., 0900) that drainage was begun on drainage bottle's adhesive tape of bottle setup or on write-on surface of disposable commercial system.	Promotes drainage. Provides a baseline for continuous assessment of type and quality of drainage.
8. Strip or milk chest tube only if indicated: a. Postoperative mediastinal chest tubes are manipulated if nursing assessment indicates obstruction of drainage secondary to clots or debris in tubing. b. Postoperative assessment is done every 15 min for the first 2 hr. This assessment interval then changes *based on client's status.*	Stripping is controversial and should be performed only if hospital policy permits and there is physician's order (Pierce, Piazza, Naftel, 1991; Johanson, et al., 1988). Stripping creates high degree of negative pressure and has potential of pulling lung tissue or pleura into drainage holes of chest tube (Duncan, Erickson, 1982; Duncan, Erickson, Weigel, 1987).
9. Wash hands.	Reduces transmission of infection.
10. Record in nurse's notes patency of chest tubes, presence of drainage, presence of fluctuations, client's vital signs, and level of comfort.	Documents accurate functioning of chest tubes and client's physical status.

Client increases walking distance or time
Client returns to resting pulse more quickly

Goal: Client maintains lung expansion.

Outcomes

Breath sounds auscultated throughout all lobes
Client's lung is free of adventitious sounds

Goal: Client maintains mobilization of pulmonary secretions.

Outcomes

Client clears airway by coughing
Sputum thin, clear

Goal: Client maintains a patent airway.

Outcomes

Client clears airway by coughing
Sputum thin, clear
Client's lung free of adventitious sounds

Goal: Client's tissue oxygenation is maintained.

Outcomes

Oxygen saturation remains above 90%
Client's skin color normal

Goal: Client's cardiopulmonary function is restored.

Outcomes

Client has spontaneous ventilation
Client's pulse is regular, within normal limits

The nurse must set priorities in the presence of several nursing diagnoses. The nurse must pay equal attention to both psychosocial and physiological findings.

SAMPLE NURSING CARE PLAN

ASSESSMENT

Clinical scenario: Mr. Marcus is 2 days post automobile accident and in *bilateral leg traction,* he has *a low-grade fever, increased pulse and respiratory rate, adventitious lung sounds are present in both bases, his sputum is yellow.*

NURSING DIAGNOSIS

Ineffective airway clearance related to thickened pulmonary secretions.

PLANNING

Goal	Expected outcomes
Client's airway secretions will be removed within 72 hours.	Adventitious lung sounds will be reduced within 24 hours. Client will maintain forceful, productive cough within 24 hours. Client's sputum will be clear, white within 48 hours.

IMPLEMENTATION

Steps	Rationale
1. Instruct client to turn and cough every 2 hours.	Major complication of reduced mobility is retained pulmonary secretions, which predisposes client to atelectasis and pneumonia (Dettenmeier, 1992).
2. Perform percussion with routine position changes.	Percussion provides mechanical force to loosen secretions adhered to walls of airways and aids secretion removal (Dettenmeier, 1992).
3. Increase fluid intake to 1500 ml within 24 hours.	Fluids and humidification help liquify secretions for easy removal (Luce, Tyler, and Pierson, 1993).

EVALUATIVE MEASURES

Auscultate client's lungs.
Observe client's cough.
Observe color of client's sputum.

The client's involvement enhances the probability of a successful outcome.

Other health care team members, such as respiratory and physical therapists, and family members can help in developing a care plan. Consulting with other health care team members or family members can result in a more concise and comprehensive approach to the care plan. This comprehensive approach is used throughout the client's hospitalization, is incorporated into the discharge plan, and is used in the home care setting. The client's level of health, age, life-style, and environmental risks affect the level of tissue oxygenation. Clients with severe impairments in oxygenation frequently require nursing interventions directed toward all six goals.

Implementation

Nursing interventions for promoting and maintaining adequate oxygenation include independent nursing actions and interdependent or dependent interventions.

Improved Activity Tolerance. Nursing interventions for improving activity tolerance primarily include measures such as dyspnea management, health promotion activities, cardiopulmonary reconditioning, and respiratory muscle training. Improved activity tolerance results in clients' increased ability of carrying out activities of daily living while not increasing their cardiac workload or work of breathing.

Dyspnea management. Dyspnea is difficult to quantify and treat. Treatment needs to be individualized, and more than one therapy is used. Ideally, the process underlying the dyspnea must be treated. After this initial phase, there are four additional therapies: drug therapy, oxygen therapy, physical techniques, and psychosocial techniques (Gift, 1990). Drug therapies may include bronchodilators, steroids, mucolytics, and antianxiety drugs. Oxygen therapy can reduce dyspnea associated with exercise. Physical techniques such as cardiopulmonary reconditioning, breathing techniques, and cough control can reduce dyspnea by decreasing the client's energy requirements while coughing, exercising, or completing hygiene measures (DeVito, 1990).

Relaxation techniques, biofeedback, and meditation are physiosocial measures that can lessen the sensation of dyspnea (Gift, 1990).

HEALTH PROMOTION ACTIVITIES. Maintaining the client's optimal level of health is important in reducing the number and/or severity of respiratory symptoms. Prevention of respiratory infections is foremost in maintaining optimal health. Nurses need to provide respiratory-related health information such as availability and interpretation of pollution indexes, how to avoid or control secondary infection exposure, and benefits of pneumonococcal pneumonia and influenza vaccines.

Second, avoiding exposure to secondhand smoke is essential to maintaining optimal cardiopulmonary function. Most businesses and restaurants now ban smoking or have separate areas designated as smoking zones. If clients are exposed to secondhand smoke in their home environments, counseling and support may be necessary to assist the smoker in successful smoking cessation.

Third, cardiopulmonary health is maintained through adequate nutritional intake. It is well documented that foods low in sodium, cholesterol, and fat reduce the risk of coronary artery disease. Clients can be taught how to use the food pyramid to restructure their diets to include more grains, fruits, and vegetables (Chapter 31).

Last, age-appropriate exercise programs achieve overall as well as cardiopulmonary conditioning. A three-time-a-week aerobic exercise plan for 20 to 30 minutes is sufficient. For clients who do not do aerobic activities, walking has also shown health promotional benefits.

CARDIOPULMONARY RECONDITIONING. The major method of cardiopulmonary reconditioning is a structured rehabilitation program. **Cardiopulmonary rehabilitation** is actively assisting the client to achieve and maintain an optimal level of health through controlled physical exercise, nutrition counseling, relaxation and stress management, prescribed medications and oxygen, and compliance. As physical reconditioning occurs, the client's cardiopulmonary complaints should decrease. The client's anxiety, depression, or somatic concerns also often decrease.

RESPIRATORY MUSCLE TRAINING. Respiratory muscle training improves muscle strength and endurance. This results in improved activity tolerance. It may prevent respiratory failure in clients with chronic obstructive pulmonary disease. One method for respiratory muscle training is the **incentive spirometer resistive breathing device (ISRBD).** Resistive breathing is achieved by placing a resistive breathing device into a volume-dependent incentive spirometer. Muscle training is achieved when the client uses the ISRBD on a scheduled routine.

Maintenance or Promotion of Lung Expansion.

Nursing interventions to maintain or promote lung expansion include noninvasive techniques such as positioning and breathing exercises, procedures using equipment such as incentive spirometers, and invasive procedures such as management of a chest tube.

POSITIONING. In the healthy, completely mobile person, adequate ventilation and oxygenation are maintained by frequent position changes during daily activities. However, when a person's illness or injury restricts mobility, there is a risk for respiratory impairment. The most effective position for clients with cardiopulmonary diseases is high-Fowler's position. It uses gravity to assist in lung expansion and to reduce pressure on the diaphragm. The nurse needs to ensure the client does not slide down in bed, which could reduce lung expansion.

BREATHING EXERCISES. Breathing exercises include techniques to improve ventilation and oxygenation. These are deep breathing and coughing exercises, pursed-lip breathing, and diaphragmatic breathing. Deep breathing and coughing exercises are routine for postoperative clients (see Chapter 36).

Pursed-lip breathing involves deep inspiration and prolonged expiration through pursed lips. This exercise keeps the alveoli from collapsing. While sitting up, the client is instructed to take a deep breath and to exhale slowly through pursed lips. Clients need to gain control of the exhalation phase so that exhalation is longer than inhalation (Dettenmeier, 1992). The client can perfect this technique by counting inhalation time and gradually increasing the count during exhalation.

Diaphragmatic breathing is more difficult and requires the client to relax intercostal and accessory respiratory muscles while taking deep inspirations. The client places one hand flat below the breastbone above the waist and the other hand 2 to 3 cm below the first hand. The client is asked to sniff. The diaphragm will expand outward, causing the client's hand to move. The client concentrates on expanding the diaphragm during controlled inspiration. The lower hand should move outward during expiration. The client observes for inward movement as the diaphragm ascends. These exercises are initially taught with the client supine and are practiced while sitting and standing. The pursed-lip breathing technique is often used. These exercises decrease air trapping and reduce the work of breathing (Luce, Tyler, Pierson, 1993). It helps clients with pulmonary disease, postoperative clients, and women in labor to promote relaxation and provide pain control.

INCENTIVE SPIROMETRY. Incentive spirometry encourages voluntary deep breathing by providing visual feedback inspiratory volume. It is used to prevent or treat atelectasis and is particularly useful for postoperative clients (Luce et al., 1993).

Flow-oriented incentive spirometers consist of one or more plastic chambers that contain freely moving colored balls. The client inhales briskly to elevate the balls and to keep them floating as long as possible. Even if a very slow inspiration does not elevate the balls, this

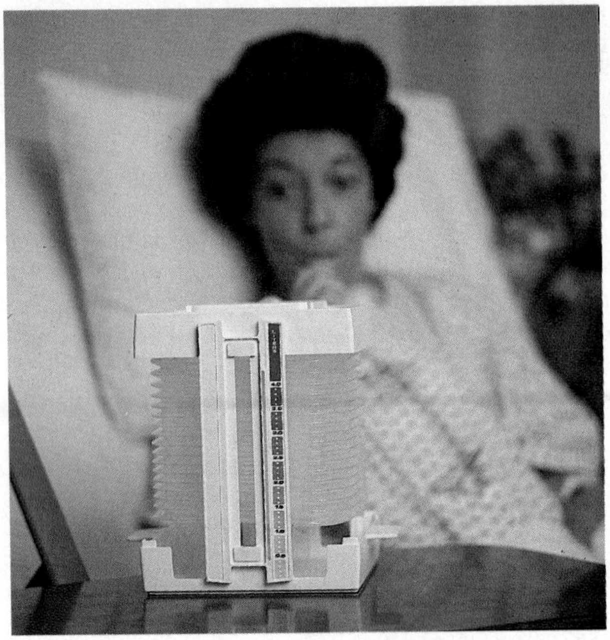

FIGURE 34-7 Volume-oriented spirometer.

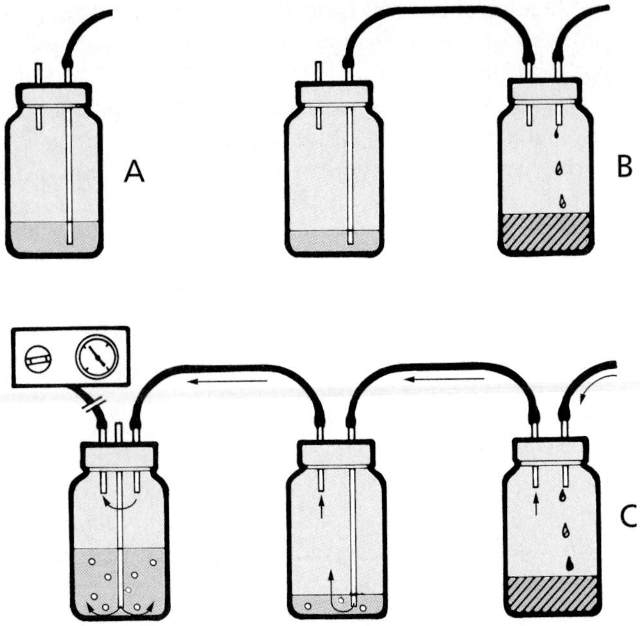

FIGURE 34-8 Chest tube drainage. **A,** One-bottle system. **B,** Two- bottle system. **C,** Three-bottle system with suction.

breathing pattern alone may achieve greater lung expansion.

Volume-oriented incentive spirometers have a bellows that is raised to a predetermined volume by an inhaled breath (Figure 34-7). An achievement light or counter is used in some devices. Some devices are constructed so the light will not turn on unless the bellows is held at a minimum desired volume for a specified period to enhance lung expansion.

Incentive spirometry encourages clients to breathe to their normal inspiratory capacities. Because of postoperative pain, a postoperative inspiratory capacity one half to three fourths of the preoperative volume is acceptable (Luce et al., 1993).

Chest tubes. Chest tubes are inserted through the thorax to remove air and fluids from the pleural space, to prevent air or fluid from reentering the pleural space, and to reestablish normal intrapleural and intrapulmonic pressures (Dettenmeier, 1992). They promote lung reexpansion. Chest tubes are used after chest surgery and chest trauma and for pneumothorax or hemothorax (see Procedure 34-2).

A **pneumothorax** is a collection of air or other gas in the pleural space, which causes the lung to collapse. It may occur spontaneously or from chest trauma, or from an invasive procedure such as thoracentesis. A client with a pneumothorax usually has pain and dyspnea.

Hemothorax is an accumulation of blood and fluid in the pleural cavity, usually as the result of trauma. It prevents the lung from full expansion. A hemothorax can also be caused by rupture of small blood vessels from pneumonia or tuberculosis. Symptoms may include pain and dyspnea, and signs and symptoms of shock can develop if blood loss is severe.

The one-bottle system is the simplest closed drainage system because the single bottle serves as a collector and a water seal (Figure 34-8, *A*). During normal respiration, fluctuations in the water-seal tube are expected. The fluid should ascend with inspiration. A two-bottle system permits the liquid to flow into the collection bottle and air flows into the water-seal bottle (Figure 34-8, *B*). Fluctuations in the water-seal tube are still normal. The two-bottle system permits more accurate measurement and observation of chest drainage (Erikson, 1981a).

A three-bottle system is used to evacuate any volume of air or fluid with controlled suction (Figure 34-8, *C*). The suction-control bottle contains a long tube, submerged under water, and two short tubes. The longer tube is vented to the atmosphere. One short tube connects bottles two and three. The second short tube is connected to an external suction source at a pressure that causes gentle, continuous bubbling in bottle three. The disposable systems, such as a Pleur-Evac system, are a one-piece molded plastic unit that duplicates the three-bottle system (Figure 34-9). The disposable units appear to be the best because they are cost effective and some facilitate autotransfusion, which is common in open-heart surgeries. Knowing the basics of chest tube management and troubleshooting maneuvers helps reduce side effects (Table 34-6).

Special considerations. The nurse should handle the bottles carefully and maintain the drainage device

table 34-6

PROBLEM SOLVING WITH CHEST TUBES

Problem	Solution
Air leak is present.	Locate leak.
Continuous bubbling is seen in water-seal bottle/chamber, indicating that leak is between client and water seal.	Tighten loose connections between client and water seal. Loose connections cause air to enter system. Leaks are corrected when constant bubbling stops.
Bubbling continues, indicating that air leak has not been corrected.	Cross-clamp chest tube close to client's chest. If bubbling stops, air leak is inside client's thorax (client centered) or at chest tube insertion site.* *Unclamp tube and notify physician immediately.* Reinforce chest dressing. Leaving chest tube clamped with client-centered leak can cause collapse of lung, mediastinal shift, and eventual collapse of other lung from buildup of air pressure within pleural cavity.
Bubbling continues, indicating that leak is not client centered.	In alternating fashion, gradually move clamps down drainage tubing away from client and toward suction-control chamber, moving one clamp at a time. When bubbling stops, leak is in section of tubing or connection that is between two clamps. Replace tubing or secure connection and release clamps.†
Bubbling continues, indicating that leak is not in tubing.	Leak is in drainage system. Change drainage system.*†
Tension pneumothorax is present.	Determine that chest tubes are not clamped, kinked, or occluded. Obstructed chest tubes trap air in intrapleural space when air leak originates within client.
Severe respiratory distress	Notify physician immediately.
Chest pain	Prepare immediately for another chest tube insertion; obtain a flutter (Heimlich) valve on large-gauge needle for short-term emergency release of air in intrapleural space; have emergency equipment (e.g., oxygen and code cart) near client.
Absence of breath sounds on affected side	
Hyperresonance on affected side	
Mediastinal shift to unaffected side	
Tracheal shift to unaffected side	
Hypotension	
Tachycardia	
Dependent loops of drainage tubing have trapped fluid.	Drain tubing contents into drainage bottle. Coil excess tubing on mattress and secure in place.
Water seal is disconnected.	Connect water seal and tape connection.
Water-seal bottle is broken.	Insert distal end of water-seal tube into sterile solution so that tip is 2 cm below surface level‡ and set up new water-seal bottle. If no sterile solution is available, double-clamp chest tube while preparing new bottle.
Water-seal tube is no longer submerged in sterile fluid.	Add sterile solution to water-seal bottle until distal tip is 2 cm under surface level† or set water-seal bottle upright so that tip is submerged.

*Data from Paulau D, Jones S: *RN* Oct. 1986.
†Data from Erickson R: *Nurs 81* 11(6):62, 1981.
‡Data from Carroll PF: *Nurs 86* 16(12):26, 1986.

below the client's chest. If the tubing disconnects from the bottles, the nurse should instruct the client to exhale as much as possible and to cough, which rids the pleural space of as much air as possible. Chest tube removal requires client preparation because it may cause burning, pain, and a pulling sensation (Gift et al., 1991).

Mobilization of Pulmonary Secretions. A client's ability to mobilize pulmonary secretions may make the difference between a short-term illness and a long period of recovery involving complications. Nursing interventions to educate the client and to promote mobilization of pulmonary secretions include hydration, humidification, nebulization, and chest physiotherapy (see box on p. 1004).

HYDRATION. Maintenance of adequate systemic hydration keeps mucociliary clearance normal. In clients with adequate hydration, pulmonary secretions are thin,

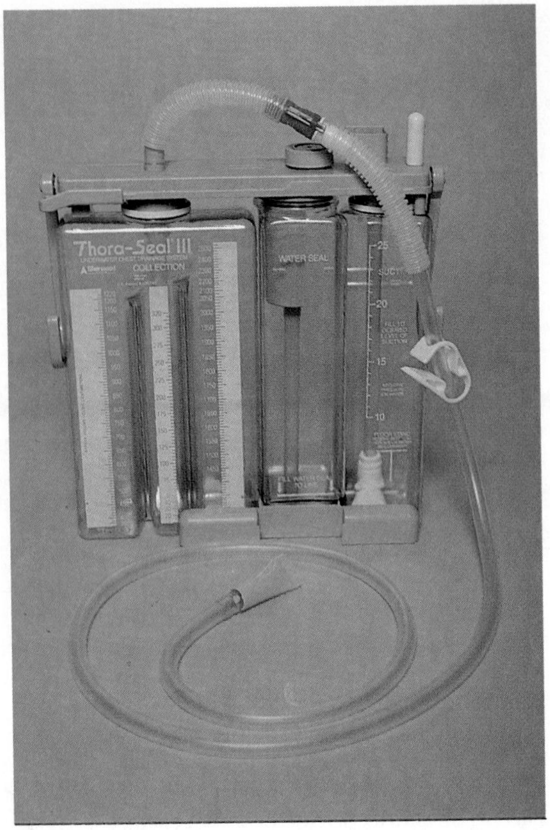

FIGURE 34-9 Disposable, commercial chest drainage system.

CLIENT TEACHING FOR PULMONARY SECRETIONS

- Teach clients to drink caffeine-free, sugar-free liquids. Drinks high in sugar and caffeine can cause dehydration.
- Instruct clients to set aside a routine time or times each day for postural drainage and coughing.
- Teach clients to assess their sputum daily and to report the following information to their physician:
  - Increases in amount of sputum
  - Changes in sputum color
  - Increased thickness of sputum
- Teach clients to cough effectively so that their cough is consistently productive without excessive expenditure of energy.
- Teach client about prescribed medications such as bronchodilators and corticosteroids: name, dosage, purpose, time of administration, and side effects.
- Teach client how to properly administer inhaled medications (see Chapter 26). Document correct administration with return demonstration of procedure.

white, watery, and easily removed with minimal coughing. Excessive coughing required to clear thick secretions is fatiguing. Unless contraindicated, most clinicians recommend a fluid intake of 1500 to 2000 ml per day (Luce et al., 1993).

HUMIDIFICATION. **Humidification** is the process of adding water to gas. Air or oxygen with a high relative humidity keeps the airways moist and loosens and mobilizes pulmonary secretions.

Oxygen delivered to the upper airways, as with a nasal catheter, nasal cannula, or face mask, can be humidified by bubbling it through water. Heating of humidifiers is impractical because condensed moisture fills the narrow tubing. Another humidification method is the humidity tent, used for infants and children with illnesses such as croup or tracheitis. These children require high humidity to liquefy secretions and help reduce fever. The nurse monitors the child's body temperature and respiratory status. Children in humidity tents require frequent changes of clothing and bed linen to remain warm and dry.

The nurse needs to ensure the right solution is used for humidification and that the solution is changed according to agency procedures. Excess humidification and reservoirs used for humidity solutions are environments that support pathogen growth, which cause nosocomial infections.

NEBULIZATION. **Nebulization** is a process of adding moisture or medications to inspired air by mixing particles of varying sizes with the air. A nebulizer uses the aerosol principle to suspend a maximum number of water drops or particles of the desired size in inspired air. The moisture added to the respiratory system improves pulmonary secretions clearance. Therefore nebulization is often used to administer bronchodilators and mucolytic agents. A jet-aerosol nebulizer uses gas under pressure. An ultrasonic nebulizer uses high-frequency vibrations to break up the water or medication into fine drops or particles.

CHEST PHYSIOTHERAPY. **Chest physiotherapy (CPT)** is a group of therapies used in combination to mobilize pulmonary secretions (see box on p. 1005). These therapies are postural drainage, chest percussion, and vibration. Chest physiotherapy should be followed by productive coughing. Suctioning is used if the client's ability to cough is inadequate.

Chest percussion involves striking the chest wall over the area being drained. The hand is positioned so that the fingers and thumb touch and the hand is cupped (Figure 34-10). Percussion on the surface of the chest wall sends waves of varying amplitude and frequency through the chest. The force of these waves can change the consistency of the sputum or dislodge it from airway walls (Luce et al., 1993). Chest percussion is performed by alternating hand motion against the

GUIDELINES FOR CHEST PHYSIOTHERAPY

Nursing care and selection of CPT skills are based on specific assessment findings. The following guidelines help the nurse in physical assessment and subsequent decision making:

Know the client's normal range of vital signs: Conditions such as atelectasis and pneumonia requiring CPT can affect vital signs. The degree of change is related to the level of hypoxia, overall cardiopulmonary status, and tolerance to activity.

Know the client's medications: Certain medications, particularly diuretics and antihypertensives, cause fluid and hemodynamic changes. These may decrease the client's tolerance to the positional changes and postural drainage. Chronic steroid use increases the client's risk of pathological rib fractures and often contraindicate rib shaking.

Know the client's medical history: Certain conditions such as increased intracranial pressure, spinal cord injuries, and abdominal aneurysm resection contraindicate the positional changes of postural drainage. Thoracic trauma or surgery may also contraindicate percussion, vibration, and rib shaking.

Know the client's level of cognitive function. Participation in controlled cough techniques requires the client to follow instructions. Congenital or acquired cognitive limitations may alter the client's ability to learn and participate in these techniques.

Be aware of the client's exercise tolerance: CPT maneuvers are fatiguing. When the client is not used to physical activity, initial tolerance to the maneuvers may be decreased. However, with gradual increases in activity and planned CPT, client tolerance to the procedure improves.

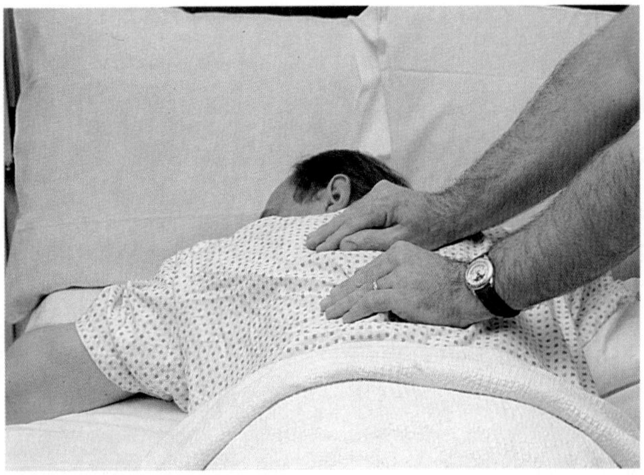

FIGURE 34-10 Hand position for chest wall percussion during physiotherapy.

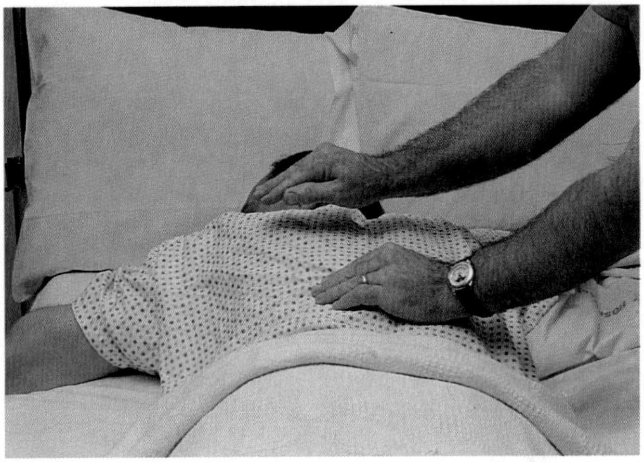

FIGURE 34-11 Chest wall percussion, alternating hand motion against the client's chest wall.

chest wall (Figure 34-11), over a single layer of clothing and not over buttons, snaps, or zippers. It is contraindicated in clients with bleeding disorders, osteoporosis, or fractured ribs. Caution should be taken to percuss the lung fields and not the scapular regions to avoid trauma to the skin and underlying structures.

Vibration is a fine, shaking pressure applied to the chest wall only during exhalation. It is thought to increase the velocity and turbulence of exhaled air, making secretion removal easier (Dettenmeier, 1992). Vibration increases the exhalation of trapped air and may shake mucus loose and induce a cough. Vibration is not recommended in infants and young children.

Postural drainage uses positioning techniques to draw secretions from specific segments of the lungs and bronchi into the trachea. Coughing or suctioning normally removes secretions from the trachea. The procedure for postural drainage can include most lung segments (Table 34-7). Because clients may not require postural drainage of all lung segments, its use depends on assessment findings.

Maintenance of a Patent Airway. The airway is patent when the trachea, bronchi, and large airways are free from obstructions. The three interventions used are coughing techniques, suctioning, and insertion of an artificial airway.

COUGHING TECHNIQUES. Coughing effectively maintains a patent airway by permitting removal of secretions from the upper and lower airways. The normal series of events in the cough mechanisms are deep inhalation, closure of the glottis, active contraction of the expiratory muscles, and glottis opening. Deep inhalation increases lung volume and airway diameter. Contraction of the expiratory muscles against the closed glottis raises intrathoracic pressure. Glottis opening re-

table 34-7

POSITIONS FOR POSTURAL DRAINAGE

Lung segment	Position of client
ADULT	
Bilateral	High Fowler's 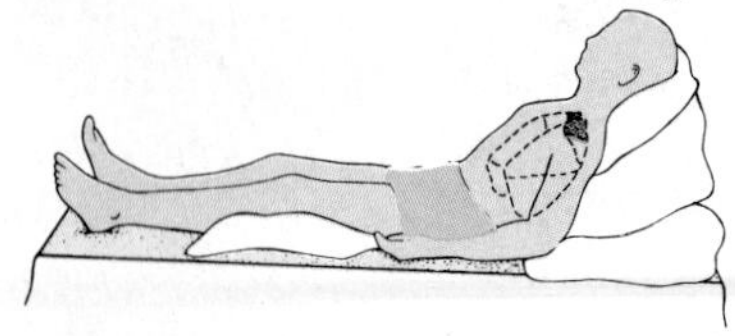
Apical segments	Sitting on side of bed
Right upper lobe—anterior segment	Supine with head elevated 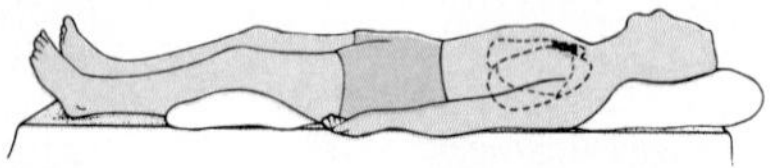
Left upper lobe—anterior segment	Supine with head elevated 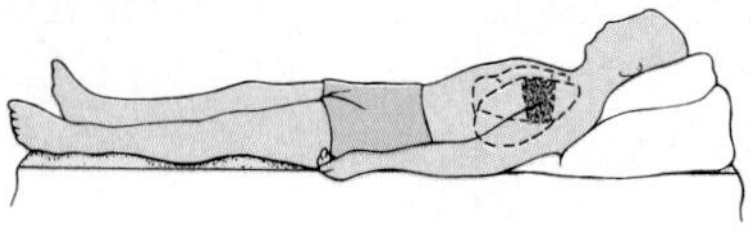
Right upper lobe—posterior segment	Side lying with right side of chest elevated on pillows 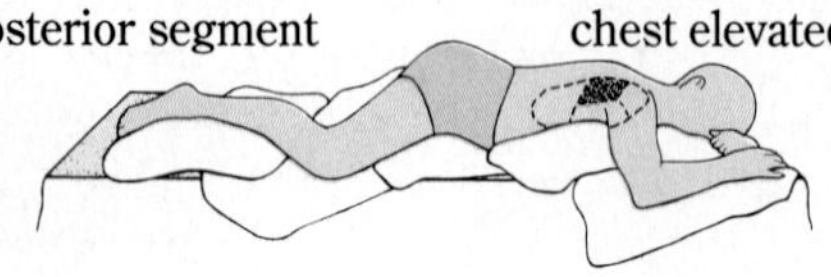
Left upper lobe—posterior segment	Side lying with left side of chest elevated on pillows 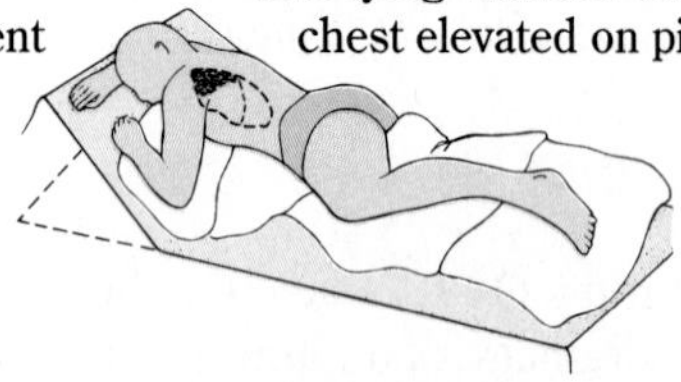
Right middle lobe—anterior segment	Three-fourths supine position with dependent lung in Trendelenburg position 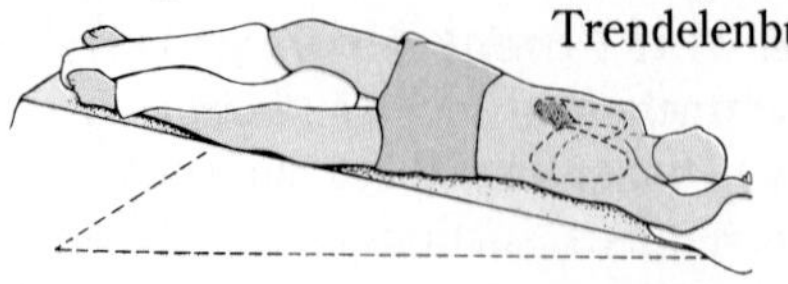
Right middle lobe—posterior segment	Prone with thorax and abdomen elevated 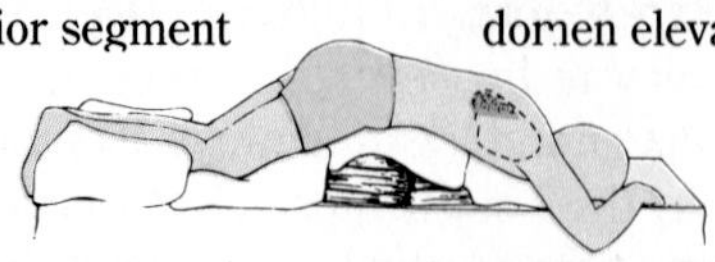
Both lower lobes—anterior segments	Supine in Trendelenburg 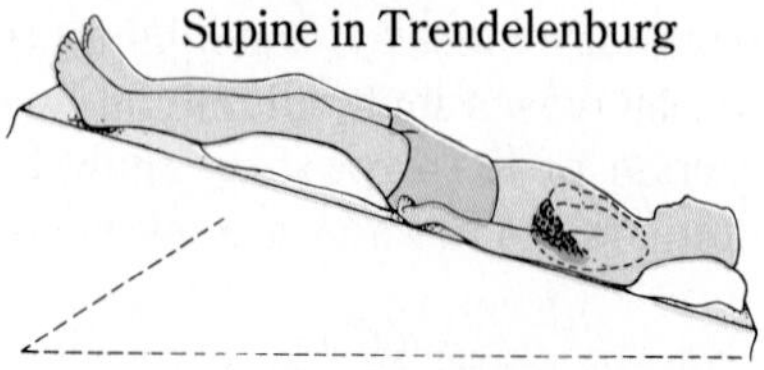
Left lower lobe—lateral segment	Right side lying in Trendelenburg position 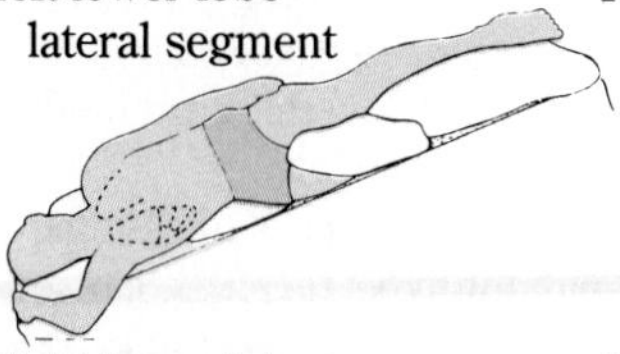
Right lower lobe—lateral segment	Left side lying in Trendelenburg position 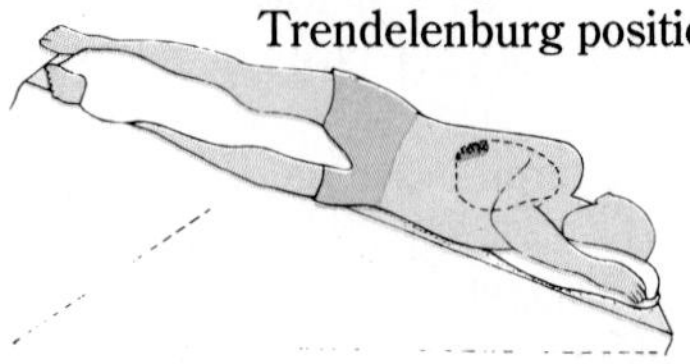
Right lower lobe—posterior segment	Prone with right side of chest elevated in Trendelenburg position 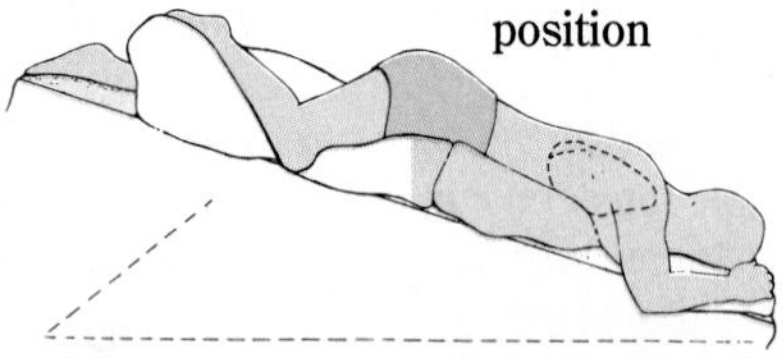
Both lower lobes—posterior segment	Prone in Trendelenburg position 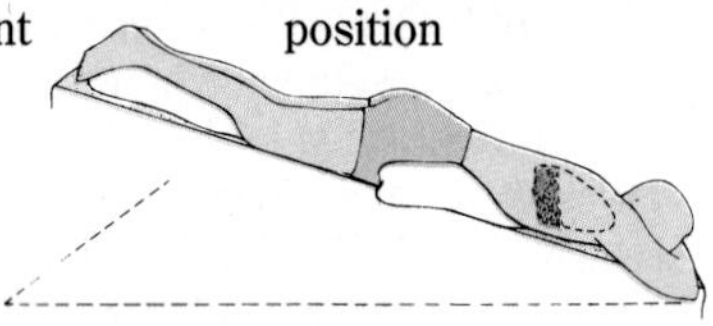
CHILD	
Bilateral—apical segments	Sitting on nurse's lap, leaning slightly forward flexed over pillow 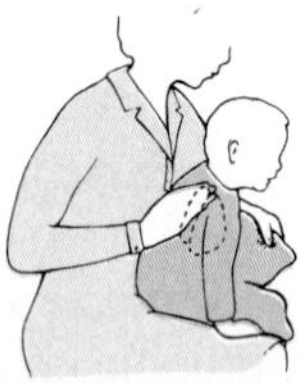
Bilateral—middle anterior segments	Sitting on nurse's lap, leaning against nurse 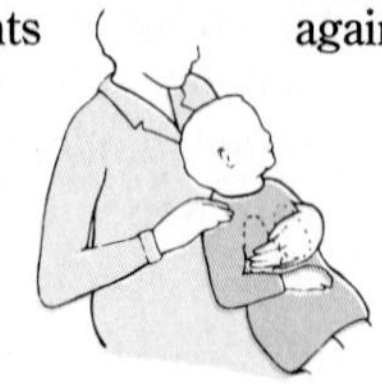
Bilateral lobes—anterior segments	Lying supine on nurse's lap, back supported with pillow 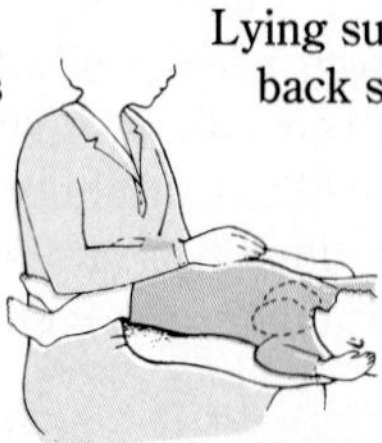

sults in larger fast expulsion of air providing momentum for mucus to move to the upper airway. After the cough the mucus can be expectorated or swallowed.

Various coughing techniques can be taught to different clients. With the cascade cough, the client takes a slow, deep breath and holds it for 2 seconds while contracting expiratory muscles. Then the client coughs several times while exhaling, thereby coughing at progressively lowered lung volumes. This technique promotes airway clearance and a patent airway in clients with large volumes of sputum.

With the huff cough the client, while exhaling, opens the glottis by saying the word "huff." It stimulates a natural cough reflex. It is generally effective only for clearing central airways, but with practice the client inhales more air and may be able to progress to the cascade cough.

The quad cough is used for clients without abdominal muscle control, such as those with spinal cord injuries. The client or nurse pushes inward and upward on the abdominal muscles toward the diaphragm while the client breathes with maximal expiratory effort, causing the cough (Luce et al., 1993).

The effectiveness of coughing is evaluated by sputum expectoration, the client's report of swallowed sputum, or clearing of adventitious sounds on auscultation. Clients with chronic pulmonary diseases, upper respiratory tract infections, and lower respiratory tract infections should cough at least every 2 hours when awake. Clients with a large amount of sputum should cough every hour while awake and every 2 to 3 hours while asleep until the acute phase of mucus production has ended.

Suctioning techniques. When a client is unable to clear respiratory tract secretions with coughing, the nurse must use suctioning to clear the airways. The three primary suctioning techniques are oropharyngeal and nasopharyngeal suctioning, orotracheal and nasotracheal suctioning, and suctioning of an artificial airway.

Because the oropharynx and trachea are considered sterile, sterile technique is required. The mouth is considered clean, so the suctioning of oral secretions should be performed after suctioning of the oropharynx and trachea. Each type of suctioning uses a beaded-tip catheter with a ring of holes along the side of the catheter at the distal end. Frequency of suctioning is determined by continued client assessment. If secretions are identified by inspection or auscultation techniques, suctioning is required. Sputum is not produced continuously or every 1 or 2 hours but occurs as a response to a pathological condition. Therefore there is no rationale for routine suctioning of all clients every 1 to 2 hours.

Oropharyngeal and nasopharyngeal suctioning. The oropharynx extends behind the mouth from the soft palate above the level of the hyoid bone and contains the tonsils. The nasopharynx is located behind the nose and extends to the level of the soft palate. Oropharyngeal or nasopharyngeal suctioning is used when the client is able to cough effectively but is unable to clear secretions by expectorating or swallowing. The suction procedure is used after the client has coughed (Procedure 34-3). As the amount of pulmonary secretions is reduced and the client is less fatigued, the client may be able to expectorate or swallow the mucus. This type of suctioning is then no longer required.

Orotracheal and nasotracheal suctioning. Orotracheal or nasotracheal suctioning is necessary when the client with pulmonary secretions is unable to cough and does not have an artificial airway (Procedure 34-3). A catheter is passed through the mouth or nose into the trachea. The nose is the preferred route because stimulation of the gag reflex is minimal. The procedure is similar to nasopharyngeal suctioning, but the catheter tip is moved farther in to suction the trachea. The entire procedure from catheter passage to its removal cannot take more than 15 seconds because oxygen does not reach the lungs during suctioning. Unless in respiratory distress, the client should be allowed to rest between catheter passes. If the client is using supplemental oxygen, the oxygen cannula or mask should be replaced during rest periods.

Artificial airway. An artificial airway is an oral airway or an endotracheal, nasotracheal, or tracheostomy tube. Indications for an artificial airway include decreased level of consciousness, airway obstruction, mechanical ventilation, and removal of tracheal secretions.

Oral airway. The oral airway, the simplest type of artificial airway, prevents tracheal obstruction by displacing the tongue into the oropharynx in the unconscious client (Figure 34-12, *A* and *B*). The oral airway extends from the teeth to the oropharynx, maintaining the tongue in the normal position. A correctly sized airway must be used. If the airway is too small, the tongue is not held in the anterior portion of the mouth. If it is too large, it may force the tongue toward the epiglottis and obstruct the airway.

The oral airway is inserted by turning the curve of the airway toward the cheek and placing it over the tongue into the oropharynx. When the airway is in the oropharynx, the nurse turns it so the opening points downward. The correctly placed airway moves the tongue forward away from the oropharynx. The flange, the flat portion of the airway, should rest against the client's teeth.

If the nurse attempts to insert the oral airway with a curve toward the tongue, the client's natural airway can be further obstructed. Incorrect insertion merely forces the tongue back into the oropharynx.

Tracheal airway. Artificial tracheal airways include endotracheal, nasotracheal, and tracheal tubes. These allow easy access to the client's trachea for deep tra-

Text continued on p. 1013.

procedure 34-3

SUCTIONING

Steps	Rationale
1. Assess for signs and symptoms indicating presence of upper airway secretions: gurgling respirations, restlessness, vomitus in mouth, drooling.	Physical signs and symptoms result from decreased oxygen to tissues as well as pooling of secretions in upper airway.
2. Explain to client how procedure will help to clear airway and relieve some breathing problems. Explain that coughing, sneezing, or gagging is normal.	Explanation of procedure relieves client's anxiety.
3. Prepare necessary equipment and supplies:	Ensures that procedure is completed quickly and efficiently.
a. Portable or wall suction unit with connecting tubing with Y-connector if needed	
b. Sterile catheter	
c. Yankauer catheter (oropharyngeal)	
d. Sterile water or normal saline, sterile basin	Cleans catheter.
e. Sterile gloves, nonsterile gloves (Yankauer only)	
f. Drape or towel	Protects linen and client's bedclothes.
g. Nasal or oral airway if indicated	Ensures access to airway.
4. Close door or pull curtain.	Ensures privacy.
5. Properly position client:	
a. Place conscious client with functional gag reflex for oral suctioning in semi-Fowler's position with head turned to one side. Place such a client for nasal suctioning in semi-Fowler's position with neck hyperextended.	Gag reflex helps prevent aspiration of gastrointestinal contents. Positioning of head to one side or hyperextending neck promotes smooth insertion of catheter into oropharynx or nasopharynx, respectively.
b. Place unconscious client in side-lying position facing nurse.	Prevents client's tongue from obstructing airway, promotes drainage of pulmonary secretions, and prevents aspiration of gastrointestinal contents.
6. Place towel on pillow or under client's chin.	Prevents soiling of bed linen or bedclothes from secretions. Secretions on towel can be discarded, thus reducing spread of bacteria.
7. Select proper suction pressure for client and type of suction unit. For wall suction units, this is 120 mm Hg in adults, 95-110 mm Hg in children, and 50-95 mm Hg in infants.	Provides safe but effective negative pressure according to client's age. Current research has demonstrated keeping negative suction pressures under 120 mm Hg reduces risk of intracranial ischemia and hypertension in head injured patients (Kerr, et al., 1993). Decreases possibility of damage to mucous membranes and hypoxemia.
8. Wash hands.	Reduces transmission of microorganisms.
9. Yankauer catheter:	
a. Apply nonsterile gloves.	Reduces transmission of microorganisms.
b. Connect one end of connecting tubing to suction machine and other to Yankauer suction catheter. Fill cup with water.	Prepares suction apparatus.
c. Check that equipment is functioning properly by placing Yankauer catheter into a small amount of water in cup or basin.	Ensures equipment function and lubricates catheter.
d. Remove oxygen mask, if present.	
e. Insert catheter into mouth along gum line to pharynx. Move catheter around mouth until secretions are cleared. Do not allow catheter to "rest" against oral mucosa.	Provides continuous suction. Care must be taken not to allow suction tip to invaginate oral mucosal surfaces.
f. Encourage client to cough. Replace oxygen mask.	Moves secretions from lower airway into mouth and upper airway.
g. Rinse catheter with water in cup or basin until connecting tubing is cleared of secretions. Turn off suction.	Rinses catheter and reduces probability of transmission of microorganisms. Clean suction tubing enhances delivery of set suction pressure.

Steps	Rationale
h. Reassess client's respiratory status.	Directs nurse to initiate or cease intervention.
i. Remove towel, place in laundry. Remove gloves and dispose in receptacle.	Reduces transmission of microorganisms.
j. Reposition client; Sims' position encourages drainage and should be used if client has decreased level of consciousness.	Facilitates drainage of oral secretions.
k. Discard remainder of water into appropriate receptacle.	Reduces transmission of microorganisms and maintains medical asepsis.
l. Rinse basin in warm soapy water and dry with paper towels. Discard disposable cup into appropriate receptacle.	
m. Place catheter in clean dry area.	
n. Wash hands.	Reduces transmission of microorganisms to other clients.
10. Nasopharyngeal or nasotracheal suction:	
a. Turn suction device on and set vacuum regulator to appropriate negative pressure.	Excessive negative pressure damages nasal pharyngeal and tracheal mucosa and can reduce greater hypoxia.
b. If indicated, increase supplemental oxygen to 100% or as ordered by physician.	Reduces suction-induced hypoxemia. (The literature is inconclusive as to the necessity of hyperoxygenation.)
c. Connect one end of connecting tubing to suction machine and place other end in convenient location.	Prepares for connection of suction catheter to suction apparatus.
d. When using suction kit:	
(1) Open package. If sterile drape is available, place it across client's chest or use towel.	Reduces transmission of microorganisms.
(2) Open suction catheter package. Do not allow suction catheter to touch any surface other than inside of its package.	Maintains medical asepsis.
(3) Unwrap or open sterile basin and place on bedside table. Be careful not to touch inside of basin. Fill with about 100 ml sterile normal saline.	Saline is used to clean tubing after each suction pass.
e. Open lubricant. Squeeze onto open sterile catheter package without touching package.	Prepares lubricant while maintaining sterility. Water-soluble lubricant is used to avoid lipoid aspiration pneumonia.
f. Apply sterile glove to each hand or apply nonsterile glove to nondominant hand and sterile glove to dominant hand.	Reduces transmission of microorganisms and allows nurse to maintain sterility of suction catheter.

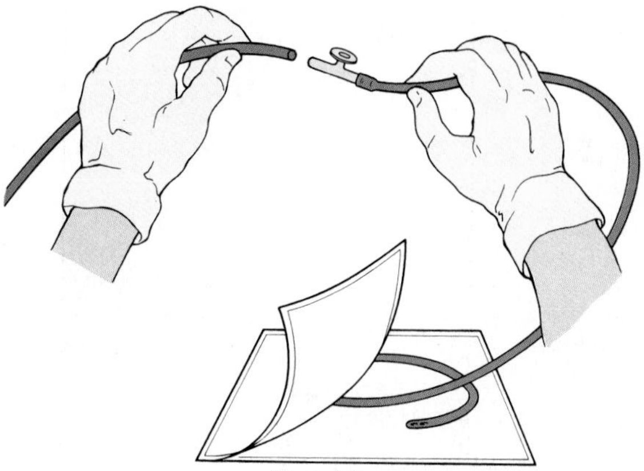

Step 10g

Continued.

procedure 34-3—cont'd

Steps	Rationale
g. Pick up suction catheter with dominant hand without touching nonsterile surfaces. Pick up connecting tube with nondominant hand. Secure catheter to tubing *(see illustration)*.	Maintains catheter sterility. Connects catheter to suction.
h. Check that equipment is functioning properly by placing distal tip of catheter into a small amount of normal saline; place thumb over suction port and remove a small amount of saline.	Ensures equipment function. Lubricates internal catheter and tubing.
i. Coat distal 6-8 cm of catheter with water-soluble lubricant.	Lubricates catheter for easier insertion.
j. Remove oxygen-delivery device, if applicable, with nondominant hand. Without applying suction, gently but quickly insert catheter with dominant thumb and forefinger into naris using slight downward slant as client breathes in. Do not force through naris. Insert a catheter 2.5 to 4 cm (1 to 1½ in); then briefly wait as client takes deep breath and quickly insert catheter to desired area (see illustration, *A* and *B*): (1) *Pharyngeal suctioning:* In adults, insert catheter about 16 cm; in older children, 8-12 cm; in infants and young children, 4-8 cm. Rule of thumb is to insert catheter distance from tip of nose to base of ear lobe. (2) *Tracheal suctioning:* In adults, insert catheter 20-24 cm; in older children, 14-20; and in young children and infants, 8-14 cm. (3) *Positioning:* In some instances turning client's head to right helps nurse suction left mainstem bronchus; turning head to left helps nurse suction right mainstem bronchus. If resistance is felt after insertion of catheter for recommended distance, nurse has probably hit carina. Pull catheter back 1 cm before applying suction.	Application of suction pressure while introducing catheter into trachea increases risk of damage to mucosa, as well as increased risk of hypoxia due to removal of oxygen present in airways. Epiglottis is open on inspiration and facilitates insertion into trachea. Client should cough. If client gags or becomes nauseated, catheter is most likely in esophagus.

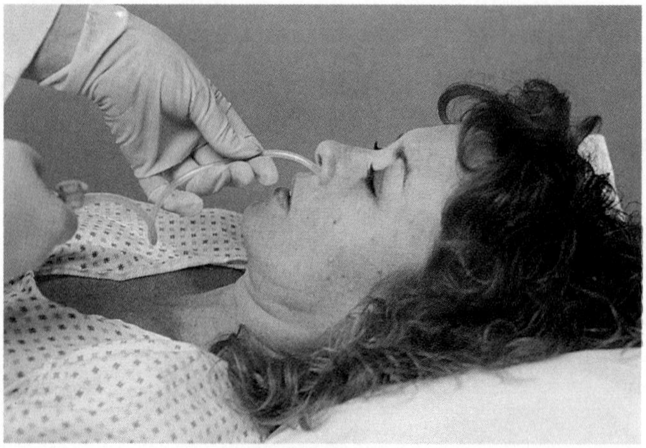

Step 10j(a)

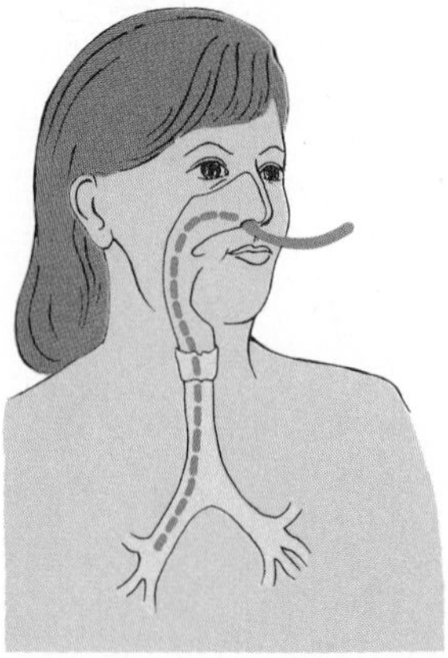

Step 10j(b)

Steps	Rationale
k. Apply intermittent suction for up to 10 sec by placing and releasing nondominant thumb over vent of catheter and slowly withdraw catheter while rotating it back and forth between dominant thumb and forefinger. Encourage client to cough. Replace oxygen device, if applicable.	Prevents injury to mucosa. If catheter "grabs" mucosa, remove thumb to release suction. Suctioning longer than 10 sec can increase the risk of cardiopulmonary compromise, increases intracranial hypertension, and cerebral ischemia (Kerr, 1993; Fiorentini, 1992).
l. Rinse catheter and connecting tubing with normal saline until cleared.	Removes secretions from catheter.
11. Artificial airway:	
a. Wash hands.	Reduces transmission of microorganisms.
b. Turn suction device on and set vacuum regulator to appropriate negative pressure (see Step 7).	Excessive negative pressure damages tracheal mucosa and can induce greater hypoxia.
c. Connect one end of connecting tubing to suction machine and place other end in convenient location.	Prepares suction apparatus.
d. Of using sterile suction kit:	
(1) Open package. If sterile drape is available, place it across client's chest.	Prevents contamination of clothing.
(2) Open suction catheter package. Do not allow suction catheter to touch any nonsterile surface.	Prepares catheter and prevents transmission of microorganisms.
(3) Unwrap or open sterile basin and place on bedside table. Be careful not to touch inside basin. Fill with about 100 ml sterile normal saline.	Prepares catheter and prevents transmission of microorganisms.
e. If indicated, open lubricant. Squeeze onto sterile catheter package without touching package.	Prepares lubricant for use while maintaining sterility.
f. Apply one sterile glove to each hand or apply nonsterile glove to nondominant hand and sterile glove to dominant hand.	Reduces transmission of microorganisms and allows nurse to maintain sterility of suction catheter.
g. Pick up suction catheter with dominant hand without touching nonsterile surfaces. Pick up connecting tubing with nondominant hand. Secure catheter to tubing.	Maintains catheter sterility.
h. Check that equipment is functioning properly by suctioning small amount of saline from basin (see Step 10h).	Ensures equipment function; lubricates catheter and tubing.
i. Coat distal 6-8 cm of catheter with water-soluble lubricant. In some situations, catheter is lubricated only with normal saline. Nursing assessment indicates need for lubrication.	Promotes easier catheter insertion. If lubricant is needed, it must be water soluble to prevent petroleum-based aspiration pneumonia. Excessive lubricant can adhere to artificial airway.
j. Remove oxygen- or humidity-delivery device with nondominant hand.	Exposes artificial airway.
k. Hyperinflate and/or oxygenate client before suctioning, using manual resuscitation (Ambu) bag or sigh mechanism on mechanical ventilator.	Decreases atelectasis caused by negative pressure. Prevents post suction hypoxemia (Lookinland, Appel, 1991; Knox, 1993). Hyperinflation also reduces risk of tachycardia and other arrhythmias (Stone et al., 1991).
l. Without applying suction, gently but quickly insert catheter with dominant thumb and forefinger into artificial airway (best to time catheter insertion with inspiration).	Places catheter in tracheobronchial tree. Application of suction pressure while introducing catheter into trachea increases risk of damage to tracheal mucosa, as well as increased hypoxia due to removal of oxygen present in airways.
m. Insert catheter until resistance is met, then pull back 1 cm.	Stimulates cough and removes catheter from mucosal wall.

Continued.

procedure 34-3—cont'd

Steps	Rationale
n. Apply intermittent suction by placing and releasing nondominant thumb over vent of catheter and slowly withdraw catheter while rotating it back and forth between dominant thumb and forefinger. Encourage client to cough.	Prevents injury to tracheal mucosal lining. If catheter "grabs" mucosa, remove thumb to release suction.
o. Replace oxygen-delivery service. Encourage client to deep breathe.	Reoxygenates and reexpands alveoli. Suctioning can cause hypoxemia and atelectasis.
p. Rinse catheter and connecting tubing with normal saline until clear. Use continuous suction.	Removes catheter secretions. Secretions left in tubing decrease suction and provide environment for microorganism growth.
q. Repeat Steps k-p as needed to clear secretions. Allow adequate time (at least 1 full min) between suction passes for ventilation and reoxygenation.	Clears airway of excessive secretions and promotes improved oxygenation.
r. Assess client's cardiopulmonary status between suction passes.	Suctioning can induce arrhythmias, hypoxia, and bronchospasm.
s. When artificial airway and tracheobronchial tree are sufficiently cleared of secretions, perform nasal and oral pharyngeal suctioning to clear upper airway of secretions. After this suctioning is performed, catheter is contaminated; do not reinsert into endotracheal or tracheostomy tube.	Removes upper airway secretions. Upper airway is considered clean, whereas lower airway is considered sterile. Therefore same catheter can be used to suction from sterile to clean areas but not from clean to sterile areas.
t. Disconnect catheter from connecting tubing. Roll catheter around fingers of dominant hand. Pull glove off inside out so that catheter remains in glove. Pull off other glove in same way. Discard into appropriate receptacle. Turn off suction device.	Reduces transmission of microorganisms.
u. Remove towel and place in laundry, or remove drape and discard in appropriate receptacle.	Reduces transmission of microorganisms.
v. Reposition client.	Promotes comfort. Sims' position encourages drainage and reduces risk of aspiration.
w. Discard remainder of normal saline into appropriate receptacle. If basin is disposable, discard into appropriate receptacle. If basin is reusable, place it in soiled utility room.	Reduces transmission of microorganisms.
x. Wash hands.	Reduces transmission of microorganisms.
12. Prepare equipment for next suctioning.	Provides ready access to suction equipment, especially if client is experiencing respiratory distress.
13. Observe client for absence of airway secretions, restlessness, oral secretions.	Indicates that secretions have been removed from oral and pharyngeal areas.
14. Record the amount, consistency, color, and odor of secretions and client's response to procedure; document client's presuctioning and postsuctioning respiratory status.	Documents that procedure was completed and client's status before and after.

*Yankauer catheters, nasopharyngeal or nasotracheal suction, artificial airway

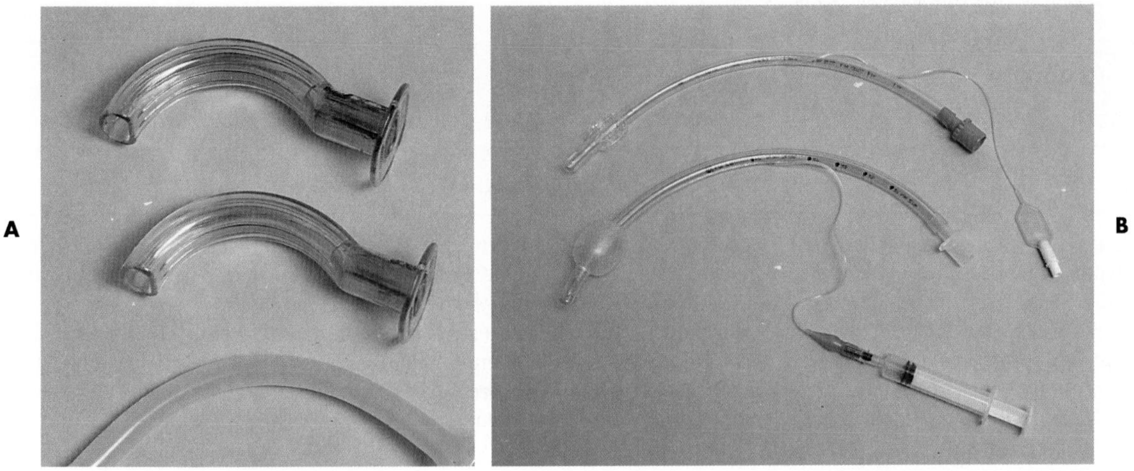

FIGURE 34-12 **A,** Artificial oral airways. **B,** Artificial nasal airways.

cheal suctioning. Because of the artificial airway, the client no longer has normal humidification of the tracheal mucosa. The nurse should ensure that humidity is being supplied to the airway through nebulization or with the oxygen delivery system. This is protective and helps remove tracheal secretions. Removal of tracheal secretions must be aseptic, atraumatic, and effective.

Maintenance and Promotion of Oxygenation.

Promotion of lung expansion, mobilization of secretions, and maintenance of a patent airway assist the client in meeting oxygenation needs. However, some clients also require oxygen therapy to keep a healthy level of tissue oxygenation.

GOALS OF OXYGEN THERAPY. The goal of oxygen therapy is to prevent or relieve hypoxia. Any client with impaired tissue oxygenation can benefit from controlled oxygen administration, but it is not a substitute for other treatment. Oxygen should be treated as a drug. It is expensive, has dangerous side effects, and must be continuously monitored. The nurse should routinely check the physician's orders to verify the client is receiving the prescribed oxygen concentration. The five rights of medication administration also pertain to oxygen (see Chapter 29).

SAFETY PRECAUTIONS WITH OXYGEN THERAPY. Oxygen is a highly combustible gas. Although it will not spontaneously burn or explode, it can easily ignite a fire on contact with a spark, such as from a cigarette or electrical equipment. Oxygen in high concentrations has a combustion potential and fuels fire readily. With increasing use of home oxygen therapy, clients and health care professionals must be aware of these dangerous combustible effects.

The nurse should promote safety by posting "no smoking" signs, explaining that smoking is not permitted in areas where oxygen is in use, ensuring that all electrical equipment in the room is functioning correctly and is properly grounded (see Chapter 29), and knowing the agency's fire procedures and the location of the closest fire extinguisher.

SUPPLY OF OXYGEN. Oxygen is supplied to the client's bedside by oxygen tanks or through a permanent wall-piped system. Oxygen tanks are transported on wide-based carriers that allow the tank to be placed upright at the client's bedside. Regulators control the amount of oxygen delivered. Common types include an upright flow meter with a flow-adjustment valve at the top or a cylinder indicator with a flow-adjustment handle.

In the hospital or home, oxygen tanks are delivered with the regulator in place. In the hospital, the respiratory therapy department usually connects the regulator. Vendors are generally responsible for connecting the oxygen tank to the regulator for home use.

METHODS OF OXYGEN DELIVERY. Oxygen can be delivered to the client by nasal cannula, nasal catheter, face mask, or mechanical ventilator.

NASAL CANNULA. A **nasal cannula** is a simple, comfortable device (Procedure 34-4). The two cannulae, about 1.5 cm ($\frac{1}{2}$ in) long, protrude from the center of a disposable tube and are inserted into the nares. Oxygen is delivered at a flow rate of up to 4 L/min. Higher flow rates dry airway mucosa and do not further increase inspired oxygen concentrations (Luce et al., 1993). The nurse must know what flow rate produces a given percentage of inspired oxygen concentration (FiO_2).

NASAL CATHETER. Nasal catheters are used less frequently than nasal cannulae. The procedure involves inserting an oxygen catheter into the nose to the nasopharynx. The catheter must be changed at least every 8 hours and inserted into the other nostril. For this reason the nasal catheter is often a less desirable method

procedure 34-4

APPLYING A NASAL CANNULA

Steps	Rationale
1. Inspect client for signs and symptoms associated with hypoxia and presence of airway secretions.	Left untreated, hypoxia can produce cardiac dysrhythmias and death. Presence of airway secretions decreases effectiveness of oxygen delivery.
2. Explain to client and family what procedure entails and purpose of oxygen therapy.	Decreases client's anxiety, which reduces oxygen consumption and increases client cooperation.
3. Assemble needed supplies and equipment: a. Nasal cannula *(see illustration)* b. Oxygen tubing c. Humidifier d. Sterile distilled water e. Oxygen source with flowmeter f. "No smoking" signs	Ensures that procedure is completed quickly and efficiently.
4. Wash hands.	Reduces transmission of infection.
5. Attach nasal cannula to oxygen tubing and attach to humidified oxygen source adjusted to prescribed flow rate.	Prevents drying of nasal and oral mucous membranes and airway secretions.
6. Place tips of cannula into client's nares *(see illustration)*.	Directs flow of oxygen into client's upper respiratory tract.
7. Adjust elastic headband or plastic slide until cannula fits snugly and comfortably *(see illustration)*.	Client is more likely to keep cannula in place if it fits comfortably.
8. Maintain sufficient slack on oxygen tubing and secure to client's clothes.	Allows client to turn head without dislodging cannula and reduces pressure on tips of nares.
9. Check the cannula every 8 hr.	Ensures patency of cannula and oxygen flow.
10. Keep humidification jar filled at all times.	Prevents inhalation of dehumidified oxygen.

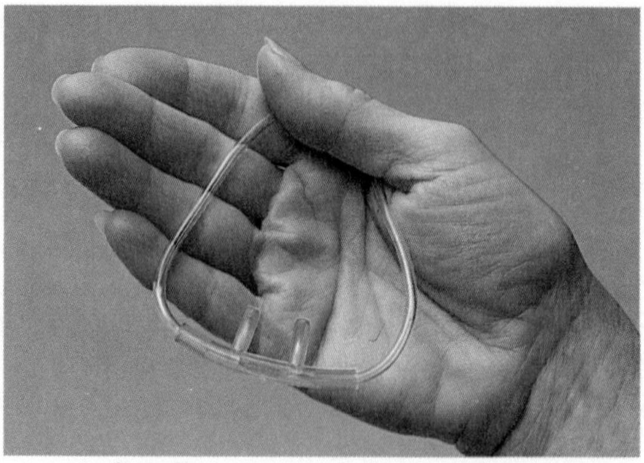

Step 3a

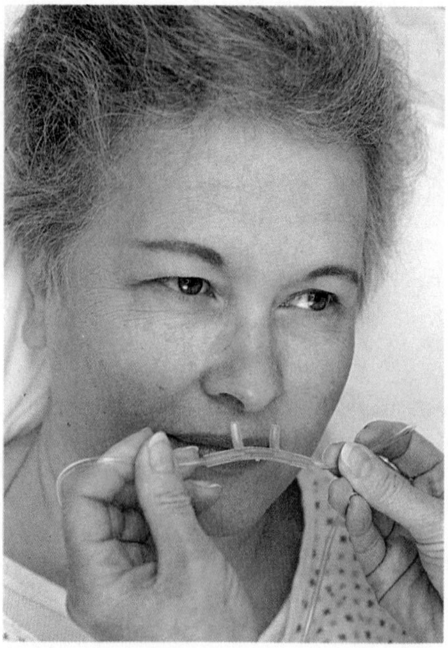

Step 6

Steps	Rationale
11. Observe client's nares and superior surface of both ears for skin breakdown.	Oxygen therapy can cause drying of nasal mucosa. Pressure on ears from cannula tubing or elastic can cause skin irritation.
12. Check oxygen flow rate and physician's orders every 8 hr *(see illustration)*.	Ensures delivery of prescribed oxygen flow rate.
13. Wash hands.	Reduces transmission of microorganisms.
14. Inspect client for relief of symptoms associated with hypoxia.	Indicates that hypoxia is corrected or reduced.
15. Record in nurses' notes method of oxygen delivery, flow rate, patency of oxygen cannula, client response, and respiratory assessment.	Documents correct use of oxygen therapy and client's response.

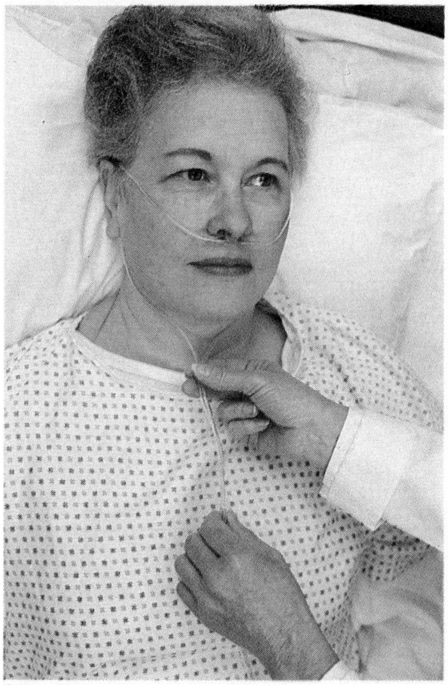
Step 7

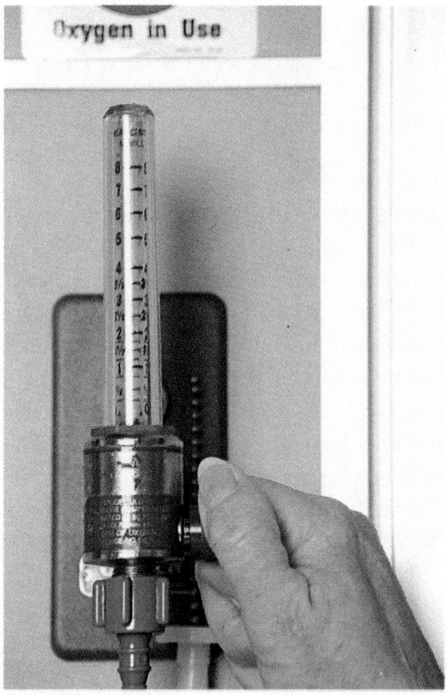

Step 12

because insertion may be painful and cause trauma to the nasal mucosa.

Transtracheal oxygen. Transtracheal oxygen is a method of oxygen delivery for clients with chronic lung diseases in which a small, intravenous-size catheter is inserted directly into the trachea through a surgical tract in the lower neck. Oxygen is delivered directly into the trachea.

The transtracheal oxygen delivery system is more advantageous in clients needing continuous oxygen for several reasons. There is no oxygen lost to the atmosphere, which is the case with a nasal cannula. Because oxygen travels directly into the trachea as opposed to through the nose to the posterior pharynx and into the trachea, clients achieve adequate oxygenation at lower flow rates. Clients are more likely to use oxygen as prescribed because of the mobility, comfort, and cosmetic improvement. Additional humidification is unnecessary because the nasopharynx, the area in most need of supplemental humidity, is bypassed (Spofford, Christopher, 1989).

Transtracheal oxygen is a potential source of danger to clients with chronic pulmonary disease who have a history of carbon dioxide retention. This therapy must

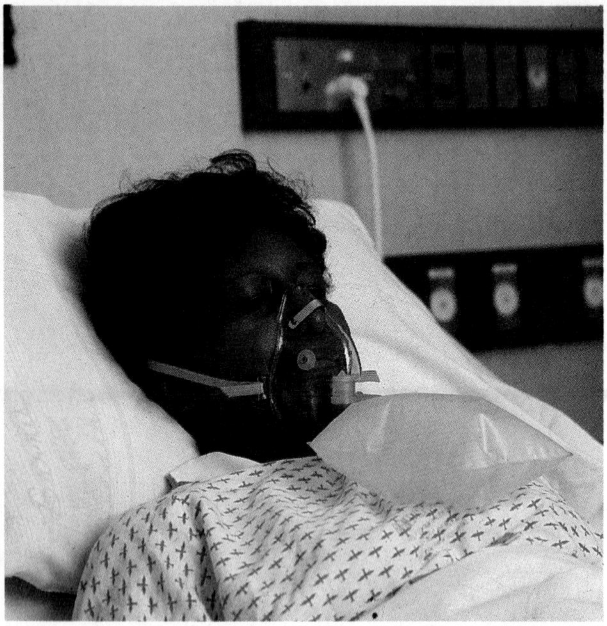

FIGURE 34-13 Plastic face mask with reservoir bag.

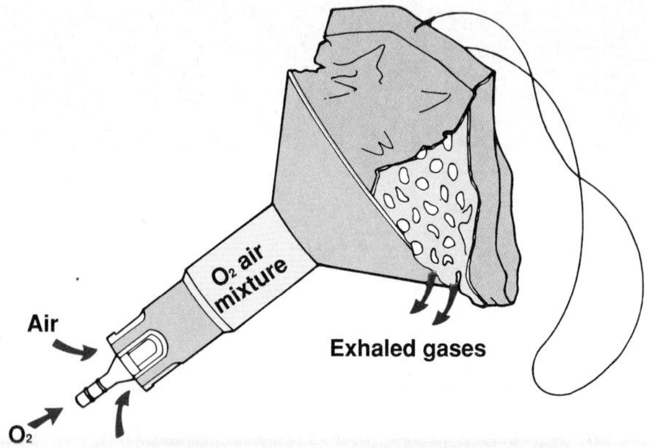

FIGURE 34-14 Venturi mask. (Courtesy Puritan-Bennett Corp., Overland Park, Kansas.)

be carefully monitored. These clients may require lower oxygen flow rates than predicted.

Use of transtracheal oxygenation occurs in four steps. First is client evaluation and selection. Not all clients requiring oxygen therapy can use this method. Some clients do not wish to have the surgical procedure, which is done with local anesthesia. Other clients are unable to care for the transtracheal equipment. The second step is surgical insertion of the stent, a stoma-type access route directly into the trachea. Third is initiation of oxygen through a number 9 French catheter into the stoma. Fourth, once the tracheal stoma is healed, the client must be taught to remove and irrigate the catheter at least 3 times a day with normal saline. This maintains catheter patency. The final oxygen flow rate, usually less than 4 L/min, is delivered through an 8 Fr catheter through the mature tract (Reinke, Hoffman, Wesmiller, 1992).

OXYGEN MASKS. An oxygen mask is a device used to administer oxygen, humidity, or heated humidity. It is shaped to fit snugly over the mouth and nose and is secured in place with a strap. The two primary types of oxygen masks are high and low concentration.

A plastic face mask with a reservoir bag (Figure 34-13) and a Venturi mask (Figure 34-14) can deliver higher concentrations of oxygen. When used as a nonrebreather, the plastic face mask with a reservoir bag can deliver from 80% to 90% oxygen (70% when used as a rebreather) with a flow rate of 10 L/min. It maintains a high-concentration oxygen supply in the reservoir bag. The nurse should frequently inspect the bag to make sure it is inflated. If it is deflated, the client may be breathing large amounts of exhaled carbon dioxide.

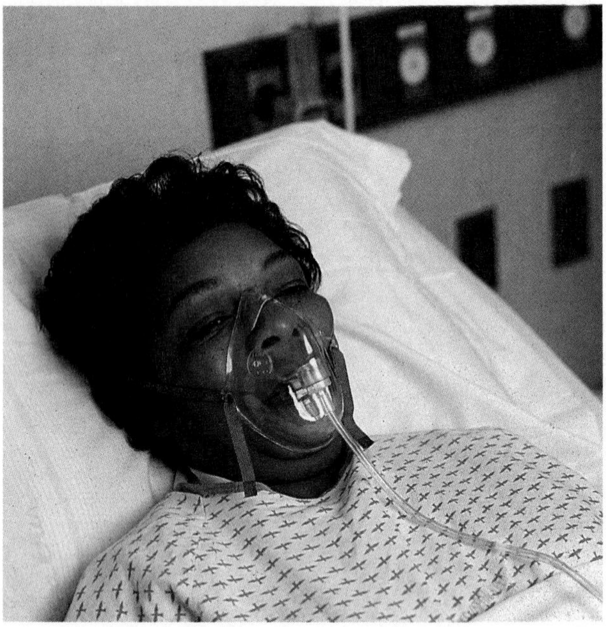

FIGURE 34-15 Simple face mask.

The Venturi mask can be used to deliver oxygen concentrations of 24% to 55% with oxygen flow rates of 2 to 14 L/min, depending on which flow control meter is selected (Dettenmeier, 1992).

The simple face mask (Figure 34-15) is used for short-term oxygen therapy. It fits loosely and delivers oxygen concentrations from 30% to 60%. The mask is contraindicated for clients with carbon dioxide retention.

HOME OXYGEN. When home oxygen is required, it is usually delivered by nasal cannula. When a client has a permanent tracheostomy, however, a T-tube or tracheostomy collar is necessary. Three types of oxygen

table 34-8
HOME OXYGEN SYSTEMS

Primary use	Advantages	Disadvantages
COMPRESSED GAS CYLINDERS		
Intermittent therapy, such as for exercise or sleep only	100% oxygen, relatively inexpensive, no loss of gas during storage, relatively portable, delivery of up to 15 L/min	Bulky, possibly unsightly, frequent refilling necessary with continuous use
LIQUID OXYGEN SYSTEMS		
High liter flows and active patients	100% oxygen, conveniently portable, portable units refilled at home, delivery of up to 6 L/min	Usually weekly delivery necessary for refill, evaporates if not used, potential for frostbite at connections and if spilled
CONCENTRATORS		
Moderate liter flows and patients with limited mobility inside or outside home	Fixed monthly cost, minimal interruption of household by supplier, no refills of "main tank," most units with delivery of up to 4 or 5 L/min	Oxygen concentration decreases as liter flow increases (usually 85% to 90%), power supply necessary, electric bill increase of $15 to $20 a month, second system for portability necessary (usually gas cylinders)

From Dettenmeier PA: *Pulmonary nursing care,* St Louis, 1992, Mosby.

used are compressed oxygen, liquid oxygen, and oxygen concentrators. The advantages and disadvantages (Table 34-8) of each type are assessed, along with the client's needs and community resources, before placing a certain delivery system in the home. In the home, the major consideration is the oxygen delivery source.

Clients requiring home oxygen need extensive teaching so they can continue oxygen therapy efficiently and safely. In preparation, the nurse must coordinate efforts of the client, primary nurse, visiting nurse, and home oxygen equipment vendor. The nurse must also allow sufficient time for teaching so the client is confident in maintaining the oxygen delivery system.

Restoration of Cardiopulmonary Functioning. Severe and prolonged hypoxia may cause cardiac arrest. When a cardiac arrest occurs, oxygen is not delivered to tissues, carbon dioxide is not transported from tissues, tissue metabolism becomes anaerobic, and metabolic and respiratory acidosis occur. Permanent heart, brain, and other tissue damage occurs within 5 minutes.

CARDIOPULMONARY RESUSCITATION. Cardiac arrest is characterized by an absence of pulse and respiration and by dilated pupils. If the nurse determines that the client has cardiac arrest, **cardiopulmonary resuscitation (CPR)** must be initiated. CPR is a basic emergency procedure of artificial respiration and manual external cardiac massage (Procedure 34-5). The three main goals of CPR are to establish an *a*irway, initiate *b*reathing, and maintain *c*irculation (the ABCs of CPR).

Evaluation

Evaluation of the expected outcomes will let the nurse know if the nursing interventions were effective. If the nursing interventions have not been effective, the nurse needs to reassess the care plan to determine what needs to be revised.

When nursing measures directed to improve oxygenation are unsuccessful, the nurse must immediately modify the nursing care plan. New interventions are then developed. The nurse should not hesitate to notify the physician about a client's deteriorating oxygenation status. Prompt notification can avoid an emergency situation or even the need for cardiopulmonary resuscitation.

Based on the general goals for clients with cardiopulmonary alterations, the nurse needs to validate whether the goals have been met.

Goal: Client achieves improved activity tolerance.
Outcome
Client reports less discomfort with exercise
Evaluative measure
Observe client exercise

procedure 34-5

CARDIOPULMONARY RESUSCITATION

Steps	Rationale
ONE NURSE	
1. Assess for unresponsiveness, observe for spontaneous respirations, palpate carotid pulse; ask victim, "Are you OK?"	Prevents injury from attempted resuscitation of person who has not suffered a cardiac or respiratory arrest.
2. Call for help: in hospital setting, call a "code"; in community setting, call emergency phone number.	Activates mechanism for additional personnel.
3. Place victim supine on firm, flat surface or use backboard.	Facilitates external compression of heart. Heart is compressed between sternum and hard surface.
4. Kneel at victim's side.	Allows performance of rescue breathing and chest compressions without moving knees.
5. Open victim's airway:	
a. Head-tilt/chin-lift maneuver (adults and children): Place one hand on victim's forehead and apply firm, backward pressure with palm to tilt head back. Place fingers of other hand under bony part of lower jaw near chin and lift to bring chin forward and teeth almost to occlusion, thus supporting jaw and helping to tilt head back *(see illustration)*. The fingers must not press deeply into the soft tissue under the chin. Thumb should not be used to lift chin.	This maneuver is more effective in opening airway than previously recommended head-tilt/neck-lift. Removes tongue or epiglottis as airway obstruction.
b. Jaw thrust maneuver (adults and children): Grasp angles of victim's lower jaw and lift with both hands, one on each side, displacing mandible forward while tilting head backward.	This technique without head-tilt is the safest first approach to opening airway of victim with suspected neck injury because it can usually be accomplished without extending neck.
6. Prepare for artificial respiration:	
a. For mouth-to-mouth resuscitation of adult, pinch victim's nose and occlude mouth. For infant, place your mouth over infant's nose and mouth.	Forms airtight seal and prevents air from escaping from nose.
b. For Ambu bag resuscitation, use proper size face mask and apply it over victim's mouth and nose.	Forms airtight seal as bag is compressed and oxygen enters client.
7. Administer artificial respiration:	
a. For mouth-to-mouth resuscitation of adult, take a deep breath and seal lips around victim's mouth, creating air-tight seal. Give two slow breaths, followed by 10 to 12 breaths per min.	In most adults this volume of air is 800 ml and is sufficient to make chest rise. Adequate ventilation is indicated by observing chest rise and fall and hearing air escape during exhalation. Excess, rapid volume causes pharyngeal pressures to exceed esophageal opening pressures, allowing air to enter stomach.

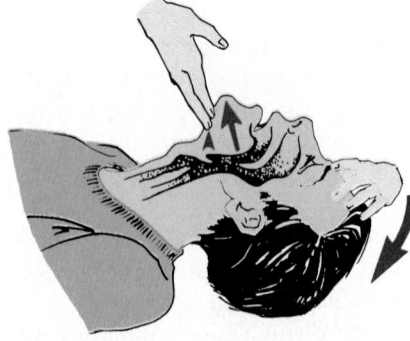

Step 5a

Data from Emergency Cardiac Care Committee and Subcommittee, American Heart Association: Guideline for cardiopulmonary resuscitation and emergency cardiac care, *JAMA* 268:2171, 1992.

Steps	Rationale
b. For mouth-to-mouth resuscitation of infant or child, administer two slow breaths, 1-1½ seconds per breath with pause between for rescuer to take a breath, followed by 20 breaths per min.	Since an infant's air passages are smaller with resistance to flow quite high, it is difficult to make recommendations about the force or volume of the rescue breaths. However, three factors should be remembered: (1) rescue breaths are the single most important maneuver in assisting a nonbreathing child, (2) an appropriate volume is one that makes the chest rise and fall, and (3) slow breaths provide an adequate volume at the lowest possible pressure, thereby reducing the risk of gastric distention.
c. For artificial respiration with an Ambu bag in an adult, compress the bag fully for two breaths.	
d. For Ambu bag resuscitation in a child, use two small compressions of bag.	Prevents overinflation of child's lungs.
8. Observe for rise and fall of chest wall with each respiration. If lungs do not inflate, reposition head and neck and check for visible airway obstruction, such as vomitus.	Ensures artificial respirations are entering lungs.
9. Suction any secretions from airway. If suction is unavailable, turn victim's head to one side.	Prevents airway obstruction. Allows gravity to drain secretions.
10. Assess for presence of carotid pulse; pulse check should take 5-10 sec.	Carotid artery pulse will persist when more peripheral pulses are no longer palpable. Performing external cardiac compressions on a victim who has a pulse may result in serious medical complications.
a. Carotid pulse is most central and accessible artery in children over 1 yr. However, in an infant the short, stubby neck makes carotid difficult to palpate; brachial artery is recommended instead.	
11. If victim is pulseless, begin external cardiac compressions.	Properly performed external chest compressions can produce systolic blood pressure peaks of more than 100 mm Hg, but diastolic pressure is low, with mean blood pressure in carotid arteries seldom exceeding 40 m Hg. Blood flow through carotid artery is only one fourth to one third of normal.
Adult	
a. Proper hand position *(see illustration)*:	
(1) Rescuer's hand locates lower margin of victim's rib cage on side next to rescuer.	
(2) Fingers are moved up rib cage to notch where ribs meet the lower sternum in center of lower part of chest.	Results in maximum compression of heart between sternum and vertebrae. If compressions occur over xiphoid process, victim's liver can be lacerated.

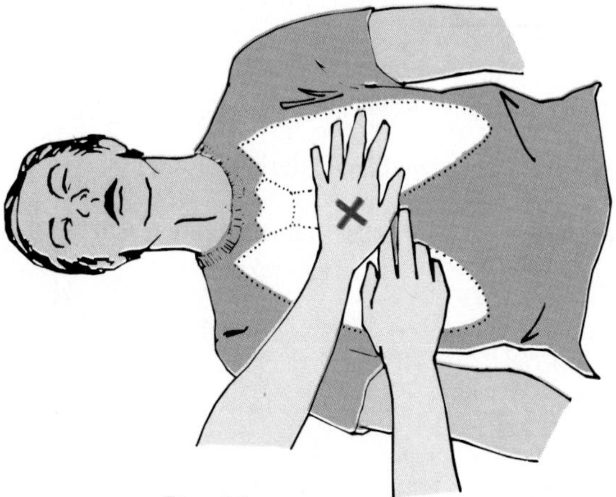
Step 11a

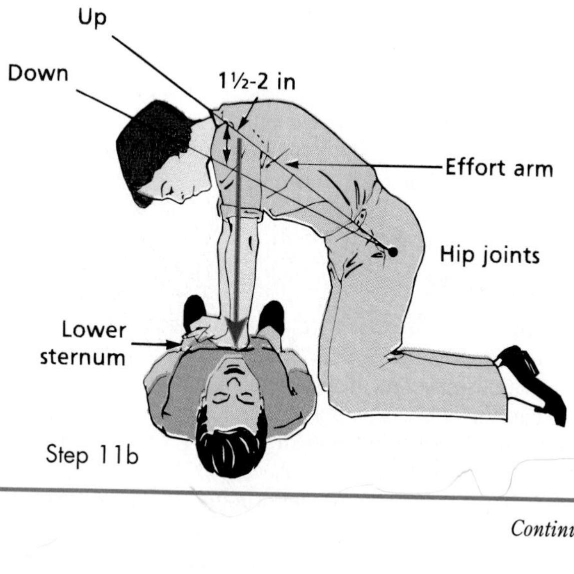

Step 11b

Continued.

Steps	Rationale
(3) Place heel of hand on lower half of sternum and place other hand on top of hand on sternum so that hands are parallel.	
(4) Fingers may be extended or interlaced but should be kept off chest.	Reduces risk of rib fracture during compression.
b. Lock elbows, maintain arms straight and shoulders directly over hands on victim's sternum (see illustration):	Thrust for each compression is straight down on sternum.
(1) Compress chest 3.8-5.0 cm (1½-2 in)	
(2) Compress chest 80-100 times/min. Perform 15 external compressions with mnemonic "one and, two and, three and . . ." to 15.	Increases blood flow with increased flow to brain and heart. Allows pause for ventilation in two-rescuer CPR.
c. Ventilate lungs with two slow rescue breaths as in Step 7a.	
d. Reassess victim after four complete cycles (15 compressions, 2 ventilations each cycle).	Determines return of pulse and respiration and need to continue CPR.
Infant (1-12 mo)	
a. Proper hand position:	Results in maximum compression.
(1) Draw imaginary line between nipples over breast bone (sternum).	
(2) Place index finger of hand farthest from infant's head just under inframammary line where it intersects sternum.	Area of compression is one finger's width below this intersection at the location of middle and ring fingers.
b. Using two or three fingers, compress 1.3-2.5 cm (½-1 in) at least 100 times/min.	Promotes adequate cardiac output.
c. At end of every fifth compression, allow a pause for ventilation (1½ seconds).	Promotes adequate ventilation during CPR.
d. Reassess victim after 10 cycles (5 compressions, 1 ventilation each cycle).	Determines return of pulse and respiration and need to continue CPR.
Child (1-7 yr)	
a. Proper hand position:	Results in maximum compressions.
(1) Locate lower margin of victim's rib cage on side next to rescuer with middle and index fingers.	
(2) Follow margin of rib cage with middle finger to notch where ribs and sternum meet.	
(3) Place index finger next to middle finger.	
(4) Place heel of hand next to point where index finger was located, with long axis of heel parallel to sternum.	
(5) Rescuer's other hand maintains child's head position.	
b. Compress sternum with one hand 2.5-3.8 cm (1-1 ½ in) at rate of 100 times/min.	Promotes adequate cardiac output.
c. At end of every fifth compression, allow a pause for a ventilation (1-1½ seconds).	Promotes adequate ventilation during CPR.
d. Reassess victim after 10 cycles (5 compressions, 1 ventilation each cycle).	Determines return of pulse and respiration and need to continue CPR.
TWO NURSES	
12. One person is positioned at victim's side and performs external cardiac compression while other remains at victim's head, maintains an open airway, and monitors carotid pulse. Compression rate is 80-100/min. The compression-ventilation ratio is 5:1 with a pause for slow rescue breath (1-1½ seconds). When compressor becomes fatigued, rescuers should exchange positions as soon as possible.	

Outcome
Client increases walking distance or time
Evaluative measure
Ask client to maintain a walking diary
Outcome
Client returns to resting pulse more quickly
Evaluative measure
Obtain client's vital signs before, during, and after exercise

Goal: Client maintains lung expansion.
Outcome
Breath sounds auscultated throughout all lobes
Evaluative measure
Auscultate for breath sounds throughout all lobes
Outcome
Client's lung free of adventitious sounds
Evaluative measure
Auscultate for adventitious sounds

Goal: Client maintains mobilization of pulmonary secretions.
Outcome
Client clears airway by coughing
Evaluative measure
Auscultate lungs after client coughs
Outcome
Sputum thin and clear
Evaluative measure
Observe sputum

Goal: Client maintains a patent airway.
Outcome
Client clears airway by coughing
Evaluative measure
Auscultate airways after client coughs
Outcome
Sputum thin, clear
Evaluative measure
Observe sputum
Outcome
Client's lung is free of adventitious sounds
Evaluative measure
Auscultate lungs for adventitious sounds

Goal: Client's tissue oxygenation is maintained.
Outcome
Oxygen saturation remains above 90%
Evaluative measure
Observe client's pulse oximeter
Outcome
Client's skin color normal
Evaluative measures
Observe client's skin color
Obtain vital signs
Assess client's level of orientation

Goal: Client's cardiopulmonary function is restored.
Outcome
Client has spontaneous ventilation
Evaluative measure
Observe for spontaneous ventilation
Outcome
Client's pulse is regular, within normal limits
Evaluative measure
Obtain pulse assessment

SUMMARY

Clients with impaired oxygenation require planned nursing care that focuses on a return to a maximal level of wellness. Many nursing interventions can be used to promote lung expansion, mobilize secretions, maintain a patent airway, promote oxygenation, and restore cardiopulmonary functioning.

Nursing interventions are individualized to the client's level of health, age, life-style, and needs. Many nursing skills are used to help the client achieve a maximal level of oxygenation.

CRITICAL THINKING ACTIVITIES

1. Mr. Havens is 65 years old and has a history of congestive heart failure. He also has poor activity tolerance. What data are important in determining the cardiac response to exercise? What criteria are used to determine when the exercise demand has exceeded cardiac workload capacity?
2. Your client has chest pain. State how to assess this pain. What are three important interventions for this client?
3. You are caring for a client who had abdominal surgery 24 hours ago. This client has a 10-year history of chronic obstructive pulmonary disease. What assessments and interventions are necessary to maintain a patent airway?
4. You are at a shopping center when a gentleman ahead of you collapses. What do you do to maintain adequate cardiopulmonary function?

KEY CONCEPTS

The heart delivers deoxygenated blood to the lungs for oxygenation and delivers oxygen and nutrients to the tissues.
Cardiac output is altered by preload, afterload, contractility, and heart rate.
Cardiac dysrhythmias are classified by cardiac activity and site of impulse origin.
The lungs transfer oxygen from the atmosphere into the alveoli and carbon dioxide out of the body as a waste product.
Ventilation is the process of providing adequate oxygenation from the alveoli to the blood.
Compliance, or the ability of the lungs to expand and contract, depends on the function of musculoskeletal and neurological systems and on other physiological factors.
The process of inspiration (active process) and expiration (passive process) is achieved with changes in lung pressures and volumes.
Respiration is controlled by the central nervous system and chemicals within the blood.
Decreased hemoglobin levels alter the client's ability to transport oxygen.
Impaired chest wall movement reduces the level of tissue oxygenation.
Hyperventilation is a respiratory rate or depth greater than that required to maintain normal levels of carbon dioxide.
Hypoventilation causes carbon dioxide retention.
Hypoxia occurs if the amount of oxygen delivered to tissues is too low.
The nursing assessment includes information about the client's cough, dyspnea, fatigue, wheezing, chest pain, environmental exposures, respiratory infection, cardiopulmonary risk factors, use of medications, and physical functioning.
Diagnostic and laboratory tests may be needed to complete the data base for a client with decreased oxygenation.
Breathing exercises improve ventilation, oxygenation, and sensations of dyspnea.
Nebulization delivers small drops of water or particles of medication to the airways.
Chest physiotherapy includes postural drainage, percussion, and vibration to mobilize pulmonary secretions.
Coughing and suctioning techniques are used to maintain a patent airway.
Oxygen therapy is delivered by nasal cannula, nasal catheter, or oxygen mask.
Cardiac arrest requires the use of cardiopulmonary resuscitation.

References

Ahrens TS: Concepts in the assessment of oxygenation, *Focus Crit Care* 14(1):36-44, 1987.
Ahrens TS: Svo_2 monitoring: is it being used appropriately? *Crit Care Nurse* 10(7):70, 1990.
Burke MM, Walsh MB: *Gerontologic nursing care of the frail elderly,* St. Louis, 1992, Mosby.
Canobbio MM: *Cardiovascular disorders,* St. Louis, 1990, Mosby.
Carroll PF: The ins and outs of chest drainage systems, *Nurs 86* 16(12):26, 1986.
Daily EK, Schroeder JS: *Techniques in bedside hemodynamic monitoring,* ed 4, St. Louis, 1989, Mosby.
Dettenmeier PA: *Pulmonary nursing care,* St. Louis, 1992, Mosby.
DeVito AJ: Dyspnea during hospitalizations for acute phase of illness as recalled by patients with chronic obstructive pulmonary disease, *Heart Lung* 19(2):186, 1990.
Duncan CR et al.: Effect of chest tube management on drainage after cardiac surgery, *Heart Lung* 16(1):1, 1987.
Duncan CR, Erickson RS: Pressures associated with chest tube stripping, *Heart Lung* 11(2):166, 1982.
Eid N, et al.: Chest physiotherapy in review, *Resp Care* 36(4):270, 1991.
Emergency Cardiac Care Committee and Subcommittee, American Heart Association: Guidelines for cardiopulmonary resuscitation and emergency cardiac care, *JAMA* 268:2171, 1992.
Erickson R: Chest tubes: they're really not that complicated, *Nurs 81* 11(5):34, 1981a.
Erickson R: Solving chest tube problems, *Nurs 81* 11(6):62, 1981b.
Farley J: About chest tubes, *Nurs 88* 18(6):16, 1988.
Fiorentini A: Potential hazards of tracheobronchial suctioning, *Intens Crit Care Nurs* 8(4): 217, 1992.
Gift AG et al.: Sensations during chest tube removal, *Heart Lung* 20(2):131, 1991.
Gift AG et al.: Psychologic and physiologic factors related to dyspnea in subjects with chronic obstructive pulmonary disease, *Heart Lung* 15:595, 1986.
Gift AG: Validation of a vertical visual analog scale as a measure of clinical dyspnea, *Rehab Nurs* 14:323, 1989.
Gift AG: Dyspnea, *Nurs Clin North Am* 25(4):955, 1990.
Gröer MW, Shekleton MS: *Basic pathophysiology: a holistic approach,* St. Louis, 1989, Mosby.
Jansen-Bjerklie S et al.: The sensation of pulmonary dyspnea, *Nurs Res* 35(3):154, 1986.
Kane RL et al.: *Essentials of clinical geriatrics,* ed 3, New York, 1994, McGraw-Hill.
Kerr ME et al.: Head-injured adults: recommendations for endotracheal suctioning, *J Neurosci Nurs* 25(2): 86, 1993.
Knox AM: Performing endotracheal suction on children: a literature review and implications for nursing practice, *Intens Crit Care Nurs* 9(1): 48, 1993.
Lookinland S, Appel PL: Hemodynamic and oxygen transport changes following endotracheal suctioning in trauma patients, *Nurs Res* 40:133, 1991.
Luce JM et al.: *Intensive respiratory care,* ed 2, Philadelphia, 1993, Saunders.
McCance KL, Huether SE: *Pathophysiology: the biologic basis for disease in adults and children,* ed 2, St. Louis, 1994, Mosby.
McDonald BR: Validation of three respiratory nursing diagnoses, *Nurs Clin North Am* 20(4):697, 1985.

Pierce JD, Piazza D, Naftel DC: Effects of two chest tube clearance protocols on drainage in patients after myocardial revascularization surgery, *Heart Lung* 20(2):125, 1991.
Reinke LF et al.: Transtracheal oxygen therapy: an alternative delivery approach, *Pers Respir Nurs* 3(3):3, 1992.
Sonnesso G: Are you ready to use pulse oximetry? *Nurs 91* 21(8):60, 1991.
Spofford B, Christopher K: *The clinician's guide for SCOOP transtracheal oxygen system,* Englewood, Colo., 1989, Transtracheal Systems.
Stone KS et al.: Effect of lung hyperinflation and endotracheal suctioning on heart rate and rhythm in patients after coronary artery bypass graft surgery, *Heart Lung* 20:443, 1991.
Walsh M: Peak expiratory flow-rate monitoring, *Perspect Respir Nurs* 3(1):1, 1992.

Bibliography

Beck GJ et al.: The relationship of respiratory symptoms and lung function loss in cotton textile workers, *Am Rev Resp Dis* 130:6, 1984.
Clinical News: Transtracheal oxygen: the nose knows the difference, *Am J Nurs* 87:421, 1987.
Dennison R: Cardiopulmonary assessment: how to do it better in 15 easy steps, *Nurs 86* 16(4):34, 1986.
Herrick TW, Yeager H: Home oxygen therapy, *Ann Fam Pract* 32(2): 157, 1989.
Kerr JAC: Adherence and self-care, *Heart Lung* 14(1):24, 1985.
Perry AG, Potter PA: *Shock: comprehensive nursing management,* St. Louis, 1983, Mosby.
Perry AG, Potter PA: *Clinical nursing skills and techniques,* ed 3, St. Louis, 1994, Mosby.
Standards and guidelines for cardiopulmonary resuscitation (CPR) and emergency cardiac care, *JAMA* 255(21):2903, 1986.
Wade JF: *Respiratory nursing care,* ed 3, St. Louis, 1982, Mosby.
Weaver TE: New life for lungs . . . through incentive spirometers, *Nurs 81* 11(2):53, 1981.
Wilson SF, Thompson JM: *Respiratory disorders,* St. Louis, 1990, Mosby.

35

Fluid, Electrolyte, and Acid-Base Balances

OBJECTIVES

Mastery of content in this chapter will enable the student to:

- Define the key terms listed.
- Describe the mechanisms by which fluids and electrolytes are moved and regulated.
- Describe the processes involved in acid-base balance.
- Discuss common disturbances in fluid, electrolyte, and acid-base balances.
- Discuss variables that affect fluid, electrolyte, and acid-base balance.
- Discuss clinical assessments for fluid, electrolyte, and acid-base imbalances.
- List and discuss nursing interventions for clients with fluid, electrolyte, and acid-base imbalances.
- Measure and record fluid intake and output.
- Describe procedures for initiating and maintaining intravenous therapy.
- Discuss complications of intravenous therapy.
- Describe the procedure for initiating a blood transfusion and the complications of blood therapy.

KEY TERMS

active transport
anions
autologous transfusion
buffer
cations
dehydration
diffusion
extracellular fluids
fluid volume deficit
fluid volume excess
hemolysis
hydrostatic pressure
hypertonic
hypervolemia
hypovolemia
infiltration
infusion pumps
interstitial fluid
intracellular fluid
intravascular fluid
isotonic
metabolic acidosis
metabolic alkalosis
milliequivalents per liter (mEq/L)
oncotic pressure
osmolality
osmoreceptors
osmosis
osmotic pressure
phlebitis
respiratory acidosis
respiratory alkalosis
transfusion reaction
vascular access device
venipuncture

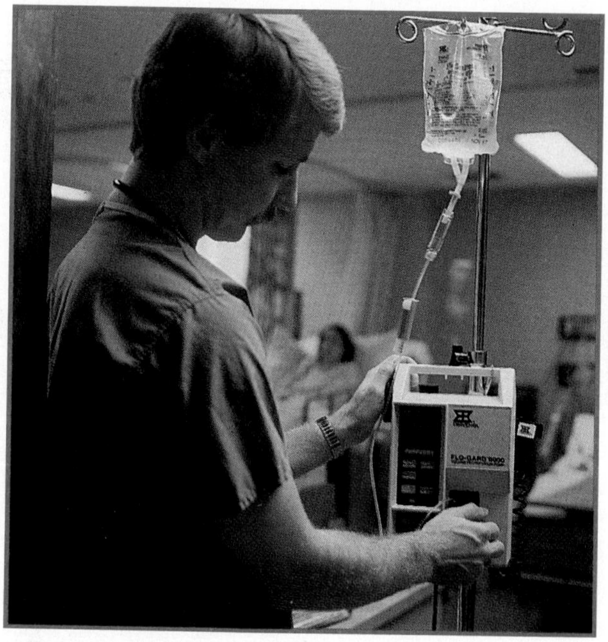

Fluid, electrolyte, and acid-base balances within the body are necessary to maintain health and function in all body systems. These are maintained by the intake and output of water and electrolytes, their distribution in the body, and the regulation of renal and pulmonary functions. Imbalances may result from many factors and are associated with illnesses; therefore nursing care includes assessment and correction of imbalances or maintenance of balance. Acid-base balance is necessary for many physiological processes, and imbalances can alter respiration, metabolism, and the function of the central nervous system.

A healthy, mobile, well-oriented adult is usually capable of maintaining normal fluid, electrolyte, and acid-base balances. This person can maintain balance because of the body's adaptive mechanisms. However, infants, severely ill adults, disoriented or immobile clients, and older adults are frequently unable to respond independently, and after a period, the body's adaptive capacities can no longer maintain balance.

ANATOMY AND PHYSIOLOGY

Distribution of Body Fluids

Body fluids are distributed in two distinct compartments, one containing intracellular fluids and the other extracellular fluids. **Intracellular fluid** (ICF) comprises all fluid within body cells. This fluid contains dissolved solutes essential to fluid and electrolyte balance and metabolism. It makes up about 40% of body weight (McCance and Huether, 1994).

Extracellular fluids (ECF) are all fluids outside a cell and are divided into two smaller compartments: interstitial and intravascular fluids. **Interstitial fluid** is the fluid between cells and outside the blood vessels, whereas **intravascular fluid** is blood plasma. Other extravascular fluids are the lymph, transcellular, and organ fluids (McCance and Huether, 1994). Extracellular fluids make up about 20% of the total body weight.

Composition of Body Fluids

Fluids that circulate through the body in the extracellular and intracellular fluid spaces are composed of electrolytes, minerals, and cells.

An **electrolyte** is an element or compound that, when melted or dissolved in water or another solvent, dissociates into ions and is able to carry an electric current. Positively charged electrolytes are **cations.** Negatively charged electrolytes are **anions.** The concentrations of electrolytes differ in extracellular and intracellular fluids. However, the total number of anions and cations in each fluid compartment should be the same.

Electrolytes are commonly measured in **milliequivalents per liter (mEq/L).** This value represents the number of grams of the specific electrolyte (solute) dissolved in 1 liter of plasma (solution). Electrolytes are vital to many body functions (e.g., neuromuscular function and acid-base balance).

Minerals, ingested as compounds, help to regulate many body functions. They are constituents of all body tissues and fluids and are important in maintaining physiological processes. Minerals are also catalysts in nerve response, muscle contraction, and the metabolism of nutrients. They also regulate electrolyte balance and hormone production and strengthen skeletal structures.

Cells, also located in body fluids, are the functional basic units of all living tissue. Examples of cells within body fluids are red and white blood cells.

Movement of Body Fluids

Fluids and electrolytes constantly shift from compartment to compartment to meet a variety of metabolic needs such as tissue oxygenation or in response to illness or drug therapies. Body fluid and electrolyte movement occurs by diffusion, osmosis, active transport, or filtration. The movement of fluids depends on cell membrane permeability.

Diffusion. **Diffusion** is a process in which solid, particulate matter in a fluid moves from an area of higher concentration to an area of lower concentration, evenly

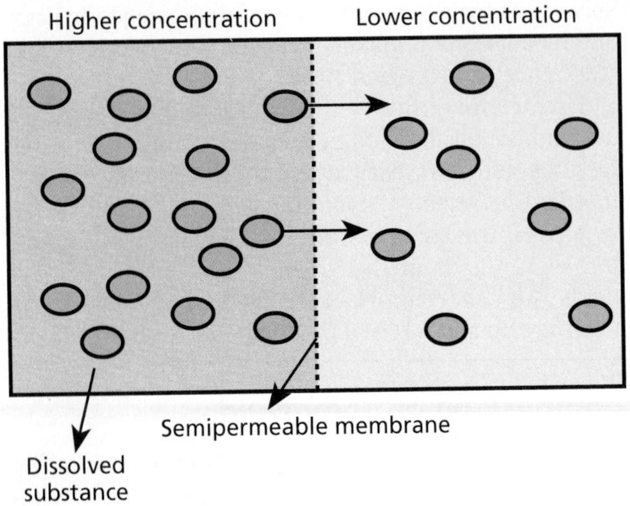

FIGURE 35-1 Diffusion is the movement of molecules across a semipermeable membrane from an area of higher concentration to an area of lower concentration (along its concentration gradient).

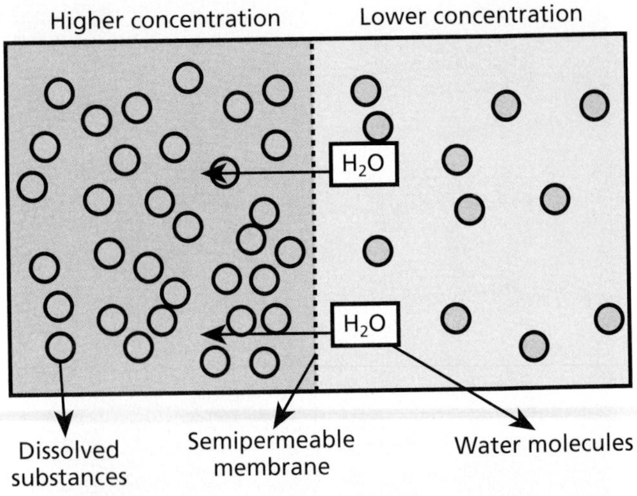

FIGURE 35-2 In osmosis, water molecules move from the less concentrated area to the more concentrated area in an effort to equalize the concentration of solutions on two sides of a membrane.

distributing particles in the fluid (Figure 35-1). The difference in the two concentrations is known as a concentration gradient. Diffusing substances therefore moves down their concentration gradient (Gröer and Shekleton, 1989). Fluids and electrolytes also diffuse across cellular membranes. For a substance to cross the membrane, the membrane must be permeable to it.

Osmosis. **Osmosis** is the movement of a pure solvent, such as water, through a semipermeable membrane from a solution that has a lower solute concentration to one that has a higher solute concentration (Figure 35-2). The membrane is permeable to the solvent but is impermeable to the solute, the particulate matter. The rate of osmosis depends on the concentrations of the solutes in the solutions, the temperature of the solutions, the electrical charges of the solutes, and the differences between the osmotic pressures exerted by the solutions.

The concentration of a solution is measured in osmols (i.e., the amount of a substance in solution in the form of molecules, ions, or both, that has the same osmotic pressure as one mole of an ideal nonelectrolyte). The osmotic pressure of a solution is expressed as **osmolality,** which is expressed in osmols or milliosmols per kilogram (mOsm/kg) of the solution. The normal osmolality of serum is 280-295 mOsm/kg.

If the concentration of the solute is greater on one side of the semipermeable membrane, the rate of osmosis is quicker and there is a more rapid transfer of solvent across the membrane, which continues until an equilibrium is reached. The osmotic pressure of the blood is affected by plasma proteins, especially albumin. Albumin exerts colloid osmotic or **oncotic pressure.**

A solution with the same osmolality as blood plasma is called **isotonic.** When fluids are isotonic, there is no net movement of fluids and electrolytes between fluid compartments. A **hypotonic** solution has a lesser concentration of solutes than is normal in body fluids. When the ECF is hypotonic, there is a net movement of water into the cells. Conversely, a **hypertonic** solution has a greater concentration of solutes than is normal in body fluids. When the ECF is hypertonic, there is a net movement of water out of the cells, resulting in cellular dehydration.

Active Transport. **Active transport** is the movement of materials across the cell membrane by chemical

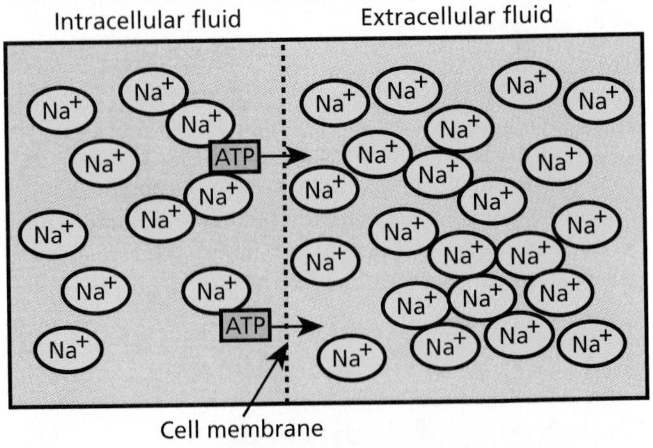

FIGURE 35-3 An example of active transport. Energy (ATP) is used to move sodium molecules across a semipermeable membrane against sodium's concentration gradient (i.e., from an area of lesser concentration to an area of greater concentration).

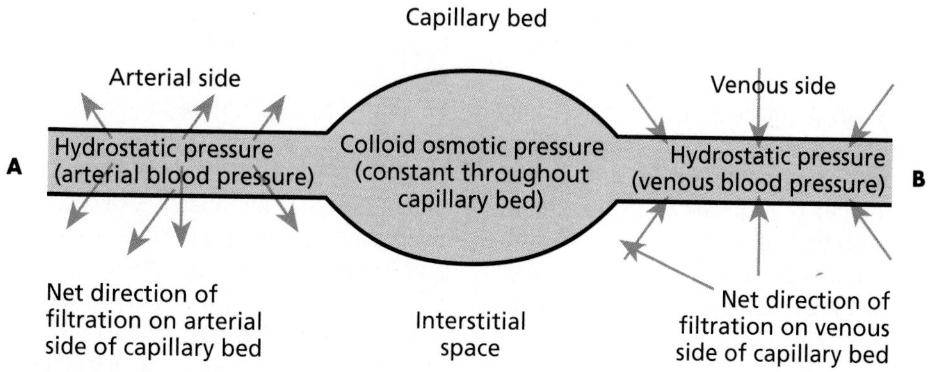

FIGURE 35-4 An example of filtration pressure changes within a capillary bed. **A,** Arterial blood pressure exceeds colloid osmotic pressure, resulting in the movement of water and dissolved substances out of the capillary into the interstitial space. **B,** Venous blood pressure is less than colloid osmotic pressure, resulting in the movement of water and dissolved substances into the capillary.

activity that allows the cell to admit larger molecules than it would otherwise be able to admit or to move molecules from areas of lesser concentration to areas of greater concentration (Figure 35-3). Unlike diffusion and osmosis, active transport requires metabolic activity and energy expenditure. An example of active transport found in the body is the sodium-potassium-ATPase pump. Active transport is enhanced by carrier molecules within a cell that bind themselves to incoming molecules. For example, oxygen binds itself to hemoglobin, which serves as a transport vehicle.

Filtration. Filtration is the process by which water and diffusible substances move together in response to fluid pressure. This process is active in capillary beds, where pressure differences determine the movement of water, electrolytes, and other dissolved substances between the capillaries and interstitial fluid.

Hydrostatic pressure is the pressure exerted by a liquid in a column. Oncotic pressure is an osmotic pressure exerted by large protein molecules in the blood. Blood and fluid entering the capillaries do so at a pressure greater than oncotic and interstitial fluid pressure, so fluid and solutes move out of the capillaries. At the venous end of the capillary bed, hydrostatic pressure is less than oncotic pressure and interstitial pressure, so fluid and waste products move back into the capillaries. (Figure 35-4).

Regulation of Body Fluids

Body fluids are regulated by fluid intake, fluid output, and hormonal controls.

Fluid Intake Regulation. Fluid intake is regulated primarily through the thirst mechanism. The sensation of thirst occurs with a loss of 0.5% of body water (Porth and Erickson, 1992). The thirst control center is located within the hypothalamus. The major physiological stimuli to the thirst center are increased plasma osmolality and decreased blood volume. The stimulation of the renin-angiotensin-aldosterone system, potassium depletion, psychological factors, and the sensation of oropharyngeal dryness also create the sensation of thirst (Figure 35-5).

Receptor cells **(osmoreceptors)** continually monitor the serum osmotic pressure and when osmolality increases, the hypothalamus is stimulated. Increased plasma osmolality can occur with any condition that interferes with the oral ingestion of fluids or it can occur with the intake of hypertonic fluids. When excess fluid is lost (e.g., with vomiting or hemorrhage), hypovolemia occurs, which also stimulates the hypothalamus.

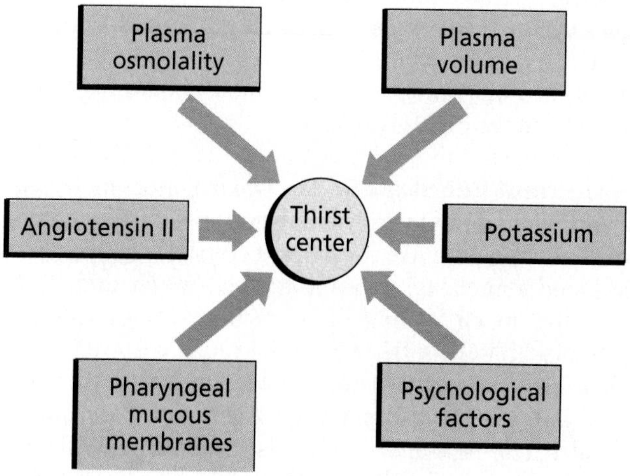

FIGURE 35-5 Stimuli affecting the thirst mechanism.

The hypothalamic stimulation results in increased secretion of ADH, increased thirst sensation, and increased drinking of fluids, especially water.

The adult male (70 kg) requires an average daily fluid intake of 2600 ml: approximately 1300 ml from fluid intake, 1000 ml from foods, and 300 ml from metabolism (Metheny, 1992). Fluid intake requires an alert state. Infants, clients with neurological or psychological problems, and some older adults are unable to perceive or respond to the thirst mechanism; they are at risk for dehydration.

Fluid Output Regulation. Fluid output occurs through four organs of water loss: kidneys, skin, lungs, and gastrointestinal tract. The kidneys are the major regulatory organs of fluid balance. They receive approximately 170 liters of plasma to filter each day and produce 1.5 liters (1500 ml) of urine. The amount of urine produced can be influenced by antidiuretic hormone (ADH) and aldosterone. These hormones affect water and sodium excretion and are stimulated by changes in blood volume.

Water loss from the skin is regulated by the sympathetic nervous system, which activates the sweat glands. Water loss from the skin can be a sensible or insensible loss. Insensible water loss is continuous and is not perceived by the person. The average insensible water loss is 600 ml per day (Metheny, 1992). Sensible water loss occurs through excess perspiration and can be perceived by the client or by the nurse through inspection. The amount of sensible perspiration is directly related to the stimulation of the sweat glands caused by increased muscular exercise, elevated environmental temperature, and increased metabolic activity (e.g., an elevation of body temperature). Sensible water loss can range up to 1000 ml depending on exercise and external and body temperatures (Metheny, 1992).

The lungs expire about 400 ml of water daily. This insensible loss may increase in response to changes in respiratory rate and depth. In addition, devices for giving oxygen can increase insensible water loss from the lungs (see Chapter 32). The average fluid loss from the gastrointestinal tract is about 100 ml/24 hours. Vomiting or diarrhea increases this loss.

Hormonal Regulation. The two major hormones affecting fluid and electrolyte balance are ADH and aldosterone. The stimulus for ADH secretion is an increase in blood osmolality, which indicates a water deficit, or decrease in circulating blood volume (McCance and Huether, 1994). ADH, released by the posterior pituitary gland, decreases the production of urine by increasing the reabsorption of water by the kidney tubules. During transient periods of fluid volume deficit (e.g., vomiting, diarrhea, or hemorrhage), the amount of ADH in the blood increases, and the water reabsorbed by the kidney tubules increases and is returned to the circulating blood volume. Urinary output declines in response to the action of the hormone.

Aldosterone is a mineralocorticoid, produced by the adrenal cortex, that regulates sodium and potassium balance. Fluid deficits (e.g., hemorrhage or gastrointestinal losses) that cause a decreased blood pressure, decreased serum sodium, increased serum potassium, and sympathetic nervous system stimulation can stimulate the secretion of aldosterone into the blood (Schauf et al., 1990). Aldosterone causes the kidney tubules to excrete potassium and reabsorb sodium; as a result, water is reabsorbed and returned to the blood volume.

Regulation of Electrolytes

Cations. Major cations within the body fluids include sodium (Na^+), potassium (K^+), calcium (Ca^{++}), and magnesium (Mg^{++}). Their actions affect neurochemical and neuromuscular transmissions, which influence muscular function, cardiac rhythm and contractility, mood and behavior, and gastrointestinal functioning as well as other processes. Cations interchange when one cation leaves the cell and is replaced by another. This occurs because cells tend to maintain electrical neutrality. Therefore one positively charged ion must be exchanged with another positively charged ion.

SODIUM REGULATION. Sodium is the most abundant cation (90%) in extracellular fluids. Sodium ions are involved in maintaining water balance through their effect on serum osmolality, transmitting nerve impulses, regulation of acid-base balance, and participation in cellular chemical reactions (McCance and Huether, 1994). The normal extracellular sodium concentration is 135 to 145 mEq/L. Sodium is regulated by dietary intake and aldosterone secretion.

POTASSIUM REGULATION. Potassium is the predominant intracellular cation. It regulates many metabolic activities and is necessary for glycogen deposits in the liver and skeletal muscle, transmission and conduction of nerve impulses, normal cardiac rhythms, and skeletal and smooth muscle contraction (McCance and Huether, 1994). The normal range for serum potassium concentrations is 3.5 to 5.3 mEq/L. Potassium is regulated by dietary intake and renal excretion. Renal excretion of potassium is affected by glomerular filtration rate, serum potassium level, aldosterone, and acid-base balance. The body does not conserve potassium well, so any condition that increases urine output (e.g., diabetes insipidus) will result in a decreased serum potassium.

CALCIUM REGULATION. Calcium is stored in bone, plasma, and body cells. The majority of calcium is located in bone. Approximately 50% of calcium in the plasma is bound to plasma proteins and 40% is ionized. Normal serum calcium is 4.0 to 5.0 mEq/L. Calcium is necessary for bone and teeth formation, blood clotting, hormone secretion, cell membrane integrity, cardiac conduction, transmission of nerve impulses, and muscle contraction.

Calcium in extracellular fluids is regulated through actions of the parathyroid hormone, calcitonin, vitamin D, and acid-base balance. Parathyroid hormone (PTH) and vitamin D control the balance among bone calcium, gastrointestinal absorption of calcium, and kidney excretion of calcium. Calcitonin from the thyroid gland and acid-base balance affect serum calcium levels by altering the rate of release of calcium from bones.

MAGNESIUM REGULATION. Magnesium is essential for enzyme activities, neurochemical activities, and cardiac and skeletal muscle excitability. Plasma concentrations of magnesium range from 1.5 to 2.5 mEq/L. Serum magnesium is regulated by dietary intake and renal mechanisms and some actions of parathyroid hormone.

Anions. The three major anions of body fluids are chloride (Cl^-), bicarbonate (HCO_3^-), and phosphate ($PO_4\equiv$) ions. Anions affect fluid, electrolyte, and acid-base balances.

CHLORIDE REGULATION. Chloride is the major anion in extracellular fluids. The transport of chloride follows sodium. Normal concentrations of chloride range from 100 to 106 mEq/L. Serum chloride is regulated by dietary intake and the kidneys. The amount of chloride excreted is related to dietary intake. A person with normal renal function who has a high chloride intake will excrete a higher amount of urine chloride.

BICARBONATE REGULATION. Bicarbonate is the major chemical base buffer within the body. The bicarbonate ion is found in extracellular and intracellular fluids. The bicarbonate ion is an essential component of the carbonic acid–bicarbonate buffering system essential to acid-base balance. The kidneys regulate bicarbonate. When the body needs to retain more base, the kidneys reabsorb greater quantities of bicarbonate and return it to extracellular fluids. Normal arterial bicarbonate levels range between 22 and 26 mEq/L; venous bicarbonate is measured as carbon dioxide content, and the normal value is 24-30 mEq/L.

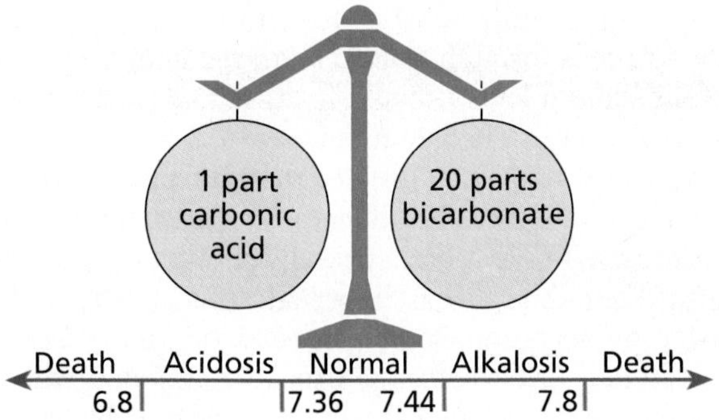

FIGURE 35-6 Carbonic acid–bicarbonate ratio and pH.

PHOSPHATE REGULATION. Phosphate is a buffer anion in intracellular and extracellular fluids assisting in acid-base regulation. Phosphate and calcium help to develop and maintain bones and teeth. Calcium and phosphate are inversely proportional; if one rises, the other falls. Phosphate also promotes normal neuromuscular action and participates in carbohydrate metabolism. Serum phosphate concentration is regulated by dietary intake, the kidneys, parathyroid hormone, and vitamin D (Gröer and Shekleton, 1989). Phosphate is normally absorbed through the gastrointestinal tract. The normal serum level is 2.5 to 4.5 mg/dl.

Regulation of Acid-Base Balance

Acid-base balance exists when the net rate at which the body produces acids or bases equals the rate at which acids or bases are excreted. This balance results in a stable concentration of hydrogen ions (H^+) in body fluids that is expressed as the pH value. Normal hydrogen ion level is necessary to maintain cell membrane integrity and the speed of cellular enzymatic reactions. The pH is a scale for measuring the acidity or alkalinity of a fluid. A pH value of 7 is neutral; below 7 is acid, and above 7 is alkaline. Normal values in arterial blood range from 7.35 to 7.45.

The human body has regulatory mechanisms for maintaining the acid-base balance and for adapting to short-term changes in H^+ concentration. Such changes occur during physical exercise, moderate anxiety states, and minor gastrointestinal alterations. The body can make adjustments for transient changes in pH (compensation). However, with severe trauma, uncontrolled diabetes mellitus, shock, or other serious illnesses, the body may not be able to maintain normal pH. In such cases, medical intervention is required.

The three general types of acid-base regulators within the body are chemical, biological, and physiological buffering systems. A **buffer** is a substance or a group of substances that can absorb or release H^+ to correct an acid-base imbalance.

Chemical Regulation. The largest chemical buffer in extracellular fluids is the carbonic acid and bicarbonate buffer system (Figure 35-6). This system can be expressed as:

$$CO_2 + H_2O \rightleftarrows H_2CO_3 \rightleftarrows H^+ + HCO_3^-$$

carbon dioxide, water, carbonic acid, hydrogen ion, hydrogen bicarbonate

The carbonic acid–bicarbonate buffer system is the first buffering system to react to change in the pH of extracellular fluids and it reacts within seconds. The excretion of carbon dioxide that results from metabolism is controlled primarily by the lungs. The excretion of hydrogen and bicarbonate ions is controlled by the kidneys. These substances can buffer a strong acid or base to maintain a relatively constant pH.

A second chemical buffering system involves inorganic phosphate, the plasma proteins albumin, fibrinogen, prothrombin, and the gamma globulins. These proteins can bind with or release hydrogen ions to correct acidosis or alkalosis. However, their capacity to maintain acid-base balance of the extracellular fluid is limited, and they cannot correct long-term imbalances.

Biological Regulation. Biological buffering occurs when hydrogen ions are absorbed or released by cells. Biological buffering occurs after chemical buffering and takes 2 to 4 hours. The hydrogen ion has a positive charge and must be exchanged with another positively charged ion, frequently potassium (K^+). In conditions with excess acid, a hydrogen ion enters the cell and a potassium ion leaves the cell and enters extracellular fluids. In another mechanism, hydrogen ions and calcium ions can exchange in the bone. Extracellular fluid is thus less acidic through either mechanism because fewer hydrogen ions are present.

A second biological buffer is the hemoglobin-oxyhemoglobin system. Carbon dioxide diffuses into the red blood cell (RBC) and forms carbonic acid. The carbonic acid dissociates into hydrogen and bicarbonate ions. The hydrogen ions attach to hemoglobin, and the bicarbonate ion becomes available for buffering by exchanging with extracellular chloride (Kokko and Tannen, 1990).

Another biological buffer is the chloride shift within red blood cells. When blood is oxygenated in the lungs, bicarbonate diffuses into the cells and chloride travels from the hemoglobin to the plasma to maintain electrical neutrality. The reverse occurs when carbon dioxide moves into the red cell in tissue capillary beds. This process is referred to as the chloride shift and is a reciprocal exchange between these anions (Gröer and Shekleton, 1989).

Physiological Regulation. The two physiological buffers in the body are the lungs and the kidneys. The lungs adapt rapidly to an acid-base imbalance; they act to return the pH to normal before the action of the biological buffers.

Ordinarily, increased levels of hydrogen ions and carbon dioxide provide the stimulus for respiration. When the concentration of hydrogen ions is altered, the lungs react to correct the imbalance by altering the rate and depth of respiration. In alkalosis, the body compensates by reducing the respiratory rate, and thus carbon dioxide is retained. Carbon dioxide combines with water in the blood to form carbonic acid, which helps to correct the alkaline excess. With acidosis, the respiratory rate increases and the lungs excrete greater amounts of carbon dioxide (McCance and Huether, 1994).

The kidneys take from a few hours to several days to regulate acid-base imbalance. They reabsorb bicarbonate in cases of acid excess and excrete it in cases of acid deficit. In addition, the kidneys use a phosphate ion ($PO_4\equiv$) to excrete hydrogen ions by forming phosphoric acid (H_3PO_4); sulfuric acid (H_2SO_4) may also be excreted. Finally, the kidneys convert ammonia (NH_3) to ammonium (NH_4) by attaching a hydrogen ion to ammonia (Price and Wilson, 1992).

DISTURBANCES IN ELECTROLYTE, FLUID, AND ACID-BASE BALANCES

Disturbances in electrolyte, fluid, or acid-base balances seldom occur alone and can disrupt normal body processes. When there is a loss of body fluids because of burns, illnesses, or trauma, the client is also at risk for electrolyte imbalances. In addition, some untreated electrolyte imbalances (e.g., potassium loss) result in acid-base disturbances.

Electrolyte Imbalances

Sodium Imbalances. Hyponatremia is a less than normal concentration of sodium in the blood, which can occur with a net sodium loss or net water excess (Table 35-1). It occurs frequently in seriously ill clients. Hyponatremia can be associated with an excess, deficit, or normal volume of extracellular fluid (Metheny, 1992). The usual situation is a loss of sodium without a loss of fluid, and this results in a decrease in the osmolality of extracellular fluid.

When a sodium loss occurs, the body initially adapts by reducing water excretion to maintain serum osmolality at near-normal levels. As the sodium loss continues, the body continues to preserve the blood and interstitial (tissue) volume. As a result, the sodium in extracellular fluids becomes diluted. However, hyponatremia caused by sodium loss can eventually result in vascular collapse and shock. When there is a sodium deficit with a distinct loss of extracellular fluid volume, the body's adaptive mechanisms may not be able to maintain blood pressure. Severe hyponatremia can result in serious neurological alterations caused by the movement of fluid into cerebral cells through osmosis. Any trend of decreasing serum sodium levels should be noted so that appropriate treatment can be instituted.

Hypernatremia is a greater than normal concentration of sodium in extracellular fluids that can be caused by excess water loss or an overall sodium excess (Table 35-1). When the cause of hypernatremia is increased aldosterone secretion, sodium is retained and potassium is excreted. Hypernatremia can be associated with an excess, deficit, or normal volume of extracellular fluid (Metheny, 1992). When hypernatremia occurs, the body

table 35-1
ELECTROLYTE IMBALANCES

Causes	Signs and symptoms
HYPONATREMIA	
Kidney disease resulting in salt-wasting Adrenal insufficiency Gastrointestinal losses Increased sweating Use of diuretics, especially when combined with low-sodium diet Psychogenic polydipsia Secretion of inappropriate ADH (SIADH)	*Physical examination:* apprehension, personality change, postural hypotension, postural dizziness, abdominal cramping, nausea and vomiting, diarrhea, tachycardia, convulsions and coma, and fingerprints remaining on sternum after palpation *Laboratory findings:* serum sodium level <135 mEq/L, serum osmolality <280 mOsm/kg, and urine specific gravity <1.010 (if not caused by SIADH)
HYPERNATREMIA	
Ingestion of large amounts of concentrated salt solutions Iatrogenic administration of hypertonic saline solution parenterally Excess aldosterone secretion Diabetes insipidus Increased sensible and insensible water loss Water deprivation	*Physical examination:* thirst, dry and flushed skin, dry and sticky tongue and mucous membranes, fever, agitation, convulsions, restlessness, and irritability *Laboratory findings:* serum sodium levels >145 mEq/L, serum osmolality >295 mOsm/kg, and urine specific gravity >1.030 (if not caused by diabetes insipidus)
HYPOKALEMIA	
Use of potassium-wasting diuretics Diarrhea, vomiting, or other gastrointestinal losses Alkalosis Excess aldosterone secretion Polyuria Extreme sweating Excessive use of potassium-free IV solutions Treatment of diabetic ketoacidosis with insulin	*Physical examination:* weakness and fatigue, decreased muscle tone, intestinal distention, decreased bowel sounds, ventricular dysrhythmias, paresthesias and weak, irregular pulse *Laboratory findings:* serum potassium level <3.5 mEq/L and electrocardiogram (ECG) abnormalities (e.g., ventricular dysrhythmias [likely when potassium level is <2.6 mEq/L*])
HYPERKALEMIA	
Renal failure Fluid volume deficit Massive cellular damage such as from burns and trauma Iatrogenic administration of large amounts of potassium intravenously Adrenal insufficiency Acidosis, especially diabetic ketoacidosis Rapid infusion of stored blood Use of potassium-sparing diuretics	*Physical examination:* anxiety, dysrhythmias, paresthesia, weakness, abdominal cramps, and diarrhea *Laboratory findings:* serum potassium level >5.3 mEq/L and ECG abnormalities (bradycardia, heart block, dysrhythmias† usually appear with serum potassium level >7 mEq/L.‡)
HYPOCALCEMIA	
Rapid administration of blood transfusions containing citrate Hypoalbuminemia Hypoparathyroidism Vitamin D deficiency Pancreatitis Alkalosis	*Physical examination:* numbness and tingling of fingers and circumoral region, hyperactive reflexes, positive Trousseau's sign (carpopedal spasm with hypoxia), positive Chvostek's sign (contraction of facial muscles when facial nerve is tapped), tetany, muscle cramps, and pathological fractures (chronic hypocalcemia) *Laboratory findings:* serum calcium level <4.0 mEq/L or 8.5 mg/100 ml and ECG abnormalities

*Data from DeAngelis R and Lessig L, 1991.
†Levels >8.5 mEq/L are frequently fatal as a result of cardiac standstill (Horne MM, Heitz UE, and Swearingen PL, 1991) (Metheny, 1987).
‡Data from Metheny NM, *Fluid and electrolyte balance: nursing considerations,* ed 2, Philadelphia, 1992, Lippincott.

Continued.

table 35-1—cont'd

ELECTROLYTE IMBALANCES

Causes	Signs and symptoms
HYPERCALCEMIA	
Hyperparathyroidism Malignant neoplastic disease Paget's disease Osteoporosis Prolonged immobilization Acidosis	*Physical examination:* anorexia, nausea and vomiting, weakness, lethargy, low back pain (from kidney stones), decreased level of consciousness, personality changes, and cardiac arrest *Laboratory findings:* serum calcium level >5 mEq/L or 10.5 mg/100 ml; x-ray examination showing generalized osteoporosis, widespread bone cavitation, radiopaque urinary stones; and elevated BUN level >25 mg/100 ml and elevated creatinine level >1.5 mg/100 ml caused by FVD or renal damage caused by urolithiasis; ECG abnormalities
HYPOMAGNESEMIA	
Inadequate intake: malnutrition and alcoholism Inadequate absorption: diarrhea, vomiting, nasogastric drainage, fistulas; diseases of small intestine Excessive loss resulting from thiazide diuretics Aldosterone excess Polyuria	*Physical examination:* muscular tremors, hyperactive deep tendon reflexes, confusion and disorientation, dysrhythmias, and positive Chvostek's and Trousseau's sign *Laboratory findings:* serum magnesium level <1.5 mEq/L
HYPERMAGNESEMIA	
Renal failure Excess oral or parenteral intake of magnesium	*Physical examination:* physical findings that are more frequent in acute elevations in magnesium levels: hypoactive deep tendon reflexes, decreased depth and rate of respirations, hypotension, and flushing *Laboratory findings:* serum magnesium level >2.5 mEq/L

attempts to conserve as much water as possible through renal reabsorption. If the hypernatremia is prolonged, however, there will be an increase in serum osmolality and in the interstitial osmotic pressure, and fluid shifts from the cells into extracellular fluids. This shift causes the cells to shrink and interrupts most of the physiological cellular processes.

Potassium Imbalances. Hypokalemia is a condition in which an inadequate amount of potassium circulates in extracellular fluids. When severe, hypokalemia can affect cardiac conduction and function especially in the client receiving digitalis preparations. Because the normal amount of potassium is so small, there is little tolerance for fluctuations in serum levels.

Hypokalemia is one of the most common alterations in electrolyte balance and can result from several conditions (see Table 35-1). The most common cause is the use of potassium-wasting diuretics such as thiazide and loop diuretics. Other factors contributing to the development of hypokalemia include deficient dietary intake and increased shift of potassium from the ECF to the ICF (with alkalosis or insulin administration) (McCance and Huether, 1994).

Hyperkalemia is a greater-than-normal amount of potassium in the blood. Severe hyperkalemia produces marked cardiac conduction abnormalities. The primary cause of hyperkalemia is renal failure because any decrease in renal function diminishes the amount of potassium the kidney can excrete. Other conditions that cause increased potassium intake or a shift of potassium from the ICF to the ECF (acidosis or insulin deficiency) also result in increased potassium (see Table 35-1).

Calcium Imbalances. Hypocalcemia represents a drop in serum and ionized calcium. It can result from several illnesses, some of which directly affect the thyroid and parathyroid glands (see Table 35-1). Signs and symptoms are directly correlated to the physiological role of serum calcium in neuromuscular function.

Hypercalcemia is an increase in the total serum concentration of calcium, as well as ionized calcium. Hypercalcemia is frequently a symptom of an underlying disease resulting in excess bone resorption with release of calcium (see Table 35-1).

Magnesium Imbalances. **Hypomagnesemia** is present when the serum concentration drops below normal. Common causes of hypomagnesemia are chronic malnutrition and alcoholism. Hypomagnesemia (see Table 35-1) produces symptoms similar to hypocalcemia by increasing neuromuscular excitability (McCance and Huether, 1994).

Hypermagnesemia occurs when the serum concentration of magnesium rises above normal and is primarily caused by renal failure and excess doses of parenterally administered magnesium (see Table 35-1). The clinical symptoms of hypermagnesemia include depressed deep tendon reflexes and respiratory depression.

Chloride Imbalances. Hypochloremia occurs when the serum chloride level falls below normal. Vomiting or prolonged and excessive nasogastric or fistula drainage can result in hypochloremia because of the loss of hydrochloric acid. A newborn can quickly develop hypochloremia as a result of diarrhea. The use of loop and thiazide diuretics also results in increased chloride excretion as sodium is excreted. When serum chloride levels fall, the body adapts by increased reabsorption of the bicarbonate ion to maintain electrical neutrality and metabolic alkalosis results.

Hyperchloremia occurs when the serum chloride level rises above normal, which usually occurs when the serum bicarbonate value falls or sodium level rises. Hypochloremia and hyperchloremia rarely occur as single disease processes but are commonly associated with acid-base imbalance. There is no single set of symptoms associated with these two alterations.

Fluid Disturbances

The basic types of fluid imbalances are isotonic and osmolar. Isotonic deficit and excess exist when water and electrolytes are gained or lost in equal proportions. In contrast, osmolar imbalances are losses or excesses of only water so that the concentration (osmolality) of the serum is affected. Table 35-2 lists the causes and symptoms of common disturbances.

Isotonic Imbalances. **Fluid volume deficit (FVD)** results when water and electrolytes are lost in isotonic proportions. Unless other imbalances are present, serum electrolyte levels remain unchanged. Clients at risk include those with gastrointestinal losses of fluid and electrolytes. The very young and old are quickly affected by these losses (Metheny, 1992). Other causes can include hemorrhage, diuretic administration, profuse sweating, fever, and increased oral intake.

Fluid volume excess (FVE) results when water and sodium are retained in isotonic proportions, resulting in hypervolemia with unchanged levels of serum electrolytes. Clients at risk include those with congestive heart failure, renal failure, cirrhosis of the liver, increased aldosterone secretion, increased levels of corticosteroids, and abnormal intake of salt (e.g., in the too-rapid administration of IV fluids containing sodium (Metheny, 1992).

Osmolar Imbalances. Hyperosmolar imbalance **(dehydration)** occurs when there is a loss of water without proportionate loss of electrolytes, especially sodium, or when there is a gain in osmotically active substances. This results in an increased serum sodium and osmolality and intracellular dehydration. Eventually neurological function is impaired, and hypovolemia can occur (McCance and Huether, 1994).

Risk factors for hyperosmolar imbalance include conditions that impair sufficient oral intake (e.g., alterations in neurological function). Frail, infirm older clients are at great risk for developing dehydration. A decrease in ADH secretion (diabetes insipidus) can lead to profound water losses. Other conditions that can cause a hyperosmolar imbalance are diabetic ketoacidosis and administration of hypertonic tube-feeding formulas or IV solutions.

Hypoosmolar imbalance (water excess) occurs when there is an excess intake of water (psychogenic polydipsia) or excess ADH secretion. Surgery or injury to the brain can cause secretion of inappropriate ADH (SIADH). The overall effect is dilution of the extracellular fluid with osmosis of water into the cells (McCance and Huether, 1994). Brain cells are particularly sensitive, and this process can lead to cerebral edema, which can cause decreased level of consciousness, coma, and even death.

Acid-Base Imbalances

The four primary types of acid-base imbalance are respiratory acidosis, respiratory alkalosis, metabolic acidosis, and metabolic alkalosis (Table 35-3).

Respiratory Acidosis. **Respiratory acidosis** is marked by an increased arterial carbon dioxide concentration ($Paco_2$), excess carbonic acid (H_2CO_3), and an increased hydrogen ion concentration (decreased pH). Respiratory acidosis is caused by hypoventilation or any condition that depresses ventilation. Decreased ventilation may begin in the respiratory system (e.g., pneumonia) or outside the respiratory system (e.g., drug overdose with a respiratory center depressant). With respiratory acidosis, the cerebrospinal fluid and brain cells become acidic, causing neurological changes. Hypoxemia occurs because of respiratory depression, result-

table 35-2
FLUID DISTURBANCES

Causes	Signs and symptoms
ISOTONIC IMBALANCES	
Fluid volume deficit (FVD)	
Losses from the gastrointestinal system such as from diarrhea, vomiting, or drainage from fistulas or tubes Loss of plasma or whole blood, such as with burns or hemorrhage Excessive perspiration Fever Decreased oral intake of fluids Use of diuretics	*Physical examination:* postural hypotension, tachycardia, dry mucous membranes, poor skin turgor, thirst, confusion, rapid weight loss, slow vein filling, lethargy, oliguria, weak pulse *Laboratory findings:* urine specific gravity >1.025, increased hematocrit level >50%, and increased blood urea nitrogen (BUN) level >25 mg/100ml (hemoconcentration)
Fluid volume excess (FVE)	
Congestive heart failure Renal failure Cirrhosis of the liver Increased serum aldosterone and steroid levels Excessive sodium intake or administration	*Physical examination:* rapid weight gain, edema (especially in dependent areas), hypertension, polyuria (if renal mechanisms are normal), neck vein distention, increased venous pressure, crackles in lungs *Laboratory findings:* decreased hematocrit level <38% and decreased BUN level <10 mg/100 ml (hemodilution)
OSMOLAR IMBALANCES	
Hyperosmolar imbalance	
Diabetes insipidus Interruption of neurologically driven thirst drive Diabetic ketoacidosis Osmotic diuresis Administration of hypertonic parenteral fluids or tube feeding formulas	*Physical examination:* dry and sticky mucous membranes, flushed and dry skin, thirst, elevated body temperature, irritability, convulsions, coma *Laboratory findings:* increased serum sodium level >145 mEq/L and increased serum osmolality >295 mOsm/kg
Hypoosmolar imbalance	
SIADH Excess water intake	*Physical examination:* decreased level of consciousness, convulsions, coma *Laboratory findings:* decreased serum sodium level <135 mEq/L and decreased serum osmolality <280 mOsm/kg

ing in further neurological impairments. Electrolyte changes such as hyperkalemia and hypercalcemia may accompany the acidosis.

Respiratory Alkalosis. Respiratory alkalosis is marked by decreased Pa_{CO_2} and increased pH. Respiratory alkalosis results from excessive exhalation of carbon dioxide or hyperventilation. Like respiratory acidosis, respiratory alkalosis can begin outside the respiratory system (e.g., anxiety with hyperventilation) or within the respiratory system (e.g., initial phase of an asthma attack).

Metabolic Acidosis. Metabolic acidosis results from a rise in hydrogen ion concentration (decreased pH) in extracellular fluids, caused by a loss of bicarbonate from the body, excess hydrogen ion production, and inability of the kidneys to excrete the acid load (Horne et al., 1991). There are many causes of metabolic acidosis. Determining the two types of metabolic acidosis (i.e., normal anion gap [hyperchloremic] and increased anion gap [lactic acidosis]) helps to determine the cause and treatment of the metabolic acidosis. The anion gap measures the difference between the measured cations (sodium and potassium) and the measured anions (chloride and bicarbonate) in the body. An increase in the anion gap indicates that the level of unmeasured anions (e.g., phosphate or lactic acid) has increased. The normal anion gap is 3-11 mEq/L (Emergency Medicine, 1990).

table 35-3

ACID-BASE IMBALANCES

Causes	Signs and symptoms
RESPIRATORY ACIDOSIS	
Hypoventilation resulting from primary respiratory problems Atelectasis (obstruction of small airways often caused by retained mucus) Pneumonia Cystic fibrosis Respiratory failure Airway obstruction Chest wall injury	*Physical examination:* confusion, dizziness, lethargy, headache, ventricular dysrhythmias, warm and flushed skin, muscular twitching, convulsions, and coma *Laboratory findings:* arterial blood gas alterations: pH <7.35, partial pressure of carbon dioxide in arterial blood ($Paco_2$) >45 mm Hg, arterial partial pressure of oxygen (Pao_2) <80 mm Hg, and bicarbonate level normal (if uncompensated) or >26 mEq/L (if compensated)
Hypoventilation resulting from factors outside of the respiratory system Drug overdose with a respiratory depressant Paralysis of respiratory muscles caused by various neurological alterations Head injury Obesity	
RESPIRATORY ALKALOSIS	
Hyperventilation resulting from primary respiratory problems Asthma Pneumonia Inappropriate mechanical ventilator settings	*Physical examination:* dizziness, confusion, dysrhythmias, tachypnea, numbness and tingling of extremities, convulsions, and coma *Laboratory findings:* arterial blood gas alterations: pH >7.45, $Paco_2$ <35 mm Hg, Pao_2 normal, and bicarbonate level normal (if short lived or uncompensated) or <22 mEq/L (if compensated)
Hyperventilation resulting from factors outside of the respiratory system Anxiety Hypermetabolic states Disorders of the central nervous system (head injuries, infections) Salicylate overdose	
METABOLIC ACIDOSIS	
High anion gap Starvation Diabetic ketoacidosis Renal failure Lactic acidosis Use of drugs (methanol, ethanol, formic acid, paraldehyde, aspirin)	*Physical examination:* headache, lethargy, confusion, dysrhythmias, tachypnea with deep respirations, abdominal cramps, and flushed skin *Laboratory findings:* arterial blood gas alterations: pH <7.35, $Paco_2$ normal (if uncompensated) or <35 mm Hg (if compensated), Pao_2 normal or increased (with rapid, deep respirations), and bicarbonate level <22 mEq/L
Normal anion gap Renal tubular acidosis Diarrhea	
METABOLIC ALKALOSIS Excessive vomiting Prolonged gastric suctioning Hypokalemia or hypercalcemia Excess aldosterone Use of drugs (steroids, sodium bicarbonate, diuretics)	*Physical examination:* dizziness, dysrhythmias, numbness and tingling of fingers, toes, and circumoral region, muscle cramps; tetany *Laboratory findings:* arterial blood gas alterations: pH >7.45, $Paco_2$ normal (if uncompensated) or >45 mm Hg (if compensated), Pao_2 normal, and bicarbonate level >26 mEq/L

Metabolic Alkalosis. Metabolic alkalosis is marked by heavy loss of acid from the body or by increased levels of bicarbonate. The most common cause is vomiting. Metabolic alkalosis also may result when a client with a gastric acidity disturbance ingests large amounts of sodium bicarbonate.

NURSING PROCESS FOR FLUID, ELECTROLYTE, AND ACID-BASE IMBALANCES

Assessment

During assessment of fluid, electrolyte, and acid-base balances, the nurse identifies clients at risk for imbalances, the presence of any alterations, and the extent to which body systems are involved. Assessment helps the nurse to anticipate the client's needs for nursing care. Gathering assessment data also helps to determine the effectiveness of therapies and any adverse reactions to them.

The assessment includes the nursing history, physical examination, measuring and recording of intake and output, laboratory studies, and consideration of factors influencing fluid, electrolyte, and acid-base balances.

Nursing History

To collect data regarding fluid, electrolyte, and acid-base status, the nurse must understand the processes involved in fluid volume and concentration alterations, electrolyte imbalances, and acid-base disturbances. The nurse also needs to identify potential or actual risk factors that increase the potential for these imbalances (see box at right). This includes the diseases, treatments, drug therapies, and diet changes that can alter balances.

RISK FACTORS FOR FLUID, ELECTROLYTE, AND ACID-BASE IMBALANCES

- Age
  - Very young
  - Very old
- Chronic diseases
  - Cancer
  - Cardiovascular disease such as congestive heart failure
  - Endocrine disease such as Cushing's disease and diabetes mellitus
  - Malnutrition
  - Chronic obstructive pulmonary disease
  - Renal disease such as progressive renal failure
  - Decreased level of consciousness
- Trauma
  - Crush injuries
  - Head injuries
  - Burns
- Therapies
  - Diuretics
  - Steroids
  - IV therapy
  - TPN
- Gastrointestinal losses
  - Gastroenteritis
  - Nasogastric suctioning
  - Fistulas

Clients with cardiovascular and renal diseases, severe burns or trauma, and endocrine disorders are at high risk for fluid, electrolyte, and acid-base disturbances. Prolonged gastrointestinal upsets, particularly in the very young and the very old, also can result in fluid, electrolyte, or acid-base imbalance.

Eventually, all types of chronic diseases can cause fluid, electrolyte, and acid-base alterations. Because the progression of these diseases is usually slow, imbalances can be controlled. However, with chronic disease, there is a loss of adaptive capacity or margin of ability to respond. Therefore nurses caring for clients with chronic illnesses need to recognize that the disease process is often no longer stabilized and that fluid, electrolyte, and acid-base disturbances are present.

Head injuries and other neurological alterations can result in cerebral edema, which can alter ADH secretion. Two alterations in fluid and electrolyte balance can occur. Diabetes insipidus occurs when too little antidiuretic hormone is secreted, and the client excretes large volumes of dilute urine with a low specific gravity. This is accompanied by hypernatremia. The secretion of inappropriate ADH (SIADH) occurs when there is excess secretion of ADH, which is seen clinically as hyponatremia. Other causes of SIADH include malignancies and pulmonary disorders (Berl and Schrier, 1992).

Head or chest trauma may also result in respiratory acidosis, as can respiratory infections especially in the client with chronic lung disease. Burns can result in the loss of plasma through the burned skin surface, causing a loss of fluid and electrolytes.

Drug therapies also increase the risk for fluid and electrolyte disturbances. Although all diuretics cause increased excretion of water, they can be potassium-sparing, such as spironolactone (Aldactone), or potassium-wasting such as furosemide (Lasix). Inappropriate use of diuretics may also result in metabolic acid-base disturbances.

Nasogastric suctioning results in the loss of sodium, potassium, magnesium, and chloride ions. Hydrogen ions are also lost and this, together with the loss of chloride ions, results in metabolic alkalosis. If excess fluid is removed along with the electrolytes lost, the client may develop fluid volume deficit.

The presence of an intestinal fistula or diarrhea (Chapter 33) can result in potassium loss. As a result, clients are at risk for hypokalemia. As with clients with other gastrointestinal disorders, the loss of potassium increases the risk for metabolic acidosis, which initially occurs because of the loss of bicarbonate. The client may also experience fluid volume deficit and hypomagnesemia. The serum sodium may decrease, increase, or remain normal depending on the amount of sodium and water lost.

Prescribed drugs (e.g., diuretics and steroids) increase the risk for fluid and electrolyte disturbances. If not delivered at the correct rate, parenteral fluids (intravenous fluids or total parenteral nutrition) increase the risk of fluid and electrolyte imbalance. In addition, some drugs and alcohol can cause respiratory depression, which can result in respiratory acidosis.

Physical Examination

Because fluid, electrolyte, and acid-base disturbances affect all systems, the nurse must identify any abnormalities during the physical examination. Tables 35-1 through 35-3 list common signs and symptoms for these imbalances.

Measuring Fluid Intake and Output

Measuring and recording all liquid intake and output (I&O) during a 24-hour period helps to complete the assessment data base for fluid and electrolyte balances. It is important to note trends in the I&O (e.g., a gradually decreasing urine output can indicate that the body is trying to adapt to a fluid volume deficit or hyperosmolar fluid imbalance). Accurate I&O measurements identify both clients at risk for and clients who are experiencing fluid, electrolyte, and acid-base disturbances. Normal oral intake of fluids from liquids and foods for the adult is 2300 ml, and normal urine output is 1 ml/kg of body weight/hour (1000 to 2000 ml/24 hours) (Metheny, 1992).

The nurse neither needs nor should wait for a physician's order to begin intake and output measurements. Generally, intake and output are routinely measured for clients after surgery and clients whose condition is unstable, who have a temperature elevation, whose fluids are restricted, or who are receiving diuretic or intravenous therapy. The nurse also measures I&O for clients with chronic cardiopulmonary or renal illnesses and clients whose health status has deteriorated.

Oral intake includes all liquids taken by mouth, such as gelatin, ice cream, soup, juice, and water. Liquid intake also includes fluids given through nasogastric or jejunostomy feeding tubes, liquids given as IV fluids, and blood or its components. Liquid output includes urine, diarrhea, vomitus, gastric suction, and drainage from post-surgical or other tubes.

Ambulatory clients' urinary output is recorded after each trip to the bathroom. These clients are instructed to save their urine in a container so that the nurse can record the amount, or clients may be instructed to measure and record their own output. When a client has an indwelling Foley catheter, drainage tube, or suction, that output is recorded at the end of each nursing shift or more frequently (e.g., every hour) as the client's condition requires. The nurse should measure, not estimate, intake and output.

In the hospital, forms for recording I&O are attached to the bedside chart or room door. The records note the type or route of intake and output and are broken down into at least 8-hour segments. At the end of each 8-hour shift, the I&O are totalled and the totals are recorded on a special form in the client's chart. The 24-hour total is calculated at midnight or 6 AM depending on agency policy.

Taking I&O measurements is a procedure requiring help from the client and family. The nurse explains the reasons that measurements are needed and instructs the client and family to not empty any container with voided fluid but to ask the nurse to do so. A client using a toilet should be instructed to use a calibrated insert, which attaches to the rim of the toilet bowl. After each urination the client notifies the nurse, who measures, records, and empties the urine and rinses the insert. Occasionally, clients may also be instructed to measure and record their own output. The output of a client who has an indwelling Foley catheter or drainage tube is recorded at the end of each shift or even more frequently as the client's condition requires. The 24-hour totals are included on the 24-hour record in the client's chart. These totals are usually recorded at midnight or 6 AM, depending on the hospital policy. The records note the type of intake and output and are broken down into 8-hour segments.

Occasionally clients receive a specific amount of a liquid medication every 1 to 2 hours. For example, antacids are commonly ordered in 30 ml doses every hour for clients who have or who are at risk for gastrointestinal bleeding. A client receiving tube feedings may receive numerous liquid medications and water may be used to flush the tube with the medications. Over a 24-hour period, these liquids can amount to a significant intake and should always be recorded on the intake record.

Recording I&O is essential for obtaining an accurate data base. This information helps to maintain an ongoing evaluation of the client's hydration status to prevent severe imbalances.

Laboratory Studies

Laboratory tests are performed to obtain further objective data about fluid, electrolyte, and acid-base balances (see box below). These tests include serum and urinary electrolyte levels, hematocrit, blood creatinine level, blood urea nitrogen levels, urine specific gravity, and arterial blood gas readings.

Serum electrolytes are measured to determine the hydration status, the electrolyte concentration of the blood plasma, and acid-base balance. Frequently measured electrolytes include sodium, potassium, chloride, and bicarbonate (venous carbon dioxide content) ions. The other electrolytes—calcium, magnesium, and phosphate—will be determined when the client's condition suggests an imbalance. The frequency with which these electrolytes are measured depends on the severity of the client's illness. Serum electrolyte tests are routinely performed on any client entering a hospital to screen for alterations and to serve as a baseline for future comparisons.

The complete blood count (CBC) is a determination of the number and type of red and white blood cells per cubic millimeter of blood. When the client does not have anemia, the hematocrit can be an indication of the hydration status of the client. The hematocrit will increase (become more concentrated) in situations where fluid is lost, whereas it will decrease in situations in which fluid is excessively retained in the vascular space.

Blood creatinine levels are useful in measuring kidney function. Creatinine is a normal by-product of muscle metabolism and is excreted by the kidneys at fairly constant levels, regardless of factors such as fluid intake, diet, or exercise. Therefore it provides a measure of renal function that is relatively independent of the hydration status of the client or the client's dietary intake.

Blood urea nitrogen (BUN) is the amount of nitrogenous substance present in the blood as urea. It is a rough indicator of kidney function. BUN is elevated in kidney failure, dehydration, and shock; it is decreased in liver disease, malnutrition, fluid volume excess, and normal pregnancy.

Serum osmolality measures the concentration of the plasma. The osmolality will decrease when the client is experiencing hypoosmolar fluid imbalance (water excess) or hyponatremia. Decreased serum osmolality results in the movement of fluid into body cells (cellular edema) by osmosis. The osmolality will increase with a hyperosmolar fluid imbalance (water deficit) or hypernatremia or other gain of solutes. This will result in the movement of fluid out of body cells into the interstitial space (cellular shrinkage). Both cellular edema and shrinkage will disrupt normal cell processes.

LABORATORY DATA FOR FLUID, ELECTROLYTE, AND ACID-BASE IMBALANCES

FLUIDS AND ELECTROLYTES

Altered concentrations of sodium, potassium, magnesium, calcium, phosphates, chloride, and bicarbonate (venous CO_2 content) ions
Increase in hematocrit, BUN, sodium, and osmolality in serum (related to loss of ECF fluid or gain of solutes)
Decrease in hematocrit, BUN, sodium, and osmolality in serum (related to gain of ECF fluid or loss of solutes)
Concentrated urine demonstrated by a urine specific gravity > 1.030
Dilute urine demonstrated by a specific gravity < 1.012

METABOLIC ALKALOSIS

pH > 7.45
$Paco_2$ normal or > 45 mm Hg if lungs are compensating
Pao_2 normal
O_2 saturation (Sao_2) normal
HCO_3^- > 26 mEq/L
K^+ < 3.5 mEq/L

METABOLIC ACIDOSIS

pH < 7.35
$Paco_2$ normal or less than 35 mm Hg if lungs are compensating
Pao_2 normal
Sao_2 normal
HCO_3^- < 22 mEq/L
K^+ > 5.3 mEq/L
K^+ < 3.5 mEq/L

RESPIRATORY ALKALOSIS

pH > 7.45
$Paco_2$ < 35 mm Hg
Pao_2 normal
Sao_2 normal
HCO_3^- normal
K^+ < 3.5 mEq/L

RESPIRATORY ACIDOSIS

pH < 7.35
$Paco_2$ > 45 mm Hg
Pao_2 normal or < 80 mm Hg, depending on cause of acidosis
Sao_2 normal or < 95%, depending on cause of acidosis
HCO_3^- normal in early respiratory acidosis or > 26 mEq/L if kidneys are compensating
K^+ > 5.3 mEq/L

The urine specific gravity test measures the urine's degree of concentration. The specific gravity can be measured at the bedside using a urinometer (see Chapter 32). Normally the specific gravity ranges between 1.010 and 1.025.

Arterial blood gas tests provide information on the status of acid-base balance and on the effectiveness of ventilatory function in providing normal oxygen–carbon dioxide exchange. The arterial pH measures the hydrogen ion concentration. A decreased pH < 7.35 is associated with acidosis, whereas an elevated pH > 7.45 is associated with alkalosis. The $Paco_2$ measures the partial pressure of carbon dioxide in the arterial blood. Alveolar hypoventilation results in an elevated $Paco_2$, whereas hyperventilation is associated with a decreased $Paco_2$. The Pao_2 is measured, which provides information concerning the effectiveness of the client's respiratory system (Chapter 34). The serum bicarbonate is another component of arterial blood gases. An elevated bicarbonate level is associated with alkalosis, whereas a decreased bicarbonate level is associated with acidosis. Bicarbonate levels reflect the renal portion of acid-base regulation.

Variables Influencing Fluid, Electrolyte, and Acid-Base Balances

A client's fluid and electrolyte status and acid-base balance are not static, nor are they separate physiological entities. Many variables can change the distribution of fluids and electrolytes and alter acid-base balance. In some instances, as with the normal changes during pregnancy and exercise, a change is a normal and expected response. However, symptoms such as vomiting or diarrhea can have more severe consequences.

During the nursing assessment, the nurse identifies altered fluid, electrolyte, and acid-base states. To assess clients effectively, the nurse considers the variables that influence fluid status, the way normal balance changes, and whether the change is a normal, anticipated change or a consequence of a pathological process (see box on pp. 1040-1041).

NURSING DIAGNOSES FOR FLUID, ELECTROLYTE, AND ACID-BASE ALTERATIONS

- Actual or high risk for fluid volume deficit
- Fluid volume excess
- Impaired or high risk for impaired skin integrity
- Impaired tissue integrity
- Impaired oral mucous membrane
- Altered peripheral tissue perfusion
- Decreased cardiac output
- Impaired gas exchange
- Ineffective breathing pattern

Nursing Diagnosis

In the areas of fluid, electrolyte, and acid-base balances, it is particularly important that the nurse be skilled in and use critical thinking to formulate nursing diagnoses (see box above). The assessment data that establishes the risk for or the actual presence of a nursing diagnosis in these areas may be subtle, and patterns and trends emerge only when the nurse consciously looks for them because many body systems will be involved. For example, relevant assessment data for the nursing diagnosis, *fluid volume deficit,* could include the presence of insufficient oral intake, weight loss, dry skin and mucous membranes, inelastic skin turgor, decreased blood pressure, and increased heart rate. The serum sodium and osmolality could be elevated. The urine could be dark, with an elevated specific gravity. The volume of the urine could be decreasing over a period of days. The omission of any of this data would result in an incomplete picture of the client's condition and could result in the identification of an incorrect diagnosis.

In addition to the accurate clustering of assessment data, the nurse must precisely identify the related factor for the nursing diagnosis to plan appropriate nursing care. For example, for the nursing diagnosis, *fluid volume deficit,* the related factor could be diarrhea, vomiting, or difficulty swallowing. This nursing diagnosis is not present if the client is NPO as part of the treatment regimen. If the related factor were diarrhea, the nurse would administer ordered antidiarrheal medications and provide oral fluids that contain electrolytes and glucose, and teach the client to use careful handwashing and to avoid dairy products. In contrast, if the related factor were vomiting, the nurse would administer antiemetics, remove sights and odors that could induce nausea, and provide a small amount of fluids containing electrolytes. Finally, if the related factor were difficulty swallowing, the nurse could ensure that the client is maximally stimulated, position the client in a high Fowler's position and perhaps to the side during times of intake, provide foods and fluids with a soft or pureed or thickened consistency, provide 5 ml amounts with each mouthful, and investigate the need for enteral or parenteral nutrition.

Planning

The first step in the planning process is priority setting. Many nursing diagnoses in the areas of fluid, electrolyte, and acid-base balance represent high-priority client responses because the consequences can be seri-

VARIABLES INFLUENCING FLUID, ELECTROLYTE, AND ACID-BASE BALANCES

FLUID AND ELECTROLYTE BALANCES

Age

Infants

Infants' proportion of total body water is greater than that of children or adults, but they are not protected from fluid loss (e.g., as a result of diarrhea) because they ingest and excrete a relatively greater daily water volume than adults (Mollohan & Riddle, 1992). They are at greater risk for FVD and hyperosmolar imbalance because body water loss is proportionately greater than per kilogram of weight.

Low-birth-weight infants are at risk for FVD and hypertonic fluid imbalances because of increased insensible water losses and immature renal function. These infants are also at risk for hypernatremia and hyperkalemia (Davis, 1992).

Children

Regulatory responses to imbalances are less stable and there is a narrow range of tolerance for severe balance changes.

Children respond to illness with high fevers.

Adolescents

Adolescents have increased metabolic processes and increased water production. Girls have greater fluid changes because of hormonal changes.

Young adults

Pregnant women have increased aldosterone secretion and excretion, which increases circulating blood volume. This increased blood volume decreases rapidly after delivery.

Older adults

In the older adult, fluid, electrolyte, and acid-base alterations can occur because of age-related changes such as decreased ability to produce a maximally concentrated urine. Older adults are at risk for decreased excretion of medications, which can affect fluid, electrolyte, or acid-base balances resulting in metabolic or respiratory acidosis, FVD and hyperosmolar imbalance, and both hyponatremia and hypernatremia (Kee, 1992).

Body size

Obese clients have proportionately less body water because fat contains no water.

Because women have more fat deposits than men, they have less total body water.

Environmental temperature

Overall body response to environmental temperatures exceeding 28 to 30° C (82.4 to 86° F) is increased water loss by sweating. The healthy adult can tolerate sweating 1 liter per hour for 2 hours, losing 5% of body weight. A body weight loss over 7% decreases the ability of the cooling mechanism to conserve water.

Exposure to excessive environmental temperatures causes an increase in peripheral vasodilation (blood comes to the surface for cooling), an increase in body fluid loss through sweating accompanied by the loss of sodium and chloride ions, an increase in cardiac output and pulse rate, and an increase in aldosterone secretion (causing sodium retention and potassium excretion by kidneys).

Life-style

Diet

When nutritional intake is inadequate, the body tries to preserve protein stores by breaking down glycogen and fat stores. Eventually, however, the body destroys protein stores, which results in hypoalbuminemia, decreased serum colloid oncotic pressure, and edema.

Stress

Causes an increase in aldosterone, resulting in sodium and water retention. Increased ADH secretion decreases urine output. The stress response increases fluid volume, cardiac output (within limits), blood pressure, and perfusion to major organs.

Exercise

Increases water loss through sweat.

Level of health

Surgery

Stress response causes fluid balance changes in the second to fifth postoperative day. Aldosterone, glucocorticoids, and ADH are increasingly secreted, causing sodium and chloride retention, potassium excretion, and decreased urinary output.

Burns

Severe second- or third-degree burns cause fluid loss by one of five routes: (1) plasma leaves the intravascular spaces and becomes trapped as edema; (2) plasma and interstitial fluids are lost as burn exudate; (3) water vapor and heat are lost because burned skin is no longer a barrier; (4) blood leaks from damaged capillaries; or (5) sodium and water shift into cells.

Heart disease

Reduced cardiac output decreases perfusion to the kidneys, glomerular filtration rate, and urinary output. Clients retain sodium and water, causing fluid volume excess and peripheral and pulmonary edema.

Renal disease

Failing kidneys cause an abnormal buildup of sodium, chloride, potassium, phosphorus, and extracellular fluid. Serum calcium will be decreased. Acute renal failure is reversible; chronic renal failure can be treated.

VARIABLES INFLUENCING FLUID, ELECTROLYTE, AND ACID-BASE BALANCES—cont'd

Cancer

All types of fluid and electrolyte imbalances can be caused by cancers. Clients with cancer may also develop third-space fluid accumulations that increase total body water, with a decrease in extracellular fluid volume.

ACID-BASE BALANCE

Age

The very young and very old are most susceptible to imbalances because of the limited adaptive reserve in these age-groups.

The aging process changes lung function and can lead to respiratory acidosis and the inability to compensate for metabolic acidosis.

Life-style

Dieting can lead to acidosis because rapid water loss can lead to hyperosmolar fluid imbalance. Near-starvation diets alter normal metabolic processes and cause metabolic acidosis.

Anxiety can lead to hyperventilation and respiratory alkalosis.

Alcoholism leads to acidosis because of its association with malnutrition.

Medications

Diuretics and steroids can cause metabolic alkalosis. Respiratory center depressants such as narcotics can cause decreased rate and depth of respirations, and stimulants can cause hyperventilation, which may result in respiratory acidosis or alkalosis, respectively.

Level of health

Clients with pulmonary disease or diabetes mellitus are at risk for acidosis.

Normal metabolism requires a 20 : 1 ratio between bicarbonate and carbonic acid. Any alteration of either element can lead to imbalances.

During illness, metabolic activities are altered and imbalances can occur rapidly.

ous, even life-threatening (e.g., convulsions, dysrhythmias, or coma).

During the planning process, the nurse will formulate nursing interventions for use to prevent or treat fluid, electrolyte, and acid-base imbalances. It is important to collaborate with the client and family during this part of the assessment and planning processes. The family will be particularly helpful in identifying the subtle changes in behavior associated with these imbalances, such as anxiety, confusion, or irritability, in a timely manner. During the planning process, it is important to remember that the client and family must know preventive measures, signs and symptoms to report, and measures that can be implemented if an imbalance occurs. When medications, special diets, or oral or IV fluids are administered in the home, the client and family need careful teaching so that these interventions are performed safely. The client's preferences and resources should be considered during each step of the planning process (e.g., if the client needs to be encouraged to increase oral intake, the nurse can determine and include the client's favorite beverages into the plan of care). In the hospital the nurse anticipates the need of the client and family for specific information and initiates teaching before discharge so that the client and family are ready for these procedures (see box on p. 1042). The home health nurse continues the teaching plan and evaluates the effectiveness of the home interventions.

The nurse will also collaborate closely with other members of the health care team, such as the physician, dietitian, or physical therapist. For example, when the client exhibits new assessment data that suggests a fluid, electrolyte, or acid-base imbalance, the nurse will consult with the physician to determine the need for dietary, pharmacological, intravenous fluid, or other therapy. The nurse also implements on-going monitoring of the client's fluid, electrolyte, and acid-base status to determine the safety of implementing physician and nursing orders and the need for a change in the plan of care. For example, the physician may order an oral potassium supplement to be given to the client three times each day. Before administering the first dose of each day, the nurse should verify that the serum potassium level is normal and that the urine output is adequate. The dose of potassium should be withheld and the physician consulted if the serum level is elevated or if the urine output has decreased.

After priority setting and collaboration with the client, family, and health care team, the nurse develops a care plan that is individualized according to the client's acute or chronic fluid, electrolyte, or acid-base status (see care plan on p. 1043). The plan is based on one or more of the following goals:

Goal: The client's fluid, electrolyte, and acid-base balance are restored and maintained.

Outcomes

- Vital signs will return to baseline normals
- The client will have normal skin turgor
- The client's weight will be stable at baseline normal

CLIENT TEACHING FOR FLUID, ELECTROLYTE, AND ACID-BASE IMBALANCES

Inform healthy clients concerning general risk factors for fluid, electrolyte, and acid-base imbalances (e.g., gastrointestinal losses) and what steps to take to prevent imbalances such as early oral rehydration therapy with isotonic fluids containing glucose and electrolytes when the client is experiencing diarrhea.

Teach clients with chronic health alterations and their care givers about the fluid, electrolyte, and acid-base imbalances for which they are at risk and how to prevent them (e.g., the client with diabetes mellitus needs to understand the dangers associated with a hyperosmolar fluid imbalance).

Instruct individuals and families on how to recognize a fluid, electrolyte, or acid-base imbalance, and on steps to take when an imbalance occurs (e.g., the parents of small children need to understand the dangers of fluid volume deficit or an osmolar fluid imbalance when the child experiences diarrhea). The parents should also be taught appropriate dietary therapy while the child has diarrhea.

Teach clients and care givers fluid, dietary, and pharmacological measures for fluid, electrolyte, and acid-base imbalances (e.g., the client with renal failure needs to understand the necessary fluid restriction both in amount of and type of fluid restricted).

Instruct clients and care givers concerning general interventions for fluid, electrolyte, and acid-base imbalances: safety measures for the client who is confused or weak, positioning to mobilize edema, skin care to prevent breakdown in the presence of edema or dry skin, and emotional support.

Teach the client and care giver important points to be implemented during IV therapy.

- If IV is positional, instruct client how to properly position arm and to avoid lying on tubing or putting pressure on the venipuncture site.
- Instruct client about signs and symptoms of infiltration, phlebitis, and infection and the need to notify the nurse immediately.
- Instruct client to inform nurse if IV flow slows or stops or blood is seen in the tubing.
- Instruct client how to ambulate with IV pole or stand maintaining correct height of IV solution.
- Teach client how to maintain the extremity with the venipuncture at an appropriate height and how to avoid dislodging the IV catheter when changing positions or changing clothes.
- Teach client how to perform hygiene measures while ensuring that the IV site remains clean and dry.
- If client will receive IV therapy at home, teach client and care giver how to maintain the IV, perform needed procedures using sterile technique, how to recognize and respond to complications, and how to obtain supplies.

The client will have no edema
The client will have clear breath sounds
Serum and urine electrolyte and chemistry results and arterial blood gas values will be normal
Urine output will equal intake

Goal: Causes of client's imbalance are identified and corrected.

Outcomes

The client will experience no vomiting, diarrhea, or other route of abnormal loss
The client will verbalize the need for and ingest increased fluids and electrolytes during times of severe stress, heat, or strenuous exercise

Goal: The client has no complications from therapies to restore balance.

Outcomes

The client will have no evidence of infiltration, phlebitis, or infection at the IV insertion site, such as redness, pain, swelling
The client will exhibit no evidence of a blood transfusion reaction: chest pain, change in vital signs

Implementation

Prevention of fluid, electrolyte, and acid-base imbalances is important. When imbalances occur, the nurse removes or treats the cause of the imbalance if possible. Other nursing interventions aim to correct the imbalances.

When a client's fluid volume is depleted, fluids and electrolytes can be replaced orally, with intravenous administration of fluids and blood components, or through total parenteral nutrition (see Chapter 31) if the fluid deficit is caused by malnutrition. For clients with FVE, the nurse implements measures to reduce fluids, such as fluid intake restrictions, reduced sodium intake, and use of diuretics. When the client has an electrolyte imbalance, the nurse provides an appropriate diet and administers supplements when ordered. For clients with acid-base imbalances, the nurse initiates such measures as reducing anxiety, improving pulmonary function, controlling the loss of gastrointestinal content, or ensuring the control of conditions such as diabetes or renal failure.

SAMPLE NURSING CARE PLAN

Fluid Volume Deficit

ASSESSMENT

Clinical scenario: Mrs. Kline is an 80-year-old woman admitted to the hospital after a *7-day history of watery diarrhea.* She reports having as many as 10 liquid bowel movements each day. Each bowel movement was accompanied by cramping. Her usual pattern is one soft, brown stool daily. Mrs. Kline's weight is 106 pounds, which is *a 5-pound loss.* When she changes from a lying to a sitting position, she complains of *dizziness, and her blood pressure falls to 90/50 from 120/70.* Her *skin turgor is poor; the mucous membranes in her mouth are dry.* After 24 hours, her *total intake is 950 ml and her output is 400 ml; the urine is dark amber with a specific gravity of 1.030.* She complains of *weakness.* Laboratory results show *serum sodium is 135 mEq/L, serum potassium is 3.5 mEq/L, serum osmolaity is 295 mOsm/kg, BUN is 25 mg/dl, hematocrit is 50%.*

NURSING DIAGNOSIS

Fluid volume deficit related to excessive diarrhea.

PLANNING

Goal

Fluid and electrolytes will return to normal by discharge.

Expected outcomes

Mucous membranes will be moist and skin turgor normal within 24 hours.
Body weight will be 110 at discharge.
Client will not experience dizziness with changes in posture within 24 hours.
Blood pressure will remain within 10% of baseline during position changes within 24 hours.
Stools will be soft and formed within 48 hours.
Urine output will equal intake within 48 hours.
Urine specific gravity will be normal within 48 hours.
Serum sodium, potassium, osmolality, BUN, and hematocrit will be normal within 48 hours.

IMPLEMENTATION

Steps	Rationale
1. Initiate intravenous line as ordered. Anticipate administration of 0.45% normal saline to infuse at 125 ml/hr.	Replacement of body fluids restores blood volume and normal serum electrolyte level; use of hypotonic fluid will allow fluid to move into body cells relieving cellular dehydration.
2. Administer antidiarrheal medications after each liquid stool as ordered.	Antidiarrheal medications decrease intestinal motility and thus periods of diarrhea.
3. Give Rehydralyte 2000 ml each day as ordered until volume of stool is less than 5 stools/24 hours or consistency of stools is not watery: 1200 ml on days 500 ml on evenings 300 ml on nights	Contains sodium and glucose with an osmolality of 310 mOsm/kg; when glucose is absorbed by the intestinal villae, sodium and water are passively absorbed, which increases serum sodium and ECF volume (Goepp and Katz, 1993; Harig & Ramaswamy, 1989).
4. Provide comfort measures:	
Apply lip balm to lips. Perform oral hygiene with mouthwash every 2 hours on the odd hour.	Keeps skin and mucous membranes moist and intact.
Assist with perianal hygiene: use Periwash and clean wash cloth for each stool; use A & D ointment on skin	Prevents irritation and skin breakdown.

EVALUATIVE MEASURES

Inspect and palpate mucous membranes; palpate skin turgor.
Weigh client daily.
Observe client for dizziness with postural changes.
Auscultate blood pressure lying, sitting, and standing.
Observe character of stool.
Measure 24-hour I & O; determine urine specific gravity.
Monitor daily diagnostic tests.

Defining characteristics are in italic type.

Interventions for Fluid and Electrolyte Imbalances

Daily Weight Measurement. When implementing specific measures to increase or reduce fluid, two nursing interventions are necessary: daily weight and intake and output measurements.

Clients with fluid and electrolyte alterations should be weighed daily. Otherwise, a client can gain 2.5 to 3.0 L of fluid in the absence of observable edema (Metheny, 1992). Weight should be determined at the same time each day with the same scale after the client voids. The scale should be calibrated each day or routinely. The client should wear the same clothes, clothes which weigh the same, or, if a bed scale is used, the same number of sheets should be used on the scale with each weighing.

Intake and Output Measurement. Intake and output records provide additional information about fluid balance. Intake and output measurements, when examined for trends, can indicate whether excess fluid volume is excreted in the urine or whether excretion of fluids through the kidneys has diminished. The intake and output is not as accurate as daily weights to assess fluid balance.

Enteral Replacement of Fluids

ORAL. Oral replacement of fluids and electrolytes is appropriate as long as the client is not so physiologically unstable that oral fluid replacement is not sufficiently rapid. Oral replacement of fluids is contraindicated when the client has a mechanical obstruction of the gastrointestinal tract. Clients unable to tolerate solid foods may still be able to ingest fluids. Oral fluid replacement is easily implemented in the home.

Mild illness such as viral diarrhea, respiratory tract infections, and fevers may cause fluid and electrolyte disturbances. In addition, clients recovering from anesthesia or gastrointestinal surgery usually first receive clear liquids and then advance to a regular diet if they tolerate the liquids. When replacing fluids by mouth in a client with a fluid deficit, it is wise to choose fluids with adequate calories and electrolyte content (Table 35-4). However, it is important to remember that liquids containing lactose or caffeine or with a low sodium content may not be appropriate when the client has diarrhea.

TUBE FEEDINGS. A feeding tube may be appropriate when the client's gastrointestinal tract is healthy but the client cannot ingest fluids (e.g., after oral surgery or with impaired swallowing). All feeding tubes require a physician's order. Fluids can also be replaced through nasogastric, gastrostomy, or jejunostomy feeding tube (Chapter 31).

table 35-4

ORAL FLUIDS

Solution	Na mEq/L	Ca mEq/L	PO_4 mEq/L	K mEq/L	Mg mEq/L	Cl mq/L	Base Buffer#	Glucose* G/L	Osmolality mOsm/L
Water†									
Gastrolyte	50-90			20		52-65	30(C)	20	NA~
Rehydralyte	75			20		65	30(C)	25	310
Lytren	50			25		45	30(C)	20	NA
Pedialyte	45			20		35	30(C)	25	250
Resol	50	4	5	20	4	50	34(C)	20	290
Infalyte	50			20		40	30(B)	20	NA
Apple juice	1-5			24-43				12-32*	870
Cola	1-7			0.1-0.6			7.3-13.4	5-12*	680
Lemon-lime soda	5			1-2				33	520
Gatorade	24			3				50	350
Ginger ale	1-7			0.1-0.4				7-12	510
Grape juice									1170
Orange juice									935
Tea					Trace				NA
Beef broth	55								NA
Jello	6-17			0.1-0.9				8	285-320

Compiled from *Drug facts and comparisons,* Philadelphia, 1992, J.B. Lippincott; Goepp JG and Katz SA: Oral rehydration therapy, *Am Fam Phys* 1993; Groer MW: *Physiology and pathophysiology of the body fluids,* St. Louis, 1981, Mosby.
*Carbohydrate source of calories is sucrose.
†Contains no calories or electrolytes.
#*B,* bicarbonate; *C,* citrate; ~*NA,* information not available.

Restriction of Fluids. Clients who retain fluids and have a fluid volume excess require restricted fluid intake.

Fluid restriction is often difficult for clients, particularly if they take drugs that dry the oral mucous membranes or if the client breathes through the mouth. The nurse should explain the reasons fluids are restricted. In addition, the client needs to know the amount of fluid permitted orally and should understand that ice chips, gelatin, and ice cream are considered fluid.

The client should help to decide the amount of fluid with each meal, between meals, before bed, and with medications. Frequently clients on fluid restriction can swallow a number of pills with as little as 1 ounce (30 ml) of liquid.

A good rule of thumb for fluid restrictions is to allow half the allotted total oral fluids between 8 AM and 4 PM, the period when clients usually are more active and receive two meals and most of their oral medications. An additional two fifths of the allotted total fluid is permitted between 4 PM and 11 PM. This permits fluids with meals and evening visitors. Between 11 PM and 8 AM, the remainder is permitted. Because the client is usually asleep during this period, fluid needs are decreased. The nurse should also make sure that clients receive the type of fluids they like best (unless contraindicated).

Parenteral Replacement of Fluid and Electrolytes. Fluid and electrolytes may be replaced through infusion directly into the blood rather than intake through the digestive system. Parenteral replacement includes total parenteral nutrition (TPN), intravenous (IV) fluid and electrolyte therapy, and blood and blood component administration.

With increasing risk to health care workers for transmission of the human immunodeficiency virus (HIV), the cause of acquired immunodeficiency syndrome (AIDS), hepatitis B virus (HBV), and other infectious diseases, the principles of body substance isolation must be practiced when administering parenteral fluids. The Centers for Disease Control and Prevention (CDC) have issued guidelines pertaining to exposure to body substances (see box at right).

Health care workers must consider all clients as potentially infected with HIV and other blood-borne pathogens and adhere rigorously to body substance isolation and universal precautions to reduce the risk of exposure to blood and body fluids. (CDC, 1987). Universal precautions should be used with all clients, especially those in obstetrical, operating room, critical care, and emergency care settings in which the risk of blood exposure is increased and infection status may be unknown (see box above). In addition, precautions for invasive procedures are followed when surgical entry into tissues, cavities, or organs or repair of major traumatic injuries occurs (CDC, 1987).

UNIVERSAL PRECAUTIONS TO PREVENT TRANSMISSION OF HIV AS THEY PERTAIN TO IV THERAPY

Gloves must be worn when there is a reasonable expectation that there may be contact with blood (e.g., during venipuncture or while changing IV administration sets).

Gloves should be changed after contact with each client.

Hands and other skin surfaces should be washed immediately and thoroughly if contaminated with blood or other body fluids (see Chapter 25). Hands should be washed immediately after gloves are removed.

To prevent needlestick injuries, needles should not be recapped, purposely bent or broken by hand, removed from disposable syringes, or otherwise manipulated by hand.

Contaminated needles, syringes, and IV fluid equipment should be placed in puncture-resistant containers that are properly labeled as a biohazard for disposal. These containers should be located as close as practical to the use area. When full, they are to be sealed and disposed of properly.

Health care workers who have exudative lesions or weeping dermatitis should refrain from all direct care and from handling invasive equipment until the condition resolves.

Pregnant health care workers are not known to be at greater risk of contracting HIV infections than health care workers who are not pregnant. However, if a health care worker develops HIV infection during pregnancy, the infant is at risk of infection resulting from perinatal transmission. Because of this risk, pregnant health care workers should strictly adhere to precautions to minimize the risk of transmission.

Modified from Centers for Disease Control: Recommendations for prevention of HIV transmission in health-care settings, *MMWR* 36(suppl 25):3s, 1987. Occupational Safety and Health Act: Bloodborne pathogens, *Federal Registry,* 56(235):64175, 1991.

VASCULAR ACCESS DEVICES. Vascular access devices are catheters, cannulas, or infusion ports designed for long-term repeated access to the vascular system (Figure 35-7). These devices are more effective than peripherally placed catheters for administering medications and solutions that are irritating to veins and for the delivery of long-term IV therapy. Recently, peripherally inserted central catheters (PICC) have begun to be used for clients with poor peripheral venous access who need infusion therapy for a period less than 3 months (Silvestri & Masoorli, 1990). Increased use of central venous catheters and implanted infusion ports require nurses to be educated in the care of these devices.

TOTAL PARENTERAL NUTRITION. Total parenteral nutrition (TPN) is a nutritionally adequate hypertonic solution consisting of glucose and other nutrients and

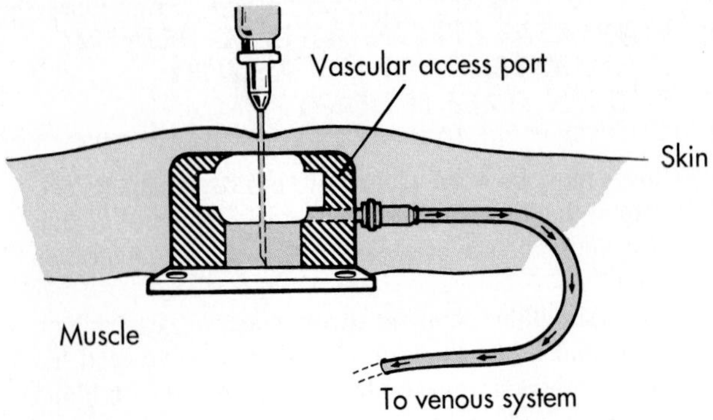

FIGURE 35-7 Example of implantable vascular access device.

electrolytes given through an indwelling peripheral or central IV catheter. TPN is used as an intervention in severe cases of malnutrition. Chapter 31 fully describes its administration.

IV THERAPY. The goal of IV fluid administration is to correct or prevent fluid and electrolyte disturbances. For example, a client with third-degree burns over 40% of the body is critically ill and has severe fluid and electrolyte imbalances. Fluid therapy must be continuously regulated because of continual changes in fluid and electrolyte balance. Another example is the client after abdominal surgery who receives IV fluid and electrolyte replacement for a period of time to prevent fluid and electrolyte imbalances while unable to ingest anything by mouth. The infusion is discontinued with resumption of normal oral intake.

When IV fluid administration is required, the nurse must know the correct solution, equipment needed, and procedures required to initiate an infusion, regulate the infusion rate, maintain the system, identify and correct problems, and discontinue the infusion.

TYPES OF SOLUTIONS. Many prepared IV solutions are available for use (Table 35-5). IV solutions fall into the following categories: isotonic, hypotonic, and hypertonic. Another method for categorizing IV solutions is based on the content of the solution: dextrose in water solutions, saline solutions, dextrose in saline solutions, and multiple electrolyte solutions. A solution is isotonic if the total electrolyte content approximates 310 mEq/L. A hypotonic solution is one in which the total electrolyte is below 250 mEq/L. A hypertonic solution has a total electrolyte content of 375 mEq/L or greater (Metheny, 1992).

In general, isotonic fluids are used for extracellular volume replacement (e.g., fluid volume deficit after prolonged vomiting). The decision to use a hypotonic or hypertonic solution is based on the specific fluid and electrolyte imbalance. For example, the client with a hypertonic fluid imbalance will generally receive a hypotonic IV in order to dilute the ECF. All IV fluids should be given carefully, especially hypertonic solutions because

table 35-5

IV SOLUTIONS

Solution	Concentration	Other names
DEXTROSE IN WATER SOLUTIONS		
Dextrose 5% in water*	Isotonic	D5W
Dextrose 10% in water	Hypertonic	D10W
SALINE SOLUTIONS		
0.45% sodium chloride (half normal saline)	Hypotonic	1/2 NS 0.45% NS
0.9% sodium chloride† (normal saline)	Isotonic	NS 0.9% NS 0.9% NaCl
3-5% sodium chloride	Hypertonic	3-5% NS 3-5% NaCl
DEXTROSE IN SALINE SOLUTIONS		
Dextrose 5% in 0.9% sodium chloride	Hypertonic	D5-0.9% NaCl D5-0.9% NS D5NS
Dextrose 5% in 0.45% sodium chloride	Hypertonic	D5-0.45% NaCl D5-0.45% NS D5-1/2NS
MULTIPLE ELECTROLYTE SOLUTIONS		
Lactated Ringer's‡	Isotonic	LR
Dextrose 5% in Lactated Ringer's	Hypertonic	D5LR

*Dextrose is quickly metabolized, leaving free water to be distributed evenly in all fluid compartments (Horne, Heitz, and Swearingen, 1991).
†Although it is isotonic because the total concentration of electrolytes equals plasma concentration, it contains 154 mEq of both sodium and chloride, which is a higher concentration of these electrolytes than is found in the plasma, which can cause fluid volume excess (Metheny, 1992).
‡Contains sodium, potassium, calcium, chloride, lactate.

these pull fluid into the vascular space by osmosis, resulting in an increased vascular volume that can lead to pulmonary edema particularly in clients with heart failure or renal failure.

Certain additives, most commonly vitamins and potassium chloride (KCl), are frequently added to IV solutions. The physician's order includes required additives, for example:

Bottle #1: 1000 ml—D5W with 20 mEq KCl and 1 ampule of multivitamins

Clients with normal renal function who are receiving nothing by mouth should have potassium added to IV solutions. If the physician's order for such a client does not include potassium, the nurse should double-check the order. The body has no conservation mechanism for potassium and even when the serum level falls the kidneys continue to excrete potassium; if there is no potassium intake orally or parenterally, hypokalemia can develop quickly. Conversely, the nurse should verify that the client has adequate urine output before administering an IV solution containing potassium because hyperkalemia can quickly develop.

The nurse collects and, if necessary, prepares the solution using the "five rights" of medication administration described in Chapter 26.

EQUIPMENT. Correct selection and preparation of equipment assists in safe and quick placement of an IV line. Because fluids are instilled into the bloodstream, sterile technique is necessary, and the nurse must therefore have all equipment organized and at the bedside. The nurse who must leave the bedside to obtain another piece of equipment must start the procedure again. Standard equipment includes IV solution and tubing, needle or catheter (Procedure 35-1, step 3), antiseptic, tourniquet, gloves, tape, dressing, and arm board.

The arm board is used to reduce movement of the extremity with the IV infusion in place and to maintain the extremity in an extended, straight position. Arm boards are often necessary when an IV line is positioned on the dorsal surface of the hand or near a joint.

Other IV equipment includes solution containers, various types of tubing, and IV pumps or volume control devices. An injectable antibiotic medication such as ampicillin may be added to a small IV solution bag and "piggybacked" into the main line to be administered over a 30- to 60-minute period (Chapter 26). The type and amount of solution depend on the medication added and the client's physiological status. For example, when ampicillin is administered parenterally, it must be infused within 1 hour after the drug was prepared. Otherwise, the medication loses its potency.

Different tubing types are used to administer medications or IV fluids. A solution given rapidly needs to be infused with macrodrip tubing, which delivers large drops (the size varies with the manufacturer) so that a rapid rate can be maintained. In contrast, microdrop tubing provides a standard drop size of 60 gtt/ml. Microdrop tubing is used to allow precise regulation of IV fluids even at slow rates. In addition, clients may require IV extension tubing to increase mobility or to facilitate changes in position. IV pumps or volume control devices are used with children, with clients with renal or cardiac failure, or with critically ill clients to prevent sudden uncontrolled rapid infusion of large volumes. (Additional information on IV pumps and volume control devices is presented in the section on regulating the infusion flow rate.)

INITIATING THE INTRAVENOUS LINE. After the equipment is collected at the bedside, the nurse prepares to place the IV line by assessing the client for the venipunc-

Text continued on p. 1054.

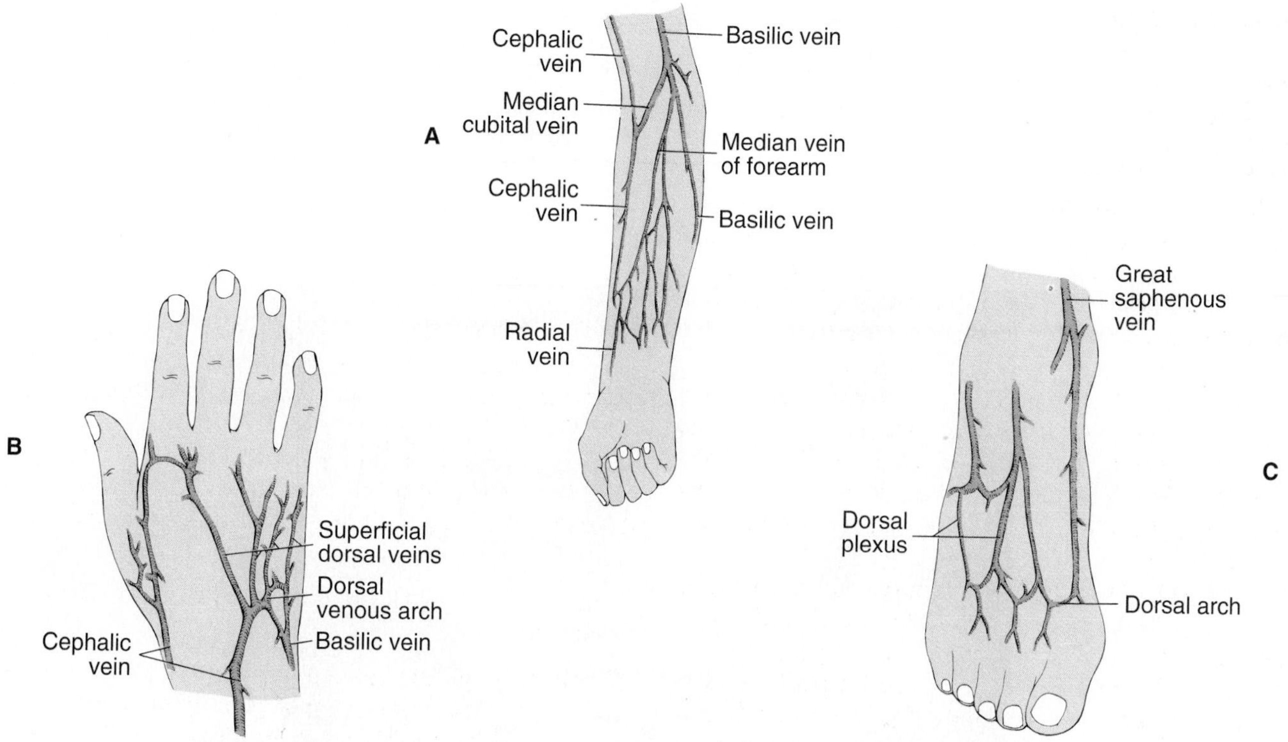

FIGURE 35-8 Common intravenous sites. **A,** Inner arm. **B,** Dorsal surface of hand, **C,** Dorsal surface of foot (used only for pediatric clients).

procedure 35-1

VENIPUNCTURE WITH AN OVER-THE-NEEDLE PLASTIC CATHETER

Steps	Rationale
1. Observe for risk factors of and signs and symptoms indicating fluid, electrolyte, and acid-base imbalances requiring intravenous therapy. a. Sunken eyes b. Edema c. Flattened neck veins d. Dry mucous membranes e. Poor skin turgor f. Change from baseline vital signs, especially hypotension and tachycardia g. Irregular pulse rhythm h. Auscultation of crackles in lungs	Many acute and chronic diseases place the client at risk for imbalances. Any abnormal route of loss of fluid and electrolytes is potentially serious, especially in the very young and the very old. Because fluid, electrolyte, and acid-base disturbances affect every system in the body, the nurse must assess the client to identify abnormalities related to such imbalances.
i. Greater than 2% decrease in body weight j. Increased or decreased bowel sounds k. Decreased urine output l. Behavioral changes m. Confusion	Changes in body weight of 1 kg correspond to 1L of fluid loss or gain.
2. Review physician's fluid replacement orders.	Venipuncture before IV therapy is an invasive technique requiring a physician's order. IV fluids are medications and require an order.
3. Assemble equipment: a. Correct IV solution b. Proper catheter for venipuncture	Assists in safe and quick placement of IV line.
c. Infusion set/IV tubing; volume control device or IV pump may be used also d. Alcohol and povidone-iodine cleansing swabs e. Tourniquet (obtain a new one for each client) f. Arm board (if necessary)	Choice will depend on type of solution, the client's age, and reason for administration.
g. Transparent dressing or gauze and povidone-iodine ointment	Transparent dressing allows for ongoing inspection of puncture site.

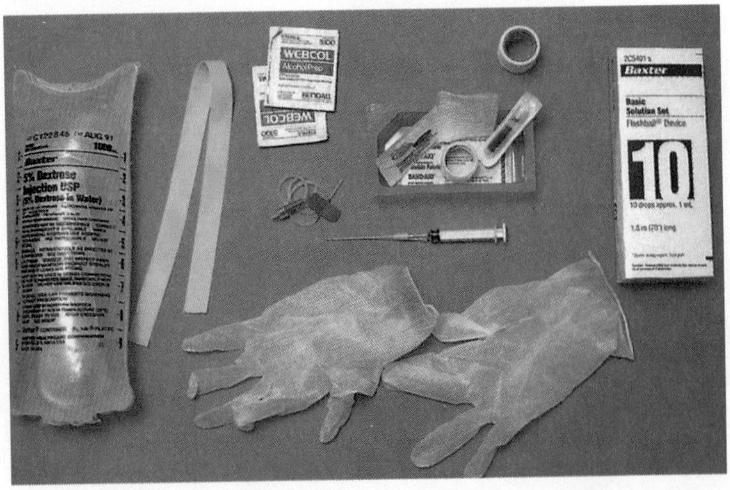

Step 5

Steps	Rationale
h. Tape (sterile and pre-cut)	
i. Towel or drape to place under client's arm	
j. IV pole	
k. Disposable gloves	
l. Special gown with snaps at shoulder	
4. Identify client and explain procedure; change client's gown to an IV gown.	Reduces anxiety and promotes cooperation. Makes removal with IV tubing easier.
5. Organize equipment on clutter-free bedside stand or overbed table (see illustration).	Increases efficiency.
6. Identify accessible vein for placement of needle or catheter (see Figure 35-8): a. Avoid bony prominences b. Use most distal portion of vein first c. Avoid placing IV catheter over wrist or in antecubital fossa d. Avoid placing IV catheter in dominant hand e. Avoid using an extremity where sensation is decreased f. Avoid inserting the needle or catheter through a rash or an infection.	Promotes ease and placement of catheter or needle. Proper placement of the IV site is especially important for the older adult (see box on p. 1059).
7. Wash hands.	
8. Open sterile packages using aseptic technique (Chapter 25).	Maintains sterility of equipment and reduces spread of microorganisms.
9. Check solution, using "five rights" of medication administration. Make sure prescribed additives, such as potassium and vitamins, have been added.	IV solutions are medications and should be carefully checked to reduce risk of error.
10. Open infusion set, maintaining sterility of both ends.	Prevents bacteria from entering infusion equipment and thus bloodstream.
11. Place roller clamp *(see illustration)* 2 to 4 cm (1 to 2 in) below drip chamber.	Close proximity of roller clamp to drip chamber allows more accurate regulation of flow rate.
12. Move roller clamp to *off* position *(see illustration)*.	Prevents accidental spillage of fluid.

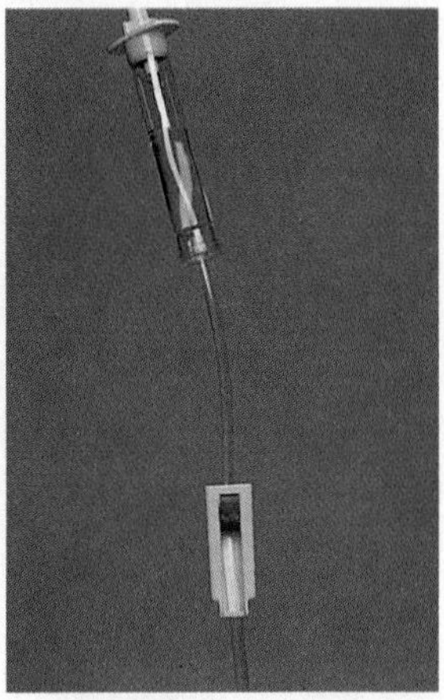

Step 11

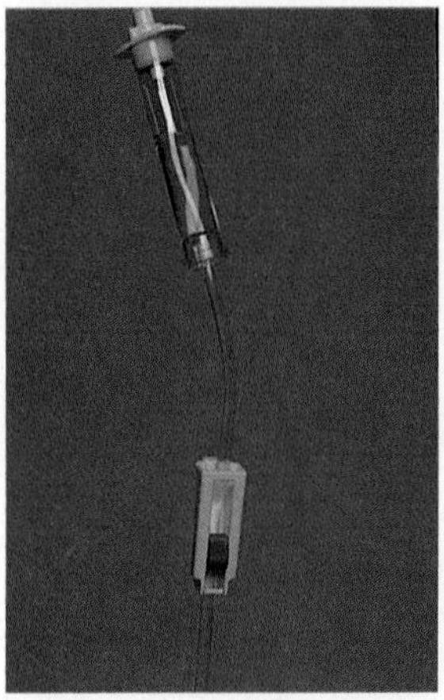

Step 12

Continued.

procedure 35-1—cont'd

Steps	Rationale
13. Insert infusion set into fluid bag:	
a. Remove protective cover from IV bag without touching opening (see illustration).	Maintains sterility of solution.
NOTE: When using bottled IV solution, remove metal cap and metal and rubber disks beneath cap.	Permits entry of infusion tubing into solution.
b. Remove protector cap from tubing insertion spike, not touching spike, and insert spike into opening of bag *(see illustration)*. Or insert spike through appropriate opening in black rubber stopper of IV bottle.	Prevents contamination of solution from contaminated insertion spike.
14. Fill infusion tubing:	
a. Compress drip chamber and release, allowing it to fill $\frac{1}{3}$ to $\frac{1}{2}$ full.	Creates suction effect; fluid enters drip chamber to prevent air from entering tubing.
b. Remove cap from end of tubing (if necessary) and release roller clamp to allow fluid to travel from drip chamber through tubing to needle adapter. Return roller clamp to *off* position after tube is filled.	Removes air from tubing and permits it to fill with solution. Closing clamp prevents accidental loss of fluid.
c. Be certain tubing is clear of air and air bubbles.	Large air bubbles (e.g., greater than 0.25 cm) can act as emboli.
d. Replace tubing cap.	Maintains system sterility.
15. Select appropriate ONC.	Used to puncture vein and allow IV fluid and medication administration.
16. Select distal site of vein to be used.	If sclerosing or damage to vein occurs, proximal site of same vein can still be used.
17. If large amount of body hair is present at needle insertion site, clip it.	Reduces risk of contamination from bacteria on hair. Also assists in maintaining intactness of dressing and makes removal of tape less painful.
18. If possible, place extremity in dependent position.	Permits venous dilation and visibility.

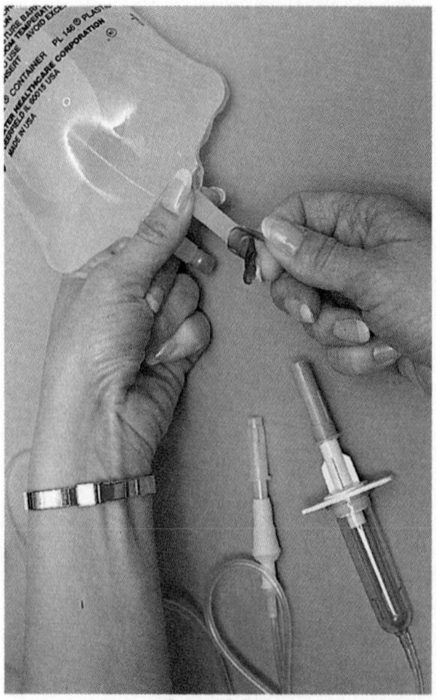
Step 13a

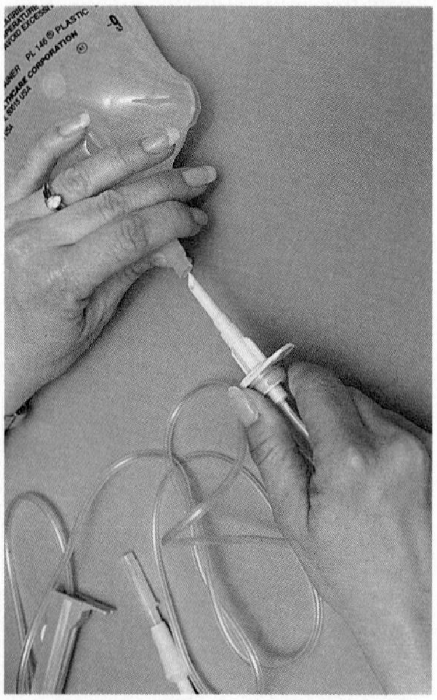
Step 13b

Steps	Rationale
19. Place tourniquet 10 to 12 cm (5 to 6 in) above insertion site (see illustration). Tourniquet should obstruct venous, not arterial, flow. Check distal pulse.	Diminished arterial flow prevents venous filling.
20. Select well-dilated vein (see illustration). Methods to foster venous dilation include stroking extremity from distal to proximal, opening and closing the fist, light tapping over the vein, applying warmth to the extremity.	Increases venous dilation.
NOTE: Be sure the needle adapter end of infusion set is nearby and on sterile gauze or towel or be able to quickly remove cap without contaminating the needle adapter end of the tubing.	Permits smooth, quick connection of infusion set to hub of catheter after vein is punctured.
21. Apply disposable gloves.	Decreases exposure to HIV, HBV, and other blood-borne organisms.
22. Cleanse insertion site with firm, concentric, circular motion outward from insertion site using povidone-iodine solution *(see illustration)*. Allow to dry.	Povidone-iodine is a topical antiinfective that reduces skin surface bacteria; it must be dry to be effective.
23. Perform venipuncture: a. Anchor vein by placing thumb over vein and by stretching skin against direction of insertion 2 to 3 in distal to site.	Stabilizes the vein so that it does not roll away from the needle.

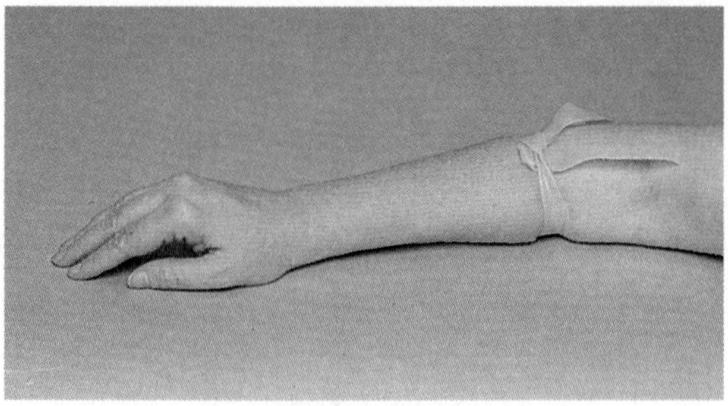
Step 19

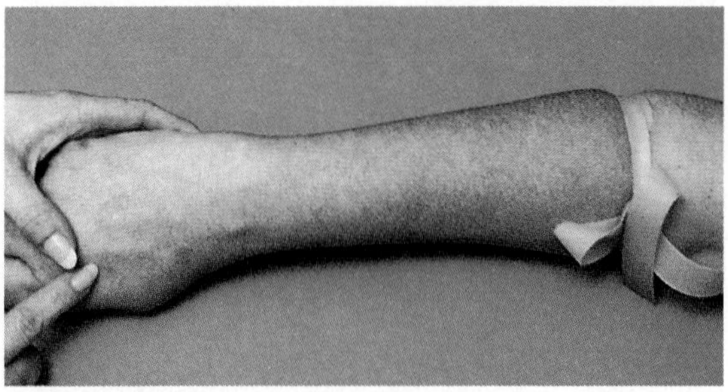
Step 20

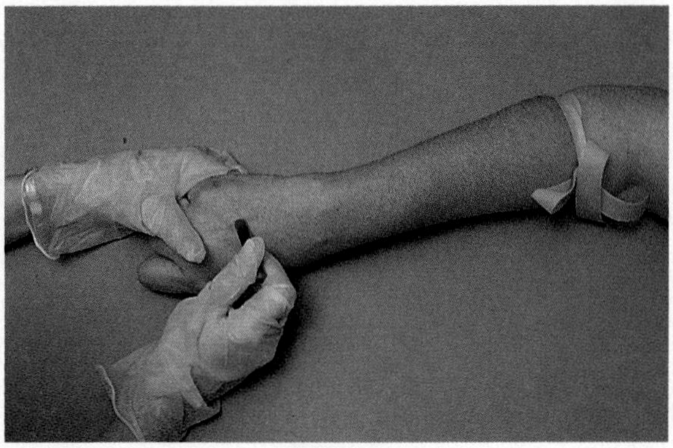
Step 22

Continued.

procedure 35-1—cont'd

Steps	Rationale
b. Place ONC at 20- to 30-degree angle with bevel up, slightly distal to actual site of venipuncture *(see illustration).*	Allows placement of needle parallel with vein. Thus when vein is punctured, risk of puncturing posterior vein wall is reduced.
24. Look for blood return through flashback chamber of ONC, indicating that needle has entered vein *(see illustration).* Lower needle until almost flush with skin. Advance ONC approximately ¼ in into vein and then loosen stylet. Advance the catheter until hub rests at venipuncture site.	Increased venous pressure from tourniquet increases backflow of blood into catheter or tubing when vein is entered. Stylet helps to puncture skin and advance catheter but must be removed to avoid puncture of the vein.
25. Stabilizing one with one hand, release tourniquet and remove stylet. **Do not** recap the stylet.	Permits venous flow, reduces backflow of blood, allows connection with administration set. Needlestick injuries are the most common occupational source of HIV and HBV infections.
26. Connect needle adapter of infusion set to hub of ONC. Do not touch point of entry of needle adapter or inside of hub of ONC *(see illustration).*	Prompt and careful connection of infusion set maintains sterility of equipment.
27. Release roller clamp to begin infusion at rate to maintain patency of IV line. Observe site for sudden swelling. Remove gloves.	Maintains patency of catheter by preventing clotting of blood in the catheter; allows infusion of solution. Indicates puncture of vein.

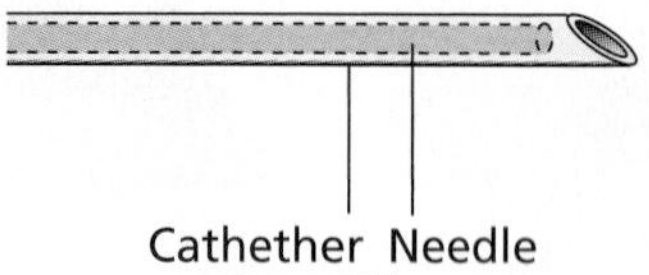

Step 23b

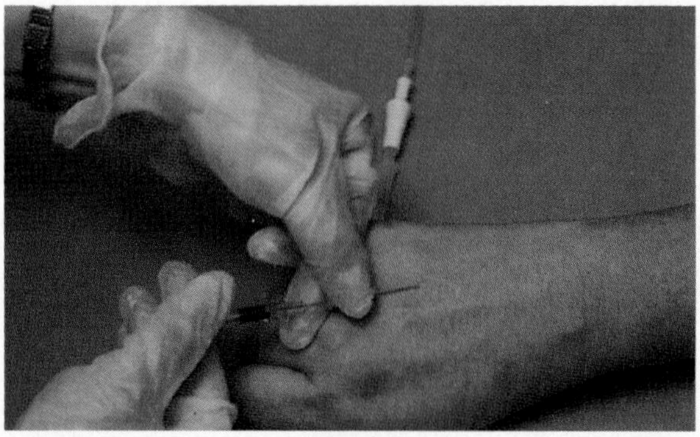
Step 24

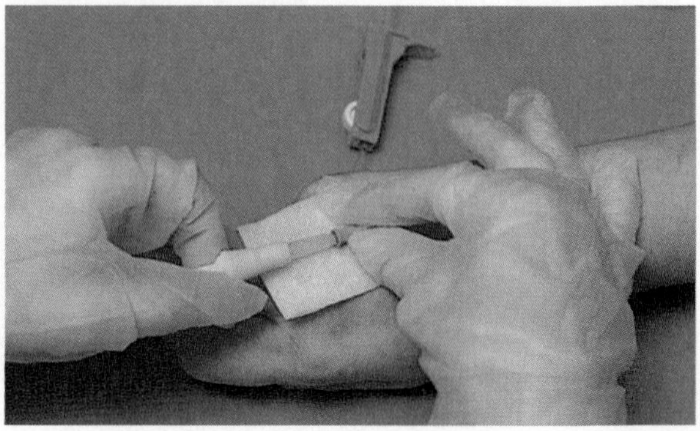
Step 26

Steps	Rationale
28. Secure IV catheter:	Prevents accidental removal of catheter from vein.
a. Place narrow piece (½ in) of tape under catheter with adhesive side up and cross tape over catheter.	
b. If a transparent dressing is used, no ointment is placed over the site. If gauze dressing is used, povidone-iodine ointment may be placed on the insertion site *(see illustration)*.	Povidone-iodine reduces bacteria on skin and may decrease risk of local or systemic infection.
c. Place second piece of narrow tape directly across catheter hub.	
d. Place transparent dressing over IV site in direction of hair growth *(see illustration)*. Place 2×2 gauze pad over insertion site and catheter hub and secure with 1 in pieces of tape. Do not cover connection between IV tubing and catheter hub.	Protects insertion site from bacteria and trauma. Transparent dressing allows inspection of the insertion site.
e. Secure infusion tubing to dressing and arm with pieces of 1 in tape.	Further stabilizes tubing, which prevents accidental disconnection of tubing from catheter and prevents weight of tubing from pulling catheter or needle out of venipuncture site.
f. Dispose of equipment and wash hands.	
29. Write date, time of placement of IV line, size and type of needle or catheter, and nurse's initials and title on IV dressing.	Provides immediate data about when line was inserted and the type of IV device used and when dressing and IV catheter need to be changed.
30. Adjust flow rate to correct drops per minute (Procedure 35-2).	Maintains correct rate of flow for IV solution.
31. Observe client every hour to determine response to therapy:	Provides continuous evaluation of type and amount of fluid delivered to client.
a. Correct amount of solution infused as prescribed.	Hourly inspection prevents accidental FVE or inadequate infusion rate and identifies early incidence of local IV site complications.
b. Proper flow rate in drops per minute or ml per hour.	
c. Patency of catheter or needle.	
d. Absence of infiltration, phlebitis, or infection.	
32. Record in nurses' notes: time infusion was begun, size and type of catheter or needle, insertion site, type of fluid, flow rate, use of volume control device or IV pump. Note response to IV fluid, amount infused, and integrity and patency of system according to agency policy.	Documents initiation of IV fluid therapy as ordered by physician. Follow-up documentation provides data about response to therapy.

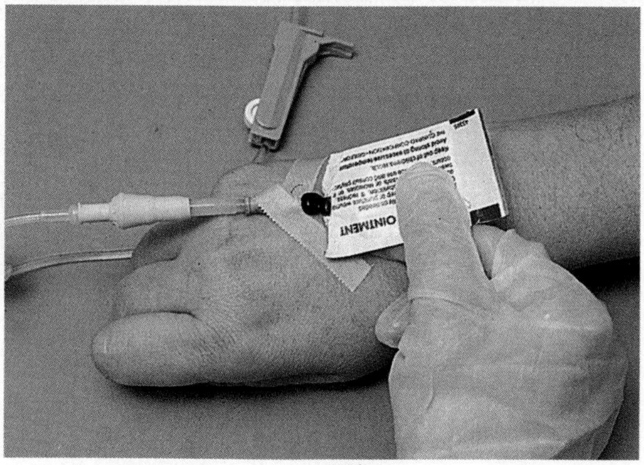

Step 28b

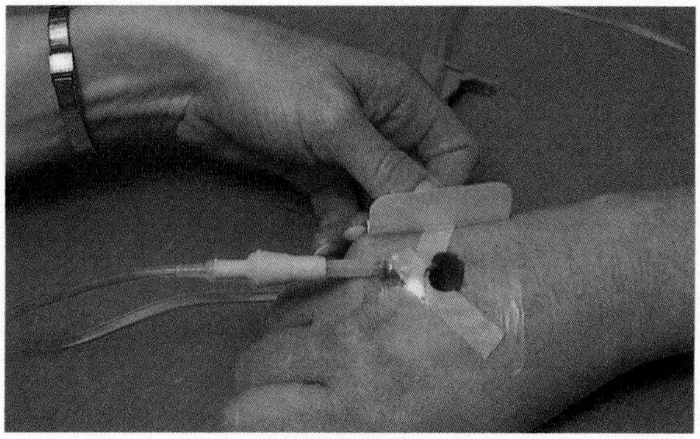
Step 28d

ture site (Procedure 35-1). A **venipuncture** is a technique in which a vein is punctured through the skin by a sharp rigid stylet (e.g., a butterfly needle or a metal needle partially covered by a plastic catheter (over-the-needle catheter or ONC) or by a needle attached to a syringe. The general purposes of venipuncture are to collect a blood specimen, to instill a medication, to start an IV infusion, or to inject a radiopaque or radioactive tracer for special examinations. Procedure 35-1 describes venipuncture for IV fluid infusion.

The nurse assessing the client for potential venipuncture sites for IV infusion should consider conditions, cautions, and contraindications that exclude certain sites. Because very young and older adults have fragile veins, the nurse should avoid sites that are easily moved or bumped such as the dorsal surface of the hand.

Common IV puncture sites include the hand and the arm (Figure 35-8, *A* and *B*). The use of the foot (Figure 35-8, *C*) for an IV site is common with pediatric clients but is avoided in the adult because of the danger of thrombophlebitis.

It is often difficult to insert an IV line in clients who have had many venipunctures because their veins may be sclerosed with scar tissue. An obese client presents problems for venipuncture because of the difficulty in locating superficial veins. The thin and emaciated client's veins are also difficult to puncture. Although they may be visible, the veins are quite fragile, and as a result, the nurse may puncture through the entire vein instead of placing the needle or catheter within it. When a client is severely dehydrated or has decreased extracellular fluids, as with shock, the veins may collapse. The collapse results from decreased circulating blood volume. When veins collapse, venipuncture becomes extremely difficult, but it is also a lifesaving measure. For these difficult clients, venipuncture should be performed by an experienced practitioner.

Venipuncture is contraindicated in a site that has signs of infection, infiltration, or thrombosis. An infected site is red, tender, swollen, and possibly warm to the touch. Exudate may be present. An infected site is not used because of the danger of introducing bacteria from the skin surface into the bloodstream.

After completing the assessment for venipuncture sites, the nurse carefully explains the procedure to the client. The nurse should explain the reason the infusion was ordered, its expected results, and the nurse's expectations of the client.

Procedure 35-1 describes the steps for using an over-the-needle catheter and a butterfly needle is used.

Large catheters placed into a central vein such as the subclavian vein are used to deliver large volumes of fluids and TPN (Chapter 31) or to administer irritating medications. Although these catheters are inserted by physicians, nurses are responsible for maintaining them.

Regulating the infusion flow rate. After the IV infusion is secured and the line is patent, the nurse must regulate the rate of infusion according to physician's orders (Procedure 35-2). An infusion rate that is too slow can lead to further cardiovascular and circulatory collapse in a client who has fluid volume deficit, hyperosmolar imbalance, or who is in shock or is critically ill. An IV that is running too slowly can also become clotted off more easily. An infusion rate that is too rapid can result in fluid volume excess. The nurse calculates the infusion rate to prevent too slow or too rapid administration of IV fluids.

Electronic infusion devices. Electronic infusion devices assist the nurse to maintain correct flow rate of IV fluids, to prevent runaway and obstructed IV infusions, and to alert the nurse when an IV bag or bottle is empty (Millam, 1990). Many electronic infusion devices (EIDs) record the volume of the fluid infused. An **infusion pump** is designed to deliver a measured amount of fluid over a period of time (i.e., ml/hr). The pump has a drop sensor and an alarm will sound if drops are not detected at the appropriate rate. There are also alarms to alert the nurse to increased system pressure that can occur with an infiltration.

A second type of EID is an IV controller that delivers fluid with the aid of gravity. IV controllers deliver fluids based on a determination of drops/minute. The rate of infusion with an IV controller depends on the height of the IV fluid container, IV tubing size, and fluid viscosity. The IV controller is less precise than the IV pump in delivering IV fluids with precision, but the client with either type of EID requires close monitoring to verify the correct infusion of the IV solution and to detect the occurrence of any complication.

Patency of the IV needle or catheter means that there are no clots at the tip of the needle or catheter and that the catheter or needle tip is not against the vein wall, which can affect the rate of infusion of the IV fluids. IV flow rates can also be affected by the patency of the IV needle or catheter, infiltration, a knot or kink in the tubing, the height of the solution, and the position of the client's extremity. The nurse can assess patency by lowering the IV bag below the level of IV insertion site and observing for a blood return. If no blood return occurs and fluid does not flow easily from the drip chamber when the roller clamp is opened, something such as a too-tight IV dressing may be impeding the flow, or a clot may be in the cannula of the IV catheter, or the tip of the catheter may be occluded against the wall of the vein. The tubing and area around the insertion site should be inspected for anything that could obstruct the flow of IV fluids. The IV tubing above the lowest medication port can be gently stripped or milked to help float the catheter tip away from the side of the vein. A sterile needle and syringe no smaller than 2 ml filled with sterile normal saline can be inserted into an injection port,

Text continued on p. 1059.

procedure 35-2

REGULATING INTRAVENOUS FLOW RATES

Steps	Rationale
1. Observe patency of IV line and needle:	For fluid to infuse at proper rate, IV line and needle must be free of kinks, knots, or clots.
a. Open drip regulator and observe for rapid flow of fluid from IV solution bag into drip chamber, then close drip regulator to prescribed rate.	Rapid flow of fluid into drip chamber denotes patency of IV line. Closing drip chamber to prescribed rate prevents FVE.
b. If fluid does not flow, lower IV fluid bag or bottle below level of infusion site and observe blood return.	Can indicate that needle is patent and in vein. Venous pressure is greater than pressure in IV tubing when bag is lowered so blood usually flows out of the vein. However, even if backflow is present, the IV may still be infiltrating and needs continual monitoring (Millam, 1987).
2. Check medical record for correct solution and additives. Usual order includes solution for 24 hr, usually divided into 2 or 3L. Occasionally, IV order contains only 1L to keep vein open (KVO). Record also shows time over which each liter is to infuse.	IV fluids are medications. Use the "Five rights" to avoid medication error.
3. Know calibration in drops per milliliter (gtt/ml) of infusion set: a. Microdrop 60gtt/ml b. Macrodrop (Roth, 1992): (1) Abbott Lab 15gtt/ml (2) Travenol Lab 10gtt/ml (3) McGraw Lab 15gtt/ml	Microdrop tubing, also called minidrip or pediatric tubing, universally delivers 60 gtt/ml and is used when small or very precise volumes are to be infused. However, macrodrop administration sets provide a variety of drop factors (drops per milliliter) sizes. Macrodrop tubing should be used when large volumes or fast rates are necessary. The nurse should consult the infusion set's packaging for information concerning drop size.
4. Calculate the flow rate (gtt/min): a. Determine the hourly volume to be infused if that is not included in the IV order: $\frac{\textbf{total volume of infusion (ml)}}{\textbf{hours of infusion}} = \textbf{ml/hr}$	For example: $\frac{\textbf{1000 ml}}{\textbf{10 hrs}} = \textbf{100 ml/hr}$
b. Choose one of the following formulas to calculate flow rate (gtt/min):	Both formulas are based on the same principles. For example for macrodrop tubing manufactured by Abbott:
(1)a. $\frac{\textbf{ml/hr}}{\textbf{60 min}} = \textbf{ml/min}$	$\frac{\textbf{100 ml/hr}}{\textbf{60}} = \textbf{1.66 ml/min}$
(1)b. **ml/min × drop factor = gtt/min**	**1.6 ml/min × 15 gtts/ml = 24.9 (25) gtts/min**
OR	
(2) $\frac{\textbf{ml/hr} \times \textbf{drop factor}}{\textbf{60 min}} = \textbf{gtt/min}$	$\frac{\textbf{100 ml/hr} \times \textbf{15 gtts/ml}}{\textbf{60 min}} = \textbf{25 gtts/min}$
5. If an infusion pump or volume control device is used, place it at the bedside.	Increases accuracy of fluid delivery rate.

Continued.

procedure 35-2—cont'd

Steps	Rationale
6. Read the physician's order: a. IV fluids are usually ordered for 24 hr and may indicate how long each bag should run or the hourly flow rate for each bag. For example, the order could state: Bag 1: 1000 ml D5W with 20 mEq KCL and an ampule of vitamin B and C Bag 2: 1000 ml LR with 20 mEq KCL Bag 3: 1000 ml NS with 20 mEq KCL Infuse these fluids over 24 hr.	Each bag is the same volume so each bag should run the same amount of time.
7. Determine the hourly rate by dividing the volume by hours: $\frac{\textbf{3000 ml}}{\textbf{24 hr}} = \textbf{125 ml/hr}$	Determining volume of fluid that should infuse hourly provides even infusion of fluid over total prescribed time.
8. Place label/tape vertically on IV bottle or bag next to volume markings. Mark tape based on hourly flow rate. For example, if 1000 ml is to be infused over 8 hours, a mark would be made indicating when each 125 ml has infused *(see illustration)*.	Marking time tape on IV bag gives nurse visual cue as to whether fluids are being administered over correct time period. Do not mark directly on bag because ink can diffuse through permeable plastic into the fluid mixture.
9. After hourly rate has been determined, calculate minute rate based on drop factor of infusion set: a. Microdrop infusion set has drop factor of 60 gtt/ml: $\frac{\textbf{125 ml/hr} \times \textbf{60 gtt/ml}}{\textbf{60 min}} = \frac{\textbf{7500 gtt}}{\textbf{60}} = \textbf{125 gtt/min}$	Allows nurse to calculate flow rate precisely and accurately.

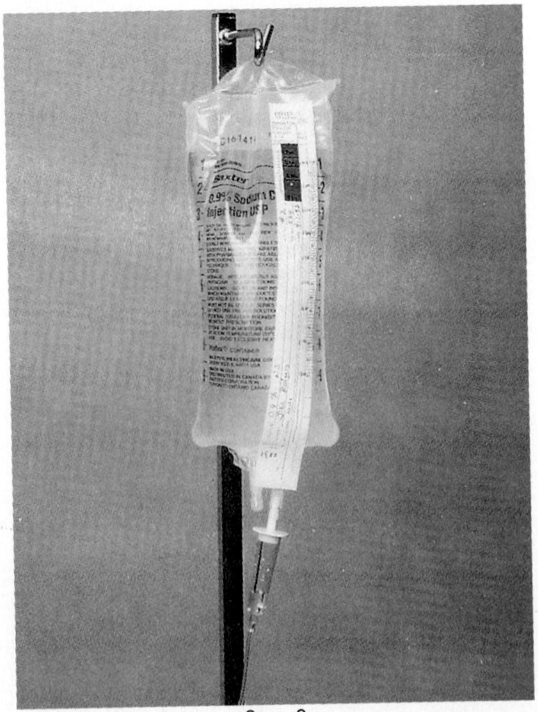

Step 8

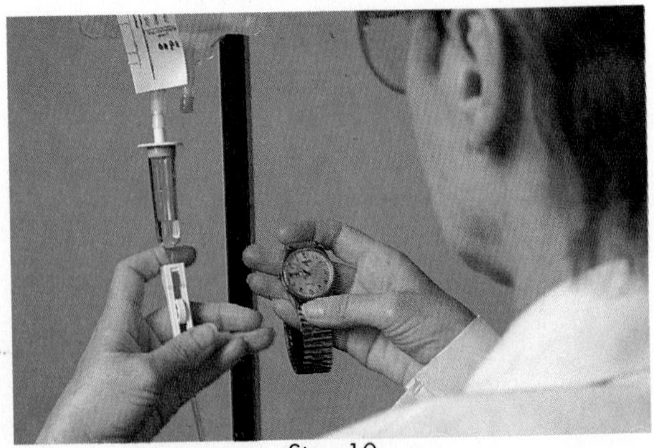

Step 10

Steps	Rationale
b. Macrodrop infusion sets have a variety of drop factors. For this example, a drop factor of 15 gtt/ml is used: $$\frac{\textbf{125 ml/hr} \times \textbf{15 gtt/ml}}{\textbf{60 min}} = \textbf{31-32 gtt/min}$$	
10. Time flow rate by counting drops entering into the drip chamber for 1 min by watch, then adjust roller clamp to increase or decrease rate of infusion *(see illustration)*.	Determines whether fluids are being administered too slowly or fast. Rate of infusion should also be checked by watch even if infusion pump is used.
11. Follow this procedure for infusion controller or IV pump:	
a. Place electronic eye on drip chamber below origin of drop and above fluid level in chamber *(see illustration)*.	The electronic eye counts the number of drops flowing from administration set to ensure that proper rate infuses.
b. Place IV infusion tubing within ridges of control box in direction of flow (i.e., portion of tubing nearest client at bottom). Required gtt/min or vol/hr is selected, door to control chamber is shut, power button is turned on, and start button is pressed *(see illustration)*.	Infusion pumps move fluid by compressing and milking tubing, thus propelling fluid through tubing. Special tubing is required for some pumps.
c. Ensure that IV drip regulator is in open position while infusion pump is in use.	
d. Monitor infusion rates at least hourly.	Infusion controllers and pumps are not infallible and do not replace frequent, comprehensive assessments; the pump may continue to infuse IV fluids after an infiltration has begun.

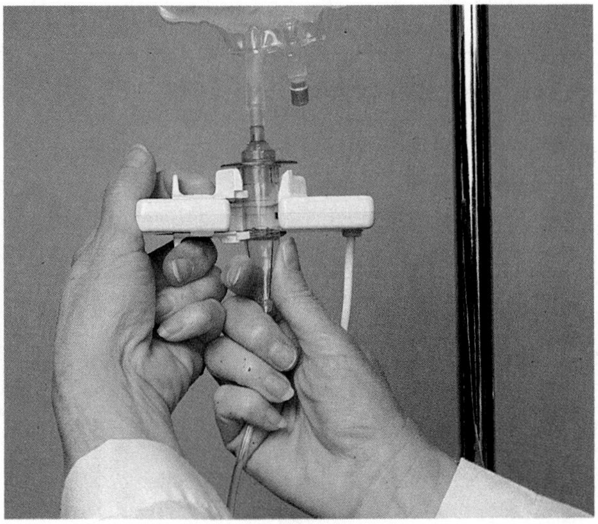

Step 11a

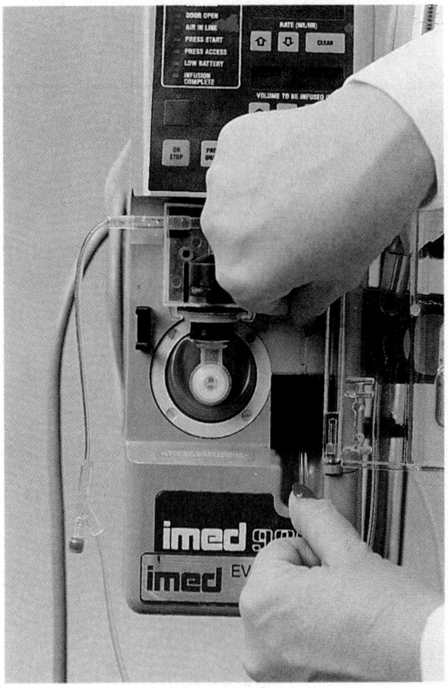

Step 11b

Continued.

procedure 35-2—cont'd

Steps	Rationale
e. Assess patency of system when alarm sounds.	Alarm indicates that electronic eye has not noted precise number of drops from drip chamber or an increase in pressure in the system. Possible causes for an alarm include empty solution bag, kink in tubing, closed drip regulator, an infiltration, or a thrombosis.
12. Follow this procedure for volume control device:	
a. Place volume control device between IV bag and insertion spike of infusion set *(see illustration)*.	Reduces risk of sudden increases in fluid volume.
b. Place 2 hours' volume of fluid into device.	Prevents IV line from running dry if nurse does not return in exactly 60 min. If accidental increase in rate occurs, client receives at most the volume equivalent to 2 hours of infusion.

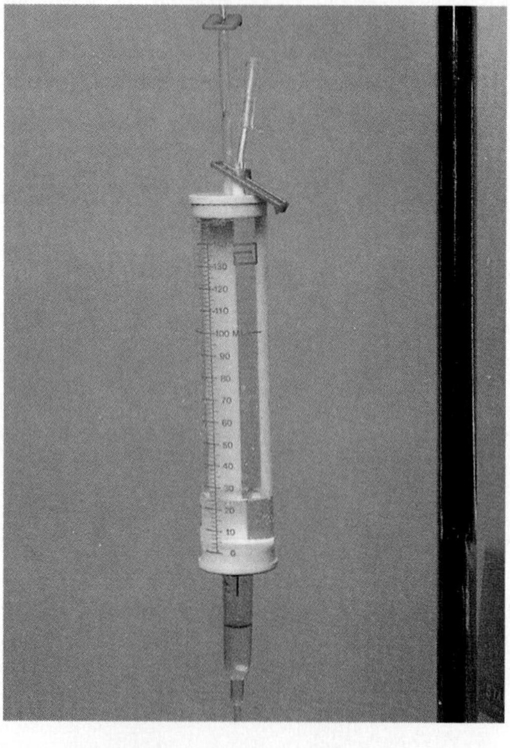

Step 12a

Steps	Rationale
c. Assess IV system at least hourly and add fluid to volume control device. Regulate flow rate.	Maintains patency of system.
13. Observe client hourly to determine response to IV therapy and restoration of fluid and electrolyte balance. Also monitor IV site for signs of infiltration, phlebitis, infection, clot in IV catheter, and kink or knot in tubing.	Signs and symptoms of FVD or FVE warrant changing rate of fluid infused. Signs of infiltration, phlebitis, or infection warrant changing the IV site. If the volume of fluids infused is excessively deficient from that ordered, the rate of the IV fluids should **not** be automatically increased because the rapid increase in vascular volume might result in fluid volume excess and pulmonary edema. When the IV fluids are behind, simply reestablish the ordered rate without attempting to rapidly infuse the deficient volume. If the fluids have infused too rapidly, the ordered rate should be reestablished and the client closely monitored for the occurrence of FVE.
14. Record rate of infusion, gtt/min, and ml/hr, in client's record as required by agency policy.	Documents that prescribed IV flow is being delivered to client.

and gentle aspiration can be used to reestablish patency of the IV needle or catheter.

A knot or kink in the tubing can decrease the flow rate. Occasionally the tubing is kinked under a dressing, which requires the nurse to remove the dressing to locate the problem. The flow rate frequently resumes after the tubing is straightened. The client may also occlude the tubing by lying or sitting on it. The height of the IV bag can also affect flow rates. Raising the bag may increase the rate because of hydrostatic pressure.

The position of the extremity, particularly at the wrist or elbow, can decrease flow rates. Occasionally the use of an arm board helps to keep the joint extended. Sometimes, it is more comfortable for the client to have an infusion started in a new location rather than dealing with a site that causes problems. However, before discontinuing the infusion hampered by an extremity position, the nurse should start the infusion in another site to verify that the client has other accessible veins.

An infiltration may be present when the insertion site is cool, clammy, swollen, and in some cases painful. An infiltration occurs when the needle or catheter has dislodged from the vein and is in the subcutaneous space. When an infiltration occurs, the IV line must be discontinued and a new line inserted.

These influences on IV flow rates can occur with any client at any time. When caring for a client with an infusion, the nurse should assess the site and the infusion rate at least every hour.

Children, older adults, clients with severe head trauma, and clients susceptible to volume overload must be protected from sudden increases in infusion volumes. The nurse needs to understand that when certain IV controller devices are opened, the IV fluid will infuse rapidly; if this is not controlled, an excessive amount of solution can infuse. Sudden increases can occur accidentally. For example, a restless client may loosen the roller clamp with a sudden movement and increase the flow rate, or the flow rate may be accidentally increased if the client ambulates. A sudden increase in IV infusion rate causes a rapid increase in vascular volume, which can make the client critically ill or even cause death. Volume control devices, such as a Volutrol or buret, can prevent sudden excessive increases in the volume of IV solution infused.

MAINTAINING THE SYSTEM. After the IV line is in place and the flow rate is regulated, the nurse maintains the system. The nurse provides assistance with hygiene and comfort measures, meals, and ambulation (see box above). IV catheters and drugs, especially those with potassium, can cause discomfort and burning sensations. Clients must be reassured that occasional discomfort is normal. Sometimes discomfort is relieved by repositioning the extremity, but occasionally it is necessary to start a new IV line in a larger vein.

GERONTOLOGIC NURSING PRACTICE FOR INTRAVENOUS THERAPY

- In older clients, use the smallest gauge catheter or needle possible (e.g., 24-26 gauge). This is less traumatizing to the vein and allows better blood flow to provide increased hemodilution of the IV fluids or medications. This gauge can be used for hourly flow rates of 75-100 ml/hr.
- Avoid the back of the older adult's hand or the dominant arm for venipuncture because these sites greatly interfere with the older adult's independence.
- If the older adult has fragile skin and veins, use minimal tourniquet pressure.
- When the older adult has lost subcutaneous tissue, the veins lose stability and will roll away from the needle. To stabilize the vein, apply traction to the skin below the projected insertion site.
- Using an angle of 5-15 degrees on insertion is helpful because the older adult's veins are more superficial.
- In the older person with fragile skin, prevent skin tears by minimizing the amount of tape used.

Modified from Coulter K: Intravenous therapy for the elder patient: implications for the intravenous nurse, *J Intraven Nurs* 15(supplement):S18, 1992.

Because a client with an infusion in the arm finds it difficult to meet hygiene needs, the nurse should help with bathing and changing gowns. It helps to use a gown specifically made with snaps along the top sleeve seam to facilitate changing the gown without disturbing the venipuncture site. Regular gowns are changed by following these six steps for maximum arm mobility and speed:

1. Remove the sleeve of the gown from the arm without the IV
2. Remove the sleeve of the gown from the arm with the IV
3. Remove the IV bottle or bag from its stand and pass it and the tubing through the sleeve. (If this involves removing the tubing from an IV pump, use the roller clamp to slow the infusion to prevent the inadvertent infusion of a volume of solution or medication too large for the client to tolerate.)
4. Place the IV bottle or bag and tubing through the sleeve of the clean gown and hang it on its stand
5. Place the arm with the IV through the gown sleeve
6. Place the arm without the IV through the gown sleeve

The client with an arm or a hand infusion is able to walk, unless contraindicated. A walking IV pole, a standard IV pole with wheels, is needed. The nurse helps the client

procedure 35-3

CHANGING IV SOLUTIONS AND TUBING

Steps	Rationale
CHANGING IV SOLUTION	
1. Identify client. Review physician's orders and client's status. Have the next solution prepared at least 1 hr before needed. If solution is prepared in pharmacy, be sure it has been delivered to floor. Check that solution is correct and properly labeled.	Ensures correct client undergoes procedure. Prevents finding empty IV bag without having replacement bag. Checking prevents medication error.
2. Prepare to change solution when 50 ml remains in the bottle or bag.	Prevents air from entering IV tubing and maintains patency of tubing and catheter or needle.
3. Be sure drip chamber is half full.	Provides IV fluid to vein while bag is changed.
4. Wash hands.	Reduces transmission of microorganisms.
5. Prepare new solution for changing. If using plastic bag, remove protective cover from entry site. If using glass bottle, remove metal cap, metal disk, and rubber disk. Maintain sterility of entry site on bag or bottle.	Permits quick, smooth, and organized change from old to new solution.
6. Move roller clamp to reduce flow rate.	Prevents solution remaining in drip chamber from emptying while changing solutions.
7. Remove old solution from IV pole; keep bag in upright position.	Brings work to nurse's eye level; keeping bag upright prevents air from getting into the tubing.
8. Turn off roller clamp, invert the bag, quickly remove spike from old IV solution, and without touching tip, spike new solution bottle.	Prevents air from entering the tubing, inverting bag prevents fluid from spilling; maintains sterility. Moving quickly prevents clotting in the catheter or needle.
9. Hang new bag or bottle of solution.	Allows gravity to assist with delivery of IV fluid into drip chamber.
10. Check for air in tubing. A few bubbles can be removed by closing the roller clamp, stretching the tubing downward, and flicking the tubing with the finger (the bubbles rise in the fluid to the drip chamber), opening the clamp. For a larger amount of air, insert a needle and syringe into a port below the air and allow the air to enter the syringe.	Reduces risk of air embolus. Use of air-eliminating filter also reduces this risk.
11. Make sure drip chamber is ⅓ to ½ full. If the drip chamber is too full, pinch off tubing below the drip chamber, invert the container, squeeze the drip chamber then release, hang up the container, and release the tubing.	Reduces risk of air entering tubing; too much fluid in the drip chamber hampers the ability to count drops.
12. Regulate flow rate to prescribed rate.	Maintains measures to restore fluid balance and deliver fluid as ordered.
13. Discard empty bag or bottle according to agency policy.	Reduces transmission of infection.
14. Observe IV system for patency and absence of infiltration, phlebitis, and infection. Observe response to therapy.	Provides ongoing evaluation of response to therapy.
CHANGING INTRAVENOUS TUBING	
15. Determine when new infusion set is warranted:	Changing tubing prevents infection.
a. Hanging first solution of day.	Procedure is simplified when tubing is changed with a bag of new solution.
b. Puncture of infusion tubing.	Punctured tubing results in leakage of fluid and contamination of solution with bacteria.
c. Contamination of tubing.	Contamination of tubing can allow entry of bacteria into bloodstream.

Steps	Rationale
d. Occlusions in tubing (e.g., after infusion of packed red blood cells, whole blood, or albumin).	Whole blood or blood component products can occlude or partially occlude IV tubing because they are thick and sticky.
e. Date on tubing indicates need for a change; frequency of tubing change is determined by agency policy and is usually every 48 to 72 hours.	Prevents bacterial growth.
16. Assemble equipment: a. Infusion tubing b. Sterile 2 × 2 gauze c. If new dressing must be applied:	Ensures efficient and safe procedure.
(1) Transparent dressing or sterile 2 × 2 gauze (2) Povidone-iodine ointment (3) Adhesive remover (4) Alcohol swabs (5) Strips of tape, sterile and pre-cut (6) Disposable gloves	Type of dressing will be determined by agency policy.
17. Explain procedure to the client.	Promotes cooperation and prevents sudden movement of extremity that could dislodge needle or catheter.
18. Wash hands.	Reduces transmission of microorganisms.
19. Open new infusion set, keeping protective coverings over infusion spike and needle adapter.	Provides nurse with ready access to new infusion set and maintains sterility of infusion set.
20. Apply nonsterile disposable gloves.	Decreases risk of exposure to HIV, HBV, and other bloodborne organisms.
21. Place sterile 2 × 2 gauze on bed near puncture site (optional).	Provides sterile field for new sterile needle adapter before connection to hub of catheter or needle.
22. If needle or catheter hub is not visible, remove IV dressing. Do not remove tape that secures needle or catheter to skin.	Needle hub must be accessible to provide smooth transition when removing old tubing and inserting new tubing.
23. Take new tubing and move roller clamp to *off* position.	Prevents spillage of solution after new bag or bottle is spiked.
24. With old tubing in place, crimp the tubing, compress drip chamber, and fill chamber.	Provides surplus of fluid in drip chamber so that there is enough fluid to maintain patency while changing tubing.
25. Close regulator clamp to old tubing, invert the bag of IV solution, remove the IV tubing spike, hang the drip chamber over IV pole or tape the drip chamber to the IV pole; open the regulator clamp to a slow rate of infusion.	Allows fluid to continue to flow through catheter while nurse prepares new tubing; slow rate prevents complete infusion of solution remaining in tubing.
26. Place insertion spike of new tubing into old bag of solution and hang solution on pole.	Permits flow of fluid from IV bag into new infusion tubing.
27. Compress and release drip chamber on new tubing.	Allows drip chamber to fill and promotes rapid, smooth flow of solution through new tubing; prevents air from entering the tubing.
28. Remove protective cap, if necessary, from needle adapter, and open roller clamp, flushing tubing with solution.	Removes air from tubing and replaces it with fluid.
29. Place needle adapter of new tubing, with protective cap off, on sterile 2×2 gauze or be prepared to quickly remove the cap while maintaining sterility of the needle adapter.	Provides smooth, quick insertion of new tubing into hub of needle or catheter, while maintaining sterility of tubing.
30. Turn roller clamp on old tubing to *off* position.	Prevents spillage of fluid as tubing is removed from needle hub.

Continued.

procedure 35-3—cont'd

Steps	Rationale
31. Stabilize hub of catheter or needle with thumb and forefinger and gently remove old tubing (may require a twisting motion of tubing); quickly insert needle adapter of new tubing into hub; careful use of a hemostat to grasp the tubing close to the insertion site may facilitate removal of the tubing from catheter hub.	Prevents accidental displacement of catheter or needle; quick implementation of this prevents clot formation in catheter or needle.
32. Open roller clamp on new tubing.	Permits solution to enter catheter and vein.
33. Regulate drip according to physician's orders and monitor rate hourly.	Maintains infusion flow at prescribed rate.
34. If necessary, apply new dressing (Procedure 35-4).	Reduces risk of bacterial infection from skin.
35. Discard old tubing and gloves in container for contaminated materials and wash hands.	Prevents transmission of microorganisms.
36. Evaluate flow rate and observe connection site for leakage.	Maintains prescribed rate of flow of IV solution, detects loss of system intactness, which can result in clot formation or bacterial contamination.
37. Record changing of tubing and solution on client's record and place piece of tape or sticker below the drip chamber with date and time of the completed tubing change or the date that the tubing should next be changed. Record fluid infused on intake and output form.	Documents procedure and records that measures to maintain sterility were carried out. Provides visual cue to all care providers of when tubing needs to be changed.

to get out of bed and places the pole next to the involved arm. The client is instructed to hold on to the pole with the involved hand and to push it while walking. The nurse should assess the equipment to make sure that the IV bag is at the proper height, that there is no tension on the tubing, and that the flow rate is correct. The nurse should instruct the client to report any blood in the tubing, a stoppage in the flow, or increased discomfort.

Because clients receiving IV therapy may require frequent changing of solutions, the nurse should allow adequate time for this. Occasionally, clients require an IV infusion to deliver a drug every 4, 6, or 8 hours rather than for fluid replacement. An hourly infusion flow of about 10 to 15 ml per hour is used to keep the vein open (KVO) using a microdrip infusion set. A new solution bag or bottle should be hung at least once every 24 hours, even if the old bag is not empty, because the sterility of the solution cannot be guaranteed for longer than a day. When an IV solution container is changed, the nurse uses sterile technique and follows an organized procedure (Procedure 35-3).

IV tubing can remain sterile for 48 to 72 hours (Maki, et al., 1987; Cohen, 1989). Each agency will have a policy determining how frequently the IV dressing, IV tubing, and IV site should be changed. These procedures are much simpler and more efficient if they are performed simultaneously (e.g., the infusion tubing can be changed when a new IV bag or bottle is hung) (Procedure 35-3). To prevent entry of bacteria into the bloodstream, sterility must be maintained during all of these procedures.

The dressing over the IV insertion site is changed according to hospital policy. Usually gauze or transparent dressings are used (Procedure 35-4). Transparent dressings enable the nurse to continually assess the venipuncture site. The dressing is usually changed at 48- to 72-hour intervals when the IV site is changed (Maki and Ringer, 1987). If the dressing becomes wet, soiled, or loose, it should be changed at that time to decrease the risk for infection.

COMPLICATIONS OF INTRAVENOUS THERAPY. Major complications of IV therapy are infiltration, phlebitis, infection, FVE, and bleeding.

An **infiltration** occurs when IV fluids enter the subcutaneous space around the venipuncture site. This is manifested as swelling (from increased tissue fluid) and pallor (caused by decreased circulation) around the venipuncture site. Fluid may be flowing through the IV line at a decreased rate or may have stopped flowing.

procedure 35-4

CHANGING IV DRESSINGS

Steps	Rationale
1. Assess need to change dressing:	
a. Determine when dressing was last changed. Many institutions require the nurse to write date and time on dressing.	Provides information regarding length of time that dressing has been in place so that nurse can plan for dressing change.
b. Observe present dressing for moisture.	Moisture is medium for bacterial growth. Moisture on sterile dressing renders dressing contaminated.
c. Observe present dressing for intactness.	Nonadhering dressing increases risk of bacterial contamination to venipuncture site or displacement of catheter.
d. Observe IV system for proper functioning or complications: kinks in infusion tubing or catheter and infiltration, phlebitis, or infection.	Unexplained decrease in flow rate or pain and swelling at venipuncture site require nurse to investigate placement and patency of catheter.
2. Assemble equipment:	Ensures efficient and safe completion of procedure.
a. Transparent dressing or sterile 2 × 2 gauze.	
b. Povidone-iodine swabs and ointment.	
c. Adhesive remover.	
d. Alcohol swabs.	
e. Strips of tape, sterile and pre-cut.	
f. Disposable gloves.	
3. Explain procedure to client. Explain that affected extremity must remain still for the entire length of the procedure.	Assists in obtaining client cooperation and gives time frame around which client can plan personal activities.
4. Wash hands.	Reduces transmission of microorganisms.
5. Apply disposable gloves.	Reduces risk of HIV, HBV, and other blood-borne organisms.
6. Remove tape and gauze or transparent dressing from IV site one layer at a time, leaving tape that secures needle or catheter in place.	Prevents accidental displacement of catheter or needle, which can occur if catheter tubing becomes tangled between two layers of dressing.
7. If infiltration, phlebitis, infection, or clotting occurs or if ordered to do so by the physician, discontinue the IV infusion:	
a. Turn roller clamp to *off* position.	Prevents spillage of IV fluid on bed, client, nurse, or floor.
b. Place gauze over venipuncture site and remove catheter or needle by pulling straight away from site.	Prevents damage to the vein.
c. Apply pressure to site for 1 to 2 min.	Controls bleeding of hematoma formation.
8. If fluid is infusing properly, gently remove tape securing needle or catheter. Stabilize needle or catheter with one hand.	Exposes venipuncture site; prevents accidental displacement of catheter or needle.
9. Use adhesive remover or alcohol to cleanse skin and remove adhesive residue or blood.	Adhesive residue decreases ability of new tape to adhere tightly to skin; blood is a medium for bacterial growth.
10. Using circular motion, cleanse insertion site with povidone-iodine solution; allow to dry.	Circular motion prevents cross-contamination from skin bacteria near venipuncture site. Povidone-iodine is a topical antiinfective that reduces skin surface bacteria; povidone-iodine must dry to be effective.
11. Replace single strip of adhesie tape under hub with adhesive side up to anchor catheter or needle.	Prevents accidental displacement of catheter or needle.
12. Place povidone-iodine ointment on venipuncture site if gauze is being used for the dressing. Place second strip of ½ in tape directly across the hub of catheter.	Povidone-iodine is a topical antiinfective that reduces skin bacteria and reduces risk or local or systemic infection.

Continued.

procedure 35-4—cont'd

Steps	Rationale
13. Place transparent dressing or sterile 2 × 2 gauze over venipuncture site. If transparent dressing is selected, apply it in direction of hair growth (See Procedure 35-1, Step 28).	Provides barrier against bacteria. Reduces discomfort when dressing is removed.
14. Anchor IV tubing with additional pieces of tape.	Prevents accidental displacement of needle or catheter of separation of tubing from needle adapter.
15. Place date and time of dressing change directly on dressing (following agency policy).	Verifies that dressing change was done.
16. Discard equipment in appropriate container, remove and dispose of gloves, and wash hands.	Reduces transmission of organisms.
17. Reassess functioning and patency of system in response to IV dressing change.	Validates that IV line is patent and functioning correctly.
18. Record in nurses' note: time dressing was changed, type of dressing used, patency of IV system, and observation of venipuncture site.	Documents that dressing was changed, that IV system is functioning, and that venipuncture site is free of infection.

Pain may also be present and usually results from edema and increases proportionately as the infiltration continues.

When infiltration occurs, the infusion must be discontinued and, if IV therapy is still necessary, the catheter or needle is reinserted into another extremity. To reduce discomfort, the nurse raises the extremity, which promotes venous drainage and helps to decrease the edema, and wraps it in a warm towel for 20 minutes, which increases circulation and reduces pain and edema.

Phlebitis is an inflammation of the vein. Selected risk factors for phlebitis include the type of catheter material; chemical irritation of additives and drugs given intravenously, (e.g., antibiotics); and the anatomical position of the catheter with position of the IV at the wrist demonstrating the highest risk (Maki and Ringer, 1991). Signs and symptoms include pain, increased skin temperature over the vein, and, in some instances, redness traveling along the path of the vein. The IV line must be discontinued, and a new line inserted in another vein. Warm, moist heat on the site of phlebitis can offer some relief to the client. Phlebitis can be dangerous because blood clots (thrombophlebitis) can occur and in some cases may result in emboli.

Fluid volume excess occurs when the client has received a too-rapid administration of IV solutions. The assessment findings include shortness of breath, crackles in the lungs, and tachycardia. The nurse should slow the rate of infusion, notify the physician, raise the head of the bed, monitor vital signs, and be prepared to give oxygen and diuretics. Prompt action is necessary to prevent worsening of the condition or even death.

Bleeding can occur around the venipuncture site during the infusion or through the catheter, needle, or tubing if these become inadvertently disconnected. Bleeding is common in clients who have received heparin or who have a bleeding disorder. If bleeding occurs around the venipuncture site and the catheter is within the vein, a pressure dressing may be applied over the site to control the bleeding. Bleeding from a vein is usually a slow, continuous seepage and is not serious.

Infusion-related infections have a higher incidence in clients who are older, immunocompromised, experiencing other infections, chronically ill, on antibiotic therapy, malnourished, or who have a loss of skin integrity. IV catheters can become colonized by contamination during venipuncture, any manipulation of the tubing or bag, through spread from the skin or other site of infection, and through administration of contaminated IV fluids (Messner and Pinkerman, 1992; Phillips, 1993). Clinical manifestations of these infections include purulent drainage, erythema, swelling, and pain at the venipuncture site. The client may also have an elevated body temperature and white blood cell count.

Infusion-related infections can be reduced by careful nursing interventions. It is important to wash hands before and after every contact with the client. Fluid containers should be changed every 24 hours. Careful aseptic technique during venipuncture is essential.

The tubing, dressing, and insertion site should be changed every 48 to 72 hours or sooner if a complication develops.

Discontinuing intravenous infusions. Discontinuing an infusion is necessary after the prescribed amount of fluid has been infused, when an infiltration occurs, if phlebitis is present, or if the infusion catheter or needle develops a clot at its tip. The nurse discontinuing an infusion first applies disposable gloves and then removes the tape and dressing in the same manner as for the daily infusion dressing changes. The nurse then moves the roller clamp to the *off/closed* position to prevent spillage of IV fluid. The nurse places a sterile 2 × 2 gauze pad over the venipuncture site and, using the other hand, withdraws the catheter needle by pulling straight back away from the puncture site. If necessary, alcohol or soap and water can be used to remove dried blood or other drainage from around the site. Alcohol is not used on the IV site because it can cause stinging and prolongs bleeding (Phillips, 1993). The nurse elevates the extremity and applies pressure to the site for 1 to 2 minutes to control bleeding and prevent hematoma formation. Clients who have received heparin require longer pressure because of the action of heparin on blood-clotting mechanisms. If needed, the nurse applies a Band-Aid over a sterile cotton ball or applies a larger sterile dressing over the venipuncture site. The nurse records the amount of fluid infused and the time of the discontinuation.

Blood replacement. Blood replacement or transfusion is the IV administration of whole blood or a component such as plasma, packed red blood cells, or platelets. The objectives for blood transfusions are:

1. To increase circulating blood volume following surgery, trauma, or hemorrhage
2. To increase the number of red blood cells and to maintain hemoglobin levels in clients with severe anemia
3. To provide selected cellular components as replacement therapy (e.g., clotting factors, platelets, albumin)

Blood groups and types. The most important grouping for transfusion purposes is the ABO system, which includes A, B, O, and AB blood types. The determination of blood groups is based on the presence or absence of A and B red cell antigens. Individuals with A antigens, B antigens, or no antigens belong to groups A, B, and O respectively. The person with A and B antigens has AB blood.

Individuals with type A blood naturally produce anti-B antibodies in their plasma. Similarly, type B individuals naturally produce anti-A antibodies. A type O individual possesses neither type A nor type B antigen, which is why a person with type O blood is considered a universal blood donor. An AB type individual produces neither antibody, which is why type AB individuals can be universal recipients. If blood that is mismatched with the client's blood is transfused, a transfusion reaction occurs. The transfusion reaction is an antigen-antibody reaction and can range from a mild response to severe anaphylactic shock.

Another consideration when matching for blood transfusions is the Rh factor, an antigenic substance in the erythrocytes of most people. A person with the factor is Rh positive, whereas a person without it is Rh negative. If Rh-positive blood is administered to an Rh-negative person, the recipient will form antibodies to the Rh factor and a second exposure to Rh-positive blood will result in **hemolysis,** or red blood cell destruction, in the recipient.

Autologous transfusion (autotransfusion). **Autologous transfusion (autotransfusion)** is the collection and reinfusion of a client's own blood. The blood for an autologous transfusion can be obtained by preoperative donation when the surgery can be planned in advance (e.g., open heart, orthopedic, plastic, or gynecological). The client donates 1 to 5 units of her/his own blood depending on the type of surgery and the ability of the client to maintain an acceptable hematocrit. The blood will be tested for human immunodeficiency virus (HIV) and hepatitis B virus (HBV). An autologous transfusion can also be obtained through perioperative blood salvage (e.g., during vascular and orthopedic surgery, organ transplant surgery, and traumatic injuries). Blood can also be salvaged postoperatively from mediastinal and chest drains and after joint and spinal surgery.

Autologous transfusions are safer for the client because they decrease the risk of complications such as mismatched blood and exposure to blood-borne infectious agents. When preoperative donation is used, the need to carefully identify the unit of blood and the client is as important as it is for a transfusion from another donor or these advantages are negated (Martin et al., 1989). When perioperative blood salvage is used, these advantages are present, plus it is not necessary to take the time to type and cross-match the client's blood. Another advantage of perioperative blood salvage is that the transfusion contains more viable red blood cells than stored blood (Peterson, 1992).

Blood transfusions. Transfusing blood or blood components is a nursing procedure. The nurse is responsible for assessment before, during, and after the transfusion and regulation of the transfusion.

If the client has an IV line in place, the nurse should assess the venipuncture site for signs of infection or infiltration. The nurse should also determine whether the venipuncture was performed with an 18- or 19-gauge catheter. The large catheter promotes flow because blood is thicker and stickier than IV fluids. The nurse should determine that the intravenous catheter is patent and functioning properly. The tubing for blood administration has an in-line filter (Figure 35-9). The tubing

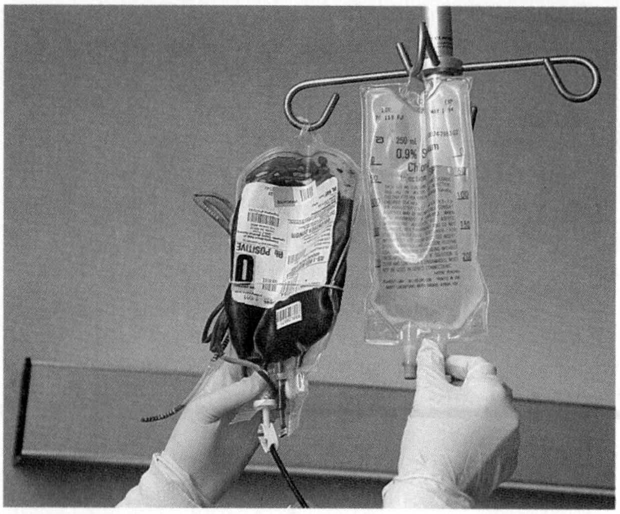

FIGURE 35-9 In-line filter infusion tubing in Y-type administration set for administration of blood allowing saline administration before, during, and after the blood transfusion.

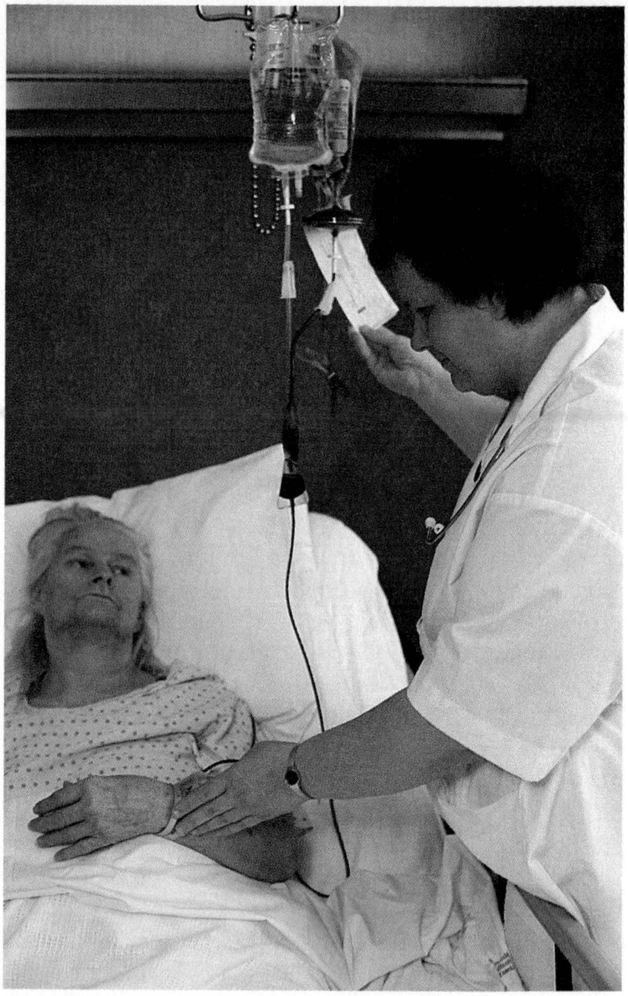

FIGURE 35-10 Nurse closely monitors client during initial period of blood transfusion.

should be primed with 0.9% normal saline to prevent hemolysis of red blood cells.

Pretransfusion assessment also includes obtaining information from the client. The nurse asks whether the client knows the reason for the blood transfusion and whether the client has ever had a transfusion or a transfusion reaction. A client who has had a transfusion reaction is usually at no greater risk for a reaction with a subsequent transfusion. However, the client may be anxious about the transfusion, necessitating nursing intervention.

The pretransfusion assessment also includes a baseline measurement of vital signs. These values must be recorded before giving any blood products because a change in vital signs can indicate a transfusion reaction.

When giving a transfusion, the nurse explains the procedure, asks the client to report any side effects, and makes sure the client has signed an informed consent. The nurse, with another registered nurse, then checks the identity of the blood products, the client, and the compatibility of the blood and the client. The transfusion begins slowly to allow the early detection of a transfusion reaction. The infusion is maintained, side effects are monitored, and the transfusion is recorded.

During the infusion of blood the client is at risk for a reaction, particularly during the first 15 minutes. Therefore the nurse should remain with the client and assess skin color and vital signs (Figure 35-10). The nurse will continue to monitor the client and obtain vital signs periodically during the transfusion as directed by agency policy (often every 15 minutes). The nurse will obtain vital signs more frequently when a transfusion reaction is anticipated or suspected (see Table 35-6). The rate of a transfusion is usually specified in the physician's orders. Ideally a unit of whole blood or packed red blood cells is transfused in 2 hours. This time can be prolonged to 4 hours if the client is at risk for FVE.

When clients have a severe blood loss such as with hemorrhage, they may receive rapid transfusions through a central venous pressure catheter. A blood warming device is often necessary because the tip of the central venous pressure catheter lies in the superior vena cava, above the right atrium. Rapid administration of cold blood can result in cardiac dysrhythmias (LaRocca and Otto, 1989).

TRANSFUSION REACTIONS. A transfusion reaction is a systemic response by the body to blood incompatible with that of the recipient. Causes include red cell incompatibility or allergic sensitivity to the leukocytes, platelets, or plasma protein components of the transfused blood or to the potassium or citrate preservative in the blood. Blood transfusion can also result in the transmission of infectious disease.

table 35-6

ADVERSE REACTIONS TO BLOOD TRANSFUSIONS

Reaction	Mechanism	Onset	Assessment	Prevention	Management
Acute hemolytic	ABO-Rh incompatibility; antibodies in recipient's plasma attach to antigens on transfused RBCs, causing those RBCs to break down.	Immediately	Fever, chills, hypotension, nausea, and vomiting; flushing; tachycardia; tachypnea; anxiety; dyspnea; hemoglobinemia and hemoglobinuria (hemoglobin molecules from the donor blood are released into the bloodstream and eliminated by the kidneys); coagulation disorder, renal failure	Careful identification of client when blood samples obtained for blood typing and when blood is released for transfusion. The most common cause is mistaken identification (Lichtor, 1989)	This is life-threatening: 1. Stop transfusion (see pp. 1068-1070). 2. Maintain IV access. 3. Notify physician and blood bank. 4. Take vital signs every 15 minutes; monitor for shock: decreased blood pressure, tachycardia, tachypnea) 5. Monitor urine output for oliguria (decreased volume and appearance of dark color secondary to hemoglobin being excreted). 6. Obtain blood and urine samples as directed by agency. 7. Return blood bag and tubing to blood bank. 8. Document reaction as directed by agency.
Delayed hemolytic	Recipient has RBC incompatibility to donor's RBC antigens other than ABO antigens because of previous exposure to blood through transfusion or pregnancy.	2 days or more	Continued anemia; hemoglobinuria	Blood bank should do careful cross-matching of donor and recipient blood for subsequent transfusions after first reaction	1. Since it occurs after the transfusion, it can be missed; monitor blood studies for continued anemia. 2. If detected, notify physician and blood bank.
Febrile, nonhemolytic	Antibodies in recipient react to antigens on donor's white blood cells, platelets, or plasma proteins; it is the most common reaction, especially with multiple transfusions or previous pregnancy.	After first 30 minutes to 6 hours after the transfusion	Fever (>1° C), flushing, chills, headache, anxiety, muscle pain	Use leukocyte-poor blood (filtered)	1. Stop transfusion. 2. Administer antipyretics as ordered. 3. Monitor temperature every 4 hours.

Continued.

table 35-6—cont'd

Reaction	Mechanism	Onset	Assessment	Prevention	Management
Circulatory overload	Too rapid infusion expands the vascular volume more than client's heart can tolerate; results in pulmonary edema	Anytime during or immediately after completion of the transfusion	Dyspnea, cough, anxiety, crackles, tachycardia, tachypnea, orthopnea, increased venous pressure	Administer blood or blood component at a rate based on client's size and health status; administer packed red blood cells rather than whole blood, if ordered; minimize amount of 0.9% normal saline used to maintain patency of IV line before and after each unit of blood; minimize the volume of 0.9% normal saline used to dilute packed red blood cells.	1. Elevate client's head. 2. Notify physician. 3. Slow or stop transfusion as ordered. 4. Administer morphine, diuretics, oxygen as ordered.
Sepsis (infection carried through the bloodstream)	Transfusion of blood or blood component contaminated by bacteria or endotoxin	Within 2 hours of transfusion	Chills, fever, vomiting, diarrhea markedly decreased blood pressure, shock	Proper care of blood or blood product from time of donation to end of administration (e.g., maintaining proper temperature of blood, beginning transfusion within 30 minutes of blood leaving blood bank, completing transfusion within 4 hours).	1. Stop transfusion. 2. Obtain culture of client's blood. 3. Monitor vital signs every 15 minutes. 4. Administer antibiotics, IV fluids, vasopressors, steroids as ordered.
Urticaria	Recipient allergy to a plasma protein	During or 1 hour after transfusion	Local flushing, hives, itching	Administer antihistamines before and during transfusion as ordered	1. Stop transfusion. 2. Notify physician and blood bank. 3. Take vital signs every 15 minutes. 4. Administer antihistamines as ordered. 5. Transfusion may be restarted if fever or if pulmonary symptoms are not present.
Anaphylactic	Administration of IgA proteins to IgA-deficient recipient who has developed IgA antibody	Immediately after transfusion begins	Anxiety, urticaria, nausea, vomiting, diarrhea, wheezing, chest pain, hypotension, cardiac arrest	Transfuse washed RBCs with plasma removed; use blood from IgA-deficient donor	This is life-threatening: 1. Stop transfusion. 2. Maintain IV access. 3. Notify physician and blood bank. 4. Take vital signs every 15 minutes.

					5. Administer epinephrine if ordered. 6. Initiate cardiopulmonary resuscitation if necessary.
Graft-versus-host-disease	Normal donor lymphocytes reproduce in a recipient who is immunocompromised (e.g., clients receiving high-dose chemotherapy); the lymphocytes attack the recipient's tissues as foreign proteins	Variable, related to rate of lymphocyte reproduction	Fever; skin rash; diarrhea; infection; liver dysfunction, manifested by jaundice; bone marrow suppression	Administer irradiated blood if ordered; administer saline-washed blood if ordered	1. Administer methotrexate, antithymocytic globulin, corticosteroids if ordered.

Modified from LaRocca J, Otto S: *Pocket guide to intravenous therapy*, St. Louis, 1989, Mosby; National Blood Resource Education Program's Nursing Education Working Group: Transfusion nursing: trends and practices for the '90's, *Am J Nurs* 91(6):42, 1991.

Several types of reactions can result from blood transfusions. General adverse reactions (Table 35-6) range from immediate onset of fever, chills, and skin rash to hypotension, shock, and a delayed reaction that may not occur until several days or weeks after the transfusion.

A second category of reactions includes diseases transmitted by infected blood donors who are asymptomatic. Diseases transmitted through transfusions are malaria, hepatitis, and acquired immunodeficiency syndrome (AIDS). Because all units of blood collected must undergo serological testing and screening for HIV and HBV, the risk of acquiring blood-borne infections from blood transfusions is reduced.

Correct administration of blood and blood products reduces the risk of transfusion reactions. The nurse, although not actually a participant in the blood labeling process, is responsible for determining that the blood delivered to the nursing unit corresponds to the client's blood type as listed in the medical record. Two nurses should check the blood against the client's identification number, blood group, and complete name. If even a minor discrepancy exists, the blood should not be given and the blood bank laboratory should be notified.

In addition to allergic reactions and the transmission of illnesses, certain risks (hyperkalemia, hypocalcemia, and circulatory overload) are associated with blood transfusions. Stored blood may cause hyperkalemia because blood cells break down during storage and potassium is released into the vascular space. The potassium level should be checked frequently for a client who receives several units of blood. If the potassium level is elevated, the client may be given an ion exchange resin such as polystyrene sulfate (Kayexalate).

In some clients, the infusion of blood can result in hypocalcemia because the citrate used as a preservative of the blood combines with the client's ionized calcium (Metheny, 1992). If hypocalcemia occurs, tetany can result. The risk for hypocalcemia increases with the number of blood transfusions the client receives.

Circulatory overload is a risk when a client receives massive whole blood or packed red blood cell transfusions for massive hemorrhagic shock or when a client with normal blood volume receives blood. Clients particularly at risk for circulatory overload are older adults and those with cardiopulmonary diseases.

Blood transfusion reactions are life threatening, but prompt nursing intervention can maintain the client's physiological stability (see Table 35-6):

1. If a blood reaction is suspected, the nurse stops the transfusion immediately.
2. The nurse keeps the IV line open by "piggybacking" 0.9% normal saline into the IV line. The nurse should not turn off the blood and turn on the 0.9% normal saline on the Y-tubing infusion set. This will infuse the blood in the tubing into the client. Even a small amount of mismatched blood can cause a major reaction.

3. The nurse notifies the physician or asks someone to do so.
4. The nurse remains with the client, observing signs and symptoms and monitoring vital signs as often as every 5 minutes.
5. The nurse prepares to administer emergency drugs such as antihistamines, vasopressors, fluids, and steroids.
6. The nurse prepares to perform cardiopulmonary resuscitation.
7. The nurse obtains a urine specimen and sends it to the laboratory.
8. The blood container, tubing, and transfusion record are saved and returned to the laboratory.
9. The nurse must document the transfusion reaction, how it was treated, and the outcome.

Although anaphylactic transfusion reactions are relatively rare, they can occur with any client. Correctly administering blood and blood products prevents reactions that would be caused by giving the client the wrong blood. When a client is having a transfusion reaction, prompt nursing actions can decrease the severity of the response.

Interventions for Acid-Base Imbalances

Nursing interventions to promote acid-base balance are performed to support prescribed medical therapies. Because acid-base disturbances can be life-threatening and require rapid correction, the nurse must maintain a functional IV line and frequently check the physician's orders for new medications or fluids. Prescribed drugs, such as insulin or sodium bicarbonate, and fluid and electrolyte replacement should be given promptly.

The nurse implements the appropriate nursing measures to promote ventilation and oxygenation (see Chapter 34). This is particularly important for the client with respiratory acidosis. Stasis of pulmonary secretions and decreased lung expansion worsen the acidotic condition. Nursing interventions to mobilize pulmonary secretions and promote lung expansion such as encouraging an effective cough and use of an incentive spirometer will be important components of the treatment plan.

For clients with respiratory alkalosis resulting from anxiety, the nurse initiates nursing measures to reduce the anxiety after first correcting respiratory alkalosis. To correct respiratory alkalosis, the nurse instructs the client to breathe into a paper bag. With this method the client rebreathes exhaled carbon dioxide, thereby providing carbon dioxide that combines with water to form carbonic acid, which increases blood acidity. After the respiratory alkalosis is corrected, the client's symptoms disappear. At this point, the nurse may be able to assist the client in determining the cause of anxiety and methods to control it. Some clients with repeated anxiety attacks need counseling, and the nurse should make an appropriate and prompt referral.

The nurse develops interventions to protect the client from complications. Clients with acid-base disturbances usually require repeated arterial blood gas analysis. This procedure provides arterial blood samples for analysis of hydrogen ion concentration.

Arterial Blood Gases. Arterial blood gas determinations require the removal of blood from an artery to determine the client's acid-base status and the adequacy of ventilation and oxygenation. Arterial blood gas samples are drawn from a peripheral artery such as the radial artery or from an arterial line. In some agencies, nurses are responsible for radial artery punctures. Beginning nursing students do not draw arterial blood gas samples but frequently assist in the sampling process and care for the client after the procedure. After the specimen is obtained, care is taken to prevent air from entering the syringe because this will affect the blood gas analysis, the syringe will be submerged in crushed ice to reduce cellular metabolism, and transported immediately to the laboratory. Pressure must be applied to the puncture site for at least 5 minutes to reduce the risk of hematoma formation.

Health Promotion/Restoration Activities for Fluid, Electrolyte, and Acid-Base Balance

Health promotion activities in the areas of fluid, electrolyte, and acid-base imbalances focus on teaching. Clients and care givers need to recognize risk factors for these imbalances and implement appropriate preventive measures. For example, parents of infants need to understand that the gastrointestinal losses of fluids, electrolytes, and bicarbonate or hydrochloric acid can quickly lead to serious imbalances because of the infant's body size and immature adaptive mechanisms. Therefore when vomiting or diarrhea occur in the infant, the parent needs to recognize the risk and promptly seek health care to restore normal balance. Another example is the healthy older adult who can quickly develop imbalances when subjected to elevated environmental temperatures. These persons need to drink appropriate beverages, maintain adequate environmental ventilation, and refrain from excessive activity during times when heat alerts are issued by the local weather department.

Clients with chronic health alterations are at particularly high risk for alterations in fluid, electrolyte, and acid-base disorders. These clients may require hospitalization for restoration of optimal health. They need to understand the risk factors for the development of fluid, electrolyte, and acid-base alterations. For example, the client with renal failure must avoid excess intake of fluid, sodium, potassium, and phosphorus. To implement this regimen and prevent further alterations, this client must recognize that many salt substitutes contain potassium, which should be avoided. Other clients such as those with chronic obstructive pulmonary disease need to understand that a respiratory infection can result in respiratory failure and respiratory acidosis because of impaired gas exchange. These clients must learn to avoid persons with respiratory infections, take flu shots, and seek health care at the first sign of a respiratory infection.

Clients with chronic health alterations also need to recognize the early signs and symptoms indicating the development of an imbalance in the areas of fluid, electrolyte, or acid-base balance. For example, a client with heart failure should be instructed to obtain an accurate body weight each day. This client should recognize that a gain in body weight can indicate fluid retention caused by a worsening of the heart failure. The client should also recognize that increasing shortness of breath, orthopnea, and dependent edema could also be associated with fluid retention.

When clients detect evidence of a developing imbalance, they should know how to treat it. For example, the client with diabetes mellitus who is hyperglycemic is at risk for hyperosmolar fluid imbalance because excess fluid is lost when the kidneys excrete glucose. Clients who can perform routine fingerstick blood glucose determinations can detect the hyperglycemia and adjust their insulin dosage based on the degree of hyperglycemia. It is also important for clients to recognize the need to contact their health care provider.

Activities related to health restoration in the areas of fluid, electrolyte, and acid-base balance can be complex and comprehensive. The first intervention must always be removing or treating the cause of the imbalance, if possible. For example, the client on a mechanical ventilator may experience respiratory alkalosis because of incorrect ventilator settings. In this situation, it would be more effective to determine and maintain optimal ventilator settings than to focus on just treating the respiratory alkalosis. General interventions for fluid, electrolyte, and acid-base disorders include safety measures, skin care, body positioning, and provision of emotional support.

There are dietary implications for most electrolyte disorders and metabolic acid-base imbalances. In addition to food, fluid intake may be encouraged or restricted (see Chapter 31). The client needs to recognize food sources to include and to avoid in the diet. The client must learn to consult lists of the nutrient content of foods and to read the labels of commercially prepared foods. For example, the client on a low-sodium diet needs to be able to consult the dietary information on the package to determine the amount of sodium in a product. The client also needs to recognize that some foods labeled low-sodium do not have added sodium but still contain the sodium naturally occurring in the product. The client must understand that a food such as green peas will have a lower sodium content when fresh (6.0 mg/cup) than canned (372 mg/cup). The nurse can consult with the dietitian to help the client and care giver plan economical meals incorporating the client's preferences and life-style as possible.

Another area involved in health restoration in fluid, electrolyte, and acid-base alterations is medication administration. Medications may be used to treat the underlying health alteration (e.g., digitalis preparations are given to strengthen the heart in heart failure, and insulin is given to lower the blood sugar in diabetes mellitus). Some medications are given as supplements (e.g., potassium, calcium, magnesium, and sodium bicarbonate). Fluids can be given by the oral, tube feeding, or intravenous routes. Another reason for medication administration in these alterations is to prevent complications (e.g., Kayexalate can be given to lower serum potassium and prevent dysrhythmias). Clients need to receive careful instruction concerning the use of over-the-counter medications. For example, certain antacids contain magnesium, which should be avoided by the client with renal failure.

Evaluation

All nursing interventions are evaluated by comparing the client's response to nursing therapy for each goal, which has objective expected outcomes.

Goal: Client's fluid, electrolyte, and acid-base balances are restored and maintained.

Outcome

Vital signs will return to baseline normals

Evaluative measure

Obtain the client's vital signs to screen for tachycardia, bradycardia, hypotension, hypertension, or orthostatic hypotension

Outcome

The client will have normal skin turgor

Evaluative measures

Palpate for poor skin turgor, edema, or weak pulse

Inspect the oral cavity for dry, sticky mucous membranes, decreased saliva, or longitudinal furrows on tongue

Outcome

The client's weight will be stable at baseline normal

Evaluative measure

Determine the client's body weight

Outcome

The client will have no edema

Evaluative measure

Inspect the client for edema or dry skin

Outcome

The client will have clear breath sounds

Evaluative measure
Auscultate for adventitious lung sounds or a third heart sound

Outcome
Serum and urine electrolyte and chemistry results and arterial blood gas values will be normal

Evaluative measures
Assess the client for signs of electrolyte and acid-base imbalance such as positive Chvostek's and Trousseau's sign, cardiac dysrhythmias, convulsions, changes in level of consciousness
Obtain laboratory findings and monitoring for fluid, electrolyte, and acid-base imbalances

Outcome
Urine output will equal intake

Evaluative measure
Measure all routes of intake and output

Goal: Client's imbalances are identified and corrected.

Outcome
The client will experience no vomiting, diarrhea, or other route of abnormal loss

Evaluative measure
Observe the client for vomiting, diarrhea, or wound drainage

Outcome
The client will verbalize the need for and ingest increased fluids and electrolytes during times of severe stress, heat, or strenuous exercise

Evaluative measure
Observe the client to determine understanding of methods to prevent and treat imbalances

Outcome
The client with a chronic illness demonstrates knowledge of methods to use to prevent fluid, electrolyte, and acid-base imbalances

Goal: The client has no complications from therapies to restore balanace.

Outcome
The client will have no evidence of infiltration, phlebitis, or infection at the IV insertion

Evaluative measures
Observe that correct type and amount of fluid has been given
Observe for patent IV catheter or needle as indicated by fluids infusing at prescribed rate and adequate blood return
Palpate IV site for pain, swelling; inspecting for redness, drainage
Inspect the infusion system for the presence of leaks or the introduction of air

Outcome
The client will exhibit no evidence of a blood transfusion reaction (chest pain, change in vital signs)

Evaluative measure
Obtain vital signs and observe for signs of FVD, FVE, or transfusion reaction

SUMMARY

Clients with altered fluid and electrolyte status require nursing care plans designed to assist in restoring normal fluid volume and electrolyte concentrations. The nurse restores fluid balance through oral fluid replacement, administration of IV fluids, or maintenance of fluid restrictions. Electrolytes can be given orally or parenterally. The nurse also treats underlying processes that may cause fluid and electrolyte imbalances.

Acid-base imbalances result from a number of underlying illnesses. With minor imbalances, the body compensates by chemical, biological, and physiological regulatory mechanisms. With more severe imbalances, however, medical and nursing interventions are required because such imbalances are life threatening. Each type of imbalance involves clinical signs and symptoms that the nurse assesses.

When providing care to clients with altered fluid, electrolyte, or acid-base balances, the nurse continually monitors for changes in the client's status and uses all components of the nursing process to maintain and restore balance.

CRITICAL THINKING ACTIVITIES

1. Mr. Jackson is 72 years old. He now has an infection and has had a fever of 102° F for 36 hours. He has been vomiting, and he reports that he has been profusely diaphoretic. What fluid imbalance is he at risk for at this time? What further assessment data is needed to confirm the type of fluid imbalance that he is experiencing?
2. Mrs. Calhoun has heart failure and is taking Lanoxin and Lasix to treat the heart failure. The nurse practitioner managing Mrs. Calhoun's care noted that her serum potassium in March is 3.6 mEq/L and, in consultation with the physician, ordered a potassium supplement to be given. In September of the same year, Mrs. Calhoun is admitted to the hospital because she has fractured her right hip and has a total hip replacement. Three days after surgery, she begins taking oral medications and the Lanoxin, Lasix, and potassium supplement are again ordered. At this time, the nurse notes that Mrs. Calhoun's heart rate is irregular, her previous 24 hour I & O showed intake of 2050 ml and output of 800 ml and that her urine now is very dark amber. What serum electrolyte level should the nurse immediately

check? What other assessment data should the nurse gather? Which medication(s) should be held until the staff nurse consults with Mrs. Calhoun's health care provider?

3. Mr. Norman is 65 years old. He has had diabetes mellitus since he was 10 years old and requires insulin injections twice each day to control the diabetes. He has had an infection for 2 days with a fever of 104° F, and he is admitted to the hospital to determine the cause of the infection. On admission, he is lethargic and arouses to answer questions only with difficulty. It is found that his blood sugar is 680 mg/dl. It is noted that his respirations are 32/minute and deep. His arterial blood gases reveal pH 7.30, $Paco_2$ 28 mm Hg, bicarbonate 15 mEq/L. Which acid-base imbalance does Mr. Norman have? Are his respiratory characteristics a cause or compensatory mechanisms for this imbalance?
4. Mr. Jones is receiving IV fluids because he is NPO after surgery earlier today. His IV fluid order is 1000 ml Lactated Ringer's with 20 mEq KCL to run over 6 hours. What IV tubing should be used to administer these fluids in terms of drop size? The nurse hangs a new bag of IV fluids at 5PM. At 8 PM, the nurse notes that 300 ml have infused from the bag. Are these fluids on time? If not, what assessments should be done to determine the reason?
5. While starting an IV, the nurse begins to advance the ONC and notes that the area immediately around the insertion site is swelling. What should the nurse do?

KEY CONCEPTS

- Body fluids are distributed in extracellular and intracellular fluid compartments.
- Body fluids are composed of electrolytes, minerals, cells, and water.
- Body fluids are regulated through fluid intake, output, and hormonal regulation.
- Volume disturbances include isotonic and osmolar deficits and excesses.
- Electrolytes are regulated by dietary intake and hormonal controls.
- Chronic and serious illnesses increase the risk of fluid, electrolyte, and acid-base imbalances.
- Clients who are very young or very old are at greater risk for fluid, electrolyte, and acid-base imbalances.
- Assessment for fluid, electrolyte, and acid-base alterations includes the nursing history; physical and behavioral assessment; measurements of intake and output; daily weights; specific laboratory data such as measurement of serum osmolality, serum electrolytes, blood urea nitrogen, urine specific gravity, and arterial blood gases.
- Fluid volume deficits and osmolar imbalances can be corrected by enteral or parenteral administration of fluid.
- Common complications of IV therapy include infiltration, phlebitis, infection, fluid volume excess, and bleeding at the infusion site.
- Blood transfusions replace fluid volume lost because of hemorrhage, treat anemia, or replace coagulation factors.
- Administration of blood or blood products requires the nurse to follow a specific procedure to identify transfusion reactions quickly.
- In addition to transfusion reactions, the risks of transfusion include hyperkalemia, hypocalcemia, fluid volume excess, and infection.
- Treatment for electrolyte disturbances includes dietary and pharmacological interventions.
- Acid-base balance depends on the hydrogen ion concentration in the blood.
- Acid-base imbalances are buffered by chemical, biological, and physiological buffering systems, especially the lungs and kidneys.
- The body's chemical buffering system responds first to acid-base abnormalities.
- Respiratory acidosis is characterized by increased carbon dioxide and hydrogen ion concentrations.
- Respiratory alkalosis is characterized by decreased carbon dioxide and hydrogen ion concentrations.
- Metabolic acidosis is characterized by a decrease in bicarbonate level and increase in hydrogen ion concentration.
- Metabolic alkalosis is characterized by an increase in bicarbonate level and decrease in hydrogen ion concentration.
- The goals of therapy for acid-base imbalances are to treat the underlying illness and to restore the arterial pH to normal.

References

Berl T and Schrier RW: Disorders of water balance. In Schrier R, editor: *Renal electrolyte disorders,* ed 3, Boston, 1992, Little, Brown and Co.

Centers for Disease Control: Recommendations for prevention of HIV transmission in health care settings, *MMWR* 36(supplement 2S), 1987.

Cohen DM: A replication study: analysis of bacterial contamination of intravenous administration sets in use for 72 hours, *J New York State Nurses Association* 20(3):12, 1989.

Coulter K: Intravenous therapy for the elder patient: implications for the intravenous nurse, *J Intraven Nurs* 15(supplement):S18-S23, 1992.

Davis M: Fluids, electrolytes, and nutrition in the low–birth-weight infant, *NAACOG's Clin Iss Perinatal Women's Health Nursing* 3(1):45-61, 1992.

DeAngelis R and Lessig L: Hypokalemia, *Critical Care Nurse* 11(7):71-75, 1991.

Drug Facts and Comparisons, St. Louis, JB Lippincott.

Emergency Medicine: New anion-gap reference values 22(9):48-49, 1990.

Goepp JG and Katz SA: Oral rehydration therapy, *Am Fam Phys* 49(4):843-848, 1993.

Gröer MW and Shekleton ME: *Basic pathophysiology: a holistic approach,* St. Louis, 1989, Mosby.

Gröer MW: *Physiology and pathophysiology of body fluids,* St. Louis, 1981, Mosby.

Harig JM and Ramaswamy K: Acute diarrhea in adults: management, with emphasis on oral rehydration therapy, *Postgrad Med* 86(8):131-146, 1989.

Horne MM et al.: *Fluid, electrolyte, and acid-base balance: a case study approach,* St. Louis, 1991, Mosby.

Kee CC: Age-related changes in the renal system: causes, consequences, and nursing implications, *Geriatric Nurs* 13(2):80-93, 1992.

Kokko JP and Tannen RL: *Fluids and electrolytes,* Philadelphia, 1990, WB Saunders.

LaRocca JC and Otto SE: *Pocket guide to intravenous therapy,* St. Louis, 1989, Mosby.

Lichtor J: Transfusion reactions, part 1: *Current Reviews for Post Anesthesia Care Nurses* 11(6):41, 1989.

Maki DG and Ringer M: Risk factors for infusion-related phlebitis with small peripheral venus catheters: a randomized controlled trial, *Ann Intern Med* 114(10):845-854, 1991.

Maki DG et al.: Prospective study of replacing administration sets for intravenous therapy at 48- vs. 72-hour intervals: 72 hours is safe and cost-effective, *JAMA* 258(13):1777-1781, 1987.

Maki DG and Ringer M: Evaluation of dressing regimens for prevention of infection with peripheral intravenous catheters: gauze, a transparent polyurethane dressing, and an iodophor-transparent dressing, *JAMA* 258(17):2396-2403, 1987.

Martin E et al.: Autotransfusion systems (ATS), *Crit Care Nurse* 9(7):65-73, 1989.

McCance KL and Huether SE: *Pathophysiology: the biologic basis for disease in adults and children,* ed 2, St. Louis, 1994, Mosby.

Messner RL and Pinkerman ML: Preventing a peripheral IV infection, *Nursing 92* 22(6):34-42, 1992.

Metheny NM: *Fluid and electrolyte balance: nursing considerations,* ed 3, Philadelphia, 1992, JB Lippincott.

Millam DA: Controlling the flow: electronic infusion devices, *Nursing 90* 20(8):65-68, 1990.

Millam DA: Tips for improving your venipuncture techniques, *Nursing 87* 17(6):46-49, 1987.

Mollohan J and Riddle II: Fluid balance in infants and children. In Metheny N, editor: *Fluid and electrolyte balance: nursing considerations,* ed 3, Philadelphia, 1992, JB Lippincott.

National Blood Resource Education Program's Nursing Education Working Group: Transfusion nursing: trends and practices for the '90's, *Am J Nurs* 91(6):42-56, 1991.

Occupational safety and health act: bloodborne pathogens, *Fed Reg* 56(235):64175, Dec. 6, 1991.

Peterson KJ: Nursing management of autologous blood transfusion, *J Intraven Nurs* 15(3):128-134, 1992.

Phillips LD: *Manual of IV therapeutics,* Philadelphia, 1993, FA Davis.

Porth CM and Erickson M: Physiology of thirst and drinking: implication for nursing practice, *Heart Lung* 21(3):273-284, 1992.

Price SA and Wilson LM: *Pathophysiology: clinical concepts of disease processes,* ed 3, St. Louis, 1992, Mosby.

Roth D: Intravenous therapy. In Metheny NM, editor: *Fluid and electrolyte balance: nursing considerations,* ed 3, Philadelphia, 1992, JB Lippincott.

Schauf CL et al.: *Human physiology: foundations and frontiers,* St. Louis, 1990, Times Mirror/Mosby College Publishing.

Silvestri A and Masoorli S: PICC lines: a new dimension in home health care, *J Home Health Care Practice* 2(4):1-28, 1990.

Bibliography

Anderson S: ABG's six easy steps to interpreting blood gases, *Am J Nurs* 90(8):42-45, 1990.

Baldwin DR: Management of intravenous hazardous materials and hazardous wastes in the work environment, *J Intraven Nurs* 15(2):90-99, 1992.

Baranowski L: Current trends in blood component therapy: the evolution of a safer, more effective product, *J Intraven Nurs* 15(3):136-151, 1992.

Batcheller J: Disorders of antidiuretic hormone secretion, *AACN's Clin Iss Crit Care Nurs* 3(20):370-378, 1992.

Bostrom-Ezrati J et al.: Intravenous therapy management: who will develop insertion site symptoms? *App Nurs Res* 3(4):146-152, 1990.

Bowles K, Lynch M: These products and procedures prevent needlesticks, *RN* 55(7):42-45, 1992.

Calhoun KA: Serum potassium concentration abnormalities, *Crit Care Nurs Q* 13(3):34-38, 1990.

Carstens VL, Earnshaw PH: Postoperative orthopedic autotransfusion, *Assoc Oper Room Nurs J* 56(2):272-280, 1992.

Frederick V: Pediatric IV therapy: soothing the patient, *RN* 54(12):40-42, 1991.

Freedman BI, Burkart JM: Hypokalemia, *Crit Care Clin* 7(1):143-153, 1991.

Friday BA, Reinhart RA: Magnesium metabolism: a case report and literature review, *Crit Care Nurse* 11(5):62-72, 1991.

Gerberding JL: Current epidemiologic evidence and case reports of occupationally acquired HIV and other bloodborne diseases, *Infect Control Hosp Epidem* 11(10):557-562, 1990.

Gloe D: Common reactions to transfusion, *Heart Lung* 20(5):506-514, 1991.

Hutchinson D: Pediatric IV therapy: starting the line, *RN* 54(12):43-48, 1991.

Innerarity SA: Hyperkalemic emergencies, *Crit Care Nurs Q* 14(4):32-39, 1992.

Johnson GM, Bowman RJ: Autologous blood transfusion: current trends, nursing implications, *Assoc Oper Room Nurs J* 56(2):282-296, 1992.

Isley WL: Serum sodium concentration abnormalities, *Crit Care Nurs Q* 13(3):82-88, 1990.

Kositzke JA: A question of balance: dehydration in the elderly, *J Gerontol Nurs* 16(5):4-11, 1992.

Kuhn MM: Colloids vs. crystalloids, *Crit Care Nurs* 11(5):37-51, 1991.

Lenox AC: IV therapy: reducing the risk of infection, *Nurs 90* 20(3):60-61, 1990.

Metheny NM: Why worry about IV fluids? *Am J Nurs* 90(6):50-57, 1990.

Millam DA: Starting IVs: how to develop your venipuncture expertise, *Nurs 92* 22(9):33-46, 1992.

Nentwich PF: Selecting the best IV site for your patient, *Nurs 91* 21(6):32C, 32F, 32H, 1991.

Oldman P: A sticky situation? microbiological study of adhesive tape used to secure IV cannulae, *Prof Nurs* 6(5):265-269, 1991.

Querin JJ, Stahl LD: 12 simple, sensible steps for successful blood transfusions, *Nurs 90* 20(10):70-81, 1990.

Rice V: Parenteral fluids: part one–an overview, *Can Intraven Nurs* 6(2):6-8, 1990.

Rice V: Parenteral fluids: part two–specifics of replacement therapy, *Can Intraven Nurs* 6(3):6-7, 1990.

Sommer M: Rapid fluid resuscitation: how to correct dangerous deficits, *Nurs 90* 20(1):52-59, 1990.

Sympson GM: CATR: a new generation of autologous blood transfusion, *Crit Care Nurs* 11(4):60-64, 1991.

Tietjen SD: Starting an infant's IV, *Am J Nurs* 90(5):44-47, 1990.

Walpert N: An orderly look at calcium metabolism disorders, *Nurs 90* 20(7):60-64, 1990.

Weldy NJ: *Body fluids and electrolytes,* ed 6, St. Louis, 1992, Mosby.

Woodtli AO: Thirst: a critical care nursing challenge, *Dimensions Crit Care Nurs* 9(1):6-15, 1990.

Workman ML: Magnesium and phosphorus: the neglected electrolytes, *AACN's Clin Iss Crit Care Nurs* 3(3):655-663, 1992.

Yeates S, Blaufuss J: Managing the patient in diabetic ketoacidosis, *Focus Crit Care* 17(3):240-248, 1990.

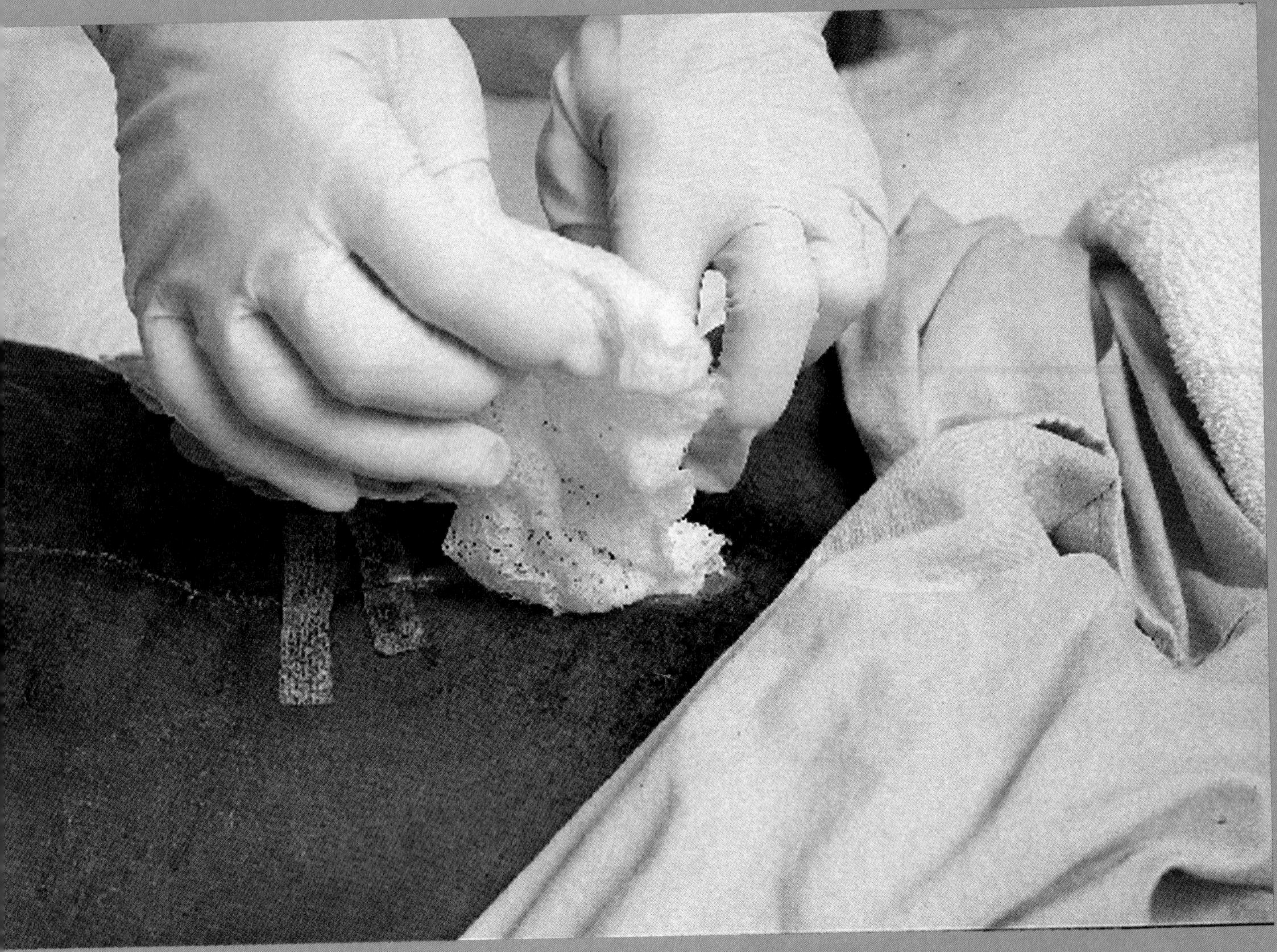

unit seven

SPECIAL NEEDS

36

Surgical Client

OBJECTIVES

Mastery of content in this chapter will enable the student to:

- Define the key terms listed.
- Explain the concept of perioperative nursing care.
- Differentiate between classifications of surgery and types of anesthesia.
- List factors to include in the preoperative assessment of a surgical client.
- Design a preoperative teaching plan.
- Prepare a client for surgery.
- Explain the differences in caring for the client undergoing outpatient surgery versus the client undergoing inpatient surgery.
- Identify key intraoperative nursing diagnoses.
- Develop an intraoperative care plan.
- Identify factors to include in the assessment of a client in postoperative recovery.
- Describe the rationale for nursing interventions designed to prevent postoperative complications.

KEY TERMS

anesthetic
antiembolism stockings
circulating nurse
endotracheal tube
general anesthesia
nasogastric tube
operating room
outpatient
perioperative nursing
postanesthesia care unit
preoperative teaching
presurgical care unit
regional anesthesia
scrub nurse

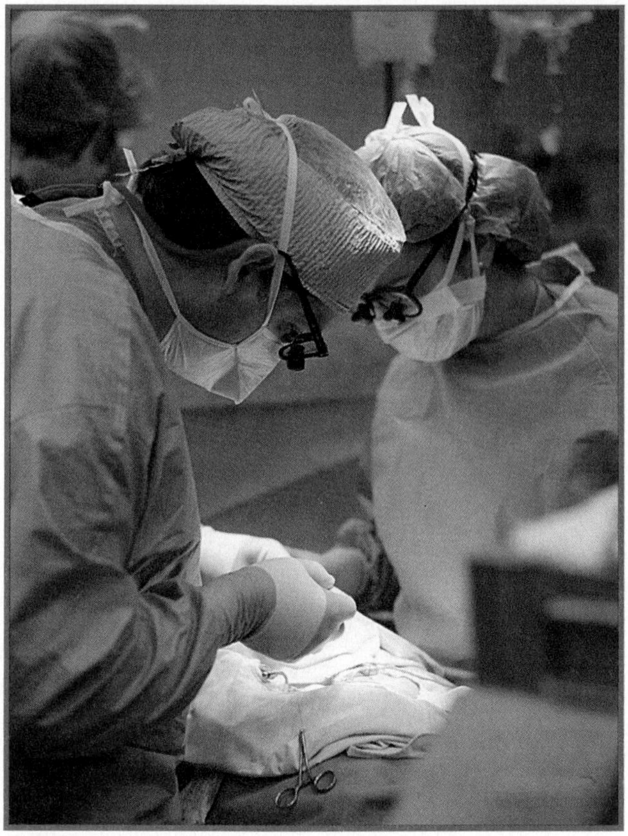

A client faces physiological and psychological stressors when confronting surgery. The trauma of surgery is physically demanding, and anesthesia alters the ability to adapt to these demands. Surgical clients require close monitoring and skilled intervention by the nurse and the physician. Anticipating surgery causes fear and anxiety for many clients, who tend to associate surgery with pain, possible disfigurement, dependence, and perhaps even loss of life. Family members may fear a disruption in their lives and feel powerless as surgery approaches. The nurse can provide psychological support for the client and family. They are better able to cooperate and participate in the care plan if the nurse has provided information about events surrounding surgery.

Surgery is performed in a variety of settings including hospitals, ambulatory surgery centers, clinics, physicians' offices, and even mobile units. The majority of surgeries are performed on an outpatient basis, with the client entering the setting, undergoing surgery, and being discharged the same day. Other clients enter the setting as outpatients and are admitted to the hospital after surgery. Only clients requiring extensive preoperative care are admitted to the hospital before surgery. Nurses working in a variety of settings must understand the principles of caring for perioperative clients.

PERIOPERATIVE NURSING CARE

Perioperative nursing refers to the role of the operating room nurse during the preoperative, intraoperative, and postoperative phases of a client's surgical experience. The concept of perioperative nursing stresses the importance of providing continuity of care for the surgical client using the nursing process. In many hospitals, perioperative nurses assess a client's health status preoperatively, identify specific client needs, teach and counsel, attend to the client's needs in the operating room, and then follow the client's recovery. However, in other institutions, different nurses care for the surgical client during each phase of the surgical experience. Involving an operating room nurse in all phases of the surgical experience ensures continuity of care for the client. The nurse's major responsibility is safe, consistent, and effective nursing care during each phase of surgery.

CLASSIFICATION OF SURGERY

Surgical procedures are classified according to the client's admission status, urgency, and purpose of surgery (Table 36-1). The same type of surgery can be found in all three classes. The classifications may also overlap: an elective procedure may be outpatient and diagnostic, or the same procedure may be performed for different reasons on different clients. The classification indicates to the nurse the type of care a client might require.

PREOPERATIVE SURGICAL PHASE

Surgical clients enter the health care setting in different stages of health. A client may enter the facility feeling relatively healthy while awaiting elective surgery or may be in much distress when facing emergency surgery. Many tests and procedures may be needed to ensure that surgery is indicated, and that the client is in optimum condition for surgery. During these tests and procedures the client meets many health care personnel, all of whom play a role in care and recovery. Family members or friends also play an important role by providing support through their presence, but they also face many of the same stressors as the client.

Clients may undergo preoperative preparation several days before the day of surgery. Preadmission testing may be done in the hospital, physician's office, or outpatient laboratory (Figure 36-1). With this testing already done, the client anticipating surgery usually enters the hospital the day surgery is performed. Many hospitals have special outpatient or "ambulatory" surgery units, where clients come to the hospital,

table 36-1

CLASSIFICATION OF SURGICAL PROCEDURES

Type	Description	Examples
ADMISSION STATUS		
Outpatient	Client enters setting, undergoes surgery, and is discharged same day	Tympanostomy, breast biopsy; cataract extraction; laparoscopy for tubal ligation
23-hour stay	Client enters hospital, undergoes surgery or procedure, released within 24 hours of the night's stay	Arthroscopy, retinal surgery, cholelaparoscopy
Same-day admit	Client enters hospital and undergoes surgery on the same day admitted to hospital	Abdominal hysterectomy, mastectomy, total hip arthroplasty, shoulder repair
Inpatient	Client is admitted to hospital, undergoes surgery, and remains in the hospital afterwards	Internal fixation of a fractured hip; kidney transplant, resection of an aortic aneurysm
URGENCY		
Elective	Performed on basis of client's choice; not essential and may not be necessary for physical health	Bunionectomy, tendon release, breast reconstruction
Urgent	Necessary for client's physical health; may prevent additional problems from developing (e.g., tissue destruction or impaired organ function)	Cholecystectomy for gallstones, vascular repair of obstructed vein, colon resection for bowel obstruction
Emergent	Must be done immediately to save client's life or to preserve body part	Removal of a ruptured appendix, repair of a traumatic amputation, control of internal hemorrhage, removal of tumor
PURPOSE		
Diagnostic	Involves surgical exploration that allows surgeon to make diagnosis; may involve removal of tissue for testing	Exploratory laparotomy, breast biopsy, bronchoscopy
Ablative	Excision or removal of diseased body part	Amputation, appendectomy, cholecystectomy; mastectomy
Palliative	Relieves or reduces intensity of disease symptoms	Colostomy, debridement of necrotic tissue, debulking of malignant tumor
Constructive	Restores function lost or reduced as result of congenital anomaly	Repair of cleft palate, closure of atrial septal heart defect
Reconstructive	Restores function or appearance reduced or lost as result of trauma or disease process.	Internal fixation of a fracture, scar revision, breast reconstruction
Transplant	Implantation of tissue or organ from another person or animal to replace malfunctioning organs or structures	Kidney, liver, heart, or cornea replacement

undergo surgery, and return home on the same day. Outpatient surgery is also done in freestanding clinics and ambulatory surgery centers. The more traditional preoperative routine involves the client entering the hospital the day before surgery. Regardless of the method of entry into the health care setting, the nurse must be able to properly prepare the client for surgery.

The nurse's role in the preoperative surgical phase is to assess the client's physical and emotional well-being, recognize the degree of surgical risk, coordinate diagnostic tests, and identify nursing diagnoses reflecting client and family needs. This information is then used to prepare the client physically and mentally for surgery, and to communicate pertinent information to surgical team members.

NURSING PROCESS

Assessment

The nurse's assessment of the surgical client involves obtaining a nursing history, performing a physical ex-

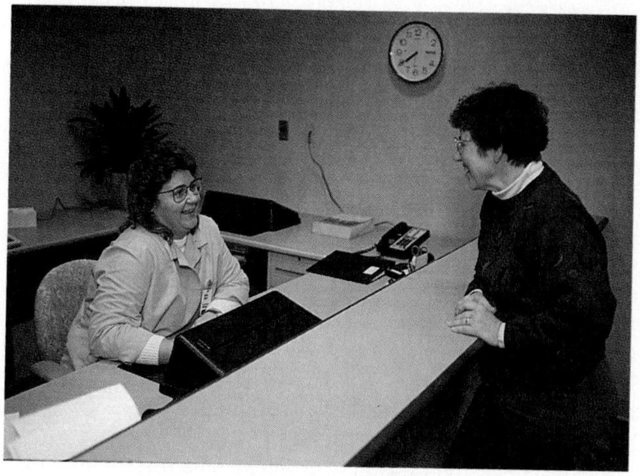

FIGURE 36-1 Client entering preadmission testing area.

amination, reviewing the client's and family members' emotional health, and analyzing risk factors and diagnostic data. The assessment establishes normal values for the client and alerts the nurse to special needs and possible postoperative complications (e.g., infection, impaired skin integrity).

Nursing History. The nurse collects a history similar to that described in Chapter 7. Key elements pertain to the surgical client's needs. In the ambulatory surgical setting, the history may be less involved than that collected when the client is hospitalized the evening before surgery. If a client is unable to relate all the necessary information, the nurse interviews family members or friends.

MEDICAL HISTORY. Preexisting illnesses can influence the client's ability to tolerate anesthesia and surgery, and reach full recovery (Table 36-2). A review of the client's medical history should include past illnesses and the primary reason for seeking medical care. Candidates for ambulatory surgery should also be screened for major medical conditions that may increase the risk of complications. If at increased risk, surgery as an outpatient may not be advisable.

PREVIOUS SURGERIES. A past experience with surgery can indicate physical and psychological responses to a procedure and alert the nurse to special needs and risk factors. Complications such as anaphylaxis or malignant hyperpyrexia (see Chapter 15) during previous surgery alert the nurse to the need for preventive measures and emergency equipment. A history of postoperative complications such as persistent vomiting or excessive pain alerts the nurse to the need for different medications. Severe anxiety before a previous surgery may indicate the need for additional emotional support.

CLIENTS' AND FAMILY MEMBERS' PERCEPTIONS AND UNDERSTANDING OF SURGERY. Identifying the client's perceptions and expectations allows the nurse to plan teaching and emotional preparation measures. When

table 36-2

MEDICAL CONDITIONS THAT INCREASE THE RISKS OF SURGERY

Type of condition	Reason for risk
Bleeding disorder (e.g., thrombocytopenia, leukemia, bone marrow depression from chemotherapy)	Increases risk of hemorrhaging during and after surgery (Murray, 1992)
Cardiac disease (e.g., recent myocardial infarction, dysrhythmias, congestive heart failure)	Stress of surgery causes increased demands on myocardium to maintain cardiac output; increases the risk of myocardial infarction (Detsky, 1986)
Chronic respiratory disease (e.g., emphysema, bronchitis, asthma)	Increases risk of hypoventilation and spasms of bronchus or larynx; reduces client's ability to compensate for acid-base alterations (Boysen, 1992)
Diabetes mellitus (advanced)	Increases susceptibility to infection and may impair wound healing from altered glucose metabolism and associated circulatory impairment; high or low blood sugar levels may cause central nervous system malfunction during surgery, including stroke (Sieber, et al., 1989; Sieber and Toung, 1989)
Liver disease	Alters metabolism and elimination of drugs administered during surgery; decreases liver function postoperatively (Greene, 1981)
Kidney disease	Increases risk of death caused by bleeding, cardiovascular dysfunction; predisposes to hypoventilation, changes in blood pressure, fluid and electrolyte imbalances, infection (Pinson, et al., 1986)
Uncontrolled hypertension	Increases risk for hypotension intraoperatively, which can lead to renal and cardiac damage (Hulyalkar and Miller, 1992)
Upper respiratory infection (during last 4 weeks)	Increases risk of bronchospasm, laryngospasm, hypoventilation (Hinkle, 1989)

table 36-3

DRUGS WITH SPECIAL IMPLICATIONS FOR THE SURGICAL CLIENT

Drug class	Effects during surgery
Antibiotics	Potentiate action of anesthetic agents
Antidysrhythmics	Can reduce cardiac contractility and impair conduction during anesthesia
Anticoagulants	Alter normal clotting factors and thus increase risk of hemorrhaging Should be discontinued at least 48 hours preoperatively Can further alter clotting mechanisms if commonly used medications, aspirin and ibuprofen, are used.
Anticonvulsants	Can alter metabolism of anesthetic agents after long-term use of certain anticonvulsants (e.g., phenytoin [Dilantin] and phenobarbital)
Antihypertensives	Interact with anesthetic agents to cause bradycardia, hypotension, and impaired circulation Inhibit synthesis and storage of norepinephrine in sympathetic nerve endings
Corticosteroids	With prolonged use, cause adrenal atrophy, which reduces body's ability to withstand stress Can temporarily increase doses before and during surgery
Insulin	Diabetic client's need for insulin preoperatively is reduced because client fasts Can increase dose requirements postoperatively because of stress response and IV administration of glucose solutions
Diuretics	Potentiate electrolyte imbalances (particularly potassium) after surgery

the nurse first assesses the client, the reasons for surgery may be unclear. A client may be admitted to a surgical nursing unit before the need for surgery has been determined. Often the client must undergo diagnostic tests before the surgeon determines the exact type of surgery required. Clients and family members may often have misconceptions about surgery.

The nurse faces an ethical dilemma when a client is unaware of the real reason for surgery. The nurse should confer with the physician before revealing specific information related to the medical diagnosis to prevent confusion and to alert the physician if clarification is needed. When a client is well prepared and knows what to expect, the nurse reinforces the client's knowledge and maintains accuracy and consistency.

MEDICATION HISTORY. If a client regularly uses prescription or over-the-counter medications, the physician may decide to temporarily discontinue the drugs before surgery or adjust the doses (Table 36-3). However, most clients undergoing outpatient surgery take their usual oral medications with a sip of water the morning of surgery. If the client is undergoing inpatient surgery, all prescription drugs taken before surgery are automatically discontinued after surgery unless a physician reorders them.

ALLERGIES. The nurse is particularly alert for allergies to drugs that may be given during any phase of the surgical experience, to antiseptics used to prepare the skin for surgery, and to latex. If one or more allergies exist, the client receives an allergy identification band to be worn before going to surgery. The nurse also makes sure that the front of the client's chart contains a list of all allergies.

SMOKING HABITS. The client who smokes is at a greater risk for postoperative pulmonary complications than a nonsmoker. The chronic smoker already has an increased amount and thickness of mucous secretions in the lungs. General **anesthetics** stimulate pulmonary secretions, which are retained due to reduced ciliary activity. Smoke also causes local irritation to the tracheobronchial mucosa, and exposure to general anesthetic agents worsens this irritation. After surgery the client who smokes has greater difficulty clearing the airways of mucous secretions and is at increased risk of a laryngospasm.

ALCOHOL INGESTION. Habitual use of alcohol predisposes the client to adverse reactions to anesthetic drugs. The client also experiences a cross-tolerance to anesthetic drugs, necessitating higher than normal doses. The physician and nurse must also be alert for an increased need for postoperative analgesics.

FAMILY SUPPORT. The nurse determines the extent of the client's support from family members or friends. Surgery often results in temporary disability that requires assistance from significant others during recovery. The client cannot always immediately assume the same level of physical activity and often returns home with dressings to change or exercises to perform following ambulatory surgery. Clients and families assume responsibility for postoperative care. The family is an important resource to the client with physical limitations and provides the emotional support needed to motivate the client to return to a previous state of health.

OCCUPATION. Surgery may result in physical alterations that hinder or prevent a person from returning to work. The nurse assesses the client's occupational history to anticipate the effects surgery might have on convalescence and eventual work performance. This prepares the nurse to explain any restrictions the client may have when returning to work. When a client is unable to return to a previous line of work, the nurse may refer the client to a social worker. The client obtains knowledge of job training programs or help in seeking economic assistance.

REVIEW OF EMOTIONAL HEALTH. Surgery causes anxiety for most clients. The client is concerned about the surgery and whether it will improve health. Hospitalization and the recovery period may be lengthy and costly. Clients often feel they have little control over their situation. Family members perceive the client's surgery as a disruption in their lives. The family may be concerned about the client's return to a normal productive life. When the client has a chronic illness, the family becomes fearful that surgery may result in further disability. To understand the impact surgery has on a client's and family's emotional health, the nurse assesses the client's feelings about surgery, self-concept, coping resources, and body image.

FEELINGS. The nurse may be able to detect the client's feelings about having surgery from many mannerisms or behaviors. A client who is fearful often asks many questions, seems uneasy when strangers enter the room, or actively seeks the company of friends and relatives.

It is often difficult to assess feelings thoroughly when ambulatory surgery is scheduled. The nurse usually has limited time for establishing a relationship with the client. In most outpatient surgical programs, the nurse telephones the client at home before surgery or interviews the client during a preadmission testing visit. For hospital inpatients, the nurse should choose a time for discussion after preliminary admitting or diagnostic tests have been completed. The nurse explains it is normal to have fears and concerns. The client's ability to share these feelings depends in part on the nurse's willingness to ask questions, listen, be supportive, and clarify misconceptions.

If the client feels powerless, the nurse determines the reason. Perhaps the client's medical diagnosis generates apprehension of increased dependence and loss of physical or mental function. The thought of being "put to sleep" with anesthesia creates concern about loss of control. Many clients need to retain the power to make decisions about treatment. The nurse reinforces the client's right to ask questions and participate in decision making.

A client may be angry about the need for surgery. For example, a young person may feel it is unfair to have a disorder that typically affects older people. Surgery may be inconvenient or potentially disruptive. The client may express anger by verbally attacking the nurse or physician or by being argumentative or overly demanding, refusing to cooperate, and criticizing the nurse's efforts to provide care.

COPING RESOURCES. Assessment of feelings and self-concept will help to reveal whether the client has the ability to cope with the stress of surgery. It is also valuable to ask the client about stress management. If the client has had previous surgery, the nurse determines the behaviors that helped to resolve past tension or nervousness. The nurse may instruct the client on relaxation exercises (see Chapter 26), which can help to control anxiety.

The nurse determines if family members or friends can provide support. The client may want a family member or friend present when the nurse provides instructions, explanations, or preoperative care. If a client is undergoing outpatient surgery, it is important that the person who will be caring for the client be taught these responsibilities also.

BODY IMAGE. Surgical removal of a diseased tissue often leaves permanent disfigurement or alteration in body function. Concern over mutilation or loss of a body part compounds a client's fears. The nurse determines the body image alterations the client perceives will result from surgery. Individuals react differently, depending on age, culture, occupation, self-image, and degree of self-esteem.

Surgery often changes the physical or psychological aspects of a client's sexuality. The excision of breast tissue, a colostomy or a ureterostomy, or the removal of the prostate gland may affect a person's sexuality. Other surgeries such as a hernia repair or a cervical conization force clients to temporarily refrain from sexual intercourse.

The nurse should encourage clients to express concerns about sexuality. The client facing even temporary sexual dysfunction requires understanding and support. Discussions about sexuality should be held with the client's sexual partner so he or she can gain a shared understanding of how to cope with limitations in sexual function.

Physical Examination. The nurse conducts a partial or complete physical examination, depending on setting and the nature of the surgery (Chapter 16). The assessment focuses on findings related to the client's medical history and on body systems that will be affected by anesthesia and surgery.

GENERAL SURVEY. The nurse observes the client's general appearance. Gestures and body movements may reflect energy or weakness caused by illness. Height and body weight are important indicators of nutritional status and are used to calculate medication dosages.

Preoperative assessment of vital signs, including blood pressure while sitting and standing, provides an important baseline with which to compare alterations that occur during and after surgery. Anxiety and fear commonly cause elevations in heart rate and blood pressure. Anesthetic agents typically depress all vital functions; however, adverse drug reactions may include elevations in heart rate and blood pressure. As the effects of anesthesia diminish after surgery, the nurse closely monitors vital signs and compares them with preoperative baselines.

Preoperative assessment of vital signs is also important to rule out fluid and electrolyte abnormalities (see Chapter 35). An elevated heart rate may result from a plasma fluid volume deficit or sodium excess. If the pulse is full and bounding, a fluid volume excess may be the cause. Cardiac dysrhythmias are commonly caused by electrolyte imbalances including potassium deficit or excess.

An elevated temperature is cause for concern. If the client has an underlying infection, surgery may be postponed until the infection has been treated. An elevated body temperature also alters drug metabolism and increases the risk of fluid and electrolyte imbalance.

Head and neck. To rule out the possibility of local or systemic infection, the nurse palpates for cervical lymph node enlargement. Inspection of the soft palate and nasal sinuses can reveal sinus drainage indicating respiratory or sinus infection.

The nurse inspects the jugular veins for distention. An excess of fluid within the circulatory system or failure of the heart to contract efficiently may lead to jugular vein distention. A client with known heart disease is at risk for dysrhythmias or other cardiovascular complications during surgery.

The condition of oral mucous membranes reveals the client's level of hydration. A dehydrated client is at risk for developing serious fluid and electrolyte imbalances during and after surgery. Loose or capped teeth must be identified because they can become dislodged during endotracheal intubation. Dentures must be noted so that they can be protected from loss or damage.

Integument. The nurse carefully inspects the skin overlying all body parts, especially bony prominences such as elbows, the sacrum, or scapula. The overall condition of the skin also reveals the client's level of hydration. During surgery a client must lie in a fixed position, often for several hours. Thus a client is susceptible to skin breakdown (see Chapter 24) if the skin is thin, dry or has poor turgor.

Thorax and lungs. Assessment of the client's breathing pattern and chest excursion will aid the nurse in determining ventilatory capacity. A decline in ventilatory function may place the client at risk for respiratory complications. Auscultation of breath sounds will indicate whether the client has pulmonary congestion or narrowing of the airways. Crackles or rales signify moisture in the bronchi or alveoli, which will be aggravated during surgery. Serious pulmonary congestion may cause postponement of surgery. If the nurse auscultates wheezing in the airways before surgery, the client is at increased risk for airway narrowing during anesthesia and surgery (Boysen, 1989).

Heart and vascular system. The nurse assesses the character of the apical pulse to assist in determining the cardiac status of the client. After surgery, the nurse compares the rate and rhythm of the pulse with preoperative baselines. Anesthetic agents, alterations in fluid balance, and stimulation from the surgical stress response can cause cardiac dysrhythmias (Detsky, 1986).

The nurse assesses peripheral pulses and the color and temperature of extremities to determine a client's circulatory status. This assessment is particularly important for the client undergoing vascular surgery, surgery on an extremity using a tourniquet, or when constricting bandages or casts will be applied to an extremity after surgery. The postoperative color changes, a change in sensation, or development of a weak or absent pulse in a client who had adequate circulation before surgery indicates impaired circulation. Prior vascular surgery with implanted grafts should be noted to plan for modified surgical positioning.

Abdomen. The nurse assesses the client's abdomen for size, shape, symmetry, and distention. If the client has abdominal surgery, the nurse makes frequent postoperative assessments of the abdominal incision and compares findings with preoperative data. Alteration in gastrointestinal function after surgery may result in decreased or absent bowel sounds and distention. The nurse should know whether the client is simply obese or the abdomen has become distended.

Assessment of preoperative bowel sounds is likewise useful as a baseline. The nurse also determines whether the client has regular bowel movements. If surgery requires manipulation of portions of the gastrointestinal tract or if a general anesthetic is used, normal peristalsis will not return and bowel sounds will be absent or diminished for several days.

Neurological status. During the health history and physical assessment, the nurse observes the client's level of orientation, alertness, and mood, noting whether the client answers questions appropriately and is able to recall recent and past events. While the client answers questions, the nurse notes the quality of the speech and any facial drooping. A client scheduled for surgery for a neurological disease (e.g., brain tumor or aneurysm) may demonstrate an impaired level of consciousness or altered behavior. A client's level of consciousness will change as a result of general anesthesia. However, after the effects of anesthesia disappear, the client should return to the preoperative level of responsiveness.

If the client will have spinal or epidural anesthesia, preoperative assessment of gross motor function and strength is important. These types of regional anesthesia cause temporary paralysis of the lower extremities. If the client enters surgery with weakness or impaired mobility of the lower extremities, the nurse should be aware of this to avoid becoming alarmed when full motor function does not return immediately after the procedure.

Risk Factors. Various conditions and factors increase the risk for physical problems during surgery. Knowledge of risk factors enables the nurse to take necessary precautions in planning a client's care.

Age. Very young and older clients are at greater surgical risk as a result of an immature or a declining physiological status. During surgery, nurses and physicians are especially concerned with maintaining normal body temperature. When compared with an adult, an infant has proportionately greater surface area and less subcutaneous fat, placing these clients at risk for wide temperature variations. Anesthesia adds to the risk, because anesthetics can cause vasodilation and heat loss. General anesthetics also inhibit shivering, a protective reflex to maintain body temperature.

During surgery, an infant has difficulty in maintaining a normal circulatory blood volume. The total blood volume of infants is considerably less than that of older children and adults. Even a small amount of blood loss can be serious. A reduced circulatory volume makes it difficult for the infant to respond to the need for increased oxygen. Fluid loss and replacement must be closely monitored. Too little fluid places the infant at risk of dehydration. However, if blood or fluids are replaced too quickly, overhydration may occur.

With advancing age a client's physical capacity to adapt to the stress of surgery is hampered because of deterioration of certain body functions. Fluid balance may be difficult to maintain because of renal or cardiopulmonary disease. Despite the risk, the majority of clients undergoing surgery are older adults. Table 36-4 summarizes physiological factors that place older adult clients at risk for surgery.

Nutrition. Normal tissue repair and resistance to infection depend on adequate nutrition. Surgery intensifies the need for nutrients. Postoperatively a client requires adequate calories to ensure a positive nitrogen balance (Chapter 31). A malnourished client is prone to improper wound healing, reduced energy stores, and infection after surgery. If a client has elective surgery, nutrient imbalances can be corrected preoperatively. However, if a malnourished client requires emergency surgery, efforts to restore necessary nutrients must occur postoperatively.

Obesity. Obesity increases surgical risk. An obese client usually has reduced ventilatory and cardiac function and has difficulty in resuming normal physical activity. The position required for surgery may further limit the obese client's ventilation. The excess weight placed on skin over bony prominences may restrict blood flow and may result in skin impairment. The obese client is susceptible to poor wound healing and wound infection because of the structure of fatty tissue, which contains a poor blood supply. The fatty tissue structure slows the delivery of essential nutrients, antibodies, and enzymes needed for healing. It is also often difficult to close the surgical wound of an obese client because of the thick adipose layer. An obese client also is at risk for dehiscence (see Chapter 37).

Radiotherapy. Radiotherapy is often given before surgery for the client with cancer to reduce the size of the cancerous tumor so it can be removed surgically. Radiation has some unavoidable effects on normal tissue, such as excess thinning of skin layers, destruction of collagen, and impaired vascularization of tissue (Frogge, 1982). Ideally the surgeon waits to perform surgery 4 to 6 weeks after the completion of radiation treatments; otherwise the client faces serious wound healing problems.

Fluid and electrolyte balance. The body responds to surgery as a form of trauma. As a result of the adrenocortical stress response, hormonal reactions cause sodium and water retention and potassium loss within the first 2 to 5 days after surgery. Protein breakdown creates a negative nitrogen balance. The severity of the stress response influences the degree of fluid and electrolyte imbalance. The more extensive the surgery, the more severe the stress. A client who is hypovolemic or who has serious electrolyte alterations preoperatively is at significant risk during and after surgery. For example, an excess or depletion of potassium preoperatively increases the chance of dysrhythmias developing during or after surgery. If the client has preexisting renal, gastrointestinal, or cardiovascular abnormalities, the risk of fluid and electrolyte alterations is even greater.

Diagnostic Screening. Before a client has surgery, diagnostic tests are ordered to screen for preexisting abnormalities. Clients scheduled for elective surgery undergo these tests as an outpatient on or before the morning of surgery. If tests reveal severe problems, the surgeon or anesthesiologist may cancel surgery until the condition is stabilized.

The nurse is responsible for coordinating the completion of tests and for verifying that the client is prepared properly. The nurse also reviews diagnostic results as they become available, alerting physicians to findings and planning appropriate therapy. Each laboratory has standards for normal laboratory values, which varies with methods and solutions used.

Screening tests depend on the condition of the client and the nature of the surgery. However, routine screening tests may include a complete blood count, serum electrolyte analysis, coagulation studies, serum creatinine test, type and cross-matched urinalysis, a 12 lead electrocardiogram, and a chest x-ray study.

Complete blood count. A complete blood count (CBC) is an analysis of a peripheral venous blood specimen that measures red blood cell count, white blood cell

table 36-4
PHYSIOLOGICAL FACTORS THAT PLACE OLDER ADULT CLIENTS AT RISK FOR SURGERY

Alterations	Risks	Nursing implications
CARDIOVASCULAR		
Degenerative change in myocardium and valves	Reduces cardiac reserve	Assess baseline vital signs.
Rigidity of arterial walls and reduction in sympathetic and parasympathetic innervation to heart	Predisposes client to postoperative hemorrhage and rise in systolic and diastolic blood pressure	Instruct client on techniques for performing leg exercises and proper turning.
Increase in calcium and cholesterol deposits within small arteries; arterial walls thickened	Predisposes client to clot formation in lower extremities	
PULMONARY		
Rib cage stiffened and reduced in size	Reduces vital capacity	Instruct client on proper technique for coughing and deep breathing exercises.
Reduced range of movement in diaphragm	Greater residual capacity or volume of air left in lung after normal breath increases, reducing amount of new air brought into lungs with each inspiration	
Lung tissue stiffened and air-spaces enlarged	Reduces blood oxygenation	
RENAL		
Reduced blood flow to kidneys	Increases danger of shock when blood loss occurs	Determine baseline urinary output for 24 hours.
Reduced glomerular filtration rate and excretory times	Limits ability to remove drugs or toxic substances	
Reduced bladder capacity	Voiding frequency increases, and larger amount of urine stays in the bladder after voiding	Instruct client to notify nurse immediately when sensation of bladder fullness develops.
	Sensation of need to void may not occur until bladder is filled	Keep call light or bedpan within easy reach.
NEUROLOGICAL		
Sensory losses, including reduced tactile sense, increased pain tolerance	Client less able to respond to early warning signs of surgical complications	Orient client to surrounding environment. Observe for nonverbal signs of pain.
Decreased reaction time	Client becomes confused easily following anethesia	
METABOLIC		
Lower basal metabolic rate	Reduces total oxygen consumption	
Reduced number of red blood cells and hemoglobin levels	Reduces ability to carry adequate oxygen to tissues	Administer necessary blood products.
Change in total amounts of body potassium and water volume	Greater risk for fluid or electrolyte imbalance	Monitor electrolyte levels.

count, platelet count, hemoglobin concentration, and hematocrit. An abnormal CBC may indicate many alterations that place the client at risk for cardiovascular and pulmonary complications or infection. The etiology of this abnormality must be identified and may require treatment before surgery.

SERUM ELECTROLYTE ANALYSIS. Analysis of serum electrolyte levels also requires the collection of a peripheral venous blood sample. Serum electrolyte tests measure sodium, potassium, chloride, and carbon dioxide content (Table 36-5). Because of the potential for fluid and electrolyte imbalances during and after surgery, the sur-

table 36-5

COMMON LABORATORY TEST VALUES

Test	Normal values*
Sodium (Na^+)	135-145 mEq/L
Potassium (K^+)	3.5-5.0 mEq/L
Chloride (Cl^-)	100-106 mEq/L
Bicarbonate (CO_2)	24-32 mEq/L
Creatinine	0.6-1.5 mg/100 ml
Prothrombin time (PT)	< 2 second deviation from control
Partial thromboplastin time (PTT)	25-27 seconds
Platelet count	150,000-350,000/mm^3

From Pagana KD and Pagana TJ: *Diagnostic testing and nursing implications: a case study approach,* ed 3, St. Louis, 1990, Mosby.
*Normal ranges vary slightly among laboratories.

geon screens preoperative electrolyte levels to determine whether electrolyte replacement is necessary preoperatively.

COAGULATION STUDY. The ability of blood to clot or coagulate is essential for minimizing the risk of hemorrhaging. The prothrombin time (PT), partial thromboplastin time (PTT), and platelet counts are routine tests for the clotting ability of blood (Table 36-5). Coagulation studies allow the nurse and physician to identify clients at risk for bleeding tendencies and thrombus formation.

SERUM CREATININE TEST. A serum creatinine test assesses renal function. Creatinine is the by-product of muscle metabolism. The body excretes a constant amount of creatinine through the kidneys, which is an excellent measure of the glomerular filtration rate. A rise in creatinine level can be a sensitive indicator of renal failure (see Table 36-5).

URINALYSIS. Analysis of a urine specimen consists of screening for urinary infection, renal disease, and diabetes mellitus. The nurse assists the client in collecting a clean voided specimen (see Chapter 32). The urinalysis measures urine color, pH, and specific gravity. It also determines the presence of protein, glucose, ketones, and blood.

CHEST X-RAY STUDY. A chest x-ray examination allows the physician to examine the condition of the heart and lungs before surgery. Although the x-ray does not always detect subtle pathological changes, it can reveal the overall size and shape of the heart, lung lesions and chest wall abnormalities, and position of the diaphragm and aorta. If abnormalities are detected, surgery may be postponed until the condition is stabilized or a different type and dose of anesthetic agents may be used. Before sending a woman for x-ray examination, the nurse should inquire as to the possibility of pregnancy. Exposure of the fetus to radiation may cause injury.

NURSING DIAGNOSES FOR THE PREOPERATIVE CLIENT

Altered role performance
Anxiety
Decisional conflict
Fear
Fluid volume deficit
Hopelessness
Ineffective family coping: compromised
Ineffective individual coping
Knowledge deficit
Powerlessness

TYPE AND CROSS-MATCH. If the client is at risk for intraoperative blood loss, the physician orders a blood specimen for type and cross-matching. This test enables the laboratory to determine the proper blood type and prepare blood products to match the client's blood. The surgeon designates the number and form of blood units to have available during surgery. An option frequently used for elective surgery is for the client to donate blood in advance of surgery; the client can then receive his or her own autologous blood, if replacement is necessary.

ADDITIONAL SCREENING TESTS. If a client is over 40 or has heart disease, an electrocardiogram (ECG) is ordered. The procedure takes less than 5 minutes and requires the client simply to lie flat and relax. It involves the painless application of electrodes to the chest and extremities. An ECG measures the heart's electrical activity to determine whether the heart rate and rhythm and other factors are normal. Depending on the type of surgery, a variety of additional diagnostic tests for specific anatomical structures and physiological functions may be ordered.

Nursing Diagnosis

The nurse clusters defining characteristics gathered during assessment to identify nursing diagnoses and related factors for the client and family (see box above). The diagnoses establish direction for care that will be provided during one or all surgical phases. For example, a client's restlessness, poor eye contact, and expressed concern about the results of surgery indicate the diagnosis of anxiety. Anxiety will influence how the nurse prepares a client preoperatively and keeps the client informed postoperatively. A diagnosis and its related factors provide the nurse with direction toward more specific interventions more likely to be effective. The related factor must be accurate. Anxiety related to knowledge deficit of perioperative routines will require the nurse to offer thorough instruction preoperatively and immediately postoperatively. Anxiety related to threat of altered role performance will require counseling and coaching during postoperative recovery. If the threat is real, a social worker may be necessary.

Preoperatively, nursing diagnoses may focus on the intraoperative and postoperative risks a client may face. Preventive care is essential to manage the surgical client effectively. The nature and type of surgery, as well as the client's health status, suggest defining characteristics for many nursing diagnoses.

Planning

It is essential to include any client, especially the surgical client, in health care planning. Involving the client early when developing the surgical plan of care minimizes surgical risks and postoperative complications. Nursing research has shown that structured preoperative teaching can reduce the client's hospital stay (Devine and Cook, 1983). A client informed about the

SAMPLE NURSING CARE PLAN
Preoperative Client: Knowledge Deficit

ASSESSMENT

Clinical scenario: Mr. Baxter, an alert, oriented, 53-year-old, married man with upper abdominal pain, has been scheduled for an elective laparoscopic cholecystectomy in 1 week. This will be Mr. Baxter's *first hospitalization for surgery,* and *he has received minimal preoperative education from his physician.* Mr. Baxter is *asking* the nurse staff many *questions* over the phone about intraoperative and postoperative events.

NURSING DIAGNOSIS

Knowledge deficit regarding implications of surgery (cholecystectomy) related to first surgical experience

PLANNING

Goals

Mr. Baxter will understand intraoperative and postoperative events before day of surgery.

Expected outcomes

Mr. Baxter and his wife will describe events that commonly occur in holding area and operating room on day before surgery.

Mr. Baxter and his wife will describe routine postoperative nursing procedures on day of admission.

Mr. Baxter and his wife will describe ways to participate in postoperative care on day of admission.

IMPLEMENTATION

Steps	Rationale
1. One week before surgery, mail Mr. Baxter the teaching booklet, *Your Surgical Experience.* Answer any questions on booklet's content.	Clients who are prepared for surgery experience less anxiety and report greater sense of psychological well-being.
2. Provide planned teaching session on day of preadmission testing with Mr. Baxter and his wife to explain events that will occur in holding area (e.g., insertion of intravenous line and vital sign check) and in operating room (e.g., positioning and anesthesia).	Teaching focused on information client will need to know on morning of admission.
3. Provide planned teaching session on day of admission with Mr. Baxter and his wife to explain common events that occur after surgery (monitoring, IV line care, actvity, diet) and demonstrate postoperative exercise.	Preoperative teaching improves client's ability to ambulate, participate in care activities, and resume activities of daily living after surgery. Demonstration is an effective method in teaching psychomotor skills.

EVALUATION

Ask Mr. Baxter and his wife to identify basic purpose of surgery and changes to expect afterward.

Ask Mr. Baxter and his wife to identify routine types of postoperative monitoring and treatment.

Have Mr. Baxter perform postoperative exercises.

Defining characteristics are shown in italic type.

surgical experience is less likely to be fearful and is able to prepare for expected outcomes. The nursing care plan box on p. 1088 provides a sample care plan for a preoperative surgical client.

For the ambulatory surgical client, the preoperative planning phase usually occurs in the outpatient surgery setting before or on the morning of surgery. Ideally, it begins in the home. This gives the client time to think about the surgical experience, make necessary physical preparations (e.g., altering diet or discontinuing medication use), and ask questions about postoperative procedures. Well-planned, preoperative care ensures the client is well informed and able to actively participate during recovery. The family or significant others may also play an active supportive role for the client.

The plan of care begins in the preoperative phase and is modified during the intraoperative and postoperative phases. The goals and expected outcomes of the preoperative care of the surgical client include:

Goal: Client understands the intended surgery and physiological and psychological responses to surgery.

Outcomes

Client describes surgical procedure (in general terms) and its purpose
Client describes expected surgical outcome
Client states reasons for postoperative exercises
Client identifies postoperative activity restrictions

Goal: Client understands preoperative, intraoperative, and postoperative routines.

Outcomes

Client states time and day of surgery
Client states unit to which he or she will be transferred postoperatively
Client and family state location of waiting room
Client identifies routine monitoring to be done intraoperatively and postoperatively

Goal: Client participates in plan of care.

Outcomes

Client demonstrates postoperative exercises before surgery
Client demonstrates care of incision site by discharge

Goal: Client achieves psychological and physical comfort and rest.

Outcomes

Client uses effective coping strategies
Client's anxiety is minimal to moderate
Client sleeps through night
Client identifies pain relief therapies
Client demonstrates correct use of PCA pump
Client states that medications should be given when pain becomes a persistent discomfort

Goal: Client returns to functional state of health within limitations posed by surgery in 6 weeks.

Outcomes

Client states the steps to activity resumption before surgery, during recovery, and at discharge
Client returns to full functioning within limitations of surgery

Goal: Client remains free of postoperative infection.

Outcome

Client's incision is clean, free of purulent drainage

Implementation

Preoperative nursing interventions provide the client with a complete understanding of surgery and prepare the client physically and psychologically for the surgical intervention.

Informed Consent

A surgeon cannot legally perform surgery or an anesthesiologist administer an anesthetic until a client understands the need for the procedure, the steps involved, risks, expected results, and alternative treatments. The primary responsibility for informing the client rests with the surgeon and anesthesiologist. Consent is not informed if the client is confused, unconscious, mentally incompetent, or under the influence of sedatives. All consent forms (Figure 36-2) must be signed before the nurse administers preoperative medications. Ideally a surgeon obtains consent before a client is admitted to the hospital or ambulatory surgery center.

The surgeon's explanation to the client should be witnessed by a qualified member of the health care team. The form's structure allows the physician to write in information related to surgery. A client's signature on a consent form implies the client has been thoroughly informed about the procedure. The nurse frequently witnesses the physician's explanation and the signing and examines the document for the correct date, time, and signature, which must be in ink. An illiterate client can sign by making a mark, as long as it is properly witnessed. As a witness, the nurse can attest the client's signature is on the form but not that the client was properly informed. In many institutions a time limit is placed on consent forms (e.g., 30 days).

Individuals must personally sign the consent form if they are of legal age (varies among states and Canadian provinces), under legal age but have a valid marriage certificate, designated as an emancipated minor (certain states), and not presently under legal guardianship. In some Canadian provinces a teenager may sign a consent form under certain conditions. If the client is a minor or legally considered to be incompetent and is not included in these categories, a parent or legal guardian signs the

G-2d$_2$ CONSENT FOR OPERATION OR PROCEDURE

(See reverse for Monitored Telephone Call)

• File most recent sheet ON BOTTOM •

DATE
HOSP. NO.
NAME
BIRTHDATE
ADDRESS

IF NOT IMPRINTED, PLEASE PRINT DATE, HOSP. NO., NAME AND LOCATION

1. I hereby authorize Doctors ______________________ (Attending and Resident Physician[s]/Dentist[s]), and such other associates as may be selected by the attending doctor to perform upon ______________ (Myself or Name of Patient) the following operation/procedure: ______________ (Technical name, followed by description in lay language)

2. In the event developments indicate that further operations/procedures may be necessary, I authorize the physicians to use their own judgment and do whatever they deem advisable during the operation/procedure for the patient's best interests, except the following ______________ (List any exclusions. If none, write "none.")

3. I consent to the administration of such anesthetics as may be considered necessary or advisable by the anesthetist, with the exception of: ______________ (List any exclusions. If none, write "none.")

4. The nature of my condition, the nature and purpose of the operation/procedure, possible alternative methods of treatment, the risks involved, and the possible consequences and complications have been explained to me by Doctor ______________. My questions concerning the operation/procedure and its possible outcome have been answered to my satisfaction.

5. I am aware that the practice of dentistry, medicine, and surgery is not an exact science and acknowledge that no guarantees have been made to me by anyone concerning the results of the operation/procedure.

6. Any tissues surgically removed may be disposed by the Hospital in accordance with accustomed practice, including use in research studies, except as follows: ______________ (If none, write "none.")

Signature: ______________ (Patient or person authorized to consent for patient)

I declare that I have personally explained to ______________ (Patient or Representative) the nature of the patient's condition, the procedures to be undertaken, the risks involved, and the alternatives, as set forth in 1 and 4 above,

on ______ (Date) at ______ (Time) a.m. p.m. ______________ (Signature of Physician/Dentist)

—Continued On Reverse—

79365/7-84/H1575 **THE UNIVERSITY OF IOWA HOSPITALS AND CLINICS**

G -2d$_2$ H PATHOLOGY I DIAGNOSIS

FIGURE 36-2 Consent for operation or procedure. (Courtesy University of Iowa Hospitals and Clinics, Iowa City, Iowa.)

MONITORED TELEPHONE CALL

Physician/Dentist Making Call ______________________

Person Called ______________________

Relationship to Patient ______________________

Concerning Permission to Operate on:

Name of Patient ______________ Hospital Number ________ Age ______

Address ______________________ Class ______

Operation or Procedure to be Performed ______________________

Permission given ☐ Yes ☐ No Time ________ Date ________

Remarks: ______________________

Call Monitored by: ______________________

FIGURE 36-2, cont'd Consent for operation or procedure.

consent form. A spouse, next of kin, or individual designated to have power of attorney signs for an unconscious or mentally incompetent adult.

In emergency situations the client may be unable to sign, and family members may be unavailable. The surgeon is legally permitted to perform surgery without consent in such a case; however, every effort must be made to obtain permission from a responsible family member by telephone, telegram, or in some states by court order. A telephone consent must be witnessed by two persons who hear the family member's oral consent. The witnesses sign the consent with the name of the family member, noting that a verbal consent was obtained. Informed consent is critical to protect the client and health personnel so the surgical team can practice without fear of legal reprisal.

After the consent form has been completed, the nurse verifies the correct date, time, and signatures are on the form and places it in the client's record. The record accompanies the client to the operating room. Chapter 6 discusses in detail the nurse's responsibilities for informed consent.

Preoperative Teaching

Structured preoperative teaching has proven benefits (Devine and Cook, 1983; Hathaway, 1986). Systematic and structural **preoperative teaching** for a client's expected postoperative behaviors has a positive influence on a client's recovery. Structured preoperative teaching can influence postoperative factors such as the following:

1. Ventilatory function. Teaching improves the ability to cough and deep breathe effectively.
2. Physical functional capacity. Teaching improves the ability to ambulate and resume activities of daily living early.
3. Sense of well-being. Clients who are prepared for surgery experience less anxiety and report a greater sense of psychological well-being.
4. Length of hospital stay. Structured preoperative teaching can reduce the client's length of hospital stay.

The most effective type of teaching program for surgical clients is planned so all clients receive the same information (Lindeman and VanAernam, 1971). This is

Text continued on p. 1095.

procedure 36-1

DEMONSTRATING POSTOPERATIVE EXERCISES

Steps	Rationale
1. Assess client's risk for postoperative respiratory complications. Review medical history to identify presence of chronic pulmonary conditions (e.g., emphysema, asthma), any condition that affects chest wall movement, history of smoking, and presence of reduced hemoglobin.	General anesthesia predisposes client to respiratory problems because lungs are not fully inflated during surgery; cough reflex is suppressed, so mucus collects within airway passages. After surgery, client may have reduced lung volume and require greater efforts to cough and deep breathe; inadequate lung expansion can lead to atelectasis and pneumonia. Client is at greater risk to develop respiratory complications if other chronic lung conditions are present. Smoking damages ciliary clearance and increases mucus secretion. Reduced hemoglobin level can lead to inadequate oxygenation.
2. Assess ability to cough and deep breathe by having client take deep breath and observing movement of shoulders and chest wall. Measure chest excursion during deep breath. Ask client to cough after taking deep breath.	Reveals maximum potential for chest expansion and ability to cough forcefully; serves as baseline to measure ability to perform exercises after surgery.
3. Assess risk for postoperative thrombus formation. (Older, immobilized clients are most at risk.) Observe for positive Homan's sign by monitoring calf pain when dorsiflexing client's foot with knee flexed. Observe for calf pain, redness, warmth, swelling, or vein distention.	After general anesthesia, circulation is slowed, and when rate of blood flow is slowed, there is greater tendency for clot formation. Immobilization results in decreased muscular contraction in lower extremities, which promotes venous stasis.
4. Prepare necessary supplies: a. Pillow (optional)	Client may prefer to use pillow to splint incision when coughing to reduce discomfort.
5. Explain postoperative exercises to client, including importance to recovery and physiological benefits.	Information allows client to attend and can motivate learning. Persons tend to learn new skills when benefits can be gained.
DIAPHRAGMATIC BREATHING	
6. Assist client to comfortable sitting or standing position. If client chooses to sit, assist to side of bed or to upright position in chair.	Upright position facilitates diaphragmatic excursion.
7. Stand or sit facing client.	Allows client to observe breathing exercise.

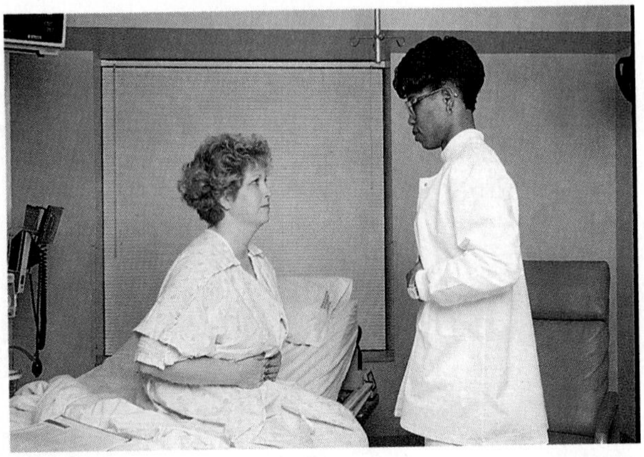

Step 8

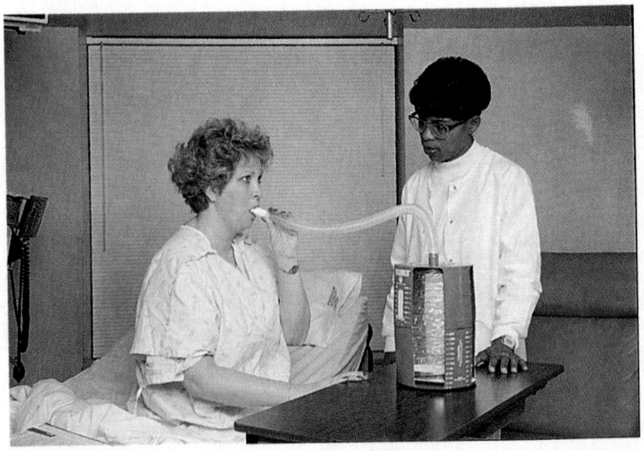

Step 17

Steps	Rationale
8. Instruct client to place palms of hands across from each other, down and along lower borders of anterior rib cage. Place tips of third fingers lightly together (see illustration). Demonstrate for client.	Position of hands allows client to feel movement of chest and abdomen as diaphragm descends and lungs expand.
9. Have client take slow, deep breaths, inhaling through nose. Tell client to feel middle fingers separate during inhalation. Demonstrate.	Slow, deep breath prevents panting or hyperventilation. Inhaling through nose warms, humidifies, and filters air. Allows client to observe slow, rhythmic breathing pattern.
10. Explain that client will feel normal downward movement of diaphragm during inspiration. Explain that abdominal organs descend and chest wall expands.	Explanation and demonstration focus on normal ventilatory movement of chest wall. Client develops understanding of how diaphragmatic breathing feels.
11. Avoid using chest and shoulders while inhaling and instruct client in same manner.	Using auxiliary chest and shoulder muscles increases useless energy expenditure.
12. Have client hold slow, deep breath for count of three and then slowly exhale through mouth. Tell client middle fingertips will touch as chest wall contracts.	Allows for gradual expulsion of all air.
13. Repeat breathing exercise 3 to 5 times.	Repetition of exercise reinforces learning.
14. Have client practice exercise. Instruct client to take 10 slow, deep breaths every 2 hr while awake during postoperative period until mobile.	Regular deep breathing prevents postoperative complications.
INCENTIVE SPIROMETRY	
15. Wash hands.	Reduces transmission of microorganisms.
16. Instruct client to assume semi-Fowler's or high Fowler's position.	Promotes optimal lung expansion during respiratory maneuver.
17. Demonstrate to client how to place mouthpiece so that lips completely cover mouthpiece (see illustration).	Demonstration is reliable technique for teaching psychomotor skill and enables client to ask questions.
18. Instruct client to inhale slowly and maintain constant flow through unit. When maximal inspiration is reached, client should hold breath for 2-3 sec and then exhale slowly. Number of breaths should not exceed 10-12 per min (Dettenmeier, 1992).	Maintains maximal inspiration and reduces risk of progressive collapse of individual alveoli. Slow breath prevents or minimizes pain from sudden pressure changes in chest (Dettenmeier, 1992).
19. Instruct client to breathe normally for short period.	Prevents hyperventilation and fatigue.
20. Have client repeat maneuver until goals are achieved.	Ensures correct use of spirometer.
21. Wash hands.	Reduces transmission of microorganisms.
CONTROLLED COUGHING	
22. Explain importance of maintaining upright position.	Position facilitates diaphragm excursion and enhances thorax expansion.
23. Demonstrate coughing. Take two slow, deep breaths, inhaling through nose and exhaling through mouth.	Deep breaths expand lungs fully so that air moves behind mucus and facilitates effects of coughing.
24. Inhale deeply third time and hold breath to count of 3. Cough fully for two or thee consecutive coughs without inhaling between coughs. (Tell client to push all air out of lungs.)	Consecutive coughs help remove mucus more effectively and completely than one forceful cough.
25. Caution client against just clearing throat instead of coughing.	Clearing throat does not remove mucus from deep in airways.
26. If surgical incision will be abdominal or thoracic, teach client to place one hand over incisional area and other hand on top of first. During breathing and coughing exercises, client presses gently against incisional area to splint or support it. Pillow over incision is optional (see illustration).	Surgical incision cuts through muscles, tissues, and nerve endings. Deep breathing and coughing exercises place additional stress on suture line and cause discomfort. Splinting incision with hands provides firm support and reduces incisional pulling. (Some clients prefer to have

Continued.

procedure 36-1—cont'd

Steps	Rationale
27. Client continues to practice coughing exercises, splinting imaginary incision. Instruct client to cough 2 to 3 times every 2 hr while awake.	Value of deep coughing with splinting is stressed to effectively expectorate mucus with minimal discomfort.
28. Instruct client to examine sputum for consistency, amount, and color changes.	Sputum consistency, amount, and color changes may indicate presence of pulmonary complication, such as pneumonia.
TURNING	
29. Instruct client to assume supine position to right side of bed. Side rails on both sides of bed should be in up position.	Positioning begins on right side of bed so that turning to left side will not cause client to roll toward bed's edge.
30. Instruct client to place left hand over incisional area to splint it.	Supports and minimizes pulling on suture line during turning.
31. Instruct client to keep left leg straight and flex right knee up and over left leg.	Straight leg stabilizes client's position. Flexed right leg shifts weight for easier turning.
32. Have client grab left side rail with right hand, pull toward left, and roll onto left side.	Pulling toward side rail reduces effort needed for turning.
33. Instruct client to turn every 2 hr while awake.	Reduces risk of vascular and pulmonary complications.
LEG EXERCISES	
34. Have client assume supine position in bed. Demonstrate leg exercises by performing passive range of motion exercises and simultaneously explaining exercise.	Provides normal anatomical position of lower extremities.
35. Rotate each ankle in complete circle. Instruct client to draw imaginary circles with big toe. Repeat 5 times.	Leg exercises maintain joint mobility and promote venous return.
36. Alternate dorsiflexion and plantar flexion of both feet. Direct client to feel calf muscles contract and relax alternately (see illustration). Repeat 5 times.	Stretches and contracts gastrocnemius muscles.
37. Have client continue leg exercises by alternately flexing and extending knees. Repeat 5 times (see illustration).	Contracts muscles of upper legs and maintains knee mobility.

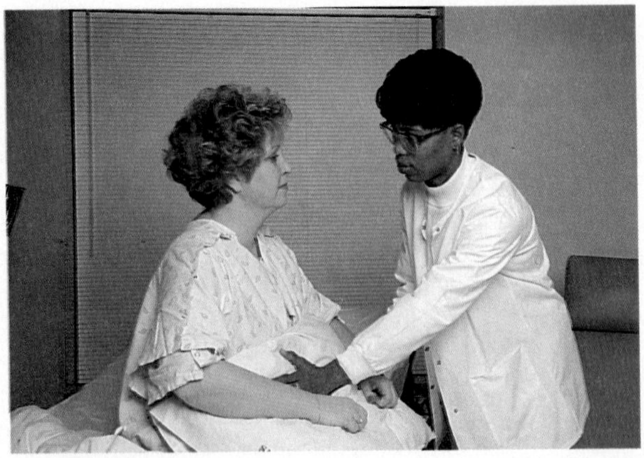

Step 26

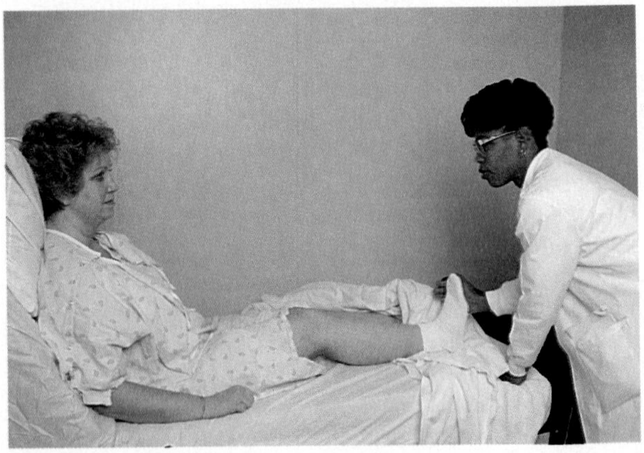

Step 36

Steps	Rationale
38. Have client alternately raise each leg straight up from bed surface, keeping legs straight. Repeat 5 times.	Promotes contraction and relaxation of quadriceps muscles.
39. Have client practice exercises at least every 2 hr while awake. Instruct client to coordinate turning and leg exercises with diaphragmatic breathing, incentive spirometry, and coughing exercises.	Repetition of sequence reinforces learning. Establishes routine for exercises that develops habit for performance. Sequence of exercises should be leg exercises, turning, breathing, incentive spirometry, and coughing.
40. Observe client's ability to perform all five exercises independently.	Ensures that client has learned correct technique.
41. Record exercises demonstrated and client's ability to perform them independently.	Documents client's education and provides data for instructional follow-up.

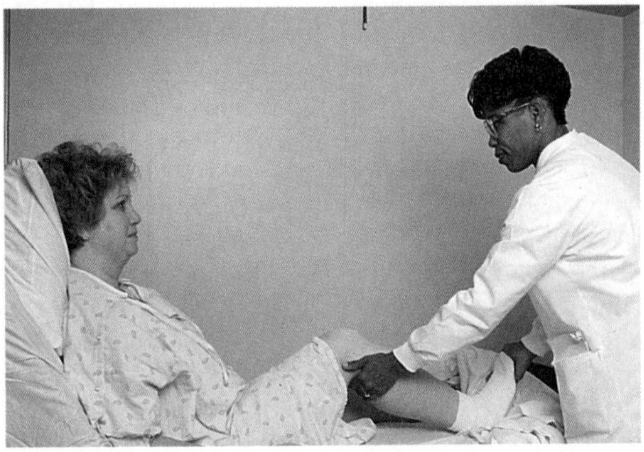

Step 37

made easier by a teaching flowsheet. Detailed discussion and demonstration of postoperative exercises are vital (Procedure 36-1). If the client understands the reasons the exercises are important to postoperative recovery and knows how to perform them correctly, the recovery period will be less complicated. Today, because many clients come to the hospital on the day of surgery, preoperative teaching may occur in the home. Printed literature and videotapes are made available to clients. Preoperatively, nurses call clients the evening before surgery to clarify questions.

Family. Including family members in preoperative preparation is valuable. A family member is often the coach for postoperative exercises when the client returns from surgery. If anxious relatives do not understand routine postoperative events, their anxiety can heighten the client's fears or concerns. Preoperative preparation of family members minimizes their anxiety and misunderstanding. However, if the client does not wish family members to be included, this sense of privacy should be honored.

Sensory Preparation. The nurse should provide the client with information about sensations typically experienced before, during, and after surgery. Preparatory information helps clients to anticipate the steps of a procedure and to form a realistic image of the surgical experience. When events occur as predicted, the client is better able to cope and attend to the experiences. For example, the operating room is very bright. A cuff for a noninvasive blood pressure monitor will be applied to the client's arm. This monitor may make a hum and a beep and the cuff tightens around the client's arm. Informing the client about these and other sensations in the operating room will reduce anxiety before the client is anesthetized. Other postoperative sensations the nurse describes include blurred vision from ophthalmic ointment, dryness of the mouth, or the sensation of a sore throat resulting from an endo-tracheal tube, pain at the incision site, and tightness of the dressings, and feeling cold.

Timing. It is best to begin preoperative teaching more than one day in advance of the scheduled surgery (Hill, 1982). If the nurse can teach a client when the client is less anxious, the client will be better able to learn. Anxiety and fear are barriers to learning, and both emotions are heightened as surgery approaches. The nurse assesses the surgical client's readiness and ability to learn. If the client is capable and receptive to learning, the nurse presents information in a logical sequence beginning with preoperative events and advancing to intraoperative and postoperative routines. Preoperative teaching checklists give nurses useful guidelines for presenting clients with comprehensive instructions.

Content. Preoperative teaching should include information to assist the client and family to prepare for the surgical experience and to participate in the plan of care. The nurse should first assess their level of understanding about the surgery and perioperative routines.

Surgical procedure. After the surgeon has explained the basic purpose of a surgical procedure and its steps, the client may ask the nurse additional questions. The nurse is careful to avoid saying anything that contradicts the surgeon's explanation. One way to avoid contradictions is to first ask what the client has been told. If the client has little or no understanding about the surgery, the nurse first checks with the physician to determine the explanations to be given.

Preoperative routines. Certain preoperative routines are expected and should be explained to the client and family. Any diagnostic tests that remain to be done should be completed. For example, the client may need to have a chest x-ray. Knowing what tests are planned will increase the client's sense of control.

The anesthesiologist will visit with the client to complete a preanesthesia assessment. The client and family need to know about this visit, so that the family can plan to be present if they have questions or are needed to provide additional information. Frequently, the incision site is prepared with an antimicrobial skin preparation. Providing this information will allow the client to plan a shower. The client is told to avoid the use of lotions and powders.

The client and family must understand that the client can have no oral intake (either food or liquids) before surgery, unless explicitly specified by the anesthesiologist. During the use of general anesthesia, the muscles relax and gastric contents can reflux into the esophagus. The anesthetic has eliminated the client's ability to gag. The client is thus at risk for aspiration from food or fluids from the stomach into the lung. The physician's orders will provide further guidance for what routines should be explained to the client (e.g., IV therapy, preoperative medications, or insertion of a urinary catheter).

Intraoperative routines. The scheduled operative time is only the anticipated time, because other surgeries may be scheduled first. Caution is exercised when discussing the anticipated length of surgery. Unanticipated delays may occur for many unharmful reasons. It must be emphasized that this time is a rough estimate, and the actual time could be much longer. Family members should be told the surgeon will speak to them in the waiting room when the surgery has been completed. Excessive delays are communicated to the family.

Postoperative routines. The client and family want to know about postoperative events. If they understand routine postoperative vital sign monitoring, they are less likely to be apprehensive when nurses perform these assessments. The nurse can also explain if the client is to have intravenous lines, dressings, or drainage tubes. It is important to neither overprepare or underprepare the client and family. The nurse cannot predict all the client's requirements, and a client may be misinformed about a therapy that may not be initiated. Contradictions between the nurse's explanations and reality can cause great anxiety.

Some hospitals use care maps or critical paths to provide guidance for the sequence of postoperative events. These maps are helpful teaching aids because they indicate the expected postoperative course following a specific surgery (e.g., the day diagnostic tests are completed or the day the client is expected to be discharged from the hospital).

Pain relief. One of the surgical client's greatest fears is pain. The family is also concerned for the client's comfort. Minimal discomfort after surgery is normal and expected. Patient controlled analgesia (PCA) is commonly used and provides the client with control over pain. The client needs to know how to operate the pump and the importance of administering medication as soon as pain becomes persistent (see Chapter 28). If a client or the nurse waits until postoperative pain becomes excruciating, an analgesic will not provide relief.

If epidural, intramuscular, or oral analgesics will be used, the client needs to know the schedule for these drugs. The client should be encouraged to inform nurses as soon as pain becomes a persistent discomfort. The client should also know it takes time for a drug to act and that all the discomfort will rarely be eliminated. The nurse informs the client and family of other therapies available for pain relief (e.g., positioning, splinting, and relaxation exercises).

Surgical clients may avoid taking pain medications for fear of becoming dependent. However, most drug dosages and the required intervals between them are not sufficient to cause dependence. The nurse should encourage the client to use analgesics as needed. Unless pain is controlled, it will be difficult for the client to participate in postoperative therapy.

Hospitalized clients initially receive parenteral analgesics. As their pain diminishes, the physician replaces these with an oral analgesic.

Postoperative exercises. Given a rationale for postoperative procedures, the client is better prepared to participate in care. Every preoperative teaching program includes explanation and demonstration of the five postoperative exercises designed to prevent postoperative complications.

When a client is under general anesthesia, the lungs do not ventilate fully. After surgery, the client has a reduced lung volume and needs greater effort to breathe. During surgery the venous blood flow to the legs slows. Stasis of the peripheral circulation may lead to the formation of thrombi or clots. A clot can break off and travel to the brain, heart, or lungs to cause potentially serious, limiting, or even fatal complications.

Diaphragmatic breathing improves lung expansion and oxygen delivery without using excess energy. The client learns to use the diaphragm during deep breathing to take slow, deep, and relaxed breaths. Eventually the client's lung volume improves. Deep breathing also helps to clear any anesthetic gases from the airways.

To facilitate deep breathing the physician often orders an incentive spirometer for the client. Incentive spirometry encourages forced inspiration. The therapy is effective in preventing atelectasis postoperatively. Incentive spirometry helps to reinflate collapsed alveoli and remove secretions.

Coughing assists in removing retained mucus in the airways. A deep, productive cough is more beneficial than merely clearing the throat. The client must anticipate postoperative discomfort and understand the importance of coughing, even when difficult. The nurse also teaches the client to splint an incision to minimize pain during coughing. Nurses direct clients to cough and deep breathe at least every 2 hours while awake.

Leg exercises and turning improve blood flow to the extremities and thus reduce stasis. Contraction of lower leg muscles promotes venous return, making it difficult for clots to form. The nurse encourages the client to perform leg exercises and turn at least every 2 hours while awake.

After explaining each exercise, the nurse demonstrates it. The nurse acts as a coach, guiding the client through each exercise. For example, the nurse assists the client to assume the proper position. The nurse then allows the client time (at least 15 minutes) for independent practice. The nurse can attend to other clients' needs before returning to watch each exercise independently. The nurse gives the client feedback, pointing out the steps done correctly and the steps needing improvement.

Activity resumption. The type of surgery a client undergoes affects the speed with which normal physical activity and regular eating habits can be resumed. The nurse explains that it is normal for the client to progress gradually in activity and eating. If the client tolerates activity and diet well, activity levels will progress more quickly.

Physical Preparation

The degree of preoperative physical preparation depends on the client's health status, the surgery to be performed, and the surgeon's preferences. A seriously ill client will receive more supportive care than the client facing a less serious elective procedure. The nurse must explain the purpose of all procedures. The nurse's responsibilities include the following:

Maintain Normal Fluid and Electrolyte Balance. The surgical client is vulnerable to fluid and electrolyte imbalances as a result of inadequate preoperative intake or excessive fluid losses during surgery. A client usually takes nothing by mouth after midnight before the morning of surgery. After 6 to 8 hours of fasting the client's gastrointestinal tract will be relatively empty, so the risks of vomiting or aspirating emesis during surgery are minimal.

The nurse removes all fluids and solid foods from the client's bedside and posts a sign over the bed to alert hospital personnel and family members about fasting restrictions. The nurse allows the client to rinse the mouth with water or mouthwash and brush the teeth as long as the client does not swallow water.

A client who is at home the evening before surgery must understand the importance of not taking food or fluids and be willing to follow restrictions. The nurse can allow the client to rinse the mouth with water or mouthwash and brush the teeth as long as the client does not swallow water. The client may also be instructed to take routine oral medications with sips of water, if the physician orders. The nurse notifies the surgeon and anesthesiologist as soon as possible if the client eats or drinks during the fasting period.

During surgery, normal mechanisms for controlling fluid and electrolyte balance are disturbed. The surgical procedure itself may cause extensive losses of blood and other body fluids. The surgical stress response aggravates any fluid and electrolyte imbalance. The nurse determines whether the client eats and drinks sufficient amounts before fasting to ensure adequate fluid and nutrition intake. The client's diet should include foods high in protein, with enough carbohydrates, fat, and vitamins. Clients have intravenous feeding until oral intake is adequate. The physician relies on serum electrolyte levels to determine the type and amount of intravenous fluids and electrolyte additives to give. Clients with severe nutritional imbalances may require supplements with concentrated protein and glucose (see Chapter 31).

Minimize Risk of Surgical Wound Infection. The risk of developing a surgical wound infection is determined by the amount and type of microorganisms contaminating a wound, susceptibility of the host, and condition of the wound at the end of the operation (largely determined by the surgeon's operative technique). All three factors interact, determining the risk of infection.

The skin is a favorite site for microorganisms to grow and multiply. Without proper skin preparation, the risk of postoperative wound infection is high. Bathing with an antimicrobial soap (e.g., chlorhexidine) the evening before surgery is believed to effectively reduce the incidence of postoperative wound infections (Larsen, 1993). Some physicians may order clients to bathe or shower more than once, whereas others may have clients give special attention to cleansing the proposed operative site. If the surgical procedure involves the head, neck, or upper chest area, the client may also be required to shampoo the hair.

Prevent Bowel and Bladder Incontinence. The client may receive a bowel preparation if surgery involves the lower gastrointestinal system. Manipulation of portions of the gastrointestinal tract during surgery results in absence of peristalsis for 24 hours and sometimes longer. Enemas and cathartics cleanse the gastrointestinal tract to prevent postoperative constipation or incontinence during surgery. An empty bowel reduces risk of injury to the intestines and minimizes contamination of the operative wound in case a portion of the bowel is incised or opened. The surgeon's order may read "give enemas until clear" (see Chapter 33). Too many enemas given over a short period of time, however, can cause serious fluid and electrolyte imbalances. Most agencies recommend a limit to the number of enemas a nurse may administer successively.

Promote Rest and Comfort. Rest is essential for normal healing. Anxiety about surgery can easily interfere with the ability to relax or sleep. The underlying condition necessitating surgery may be painful, further impairing rest.

The client may feel like part of an assembly line during the preoperative surgical phase. Frequent visits by staff members, diagnostic testing, and physical preparation for surgery consume a large amount of time, and the client has few opportunities to reflect on events. The nurse makes sure that the client feels like an individual. The client and family need time to express feelings about surgery either together or separately. The client's level of anxiety influences the frequency of discussions, and the nurse encourages expression of these concerns.

The nurse should attempt to make the client's environment quiet and comfortable. Frequently, the physician orders a sedative-hypnotic or antianxiety agent for the night before surgery. Sedative-hypnotics (e.g., flurazepam [Dalmane]) affect and promote sleep. Antianxiety agents (e.g., alprazolam [Xanax] and diazepam [Valium]) act on the cerebral cortex and limbic system to relieve anxiety.

An advantage to ambulatory surgery or same-day surgical admissions is that the client is able to sleep at home the night before surgery. The client will probably get more rest in a familiar environment.

Day of Surgery

On the morning of surgery the nurse completes routine procedures before releasing the client for surgery, as follows:

Documentation. Before the client goes to the operating room, the nurse checks the medical record to be sure all pertinent laboratory and test results are present. The nurse checks all consent forms for completeness and accuracy of information. A preoperative checklist (Figure 36-3) provides guidelines for ensuring completion of all nursing interventions. The nurse also checks the nurses' notes to be sure documentation is current. This is especially important if the client experienced unpredicted problems the night before surgery.

Assess Vital Signs. The nurse makes a final assessment of vital signs. If the preoperative vital signs are abnormal, surgery may need to be postponed. Therefore the nurse notifies the physician of abnormalities before sending the client to surgery. The anesthesiologist compares preoperative values with the client's intraoperative vital signs.

Provide Necessary Hygiene. Basic hygiene measures remove contamination and give the client an additional level of comfort. If the client is unwilling to take a complete bath, a partial bath is refreshing and removes irritating secretions or drainage from the skin. Because the client cannot wear personal nightwear to the operating room, the nurse provides a clean hospital gown. After being allowed nothing by mouth throughout the night, the client usually has a very dry mouth. The nurse may offer mouthwash and toothpaste, again cautioning the client not to swallow water.

Prepare the Hair and Remove Cosmetics. During surgery using general anesthesia, the anesthesiologist positions the client's head to put an **endotracheal tube** into the airway (see Chapter 34). This may involve manipulation of the hair and scalp. To avoid injury, the nurse asks the client to remove hairpins or clips. Clients

A-1c PREOPERATIVE/PREPROCEDURAL CHECKLIST

• File with other A-1c's of same date. •

PROCEDURE: ______________________________

DATE OF PROCEDURE: ______________________________

1. Place initials in appropriate box: YES, NO, N/A (not applicable, or was not ordered). Each item must have an entry.
2. Explain any "No." This can be done in the space after the item or in the "Comments" section. Use back of form, if needed.
3. To give more information on any item, use the space after the item. If more space needed, use the "Comments" section or back of form.

DATE

HOSP. NO.

NAME

BIRTHDATE

ADDRESS

IF NOT IMPRINTED, PLEASE PRINT DATE, HOSP. NO., NAME AND LOCATION

YES	NO	N/A	
			Special Information (e.g., blind, O_2, combative)
			Preoperative orders written.
			(If "NO", Dr. ____________ notified at ____________ date/time.)
			Consent complete and in medical record.
			Allergies (or NKA) labelled on cover of medical record.
			Specify Allergies:
			Isolation label on cover of medical record. Specify type:
			Ordered lab results in medical record.
			Urinalysis results in medical record.
			Chest x-ray completed. (Report in medical record: Yes ____ No ____)
			EKG in medical record.
			Type and cross/screen (circle) done. Date drawn:
			History and physical in medical record.
			Forms complete and in medical record:
			1. Nursing documentation with assessment, VS, and wt./ht.
			2. IV Solution Administration Cardex.
			3. Medication Administration Cardex.
			Addressograph plate on cover of medical record. All volumes to procedure, if required.
COMMENTS:			
			Blood band on patient and legible. Specify location ____________ and blood band # ____________
			Identification band on patient and legible. Specify location:
			Bathed and in proper attire.
			Nail polish, makeup, and hairpins removed.
			Jewelry removed. Specify item(s) removed and disposition:
			Prosthesis removed: hearing aid, dentures, eye glasses, contact lenses (circle).
			Other: Disposition:
			Anti-embolism stockings on.
			Sequential compression device sleeves on and controller to OR.
			NPO since:
			Teaching completed and documented.
			Preps/tests completed as ordered. Specify:
			Voided/catheterized (circle). Time:
			Medication(s) given.
			Medication(s)/article(s) sent with patient. Specify:
COMMENTS:			

Date	Initials	Signature and Title of Individuals Filling Out Form

Date	Initials	Signature of RN Sending Patient to Procedure

41006/4-93/H7528 THE UNIVERSITY OF IOWA HOSPITALS AND CLINICS

A 1c | B CLIN. NOTES | C LABORATORY | D X-RAY EXAM | E CONSULTATION | F SPEC. EXAM | G THERAPY | H PATHOLOGY | I DIAGNOSIS

FIGURE 36-3 Preoperative/preprocedural checklist. (Courtesy University of Iowa Hospitals and Clinics, Iowa City, Iowa.)

should also remove hairpieces or wigs. Long hair can be braided. The client will be asked to wear a disposable hat to contain hair before entering the operating room. During and after surgery, the anesthesiologist and nurses assess skin and mucous membranes to determine the client's level of oxygenation and circulation. Therefore all makeup (lipstick, powder, blush, and nail polish) and artificial fingernails should be removed to expose normal skin and nail coloring. Anything in or around the eye may irritate or injure the eye during surgery. Therefore contact lenses, false eyelashes, and eye makeup must also be removed. Glasses usually remain in the room or are given to the family immediately before entering the operating room.

Removal of Prostheses. It is easy for any type of prosthetic device to become lost or damaged during surgery. The client must remove for safekeeping all removable prosthetics including partial or complete dentures, artificial limbs, and artificial eyes. If the client has a brace or splint, the nurse checks with the physician to determine whether it should remain with the client, to be reapplied after surgery.

Although hearing aids and eyeglasses must also be removed, this should not be done until immediately before the client is taken to surgery. Allowing the client to wear these aids facilitates communication and increases the client's sense of control. The nurse should refer to institution's policies for clarification.

Having dentures in place provides a better seal for ventilation during intubation in the operating room. Therefore in some settings, dentures are left in place until after the first stages of anesthesia. For many clients, removing dentures is embarrassing. Therefore if the dentures are to be removed before surgery, privacy should be offered. Dentures, placed in special containers, are labeled with the client's name for safekeeping to prevent breakage. The client is assessed for loose teeth. A broken tooth can become dislodged during insertion of an endotracheal tube and obstruct the airway.

In some agencies nurses inventory and secure all prosthetic devices. It is also common for nurses to give prosthetics to family members or to keep the devices at the client's bedside.

Prepare Bowel and Bladder. The client may require an enema or cathartic the morning of surgery. If so, it should be given at least 1 hour before the client is scheduled to leave, allowing time for the client to defecate and void without rushing. The nurse verifies that the client has emptied his or her bladder immediately before the surgery. If the client is unable to void, it should be noted on the preoperative checklist.

The bladder is not prepared until the morning of surgery. The nurse instructs the client to void just before entering the operating room. An empty bladder minimizes incontinence during surgery. This is particularly important during abdominal surgery, when it may become necessary for the surgeon to manipulate the bladder. An empty bladder also makes abdominal organs more accessible during surgery. Therefore for abdominal procedures, operating room nurses sometimes insert a Foley catheter to maintain an empty bladder. However, because indwelling catheters increase the risk of urinary tract infections, they are not routinely inserted for most procedures.

Apply Antiembolism Stockings. Many physicians order **antiembolism stockings** for wear during surgery. Designed to support the lower extremities, they maintain compression of small veins and capillaries. The constant compression forces blood into larger vessels, thus promoting venous return and preventing circulatory stasis. When correctly sized and properly applied, antiembolism stockings can reduce the risk of thrombi (see Chapter 23). Pneumatic antiembolism stockings are also used for encouraging venous return. These stockings are attached to an air pump that inflates and deflates them, applying intermittent pressure sequentially up the leg.

Promote the Client's Dignity. During preoperative preparations, care can become depersonalized unless the nurse maintains the client's privacy and reduces sources of anxiety. Ambulatory and same-day surgical admission clients often must sit in a waiting room before surgery. To protect clients' modesty, the nurse allows clients to wear underclothes when possible and provides cover robes. Hospitalized clients should be ensured privacy by closing room curtains or doors during preoperative preparation. Family may be allowed to stay until transport to the operating room.

Perform Special Procedures. A client's condition may warrant special interventions before surgery. The surgeon's orders inform nurses of the need to start intravenous infusions, insert Foley catheters or nasogastric tubes (Procedure 36-2), or administer medications.

Safeguard Valuables. If a client has valuables, the nurse turns them over to family members or secures them for safekeeping. Many facilities require clients to sign a release to free the institution of responsibility for lost valuables. Valuables can usually be stored and locked in a designated location. Clients are often reluctant to remove wedding rings or religious medals. A wedding band can be taped in place; however, if there is a risk that the client will experience swelling of the hand or fingers, the band should be removed. Many hospitals allow clients to pin religious medals to their gowns, although the risk of loss increases.

Administer Preoperative Medications. The anesthesiologist or surgeon may order preanesthetic drugs. Tranquilizers reduce anxiety and relax skeletal

Text continued on p. 1105.

procedure 36-2

INSERTING AND MAINTAINING AN NG TUBE

Steps	Rationale
1. Inspect condition of client's oral cavity. (Use of gloves is recommended.)	Baseline condition determines need for special nursing measures for oral hygiene after tube placement.
2. Palpate client's abdomen.	Baseline determination will later serve as comparison after tube is inserted.
3. Check medical record for surgeon's order, type of NG tube to be placed, and whether tube is to be attached to suction or drainage bag.	Procedure requires physician's order. Adequate decompression depends on suction.
4. Prepare equipment and supplies:	
a. 14 or 16 Fr NG tube (smaller lumen for child)	For decompression, smaller lumen catheters are not used because they cannot remove thick secretions.
b. Water-soluble lubricating jelly	Used to lubricate tube for insertion.
c. pH test strips	Used to measure gastric aspirate acidity.
d. Tongue blade	
e. Flashlight	
f. Asepto bulb or cone-tip syringe	Used to irrigate or instill fluid into tube.
g. 2.5-cm (1-in) wide hypoallergenic tape	Less adhesive than regular tape and reduces loss of skin on nose.
h. Safety pin and rubber band	
i. Clamp, drainage bag, or suction machine	Tube may be open or closed to drainage.
j. Bath towel	
k. Glass of water with straw	
l. Facial tissues	
m. Normal saline	Used for irrigation of tube.
n. Tincture of benzoin (optional)	Increases adhesion of tape to nose.
o. Disposable gloves	
5. Identify client and explain procedure.	Prevents error and gains client's cooperation to facilitate passage of tube and lessen possibility that client will remove tube.
6. Wash hands and don gloves.	Reduces transmission of microorganisms.
7. Position client in high Fowler's position with pillows behind head and shoulders. Raise bed to its highest horizontal level.	Promotes client's ability to swallow during procedure. Good body mechanics prevent injury to nurse or client.
8. Assemble all equipment at bedside and place on your side of bed. Pull curtain around bed or close room door.	Procedure should be organized to limit discomfort. Provides privacy.
9. Stand at right side of bed if right-handed and left side if left-handed.	Allows easiest manipulation of tubing.
10. Place bath towel over chest; give tissues to client.	Prevents soiling of gown. Tube insertion through nasal passages may cause tearing.
11. Instruct client to relax and breathe normally while occluding one naris. Then repeat this action for other naris. Select nostril with greater air flow.	Tube passes more easily through naris that is more patent.
12. Measure distance to insert tube:	Tube should extend from nares to stomach; distance varies with each client. Length provides distance from nose to stomach in 98% of clients (Grant, Kennedy-Caldwell, 1988).
a. Traditional method: measure distance from tip of nose to earlobe to xiphoid process to sternum (see illustration).	
b. Hanson method: first mark 50-cm (20-in) point on tube and then do traditional measurement. Tube insertion should be to midway point between 50 cm and traditional mark.	

Continued.

procedure 36-2—cont'd

Steps	Rationale
13. Mark length of tube to be inseted with piece of tape or note distance from next tube marking.	Marks amount of tube to be inserted from nares to stomach.
14. Cut 10-cm (4-in) long piece of tape. Split one end lengthwise 5 cm (2 in).	Tape will be used after tube insertion to anchor tube securely.
15. Curve 10-15 cm (4-6 in) of end of tube tightly around index finger; release.	Curving tube tip aids insertion.
16. Lubricate 7.5-10 cm (3-4 in) of end of tube with water-soluble lubricating jelly.	Minimizes friction against nasal mucosa.
17. Initially instruct client to extend neck back against pillow; insert tube slowly through naris with curved end pointing downward (see illustration).	Facilitates initial passage of tube through naris and maintains clear airway for open naris.
18. Continue to pass tube along floor of nasal passage, aiming down toward ear. When resistance is felt, apply gentle downward pressure to advance tube (do not force past resistance).	Minimizes discomfort of tube rubbing against upper nasal turbinates. Resistance is caused by posterior nasopharynx. Downward pressure helps tube to curl around corner of nasopharynx.
19. If resistance is met, withdraw tube, allow client to rest, relubricate tube, and insert into other naris.	Forcing against resistance can cause trauma to mucosa. Helps relieve anxiety.
20. Continue insertion of tube until just past nasopharynx by gently rotating tube toward opposite naris:	
a. Stop the advancement, allow client to relax, and provide tissues.	Relieves anxiety; tearing is natural response to mucosal irritation.
b. Explain that next step requires swallowing.	Tube is about to enter esophagus.
21. With tube just above oropharynx, instruct client to flex head forward and dry swallow or suck in air through straw. Advance tube 2.5-5 cm (1-2 in) with each swallow. If client has trouble swallowing and is allowed fluids, offer glass of water. Advance tube with each swallow of water.	Flexed position closes off upper airway to trachea and opens esophagus. Swallowing closes epiglottis over trachea and helps to move tube into esophagus. Swallowing water reduces gagging or choking.
22. If client begins to cough, gag, or choke, stop tube advancement. Instruct client to breathe easily and take sips of water.	Tubing may accidentally enter larynx and initiate cough reflex. Gagging is eased by swallowing water.

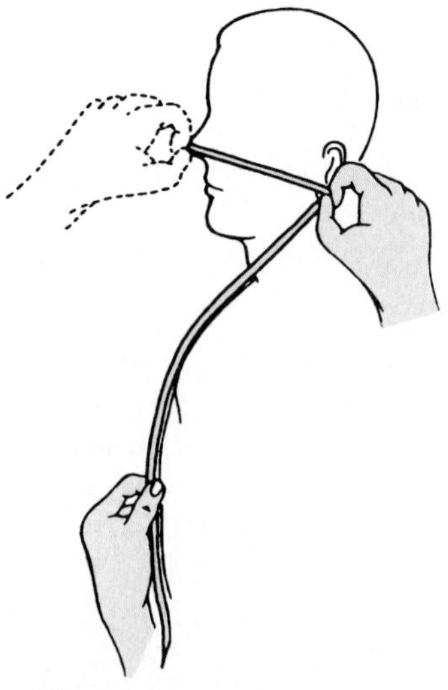
Step 12a

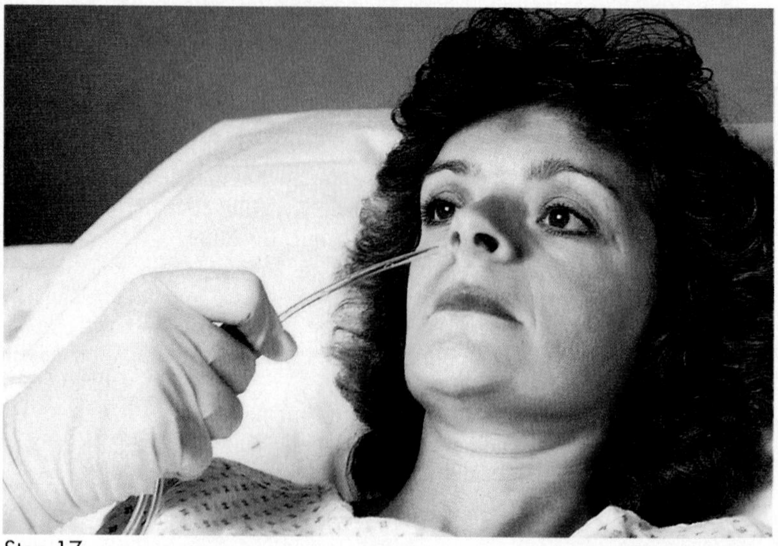
Step 17

Steps	Rationale
23. If client continues to cough, pull tube back slightly.	Tube may enter larynx and obstruct airway.
24. If client continues to gag, check back of pharynx using flashlight and tongue blade.	Tube may coil around itself in back of throat.
25. After client relaxes, continue to advance tube desired distance.	Tip of tube should be within stomach to decompress properly.
CHECKING TUBE PLACEMENT	
26. Ask client to talk.	Client would be unable to talk if tube passed through vocal cords.
27. Check posterior pharynx for presence of coiled tube.	Tube is pliable and can coil up in back of pharynx instead of advancing into esophagus.
28. Attach cone-tipped syringe to end of tube. Aspirate gently back on syringe to obtain gastric contents. (Insufflation of air into tube followed by auscultation of sounds is no longer considered most effective in determining tube placement.)	Aspiration of contents provide means to measure fluid pH and thus determine tube tip placement in gastrointestinal tract. (Sounds transmitted by insufflation of air may be transmitted from pleural space to upper abdomen, giving false impression of placement [Metheny, 1988; Metheny, et al., 1989b]).
29. Measure pH of aspirate with color-coded pH paper with range of whole numbers from 1-11.	Gastric aspirates have decidedly acidic pH values, preferably 4 or less (Metheny, et al., 1989).
30. If tube is not in stomach, advance another 2.5-5 cm (1-2 in) and repeat Steps 29 and 30 to check tube position.	Tube must be in stomach to provide decompression.
ANCHORING TUBE	
31. After tube is properly inserted, clamp end or connect it to drainage bag or suction machine.	Drainage bag is used for gravity drainage. Intermittent suction is most effective for decompression. Tube is often clamped in client going to operating room.
32. Tape tube to nose; avoid putting pressure on nares.	Prevents tissue necrosis. Tape anchors tube securely. Benzoin prevents loosening of tape if client perspires.

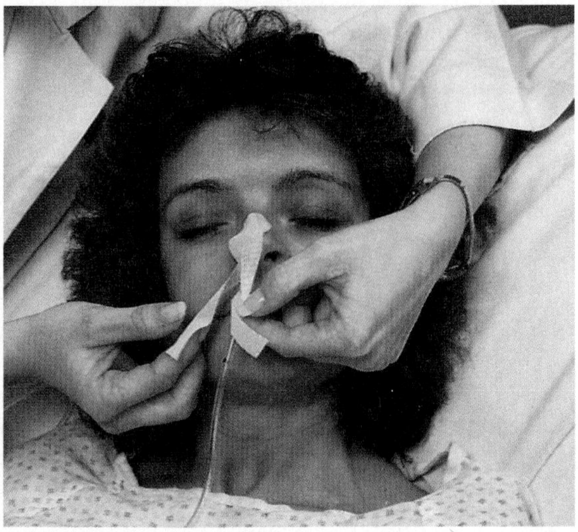
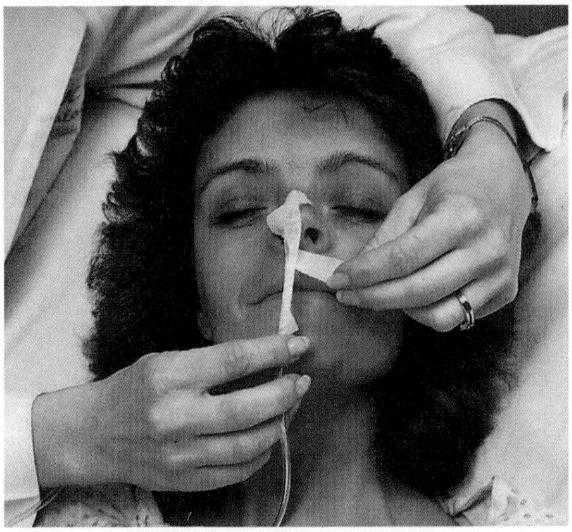

Step 32b

Continued.

procedure 36-2—cont'd

Steps	Rationale
a. OPTIONAL: Apply small amount of tincture of benzoin to lower end of nose and allow to dry. Place top end of tape over nose.	
b. Carefully wrap two split ends around tube (see illustrations).	
33. Fasten end of tube to gown by looping rubber band around tube in slip knot. Pin rubber band to gown.	Reduces pressure on nares if tube moves. Pinning provides slack for movement.
34. Unless physician orders otherwise, head of bed should be elevated 30 degrees.	Helps prevent esophageal reflux and minimizes irritation of tube against posterior pharynx.
35. Explain that sensation of tube will decrease somewhat.	Helps adaptation to continued sensory stimulus.
36. Wash hands.	Reduces transmission of microorganisms.
37. Record in nurses' notes time and type of tube inserted, tolerance to procedure, confirmation of placement, character of gastric contents, and whether tube is changed or connected to drainage device.	Documents that procedure was performed correctly. Description of gastric contents provides baseline to determine change.
TUBE IRRIGATION	
38. Check tube placement if it remains patent.	Prevents accidental entrance of irrigating solution into lungs.
39. Draw up 30 ml of normal saline into Asepto or cone-tipped syringe.	Minimizes loss of electrolytes from stomach fluids.
40. Clamp connection tubing proximal to connection site for drainage or suction apparatus. Disconnect tubing and lay end on towel.	Reduces backflow of secretions and soiling of gown and bed linen.
41. Insert tip of irrigating syringe into end of tube. Hold syringe with tip pointed at floor and inject saline slowly and evenly. (Do not force solution.)	Position prevents introduction of air into vent tubing, which could cause gastric distention. Solution introduced under pressure can cause trauma.
42. If resistance occurs, check for kinks in tubing. Turn client onto left side. Repeated resistance should be reported to surgeon.	Tip of tube may lie against stomach lining. Buildup of secretions causes distention.
43. After instilling saline, immediately aspirate or pull back slowly on syringe to withdraw fluid. Measure volume returned as output.	Irrigation clears tubing, so stomach should remain empty. Fluid remaining in stomach is measured as intake.
44. Reconnect tube to drainage or suction. (If solution does not return, repeat irrigation.)	Reestablishes drainage collection; may repeat irrigation or repositioning of tube until drains tube properly.
45. Wash hands.	Reduces transmission of microorganisms.
46. Record each irrigation: type and amount of solution used and character and volume of aspirate.	Documents procedure and results.
DISCONTINUATION OF TUBE	
47. Apply nonsterile gloves.	Reduces transmission of microorganisms.
48. Turn off suction and disconnect tube from drainage bag or suction. Remove tape from bridge of nose and unpin tube from gown.	Tube is free of connections before removal.
49. Explain procedure to client and reassure that removal is less distressing than insertion.	Minimizes anxiety and increases cooperation. Tube passes out smoothly.
50. Hand client facial tissue; place clean towel across chest. Instruct client to take and hold deep breath.	Airway will be temporarily obstructed during removal. Client may wish to blow nose after removal.
51. Clamp or kink tubing securely and pull tube out steadily and smoothly while client holds breath.	Clamping prevents tube contents from draining into oropharynx.

Steps	Rationale
52. Measure unit of drainage and note character of content. Dispose of tube and drainage equipment.	Provides accurate measure of fluid output. Reduces transfer of microorganisms.
53. Wash hands.	Reduces transmission of microorganisms.
54. Clean nares and provide mouth care.	Promotes comfort.
55. Position client comfortably and explain procedure for drinking fluid, if not contraindicated.	Depends on physician's order; usually begins with small amount of ice chips each hour and increases as client is able to tolerate more.
56. Clean equipment and return to proper place. Place soiled linen in "dirty" utility room or proper receptacle.	Proper disposal of equipment prevents spread of microorganisms and ensures proper exchange procedures.
57. Remove gloves, dispose in receptacle, and wash hands.	Reduces transmission of microorganisms.
58. Palpate abdomen periodically, noting distention.	Determines success of abdominal decompression.
59. Inspect condition of nares and nose.	Evaluates onset of skin and tissue irritation.
60. Record removal of NG tube, client's tolerance of procedure, presence of bowel sounds, and abdominal assessment.	Documents procedure and provides baseline information regarding abdominal assessment and bowel sounds.

muscles. Narcotic analgesics provide sedation, reduce pain and anxiety, and reduce the amount of anesthetic required during surgery. Anticholinergic drugs inhibit mucous secretions in the oral and respiratory passages and prevent spasm of laryngeal muscles. Typically the physician orders preoperative drugs to be given before the client leaves for the operating room. The nurse provides all nursing care measures before giving the drugs. Because the drugs cause sedation, the client should not be allowed to leave the bed until the surgical nursing assistant or transporter arrives to take the client to the operating room. The client should be warned to anticipate drowsiness and dry mouth, although the drugs usually do not induce sleep. The bed side rails should be raised and the bed kept in the low position for client safety.

Evaluation

Evaluation of the preoperative goals and outcomes of the nurse's preoperative plan of care begins before surgery and extends into the postoperative period, providing direction for future interventions. The client's surgery may be an emergency, or procedures may be required up until the time the client is taken to surgery. This leaves little time for evaluation. For some measures, such as those to prevent infection, evaluation is done postoperatively when the outcome can be determined.

The following are examples of goals, expected outcomes, and corresponding evaluative measures:

Goal: Client understands the intended surgery and the physiological and psychological responses to surgery.

Outcome

Client describes surgical procedure (in general terms) and its purpose

Evaluative measure

Ask client to explain reason for having surgery and what the procedure involves

Outcome

Client describes expected surgical outcome

Evaluative measure

Have client and family describe the anticipated result of surgery

Outcome

Client states reasons for postoperative exercises

Evaluative measure

Ask client to explain the purpose for deep breathing, spirometry, coughing, turning, and leg exercises during recovery

Outcome

Client identifies postoperative activity restrictions

Evaluative measure

Ask client and family to explain the activities to avoid following surgery

Goal: Client understands preoperative, intraoperative, and postoperative routines.

Outcome

Client states time and day of surgery and unit to be transferred postoperatively

Evaluative measure
Ask client to recall when surgery is scheduled and the unit in which he or she will be taken after surgery
Outcome
Family states location of waiting room
Evaluative measure
Have family describe where to wait during surgery
Outcome
Client identifies routine monitoring to be done intraoperatively and postoperatively
Evaluative measure
Ask client to describe the activities nurses will be performing during and immediately after surgery to monitor his or her progress

Goal: Client participates in plan of care by evening of surgery.
Outcome
Client demonstrates postoperative exercises before surgery
Evaluative measure
Have client demonstrate deep breathing, spirometry, and coughing; perform leg exercises; and turn in bed

Goal: Client achieves psychological and physical comfort and rest.
Outcome
Client uses effective coping strategies
Evaluative measure
Observe client's behavior and reaction to accepting assistance in self-care
Outcome
Client's anxiety is minimal to moderate
Evaluative measure
Observe client's nonverbal responses during treatments
Outcome
Client sleeps through night
Evaluative measure
Observe client at select times during the night and ask client to report quality of sleep the following morning
Outcome
Client demonstrates correct use of PCA pump
Evaluative measure
Have the client manipulate the PCA control device before receiving an analgesic or sedative
Outcome
Client states that medications should be given when pain becomes a persistent discomfort
Evaluative measure
Ask client to describe when is the best time to request something for pain

Goal: Client returns to functional state of health within limitations posed by surgery in 6 weeks.
Outcome
Client states the steps to activity resumption before surgery, during recovery, and at discharge
Evaluative measure
Ask client and family to describe the activity client will be allowed to perform the evening of surgery, a day later, and at progressive intervals

Evaluation of other goals is deferred until after surgery (e.g., remain free of postoperative infection).

Transport to the Operating Room

Personnel in the **operating room** notify the nursing unit when it is time for surgery. In many hospitals a nursing assistant or transporter brings a stretcher for transporting the client. The transporter checks the client's identification bracelet against the client's medical record to be sure the correct person is going to surgery. When a client is to be transported by a stretcher, the nurses and transporter assist the client in safely transferring from bed to stretcher. The ambulatory surgery client may walk to the operating room, providing more control over the event.

The family is provided an opportunity to visit before the client is transported to the operating room. The nurse then directs the family to the appropriate waiting area. If the client has been hospitalized before surgery and will be returning to the same nursing unit, the nurse prepares the bed and room for the client's return. A postoperative bedside unit should include:

1. Sphygmomanometer, stethoscope, and thermometer
2. Emesis basin
3. Clean gown
4. Washcloth, towel, and facial tissues
5. Intravenous pole
6. Suction equipment
7. Oxygen equipment
8. Extra pillows for positioning
9. Bed pads to protect bed linen from drainage
10. Intravenous pump
11. Patient controlled analgesia pump (see Chapter 28)

The nurse will be better prepared for postoperative care if the room is readied before the client's return.

Holding Area

In many hospitals the client enters a **preanesthesia care unit (PSCU)** (sometimes called a holding area) outside the operating room, where the nurse completes the preoperative preparations. Nurses in the PSCU are usually part of the operating room staff and wear surgical scrub suits.

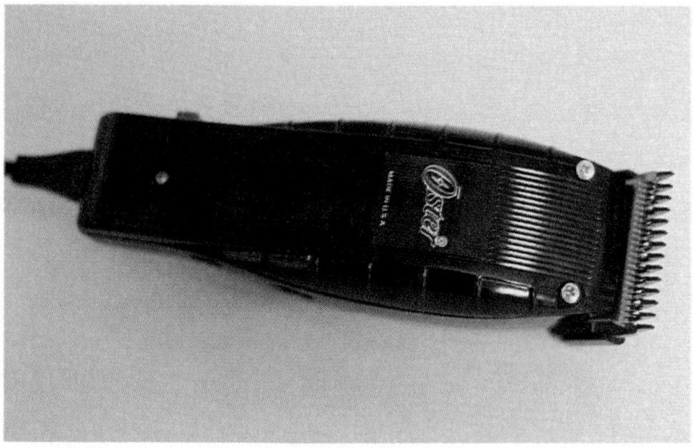

FIGURE 36-4 Clippers used to remove body hair over surgical site.

The nurses or anesthesiologist will insert an intravenous catheter into the client's vein to establish a route for fluid replacement and intravenous drugs. A large-bore intravenous catheter is used for optimal infusion of all fluids. Preoperative medications are administered.

If hair around the surgical site needs to be removed, this is done in a private area near the operating room immediately before surgery. Clippers (Figure 36-4) are preferred over a razor because they minimize the risk of small cuts, which predispose the client to infection (Garner, 1985). Studies have shown that shaving the surgical site increases the risk of infection (Cruse and Ford, 1980). The nurse should consult the physician's order sheet and the institution's policy and procedure manual.

Because the temperature in the operating room suite is usually cool, the client should be offered an extra blanket for warmth and relaxation. The client's stay in the holding area is brief.

INTRAOPERATIVE SURGICAL PHASE

Care of the client during surgery requires careful preparation and knowledge of the events that will occur during the surgical procedure.

Nurse's Role During Surgery

The nurse usually assumes one of two roles in the operating room: circulating nurse or scrub nurse. The **circulating nurse** cares for the client while in the operating room by completing the preoperative assessment, establishing and implementing the intraoperative plan of care, evaluating the care, and providing for the continuity of care postoperatively. The circulating nurse assists the anesthesiologist with endotracheal intubation, calculating blood loss and urinary output, and administering blood. This nurse monitors sterile technique and a safe operating room environment and assists the surgeon and scrub nurse by operating nonsterile equipment and providing additional instruments and supplies.

The **scrub nurse** is responsible for maintaining a sterile field during the surgical procedure, adhering to strict surgical asepsis (see Chapter 25). This nurse assists with applying surgical drapes and provides the surgeon with instruments, sponges, sutures, and other supplies. The scrub nurse keeps close count of all sponges, needles, and instruments used on the sterile field. This requires a detailed understanding of the surgical procedure, techniques, and instruments necessary.

Admission to the Operating Room

The circulating nurse transfers the client to the operating room. The client is usually still awake and will notice nurses and physicians wearing complete surgical masks, protective eyewear, and gowns. The staff members carefully transfer the client to the operating table, being sure the stretcher and table are locked in place. After the client is on the table, the nurse fastens a safety strap around the client's legs.

NURSING PROCESS

Assessment

The circulating nurse conducts a special preoperative assessment to verify the client is ready for surgery and to use as a basis for planning intraoperative care. In some settings, the operating room nurse does this in the PSCU. The client is asked his or her name, and this is compared with the identification band and chart. The nurse reviews consent forms, allergies, medical history, physical assessment findings, and test results. The nurse verifies with the client what surgery is to be performed and the surgical site. A brief assessment of the respiratory, circulatory, neurological, and musculoskeletal systems is performed. The condition of the skin is assessed, with attention paid to any bruises or redness. If any prosthetic devices or valuables are with the client, the nurse makes arrangements for their safekeeping. Special attention is also paid to the psychological comfort of the client.

Nursing Diagnosis

Preoperative nursing diagnoses are reviewed and, based on this assessment, modified to individualize the care plan for the client in the operating room. Additional diagnoses and related factors are added (see box on p. 1108). These diagnoses provide direction for postoperative care of the client.

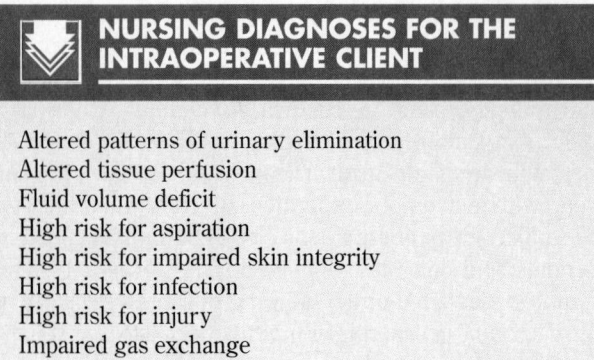

NURSING DIAGNOSES FOR THE INTRAOPERATIVE CLIENT

Altered patterns of urinary elimination
Altered tissue perfusion
Fluid volume deficit
High risk for aspiration
High risk for impaired skin integrity
High risk for infection
High risk for injury
Impaired gas exchange
Ineffective thermoregulation

Planning

Based on identified nursing diagnoses, the nurse completes a plan of care for the client. Although most of the preparation for care in the operating room has already been accomplished, changes may be made to meet individualized needs.

Some goals of preoperative care extend into the intraoperative phase. These include remaining free of infection and achieving psychological and physical comfort. Additional goals and outcomes include the following:

Goal: Client maintains skin integrity.
Outcome
The client's skin over bony prominences and under grounding pad is intact, without redness or signs of pressure

Goal: The client maintains a therapeutic body temperature.
Outcome
Client's body temperature remains as desired

Goal: Client maintains fluid and electrolyte balance
Outcomes
Client will remain hydrated
Client's vital signs will remain stable

Implementation

A major focus of intraoperative care is to prevent injury and complications related to anesthesia, surgery, positioning, and equipment used. The nurse acts as an advocate for the client during surgery. The client's dignity and rights are protected at all times.

Physical Preparation

After securing the client's safety, the circulating nurse completes the physical preparation. Clients undergo continuous electrocardiographic monitoring during surgery. The nurse applies small, plastic electrodes on the chest and extremities to record the electrical activity of the heart. A monitor displays the heart's electrical activity. Next, the nurse applies a blood pressure cuff from a noninvasive blood pressure monitor around the client's arm to allow the anesthesiologist to measure the blood pressure while using both hands to ventilate the client. A pulse oximeter probe is attached to the client's finger or ear lobe, allowing measurement of the oxygen saturation in the blood and an evaluation of ventilation.

table 36-6

STAGES OF GENERAL ANESTHESIA

Stage	Client response
Stage 1	Begins with client being awake; client gradually becomes drowsy and loses consciousness; state of analgesia begins
Stage 2	Stage of excitement; client's muscles are often tense and almost spasmodic; swallowing and vomiting reflexes remain intact; client may breathe irregularly
Stage 3	Begins with onset of regular rhythmical breathing; vital functions depressed; client's reflexes depressed or temporarily lost; surgeon begins operation during this phase
Stage 4	Stage of complete respiratory depression requiring respiratory support; can be fatal

Psychological Support

Entering the operating room is stressful for most clients. The nurse reassures the client and should remain at the client's side until after anesthesia is induced. Offering a hand to hold is often helpful. If the client is awake during surgery, this support is given throughout the surgical procedure.

Introduction of Anesthesia

One of three types of anesthesia is used during surgical procedures: general, regional, or local.

General Anesthesia. Under **general anesthesia** a client loses all sensation and consciousness. Muscles relax to ease manipulation of body parts. The client also experiences amnesia of all surgical events. Surgery using general anesthesia includes major procedures requiring extensive tissue manipulation. An anesthesiologist or certified registered nurse anesthetist (CRNA) administers general anesthetics by intravenous and inhalation routes. The client's response to these agents progresses through stages (Table 36-6).

To move the client quickly from stage 1 to stage 3 of general anesthesia an intravenous dose of a barbiturate is given. To prevent possible aspiration and other respiratory complications the anesthesia provider places an endotracheal tube into the airway. A depolarizing muscle relaxant (e.g., succinylcholine) is used, causing temporary paralysis of vocal cords and respiratory muscles while the client is intubated. The anesthesia provider then artificially ventilates the client until the muscle relaxant is metabolized and the client again breathes spontaneously. From that point, anesthetic gases or vapors are usually delivered by inhalation through the endotracheal tube. The client also receives a continuous supply of oxygen. The duration of anesthesia desired depends on the length of surgery. The greatest risks from general anesthesia are the side effects of anesthetic agents, including cardiovascular depression or irritability, respiratory depression, and liver and kidney damage.

Regional Anesthesia. Induction of **regional anesthesia** results in loss of sensation in an area of the body. The method of induction influences the portion of the sensory pathways anesthetized. The anesthesiologist gives regional anesthetics by infiltration and local application (see Chapter 28). In some surgeries such as a hernia repair or vascular repair of leg blood vessels only infiltrative induction is used. Infiltration of anesthetic agents may involve any one of the following induction methods: nerve block and spinal and epidural anesthesia.

There are risks involved with infiltrative anesthetics, particularly in the case of spinal anesthesia because the level of anesthesia may extend. The client may experience a sudden fall in blood pressure, which results from extensive vasodilation caused by the anesthetic block to sympathetic vasomotor nerves, pain, and motor fibers. If the level of anesthesia rises, respiratory paralysis may develop, requiring resuscitation by the anesthesiologist. The client requires careful monitoring during and immediately after regional anesthesia.

The client under regional anesthesia is awake throughout surgery unless a sedative is administered. Because the client is responsive and breathing voluntarily, it is not necessary for the anesthesiologist to use an endotracheal tube. Operating room personnel are aware that the client is awake and can hear communication between team members. Therefore they need to be especially careful not to say something that may be misunderstood or be stressful for the client.

Local Anesthesia. Local anesthesia involves loss of sensation at the desired site (e.g., a growth on the skin or a cyst in the breast). The anesthetic agent (e.g., lidocaine) inhibits peripheral nerve conduction until the drug diffuses into the circulation. The client experiences a loss in pain sensation, touch, and motor function. Autonomic activities (e.g., bladder emptying) can be lost when extensive anesthesia is used. Local anesthesia is commonly used for minor procedures performed in ambulatory surgery.

Local anesthetics are also administered to clients receiving general anesthesia. Long-acting local anesthetics (e.g., bupivicaine) are frequently injected into the incision at the end of the client's surgery for postoperative pain relief.

When a local anesthetic is used, an anesthesia provider may administer intravenous sedation and monitor the client (monitored anesthesia care). The registered nurse assumes this responsibility when an anesthesia provider is not present. The nurse supports the client by explaining procedures and encouraging questions. Sights and sounds in the operating room may frighten clients. Therefore the nurse warns the client when unpleasant sensations will be experienced (e.g., injections or a tightening blood pressure cuff). Emotional support is given throughout the procedure, and conversation can be an effective distraction. In some settings, the client listens to music to mask unpleasant sounds and to promote relaxation.

Positioning

The choice of position is usually determined by the surgical approach. Ideally the client's position provides good access to and exposure of the operative site and sustains adequate circulatory and respiratory function; it should not impair neuromuscular structures or skin integrity. The client's comfort and safety must be considered. When general anesthesia is used, the nursing personnel and surgeon usually do not position the client until the stage of complete relaxation. It is sometimes difficult for nurses caring for clients postoperatively to appreciate the discomfort a client may feel after surgery. Normal range of motion is maintained by the alert person by pain and pressure receptors. If a joint is extended too far, pain stimuli warn that muscle and joint strain are too great. In a client who is anesthetized, normal defense mechanisms cannot guard against joint damage, muscle stretch, and strain. The client's muscles are so relaxed that it is relatively easy to place the client in a position he or she normally could not assume while awake. The client often remains in a given position for several hours. Although it may be necessary to place a client in an unusual position, the nurse should attempt to maintain correct physiological alignment and protect the client from pressure, abrasion, and other injuries. Special positioning devices allow for proper support and protection and dispersement of pressure over bony prominences. Positioning should not impede normal movement of the diaphragm or interfere with circulation to body parts. Restraints should not impair circulation or skin integrity.

Prevention of Infection

Prevention of infection is a primary responsibility of operating room nurses. Both the circulating nurse and the scrub nurse closely monitor surgical asepsis (see Chapter 25) and correct any breaks in technique. Universal precautions are followed to protect clients and staff members from possible infections.

Once the client is positioned, the circulating nurse prepares the skin for the surgical incision. First, the skin is carefully assessed and allergies reviewed. Next, an antimicrobial solution is applied to the skin (e.g., chlorhexidine or povidone-iodine) to reduce the microorganisms normally located on the skin and to minimize their entry into the surgical wound (Larsen, 1993). The nurse must be careful not to allow any of the solution to pool under the client, because it may irritate or burn the skin. The scrub nurse and the surgeon apply sterile surgical drapes to create a sterile field for the surgical procedure.

Prevention of Injury

Prevention of injury to the client is an extremely important part of the nurse's role. Before the beginning and at the end of the surgical procedure, together the scrub and circulating nurses count all of the sponges, needles, and instruments brought to the sterile field. During the procedure, these nurses keep close count of these items to prevent accidental loss of any item inside the surgical wound. The nurse who fails to accurately count items can be held legally accountable and found negligent if a client is injured by a misplaced item (see Chapter 6). The operating room nurse must also be aware of the risks to the client when using special equipment (e.g., electrosurgical cautery and lasers). Use of this equipment requires additional interventions to protect the client. If electrosurgical cautery is used, the nurse applies a grounding pad to the client to protect against burns. Lasers pose an increased risk of a fire and client injury. The laser beam generates intense heat and can be reflected. Of particular concern is the oxygen-rich environment of the airway. Specific protective measures are taken to protect the client and operating room staff (e.g., using water-soaked drapes and sponges, nonreflective instruments, and eye protection). If laser surgery is near the airway, a special endotracheal tube is used.

Maintenance of Fluid and Electrolyte Balance

Maintenance of fluid and electrolyte balance is the responsibility of the nurse and the anesthesiologist. Blood loss and urinary and nasogastric drainage are monitored during surgery; intravenous solutions and sometimes blood products are administered to replace lost fluids.

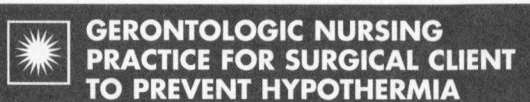

GERONTOLOGIC NURSING PRACTICE FOR SURGICAL CLIENT TO PREVENT HYPOTHERMIA

- Set the room temperature between 18° and 21° C
- Place a thermoregulating blanket under the client
- Apply a reflective head cover and blanket
- Warm IV solutions and transfusions
- Warm irrigating solutions

Temperature Control

The client under general anesthesia lacks the ability to regulate body temperature. The anesthetic agents used block the reflex to shiver and cause vasodilation. These effects, combined with surgical exposure and a cool room, can cause hypothermia. Therefore the client's temperature is continuously monitored throughout surgery by the anesthesiologist. The nurse takes measures to prevent heat loss (see box above). The room should be kept warm until the surgical drapes are in place. A warming blanket may be placed under the client on the operating table. A reflective hat or blanket may be used to prevent heat loss. Some hospitals use a hot air blanket or heating lamp on top of the client, under the surgical drapes. Irrigating solutions and blood are warmed before administration. For some surgeries (e.g., coronary artery bypass) hypothermia is planned and induced to reduce the oxygen demands of vital organs (Thelan, et al., 1992). The nurse then uses a cooling blanket to maintain hypothermia.

Emergencies

In rare instances, emergencies occur while the client is in the operating room. These are usually related to the client's preoperative health status. Respiratory complications can occur when the airway is irritated by anesthetic agents. Cardiac dysrhythmias can occur in response to anesthetic agents, the surgical procedure, or fluid and electrolyte shifts. Malignant hyperpyrexia (hyperthermia) is a genetically transmitted life-threatening complication of anesthesia. When exposed to a triggering agent, a high fever, tachycardia, metabolic changes, and an acid-base imbalance occur. If not detected and treated early, it is fatal.

All operating room team members pay close attention to the client's condition and the need to be prepared for emergencies. The nurse must know what emergency equipment and supplies are needed and where they are located. A nurse must be ready to respond appropriately.

Documentation of Intraoperative Care

During the intraoperative phase, the nursing staff continue the established plan of care, and modify it as needed. Throughout the surgical procedure, the circulating nurse keeps an accurate record of client care activities and procedures performed by operating room personnel; this record provides useful data for the nurse who cares for the client postoperatively.

Evaluative Measures

At the end of the surgical procedure, the nurse performs a postoperative assessment of the client. This assessment forms the basis for the initial evaluation of the nursing care provided during the intraoperative phase. Only part of the evaluation can be completed in the operating room because some complications (e.g., infection) can arise days after surgery.

Evaluative measures to identify the effectiveness of intraoperative interventions include:

Goal: Client maintains skin integrity.

Outcome

The client's skin over bony prominences and under grounding pad is intact, without redness or signs of pressure.

Evaluative measure

Inspect skin under grounding pad and inspect areas of skin where pressure may be exerted because of positioning.

Goal: Client maintains a therapeutic body temperature.

Outcome

Client's body temperature remains as desired (depends on surgical procedure)

Evaluative measure

Measure client's body temperature during procedure, immediately postoperatively, and at ordered intervals

Goal: Client maintains fluid and electrolyte balance.

Outcomes

Client will remain hydrated

Client's vital signs will remain stable

Evaluative measure (may be evaluated by the anesthesiologist)

Obtain vital signs and auscultate lung sounds

Many interventions taken during the intraoperative phase are directed toward prevention of injury or complication. These interventions are comprehensively evaluated postoperatively.

POSTOPERATIVE SURGICAL PHASE

Postoperative care of the client is challenging because of complex physiological changes. To assess the client's postoperative condition the nurse relies on information from the preoperative nursing assessment and on information regarding the surgical procedure and events occurring during surgery. The nurse must be skilled at noticing change. A variation from the norm may indicate the onset of complications.

The postoperative course involves the immediate postoperative period and convalescence. For an ambulatory surgical client the immediate postoperative period normally lasts only 1 to 2 hours and convalescence will occur at home. For a hospitalized client the immediate postoperative period may last a few hours, with convalescence taking 1 or more days, depending on the extent of surgery and the client's response.

NURSING PROCESS

Assessment–Postanesthesia

Immediately after surgery, the client is transferred to the postanesthesia care unit (PACU), formerly called the recovery room, for close monitoring (Figure 36-5). Before the arrival of the client, the PACU nurse receives a report from the surgical team in the operating room to determine the client's general status and the need for special equipment and nursing care.

When the client enters the PACU, the nurse performs a rapid assessment of the respiratory and circulatory status of the client and attaches electronic monitors. Then the nurse and members of the surgical team

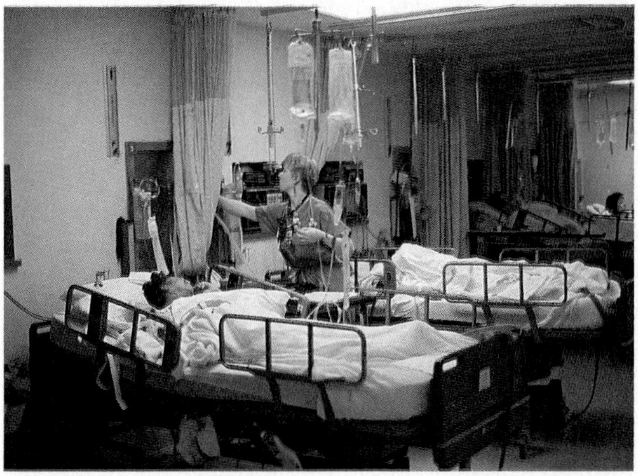

FIGURE 36-5 In postanesthesia care units, clients are closely monitored following surgery.

confer about the client's status. During this report, the client is continuously monitored. The anesthesiologist's report includes a review of anesthetic agents given so the PACU nurse can anticipate the course with which a client should recover. A report on intravenous fluids or blood products given during surgery alerts the nurse to the fluid and electrolyte balance. The operating room nurse reports any allergies, drainage devices (e.g., Foley catheter or wound drain), and whether the client had any surgical complications such as excessive blood loss. The surgeon often reports any special concerns (e.g., whether the client is at risk for hemorrhage or infection).

After reviewing events occurring in the operating room, the PACU nurse assesses the client's status, starting with respiratory and circulatory systems. Interventions are initiated immediately, as needed.

Respiration. The nurse assesses the quality of the respirations and the patency of the airway. A client receiving a general anesthetic often has an artificial airway in place when arriving in the PACU. Certain anesthetic agents may continue to cause respiratory depression. Thus the nurse is especially alert for shallow, slow breathing. The nurse assesses respiratory rate, rhythm, depth of ventilation, symmetry of chest wall movement, breath sounds, and color of mucous membranes. Lung sounds are auscultated to identify any abnormalities such as rales or wheezing. If breathing is unusually shallow, placement of the nurse's hand over the client's face or mouth allows the nurse to feel exhaled air. Pulse oximetry is used to continuously monitor the oxygen saturation of the blood (Chapter 15).

Circulation. The client is at risk for cardiovascular complications from blood loss at the surgical site, side effects of anesthesia, electrolyte imbalances, and depression of normal circulatory regulating mechanisms. Therefore continuous electrocardiograph monitoring is used routinely for clients in the PACU. Careful assessment of heart rate and rhythm and blood pressure reveals the client's cardiovascular status. The nurse compares preoperative vital signs with postoperative values to determine the client's status.

The nurse assesses circulatory perfusion by noting the color of nail beds and skin. If the client has had vascular surgery, a tourniquet has been used, or has casts or tight dressings that may impair circulation, the nurse assesses peripheral pulses distal to the site of surgery.

The PACU nurse must always be alert to the amount of bleeding that occurs after surgery and the possibility of hemorrhage. Blood loss may occur externally through a drain or incision, or internally within the surgical wound. Either type of hemorrhage may manifest itself by a fall in blood pressure, elevated heart and respiratory rate, diminished pulse, cool, clammy, pale skin, and restlessness.

Temperature Control. The operating room environment is cool. The client's depressed level of body function results in a lowering of metabolism and fall in body temperature. When clients begin to awaken, they may complain of feeling cold and uncomfortable. Shivering may not be a sign of hypothermia but rather a side effect of certain anesthetic agents. The nurse measures body temperature to provide direction for interventions.

Neurological Functions. On arrival in the PACU the client is usually drowsy and reacting to verbal commands. However, drugs, electrolyte and metabolic changes, pain, and emotional factors influence level of consciousness. As anesthetic agents are metabolized, the client's reflexes return, muscle strength is regained, and a normal level of orientation returns. The nurse can easily check for pupillary and gag reflexes (see Chapter 16). If a client has had surgery involving a portion of the neurological system, the nurse will conduct a more thorough neurological assessment.

Skin Integrity and Condition of Wound. The PACU nurse assesses the condition of the client's skin. A rash may indicate a drug sensitivity or allergy. Abrasions or petechiae may result from inadequate padding during positioning or restraining that injures skin layers. Burns or serious injury to the skin should be communicated by an incident report. Most surgical wounds are covered with a dressing that protects the wound site and collects drainage. The nurse observes the amount, color, odor, and consistency of drainage on dressings and estimates the amount of drainage by noting the number of saturated gauze sponges. If drainage appears on the outer surface of a dressing, another way of assessing drainage is by drawing a circle around the outer perimeter of the drainage. If the perimeter expands, drainage is increasing. However, this is not the most accurate measure of fluid volume lost.

Genitourinary Function. A spinal anesthetic may prevent the client from feeling bladder fullness or distention and cause urinary retention for up to 6 to 8 hours. The nurse palpates the lower abdomen just above the symphysis pubis for bladder distention. A full bladder can be painful and is often the cause of a client's restlessness, agitation, or high blood pressure in the PACU. If the client has a Foley catheter (see Chapter 32), there should be a continuous flow of urine of at least 30 cc/hr in adults. The nurse observes the color and odor of urine. Surgery involving portions of the urinary tract normally causes bloody urine for at least 12 to 24 hours, depending on the type of surgery.

Gastrointestinal Function. Anesthetic agents slow gastrointestinal motility and may cause nausea. A nurse will normally hear faint or absent bowel sounds in all four quadrants during the immediate recovery phase.

Inspection of the abdomen rules out distention that may be caused by the accumulation of gas. Distention may develop if internal bleeding occurs in a client who has had abdominal surgery. If a nasogastric tube is in place, the nurse assesses the patency of the tube, and the color and amount of any drainage.

Fluid and Electrolyte Balance. Because of the surgical client's risk for fluid and electrolyte abnormalities, the nurse assesses the hydration status and monitors cardiac and neurological function for signs of electrolyte alterations (see Chapter 35). The nurse inspects the intravenous catheter insertion site to be sure it is patent, and that there are no signs of infiltration. The physician orders a prescribed rate for each infusion.

Monitoring and accurate recording of intake and output helps to assess the fluid and electrolyte balance, as well as renal and cardiac function. The nurse measures all sources of output, including urine, gastric drainage, and wound drainage and consults with the physician if appropriate.

Comfort. As a client awakens from general anesthesia, the sensation of discomfort can become prominent. Pain can be perceived before full consciousness is regained. Acute incisional pain causes the client to become restless and may cause changes in vital signs. It is difficult for clients to begin coughing and deep breathing exercises when they have pain. The client who had regional or local anesthesia usually does not experience pain initially because the incisional area is still anesthetized. The PACU nurse must be skilled at assessing levels of pain (Chapter 28) and alert to the need for medication for treatment.

Respiratory status is evaluated continuously while the client is in the PACU. However, after the initial assessment, the nurse evaluates blood pressure and other key observations every 15 minutes, or more frequently if indicated. Based on these assessments, the plan of care is modified to meet the immediate needs of the client.

NURSING DIAGNOSES FOR THE POSTOPERATIVE CLIENT

Activity intolerance
Altered patterns of urinary elimination
Altered role performance
Body image disturbance
High risk for fluid volume deficit
High risk for infection
Ineffective breathing pattern
Impaired physical mobility
Impaired verbal communication
Ineffective airway clearance
Pain

Nursing Diagnosis

Based on the postanesthesia assessment, and reports given by the operating room nurse, surgeon, and anesthesiologist, postoperative nursing diagnoses are identified for the client. These diagnoses give direction to the continuing care of the client in the PACU and the postoperative nursing unit (see box below).

Planning

Based on these diagnoses, a plan of care is established. Because of the critical nature of the immediate postoperative period, this plan always involves close monitoring of the client and frequent assessments. Goals and outcomes identified for the client immediately postoperatively include:

Goal: Client achieves physical and psychological comfort.

Outcomes

Client verbalizes relief or reduction of pain
Client's anxiety is low or moderate

Goal: Client returns to normal physiological functioning.

Outcomes

Client has oxygen saturation over 95% (or within preoperative baseline range)
Client has patent airway
Client has stable blood pressure
Client has palpable peripheral pulses
Client is able to move all extremities
Client is awake and oriented to PACU environment
Client's temperature is 35.5° to 38.5° C

Goal: Client maintains fluid and electrolyte balance.

Outcomes

Vital signs are stable
Wound drainage is minimal
Intake and output remain balanced

Goal: Client remains free of postoperative infection.

Outcome

Client's incision is clean, free of purulent drainage

Implementation

Respiration. Following general anesthesia, the client often has an oral or nasal airway inserted to maintain a patent airway until regular breathing at a normal rate resumes. As respiratory function returns, the nurse will ask the client to expel the airway. The client's ability to do so signifies a return of a normal gag reflex.

One of the nurse's greatest concerns is airway obstruction resulting from aspiration of emesis, accumulation of mucous secretions in the pharynx, or swelling or spasm of the larynx. The following measures maintain airway patency:

1. The nurse positions the client on one side with the face down and the neck slightly extended. A small, folded towel supports the head. The neck extension prevents occlusion of the airway at the pharynx. When the face is kept turned downward, the tongue moves forward and mucous secretions flow out of the mouth instead of accumulating in the pharynx. If the nature of the surgery prevents turning the client on one side, the head of the bed is slightly elevated and the client's neck slightly extended, with the head turned to the side. The client should never be positioned with arms over or across the chest because this reduces maximum chest expansion.
2. The nurse suctions artificial airways and the oral cavity for mucous secretions, as necessary. Care must be taken to avoid continually eliciting the gag reflex, which might cause vomiting. Before removing an airway, the back of the airway should be suctioned so that mucous plugs and secretions are not retained.
3. The nurse begins any coughing and deep breathing exercises as soon as the client can respond to instructions.
4. The nurse administers oxygen as ordered, by mask or nasal prongs. In many PACU settings, oxygen is routinely administered.

Circulation. The nurse must be aware of changes in blood pressure or heart rate. The physician may have written an order indicating which changes are to be reported. However, the nurse must use judgment and notify the physician when there is a significant change or a continuous trend in vital signs.

If hemorrhage is external, the nurse should observe for increased bloody drainage on dressings or through drains. If a dressing becomes saturated, the blood will ooze down the client's sides and collect in a pool under bedclothes. When hemorrhage is internal, the operative site becomes swollen, tight, and a hematoma may develop. The first signs of suspected hemorrhaging should be reported to the physician immediately. The nurse closely monitors vital signs until the client's condition stabilizes.

Temperature Control. The client is usually cool when arriving in the PACU. Therefore the nurse provides specially warmed blankets or other warming devices (e.g., a hot air blanket). Increasing body warmth causes the client's metabolism to rise and circulatory and respiratory functions to improve.

Neurological Functioning. Deep breathing and coughing will help to expel retained anesthetic gases, and promote return of the client's level of consciousness. The nurse arouses the client by calling his or her name in a moderate tone of voice. The nurse notes whether the client responds appropriately or seems confused and disoriented. If the client remains asleep or unresponsive, the nurse attempts arousal through touch or by gently moving a body part. If a painful stimulus is needed to arouse the client, the nurse should notify the anesthesiologist. Orientation to the PACU environment is important in maintaining alertness. The nurse explains that surgery is completed and describes all procedures and nursing measures performed.

Wound and Dressing Care. Dressings should be left in place to reduce the risk of infection. Therefore the PACU nurse may simply add an extra layer of gauze on top of the original dressing. Notify the physician if bleeding is excessive.

Gastrointestinal. To minimize nausea the nurse avoids sudden movement of the client. If the client has a nasogastric tube, the nurse maintains the tube patency. Occlusion of a nasogastric tube results in the accumulation of gastric contents within the stomach. Because stomach emptying slows under anesthesia, the accumulated contents cannot escape, and nausea and vomiting develop. Normally a client does not receive fluids to drink in the PACU because of the risk of vomiting. A moist cloth or swab is sometimes used to relieve dryness of the client's lips and mouth.

Genitourinary. A full bladder is painful and can cause the client to be restless or agitated. If the bladder becomes distended, the nurse will probably need to obtain a physician order to insert a catheter. If a catheter is already in place and urinary output is less than 30 cc/hr in an adult client, the nurse notifies the surgeon.

Fluid and Electrolyte Balance. The nurse maintains patency of intravenous infusions. The client's only source of fluid intake immediately after surgery is through intravenous catheters. The client may also receive blood products, depending on the amount of blood lost during surgery.

Comfort. The anesthesiologist orders medications for pain management in the PACU. Intravenous opioid analgesics such as morphine sulphate are the drugs of choice for the immediate postoperative period (AHCPR, 1992). The nurse administers morphine intravenously, titrating it until pain relief is achieved. Morphine may depress vital signs and level of consciousness. However, a low blood pressure may be caused by acute pain. In such a situation an analgesic may improve vital sign values. The PACU nurse is skilled at determining the proper dose of an analgesic.

CLIENT TEACHING FOR AMBULATORY SURGICAL CLIENTS

Physician's office telephone number (24-hour answer)
Surgery center's telephone number
Follow-up appointment, date, time
Review of prescribed medications
Guidelines related to specific surgery
- Dressing and wound care
- Activity restrictions

Guidelines related to anesthesia
- Dietary
- Activity restrictions

Warning signs of complications

Postanesthesia Care in Ambulatory Surgery

The postanesthesia care of ambulatory surgery clients occurs in two phases, in two separate areas. Phase I is essentially the same as described for hospitalized clients. Phase II, however, prepares the client for discharge and self-care. The client receiving only local anesthesia may be admitted directly to the Phase II area. In Phase II, clients are encouraged to gradually sit up on the stretcher or recliner and begin to take ice chips or sips of water after regaining full alertness.

Phase II postanesthesia care occurs in a room equipped with medical recliner chairs, side tables, and footrests. Kitchen facilities for preparing light snacks and beverages are located in the area, along with bathrooms. The Phase II environment promotes the client's and families' comfort and well-being until discharge. The nurse monitors clients but not at the same intensity as Phase I. In Phase II, the nurse initiates postoperative teaching with clients and family members (see box above). After the client's condition becomes stable, he or she is discharged.

Evaluation

The nurse continuously evaluates the effectiveness of interventions. The client's condition can change quickly. The nurse may need to increase frequency of select interventions or choose totally new interventions. Examples of goals, outcomes, and corresponding evaluative measures include:

Goal: Client achieves physical and psychological comfort.
- **Outcome**
  - Client verbalizes relief or reduction of pain
- **Evaluative measure**
  - Observe client's facial expressions and posture when moving painful body part
  - Ask client to rate pain relief (when alert) on same scale used preoperatively
- **Outcome**
  - Client's anxiety is low or moderate
- **Evaluative measures**
  - Assess client's blood pressure and heart rate
  - Observe for nonverbal behavior and note client's expression of feelings and concerns

Goal: Client returns to normal physiological functioning.
- **Outcomes**
  - Client has oxygen saturation over 95% (or at preoperative baseline)
  - Client has patent airway
- **Evaluative measures**
  - Perform pulse oximetry and assess respiratory rate and rhythm
  - Auscultate lung sounds
- **Outcome**
  - Client has palpable peripheral pulses
- **Evaluative measure**
  - Palpate pulses distal to operative site
- **Outcomes**
  - Client is able to move all extremities
  - Client is awake and oriented to PACU environment
- **Evaluative measures**
  - Assess Glascow Coma Scale status (Chapter 16)
  - Ask client to move all extremities slowly
- **Outcome**
  - Client's temperature is 35.5° to 38.5° C
- **Evaluative measure**
  - Assess body temperature per ordered frequency

Goal: Client maintains fluid and electrolyte balance.
- **Outcome**
  - Vital signs are stable
- **Evaluative measure**
  - Measure vital signs per ordered frequency or more often if client's condition changes
- **Outcome**
  - Intake and output remain balanced
- **Evaluative measure**
  - Measure all sources of output and monitor intravenous fluid infusion

Goal: Client remains free of postoperative infection.
- **Outcome**
  - Client's incision is clean, free of purulent drainage
- **Evaluative measures**
  - Inspect incision for closure and drainage
  - Inspect character of drainage in drainage device

Documentation. Documentation in the PACU is done on the PACU record or flowsheet. It includes all assessment findings, interventions, and the client's response to these interventions. A graph is used to plot vital signs so the nurse can easily identify a trend in the client's status.

Discharge from the PACU. The nurse evaluates a client's readiness for discharge from the PACU on the basis of achieved outcomes. If the client's condition is still unstable after 2 to 3 hours, the anesthesia provider may transfer the client to an intensive care unit (ICU).

When a hospitalized client's condition stabilizes, it is time for transfer from the PACU to the postoperative nursing unit. Nursing care focuses on returning the client to a functional level of wellness as soon as possible. The speed of recovery depends on the extent of surgery, type of anesthesia, risk factors, postoperative complications, and the effectiveness of the nurse's care plan.

The client discharged from the PACU is transported to the postoperative unit on a stretcher. Staff members assist in safely transferring the client to a bed. The PACU nurse reviews the client's course and the PACU record, with the nurse caring for the client postoperatively. This report includes a review of physician orders requiring attention. Before the PACU nurse leaves, the unit nurse takes a complete set of vital signs to compare with postanesthesia findings. Minor vital sign variations normally occur after transporting the client. In some settings, when the client is stable, a transporter may take the client to the postoperative unit. In this situation, the PACU nurse telephones a report to the nurse on the postoperative unit.

Family. The preoperative nurse usually advises the family to remain in the waiting room while the client is in the operating room, so the surgeon can report to them at the end of the surgery. Waiting is stressful for family members, and they can become anxious if surgery takes longer than expected. Nurses can help to relieve this concern by explaining the reasons for normal delays, such as room preparation or delay in the previous surgery. Family members usually remain in the waiting room while the client is in the PACU. However, under select circumstances a family member may visit the client in the PACU. In some facilities, a parent may remain with pediatric clients in the PACU to provide emotional support. If the client's stay in the PACU is extended, the nurse can explain the client is being held longer for observation.

Communication with the family while the client is in the operating room and PACU is very important. Family members indicate that having questions answered honestly and knowing facts about the client's progress are important to them (Norheim, 1989). Progress reports reduce the anxiety of family members (Leske, 1993). However, while the client is in surgery, the nurse should confer with the surgeon before giving progress reports to the family. This will avoid any miscommunications. When the surgery is complete, the surgeon reports to the family the client's status, the results of surgery, and the occurrence of any complications. The nurse should listen to the family's concerns and feelings, and assess the ability of the family to cope with this information. The nurse can reinforce adaptive coping and give emotional support by listening to their concerns and assisting them with obtaining answers to their questions. In some PACU settings, a parent is allowed to stay in the PACU with a child for emotional support.

NURSING PROCESS

Assessment–Post Recovery

Once the client arrives at the postoperative unit and the first set of vital signs have been measured, the nurse's assessment includes an initial check of the client's general condition, including level of consciousness, condition of dressings and drains, intravenous fluid status, comfort level, and skin integrity. The physical measurements and observations performed in the PACU are also continued in the postoperative unit. The nurse routinely assesses the client at least every 15 minutes the first hour, every 30 minutes for 1 to 2 hours, every hour for 4 hours, and then every 4 hours. Assessments may be more frequent, depending on the client's condition. If the client appears normal during the initial assessment, the nurse should not assume that further monitoring is unnecessary. A client's condition can change rapidly. A nurse is guilty of neglect when failing to follow the assessment schedule. The nurse documents the initial assessment and makes entries in the nurses' notes. Vital signs, intravenous fluid intake, and urinary output are entered on flowsheets. The initial findings are a baseline for identifying any postoperative changes.

After the nurse completes the first assessment of the client and has attended to the immediate needs, the family is allowed to visit. The nurse should explain the purpose of postoperative procedures. The family will want to know how the client is doing. The nurse tells them when vital signs are stable and the client seems to be awakening without difficulty. The family should know that the client will fall in and out of sleep for most of the day. The nurse should also remind the family that frequent assessments of the client's condition are to be expected, and if the client had spinal anesthesia, loss of sensation and movement in the extremities can remain for several hours.

Nursing Diagnosis

The nurse determines the status of problems identified from preoperative, intraoperative, and immediate postoperative diagnoses and clusters new relevant data to identify additional postoperative diagnoses (see box on p. 1113). Previously defined diagnoses such as "impaired skin integrity" may continue as a postoperative problem. For example, an older adult client who has had lengthy abdominal surgery and who has a preexisting problem of dehydration and malnutrition is at *high risk for impaired skin integrity.* The nurse also considers needs of a client's family when making diagnoses. For example, the inability of the family to cope with the client's condition requires nursing intervention.

Planning

During the convalescent phase, the nurse has much information to use for planning the client's care. Postoperative physical assessment data and analysis of the preoperative nursing history allow the nurse to plan specific nursing interventions. The surgeon's postoperative orders also provide guidelines. Typical postoperative orders include the following:

1. Frequency of special assessments
2. Types of intravenous fluids and rate of infusion
3. Postoperative drugs
4. Oxygen therapy or incentive spirometry
5. Dietary restrictions
6. Level of activity the client is allowed to resume
7. Positioning in bed
8. Intake and output
9. Laboratory tests and x-ray studies
10. Special directions

The nurse considers effects of the stress of surgery and limitations it produces when establishing goals of care for the client. Likewise, the nurse considers goals of care established during the preoperative and intraoperative phases. Typical postoperative goals and outcomes include the following:

Goal: Client participates in care activities.

Outcomes

Client coughs, deep breathes as instructed
Client performs leg exercises
Client ambulates as planned

Goal: Client achieves physical and psychological comfort.

Outcomes

Client verbalizes relief of pain
Client's anxiety is low or moderate

Goal: Client gains a return of normal physiological function.

Outcomes

Airways are clear with normal ventilation
Client's vitals signs remain stable
Peripheral pulses are palpable with normal capillary refill
Client is awake and oriented
Bowel sounds are audible
Client voids voluntarily
Wound drainage ceases
Client resumes full diet

Goal: Client remains free of postoperative infection.

Outcomes

Incision is clear, free of exudate
Temperature within normal limits

Goal: Client maintains self-concept.

Outcomes

Client inspects wound or dressing
Client discusses wound care at home
Client is well groomed

Goal: Client returns to functional state of health within limitations posed by surgery.

Outcomes

Client independently participates in self-care activities
Client progresses in exercise and ambulation

The nursing care plan outlines a typical sample care plan for a postoperative surgical client (see p. 1118).

Implementation

Regaining Normal Physiological Function. A surgical wound, the effects of prolonged immobilization during surgery and convalescence, and the influence of anesthesia and analgesics are the principal causes for postoperative complications. Failure of the client to become actively involved in recovery adds to the risk of complications (Table 36-7). Virtually any body system can be affected by complications. The nurse must thus consider the interrelationship of all systems, as well as therapies provided.

MAINTAINING RESPIRATORY FUNCTION. To prevent respiratory complications the nurse begins aggressive pulmonary hygiene measures early. The benefits of thorough preoperative teaching are realized when the client can participate actively. The following measures promote expansion of the lung:

1. Encourage diaphragmatic breathing exercises at least every 2 hours while the client is awake. Maximal inspirations lasting 3 to 5 seconds open alveoli.
2. Instruct the client to use an incentive spirometer for maximum inspiration (see Chapter 34).
3. Encourage early ambulation. Walking causes the client to assume a position that does not restrict

SAMPLE NURSING CARE PLAN

Postoperative Client: Ineffective Airway Clearance

ASSESSMENT

Clinical scenario: Ms. Cooper is a 67-year-old obese female who is *complaining of incisional pain* from the previous day's umbilical hernia repair. Ms. Cooper is also complaining of *shortness of breath with exertion,* and her *resting respiratory rate is 30 breaths/min.* Ms. Cooper's *respirations are shallow,* and *scattered rales* are heard in both lungs. Her *cough is weak,* and she is *unable to cough out secretions.*

NURSING DIAGNOSIS

Ineffective airway clearance related to incisional pain.

PLANNING

Goals	Expected outcomes
Ms. Cooper will achieve normal ventilatory function with patent airway within 24 hours.	Client will demonstrate adequate use of an incentive spirometer within 8 hours. Client will breathe deeply. Client's cough will be clear and nonproductive. Client's lung sounds will be clear within 24 hours.

IMPLEMENTATION

Steps	Rationale
1. Administer analgesics before coughing exercises.	Reduces discomfort sensed from pulling of abdominal muscles.
2. Have Ms. Cooper perform diaphragmatic breathing using incentive spirometer every 2 hours while awake.	Slow, deep breaths prevent panting or hyperventilation and allow for lung expansion so that air moves behind mucus and facilitates coughing.
3. Have Ms. Cooper splint abdominal incision with pillow while performing consecutive coughing exercises.	Splinting incision with pillow reduces discomfort when coughing. Consecutive coughs helps to remove mucus more effectively and completely from airways.
4. Turn Ms. Cooper side to side every 1 to 2 hours while awake.	Turning reduces risk of pulmonary (atelectasis and pneumonia) and vascular (clot formation) postoperative complications.

EVALUATIVE MEASURES

Observe Ms. Cooper's chest excursion.
Auscultate Ms. Cooper's lung sounds.
Assess Ms. Cooper's vital signs.
Assess Ms. Cooper's pulmonary function using an incentive spirometer.

Defining characteristics are shown in italic type.

chest wall expansion and stimulates an increased respiratory rate and circulation.

4. Assist clients who are restricted to bed to turn side-to-side every 1 to 2 hours while awake and sit when possible. Turning permits expansion of the lungs. Sitting causes lowering of abdominal organs, thus facilitating diaphragmatic movement and lung expansion.

The following measures promote the removal of pulmonary secretions:

1. Encourage coughing exercises every 2 hours while the client is awake and maintain pain control to promote a full productive cough.
2. Provide oral hygiene to expectorate mucus. Oral mucosa becomes dry when the client is allowed nothing by mouth or placed on limited fluid intake.
3. Initiate orotracheal or nasotracheal suction for clients too weak or unable to cough (see Chapter 34).

PREVENTING CIRCULATORY STASIS. Early measures directed at preventing circulatory complications prevent circulatory stasis. Some clients are at greater risk of ve-

table 36-7

POSTOPERATIVE COMPLICATIONS

Complication	Cause
RESPIRATORY SYSTEM	
Atelectasis is collapse of alveoli with retained mucous secretions. Signs and symptoms include elevated respiratory rate, dyspnea, fever, crackles auscultated over involved lobes of lungs, and productive cough.	Inadequate lung expansion Anesthesia, analgesics, and immobilized position preventing full lung expansion Greater risk in clients with upper abdominal surgery who have pain during inspiration and repress deep breathing
Pneumonia is inflammation of alveoli caused by infectious process; it may involve one or several lobes of lung, and development in lower dependent lobes of lung is common in immobilized surgical client. Signs and symptoms include fever, chills, productive cough, chest pain, purulent mucus, and dyspnea.	Poor lung expansion with retained secretions Common resident bacteria in respiratory tract, *Diplococcus pneumoniae,* which causes most cases of pneumonia
Hypoxia is inadequate concentration of oxygen in arterial blood. Signs and symptoms include restlessness, dyspnea, high blood pressure, tachycardia, diaphoresis, and cyanosis.	Respirations depressed by anesthetics or analgesics Increased retention of mucus with impaired ventilation because of pain or poor positioning
Pulmonary embolism is embolus blocking pulmonary artery and disrupting blood flow to one or more lobes of lung. Signs and symptoms include dyspnea, sudden chest pain, cyanosis, tachycardia, and drop in blood pressure.	Same factors that lead to formation of thrombus or embolus High risk to immobilized surgical client with preexisting circulatory or coagulation disorders
CIRCULATORY SYSTEM	
Hemorrhage is loss of large amount of blood externally or internally in short period of time. Signs and symptoms are same as hypovolemic shock.	Slipping of suture or dislodged clot at incisional site Clients with coagulation disorders at greater risk
Hypovolemic shock is inadequate perfusion of tissues and cells from loss of circulatory fluid volume. Signs and symptoms include hypotension, weak and rapid pulse, cool clammy skin, rapid breathing, restlessness, and reduced urine output.	In surgical client, usually caused by hemorrhage
Thrombophlebitis is inflammation of vein often accompanied by clot formation; leg veins are most commonly affected. Signs and symptoms include swelling and inflammation of involved site, aching or cramping pain; vein feels hard, cordlike, and sensitive to touch, and there is pain in calf when client walks or places foot in dorsiflex position (Homans' sign).	Venous stasis aggravated by prolonged sitting or immobilization Trauma to vessel wall and hypercoagulability of blood increasing risk of vessel inflammation
Thrombus is formation of clot attached to interior wall of a vein or artery, which can occlude vessel lumen. Embolus is piece of thrombus that has dislodged and circulates in bloodstream until it lodges in another vessel, commonly lungs, heart, or brain.	Venous stasis (see *thrombophlebitis*) and vessel trauma Venous injury common after surgery of legs, abdomen, pelvis, and major vessels Thrombi also forming from increased coagulability of blood (e.g., polycythemia and use of birth control pills containing estrogen)
GASTROINTESTINAL SYSTEM	
Abdominal distention is retention of air within intestines. Signs and symptoms include increased abdominal girth and tympanic percussion note over abdominal quadrants; client complains of fullness and "gas pains."	Slowed peristalsis from anesthesia, bowel manipulation, or immobilization
Constipation is infrequent passage of stools; it should not be concern immediately after surgery, especially if client has preoperative bowel preparation. After client resumes solid diet, failure to pass stool within 48 hours is cause for concern.	Slowed peristalsis (see *distention*) and delay in resuming normal diet

Continued.

table 36-7

POSTOPERATIVE COMPLICATIONS

Complication	Cause
Nausea and vomiting are symptoms of improper gastric emptying or chemical stimulation of vomiting center. Client complains of gagging, feeling full or sick to stomach.	Severe pain, abdominal distention, fear, medications, eating or drinking before peristalsis returns, initiating gag reflex
GENITOURINARY SYSTEM	
Urinary retention is involuntary accumulation of urine in bladder as result of loss of muscle tone. Signs and symptoms include inability to void, restlessness, bladder distention; it is common 6 to 8 hours after surgery.	Effects of anesthesia and narcotic analgesics Local manipulation of tissues around bladder and edema interfering with bladder tone Poor positioning of client impairing voiding reflexes
INTEGUMENTARY SYSTEM	
Wound infection is invasion of deep or superficial wound tissues by pathogenic microorganisms. Signs and symptoms include warm, red, and tender skin around incision, and client may have fever and chills; purulent material may exit from drains or from separated wound edges. It appears 3 to 6 days postoperatively.	Contamination of wound Contaminated wound before surgical exploration
Wound dehiscence is separation of wound edges at suture line. Signs and symptoms include increased drainage and appearance of underlying tissues. It usually occurs 6 to 8 days after surgery.	Malnutrition Obesity Preoperative radiation to surgical site Old age Poor circulation to tissues Unusual strain on suture line from coughing
Wound evisceration is protrusion of internal organs and tissues through incision. It usually occurs 6 to 8 days after surgery.	See *dehiscence* Client with dehiscence at risk for developing evisceration
Skin breakdown	Prolonged immobilization and pressure

nous stasis because of the nature of their surgery. The following measures promote normal venous return and peripheral blood flow:

1. Encourage clients to perform leg exercises at least every hour while awake. Exercise may be contraindicated in an affected extremity involving vascular repair, skin graft, or realignment of fractured bones and torn cartilage.
2. Apply elastic antiembolism stockings as ordered by the physician. The stockings should be removed every 8 hours and left off for 1 hour.
3. Apply pneumatic antiembolism stockings. Each stocking wraps around a client's leg and is kept in place with a Velcro attachment. Compressed air inflates the padded plastic stocking systematically from ankle to calf to thigh and then deflates. The stocking reduces venous stasis.
4. Encourage early ambulation. Most clients are ordered to ambulate the evening of surgery, depending on the severity of surgery and the client's condition. The degree of activity allowed progresses as the client's condition improves. Before ambulation, the nurse assesses vital signs. Abnormalities may contraindicate ambulation. If vital signs are normal, the nurse first assists the client to sit on the side of the bed. Dizziness is a sign of postural hypotension (see Chapter 15). A recheck of blood pressure determines whether ambulation is safe. The nurse assists with ambulation by standing at the client's side, making sure the client is able to walk steadily. During the first few times out of bed, the client may be able to walk only a few feet. Tolerance will improve each time. The nurse evaluates the client's tolerance to activity, periodically assessing pulse rate.
5. Avoid positioning the client in a manner that interrupts blood flow to the extremities. While in bed, the client should not have pillows or rolled blankets placed under the knees. Compression of the popliteal vessels can cause a thrombus. When sitting in a chair, the client should elevate the legs on a footstool. The client should never be allowed to sit with one leg crossed over the other.
6. Give anticoagulant drugs as ordered. Physicians

often order small doses of anticoagulants such as heparin for clients at greatest risk for thrombus formation. Orthopedic clients often receive aspirin for anticoagulation.

7. Promote adequate fluid intake orally or intravenously. Adequate hydration prevents the concentration of formed blood elements such as platelets and red blood cells. When the plasma volume is low, these may gather to form small clots within blood vessels. Adequate hydration also promotes tissue healing.

Promoting normal elimination and adequate nutrition. Interventions for preventing gastrointestinal complications promote the return of normal elimination and faster resumption of normal nutritional intake. It takes several days for a client who has had surgery on gastrointestinal structures to resume a normal dietary intake. Normal peristalsis may not return for 2 to 3 days. In contrast, the client whose gastrointestinal tract is unaffected directly by surgery must simply endure the effects of anesthesia before resuming dietary intake. The following measures promote return of normal elimination:

1. Assess for return of peristalsis. The nurse routinely auscultates the abdomen to detect the return of normal bowel sounds. Five to thirty loud gurgles per minute over each quadrant usually indicate that peristalsis has returned. It may take as long as a minute to hear bowel sounds. High-pitched tinkling sounds accompanied by abdominal distention suggest that the bowel is not functioning properly. The nurse asks whether the client is passing flatus, an important sign indicating normal bowel function.
2. Maintain a gradual progression in dietary intake. Immediately after surgery, a client receives only intravenous fluids. If the physician orders a normal diet the first evening after surgery, the nurse first provides clear liquids such as water, apple juice, or tea after nausea subsides. Overloading with large amounts of fluids may lead to distention and vomiting. If the client tolerates liquids without nausea, the diet is advanced as ordered. Clients who have had abdominal surgery are usually not allowed anything by mouth (NPO) the first 24 to 48 hours. As peristalsis returns, the nurse provides clear liquids, followed by full liquids, a light diet of solid foods, and finally a regular diet.
3. Promote ambulation and exercise. Physical activity stimulates a return of peristalsis. The client who suffers abdominal distention and "gas pain" will often obtain relief while walking.
4. Maintain an adequate fluid intake. Fluids keep fecal material soft for easy passage. Fruit juices and warm liquids are especially effective.
5. Administer fiber supplements, stool softeners, enemas, rectal suppositories, and rectal tubes as ordered. Constipation or distention can develop postoperatively.

The following measures assist the client to maintain an adequate dietary intake:

1. Remove sources of noxious odors.
2. Assist the client to sit (if possible) during mealtime to minimize pressure on the abdomen.
3. Provide small servings of nonspicy food.
4. Provide frequent oral hygiene to eliminate dryness and bad tastes in the mouth.
5. Provide meals when the client is rested and free from pain. A client will often lose interest in eating if mealtime has been preceded by exhausting activities such as ambulation or postoperative exercises. When a client has pain, the associated nausea causes a loss of appetite.

Promoting urinary elimination. The depressant effects of anesthesia and analgesics impair the sensation of bladder fullness. If bladder tone is reduced, the client has difficulty starting urination. Clients who undergo surgery of the urinary system frequently have Foley catheters inserted to maintain free urinary flow until voluntary control of urination returns. The following measures promote normal urinary elimination (see Chapter 32):

1. Assist the client to assume normal positions during voiding.
2. Check the client frequently for the need to void. A surgical client restricted to bed will need assistance in handling and using bedpans or urinals. The feeling of bladder fullness and urgency to void is often sudden, and the nurse must respond promptly when the client calls for assistance.
3. Assess for bladder distention. If a client does not void within 8 hours of surgery, it may be necessary to insert a straight urinary catheter. A physician's order is required. Continued difficulty may necessitate a Foley catheter, although the risk for urinary tract infection increases.
4. Monitor intake and output. An accepted level of urine output is a minimum of 30cc/hr for adults. If the client's urine is dark, concentrated, and low in volume, a physician should be notified. A client can easily become dehydrated as a result of fluid loss from the surgical wound. The nurse measures intake and output for several days until normal fluid intake and urinary output are achieved.

Promoting Wound Healing. A surgical wound undergoes considerable stress during convalescence. The stress of inadequate nutrition, impaired circulation, and metabolic alterations increases the risk for delayed healing. A wound may also undergo considerable physical stress (e.g., strain on sutures from coughing, vomiting, distention, and movement of body parts). The nurse protects the wound and promotes healing. A critical time for wound healing is 24 to 72 hours after surgery. If a wound becomes infected, it usually occurs 3 to 6 days after surgery. A clean surgical wound usually does not regain strength against normal stress for 15 to 20 days after surgery (see Chapter 37). The nurse uses aseptic technique during dressing changes and wound care. Surgical drains must remain patent so that accumulated secretions may escape from the incision site. Ongoing observation of the wound identifies early signs and symptoms of infection.

Promoting Rest and Comfort. A surgical client's pain increases as the effects of anesthesia wear off. The client becomes more aware of surroundings and more perceptive of discomfort. The incisional area may be only one source of pain. Irritation from drainage tubes, tight dressings, or casts and the muscular strains caused from positioning on the operating room table are factors that can make the client feel miserable.

Pain can significantly slow recovery. The client becomes reluctant to perform necessary postoperative exercises. The nurse should assess the pain thoroughly (see Chapter 28). It should not be assumed that the pain is incisional. When the client calls for a pain drug, the nature and character of the pain should be determined. Clients have the most surgical pain during the first 24 to 48 hours. The nurse should provide analgesics as often as allowed during this time. The patient-controlled analgesia system allows clients to administer their own intravenous analgesics from a specially prepared intravenous pump (Bast and Hayes, 1986). The clients gain a sense of control over their pain and are able to administer analgesics before the pain becomes too intense. Epidural infusion of narcotics such as morphine, fentanyl, and meperidine is also a popular method of postoperative analgesia for many surgical clients (Powell and Bora, 1989). Epidural narcotics relieve severe pain, often without the central nervous system depression that usually occurs with systemic narcotics.

Maintaining Self-Concept. The appearance of wounds, bulky dressings, and extruding drains and tubes threaten a client's self-concept. The nature of the surgery may also create permanent change in body image. If surgery leads to impairment in body function, the client's role within the family can change significantly. The nurse should observe the client for alterations in self-concept. Clients may show a revulsion toward their appearance by refusing to look at an incision or carefully covering dressings with bedclothes. The fear of not being able to return to a functional role in the family may even cause the client to avoid participating in the care plan.

The family plays an important role in the efforts to improve the client's self-concept. The nurse explains the client's appearance and ways to avoid nonverbal expressions of revulsion or surprise. The family needs to be accepting of the client's needs and still encourage independence. If the condition is terminal, the family learns to assist the client through the grieving process so that the client and family can reach a phase of acceptance. The following measures maintain the client's self-concept:

1. Provide privacy during dressing changes or wound inspection. Room curtains are kept closed around the bed, and the client is draped so that only the dressing and incisional area are exposed.
2. Maintain the client's hygiene. Wound drainage and antiseptic solutions may dry on the skin's surface, causing irritation. A complete bath the first day after surgery can make the client feel renewed. The nurse offers a clean gown and washcloth when the gown becomes soiled. The nurse keeps the client's hair neatly combed and offers frequent oral hygiene, especially for the client who is allowed nothing by mouth.
3. Prevent drainage sets from overflowing. Typically the drainage sets are measured every 8 hours for output recording. The client sometimes becomes preoccupied with observing the gradual collection of drainage, and some drainage sets can leak contents if they become too full. The nurse should empty the sets periodically to prevent hampering the client's movement and accidental spills.
4. Maintain a pleasant environment. Self-concept is heightened by pleasant, comfortable surroundings. The nurse should store or remove all unused supplies and keep the bedside orderly and clean.
5. Offer opportunities for the clients to discuss feelings about appearance. A client having surgery for the first time is often more anxious than a client who has had multiple surgeries. Clients worry about permanent scarring. A client is more apt to look at an incision several days after surgery when healing is occurring and the client begins to gain energy and a feeling of well-being. If the client chooses to look at an incision for the first time, the area should be clean. Eventually the client should be able to care for the incision site by applying simple dressings or bathing.
6. Provide the family with opportunities to discuss ways to promote the client's self-concept. Encouraging independence can be difficult for a family member who has a strong desire to assist the client in any way. By knowing about the appearance of a wound or incision, family members can be supportive during dressing changes. The topic or tone of a conversation can also help family members to distract a client from dwelling on fears and concerns. Family members should not avoid discussing the future. However, the nurse

must help them to know when it is appropriate to discuss future plans. Then the client and family can work together to discuss realistic plans for the client's return home.

Promoting Return to a Functional State of Health. Throughout the postoperative convalescent period the nurse promotes the client's independence and active participation in care. When a client is in pain or suffers from postoperative complications, there is little motive for self-care. The nurse must balance provision of client needs and promotion of involvement when a client's condition allows. The goals a nurse sets for a client's involvement must be realistic. Surgery may limit the ability to participate effectively. It is unrealistic for the nurse to involve the client if movement is highly restricted or if participation increases the discomfort.

The nurse should keep the client and family informed of progress made toward recovery. Many clients become depressed if they think recovery is slow. The nurse explains the length of time expected to reach a level of maximal recovery. When using a Care Map, the nurse may show the client progress compared with the Care Map and explain any alterations. Surgery may also cause permanent physical limitations that will require time for the client to accept.

The nurse plans care daily, keeping in mind the ultimate goals for recovery. From the moment the client enters the hospital, through surgery, and during the postoperative phase, the nurse anticipates and plans for the client's return home.

Involvement of family members in the care plan can facilitate recovery. If the client requires additional care at home, such as dressing changes, assistance with ambulation, or drug administration, the nurse instructs family members about proper care techniques. If family members are unable to assist the client, the nurse works with the physician, social worker, or discharge planner to make plans for home care. The client will be more able to assume a functional state of health when family members understand the client's limitations.

Evaluative Measures

The nurse evaluates effectiveness of care on the basis of expected outcomes resulting from nursing interventions. In all surgical settings the nurse consults with the client and family to gather data. The nurse can evaluate the ambulatory surgical client's outcomes by making a postoperative telephone call to the client's home. The call is usually placed 24 hours after surgery, reassures the client that the nurse is concerned, and allows the nurse to evaluate the progress of recovery. In the inpatient setting the nurse monitors the client's progress over several days. The use of evaluative measures determines whether outcomes are achieved.

Examples of goals, outcomes, and corresponding evaluative measures include:

Goal: Client participates in care activities.

Outcome

Client coughs and deep breathes as instructed

Evaluative measure

Observe client perform coughing and deep breathing exercise

Outcome

Client performs leg exercises

Evaluative measure

Observe client do leg exercises during bathing

Outcome

Client ambulates as planned

Evaluative measure

Accompany client during ambulation in room or down hallways

Outcome

Client complies with limitations of surgery

Evaluative measure

During meals, bathing, or treatments, observe if client refrains from those activities contraindicated by surgery

Goal: Client achieves physical and psychological comfort.

Outcome

Client verbalizes pain reduced or relieved

Evaluative measures

Observe for nonverbal signs of discomfort

Assess number of requests for analgesia or use of PCA pump

Outcome

Client's anxiety is low or moderate

Evaluative measures

Question client regarding perceptions regarding recovery

Observe client's nonverbal signs of anxiety

Goal: Client gains a return of normal physiological functioning.

Outcome

Airways are clear with normal ventilation

Evaluative measures

Auscultate lung sounds

Palpate chest excursion

Outcome

Vital signs remain stable

Evaluative measure

Assess vital signs per ordered frequency

Outcome

Peripheral pulses are palpable with normal capillary refill

Evaluative measures

Palpate peripheral pulses bilaterally

Measure capillary refill time in fingers

Outcome
Client is awake and oriented
Evaluative measure
Observe client during conversation over meal or during medication administration
Outcome
Bowel sounds are audible and client voids voluntarily
Evaluative measures
Auscultate abdomen for normal bowel sounds
Measure frequency of voiding and volume of urine with each void
Outcome
Wound drainage ceases
Evaluative measures
Inspect surgical drains and drainage collection devices
Inspect dressings over wound
Outcome
Client resumes full diet
Evaluative measures
Observe client eating meals and nutritional supplements
Perform a calorie count

Goal: Client remains free of postoperative infection.
Outcome
Incision is clear, free of exudate
Evaluative measure
Inspect surgical incision during each dressing change and following permanent removal of dressing
Outcome
Temperature within normal limits
Evaluative measure
Measure body temperature per routine orders

Goal: Client maintains self-concept.
Outcome
Client inspects wound or dressing
Evaluative measure
Watch client's nonverbal behavior during dressing change
Outcome
Client discusses wound care at home
Evaluative measure
Ask client to explain how wound care is to be performed in the home setting
Outcome
Client is well groomed
Evaluative measure
Once client initiates grooming activities, observe appearance

Goal: Client returns to functional state of health within limitations posed by surgery.
Outcome
Client independently participates in self-care activities
Evaluative measure
Observe client perform hygiene activites and exercise
Outcome
Client progresses in exercise and ambulation
Evaluative measures
Monitor client's progression from sitting in chair, to ambulating with assistance, to walking independently
Observe coordination and ease of movement during activity

SUMMARY

Care for the client during all phases of the surgical experience needs to be continuous and integrated. These principles apply for hospitalized clients, as well as for those who have surgery as outpatients. Before surgery, the nurse prepares the client and family for surgery and performs diagnostic tests and assessments. During surgery, the nurse assists surgeons and other operating room nurses to ensure the client receives optimal care. After surgery, the nurse assists the client to physiological stability, wakefulness, and institutes measures to help the client to achieve maximal recovery. Through all phases of care, the nurse involves the client and family in the care plan while maintaining the client's dignity.

CRITICAL THINKING ACTIVITIES

1. Mr. Wilson is a 76-year-old client admitted for a fractured hip. He has a history of emphysema. What risk does Mr. Wilson face as a result of surgery and why?
2. Mrs. Tice is a 40-year-old mother of two entering the outpatient surgery clinic for a breast biopsy. She has not had surgery before. She is a smoker and takes medication for high blood pressure. What factors will the nurse assess preoperatively in developing a plan for surgical care?
3. Joseph is the nurse working in the 3rd floor PACU. Mr. Sennett is admitted following abdominal surgery for removal of a colonic tumor. What should Joseph assess first when the client enters the PACU?
4. Ms. Lyons is recovering from surgery on the first postoperative day. The nurse finds that the client's abdomen is distended. What might this indicate?

KEY CONCEPTS

- Perioperative nursing is professional nursing care afforded the surgical client before, during, and after surgery.
- In addition to the nature of nursing care provided, previous illnesses and past surgeries influence the ability to tolerate surgery.
- Older adult clients are at surgical risk from their declining physiological status.
- All medications taken before surgery are automatically discontinued after surgery unless a physician reorders the drugs.
- Family members are important in assisting clients with physical limitations and in providing emotional support during the postoperative recovery.
- Preoperative assessment of vital signs and physical findings provides an important baseline with which to compare postoperative assessment data.
- A client's feelings about surgery can have a significant impact on relationships with nursing staff and the client's ability to participate in care.
- Surgical removal of a body part may permanently alter body image and sexuality.
- Nursing diagnoses of the surgical client may pose implications for nursing care during one or all phases of surgery.
- Primary responsibility for informed consent rests with the surgeon.
- Informed consent should not be obtained if a client is confused, unconscious, mentally incompetent, or under the influence of sedatives.
- Structured preoperative teaching positively influences postoperative recovery.
- If hair around the incision must be removed, it should be clipped as close as possible to the time of surgery to minimize infection.
- In ambulatory surgery, nurses must use the limited time available to educate clients, assess their health status, and prepare them for surgery.
- The responsibility of nurses within the operating room focuses on protecting the client from potential harm.
- Assessment of the postoperative client centers on the body systems most likely to be affected by anesthesia, immobilization, and surgical trauma.
- Because a surgical client's condition may change rapidly during recovery, the nurse monitors the client's status at least every 15 minutes.
- The PACU nurse reports to the nurse on the postoperative unit information pertaining to the client's current physical status and risk for postoperative complications.
- From the time of admission, the nurse plans for the surgical client's discharge.

References

AHCPR, Acute pain management guideline panel: acute pain management in infants, children, and adolescents: operative or medical procedures and trauma. *Clinical practice guideline,* AHCPR Pub No. 92-0032. Rockville, Md.: Agency for Health Care Policy and Research, PHS, USDHHS, Feb., 1992.

Bast C and Hayes P: Patient-controlled analgesia, *Nurs 86* 16:25, 1986.

Biddle C, Cannady J: Surgical positions: their effects on cardiovascular, respiratory systems, *AORN J* 52:350, 1990.

Boysen PG: Evaluation of the patient with pulmonary disease. In Rogers MC, Tinker JH, et al., editors: *Principles and practice of anesthesia,* St. Louis, 1992, Mosby.

Detsky AS, et al.: Predicting cardiac complications in patients undergoing noncardiac surgery, *J Gen Intern Med* 1:211, 1986.

Dettenmeier PA: *Pulmonary nursing care,* St. Louis, 1992, Mosby.

Devine EC and Cook TD: A meta-analysis of effects of psychoeducational interventions on length of postsurgical hospital stay, *Nurs Res* 32:267, 1983.

Frogge MH: Promoting wound healing in the irradiated patient, *AORN J* 35:1088, 1982.

Garner JS: *Guidelines for prevention of surgical wound infections,* 1985, Hospital infections program, CDC, PHS, US Department of Health and Human Services.

Grant JA, Kennedy-Caldwell C: *Nutritional support in nursing,* New York, 1988, Grune & Stratton.

Greene NM: Anesthesia risk factors in patients with liver disease, *Contemp Anesth Pract* 4:87, 1981.

Hathaway A: Effect of preoperative instruction on postoperative outcomes: a meta-analysis, *Nurs Res* 35:269, 1986.

Hill BJ: Sensory information, behavioral instructions, and coping with sensory alteration surgery, *Nurs Res* 31:17, 1982.

Hinkle AJ: What wisdom is there in administering elective general anesthesia to children with active respiratory tract infection? *Anesth Analg* 68:413, 1989.

Hulyalkar AR and Miller ED: Evaluation of the hypertensive patient. In Rogers MC, Tinker JH, et al., editors: *Principles and practice of anesthesia,* St. Louis, 1992, Mosby.

Larsen E: Skin cleansing. In Wenzel RP, editor: *Prevention and control of nosocomial infections,* ed 2, Baltimore, 1993, Williams & Wilkins.

Leske JS: *Effects of "progress reports" on anxiety levels of elective surgical patients' family members.* Paper presented at Midwest Nursing Research Society: Nursing Research and its Multidisciplinary Dimensions, March 27-30, 1993.

Lindeman C and VanAernam B: Nursing intervention with the presurgical patient: the effects of structured and unstructured preoperative teaching, *Nurs Res* 20:319, 1971.

Metheny N: Measures to test placement of nasogastric and nasointestinal feeding tubes: a review, *Nurs Res* 37:324, 1988.

Metheny N, et al.: Effectiveness of pH measurements in predicting feeding tube placement, *Nurs Res* 38:280, 1989.

Murray DJ: Evaluation of the patient with anemia and coagulation disorders. In Rogers MC, Tinker JH, et al., editors: *Principles and practice of anesthesia,* St. Louis, 1992, Mosby.

Norheim C: Family needs during coronary artery bypass graft surgery during the intraoperative period, *Heart Lung* 18:622, 1989.
Pagana KD and Pagana TJ: *Diagnostic testing and nursing implications: a case study approach,* ed 3, St. Louis, 1990, Mosby.
Pinson CW, et al.: Surgery in long-term dialysis patients: experience with more than 300 cases, *Am J Surg* 151:567, 1986.
Powell AH and Bora MB: How do you give continuous epidural fentanyl? *Am J Nurs* 89:1107, 1989.
Sieber FE, et al.: Effect of hypoglycemia on cerebral metabolism and carbon dioxide responsiveness, *Am J Physiol* 256:H697, 1989.
Sieber FE and Toung TJ: Hyperglycemia and stroke outcomes following carotid endarterectomy, *Anesthesiology* 71:A1136, 1989.
Steelman VM: Intraoperative music therapy: effects on anxiety, blood pressure, *AORN J* 52:1026, 1990.
Thelan T, et al.: Temperature and temperature measurement after induced hypothermia, *Nurs Res* 41:296, 1992.

Bibliography

Andrews AJ: Inadvertent hypothermia: a comparison of postoperative cholecystectomy patients by age, *AORN J* 52(5):987, 1990.
Association of Operating Room Nurses: *1993 standards and recommended practices,* Denver, AORN, 1993.
Ayliffe GA, et al.: A comparison of preoperative bathing with chlorhexidine-detergent and non-medicated soap in the prevention of wound infection, *J Hosp Infect* 4(3):237, 1983.
Boyes RJ and Kruse JA: Nasogastric and nasenteric intubation, *Crit Care Clin* 8:865, 1992.
Carpenito L: *Nursing diagnosis: application to clinical practice,* New York, 1992, JB Lippincott.
Cooper DM: Optimizing wound healing: a practice within nursing's domain, *Nurs Clin North Am* 15:165, 1990.
Cruse PJE and Ford R: The epidemiology of wound infection: a ten-year prospective study of 62,939 wounds, *Surg Clin North Am* 60:1, 1980.
Cullins L: Interventions related to fluid and electrolyte balance, *Nurs Clin North Am* 27:569, 1992.
Cummings C: Taking the fear out of surgery, *Nurs 87* 17:64b, 1987.
Fortin F and Kirovac S: A randomized controlled trial of preoperative patient education, *Int J Nurs Stud* 13:11, 1976.
Frost AM: *Post anesthesia care unit,* ed 2, St. Louis, 1990, Mosby.
Garibaldi RB, et al., Risk factors for postoperative infection, *Am J Med* 91 (suppl 3B):152S, 1991.
Garner JS: *Guidelines for prevention of surgical wound infections,* 1985, Hospital Infections Program, CDC, PHS, and US Department of Health and Human Services.
Gilliss CL: Family nursing research, theory and practice, *Image* 23:19, 1991.
Horsley J and Crane J: *Structured preoperative teaching,* New York, 1981, Grune & Stratton.
Jackson DC, et al.: Endoscopic laser cholecystectomy: a new approach to gall bladder removal, *AORN J* 51:1546, 1990.
Kneedler J and Dodge G: *Perioperative patient care,* Boston, 1987, Blackwell Scientific Publications.
Litwack K: *Post anesthesia care nursing,* St. Louis, 1991, Mosby.
Lynch S: Ambulatory surgery: families can watch surgery while they wait, *AORN J* 46:522, 1987.
Mayhall GG: Surgical infection including burns. In Wenzel RP, editor: *Prevention and control of nosocomial infections,* ed 3, Baltimore, 1993, Williams & Wilkins.
McHugh NG, et al.: Preparatory information: what helps and why, *Am J Nurs* 82:780, 1982.
Meeker MH and Rothrock JC: *Alexander's care of the patient in surgery,* ed 9, St Louis, 1991, Mosby.
Miller F: Evaluation of the patient with endocrine disease and diabetes mellitus. In Rogers MC, Tinker JH, et al., editors: *Principles and practice of anesthesia,* St. Louis, 1992, Mosby.
Moddeman G: The elderly surgical patient—a high risk for hypothermia, *AORN J* 53:1270, 1991.
Ross R: Overcoming fear: a review on research on patient, family instruction, *AORN J* 43:1107, 1986.
Rothrock JC: Preoperative psychoeducational interventions. In AORN: Perioperative nursing research, a ten year review, Denver, 1989, AORN.
Rothrock JC: *Perioperative nursing care planning,* St. Louis, 1990, Mosby.
Schoessler M: Perceptions of preoperative education in patients admitted the morning of surgery, *Patient Educ Couns* 14:127, 1989.
The American Society of Post Anesthesia Nurses: *Standards of postanesthesia nursing practice 1992,* Richmond Va., 1992, ASPAN.
United States Department of Health and Human Services, Centers for Disease Control: Recommendations for prevention of HIV transmission in health care setting, *MMWR* 36:S2, 1987.
United States Department of Health and Human Services, Public Health Services, Agency for Health Care Policy and Research: *Pressure ulcers in adults: prediction and prevention,* Pub. No. 92-0047, Rockville, Md., AHCPR, May, 1992.
United States Department of Health and Human Services, Public Health Services, Agency for Health Care Policy and Research. *Acute pain management: operative or medical procedures and trauma.* Pub. No. 92-0032, Rockville, Md., AHCPR, Feb. 1992.
Ziemer MM: Effects of information on postsurgical coping, *Nurs Res* 32:232, 1983.

37

Wound Care

OBJECTIVES

Mastery of content in this chapter will enable the student to:

- Define the key terms listed.
- Discuss the body's response during each stage of the wound healing process.
- Classify a wound according to the state of skin integrity, severity, cleanliness, and descriptive qualities.
- Differentiate healing by primary and secondary intention.
- Discuss common complications of wound healing.
- Explain factors that impair or promote normal wound healing.
- Conduct an assessment of a surgical and open wound.
- Apply a sterile, dry, and wet-to-dry dressing using sterile technique.
- Describe the purposes of and precautions taken with applying bandages and binders.
- Administer a wound irrigation.
- Apply a warm and a cold compress safely to an injured body part.
- Describe the differences in therapeutic effects of heat and cold.

KEY TERMS

abrasion
approximate
binders
collagen
compress
dehiscence
drainage evacuators
ecchymosis
evisceration
fibrin
fistula
granulation tissue
hematoma
hemostasis
laceration
primary intention
secondary intention
sitz bath
wound culture

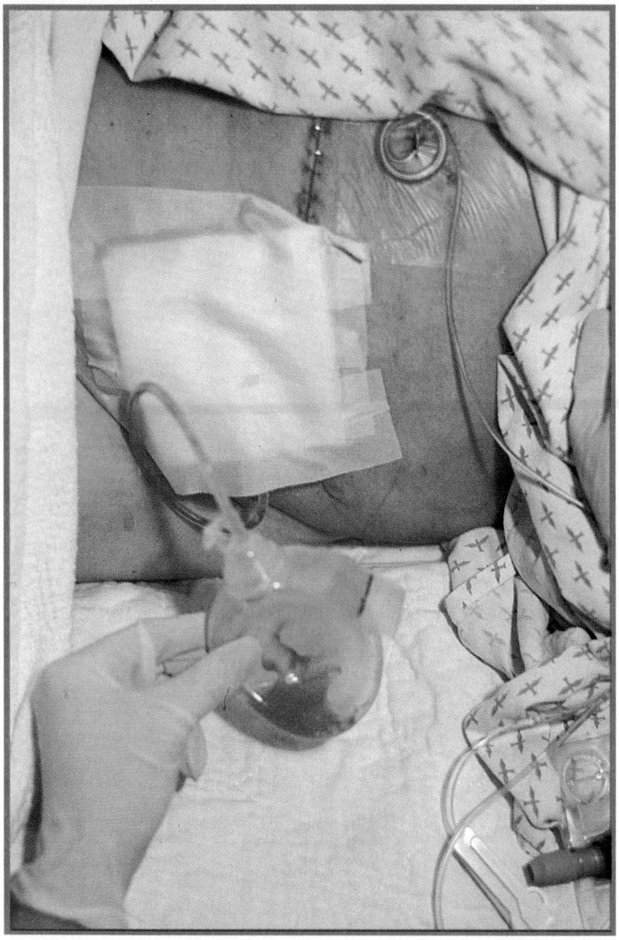

The integument is the body's protective barrier against injury and disease-causing organisms and is a sensory organ for pain, temperature, and touch. Injury to the integument causes risks to safety and precipitates a complex healing response. Knowing the normal healing pattern helps the nurse to recognize alterations requiring intervention. The nurse's primary responsibilities are to prevent the invasion of microorganisms into wounds and to support the body's defenses in achieving wound repair. In choosing interventions, the nurse must consider the type of wound, the pain associated with it, conditions that affect healing, and the client's psychological well-being.

WOUND CLASSIFICATIONS

Wound classifications focus on the status of skin integrity, the cause of the wound, the severity of tissue injury, the cleanliness of the wound, or the descriptive qualities of the wound (Table 37-1). These overlapping classifications help to define the risks and care implications associated with particular types of wounds. For example, a penetrating knife wound is also an open wound, which presents a greater risk of infection than a closed wound.

WOUND HEALING PROCESS

The process of wound healing involves an orderly series of integrated physiological responses that result in healing in the healthy individual. The process is basically the same for all wounds but is affected by the location, severity, extent of injury, and the ability of the injured cells to regenerate. A wound with little or no tissue loss, such as a clean surgical incision, heals by **primary intention;** the skin edges **approximate,** or close together, and the risk of infection developing is slight. In contrast, a wound involving loss of tissue, such as a pressure ulcer or severe laceration, heals by **secondary intention;** the edges do not approximate, the wound is left open until filled by scar tissue, the longer healing period increases the chance of infection, and, where scarring is severe, there may be permanent loss of tissue function. There are also instances in which a surgical wound is initially closed in the deep tissue layers, however the subcutaneous fat and skin layers are left open. This method of wound closure is called **delayed primary;** the wound heals with a layer of granulation tissue at the edges and base, and several days after the initial wounding, the wound edges are brought together with sutures or adhesive closures and the wound goes on to heal by primary intention.

Healing by Primary Intention

The healing process occurs in the following stages as described by Westaby (1986), Gilmore (1991), and Gogia (1992): defensive (inflammatory), reconstructive or fibroblastic (destructive and proliferative), and maturative (maturation). The defensive stage begins immediately after the injury, lasts about 4 days, and includes hemostasis, inflammation, and epithelial cell migration. During **hemostasis** (termination of bleeding), injured blood vessels constrict, platelets gather, thrombin acts on fibrinogen to form a protein matrix called **fibrin,** and a scab consisting of clotted blood and dead tissue forms to protect against infectious organisms. During the inflammatory phase, complex chemical reactions result in white blood cells, initially *neutrophils* and *monocytes* to enter the wound and begin wound cleansing. These phagocytic cells remove cellular debris and protect the wound from bacterial invasion. Then epithelial cells migrate from the wound mar-

table 37-1
WOUND CLASSIFICATIONS

Type and description	Causes	Implications for healing
STATUS OF SKIN INTEGRITY		
Open wound involving break in skin or mucous membranes	Trauma by sharp object (e.g., surgical incision, venipuncture, or gunshot wound)	Exposes body to invasion by microorganisms Loss of blood and body fluids through wound Reduces function of body part
Closed wound involving no break in skin integrity	Part of body being struck by blunt object Twisting, straining, or deceleration force against body (e.g., bone fracture or tear of visceral organ)	May predispose person to internal hemorrhage Reduces function of affected body part
CAUSE		
Intentional wound resulting from therapy	Surgical incision Introduction of needle into body part	Usually performed under aseptic technique, which minimizes chances of infection Wound edges usually smooth and clean
Unintentional wound occurring unexpectedly	Traumatic injury (e.g., knife wound, burn, or pressure ulcer)	Occurs under unsterile conditions Wound edges often jagged
SEVERITY OF INJURY		
Superficial wound involving only epidermal layer of skin	Result of friction applied to skin surface (e.g., abrasion or first-degree burn)	Creates risk of infection Does not involve underlying injury to tissues or organs Blood supply to area intact
Penetrating wound involving break in epidermal skin layer and dermis and deeper tissues or organs	Foreign object or instrument entering deep into body tissues, usually unintentional (e.g., gunshot or stab wound)	High risk of infection because foreign object is contaminated May cause internal and external hemorrhage Damage to organs causes temporary or permanent loss of function
Perforating penetrating wound in which foreign object enters and exits internal organ	Same as penetrating wound	High risk of infection Nature of injury depends on organ perforated: Lung—compromised oxygenation Major vessel—serious hemorrhage Intestine—contamination of abdominal cavity by feces
CLEANLINESS		
Clean wound containing no pathogenic organisms	Surgical wound that does not enter the gastrointestinal tract, respiratory tract, or oropharyngeal cavity	Low risk of infection
Clean-contaminated wound made under aseptic conditions but involving entrance into body cavity that normally harbors microorganisms	Surgical wound entering gastrointestinal or respiratory tract or oropharyngeal cavity	Greater risk of infection than with clean wound
Contaminated wound existing under conditions in which presence of micororganisms is likely	Open, traumatic wounds Surgical wound in which break in asepsis occurred	Tissues often not healthy and show inflammation High risk of infection
Infected wound involving bacterial organisms in wound site	Any wound that does not properly heal and grows organisms Old traumatic wound Surgical incision into area infected (e.g., ruptured bowel)	Wound presents signs of infection (e.g., inflammation, purulent drainage, and skin separation)

Continued.

table 37-1—cont'd

WOUND CLASSIFICATIONS

Type and description	Causes	Implications for healing
Colonized wound containing microorganisms (usually multiple)	Chronic wound (e.g., vascular wound or stasis or pressure ulcer)	Wound healing slow High risk of infection
DESCRIPTIVE QUALITIES		
Laceration: tearing of tissues with irregular wound edges	Severe traumatic injury (e.g., knife wound, industrial accident involving machinery, or tissues cut by broken glass)	Wound usually created by contaminated object Depth determines other complications
Abrasion: superficial wound involving scraping or rubbing of skin's surface by friction	Fall (e.g., skinned knee or elbow) Dermatological procedure for removing scar tissue	Painful from exposure of superficial nerves Deeper tissues uninvolved Risk of infection from exposure to contaminated surface
Contusion: closed wound caused by blow by blunt object; contusion by bruise characterized by swelling, discoloration, and pain	Bleeding in underlying tissues caused by blunt force against body part	More severe if internal organ contused May cause temporary loss of function of body part Localized bleeding into tissues may form hematoma, or collection of blood

gins toward the base of the clot or scab until, after about 48 hours, a thin layer of epithelial tissue forms over the wound to exclude infectious organisms and toxic materials.

Reconstruction begins on the third or fourth day after injury and lasts from 2 to 3 weeks. During this stage, monocytes that have become **macrophages** continue to clear the wound of unwanted debris (destructive process), attracting further macrophages and stimulating formation of fibroblasts, cells that synthesize **collagen** (proliferative process). Collagen can be found as early as the second day and is the main component of scar tissue. Fibroblasts require vitamins B and C, oxygen, and amino acids to function properly. As reconstruction progresses, new capillary networks form to provide oxygen and nutrients for the continued synthesis and support of collagen. As collagen fibers and capillary networks continue to synthesize and increase in size *(proliferate)*, the wound begins to close with new tissue. The amount of scar tissue formed is influenced by the degree of stress on the wound. As the tensile strength of the wound increases, the risk of wound separation or rupture is less likely. After 15 to 20 days the wound can resist normal stress such as tension or twisting. Impairment of healing during this stage usually results from factors such as age, anemia, hypoproteinemia, and zinc deficiency (see box on p. 1131).

Maturation, the final stage of healing, may take more than a year, depending on the depth and extent of the wound. The collagen scar continues to gain strength for several months but will remain weaker and lighter in color than the tissue it replaces.

An important concept in wound healing is that the stages of wound healing, while progressive, do not occur in a linear fashion, but they occur in an integrated, overlapping pattern. Therefore a normally healing wound could simultaneously be in all three stages of wound healing. The stages described previously provide a model for acute wound healing.

Healing by Secondary Intention

When tissue loss in a wound is extensive, healing takes longer. Inflammation is often chronic, and tissue defects become filled with fragile granulation tissue rather than collagen. **Granulation tissue** is a form of connective tissue (scar) that has a more abundant blood supply than collagen. Because the wound is larger, it takes much longer to fill and the amount of connective tissue scarring is larger. Formulation of granulation tissue occurs at the same time as wound contraction. The tissue and skin surrounding the defect are mobilized and pulled together, thus reducing the size of the defect (Bryant, 1992). Contraction speeds healing because it reduces the amount of scar tissue required for repair. The degree of contraction is limited by the mobility of surrounding tissue (Bryant, 1992). In some areas of the body, such as wounds on the face, sternum, and anterior

FACTORS INFLUENCING WOUND HEALING

AGE

Blood circulation and oxygen delivery to the wound, clotting, inflammatory response, and phagocytosis may be impaired in the very young and the aged. Risk of infection is greater.

Cell growth and differentiation in reconstruction are slower with advancing age.

Scar tissue is more taut and less pliable, increasing the risk of altered body part function in older adults.

NUTRITION

Tissue repair and infection resistance depend on balanced diet. Surgery, severe wounds, serious infections, and preoperative nutritional deficits increase nutritional requirements.

OBESITY

The less abundant supply of blood vessels in fatty tissue impairs delivery of nutrients and cellular elements needed for healing.

Suturing of adipose tissue is more difficult. If the wound heals by secondary intention, dehiscence or evisceration and subsequent infection are greater.

EXTENT OF WOUND

Deeper wounds with more tissue loss heal more slowly and by secondary intention and thus are more vulnerable to complications.

OXYGENATION

Reduced oxygen delivery to the wound inhibits repair.

Low arterial oxygen tension alters the synthesis of collagen and the formation of epithelial cells.

A wound heals more slowly when local blood flow is reduced and the wound is not exposed to oxygen.

The low hemoglobin levels exhibited in severe anemia reduce oxygenation and impede tissue repair.

SMOKING

Functional hemoglobin levels decrease; oxygen release in the tissues is impaired.

IMMUNOSUPPRESSION

Reduced immune response contributes to poor healing.

Cortisone depresses fibroblast activity and capillary growth and thereby impairs wound closure.

Because steroids mask an inflammatory response, the nurse may not be able to detect early signs of inflammation or infection.

Chemotherapeutic drugs and certain cancerous diseases interfere with leukocyte production and the immune response.

DIABETES MELLITUS

The diabetic client has small vessel disease that impairs tissue perfusion; thus oxygen delivery may be poor.

An elevated blood glucose level impairs macrophage function.

Risk of infection is increased due to poor wound healing.

RADIATION

Radiotherapy, which eventually results in fibrosis and vascular scarring, interferes with postoperative wound healing when surgery is delayed more than 4 to 6 weeks and irradiated tissues have become fragile and poorly perfused.

WOUND STRESS

Sustained stress (e.g., vomiting, abdominal distention, and coughing) disrupts wound layers and tissue repair.

lower leg, contraction gives poor cosmetic results. Wound contraction is not the same as a contracture or deformity resulting from muscle shortening and joint fixation. Special attention should be paid to maintaining joint mobility when wounding has occurred within a joint to prevent or minimize cosmetic deformities or flexion contractures.

COMPLICATIONS OF WOUND HEALING

Hemorrhage

Bleeding from a wound is normal during and immediately after initial trauma, but hemostasis usually occurs within several minutes. Hemorrhage occurring later indicates a slipped surgical suture, a dislodged clot, infection, or the erosion of a blood vessel by a foreign object (e.g., a drain). Hemorrhage may be external or internal. Symptoms of internal bleeding are hypovolemic shock and swelling of the affected body part. A **hematoma** is a localized collection of blood underneath tissues, often appearing as a bluish swelling or mass. External hemorrhaging is more obvious because dressings covering the wound soon become saturated with blood. Surgical drains also drain blood. The nurse observes wounds closely, particularly surgical wounds in which the risk of hemorrhage is greatest during the first 24 to 48 hours.

Infection

Bacterial wound infection inhibits healing by increasing tissue damage and altering the healing process. The chances of wound infection are greater when the wound contains dead or necrotic tissue, when foreign bodies are in or near the wound, and when the blood supply and local tissue defenses are reduced.

A contaminated or traumatic wound infection may develop within 2 to 3 days; a surgical wound infection may develop within 4 to 5 days. The distinction between contamination and true infection is difficult to determine clinically (Mulder, 1991). Locally, drainage may be yellow, green, or brown and may be odorous, depending on the causative organism. The wound edges may appear tense, swollen, painful, and with redness extending beyond the immediate wound edge. Other systemic signs include fever, general malaise, and an elevated white blood cell count. Remember that in some client populations, the inflammatory and immune responses are reduced, so that signs of infection are subtle or absent (see box on p. 1131).

Dehiscence

When an acute wound fails to heal properly, the layers of skin and tissue may separate. This most commonly occurs before collagen formation (3 to 11 days after injury). **Dehiscence** is the partial or total separation of layers of skin and tissue above the fascia in a wound that is not healing properly. A client with poor wound healing is at risk for dehiscence. However, obese clients have a high risk because of constant strain on their wounds and the poor vascularity of fatty tissue. Dehiscence occurs most often in abdominal surgical wounds after a sudden strain such as coughing, vomiting, or sitting up in bed. Clients often report feeling as though something has given way. When serosanguineous drainage increases from a wound, the nurse should be alert for dehiscence.

Evisceration

When wound layers separate, visceral organs may protrude through the wound opening. This condition, called **evisceration,** is a medical emergency requiring placement of sterile towels soaked in sterile saline over the extruding tissues to reduce chances of bacterial invasion and drying before surgical repair occurs.

Fistulas

A **fistula** is an abnormal passage between two organs or between an organ and the outside of the body. A surgeon may create a fistula for therapeutic purposes (e.g., making an opening between the stomach and the outer abdominal wall to insert a gastrostomy tube for feeding). Most fistulas result from poor wound healing caused by trauma, infection, radiation exposure, or disease such as cancer. Fistulas increase the risks of infection, fluid and electrolyte imbalances, and skin breakdown from chronic drainage.

NURSING PROCESS

Assessment

The nurse assesses wounds at the time of injury, before the initiation of treatment, and after therapy, when the wound is relatively stable. Each condition requires different observations and actions.

Emergency Setting

In an emergency the type of wound determines the criteria for inspection. After a client's cardiopulmonary status is stabilized (Chapter 34), the nurse inspects the wound for bleeding. An **abrasion** is usually superficial with little bleeding but some weeping (plasma leakage from damaged capillaries). The depth and location of a **laceration** (torn, jagged wound) affect the extent of bleeding, with serious bleeding possible in lacerations greater than 5 cm (2 inches) long or 2.5 cm (1 inch) deep.

Puncture wounds bleed in relation to the depth and size of the wound; internal bleeding and infection are the primary dangers. The nurse next inspects the wound for contaminant material such as soil, broken glass, shreds of cloth, and foreign substances clinging to penetrating objects. The nurse then assesses the size of the wound and the need for suturing or surface protection. When the injury is the result of trauma from a dirty penetrating object, the nurse asks if the client has received a tetanus toxoid injection within the last year.

Stable Setting

Once a wound is stable after surgery or treatment, the nurse assesses its progress toward healing. If the wound is covered by a dressing that the physician has written orders not to change, the nurse inspects only the dressing and any external drains. Should a dressing appear saturated with drainage, the nurse may reinforce the secondary dressing pending a definitive response and orders from the physician. Saturated dressings provide an excellent environment for bacterial growth, and the physician will need to be informed of the color, odor, and estimate of drainage amount.

When a dressing change is planned, it may help to administer an analgesic at least 30 minutes before exposing a wound. The nurse must avoid accidentally removing or displacing underlying drains.

The nurse first inspects the appearance of the wound, noting the approximation of wound edges, the presence of exudate, the condition of underlying tissue in an open wound, and signs of dehiscence, evisceration, or infection. The nurse also notes **ecchymosis,** skin discoloration or bruising caused by blood leakage into subcutaneous tissues after trauma to underlying vessels. The outer edges of a wound normally appear inflamed for the first 2 to 3 days, but this slowly disappears. If infection develops, the wound edges usually become brightly inflamed, warm, tender, and swollen.

The nurse next assesses the character of wound drainage by noting the amount, color, odor, and consistency. The amount of drainage depends on the location and extent of the wound and can be measured by comparing the weights of wet and dry dressings. A rule of thumb is 1 g of drainage equals 1 ml. Another simple method for estimating the volume of wound drainage is to report the number and type of dressings used and saturated over what interval of time. The color and consistency of drainage vary, depending on its components. Types of drainage include the following:

1. Serous: clear, watery plasma
2. Sanguineous: fresh bleeding
3. Serosanguineous: pale, more watery, a combination of plasma and red cells, may be blood-streaked
4. Purulent: thick, yellow, green, or brown, indicating the presence of dead or living organisms and white blood cells

If the drainage has a pungent or strong odor, an infection is likely. The nurse objectively documents the integrity of the wound and the character of drainage, describing the appearance by observable characteristics.

The presence of drains is another important assessment criterion. A drain is used in a surgical wound if a large amount of drainage is expected and if keeping wound layers closed is especially important because accumulated fluid under the tissues prevents closure. A drain may lie under a dressing, extend through a dressing, or be connected to a drainage bag or suction apparatus. A pin or clip through the drain prevents it from slipping farther into a wound (Figure 37-1). As wound drainage decreases, the physician slowly withdraws the drain or leaves orders for the nurse to withdraw the drain a specified length over several days. The nurse first observes the security of the drain and its location with respect to the wound. Next the nurse notes the character and amount of drainage if there is a collecting device. The nurse pays particular attention to the flow of drainage through the tubing and notifies the physician of any sudden decrease that might indicate a blocked drain or an increase indicating bleeding or infection.

In the case of a surgical wound, the nurse inspects the staples, sutures, or wound closures for irritation and notes whether the closures are intact. The nurse may choose to count sutures when the physician has removed a portion of them. After the first few days when normal swelling around closures usually has subsided, continued swelling may indicate overly tight closures, which can cause wound separation or dehiscence. Early suture removal reduces formation of defects along the suture line and minimizes chances of unattractive scar formation.

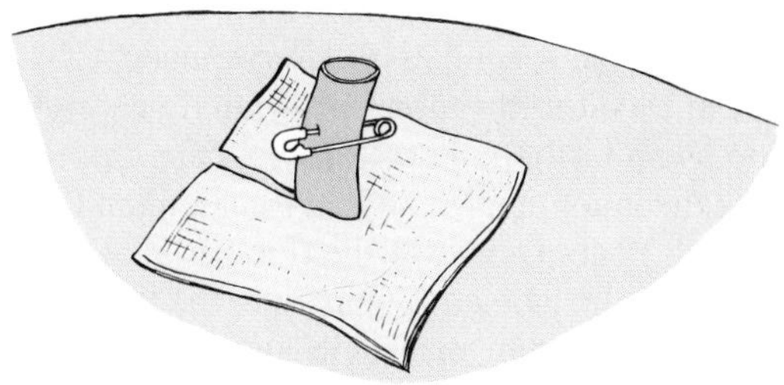

FIGURE 37-1 Penrose drain.

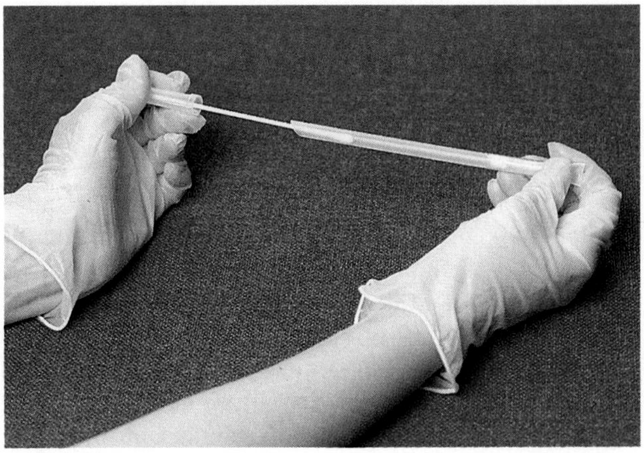

FIGURE 37-2 Wound culturette tube.

When a wound exhibits swelling or separation of its edges, the nurse can use light palpation to detect localized areas of tenderness or collection of drainage. Wearing sterile gloves, the nurse gently applies the fingertips along the wound edges. If pressure causes fluid to be expressed from the wound, the nurse notes the character of the drainage and collects it for culturing if necessary. Sensitivity to such palpation is normal, but extreme tenderness may indicate infection.

Pain assessment is an important component of wound assessment for detecting complications and planning future wound care. Serious discomfort during inspection or palpation of the wound suggests underlying problems, whereas discomfort related to dressing removal or application calls for administration of analgesics before future dressing changes.

Wound Cultures

If the nurse detects purulent or suspicious-looking drainage, a **wound culture** may be ordered by the physician. The nurse should never collect a wound culture sample from old drainage because resident colonies of bacteria grow in exudate. The nurse first cleans the wound to remove skin flora. Aerobic organisms grow in superficial wounds exposed to the air, and anaerobic organisms tend to grow within body cavities. To collect an aerobic specimen, the nurse inserts a sterile swab from a culturette tube into wound secretions, returns the swab to the culturette tube, caps the tube, and crushes the inner ampule so that the medium for organism growth coats the swab tip (Figure 37- 2). The nurse then sends the labeled specimen to the laboratory immediately. To collect an anaerobic specimen deep in a body cavity, the nurse uses a sterile syringe tip to aspirate visible drainage from the inner wound, expels any air from the syringe, and injects contents into a special vacuum container with culture medium. In some institutions, the nurse may place a cork over the needle to prevent entrance of air and sends the syringe to the lab.

NURSING DIAGNOSES FOR WOUND HEALING

Impaired skin integrity
High risk for impaired skin integrity
High risk for infection
Acute pain
Impaired physical mobility
Altered nutrition: less than body requirements
Ineffective breathing pattern
Altered peripheral tissue perfusion
Self-esteem disturbance

Nursing Diagnosis

After gathering appropriate assessment data the nurse clusters defining characteristics to establish nursing diagnoses. For example, the destruction of the skin's surface clearly allows the nurse to diagnose impaired skin integrity. The identification of nursing diagnoses related to wound healing helps the nurse to anticipate the need for supportive or preventive care (see box above).

The nurse assesses related factors contributing to each diagnostic statement. These related factors become the focus of the nurse's interventions. For example, the client with impaired skin integrity related to a surgical incision requires a different set of interventions than the client with impaired skin integrity related to pressure and nutritional deficiency. The client whose surgical incision causes drainage will require different and perhaps more frequent skin cleansing and dressings chosen to contain more drainage (Palamand, et al., 1992; Ryan, 1993). The client with a pressure ulcer will require nutritional support and measures to relieve or eliminate pressure over the wound site.

The nature and extent of a wound can also cause clients other health problems. Acute pain, impaired physical mobility, and ineffective breathing patterns are problems that can affect the client's recovery. In these cases, impaired wound healing becomes the related factor.

Planning

After identification of appropriate nursing diagnoses, the nurse establishes a plan of care that reflects the client's health care needs (see nursing care plan on p. 1135). Priorities in wound care depend on whether the client's condition is stable or emergent. Similarly, the type of wound care administered depends on the type of wound, its size and its location, and any complications. The nurse establishes with the client expected outcomes based on the goals of care. Nursing interventions are dependent and independent. Dependent interventions result from the physician's specific wound care orders. Independent nursing interventions may include, but are not limited to, the method utilized to secure the dressings, the time of the dressing change, the client position for dressing change, and the plan for client education.

With the trend toward earlier discharge from health care settings, it is important to consider the client's plan for discharge. Clients and their families may need to continue the objectives of wound management after discharge. Thus they may need to discuss the likelihood of the client returning home, returning home with the assistance of home nursing or transferring to a skilled nursing facility for more care and observation. The nurse and client work together to establish ways of maintaining client and family involvement and promotion of healing whether the client is in the hospital or home.

Examples of goals and expected outcomes for clients with wounds include the following:

Goal: Client's wound heals by primary intention.

Outcomes

Client's wound is closed and without drainage within 4 days

Wound scar forms without limiting client's function

Goal: Client's wound is free of infection.

Outcome

No purulent drainage or separation during healing

Goal: Client's skin remains intact.

Outcome

Client's skin is supple and without breakdown

Goal: Client regains normal function of involved body part within 4 weeks.

Outcomes

Client resumes baseline level of activity in 2 weeks

Client reports acceptable level of energy in 4 weeks

SAMPLE NURSING CARE PLAN
Impaired Skin Integrity

ASSESSMENT

Clinical scenario: Mr. Clark underwent an *exploratory laparotomy 24 hours ago.* A *6-inch incision* extends along the *midline;* it is *closed* with *intermittent* sutures. The *suture line* is *swollen* with minimal oozing of *serous fluid.* A small *drain extends through* a small *stab wound* lateral to the incision. The drain is connected to a Jackson-Pratt drainage device, which contains 50 ml of serosanguineous fluid. A *small amount* of *serosanguineous* drainage is seen *along the stab wound.* The incision is covered with four gauze 4 × 4 dressings and one abdominal pad. The *gauze* is *soiled* with *serosanguineous* drainage.

NURSING DIAGNOSIS

Impaired skin integrity related to abdominal incision and wound drainage

PLANNING

Goal

Client's incision will close without complication by discharge (planned for 7/24).

Expected outcomes

Wound drainage will be contained in dressing and Jackson-Pratt device with daily reduction in volume.
Client will deny irritation around incisional site daily.
Wound will be free of infection by 7/24.

IMPLEMENTATION

Steps	Rationale
1. Change or reinforce dressings when drainage accumulates. Use Montgomery ties to secure dressings.	Early recognition of need to change dressing may prevent maceration of skin over incision. Montgomery ties reduce need to apply tape with each dressing change, thus minimizing skin irritation. Wound healing depends on clean, moist environment for epithelialization and granulation (Cooper, 1990).
2. Use sterile technique while emptying Jackson-Pratt device.	Contamination of inside of bulb may result in wound contamination (Jermier and Treloar, 1986).
3. Cleanse skin around abdominal incision and drain to remove drainage. Use antimicrobial solution as ordered.	Cleansing reduces number of microorganisms in contact with incision line and stab wound.

EVALUATIVE MEASURES

Observe appearance of surrounding skin, incision, and character of drainage.
Measure volume of drainage in Jackson-Pratt device.
Ask client whether discomfort is experienced at wound site.
Monitor client's body temperature for elevation.

Defining characteristics are shown in italic type.

Goal: Client achieves comfort.

Outcomes

Client reports acceptable level of pain with dressing changes

Client's use of pain medication lessens as wound heals

Implementation

In an emergency setting the nurse uses first aid measures for wound care. Under more stable conditions the nurse is able to use a variety of interventions for wound healing.

First Aid for Wounds

When a client suffers a traumatic wound, first aid interventions include stabilizing cardiopulmonary function (see Chapter 34), promoting hemostasis, cleansing the wound, and protecting the wound from further injury.

Hemostasis. After assessing the type and extent of the wound, the nurse controls bleeding of a laceration by applying direct pressure on the wound with a sterile or clean dressing, such as a washcloth. After bleeding subsides, an adhesive bandage strip or gauze dressing taped over the laceration allows skin edges to close and a blood clot to form. If a dressing becomes saturated with blood, the nurse adds another layer of dressing, continues to apply pressure, and elevates the affected part. Serious lacerations should be sutured by a physician in an emergency clinic or hospital.

A puncture wound is allowed to bleed to remove dirt and other contaminants. If a penetrating object such as a knife blade is in a client's body, removal could cause massive, uncontrolled bleeding. The nurse may apply pressure around the object but not on it or on adjacent tissues.

Cleansing. Gentle cleansing of a wound removes contaminants that serve as sources of infection. However, vigorous cleaning can cause bleeding or further injury. For abrasions, minor lacerations, and small puncture wounds the nurse first rinses the wound in running water, cleans it with mild soap and water, and may apply an over-the-counter antiseptic. When a laceration is bleeding profusely, the nurse should only brush away surface contaminants and concentrate on hemostasis until the client can be cared for in a clinic or hospital.

Protection. Regardless of whether bleeding has stopped, the nurse protects the wound by applying sterile or clean dressings and immobilizing the body part. A light dressing applied over minor wounds prevents entrance of microorganisms. In the case of small abrasions, it is acceptable to leave the wound open to air so that a scab can form.

The more extensive the wound, the larger the bandage required. In the home a clean towel or diaper may be the best dressing. A bulky dressing applied with pressure minimizes movement of underlying tissues and helps to immobilize the entire body part. A bandage or cloth wrapped around a penetrating object should immobilize it adequately.

Dressings

The use of dressings requires an understanding of wound healing as well as factors influencing healing (see box on p. 1131). A variety of dressing materials are commercially available. Unless a dressing is suited to the characteristics of a wound, the dressing can hinder wound repair.

The choice of dressings and the method of dressing a wound influence healing. The proper dressing should not allow a draining wound to become overly dry with extensive scab formation. When this occurs, the dermis dehydrates and crusts. As a result, a barrier forms against normal epidermal cell growth, leaving a depression or defect in the new epidermal surface. Furthermore, dryness may increase discomfort. Ideally a dressing leaves a wound slightly moist to promote normal epidermal cell migration. The dressing should also absorb drainage to prevent pooling of exudate that may promote bacterial growth and to prevent wound drainage from coming into contact with intact skin.

For surgical wounds that heal by primary intention, dressings are commonly removed as soon as drainage stops. The primary dressing placed in the operating room is frequently removed by the physician 2 to 3 days postoperatively. This coincides with initial epithelialization so when the primary dressing is removed, the risk of infection is less. In contrast, when the nurse dresses an open wound healing by secondary intention, the dressing material becomes a means for mechanically removing exudate and necrotic tissue.

Purposes. A dressing may serve several purposes. It discourages exposure to microorganisms. However, if a wound has minimal drainage, the natural formation of a fibrin seal eliminates the need for a dressing. A pressure dressing promotes hemostasis by exerting localized, downward pressure over an actual or potential bleeding site and fosters normal healing by eliminating dead space in underlying tissues. The nurse must assess skin color, pulses in distal extremities, client comfort, and any changes in sensation to ensure that pressure dressings do not interfere with circulation. A dressing also promotes healing by absorbing drainage, preventing drying of the wound surface, and debriding the wound. Contact dressings may stick to underlying tissue; removal of such dressings disturbs healing surfaces but

GERONTOLOGIC NURSING PRACTICE FOR CLIENT WITH SKIN INTEGRITY ALTERATIONS

- The epidermis of older adults may be less tolerant of adhesives used to secure dressings. Use gentle adhesives when needed, or wrap to secure. Minimize tape to skin.
- Wound healing time may be longer because of the increased cellular repair and replacement time.
- Avoid frequent dressing changes, which may disrupt the healing wound and increase the skin stripping effects of removing tape.
- Monitor the ability of the client to manipulate the wound dressings and reach the wound in determining ability to perform self-care.
- Ensure potential sensory deficits are minimized (e.g., make certain that client is wearing eyeglasses or hearing aid during teaching sessions, if indicated).

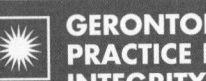

also cleans debris, exudate, and necrotic tissue from wounds that require debridement.

A firmly taped or wrapped dressing supports or immobilizes a body part, minimizing movement of the underlying incision and traumatized tissues. A dressing also serves to protect the client from seeing the wound, which may be unpleasant and cause anxiety. Finally, a dressing promotes thermal insulation to the wound surface and protects it from the dehydrating effects of air.

Types. Dressings vary by type of material and mode of application (dry, wet to dry, and moist). They should be easy to apply, comfortable, and made of materials that promote wound healing (Figure 37-3).

Gauze dressings are the most common type. They do not interact with wound tissues and thus cause little wound irritation. Gauze is available in different textures and in squares, rectangles, and rolls of various lengths and widths. Gauze dressings are best used for exudative wounds, wounds with dead space or sinus tracts, and wounds with a combination of exudate and necrotic tissue (Bryant, 1992). The nurse applies dry gauze such as a 4×4 pad or Telfa to wounds with moderate drainage. For wounds requiring debridement, a wet-to-dry dressing may be effective. The nurse moistens the contact dressing and applies it as a single layer against the wound surface. Moistening the contact layer increases the ability of the gauze to collect exudate and wound debris. Another dry layer of a fluffy, absorbent gauze is then applied. This type of dressing should be removed abruptly from the wound surface during the dressing change procedure and may be quite painful. Increasing awareness and acceptance of moist wound healing encourages the use of a moist dressing that must remain damp along the wound surface. It is critical that the first layer remain damp because wounds heal more quickly and **autolytic debridement** is enhanced in a moist environment. Autolysis involves the breakdown of necrotic tissue provided by the body's own white blood cells. If a moist dressing begins to dry, it must be changed.

A

B

C

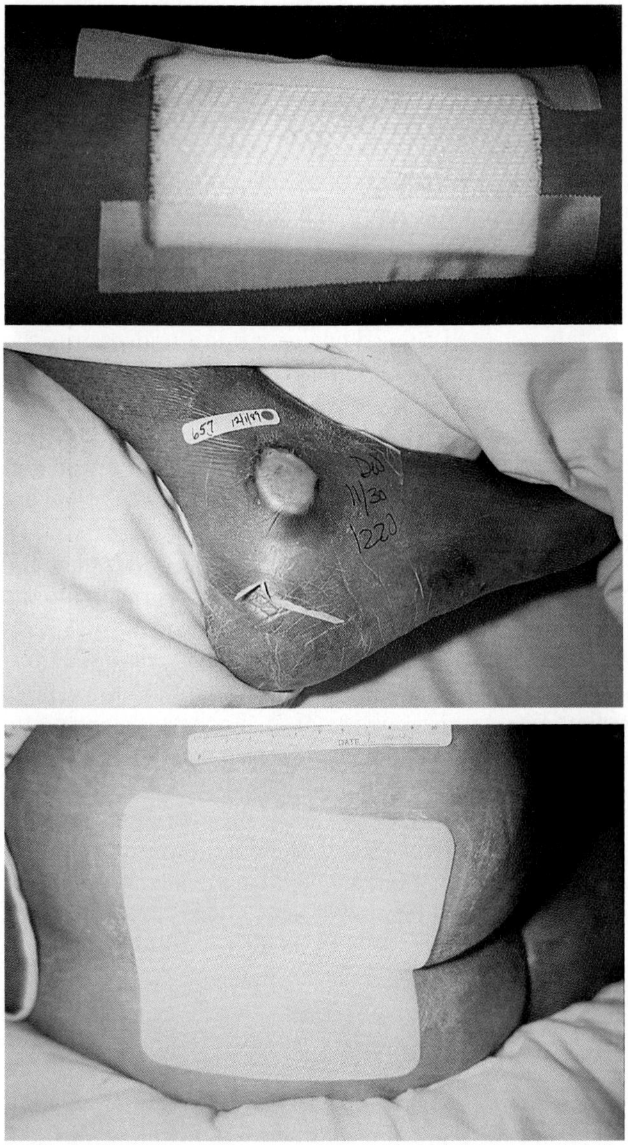

FIGURE 37-3 Variety of dressing materials are used for wound care **A,** Gauze dressings. **B,** Transparent dressing. **C,** Hydrocolloid dressing.

Another type of dressing is a self-adhesive, transparent film, a synthetic permeable membrane that acts as a temporary second skin. It has several advantages. It adheres to undamaged skin to contain exudate and minimize wound contamination. It also serves as a barrier to external fluids and bacteria yet still allows the wound to breathe. It promotes a moist environment that speeds epithelial cell growth. It also permits visualization of the wound. The transparent dressing is ideal for small, superficial wounds or wounds requiring minimal debridement. Under a transparent dressing, debridement occurs through rehydration and liquefaction of necrotic tissue; when used in this manner, the dressing should be changed more frequently, or a "pouch" dressing should be used. The transparent dressings may also be used over an island dressing such as Telfa gauze.

Hydrocolloid (HCD) and **hydrogel** dressings are occlusive (HCD) and semi-occlusive (gel) dressings that contain hydroactive particles. Both are moldable and easy to apply. Hydrocolloid and gel dressings are autolytic because they maintain wound humidity, slowly liquefy necrotic debris, and provide protective cushioning. The occlusive HCD dressings are not recommended for infected wounds, but they may protect clean wounds from secondary infection (Bryant, 1992). This type of dressing is most useful on shallow to moderately deep dermal ulcers. Dressings of this category include calcium alginates (Kaltostat), DuoDerm granules, Bard's absorption dressing, and Comfeel Ulcus powder. An advantage of many of the specialty dressings is that they need to be changed less frequently than traditional gauze dressings, often as infrequently as once or twice weekly. This minimizes disruption of the healing wound tissues, maintains a moist wound healing environment, and allows valuable nursing time to be spent on other care issues.

Changing Dressings. To prepare for changing a dressing, the nurse must know the type of dressing, any underlying drains or tubing used, and the type of supplies needed for wound care. The nurse can adjust the type and amount of dressings if the character or amount of drainage changes or if a wound becomes deeper. Notifying the physician of any change is essential.

The physician's order for changing a dressing should indicate the dressing type, frequency of changing, and solutions or ointments to be applied. An order to "reinforce dressing prn" (add dressings without removing existing ones) is common immediately after surgery, when the physician does not want accidental disruption of the suture line or loss of hemostasis. A client's medical or operating room record usually reveals whether drains are present. After the initial dressing change, the nurse communicates on the care plan the type of dressing materials and solutions to use, as well as the type and location of drains.

The most important principles to follow during dressing change procedures are those of aseptic technique, including use of a face mask and protective eyewear when necessary, thorough handwashing, and use of sterile gloves for handling sterile supplies and solutions (see Chapter 25). Also essential is ensuring that the client understands the steps of the procedure beforehand so less anxiety is experienced, describing normal signs of the healing process and offering to answer questions about the procedure or wound.

If wound care is needed in the home, the nurse must demonstrate dressing changes to the client and family and then provide an opportunity for practice (see box above). In the home, wound healing stabilizes so that sterile technique is usually unnecessary. However, clients must learn clean technique. The client should be able to change a dressing independently or with assistance from a family member before discharge unless home health care is to be provided. Procedure 37-1 outlines the steps for changing dry and wet-to-dry dressings.

Securing Dressings. The nurse uses tape, ties, or bandages and cloth binders to secure a dressing over a wound site. The choice of anchoring depends on the wound size, location, drainage, frequency of dressing changes, and the client's level of activity. The nurse most often uses strips of tape to secure dressings if the client is not allergic to them. Nonallergenic paper, plastic, and woven fabric tapes minimize skin reactions. Adhesive tape, the most likely anchor to cause skin irritation, adheres well to the skin's surface, whereas elastic adhesive tape compresses closely around pressure bandages and permits more movement of a body part.

Tape is available in various widths; the nurse chooses a size that sufficiently secures the dressing. The tape should cross the dressing and adhere to several inches of skin on each side. When securing the dressing, the nurse presses the tape gently, exerting pressure away from the wound. Tape is never applied over irritated skin. An adhesive skin barrier wafer such as Stomahesive may be applied to the skin around the wound so that the tape is secured to the skin barrier wafer and not sensitive skin. To remove tape safely, the nurse loosens the tape ends and gently pulls the outer end toward the wound, parallel to the skin, applying light traction to the skin away from the wound.

To avoid repeated removal of tape from sensitive skin, the nurse can secure dressings with reusable Montgomery ties (Figure 37-4). Each tie consists of a long strip; half contains an adhesive backing to apply to the skin, and the other half folds back and contains a cloth tie to be tied across a dressing and untied at dressing changes. A large, bulky dressing may require two or more sets of Montgomery ties. To provide even support to a wound and immobilize a body part, the nurse may apply elastic gauze or cloth bandages and binders over a dressing.

CLIENT TEACHING FOR DRESSINGS

- Instruct client on the importance of washing hands before and after dressing change.
- Have client practice cleansing of the skin around the wound with mild soap and water. Explain that this can be accomplished in a shower if the physician's order permits.
- Explain that the skin should be dried thoroughly after washing to prevent maceration.
- Instruct client on the importance of keeping dressing materials dry.
- Emphasize that the physician should be notified for signs of wound infection, including inflammation along incision, wound drainage (green, yellow, or brown), tenderness, and fever.

Comfort Measures

Any wound can be painful, depending on the extent of tissue injury. The nurse uses several techniques to minimize discomfort. Careful removal of tape, gentle cleansing of wound edges, and careful manipulation of dressings and drains minimize stress on sensitive tissues.

procedure 37-1

APPLYING DRY, WET-TO-DRY, AND MOIST DRESSINGS

Steps	Rationale
1. Assess size and location of wound to be dressed.	Assists nurse to plan for proper type and amount of supplies needed. Alerts nurse when assistance is needed to hold dressings in place.
2. Assess client's level of comfort.	Removal of dry dressing can be painful; client may require pain medication.
3. Review medical orders for dressing change procedure.	Indicates type of dressing or applications to use.
4. Prepare equipment and supplies:	
a. Sterile gloves	
b. Dressing set (sterile); scissors; forceps	Used to apply dressing and cut gauze to size.
c. Sterile drape (optional)	
d. Variety of gauze dressings and pads	
e. Fine mesh gauze (wet to dry only)	
f. Sterile basin	Used for antiseptic or cleansing solution.
g. Antiseptic ointment (optional for dry dressing)	
h. Cleansing solution	
i. Sterile solution (wet to dry only)	
j. Clean, disposable gloves	
k. Tape, ties, or bandage as needed	
l. Waterproof bag	Used for disposal of old dressing and supplies.
m. Extra gauze dressings, Surgipads, or ABD pads	
n. Bath blanket	
o. Adhesive remover (optional)	
p. Disposable mask (optional)	
5. Explain procedure to client and instruct client not to touch wound area or sterile supplies.	Decreases anxiety. Sudden, unexpected movement on client's part could result in contamination of wound and supplies.
6. Close room or cubicle curtains and windows.	Provides privacy and reduces airborne microorganisms.
7. Position client comfortably and drape with bath blanket to expose only wound site.	Provides access to the wound, yet minimizes unnecessary exposure.
8. Place disposable bag within reach of work area. Fold top of bag to make cuff.	Ensures easy disposal of soiled dressings. Prevents soiling of bag's outer surface.
9. Apply face mask and protective eyewear, if required, and wash hands thoroughly.	Reduces transmission of pathogens to exposed tissues. Protects nurse from splashes.
10. Put on clean, disposable gloves and remove tape, bandage, or ties.	Prevents transmission of infectious organisms from soiled dressings to nurse's hands.
11. Remove tape: pull parallel to skin; pull toward dressing; remove remaining adhesive from skin.	Pulling tape toward dressing reduces stress on suture line or wound edges.
12. With gloved hand carefully remove gauze dressings one layer at a time, taking care not to dislodge drains or tubes. Keep soiled undersurface away from client's sight.	Appearance of drainage may be upsetting to client. Removal of one layer at a time reduces the chance of accidental removal of underlying drains.
a. If dressing sticks on a wet-to-dry dressing, do not moisten it; instead gently free dressing and alert client of potential discomfort.	Wet-to-dry dressing should debride wound.
13. Observe character and amount of drainage on dressing and appearance of wound.	Provides estimate of drainage amount and assessment of wound's condition.
14. Dispose of soiled dressings in disposable bag.	Reduces transmission of microorganisms.
15. Remove gloves by pulling them inside out. Dispose in bag.	Prevents contact of nurse's hands with material on gloves.
16. Open sterile dressing tray or individually wrapped sterile supplies. Place on bedside table (see illustration).	Sterile dressings remain sterile while on or within sterile surface. Preparation of supplies prevents break in technique during dressing change.

Continued.

procedure 37-1—cont'd

Steps	Rationale
17. Apply dry dressing:	
a. Open bottle of antiseptic solution (if ordered) and pour into sterile basin.	Keeps supplies sterile.
b. Apply sterile gloves.	Allow handling of sterile supplies without contamination.
c. Inspect wound for appearance, drains, drainage, and integrity. Avoid contact with contaminated material.	Indicates status of wound healing.
d. Cleanse wound with antiseptic solution:	
(1) Use separate swab for each cleansing stroke.	Prevents contamination of previously cleaned area.
(2) Clean from least contaminated area to most contaminated.	Prevents introduction of organisms into wound.
e. Use dry gauze to swab in same manner as Step 17d to dry wound.	Reduces excess moisture, which could eventually harbor microorganisms.
f. Apply antiseptic ointment if ordered, using same technique as for cleansing.	Helps to reduce growth of microorganisms. Ointment may be applied to dressing if direct application causes discomfort.
g. Apply dry sterile dressings to incision or wound:	
(1) Apply loose, woven gauze as contact layer.	Promotes proper absorption of drainage.
(2) Cut 4×4 gauze flat to fit around drain, if present. Precut gauze is also available.	Secures drain and promotes drainage absorption at site.
	Ensures proper coverage and optimal absorption.
(3) Apply second layer of gauze.	Protects wound from external environment.
(4) Apply thicker woven pad (Surgipad).	Protects wound from microorganisms
18. Apply wet-to-dry dressing:	
a. Pour prescribed solution into sterile basin and add fine-mesh gauze.	Contact layer must be totally moistened to increase dressing's absorptive abilities.
b. Apply sterile gloves.	Allows handling of sterile supplies without contamination.
c. Inspect wound for color, character of drainage, type of sutures, and drains (see illustration).	Provides assessment of wound healing.
d. Cleanse wound with prescribed antiseptic solution or normal saline. Clean from least to most contaminated area.	Assists in debridement and cleanses wound of debris.

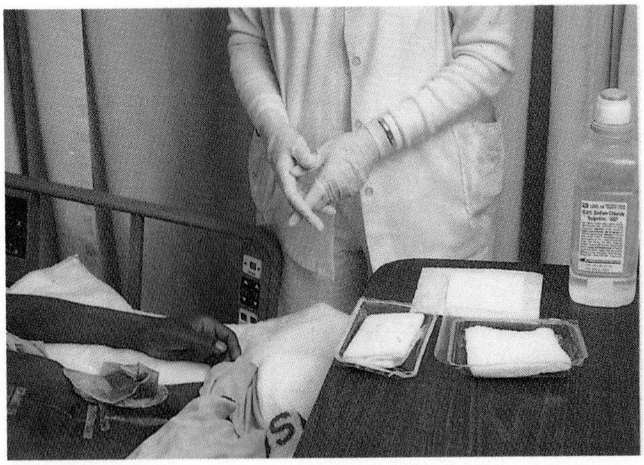
Step 16

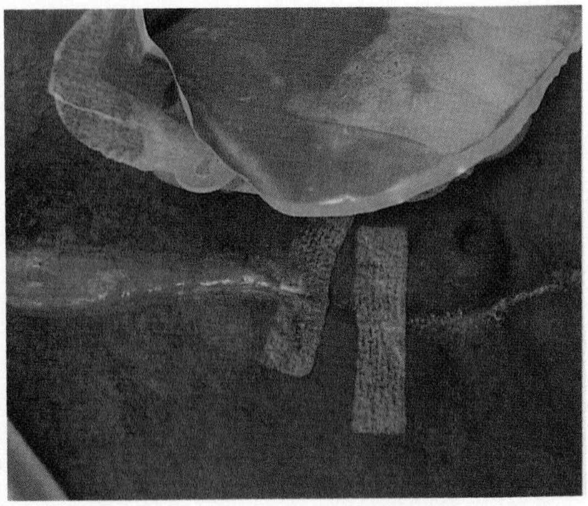
Step 18c

Steps	Rationale
e. Apply moist fine-mesh gauze as a single layer directly onto wound surface. If wound is deep, gently pack gauze into wound with forceps until all wound surfaces are in contact with moist gauze (see illustrations).	Absorbs drainage and adheres to debris. Wound should be loosely packed to facilitate wicking of drainage into absorbent outer layer of dressing.
f. Apply dry sterile 4 × 4 gauze over wet gauze.	Pulls moisture from wound.
g. Cover with ABD pad, Surgipad, or gauze.	Protects wound from the entrance of microorganisms.
19. Apply tape over dressing, Kling roll (for circumferential dressings), or Montgomery ties. For application of Montgomery ties:	Secures dressing in place.
a. Expose adhesive surface of tape on end of each tie.	Montgomery tie allows for frequent dressing changes without removal of adhesive tape.
b. Place ties on opposite sides of dressing.	
c. Place adhesive directly on skin or use skin barrier.	
d. Secure dressing by lacing ties across it.	Ensures dressing remains intact and covers wound.
20. Remove gloves and dispose in bag. Remove mask and eyewear.	Reduces transmission of infection.
21. Assist client to comfortable position.	Promotes client's sense of well-being. Enhances comfort.
22. Dispose of supplies and wash hands.	Reduces transmission of infection.
23. Evaluate client to determine response to dressing change.	Determines client's comfort level.
24. Monitor status of dressing at least every shift.	Evaluates extent of drainage and integrity of dressing.
25. Document appearance of wound and drainage, client's tolerance, and type of dressing applied in nurses' notes.	Documents progress of wound healing and promotes continuity in dressing change techniques.
26. Document frequency of dressing change and supplies needed on Kardex or care plan.	Alerts staff members to dressing change times and supplies needed.

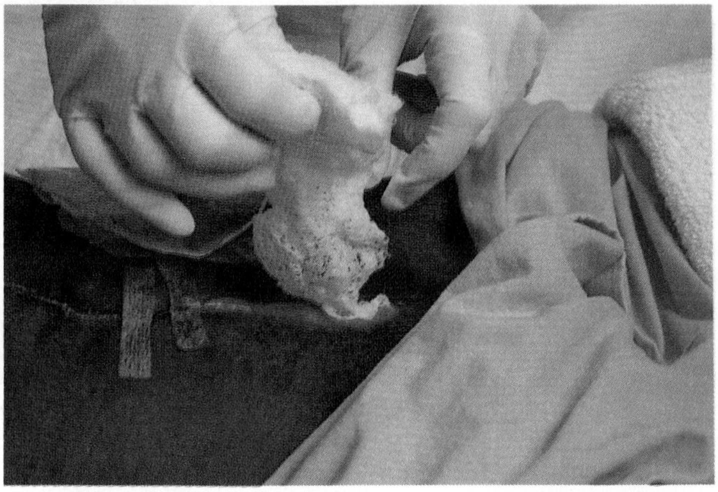

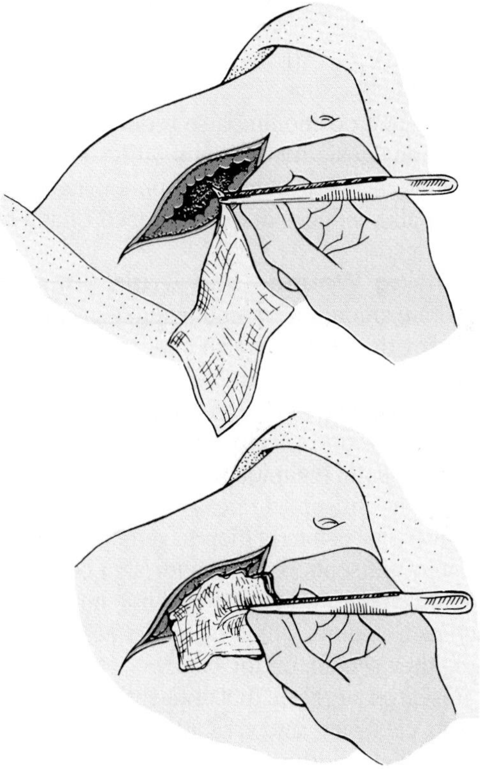

Step 18e

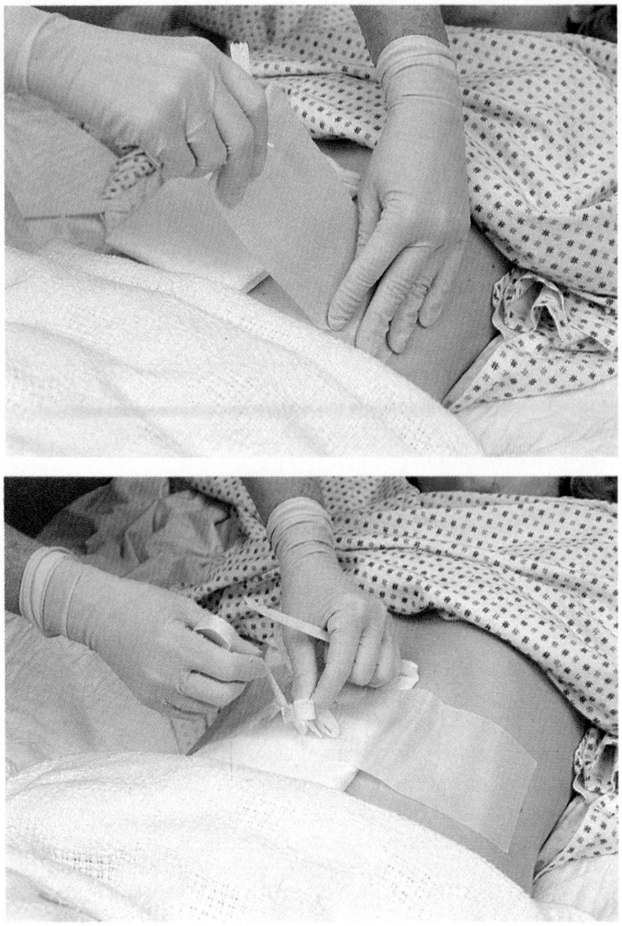

FIGURE 37-4 Montgomery ties.

Turning and positioning also reduce strain. Administration of analgesic medications 30 to 60 minutes before dressing changes (depending on a drug's time of peak action) also reduces discomfort (see Chapter 28).

Cleansing Wounds and Drain Sites. Although a moderate amount of wound exudate promotes epithelial cell growth, the physician may order cleansing of a wound or drain site if a dressing does not properly absorb drainage or if an open drain deposits drainage onto the skin. Wound cleansing requires good handwashing and aseptic techniques (see Chapter 25). The nurse may apply antiseptics locally to intact skin to remove pathogens or use irrigation to remove debris. The most effective antiseptic solutions for skin cleansing are tincture of chlorhexidine (Hibiclens) and the iodophors such as Betadine, which persist in acting against bacteria as they remain on the skin.

Research suggests that antiseptics commonly used in wound cleansing and irrigation (Table 37-2) are cytotoxic and should be used with caution only under very specific conditions. Such solutions require a physician's order for use in wound care (Lineaweaver, Howard, et al., 1985).

Diluted hydrogen peroxide may be useful when cleaning open wounds containing necrotic debris. The oxidizing property of peroxide exerts a mechanical cleansing effect, although its antiseptic action is slight. Its use should be avoided in the presence of granulation tissue and should **not** be used as an irrigating solution for deep wounds. The use of hydrogen peroxide in deep wounds or blind cavities may result in air embolus (Lineaweaver, Howard, et al., 1985). Normal saline is not irritating to wounded tissues and is frequently ordered for wound cleansing and irrigation.

Preoperative Skin Preparation. The CDC recommends that preoperative preparation of the skin includes bathing the operative site with antiseptics and hair removal, which, if necessary, should be done with clippers or a depilatory just before the operation (Garibaldi, et al., 1988; Mackenzie, 1988; Gilliam, 1990). Hair removal reduces entry of microorganisms into a surgical incision. In the operating room the nurse scrubs the skin thoroughly with a detergent solution and then applies an antiseptic solution to kill more adherent and deeper-residing bacteria. The surgeon may place a special transparent sterile drape directly over the skin before making an incision.

Basic Wound Cleansing. The basic principles of wound cleaning are to remove bacteria and surface contaminants and to protect the healing wound (Bryant, 1992). When cleansing surgical or traumatic wounds, the nurse applies antiseptic solutions with sterile gauze or by irrigation. The following principles are important when cleaning an incision or the area around a drain:

1. Cleanse in a direction from the least contaminated area to the most contaminated such as from the wound or incision to the surrounding skin or drain site (Figure 37-5) or from an isolated drain site to the surrounding skin (Figure 37-6).
2. Use friction when applying antiseptics locally to the skin.
3. When irrigating, allow the solution to flow from the least contaminated to the most contaminated area.

Irrigations. Irrigations are a special means of cleansing wounds of exudate and debris. The nurse uses an irrigating syringe to flush the area with a constant flow of solution. Irrigations are useful for cleaning open deep wounds or sensitive or inaccessible body parts. Through irrigations, cleansing or locally acting medications can be applied to an affected area. The nurse administers the prescribed solution (usually sterile water,

table 37-2

CLEANSING AGENTS

Solution	Indications	Effects
Acetic acid (bactericidal)	Effective against *Pseudomonas aeruginosa* in superficial wounds	May change color of wound exudate, does not significantly aid healing. Toxic to fibroblasts in normal dilution.
Povidone-iodine (antibacterial)	Reported to be active against bacteria, spores, fungi, and viruses when used on intact skin or small clean wounds	Liberates 10% free iodine. Toxic to fibroblasts in normal dilution.
Sodium hypochloride (antimicrobial)	Effective against staphylococci, streptococci, controls odors	Releases elemental chlorine, which is tissue irritant. Toxic to fibroblasts in normal dilution.
Chlorhexidine (bactericidal)	Effective against gram-negative and gram-positive organisms and some fungi	Should not be used in presence of granulation tissue
Hydrogen peroxide (oxidizing agent)	Useful for softening and removing crusted exudate and debris	Can cause ulceration of newly formed tissue. Toxic to fibroblasts. Never use to pack sinus tracts; can cause air embolism (Cooper, 1983; Lineaweaver, et al., 1985).
Normal saline (irrigant)	Useful for irrigation of clean or noninfected wounds	May be used under gentle pressure (35-ml syringe with 19-gauge needle) to assist in wound debridement
Cara-Klenz (cleanser) PharmaClens (cleanser)	Useful for cleaning dead tissue and secretions	Does not delay wound healing

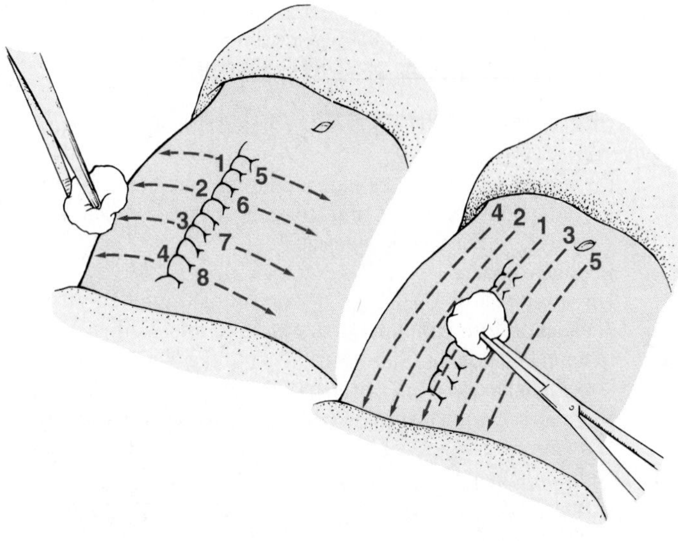

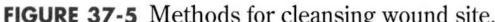

FIGURE 37-5 Methods for cleansing wound site.

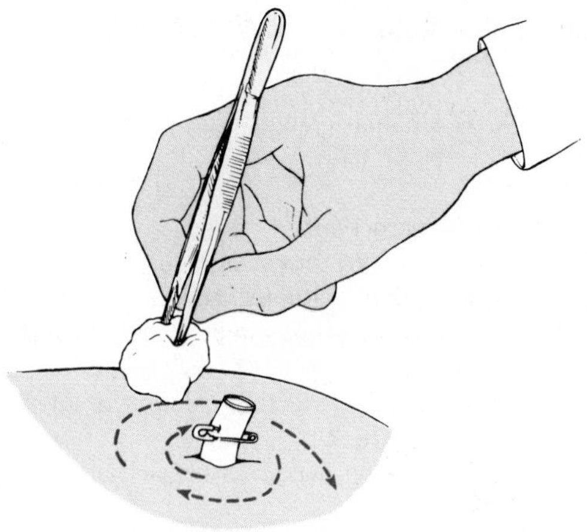

FIGURE 37-6 Cleansing of drain site.

procedure 37-2

PERFORMING WOUND IRRIGATION

Steps	Rationale
1. Assess client's level of pain.	Discomfort may be related directly to wound or indirectly to muscle tension or immobility.
2. Review medical record for physician's prescription for irrigation of open wound and type of solution to be used.	Open wound irrigation requires medical order including type of solutions to use.
3. Identify recent recording of signs and symptoms related to client's open wound:	Data are used as baseline to indicate change in condition of wound.
a. Condition of skin and wound	
b. Elevation of body temperature	May indicate response to infection.
c. Drainage from wound (amount, color)	Amount will decrease as healing takes place; serous drainage is clear; bright red drainage indicates fresh bleeding; purulent drainage is thick and yellow, pale green, or white.
d. Odor	Strong odor indicates infectious process.
e. Consistency of drainage	Leukocytes produce thick drainage.
f. Size of wounds, including depth, length, and width	Determines stage of healing.
4. Administer prescribed analgesic 30-45 min before starting wound irrigation procedure.	Increased comfort level will permit client to move more easily and be positioned to facilitate infection control during irrigation.
5. Gather equipment at bedside:	Increases efficiency.
a. Sterile basin	Used to hold sterile irrigation solution in preparation for irrigation.
b. 150- to 500-ml prescribed sterile irrigating solution warmed to body temperature	Warming adds to comfort level.
c. Sterile 35cc irrigation syringe, sterile soft catheter, if needed	Prevents introduction of additional pathogens during procedure; soft catheter is used to irrigate deep wounds with small openings.
d. 19-gauge needle	Used to irrigate infected wound.
e. Clean basin	Used to collect contaminated irrigating solution.
f. Clean gloves (check policy of institution)	Protect nurse from infection while removing wound dressing.
g. Sterile gloves	Used to maintain asepsis during irrigation and redressing procedures.
h. Waterproof underpad	Prevents soiling of bed linen; is cost and time effective.
i. Sterile dressing tray and supplies for dressing change, including packing, if ordered	Prevents infection and promotes wound healing.
j. Leakproof refuse bag	Used to gather soiled and contaminated dressings and prevent cross-infection.
k. Gown, mask, and goggles	Gown may or may not be indicated to protect uniform from contamination. Mask and goggles may be indicated if spraying of drainage is possible.
6. Explain procedure.	Reduces anxiety.
7. Position client comfortably to permit gravitational flow of irrigating solution through wound and into collection basin. Position client so that wound is vertical to collection basin.	Directing solution from top to bottom of wound and from clean area to contaminated area prevents further infection. Positioning client during planning stage provides bed surfaces for later preparation.
8. Warm sterile irrigating solution to approximate body temperature.	Increases comfort and reduces vascular constriction response in tissues.
9. Form cuff on leakproof refuse bag and place it near bed.	Helps maintain large opening, thereby permitting placement of contaminated dressing without soiling bag's outer surface.
10. Close room door or bed curtains.	Maintains privacy.

Steps	Rationale
11. Place waterproof underpad on bed surface in front of wound.	Eliminates need to change linens.
12. Place clean basin or thick towel directly under wound.	Collects contaminated irrigating solution.
13. Wash hands.	Prevents infection.
14. Apply gown, mask, goggles as needed.	Protects nurse's clothing and prevents exposure to splash.
15. Prepare sterile field using sterile dressing set and supplies.	Reduces risk of introducing microorganisms into wound.
16. Add sterile basin and pour in estimated volume of warm sterile irrigating solution and set irrigating syringe in basin with solution.	Prepares solution for wound irrigation.
17. Place several strips of adhesive tape within reach and not on sterile field.	Provides easy access to tape for securing dressing.
18. Put on clean gloves and remove soiled dressing and discard in leakproof refuse bag.	Reduces transmission of microorganisms.
19. Remove and discard gloves.	
20. Inspect wound and make mental note of healing process, inflammation, drainage, or purulent matter.	Provides accurate description later during charting.
21. Put on sterile gloves.	
22. Irrigate wound with wide opening:	Aids in removal of debris and facilitates healing by secondary intention.
a. Fill syringe with irrigating solution.	
b. Hold syringe tip 2.5 cm (1 in) above upper end of wound.	Prevents trauma to granulation tissue from syringe.
c. Using slow, continuous pressure, flush wound.	Ensures removal of all debris.
d. Repeat Steps 22a through 22c until solution draining into basin is clear.	
23. Irrigate deep wound with very small opening:	
a. Attach soft catheter to filled irrigating syringe.	Permits direct flow of irrigant into wound.
b. Lubricate tip of catheter with irrigating solution; then gently insert tip of catheter and pull out about 1.2 cm (½ in) to remove tip from fragile inner wall of wound.	
c. Using slow, continuous pressure, flush wound.	Ensures removal of debris without traumatizing new granulation tissue.
d. Pinch off catheter just below syringe.	
e. Fill syringe and reattach to catheter; repeat process until return is clear.	Avoids contamination of sterile solution or basin.
24. Irrigate infected, exudative, or necrotic wounds:	
a. Attach 19-gauge needle to 35 cc syringe.	Permits direct flow of irrigant into wound
b. Using continuous pressure, direct spray to wound base or edge of necrotic tissue.	Ensures removal of debris without trauma to new tissue.
c. Repeat until solution is clear or prescribed amount has been used.	
25. Dry wound edges with sterile gauze.	Prevents maceration of surrounding tissue from excess moisture.
26. Apply sterile dressing.	Maintains sterile protective barrier over wound.
27. Remove and dispose of gloves in proper receptacle.	Facilitates placement of adhesive tape.
28. Secure dressing with adhesive tape.	
29. Assist client to comfortable position.	
30. Remove goggles, mask, and gown and dispose of equipment and refuse; retain remaining bottle of sterile solution.	Sterile solution can be used for subsequent irrigations for 24 hours.

Continued.

procedure 37-2—cont'd

Steps	Rationale
31. Wash hands.	Reduces transmission of microorganisms.
32. Inspect dressing periodically.	Determines response to wound irrigation and need to modify plan of care.
33. Evaluate skin integrity.	Determines whether extension of wound has occurred.
34. Record wound appearance, irrigation, and response on nurses' notes.	Recording fulfills legal responsibility of nurse and provides information needed to ensure continuity of care.

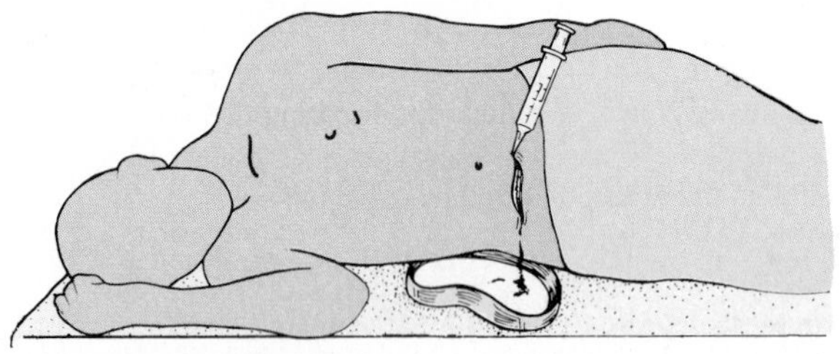

FIGURE 37-7 Position of client for abdominal wound irrigation.

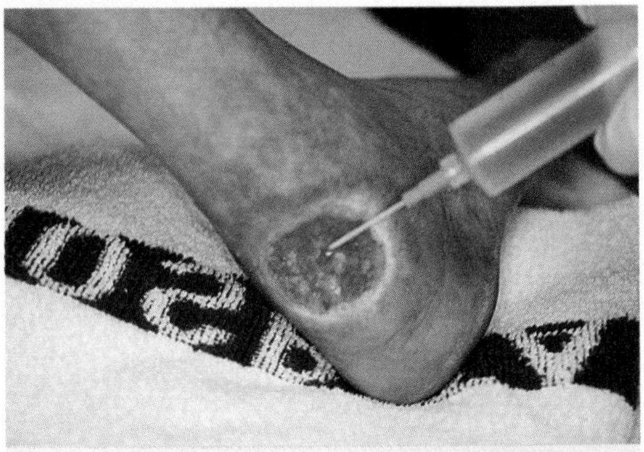

FIGURE 37-8 Wound irrigation by 35 cc syringe and 19-gauge catheter to facilitate removal of necrotic slough.

normal saline, or an antiseptic solution) at body temperature to enhance comfort and provide local cleansing application.

Wound irrigations. When irrigating clean proliferative wounds, the nurse uses sterile technique and a large, cone-tipped syringe to irrigate a wound, being careful never to occlude the wound opening with the syringe, so that irrigating fluid enters a closed space. The syringe tip should be over but not in the drainage site, and fluid should not flow over a contaminated area before entering the wound (Figure 37-7). For infected or necrotic wounds, an alternative method for wound cleansing and irrigation is the use of a 35cc syringe and a 19-gauge needle. This method provides an ideal solution pressure for cleansing wounds while minimizing tissue trauma (Rogness, 1985) (Figure 37-8).

In some situations a client may require continuous wound irrigation. The physician orders the rate of flow and the type of solution to be used. In this case, the irrigating fluid should be warmed to body temperature and will be instilled through an implanted irrigation catheter. Procedure 37-2 lists steps for wound irrigation.

Ear irrigations. Using a small syringe and solution at body temperature, the nurse can cleanse a client's external auditory canal of excess cerumen or exudate from a lesion or inflamed area. The use of solution at body temperature prevents discomfort and severe dizziness. The nurse should avoid irritating the canal's sensitive skin lining by not pulling the auricle excessively, nor introducing the tip of the irrigating syringe into the canal. The auditory canal should never be occluded with the syringe tip because introducing fluid under pressure could rupture the tympanic membrane. A slow, gentle irrigation works best. Procedure 37-3 describes the technique for ear irrigations.

Eye irrigations. Irrigations of the eye are usually not for actual wound care but rather to relieve local inflammation of the conjunctiva, apply antiseptic solution, or flush out exudate or caustic or irritating solutions. Warm normal saline and a small syringe or eye dropper are usually used to instill a few hundred milliliters of solution. Irrigation should always be done in a direction from the inner to the outer canthus to reduce absorption of contaminants through the nasolacrimal duct. The nurse should never allow the syringe top to touch the eye. When caustic chemicals enter the eye, however, the nurse must gently flush the eye continuously for at least 15 minutes with tap water to prevent burning of the

procedure 37-3

EAR IRRIGATION

Steps	Rationale
1. Inspect condition of external auditory canal. Assess client's level of comfort. If indicated, use otoscope to check condition of tympanic membrane.	Provides baseline data to determine change after irrigation. Ruptured tympanic membrane contraindicates irrigation.
2. Check physician's order for type of irrigating solution to order.	Certain solutions may have specific medicinal properties.
3. Prepare equipment and supplies:	
a. Warmed irrigating solution prescribed (volume depends on purpose; 200 to 500 ml.	Fluid at body temperature prevents adverse reaction.
b. Sterile basin for solution	
c. Asepto or small bulb syringe	
d. Curved emesis basin	
e. Moisture-proof towel or pad	
f. Cotton-tip applicators	Used to remove cerumen in outer ear canal.
g. Cotton balls	
h. Clean gloves, mask, and goggles or eyewear	Masks and eyewear protect from splashes.
4. Explain steps of procedure and warn client about sensations that might be experienced (wet, warm flow of fluid).	Relieves anxiety.
5. Wash hands; apply gloves, mask, and eyewear.	Reduces transmission of microorganisms.
6. Assist client to lying or sitting position with head tilted toward affected ear. Position emesis basin under affected ear. (Client may help hold basin.)	Irrigating solution will flow from auditory canal into basin.
7. Place towel over shoulder just under ear and emesis basin.	Prevents soiling of client's gown and bed linen.
8. Inspect ear canal for accumulation of cerumen or debris. Remove with cotton applicator. (Do not force cerumen into canal.)	Prevents reentrance into canal during irrigation.
9. Check the irrigating solution for proper temperature by allowing small amount to run over inner aspect of forearm. Fill bulb syringe with appropriate volume.	Irrigating solution at body temperature minimizes onset of dizziness and discomfort.
10. Straighten auditory canal for introduction of solution. In infants, pull auricle or pinna down and back. In adults, pull auricle or pinna up and back.	Facilitates entrance and flow of irrigating solution.
11. With the tip of syringe just above canal opening, irrigate gently by creating steady flow of solution against roof of auditory canal.	Occlusion of canal with syringe causes pressure against tympanic membrane during irrigation. Flow of solution drains safely out of canal while loosening debris.
12. Continue irrigation until all debris has been removed or all solution has been used.	Purpose of irrigation may be to cleanse canal, instill antiseptics, or provide local heat.
13. Assess client for onset of dizziness or nausea. Onset of symptoms may require temporary cessation of procedure.	Irritation of semicircular canals from irrigant may cause dizziness and nausea.
14. Dry off external ear and apply cotton ball to auditory meatus.	Promotes comfort. Cotton ball collects excess drainage.
15. Position client on side of affected ear for 10 min.	Allows solution remaining in auditory canal to drain.
16. Remove equipment.	Controls transfer of microorganisms.
17. Remove gloves, mask, and eyewear and dispose in receptacle.	
18. Wash hands.	Reduces transmission of microorganisms.
19. Return to client to evaluate character and amount of drainage and determine client's level of comfort.	Enables nurse to identify client's tolerance of procedure.
20. Document response to irrigation and note type, temperature, and volume of solution used and character of the drainage.	Timely recording provides accurate documentation of response to procedure.
21. Return to client after 10 min to remove cotton ball and evaluate drainage (gloves may be needed). Client may return to normal level of activity.	Increase in drainage or onset of pain may indicate injury to tympanic membrane.

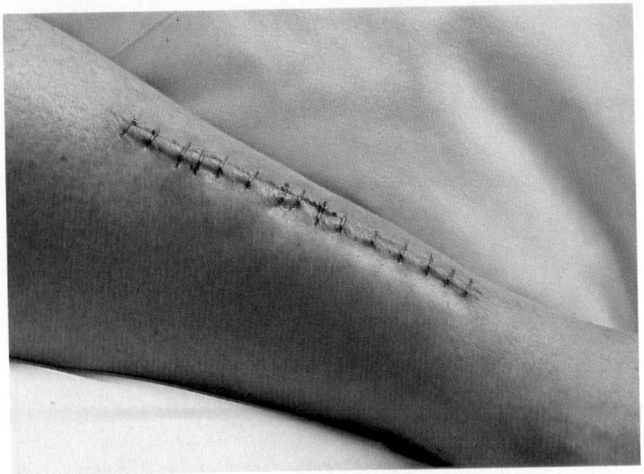

FIGURE 37-9 Wound sutured with staples.

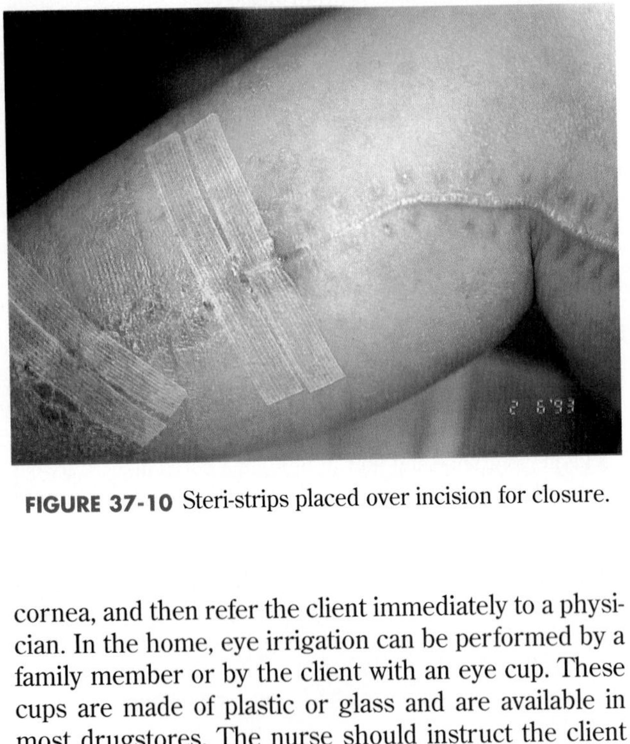

FIGURE 37-10 Steri-strips placed over incision for closure.

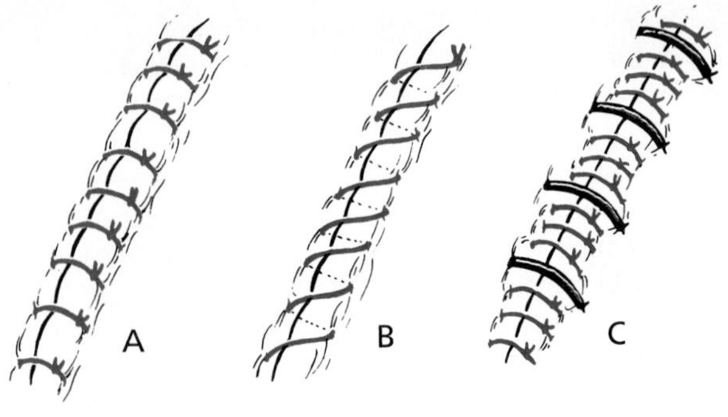

FIGURE 37-11 Examples of suturing methods. **A,** Intermittent. **B,** Continuous. **C,** Retention.

cornea, and then refer the client immediately to a physician. In the home, eye irrigation can be performed by a family member or by the client with an eye cup. These cups are made of plastic or glass and are available in most drugstores. The nurse should instruct the client about proper cleansing of the cup between uses and on the need to check for chipped glass.

Suture Care. A surgeon closes a wound by bringing the edges as close together as possible to reduce the formation of scar tissue while minimizing trauma and tension and controlling bleeding. Sutures are threads or wires used to sew body tissues together. They are available in a variety of materials including silk, steel, cotton, nylon, and polyester (Dacron), and they come with or without sharp surgical needles. The client's history of wound healing, the site of surgery, tissues involved, and purpose of the sutures determine the material to be used. For example, if a client has had repeated surgery for an abdominal hernia, the physician might choose wire sutures to provide greater strength for wound closure. In contrast, a small laceration of the face calls for the use of very fine Dacron sutures to minimize scar formation. Steel staples, a type of outer skin closure, are frequently used because they result in less trauma to tissues while providing extra strength (Figure 37-9). It is also common to see wounds closed with Steri-strips, a sterile butterfly tape applied along both sides of a wound to keep the edges closed (Figure 37-10).

Sutures are placed within tissue layers in deep wounds and superficially to complete wound closure. Deeper sutures are usually made of an absorbable material that disappears in several days. Sutures are foreign bodies and thus capable of causing local inflammation.

Policies vary at institutions as to who may remove sutures. If the nurse removes sutures, a physician's order is required. The method of suturing used by the physician determines the method of removal. Examples of suturing methods are intermittent or interrupted (individual, knotted sutures), continuous (a series of sutures knotted only at the beginning and the end of the suture line), and retention (Figure 37-11). The nurse should never pull the visible, contaminated portion of the suture through underlying tissue because infection could result (Figure 37-12). If staples have been used, the nurse inserts the tips of the staple remover (Figure 37-13) under each staple. While the ends of the staple remover are slowly closed, the tips squeeze the center, freeing the staple from the skin.

Drainage Evacuation. When drainage interferes with healing, drainage evacuation can be achieved by using a drain or a drainage tube with continuous suction. **Drainage evacuators** are convenient, portable units that connect to tubular drains within a wound bed and exert a safe, constant, low-pressure vacuum to remove and collect drainage (Figure 37-14). The nurse ensures that suction is exerted and that all connection

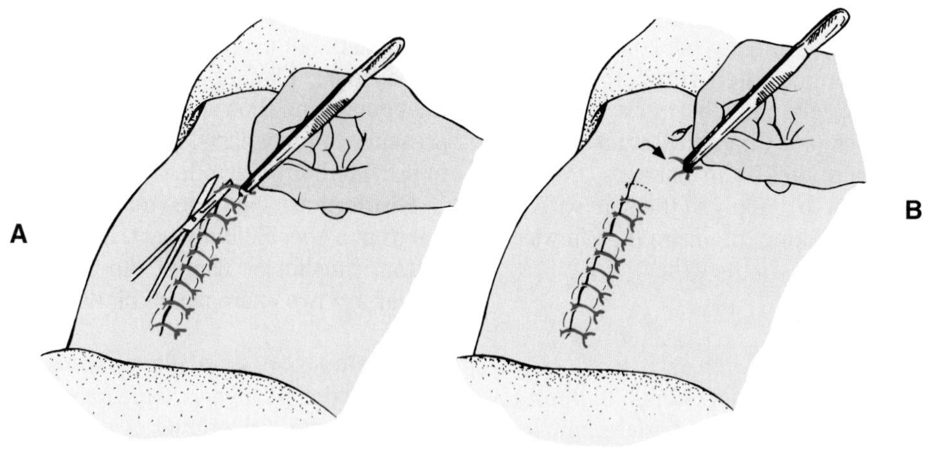

FIGURE 37-12 Removal of intermittent suture. **A,** Nurse cuts suture as close to skin as possible, away from knot. **B,** Nurse removes suture and never pulls contaminated stitch through tissues.

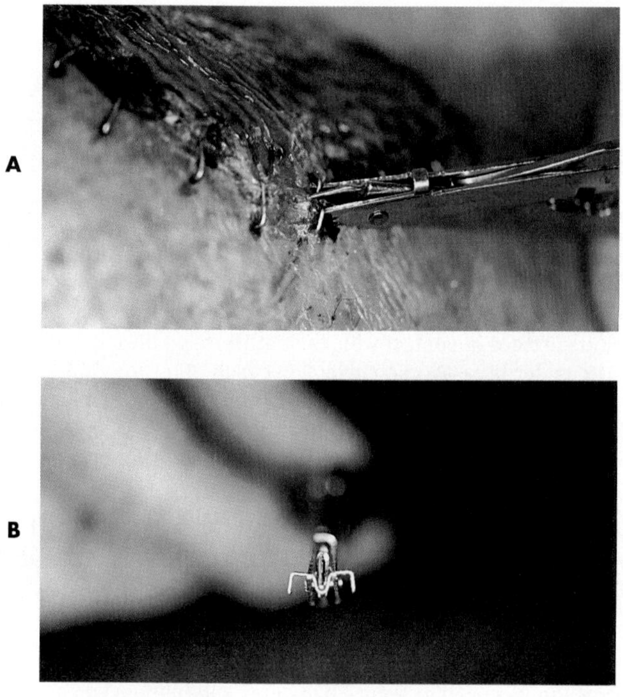

FIGURE 37-13 A, Staple remover placed under staple. **B,** Staple removed.

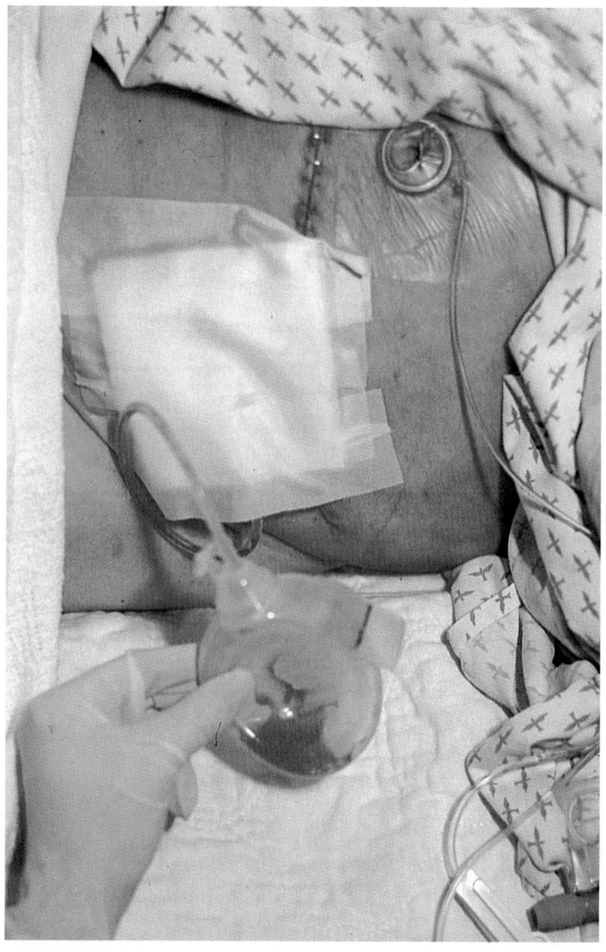

FIGURE 37-14 Jackson-Pratt drainage tubes and reservoir.

points between the evacuator and tubing are intact. The evacuator collects drainage that the nurse assesses for volume and character. When the evacuator fills, the nurse measures output by emptying the contents into a graduated cylinder and immediately resets the evacuator to apply suction. Special skin barriers, similar to those used with ostomies (see Chapters 32 and 33), may be applied around drain sites. The barriers are soft, waferlike, plastic material that apply to the skin with adhesive. If drain sites are leaking, drainage then flows on the barrier but not directly onto the skin.

Bandages and Binders

A simple gauze dressing is often not enough to immobilize or provide support to a wound. Binders and bandages applied over or around dressings can provide extra protection and therapeutic benefits by creating pressure over a body part (e.g., an elastic pressure bandage applied over an arterial puncture site), immobilizing a body part (e.g., an elastic bandage applied around a sprained ankle), supporting a wound (e.g., an abdominal binder applied over a large abdominal incision and dressing), reducing or preventing edema (e.g., a breast binder used to minimize swelling between skin and tissue layers after a mastectomy), securing a splint (e.g., a bandage applied around hand splints for correction of deformities), or securing dressings (e.g., elastic webbing applied around leg dressings after a vein stripping).

Bandages are available in rolls of various widths and materials including gauze, elasticized knit, elastic webbing, flannel, and muslin. Gauze bandages are lightweight and inexpensive, mold easily around contours of the body, and permit air circulation to underlying skin to prevent maceration. Elastic bandages conform well to body parts but can also be used to exert pressure over a body part. Flannel and muslin bandages are thicker than gauze and thus stronger for supporting or applying pressure to body parts. A flannel bandage also insulates to provide body warmth.

Binders are bandages made of large pieces of material to fit a specific body part. Most binders are made of cotton, muslin, or flannel. An arm sling and a breast binder are two examples of binders.

Principles for Applying Bandages and Binders. Correctly applied bandages and binders do not cause injury to underlying or nearby body parts or create discomfort for the client. Before applying a bandage or binder, the nurse performs the following steps:

1. Inspect the skin for abrasions, edema, discoloration, or exposed wound edges
2. Cover exposed wounds or open abrasions with a sterile dressing
3. Assess the condition of underlying dressings and change them if they are soiled
4. Assess the skin of underlying body parts and parts that will be distal to the bandage for signs of circulatory impairment (coolness, pallor or cyanosis, diminished or absent pulses, swelling, numbness, and tingling) to provide a means for comparing changes in circulation after bandage application

Table 37-3 outlines the principles of bandage and binder application. After a bandage is applied, the nurse as-

table 37-3

PRINCIPLES FOR BANDAGE AND BINDER APPLICATION

Principle	Rationale
Position body part to be bandaged in comfortable position of normal anatomical alignment.	Bandages cause restriction in movement. Immobilization in normal functioning position reduces risks of deformity or injury.
Prevent friction between and against skin surfaces by applying gauze or cotton padding.	Skin surfaces in contact with each other (e.g., between toes or under breasts) can rub against each other to cause abrasion or chafing. Bandages over bony prominences may rub against skin to cause breakdown.
Apply bandages securely to prevent slippage during movement.	Friction between bandage and skin can cause skin breakdown.
When bandaging extremities, apply bandage first at distal end and progress toward trunk.	Gradual application of pressure from distal toward proximal portion of extremity promotes venous return and minimizes risk of edema or circulatory impairment.
Apply bandages firmly, with equal tension exerted over each turn or layer. Avoid excess overlapping of bandage layers.	Equal tension prevents unequal pressure distribution over bandaged body part. Localized pressure causes circulatory impairment.
Position pins, knots, or ties away from wound or sensitive skin areas.	Pins and ties used to secure bandages and binders can exert localized pressure and irritation.

procedure 37-4

APPLYING AN ABDOMINAL BINDER, T BINDER, OR BREAST BINDER

Steps	Rationale
1. Observe client with need for support of thorax or abdomen. Observe ability to breathe deeply and cough effectively.	Baseline assessment determines client's ability to breathe and cough. Impaired ventilation of lung can lead to alveolar atelectasis and inadequate arterial oxygenation.
2. Inspect skin for actual or potential alterations in integrity. Observe for irritation, abrasions; skin surfaces that rub against each other; allergic response to adhesive tape used to secure dressing.	Actual impairments in skin integrity can be worsened with application of binder. Binder can cause pressure and excoriation.
3. Review medical record if medical prescription for particular binder is required and reasons for application.	Application of supportive binders may be based on nursing judgment. In some situations, physician input is required.
4. Gather necessary data regarding size of client and appropriate binder.	Ensures proper fit of binder.
5. Prepare necessary equipment and supplies:	
a. Abdominal binder:	
(1) Correct size cloth or elastic straight binder (2) Safety pins (unless Velcro closure is attached)	Binder must be large enough to surround abdomen and overlap to secure closure.
b. T and double-T binder: (1) Correct size binder (2) Safety pins: 2 pins for T binders; 3 pins for double-T binder	One pin secures horizontal waistband. Second pin secures each tail, placing pin through all thicknesses at horizontal level.
c. Breast binders:	
(1) Correct size binder	Binder must be large enough to overlap to secure Velcro closure.
d. Disposable gloves (required if binder placed over open wound).	
6. Explain procedure to client and close curtains or room door.	Promotes understanding. Provides privacy.
7. Wash hands (apply gloves if needed).	Maintains medical asepsis and infection control.
8. Apply abdominal binder:	
a. Position client in supine position with head slightly elevated and knees slightly flexed.	Minimizes muscular tension on abdominal organs.
b. Fanfold far side of binder toward midline of binder.	Reduces time client remains in uncomfortable position.
c. Instruct and assist client to roll away from you toward raised side rail while firmly supporting abdominal incision and dressing with hands.	Splinting reduces pain and discomfort.
d. Place fanfolded ends of binder under client.	Permits placement and centering of binder with minimal discomfort.
e. Instruct and assist client to roll over folded ends.	
f. Unfold and stretch ends out smoothly on far side of bed. (Binder should extend from just above symphysis pubis to just below costal margin.)	Maintains skin integrity and comfort.
g. Instruct client to roll back into supine position.	Facilitates chest expansion and adequate wound support when binder is closed.
h. Adjust binder so that supine client is centered over binder using symphysis pubis and costal margins as lower and upper landmarks.	Centers support from binder over abdominal structures.
i. For a straight binder, pull distal end of binder over center of client's abdomen. While maintaining tension on that end of binder, pull opposite end of binder over center and secure with Velcro closure tabs or safety pins.	Provides continuous wound support and comfort.
j. Assess client's ability to breathe deeply and cough effectively.	Determines ventilation and clears airways of pulmonary secretions.

Continued.

procedure 37-4—cont'd

Steps	Rationale
k. Ask client about comfort level.	Excess discomfort may inhibit expirations.
l. Adjust binder as necessary.	
9. Apply T and double-T binders:	
a. Assist client to dorsal recumbent position.	
b. Have client raise hips and place horizontal band around waist (or above iliac crests) with vertical tails extending past buttocks. Overlap waistband in front and secure with safety pins.	Minimizes muscular tension on perineal organs. Secures binder around client.
c. Complete binder application:	Single-T binders and double-T provide support to perineal muscles and organs.
(1) *T binder:* Bring remaining vertical strip over perineal dressing and continue up and under center front of horizontal band. Bring ends over waistband and secure all thicknesses with safety pin.	
(2) *Double-T binder:* Bring remaining vertical strips over perineal or suprapubic dressing with each tail supporting one side of scrotum and proceeding upward on either side of penis. Continue upward on either side of penis. Continue drawing ends behind and then downward in front of horizontal band. Secure all thicknesses with one safety pin.	
d. Assess comfort level with client in lying, sitting, and standing positions. Readjust front pins as necessary. Increase padding if any area rubs against surrounding tissues.	Determines efficacy of binder to maintain dressings and support perineal structures.
e. Instruct client regarding removal of binder before defecating or urinating and need to replace binder after these bodily functions.	Cleanliness of binder reduces infection risk.
10. Apply breast binder:	
a. Assist client in placing arms through binder's armholes.	Positions binder for application.
b. Assist client to supine position in bed.	Facilitates normal anatomical position of breasts. Facilitates healing and comfort.
c. Pad area under breasts if necessary.	Prevents skin contact with undersurface.
d. Using Velcro closure tabs, secure binder at nipple level first. Continue closure process above and then below nipple line until entire binder is closed.	Reduces risk of uneven pressure or localized irritation.
e. Make appropriate adjustments including individualizing fit of shoulder straps.	Maintains support to client's breasts.
f. Instruct and observe skill development in self-care related to reapplying breast binder.	Self-care is an integral aspect of discharge planning. Skin integrity and comfort level goals are ensured.
11. Wash hands.	Prevents cross-infections.
12. Observe site for skin integrity, circulation, and characteristics of the wound. Note comfort level of client.	Determines that binder has not resulted in irritation to skin or underlying organs. Binders should not impede breathing or increase discomfort.
13. Record application of binder, condition of skin and circulation, integrity of dressings, and comfort level.	Documents procedure. Baseline data ensure continuity of care.

sesses, documents, and immediately reports any changes in circulation, comfort level, body function such as ventilation, and skin integrity. The nurse who applies a bandage can loosen or readjust it as necessary, but the nurse should seek an order before loosening or removing a bandage applied by the physician. The nurse explains to the client that any bandage or binder will feel relatively firm or tight, assesses the bandage carefully to be sure it is applied properly and is providing therapeutic benefit, and replaces bandages as they become soiled.

Binder Application. Binders are especially designed for the body part to be supported. The most common types of binders are the breast binder, abdominal binder, T binder, and sling.

Breast binder. A breast binder looks like a tight-fitting sleeveless vest. It conforms to the shape of the chest wall and is available in different sizes. Breast binders can provide support after breast surgery or exert pressure to reduce lactation after childbirth. It is essential, however, that excess pressure be avoided when clients or family members are learning how to apply a breast binder. Chest expansion should be unimpaired, but if pulmonary secretions increase, the nurse must encourage active pulmonary hygiene exercises. Procedure 37-4 outlines steps for binder application.

Abdominal binder. An abdominal binder supports large incisions that are vulnerable to stress when the client moves or coughs. It is a rectangular piece of cotton or elasticized material with many tails attached to the two longer sides or long extensions on each side to surround the abdomen (Figure 37-15). Procedure 37-4 describes steps for an abdominal binder application.

T binders. A T binder looks like the letter T (Figure 37-16) with either a single or double tail. T binders secure rectal or perineal dressings. The belt of the binder fits securely around the waist, with the tail passing between the legs from back to front. T binders are easily soiled and require frequent changing. Irritation to the urethra or scrotum must be avoided.

Slings. Slings support arms with muscular sprains or fractures. A commercially made sling consists of a long sleeve that extends to the elbow and a strap that fits around the neck. In the home a large triangular piece of cloth can be used as a sling. The client may sit or lie supine for a sling application (Figure 37-17). The nurse instructs the client to bend the affected arm, bringing the forearm straight across the chest. The open sling fits under the client's arm and over the chest, with the base of the triangle under the wrist and the triangle's point at the elbow. One end of the sling fits around the back of the neck. The nurse brings the other end up over the affected arm while supporting the extremity. The nurse ties the two ends at the side of the neck so that the knot does not press against the cervical spine.

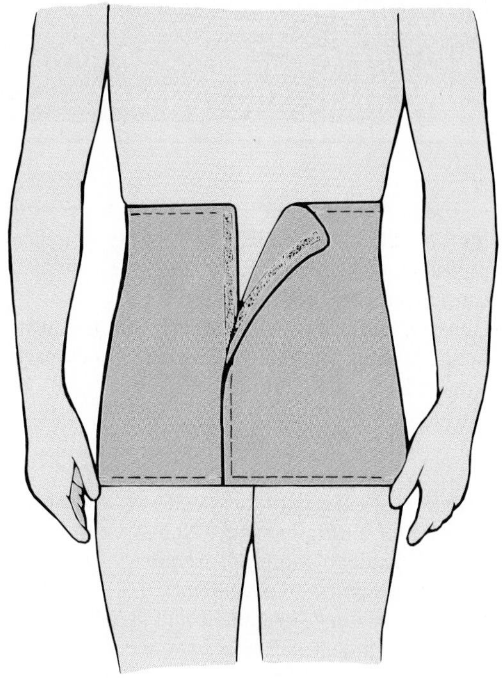

FIGURE 37-15 Abdominal binder secured with velcro.

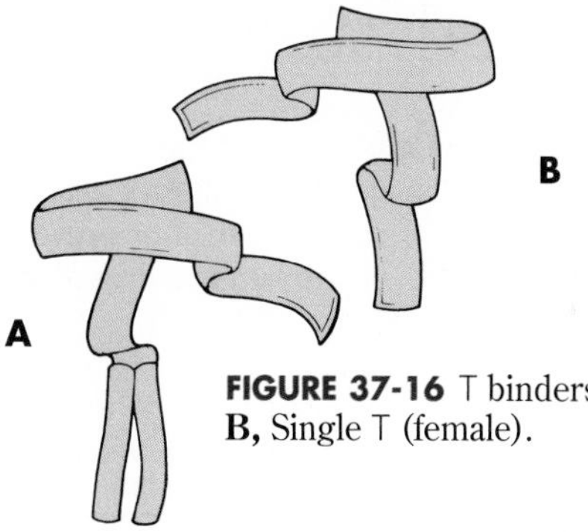

FIGURE 37-16 T binders. **A,** Double T (male). **B,** Single T (female).

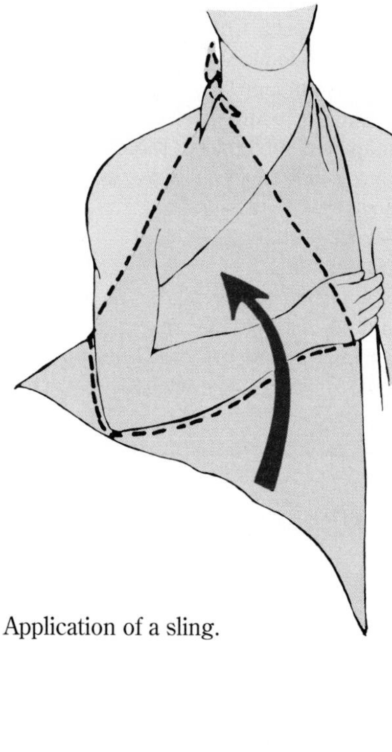

FIGURE 37-17 Application of a sling.

procedure 37-5

APPLYING AN ELASTIC BANDAGE

Steps	Rationale
1. Inspect skin for alterations in integrity as indicated by abrasions, discoloration, chafing, or edema. (Look carefully at bony prominences.)	Altered skin integrity contraindicates the use of elastic bandage.
2. Observe adequacy of circulation by noting surface temperature, skin color, and sensation of body parts to be wrapped.	Comparison of area before and after application of bandage is necessary to ensure continued adequate circulation. Impairment of circulation may result in coolness to touch when compared with opposite side of body, cyanosis or pallor of skin, diminished or absent pulses, edema or localized pooling, and numbness or tingling of part.
3. Review medical record for specific orders related to application of elastic bandage. Note area to be covered, type of bandage required, frequency of change, and previous response to treatment.	Specific prescription may direct procedure, including factors such as extent of application (e.g., toe to knee, toe to groin) and duration of treatment.
4. Obtain necessary equipment and supplies (determine if present bandage will be reused or replacement be obtained):	
a. Correct widths and number of bandages (Elastic bandages are available in 2, 2½, 3, 4, 6, and 8 in and 1½ and 3 yd [5, 6.25, 7.5, 10, 15, and 20 cm and 135 and 270 cm]; 7.5- and 10-cm bandages are most often appropriate.)	Increasingly wider bandages are used as size of body part increases (e.g., 7.5-, 10-, and 15-cm bandages may be used to cover foot, calf, thigh).
b. Safety pins, tape	Secures bandage in place.
5. Explain procedure. Reinforce teaching that smooth, even, light pressure will be applied to improve venous circulation, prevent clot formation, reduce or prevent swelling, immobilize arms, secure surgical dressings, and provide pressure.	Promotes cooperation and reduces anxiety. Improves knowledge level regarding need for elastic bandages.
6. Wash hands.	Reduces transmission of infection.
7. Close room door or curtains. Assist client to assume comfortable, anatomically correct position.	Maintains comfort and dignity. Maintains alignment. Prevents musculoskeletal deformity.
8. Hold roll of elastic bandage in dominant hand and use other hand to lightly hold beginning of bandage at distal body part. Continue transferring roll to dominant hand as bandage is wrapped.	Maintains appropriate and consistent bandage tension.
9. Apply bandage from distal point toward proximal boundary using variety of turns to cover various shapes of body parts (Table 37-4).	Bandage is applied in manner that conforms evenly to body part and promotes venous return.
10. Unroll and very slightly stretch bandage. Overlap turns.	Maintains uniform bandage tension. Prevents uneven bandage tension and circulatory impairment.
11. Secure first bandage before applying additional rolls.	Prevents wrinkling or loose ends.
12. Wash hands.	Reduces transmission of microorganisms.
13. Evaluate distal circulation as application is completed and at least twice during 8-hr period (note color, warmth, pulses, and numbness).	Early detection of circulatory difficulties ensures healthy neuromuscular status.
14. Record bandage application and client's response in nurses' notes.	Documents procedures and ensures continuity of care.

table 37-4

TYPES OF BANDAGE TURNS

Type	Description	Purpose or use
Circular	Bandage turn overlapping previous turn completely 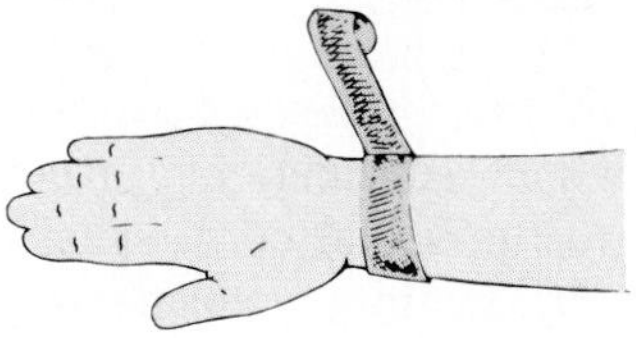	Anchors bandage at the first and final turn; covers small part (finger, toe)
Spiral	Bandage ascending body part with each turn overlapping previous one by one-half or two-thirds width of bandage 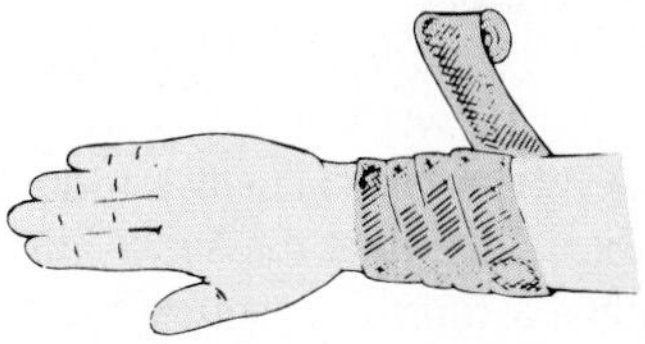	Covers cylindrical body parts such as wrist or upper arm
Spiral—reverse	Turn requiring twist (reversal) of bandage halfway through each turn 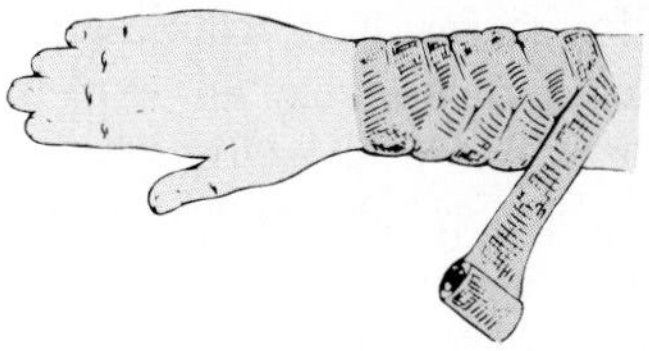	Covers cone-shaped body parts such as the forearm, thigh, or calf; useful with nonstretching bandages such as gauze or flannel
Figure eight	Oblique overlapping turns alternately ascending and descending over bandaged part; each turn crossing previous one to form figure eight 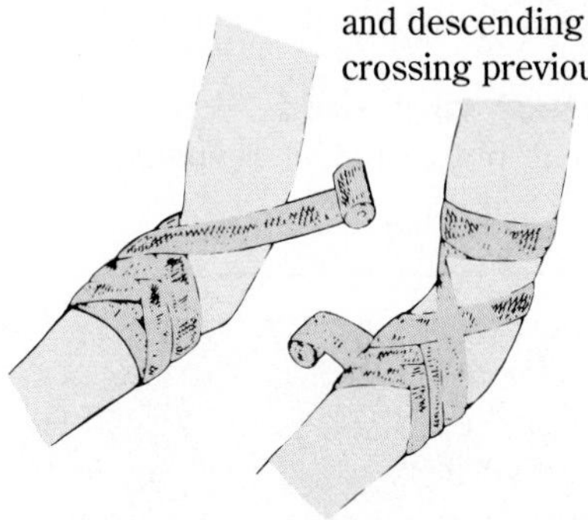	Covers joints; snug fit provides excellent immobilization
Recurrent	Bandage first secured with two circular turns around proximal end of body part; half turn made perpendicular up from bandage edge; body of bandage brought over distal end of body part to be covered with each turn folded back over on itself 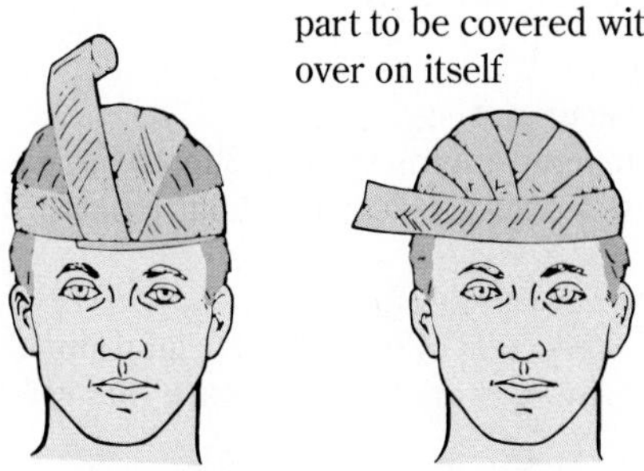	Covers uneven body parts such as head or stump

The loose fold at the elbow can be folded evenly around the elbow and pinned. The lower arm should always be supported at a level above the elbow to prevent the formation of dependent edema.

Bandage Application. Rolls of bandage can secure or support dressings over irregularly shaped body parts. Each roll has a free outer end and a terminal end at the center. The rolled portion of the bandage is its body, and its outer surface is placed against the client's skin or dressing. Procedure 37-5 describes the steps for applying an elastic bandage. The nurse may use a variety of bandage turns depending on the body part to be bandaged (Table 37-4).

Heat and Cold Therapy

The local application of heat and cold to an injured body part provides therapeutic benefits. Before using these therapies, however, the nurse must understand normal body responses to local temperature variations, assess the integrity of the body part, determine the client's ability to sense temperature variations, and ensure proper operation of equipment. The nurse is legally responsible for the safe administration of all heat and cold applications.

Body Responses to Heat and Cold. Exposure to heat and cold can cause systemic and local responses. Systemic responses occur through heat loss mechanisms (sweating or vasodilation) or mechanisms promoting heat conservation (vasoconstriction or piloerection) and heat production (shivering) (see Chapter 15). Local responses to heat and cold occur through stimulation of temperature-sensitive nerve endings within the skin. This stimulation sends impulses from the periphery to the hypothalamus, which becomes aware of local temperature sensations and triggers adaptive responses for the maintenance of normal body temperature. If alterations occur along temperature-sensation pathways, the reception and eventual perception of stimuli are altered.

The body also has a protective reflex response so that, when a person touches an extremely hot or cold stimulus, impulses travel to the spinal cord, synapse within the cord, and return by way of a motor nerve to cause withdrawal from the stimulus. The person simultaneously becomes aware of discomfort.

The body can tolerate wide variations in temperature. The normal temperature of the skin's surface is 34° C (93.2° F), but temperature receptors usually adapt quickly to local temperatures between 45° C (113° F) and 15° C (59° F). Pain develops when local temperatures exceed this range. Excessive heat causes a burning sensation. Cold produces a numbing sensation before the pain.

The body's adaptive ability creates the major problem in protecting clients from injury resulting from temperature extremes. A person initially feels an extreme change in temperature but within a short time hardly notices the temperature variation. This phenomenon can be dangerous because a person insensitive to heat and cold extremes can suffer serious tissue injury. The nurse must recognize clients most at risk for injuries from heat and cold applications (Table 37-5).

Local Effects of Heat and Cold. Heat and cold stimuli create different physiological responses. The

table 37-5

CONDITIONS THAT INCREASE RISK OF INJURY FROM HEAT AND COLD APPLICATION

Condition	Risk factors
Very young; older adults	Thinner skin layers in children and aged increase risk of burns; older adults have reduced sensitivity to pain.
Open wounds, broken skin, stomas	Subcutaneous and visceral tissues are more sensitive to temperature variations; they also contain no temperature and fewer pain receptors.
Areas of edema or scar formation	There is reduced sensation to temperature stimuli because of thickening of skin layers from fluid buildup or scar formation.
Peripheral vascular disease (e.g., diabetes or arteriosclerosis)	Body's extremities are less sensitive to temperature and pain stimuli because of circulatory impairment and local tissue injury; cold application would further compromise blood flow.
Confusion or unconsciousness	There is reduced perception of sensory or painful stimuli.
Spinal cord injury	Alterations in nerve pathways prevent reception of sensory or painful stimuli.
Abscessed tooth or appendix	Infection is highly localized; application of heat may cause rupture with spread of microorganisms systemically.

choice of heat or cold therapy depends on the local responses desired for wound healing.

EFFECTS OF HEAT APPLICATION. Table 37-6 summarizes the benefits of heat application. Heat generally is therapeutic, improving blood flow to an injured part. If heat is applied for 1 hour or more, however, blood flow is reduced by a reflex vasoconstriction as the body attempts to control heat loss from the area. The periodic removal and reapplication of local heat will restore vasodilation. Continuous exposure to heat damages epithelial cells, causing redness, localized tenderness, and even blistering of the skin.

EFFECTS OF COLD APPLICATION. Table 37-6 also summarizes the benefits of cold application. Prolonged exposure of the skin to cold results in a reflex vasodilation. The cell's inability to receive adequate blood flow and nutrients results in tissue ischemia. The skin initially takes on a reddened appearance, followed by a bluish purple mottling with numbness and a burning type of pain. Tissues can actually freeze from exposure to extreme cold.

Factors Influencing Heat and Cold Tolerance. The body's response to heat and cold therapies depends on the following factors:

1. Duration of application. A person is better able to tolerate short exposures to any temperature extremes.
2. Body part. The neck, inner aspect of the wrist and forearm, and perineal regions are more sensitive to temperature variations. The foot and the palm of the hand are less sensitive.

table 37-6

THERAPEUTIC EFFECTS OF HEAT AND COLD APPLICATIONS

Physiological response	Therapeutic benefit	Examples of conditions treated
HEAT THERAPY		
Vasodilation	Improves blood flow to injured body part Promotes delivery of nutrients and removal of wastes Lessens venous congestion in injured tissues	Inflamed or edematous body part New surgical wound Infected wound Arthritis or degenerative joint disease Localized joint pain or muscle strains Low back pain Menstrual cramping Hemorrhoidal, perianal, and vaginal inflammation Local abscesses
Reduced blood viscosity	Improves delivery of leukocytes and antibiotics to wound site	
Reduced muscle tension	Promotes muscle relaxation Reduces pain from spasm or stiffness	
Increased tissue metabolism	Increases blood flow Provides local warmth	
Increased capillary permeability	Promotes movement of waste products and nutrients	
COLD THERAPY		
Vasoconstriction	Reduces blood flow to injured site, preventing edema formation Reduces inflammation	Immediately after direct trauma (e.g., sprains, strains, fractures, and muscle spasms) Superficial laceration or puncture wound Minor burn Suspected malignancy in area of injury or pain After injections Arthritis or joint trauma
Local anesthesia	Reduces localized pain	
Reduced cell metabolism	Reduces oxygen needs of tissues	
Increased blood viscosity	Promotes blood coagulation at injury site	
Decreased muscle tension	Relieves pain	

3. Damage to body surface. Exposed skin layers are more sensitive to temperature variations.
4. Prior skin temperature. The body responds best to minor temperature adjustments.
5. Body surface area. A person is less tolerant of temperature changes over a large area of the body.
6. Age and physical condition. The very young and old are most sensitive to heat and cold. If a client's physical condition reduces the reception or perception of sensory stimuli, the tolerance to temperature extremes is high, but the risk of injury is also high.

Assessment for Temperature Tolerance. Before applying heat or cold therapies, the nurse assesses the client's physical condition for signs of potential intolerance to heat and cold. The nurse first observes the area to be treated so that therapy-related skin changes can later be evaluated. Alterations in skin integrity, such as abrasions, open wounds, edema, bruising, bleeding, or localized areas of inflammation, increase the risk of thermal injury.

The nurse identifies conditions that contraindicate heat or cold therapy. Heat should not be applied over an active area of bleeding (risk of continued bleeding) or an acute localized inflammation such as appendicitis (risk of rupture). If the client has cardiovascular problems, it is unwise to apply heat to large portions of the body because massive vasodilation may disrupt blood supply to vital organs. Cold is contraindicated if the site of injury is edematous or the client has impaired circulation or is shivering (may intensify shivering and reduce blood flow).

The nurse also assesses the client's ability to recognize when heat or cold becomes excessive. If a client has peripheral vascular disease, the nurse particularly observes circulation to the extremities. If a client is confused or unresponsive, the nurse checks skin integrity frequently after therapy begins.

Finally, the nurse assesses the condition of all equipment used, checking for cracked cords, frayed wires, damaged insulation, exposed heating components, leaks, and evenness of temperature distribution.

Client Education and Safety. Before application of heat or cold therapy, the client should understand its purpose, the symptoms of temperature exposure, and the precautions taken to prevent injury. The box above provides hints for safely applying heat and cold therapy.

Applying Heat and Cold. A prerequisite to using heat or cold application is a physician's order, which should include the body site to be treated and the type, frequency, and duration of application. The correct temperature to use for heat and cold applications varies according to agency policy.

SAFETY SUGGESTIONS FOR APPLYING HEAT OR COLD THERAPY

Explain to the client the sensations to be felt during procedure.
Instruct the client to report changes in sensation or discomfort immediately.
Provide a timer, clock, or watch so that the client can help the nurse to time the application.
Keep the call light within the client's reach.
Refer to the institution's policy and procedure manual for safe temperatures.
Do not allow the client to adjust temperature settings.
Do not allow the client to move an application or place his or her hands on the wound site.
Do not place the client in a position that prevents movement away from the temperature source.
Do not leave unattended a client who is unable to sense temperature changes or move from the temperature source.

CHOICE OF MOIST OR DRY. Heat and cold applications can be administered in dry or moist forms. The type of wound or injury, location of the body part, and presence of drainage or inflammation are considered when selecting dry or moist applications. Table 37-7 summarizes advantages and disadvantages of both.

WARM MOIST COMPRESSES. For open wounds, sterile, warm, moist compresses improve circulation, relieve edema, and promote concentration of pus and drainage. A **compress** is a piece of gauze dressing moistened in a prescribed warmed solution. A pack is a larger cloth or dressing applied to a larger body area.

Heat from warm compresses evaporates quickly. To maintain a constant temperature, the nurse must change the compress frequently or apply a warm aquathermic pad, or waterproof heating pad over the compress. Because moisture conducts heat, any device's temperature setting should be lower for a moist compress than for a dry application. A layer of plastic wrap or a dry towel can also be used to insulate the compress and retain heat. Moist heat promotes vasodilation and evaporation of heat from the skin's surface. For this reason a client may feel chilly. The nurse controls drafts and keeps the client covered with a blanket or robe. Procedure 37-6 describes the steps for applying a warm compress.

WARM SOAKS. Immersion of a body part in a warmed solution promotes circulation, lessens edema, increases muscle relaxation, and can provide a means to debride wounds and apply medicated solution. A soak can also be accomplished by wrapping the body part in dressings and saturating them with the warmed solution.

The nurse positions the client comfortably, places waterproof pads under the area to be treated, and heats the solution to the client's tolerance. The nurse checks the

procedure 37-6

APPLYING A HOT, MOIST COMPRESS TO AN OPEN WOUND

Steps	Rationale
1. Inspect condition of exposed skin and/or wound on which compress is to be applied.	Provides baseline to determine changes in skin during heat application. Very thin or damaged skin is more susceptible to injury from heat.
2. Assess client's extremities for sensitivity to temperature and pain by measuring light touch, pinprick, and temperature sensation tests.	Determines whether client is insensitive to heat and cold extremes.
3. Refer to physician's order for type of compress, location and duration of application, and desired temperature.	Ensures likelihood of safe application.
4. Prepare necessary equipment and supplies:	
a. Prescribed solution warmed to client's tolerance.	Correct temperature prevents accidental burns.
b. Sterile gauze dressings	
c. Sterile container for solution	
d. Commercially prepared compresses (optional)	Premoistened compress reduces preparation.
e. Sterile gloves (used for open wound)	
f. Petrolatum jelly, if desired	Protects untreated skin surface.
g. Sterile cotton swabs	
h. Waterproof pad	Prevents soiling of bed linen.
i. Tape or ties	
j. Dry bath towel	
k. Aquathermic or heating pad (optional)	Provides continuous source of heat.
l. Disposable gloves	
m. Bath blanket	
5. Explain steps of procedure and purpose. Describe sensation to be felt (e.g., feeling of warmth and wetness). Explain precautions to prevent burning.	Minimizes anxiety and promotes cooperation.
6. Assist client in assuming comfortable position in proper body alignment.	Compress remains in place for several minutes. Limited mobility in uncomfortable position causes muscular stress.
7. Place waterproof pad under area to be treated.	Prevents soiling of bed linen.
8. Expose body part to be covered with compress and drape client with bath blanket. Close bedside curtains.	Prevents unnecessary cooling and exposure of body part. Provides privacy.
9. Wash hands.	Reduces transmission of infection.
10. Assemble equipment. Pour warmed solution into sterile container. (If using portable heating source, keep solution warm. Commercially prepared compresses may remain under infrared lamp until just before use.) Open sterile packages and drop gauze into container to become immersed in solution. Turn aquathermia pad (if desired) to correct temperature.	Compresses must retain warmth for therapeutic benefit. (Note: if compress is applied to intact skin, clean technique is acceptable.)
11. Apply disposable gloves. Remove any existing dressing covering wound. Dispose of gloves and dressing in proper receptacle.	Reduces transmission of microorganisms.
12. If wound was covered, assess condition of it and surrounding skin.	Provides baseline to determine skin changes after compress application.
13. Apply sterile gloves (for wound application).	Allows nurse to manipulate sterile dressing and touch open wound.
14. Apply sterile petrolatum jelly, if desired, with cotton swab to skin surrounding wound. Do not apply jelly on broken areas of skin.	Protects skin from possible burns and maceration.

Continued.

procedure 37-6

Steps	Rationale
15. Pick up one layer of immersed gauze and wring out excess water.	Excess moisture macerates skin and increases risk of burns and infection.
16. Apply gauze lightly to open wound. Watch response and ask whether client feels discomfort. In a few seconds, lift edge of gauze to assess for redness.	Skin is sensitive to sudden change in temperature. Redness indicates burn.
17. If client tolerates compress, pack gauze snugly against wound. Be sure all wound surfaces are covered by hot compress.	Prevents rapid cooling from underlying air currents.
18. Wrap or cover moist compress with dry bath towel. If necessary, pin or tie in place.	Insulates compress to prevent heat loss.
19. Change hot compress every 5 min or as ordered.	Prevents cooling and maintains therapeutic benefit of compress.
20. Apply aquathermic or waterproof heating pad over towel (optional). Keep it in place for desired duration of application (about 20-30 min).	Provides constant temperature to compress. Local application of heat for more than 60 min often results in reflex vasoconstriction. Removing hot compress after 30 min and then reapplying in 15 min, if desired, maintains vasodilation and positive therapeutic effects.
21. Ask client periodically whether there is discomfort or burning sensation. Observe area of skin not covered by compress.	Continued exposure to heat can cause burning of skin.
22. Remove pad, towel, and compress in 30 min. Again assess wound and condition of skin.	Continued exposure to moisture will macerate skin.
23. Replace dry sterile dressing as ordered.	Prevents entrance of microorganisms into wound site.
24. Assist client to preferred comfortable position.	Maintains comfort.
25. Dispose of equipment and soiled compress. Wash hands.	Reduces transmission of infection.
26. Inspect affected area covered by compress and heating pad.	Assists in determining effects of application.
27. Ask client whether an unusual burning sensation is noticed that was not felt before.	It may be difficult to assess burn merely by color changes if wound is inflamed or drainage is present.
28. Record type, location, and duration of application. Note temperature used in nurses' notes.	Documents therapy administered.
29. Describe condition of wound, skin, and response.	Documents response to therapy.

temperature by placing a small amount of solution on the forearm. After immersing the body part, the nurse covers the container and extremity with a towel to reduce heat loss. It is usually necessary to remove the cooled solution and the body part and add heated solution after about 10 minutes. The problem is to keep the solution at a constant temperature. Never add a hotter solution while the body part remains immersed. After any soak, the nurse dries the body part thoroughly to prevent maceration.

SITZ BATH. The client who has had rectal surgery or an episiotomy during childbirth or who has painful hemorrhoids or vaginal inflammation may benefit from a **sitz bath,** a bath in which only the pelvic area is immersed in warm fluid. The client sits in a special tub or chair or in a basin that fits on the toilet seat so that the legs and feet remain out of the water. Immersing the entire body causes widespread vasodilation and negates the effect of local heat to the pelvic area.

The desired temperature for a sitz bath depends on whether the purpose is to promote relaxation or to clean a wound. It may be necessary to carefully add hot water during the procedure, which usually lasts 20 minutes. A disposable basin contains an attachment that resembles an enema bag and allows the gradual introduction of warmer water.

The nurse should prevent overexposure by draping bath blankets around the client's shoulders and thighs and controlling drafts. The client should be able to sit in the basin or tub with feet flat on the floor and without

table 37-7

CHOICE OF DRY OR MOIST APPLICATIONS

Advantages	Disadvantages
MOIST APPLICATIONS	
Moist application reduces drying of skin, softens wound exudate, and comforms well to body area being treated.	Prolonged exposure can cause maceration of skin. Moist heat will cool rapidly because of moisture evaporation.
Moist heat penetrates deeply into tissue layers.	Moist heat creates greater risk for burns to skin because moisture conducts heat.
Warm, moist heat does not promote sweating and insensible fluid loss.	
DRY APPLICATIONS	
Dry heat has less risk of burns to skin than moist applications.	Dry heat increases body fluid loss through sweating.
Dry application does not cause skin maceration.	Dry applications do not penetrate deep into tissues.
Dry heat retains temperature longer because it is not influenced by evaporation.	Dry heat causes increased drying of skin.

pressure on the sacrum or thighs. Because exposure of a large portion of the body to heat causes extensive vasodilation, the nurse should assess the client's pulse and facial color and ask whether the client feels light-headed or nauseated.

Paraffin baths. A paraffin bath consists of a mixture of heated paraffin wax and mineral oil (1 part oil to 5 parts paraffin). Clients with painful arthritis or other joint discomforts of the hands and feet benefit most from the baths. In many institutions only physical therapists administer the applications. Clients often heat paraffin baths at home in double boilers (53.3° to 54.4° C [128° to 130° F]).

Aquathermia (water-flow) pads. The aquathermia (water-flow) pad (Figure 37-18) is useful for treating muscle sprains and areas of mild inflammation or edema. The unit consists of a waterproof plastic or rubber pad connected by two hoses to an electrical control unit that has a heating element and motor. Distilled water circulates through hollowed channels within the pad to the control unit where water is heated or cooled (depending on temperature setting). Although the units are safer than the conventional heating pad, the nurse should still check for equipment malfunctions. The temperature setting is fixed by inserting a plastic key into the temperature regulator. If the water in the unit runs low, the nurse simply adds distilled water to the reservoir at the top of the control unit.

To avoid burning the client's skin, the nurse folds a thin cloth or pillow case over the heating pad; tape, ties, or a gauze roll holds the pad in place. Pins are never used. The nurse checks the skin frequently for signs of burning. An application should last only 20 to 30 minutes, and the client must not lie on the pad.

Commercial hot packs. Commercially prepared, disposable hot packs apply warm dry heat to an injured area. By striking, kneading, or squeezing the pack, chemicals that release heat are mixed. Package directions recommend the time for heat application.

Hot water bottles. The hot water bottle is an economical means of applying heat to an injured body part. Many clients use them in the home. Nurses must give clients and family members the following instructions about the safe use of water bottles:

1. Ensure no leaks. Fill the bottle with tap water, secure the cap, and turn the bottle upside down.
2. Use warm tap water.
3. Fill the bag only two-thirds full, expel air at the top, and secure the cap. The bag is then easier to mold over a body part.

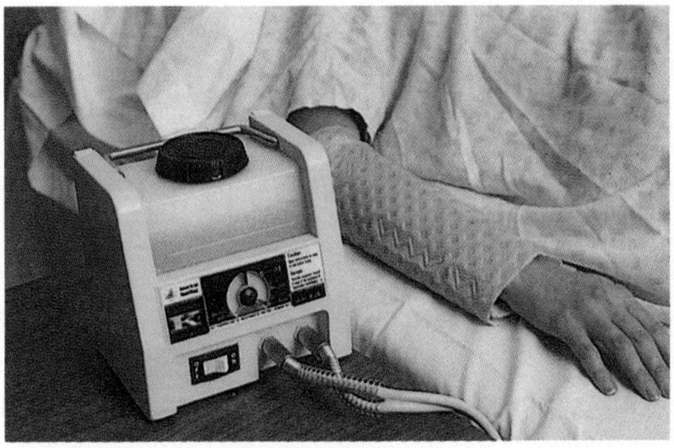

FIGURE 37-18 Aquathermia pad.

4. Wipe off moisture on the outside of the bag.
5. Never apply a water bottle directly to the skin surface. Cover it with a towel or pillow case.
6. Keep the bottle in place for 20 to 30 minutes.

ELECTRIC HEATING PADS. Another conventional form of heat therapy is the heating pad, an electric coil enclosed within a waterproof pad covered with cotton or flannel cloth. The pad is connected to an electric cord that has a temperature-regulating unit for a high, medium, or low setting. Nurses should advise clients to avoid using the high setting and to never lie on the pad. Another precaution to note is that a safety pin inserted through a pad can result in an electrical shock.

COLD MOIST COMPRESSES. The procedure for applying cold moist compresses is the same as that for warm compresses. Cold compresses should be applied for 20 minutes at a temperature of 15° C (59° F) to relieve inflammation and swelling. They may be clean or sterile. The nurse observes for adverse reactions such as burning or numbness, mottling of the skin, redness, extreme paleness, or a bluish skin discoloration.

COLD SOAKS. The procedure for preparing cold soaks and immersing a body part is the same as for warm soaks. The desired temperature for a 20-minute soak is 15° C (59° F). The nurse takes precautions to protect the client from chilling.

ICE BAG OR COLLAR. For a client who has a muscle sprain, localized hemorrhage, or hematoma or has undergone dental surgery, an ice bag is ideal to prevent edema formation, control bleeding, and anesthetize the body part. Proper use of the bag requires the following:

1. Fill the bag with water, secure the cap, invert to check for leaks, and pour out the water.
2. Fill the bag two-thirds full with crushed ice so that the bag can mold easily over a body part.
3. Release air from the bag by squeezing its sides before securing the cap (because excess air interferes with conduction of cold).
4. Wipe off excess moisture.
5. Cover the bag with a flannel cover, towel, or pillow case.
6. Apply the bag to the injury site for 30 minutes; the bag can be reapplied in an hour.

COLD PACKS. Commercially prepared single-use ice packs come in various sizes and shapes. When the pack is squeezed or kneaded, an alcohol-based solution is released inside to create the cold temperature. The soft outer coverings can usually be safely applied directly to the skin surface.

Health Promotion/Restoration Activities

Despite the nurse's efforts with wound care, wound healing will not occur if the client is malnourished. Tissue repair requires more protein, carbohydrates, fats, vitamins, minerals, water, and oxygen than normal tissue metabolism (Table 37-8). In addition, the delivery of nutritional substances to tissues depends on a healthy circulatory system. Malnutrition causes an insufficient supply of the necessary nutritional elements and alterations in blood vessel integrity. The nurse therefore works closely with dietitians to provide a well-balanced diet and educates the client about the importance of good dietary habits (see Chapter 31). For clients weakened or debilitated by illness, supportive nutritional therapies may become necessary. The surgical client who is well nourished and has no complications requires at least 0.8 g of protein per kilogram daily for nutritional maintenance (Konstantinides, 1992). Supplemental tube feedings (enteral feedings) introduce nutrients directly into the gastrointestinal tract. If a client is unable to tolerate enteral feedings, the physician may order parenteral (intravenously administered) nutrition.

table 37-8

NUTRIENTS FOR WOUND HEALING

Nutrient	Function in wound repair
Protein	Angiogenesis (new blood vessel formation) Fibroblast proliferation Synthesis of collagen
Carbohydrate	Provision of spare protein for healing Energy for cell metabolism
Fat	Component of cell membranes
Vitamin C	Infection resistance Optimal fibroblast function Collagen synthesis
Vitamin A	Possible mediation of the stress response
Copper	Collagen cross-linkage for scar strength
Zinc	Epithelialization Collagen synthesis

The client with a wound that restricts mobility or has the potential to compromise the function of a joint may require additional physical and/or occupational therapy. The nurse works closely with the physical therapist in monitoring the client's activity and tolerance for exercise. It is important to optimize activity within the client's physical limitations and return function as rapidly as possible.

Some chronic wounds are the result of underlying pathology that may continue long after wound healing occurs. Examples of this include the client with peripheral neuropathy who remains at risk for injury and the client with peripheral venous disease resulting in chronic edema of the lower extremities. For these clients, special attention should be given to teaching preventive skin care and assistive devices to normalize daily living. Orthotic devices are available to protect the feet from injury secondary to pressure as are shoes with added depth. Supportive compression garments and pumps can be used by the client with edema to keep the skin healthy. These devices do not in themselves correct the problem but support the client in practicing preventive skin care.

Evaluation

The evaluation of the effectiveness of wound care involves an analysis of the techniques used in wound care management and their success in maintaining wound integrity and the well-being of the client. The nurse must recognize the phases of wound healing and the client's response throughout recovery. Wound healing is evaluated with each dressing change, after application of heat and cold therapies, after wound irrigations, and after any stress to the wound site.

To evaluate the effectiveness of nursing interventions in meeting goals of care, the nurse uses evaluative measures to identify actual outcomes. These outcomes are compared with expected outcomes to determine the client's health status. The following are examples of goals, expected outcomes, and corresponding evaluative measures:

Goal: Client's wound heals by primary intention.

Outcome

Client's wound is closed and without drainage within 4 days

Evaluative measures

Inspect wound edges for gradual closure or approximation

Inspect the wound and surrounding skin for reduction in the initial inflammatory response

Observe the wound bed and presence of any dressing drainage

Outcome

Wound scar forms without limiting client's function

Evaluative measure

Have client move involved body part through normal range of motion

Goal: Client's wound is free of infection.

Outcome

No purulent drainage from wound site during healing

Evaluative measures

Inspect the wound bed or dressings for a foul, pungent odor and yellow, green, or brown drainage

Palpate the surrounding skin for tenderness

Inspect the wound edges for inflammation

Goal: Client's skin remains intact.

Outcome

Skin is supple and without breakdown

Evaluative measures

Observe skin surrounding the wound for excoriation, inflammation, or maceration

Inspect the skin under heat or cold applications for a normal vascular response

Goal: Client regains normal function of involved body part within 4 weeks.

Outcome

Client resumes baseline level of activity in 2 weeks

Evaluative measures

Observe the client's ability to maintain movement of the body part affected by the wound

Assess client for level of discomfort when moving body part

Outcome

Client reports acceptable level of energy in 4 weeks

Evaluative measure

Ask client to describe how he or she feels after course of ambulation

Goal: Client achieves comfort.

Outcome

Client reports acceptable level of pain with dressing changes

Evaluative measures

Ask the client to rate discomfort along the suture line or wound edges using a visual analog scale (see Chapter 28)

Observe the client for nonverbal signs of discomfort during bandage or dressing application

Ask if client feels a burning or tingling sensation during hot or cold applications

Outcome

Client's use of pain medication lessens as wound heals

Evaluative measure

Compare dosage and frequency of pain medication delivered over recovery period

SUMMARY

The nurse administers various forms of therapy to clients with surgical or traumatic wounds. The type of wound determines the type of dressing used and its method of application, the manner of caring for drains and sutures, the use of hot or cold applications, and the observations to make for monitoring wound repair. Clients at risk for impaired wound healing require close observation and may benefit from the use of bandages and binders to support and protect wounds.

The nurse follows several principles to promote wound healing, including use of aseptic technique, protection of the wound and surrounding skin from further injury, and promotion of the stages of healing. The successful healing of any wounds depends on provision of a balanced diet to meet increased energy and nutritional requirements.

KEY CONCEPTS

- A clean surgical incision with little tissue loss heals by primary intention, which proceeds through the defensive, reconstruction, and maturation stages.
- When there is extensive tissue loss, a wound heals by secondary intention.
- The chances of wound infection are greater when the wound contains dead or necrotic tissue, when foreign bodies lie on or near the wound, and when blood supply and tissue defenses are reduced.
- A wound assessment requires a description of the appearance of the wound, character of drainage, presence of drains and wound closures, and presence of pain.
- Wound drains remove secretions within tissue layers to promote wound closure.
- Principles of wound first aid include control of bleeding, wound cleansing, and wound protection.
- The layers of a dry dressing protect the wound edges, absorb drainage, and prevent entrance of bacteria.
- The wet-to-dry dressing mechanically removes dead tissue and wound exudate to cleanse the wound.
- When cleaning wounds or drain sites, the nurse should clean from the least to the most contaminated area, away from wound edges.
- The type of suture securing a wound influences the method of suture removal.
- The safe use of heat and cold therapy requires assessment of the client's sensory function, identification of risk factors, and understanding of the physiological effects of heat and cold.
- An acute sprain, fracture, or bruise responds best to cold applications.
- Warm applications are effective for improving circulation to wound sites and promoting muscle relaxation.
- The choice of moist or dry applications depends on the type of wound, location of body part, and presence of drainage or inflammation.

CRITICAL THINKING ACTIVITIES

1. Explain the correct first aid procedures for an abrasion, laceration, and puncture wound. Include application of dressing, if appropriate.
2. Your client presents with a 3 cm left trochanteric ulcer, full thickness, as evidenced by necrotic slough in the base. The edges of the ulcer are smooth and rounded with the necrotic tissue lifting. What method of wound cleansing would be best suited to this situation with a bedfast client.
3. Your client is admitted for abdominal pain. Upon visual inspection, you identify a red, blistering area over the lower abdomen. The client reports having used a hot water bottle at home. Please list additional assessment parameters needed and identify a treatment and teaching plan.
4. There is an order to cleanse a lower abdominal wound with normal saline with each dressing change. Upon inspection, you identify a 1 cm diameter wound with a depth of 4.5 cm; you are unable to visualize the base. What steps should you take in caring for this client?
5. Your client has been instructed to wear an Ace bandage on the right lower extremity to assist with edema control. Your client presents to the outpatient clinic with complaint of increased swelling of the toes as well as numbness and tingling. List your interventions.

References

Bryant RA: *Acute and chronic wounds: nursing management,* St. Louis, 1992, Mosby.

Cooper D: Fundamental products and their usage. In *Guide to wound care,* Chicago, 1983, Hollister.

Cooper DM: Optimizing wound healing: a practice within nursing domain, *Nurs Clin North Am* 25:165, 1990.

Garibaldi RA, Skolnick D, et al.: The impact of preoperative skin disinfection on preventing intraoperative wound contamination, *Infect Control Hosp Epidem* 9(3):109-113, 1988.

Gilliam DL, Nelson CL: Comparison of a one-step iodophor skin preparation versus traditional preparation in total joint surgery, *Clin Orthop Rel Res* (250):258-260, 1990.

Gilmore MA: Phases of wound healing, *Dimensions in Oncol Nurs* 5(3):32-34, 1991.

Gogia PP: The biology of wound healing, *Ostomy-Wound Manage* 38(9):12, 14-16, 18-22, 1992.

Konstantinides NN: Principles of nutritional support. In Bryant RA: *Acute and chronic wounds*, St. Louis, 1992, Mosby.

Lineaweaver W, Howard R, et al.: Topical antimicrobial toxicity, *Arch Surg* 120:267-270, 1985.

Mackenzie I: Preoperative skin preparation and surgical outcome, *J Hosp Infect* 11(suppl B): 27-32, 1988.

Mulder GD, Jeter KF and Fairchild PA: *Clinicians' pocket guide to chronic wound repair,* Spartanburg, 1991, Wound Healing Publications.

Palamand S, Reed AM, and Weimann LJ: Testing intelligent wound dressings, *J Biomaterials Applications* 6(3):198-215, 1992.

Rogness: High-pressure wound irrigation, *J Enterostom Ther* 12:27-28, 1985.

Ryan TJ: Wound dressing, *Dermatol Clin* 11(1):207-213, 1993.

Westaby S: *Wound care,* St. Louis, 1986, Mosby.

Bibliography

Alterescu V: Toward a physiologic approach to the topical treatment of opened wounds, *J Enterostomal Ther* 10:101, 1983.

Cooper DM: Wound assessment and evaluation of healing. In Bryant RA: *Acute and chronic wounds: nursing management,* St. Louis 1992, Mosby.

Ehrlichman RJ, et al.: Common complications of wound healing, *Surg Clin North Am* 71(6):1323-1351, 1991.

Fylling CP: Comprehensive wound management with topical growth factors, *Ostomy-Wound Manage* 22:62, 1989.

Holt DR, et al.: Effect of age on wound healing in healthy human beings, *Surgery* 112(2):293-297, 1992.

Jensen JA, Hunt TK: The wound healing curve as a practical teaching device, *Surgery, Gynecology and Obstetrics* 173(1):63-64, 1991.

Mash N: Protocols for wound management, *Ostomy-Wound Manage* 23:42, 1989.

Moncada GA: The healing wound: clinical management. *Plastic Surg Nurs* 12(2):56-60, 1992.

Neuberger GB, Reckling JB: Preventing wound complications in an age of DRGs, *Ostomy-Wound Manage* 17:20, 1987.

Newsom SW, Rowland C: Studies on perioperative skin flora, *J Hosp Infect* 11(suppl B):21-26, 1988.

Pollack S: Wound healing: a review. I. The biology of wound healing, *J Enterostomal Ther* 8:16, 1981.

Pollack S: Wound healing: a review. II. Environmental factors affecting wound healing, *J Enterostomal Ther* 9:14, 1982.

Pollack S: Wound healing: a review. III. Nutritional factors affecting wound healing, *J Enterostomal Ther* 9:28, 1982.

Robles CR, et al.: Management of the perineal wound following abdominoperineal resection: prospective study of three methods, *Brit J Surg* 79(1):29-31, 1992.

Rubio PA: Use of semiocclusive, transparent film dressings for surgical wound protection: experience in 3637 cases, *Int Surg* 76(4):253-254, 1991.

Seaman M, Lammers R: Inability of patients to self-diagnose wound infections, *J Emerg Med* 9(4):215-219, 1991.

Simmons BP: CDC guidelines for prevention of surgical wound infections, *Am J Infect Control* 11:133, 1983.

38

Sensory Alterations

OBJECTIVES

Mastery of content in this chapter will enable the student to:

- Define the key terms listed.
- Differentiate among the processes of reception, perception, and reaction to sensory stimuli.
- Discuss common causes and effects of sensory alterations.
- Discuss common sensory changes that occur with aging.
- Identify factors to assess in determining sensory status.
- Describe behaviors indicating sensory alterations.
- Develop a care plan for clients with visual, auditory, tactile, speech, gustatory, and olfactory alterations.
- Describe nursing interventions that promote effective communication with clients who have sensory alterations.
- Describe conditions in the health care agency or client's home that can be adjusted to promote meaningful sensory stimulation.
- Discuss ways to maintain a safe environment for clients with sensory alterations.

KEY TERMS

aphasia
auditory
expressive aphasia
global aphasia
gustatory
kinesthetic
olfactory
ototoxicity
receptive aphasia
refractive error
sensory deficit
sensory deprivation
sensory overload
tactile
tinnitus

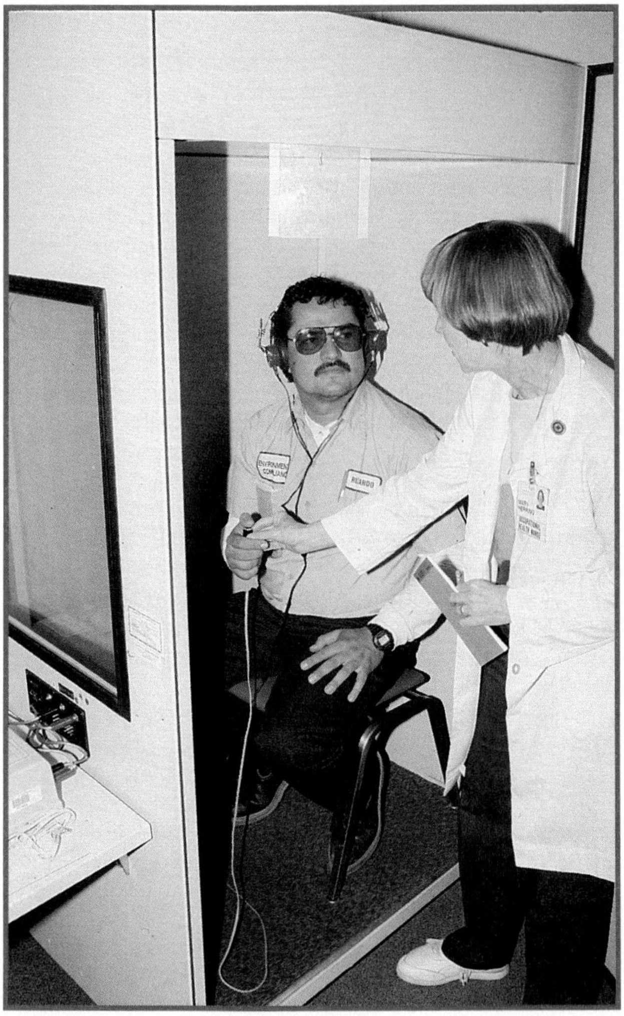

Part of the uniqueness of human beings is the ability to sense various stimuli caused by changes in their internal and external environment, perceive and organize those stimuli, and respond appropriately. The ability to see, for example, provides the necessary warning to avoid injury from the danger of slipping on a wet floor. The sense organs of sight **(visual),** hearing **(auditory),** touch **(tactile),** smell **(olfactory),** taste **(gustatory),** and balance function to produce the special senses and to initiate reflexes important for homeostasis. The body also has a **kinesthetic** sense of its position and movement in space. Meaningful stimuli from sensory organs allow a person to learn about the environment and are necessary for healthy functioning and normal development of the sensory organs. When sensory function is altered, the client's ability to relate to and function within the environment changes drastically. The nurse must understand and help to meet the needs of clients with sensory alterations, as well as recognize clients most at risk for developing sensory problems. The nurse helps clients with sensory alterations learn to react safely and effectively in their environment.

Courtesy Philip James Acker, Motorola, Inc.

NORMAL SENSATION

The nervous system continually receives thousands of bits of information from sensory nerve organs. It relays the information through appropriate channels and integrates the information into a meaningful response. The nervous system must be intact for sensory stimuli to reach appropriate brain centers and for the individual to perceive the sensation. After interpreting the sensation, the person can react to the stimulus.

Reception, perception, and reaction comprise any sensory experience (see Chapter 28). Reception begins with stimulation of a nerve cell called a receptor, which is usually specifically designed for only one type of stimulus. In the case of special senses, the receptors are grouped close together or located in specialized organs (Thibodeau and Patton, 1993) such as the taste buds of the tongue or the retina of the eye. Once a nerve impulse is created it travels along pathways to the spinal cord or directly to the brain. For example, light waves stimulate receptors within the retina of the eye, which cause impulses to travel along the optic nerve to the occipital lobe of the brain. Sensory nerve pathways usually cross over to send stimuli to opposite sides of the brain. The actual perception or awareness of unique sensations depends on the receiving region of the cerebral cortex, where specialized brain cells interpret the quality and nature of the sensory stimuli. For example, visual images pass from the retina of the eye to the visual cortex in the occipital lobe of the brain. When the person becomes conscious of the stimuli and receives the information, perception takes place. Perception includes an integration and interpretation of the stimuli based on the person's experiences. If sensation is incomplete, such as blurred vision, or if past experience is inadequate for understanding stimuli such as pain, the person may react inappropriately.

It is impossible to react to each of the multiple stimuli entering the nervous system. The brain is normally capable of discarding or storing sensory information to prevent sensory bombardment. A person usually reacts to stimuli that are most meaningful or significant at the time. After continued reception of the same stimulus, however, a person stops responding, and the sensory experience goes unnoticed. This adaptability phenomenon occurs with most sensory stimuli.

The balance between sensory stimuli entering the brain and those that actually reach conscious awareness

FACTORS THAT INFLUENCE SENSORY FUNCTION

AGE

Infants

Infants have immature nerve pathways and are initially unable to discriminate sensory stimuli. Binocular vision begins at 6 weeks of age and is well established by 4 months. During the second year of life, the infant can discriminate shapes, objects, and colors. A neonate will initially respond generally to loud noises. Within a year the infant can locate sounds.

Children

Refractive errors are the most common types of visual disorders in children and can be treated with corrective lenses. More serious visual impairment affects a child's ability to play and socialize. A blind child cannot imitate others.

Hearing loss in infants can occur from a variety of prenatal and postnatal conditions. Discovery of hearing impairments within the first 6 to 12 months of life is essential. Hearing loss can impair speech development.

Adults

Visual changes during adulthood include presbyopia (inability to focus on near objects) and the need for glasses for reading (ages 40 to 50).

Older adults

Hearing changes, which begin at age 30, include decreased hearing acuity, speech intelligibility, and pitch discrimination, which is referred to as **presbycusis.**

Older adults have reduced visual fields, increased glare sensitivity, impaired night vision, reduced accommodation, and depth perception, and reduced color discrimination. Older adults require three times as much light to see objects as they did when they were in their 20s (Ebersole and Hess, 1990).

Older adults hear low-pitched sounds the best but have difficulty hearing conversation over background noise.

Older adults have difficulty discriminating the consonants (*f, z, s, th, ch, p, k, t* and *g*). Vowels that have a low pitch are more easy to hear. Speech sounds are garbled, and there is a delayed reception and reaction to speech.

Cerumen is normally absorbed in a young adult's ear but becomes hard and collects in the aurel meatus of an older adult (Bernardini, 1985).

Older adults experience olfactory changes including a loss of cells in the olfactory bulb of the brain and a decrease in the number of sensory cells in the nasal lining (Ebersole and Hess, 1990). This change begins around age 50. Reduced sensitivity to odors is common.

Aging causes taste buds to atrophy, to lose efficiency in relaying flavor, and to reduce in number (Ebersole and Hess, 1990). Reduced taste discrimination is common.

Proprioceptive changes include an increased difficulty with balance, spatial orientation, and coordination (age 60). The aged cannot avoid obstacles as quickly nor are they able to prevent an accident from happening to themselves when fast action is needed. The automatic response to protect and brace oneself when falling is slower (Ebersole and Hess, 1990).

Older adults experience tactile changes including declining sensitivity to pain, pressure, and temperature.

MEDICATIONS

Many medications cause **ototoxicity** which may affect hearing, balance, or both (see box on p. 1169). The most common symptom reported is **tinnitus.** Ototoxicity causes a progressive or continuing hearing loss. Most clients are not aware it is occurring (McKenry and Salerno, 1992).

Chloramphenicol is an antibiotic that can irritate the optic nerve.

Narcotic analgesics, sedatives, and antidepressant medications can alter the perception of stimuli.

ENVIRONMENT

Excessive environmental stimuli (e.g., hospital equipment, staff conversation) can result in sensory overload, marked by confusion, disorientation, and inability to make decisions. Restricted environmental stimulation (e.g., bed rest and isolation) can lead to sensory deprivation. Poor quality of environment (e.g., reduced lighting, narrow walkways, background noise) can worsen sensory impairment.

PREEXISTING ILLNESSES

Peripheral vascular disease can cause reduced sensation in the extremities and impaired cognition. Chronic diabetes can cause reduced vision or blindness or peripheral neuropathy. Some neurological disorders such as stroke impair sensory reception.

SMOKING

Chronic tobacco use can atrophy the taste buds, lessening the perception of flavors.

Long-term exposure to tobacco smoke and other toxins interferes with olfactory function.

NOISE LEVELS

Constant exposure to high noise levels (e.g., construction work) can cause hearing loss.

maintains a person's well-being. If an individual attempts to react to every stimulus within the environment or if the variety and quality of stimuli are lacking, sensory alterations occur.

TYPES OF SENSORY ALTERATIONS

Many factors alter the capacity to receive or perceive sensations (see box below). The general types of sensory alterations commonly seen by the nurse are sensory deficits, sensory deprivation, and sensory overload. When a client suffers from more than one sensory alteration, the ability to function and relate effectively is seriously impaired.

Sensory Deficits

A defect in the normal function of sensory reception and perception is a **sensory deficit.** As a result a client may not be able to receive certain stimuli (e.g., deafness) or the stimuli are distorted (e.g., blurred vision from cataracts). A sudden sensory loss can cause fear, anger, and feelings of helplessness. The client may withdraw socially to cope with the sensory loss. The client's safety is threatened due to an inability to respond normally to stimuli in the environment. When a deficit develops gradually or when considerable time has passed since the onset of an acute sensory loss, the client learns to rely on unaffected senses. Certain senses may even become more acute to compensate for an alteration. For example, a blind client often develops an acute sense of hearing. Clients with sensory deficits may change their behaviors in adaptive or maladaptive ways.

Sensory Deprivation

Sensory stimulation must be of sufficient quality and quantity to maintain awareness. When an inadequate quality or quantity of stimulation impairs perception, **sensory deprivation** occurs. A person suffers from inadequate cerebral cortical arousal. Three types of sensory deprivation (Ebersole and Hess, 1990) are reduced sensory input such as hearing loss, elimination of order or meaning from input such as that which occurs from confusion, and restriction of the environment such as bed rest that produces monotony and boredom.

The effects of sensory deprivation can be far reaching (see box below). Behaviors in children are often demonstrated by a higher than normal level of anxiety that leads to restlessness, difficulty with problem solving, and depression (Whaley and Wong, 1991). Children will often regress and revert to earlier developmental behaviors such as increased reliance on parents. In adults the symptoms of sensory deprivation can easily cause nurses or physicians to believe that a client is psychologically ill, suffering from severe electrolyte imbalance or organic brain syndrome, or under the influence of psychotropic drugs. Therefore the nurse must always be aware of the client's baseline sensory function and the quality of stimuli within the environment.

EFFECTS OF SENSORY DEPRIVATION

COGNITIVE

Reduced capacity to learn, inability to solve problems, poor task performance, disorientation, bizarre thinking, regression.

AFFECTIVE

Boredom, restlessness, increased anxiety, emotional lability, increased need for physical stimulation and socialization.

PERCEPTUAL

Reduced attention span, disorganized visual and motor coordination, temporary loss of color perception, disorientation, confusion of sleeping and waking states.

MEDICATIONS REPORTED TO CAUSE OTOTOXICITY

ANTIBIOTICS

aminoglycosides (amikacin, gentamicin, neomycin, streptomycin)
minocycline
vancomycin

DIURETICS

ethacrynic acid
furosemide

CARDIAC DRUGS

quinidine

ANALGESICS

NSAIDs
aspirin
indomethacin
ibuprofen

ANTINEOPLASTIC AGENTS

bleomycin
cisplatin
dactinomycin
mechlorethamine

Sensory Overload

When a person receives multiple sensory stimuli and the brain cannot perceptually disregard or selectively ignore some stimuli, **sensory overload** occurs. Because of the multitude of stimuli leading to overload, the person no longer perceives the environment in a way that makes sense. Overload prevents meaningful response by the brain. Thoughts race, attention moves in many directions, and restlessness occurs. A client can demonstrate panic, confusion, aggressiveness, and combativeness. Sleep loss is common. Overload thus causes a state similar to that associated with sensory deprivation.

The acutely ill client may easily develop sensory overload. Sleep loss is a risk factor, along with loss of control for the client. Individual clients will vary as to their risk for sensory overload. The point at which stimuli become enough to tax a client's endurance changes according to level of fatigue, attitude, and physical well-being.

NURSING PROCESS AND SENSORY ALTERATIONS

Assessment

When assessing clients with or at risk for sensory alterations, the nurse considers all factors that influence sensory function (see box on p. 1169), particularly age. The nurse assesses the degree to which a sensory deficit affects life-style, psychosocial adjustment, and a client's safety. The assessment must also focus on the quality and quantity of environmental stimuli.

Persons at Risk. A nurse can quickly assess sensory function for clients most at risk. Older adults are at a high risk because of normal physiological changes involving sensory organs. Clients who are immobilized by bed rest, physical encumbrances (e.g., casts or traction), or chronic disability are unable to experience all the sensations of free movement. A client isolated in a health care setting or at home is also at risk. For example, the client in isolation as a result of tuberculosis (see Chapter 25) is often restricted to a hospital room and is unable to enjoy normal interactions with visitors.

A client with a known sensory deficit resulting from visual and hearing losses, spinal cord injury, or peripheral **neuropathies** is at risk for sensory alterations (see box above). The length of time a client has had a sensory deficit may not help in coping with the limitation or the environment. Magilvy (1985) found that women with late onset hearing loss considered themselves to have a lowered quality of life compared with women who experience hearing loss at a younger age. Walsh and Eldredge (1989) warn that people who lose their hearing at an early age have cumulative developmental effects and socialization problems compounded by aging.

A hospital environment is full of stressors. Therapeutic isolation, disruption of sleep cycles, medication effects, and electrolyte imbalances are just a few. A healthy person can change an environment or seek a different one. As a result of illness or hospitalization, a client is often confined to an unfamiliar and unresponsive environment. This does not mean that all hospitalized clients suffer from sensory alterations. However, the nurse must assess more carefully those clients subjected to high stress levels (e.g., ICU environment, long-

COMMON SENSORY DEFICITS

VISUAL

Presbyopia—loss of accommodation of the lens to near objects. Individual is unable to see near objects clearly. Glasses with bifocal lenses can be prescribed.

Cataract—opacity of the lens resulting in blurred vision. Occurs to some degree in more than 95% of persons over age 65 (Bernardini, 1985).

Open-angle glaucoma—an increase in intraocular pressure caused by an obstruction to the normal flow of aqueous humor through the canal of Schlemm. Causes progressive pressure against optic nerve if untreated.

Diabetic retinopathy—pathological changes occur in the blood vessels of the retina. Small hemorrhages and aneurysms affect capillary walls. Bleeding into the vitreous humor develops.

HEARING

Presbycusis—hearing loss associated with aging. An inner ear disorder that interferes with the ability to hear high-frequency sounds. Speech discrimination is reduced.

Cerumen accumulation—build up of ear wax in the external auditory canal. Cerumen, which is normally absorbed in a younger person's ear, becomes hard and collects in the canal. Causes a conduction deafness.

NEUROLOGICAL

Stroke—cerebrovascular accident caused by clot, hematoma, or hemorrhage of blood vessel leading to or within the brain. Creates altered proprioception demonstrated by marked incoordination and imbalance. Loss of sensation and motor function in affected extremities also occurs.

Peripheral neuropathy—disorder of the peripheral nervous system. Commonly caused in older adults by diabetes, Guillain-Barré syndrome, and neoplasms (Ebersole and Hess, 1990). Symptoms include numbness and tingling of affected area and stumbling gait.

term hospitalization, multiple therapies) and those who have other risk factors for sensory alterations.

Nursing History. The nursing history allows for assessment of the nature and characteristics of any sensory alteration or any problem related to a sensory alteration. The nurse begins by asking the client to describe the sensory deficit. For example:

Describe your visual loss for me.

Describe how your hearing is affected.

Explain how your ability to feel things has changed.

Knowledge about the onset and duration of the sensory alteration can be helpful. The nurse begins to learn how long the client has taken measures to adjust to the alteration.

How long have you been experiencing a visual problem?

When did you begin to feel numbness in your legs?

How long have you been unable to hear conversations normally?

It is also useful to assess the client's self-rating for a sensory deficit. Janken and Cullinan (1990) found that a client's self-rating for hearing was one of the most important defining characteristics for accurately diagnosing auditory sensory/perceptual alteration. The nurse can simply ask the client:

"Rate your hearing as either excellent, good, fair, poor, or bad."

Based on a client's self-rating the nurse may explore more fully the client's perception of a sensory loss. This provides a more in-depth look at how the client's quality of life has been influenced. The nurse can ask:

What problems are you experiencing as a result of your hearing/visual loss?

What problem does loss of sensation cause for you?

Tell me how you have adjusted to the loss.

What has changed because of the loss of vision/hearing/sensation?

A nursing history can also reveal any recent changes in a client's behavior. Frequently family or friends are the best resources for this information as the client may be unaware of any change.

Has the client been displaying any recent mood swings (e.g., outbursts of anger, depression, fear or irritability)?

Has the client shown signs of lack of concentration, confusion, or disorientation?

Ability to Perform Self-Care. The nurse assesses the client's ability to perform activities of daily living. Can the client with altered vision find items on a meal tray? Can the client with diminished tactile perception button a shirt or dress? If the client seems sensorially deprived, is concern shown for grooming? Does a client's loss of balance prevent rising from a toilet seat safely? Any impairment in the ability to perform self-care has implications for planning discharge from an acute care setting and in providing resources within the home.

Environment. The environment can either minimize or heighten sensory alterations. In some cases it is the cause of the problem. The nurse assesses the quality and quantity of stimuli within the health care and home environments.

Hazards. A client with sensory alterations may be at risk for injury if the environment is unsafe. Cluttered furniture, dimly lit corridors, and torn carpets are dangers for clients with visual impairments. Because an older adult experiences more glare in light, shiny objects such as highly waxed floors can pose problems. If a client has a hearing impairment, the nurse assesses if the sounds of a doorbell, telephone, smoke alarm, and alarm clock are audible.

Meaningful stimuli. Meaningful stimuli reduce the incidence of sensory deprivation. The nurse observes the environment for presence of pets, family pictures, television, and a clock or calendar. In a health care setting the nurse notes if clients have roommates or visitors who can offer positive stimulation. A roommate who persistently talks or continuously keeps lights on can contribute to sensory overload. A client can become disoriented in an environment that gives few signals for normal sensory perception. The presence or absence of meaningful stimuli influences alertness and the ability to participate in care. In the home or health care setting the nurse checks for bright colors, comfortable furnishings, adequate lighting, good ventilation, and clean surroundings.

With infants and young children the nurse assesses the toys available. The play area should have age-appropriate toys of different sizes, shapes, and colors and should be clean, pleasantly lit, and decorated attractively.

Amount of stimuli. Excessive environmental stimuli can cause sensory overload. In an acute care setting the nurse assesses the level of care required. The frequency of observations, tests, and procedures may be stressful to the client. The location of a client's room may be near repetitive or loud noises (e.g., an elevator or supply room). There may be an abundance of equipment that creates noise in the client's room. Clients in pain may also be at risk for overstimulation.

Socialization. The amount and quality of contact with supportive family members or significant others can influence a client's degree of isolation. The nurse assesses if a client lives alone and if family, friends, or neighbors frequently visit. The absence of visitors during hospitalization can also affect sensory status. Social isolation can result from or contribute to sensory changes.

It is important for the nurse to know the client's so-

table 38-1

ASSESSMENT OF SENSORY FUNCTION

Assessment	Behavior indicating deficit (children)	Behavior indicating deficit (adults)
VISION		
Ask client to read newspaper, magazine, or lettering on menu. Measure visual acuity with Snellen chart (see Chapter 16). Assess visual fields and depth perception. Assess pupil size, reaction to light, and accommodation. Ask client to identify colors on color chart or crayons.	Self-stimulation, including eye rubbing, body rocking, sniffing or smelling, arm twirling; hitching (using legs to propel while in sitting position) instead of crawling	Poor coordination, squinting, underreaching or overreaching for objects, persistent repositioning of objects, impaired night vision, accidental falls
HEARING		
Perform conventional assessment, including ticking watch, whisper, and tuning fork (see Chapter 16). Perform audiometry using an AudioScope. Observe client conversing with others. Compare client's ability to recognize consonants with ability to distinguish vowels. Assess client's perception of hearing ability and history of tinnitus. Inspect external ear canal for hardened cerumen.	Frightened when unfamiliar people approach, no reflex or purposeful response to sounds, failure to be awakened by loud noise, slow or absent development of speech, greater response to movement than to sound, avoidance of social interaction with other children	Blank looks, decreased attention span, lack of reaction to loud noises, increased volume of speech, positioning of head toward sound, smiling and nodding of head in approval when someone speaks, use of other means of communication such as lip reading or writing, complaints of ringing in ears
TOUCH		
Assess client for sensitivity to light touch and temperature (see Chapter 16). Check client's ability to discriminate between sharp and dull stimuli. Assess whether client can distinguish objects (coin or safety pin) in the hand with eyes closed. Ask whether client feels unusual sensations.	Inability to perform developmental tasks related to grasping objects or drawing, repeated injury from handling of harmful objects (e.g., hot stove, sharp knife)	Clumsiness, overreaction or underreaction to painful stimulus, failure to respond when touched, avoidance of touch, sensation of pins and needles, numbness
SMELL		
Have client close eyes and identify several nonirritating odors (e.g., coffee, vanilla).	Difficult to assess until child is 6 or 7 years old, difficulty discriminating noxious odors	Failure to react to noxious or strong odor, increased body odor, increased sensitivity to odors
TASTE		
Ask client to sample and distinguish different tastes (e.g., lemon, sugar, salt). (Have client drink or sip water and wait 1 min between each taste.) Ask client if recent weight change has occurred.	Inability to tell whether food is salty or sweet, possible ingestion of strange-tasting things	Change in appetite, excessive use of seasoning and sugar, complaints about taste of food, weight change

*AudioScope has been found to be a valid instrument for detecting hearing impairment (Bienvenue, et al., 1985: Hawke and Mansfield, 1984).

table 38-1—cont'd

Assessment	Behavior indicating deficit (children)	Behavior indicating deficit (adults)
POSITION SENSE		
Perform conventional tests for balance and position sense (see Chapter 16).	Clumsiness, extraneous movement, excessive arm swinging in those with hyperactivity or learning difficulty	Poor balance and spatial orientation, shuffling gait, reduced response to brace self when falling, more precise and deliberate movements

cial skills and level of satisfaction in the support given by family and friends. Is the client satisfied with the support made available by friends? Is the client able to solve problems with family members? Does the family offer the support needed when the client requires assistance as a result of a sensory loss? The long-term effects of sensory alterations can significantly influence family dynamics and a client's willingness to remain active in society.

Communication Methods. Clients with existing sensory deficits often develop alternative ways of communicating. The nurse must understand the client's method of communication to interact effectively with the client. A deaf or hearing-impaired client may read lips, use sign language, use a hearing aid, or read and write notes. Vision becomes almost a primary sense for the hearing impaired. The visually impaired learn to detect voice tones and inflections to acquire the emotional tone of a conversation. Some may also learn to read braille.

Physical Examination. To identify sensory deficits, the nurse assesses vision, hearing, olfaction, and taste, and the ability to discriminate touch, temperature, pain, and position (see Chapter 16). Table 38-1 summarizes assessment techniques for identifying sensory deficits. In all examples, the nurse will gather more accurate data if the examination room is private, quiet, and comfortable for the client.

Janken and Cullinan (1990) have reported use of the AudioScope as an easy to use and effective instrument for assessing the hearing frequencies commonly used to screen for a hearing loss. In many clinics or hospitals, specially trained personnel gather audiometry data.

The nurse also assesses if the client uses sensory aids (e.g., a hearing aid) and if they are in proper working order. For hospitalized clients it is important to know if sensory aids have been brought to the hospital. If not, the nurse may request that family bring the aids for the client's use.

An assessment of mental status is valuable if the nurse suspects sensory deprivation is present (see box below). Observation of the client during history taking, physical examination, or during care can provide data that reveals key client behaviors. The nurse will observe the client's physical appearance and behavior, measure cognitive ability, and assess the client's emotional stability. The MMSE (Mini-Mental Status Examination) is an example of a tool that can be used to measure disorientation, altered conceptualization and abstract thinking, and change in problem-solving abilities. The mental status test provides the nurse data to assess orientation, memory, and attention.

ASSESSMENT OF MENTAL STATUS

PHYSICAL APPEARANCE AND BEHAVIOR

Motor activity
Posture
Facial expression
Hygiene

COGNITIVE ABILITY

Level of consciousness
Abstract reasoning
Calculation
Attention
Judgment
Ability to carry on a conversation
Ability to read, write, and copy figures
Recent and remote memory

EMOTIONAL STABILITY

Agitation, euphoria, irritability, hopelessness, or wide mood swings
Auditory, visual, or tactile hallucinations
Illusions
Delusions

Nursing Diagnosis

After assessment, the nurse reviews all available data and looks for patterns and trends suggestive of a health problem relating to sensory alterations. For example, the advanced age of a client, along with apathy, the client's inattentiveness during conversations, and the client's self-rating of hearing as "poor," are all defining characteristics for the nursing diagnosis, auditory sensory/perceptual alteration (Janken and Cullinan, 1990). The nurse will validate findings to ensure accuracy of the diagnosis. A colleague may be asked to examine the auditory canal or the nurse may discuss further with the client the self-rating for hearing.

The nurse determines the factor that likely causes the client's health problem. In the previous example, impacted cerumen is the etiology for the client's hearing alteration. The etiology of a nursing diagnosis is a condition that can be affected by nursing intervention. The etiology must be accurate; otherwise nursing therapies will be ineffective. For a client with impacted cerumen, regular irrigations of the ear canal have the potential for improving auditory perception (Cullinan and Janken, 1990). In contrast, if the client's auditory sensory/perceptual alteration was related to hearing loss from nerve deafness, nursing interventions would include alternative communication methods to enhance use of remaining sensory function.

The nurse will also review assessment data for diagnoses in which sensory alteration is the etiology (see box below). For example, hopelessness, characterized by decreased response to stimuli, lack of involvement in care, and passivity may be associated with a visual loss. The nurse must recognize patterns of data that reveal health problems created by the client's sensory alteration.

NURSING DIAGNOSES FOR SENSORY ALTERATIONS

- Visual sensory/perceptual alteration
- Auditory sensory/perceptual alteration
- Tactile sensory/perceptual alteration
- Gustatory sensory/perceptual alterations
- Olfactory sensory/perceptual alteration
- Dressing/grooming self-care deficit
- High risk for injury
- Bathing/hygiene self-care deficit
- Social isolation
- Hopelessness
- Altered thought processes
- Impaired social interaction

Planning

The plan of care (see care plan on p. 1175) depends on the nurse's assessment of the client's perception and acceptance of the sensory alteration. It also depends on the extent to which the client has adjusted to sensory loss. The nurse tries to provide care that will enable the client to adapt to the health care setting and to the home. The client must actively participate in choosing therapies for the plan of care. This is especially important in the case of blind clients who need to be able to control whatever part of their care they can (Norris, 1989). Clients who have sensory alterations at the time of entering a health care setting are usually most informed about how to adapt interventions to their lifestyles.

Priorities of care must be set with regard to the extent a sensory alteration affects a client. Safety is a top priority. The client can assist in prioritizing by choosing aspects of care that are most important. For example, the client may prefer to learn more about ways to prevent additional sensory loss than how to communicate more effectively.

Some sensory alterations are short term (e.g., a client suffering sensory/perceptual alterations as a result of sensory overload in an intensive care unit). Appropriate interventions are thus likely to be only temporary. Sensory alterations such as permanent visual loss require long-term goals of care. Sometimes the client must make major changes in the way self-care activities, communication, and socialization are performed.

When developing a care plan the nurse reviews all resources available to clients. The family can play a key role in providing meaningful stimulation and learning ways to help a client adjust to any limitations. The nurse may refer the client to other health care professionals such as occupational or speech therapists. There are also numerous community-based resources (such as the Society for the Blind and Visually Impaired, and local Institutes for the Deaf) and organizations whose volunteers assist the deaf. The nurse may be able to arrange a volunteer to visit a client or have printed materials made available that describe ways to cope with sensory problems.

When the client has a known sensory alteration, common goals and expected outcomes in the plan of care may include:

Goal: The client maintains optimal function of existing senses.

Outcomes

Client uses available sensory aids correctly within 1 week

Client will report improved sensory function within 2 weeks

SAMPLE NURSING CARE PLAN
Sensory and Perceptual Alterations

ASSESSMENT

Clinical scenario: Mrs.Whittaker is a *70*-year-old woman who resides in a skilled nursing facility. She has been observed to *avoid conversation* with other residents during mealtime. At night she occasionally becomes *disoriented,* and staff say she can become *irritable.* On examination the *external auditory canal* is *occluded with cerumen.* Mrs. Whittaker's *hearing acuity* was measured and found to be *reduced* as she could hear only 4 of the 8 tones tested. When asked to *self rate* her *hearing,* Mrs. Whittaker described it as *poor.*

NURSING DIAGNOSIS

Auditory sensory/perceptual alteration related to altered sensory reception

PLANNING

Goals

Client will acquire improved hearing acuity within 1 week.
Client will engage routinely in conversation with fellow residents within 1 month.

Expected outcomes

Client will be able to hear more than 4 tones/frequencies on audiometry.
Client will remain oriented to day, place and time.
Client will describe techniques that improve ability to hear conversations within 1 week.
Client will use communication techniques to converse with residents within 2 weeks.

IMPLEMENTATION

Steps	Rationale
1. Irrigate the external auditory canal daily, for 3 days. Use tepid water in a 60 ml syringe and irrigate canal gently.	Removal of impacted cerumen can significantly improve hearing (Cullinan and Janken, 1990).
2. Instill cleansing ear drops twice daily into external auditory canal of both ears.	Over time, drops loosen and remove hardened, tightly packed cerumen (Bernardini, 1985).
3. Refer client for formal audiometry testing to determine the extent of the hearing defict.	If a deficit exists, fitting with hearing aid may improve reception of sound.
4. Instruct client on ways to improve hearing reception during a conversation: look at face of speakers, be attentive to speaker, keep eyeglasses clean, ask speaker to speak in normal voice tones, and have conversation in quiet setting.	Communication techniques help listener attend to conversation and uses visual stimuli to enhance message reception (Chovaz, 1989).

EVALUATION

Measure client's hearing acuity before and after each cleansing of the canal and routinely with each examination.
Ask client to identify his/her name, the day of week, and current location.
Ask client to rate hearing on scale of excellent, good, fair, poor, or bad following cleansing (Janken and Cullinan, 1990).
Observe client interactions with residents.
Ask client to describe ways to improve ability to hear conversation in a group.

Defining characteristics are in italic type.

Goal: Client's environment contains meaningful sensory stimuli.

Outcomes

Client remains oriented to environment daily
Client achieves regular rest and sleep patterns within 1 week

Goal: Client interacts in an environment safe, and free of hazards.

Outcomes

Visually impaired client can negotiate hospital room without injury by second hospital day
Hearing impaired client identifies safety precautions adapted within home within 1 week
Client (with reduced tactile sensation) experiences no impairment in skin integrity during hospitalization

Goal: Client experiences no additional sensory loss.

Outcomes

Client explains ways to avoid exposure to environmental hazards

Client's hearing/vision acuity remains stable

Goal: Client communicates effectively within limitations of sensory loss.

Outcomes

Client reports hearing verbal conversation among family members by discharge

Client demonstrates alternative communication method (e.g., speechreading) within 1 month

Goal: Client is able to perform self-care by discharge.

Outcomes

Client with visual impairment demonstrates ability to feed self by second hospital day

Client with tactile impairment is able to dress independently by discharge from hospital

Goal: Client engages in regular social activities within 2 months.

Outcome

Client will attend local community activities with friends.

TIPS FOR PREVENTING EYE INJURY IN CHILDREN

INFANTS AND TODDLERS

Avoid toys with long pointed handles or projections.
Do not allow child to walk or run with pointed object in the hand.
Keep pointed instruments and tools out of reach.

PRESCHOOLERS

Supervise use of sharp or pointed objects such as scissors.
Teach child to walk carefully when carrying pointed objects.
Keep child away from projectile activities.
Begin to teach respect for firearms.

SCHOOL AGERS AND ADOLESCENTS

Teach proper use of potentially dangerous equipment such as power tools, fireworks, and sports equipment.
Stress use of eye protection when playing ball and racquet sports, shooting, using power tools, and riding motorcycles.
Warn children not to look directly at the sun even when wearing sunglasses.

Modified from Whaley LF and Wong DL: *Nursing care of infants and children,* ed 4, St. Louis, 1991, Mosby.

Implementation

Nursing interventions involve the client and family to maintain a safe, pleasant, and stimulating sensory environment. The most effective interventions enable the client to function safely with existing deficits. The client generally is able to continue a normal life-style. Nursing interventions depend on the nursing diagnosis and the related factors contributing to the client's problem.

Health Promotion and Illness Prevention

The nurse plays an important role in preventing visual impairments from developing. In addition, when clients have sensory deficits, the nurse selects measures that enhance a client's remaining sensory function or maximize other senses. Sensory testing detects problems early so corrective devices can be made available.

VISION. The prevention of visual impairment in children requires screening of women considering pregnancy for rubella or syphilis. Adequate prenatal care is needed to prevent prematurity of an infant and the danger of exposure to excessive oxygen administration (Whaley and Wong, 1991). Children should receive immunization early for rubella.

Trauma is a common cause of blindness in children. Penetrating injury from propulsive objects such as firecrackers, slingshots, rocks, or penetrating wounds from scissors are just a few examples. Parents and children require counseling on ways to avoid eye trauma (see box at left and Figure 38-1).

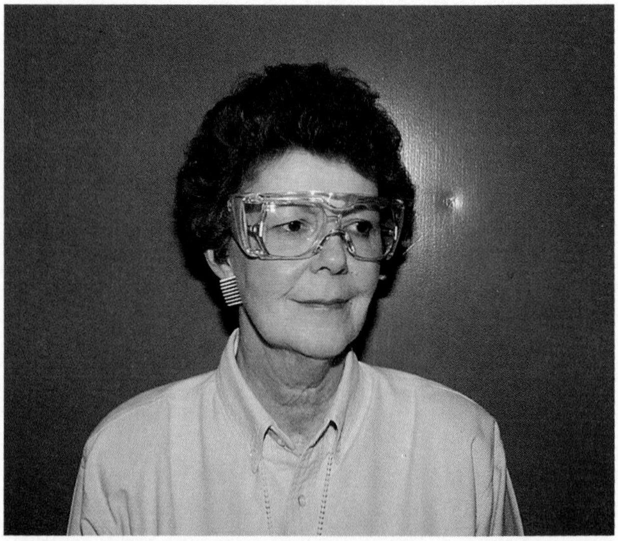

FIGURE 38-1 Safety glasses protect against accidental eye injury. (Courtesy Philip James Acker, Motorola, Inc.)

Visual impairments are common during childhood. The most common visual problem is a **refractive error** such as nearsightedness. The nurse's role is one of detection and referral. Parents should be informed as to behaviors that suggest visual problems. Blindness can be suspected when a newborn fails to react to light and parents express concerns (Whaley and Wong, 1991). Vision screening of school-age children and adolescents can detect visual impairment early. The school nurse is usually responsible for vision testing.

Because adults develop visual changes with aging, the nurse uses several strategies to help clients adapt to these changes. A client who wears corrective contact lenses or eyeglasses should make sure they are kept clean, accessible, and functional. Regular eye examinations ensure a client wears proper lenses. The nurse can instruct clients on ways to maintain existing visual function (see box below). The client can learn to strengthen visual stimuli, use other senses and sharp visual contrasts, and minimize the effects from glare.

HEARING. Hearing impairment is one of the most common disabilities in the United States (Whaley and Wong, 1991). Children at risk include those with a family history of childhood hearing impairment, perinatal infection (rubella, herpes, cytomegalovirus), low birth weight, chronic ear infection, and Down syndrome. Nurses should advise pregnant women of the importance of early prenatal care, avoidance of ototoxic drugs, and testing for syphilis or rubella.

Children with chronic middle ear infections—a common cause of impaired hearing—should receive periodic auditory testing. Parents must be warned of the risks and should seek medical care when the child has symptoms of earache or respiratory infection. Exposure to loud noise is also a risk factor for hearing loss. The nurse advises children and parents to take precautions when involved in activities associated with high-intensity noise. Earplugs and earmuffs can afford protection.

Children should also be immunized against childhood diseases capable of causing hearing loss (e.g., rubella, mumps, and measles) and should not be treated with **ototoxic** drugs. Nurses who work in physician offices, schools, and community clinics should reinforce the importance of early and timely immunization.

Christian, et al. (1989) report that between 28% and 55% of people over 65 years of age have some degree of hearing impairment. Screening for hearing loss is an important step in detecting and treating a hearing impairment. The nurse should encourage older adults to follow through with recommendations for hearing aids. Christian, et al. (1989) found that older adults fitted with hearing aids often avoid using the aids in social situations.

Older adults often develop a hearing loss as a result of impacted cerumen, which thickens and builds up in the ear canal. Excessive cerumen blocking the ear canal can cause a **conductive hearing loss.** Irrigating the canal with tepid water in a 60-ml syringe will remove

CLIENT TEACHING FOR VISUAL FUNCTION

STRENGTHENING VISUAL STIMULI

Teach client to use assistive devices (e.g., pocket magnifiers, near-vision microscopic glasses, and large-print wristwatch, phone dialers, and books).

Tell client to install two side mirrors on cars for enhancing visual field.

USING OTHER SENSES

Encourage client to listen to books on taped cassettes.

Instruct client to install textual cues on walkways or ramps to alert person to intersections.

Teach client to pour salt and pepper into the hand before adding it to food.

Instruct client to fold money according to value and place in different wallet compartments.

USING SHARP VISUAL CONTRASTS

Direct client to use warm colors to highlight visual targets. Orange, red, or yellow can be used on handrails or light switches.

Encourage client to color-code the control dials of irons, stoves, dryers, washers, and thermostats and to mark a reference point on dials and their desired settings.

Instruct client to use colored rims around dishes and cups to reduce spills.

MINIMIZING GLARE

Direct client to decrease light contrasts by using diffuse, soft lighting.

Tell client to avoid waxed floors and exposure to bright sunlight.

Instruct client to install tinted glass windows with adjustable shades or sheer curtains in large windows.

Teach client to shield eyes with sunglasses, visors, or hats with brims.

Advise client to avoid driving at dusk or night.

cerumen. To perform the procedure the nurse wears gloves if drainage is suspected. The nurse positions the client in a side-lying position. The irrigating solution flows in and out of the ear freely into an emesis basin held below the ear. Assessment of the solution reveals if cerumen or other drainage was successfully removed.

Use of ear drops to cleanse the outer ear and aid in the removal of hardened, packed cerumen can prevent or control the problem. Removing cerumen can improve the client's hearing. In a study involving 226 older adult clients, Lewis-Cullinan and Janken (1990) found improvement in the hearing test scores in 75% of the ears after cerumen removal.

To maximize residual hearing function, the nurse suggests ways to modify the environment. Telephone rings can be amplified. Special handsets are available if incoming voices cannot be heard. Important environmental sounds (e.g., smoke alarms, doorbells, and alarm clocks) may be heard best if amplified or changed to a more low-pitched, buzzerlike sound. The older adult may not be able to hear with background noise. The nurse can suggest that clients turn off radios, televisions, or appliances during conversations. Bernardini (1985) found it helpful to have conversations in areas where floor covering and drapes muffle background noises.

Taste. The nurse can easily promote the sense of taste by using measures to enhance remaining taste perception. Good oral hygiene keeps the taste buds well hydrated. Taste perception will be heightened if foods are well seasoned, differently textured, and eaten separately. Vinegar and lemon juice can add tartness to food. If taste perception is improved, food intake and appetite also improve. Stimulation of the sense of smell with pleasant aromas can also heighten taste sensation. Clients should avoid mixing foods because it makes it difficult to identify separate food tastes.

Touch. Clients with reduced tactile sensation usually have the impairment over a limited portion of their bodies. The nurse can stimulate existing function by providing touch therapy. If the client is willing to be touched, hairbrushing and combing, backrubs, and touching the arms or shoulders are ways of increasing tactile contact. When sensation is reduced, a firm pressure may be necessary for the client to feel the nurse's hand. Turning and repositioning can also improve the quality of tactile sensation.

If a client is overly sensitive to tactile stimuli (hyperesthesia), the nurse must minimize irritating stimuli. Keeping bed linens loose to reduce direct contact with the client and protecting the skin from exposure to irritants are helpful.

Smell. Smell can be improved through pleasant olfactory stimulation in the environment. Fragrant flowers and sachets are useful. The nurse encourages clients to smell food before eating. When the nurse assists clients with eating or sets up a meal tray, naming the foods may help clients imagine the aromas. Certain aromas, however, may actually cause clients to lose their appetites. Removing unpleasant odors improves the quality of the environment. The nurse should keep a client's room clean, empty bedpans or urinals, and keep bathroom doors closed.

Maintaining Meaningful Stimulation

When the environment presents risks of sensory understimulation or overstimulation, the nurse should provide meaningful stimuli or eliminate confusing or irritating stimuli (see box below). For the client with sensory deprivation, the nurse should introduce meaningful stimuli for all senses based on client preferences. The nurse does not force stimulation if the client is more concerned with basic functions such as comfort or nutrition.

The nurse controls excessive stimuli for clients at

MEANINGFUL ENVIRONMENTAL STIMULI

VISUAL

Open the drapes to the client's room so outside sights can be seen.

Raise the head of the bed and draw back dividing curtains or partitions so the client can see a roommate or movement in the hallway.

Provide attractive decorations on tables or cabinets, such as fresh flowers, plants, a picture, or greeting cards.

Stimulate vision with bright colors and pictures hanging at eye level.

Encourage family to enrich the client's home with clean curtains, familiar objects or keepsakes, and perhaps a fresh coat of paint on bedroom walls.

Provide talking books and large-print reading material.

AUDITORY

Sit down and speak with the client. Listen to the client's thoughts and experiences. Make the conversation meaningful.

Turn on a radio with pleasant music of the type the client (not the nurse) enjoys. A favorite radio or television program can also be stimulating.

TASTE AND SMELL

Provide attractive, taste-appealing meals. Be sure tableware and glasses are clean. Foods meant to be served warm should be warm and cold foods cold.

Provide a variety of textures, aromas, and flavors to enhance the client's appetite.

TOUCH

Use the same measures that promote existing sensory function (see text at left).

risk for sensory overload. Clients need time for rest and freedom from stresses caused by frequent monitoring and repeated tests. The nurse may sit quietly with clients or involve them in undemanding repetitive activities such as combing hair or brushing teeth. A client under stress at home may find relief in simple activities such as meal planning and household chores.

Reorientation to the institutional environment may be provided through wearing name tags on uniforms, addressing the client by name, or using conversational cues as to time or location. The tendency for clients to become confused can be reduced by offering short and simple repeated explanations and reassurance. Helping clients to become as mobile and independent as possible within safe limits also provides meaningful stimulation. The nurse can encourage the family not to argue with or contradict the confused client but to explain calmly their location, identity, and the time of day.

The nurse can reduce sensory overload by organizing the care plan. Combining activities such as dressing changes, bathing, and vital sign assessment in one visit prevents the client from becoming overly fatigued. Coordination with laboratory and radiology departments reduces the amount of time needed for tests and examinations. Anticipating client needs such as voiding helps reduce uncomfortable stimuli. The nurse can also try to control extraneous noise in and around the client's room, such as television volume and visitors. Routine nursing procedures should be done as quietly as possible.

Faulty perception of the environment may be a cause for seemingly inappropriate behavior in older adults. Proper lighting can influence a person's perception and therefore behavior (Kolanowski, 1992). Use of bright lighting can cause glare in older clients. Glare is the dazzling effect created by bright lighting. Sensory overload, fatigue, eye strain, and tension can be attributed to glare (Kolanowski, 1992).

Proper environmental lighting can improve a person's color discrimination, perceptual satisfaction, and general sense of relaxation. Kolanowski (1990, 1992) has conducted research and recommends the following lighting for care of older adults:

- Bright, nonglaring, indirect sources of light facilitate vision.
- Broad spectrum lighting that simulates natural sunlight provides a more satisfying, calming environment.
- Sufficient exposure to light may lift mood in depressed clients.

Providing a Safe Environment

Clients with existing sensory loss must be protected from injury, whereas clients at risk for sensory loss must learn to avoid injury. The nature of the actual or potential sensory loss determines the safety precautions taken.

Visual loss. A client with a serious visual impairment needs to be oriented to the immediate environment. Normally we see physical boundaries within a room. The blind or severely visually impaired must touch the boundaries to make them real (Norris, 1989). The client needs to walk through a room and feel the walls to establish a sense of direction. The nurse can help by explaining objects within the room such as furniture or appliances. It takes time for the client to absorb a room's arrangement. The client may need to reorient again with the nurse explaining the location of key items (e.g., call light, telephone, chair, etc.). It is also helpful to always approach a blind client from the front.

It is very important to keep all objects in the same position and place (Norris, 1989). After moving an object even a short distance, it no longer exists for a blind person. Simply moving a chair aside may create a dangerous safety hazard. The nurse should ask the client if any item should be arranged to make ambulation easier. Keep traffic patterns clear and avoid use of furniture with sharp edges. The nurse should also remember to give blind clients extra time to perform any task. The client will need a detailed description of how to perform an activity and will move slowly in order to remain safe.

The client with recent visual impairment often requires help with walking. The nurse should stand at the

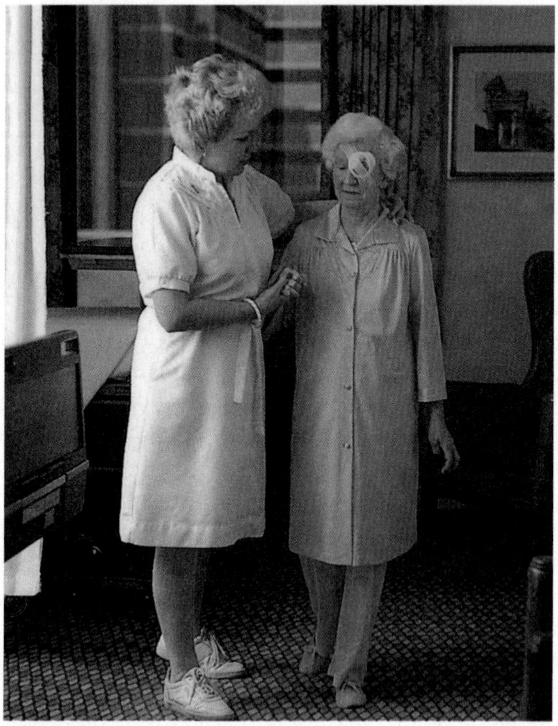

FIGURE 38-2 Nurse assists in ambulation of client wearing eye patch.

client's nondominant side approximately one step in front (Figure 38-2). The client can use the nondominant hand to grasp the nurse's arm and reach forward with the dominant hand to feel for any barriers or landmarks. The nurse should describe the course of movement and ensure that obstacles have been removed. A client with a visual impairment, unaccustomed to the sensory loss, should not be left alone in an unfamiliar area.

A visually impaired client who spends considerable time in bed should have a call light close by. Necessary objects should be placed in front of the client to prevent accidental falls caused by reaching over the bedside. Side rails are also important. At night a nightlight with a red bulb can help to reduce falls (Matteson, McConnell, 1988). The red light reduces the time required for the eyes to adapt to the dark.

If the client has reduced peripheral vision and difficulty driving in darkness, the nurse should emphasize precautions such as looking to both sides before passing cars or while turning a corner and driving only during the day. When a client's depth perception is poor, the edges of steps, baseboards, and driveway curbs should be painted a bright contrasting color to delineate floors from walls and stairs. The use of throw rugs is not recommended. Area rugs should be a bright color to contrast with woodwork and walls.

Hearing loss. Nurses often rely on clients to report unusual sounds, such as a suction apparatus running improperly or an intravenous pump alarm sounding. However, the client with a hearing loss may not hear such sounds and thus requires more frequent visits by the nurse. The client can also benefit from learning to use the sense of vision to discover sources of danger. The nurse ensures the client's glasses are clean and easy to reach.

In the home, light-signaling devices for burglar alarms, doorbells, alarm clocks, smoke detectors, and telephones are available with red or green flashing lights. Signaling devices allow for greater independence. Anyone who calls the client regularly should learn to let the phone ring for a longer period. A telecommunications device for the deaf (TDD) is a computer and printer that transfers written words over the telephone to the hearing impaired. Both a sender and a receiver must have a TDD to complete a call (Walsh, Eldredge, 1989).

Reduced olfaction. A reduced sensitivity to odors means the client may be unable to smell leaking gas, a smoldering cigarette or fire, or tainted food. The client should use smoke detectors and other alternative precautions such as visually checking pilot gas flames and ashtrays, placing cigarette butts in water, or observing the color and consistency of leftover foods.

Reduced tactile sensation. Clients with reduced tactile sensation risk injury when their condition confines them to bed because they are unable to sense pressure on bony prominences or the need to change position. These clients rely on nurses for timely repositioning and turning to prevent pressure sore formation (Chapter 24).

When a client's ability to sense temperature variations is reduced, the nurse should use extra caution in applying heat and cold therapies (see Chapter 37) and frequently check the condition of the client's skin.

GUIDELINES FOR CHECKING HEARING AID FUNCTION

Check the battery. Turn off the aid and remove from client's ear. Cup the aid between your hands and turn the volume up full. A whistle should be heard. If not, the battery is low.

The hearing aid should not produce feedback (whistling sound heard when the client talks with others). If it does, check the position of the aid in the ear. Note if a hole is in the tubing or if hair or cloth interferes with the microphone.

The hearing aid should not emit scratchy sounds or work intermittently. Look for dirt or dust blocking battery contact in the case. See if dirt or dust is found around the volume control.

The hearing aid should be intact. Check for cracks or separation of the case or receiver and cracks or fraying of the cord or tubing.

Promoting Communication

A sensory deficit can cause a client to feel isolated because of an inability to communicate with others. The nature of the sensory loss influences the methods and styles of communication nurses can use with clients. The methods described can be taught to family members and significant others.

The hearing-impaired client may be able to speak normally. However, the deaf client's inability to hear his or her own words may cause serious speech alterations. A child born deaf will require extensive rehabilitation and training to learn how to speak. A client may use sign language, speechreading, or write with a pad and pencil. Special communication boards containing common terms used in nursing care help a client to express needs. If a client has a hearing aid, some procedures can help ensure the aid works properly (see box above). The nurse should not rush a client to communicate and should show interest in the client's ideas and opinions. The box on p. 1181 contains suggestions for communicating with the hearing impaired.

The family can add to communication problems by trying to speak for the hearing-impaired client rather than giving the client a chance at self-expression. The nurse should share communication-promoting tech-

COMMUNICATION GUIDELINES

CLIENTS WITH HEARING IMPAIRMENTS

If a client has a hearing aid, make sure the aid is in place and working before speaking.

Get the client's attention. Do not startle when entering a room. Be sure the client knows you wish to speak.

Face the client before beginning to speak. Be sure your face and lips are illuminated. Avoid speaking with something in your mouth (gum, pencil, etc.) and do not cover your mouth.

If the client wears glasses, be sure they are clean so your gestures and face can be seen.

Speak slowly and articulate clearly. Use normal tones of voice and inflections of speech. Do not exaggerate lip movements, since this interferes with speechreading.

When you are not understood, rephrase rather than repeat the conversation.

Do not shout. Loud sounds are usually of a higher pitch. If it is necessary to raise your voice, speak in lower tones.

Talk toward the client's best or normal ear.

Use visible aids. Speak with your hands, your face, and your eyes.

Avoid using an intercom to speak with a client. The sounds will often be faint and distorted.

Do not restrict a deaf client's hands. Never have intravenous lines in both of the client's hands if the preferred method of communication is sign language.

*Data from Chovaz C: *Can Nurs* 85(3):34, 1989.

niques with the family and explain the importance of giving clients time to communicate.

Client instruction is one aspect of communication. There are teaching booklets available in large print for clients with visual loss. The client who is blind may require more frequent and detailed verbal descriptions of information. This is particularly true if there are no instructional booklets written in braille. The visually impaired can learn by listening to audiotapes or the sound portion of a televised teaching session. Clients with hearing impairment benefit from a variety of written instructional materials and the use of visual teaching aids (posters, graphs, etc.) Demonstrations by the nurse are also very useful.

All staff within a health care setting should be alerted to clients with hearing or visual impairment. A notation on the care plan or on the front of the chart is useful. Hospitals are required to make interpreters available to read sign language of deaf clients.

SOCIALIZATION. Sensory alterations are a factor in the development of loneliness. Christian, et al. (1989) have reported studies in which hearing impairment contributes to withdrawal and social restriction. The inability to follow conversations in a group causes the hearing impaired to withdraw. The visually impaired become restricted by the limitation of being unable to see objects in their surroundings. Being able to interact with others becomes a burden for many clients with sensory alterations and thus they lose the motivation to engage in social situations.

GERONTOLOGIC NURSING PRACTICE

NURSING THERAPIES FOR LONELINESS

- Spend time with clients in silence or conversation.
- Assist in recommending alterations in living arrangements if physical isolation is a factor.
- Give older adults extra time to communicate.
- Assist clients in keeping contact with people important to them.
- Help clients acquire information about mutual help groups.
- Arrange for security escort services as needed.
- Link clients with religious organizations attuned to the social needs of older adults.

The nurse should be sure to have assessed if clients are truly lonely or prefer to be alone. The nurse can introduce therapies to reduce the sense of loneliness (see box above) if they match the clients' needs. The client's perceptions should direct the choice of nursing therapies.

Promoting Self-Care

The ability to perform self-care is essential for self-esteem. Frequently, family members and nurses believe sensorially impaired persons require assistance when they can actually help themselves. The following suggestions may help clients with visual or tactile impairment to carry out activities of daily living.

A meal tray can be set up as though food on the tray and condiments or drinks around the tray are numbers on the face of a clock. The visually impaired client can easily become oriented to the items after the nurse explains each item's location.

If tactile sense is diminished, the client will dress more easily with zippers or Velcro strips, pullover sweaters or blouses, and elasticized waists. If a client has partial paralysis and reduced sensation, the affected side should be dressed first.

Family members responsible for selecting clothing for visually impaired clients should be encouraged to follow the client's preferences. Any sensory impairment influences body image, and the client needs to feel well groomed and attractive. The nurse should offer assistance if needed in brushing, combing, and shampooing of hair.

CRITICAL THINKING ACTIVITIES

1. Mrs. Wilson enters the community clinic to have her 4-year-old child's hearing tested. As the nurse you learn that Mrs. Wilson also has a 6-year-old and that both children are very active. Approximately 6 months ago the 4-year-old entered the clinic with a ruptured ear drum following a fireworks incident. Describe nursing interventions designed to prevent additional sensory loss for the 4-year-old and the 6-year-old.
2. Mr. Thomas is a 72-year-old client who presents a blank, dull affect, a hesitancy to communicate, and a tendency to speak loudly when spoken to. Physical examination should be focused on what potential problem area for this client?
3. Explain how you as the nurse would communicate with a client who has undergone cataract surgery and wears a hearing aid?
4. Mrs. Tillis lives in a two-room apartment on the second floor. During your home visit you notice there is a single light over the stairwell. The client's apartment is painted in a dull gray, with throwrugs throughout. Mrs. Tillis is 80 years old and lives alone. What recommendations might you make to improve the safety of Mrs. Tillis's environment.

References

Bienvenue G, et al.: The audioscope: a clinical tool for otoscopic and audiometric examination, *Ear and Hearing* 6:251-254, 1985.

Bernardini L: Effective communication as an intervention for sensory deprivation in the elderly client, *Top Clin Nurs* 6(4):72, 1985.

Campbell SD: The AudioScope: a valuable hearing assessment tool, *J Gerontol Nurs* 12:28-32, 1986.

Chovaz C: Nursing the hearing impaired patient, *Can Nurse* 85(3):34, 1989.

Christian E, et al.: Sounds of silence: coping with hearing loss and loneliness, *J Gerontol Nurs* 15(11):4, 1989.

Ebersole P, Hess P: *Toward healthy aging,* ed 3, St. Louis, 1990, Mosby.

Hawke M, Mansfield D: Clinical evaluation of a screening audiometer and integral otoscope, *Mod Med Canada* 39:200-203, 1984.

Heidt P: Effect of therapeutic touch on anxiety level of hospitalized patients, *Nurs Res* 30(1):32, 1981.

Hutton J: Aging and the glare problem, *J Gerontol Nurs* 3(5):38-44, 1977.

Janken JK, Cullinan CL: Auditory sensory/perceptual alteration: suggested revision of defining characteristics, *Nurs Diag* 1(4): 147-153, 1990.

Kolanowski A: The clinical importance of environmental lighting to the elderly, *J Gerontol Nurs* 18(1):10-14, 1992.

Kolanowski A: Restlessness in the elderly: the effect of artifical lighting, *Nurs Res* 39:181-183, 1990.

Lewis-Cullinan C, Janken JK: Effect of cerumen removal on the hearing ability of geriatric patients, *J Adv Nurs* 15:594, 1990.

Magilvy JK: Quality of life of hearing-impaired older women, *Nurs Res* 34:140, 1985.

Matteson MA, McConnell ES: *Gerontological nursing: concepts and practice,* Philadelphia, 1988, Saunders.

McKenry LM, Salerno E: *Mosby's pharmacology in nursing,* ed 18, St. Louis, 1992, Mosby.

Norris RM: Commonsense tips for working with blind patients, *AJN* 89:360-361, 1989.

Thibodeau GA, Patton KT: *Anatomy and physiology,* ed 2, St. Louis, 1993, Mosby.

Walsh C, Eldredge N: When deaf people become elderly, *J Gerontol Nurs* 15(12):27, 1989.

Whaley LF, Wong DL: *Nursing care of infants and children,* ed 4, St. Louis, 1991, Mosby.

Bibliography

Brinkman K: Why can't your patient hear you? *RN* 54:46, 1991.

Kee CC: Sensory impairment: factor X in providing nursing care to the older adult, *J Community Health Nurs* 7(1):45, 1990.

Kim, JM, McFarland GK, McLane AM: *Pocket guide to nursing diagnoses,* ed 5, St. Louis 1993, Mosby.

Palumbo MV: Hearing access 2000: increasing awareness of the hearing impaired, *J Gerontol Nurs* 16(9):26, 1990.

Steffee DR, et al.: More than a touch: communicating with a blind and deaf patient, *Nurs 85* 37-39, Aug., 1985.

Uhlmann RF, et al.: Relationship of hearing impairment to dementia and cognitive dysfunction in older adults, *JAMA* 261(13):1916, 1989.

Zegeer LJ: The effects of sensory changes in older persons, *J Neurosci Nurs* 18:325, 1986.

appendix A
Normal Reference Laboratory Values

BLOOD, PLASMA, OR SERUM VALUES

Determination	Reference range: Conventional	Reference range: SI
Acetoacetate plus acetone	0.3-2.0 mg/100 ml	3-20 mg/l
Aldolase	1.3-8.2 mU/ml	12-75 nmol · s^{-1}/l
Alpha amino nitrogen	3.0-5.5 mg/100 ml	2.1-3.9 mmol/l
Ammonia	80-110 μg/100 ml	47-65 μmol/l
Ascorbic acid	0.4-1.5 mg/100 ml	23-85 μmol/l
Barbiturate	0	0 μmol/l
	Coma level: phenobarbital, approximately 10 mg/100 ml; most other drugs, 1-3 mg/100 ml	
Bicarbonate	24-32 mEq/L	
Bilirubin (van den Bergh test)	One minute: 0.4 mg/100 ml	Up to 7 μmol/l
	Direct: 0.4 mg/100 ml	
	Total: 1.0 mg/100 ml	
	Indirect is total minus direct	Up to 17 μmol/l
Blood volume	8.5-9.0% of body weight in kg	80-85 ml/kg
Bromide	0	0 mmol/l
	Toxic level: 17 mEq/l	
Bromsulfalein (BSP)	Less than 5% retention 45 min after 5 mg/kg IV	<0.051
Calcium	8.5-10.5 mg/100 ml (slightly higher in children)	2.1-2.6 mmol/l
Carbon dioxide content	24-30 mEq/l	24-30 mmol/l
	20-26 mEq/l in infants (as HCO_3^-)	
Carbon monoxide	Symptoms with over 20% saturation	0(1)
Carotenoids	0.8-4.0 μg/ml	1.5-7.4 μmol/l
Ceruloplasmin	27-37 mg/100 ml	1.8-2.5 μmol/l
Chloride	100-106 mEq/l	100-106 mmol/l
Cholinesterase (pseudocholinesterase)	0.5 pH U or more/h	0.5 or more arb unit
	0.7 pH U or more/h for packed cells	
Copper	Total: 100-200 μg/100 ml	16-31 μmol/l
Creatine phosphokinase (CPK)	Female 5-35 mU/ml	0.08-0.58 μmol · s^{-1}/l
	Male 5-55 mU/ml	
Creatinine	0.6-1.5 mg/100 ml	60-130 μmol/l

Modified from Kaye DA and Rose LF: *Fundamentals of internal medicine,* St Louis, 1983, Mosby. Adapted by permission from the New England Journal of Medicine, Vol 302, pages 37-48, 1980.

Abbreviations used: *SI,* Système international d'Unités (The SI for the Health Professions. World Health Organization, Office of Publications, Geneva, Switzerland, 1977); *d,* 24 hours; *P,* plasma; *S,* serum; *B,* blood; *U,* urine; *l,* liter; *h,* hour; and *s,* second.

Determination	Reference range: Conventional	Reference range: SI
Ethanol	0.3-0.4%, marked intoxication; 0.4-0.5%, alcoholic stupor; 0.5% or over, alcoholic coma	65-87 mmol/l 87-109 mmol/l >109 mmol/l
Glucose	Fasting: 70-110 mg/100 ml	3.9-5.6 mmol/l
Iron	50-150 μg/100 ml (higher in males)	9.0-26.9 μmol/l
Iron-binding capacity	250-410 μg/100 ml	44.8-73.4 μmol/l
Lactic acid	0.6-118 mEq/l	0.6-1.8 mmol/l
Lactic dehydrogenase	60-120 U/ml	1.00-2.00 μmol · s^{-1}/l
Lead	50 μg/100 ml or less	Up to 2.4 μmol/l
Lipase	2 U/ml or less	Up to 2 arb, unit
Lipids		
Cholesterol	120-220 mg/100 ml	3.10-5.69 mmol/l
Cholesterol esters	60-75% of cholesterol	
Phospholipids	9-16 mg/100 ml as lipid phosphorus	2.9-5.2 mmol/l
Total fatty acids	190-420 mg/100 ml	1.9-4.2 g/l
Total lipids	450-1000 mg/100 ml	4.5-10.0 g/l
Triglycerides	40-150 mg/100 ml	0.4-1.5 g/l
Lithium	Toxic level 2 mEq/l	2 mmol/l
Magnesium	1.5-2.0 mEq/l	0.8-1.3 mmol/l
5′Nucleotidase	0.3-3.2 Bodansky U	30-290 nmol · s^{-1}/l
Osmolality	285-295 mOsm/kg water	285-295 mmol kg
Oxygen saturation (arterial)	96%-100%	0.96-1.00 1
Pco_2	35-43 mm Hg	4.7-6.0 kPa
pH	7.35-7.45	Same
Po_2	75-100 mm Hg (dependent on age) while breathing room air Above 500 mm Hg while on 100% O_2	10.0-13.3 kPa
Phenylalanine	0-2 mg/100 ml	0.120 μmol/l
Phenytoin (Dilantin)	Therapeutic level, 5-20 μg/ml	19.8-79.5 μmol/l
Phosphorus (inorganic)	3.0-4.5 mg/100 ml (infants in 1st yr up to 6.0 mg/100 ml)	1.0-1.5 mmol/l
Potassium	3.5-5.0 mEq/l	3.5-5.0 mmol/l
Primidone (Mysoline)	Therapeutic level 4-12 μg/ml	18-55 μmol/l
Protein: Total	6.0-8.4 g/100 ml	60-84 g/l
Albumin	3.5-5.0 g/100 ml	35-50 g/l
Globulin	2.3-3.5 g/100 ml	23.35 g/l
Electrophoresis	*% of total protein*	*Of total protein*
Albumin	52-68	0.52-0.68
Globulin:		
$Alpha_1$	4.2-7.2	0.042-0.072
$Alpha_2$	6.8-12	0.068-0.12
Beta	9.3-15	0.093-0.15
Gamma	13-23	0.13-0.23
Pyruvic acid	0-0.11 mEq/l	0.0.11 mmol/l
Quinidine	Therapeutic: 1.5-3 μg/ml	4.6-9.2 μmol/l
Salicylate:		
Therapeutic	20-25 mg/100 ml; 25-30 mg/100 ml to age 10 yr, 3 h post dose	1.4-1.8 mmol/l 1.8-2.2 mmol/l
Toxic	Over 30 mg/100 ml Over 20 mg/100 ml after age 60	Over 2.2 mmol/l Over 1.4 mmol/l
Sodium	135-145 mEq/l	135-145 mmol/l
Sulfate	0.5-1.5 mg/100 ml	0.05-1.2 mmol/l
Sulfonamide	0 mg/100 ml Therapeutic: 5-15 mg/100 ml	0 mmol/l
Transaminase (SGOT) (asparatate amino-transferase)	10-40 U/ml	0.08-0.32 μmol · s^{-1}/l
Urea nitrogen (BUN)	8.25 mg/100 ml	2.9-8.9 mmol/l
Uric acid	3.0-7.0 mg/100 ml	0.18-0.42 mmol/l
Vitamin A	0.15-0.6 μg/ml	0.5-2.1 μmol/l
Vitamin A tolerance test	Rise to twice fasting level in 3 to 5 h	

URINE VALUES

Determination	Reference range: Conventional	SI
Acetone plus acetoacetate (quantitative)	0	0 mg/l
Alpha amino nitrogen	64-199 mg/d not over 1.5% of total nitrogen	4.6-14.2 mmol/d
Amylase	24-76 U/ml	24-76 arb, unit
Calcium	150 mg/d or less	3.8 or less mmol/d
Catecholamines	Epinephrine: under 20 µg/d	<55 nmol/d
	Norepinephrine: under 100 µg/d	<590 nmol/d
Copper	0-100 µg/d	0-1.6 µmol/d
Coproporphyrin	50-250 µg/d	80-380 nmol/d
	Children under 80 lb 0-75 µg/d	0-115 nmol/d
Creatine	Under 100 mg/d or less than 6% of creatinine. In pregnancy: up to 12%. In children under 1 yr: may equal creatinine. In older children: up to 30% of creatinine	<0.75 mmol/d
Crystine or cysteine	0	0
Follicle-stimulating hormone:		
Follicular phase	5-20 IU/d	Same
Midcycle	15-60 IU/d	
Luteal phase	5-15 IU/d	
Menopausal	50-100 IU/d	
Men	5-25 IU/d	
Hemoglobin and myoglobin	0	
5-Hydroxyindole acetic acid	2-9 mg/d (women lower than men)	10-45 µmol/d
Lead	0.08 µg/ml or 120 µg or less/d	0.39 µmol/l or less
Phenolsulfonphthalein (PSP)	At least 25% excreted by 15 min; 40% by 30 min; 60% by 120 min	0.25 l
Phosphorus (inorganic)	Varies with intake; average 1 g/d	32 mmol/d
Porphobilingen	0	0
Protein:		
Quantitative	<150 mg/d	<0.15 g/d
Steroids		

17-Ketosteroids (per day)	*Age* (64)	*Male* (mg)	*Female* (mg)	*Male* (µmol/d)	*Female* (µmol/d)
	10	1-4	1-4	3-14	3-14
	20	6-21	4-16	21-73	14-56
	30	8-26	4-14	28-90	14-49
	50	5-18	3-9	17-62	10-31
	70	2-10	1-7	7-35	3-24

Determination	Conventional	SI
17-Hydroxysteroids	3-8 mg/d (women lower than men)	8-22 µmol/d as hydrocortisone
Sugar:		
Quantitative glucose	0	0 mmol/l
Identification of reducing substances:		
Fructose	0	0 mmol/l
Pentose	0	0 mmol/l
Titratable acidity	24-40 mEq/d	20-40 mmol/d
Urobilinogen	Up to 1.0 Ehrlich U	To 1.0 arb. unit
Uroporphyrin	0	0 nmol/d
Vanillylmandelic acid (VMA)	Up to 9 mg/d	Up to 45 µmol/d

SPECIAL ENDOCRINE TESTS

Determination	Reference range: Conventional	Reference range: SI
STEROID HORMONES		
Aldosterone	Excretion: 5-19 μg/d	14-53 nmol/d
Fasting, at rest, 210 mEq sodium diet	Supine: 48 ± 29 pg/ml	180 ± 64 pmol/l
	Upright: (2 h) 65 ± 23 ¶/ml	
Fasting, at rest, 110 mEq sodium diet	Supine: 107 ± 45 pg/ml	279 ± 125 pmol/l
	Upright: (2 h) 239 ± 123 pg/ml	663 ± 341 pmol/l
Fasting, at rest, 10 mEq sodium diet	Supine: 175 ± 75 pg/ml	485 ± 108 pmol/l
	Upright: (2 h) 523 ± 228 pg/ml	1476 ± 632 pmol/l
Cortisol		
Fasting	8 AM: 5-25 ≈g/100 ml	0.14-0.69 μmol/l
At rest	8 PM: Below 10 μg/100 ml	0-0.28 μmol/l
20 U ACTH	4 h ACTH test: 30-45 μg/100 ml	0.83-1.24 μmol/l
Dexamethasone at midnight	Overnight suppression test: Below 5 μg/100 ml	<0.14 nmol/l
	Excretion: 20-70 μg/d	
11-Deoxycortisol	Responsive; over 7.5 μg/100 ml (after metyrapone)	≥ 0.22 ≈ mol/l
Testosterone	Adult male: 300-1100 ng/100 ml	10.4-38.1 nmol/l
	Adolescent male: over 100 ng/100 ml	>3.5 nmol/l
	Female: 25-90 ng/100 ml	0.87-3.12 nmol/l
Unbound testosterone	Adult male: 3.06-24.0 ng/100 ml	106-832 pmol/l
	Adult female: 0.09-1.28 ng/100 ml	3.1-44.4 pmol/l
POLYPEPTIDE HORMONES		
Adrenocorticotropin (ACTH)	15-70 pg/ml	3.3-15.4 prmol/l
Calcitonin	Undetectable in normals	0
	>100 pg/ml in medullary carcinoma	>29.3 pmol/l
Growth hormone		
Fasting, at rest	Below 5 ng/ml	<233 pmol/l
After exercise	Child: over 10 ng/ml	>465 pmol/l
	Male: Below 5 ng/ml	<233 pmol/l
	Female: Up to 309 ng/ml	0-1395 pmol/l
After glucose	Male: Below 5 ng/ml	<233 pmol/l
	Female: Below 10 ng/ml	0-465 pmol/l
Insulin		
Fasting	6-26 μU/ml	43-187 pmol/l
During hypoglycemia	Below 20 μU/ml	<144 pmol/l
After glucose	Up to 150 μU/ml	0-1078 pmol/l
Leuteinizing hormone	Male: 6-18 mU/ml	6-18 μ/l
Preovulatory or postovulatory	Female: 5-22 mU/ml	5-22 μ/l
Midcycle peak	30-250 mU/ml	30-250 μ/l
Parathyroid hormone	<10 μl equiv/ml	<10 ml equiv/l
Prolactin	2-15 ng/ml	0.08-6.0 nmol/l
Renin activity		
Normal diet	Supine: 1.1 ± 0.8 ng/ml/h	0.9 ± 0.6 (nmol/l)h
	Upright: 1.9 ± 17 ng/ml/h	1.5 ± 1.3 (nmol/l)h
Low-sodium diet	Supine: 2.7 ± 118 ng/ml/h	2.1 ± 1.4 (nmol/l)h
	Upright: 6.6 ± 2.5 ng/ml/h	5.1 ± 1.9 (nmol/l)h
Low-sodium diet	Diuretics: 10.0 ± 3.7 ng/ml/h	7.7 ± 2.9 (nmol/l)h
THYROID HORMONES		
Thyroid-stimulating hormone (TSH)	0.5-3.5 μU/ml	0.5-3.5 mU/l
Thyroxine-binding globulin capacity	15-25 μg T_4/100 ml	193-322 nmol/l
Total triiodothyronine by radioimmunoassay (T_3)		
Total thyroxine by RIA (T_4)	4-12 μg/100 ml	52-154 nmol/l
T_3 resin uptake	25-35%	0.25-0.35
Free thyroxine index (FT$_4$l)	1-4 ng/100 ml	12.8-51.2 pmol/l

CEREBROSPINAL FLUID VALUES

Determination	Reference range: Conventional	Reference range: SI	Determination	Reference range: Conventional	Reference range: SI
Bilirubin	0	0 μmol/l	Glucose	50-75 mg/100 ml (30-50% less than blood)	2.8-4.2 mmol/l
Chloride	120-130 mEq/l (20 mEq/l higher than serum)		Pressure (initial)	70-180 mm of water	70-80 arb. units
Albumin	Mean: 29.5 mg/100 ml ±2 SD: 11-48 mg/100 ml	0.295 g/l ±2 SD: 0.11-48	Protein:		
			Lumbar	15-45 mg/100 ml	0.15-0.45 g/l
IgG	Mean: 4.3 mg/100 ml ±2 SD: 0-8.6 mg/100 ml	0.043 g/l ±2 SD: 0-0.086	Cisternal	15-25 mg/100 ml	0.15-0.25 g/l
			Ventricular	5-15 mg/100 ml	0.05-0.15 g/l

HEMATOLOGIC VALUES

Determination	Reference range: Conventional	Reference range: SI
Coagulation factors:		
Factor I (fibrinogen)	0.15-0.35 g/100 ml	4.0-10.0 μmol/l
Factor II (prothrombin)	60-140%	0.60-1.40
Factor V (accelerator globulin)	60-140%	0.60-1.40
Factor VII-X (proconvertin-Stuart)	70-130%	0.70-1.30
Factor X (Stuart factor)	70-130%	0.70-1.30
Factor VIII (antihemophilic globulin)	50-200%	0.50-2.0
Factor IX (plasma thromboplastic cofactor)	60-140%	0.60-1.40
Factor XI (plasma thromboplastic antecedent)	60-140%	0.60-1.40
Factor XII (Hageman factor)	60-140%	0.60-1.40
Coagulation screening tests:		
Bleeding time (Simplate)	3-9 min	18-540 s
Prothrombin time	Less than 2-s deviation from control	Less than 2-s deviation from control
Partial thromboplastin time (activated)	25-37 s	25-37 s
Whole-blood clot lysis	No clot lysis in 24 h	0/d
Fibrinolytic studies:		
Euglobin lysis	No lysis in 2 h	0 (in 2 h)
Fibrinogen split products	Negative reaction at greater than 1:4 dilution	0 (at >1:4 dilution)
Thrombin time	Control ± 5 s	Control ± 5 s
Complete blood count:		
Hematocrit	Male: 45-52% Female: 37-48%	Male: 0.42-0.52 Female: 0.37-0.48
Hemoglobin	Male: 13-18 g/100 ml Female: 12-16 g/100 ml	Male: 8.1-11.2 mmol/l Female: 7.4-9.9 mmol/l
Leukocyte count	4300-10,800/mm3	$4.3\text{-}10.8 \times 10^9$/l
Erythrocyte count	4.2-5.9 million/mm^3	$4.2\text{-}5.9 \times 10^{12}$/l
Mean corpuscular volume (MCV)	80-94 μm^3	80-94 fl
Mean corpuscular hemoglobin (MCH)	27-32 pg	1.7-2.0 fmol
Mean corpuscular hemoglobin	32%-36%	19-22.8 mmol/l
Mean corpuscular hemoglobin concentration (MCHC)		
Erythrocyte sedimentation rate (Westergren method)	Male: 1-13 mm/h Female: 1-20 mm/h	Male: 1-13 mm/h Female: 1-20 mm/h

HEMATOLOGIC VALUES—cont'd

Determination	Reference range: Conventional	SI
Erythrocyte enzymes:		
Glucose-6-phosphate dehydrogenase	5-15 U/gHb	5-15 U/g
Pyruvate kinase	13-17 U/gHb	13-17 U/g
Ferritin (serum)		
Iron deficiency	0.20 ng/ml	0-20 μg/l
Iron excess	Greater than 400 ng/l	>400 μg/l
Folic acid		
Normal	Greater than 1.9 ng/ml	>4.3 mmol/l
Borderline	1.0-1.9 ng/ml	2.3-4.3 mmol/l
Haptoglobin	100-300 mg/100 ml	1.0-3.0 g/l
Hemoglobin studies:		
Electrophoresis for A_2 hemoglobin	1.5-3.5%	0.015-0.035
Hemoglobin F (fetal hemoglobin)	Less than 2%	<0.02
Hemoglobin, met- and sulf-	0	0
Serum hemoglobin	2-3 mg/100 ml	1.2-1.9 μmol/l
Thermolabile hemoglobin	0	0
LE (lupus erythematosus) preparation:		
Heparin as anticoagulant	0	0
Defibrinated blood	0	0
Leukocyte alkaline phosphatase:		
Quantitative method	1-40 mg of phosphorus liberated/h/ 10^{10} cells	15-40 mg/h
Qualitative method	Males: 33-188 U	33-188 U
	Females (off contraceptive pill): 30-160 U	30-160 U
Muramidase	Serum, 3-7 μg/ml	3-7 mg/l
	Urine, 0-2 ≈ g/ml	0-2 mg/l
Osmotic fragility of erythrocytes	Increased if hemolysis occurs in over 0.5% NaCl; decreased if hemolysis is incomplete in 0.3% of NaCl	
Peroxide hemolysis	Less than 10%	<0.10
Platelet count	150,000-350,000/mm^3	150-350 × 10^9/l
Platelet function tests:		
Clot retraction	50-100%/2 h	0.50-1.00/2 h
Platelet aggregation	Full response to ADP, epinephrine, and collagen	1.0
Platelet factor 3	33-57 s	33-57 s
Prothrombin time	Less than 2 sec deviation from control	
Reticulocyte count	0.5-1.5% red cells	0.005-0.015
Vitamin B_{12}	90-280 pg/ml (borderline: 70-90)	66-207 pmol/l (borderline: 52-66)

MISCELLANEOUS VALUES

Determination	Reference range: Conventional	SI
Autoantibodies in serum		
Thyroid collaid and microsomal antigens	Absent	
Stomach parietal cells	Absent	
Smooth muscle	Absent	
Kidney mitochondria	Absent	
Rabbit renal collecting ducts	Absent	
Cytoplasm of ova, theca cells, testicular interstitial cells	Absent	
Skeletal muscle	Absent	
Adrenal gland	Absent	

Continued.

MISCELLANEOUS VALUES—cont'd

Determination	Reference range: Conventional	Reference range: SI
Carcinoembryonic antigen (CEA) in blood	0-2.5 ng/ml, 97% healthy nonsmokers	0-2.5 μg/l, 97% healthy nonsmokers
Cryoprecipitable proteins in blood	0	0 arb unit
Digitoxin in serum	17 ± 6 ng/ml	22 ± 7.8 nmol/l
Digoxin in serum		
0.25 mg/d	1.2 ± 0.4 ng/ml	1.54 ± 0.5 nmol/l
0.5 mg/d	1.5 ± 0.4 ng/ml	1.92 ± 0.5 nmol/l
Duodenal drainage:		
pH	5.5-7.5	5.5-7.5
Amylase	Over 1200 U/total sample	>1.2 arb. unit
Trypsin	Values from 35 to 160% "normal"	0.35-1.60
Viscosity	3 min or less	180 s or less
Gastric analysis	Basal:	
	Females 2.0 ± 1.8 mEq/h	0.6 ± 0.5
	Males: 3.0 ± 2.0 mEq/h	0.8 ± 0.6 μmol/s
	Maximal: (after histalog or gastrin)	
	Females 16 ± 5 mEq/h	
	Males 23 ± 5 mEq/h	6.4 ± 1.4 μmol/s
Gastrin-I in blood	0-200 pg/ml	0-95 pmol/l
Alpha-feto-globulin	Abnormal if present	
Alpha 1-antitrypsin	200-400 mg/100 ml	2.0-4.0 g/l
Antinuclear antibodies	Positive if detected with serum diluted 1:10	
Anti-DNA antibodies	Less than 15 units/ml	
Complement, total hemolytic	150-250 U/ml	
C3	Range 55-120 mg/100 ml	0.55-1.2 g/l
C4	Range 20-50 mg/100 ml	0.2-0.5 g/l
Immunoglobulins in blood:		
IgG	1140 mg/100 ml	11.4 g/l
	Range 540-1663	5.5-16.6 g/l
IgA	214 mg/100 ml	2.14 g/l
	Range 66-344	0.66-3.44 g/l
IgM	168 mg/100 ml	1.68 g/l
	Range 39-290	0.39-2.9 g/l
Viscosity	1.4-1.8 expressed as relative viscosity of serum compared with water	
Iontophoresis	Children: 0-40 mEq sodium/l	0-40 mmol/l
	Adults: 0-60 mEq sodium/l	0-60 mmol/l
Propranolol (includes bioactive 4-OH metabolite) in serum 4h after last dose		
Stool fat	Less than 5 g in 24 hr or less than 4% of measured fat intake in 3-d period	<5 g/d
Stool nitrogen	Less than 2 g/d or 10% of urinary nitrogen	<2 g/d
Synovial fluid:		
Glucose	Not less than 20 mg/100 ml lower than simultaneously drawn blood sugar	See blood glucose mmol/l
Mucin	Type 1 or 2	1-2 arb. unit
	Grades as:	
	Type 1-tight clump	
	Type 2-soft clump	
	Type 3-soft clump that breaks up	
	Type 4-cloudy, no clump	
D-Xylose absorption	5-8 g/5 h in urine	33-53 mmol
	40 mg/100 ml in blood 2 h after ingestion of 25 g of D-xylose	2.7 mmol/l

appendix B

Common Abbreviations

NOTE: Abbreviations in common use can vary widely from place to place. Each institution's list of acceptable abbreviations is the best authority for its records.

°C	degrees Centigrade
°F	degrees Farenheit
μg	microgram
μm	micrometer
ʒ	dram
@	at
A	
aa	of each
ABG	arterial blood gas
ac	before meals
ad lib	freely as desired
ADL	activities of daily living
Ag	silver, antigen
AIDS	acquired immunodeficiency syndrome
ALS	amyotrophic lateral sclerosis
AM	morning
ama	against medical advice
AMI	acute myocardial infarction
amp	ampule
ARC	AIDS-related complex
ARDS	adult respiratory distress syndrome
AS	aortic stenosis
ASD	atrial septal defect
B	
Ba	barium
BE	barium enema
bid	two times a day
BM, bm	bowel movement
BMR	basal metabolic rate
BP	blood pressure
BPH	benign prostatic hypertrophy
BRP	bathroom privileges
BSA	body surface area
BUN	blood urea nitrogen
C	
c̄	with
c/o	complains of
Ca	calcium, cancer, carcinoma
CAD	coronary artery disease

cap	capsule
CAT	computed axial tomography
cath	catheter, catheterize
CBC	complete blood count
CBR	complete bed rest
CC	chief complaint
cc	cubic centimeter
CCU	coronary care unit, critical care unit
CDC	Centers for Disease Control and Prevention
CEA	carcinoembryonic antigen
CFT	complement-fixation test
cg	centigram
CHF	congestive heart failure
CHO	carbohydrate
Cl	chlorine
cm	centimeter
cm^3	cubic centimeter
CNS	central nervous system
CO	carbon monoxide
CO_2	carbon dioxide
COPD	chronic obstructive pulmonary disease
CPK	creatine phosphokinase
CPR	cardiopulmonary resuscitation
CSF	cerebrospinal fluid
CT	computed tomography
CVA	cerebrovascular accident, costovertebral angle
CVP	central venous pressure
D	
D&C	dilation and curettage
D5W	5% dextrose in water
db, dB	decibels
dc	discontinue
DIC	disseminated intravascular coagulation
diff	differential blood count
dil	dilute
DJD	degenerative joint disease
dl	deciliter

DM	diastolic murmur
DNR	do not resuscitate
DOE	dyspnea on exertion
dx, Dx	diagnosis
E	
EBV	Epstein-Barr virus
ECF	extracellular fluid
ECG	electrocardiogram
ECHO	echocardiography
ECT	electroconvulsive therapy
EDC	estimated date of confinement
EDD	estimated date of delivery
EEG	electroencephalogram
EKG	electrocardiogram
elix	elixer
EMG	electromyogram
ENG	electronsystagmography
ER	emergency room
ERG	electroretinogram
ESRD	end-stage renal disease
EST	electroshock therapy
F	
℥	fluid ounce
FANA	fluorescent antinuclear antibody test
FBS	fasting blood sugar
Fe	iron
FEV	forced expiratory volume
FHR	fetal heart rate
FRC	functional residual capacity
FSH	follicle-stimulating hormone
FUO	fever of unknown origin
Fx, fx	fracture, fractional urine test
G	
g, gm, Gm	gram
Gc,GC	gonococcus
GI	gastrointestinal
gr	grain
grav I, II, III, etc	pregnancy one, two, three, etc
gt, gtt	drop, drops
GTT	glucose tolerance test
GU	genitourinary
GYN, Gyn	gynecological
H	
H_2O	water
h	hour
H^+	hydrogen ion
h/o	history of
H&P	history and physical examination
HAV	hepatitis A virus
Hb	hemoglobin
HBAg	hepatitis B antigen
HBV	hepatitis B virus
Hct, HCT	hematocrit
HDL	high-density lipoprotein
Hg	mercury
Hgb	hemoglobin
HIV	human immunodeficiency (AIDS) virus
HLA	human lymphocyte antigen
HSV2	herpes simplex virus, type 2
I	
I&O	intake and output

IC	inspiratory capacity
ICP	intracranial pressure
ICU	intensive care unit
IDDM	insulin-dependent diabetes mellitus
IE	immunoelectrophoresis
Ig	immunoglobulin
IgA, etc	immunoglobulin A, etc
IM	intramuscular
IOP	intraocular pressure
IPPB	intermittent positive pressure breathing
IV	intravenous
IVP	intravenous push; intravenous pyelogram
IVU	intravenous urogram
J	
JRA	juvenile rheumatoid arthritis
K	
K	potassium
kg	kilogram
KUB	kidney, ureters, and bladder (radiograph)
KVO	keep vein open
L	
L	liter
L&A	light and accommodation
LBBB	left bundle branch block
LE	lupus erythematosus
LGV	lymphogranuloma venereum
LLL	left lower lobe
LLQ	left lower quadrant
LMP	last menstrual period
LNMP	last normal menstrual period
LP	lumbar puncture
LUL	left upper lobe
LUQ	left upper quadrant
LVH	left ventricular hypertrophy
M	
m	meter
m, min, ♏	minum
MAP	mean arterial pressure
mcg	microgram
MCH	mean corpuscular hemoglobin
MCHC	mean corpuscular hemoglobin concentration
MCV	mean cell volume, mean corpuscular volume
mg	milligram
Mg	magnesium
MG	myasthenia gravis
MI	myocardial infarction
MICU	medical intensive care unit
ml	milliliter
mm	millimeter
mm^3	cubic millimeter
mm Hg	millimeters of mercury
MRI	magnetic resonance imaging
MS	multiple sclerosis
MW	molecular weight
N	
N	nitrogen
Na	sodium
NICU	neonatal intensive care unit
NIH	National Institutes of Health

nm	nanometer
NMR	nuclear magnetic resonance
NPO	nothing by mouth
NS	normal saline
O	
O_2	oxygen
OD	right eye; optical density; overdose
OL	left eye
OOB	out of bed
ORIF	open reduction and internal fixation
OS	left eye
OT	occupational therapy
OTC	over-the-counter
ou	both eyes
oz, ℥	ounce
P	
P&A	percussion and auscultation
PaCO_2	partial pressure of carbon dioxide (arterial blood)
PaO_2	partial pressure of oxygen (arterial blood)
para I, II, etc	unipara, bipara, etc
PAT	paroxysmal atrial tachycardia
pc	after meals
PCG	phonocardiogram
PCO_2	partial pressure of carbon dioxide
PCP	pulmonary capillary pressure, phencyclidine
PCV	packed cell volume
PCWP	pulmonary capillary wedge pressure
PD	interpupillary distance; postural drainage
PE	pulmonary embolism, physical examination
PEEP	positive end expiratory pressure
PEG	pneumoencephalography
per	through, by way of
PERRLA	pupils equal, round, and reactive to light and accommodation
PET	positron emission tomography
PG	prostaglandin
pH	hydrogen ion concentration (acidity and alkalinity)
PID	pelvic inflammatory disease
PKU	phenylketonuria
PM	postmortem
PM	evening
PMS	premenstrual syndrome
PND	paroxysmal nocturnal dyspnea, postnasal drip
PO_2	partial pressure of oxygen
PO, po	orally
PPD	purified protein derivative
ppm	parts per million
prn	when required, as often as necessary
PT	physical therapy; prothrombin time
PTT	partial thromboplastin time
PUO	pyrexia of unknown origin
PVC	premature ventricular contraction
Q	
q	every
q2h	every 2 hours
q3h	every 3 hours
q4h	every 4 hours
qd	every day
qh	every hour
qid	four times a day
qn	every night
qod	every other day
qns	quantity not sufficient
R	
R/O	rule out
RBBB	right bundle branch block
RBC	red blood cell
RDS	respiratory distress syndrome
Rh+	positive Rh factor
Rh−	negative Rh factor
RHD	rheumatic heart disease
RLL	right lower lobe
RLQ	right lower quadrant
RML	right middle lobe
ROM	range of motion
ROS	review of systems
RS	Reiter's syndrome
RSV	Rous sarcoma virus
RUL	right upper lobe
RUQ	right upper quadrant
Rx	take; treatment
S	
$\bar{s}$	without
SB	sternal border
SC	subcutaneous
sib	sibling
SICU	surgical intensive care unit
SIDS	sudden infant death syndrome
Sig	write on label
SLE	systemic lupus erythematosus
sol	solution, dissolved
sos	if necessary
sp gr, SG, sg	specific gravity
SQ, subq	subcutaneous
SR	sedimentation rate
ss	half
SSS	sick sinus syndrome, specific soluble substance, short-stay surgery
stat	immediately
STD	sexually transmitted disease
STS	serologic test for syphilis
susp	suspension
SV	stroke volume
T	
T_3	triiodothyronine
T_4	tetraiodothyronine
T&A	tonsillectomy and adenoidectomy
TAB	typhoid and paratyoid A and B
TAH	total abdominal hysterectomy
TAT	tetanus antitoxin; thermatic apperception test
TB, TBC	tuberculosis
TBG	thyroxin-binding globulin
TG	triglyceride
TIA	transient ischemic attack
TIBC	total iron-binding capacity

tid	three times a day
TKO	to keep open
TLC	total lung capacity; thin layer chromatography
TPN	total parenteral nutrition
TPR	temperature, pulse, and respirations
tr, tinct	tincture
TST	triple sugar iron test
TSH	thyroid-stimulating hormone
U	
UA	urinalysis
UGI series	upper gastrointestinal series
UIBC	unsaturated iron-binding capacity
URI	upper respiratory infection
US	ultrasound
UTI	urinary tract infection
V	
V&T	volume and tension
VC	vital capacity
VD	venereal disease
VDA	visual discriminatory acuity
VDH	valvular disease of the heart
VDRL	Venereal Disease Research Laboratory
VLDL	very low-density lipoprotein
VS	vital signs
VSD	ventricular septal defect
V_T	Tidal volume
W	
W/V	weight/volume
WBC	white blood cell, white blood count
WNL	within normal limits
WR	Wasserman reaction

Glossary

abduction Movement of a limb away from the body.

abnormal reactive hyperemia Hyperemia over a pressure site lasting longer than 1 hour following removal of pressure; surrounding skin does not blanch.

abrasion Scraping or rubbing away of epidermis; may result in localized bleeding and later weeping of serous fluid.

absorption Passage of drug molecules into the blood. Factors influencing drug absorption include route of administration, ability of the drug to dissolve, and conditions at the site of absorption.

accessory muscles Muscles in the thoracic cage that assist with respiration.

accountability State of being answerable for one's actions—the professional nurse answers to herself, the client, the profession, the employing institution, and society for the effectiveness of nursing care performed.

accreditation A process whereby a professional association or nongovernmental body grants recognition to a school or institution for demonstrated ability in a special area of practice or training.

acculturation Process of intercultural borrowing between diverse peoples, resulting in new and blended patterns.

acne Inflammatory, papulopustular skin eruption, usually occurring on the face, neck, shoulders, and upper back.

active range of motion (ROM) The range of movement through which a joint can be moved without assistance.

active strategies of health promotion Activities that depend on the client being motivated to adopt a specific health program.

active transport Movement of materials across the cell membrane by means of chemical activity that allows the cell to admit larger molecules than would otherwise be possible.

activities of daily living (ADLs) Activities usually performed in the course of a normal day in the client's life, such as eating, dressing, bathing, brushing the teeth, or grooming.

activity The amount of independent movement; ability to ambulate, change positions, perceive, and relieve pressure.

activity tolerance Kind and amount of exercise or work that a person is able to perform.

actual problems Problems that the client is currently experiencing.

acute illness Illness characterized by symptoms that are of relatively short duration, are usually severe, and affect the functioning of the client in all dimensions.

adaptation Process by which changes occur in any of a person's dimensions in response to stress.

adduction Movement of a limb toward the body.

adolescence The period of development between the onset of puberty and adulthood.

adventitious sounds Abnormal lung sounds heard with auscultation.

adverse reaction Harmful or unintended effect of a medication, diagnostic test, or therapeutic intervention.

advocacy Process whereby a nurse objectively provides a client with the information he or she needs to make decisions and supports the client in whatever decisions he or she makes.

aerosolization Providing medication by way of nebulized particles suspended in a gas or air.

afebrile Without fever.

affective learning Acquisition of behaviors involved in expressing feelings in attitudes, appreciations, and values.

afterload The resistance to ventricular ejection.

afternoon care Hygiene measures provided by the nurse that include washing the hands and face, assisting with oral care, offering a bedpan or urinal, and straightening bed linen.

agent-host-environment model Model of health and illness for an individual or community that states that the level of health of the client depends on the relationship between agent, host, and environment.

agents Elements of the agent-host-environment model of health and illness; biological, chemical, physical or mechanical, or psychosocial factors whose presence or absence can lead to disease or illness.

AHCPR Agency for Health Care Policy and Research, which synthesizes research and develops standards of practice.

air pollution Contamination of the environmental atmosphere with substances known as pollutants that are not normally found in the air.

airway resistance The pressure difference between the mouth, nose, or other airway opening and the alveoli.

alarm reaction Reaction in response to stress characterized by the mobilization of the various defense mechanisms of the body or mind to cope with the stressor.

alveolar hypoventilation Respiratory rate insufficient to prevent carbon dioxide retention.

alveolar hyperventilation Respiratory rate in excess of that required to maintain normal carbon dioxide levels in the body tissues.

Alzheimer's disease Disease of the brain parenchyma that causes a gradual and progressive decline in cognitive functioning.

AM care Routine hygiene care performed before breakfast or early in the morning.

analgesics Relieving pain; drugs that relieve pain.

anaphylactic reaction A hypersensitive condition induced by contact with certain antigens.

anemia Disorder characterized by a decrease in hemoglobin of the blood.

anesthesics Drugs causing absence of normal sensation, especially sensitivity to pain.

angina pectoris Episodic chest pain caused most often by myocardial anoxia, resulting from atherosclerosis of the coronary arteries. Pain radiates down the inner aspect of the left arm and is often accompanied by feeling of suffocation and impending death.

angiography A radiographic visualization of internal anatomy of the heart and blood vessels after the introduction of a radiopaque contrast medium.

anions Negatively charged electrolytes.

anorexia Lack or loss of appetite resulting in the inability to eat.

antagonistic muscles Group of muscles that work together to bring about movement at the joint.

anthropometric Relating to measurement of various body parts to determine nutritional and caloric status, muscular development, brain growth, and other parameters.

anthropometry Measurement of various body parts to determine nutritional and caloric status, muscular development, brain growth, and other parameters.

antibodies Immunoglobulins, essential to the immune system, that are produced by lymphoid tissue in response to bacteria, viruses, or other antigens.

anticipatory grief Grief response in which the person begins the grieving process before an actual loss.

antiembolic stockings Elasticized stockings that prevent formation of emboli and thrombi, especially after surgery or during bed rest.

antigen Substance, usually a protein, that causes the formation of an antibody and reacts specifically with that antibody.

antipyretic Substance or procedure that reduces fever.

Apgar scale Assessment tool that rates the newborn's physiological status 1 to 5 minutes after birth.

aphasia Abnormal neurological condition in which language function is defective or absent; related to injury to speech center in cerebral cortex, causing receptive or expressive aphasia.

apical pulse The heartbeat taken with the bell or diaphragm of a stethoscope placed on the apex of the heart.

apnea Cessation of airflow through the nose and mouth.

apocrine gland Large, deep exocrine glands located in the axillary, anal, genital, and mammary areas of the body; secrete sweat having a strong odor.

apothecary system System of measurement; basic unit of weight is a grain. Weights derived from the grain are the gram, ounce, and pound. The basic measure for fluid is the minim. The fluidram, fluid ounce, pint, quart, and gallon are measures derived from the minim.

approximate To come close together, as in the edges of a wound.

asepsis Absence of germs or microorganisms.

assault Unlawful threatening or inflicting of harm on another.

assessment First step of the nursing process; activities required in the first step are data collection, data validation, data sorting, and data documentation. The purpose is to gather information for health problem identification.

assimilation To become absorbed into another culture and to adopt its characteristics.

assistive care Measures provided to assist the client with hygiene measures. The level of assistive care is individualized based on assessment of client's self-care abilities.

associative play A form of play in which a group of children participate in similar or identical activities without formal organization, direction, interaction, or goals.

atelectasis Collapse of alveoli, preventing the normal respiratory exchange of oxygen and carbon dioxide.

atrioventricular (AV) node A portion of the cardiac conduction system located on the floor of the right atrium, it receives electrical impulses from the atrium and transmits them to the bundle of His.

attachment Initial psychosocial relationship that develops between parents and the neonate.

attentional set Internal state of the learner that allows focusing and comprehension.

auditory Related to, or experienced through, hearing.

auscultation Method of physical examination; listening to the sounds produced by the body, usually with a stethoscope.

auscultatory gap Disappearance of sound when obtaining a blood pressure; typically occurs between the first and second Korotkoff's sounds.

autologous transfusion The collection of the client's blood for reinfusion after a surgical procedure.

autonomy Ability or tendency to function independently.

autopsy Postmortem examination performed to confirm or determine the cause of death.

autotransfusion The collection, anticoagulation, filtration, and reinfusion of blood from an active bleeding site.

bacteriuria Presence of bacteria in the urine.

balance Position when the person's center of gravity is correctly positioned so that falling does not occur.

basal metabolic rate (BMR) Amount of energy used in a unit of time by a fasting, resting subject to maintain vital functions.

battery Legal term for touching of another's body without consent.

bed boards Boards placed under the mattress of a bed that provide extra support to the mattress surface.

bed rest Placement of the client in bed for therapeutic reasons for a prescribed period.

bereavement Response to loss through death; a subjective experience that a person suffers after losing a person with whom there has been a significant relationship.

binder Bandages made of large pieces of material to fit specific body parts.

bioavailability The degree of activity or amount of an administered drug or other substance that becomes available for activity in the target tissue.

biological clock Cyclical nature of body functions; functions controlled from within the body are synchronized with environmental factors; same meaning as biorhythm.

biotransformation The chemical changes that a substance undergoes in the body, such as by the action of enzymes.

blanching Whitening of the skin from pressure, vasoconstriction, hypotension.

body image Person's subjective concept of his or her physical appearance.

body mechanics Coordinated efforts of the musculoskeletal and nervous systems to maintain proper balance, posture, and body alignment.

bolus Round mass of chewed food ready to be swallowed.

bonding The parents' emotional tie to their child that usually develops soon after birth as a result of their interaction.

bone resorption Destruction of bone cells and release of calcium into the blood.

brachial pulse Rhythmic beating palpated over the brachial artery.

bradycardia Slower than normal heart rate; heart contracts fewer than 60 times per minute.

bradypnea An abnormally slow rate of breathing.

bronchoscopy Visual examination of the tracheal and bronchial tree using a flexible fiberoptic bronchoscope.

bruit Abnormal sound or murmur heard while auscultating an organ, gland, or artery.

buccal Of or pertaining to the inside of the cheek or the gum next to the cheek.

buffer Substance or group of substances that can absorb or release hydrogen ions to correct an acid-base imbalance.

bulbar synchronizing region (BSR) Area in the pons and medial forebrain region releasing serotonin from specialized cells believed to aid in sleep.

bulimia Craving for food, resulting in episodes of continuous eating, followed by periods of guilt and depression.

bundle of His A portion of the cardiac conduction system that arises from the distal portion of the AV node and extends across the AV groove to the top of the intraventricular septum, where it divides into right and left bundle branches.

burnout Popular term for the condition of mental or physical energy depletion after a period of chronic, unrelieved job-related stress sometimes characterized by physical illness.

cachexia Malnutrition marked by weakness and emaciation, usually associated with severe illness.

calorie Amount of heat required to raise 1 gram of water 1° centigrade at atmospheric pressure; a kilocalorie or large calorie, used to represent energy values of food, is 1000 times as large as the small calorie, the unit used in physics to describe energy exchange in the body.

carbohydrates Dietary classification of foods comprising sugars, starches, cellulose, and gum.

carbon monoxide Colorless, odorless, poisonous gas produced by the combustion of carbon or organic fuels.

carcinogen Substance or agent that causes the development or increases the incidence of cancer.

cardiac catheterization A diagnostic procedure in which a catheter is introduced into a large vein, usually of an arm or leg, and threaded through the circulatory system to the heart.

cardiac output Volume of blood expelled by the ventricles of the heart, equal to the amount of blood ejected at each beat, multiplied by the number of beats in the period of time used for computation (usually 1 minute).

cardiopulmonary resuscitation (CPR) Basic emergency procedures for life support consisting of artificial respiration and manual external cardiac massage.

career roles Specific employment positions within nursing.

carotid pulse Rhythmic beating palpated over the carotid artery.

carriers Animals or persons who harbor and spread disease-causing organisms but who do not become ill.

cartilage Nonvascular, supporting connective tissue located mainly in the joints and in the thorax, trachea, larynx, nose, and ear.

cartilaginous joint Slightly movable, highly elastic cartilage that unites bony surfaces.

case management Organized system for delivering health care to an individual client or group of clients across an episode of illness and/or a continuum of care; includes assess-ment and development of a plan of care, coordination of all services, referral, and follow-up; usually assigned to one profes-sional.

cathartics Drugs that act to promote bowel evacuation.

catheterization Introduction of a catheter into a body cavity or organ to inject or remove fluid.

cations Positively charged electrolytes.

center of gravity Midpoint or center of the weight of a body or object.

Centers for Disease Control and Prevention (CDC) Agency of the U.S. government that provides facilities and services for the investigation, identification, prevention, and control of disease.

Centigrade Denotes temperature scale in which 0 degrees is the freezing point of water and 100 degrees is the boiling point of water at sea level; also called Celsius.

central sleep apnea Sleep disorder characterized by the absence of attempts to breathe; person is momentarily unable to move respiratory muscles or maintain airflow through the nose and mouth.

certification A process in which an individual, an institution, or an educational program is evaluated and recognized as meeting certain predetermined standards.

cerumen Yellowish or brownish waxy secretion produced by sweat glands in the external ear.

change-of-shift reports Reports that occur between two scheduled nursing work shifts. Nurses communicate information about their assigned clients to nurses working on the next shift of duty.

channels Method used in the teaching-learning process to present content: visual, auditory, taste, smell. In the communication process, a method used to transmit a message: visual, auditory, touch.

chest percussion Striking of the chest wall with a cupped hand to promote mobilization and drainage of pulmonary secretions.

chest physiotherapy (CPT) Group of therapies used to mobilize pulmonary secretions for expectoration.

chest tube A catheter inserted through the thorax into the chest cavity for removing air or fluid, used following chest or heart surgery or pneumothorax.

chronic illness Illness that persists over a long period of time and affects physical, emotional, intellectual, social, and spiritual functioning.

chyme Viscous, semifluid contents of the stomach present during digestion of a meal, which eventually pass into the intestines.

climacteric Physiological, developmental change that occurs in the male reproductive system between the ages of 45 to 60.

circadian rhythm Repetition of certain physiological phenomena within a 24-hour cycle.

circulating nurse Assistant to the scrub nurse and surgeon whose role is to provide necessary supplies, dispose of soiled instruments and supplies, and keep an accurate count of instruments, needles, and sponges used.

circulatory overload or fluid volume excess Excess of extracellular fluid.

civil law Statutes concerned with protecting a person's rights.

client-centered goal Specific measurable objective designed to reflect the client's highest level of wellness and independence in function.

code of ethics Formal statement that delineates a profession's guidelines for ethical behavior; a code of ethics sets standards or expectations for the professional to achieve.

cognitive learning Acquisition of intellectual skills that encompass behaviors such as thinking, understanding, and evaluating.

collaboration The working together of health team members in the delivery of care to a client or group of clients.

collagen Substance that combines to form the white, glistening, inelastic fibers of tendons, ligaments, and fasciae.

colonized Referring to the establishment of a mass of microorganisms, often nonpathogenic, in or on the body.

common law One source for law that is created by judicial decisions as opposed to those created by legislative bodies (statutory law).

communicable disease Any disease that can be transmitted from one person or animal to another by direct or indirect contact, or by vectors.

communication Ongoing, dynamic series of events that involves the transmission of meaning from sender to receiver.

community-based nursing Nursing care directed toward the health of the community and the interaction of individuals within that community.

complete bed bath Bath in which the entire body of a client is washed in bed.

compliance Person's fulfillment of the prescribed course of treatment.

compress Soft pad of gauze or cloth used to apply heat, cold, or medications to the surface of a body part.

concentration Relative content of a component within a substance or solution.

concrete operation A thought process based on concrete rather than abstract points of reference.

conduction Process in which heat is transferred from one substance to another because of a difference in temperature.

connotative Meaning of a word assumes apart from what it explicitly describes.

constipation Condition characterized by difficulty in passing stool or an infrequent passage of hard stool.

consultation Process in which the help of a specialist is sought to identify ways to handle problems in client management or in the planning and implementing of programs.

contaminated Process by which an object becomes unclean or unsterile.

continuing education Formal educational programs designed to further the knowledge, skills, and professional attitudes of practicing nurses.

contracture Permanent shortening of a muscle and the eventual shortening of associated ligaments and tendons.

convection Transfer of heat through a gas or liquid by the circulation of heated particles.

core temperature Temperature of deep body tissues and organs.

counseling Implementation method that helps the client recognize and manage stress and that facilitates interpersonal relationships between the client and the family, significant others, or the health care team.

crackles Fine bubbling sounds heard on auscultation of the lung; produced by air entering distal airways and alveoli, which contain serous secretions.

credentialing Achieving a predetermined set of standards, such as licensure or certification, establishing that a person or institution has achieved professional recognition in a specific field of health care.

crime Act that violates a law and that may include criminal intent.

criminal law Concerned with acts that threaten society but may involve only an individual.

crisis intervention Use of therapeutic techniques directed toward helping a client resolve a particular and immediate problem.

criteria Standards, principles, or requirements established for accomplishing or evaluating an activity or condition, such as formulating a nursing diagnosis.

crutch gait Gait assumed by a person on crutches by alternately bearing weight on one or both legs and on the crutches.

culture Nonphysical traits, such as values, beliefs, attitudes, and customs, that are shared by a group of people and passed from one generation to the next.

cutaneous stimulation Stimulation of a person's skin to prevent or reduce pain perception. A massage, warm bath, hot and cold therapies, and transcutaneous electric nerve stimula-tion are some ways to reduce pain perception.

cyanosis Bluish discoloration of the skin and mucous membranes caused by an excess of deoxygenated hemoglobin in the blood or a structural defect in the hemoglobin molecule.

data analysis Logical examination of and professional judgment about client assessment data; used in the diagnostic process to derive a nursing diagnosis.

data collection Part of the assessment step of the nursing process when all pertinent subjective and objective information about the client is gathered. Data collection includes the nursing history, physical examination, laboratory data and diagnostic tests, and information from health team members and the client's family and significant others.

data clustering Categorizing of related data into groups.

death Cessation of life as indicated by the absence of heartbeat or respiration. Legally, death is total absence of activity in the brain and central nervous, cardiovascular, and respiratory systems.

debridement Removal of dead tissue from a wound.

decibels Units of measure of the intensity of sound.

defamation of character Communication disseminated about a person that injures his reputation.

defecation Passage of feces from the digestive tract through the rectum.

defining characteristics Related signs and symptoms, or clusters of data that support the nursing diagnosis.

dehiscence Separation of a wound's edges, revealing underlying tissues.

dehydration or fluid volume deficit Excessive loss of water from the body tissues, accompanied by a disturbance of body electrolytes.

delegation The process of assigning another member of the health care team aspects of client care; for example, assigning nurse assistants to bathe a client.

delivery-of-care model System used by nurses in the delegation of authority and responsibility for the direct care of clients.

dementia Irreversible mental state characterized by decreased intellectual function, changes in personality, impaired judgment, and often changes in affect as a result of permanently altered cerebral metabolism.

demography Focusing on the distribution, density, and vital information about a population.

denotative Meaning of a word or phrase shared by individuals who use a common language.

dental caries Abnormal destructive condition in a tooth caused by a complex interaction of food, especially starches and sugars, with bacteria that form dental plaque.

dependent interventions Actions based on the instruction or written orders of another professional.

dermis Sensitive vascular layer of the skin directly below the epidermis; is composed of collagenous and elastic fibrous connective tissues that give the dermis strength and elasticity.

detoxify To remove the toxic quality of a substance; the liver acts to detoxify chemicals in drug compounds.

development Qualitative or observable aspects of the progressive changes one makes in adapting to the environment.

developmental crises Occur when a person is unable to complete the developmental tasks of a psychosocial stage and is therefore unable to continue developing.

diagnostic process Mental steps (data clustering and analysis, problem identification) that follow assessment and lead directly to the formulation of a diagnosis.

diagnostic related groups Group of clients classified to establish a mechanism for health care reimbursement based on length of stay; classification is based on the following variables: primary and secondary diagnosis, comorbidities, primary and secondary procedures, and age.

diaphoresis Secretion of sweat, especially profuse secretion associated with an elevated body temperature, physical exertion, or emotional stress.

diaphragmatic breathing Respiration in which the abdomen moves out while the diaphragm descends on inspiration.

diarrhea Increase in the number of stools and the passage of liquid, unformed feces.

diastole Period of time between contractions of the atria or the ventricles during which blood enters the relaxed chambers.

diffusion Movement of molecules from an area of high concentration to an area of lower concentration.

digestion Breakdown of nutrients by chewing, churning, mixing with fluid, and chemical reactions.

diplopia Double vision caused by an abnormality of the extraocular muscles or nerves that innervate the muscles.

discharge summary Record of the client's remaining problems, future proposed therapy, and need for additional resources before and after returning home.

disinfection Process of destroying all pathogenic organisms, except spores.

disuse osteoporosis Reductions in skeletal mass routinely accompanying immobility or paralysis.

documentation Written entry into the client's medical record of all pertinent information about the client. These entries validate the client's problems and care and exist as a legal record.

dorsalis pedis pulse Rhythmic beating palpated over the dorsalis pedis artery.

dorsiflexion Flexion toward the back.

drainage evacuators Convenient portable units that connect to tubular drains lying within a wound bed and exert a safe, constant, low-pressure vacuum to remove and collect drainage.

drug abuse Use of a chemical substance for nontherapeutic purposes that do not comply with cultural or social standards.

drug allergy Response to a drug, its chemical preservatives, or a metabolite; drug or chemical acts as an antigen, triggering the release of the body's antibodies, which trigger an allergic reaction.

drug interaction When one drug modifies the action of another. A drug may potentiate or diminish the action of other drugs and may alter the way in which another drug is absorbed, metabolized, or eliminated from the body.

drug toxicity Ability of a drug to create poisonous or lethal effects as a result of excessive administration, high dose use, or altered drug metabolism, absorption, and excretion.

durable medical equipment (DME) Equipment leased or sold to clients for use in their homes (for example, wheel-chairs, hospital beds, walkers, canes, etc.).

dysmenorrhea Painful menstruation.

dyspnea Sensation of shortness of breath.

dysrhythmia Deviation from the normal pattern of the heartbeat.

dysuria Painful urination resulting from bacterial infection of the bladder and obstructive conditions of the urethra.

ecchymosis Discoloration of the skin or bruise caused by leakage of blood into subcutaneous tissues as a result of trauma to underlying tissues.

eccrine glands Two types of sweat glands; eccrine glands are present throughout the body and promote cooling by evaporation of their secretions.

echocardiography A diagnostic procedure, which uses ultrasonic waves, for studying the structure and motion of the heart.

edema Abnormal accumulation of fluid in interstitial spaces of tissues.

ego-defense mechanisms Unconscious behaviors that protect a person from emotional stress.

egocentricity Regarding of the self as the center, object, and norm of all experience and having little regard for the needs, interests, ideas, and attitudes of others.

electrocardiogram A graphic record of the electrical activity of the myocardium.

empathy Understanding and acceptance of a person's feelings and the ability to sense the person's private world.

endogenous infections Infections produced within a cell or organism.

endorphins Naturally occurring neuropeptides composed of amino acids and secreted within the central nervous system to reduce pain.

endoscope Instrument used to visualize the interior of body organs and cavities with an endoscope.

endotracheal tube Artificial airway inserted into a client's mouth or nose.

enema Procedure involving introduction of a solution into the rectum for cleansing or therapeutic purposes.

enuresis Involuntary passage of urine; incontinence.

environmental factors Characteristics of a person's physical or social environments that can increase or decrease the person's susceptibility to disease.

enzymes Proteins produced by living cells that catalyze chemical reactions in organic matter.

epidermis Outer layer of the skin that has several thin layers of skin in different stages of maturation; shields and protects the underlying tissues from water loss, mechanical or chemical injury, and penetration by disease-causing microorganisms.

epidural infusion A type of nerve block anesthesia in which an anesthetic is intermittently or continuously injected into the lumbosacral region of the spinal cord.

error of commission Mistake resulting from over-diagnosis or diagnosing a nonexistent health problem.

error of omission Mistake resulting from failure of the nurse to diagnose a health problem.

eschar Scab or dry crust that results from excoriation of the skin.

ethics Principles or standards that govern proper conduct.

ethic of care The delivery of health care based on ethical principles and standards of care.

ethnicity Cultural group's sense of identification associated with the group's common social and cultural heritage.

ethnocentrism Tendency of members of one cultural group to view the members of other cultural groups in terms of the standards of behavior, attitudes, and values of their own group.

eupnea Normal respirations that are quiet, effortless, and rhythmical.

euthanasia Deliberately bringing about the death of a person who has an incurable disease or condition, either actively, by administering a lethal drug, or passively, by withholding treatment and allowing the person to die.

evaluation Determination of the extent to which established client goals have been achieved.

eversion Movement of a limb turning outward from the body.

evisceration Protrusion of visceral organs through a surgical wound.

exacerbations Increases in the seriousness of a disease or disorder as marked by greater intensity in signs or symptoms.

exercise stress test An evaluation of the client's cardiopulmonary endurance during physical activity. An ECG and analysis of respiratory function is usually performed during the test.

exhaustion stage Phase that occurs when the body can no longer resist the stress; when the energy necessary to maintain adaptation is depleted.

exogenous infection Infection originating outside an organ or part.

exophthalmos Abnormal protrusion of one or both eyeballs.

expected outcomes Expected conditions of a client at the end of therapy or of a disease process, including the degree of wellness and the need for continuing care, medications, support, counseling, or education.

expressive aphasia Inability to name common objects or to express simple ideas in words or writing.

extension Movement by certain joints that increases the angle between two adjoining bones.

extracellular fluids Portion of body fluids comprised of the interstitial fluid and blood plasma.

exudate Fluid, cells, or other substances that have been slowly discharged from cells or blood vessels through small pores or breaks in cell membranes.

Fahrenheit Denotes temperature scale in which 32 degrees is the freezing point of water and 212 degrees is the boiling point of water at sea level.

family Group of interacting individuals composing a basic unit of society.

family as client Nursing perspective in which the family is viewed as a unit of interacting members having attributes, functions, and goals separate from those of the individual family members.

family as context Nursing perspective in which the primary focus of care is on an individual within a family.

family functioning Processes families use to achieve their goals.

family health Determined by the effectiveness of the family's structure, the processes that the family uses to meet its goals, and internal and external resources.

family structure Ongoing membership of the family and the pattern of relationships (organization).

febrile Pertaining to or characterized by an elevated body temperature.

fecal impaction Accumulation of hardened fecal material in the rectum or sigmoid colon.

fecal incontinence Inability to control passage of feces and gas from the anus.

feces Waste or excrement from the gastrointestinal tract.

feedback Process in which the output of a given system is returned to the system.

felony Crime of serious nature that carries a penalty of imprisonment or death.

femoral pulse Rhythmic beating palpated over the femoral artery.

fertilization The union of the male and female gametes to form a zygote from which an embryo develops.

fever Elevation in the hypothalamic set-point, so that body temperature is regulated at a higher level.

fibrin Protein product formed from the action of thrombin on fibrinogen in the clotting process.

fissures Cleft or groove on the surface of an organ, often marking division of the organ into parts.

fistula Abnormal passage from an internal organ to the body surface or between two internal organs.

flatus Intestinal gas.

flexion Movement by certain joints that decreases the angle between adjoining bones.

"flight-or-fight" response Set of physiological responses to a stressor that prepares a person to attempt to overcome or avoid stress.

flow sheet Document on which frequent observations or specific measurements are recorded.

fluid overload Excess extracellular fluid volume.

focus charting A charting methodology for structuring progress notes according to the focus of the note, for example, symptoms and nursing diagnosis. Each note includes data, actions, and client response.

Food and Drug Administration (FDA) Federal agency responsible for the enforcement of federal regulations regarding the manufacture and distribution of food, drugs, and cosmetics to ensure protection against the sale of impure or dangerous substances.

food poisoning Toxic processes resulting from the ingestion of a food contaminated by toxic substances or by bacteria-containing toxins.

footboard Board placed perpendicular to the mattress, parallel to and touching the plantar surface of the client's foot, and used to maintain dorsiflexion of the feet.

footdrop An abnormal neuromuscular condition of the lower leg and foot, characterized by an inability to dorsiflex, or evert, the foot.

fracture Breakage of bone caused by violence to the body; disruption of bone tissue continuity.

friction Effects of rubbing or the resistance that a moving body meets from the surface on which it moves; a force that occurs in a direction to oppose movement.

frostbite Traumatic effect of extreme cold on the skin and subcutaneous tissues, first manifested by distinct pallor.

functional health patterns a method for organizing assessment data based on the level of client function in specific areas, for example mobility.

functional nursing system Method of client care delivery in which each staff member is assigned a task that is completed for all clients on the unit.

gait Manner or style of walking, including rhythm, cadence, and speed.

gastrostomy feeding tube The insertion of a feeding tube, through a stoma, into the stomach for the purpose of providing enteral nutrition.

gender identity Individual's sense of being feminine or masculine that develops from infancy.

gender role Individual's behavioral expression of masculinity or femininity. Society's definition of appropriate male or female behaviors.

general adaptation syndrome (GAS) Generalized defense response of the body to stress, consisting of three stages: alarm, resistance, and exhaustion.

general anesthesia Intravenous or inhaled medications that cause the client to lose all sensation and consciousness.

gingiva Gum of the mouth; a mucous membrane with supporting fibrous tissue that overlies the crowns of unerupted teeth and encircles the necks of those teeth that have erupted.

global aphasia Abnormal neurological condition in which language function is defective or absent, affecting the client's ability to understand and to speak.

glomerulus Cluster or collection of capillary vessels within the kidney involved in the initial formation of urine.

goals Desired results of nursing actions, set realistically by the nurse and client as part of the planning stage of the nursing process.

good samaritan laws Legislation enacted in some states to protect health care professionals from liability in rendering emergency aid, unless there is proven willful wrong or gross negligence.

granulation tissue Soft, pink, fleshy projections of tissue that form during the healing process in a wound not healing by primary intention.

grieving process Sequence of affective, cognitive, and physiological states through which the person responds to and finally accepts an irretrievable loss.

guaiac test Test of feces for the presence of occult (hidden) blood.

guided imagery Method of pain control in which the client creates a mental image, concentrates on that image, and gradually becomes less aware of pain.

gurgles Abnormal coarse sounds heard during auscultation of the lung; produced by air entering large mucus-containing airways. Also called rhonchi.

gustatory Pertaining to the sense of taste.

hand-wrist splints Splints individually molded for the client to maintain proper alignment of the thumb, slight adduction of the wrist, and slight dorsiflexion.

hand rolls A roll of cloth that keeps the thumb slightly adducted and in opposition to the fingers.

Harris flush A return flow enema that helps to expel flatus.

Haustral contractions Segmental contractions of the colon, creating an increase in surface area for absorption.

healing Holistic or three-dimensional phenomenon that results in the restoration of balance or harmony to the body, mind, and spirit.

health Dynamic state in which an individual adapts to his or her internal and external environments so that there is a state of physical, emotional, intellectual, social, and spiritual well-being.

health behaviors Activities through which a person maintains, attains, or regains good health and prevents illness.

health belief Client's personal beliefs about levels of wellness, which can motivate or impede participation in changing risk factors, participating in care, and selecting care options.

health belief model Conceptual framework that describes a person's health behavior as an expression of his or her health beliefs.

health care problems Any conditions or dysfunctions that the client experiences as a result of illness or treatment of an illness.

health care team All those people, departments, and ancillary services that collectively render care and services to the client.

health history Subjective and objective data about the client's prior health status gathered by the nurse during the interview.

health promotion Activities directed toward maintaining or enhancing the health and well-being of clients.

health-illness continuum model Scale by means of which a person's level of health can be described, ranging from high-level wellness to severe illness. The scale takes into account risk factors.

heat stroke Continued exposure to extreme heat raising the core body temperature to 47° C (105° F) or higher.

hematemesis Vomiting of blood indicating upper gastrointestinal bleeding.

hematocrit Measure of the packed cell volume of red blood cells, expressed as a percentage of the total blood volume.

hematoma Collection of blood trapped in the tissues of the skin or an organ.

hematuria Abnormal presence of blood in the urine.

hemolysis Breakdown of red blood cells and release of hemoglobin that may occur following administration of hypotonic intravenous solutions, causing swelling and rupture of erythrocytes.

hemoptysis Coughing up blood from the respiratory tract.

hemorrhoids Permanent dilation and engorgement of veins within the lining of the rectum.

hemostasis Termination of bleeding by mechanical or chemical means or by the coagulation process of the body.

hemothorax Accumulation of blood and fluid in the pleural cavity between the parietal and visceral pleurae.

heritage consistency Theoretical model that assesses a client's acculturation to a new culture on a continuum.

hernias Protrusions of an organ through an abnormal opening in the muscle wall of the cavity that surrounds it.

high-level wellness model Theory of health as a state in which all aspects of a person's functioning are balanced, purposeful, and directed toward attaining full potential.

hirsutism Excessive body hair in a masculine distribution caused by heredity, hormonal dysfunction, or medication.

Holter monitor A device for making prolonged electrocardiograph recordings on a portable recorder while the client continues normal daily activities.

home health care Professional and paraprofessional services and equipment provided to clients and families in their place of residence for purposes of health promotion and maintenance, client and family education, illness prevention, diagnosis and treatment of disease, and palliation and rehabilitation.

home health care agencies Organizations providing skilled, intermittent health care services usually in the form of nursing, home care aides, or rehabilitative therapies.

home IV therapies The delivery of intravenous (IV) therapy to the client in the home, usually provided by professional nurses through home care agencies.

homeostasis State of relative constance in the internal environment of the body, maintained naturally by physiological adaptive mechanisms.

hope Confident, yet uncertain, expectation of achieving a future goal.

hospice System of family-centered care designed to help terminally ill persons be comfortable and maintain a satisfactory life-style throughout the terminal phase of their illness.

hospice care Philosophy of client care that advocates physical and psychosocial support for palliative care of persons in the last months of an incurable illness so that life can be lived as fully and comfortably as possible.

host Elements of the agent-host environment model of health and illness. A host is a person or group who, because of risk factors, may be susceptible to disease or illness.

hydrostatic pressure A pressure caused by a liquid.

hypercapnia Greater than normal amounts of carbon dioxide in the blood; also called hypercarbia.

hypercarbia Greater than normal amounts of carbon dioxide in the blood; also called hypercapnia

hyperextension A position of maximal extension of a joint.

hyperglycemia Elevated serum glucose levels.

hypertension Disorder characterized by an elevated blood pressure persistently exceeding 150/90 mm Hg.

hyperthermia Situation in which body temperature exceeds the set-point.

hypertonic The situation in which one solution has a greater concentration of solute than another solution; therefore the first solution exerts greater osmotic pressure.

hyperventilation Respiratory rate in excess of that required to maintain normal carbon dioxide levels in the body tissues.

hypervolemia Increase in the amount of fluid in the circulating blood volume.

hypoglycemia Reduced serum glucose levels.

hypotension Abnormal lowering of blood pressure, which is inadequate for normal perfusion and oxygenation of tissues.

hypothalamus Portion of the diencephalon of the brain that activates, controls, and integrates the peripheral autonomic nervous system, endocrine processes, and many bodily functions such as body temperature, sleep, and appetite.

hypothermia Abnormal lowering of body temperature below 93° F or 35° C, usually caused by prolonged exposure to cold.

hypotonic A situation in which one solution has a smaller concentration of solute than another solution; therefore the first solution exerts less osmotic pressure.

hypoventilation Respiratory rate insufficient to prevent carbon dioxide retention.

hypovolemia An abnormally low circulating blood volume.

hypoxia Inadequate cellular oxygenation that may result from a deficiency in the delivery or use of oxygen at the cellular level.

iatrogenic infection Infection caused by a treatment or diagnostic procedure.

identity Component of self-concept—one's persisting consciousness of being oneself, separate and distinct from others.

idiosyncratic reactions An individual sensitivity to effects of a drug caused by inherited or other bodily constitution factors.

illness Abnormal process in which any aspect of a person's functioning is diminished or impaired as compared with his or her previous condition.

illness behavior Ways in which people monitor their bodies, define and interpret their symptoms, take remedial actions, and use the health care system.

illness prevention Health education programs or activities directed toward protecting clients from threats or potential threats to health and toward minimizing risk factors.

immobility inability to move about freely, caused by any condition in which movement is impaired or therapeutically restricted.

immunity The quality of being insusceptible to or unaffected by a particular disease or condition.

implementation Initiation and completion of the nursing actions necessary to help the client achieve health care goals.

in-service education Instruction or training provided by an agency or institution to nurses practicing within the agency or institution.

incentive spirometry Method of encouraging voluntary deep breathing by providing visual feedback to clients of the inspiratory volume they have achieved.

incident report Confidential document that describes any client accident while the person is on the premises of a health care agency.

independent interventions Actions pertaining to certain aspects of professional nursing practice that are encompassed by applicable licensure and law and require no supervision or direction from others.

induration Hardening of a tissue, particularly the skin, because of edema or inflammation.

infancy Stage of life from 1 month to 1 year of age

infertility Man's, woman's, or couple's involuntary inability to conceive.

infiltration Dislodging an intravenous catheter or needle from a vein into the subcutaneous space.

inflammation Protective response of body tissues to irritation or injury.

inflammatory response Localized response to trauma to prevent the spread of infection and to promote wound healing.

informed consent Process of obtaining permission from a client to perform a specific test or procedure, after describing all risks, side effects, and benefits.

infusion Introduction of fluid into the vein, giving intravenous fluid over time.

infusion pump Device that delivers a measured amount of fluid over a period of time.

inhalers Aerosol sprays, mists, or powders that penetrate lung airways, which the client inhales through his or her mouth.

injection Parenteral administration of medication; four major sites of injection: subcutaneous, intramuscular, intravenous, and intradermal.

insomnia Condition characterized by chronic inability to sleep or remain asleep through the night.

inspection Method of physical examination by which the client is visually systematically examined for appearance, structure, function, and behavior.

instillation To cause to enter drop by drop, or very slowly.

integument Skin and its appendages: hair, nails, and sweat and sebaceous glands.

interdependent interventions Actions carried out by the nurse in collaboration with another health care professional.

interpersonal communication Exchange of information between two persons or among persons in a small group.

interstitial fluid Fluid that fills the spaces between most of the cells of the body and provides a substantial portion of the liquid environment of the body.

interventions Actions performed to prevent harm to a client or to improve the mental, emotional, physical, or social function of a client.

interview Organized, systematic conversation with the client designed to obtain pertinent health-related subjective information.

intimate zone Personal space between client and care giver; 18 inches or less.

intonation Rise and fall in pitch of the voice in speech.

intracellular fluid Liquid within the cell membrane.

intractable pain Pain not easily relieved, such as that which occurs with some types of cancer.

intradermal Injection given between layers of the skin, into the dermis. Injections are given at a 5- to 15-degree angle.

intramuscular (IM) Injections given into muscle tissue. Intramuscular route provides a fast rate of absorption that is related to the muscle's greater vascularity. Injections are given at a 90-degree angle.

intrapersonal communication Communication that occurs within an individual, for example, a person "talks with himself" silently or forms an idea in his or her own mind.

intravascular Fluid contained within the vessels of the circulatory system.

intravenous Injection directly into the bloodstream. Action of the drug begins immediately when given intravenously.

invasion of privacy Release of personal information (e.g., health records, financial statements, or employment history) without the person's permission.

inversion Movement of a limb by turning inward toward the body.

irrigation Process of washing out a body cavity or wounded area with a stream of fluid.

ischemia Decreased blood supply to a body part such as skin tissue, or to an organ such as the heart.

isolation Separation of a client from other clients to prevent the spread of infection or to protect the client from irritating environmental factors.

isometric Related to increased muscle tension without muscle shortening.

isometric contraction Increased muscle tension without muscle shortening.

isotonic The situation in which two solutions have the same concentration of solute; therefore both solutions exert the same osmotic pressure.

isotonic contraction Increased muscle tension resulting in muscle contraction and muscle shortening.

jejunal feeding tube The insertion of a feeding tube, usually by the nasal route, and allowing the tube to pass into the client's jejunum for the purpose of providing enteral nutrition.

joint contracture Abnormal and usually permanent condition of a joint, characterized by flexion and fixation and caused by disuse, atrophy, and shortening of muscle fibers.

joints Connections between bones; classified according to structure and degree of mobility.

Kardex Trade name for card-filing system that allows quick reference to the particular need of the client for certain aspects of nursing care.

kinesthesic Relating to perception of position of body parts, weight, and movement.

Korotkoff sounds Sounds heard during the taking of blood pressure using a sphygmomanometer and stethoscope.

laceration Torn, jagged wound.

lactation Process and period in which the mother produces milk for a child.

learning Acquisition of new knowledge and skills as a result of reinforcement, practice, and experience.

learning objective Written statement that describes the behavior a teacher expects from an individual following a learning activity.

legalism An often strict and literal adherence to law or code.

leukocytosis Abnormal increase in the number of circulating white blood cells.

leukoplakia Thick, white patches observed on oral mucous membranes.

libel Written false statement about a person that may injure his or her reputation.

licensed practical or vocational nurse Person trained in basic nursing techniques and direct client care who practices under the supervision of a registered nurse.

life-saving measure Independent, dependent, or interdependent nursing intervention that is implemented when a client's physiological or psychological status is threatened.

lipids Compounds that are insoluble in water but soluble in organic solvents.

living wills Instruments by which a dying person makes wishes known.

local adaptation syndrome (LAS) Localized response of tissue, an organ, or a system that occurs as a direct reaction to stress.

local anesthesia Loss of sensation at the desired site of action.

loss Absence of a significant other, object, or state of health to which the person must adapt through the grieving process.

lymphocyte One type of leukocyte developing in the bone marrow; responsible for synthesizing antibodies and T cells that attack antigens.

maceration Softening and breaking down of skin from prolonged exposure to moisture.

macrophages Large phagocytic cells of the reticuloendothelial system.

malignant hyperthermia An autosomal dominant trait characterized by often fatal hyperthermia in affected people exposed to certain anesthetic agents.

malnutrition Any nutritional disorder such as unbalanced, insufficient, or excessive diet or impaired absorption, assimilation, or utilization of food.

malpractice Injurious or unprofessional actions that harm another.

malpractice insurance A type of insurance to protect the health care professional. In case of a malpractice claim, the insurance pays the award to the plaintiff.

masticate To chew or tear food with the teeth while it becomes mixed with saliva.

maturational loss Loss, usually of an aspect of self, resulting from the normal changes of growth and development.

medical asepsis Procedures used to reduce the number of microorganisms and prevent their spread.

medical diagnosis Formal statement of the disease entity or illness made by the physician.

medical record Client's chart; a legal document.

melena Abnormal black, sticky stool containing digested blood; indicative of gastrointestinal bleeding.

menarche Onset of a girl's first menstruation.

menstrual cycle Recurring cycle of changes in the ovaries, and hormone levels, involving the development of an egg, ovulation, and implantation of the egg or sloughing of the corpus luteum and lining. The cycle can be divided into proliferative and secretory phases by uterine changes or follicular, ovulation, and luteal phases based on ovarian activity.

message Information sent or expressed by sender in the communication process.

metabolic acidosis Abnormal condition of high hydrogen ion concentration in the extracellular fluid caused by either a primary increase in hydrogen ions or a decrease in bicarbonate.

metabolic alkalosis Abnormal condition characterized by the significant loss of acid from the body or by increased levels of bicarbonate.

metabolism Aggregate of all chemical processes that take place in living organisms, resulting in growth, generation of energy, elimination of wastes, and other functions concerned with the distribution of nutrients in the blood after digestion.

metacommunication system Dependent not only on what is said but also on the relationship to the other person involved in the interaction. It is a message that conveys the sender's attitude toward the self and the message and the attitudes, feelings, and intentions toward the listener.

metered dose inhaler A device designed to deliver a measured dose of an inhalation drug.

metric system Logically organized decimal system of measurement; metric units can easily be converted and computed through simple multiplication and division. Each basic unit of measurement is organized into units of 10.

microorganisms Microscopic entities capable of carrying on living processes, such as bacteria, viruses, and fungi.

micturition Urination; act of passing or expelling urine voluntarily through the urethra.

middle adulthood Transitional stage between young adult and older adult.

milliequivalent per liter (mEq/L) Number of grams of a specific electrolyte dissolved in 1 liter of plasma.

mind-body interaction Belief that a person's state of mind can have a negative or beneficial effect on level of health.

minerals Inorganic elements essential to the body because of their role as catalysts in biochemical reactions.

misdemeanor Lesser crime than a felony; the penalty is usually a fine or imprisonment for less than 1 year.

mobility Person's ability to move about freely.

modern approach Present-day beliefs and practices provided within the American, or Western, health care delivery system.

monamine oxidase inhibitor A heterogenous group of drugs used primarily to treat depression.

moral development The acquisition of moral principles as an individual goes through growth and development, crises, life experiences, etc.

moral reasoning Decision making based or moral principles and standards.

morals Personal conviction that something is absolutely right or wrong in all situations.

morning care Hygienic care typically offered to clients in the morning (for example, toileting assistance, bath, oral care, and hair care).

motivation Internal impulse that causes a person to take action.

mourning A psychological process of reaction activated by an individual to assist in overcoming a great personal loss.

multicultural nursing A framework for broadening nurses' understanding of health-related beliefs, practices, and issues that are part of the lived experiences of people from diverse cultural backgrounds.

murmurs Blowing or whooshing sounds created by changes in blood flow through the heart or by abnormalities in valve closure.

muscle tone Normal state of balanced muscle tension.

mutual goal setting Establishing health care outcomes by both the nurse and the client; client being the individual, family, or group.

myocardial infarction Necrosis of a portion of cardiac muscle caused by obstruction in a coronary artery.

NANDA North American Nursing Diagnosis Association, organized in 1973, which formally identifies, develops, and classifies nursing diagnoses.

narcolepsy Syndrome involving sudden sleep attacks that a person cannot inhibit; uncontrollable desire to sleep may occur several times during a day.

narcotic Drug substance, derived from opium or produced synthetically, that alters perception of pain and that with repeated use may result in physical and psychological dependence.

nasal cannula A device for delivering oxygen by way of two small tubes inserted into the nares.

nasogastric tube Tube passed into the stomach through the nose for the purpose of emptying the stomach of its contents or for delivering medication and/or nourishment.

nebulization Process of adding moisture to inspired air by the addition of water droplets.

necrotic Of or pertaining to the death of tissue in response to disease or injury.

negative nitrogen balance Condition occurring when the body excretes more nitrogen than it takes in.

negligence Careless act of omission or commission that results in injury to another.

neonate Stage of life from birth to 1 month of age.

nephrons Structural and functional units of the kidney containing renal glomeruli and tubules.

neurotransmitter Chemical that transfers the electrical impulse from the nerve fiber to the muscle fiber.

nitrogen balance Relationship between the nitrogen taken into the body, usually as food, and the nitrogen excreted from the body in urine and feces. Most of the body's nitrogen is incorporated into protein.

nociceptors Somatic and visceral free nerve endings of thinly myelinated and unmyelinated fibers. They usually react to tissue injury but may also be excited by endogenous chemical substances.

nocturnal enuresis Incontinence of urine during the night.

noise pollution Noise level in an environment when it becomes uncomfortable to its inhabitants.

nonREM sleep Abbreviation for nonrapid eye movement, which occurs during the first four stages of normal sleep.

nonverbal communication Communication using expressions, gestures, body posture, and positioning rather than words.

normal reactive hyperemia Hyperemia over a pressure site lasting 1 hour or less following removal of pressure; surrounding skin does blanch.

normal sinus rhythm (NSR) The wave pattern on an electrocardiogram that indicates normal conduction of an electrical impulse through the myocardium.

nosocomial infections Infections acquired during hospitalization or stay in a health care facility.

NPUAP National pressure ulcer advisory panel.

nurse practice acts Statutes enacted by the legislature of any of the states or by the appropriate officers of the districts or possessions that describe and define the scope of nursing practice.

nursing care plan Written outline, or schema, that includes identification of the client's expected outcomes for problem resolution and specific interventions and nursing orders. The care plan, a legal document that is part of the client's chart, documents and ensures use of the nursing process.

nursing diagnosis Formal statement of an actual or potential health problem that nurses can legally and independently treat. The second step of the nursing process during which the client's actual and potential unhealthy responses to an illness or condition are identified.

nursing health history Data collected about a client's present level of wellness, changes in life patterns, sociocultural role, and mental and emotional reactions to illness.

nursing intervention Nursing action performed to prevent harm from occurring to a client or to improve the mental, emotional, physical, or social function of a client.

nursing process Systematic problem-solving method by which nurses individualize care for each client. The five steps of the nursing process are assessment, diagnosis, planning, implementation, and evaluation.

nutrients Foods that contain elements necessary for body function, including water, carbohydrates, proteins, fats, vitamins, and minerals.

nystagmus Involuntary, rhythmic movements of the eyes; the oscillations may be horizontal, vertical, rotatory, or mixed. May be indicative of vestibular, neurological, or vascular disease.

obesity Abnormal increase in the proportion of fat cells, mainly in the viscera and subcutaneous tissues of the body.

objective data Information that can be observed by others; free of feelings, perceptions, prejudices.

obstructive sleep apnea Temporary cessation of airflow (apnea) but with continuation of chest and abdominal movements; occurs while a person is sleeping.

older adulthood Stage of life beyond middle adulthood.

olfactory Pertaining to the sense of smell.

oncotic pressure The total influence of the protein on the osmotic activity of plasma fluid.

operating room (1) A room in a health care facility in which surgical procedures requiring anesthesia are performed; (2) *informal* a suite of rooms or an area in a health care facility in which patients are prepared for surgery, undergo surgical procedures, and recover from the anesthetic procedures required for the surgery.

ophthalmic Drugs given into the eye, in the form of either eye drops or ointments.

oral hygiene Condition or practice of maintaining the tissues and structures of the mouth.

organic brain syndrome Any psychological or behavioral abnormality associated with transient or permanent brain dysfunction caused by a disturbance of the physiological functioning of brain tissue.

orthopnea Abnormal condition in which a person must sit or stand up to breathe comfortably.

orthostatic hypotension Abnormally low blood pressure occurring when a person stands up.

osmolality The concentration or osmotic pressure of a solution expressed in osmols or milliosmols per kilogram of water.

osmoreceptors Receptors that are sensitive to fluid concentration in the blood plasma and regulate the secretion of antidiuretic hormone.

osmosis Movement of a pure solvent through a semipermeable membrane from a solution with a lower solute concentration to one with a higher solute concentration.

osmotic pressure Drawing power for water, which depends on the number or molecules in the solution.

ostomy Surgical procedure in which an opening is made into the abdominal wall to allow the passage of intestinal contents from the bowel (colostomy) or urine from the bladder (urostomy).

ototoxicity Having a harmful effect on the eighth cranial (auditory) nerve or the organs of hearing and balance.

outcome indicators Condition of a client at the end of treatment, including the degree of wellness and the need for continuing care, medication, support, counseling, or education.

outpatient Client who has not been admitted to a hospital but receives treatments in a clinic or facility associated with the hospital.

oximeter, oximetry A device used to measure oxyhemoglobin in the blood.

oxygen saturation The amount of hemoglobin fully saturated with hemoglobin, given as a percent value.

pain Subjective, unpleasant sensation caused by noxious stimulation of sensory nerve endings.

palliative Relating to treatment designed to relieve or reduce intensity of uncomfortable symptoms but not to produce a cure.

pallor Unnatural paleness or absence of color in the skin.

palpation Method of physical examination whereby the fingers or hands of the examiner are applied to the client's body for the purpose of feeling body parts underlying the skin.

palpitations Bounding or racing of the heart associated with normal emotions or a heart disorder.

parainsomnias Group of sleep disorders, including somnambulism, night terrors, and nocturnal enuresis.

parallel play A form of play among a group of children, primarily toddlers, in which each one engages in an independent activity that is similar but not influenced by or shared with the others.

parasite Organism living in or on another organism and obtaining nourishment from it.

parenteral administration Giving medication by a route other than the gastrointestinal tract.

partial bed bath Bath in which body parts that might cause the client discomfort if left unbathed (that is, face, hands, axillary areas, back, and perineum) are washed in bed.

parturition The process of giving birth.

passive range of motion (ROM) The range of movement through which a joint is moved with assistance.

passive strategies of health promotion Activities that involve the client as the recipient of actions by health care professionals.

pathogens Microorganisms capable of producing disease.

pathological fractures Fractures resulting from weakened bone tissue; frequently caused by osteoporosis or neoplasms.

patient-controlled analgesia (PCA) Drug delivery system that allows clients to self-administer analgesic medications when they want.

perception Person's mental image or concept of elements in his or her environment, including information gained through the senses.

percussion Method of physical examination whereby the location, size, and density of a body part is determined by the tone obtained from the striking of short, sharp taps of the fingers.

perfusion (1) Passage of a fluid through a specific organ or an area of the body. (2) Therapeutic measure whereby a drug intended for an isolated part of the body is introduced via the bloodstream.

perineal care Procedure prescribed for cleaning the genital and anal areas as part of the daily bath or after various obstetrical and gynecological procedures.

perioperative nursing Refers to the role of the operating room nurse during the preoperative, intraoperative, and postoperative phases of surgery.

peripheral Pertains to the outside, surface, or surrounding area of an organ, structure, or field of vision.

peristalsis Rhythmic contractions of the intestine that propel gastric contents through the length of the gastrointestinal tract.

personal space Culturally influenced set of attitudes and behaviors related to one's use of the physical space about oneself.

pharmacokinetics Study of how drugs enter the body, reach their site of action, are metabolized, and exit from the body.

phlebitis Inflammation of a vein.

photophobia Abnormal sensitivity of the eyes to light.

physical examination Assessment of the client's body using the techniques of inspection, auscultation, palpation, and percussion for the purpose of determining physical abnormalities.

PIE note Problem-oriented medical record; the four interdisciplinary sections are the data base, problem list, care plan, and progress notes.

pigmentation Organic coloring material, such as melanin, that gives color to the skin.

placebo Dosage form that contains no pharmacologically active ingredients but may relieve pain through psychological effects.

planning The process of designing interventions to achieve the goals and outcomes of health care delivery.

plantar flexion A toe-down motion of the foot at the ankle.

pleural friction rub Adventitious lung sound caused by an inflamed parietal and visceral pleura rubbing together on inspiration.

PM care Routine hygiene care performed before bedtime.

pneumothorax Collection of air or gas in the pleural space.

point of maximal impulse (PMI) Point where the heartbeat can most easily be palpated through the chest wall.

poison Any substance that impairs health or destroys life when ingested, inhaled, or absorbed by the body in relatively small amounts.

poison control center One of a network of facilities that provides information regarding all aspects of poisoning or intoxication, maintains records of their occurrence, and refers clients to treatment centers.

pollutant A harmful chemical or waste material discharged into the water or atmosphere.

polysomnogram Monitoring device that involves placement of electrodes on the scalp, face, chin, and legs to measure brain waves, eye movements, and muscle activity; used to diagnose sleep disorders.

popliteal pulse Pulse of the popliteal artery, palpated behind the knee of a person lying prone with the knee flexed.

postanesthesia care unit An area adjoining the operating room to which surgical clients are taken while still under anesthesia.

posterior tibial pulse Pulse of the posterior tibial artery, palpated on the medial aspect of the ankle, just posterior to the prominence of the ankle bone.

postural drainage Use of positioning along with percussion and vibration to drain secretions from specific segments of the lungs and bronchi into the trachea.

postural hypotension Abnormally low blood pressure occurring when an individual assumes the standing posture; also called orthostatic hypotension.

potential problems Status placed before a nursing diagnosis statement when the problem does not yet actually exist but is likely to occur unless preventive action is taken; written when high-risk factors associated with the problem exist.

preload The volume of blood in the ventricles at the end of diastole, immediately before ventricular contraction.

prenatal care The health care provided the mother and fetus before childbirth.

preoperational thought Children can think about things not physically present by using mental representations but are limited by their inability to use logic.

preoperative teaching Instruction regarding a client's anticipated surgery and recovery given before surgery. Instruction includes, but is not limited to, dietary and activity restrictions, anticipated assessment activities, postoperative procedures, and pain relief measures.

prescriptions Written directions for a therapeutic agent (e.g., medication, drugs).

pressure ulcer Inflammation, sore, or ulcer in the skin over a bony prominence.

preventive nursing actions Nursing actions directed toward preventing illness and promoting health to avoid the need for primary, secondary, or tertiary health care.

primary intention Primary union of the edges of a wound, progressing to complete scar formation without granulation.

primary nursing system A method of nursing practice in which the client's care is managed, for the duration, by one nurse, who directs and coordinates other nurses and health care personnel. When on duty the primary nurse cares for the client directly.

primary preventive care First contact in a given episode of illness that leads to a decision regarding a course of action to prevent worsening of the health problem.

prioritization Act of listing nursing diagnoses in their order of importance of client health and well-being.

private duty agencies Organizations that provide professional and paraprofessional home health care services on a continuous basis.

problem Question proposed for solution or consideration.

problem identification One of the steps of the diagnostic process in which the client's health care problem is recognized as a result of data analysis based on professional knowledge and experience.

problem-oriented medical record (POR or POMR) Method of recording data about the health status of a client that fosters a collaborative problem-solving approach by all members of the health care team.

productive cough A sudden expulsion of air from the lungs that effectively removes sputum from the respiratory tract and helps clear the airways.

professionalism Conduct or qualities that characterize or mark a professional person.

progress notes Notes made by a nurse and physician that describe the client's condition and the treatments given or planned. Progress notes may follow the problem-oriented medical record format.

prolapse Falling, sinking, or sliding of an organ from its normal position or location in the body, as a prolapsed uterus.

pronation Position of the hand in which the palm of the hand faces downward and backward.

prostaglandins Potent hormone-like substances that act in exceedingly low doses on target organs. They can be used to treat asthma and gastric hyperacidity.

protein Any of a large group of naturally occurring, complex, organic nitrogenous compounds. Each is composed of large combinations of amino acids containing the elements carbon, hydrogen, nitrogen, oxygen, usually sulfur, and occasionally phosphorus, iron, iodine, or other essential constituents of living cells. Protein is the major source of building material for muscles, blood, skin, hair, nails, and the internal organs.

proteinuria Presence in the urine of abnormally large quantities of protein, usually albumin. Persistent proteinuria is usually a sign of renal disease or renal complications of another disease, or hypertension or heart failure.

protocol Written and approved plan specifying the procedures to be followed during an assessment or in providing treatment.

psychomotor learning Acquisition of ability to perform motor skills.

ptosis Abnormal condition of one or both upper eyelids in which the eyelid droops, caused by weakness of the levator muscle or paralysis of the third cranial nerve.

ptyalin A digestive enzyme secreted by the salivary glands.

puberty Developmental period of emotional and physical changes, including the development of secondary sex characteristics and the onset of menstruation and ejaculation.

puerperium Period of approximately 6 weeks after childbirth during which the woman's reproductive system is in transition to the nonpregnant state.

pulmonary function test A procedure for determining the capacity of the lungs to exchange oxygen and carbon dioxide efficiently.

pulse deficit Condition that exists when the radial pulse is less than the ventricular rate as auscultated at the apex or seen on an electrocardiogram. The condition indicates a lack of peripheral perfusion for some of the heart contractions.

pulse pressure The difference between the systolic and diastolic pressures, normally 30 to 40 mmHg.

Purkinje network A complex network of muscle fibers that spread through the right and left ventricles of the heart and carry the impulses that contract those chambers almost simultaneously.

pursed-lip breathing Deep inspiration followed by prolonged expiration through pursed lips.

pyrexia Abnormal elevation of the temperature of the body above 37° C (98.6° F) because of disease. Same as fever.

pyrogens Substances that cause a rise in body temperature, as in the case of bacterial toxins.

quality assurance Evaluation of nursing services provided and the results achieved as compared with accepted standards.

quality improvement The monitoring and evaluation of processes and outcomes in health care or any other business to identify opportunities for improvement.

radial pulse Pulse of the radial artery palpated at the wrist over the radius. The radial pulse is the one most often taken.

radiation A method of temperature regulation used by the body to lower body temperature.

range of motion The range of movement of a joint, from maximum extension to maximum flexion, as measured in degrees of a circle.

rapid eye movement (REM) sleep Stage of sleep in which dreaming and rapid eye movements are prominent; important for mental restoration.

Raza-Latina A popular term used as a reference group name for people of Latin-American descent.

reaction Component of the pain experience that may include both physiological responses such as in the general adaptation syndrome and behavioral responses.

reactive hyperemia Condition characterized by an increased blood flow to part of the body, as in the inflammatory response, local relaxation of arterioles, or obstruction of the outflow of blood from an area.

reality orientation Therapeutic modality for restoring an individual's sense of the present.

receiver Person to whom message is sent during the communication process.

reception Neurophysiological components of the pain experience, in which nervous system receptors receive painful stimuli and transmit them through peripheral nerves to the spinal cord and brain.

receptive aphasia Abnormal neurological condition in which language function is defective because of an injury to certain areas of the cerebral cortex; specifically language is not understood.

recommended daily allowances (RDAs) Suggested or recommended amounts of various nutrients used in planning diets.

record Written form of communication that permanently documents information relevant to health care management.

referent Factor that motivates a person to communicate with another individual.

reflex pain response Reflected, involuntary withdrawal of a body part away from a noxious or painful stimulus.

refractive error Defect in the ability of the lens of the eye to focus light, such as occurs in nearsightedness and farsightedness.

regional anesthesia Loss of sensation in an area of the body supplied by sensory nerve pathways.

registered nurse Health care professional who has completed a course of study at an accredited school of nursing and has passed a licensure examination administered by NCLEX or the Canadian Nurses' Association Testing Service.

regression A return to an earlier developmental stage or behavior.

regulatory agencies Local, state, province, or national agencies that inspect and certify health care agencies as meeting specified standards. These agencies can also determine the amount of reimbursement for health care delivered.

reinforcement Provision of a contingent response to a learner's behavior that increases the probability of the behavior recurring.

related factor Any condition or event that accompanies or is linked with the client's health care problem.

relative humidity Amount of moisture in the air as compared with the maximum amount that the air could contain at the same temperature.

relaxation Act of being relaxed or less tense.

religious Relating to specific practices, rites, and rituals of one's professed religion.

reminiscence Recalling the past for the purpose of assigning new meaning to past experiences.

remissions Partial or complete disappearances of the clinical and subjective characteristics of chronic or malignant disease; remission may be spontaneous or the result of therapy.

renal calculi Calcium stones in the renal pelvis.

report Transfer of information from the nurses on one shift to the nurses on the following shift. Report may also be given by one of the members of the nursing team to another health care provider, for example, physician or therapist.

residual urine Volume of urine remaining in the bladder after a normal voiding; the bladder normally is almost completely empty after micturition.

resistance stage Third stage of the stress response when the person attempts to adapt to the stressor. The body stabilizes, hormone levels stabilize, and heart rate, blood pressure, and cardiac output return to normal.

respiratory acidosis Abnormal condition characterized by increased arterial carbon dioxide concentration, excess carbonic acid, and increased hydrogen ion concentration.

respiratory alkalosis Abnormal condition characterized by decreased arterial carbon dioxide concentration and decreased hydrogen ion concentration.

respite care Short-term health services to the dependent older adult either in his or her home or in an institutional setting.

responsibility Carrying out duties associated with a particular role.

restraints Devices to aid in the immobilization of a client or client's extremity.

reticular activating system (RAS) Group of specialized nerve cells located in the brainstem, upper spinal cord, and cerebral cortex.

rhonchi Abnormal lung sound auscultated when the client's airways are obstructed with thick secretions.

risk factor Any internal or external variable that makes a person or group more vulnerable to illness or an unhealthy event.

role Set of behaviors by means of which a person participates in a social group.

sagittal plane Line that passes through the body from front to back, dividing the body into left and right sides.

school-age A developmental stage referring to children between toddler and adolescence.

scientific rationale Reason, based on supporting literature, why a specific nursing action was chosen.

scintigraphy A diagnostic technique that produces a photographic recording that shows the distribution and intensity of radioactivity in various tissues and organs after the administration of a radiopharmaceutical.

scrub nurse Registered nurse or operating room technician who assists surgeons during operations.

sebum Normal secretion of the sebaceous glands of the skin; when combined with sweat, forms a moist, oily, acidic film that protects the skin from drying.

secondary intention Wound closure in which the edges are separated, granulation tissue develops to fill the gap, and finally, epithelium grows in over the granulation, producing a larger scar than results with primary intention.

secondary preventive care Level of preventive medicine that focuses on early diagnosis, use of referral services, and rapid initiation of treatment to stop the progress of disease processes.

segmentation Alternating contraction and relaxation of gastrointestinal mucosa.

self-concept Complex, dynamic integration of conscious and unconscious feelings, attitudes, and perceptions about one's identity, physical being, worth, and roles; how a person perceives and defines self.

self-esteem Feeling of self-worth characterized by feelings of achievement, adequacy, self-confidence, and usefulness.

sender Person who initiates interpersonal communication by conveying a message.

sensorimotor period The development phase of childhood, encompassing the period from birth to 2 years of age.

sensory deficit Defect in the function of one or more of the senses, resulting in visual, auditory, or olfactory impairments.

sensory deprivation State in which stimulation to one or more of the senses is lacking, resulting in impaired sensory perception.

sensory overload State in which stimulation to one or more of the senses is so excessive that the brain disregards or does not meaningfully respond to stimuli.

serum half-life Time needed for excretion processes to lower the serum drug concentration by half.

sexual dysfunction Inability or difficulty in sexual functioning caused by physiological or psychological factors or both.
sexual orientation Clear, persistent erotic preference for a person of one sex or the other.
sexual response cycle Phases of biological sexual response: excitement, plateau, orgasm, and resolution as defined by Masters and Johnson.
sexuality "A function of the total personality . . . concerned with the biological, psychological, sociological, spiritual and culture variables of life . . ." (Sex Information and Education Council of the United States, 1980).
shearing force Friction exerted when a person is moved or repositioned in bed by being pulled or allowed to slide down in bed.
shivering A process used by the body to raise body temperature.
side rails Bars positioned along the sides of the length of the bed or stretcher to reduce the client's risk of falling.
situational crisis Crisis occurring suddenly in response to a specific external event or conflict.
situational loss Loss of a person, thing, or quality resulting from a change in a life situation, including changes related to illness, body image, environment, and death.
sitz bath Bath in which only the hips or buttocks are immersed in fluid.
slander Utterance of a false statement about another that harms his or her reputation.
sleep State marked by reduced consciousness, diminished activity of the skeletal muscles, and depressed metabolism.
sleep deprivation Condition resulting from a decrease in the amount, quality, and consistency of sleep.
sleep disorder Condition that interrupts the integrity of a normal sleep pattern, for example, the ability to fall or stay asleep.
sloughing Shedding of dead tissue cells.
SOAP note Progress notes that focus on a single client problem and include subjective and objective data, analysis, and planning; most often used in the POMR.
social isolation Aloneness experienced by an individual and perceived as imposed by others and as a negative or threatened state.
social zone Distance maintained by people within a group as they engage in communicating with one another. Social distance is generally considered to be 4 to 12 feet.
socialization Process of being raised within a culture and acquiring the characteristics of the given group.
solution Mixture of one or more substances dissolved in another substance. The molecules of each of the substances disperse homogeneously and do not change chemically. A solution may be a liquid, gas, or a solid.
sphygmomanometer Device for measuring the arterial blood pressure that consists of an arm or leg cuff with an air bladder connected to a tube and a bulb for pumping air into the bladder and a gauge for indicating the amount of air pressure being exerted against the artery.
spiritual Things of a religious or sacred nature.
spiritual distress State of being out of harmony with a system of beliefs, a Supreme Being, or God.
spiritual health Awareness and openness to a system of beliefs, a Supreme Being, or God; a presence with or in each person and in the world.
spirituality Spiritual dimension of a person, including the relationship with humanity, nature, and a Supreme Being.
standardized care plans Written care plans used for groups of clients that have similar health care problems.
standards of care The minimum level of care accepted to ensure high quality of care to clients. Standards of care define the types of therapies typically administered to clients with defined problems or needs.
standing order Written and approved documents containing rules, policies, procedures, regulations, and orders for the conduct of client care in various stipulated clinical settings.
statutory law Of or related to laws enacted by a legislative branch of the government.
sterilization (1)Rendering a person unable to produce children; accomplished by surgical, chemical, or other means; (2) a technique for destroying microorganisms using heat, water, chemicals, or gases.
stoma Artificially created opening between a body cavity and the body's surface; for example, a colostomy, formed from a portion of the colon pulled through the abdominal wall.
strabismus Abnormal ocular condition in which the eyes are crossed.
stratum corneum Horny outermost layer of skin, composed of dead cells converted to keratin, which continually flakes away.
stress Physiological or psychological tension that threatens homeostasis or a person's psychological equilibrium.
stressor Any event, situation, or other stimulus encountered in a person's external or internal environment that necessitates change or adaptation by the person.
striae Streaks or linear scars that result from rapid development of tension in the skin.
stroke volume The amount of blood ejected by the ventricles with each contraction.
subcutaneous Injection given into the connective tissue, under the dermis. The subcutaneous tissue absorbs drugs more slowly than those injected into muscle. Injections are *usually* given at an angle of 45 degrees.
subcutaneous layer Continuous layer of connective tissue over the entire body between the skin and the deep fascia.
subjective data Information gathered from client statements; the client's feelings and perceptions. Not verifiable by another except by inference.
sublingual A route of medication administration in which the medication is placed underneath the client's tongue.
supination Position of the hand in which the palm of the hand faces upward.
supportive care Nursing treatments designed to assist the client in maintaining the optimal comfort level and a maximum level of functioning.
surgical asepsis Procedures used to eliminate any microorganisms from an area. Also called sterile technique.
synapse Region surrounding the point of contact between two neurons or between neuron and an effector organ.
synergistic effect When two drugs act synergistically, the effect of the two drugs combined is greater than the effect that would be expected if the individual effects of the two drugs acting alone were added together.
systole Contraction of the heart, driving blood into the aorta and pulmonary arteries. The occurrence of systole is indicated by the first heart sound heard on auscultation and by the palpable apex beat.
tachycardia Rapid regular heart rate ranging between 100 and 150 beats per minute.
tachypnea An abnormally rapid rate of breathing.
tactile Relating to the sense of touch.
tactile fremitus A tremulous vibration of the chest wall during breathing that is palpable on physical examination.
task-oriented behavior Actions involving a person's cognitive abilities in an attempt to solve problems, resolve conflicts, and gratify the person's needs in order to reduce or avoid stress.
taxonomy Framework for categorizing nursing diagnosis labels into broad groups of human response patterns.
teaching Implementation method used to present correct principles, procedures, and techniques of health care; to inform the client about his or her health status; and to refer the client and family to appropriate health or social resources in the community.
team nursing system Method of client care delivery in which a small group of staff together provide client care to an assigned number of clients.

tepid sponging Washing a client with a damp washcloth moistened in lukewarm water.

teratogens Chemical or physiological agents that may produce adverse effects in the embryo or fetus.

territoriality Persistent attachment of a person to a specific area or space.

tertiary prevention Activities directed toward rehabilitation rather than diagnosis and treatment.

therapeutic communication Process in which the nurse consciously influences a client or helps the client to a better understanding through verbal and/or nonverbal communication.

therapeutic effect The desired benefit of a medication, treatment, or procedure.

thermoregulation Internal control of body temperature.

thoracentesis Surgical perforation of the chest wall and pleural space with a needle for the aspiration of fluid or to obtain a specimen for diagnostic or therapeutic purposes.

threshold Point at which a person first perceives a painful stimulus as being painful.

thrombosis Abnormal vascular condition in which a thrombus develops with a blood vessel of the body.

thrombus Accumulation of platelets, fibrin, clotting factors, and the cellular elements of the blood attached to the interior wall of a vein or artery, sometimes occluding the lumen of the vessel.

time orientation Value that a client places on promptness, future planning, and keeping appointments, which are important in the planning of long-term care and self-care discharge therapies.

tinnitus Ringing heard in one or both ears.

tissue ischemia The point at which tissues receive insufficient oxygen and perfusion.

toddlerhood Stage of life from 1 to 3 years of age.

tolerance Point at which a person is not willing to accept pain of greater severity or duration.

tort Act that causes injury for which the injured party can bring civil action.

total client care A type of nursing assignment in which a nurse is responsible for the total care of a group of clients through a shift.

total parenteral nutrition (TPN) Administration of a nutritionally adequate hypertonic solution consisting of glucose, protein, minerals, and vitamins through an indwelling catheter into the superior vena cava. Used for clients in prolonged coma, severe uncontrolled malabsorption, extensive burns, GI fistulas, and other conditions in which feeding by mouth cannot provide adequate nutrients.

toxic effect An effect of a medication that results in an adverse response.

traditional approach Ancient ethnocultural and religious beliefs and practices that have been handed down through the generations.

transcutaneous electrical nerve stimulation (TENS) Technique in which a battery-powered device blocks pain impulses from reaching the spinal cord by delivering weak electrical impulses directly to the skin's surface.

transfusion reaction A systemic response by the body to the administration of blood incompatible with that of the recipient.

transverse plane Any one of the planes that cut across the body perpendicular to the sagittal and the frontal planes, dividing the body into caudal and cranial portions.

trapeze bar Metal triangular-shaped bar that can be suspended over a client's bed from an overhanging frame; permits clients to move up and down in bed while in traction or some other encumbrance.

trimester Referring to one of the three phases of pregnancy.

trochanter roll Rolled towel support placed against the hips and upper leg to prevent external rotation of the legs.

turgor Normal resiliency of the skin caused by the outward pressure of the cells and interstitial fluid.

ulnar pulse Pulse of the ulnar artery, palpated along the ulnar side of the forearm.

universal precautions Set of precautions recommended to be followed by health care workers to prevent exposure to bloodborne pathogens such as hepatitis and HIV.

ureterostomy Diversion of urine away from a diseased or defective bladder through an artificial opening in the skin.

urinary incontinence Inability to control urination.

urinary reflux Abnormal, backward flow of urine.

urinary retention Retention of urine in the bladder; condition frequently caused by a temporary loss of muscle function.

urticaria An itchy skin eruption characterized by transient wheals of varying shapes and sizes with well-defined erythematous margins and pale centers.

validation Act of confirming, verifying, or corroborating the accuracy of assessment data or the appropriateness of the care plan.

Valsalva maneuver Any forced expiratory effort against a closed airway as when an individual holds the breath and tightens the muscles in a concerted, strenuous effort to move a heavy object or to change positions in bed.

value Personal belief about the worth of a given idea or behavior.

varicosities Abnormal conditions of a vein, characterized by swelling and irregular shape or course.

vascular access device Catheters, cannulas, or infusion ports designed for long-term, repeated access to the vascular system.

vasoconstriction Narrowing of the lumen of any blood vessel, especially the arterioles and the veins in the blood reservoirs of the skin and abdominal viscera.

vasodilation An increase in the diameter of a blood vessel caused by inhibition of its vasoconstrictor nerves or stimulation of dilator nerves.

venipuncture Technique in which a vein is punctured transcutaneously by a sharp rigid stylet (such as a butterfly needle), a cannula (such as an angiocatheter that contains a flexible plastic catheter), or a needle attached to a syringe.

ventilation Respiratory process by which gases are moved into and out of the lungs.

ventricular gallop An abnormal low-pitched extra heart sound (S_4) heard in early diastole.

verbal communication The sending of messages from one individual to another or to a group of individuals through the spoken word.

vertigo A sensation of dizziness or the clients feel as though they are spinning.

vibration Fine, shaking pressure applied by hands to the chest wall only during exhalation.

virulence A very pathogenic or rapidly progressive condition.

vital signs Temperature, pulse, respirations, and blood pressure.

vitamins Organic compound essential in small quantities for normal physiological and metabolic functioning of the body. With few exceptions, vitamins cannot be synthesized by the body and must be obtained from the diet or dietary supplements.

vocal fremitus Vibration of the chest wall as the person speaks or sings that allows the person's voice to be heard by the examiner during auscultation of the chest with a stethoscope.

water pollution Contamination of lakes, rivers, and streams by industrial pollutants.

wellness Dynamic state of health in which an individual progresses toward a higher level of functioning, achieving an optimum balance between internal and external environments.

wheezes Adventitious lung sound caused by a severely narrowed bronchus.

young adulthood Stage of life from 22 to middle adulthood.

Z-track injection A technique for injecting irritating preparations into muscle without tracking residual medication through sensitive tissues.

zygote Fertilized ovum created by joining of the ovum and sperm.

Index

D

F

I

M

T

U

V